PRiMEs™

PG Review in Minimum Efforts

The Smart & Completely Different Approach to Crack

NEET/NEXT
Exams

| Third Edition |

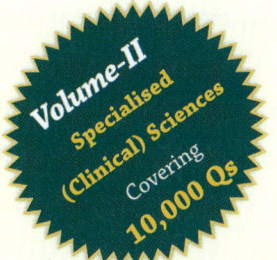

Volume-II
Specialised (Clinical) Sciences
Covering **10,000 Qs**

VD Agrawal DCH
Paediatrician, Saraswati Vihar, Pitampura, New Delhi
Consultant, Paediatrics, Max Hospital, Shalimar Bagh, New Delhi

Reetu Agrawal DNB, MNAMS
Consultant (Anaesthesiology), Max Hospital, Shalimar Bagh, New Delhi

Mohammed Shakeel Sillat DNB
Internal Medicine, Indraprastha Apollo Hospital, Sarita Vihar, New Delhi
Ex Senior Resident, Baba Saheb Ambedkar Hospital & Medical College, Rohini, New Delhi

Subject Specialist Reviewers

Shailendra Kumar Gupta	Dinesh Chaudhary	Shipra Srivastava
Pooja Lal	Sameer Arora	Latika Singh
Meraj Ahmed	Shrey Gupta	Vaishakhi Rustagi
Vikas Agrawal	Tarush Rustagi	Lokesh Singh
Tanvi Aggarwal	Gishita Gulati	Geetika Sinha
Gaurav Mandhan	Shailabh Gupta	Mohd Ishaque Qureshi

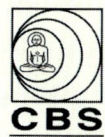

CBS
Dedicated to Education

CBS Publishers & Distributors Pvt Ltd

• New Delhi • Bengaluru • Chennai • Kochi • Kolkata • Mumbai
• Hyderabad • Nagpur • Patna • Pune • Vijayawada

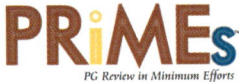

ISBN: 978-93-89941-94-4

Copyright © Authors and Publishers

Third Edition: 2020

Published by **Satish Kumar Jain** and produced by **Varun Jain** for
CBS Publishers & Distributors Pvt Ltd

4819/XI Prahlad Street, 24 Ansari Road, Daryaganj, New Delhi 110 002, India.
Ph: +91-11-23289259, 23266861, 23266867   Website: www.cbspd.com
Fax: 011-23243014
e-mail: delhi@cbspd.com; cbspubs@airtelmail.in.

Corporate Office: 204 FIE, Industrial Area, Patparganj, Delhi 110 092
Ph: +91-11-4934 4934   Fax: 4934 4935
e-mail: feedback@cbspd.com; bhupesharora@cbspd.com

Branches

- **Bengaluru:** Seema House 2975, 17th Cross, K.R. Road, Banasankari 2nd Stage, Bengaluru 560 070, Karnataka
  Ph: +91-80-26771678/79   Fax: +91-80-26771680   e-mail: bangalore@cbspd.com

- **Chennai:** 7, Subbaraya Street, Shenoy Nagar, Chennai 600 030, Tamil Nadu
  Ph: +91-44-26680620, 26681266   Fax: +91-44-42032115   e-mail: chennai@cbspd.com

- **Kochi:** 68/1534, 35, 36-Power House Road, Opp. KSEB, Cochin-682018, Kochi, Kerala
  Ph: +91-484-4059061-65   Fax: +91-484-4059065   e-mail: kochi@cbspd.com

- **Kolkata:** 6/B, Ground Floor, Rameswar Shaw Road, Kolkata-700 014, West Bengal
  Ph: +91-33-22891126, 22891127, 22891128   e-mail: kolkata@cbspd.com

- **Mumbai:** 83-C, Dr E Moses Road, Worli, Mumbai-400018, Maharashtra
  Ph: +91-22-24902340/41   Fax: +91-22-24902342   e-mail: mumbai@cbspd.com

Representatives

- **Hyderabad**   +91-9885175004
- **Pune**   +91-9623451994
- **Patna**   +91-9334159340
- **Vijayawada** +91-9000660880

Printed At : Goyal Offset Works (P) Limited

SPECIAL CONTRIBUTORS

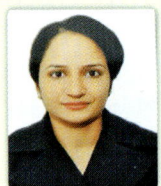
Shweta Dixit
MDS (Orthodontics)
Consultant, Andheri, Mumbai
(Special contributor 2017-2020)

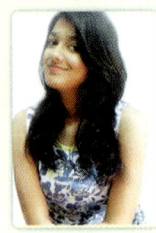
Masum Goel
MBBS, Goa Medical College, Goa
(Special contributor 2017-2020)

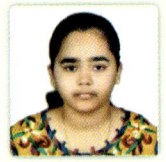
Ruhi Anjum
MBBS (Govt Medical College, Jagdalpur)
(Special contributor 2020)

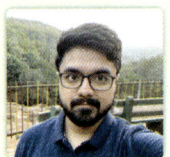
Vaibhav Vishal
MBBS (Pt. JNM Medical College, Raipur)
(Special contributor 2020)

Yugal Kumar Agrawal
MD (Radiodiagnosis) std., Sion,
MBBS (LTMC), Sion, Mumbai, Maharashtra
(Special contributor 2017)

Chaitali Chikhale
MBBS (Sion Medical College, Mumbai)
MS (ENT) std., T N Medical College, Nair Hospital
Mumbai, Maharashtra
(Special contributor 2017)

Surbhi Singh
MBBS Manipal Medical Collegea, Sikkim

Veenu Gupta MD
Consultant Internal Medicine,
St. Stephen's Hospital, New Delhi
Contributed in General Medicine

Parul Agrawal
MBBS, Medical College, Durg, Chhattisgarh

Meenu
Special Technical Support

SUBJECT SPECIALIST REVIEWERS

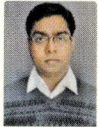

Shailendra Kumar Gupta MS (ENT)
Ex Assistant Prof. FH Medical College
Tundla, Firozabad (UP)
Consultant at Vijay ENT Clinic, Agra (UP)
Contributed in ENT

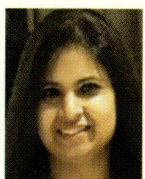

Pooja Lal DNB (Ophthalmology)
SR in Ophthalmology
DDU, Harinagar, Delhi
Contributed in Ophthalmology

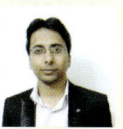

Meraj Ahmed MBBS, MS (General Surgery)
AMU, Aligarh (Uttar Pradesh)
Contributed in General Surgery

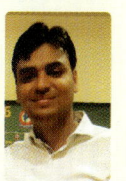

Vikas Agrawal MBBS, DNB
(General Surgery)
FMAS, FISCP, MNAMS, PDF Surgical
Oncology (Tata Hospital)
Contributed in General Surgery

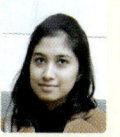

Tanvi Aggarwal MBBS, DNB
Attending Consultant,
Max Supers Peciality Hospital
Shalimar Bagh, New Delhi
Contributed in Pediatrics and Neonatology

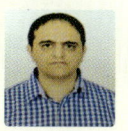

Gaurav Mandhan MD, DM (Std.)
Ex. Neonatologist
Max Super Speciality Hospital
Shalimar Bagh, New Delhi
Contributed in Pediatrics and Neonatology

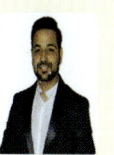

Dinesh Chaudhary DNB
(Internal Medicine)
Associate Consultant, Neurology
Indraprastha Apollo Hospitals, New Delhi
*Reviewed Neurosciences and
Rheumatology (2nd/ed.)*

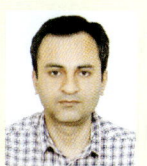

Sameer Arora
DMRD, JNMC Belgaum
DNB - Vikram Hospital, Mysore
Attending Consultant
Max Super Speciality Hospital
Shalimar Bagh, New Delhi

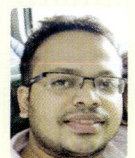

Shrey Gupta MD
Pediatrician, Delhi Newborn Centre
Pitampura, New Delhi
*Contributed in Pediatrics and Neonatology
(2nd/ed.)*

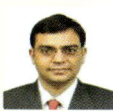

Tarush Rustagi MS (Orthopedics)
Consultant
Indian Spinal Centre
Vasant Kunj, New Delhi
Contributed in Orthopedics

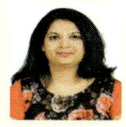

Gishita Gulati MD (Dermatology)
PGIMER, RML Hospital, New Delhi
Consultant Dermatologist
Max Multi Speciality Centre,
Pitampura, New Delhi
Contributed in Dermatology

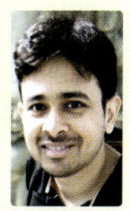

Shailabh Gupta MBBS, DNB, FNNF
Consultant
Neonest Hospital, Delhi
Contributed in Pediatrics & Neonatology

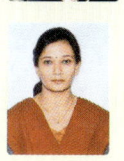

Shipra Srivastava DNB (Obs and Gyne)
Fellow in Reproductive Medicine
St Stephen's Hospital, Delhi
Contributed in Obstetrics

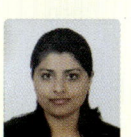

Latika Singh MBBS, DGO, DNB
(Obs and Gynae)
Consultant Obs & Gynae
Yatharth Super Speciality Hospital
Greater Noida
Contributed in Gynecology

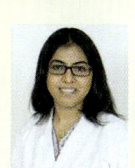

Vaishakhi Rustagi MD, FNB (Pune)
Endocrinologist
Max Hospital Shalimar Bagh & Pitampura
New Delhi
Contributed in Endocrinology

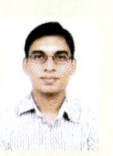

Lokesh Singh MD
Consultant Psychiatry
AIIMS, Raipur, Chhattisgarh
Contributed in Psychiatry

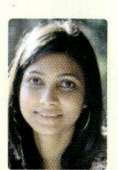

Geetika Sinha MBBS
DNB (General Surgery)
Vivekananda Hospital, Lucknow (UP)
SR, Medanta Hospital, Lucknow (UP)
Contributed in Oncology

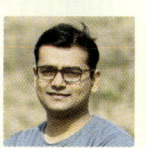

Mohd Ishaque Qureshi
MD Psychiatry Resident
Command Hospital, Kolkata (WB)
Contributed in Psychiatry (2nd/ed.)

From Publisher's Desk

Dear Readers,

I extend my warm welcome and convey my heartfelt thanks for appreciating the CBS Exam Books for another successful year. It has been an amazing journey so far and I am highly grateful for your support and cooperation to help us achieve various milestones in this whole span of time. The mission with which we started in the year 2015 was to bring nothing but the best of everything to our target audience and today I can proudly say that we have maintained that standard and are committed to continue the same in future as well.

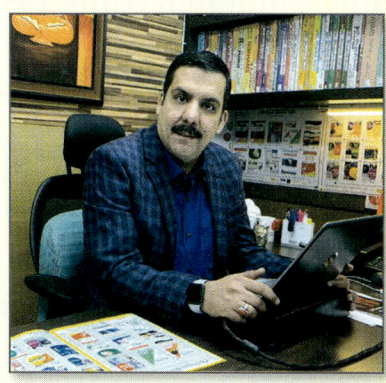

Every single title under the banner of CBS Exam Books has been developed and nurtured like an infant. The authors and our entire team work day and night to bring the best in everything for you. Be it content, presentation, social media contests and offers, we strive to meet your expectations with every passing year. Your trust has motivated us to maintain and upgrade ourselves during this period. I am extremely thankful to all our authors who are the real pillars of the complete series of CBS Exam Books. The contributions of our esteemed authors have laid the foundations of CBS Exam Books.

At this juncture, I can recall these lines by Drake,

> "Sometimes it's the journey that teaches you a lot about your destination".

We have grown and changed with the passage of time to upgrade our ways of providing our readers with maximum benefits and help them manage their time and efforts in effective manner. Previous year was the year of great achievements. Let me show you a glimpse of our successful journey:

- Most of the titles of CBS Exam Books received wide acceptance and recognition by the readers of proving their usefulness and supremacy. To mention a few, SARP Anatomy, CRISP, Surgery Sixer, Complete Review of Pathology, Conceptual Review of Pharmacology, SOCH, Forensic Medicine, Complete Review of Medicine, Conceptual Review of PSM, MICRONS, My PGMEE Notes, AIIMS MedEasy, and PRIMEs. With your constant support and our consistent efforts, I am sure that we will together witness an exponential acceptance of all CBS Exam Books in coming future as well.

- The presence of CBS Exam Books has broadened through our various social media platforms. We have received great appreciation for our regular Facebook activities such as online test series, giveaways, scientific content for knowledge enhancement, authors' live sessions, and various contests, like Bid 2 Win, Fastest Finger First, Book Fair and Facebook Community Awards. Join us on all these platforms to avail and enjoy our exciting offers and benefits.

A book is incomplete if it does not have the right readers. We value you and your feedback. Please share your feedback and suggestions directly with me at **bhupesharora@cbspd.com**. We promise to deliver in our books, what you desire to see.

I would like to sum up with these eternal lines of Robert Frost:

> Woods are lovely dark and deep,
> But I have promises to keep.
> And miles to go before I sleep,
> And miles to go before I sleep!
> Wishing you success in all your endeavors!

Bhupesh Arora
Vice President – Publishing & Marketing
(PGMEE and Nursing Division)
Email: bhupesharora@cbspd.com
Mobile: (+91) 9555590180

PREFACE

In today's era of cut-throat competition, it is very difficult to find out the ideal way to prepare for PG entrance. We have experienced that a PG aspirant has to go through a number of books, notes and what not. And when the testing moment comes, where exam is round the corner, one feels completely lost in those thousands of pages of theories and MCQs. He gets confused and finds it difficult to memorize too many things at a time.

With all these confusions going on in the mind, he keeps on turning those pages finding himself completely lost and this is the time when he feels that his confidence level is going down. He/she starts getting depressed about his/her preparation and many negative thoughts start haunting his/her mind.

One question which occupies the center of an aspirant's thought process is how to utilize the last few weeks before exams. He/she finds it bewildering and fails to decide whether he/she should revise the theory or practice the MCQs. The fact however is that both theory and MCQs play a vital role in securing a rank. The concept of PRIMES that came into existence last year, proved successful in catering to the needs of the students. The book is a perfect balance of both the theory and MCQs parts. One needs to revise not only all the important topics and one liners but also he needs to master the frequently-asked questions as well as questions based on recent pattern. We as a student and author believe that success lies far from us not because what we do not know rather because we are unable to recall what we know. PRIMES is uniquely developed so that it could simplify the approach during last few days and it could prove itself as a savior of one's yearlong hard work. It is not meant to replace any standard textbook rather it should be utilized as a quick revision tool before any entrance exam.

Our latest creation under the title "PRIMES", the **P**G **R**eview **I**n **M**inimum **E**fforts is written with a completely different approach to PGMEE. You do not need to prepare in haphazard manner. We have organized this book in your way and hope it will fulfill all your expectations. Your efficiency will get wings for maximum with minimum efforts. The third edition of this extremely useful book also contains, explanations of those questions which are not covered elsewhere. It includes recent pattern question 2020 along with detailed explanation of elaborative questions.

Constructive suggestions for the improvement of the book will be highly appreciated. Readers are requested to mail their suggestions/corrections on the given e-mail id: *primesbook@gmail.com*

VD Agrawal
Reetu Agrawal
Mohammed Shakeel Sillat

ACKNOWLEDGEMENTS

Organizing all the important questions subjectwise, chapterwise, topicwise and sub topicwise was a marathon job and it became possible only because contributors put their best efforts in this project. We would like to extend our sincere thanks to all of them.

We are highly indebted to all the consultants of Max Hospital, Shalimar Bagh and Indraprastha Apollo Hospital, Sarita Vihar for their guidance as well as for providing necessary input and also for their support in completing the book.

Beside we would like to express our sincere thanks and acknowledge these contributors who have willingly helped us in this project.

- Dr Anil Murarka [Plastic Surgeon, B L Kapoor Hospital, New Delhi]
- Dr Rajeev Malhotra [Sr. Radiologist, Max Hospital, Shalimar Bagh, New Delhi]
- Dr Anuj Thukral [Sr. Radiologist, Max Hospital, Shalimar Bagh]
- Dr Sparsh Gupta MD (Pharmacology) [Consultant Safdarjung Hospital, New Delhi]
- Dr Vishwas Gulati [MD (Gen. Medicine) RML, PGIMER, New Delhi]
- Dr Gaurav Garg [Pediatric Cardiologist, Max Hospital, Shalimar Bagh, New Delhi]
- Dr Ashish Gupta [Oncosurgeon, DNB Oncosurgery, Mahaveer Cancer Sansthan, Patana, New Delhi]
- Dr Simon Thomas [Orthopedic Surgeon, Sant Parmanad Hospital, New Delhi]
- Dr Anand Singh Kushwaha [Pediatric Surgeon, Action Balaji Hospital, Paschim vihar, and Mata Chaanan Devi Hospital, New Delhi]
- Dr Rehan Ul Haq [Consultant (Orthopedics), UCMS & GTB Hospital, New Delhi]

- Dr Pankaj Agrawal [Paediatrician, Childcare Hospital, Ireland]
- Dr Sushil Kumar Shukla [Paediatric Cardiologist, Max Hospital, Shalimar Bagh, New Delhi]
- Dr Supriya Rustogi [Neonatologist, Faridabad]
- Dr Nitin Bajaj [AC, Paediatrics, Max Hospital, Shalimar Bagh, New Delhi]
- Dr Vipra Bhagat [AC, Paediatrics, Max Hospital, Shalimar Bagh, New Delhi]
- Dr Madhu Garg [AC, Paediatrics, Max Hospital, Shalimar Bagh, New Delhi]
- Dr Neelesh Agrawal [MS (General Surgery) SR MAMC, New Delhi]
- Dr Pragya Agrawal [BDS]
- Gurpreet Singh Kapoor [MBBS std., Manipal Medical College]
- Arjun Sehgal [MBBS std., HIMS, Jolly Grant, Dehradun]
- Mudit Murarka [Liberal Arts student, USA]
- Rameshwaram Publication, Sitapur, Surguja (Chhattisgarh)

We hope, we are not overstepping our bounds but it is a fact that this was not possible without the blessings of Tauji Shri Ramdas Agrawal .

To our family members Ajay and Preeti, Vicky and sisters Sunita, Rekha and Asha and sister in law Vineeta for their guidance and advice throughout the preparation of this book.

VD Agrawal
Reetu Agrawal

- Dr Abhijeet Prasad [DNB Medicine, Jaslok Hospitals, Mumbai]
- Dr (Major) Mohd. Ishaque Qureshi [MD Psychiatry, Command Hospital, Kolkata]
- Dr Dinesh Chaudhary [Associate Consultant, Neurology, Indraprastha Apollo Hospitals, New Delhi]
- Dr Abhas Kumar [DNB Neurology, Indraprastha Apollo Hospitals, New Delhi]
- Dr Vasanti Namala [DNB Medicine, Indraprastha Apollo Hospitals, New Delhi]
- Dr Mithilesh Yadu [DNB Paediatrics, Chandulal Chandrakar Hospital, Bhilai]
- Dr Hemant Gajendra [DNB ENT, Northern Railway Central Hospital, New Delhi]
- Dr Puja Singh [FNB Reproductive Medicine, Nova IVF Fertility, Ahmedabad]
- Dr Sunil Mall [MS Ophthalmology, AIIMS, New Delhi]
- Dr Rakesh Jha [Consultant Anaesthesiologist, Ramakrishna Care Hospital, Raipur]
- Dr Gajendra Gupta [DNB Cardiology, Yashoda Hospital, Secundrabad]
- Dr Rachit Singhania [MBBS, North Bengal Medical College, Darjeeling]

- Dr Ruhi Anjum [MBBS, Late Baliram Kashyap Govt Medical College, Jagdalpur]
- Dr Vaibhav Vishal [MBBS, Pt JNM Medical College, Raipur]

I would like to thank **Mr Satish Kumar Jain** (Chairman) and **Mr Varun Jain** (Managing Director), M/s CBS Publishers and Distributors Pvt Ltd for providing me the platform in bringing out the book. I have no words to describe the role, efforts, inputs and initiatives undertaken by **Mr Bhupesh Arora,** (Vice President – Publishing & Marketing, PGMEE and Nursing Division) for helping and motivating me.

I sincerely thank the entire CBS team for bringing out the book with utmost care and attractive presentation. I thank Dr Mrinalini Bakshi (Editorial Head & Content Strategist) for her editorial support and Ms Nitasha Arora (Production Head & Content Strategist), Dr Anju Dhir (Project Manager & Senior Scientific Coordinator), Mr Shivendu Bhushan Pandey (Senior Editor), Mr Ashutosh Pathak (Senior Proof Reader) and all the production team members Mr Prakash Gaur, Mr Phool Kumar, Mr Bunty Kashyap, Mr Chaman Lal, Mr Chander Mani, Ms Tahira Parveen, Ms Manorama Gupta, Ms Babita Verma, Mr Raju Sharma, Mr Manoj Chaudhary, Mr Vikram Chaudhary, Mr Manoj Malakar, Mr Arun Kumar and Mr Rahul Negi for devoting laborious hours in designing and typesetting of the book.

Mohammed Shakeel Sillat

REFERENCES USED IN THE BOOK
[Suggested Books for Readers]

- Gray's Anatomy (Barnes & Noble Collectible Editions) by Henry Gray, H.V. Carter, 40th Edition
- B.D. Chaurasia's Human Anatomy, 8th Edition
- B.D. Chaurasia's Handbook of General Anatomy 5th Edition
- Langman's Medical embryology by *T.W. Sadler* 12th Edition
- Textbook of Histology by *Krishna Garg, Indira Bahl, Mohini Kaul,* 2nd Edition
- Ganong's Review of Medical Physiology 26th Edition by *William F. Ganong*
- Guyton & Hall Textbook of Medical Physiology, Second South Asia Edition
- Harper's Illustrated Biochemistry, 31st Edition
- Biochemistry for Medical Students 7th Edition by *DM Vasudevan*
- Robbins & Cotran Pathologic Basis of Disease (9th Edition = First South Asia Edition)
- Ananthanarayan & Paniker's Textbook of Microbiology, 9th Edition
- Parasitology (Protozoology & Helminthology) by *K.D. Chatterjee, 13th Edition*
- Medical Parasitology by D.R. Arora & Brij Bala Arora, 4th Edition
- Essentials of Medical Pharmacology by K.D. Tripathi, 8th Edition
- The Essentials of Forensic Medicine & Toxicology by *K.S. Narayan Reddy*, 33rd Edition
- Park's Textbook of Preventive & Social Medicine, 25th Edition
- Harrison's Principles of Internal Medicine, 20th Edition
- Sabiston Textbook of Surgery, 20th Edition = First South Asia Edition)
- Bailey & Love's Short Practice of Surgery, 27th Edition
- Schwartz's Principles of Surgery, 10th Edition
- Textbook of Obstretics *by D.C. Dutta,* 9th Edition
- Holland & Brew's Manual of Obstetrics, 4th Edition
- Howkins & Bourne Shaw's Textbook of Gynaecology by *Shirish N. Daftary*, 16th Edition
- Howkins & Bourne Shaw's Textbook of Gynaecology by *Shirish N. Daftary*, 16th Edition
- Jeffcoate's Principles of Gynaecology, 8th Edition
- Berek & Novak's Gynecology, 15th Edition
- Williams Obstetrics, 24th and 25th Edition
- Parsons' Diseases of the Eye, 23rd Edition
- Textbook of Ophthalmology by H.V. Nema & Nitin Nema
- Comprehensive Ophthalmology by *A K Khurana,* 6th Edition
- Fundamentals of Ear, Nose, Throat and Head neck Diseases by *S.K. De*
- Logan Turner's Nose, Throat & Ear
- Diseases of Ear, Nose and Throat & Head and Neck Surgery by *P L Dhingra & Shruti Dhingra*, 7th Edition
- Essential Orthopaedics (Including Clinical Methods) by Maheshwari and Mhaskar, 6th Edition
- Nelson Textbook of Pediatrics, 21st Edition
- Ghai Essential Paediatrics by Paul and Bagga, 8th Edition
- Chapman's Synopsis of Radiology
- Radiology Review Manual by *Wolfgang Dahnert*
- Morgan & Mikhail's Clinical Anaesthesiology, 6th Edition
- Marino's The ICU Book by *Paul L. Marino*, 4th Edition
- Lee's Synopsis of Anaesthesia, 13th Edition
- Short Textbook of Anaesthsia by *Ajay Yadav,* 5th Edition
- Kaplan & Sadock's Synopsis of Psychaitry, 11th Edition
- A Short textbook of Psychaitry by *Niraj Ahuja*, 7th Edition
- IADVL's Concise Textbook of Dermatology by *Vishalakshi Vishwanath*, First Edition
- Pediatric Endocrine Disorders by *Meena P. Desai, P.S.N. Menon and Vijaylakshmi Bhatia*, 3rd Edition

ABBREVIATIONS/SHORT FORMS USED IN THE BOOK

Mn	:	**Mnemonic**
Aka or aka	:	**Also known as**
Ca	:	Carcinoma/Cancer
~	:	denotes heading
D/to	:	due to
↑	:	Increase, High
n.or nv	:	Nerve
↓	:	Decrease , low
D/g, Dx	:	Diagnosis
A/E	:	All except
DOC	:	Drug of choice
R_x or T/t	:	Treatment
Sx	:	Surgery
Hx	:	History
P/g	:	**Prognosis**
IOC	:	Investigation of choice
P_x	:	**Prophylaxis**
TOC	:	Treatment of choice
C/c	:	Complication
Acc/ to	:	According to
C_T	:	Chemotherapy
Mc, m/c	:	Most common
R_T	:	Radiotherapy
Vs	:	Versus (= against)
Supf.	:	Superficial
Ds, d/s	:	Disease or Disease
——	:	Reaction block by, inhibited by
Ms, m/s	:	Muscle
B/L or b/L	:	Bilateral
Ipsi/L	:	Ipsilateral
U/L or u/L	:	Unilateral
Cont./L	:	Contralateral
A/w	:	Associated with
K/as	:	Known as
V/s	:	Vessel
Ad/E, ad/e	:	Adverse effects
C/I	:	Contraindication
A/w or a/w	:	Associated with
M/m	:	Management
b/n or b/w	:	Between

e/o	:	Evidence of
F/H	:	Family history
Cl/f	:	Clinical features
C/by	:	Characterized by, caused by
FA	:	Fatty Acid
AD	:	Autosomal dominant
FFA	:	Free fatty acid
FTT	:	Failure to thrive
DM	:	Diabetes mellitus
CTD	:	Connective tissue disease
Cx	:	Cervix
SCLC	:	Small cell lung carcinoma
MN	:	Malnutrition
SM	:	Smooth muscle
HCC	:	Hepato cellular carcinoma
BM	:	Bone marrow, basement membrane
IOT	:	Intraocular tension
HS	:	Hereditary spherocytosis
HD	:	Hodgkin's disease
BM	:	Bone marrow, basement membrane
WT	:	Wilm's tumour
HS	:	Hereditary spherocytosis
NHL	:	Non-Hodgkin's lymphoma
ICT	:	Intracranial tension
SqCC	:	Squamous cell carcinoma
LN	:	Lymph node
PBC	:	Primary biliary cirrhosis
MG	:	Myasthenia gravis
MN	:	Malnutrition
WG	:	Wegner's granulomatosis
ILD	:	Interstitial lung disease
Ix	:	Indication
AR	:	Autosomal recessive
HDN	:	Hemorrhagic disease of newborn
HMD	:	Hyaline membrane disease
NEC	:	Necrotising enterocolitis
PVL	:	Periventricular leucomalacia
IVH	:	Intraventricular Hemorrhage
BAL	:	Broncho-alveolar lavage
CST	:	Cortco spinal tract
ASA	:	Anterior spinal artery

CONTENTS

1.   General Medicine

THEORY 1, **MCQs** (Ch. 1. General Medicine 16; Ch. 2. Emergency Medicine 24)

2.   Neurosciences

THEORY 27, **MCQs** (Ch. 1. Neurosciences 44)

3.   Ophthalmology

THEORY 67, **MCQs** (Ch. 1A. Anatomy and Development 77; Ch. 1B. Optics and Refraction 78; Ch. 2. Conjunctiva 83; Ch. 3. Cornea and Sclera 88; Ch. 4. Uveal Tract 93; Ch. 5. Lens 97; Ch. 6. Glaucoma 103; Ch. 7. Vitreous and Retina 107; Ch. 8. Neuro-ophthalmology 113; Ch. 9. Diseases of Orbit, Lids and Lacrimal Apparatus 117; Ch. 10. Ocular examination & Investigations 123; Ch. 11. Systemic Disease in Eyes & Preventive Ophthalmology 127; Ch. 12. Tumors 129; Ch. 13. Ocular Trauma 131; Ch. 14. Ocular Motility and Squint (Strabismus) 133; Ch. 15. Lasers, Anaesthesia and Drugs 136)

4.   Diseases of Ear, Nose and Throat

THEORY 138, **MCQs** (Ch. 1. EAR 155; Ch. 2. The Nose, Nasopharynx and PNS 179; Ch. 3. The Larynx, Trachea and Bronchi 196; Ch. 4. The Oral Cavity, Pharynx and Esophagus 204; Ch. 5. Head and Neck 210)

5.   Endocrinology

THEORY 211, **MCQs** (Ch. 1. Hypothalamic and Pituitary Hormones Endocrinology 224; Ch. 2. Thyroid and Parathyroid Hormones 228; Ch. 3. Diabetes Mellitus, DM, Obesity and Metabolic Syndrome 233; Ch. 4. Adrenal Gland, CAH and Reproductive Endocrinology 239; Ch. 5. Endocrine Tumors 243)

6.   Pulmonology

THEORY 245, **MCQs** (Ch. 1. Pulmonology 256)

7.   Cardiology

THEORY 272, **MCQs** (Ch. 1. Cardiology 294; Ch. 2. Coronary and Peripheral Vascular Diseases 310; Ch. 3. Pediatric Cardiology 317)

8.   Gastroenterology

THEORY 320, **MCQs** (Ch. 1. Esophagus 327; Ch. 2. Stomach 333; Ch. 3. Intestine 337; Ch. 4. GI Surgery Abdomen and Peritoneum 343)

RECENT PATTERN QUESTIONS 2020

GENERAL MEDICINE

1. A female from a tribal area of Jharkhand reports with fever for last 3 days. Peripheral blood is collected and stained with Giemsa. A diagnosis of malaria is made. The smear is shown in the figure. What is the likely cause?

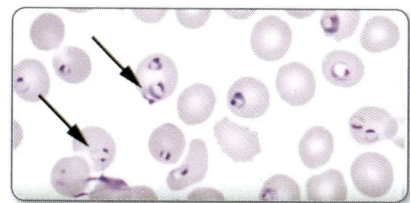

  a. P. falciparum   b. P. vivax
  c. P. knowlesi/ P. malariae   d. P. ovale

[Ref: Harrison's 20th/e pg. 1576, 1581; Park's 25th/e pg. 280]

Explanation

- Ring forms and banana shaped gametocytes are visible in peripheral blood smear which are typical of P. falciparum infection.
- P. falciparum is highly prevalent in Jharkhand, In India about 21.98 per cent population lives in malaria high transmission (~1 case/1000 population) areas. About 91 per cent of malaria cases and 99% of deaths due to malaria is reported from North-eastern states, Chhattisgarh, Jharkhand, Madhya Pradesh, Odisha, Andhra Pradesh, Maharashtra, Gujarat, Rajasthan, West Bengal and Karnataka.

2. An HIV positive patient with a CD4 count of 300/cumm presents with mucosal lesions in the mouth as shown in the figure. On microscopy budding yeasts and pseudohyphae are seen. What is the likely diagnosis?

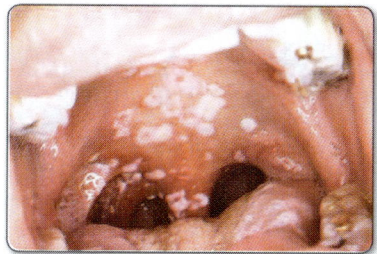

  a. Lichen planus   b. Oral Candidiasis
  c. Aphthous ulcers   d. Oral hairy leukoplakia

[Ref: Harrison's 20th/e pg. 1435]

Explanation

- History of Immunocompromised status as in HIV with presence of widespread white plaques on oral mucosa of palate, uvula and tonsillar fossa in the image clearly points towards oral candidiasis.
- Oral lesions, including thrush, hairy leukoplakia, and aphthous ulcers are particularly common in patients with untreated HIV infection. Thrush due to Candida

albicans are usually indicative of fairly advanced immunological decline; they generally occur in patients with CD4 counts < 300/μL.

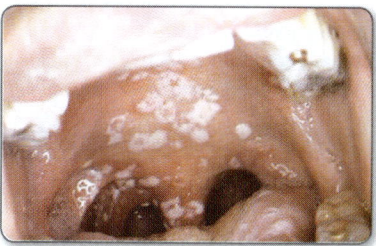

- ***Lichen Planus*** is a chronic inflammatory condition affecting oral mucosa and appears as white, lacy patches; red, swollen tissues; or open sores. These lesions may cause burning, pain or other discomfort.

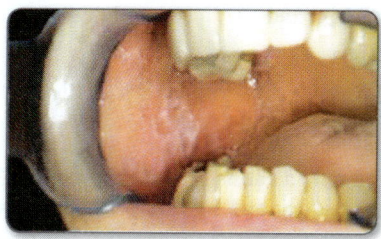

- ***Leukoplakia*** is found in smokers and presents as a white patch or plaque that cannot be rubbed off.

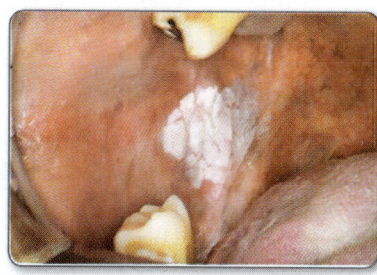

- ***Aphthous ulcers*** are recurrent round or oval sore or ulcer in the mouth on an area where the skin is not tightly bound to the underlying bone, such as on the inside of the lips and cheeks or underneath the tongue. It has a red ring of inflammation on its margins.

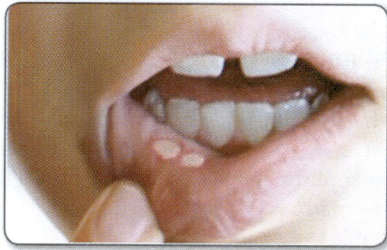

3. Woman sleeping in the night develops pain and funny feelings in the legs which is relieved by shaking her legs. Which of the following drug is used as first line?

  a. Iron therapy   b. Pramipexole
  c. Levodopa   d. No specific treatment

[Ref: Harrison's 20th/e pg. 3140]

1.   a
2.   b
3.   b

Explanation

- Clinical scenario given in the question is consistent with restless leg syndrome

Restless Leg Syndrome (RLS)

- Most RLS sufferers have mild symptoms & does not require any treatment.
- If symptoms persist, low doses of dopamine agonists e.g., **pramipaxole**, ropinirole or rotigotine patch, before bedtime are generally effective.
- Iron therapy is used for anemic patients.

4. The blood gas reports of a patient given below: pH = 7.2; HCO₃ = 10 mEq/L; PCO₂ = 30 mmHg This exemplifies which of the following partially compensated disorder?

- a. Respiratory acidosis
- b. Respiratory alkalosis
- c. Metabolic acidosis
- d. Metabolic alkalosis

[Ref: Harrison's 20th/e pg. 316]

Explanation

- pH , HCO_3^- and CO_2 all three low indicates metabolic acidosis.

5. A 55-year-old male presents with tachypnea and confusion. Blood glucose 350 mg/dl pH=7.0. What is the most likely acid base disorder?

- a. Respiratory acidosis
- b. Respiratory alkalosis
- c. Metabolic acidosis
- d. Metabolic alkalosis

[Ref: Harrison's 20th/e pg. 316]

Explanation

- It is a case of diabetic ketoacidosis, which is an example of metabolic acidosis.

6. A 23-year-old male presented with history of fatigue and tiredness. On investigating, he had a hemoglobin of 8 g/dL, MCV of 101fl and hematocrit of 33% . Peripheral smear is showing macrocytes and hypersegmented neutrophils. Which of the following is the most likely cause of the findings in this patient?

- a. Lead poisoning
- b. Chronic alcoholism
- c. Chronic renal failure
- d. Hemolytic anemia

[Ref: Harrison's 20th/e pg. 1631]

Explanation

- Ethanol causes:-
  - ↑ **in RBC size (↑MCV)**, which reflects its effects on stem cells.
  - If heavy drinking is accompanied by folic acid deficiency, there can also be **hypersegmented neutrophils**, reticulocytopenia, and a hyperplastic bone marrow.
  - Anemia
- If malnutrition is present, sideroblastic changes can be observed.

7. A 29-year-old women came with the complaints of easy fatigability, exertional dyspnea and weight loss. She also complaints of frequent fall. Physical examination revealed that there was bilateral decrease in vibration sense. Her hemoglobin levels were 8.2 gm%. She received folate treatment which improved her anemia but her neurological symptoms worsened. Which of the following is the most probable reason for her condition?

- a. Folate not absorbed
- b. Unmasked pyridoxine deficiency
- c. Deficiency of folate reductase in CNS
- d. Folate therapy caused depletion of B12 stores aggravating symptoms

[Ref: Harrison's 20th/e pg. 707-708]

Explanation

- The clinical picture in above question is typical of sub acute combined degeneration (SACD).
  - SACD is a frequent consequence of cobalamin deficiency.
  - It is usually associated with **pernicious anemia** (vitamin B12 deficiency).
  - There is degeneration of the posterior and lateral columns of the spinal cord. This might lead to ataxia, paresis, hyperreflexia, and bladder dysfunction
- Folate therapy alone depletes vitamin B12 stores so further aggravating symptoms of B12 deficiency.

8. Patient with atrial fibrillation which is false:

- a. Brain imaging not done
- b. Major source of thromboembolism is from left atrium
- c. Electric cardioversion is required for new onset atrial fibrillation which produces hypotension, pulmonary edema or angina.
- d. Acute rate control can be achieved by beta blockers or calcium channel blockers.

[Ref: Harrison's 20th/e pg. 1746]

9. All trans retinoic acid (ATRA) is used in the treatment of tumor associated with which of the following gene mutation?

- a. BCR-ABL
- b. PML- RARA
- c. cMYC
- d. CEBPA

Explanation

- AML FAB M3 is now designated acute promyelocytic leukemia (APL), based on the presence of either the t(15;17)(q22;q12) cytogenetic rearrangement or the **PML-RARA** fusion product of the translocation.
  - ATRA is superior to idarubicin and is new standard in treatment of low risk APL (acute promyelocytic leukemia) patients.
- AML with abnormal bone marrow eosinophils is a/w inv(16)(p13q22) or t(16;16)(p13;q22);**CBFB/MYH11** mutation.
- AML with translocation t(8;21)(q22;q22) is a/w RUNX1/RUNX1T1 mutations.

10. A 5-year-old male child presented to the clinic with history of recurrent infections. On examination the child had eczematous rashes as shown below. Routine blood investigations revealed the patient had low platelets. Which of the following is the probable diagnosis in the child?

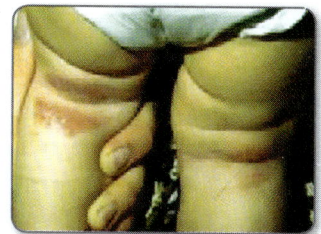

a. Job syndrome
b. Wiskott-Aldrich syndrome
c. Henoch scholein purpura
d. Hyper IgM syndrome

[Ref: Robbins 9th/e pg. 198; 242;Harrison's 20th/e pg. 2494]

Explanation

- The clinical picture is of Wiskott Aldrich syndrome.
- Wiskott Aldrich syndrome is a complex, rare X-linked recessive disease characterized by eczema, thrombocytopenia (low platelet count), immune deficiency, and bloody diarrhea (secondary to the thrombocytopenia).
- Immunodeficiency poses risk of recurrent respiratory infections.
- Mutations are found in in WASP gene.

11. A patient with h/o diabetes mellitus and hypothyroidism now present with passing stools and not gaining weight. Which of the following investigation you would like to order next:
a. Anti gliadin antibody
b. Biopsy
c. Anti-endomysial antibody
d. Anti TTG

[Ref: Harrison's 20th/e pg. 2253]

Explanation

- The clinical picture arouse suspicion of celiac disease. Anti-tTG antibody titres are required as initial work up.

12. A 23-year-old lady presented with diarrhoea, vomiting and poor appetite. Biopsy showed crypt hyperplasia, villous atrophy and CD8+ cells in the lamina propria. Most likely diagnosis is?
a. Whipple's disease
b. Chronic pancreatitis
c. Tropical sprue
d. Celiac disease

[Ref: Harrison's 20th/e pg. 2253]

Explanation

- This is a clinical picture is of celiac disease. (For details see theory section)

13. Recurrent oral ulcer with venous thrombosis are seen in:
a. Behcet's disease   b. Reiter's syndrome
c. Felty syndrome   d. None of the above

[Ref: Harrison's 20th/e pg. 2589]

Explanation

- Behcet's disease patients must present with:
  ○ Recurrent oral ulcerations (apthous or herpetiform) at least three times in one year.
  ○ Recurrent genital ulcerations.
  ○ Eye lesions (uveitis or retinal vasculitis)

14. A known case of COPD patient presents with acute exacerbation. On examination patient is conscious and alert, her pulse is 110/min. On auscultation bilateral wheeze is present. Which of the following is not true in this patient?
a. IV Steroids
b. Inhalation with salbutamol
c. Permissible hypercapnia allowed
d. Non-invasive ventilation not indicated

[Ref: Harrison's 20th/e pg. 1998]

Explanation

T/t of Acute Exacerbations of COPD patient

- Typically, patients are treated with an inhaled agonist, such as salbutamol often with the addition of an anticholinergic agent.
- Use of **glucocorticoids** has been demonstrated to reduce the length of stay, hasten recovery, and reduce the chance of subsequent exacerbation or relapse for a period of up to 6 months.
- The initiation of noninvasive positive pressure ventilation (NIPPV) in patients with respiratory failure, defined as $PaCO_2 > 45$ mmHg, results in a significant reduction in mortality.
- Invasive (conventional) mechanical ventilation is indicated for patients with severe respiratory distress despite initial therapy, life-threatening hypoxemia, severe hypercapnia and/or acidosis, markedly impaired mental status, respiratory arrest, hemodynamic instability, or other complications.

15. Which of the following is not seen in pituitary apoplexy?
a. Hypotension   b. Hypoglycemia
c. Hypertension   d. Headache

[Ref: Harrison's 20th/e pg. 189,2665]

Explanation

- Pituitary apoplexy is caused by acute intrapituitary hemorrhagic vascular event.
- It is characterized by a sudden onset of headache, visual symptoms, altered mental status, and hormonal dysfunction due to acute hemorrhage or infarction of a pituitary gland.
- Apoplexy is an endocrine emergency which may result in severe hypoglycemia, hypotension and shock.

10.	b
11.	d
12.	d
13.	a
14.	d
15.	c

16. Patient with low TSH. But on administering TRH, TSH improved. Likely cause:
   a. Thyroid hormone resistance
   b. Subclinical hypothyroidism
   c. Subclinical hyperthyroidism
   d. Hypothalamic lesion

[Ref: Harrison's 20th/e pg. 2705]

17. Water hammer pulse is seen in:
   a. Aortic regurgitation
   b. Mitral stenosis
   c. Aortic stenosis
   d. Left ventricular failure

[Ref: Harrison's 20th/e pg. 1670]

Explanation

- With chronic severe AR, the carotid upstroke has a sharp rise and rapid fall-off (*Corrigan's or Water-hammer pulse*).
- Some patients with AS may also have a slow, notched or interrupted upstroke with a thrill (*Anacrotic pulse*).

18. A 60-year-old patient with history of hypertension and diabetes developed the following rhythm. His BP was 80/60 mm of Hg and pulse was feeble. On giving IV medication he became unstable and ECG showed no change. Next line in management?

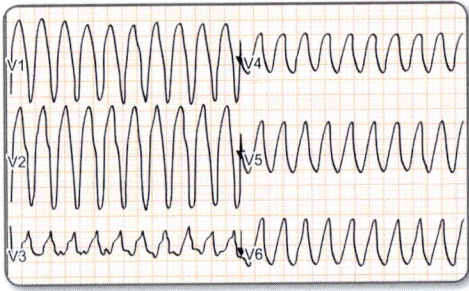

   a. Iv flecainide
   b. Iv ibulitide
   c. Iv diltiazem
   d. DC cardioversion

[Ref: Harrison's 20th/e pg. 1736, 1742]

Explanation

- This is a case of SVT and was treated by IV adenosine.
- DC cardioversion is indicated in refractory SVT

19. A patient presents to OPD with b/l chest rales, dyspnea, pedal edema, distended jugular vein and positive hepato-jugular reflex. All of the following are seen in chest X-ray of this patient, except?
   a. Pedal edema
   b. Rales
   c. Kerley B lines
   d. Lung oligemia

[Ref: Harrison's 20th/e pg. 1766]

Explanation

- This is a clinical picture of left ventricular failure/CHF.
- DC cardioversion is indicated in refractory SVT

Findings seen in LVF:

- Symptoms
  - Dyspnea, orthopnea or paroxysmal nocturnal dyspnea
  - Cheyne Stroke respirations
  - GI symptoms: anorexia, nausea, early satiety etc.

- Physical findings
  - Sinus tachycardia
  - Pulmonary crackles (Rales or crepitations)
  - Raised jugular venous pressure
  - Hepatomegaly
- Radiological findings
  - Pulmonary hypertension
  - Pulmonary edema, interstitial edema, plethora

20. A boy met with a motor bike accident. CT brain shows infarction at posterior end of superior temporal gyrus. He is likely to suffer from?
   a. Global aphasia
   b. Fluent aphasia
   c. Transcortical motor aphasia
   d. Non fluent aphasia

[Ref: Harrison's 20th/e pg. 159]

Explanation

- Lesions of the posterior end of superior temporal gyrus results in Wernicke's aphasia.
- Broca's aphasia or motor aphasia is MC due to infarction of Broca's area (Inferior frontal convolutions).
- ***Fluent aphasias include:-***
  - Wernicke's aphasia
  - Transcortical sensory aphasia
  - Conduction aphasia
  - Anomic aphasia
- ***Non- fluent aphasias include:-***
  - Broca's aphasia
  - Transcortical motor aphasia
  - Mixed transcortical aphasia
  - Global aphasia

21. Broad base gait with enuresis is a feature of:
   a. Normal pressure hydrocephalus
   b. Alcohol withdrawal syndrome
   c. Cerebellar lesion
   d. Parkinsonism

[Ref: Harrison's 20th/e pg. 144]

Explanation

- Normal pressure (Communicating) hydrocephalus in the adult may presents with a frontal gait disorder.
- The diagnostic triad (mental change, incontinence) may be absent in the initial stages. MRI demonstrates ventricular enlargement, an enlarged flow void about the aqueduct, and a variable degree of periventricular white matter change.
- A lumbar puncture is necessary to confirm the presence of hydrocephalus

22. As per NCEP- ATP III, which is not included in metabolic syndrome:
   a. Hypertrigliceridemia
   b. High LDL
   c. Central obesity
   d. Hypertension

[Ref: Harrison's 20th/e pg. 2903]

16.	d
17.	a
18.	d
19.	d
20.	b
21.	a
22.	b

Explanation

- *Diagnostic criteria for Metabolic syndrome[a]:*

Criterion	Definition
Abdominal obesity	Waist circumference: men, >40 in. (>102 cm); women, >35 in. (> 88 cm)
Hypertriglyceridemia	≥ 150 mg/dL
Low HDL-C	Men, <40 mg/dL; women <50 mg/dL
High blood pressure	≥ 130/85 mmHg
High fasting glucose	≥ 110 mg/dL

[a] Diagnosis based on presence of three of five factors.

23. While accent to high altitude patient developed high altitude reaction. Which of the following should not be done in this patient?

a. Acetazolamide   b. Rapid descent
c. IV Digoxin   d. Oxygen

[Ref: Harrison's 20th/e pg. 3334]

Explanation

- T/t of Altitude mountain sickness (AMS)
  - For the mild AMS, rest along with analgesics.
  - Descent or simulation of descent in a portable hyperbaric chamber
  - Use of acetazolamide
  - Oxygen
  - Dexamethasone for moderate AMS
- Nifedipine, phosphodiesterase-3 inhibitor and IV digoxin have no role in t/t .

24. Which of the following is the site of defect in multiple sclerosis?

a. Oligodendrocyte   b. Node of Ranvier
c. Myelin sheath   d. Basket cells

[Ref: Harrison's 20th/e pg. 3190]

Explanation

- Axonal damage occurs in every newly formed MS lesion, and cumulative axonal loss is considered to be the major cause of progressive and irreversible neurological disability in MS.
- Demyelination is a prerequisite for axonal injury in MS. Demyelination is the pathological hallmark and evidence of myelin degeneration is found at the earliest time points of tissue injury.

25. A patient presented with clinical features of scleroderma and acute onset respiratory distress. X-ray shows reticular basilar shadow. Next line of investigation is:-

a. Pulmonary function test
b. CECT
c. HRCT
d. Echo to look for cor pulmonale

[Ref: Harrison's 20th/e pg. 2005; 2550]

Explanation

- The most common histologic pattern of lung involvement in scleroderma is **nonspecific interstitial pneumonitis**. Progressive thickening of the alveolar septae results in obliteration of the airspaces and honeycombing, as well as loss of pulmonary blood vessels.
- Investigations:-
  - While evidence of ILD can be found in up to 65% of SSc patients by **HRCT**, clinically significant ILD develops in 16–43% of patients.
  - On **PFT** there is decreased FVC and DLCO but unaffected flow rates.
  - CXR can be used as initial screening tool to rule out infection .
  - HRCT chest is more sensitive and may show reticular linear opacities predominantly in the lower lobes, even in early disease. Additional findings include mediastinal lymphadenopathy, nodules, and honeycombing. **HRCT is a predictor of ILD progression & mortality.**

26. Loss of pain/temperature sensation on ipsilateral face & contralateral body are due to thrombosis in?

a. PICA
b. Posterior cerebral artery
c. Superior cerebellar artery
d. All of the above

[Ref: Harrison's 20th/e pg. 3074, 3076]

Explanation

- Embolic occlusion or thrombosis of **vertebral > PICA** artery or V4 segment causes ischemia of the lateral medulla. The constellation of vertigo, numbness of the ipsilateral face and contralateral limbs, diplopia, hoarseness, dysarthria, dysphagia, and ipsilateral Horner's syndrome is called the *lateral medullary (or Wallenberg's) syndrome.*
- Occlusion of the medullary penetrating branches of the vertebral artery or PICA results in partial syndromes. Hemiparesis is not a feature of vertebral artery occlusion, however, quadriparesis may result from occlusion of the anterior spinal artery.
- Rarely, a *medial medullary syndrome* occurs with infarction of the pyramid and contralateral hemiparesis of the arm and leg, sparing the face. If the medial lemniscus and emerging hypoglossal nerve fibers are involved, contralateral loss of joint position sense and ipsilateral tongue weakness occur.
- *Lateral inferior pontine syndrome* is due to occlusion of anterior inferior cerebellar artery (**AICA**). It is characterized by:-
  - On the side of lesion: Horizontal and vertical nystagmus, vertigo, nausea, vomiting, oscillopia: Vestibular nerve or nucleus; Facial paralysis: Seventh nerve; Paralysis of conjugate gaze to side of lesion: Center for conjugate lateral gaze; Deafness, tinnitus: Auditory nerve or cochlear nucleus; Ataxia: Middle cerebellar peduncle and cerebellar hemisphere; Impaired sensation over face: Descending tract and 5th nerve nucleus.
  - On side opposite to lesion: Impaired pain and thermal sense over half the body (may include face): Spinothalamic tract

23.	c
24.	c
25.	c
26.	a

27. A patient, after cerebrovascular accident, presents with nystagmus, ataxia and dysdiadochokinesia. Most likely artery involved is

a. PICA
b. AICA
c. Vertebral artery
d. Internal carotid artery

[Ref: Harrison's 20th/e pg. 3074, 3076]

Explanation

- CVA resulting in cerebellar injury is characterized by signs and symptoms of cerebellar dysfunction (ataxia, dysdiadochokinesia, nystagmus).
- Occlusion of arteries which supply cerebellum produce cerebellar signs.

28. A patient has fatigue with no increase in weight. On examination his body was warm. Investigation will show?

a. High TSH with euthyroid
b. High TSH with normal T3/T4
c. Increase uptake of T3, decrease T4
d. Low TSH with high T3/T4

[Ref: Harrison's 20th/e pg. 2698]

Explanation

- Clinical features are suggestive of hypothyroidism.
- Lab/F: **Low TSH with high T3/T4**

29. Which of the following differentiates between IBS and organic GI disease (IBD)?

a. Mucus in stools
b. Stool calprotectin
c. Abdominal pain
d. Diarrhoea

Explanation

- Stool Calprotectin is a is readily available non-invasive laboratory test
- It is a helpful diagnostic tool to monitor individuals with inflammatory bowel disease (Crohn's disease, ulcerative colitis, indeterminate colitis) and to distinguish from irritable bowel syndrome.

30. When compared to normal healthy person in the evening time, which of these will have elevated ACTH and elevated cortisol?

a. Addison's disease
b. Cushing's disease
c. After exercise
d. Normal healthy person/ Normal healthy person in the morning

[Ref: Harrison's 20th/e pg. 2720; 2726]

Explanation

- ACTH secretion is pulsatile and exhibits a characteristic circadian rhythm, peaking at 6 A.M. and reaching a nadir about midnight. Adrenal glucocorticoid secretion, which is driven by ACTH, follows a parallel diurnal pattern.
- ACTH circadian rhythmicity is determined by variations in secretory pulse amplitude rather than changes in pulse frequency. Superimposed on this endogenous rhythm, ACTH levels are increased by AVP, physical stress, exercise, acute illness, and insulin- induced hypoglycemia

31. Patient underwent bilateral adrenalectomy in view of bilateral phaeochromocytoma. On the 1st post op day, the patient developed fatigue and lethargy. His BP and pulse are normal. What could be the most likely cause?

a. Cortisol deficiency
b. Cardiogenic shock
c. Hypovolemic shock
d. Septic shock

[Ref: Sabiston 1st SEA edition pg. 983; Harrison's 20th/e pg. 2733]

Explanation

- Bilateral adrenalectomy is increasingly used to treat patients with Cushing's disease. Since the absence of adrenal glands leads to a sharp drop in cortisol, this treatment implies lifelong glucocorticoid replacement therapy and increases the risk of developing Nelson syndrome.
- After adrenalectomy post op hypotension may be profound which results from a state of hypovolemia (hypovolemic shock) created by presence of excess circulating catecholamines. Sudden withdrawal of this stimulus after tumour removal leads to peripheral arteriolar vasodilation and a dramatic increase in venous capacitance, which together may precipitate cardiovascular collapse.

32. Which of the following is the correct statement related to Huntington's Chorea?

a. It is a tri-nucleotide expansion mutation related disorder
b. There is loss of function type of mutation
c. There are abnormal repeats of CUG
d. Abnormality is seen due to mutation in Chromosome 6

[Ref: Harrison's 20th/e pg. 3048; 3136]

Explanation

Huntington's Disease

- HD is a progressive fatal, highly penetrant autosomal dominant disease characterized by motor, behavioural, oculomotor, and cognitive dysfunctions.
- HD is caused by an expansion in **CAG** triplet repeats in the huntingtin gene which leads to an expanded polyglutamine tract in the huntingtin protein.

OPHTHALMOLOGY

33. Which vitamin toxicity leads to macular cyst and macular edema?

a. Retinol
b. Vitamin B3
c. Vitamin C
d. Vitamin D

[Ref: Harrison's 20th/e pg. 2312; Nema's 6th/e pg. 105]

Explanation

- Vitamin B3 is niacin or nicotinic acid.
- Toxicity manifestations include:-
  ○ Prostaglandin-mediated flushing at daily doses as low as 50 mg
  ○ There is no evidence of toxicity from niacin derived from food sources. Flushing always starts in the face and may be accompanied by skin dryness, itching,

27.	a
28.	d
29.	b
30.	b
31.	a
32.	a
33.	b

paresthesia, and headache. Premedication with aspirin may alleviate these symptoms. Flushing is subject to tachyphylaxis and often improves with time.
- Nausea, vomiting, and abdominal pain
- Hepatic toxicity (raised AST & ALT levels) is the most serious toxic reaction due to niacin. Fulminant hepatitis is rare.
- Glucose intolerance, hyperuricemia, **macular edema, and macular cysts**.
- The upper limit for daily niacin intake has been set at 35 mg.

34. Satellite lesions in eye are seen in:
a. Viral keratitis
b. Bacterial keratitis
c. Fungal keratitis
d. All of the above

[Ref: Parsons' 23rd/e pg. 176]

Explanation
- The filamentary fungi produce corneal lesions with white/gray infiltrate and feathery borders.
- There might be satellite lesions with hypopyon and conjunctival injection as well as purulent secretions

35. Layer of cornea which helps in maintaining the hydration of stroma:
a. Endothelium
b. Epithelium
c. Epithelium and endothelium both
d. Bowman's layer

[Ref: Parsons' 23rd/e pg. 108]

Explanation
- The corneal epithelium & endothelium maintain a steady fluid content of the corneal stroma.

36. Esotropia is more common in:
a. Astigmatism
b. Myopia
c. Hypermetropia
d. Emmetropia

[Ref: Parsons' 23rd/e pg. 377; Nema 6th/e pg.324]

Explanation
- Esodeviation (convergent strabismus is generally more common in hypermetropies.
- *Classification of esodeviation*

Type	Criterion
Nonaccommodative	Esotropia at distance = near fixation; no change with refractive correction
Accommodative ■ Refractive (normal AC/A ratio) ■ Nonrefractive (high AC/A ratio) ■ Mixed	Esotropia at distance ⩾ near fixation; fully corrected by hyperopic correction for distance Esotropia at near fixation > distance or manifesting only at near; fully corrected by an additional hyperopic correction for near work
Partially accommodative	Esotropia partly corrected by the use of refractive correction

37. Shifting fluid sign is seen in
a. Retinal dialysis
b. Tractional RD
c. Exudative RD
d. Rhegmatogenous RD

[Ref: Parsons' 23rd/e pg. 306; Nema 6th/e pg.324]

Explanation
- A shift in subretinal fluid with changing the position of head is hallmark of an exudative RD.
- Fundus examination reveals a smooth bullous RD without any retinal folds.

38. Photostress test used to differentiate between:
a. Macula and optic nerve
b. Cataract and glaucoma
c. Retinal and vitreoul diseases
d. Cornea and lens diseases

[Ref: Parsons' 23rd/e pg. 90; Nema 6th/e pg.83]

Explanation
- The photostress recovery test is a simple clinical technique that can differentiate between retinal (macular) and postretinal (e.g. optic nerve) disease.
- Of all the known macular function tests, Photostress is the easiest test of macular function. It can be performed quickly as an OPD procedure
- The basis of this test is to utilise an induced fatigue of macula.
  - In normal people & those with optic nerve disease, there is no significant difference in the time taken for the two eyes to recover from photostress.
  - In a subject with macular disease, the recovery time is prolonged.
- The test is useful in early macular disease, particularly central serous retinopathy.

39. Incongruous homonymous hemianopia with Wernicke's hemianopia pupil. What is the site of lesion?
a. Visual cortex/Anterior occipital cortex
b. Optic tract
c. Optic nerve/Lateral geniculate body
d. Optic radiations

[Ref: Parsons' 23rd/e pg. 456; Nema 6th/e pg. 342]

Explanation
- Hemianopia is due to a lesion situated in any part of the visual paths from the chiasma to the occipital lobe.
- More proximal the lesion, hemianopia is more congruous. Lesion of optic tract are distal so incongruous.
- The optic tract carries uncrossed temporal fibres of the same side & more crossed nasal fibres of the opposite side, therefore, a lesion of the tract results in homonymous hemianopia. As the arrangement of the nerve fibres is not regular in the tract, lesions of the optic tract give asymmetrical or incongruous (dissimilarities in the size, shape & location of the visual field of each eye) homonymous hemianopia. Optic tract lesions are a/w Wernicke's hemianopic pupil.
- The association of hemianopia with contralateral 3rd CN palsy & ipsilateral hemiplegia indicates an optic nerve lesion.

34.	c
35.	a
36.	c
37.	c
38.	a
39.	b

40. A 40-year-old women presents with bilateral painful proptosis, with restricted ocular movement and chemosis. What is your probable diagnosis?

a. Orbital lymphoma
b. Orbital cellulitis
c. Pseudotumor of orbit
d. Thyroid eye disease

[Ref: Parsons' 23rd/e pg. 435; Nema 6th/e pg. 458]

Explanation

- Bilateral thyroid ophthalmopathy involves multiple extraocular muscles and restricts the ocular movements.
- Graves' ophthalmopathy most commonly involves the inferior rectus muscle causing its fibrosis and restriction of elevation.

41. A patient with history of diabetes mellitus and hypertension complaints of diplopia and squint. On examination secondary deviation is more common than primary deviation. Diagnosis is:-

a. Concomitant squint
b. Paralytic squint
c. Accommodative esotropia
d. Convergence insufficiency

[Ref: Parsons' 23rd/e pg. 386; Nema 6th/e pg. 393]

Explanation

- Incomitant or paralytic strabismus (paralytic squint) is characterized by impaired action of one or more extraocular muscles a/w diplopia & variation in the angle of deviation in different directions of gaze.
  - Secondary deviation is always greater than the primary deviation in incomitant (paralytic) strabismus.
  - In non-paralytic (comitant) squint secondary deviation is = the primary deviation.
  - In all phorias the deviation is equally shared between the two eyes.
- The sign & symptoms a/w paralytic squint:-
  - Squint
  - Diplopia
  - Limitation of ocular movement
  - False orientation
  - Abnormal head position
  - Vertigo

		Paralytic Incominant)	Non-paralytic (cominant)
1	Occurrence	Less common (15%)	More common (85%)
2	Onset	Usually acquired & sudden; usually a sign of neurological or orbital disease; any age	Usually congenital
3	Deviation	Secondary deviation > primary deviation	Primary deviation = secondary deviation
4	Limitation of movement	+	-

42. Patient presented with unilateral proptosis with restriction of eye movement but euthyroid. What can be the cause:

a. Thyroid ophthalmopathy
b. Orbital cellulitis
c. Orbital pseudotumor
d. Orbital lymphoma

[Ref: Parsons' 23rd/e pg. 435; Nema 6th/e pg. 458]

Explanation

- Ocular movements can get restricted in a specific directional of gaze by an orbital mass.

43. These marked eye movements are lost in

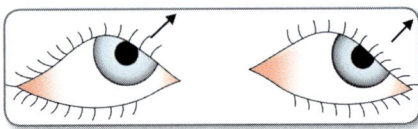

a. 4th nerve palsy
b. 6th nerve palsy
c. 7th nerve palsy
d. 3rd nerve palsy

[Ref: Parsons' 23rd/e pg. 359]

Explanation

- The movements shown in the image are carried out by right inferior oblique and left superior rectus muscle.
- These muscles are supplied by 3rd CN. So the most likely cause is 3rd nerve palsy.

44. Presence of extra layer of cilia posterior to grey line is called

a. Trichiasis
b. Distichiasis
c. Poliosis
d. Madarosis

[Ref: Parsons' 23rd/e pg. 420]

Explanation

- *Trichiais*: Misdirected cilia (e.g. in trachoma & spastic entropion)
- *Distichiais*: Extra posterior row of cilia. Treated by lid splitting with cryotherapy.
- *Poliosis*: A patch of white hair due to lack of melanin in the hair shafts of the affected area. It is most often seen in scalp hair, but may also affect eyebrows, eyelashes.
- *Madarosis*: Loss of eyelashes & sometimes eyebrows.

45. Prerequisite to sympathetic ophthalmitis is:-

a. Blunt trauma
b. Penetrating trauma
c. Chemical injury
d. Retained intra ocular Iron foreign body

[Ref: Parsons' 23rd/e pg. 506]

Explanation

- Sympathetic ophthalmitis or sympathetic ophthalmia almost always results from a penetrating wound o, occurring in 0.2%-0.5% of such cases.

Answer key

40. d
41. b
42. c
43. d
44. b
45. b

46. A patient diagnosed with rheumatoid arthritis was on monotherapy for long time. After 2 years, he developed blurring of vision and was found to have corneal opacity. Which drug is most likely culprit in this case?
  a. Sulfasalazine   b. Chloroquine
  c. Methotrexate   d. Leflunomide

[Ref: KDT Essential of medical pharmacology 8th/e pg. 880]

Explanation

- Prolonged use of high doses of chloroquine (as required for RA, DLE, etc.) may cause loss of vision due to retinal damage. **Corneal deposits** may also occur and affect vision, but are reversible on discontinuation.
- Sulfasalazine, methotrexate and leflunomide are used in Rheumatoid arthritis but does not cause blurring of vision due to corneal opacity.

ENT

47. Tubercular otitis media is characterized by all the following except?
  a. Multiple perforations of tympanic membrane are seen
  b. Pale granulations
  c. ATT should be started
  d. Painful otorrhea is seen

[Ref: Dhingra's 7th/e pg. 81]

Explanation

Tubercular Otitis Media

- CF: Typical presentation is **chronic painless foul smelling otorrhea**, severe conductive type hearing loss (out of proportion to symptoms), involvement of labyrinth can lead to SNHL, Facial nerve palsy.
- O/E: Multiple perforations in tympanic membrane which are later coalesce into single large perforation (Sieve like tympanic membrane). Middle ear and mastoid are filled with pale granulation tissue
- Treatment- ATT for Primary disease, Oral toilet, Mastoid surgery

48. Surgery to widen the cartilaginous part of external auditory canal (EAC) is called:
  a. Myringoplasty   b. Meatoplasty
  c. Otoplasty   d. Tympanoplasty

[Ref: Dhingra's 7th/e pg. 455]

Explanation

- **Meatoplasty** is an operation to widen the meatus. In this crescent of conchal cartilage is excised. It is invariably combined with all canal wall down procedures e.g. radical mastoidectomy & modified radical mastoidectomy.
- Myringoplasty is repair of a perforation of the tympanic membrane (the pars tensa).
- Tympanoplasty is ossicular reconstruction with myringoplasty. (TYMPANUM=Middle ear)
- Otoplasty is reconstruction of pinna

49. A 6-year-old boy presented with fever with pain in the throat and difficulty in deglutition. On examination of throat following finding are seen. Most likely diagnosis is / Pt. came to the OPD with the history of fever ,sore throat. On examination the throat shows the following appearance. Diagnosis is

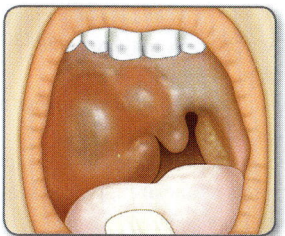

  a. Peritonsillar abscess   b. Parapharyngeal abscess
  c. Ludwig's angina   d. Retropharyngeal abscess

[Ref: Dhingra's 7th/e pg. 298]

Explanation

- The clinical presentation and examination findings are typical of *peritonsillar abscess*.
  ○ Peritonsillar abscess or Quinsy is collection of pus in the peritonsillar space which lies between the fibrous capsule of the tonsil, and the superior constrictor muscle of the pharynx.
  ○ Usually follows acute tonsillitis.
  ○ Usually the largest crypt, crypta magna is affected first.
  ○ Condition is generally unilateral. Tonsil is swollen, red, hot & congested.
  ○ Uvula and soft palate are pushed to opposite side. Uvula Points towards Normal side as shown in the image.
  ○ Common organism are Streptococcus, Staph aureus, anaerobic organism, more often mixed growth is seen.
- ***Parapharyngeal abscess*** (abscess of lateral pharyngeal space, pterygomaxillary space, pharyngomaxillary space): Swelling is on lateral wall of Pharynx pushing tonsils towards midline. Patient may also have a swelling in neck, posterior to SCM muscle. Patient may also present with Trimus.
- ***Ludwig's angina*** is cellulitis of submandibular space.

50. A 2-year-old child presented with hoarseness and following X-ray finding on AP view neck. What is the most likely diagnosis?

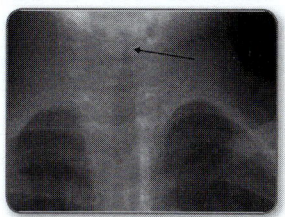

  a. Croup
  b. Acute epiglottitis
  c. Laryngomalacia
  d. Foreign Body in the trachea

[Ref: Dhingra's 7th/e pg. 328]

46. b
47. d
48. b
49. a
50. a

Explanation

- The given radiograph of neck is showing "Steeple sign"/pencil tip sign, which is classical of croup/ Acute Laryngotracheobronchitis (ALTB) –
  - Occurs due to subglottic inflammation, most commonly a result of infection with parainfluenza virus.
  - Typically occurs in children between 6 months and 3 years of age.
  - Croup is the most common cause of airway obstruction in young children.
  - Younger patients have a characteristic "barking" cough that is worse at night and when crying.
- Clinical Features
  - Onset of croup is gradual with prodrome of upper respiratory symptoms.
  - Fever is usually of low grade, painful croupy cough (barking cough or seal barks cough) is associated with hoarseness and stridor.
- Imaging Features:
  - Frontal radiograph of the neck is most helpful. Subglottic larynx with smooth lateral convex shoulders is normal finding.
  - **Steeple Sign (Inverted V sign):** Loss of these lateral convexities leading to **narrowing of the tracheal air column** resembling a church steeple.
  - Subglottic region is most narrowed because conus elasticus is particularly susceptible to edema.
  - Lateral soft-tissue neck radiograph: Subglottic narrowing and increased density of the subglottic region.
  - Always identify the normal epiglottis on every lateral radiograph, because this identification will exclude epiglottitis, a more sinister diagnosis, from the differential diagnosis.
- Treatment: supportive because the symptoms are usually self-limited.

Differential Diagnosis

- *Acute epiglottis (Supraglottic laryngitis)* is an acute inflammatory condition of the supraglottic structures epiglottis, aryepiglottic fold and arytenoids.
  - Child prefers sitting position with hyperextended neck (**tripod sign**) which relieves stridor
  - Drooling of saliva is found as child has dysphagia
  - Lateral soft tissue X-ray of neck shows: Swollen epiglottis (**Thumb sign**), Absence of deep well-defined vallecula (**vallecula sign**).

51. Saccule of ear develops from

a. Pars superior
b. Pars inferior
c. Sacculus anterior
d. Saculus posterior

[Ref: Dhingra's 7th/e pg. 13]

Explanation

- Development of pars superior (semicircular canals and utricle) takes place earlier than pars inferior (saccule and cochlea).
- The pars superior is phylogenetically older part of labyrinth.

52. After an RTA patient presents with multiple contusions all over the body and blue purplish colour behind mastoid as shown in the image. This signifies:

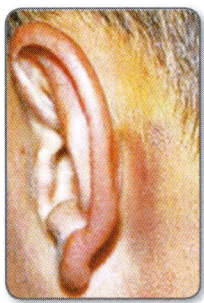

a. Battle sign
b. Bezold abcess
c. Raccoon sign
d. Guerin,s sign

[Ref: Dhingra's 7th/e pg. 507; Essentials of Forensic Medicine & toxicology, KS Narayana Reddy 33rd/e pg. 247]

Explanation

Battle sign	▪ Ecchymosis or hematoma over mastoid ▪ Seen in # of temporal bone, # posterior cranial fossa ▪ Suggestive of underlying brain trauma	
Racoon sign	▪ Periorbital ecchymosis ▪ Seen in # of orbital floor. ▪ Bruising in the palate in the region of the greater palatine arteries	
Guerin's sign	▪ Bruising in the palate in the region of the greater palatine arteries. ▪ Seen in midfacial/Le Fort I #.	
Bezold's abscess	▪ Pus passes through the tip of mastoid into the sternocleidomastoid muscle in the upper part of neck	
Citelli's abscess	▪ Pus is seen in digastric triangle.	

53. A child presented with fever and dysphagia. Examination showed the following. What could be your diagnosis?

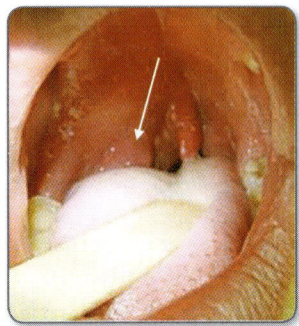

a. Infectious mononucleosis
b. Tonsillar growth
c. Parapharyngeal mass
d. Quinsy

54. While doing parotid Surgery, the following landmarks are used to identify the facial nerve trunk except:
a. Inferior belly of omohyoid
b. Dissecting from peripheral branches
c. Posterior belly of digastric insertion
d. Tragal pointer

[Ref: Dhingra's 7th/e pg. 100]

Explanation

- *Surgical landmarks of facial nerve for parotid surgery*
  - Cartilaginous pointer. The nerve lies 1 cm deep and slightly anterior and inferior to the pointer. Cartilaginous pointer is a sharp triangular piece of cartilage of the pinna and "points" to the nerve.
  - Tympanomastoid suture. Nerve lies 6–8 mm deep to this suture.
  - Styloid process. The nerve crosses lateral to styloid process.
  - Posterior belly of digastric. If posterior belly of digastric muscle is traced backwards along its upper border to its attachment to the digastric groove, nerve is found to lie between it and the styloid process.

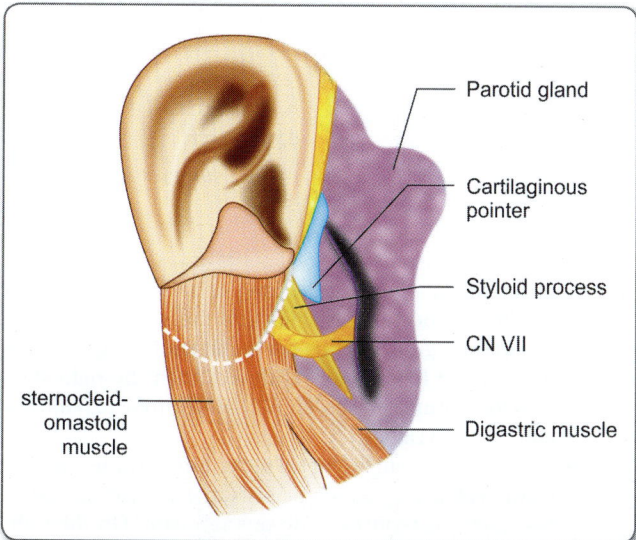

- *Surgical landmarks of facial nerve for ear & mastoid surgery*
  - Processus cochleariformis
  - Oval window & horizontal canal
  - Incus short process
  - Pyramid
  - Tympanomastoid suture
  - Digastric ridge

55. Partial closure of nostril is done in which condition
a. Allergic rhinitis
b. Atrophic rhinitis
c. Vasomotor rhinitis
d. Occupational rhinitis

[Ref: Dhingra's 7th/e pg. 10073]

Explanation

- Atrophic Rhinitis: Atrophic chronic inflammatory disease characterized by progressive atrophy of the nasal mucosa and the underlying bone of the turbinates associated with excessive crusting which leads to nasal obstruction.
- Young's operation & modified Young's operation are surgical treatment modalities for Atrophic rhinitis patients.
  - In Young's operation: Both the nostrils are closed **completely**. after elevation of the nasal vestibular folds. They are opened after 6 months.
  - In Modified Young's operation: To avoid the discomfort of bilateral nasal obstruction, partial closure of the nostril is done leaving behind a 1- 3 mm hole. It is kept for a period of 2 years.

56. Occipito- mental X-ray view of paranasal sinuses with open mouth as shown below is also known as?

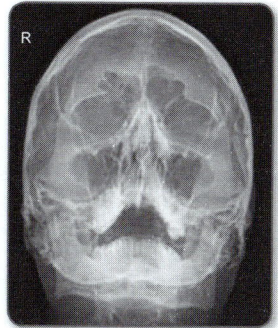

a. Pierre's view   b. Towne's view
c. Caldwell view   d. Water's view

[Ref: Dhingra's 7th/e pg. 493, 497]

Explanation

Water's view	▪ Occipito-mental view or nose chin position
	▪ For maxillary sinus & anterior ethmoid sinuses
	▪ Sinuses not seen in water's view → Post. ethmoidal > sphenoid
Caldwell's view	▪ Occipito-frontal view or nose forehead position
	▪ Best view for frontal sinus
Rhese view	▪ Oblique view.
	▪ For ethmoid sinus.
Base skull view	▪ For sphenoid sinus
Pierre's view	▪ Occipito-mental or Water's view with mouth wide open

- Waters' view (also known as the Occipitomental view) is a radiographic view, where an X-ray beam is angled at 37° to the orbitomeatal line.
- Air fluid levels are seen in acute sinusitis.
- Mucosal thickening is a feature of chronic sinusitis.

57. A 70 yrs old patient presented with history of fever, repeated aspiration, halitosis and coughing in the night. On examination there is a swelling on left side of neck which produces gurgling sound on compression. Following is the barium swallow study of the patient. What is the most likely Diagnosis?

a. Zenkers diverticulum
b. Laryngocoele
c. Plummer Vinson Syndrome & Schatzki's ring
d. Dysphagia lusoria

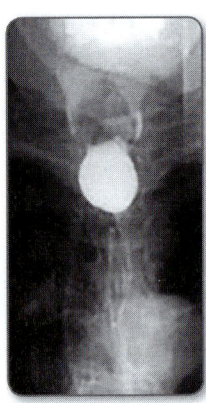

[Ref: Dhingra's 7th/e pg. 310]

Explanation

- **■ *Zenker's Diverticulum***
  - It is a pharyngeal pouch and also called hypopharyngeal diverticulum.
  - It is a type of pulsion diverticulum where pharyngeal mucosa herniates through the Killian's dehiscence.
  - Patient present with intermittent dysphagia, regurgitation of food and foul smelling breath. Gurgling sound is produced on swallowing
  - May have associated hiatus hernia.
  - Rx: Cricopharyngeal myotomy, Dohlman's procedure & endoscopic surgery.
- **■ *Laryngocele*** is an air-filled cystic swelling due to dilatation of saccule. It is a diverticulum of mucosa which starts from the anterior part of ventricular cavity and extends upward between vestibular folds and lamina of thyroid cartilage .

58. A patient presented to OPD with multiple contusion marks and scratches after being beaten. He starts coughing whenever he scratches over the post-auricular contusion marks. Most likely nerve involved is?

a. Auricular Branch of vagus
b. Auriculo temporal nerve
c. Greater auricular nerve
d. Facial nerve

[Ref: Dhingra's 7th/e pg. 5]

Explanation

- ■ Mechanical stimulation (e.g. during scratching or syringing) of the external auditory meatus (EAM or EAC) can activate the auricular branch of the vagus nerve (Arnold's nerve) and evoke reflex cough.
- ■ *Nerve supply of EAC:-*
  - Anterior wall and roof by auriculotemporal nerve

- Posterior wall and floor by auricular branch of vagus nerve (Arnold N).
- Posterior wall of auditory canal also receives innervations by facial nerve through auricular branch of vagus.

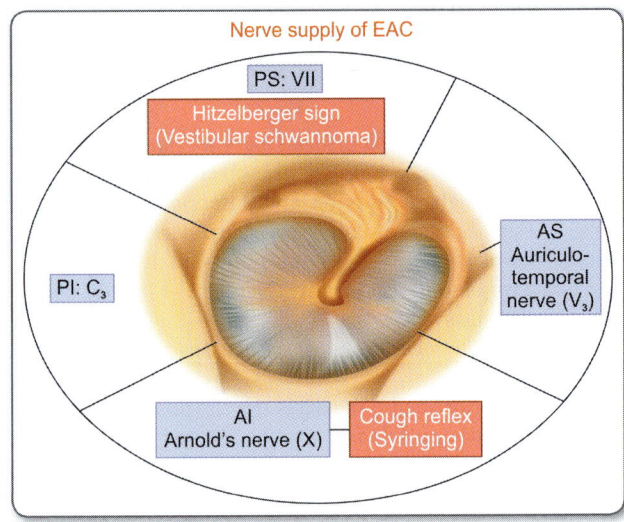

Nerve supply of EAC

59. Left recurrent laryngeal nerve has a longer course than right because of which arch artery:

a. 1st arch   b. 2nd arch
c. 4th arch   d. 6th arch

[Ref: Dhingra's 7th/e pg. 310]

Explanation

- ■ The Left recurrent laryngeal nerve arises from the vagus in the mediastinum at the level of arch of aorta, loops around it, and then ascends into the neck in tracheo-esophageal groove. Thus left recurrent laryngeal nerve has a much longer course in neck than the right side. This long course makes left RLN more prone to paralysis compared to right RLN.
- ■ The Left recurrent laryngeal nerve **hooks under the left sixth arch artery** which persists in extra-uterine life as the ductus arteriosus, a fibrous remnant. On the right side, neither the 6th nor 5th arch arteries persist and so the recurrent laryngeal nerve is restrained by the next most superior structure which is the fourth branchial arch artery (Right Subclavian Artery).
- ■ Rarely, the right recurrent laryngeal nerve is no longer restrained by a subclavian artery and so it divides from the vagus more superiorly to run inferiorly on the larynx. This anomalous nerve (Non Recurrent Laryngeal nerve) may be transected during thyroid surgery.

DERMATOLOGY

60. An elderly female with a long-standing mole over face for many years, now presents with suddenly increase in the size & irregular borders of the mole. What is the cause?

a. Superficial spreading melanoma
b. Lentigo maligna melanoma
c. Acral Lentiginous
d. Nodular melanoma

[Ref: Bailey & Love's 27th/e pg. 609]

57. a
58. a
59. d
60. a

Explanation

- Superficial spreading melanoma: This is the MC type (70 %), of malignant melanoma and it is also the most common type which occurs in a patient with a pre-existing mole (naevus), after several years of slow change, followed by rapid growth in the preceding months before presentation.
- Borders are usually irregular.

61. Image showing grouped lesion on lips?

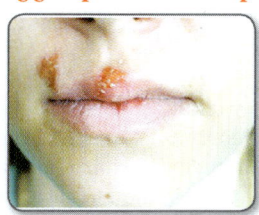

a. Impetigo contagiosa   b. Pemphigus vulgaris
c. Herpes labialis   d. Varicella zoster

[Ref: Nelson's 21st/e pg. 1703]

Explanation

Herpes labialis

- Grouped lesions shown in the image are typical of herpes labialis. It is characterized by:-
  - **Fever blisters:** Fever blisters (cold sores) are the MC manifestations of recurrent HSV-1 infections.
  - MC site is vermilion border of lip.
  - The lesions begin as small grouped papules that progress to vesicles over few hours.
  - Complete healing without scarring occurs usually within 6-10 days.

62. Identify the phenomenon shown in the image:

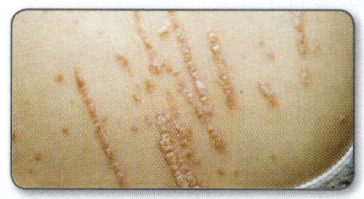

a. Isomorphic phenomenon
b. Reverse isomorphic phenomena
c. Nikolsky sign
d. Gottron's papule

[Ref: Nelson's 21st/e pg. 3497]

Explanation

- Lesion aggravates on trauma in isomorphic phenomena
- Lesions disappear in Reverse isomorphic
  [For Details: See Dermatology theory]

63. Identify the condition with scarring as shown in the image:

a. DLE   b. SLE
c. Rosaceae   d. Vitiligo

[Ref: Harrison's 20th /e pg. 361; Nelson's 21st/e pg. 3445]

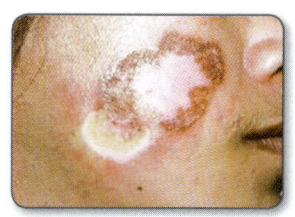

Explanation

- The characteristic finding in DLE (Discoid lupus erythematosus) is chronic, erythematous, scaly and atrophic plaques on sun exposed skin area which frequently heal with scarring. and dyspigmentation.
- Nasal, oral mucosa, eyes may be involved.

64. Identify the lesion associated with scaling and itching:

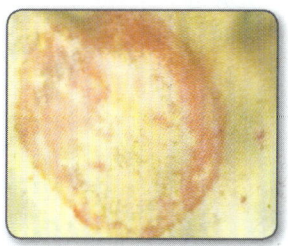

a. Granulum annulare   b. Tinea corporis
c. Pyoderma granulosum   d. Icthyosis vulgaris

[Ref: Nelson's 21st/e pg. 3562]

Explanation

- Tinea corporis, aka ringworm, is a superficial dermatophytosis of the arms and legs, especially on glabrous skin; however, it may occur on any part of the body. It usually does not affect palm, soles, groin.
- *T. rubrum & Trichophyton mentagrophytes* are the MC species .
- Acquired by direct contact.
- Typical lesion is dry, mildly erythematous, elevated , **scaly** papule/plaque which spreads centrifugally & clears centrally to form the characteristic **annular** lesion. (hence called "ringworm").

65. A patient presented to the OPD with complaints of papular lesions over the extremities. On examination the lesions were soft and non tender. Image of the lesion is provided below. What is the probable diagnosis of this case?

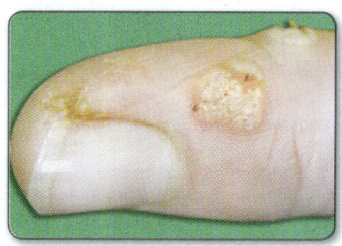

a. Condylomata lata
b. Molluscum contagiosum
c. Condylomata accuminata
d. Common warts

[Ref: Nelson's 21st/e pg. 3566]

61.	c
62.	a
63.	a
64.	b
65.	d

Explanation

- Warts (Verruca) are caused by HPV.
- Common warts (Verruca vulgaris) are, caused MC by HPV type 2 and 4 and occurs most frequently on the fingers, dorsum of the hands, face, knees & elbows.
- They are well-circumscribed papules with an irregular, roughened, keratotic surface.
- Uncinate process cancer is more likely to invade blood vessel and has worse prognosis due to the earlier and more frequent locoregional recurrence.

66. A patient with history of contact with tuberculosis presents with following lesion over chest . There is central scarring. What is true about this patient?

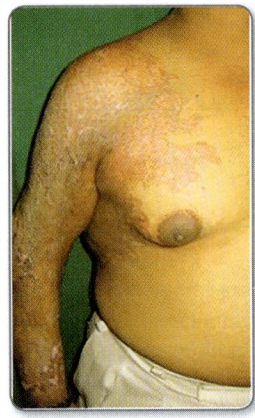

[Ref: Nelson's 21st/e pg. 3558; Harrison's 20th/e pg. 352]

a. This is a case of sarcoidosis , start steroids immediately
b. It is a case of lupus vulgaris, start on ATT
c. Start antifungals
d. None of the above

66. b
67. c
68. c
69. c

Explanation

- Lupus vulgaris is a form of cutaneous TB that is seen in previously infected and sensitized individual. There is often an underlying active TB in the lungs or lymph nodes.
- Typical lesions are **red brown plaques which show secondary central scarring.**

GENERAL SURGERY

67. A patient was diagnosed as Carcinoma uncinate process presents with sudden abdominal pain on one day. The tumor has infiltrated into

a. Portal vein
b. Inferior mesenteric artery
c. Superior mesenteric artery
d. Splenic Vein

[Ref: Bailey & Love's 27th/e pg. 1236]

Explanation

- Uncinate process cancer is more likely to invade blood vessel and has worse prognosis due to the earlier and more frequent locoregional recurrence.

- The uncinate process is a hook like extension from the lower part of the head of the pancreas, and it extends supero- posteriorly behind the superior mesenteric vein (SMV). Invasion of the **root of the superior mesenteric artery** is also noted.

68. Which of the following is not a part of ASEPSIS wound scoring system?

a. Serous discharge
b. Isolation of Bacteria
c. Induration
d. Erythema

[Ref: Bailey & Love's 27th/e pg. 48]

Explanation

- In ASEPSIS wound score the points are given for the need for **A**dditional treatment, the presence of **S**erous discharge, **E**rythema, **P**urulent exudate, and **S**eparation of the deep tissues, the **I**solation of bacteria, and the duration of inpatient **S**tay (ASEPSIS).

Criterion	Description	Points
A Additional treatment	Antibiotics	10
	Drainage of pus under local anaesthetics	5
	Debridement of wound (General anaesthetics)	10
S Serous discharge	Daily	0-5
E Erythema	Daily	0-5
P Purulent exudates	Daily	0-10
S Separation of deep tissues	Daily	0-10
I Isolation of bacteria		10
S Stay in hospital prolonged over 14 days		5

69. Management of an RCC less than 4 cm in size?

a. Chemotherapy
b. Surgery followed by chemotherapy
c. Partial nephrectomy
d. Radical nephrectomy

[Ref: Bailey & Love's 27th/e pg. 1420]

Explanation

Treatment for Renal Tumours

- Surgery is the mainstay of treatment for organ confined RCC.
  - Partial nephrectomy is done for T1 lesions (≤ 7 cm).
  - Cytoreductive nephrectomy (removal of kidney in presence of metastatic disease) is performed in a patient with good performance status.
  - Radical nephrectomy is the treatment of choice for localized RCC.
- Tyrosine kinase inhibitors can be used for treatment of metastatic RCC.

70. A male patient on follow up of recurrent abdominal pain, incidentally detected with an abdominal aortic aneurysm with diameter of 44 mm. What is the appropriate management of this patient:
a. Immediate surgery
b. Medical treatment using anti-hypertensives
c. Serial USG monitoring till size of the aneurysm reaches 77 mm
d. Operate when size reaches 55 mm

[Ref: Bailey & Love's 27th/e pg. 961]

Explanation

- 55 mm is the critical diameter of an abdominal aortic aneurysm and surgery should be done even in asymptomatic patients at this level.

71. True statement about intermittent claudication:
a. Felt at rest
b. Claudication distance can vary from day to day
c. Relieved after getting out of bed and walking
d. Most common site is the calf

[Ref: Bailey & Love's 27th/e pg. 943]

Explanation

Intermittent Claudication

- Intermittent claudication is a cramp-like pain felt in the muscles that is:
  - **pain is brought on by walking**;
  - not present on taking the first step (unlike osteoarthritis);
  - relieved by standing still (unlike nerve compression from a lumbar intervertebral disc prolapse or osteoarthritis of the spine or spinal stenosis).
- Claudication distance: distance that a patient is able to walk without stopping varies only slightly from day to day.
  - It is altered by walking up hill, the speed of walking, carrying heavy weights and changes in general health, such as anaemia or heart failure.
  - Claudication pain is increased after getting out of bed and walking.
- The pain of claudication is usually felt in the **calf** because the superficial femoral artery is the most commonly affected (70 %) > aortoiliac disease (30%).
- Rarely buttock claudication is associated with sexual impotence resulting from arterial insufficiency, known as *Leriche's syndrome*.

72. A 70-years-old male smoker comes to hospital with cramping gluteal pain after walking 500 meter. Pain in both the calf and in the buttock, claudication is present. What is the most common site of atherosclerosis?
a. Arterial disease with Aortoiliac obstruction
b. Arterial disease with femoral obstruction
c. Iliac obstruction
d. Distal obstruction

[Ref: Bailey & Love's 27th/e pg. 943]

Explanation

- Arterial disease with aorto-iliac involvement is seen in 30% cases of intermittent claudication.
- Aks Leriche's syndrome.
- Patient presents with gluteal claudication and sexual impotence.

73. Barium image is showing bird's beak appearance. Diagnosis is:
a. Achalasia cardia   b. Esophageal stricture
c. Jackhammer esophagus d. Normal esophagus

[Ref: Bailey & Love's 27th/e pg. 1085]

Explanation

- Bird's beak and rat tail appearance are seen in → Achalasia cardia. Other important points regarding achalasia are:-
  - Megaesophagus
  - Manometry is gold standard
  - Secondary achalasia is seen in Chagas disease.

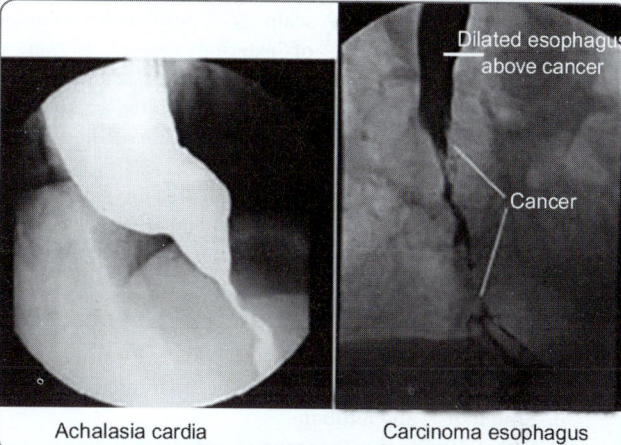

Achalasia cardia   Carcinoma esophagus

- Pseudoachalasia is an achalasia-like disorder that is usually produced by adenocarcinoma of the cardia.
- The two main methods of treatment are forceful dilatation of the cardia and Heller's myotomy.

74. A barium swallow image is given, Most Likely Diagnosis is:

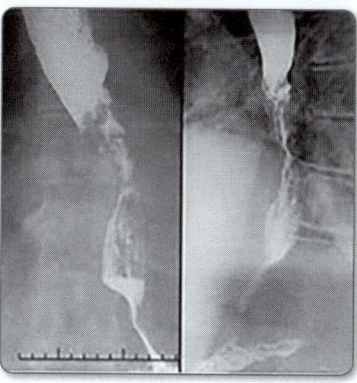

a. Achalasia cardia
b. Ca esophagus
c. Esophageal stricture
d. GERD

70.	d
71.	d
72.	a
73.	a
74.	b

75. A middle aged man presented with a swelling over neck since childhood. Neck swelling has a bag of worm appearance and a bruit heard over the swelling on auscultation. What is your diagnosis?

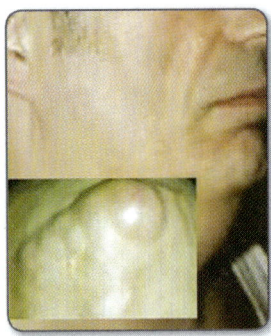

a. Cirsoid aneurysm
b. Plexiform neurofibroma
c. Vasculitis
d. Lymphangioma

Explanation

- Cirsoid aneurysm of scalp is a rare arteriovenous malformation (AVM) of external carotid branches and scalp veins. This malformation of scalp is also synonymously called as plexiform angioma, aneurysma racemosum, and aneurysm cirsoide, aneurysma serpentinum.
- Plexiform neurofibromas can be present since early childhood and can be seen in the head and neck region.

76. A 20-year-old boy is brought to the emergency following an RTA with shortness of breath and hypotension. He has subcutaneous emphysema and no air entry on the right side. What is the next best step in the management:
a. Wide bore Needle insertion in the 5th intercostal space
b. Shift to ICU and intubate
c. Start IV fluids after insertion of wide bore IV line
d. Positive pressure ventilation

[Ref: Bailey & Love's 27th/e pg. 919]

Explanation

- History and clinical examination is suggestive of tension pneumothorax- according to trauma updates, needle decompression in adults should be done in the 5th intercostal space.

77. Patient presents with purulent peritonitis. During exploratory laparotomy a diverticular perforation is seen in sigmoid colon with fecal peritonitis. What is the Hinchey's stage:
a. Stage 1
b. Stage 2b
c. Stage 3
d. Stage 4

[Ref: Bailey & Love's 27th/e pg. 1274]

Explanation

Modified Hinchey Classification of Diverticulitis

- Hinchey Classification is used to describe perforations of the colon due to diverticulitis.
- Fecal peritonitis is stage 4 according to Hinchey's classification.

Stage	Features
Stage 0	Mild clinical diverticulitis
Stage 1a	Confined pericolic inflammation or phlegmen
Stage 1b	Confined pericolic abscess
Stage 2	Pelvic distant intra-abdominal or retroperitoneal abscess
Stage 3	Generalised purulent peritonitis
Stage 4	Fecal peritonitis

78. In a patient with parathyroid adenoma, to confirm the removal of the correct gland after surgery, Miami criteria is used. Regarding Miami criteria which is correct?
a. 50% reduction in PTH within 10 mins of gland removal
b. 50% reduction in PTH within 5 mins of gland removal
c. 25% reduction in PTH within 10 mins of gland removal
d. 25% reduction in PTH within 5 mins of gland removal

[Ref: Bailey & Love's 27th/e pg. 830]

Explanation

- The Miami criteria were developed to determine the extent of parathyroid resection during minimally invasive parathyroidectomy.
- According to this criteria, iPTH drop ⩾50% from the highest of either pre-incision or pre-excision level at 10 minutes after gland excision.

79. During evaluation of dysphagia in a 30 years old patient high resolution esophageal manometry was performed, which revealed abnormal spastic contractions in esophagus, integrated relaxation pressure >450 mm Hg in the body of stomach & panesophageal pressurization. Diagnosis is:
a. Type 1 achalasia
b. Type 2 achalasia
c. Type 3 achalasia
d. Jackhammer esophagus

[Ref: Bailey & Love's 27th/e pg. 1096]

Explanation

The Chicago Classification of Esophageal Motility

Achalasia & EGJ ouflow obstruction	Criteria
Type 1 achalasia (Classic achalasia)	(Classic) with minimal contractility in the esophageal body, 100% failed peristalsis
Type II	Intermittent periods of panesophageal pressurization, 100% failed peristalsis
Stage III	Spastic achalasia with premature or spastic distal esophageal contractions, no normal peristalsis

- Achalasia type 1,2,3 & esophagogastric junction obstruction all are a/w ↑ median IRG (integrated relaxation pressure) > 15 mm Hg.

75.	a
76.	a
77.	d
78.	a
79.	c

80. What is the name of the Flap reconstruction shown in the image below:

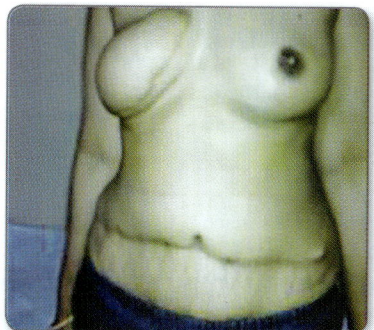

a. DIEP flap - deep inferior epigastric artery perforator flap
b. PMMC Flap
c. DP flap
d. LD flap

[Ref: Bailey & Love's 27th/e pg. 880]

Explanation

- A DIEP flap is similar to a muscle-sparing free TRAM flap, except that no muscle is used to rebuild the breast. It is based on deep inferior epigastric vessels.
- In a DIEP flap, fat, skin, and blood vessels are cut from the abdominal wall /lower belly and moved up to your chest to rebuild your breast (Tummy tuck operation).
- This flap may be preferable to the older TRAM flap .

81. A child presented with evisceration of bowel loops without coverings. Visceras were coming out of the defect in abdominal wall right to the umbilicus. The possible diagnosis is:

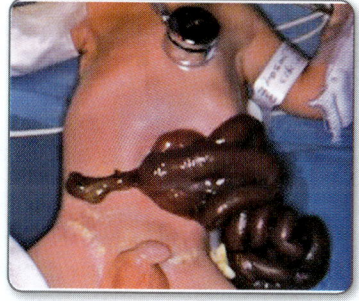

a. Omphalocele
b. Gastrochisis
c. Spigelian hernia
d. Prune belly syndrome

[Ref: Bailey & Love's 27th/e pg. 135, 1041]

Explanation

- *Gastroschisis* is an abdominal wall defect in this the bowel herniates out adjacent to the umbilicus and the bowel is not covered with any peritoneum.
- *Spigelian hernia (or lateral ventral hernia)* occurs through slit like defect in the anterior abdominal wall adjacent to the semilunar line.
- *Prune belly syndrome* is a condition characterized by a lack of abdominal muscles, causing the skin on the abdominal area to wrinkle and appear "prune-like"; undescended testicles in males

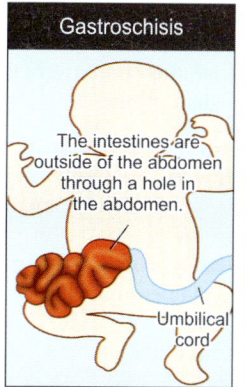
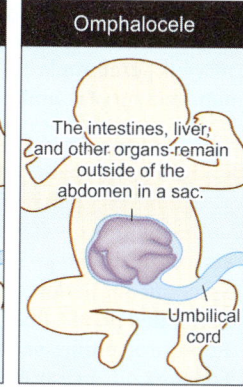

82. Which of the following statements is true regarding retrosternal goitres:

a. Median sternotomy /sternal incision is always required
b. All should undergo CT chest
c. Majority of the goitres derive their blood supply from thoracic vessels
d. Requires immediate surgery

[Ref: Bailey & Love's 27th/e pg. 810]

Explanation

- Majority of the retrosternal goitres are secondary goitres.
- Mostly arise from the lower pole of a nodular goitre.
- Often symptomless and discovered on a routine chest radiograph.
- Surgical T/t:
  - Resection can almost always be carried out from the neck via a neck/cervical incision, but median sternotomy is sometimes necessary.
  - Early division of the isthmus is often helpful.

83. A man was brought to the emergency after he fell into a man hole and injured his perineum. He feels the urge to micturate but is unable to pass urine. O/e there is blood at the tip of the urethral meatus with extensive swelling of the penis and scrotum. What is the location of the injury:

a. Urinary bladder
b. Prostatic urethra
c. Bulbar urethra
d. Membranous urethra

[Ref: Bailey & Love's 27th/e pg. 1479]

Explanation

- Question stem is representative of a distal urethral/ straddle injury with a haematoma in the penis and scrotum. Therefore most likely it is a case of injury of bulbar urethra.
- There is a history of a **blow to the perineum**, usually due to a fall astride injury. The bulbar urethra is crushed upwards onto the pubic bone, typically with significant bruising.
- Cycling accidents, **loose manhole covers** and gym accidents astride the beam account for a number of cases.
- CF: perineal bruising and butterfly shaped haematoma, extravasation of urine is common. There is usually bleeding from the urethral meatus and retention of urine is also typically present.
- Rupture of bulbar urethra leads to extravasation of urine in
  - Penis
  - Scortum

80.	a
81.	b
82.	b
83.	c

○ Superficial perineal pouch
○ Anterior abdominal wall
■ Delayed urethroplasty is the preferred definitive management of complete disruptions.

84. A 25-year old male after a full stomach meal presents with abdominal pain following a sudden vomiting. There is tenderness in the upper abdomen and on X-ray, widening of the mediastinum is seen with pneumo-mediastinum. What is the most probable diagnosis:

a. Spontaneous perforation of the esophagus
b. Perforated peptic ulcer
c. Rupture of emphysematous bulla
d. Foreign body in esophagus

[Ref: Bailey & Love's 27th/e pg. 1072]

Explanation

■ Clinical picture is suggestive of spontaneous perforation of esophagus/ Boerhaave's syndrome.
○ Patient can present with retching, subcutaneous emphysema and pain.
○ A chest x-ray is often confirmatory with air in the mediastinum (pneumo-mediastinum), pleura or peritoneum..
○ This occurs classically when a person vomits against a closed glottis. The pressure in the oesophagus increases rapidly, and the oesophagus bursts at its weakest point in the lower one third.
■ The clinical history is usually of severe pain in the chest or upper abdomen following a meal or a bout of drinking. Associated shortness of breath is common. Many cases are misdiagnosed as myocardial infarction, perforated peptic ulcer or pancreatitis if the pain is confined to the upper abdomen.

Boerhaave Syndrome

■ MC in middle aged men.
■ Mackler Triad:
○ a) Episode of severe retching + forceful vomiting
○ b) Sudden excruciating chest pain
○ c)Subcutaneous emphysema
■ Chest radiographic findings: mediastinal widening; air fluid level in mediastinum, extravasation of contrast into mediastinum/ pleura, pneumomediastinum (single most important finding), pneumopericardium & subcutaneous air; pleural effusion (left > right);
■ V sign of Naclerio: Localized mediastinal emphysema with air between lower thoracic aorta and diaphragm.

85. Patient underwent LSCS. Post operatively patient developed abdominal distension and obstipation. Examination showed absence of bowel sounds and Soft consistency of palpation. What is your diagnosis?

a. Uterine Rupture
b. Paralytic ileus
c. Appendicitis
d. **Amniotic fluid peritonitis.**

[Ref: Bailey & Love's 27th/e pg. 1296-97]

Explanation

■ Clinical features of abdominal distension and obstipation along with absent bowel sounds are suggestive of paralytic ileus.
■ Post operative paralytic ileus is common after LSCS.

86. Which one of the following is not a component of THORACOSCORE:

a. Performance status
b. Complication of surgery
c. ASA grading
d. Priority of surgery

[Ref: Bailey & Love's 27th/e pg. 915]

Explanation

■ Thoracoscore is a score used to predict the in-hospital mortality in a patient requiring thoracic surgery

Table: Parameters of thoracoscore for predicting in-hospital mortality for patients requiring thoracic surgery.
Age (<55, 55-65, >65 years)
Sex
ASA score (≤2, ≥3)
Performance status according to Zubrod scale (≤2, ≥3)
Dyspnea score(≤2, ≥3)
Priority of surgery (elective, urgent/emergency)
Extent of resection (pneumonectomy, other)
Diagnosis (malignant, benign)
Composite comorbidity score

87. Which is the most common pancreatic endocrine neoplasm:

a. Insulinoma
b. Gastrinoma
c. VIPoma
d. Glucagonoma

[Ref: Bailey & Love's 27th/e pg. 849]

Explanation

■ Insulinoma is the most frequent of all the functioning pancreatic endocrine tumors (PETs) with reported incidence of 2-4 cases per million population per year.

88. What is the most common site of gastrinoma in MEN 1 syndrome:

a. Jejunum
b. Stomach
c. Duodenum
d. Ileum

[Ref: Bailey & Love's 27th/e pg. 851]

Explanation

■ Wall of the first part of duodenum is the most common site of gastrinoma. Pancreatic gastrinomas are mainly found in sporadic disease; most are found in the head of the pancreas. >70 per cent of the gastrinomas in MEN 1 syndrome and most sporadic gastrinomas are located in the first and second part of the duodenum.

89. 80 yrs old female presented with abdominal colic, jaundice. On further work up LFT showed: increased SGOT, SGPT, Alkaline phosphatase, serum bilirubin levels are elevated, GGT is increased. She has the following findings in Ultrasound abdomen:-scleroatrophic Gall bladder, dilated CBD with large impacted stone, with dilated intrahepatic radicles. What is next step of management:

a. Cholecystectomy
b. ERCP
c. CECT abdomen
d. Observation

[Ref: Bailey & Love's 27th/e pg. 1205]

84.	a
85.	b
86.	b
87.	a
88.	c
89.	b

Explanation

- ERCP should be the next step to retrieve the stones. Cholecystectomy should be done a few days after ERCP if CBD stones are detected along with gall stones.

90. **What is the T stage of a 2.5 cm lung primary lung tumour, which is not involving the pleura, as per AJCC classification?**
    a. T1a
    b. T2
    c. T1b
    d. T1c

[Ref: Bailey & Love's 27th/e pg. 927]

Explanation

	TNM 8th - Primary tumor characteristics
T_x	Tumor in sputum/bronchial washings but bot be assessed in imaging or bronchoscopy
T_0	No evidence of tumor
T_{is}	Carcinoma in situ
T_1	3 cm surrounded by lung/visceral pleura, not involving main bronchus
$T_{1a(mi)}$	Minimally invasive carcinoma
T_{1a}	1 cm
T_{1b}	<1 to ≤ 2 cm
T_{1c}	>2 to ≤ 3 cm in greatest dimension
T_2	>3 to ≤ 5 cm or Involvement of main bronchus without carina, regardless of distance from carina or invasion visceral pleural or atelectasis or post obstructive pneumonitis extending to hilum
T_{2a}	>3 to ≤4 cm
T_{2b}	>4 to ≤5 cm
T_3	>5 to 7 cm in greatest dimension or tumor of any size that involves chest wall, pericardium, phrenic nerve or satellite nodules in the same lobe
T_4	>7 cm in greatest dimension or any tumor with invasion of mediastinum, diaphragm, heart, great vessels, recurrent laryngeal nerve, carina, trachea, oesophagus, spine or separate tumor in different lobe of ipsilateral lung
N_1	Ipsilateral peribronchial and/or hilar nodes and intrapulmonary nodes
N_2	Ipsilateral mediastinal and/or subcarnial nodes
N_3	Contralateral mediastinal or hilar, ipsilateral/ contralateral scalene/supraclavicular
M_1	Distant metastasis
M_{1a}	Tumor in contralateral lung or pleural/pericardial/ contralateral scalene/supraclavicular
M_{1b}	Single extrathoracic metastasis, including signal non-regional lymphnode
M_{1c}	Multiple extrathoracic metastases in one or more organ-

91. **A patient presented in emergency room with a stab injury in left lower chest, with low BP and Pulse rate. After IV fluid resuscitation in trauma center patient's BP became normal. X-ray chest shows clear lung fields. What will be your next step in management:**
    a. CECT Abdomen
    b. Immediate intercostal chest drain insertion
    c. CECT chest
    d. E-fast

[Ref: Bailey & Love's 27th/e pg. 366]

Explanation

- E-fast. This question covers two concepts-
  - Injury to lower chest (esp below the nipples) can also lead to abdominal injury and this has been highlighted by the fact that the lung fields are clear
  - Next step in the management of the patient with suspected abdominal injury would be e-fast.

92. **Which of the following is not included in primary survey of a Trauma patient?**
    a. CECT to look for bleeding
    b. Airway, Breathing, Circulation
    c. Recording BP
    d. Exposure of whole body

[Ref: Bailey & Love's 27th/e pg. 323]

Explanation

- The primary survey comprises the fundamental principles of the ATLS system, the 'ABCDE' of trauma care:-
  - **A**, Airway with cervical spine protection
  - **B**, Breathing and ventilation
  - **C**, Circulation (BP recording) with haemorrhage control
  - **D**, Disability: neurological status
  - **E**, Exposure: completely undress the patient and assess for other injuries

93. **A 50-years-old female patient presented with a midline swelling in the neck 2 cm in size. FNAC from the swelling showed Orphan Annie eyed nuclei. Most likely diagnosis is?**
    a. Papillary thyroid carcinoma
    b. Medullary thyroid carcinoma
    c. Toxic nodular goitre
    d. Follicular thyroid carcinoma

[Ref: Bailey & Love's 27th/e pg. 818]

Explanation

- Histologically the tumour shows papillary projections and characteristic pale, empty nuclei (**Orphan Annie-eyed nuclei**).
- Papillary carcinomas are very seldom encapsulated.
- Papillary microcarcinoma term is used to describe PTC that is <10 mm in size.

90. d
91. d
92. a
93. a

94. Buffalo hump appearance of foot as shown below is seen in:

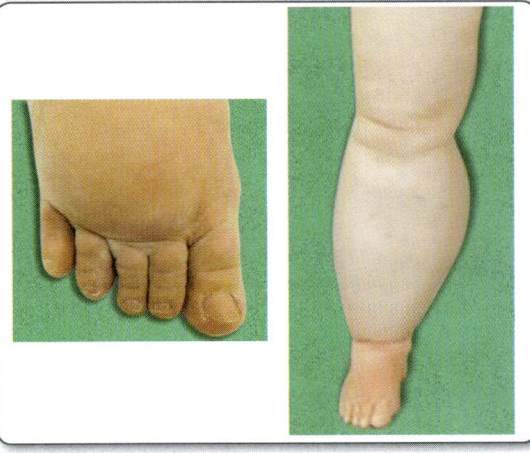

a. Varicose insufficiency
b. Seen in chronic lymphoedema
c. Congestive cardiac failure
d. Arterial obstruction

[Ref: Bailey & Love's 27th/e pg. 1005]

95. 25-year-old female presented with disffuse swelling in front of neck. She also complaints of lethargy and cold intolerance. TSH levels were elevated. HPE reports of biopsy specimen showed lymphocytic infiltration and Hurthle cells. Which of the following is the possible diagnosis?

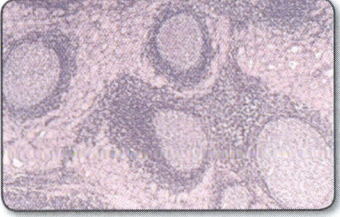

a. Graves' disease
b. Hashimoto's thyroiditis
c. Medullary carcinoma thyroid
d. Follicular carcinoma thyroid

[Ref: Bailey & Love's 27th/e pg. 821; Robbins 9th/e pg. 1087]

Explanation

- Lethargy and cold intolerance points towards hypothyroidism.
- Hashimoto's thyroiditis is the most common type of thyroiditis. It is also known as lymphcytic thyroiditis due to an intense lymphocytic infiltration of the gland.
- Not infrequently there is a family history of other autoimmune disease. It commonly presents as a goitre, which may be diffuse or nodular with a characteristic 'bosselated' feel or with established or subclinical thyroid failure.
- Significantly, raised serum levels of one or more thyroid antibodies are present in over 85% of cases.
- FNAC is the IOC. Abundant lymphocytes are seen.

94. **b**
95. **b**
96. **d**
97. **a**
98. **d**

96. Mr. Kumar, a 60-year-old male with H/o Bladder cancer, while travelling by flight complained of leg pain and hemoptysis. On examination- Pulse rate was 102/minute. On enquiry he had previous history of hospitalization for pulmonary embolism. He had undergone surgical procedure 3 weeks back, what is the clinical probability of thrombotic risk with Modified Well's Criteria.

a. Well's score cannot be calculated as D -dimer levels are not given
b. Low risk
c. Moderate risk
d. High risk

[Ref: Bailey & Love's 27th/e pg. 989]

Explanation

- **Modified Well's Criteria** are used to predict the risk of pulmonary thromboembolism in DVT patient.
- A score <4 means PE is unlikely & > 4 is suggestive of PE.
- In the given clinical scenario score is >4 , so risk of PE developing is high.

Variable	Score
▪ Clinical signs and symptoms of DVT (minimum of leg swelling and pain on palpation of deep veins)	3
▪ Alternative diagnosis less likely than PE	3
▪ **HR >100 bpm**	1.5
▪ Immobilisation >3 days or surgery within past 4 weeks	1.5
▪ Previous DVT or PE	1.5
▪ Haemoptysis	1
▪ Malignancy (treatment of palliation within past 6 months)	1

97. The instrument shown below are used for

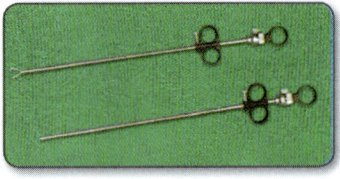

a. Laparoscopic sterilization
b. Removal of ectopic pregnancy
c. Uterine artery ligation/Biopsy
d. Laparoscopic cystectomy

[Ref: D.C. Dutta's Textbook of Obstetrics 9th/e pg. 515]

98. A 20-years-old male underwent a major accident and injury in abdomen. For him the entire ileum and part of the jejunum is resected. Which of the following problem the patient will suffer from?

a. Constipation
b. Bleeding in GIT
c. Gastric Ulcer
d. Vitamin B12 deficiency

[Ref: Sabiston's 1st SEA ed pg. 1291]

Explanation

- Patient will develop small bowel syndrome resulting in vitamin B12 deficiency.

99. **A 5-year-old child with fulminant acute liver failure. Which one of the following criteria are not included in the King's college criteria for liver transplantation?**
    a. Age <10 years
    b. INR >6.5
    c. Bilirubin >17 mg/dl
    d. Jaundice less than 7 days before development of encephalopathy

Explanation

King's College Criteria for Liver Transplantation	

ALF due to acetaminophen toxicity	■ pH <7.3 or arterial serum lactate >3.0 mmol/L
	■ ALL three following conditions occur within a 24-hour period:
	  ○ Presence of grade 3 or 4 hepatic encephalopathy
	  ○ INR >6.5
	  ○ Serum creatinine >3.4 mg/dL

ALF due to other etiologies	■ INR >6.5 and encephalopathy present (irrespective of grade)
	■ ANY three of the following conditions are present:
	  ○ Age <10 or >40 years
	  ○ Jaundice >7 days before development of encephalopathy
	  ○ INR ≥3.5
	  ○ Serum bilirubin ≥17 mg/dL
	  ○ Unfavorable etiology such as:
	    - Wilson disease
	    - Idiosyncratic drug reaction
	    - Seronegative hepatitis

100. **A patient presents with painless cancerous mass lesion and inguinal nodes. Likely diagnosis is?**
     a. Cancer anal canal
     b. Cancer testis
     c. Cancer prostate
     d. Cancer Bladder

     [Ref: Bailey & Love's 27th/e pg. 1507, 1341]

Explanation

- Lymph from lower half of anal canal is drained on each side , first into superficial inguinal nodes and then into the deep inguinal nodes.
- Usually the testicular tumour patient present with a painless mass.

101. **In a patient with Frost Bite what is the temperature of water that must be used to rewarm the patient:**
     a. 37 degrees   b. 42 degrees
     c. 48 degrees   d. 52 degrees

     [Ref: Harrison's 20th/e pg. 3342;
     Bailey & Love's 27th/e pg. 422]

Explanation

- Warming should be gentle as the heat used may actually cause a burn.
- Frozen tissue should be thawed rapidly and completely by immersion in circulating water at 37°C - 40°C (99°F to 100 °F) for 30-60 min.

102. **What is the child pugh class for patient who has a serum bilirubin of 2.5 mg/dl, S albumin – 3 g/dl, INR of 2. Mild ascites is present but there is no encephalopathy:**
     a. CTP A
     b. CTP B
     c. CTP C
     d. CP D

     [Ref: Bailey & Love's 27th/e pg. 1156]

Explanation

Child-Turcotte-Pugh (CTP) Classification of hepatocellular functions in cirrhosis

- CTP B as score is 9

Clinical and Lab Criteria	Points		
	1	2	3
Encephalopathy	None	Mild to moderate (grade 1 to 2)	Severe (grade 3 or 4)
Ascites	None	Mild to moderate (diuretic responsive)	Severe (diuretic refractory)
Bilirubin (mg/dL)	<2	2-3	>3
Albumin (g/dL)	>3.5	2.8-3.5	<2.8
Prothrombin time Seconds prolonged	<4	4-6	>6
International normalized ratio	<1.7	1.7-2.3	>2.3

Child-Turcotte-Pugh Class obtained by adding score for each parameter (total points)
Class A = 5 to 6 points (least severe liver disease)
Class B = 7 to 9 points (moderately severe liver disease)
Class C = 10 to 15 points (most severe liver disease)

103. **A 40-year-old man with diagnosis of ADPKD dependent on Tolvaptan now presents with abdominal pain. What is the cause?**
     a. Colonic perforation   b. Side effects of Tolvaptan
     c. Colonic diverticulitis   d. Appendicitis

     [Ref: Harrison's 20th/e pg. 2153; 2154]

Explanation

- The prevalence of colonic diverticulae and abdominal wall hernias are also increased in ADPKD patients.
- Liver function impairement, polydipsis, and diarrhoea, have been observed side effects of tolvaptan.

99. d
100. b
101. a
102. b
103. c

ORTHOPEDICS

104. Patient present with pain in base of thumb. A test was performed as shown in the image. Which tendons are involved?

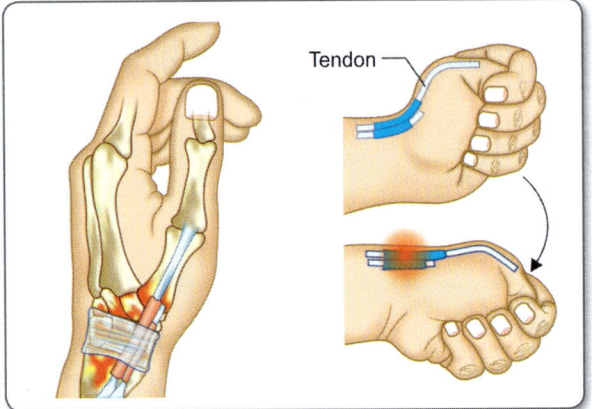

a. Abductor pollicis longus and Extensor pollicis brevis (APL & EPB)
b. Abductor pollicis brevis and Extensor pollicis brevis (APB and EPB)
c. Abductor pollicis longus and Extensor pollicis longus (APL & EPL)
d. Abductor pollicis brevis and Extensor pollicis longus (APB and EPL)

[Ref: Maheshwari & Mhaskar 6th/e pg 303]

Explanation

- Finkelstein test has been shown which helps to diagnose deQuervains tenosynovitis (Inflammation of Abductor Pollicis Longus and Extensor Pollicis brevis).

de Quervain's Disease

- Condition characterized by pain and swelling over the radial styloid process (base of thumb).
- Pathology: The abductor pollicis longus and extensor pollicis brevis tendons may become inflamed beneath the retinacular pulley at the radial styloid with in the first extensor compartment.
- Pathognomic sign is Finkelstein's test. The examiner places patients' thumb across the palm in full flexion, and then holding the patient's hand firmly, turns the wrist sharply into adduction. In positive test this is acutely painful; repeating the movement with the thumb left free is relatively painless.

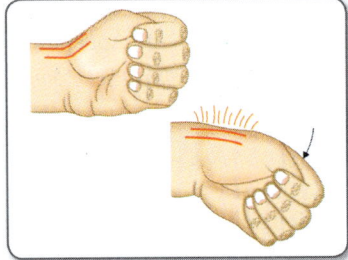

Fig. Finkelstein's test—de Quervain's tenosynovitis

- Differential diagnosis includes scaphoid non-union, arthritis at the base of thumb and intersection syndrome.

- Treatment
  ○ NSAIDs with splint if it fails than steroid injection into tendon

105. A child presented with some skeletal deformity and the radiograph was obtained and an angle is being measured. What is the name of the angle measured in this image:

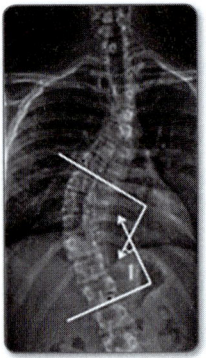

a. Fergusons angle   b. Cobb's angle
c. Bohlers angle   d. Pauwels angle

[Ref: Maheshwari & Mhaskar 6th/e pg 281]

Explanation

- X-ray lateral view spine shows lateral curvature (scoliosis) and angle marked is for its measurement - Cobb's angle.

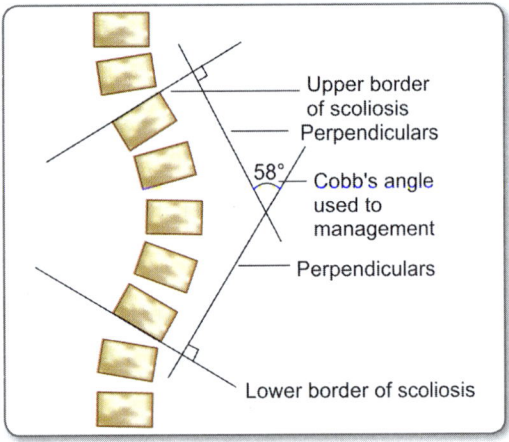

Fig. Cobb's angle

106. Which drug is used as a first line management for postmenopausal female with osteoporosis?

a. Bisphosphonates   b. Raloxifene
c. Estrogens   d. Combined OC pills

[Ref: Harrison's 2953; KDT's 8th/e pg. 370]

Explanation

- Estrogens are first line treatment for postmenopausal osteoporosis. They reduce bone turnover, prevent bone loss and induce small increase in bone mass.
- The second and 3rd generation bisphosphonates , risedronate & zoledronate are effective for prevention of steroid induced osteoporosis.

104.	a
105.	b
106.	c

107. A 55-year-old lady complains of chronic low back pain since a few months. X-ray LS spine is shown below. Her BMD score is 2.4. What is the probable cause of her condition?

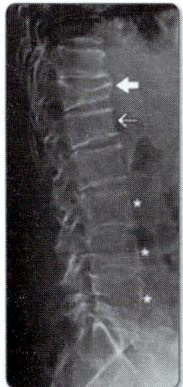

a. Hurler syndrome
b. Paget's disease
c. Renal osteodystrophy
d. Osteoporosis

[Ref: Maheshwari & Mhaskar 6th/e pg 309; RSNA article: Integrated Imaging Approach to Osteoporosis: State-of-the-Art Review and Update.]

Explanation

- The X-ray lateral view is showing " codfish/fishmouth" vertebra, which is seen in osteoporosis. This X-ray picture with along with chronic back pain in a 65 yr old lady is suggestive of osteoporosis.

Osteoporosis

- Osteoporosis is the MC metabolic bone disease. It is characterized by low bone mass and microarchitectural deterioration of bone tissue, with a consequent ↑ in bone fragility and susceptibility to fractures.
- Type I osteoporosis occurs in a subset of postmenopausal women, typically between 50 and 65 years of age. Fracture pattern in this group primarily involves the spine and wrist. **Vertebral compression fractures** are recognized as the hallmark of osteoporosis and they **typically** occur at the **thoracolumbar** junction.
- Bone Mineral Density (BMD) is measured by DEXA (Dual Emission X-ray Absorptiometry) Scan and it is matched to Dexa scan of 30-year-old individual and T score is calculated. WHO classifies BMD on the basis of the T score as.
  - T score 0 to –1 is normal
  - T score –1 to –2.5 is osteopenia
  - T score less than –2.5 is osteoporosis
  - Osteoporosis with (≤ –2.5 with a fragility fracture) is severe osteoporosis
- Etiologies
  - Inherited, e.g. osteogenesis imperfecta, Marfan syndrome.
  - Nutritional, e.g. malnutrition, malabsorption
  - Drugs, e.g. Anticonvulsants, Alcohol, Heparin, Lithium, aluminium, cytotoxic drugs, excessive thyroxine.
  - Endocrine: hyperparathyroidism, thyrotoxicosis, IDDM, Cushing syndrome
  - Rheumatological: Rheumatoid arthritis, Ankylosing spondylitis
- Lab: Osteoporosis characteristically has normal calcium, phosphate and alkaline phosphatase levels.
- Radiological features: Loss of vertical height of vertebrae (collapse), codfish appearance of vertebrae.
  - "EMPTY BOX: As a result of loss of adjacent trabecular bone, the thinning of the cortex usually remains sharp and clear in osteoporosis, thus giving rise to a well demarcated outline of the vertebral body resulting in empty box appearance.
  - PUZZLE SIGN: Presence of sharp fracture line without cortical disruption so that the displaced bone fragments could be reconstructed into their original position to complete the "puzzle". Reference of puzzle sign: Review of the Imaging Features of Benign Osteoporotic and Malignant Vertebral Compression Fractures
- Singh's Index is used for osteoporosis grading.
- Treatment
  - Drug used in osteoporosis
    Inhibit resorption: Bisphosphonates (drug of choice), Denosumab, calcitonin, estrogen, SERMS, gallium nitrate.
  - Drugs which stimulate bone formation: Teriparatide (PTH analogue), calcium, calcitriol, fluorides.
  - Both actions: Strontium ranelate.

108. A 30-year-old male presents with swelling over knee joint. Biopsy reveals giant cells interspersed with mononuclear cells. What is the most probable diagnosis?

a. Chondrosarcoma
b. Osteoclastoma
c. Osteosarcoma
d. Chondroblastoma

[Ref: Maheshwari & Mhaskar 6th/e pg 237]

Explanation

- Lesion around femur with giant cells and mononuclear cell in skeletally mature, is suggestive of osteoclastoma (GCT).

Giant Cell Tumor (Osteoclastoma)

- Age group: 20–40 years . A slight female predominance.
- The MC location for this tumor is the distal femur, followed closely by the proximal tibia.
- Tumor of lower end radius is GCT till proved otherwise.
- Multiple giant cell like bone tumors—Goltz syndrome. GCT has egg shell crackling on palpation.
- Although these tumors typically are benign, pulmonary metastases occur in approximately 3% of patients.
- Malignant GCTs represent < 5% of total GCT. They turn into osteosarcoma, malignant fibrous histiocytoma or fibrosarcoma.
- Radiographically the lesions are eccentrically located in the epiphyses of long bones and usually about the subchondral bone. Although rare in skeletally immature patients, giant cell tumors arise in the metaphysis in this age group. Radiographically, the lesions are purely lytic. The lesion frequently expands or breaks through the cortex; however, intraarticular extension is rare because the subchondral bone usually remains intact.

107. d
108. b

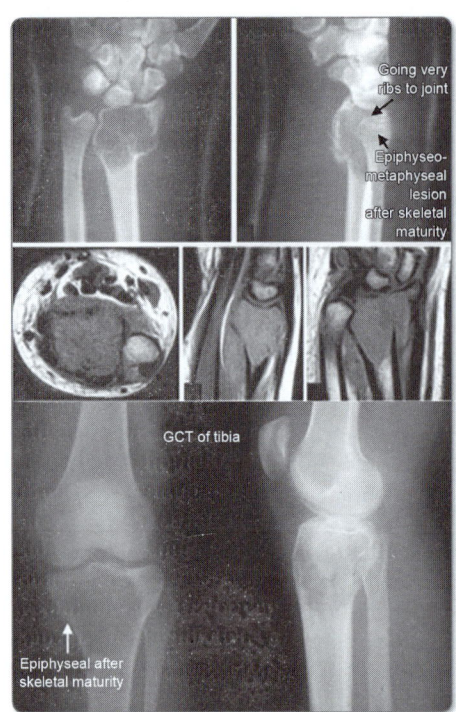

Fig. Giant cell tumor of lower end radius (F) Giant cell tumor of upper end tibia

- Micro: GCTs are composed of many multinucleated giant cells (typically 40–60 nuclei per cell) in a sea of mononuclear stromal cells (malignant cells). The nuclei of the mononuclear cells are identical to the nuclei of the giant cells, a feature that helps to distinguish giant cell tumors from other tumors that may contain many giant cells.
- **Giant cell variants (Tumor with giant cells)**
  - Brown tumor of hyperparathyroidism
  - Aneurysmal bone cyst (closest) and unicameral bone cyst
  - Non-ossifying fibroma (commonest) and Fibrous dysplasia
  - Osteoblastoma and Osteosarcoma
  - Metastatic carcinoma with giant cells
  - Chondromyxoid fibroma and Chondroblastoma
  - Pigmented villonodular synovitis (mostly occurring in knee)
  - Benign fibrous histiocytoma
  - Malignant fibrous histiocytoma
  - Fibrosarcoma
  - Clear cell chondrosarcoma

Treatment of Osteoclastoma (GCT)

- Extended Curettage by PMMA or phenol or liquid nitrogen and bone grafting
  - It is procedure of choice for most lesions.
- Excision
  - Lower end of ulna
  - Upper end of fibula
- Excision and replacement by vascularized bone graft
  - Lower end of radius where upper end of fibula is grafted

- Excision and arthrodesis or prosthetic replacement or Turn -
  - O – Plasty (Bone ends are cut and rotated)
  - Lower end femur and upper end tibia
- Treatment of recurrent lesions is the same as for primary lesions. After biopsy shows that the tumor is still benign, repeat curettage or resection should be performed.
- Amputation
  - Malignant recurrent GCT of extremity
- Radiotherapy
  - Spine (RT may cause malignant transformation of GCT).

109. A 4 year child, while playing with her maid, spinned around his elbow. Immediately after, the child started crying. On examination, his arm was pronated. X-ray is given below. What is the likely diagnosis?

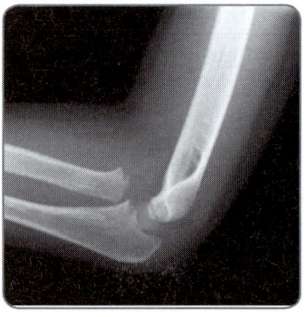

a. Dislocation of elbow   b. Pulled elbow
c. Fracture head of radius   d. Fracture coronoid process

[Ref: Maheshwari & Mhaskar 6th/e pg 105]

Explanation

- History of traction on elbow forearm pronated is classical of pulled elbow.
- Pulled elbow usually occurs in children 2-5 yrs of age..
- In this the head of radius is pulled partly out of the annular ligament when a child is lifted by the wrist.
- CF: The child starts crying & is unable to move the limb.
- T/t: The head is reduced by fully supinating the forearm and applying direct pressure over the head of radius.

Pulled Elbow/Nurse Maid's Elbow

- It is subluxation of radial head or more accurately subluxation of the annular (orbicular) ligament which slips up over the head of radius into the radiocapitellar joint.

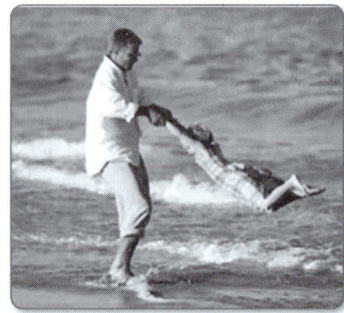

Fig. Violent force to elbow – pulled elbow

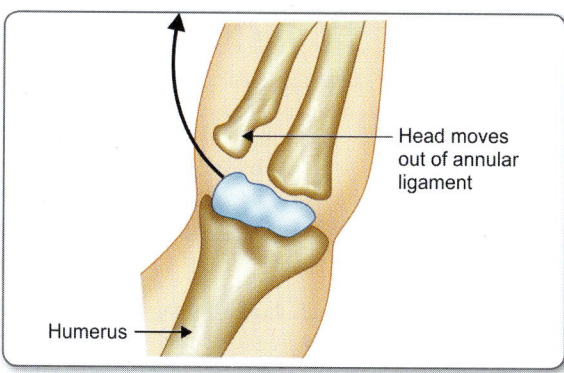

Fig. Pulled elbow

Actinomycosis*	Mandible
Hemophilic arthritis*	Knee (children-ankle)
Acute Osteomyelitis*	Lower end of femur (Metaphysis)
Brodie's abscess*	Upper end of tibia

- Mechanism of Injury
  - Traction to elbow.
- Clinical Features
  - Maximum incidence in 1–4 years age group.
  - The child holds the elbow in slight flexion with the forearm pronated.
- X-rays are normal
- Treatment
  - Reduced by flexing the elbow to 90° and rapidly and firmly rotating the forearm into full supination on outdoor basis without anaesthesia Immobilization is not necessary.
  - Supination is a gravity assisted movement and pulled elbow may be reduced spontaneously by gravity, but this may take time.

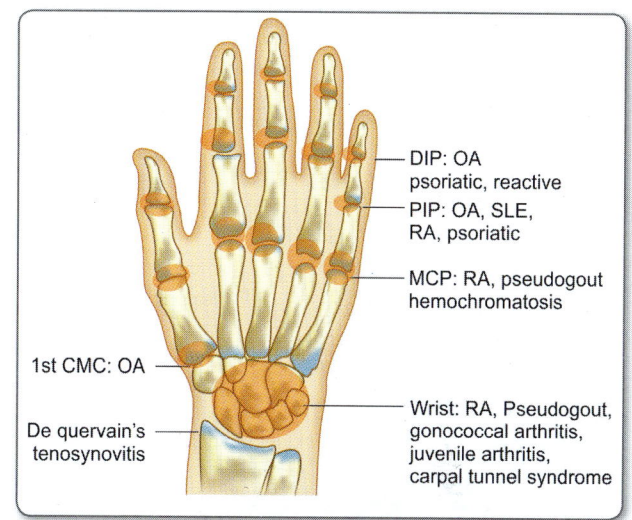

Fig. 'The hand' (to diagnose arthritis)

110. A 55-year-old female patient presents with pain and stiffness in fingers. DIP, PIP, 1st CMC joints are involved, MCP and wrist are spared. Likely diagnosis is?

a. Rheumatoid arthritis
b. Osteoarthritis
c. Ankylosing spondylitis
d. Osteophytoses

[Ref: Maheshwari & Mhaskar 6th/e pg 295]

Explanation
- Sparing of wrist and MCP is a feature of Osteoarthritis.
- RA spares DIP and involves PIP, MCP and Wrist
- ***Diseases and usual joints affected:***

Septic	Knee
Syphilitic arthritis*	Knee
Gonococcal arthritis*	Knee
Gout	MTP joint of Great toe
Pseudoguot*	Knee
Rheumatoid arthritis	Metacarpophalangeal joint
Ankylosing spondylitis*	Sacroiliac joint
Diabetic charcot joint*	Foot joint (midtarsal)
Senile osteoporosis*	Vertebra
Paget's disease*	Pelvic bones > Femur > Skull > Tibia
Osteochondritis dissecans*	Knee > elbow

Contd...

111. A female presents with pain and swelling over multiple peripheral small joints and deformity, in which PIP is involved and DIP is spared, is shown below. What is the likely diagnosis?

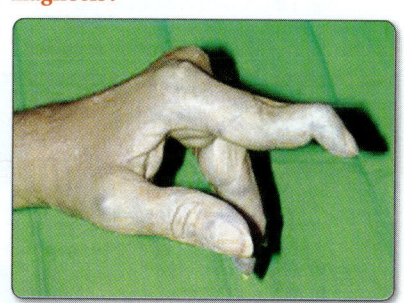

a. Rheumatoid arthritis   b. Psoriatic arthropathy
c. Osteoarthritis   d. Scleroderma

[Ref: Maheshwari & Mhaskar 6th/e pg 288]

Explanation
- The image shows swan neck deformity seen in RA (for detailed explanation: Chapter 16 Page no. 212)
- Characteristic Deformities of Hand and Foot in RA
  - 'Z-deformity', i.e. radial deviation of the wrist with ulnar deviation of the digits, often with palmar subluxation of proximal phalanges.
  - 'Swan-neck deformity', i.e. hyperextension of PIP joints with compensatory flexion of the distal interphalangeal joints.
  - Boutonniere deformity is due to rupture of extensor tendon. There is flexion contracture of PIP joints and hyperextension of DIP joints.

110. b
111. a

○ Hyperextension of 1st interphalangeal joint and flexion of MP joint with a consequent loss of thumb mobility and pinch - Swan Neck deformity of thumb.

○ Eversion at hindfoot (subtalar joint), plantar subluxation of metatarsal heads, widening of forefoot, hallux valgus, and lateral deviation and dorsal subluxation of toes; hammer toe. (Fexion of PIP).

○ Wind swept deformities of toes, i.e. valgus deformities of toes in one foot and varus in other (as wind sweeps all the structure in one direction).

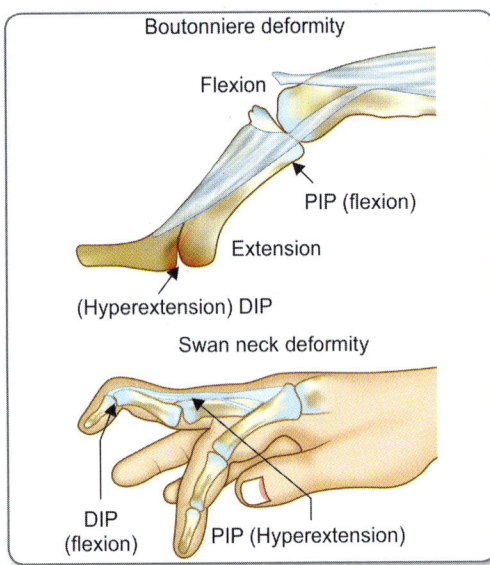

Fig. Finger deformities in RA

112. The sign shown in following image is called?

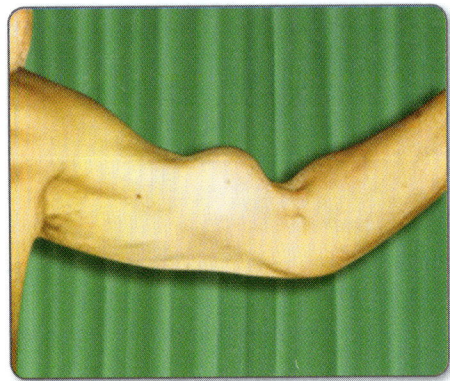

a. Popeye sign
b. Inverted champagne bottle sign
c. Biceps hematoma
d. Waddell sign

[Ref: Bailey & Love's 27th/e pg. 496]

Explanation

■ **Th**e Popeye is a cartoon character with bulging muscles. Hence his name.

■ Popeye sign or Popeye deformity is caused by bulging of the biceps muscle belly after rupture of the biceps tendon.

112. a
113. a

---

113. A patient presented to ER after 12 hrs of trauma with fracture tibia. His PaO2 was 60% and rebreathing unit maintaining the saturation of 100% but confused. He was dyspneic and had rashes over body. Patients chest is clear. What is the likely diagnosis?

a. Fat embolism   b. Air embolism
c. Pulmonary embolism   d. DIC

[Ref: Maheshwari & Mhaskar 6th/e pg 43]

Explanation

■ Fat embolism although should be diagnosed with trauma to long bone, usually Femur and clinical presentation of pulmonary involvement, CNS depression and skin involvement (Petechiae).The diagnosis is considered usually after 48 hours. But out of given options Fat embolism is the best possible answer.

FAT Embolism Syndrome

■ Fracture Femur with Breathlessness after 48 hours think of it!

■ Fat embolism refers to the presence of fat globules in vital organs and peripheral circulation after fracture of a long bone or other major trauma. Fat embolism syndrome reflects a serious systemic manifestation as a consequence to these emboli.

■ Fat embolism is a common phenomenon. It is more commonly seen in patients with multiple **fractures and in fractures i**nvolving lower limbs especially femur.

■ Fat originates from the site of trauma, particularly from the injured marrow. Fat globules > 10 mm are considered significant.

■ Clinical Presentation
○ Early warning signs are a slight rise in temperature and pulse rate (tachycardia)

■ The classical triad of fat embolism syndrome is:
1. Respiratory symptoms: Dyspnea or tachypnea.
2. Neurological symptoms: Confusion or disorientation.
3. Petechial rash: In axilla, neck, periumbilical area, conjunctiva of lower lid, front and back of chest, shoulder.

○ Fat embolism is rare in children.

■ Diagnostic Criterion for Fat Embolism

■ Gurd's Major Criteria (4)
○ Axillary or subconjunctival petechia
○ PaO2 below 60 mm Hg
○ CNS depression
○ Pulmonary oedema

■ Gurd's Minor Criteria (8)
○ Tachycardia
○ Fever
○ Anemia
○ Thrombocytopenia
○ Fat globules in sputum
○ Fat globules in urine (Gurd Test)
○ Increasing ESR
○ Retinal emboli
○ 1 major + 4 minor = fat embolism

■ Prevention
○ Fracture stabilization

- Removing fat emboli from circulation by:
  - Lipolytic agents as heparin (increase serum lipase activity)
  - Hypertonic glucose (decrease FFA production)
- Offset its effect by:
  - Dextran (expand plasma volume, reduces RBC aggregation and platelet adherence)
  - Aprotinin (protease inhibitor) decreases platelet aggregation and serotonin release.
  - Alcohol has vasodilator and lipolytic effect.
- Treatment
  - The aim of treatment is maintaining adequate oxygen level in the blood. If necessary by using intermittent positive pressure ventilation. Oxygen is the only therapeutic tool of proven use.
  - It should be administered in sufficient amount to maintain arterial
  - PO2 > 80 mm Hg. O2 toxicity (pneumonitis) is avoided by using O2 conc. below 40%.
  - Steroids are given to avoid pneumonitis.
  - Waddell's triad: Head injury; Fracture shaft femur and intra-abdominal/intra-thoracic injury.

ANAESTHESIA

114. 60-year-old female patient was on ACE inhibitors for hypertension. She had CABG 4 years back. Now the patient is scheduled for hernia surgery. She has BP under control and has been symptom free since surgery. What is the proper investigation to be ordered?
a. Routine preop, clinical evaluation and V/Q scan
b. Routine preop, clinical evaluation and angiography to look for patency
c. Routine preop, clinical evaluation and stress testing
d. Routine preop, clinical evaluation

[Ref: Morgan's 6th/e. pg. 386]

Explanation

- Routine preop investigations and clinical evaluation only required. Stress testing is NOT required as it is a small surgery.

115. What does the following capnograph depict?

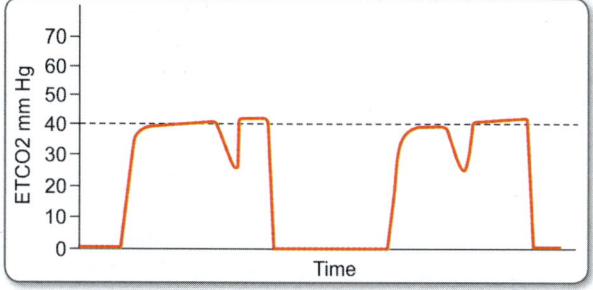

a. Esophageal intubation
b. Spontaneous efforts
c. Bronchospasm
d. Normal surgical stage

[Ref: Morgan's 6th/e pg.123]

Explanation

- Notch is slightly right (in later phase) in spontaneous breathing.

116. In an orthopedic surgery, a patient was given a muscle relaxant that competitively blocks nicotinic receptors. Which of the following drug is used for reversal of muscle relaxation after surgery?
a. Neostigmine
b. Carbachol
c. Succinylcholine
d. Physostigmine

[Ref: Morgan's 6th/e pg.222; KDT Essential of medical pharmacology 8th/e pg. 122]

Explanation

- Neostigmine is water soluble reversible anticholilnesterases used to reverses muscle paralysis induced by competitive neuromuscular blockers
- Carbachol is a parasympathomimetic that mimics the effect of acetylcholine on both the muscarinic and nicotinic receptors. This drug is administered ocularly to induce miosis to reduce intraocular pressure (IOT) in the treatment of glaucoma.
- Succinyl choline is a depolarising muscle relaxant.
- Physostigmine is lipid soluble Reversible anticholilnesterases can cross blood brain barrier therefore not used in reversal muscle relaxation.

117. Patient presented in emergency with biliary colic. On duty intern given her IM drug after which intensity of pain increased. Which is the most likely injection given?
a. Acetaminophen
b. Diclofenac
c. Nefopam
d. Morphine

[Ref: Morgan's 6th/e pg.193; KDT Essential of medical pharmacology 8th/e pg. 502]

Explanation

- Morphine and related opioid causes spasm of sphincter of Oddi and hence they can aggravate certain condition, e.g., biliary colic, pancreatitis, diverticulitis. Inflamed appendix may rupture. Morphine can be given after the diagnosis is established.
- Diclofenac, Nefopam, acetaminophen and Etoricoxib have no effect on sphincter of Oddi, so they do not precipitate biliary colic.

RADIOLOGY

118. Remote after loading is done in?
a. Stereotactic radiotherapy
b. Proton beam radiotherapy
c. Cyber knife therapy
d. Brachytherapy

[Ref: Harrison's 20th/e pg. 483]

Explanation

- Remote afterloading of radioactive sources for brachytherapy is becoming increasingly popular.
- By remote afterloading for uterus applicators and for other intracavitary and interstitial techniques, radiation exposure during insertion of the applicator can be avoided.

114. d
115. b
116. a
117. d
118. d

119. The sign seen on ultrasound when the common femoral vein meets the GSV and femoral artery at the saphenofemoral junction is called:

a. Stemmers sign
b. Tillaux sign
c. Mickey mouse sign
d. String sign

[Ref: Bailey & Love's 27th/e pg. 976; Internet]

Explanation

- "The Mickey Mouse sign" is a medical sign resembling the head of Mickey Mouse, the Walt Disney character.
- This sign has been described as the image at the groin when a dilated accessory saphenous vein (ASV) exists: the common femoral vein (CFV) represents the head of Mickey Mouse while the great saphenous vein (GSV) and the dilated accessory saphenous vein (ASV) represent the ears.
- The presence of this sign has been a great diagnostic clue to check ASV insufficiency.
- Mickey **Mouse appearance** can be seen in following conditions also:
  ○ Anencephaly
  ○ Progressive supranuclear palsy
  ○ Synonymously with a finger in glove sign
  ○ Flared shape of the iliac wings on pelvic radiograph in Down syndrome
  ○ Paget disease: if there is increased radiotracer uptake on the bone scan in the spinous process and pedicles.
  ○ Configuration of the portal triad in short axis on a biliary ultrasound scan, with the portal vein comprising Mickey's "head" and the common bile duct and hepatic artery as his right and left "ears", respectively.
  ○ Hutch diverticulum: in delayed contrast study (IVU/CT): appearance of bilateral smooth, walled posterolateral outpouching from urinary bladder adjacent to the vesicoureteric junction.

120. Radiation dose monitoring in occupational personnel is done by:

a. TLD badge
b. Linear accelerator
c. Collimators
d. Grid
e. Gamma camera & GM counters

[Ref: Harrison's 20th/e pg. 483; Internet]

Explanation

- " Thermoluminescence Dosimeter (TLD) badge are used for monitoring beta and gamma doses of radiation workers.
- Personal Monitoring Devices.
  ○ Film badge are of 2 types:– Chest badge and Extremity Badge (Consists of Photographic film + Filters + Badge holder). Minimum dose detected can be 0.2mSv. Range of film badge is 10KeV to 2 MeV.
  ○ TLD badge are currently used in India. Based on phenomenon of Thermo luminescence – phenomenon of emission of light when certain

materials are heated after radiation exposure. Range 0.2 mSv to 10 Sv. Consists of Card and cassette. Card consists of three CaSo4: Dy-teflon Disc. Card is made of Nickle coated Aluminium. Three types of chest badge, wrist badge and Finger Dosimeter. Reusable and can be used 100 times.
  ○ OSL (Optically Stimulated Luminescence): Uses thin layer of Aluminium oxide (Al2 O3:C). Range 5KeV to 40 MeV.
  ○ RPL (Radiophotoluminescence). Material used is silver activated phosphate glass.
  ○ Pocket Dosimeter

121. A 25-year-old female with hypertension has the following chest X-ray with prominent aortic notch. What could be the likely cause?

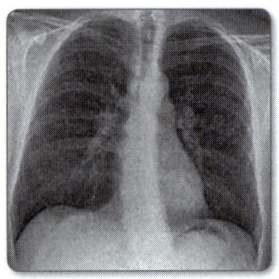

a. Persistent truncus arteriosus
b. Mitral stenosis
c. Coarctation of aorta
d. Transposition of great arteries

[Ref: Harrison's 20th/e pg. 1837;

www.bcm.edu › radiology › cases › pediatric › text]

Explanation

- Hypertension along with 3 signs as shown in CXR is suggestive of aortic coarctation.
  ○ In a**dult: Characterized by a short segment a**brupt obstruction in the just post ductal/ligamentum arteriosum region secondary to localized thickening of the aortic media.
  ○ Infantile coarctation (preductal): Characterized by a diffuse narrowing or hypoplasia of the aorta also in the presence of a discrete area of constriction in the aorta just beyond the origin of the left subclavian artery but proximal to the ductus arteriosus.
- Associations:
  ○ Bicuspid aortic valve in up to 85% of cases.
  ○ VSD (all types).
  ○ Mitral valve lesions including hypoplastic mitral valve, parachute mitral valve and abnormal papillary muscles
  ○ Shone's syndrome (multiple left sided obstructions; supravalvular mitral ring, mitral valve stenosis, subaortic membrane/stenosis, aortic valve stenosis, coarctation).
- CXR findings: Characteristics findings
  ○ Post-stenotic dilation of the descending aorta
  ○ "figure 3" sign,
  ○ Development of rib notching secondary to dilated intercostal collateral vessels.

119. c
120. a
121. c

122. Identify the disease shown in the X-ray.

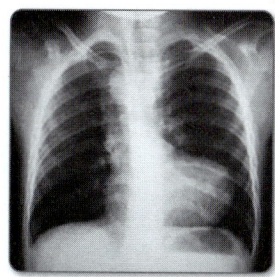

a. Tetralogy of fallot
b. Truncus arteriosus
c. Total anomalous pulmonary venous return
d. Coarctation of aorta.

[Ref: Nelson's 21st /e pg. 2397-98; Radiology Review Manual 8th/e]

Explanation

- Typical boot shaped heart is characteristic CXR finding in TOF.
- TOF includes:
  ○ Large VSD immediately below aortic arch
  ○ Right ventricular Hypertrophy
  ○ Overriding of Arch of aorta
  ○ Pulmonic Stenosis
- Chest Radiograph findings:
  ○ Boot shaped heart (Coeur en sabot)
  ○ Pronounced concavity in pulmonary bay
  ○ Reduction in caliber and number of pulmonary arteries
  ○ Enlarged aorta
  ○ Right sided aortic arch.

123. CT scan of a child with cystic lesion with calcification in suprasellar region is given, Probable diagnosis is:

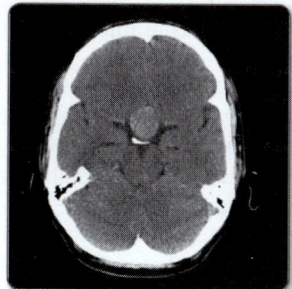

a. Pituitary adenoma   b. Meningioma
c. Oligodendroglioma   d. Craniopharyngioma

[Ref: Harrison's 20th /e pg. 2673; Osborn]

Explanation

- Craniopharyngioma is suprasellar cystic mass, many of them are partly calcified. They arise from Rathke's pouch near the pituitary stalk.
  ○ Approximately >50% arise before the age of 20.
  ○ Primarily suprasellar tumors (75%).
  ○ Most common nonglial neoplasm in children.
  ○ Adamantinomatous type: Rule of ninety - 90% mixed cystic and solid, 90% calcify and 90% enhance.

○ "Machinery Oil fluid" - Fluid rich in cholesterol crystals, in cystic craniopharyngiomas.
○ Papillary: Often or mostly solid and rarely calcify.
○ "Stalk effect"- Clinical presentation.

124. A 45-year-old female presents with sudden onset headache and neck rigidity. There is no history of trauma. The CT image is shown below. What could be the likely diagnosis?

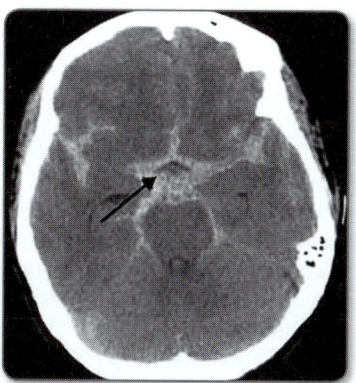

a. Hemorrhagic stroke
b. Subarachnoid hemorrhage (SAH)
c. Sub dural hematoma
d. Meningitis

[Ref: Harrison's 20th /e pg. 2085; Radiology Review Manual 8th/e]

Explanation

- Clinical history is typical of aneurysmal rupture. Aneurysmal rupture with major SAH leads to → rise of ICP → sudden transient loss of unconsciousness, brief excruciating headache, but most patients first complain of headache upon regaining consciousness.
- On imaging, blood is found in the CSF if NCCT head obtained within 72 hr.

Subarachnoid hemorrhage (Blood between pia and arachnoid membrane)

- Causes:
  ○ Spontaneous: Ruptured Aneurysm, AV malformation, Hypertensive hemorrhage, Blood dyscrasia.
  ○ Trauma: Injury to leptomeningeal vessels. Rupture of major intracerebral vessels.
- Imaging:
- NECT:
  ○ Increased density in basal cisterns, superior cerebellar cistern, sylvian fissure, cortical sulci, intraventricular and along interhemispheric fissure.
  ○ Cortical vein Sign: Visualization of cortical vein passing through extra axial fluid collection.
- MRI (Depending on stage of bleed):
  ○ Hyperintense sulci and cisterns on FLAIR
  ○ Dirty CSF – isointense to brain on TI and T2
  ○ Blooming: Low signal intensity on brain surface
- Complications:
  ○ Hydrocephalus, Cerebral vasospasm + infarct, Transtentorial herniation.

122. a
123. d
124. b

125. A 24-year-old lady with 7-week pregnancy was accidentally exposed to chest X-ray in the hospital. What will you advise her regarding pregnancy management?

a. To continue pregnancy

b. Immediately terminate pregnancy.

c. Do chromosomal analysis to check for chromosomal anomalies.

d. Pre-invasive diagnostic testing.

[Ref: Nelson's 21st/e pg. 888]

Explanation

- **Accidental expos**ure of a pregnant woman to radiation is a common cause of anxiety for her. It is unlikely that exposure to diagnostic radiation (which is CXR here) will cause gene mutations.

- The estimated radiation dose for most radiographs is 0.1 rad. and for most CT scans <5 rad (which is maximum recommended radiation exposure in pregnancy).

- Thus single diagnostic studies do not result in radiation doses high enough to affect embryo or fetus.

- At 2-8 weeks gestation, doses >20 rad have been a/w congenital anomalies and IUGR. Here chromosomal analysis is advisable.

126. A Patient presenting with abdominal pain, blood in stools and a palpable mass on examination. The following barium image was obtained from the patient, probable diagnosis is?

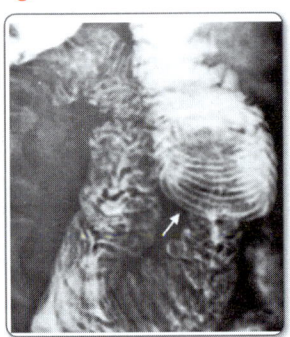

a. Sigmoid diverticulum   b. Intussusception

c. Cancer colon   d. Volvulus

[Ref: Bailey & Love's 27th/e pg. 1289]

Explanation

- *It is a* colo-colic intussusception
- Claw sign is diagnostic of iliac intussusception. The barium in the intussusception is seen as a claw around a negative shadow.
- Plain radiographic signs
  - Target Sign: Soft tissue mass containing concentric circular or nearly circular areas of lucency due to mesenteric fat of intussusceptum.
  - Meniscus Sign: Crescent of gas within the colonic lumen that outlines the apex of intussusceptum.
- Barium Enema Signs:
  - Meniscus sign: Rounded Apex of intussusceptum protruding into the column of contrast material.
  - Coiled Spring Sign: When edematous mucosal folds of returning limb of intussusceptum are outlined by contrast material in the lumen of colon.

127. Identify the Investigation being performed and possible diagnosis.

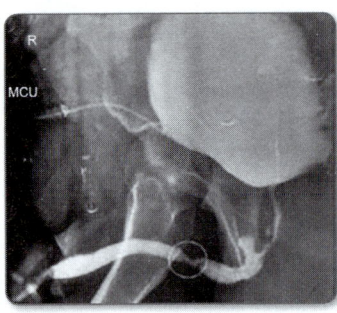

a. MCU with bulbar urethral stricture

b. MCU with penile urethral stricture

c. RGU with membranous urethral stricture

d. RGU with prostatic stricture

[Ref: Bailey & Love's 27th/e pg. 1483; RSNA Article Imaging of Urethral Disease: A Pictorial Review]

Explanation

- It is a micturating cystourethrogram (MCU) or voiding cystourethrography.
- Stricture is visible at the root of penis which is a site of bulbar urethral injury.

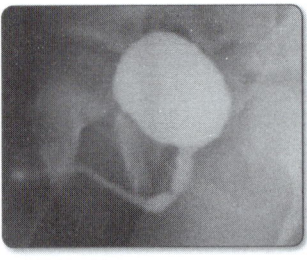

- MCU with bulbar stricture:-
  - In general, the term urethral stricture refers to a fibrous scarring of the anterior urethra.
  - Anterior urethral injury following blunt trauma - Type V urethral injury.
  - Type V urethral injuries are caused by straddle injury and occur in the bulbous urethra.
  - The most common external cause of traumatic stricture is straddle injury.
  - Other causes of anterior urethral strictures may be inflammatory (e.g. infectious urethritis, balanitis xerotica obliterans), traumatic (iatrogenic instrumentation) or congenital.

128. Pulmonary plethora is seen in:

a. TOF   b. TAPVC

c. CoA   d. Tricuspid Atresia

[Ref: Radiopedia]

Explanation

Pulmonary Plethora

- Pulmonary plethora is a term used to describe the appearances of ↑ pulmonary perfusion on chest radiographs. It is seen in Left to right shunt lesions:-
- Other causes of pulmonary plethora include:
  - Left to right cardiac shunts – ASD, VSD, PDA

125. a

126. b

127. a

128. b

- ○ Transposition of great arteries with ASD or VSD
- ○ Truncus arteriosus
- ○ Coronary artery fistula into right heart
- ○ Aortopulmonary window
- ○ Vein of Galen malformation
- ○ Total anomalous pulmonary venous connection (TAPVC or TAPVR)
- TAPVR is thought to result from failure of the common pulmonary vein to connect to the left atrium, with persistence of the primitive splanchnic connections of the pulmonary veins to the cardinal systemic veins and thence to the right atrium. Four broad categories of TAPVR according to where the anomalous veins drain: supracardiac, cardiac, infracardiac and mixed.
  - ○ Supracardiac type is the most common form of TAPVR.
  - ○ Cardiac type: Pulmonary venous confluence connects directly to the right atrium, usually through the coronary sinus. The pulmonary veins and coronary sinus are significantly dilated, and echocardiography shows a characteristic "whale's tail" appearance.
  - ○ Infracardiac type: Pulmonary venous confluence drains to systemic veins below the diaphragm. The confluence is usually posterior to the left atrium and vertically oriented (sometimes described as an "inverted fir tree").

Pulmonary Oligemia

- Pulmonary oligemia is a term used to describe the appearances of ↓ pulmonary perfusion on chest radiographs.
- Cause of Generalized oligemia (reduction in pulmonary blood volume): aortic valve disease, over penetration of film (artifact).
- Causes of Regional Oligemia
  - ○ ↓ in blood volume: pulmonary arterial hypoplasia, mitral valve disease, pulmonary embolism.
  - ○ ↑se in air space: Regional emphysema, Swyer-James syndrome.
- Oligemia a/w cyanosis is seen in right to left shunt lesions:-
  - ○ TOF
  - ○ PA
  - ○ PS+ASD + VSD
  - ○ PS+TGA/ DORV/ DOLV

129. A cancer patient undergoes radiotherapy, pick the true statement regarding radio sensitivity of tissues:
- a. Rapidly dividing cells are resistant to radiation
- b. GI mucosa is one of the most radio resistant tissue in the body
- c. The intensity of radiation is inversely proportional to the square of distance from the source
- d. Small blood vessels are least resistant to radiation

[Ref: Harrison's 20th/e pg. 482-483]

Explanation
- Rapidly dividing cells are more sensitive to radiation than non dividing cells.
- GI mucosa is highly sensitive to radiation.

- According to inverse square law: The radiation intensity is inversely proportional to the square of the distance from the source.
- In radiation resistant organs, the vascular endothelium is the most sensitive component.

130. A 26-year-old female with married life of 2 year was under IVF treatment for infertility. She was put on injection hMG. Now she presents with abdominal distension, dyspnea, vomiting, nausea, and headache. The USG is shown below, what is the diagnosis?

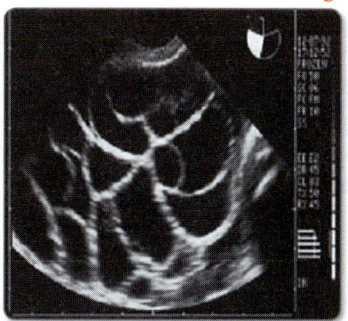

- a. Polycystic ovarian disease
- b. Ovarian hyperstimulation Syndrome
- c. Theca Leutein cysts
- d. Granulosa cell tumor

[Ref: Shaw's Textbook of Gynaecology 16th/e pg. 552]

Explanation
- Ovarian hyperstimulation syndrome (OHSS) is a complication of assisted reproductive techniques like IVF.
- It results from induction of ovulation in infertility cases.
- It is more common with FSH/LH (gonadotropin) therapy than clomiphene and GnRH analogues.
- Risk factors for OHSS:-
  - ○ Young age
  - ○ PCOS
  - ○ Previous h/o OHSS
  - ○ Previous estradiol levels > 3000 pg/ml
  - ○ ⩾20 small follicles
  - ○ ↑renin and angiotensin levels
- T/t: Hospitalization.

131. A 60 yr old female with history of intermenstrual bleeding per vagina, endometrial collection and with thickening and anterior bulging of the fundal area. On ultrasound showing a feeding vessel sign. Diagnosis is:

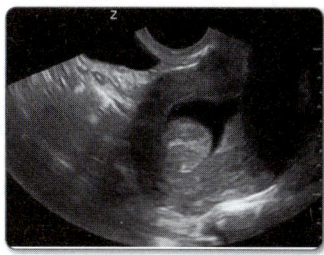

- a. Endometrial polyp
- b. Endometrial cancer
- c. Submucous fibroid
- d. Leiomyosarcoma

[Ref: Shaw's Textbook of Gynaecology 16th/e pg. 391; Radiopedia]

129. c
130. b
131. a

Explanation

Estrogenic effects

- **Endometrium → Proliferativ**e growth (in preovulatory period).
- Hair → Feminine pattern hair growth
- Breast → Hypertrophy of ducts & parenchyma, vascularity.

142. During episiotomy, incision extended posteriorly beyond perineal body towards rectum. Which structure is at risk of damage:

   a. External anal sphincter b. Bulbospongious muscle
   c. Ischiocavernosus   d. Bulbocavernosus

[Ref: D.C. Dutta's Textbook of Obstetrics 9th/e pg. 531]

Explanation

- Immediate complications of episiotomy:-
  ○ Extension of incision to involve rectum in median episiotomy → May damage
  ○ Vulval hematoma
  ○ Infection
- Remote complications of episiotomy:-
  ○ Dyspareunia
  ○ Perineal lacerations
- The levator ani, bulbocavernosus, and transverse vaginal muscles all have attachments to or near the perineal body but do not actually cross the midline. If the perineal body is transected and not repaired, the important connections between the two sides of each of these structures are lost. The continuity of structures across the midline in the perineal body can be appreciated by feeling the ridge that is palpable just inside the hymenal ring as the perineum is distended.
- The median episiotomy incision is made in the perineal body from the midline of the hymenal ring through the connective tissue that unites the bulbocavernosus muscle, the superficial transverse perineal muscles, and the perineal membrane (urogenital diaphragm). The incision is made down to but not including the anal sphincter.
- Episioproctotomy carries the risk of fistula and anal incontinence, whereas a mediolateral episiotomy causes greater blood loss and may be more painful. Mediolateral episiotomy, because it can be extended to incise the levator ani (which episioproctotomy does not), provides more room for delivering impacted shoulders or for managing breech delivery.
- Extension of the episiotomy involving the anal sphincter or rectum has been reported to be increased with midline episiotomy. Rarely the rectum may be unexpectedly incised.

143. A 35-year-old female attends gynae OPD with h/o excessive bleeding since 6 months, not controlled with non hormonal drugs. USG and clinical examinations reveal no abnormality. Next step is?

   a. Endometrial sampling b. Endometrial ablation
   c. Hormonal therapy   d. Hysterectomy

[Ref: Shaw's Textbook of Gynaecology 16th/e pg. 338, 343]

142. a
143. a
144. b
145. b
146. a

Explanation

- **Chronic AUB (abnormal uter**ine bleeding) is described as abnormal menstrual bleeding related to volume, timing, regularity and duration of bleeding that lasts for ≥6 months , and require thorough investigations.
- First line of treatment is medical therapy. If it fails, D& C may be helpful. If hormonal therapy fails, many prefers Mirena IUCD. Failing this decision should be taken regarding conservative surgery or hysterectomy.
- Postmenopausal women if any endometrial thickening is found do sampling.

144. Image given below is of which contraceptive?

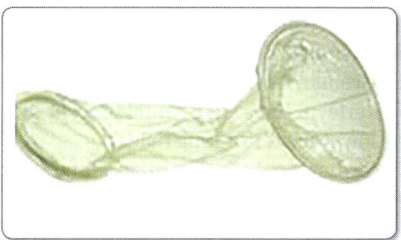

   a. Male condom   b. Female condom
   c. Vaginal sponge   d. Cervical cap

[Ref: Shaw's Textbook of Gynaecology 16th/e pg. 267]

145. Fetal condition (as shown in image below) in the mother is associated with-

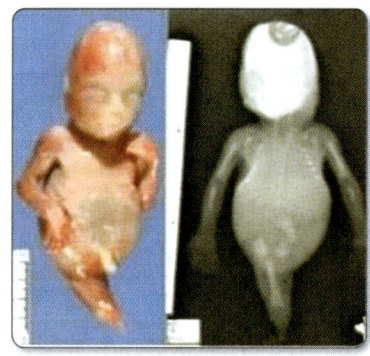

   a. Overt diabetes mellitus
   b. Pregestational diabetes mellitus
   c. Intake of ACE inhibitors
   d. Intake of sodium valproate
   e. Autoamputation oligo, IUGR baby

[Ref: D.C. Dutta, Textbook of Obstetrics 9th/ed pg. 262]

Explanation

- Pregestational (pre-existing) DM is a/w congenital anomalies (e.g. absent limbs due to autoamputation), IUGR.

146. A 22-year-old primigravida with sure of dates attends ANC OPD with 20 weeks POG. On further obstetric examination fundal height reveals 16 weeks uterine size. Obstetric USG shows reduced liquor. What is the probable cause?

   a. Renal agenesis   b. Fetal anemia
   c. Barters syndrome   d. Liddle syndrome

[Ref: D.C. Dutta's Textbook of Obstetrics 9th/e pg. 203]

Explanation

- Oligohydramnios (or oligmnios) is caused by renal agenesis and ureteric atresia in fetus.
- Renal agenesis → Fetal urine is not formed → Less amniotic fluid → Oligohydramnios.
- Conversely esophageal atresia → Amniotic fluid is not swallowed by fetus → More amniotic fluid in sac → Polyhydramnios.

147. A mother brings her 16-year-old daughter to gynae OPD with complaints of not attaining menarche. She gives h/o cyclical abdominal pain. On further examination, midline abdominal swelling seen. Per rectal examination reveals bulging mass in vagina. Which of the following do you suspect?

a. Transverse vaginal septum
b. Androgen insensitivity syndrome
c. Hematocalpos
d. Vaginal atresia

[Ref: Shaw's Textbook of Gynaecology 16th/e pg. 131]

Explanation

- *Hemato*calpos: Blood-filled distended vagina due to menstrual blood in the setting of an anatomical obstruction, usually an imperforate hymen. When there is concurrent uterine distention, the term hematometrocolpos is used. Patients may present with amenorrhea or vague abdominal pain. Causes
- Causes:-
  - Imperforate hymen: the most frequent cause
  - Transverse vaginal septum

148. A 35-year old primigravida, who has conceived after IVF, attends ANC check-up at 38 weeks POG. Her obstetric details reveal dichorionic diamniotic (DCDA) twins with first twin being a breech. On examination her BP >140/90 mm Hg on two occasions with proteinuria +1. How will you manage this patient?

a. Watch for BP and terminate when BP gets elevated.
b. BP monitoring and induction on EDD
c. Immediate C section
d. Induction of labour

[Ref: D.C. Dutta's Textbook of Obstetrics 9th/e pg. 196, 198]

Explanation

- This is an obstetric indication of C section as it is a case of precious pregnancy with first twin breech, so immediate C section

149. A 24-year-old female with married life of 4 years attends infertility clinic with h/o recurrent abortions. On further workup, she was found to have "septate uterus". Which of the following surgery is best for reproductive outcomes?

a. Strassmann's metroplasty
b. Tompkins metroplasty
c. Transcervical hysteroscopic resection of septum.
d. Jones metroplasty

[Ref: Shaw's Textbook of Gynaecology 16th/e pg. 103]

Explanation

- Uterine septum is the MC Müllerian fusion defect.
- T/t of Septate uterus: Uterine septum is cut with scissors, cautery or laser or resectoscope. Usually done under hysteroscopic visualisation. 70% success rate is there.
- Metroplasty: Surgery to reconstruct uterus . Used to repair congenital anomalies of uterus.
  - Bicornuate uterus is managed with laparoscopic Strassman metroplasty.
  - Tompkins metroplasty is sometimes used for septate uterus.
  - Jones metroplasty and the 'Baghdad' techniques are used for double uterus.

150. A sexually active female came with profuse frothy foul-smelling discharge with intense itching. On examination, strawberry cervix revealed. What condition she belongs to?

a. Trichomonas vaginalis   b. Candidiasis
c. Bacterial vaginosis   d. Gardernella vaginalis

[Ref: Shaw's Textbook of Gynaecology 16th/e pg. 385]

Explanation

- The characteristic vaginal discharge white , foul smelling & the presence of strawberry vagina/cervix points out towards Trichomoniasis.

151. Distention media for hysteroscopy with bipolar cautery:

a. Normal saline   b. Hypertonic saline
c. Distilled water   d. Mannitol

[Ref: Shaw's Textbook of Gynaecology 16th/e pg. 104]

Explanation

- The popular liquid media include- normal saline, 5% dextrose & ringer lactate.
- More sophisticated pressure systems are available when prolonged hysteroscopic procedures such as myomectomy, septum cutting or endometrial ablation are performed. In such cases, the distension media must be non-ionic (not normal saline).The distending media in common use are Hyskon or glycine.
- Preferred gaseous media is CO_2.
- Mini-hysteroscopes with bipolar electrodes with use of isotonic saline reduce the risk of electrical burns due to proximity of the electrodes and electrolyte imbalance.

152. Identify the hysterosalpingogram image of a female who presented for infertility work up?

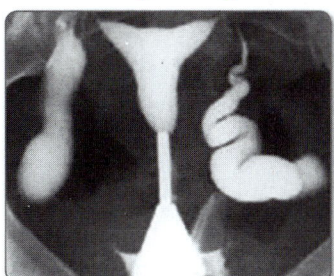

a. Normal HSG   b. B/L hydrosalpinx
c. B/L cornual block   d. Extravasation of dye

[Ref: Shaw's Textbook of Gynaecology 16th/e pg. 180]

147. c
148. c
149. c
150. a
151. a
152. b

Explanation

- Fallopian tube abnormalities are the MC cause of female infertility, accounting for 30%–40% of cases. Hysterosalpingography provides optimal depiction of the fallopian tubes, allowing detection of tubal patency, tubal occlusion, tubal irregularity and peritubal disease.
- Radiologically: Fallopian tubes have three segments visible at HSG:
  o Interstitial portion: It traverses the myometrium
  o Isthmic portion: It courses within the broad ligament
  o Ampullary portion: It is adjacent to the ovary.
- Hydrosalpinx results from occlusion at the ampullary end of the fallopian tube, a condition MC caused by pelvic inflammatory disease. Dilated tubes with absence of intraperitoneal spillover of contrast material are the HSG findings.
- If hydrosalpinx is seen at hysterosalpingography, it is important to prescribe postprocedural antibiotic prophylaxis, typically doxycycline, to prevent procedure-related infection due to stasis of contrast material within the obstructed fallopian tube.

153. Mrs Rekha having her child of 2 years of age presents to her family obstetrician with c/o pruritus vulvae, visual complaints and amenorrhoea. She gives h/o severe blood loss during delivery and failure of lactation subsequently. She also complaints of fatigue and cold intolerance. She has got multiple skin infections and anaemia. What is the diagnosis?

a. Sheehan's syndromes   b. Asherman's syndrome
c. Prolactinomas   d. Premature ovarian failure
e. Lymphocytic hypophysitis

153. a
154. b
155. b
156. d

[Ref: Shaw's Textbook of Gynaecology 16th/e pg. 328; D.C. Dutta's Textbook of Obstetrics 9th/e pg. 241]

Explanation

- *Sheehan's syndrome, aka postpartum pituitary necrosis,* is hypopituitarism (↓ functioning of the pituitary gland), caused by ischemic necrosis due to blood loss and hypovolemic shock during and after parturition.
- CF:
  o Panhypopituitarism
  o Signs of hypothyroidism, cortisol deficiency
  o Lactational failure
- Sheehan's syndrome/ Simmond's disease is an important cause of secondary amenorrhoea.

154. Serum prolactin levels are highest in?

a. REM sleep
b. 24 hrs after parturition
c. 1 hrs after running
d. After 24 hours of ovulation/when estrogens are high

Explanation

- PRL secretion is pulsatile, with the highest secretory peaks occurring during rapid eye movement sleep. (Harrison' 20th pp 2660).
- Immediately after postpartum, prolactin surge occurs within 2 hour postpartum. Thereafter, PRL level decline reaching a nadir at -9 hour postpartum and this low level is maintained for 9-24 hour postpartum.

155. Interpret the partogram.

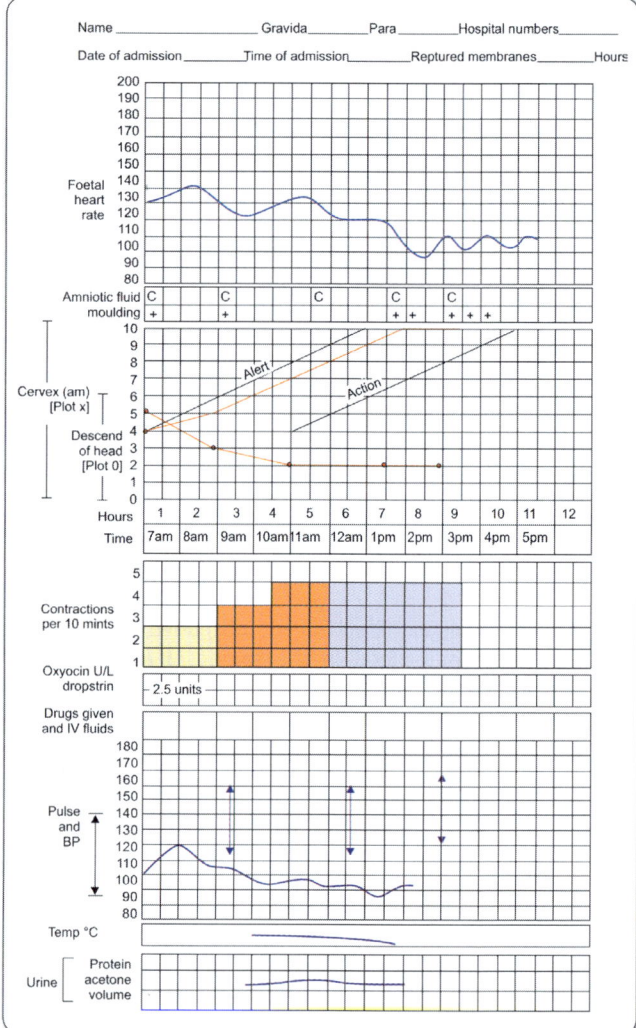

a. Inadequate uterine contraction
b. Cephalopelvic disproportion
c. Maternal Exhaustion
d. Uterine rupture

[Ref: D.C. Dutta's Textbook of Obstetrics 9th/e pg. 330, 378]

156. A 50-year-old woman diagnosed to be Ca cervix stage 2B advised for chemoradiation. Which of the following is true statement?

a. Small bowel is most radioresistant.
b. Small bowel vessel is most radioresistant.
c. Rapidly proliferating cells are most radioresistant.
d. Dose/intensity of radiation is inversely proportional to the square of distance of the source.

[Ref: Shaw's Textbook of Gynaecology 16th/e pg. 503; Protection against Radiation Hazard; IJRI Article]

Explanation

Radiation protection actions

- The triad of radiation protection actions comprise of "time-distance-shielding".

- Reduction of exposure time; increasing distance from source; shielding of patients and occupational workers.
  - Time: The exposure time is related to radiation exposure and exposure rate (exposure per unit time) as follows:
  - Exposure = Exposure rate x Time; Simply implying that if the exposure time is kept short, then the resulting dose to the individual is small.
- Distance: The exposure to the individual decrease inversely as the square of the distance (inverse square law). It means when distance is doubled exposure is reduced by factor of four.
- Shielding: Shielding implies that certain materials (concrete, lead) will attenuate radiation (reduce its intensity) when they are placed between the source of radiation and the exposed individual. The aspects of shielding in diagnostic radiology include:-
  - X-ray tube shielding
  - Room shielding: X-ray equipment room shielding and Patient waiting room shielding.
  - Personnel shielding.
  - Patient shielding (of organs not under investigation).

157. Which of the following is not oestrogen dependent pubertal change?
a. Hair growth   b. Menstruation
c. Vaginal cornification   d. Cervical mucous

158. A 13-year-old child attends gynae OPD with complaints of failure to attend menarche with karyotype 46XX. On examination there is clitoromegaly. What enzyme likely to be deficient in the above condition?
a. 21 alpha hydroxylase
b. 11 beta hydroxylase
c. 17 alpha hydroxylase
d. 3 beta hydroxysteroid dehydrogenase

[Ref: Shaw's Textbook of Gynaecology 16th/e pg. 148; Nelson's 21st /e pg. 2972]

Explanation
- Above clinical scenario is classical of CAH or adrenogenital syndrome. Primary amenorrhoea with clitoromegaly in a phenotypic female and 46 XX karyotype indicates 3 beta hydroxysteroid dehydrogenase deficiency.
- See theory section for details.

159. In current obstetric advanced era, best test for obstetric monitoring of sensitized Rh negative mother?
a. Middle cerebral artery doppler wave forms. (MCA PSV)
b. Amniotic fluid spectrometric analysis
c. Fetal blood sampling
d. Biophysical profile.

[Ref: D.C. Dutta's Textbook of Obstetrics 9th/e pg. 316]

Explanation
- Currently, MCV PSV is the mainstay of fetal surveillance in case with red cell alloimmunization. It can be started as early as 18 weeks and may be repeated at interval of 1-2 weeks or as clinically indicated.
- Assessment of fetal anemia is more accurate by doing fetal blood sampling.

160. An 18 years old girl presented to gynae OPD with 6 months of amenorrhea. She has history of low grade fever, pain abdomen, weight loss and generalized weakness. On examination, pelvic mass was felt on the left side with features of ascites. What is the diagnosis?
a. Ectopic pregnancy
b. Granulosa cell tumour/ Ovarian malignancy
c. Fibroid with degeneration
d. Tuberculosis of pelvis with tubo-ovarian mass

[Ref: Shaw's Textbook of Gynaecology 16th/e pg. 188]

Explanation
- History of low grade fever, pain abdomen, weight loss and generalized weakness all are in favour of tubercular etiology.
- Oligo-amenorrhoea, infertility may be seen.
- The five characteristic features of Kawasaki disease are: bilateral bulbar conjunctival injection, usually without exudate; erythema of the oral and pharyngeal mucosa with strawberry tongue and dry, cracked lips, and without ulceration; edema and erythema of the hands and feet; rash of various forms (maculopapular, erythema multiforme, or scarlatiniform) with accentuation in the groin area; and nonsuppurative cervical lymphadenopathy, usually unilateral, with node size of ≥1.5 cm

PEDIATRICS

161. A child presents with fever, rash with desquamation with cervical lymphadenopathy. Most likely diagnosis is?
a. Measles
b. Scarlet fever
c. Kawasaki disease
d. Staphylococcal disease

[Ref: Nelson's Textbook of Pediatrics 21st /e pg. 1310]

Explanation
- The five characteristic features of Kawasaki disease are:
  - Bilateral bulbar conjunctival injection, usually without exudate;
  - Erythema of the oral and pharyngeal mucosa with strawberry tongue and dry, cracked lips, and without ulceration; edema and erythema of the hands and feet; rash of various forms (maculopapular, erythema multiforme, or scarlatiniform) with accentuation in the groin area; and nonsuppurative cervical lymphadenopathy, usually unilateral, with node size of ≥1.5 cm.

162. Term AGA baby presented on day 5 of life with serum bilirubin of 14 mg/dl. What will you advise to mother?
a. Phototherapy
b. Ultrasound abdomen
c. Routine care
d. Exchange transfusion

[Ref: Nelson's Textbook of Pediatrics 21st /e pg. 959]

157. a
158. a,d
159. a
160. d
161. c
162. c

163. Supravalvular aortic stenosis is seen in:
a. Noonan's syndrome
b. Williams syndrome
c. Turner syndrome
d. Shone syndrome

[Ref: Nelson's Textbook of Pediatrics 21st /e pg. 2387]

Explanation
- Types of aortic stenosis

Valvular	MC form
Subvalvular (subaortic)	in LVOT obstruction, Shone syndrome, hypertrophic cardiomyopathy
Supravalvular	Least common type, A/w William syndrome

- William syndrome is a s a rare genetic disorder that causes a variety of symptoms and learning issues. It is characterized by "Elfin facies", supravalvular AS, idiopathic hypercalcemia of infancy, stenosis of other arteries.

164. Normal value of these rules out malnutrition:
a. Lean body mass
b. Mid upper arm circumference
c. Hand grip strength
d. None of the above

[Ref: Nelson's Textbook of Pediatrics 21st/e pg. 344]

165. An 18-month-old child presents in OPD. Mother gives history of consuming rice milk. On examination he is lethargic, his weight is 6 kg, prominent abdomen/ pot belly. Lab values are given below:
i) S. albumin 2.9 gm%
ii) Hb 8 gm%
iii) Urine albumin -nil
Most likely diagnosis is
a. Marasmus
b. Iron deficiency anemia
c. Kwashiorkor
d. Indian childhood cirrhosis

[Ref: Nelson's Textbook of Pediatrics 21st /e pg. 1346, 3589]

Explanation
- Low serum albumin, weight loss, h/o rice milk consumption (hence inadequate protein intake) all points towards malnutrition.
- Pot belly abdomen goes in favour of Kwashiorkor.

166. A 10-year-old boy, after playing football, complaints of fatigue and abdominal pain. He also had a history of painful swelling of hands in the past. USG abdomen showed a small shrunken spleen. Which of the following is the most likely diagnosis:
a. Hereditary spherocytosis
b. Thalassemia
c. Sickle cell anemia
d. Acute pancreatitis

[Ref: Nelson's Textbook of Pediatrics 21st /e pg. 2543]

Explanation
- Dactylitis and autosplenectomy are clues to SCD.
- Dactylitis, often referred to as hand-foot syndrome, is frequently the 1st manifestation of pain in children with sickle cell anemia, occurring in 50% of children by 2 yr of age. Dactylitis often presents with symmetric swelling of the hands and/or feet.
- The cardinal clinical feature of sickle cell anemia is pain from vaso-occlusive episode. The pain is characterized as unremitting discomfort that may occur in any part of the body, but most often occurs in the chest, abdomen, or extremities. These painful episodes are often abrupt and can disrupt daily life activities.

167. A 5-year-old boy presents with sore throat for the last two days. On examination he has a grayish white pseudomembrane around his tonsils (image shown). Diphtheria is suspected. What prophylactic step should be taken for the 3 years old younger sibling who has received immunization as per the immunization schedule?
a. Booster dose of DPT
b. Chemoprophylaxis with erythromycin
c. Nothing to be done
d. Both chemoprophylaxsis and booster vaccine

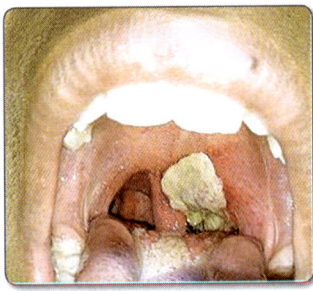

[Ref: Nelson's Textbook of Pediatrics 21st /e pg. 1461]

Explanation
- All household contacts and those who have had intimate respiratory or habitual physical contact with a patient are closely monitored for illness through the 7 day incubation period. Cultures of the nose, throat, and any cutaneous lesions are performed.
  - Antimicrobial prophylaxis is presumed effective and is administered regardless of immunization status using erythromycin (40–50 mg/kg/day divided qid PO for 7 days; maximum 2 g/day) or a single injection of benzathine penicillin G (600,000 U IM for <30 kg, 1,200,000 U IM for ≥30 kg).
  - Diphtheria toxoid vaccine, in age-appropriate form, is given to immunized individuals who have not received a booster dose within 5 yr. Children who have not received their 4th dose should be vaccinated.
  - Those who have received fewer than 3 doses of diphtheria toxoid or who have uncertain immunization status are immunized with an age-appropriate preparation on a primary schedule.

168. A child develops septic shock following acute meningitis. On examination the child has a petechial rash as shown in the picture. Gram stain of the exudates from lesion revealed gram negative diplococci. Causative organism in this case could be:

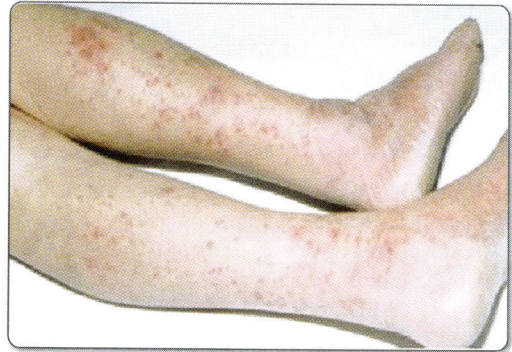

- a. Group B streptococcus
- b. Pneumococcus
- c. H. influenzae
- d. Meningococcus

[Ref: Nelson's Textbook of Pediatrics 21st /e pg. 1476]

Explanation

- In fulminant meningococcemia, the disease progresses rapidly over hours to septic shock characterized by prominent petechiae and purpura (purpura fulminans), hypotension, DIC, acidosis, adrenal hemorrhage, renal failure, myocardial failure, and coma. Meningitis may or may not be present.
- The rash is maculopapular, nonhemorrhagic & non blanching.

169. Meconium is passed
- a. Soon after birth
- b. Within 12 hrs of birth
- c. Within 24 hrs of birth
- d. Within 48 hrs of birth

[Ref: Nelson's Textbook of Pediatrics 21st /e pg. 942]

Explanation

- More than 90% of full-term newborn infants pass meconium within the 1st 24 hr. The possibility of intestinal obstruction should be considered in any infant who does not pass meconium by 24–36 hr.
- Meconium consist of bile salts, bile acids, and debris shed from the intestinal mucosa in the intrauterine period.

170. Greenish black colour in newborn stool is due to:
- a. Biliverdin
- b. Bilirubin
- c. A combination of amniotic fluid, bile and mucus
- d. Stercobilin

Explanation

- During pregnancy, all the baby's bilirubin is cleared by Mother's liver via the placenta.
- In babies, faeces can be a much darker colour (bordering on black) when the baby is first born. It's actually just the result of the waste present in the baby's bowel at birth being expelled – a combination of amniotic fluid, bile and mucus.

- Biliverdin is a green tetrapyrrolic bile pigment, and is a product of heme catabolism.
  - This pigment is responsible for a greenish color of neonatal stools
  - Sometimes seen in bruises.
- Bilirubin is a brownish bile pigment, which gives turmeric yellow tinge to neonatal skin in jaundice.
- Urobilinogen is oxidised into urobilin in bloodstream and excreted by kidney which gives yellow color to urine.
- Urobilinogen produced by breakdown of bilirubin in the intestine can be continued down and be reduced to stercobilin, which is responsible for brownish color of stools. If stercobilin is absent, faeces would be more of a pale clay-coloured hue.

171. A 24-month-old child was brought by mother with complaints of fever and cough. . On general physical examination there was chest indrawing, RR 38/min. What is the next line of management?
- a. Antibiotics for 5 days
- b. Antibiotic and refer to tertiary care center
- c. Intravenous antibiotics
- d. No treatment needed

Explanation

- According to 2019 guidelines this is a case of severe pneumonia, so best way to manage this child is give antibiotic shot and refer to tertiary care.

172. A 2-year-old boy presented with history of fever for 2 days, redness of the eyes and rashes. He developed oral lesion as shown in the image below. What complications is anticipated in the acute phase of this disease.

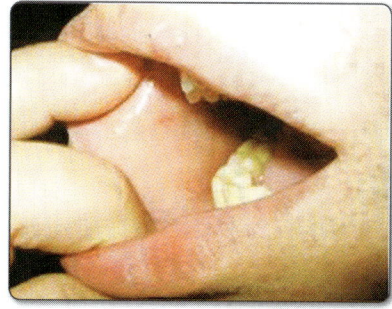

- a. Pancreatitis
- b. GBS
- c. Acute myocarditis
- d. Septic meningitis

[Ref: Nelson's Textbook of Pediatrics 21st /e pg. 942]

Explanation

- Koplik spots have been shown in the oral mucosa which aids to diagnosis of measles.
- Acute myocarditis is a complication of measles.

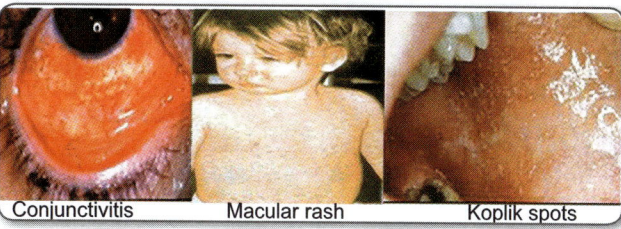

Conjunctivitis   Macular rash   Koplik spots

168. d
169. c
170. c
171. b
172. c

PSYCHIATRY

173. A patient of BPD was on lithium therapy for 6 months. After fasting for a day she presents with seizures, coarse tremors, confusion and weakness of limbs. What is the most accurate to diagnose her condition?
a. Serum lithium level
b. Serum electrolytes
c. Perform an ECG
d. None of the above

[Ref: Niraj Ahuja 7th/e pg. 78]

Explanation
- Seizures and coarse tremors, confusion all are neurological manifestation of lithium toxicity. Weakness of the limb may be because of hypotonia a/w lithium toxicity. So, serum electrolyte levels must be ordered.

174. A lady presents with recurrent history of irritability, frequent mood swings, sometimes lack of interest in surroundings and general dissatisfaction with everything. There is no significant disruption in his sleep or appetite. There was history of depressed mood for few months. She is likely to be suffering from:
a. Manic depressive psychosis
b. Persistent mood disorder
c. Hypomania
d. Schizo-affective disorder

[Ref: Niraj Ahuja 7th/e pg. 73]

Explanation
- Clinical h/o dysthymia is there, so it is most likely persistent mood disorder.
- Clinical features are consistent with bipolar mood disorder

175. MBBS 1st year girl complains of sudden onset of breathlessness, palpitation and feeling of impending doom. Physical examination is normal. What is her most probable condition?
a. Conversion reaction
b. Acute psychosis
c. Generalized Anxiety disorder
d. Panic attack

[Ref: Niraj Ahuja 7th/e pg. 90]

Explanation
- In panic attack, the attack often begins with extreme anxiety and a sense of impending doom. The symptoms rapidly increase over a period of 10 minutes. There may be palpitations, tachycardia, dyspnea and sweating. Usually GPE is normal except for sinus tachycardia.
- GAD (Generalized Anxiety disorder) will not present with acute attack & is characterized by persistent symptoms not acute symptoms.

176. A patient was put on imipramine for depression. She developed clinical features of mania, what is the next appropriate step:
a. Stop imipramine and start on valproate
b. Continue imipramine and add on valproate
c. Give Anti-psychotic continue imipramine for the time being
d. Stop imipramine and give him ECT

[Ref: Niraj Ahuja 7th/e pg. 78]

Explanation
- If a patient is on antidepressant develops manic symptoms it's called as manic switch. It must be treated as bipolar disorder. So stop antidepressants and start a mood stabilizer like valproate.

173. a
174. b
175. d
176. c

General Medicine

FACTS

- The most useful test for distinguishing proximal and distal RTA is measurement of urinary pH.
- In salicylates (Aspirin) overdose there is metabolic acidosis with respiratory alkalosis.
- Urinary anion gap is an indication of NH_4^+ ion excretion.
- Most frequently encountered acid base disorder → Respiratory alkalosis.
- Acid base disorder seen in normal pregnancy → Respiratory alkalosis.
- Body temperature is controlled by the hypothalamus – Preoptic anterior hypothalamus and the posterior hypothalamus
- **R**ectal temperature is generally 0.4°C (0.7°F) higher than **O**ral temperature which is 0.6°C (1°F) higher than the **A**xillary temperature [**Mn:** ROAms].
- Core temperature monitoring is used to monitor intraoperative hypothermia.
- *Sites for measuring core temperature are:*
  - Pulmonary artery (Best site/Gold standard)
  - Tympanic membrane
  - Distal esophagus, and
  - Nasopharynx.
- Temperature-pulse dissociation (relative bradycardia) occurs in typhoid fever, brucellosis, leptospirosis, some drug-induced fevers, and factitious fever.
- A fever of >41.5°C (>106.7°F) is called hyperpyrexia.
- Hyperthermia (heat stroke) is characterized by an uncontrolled increase in body temperature due to exogenous source that exceeds the body's ability to lose heat.
- The pyrogenic cytokines include IL-1, IL-6, tumor necrosis factor (TNF), Ciliary Neurotrophic Factor, and Interferons (IFNs), particularly IFN-α.
- The elevation of **PGE_2** in the brain raises the hypothalamic set point for core temperature.
- **Malignant hyperthermia** is triggered by use of inhalation anesthetics (Halothane, Cyclopropane) and muscle relaxants (Succinylcholine).
- Central muscle relaxant (Dantrolene sodium) is helpful in malignant hyperthermia and Neuroleptic malignant syndrome.
- Targeted temperature management (Therapeutic Hypothermia) is recommended for comatose cardiac arrest patients.

SYNDROMES

	Neuroleptic Malignant Syndrome	Malignant Hyperthermia	Serotonin Syndrome
Precipitant	▪ An idiosyncratic reaction ▪ Haloperidol, Phenothiazines	▪ Halothane, Cyclopropane, Succinylcholine	▪ SSRIs, MAO inhibitors and other serotonergic drugs
Features	▪ **F**ever/Hyperthermia ▪ **A**utonomic dysfunction ▪ Muscle **R**igidity ▪ Altered **M**ental status	▪ Hyperthermia ▪ Rigidity ▪ High end tidal CO_2 levels – earliest sign	▪ Hyperthermia ▪ Diarrhea ▪ Tremor ▪ Myoclonus
Treatment	▪ Dantrolene >Bromocriptine	▪ Dantrolene sodium	▪ Cyproheptadine

SODIUM IMBALANCE

	Hyponatremia	Hypernatremia
Definition	▪ Plasma sodium <135 mEq/L	▪ Plasma sodium >145 mEq/L

Etiology	▪ **Pseudo hyponatremia:**
	○ Normal osmolality –
	  – Hyperlipidemia, Hyperproteinemia
	○ High osmolality –
	  – Hyperglycemia, Mannitol
	▪ **True/hypo-osmolar hyponatremia:**
	○ With ECF volume depletion
	○ With normal ECF volume
	○ With increased ECF volume
		▪ Excess water loss
		▪ Heat exposure, Severe burn, Severe exercise
		▪ Diabetes insipidus – Urine output of >3 L/day
		▪ Excess of diuretics
		▪ Uncontrolled diabetes mellitus
		▪ Impair thirst
		▪ Primary hypodypsia
		▪ IV hypertonic saline or $NaHCO_3$

Clinical features	▪ Anorexia, Nausea, Vomiting, Lethargy ▪ Weakness, Confusion, Altered sensorium ▪ Brain swelling or cerebral edema ▪ Drowsiness, Convulsion, Coma, Death	▪ Dehydration, Nausea, Weakness ▪ Altered mental status ▪ Focal neurological deficit, Coma, Seizure ▪ Intracerebral and SAH due to brain shrinkage
Treatment	▪ **With ECF volume depletion:** ○ Acute and symptomatic: 3% saline ○ IV isotonic saline/Oral salt supplementation ○ Free fluid restriction ▪ **With normal ECF volume:** ○ Fluid restriction; Tolvaptan ▪ **With increased ECF volume:** ○ Diuretics ○ Salt and fluid restriction ○ V2 receptor antagonist (Tolvaptan)	▪ Calculate the free water deficit and administer the deficit fluid in 48-72 hours. ▪ **Fluid of choice :** ○ Acute hypernatremia: 5% Dextrose ○ Hypernatremia with ECF contraction: Isotonic saline followed by 5% D or ½ NS or Oral fluids. ▪ **Central DI :** Vasopressin ▪ **Nephrogenic DI :** Thiazides, Indomethacin ▪ **Lithium induced DI:** <u>Ami</u>loride [**Mn:** AmiLi]
Extra Edge	Na^+ req. = (Desired Na – Actual Na) × TBW Rate of correction = <0.5 mEq/L/hr	Free water deficit = [(Na – 140)/140] × TBW Rate of correction = 0.5 – 1.0 mEq/L/hr

- In acute hyponatremia, symptoms develop at serum Na^+ level of ~ 120 mEq/L.
- In chronic hyponatremia, symptoms develop at serum Na^+ level of ~ 110 mEq/L.

CENTRAL PONTINE MYELINOSIS

- Aka Osmotic Demyelination Syndrome
- Complication of severe hyponatremia occurring as a result of rapid correction of serum Na^+ with hypertonic saline
- *Risk factors:*
  ○ Serum Na <120 mEq/L for >48 hr
  ○ Aggressive Na^+ correction with hypertonic saline
- Clinical features: Confusion, Horizontal gaze palsy, Spastic Quadriplegia, Increased Tone, Babinski positive
- IOC: MRI – Demyelination in pons and extrapontine regions is characteristic

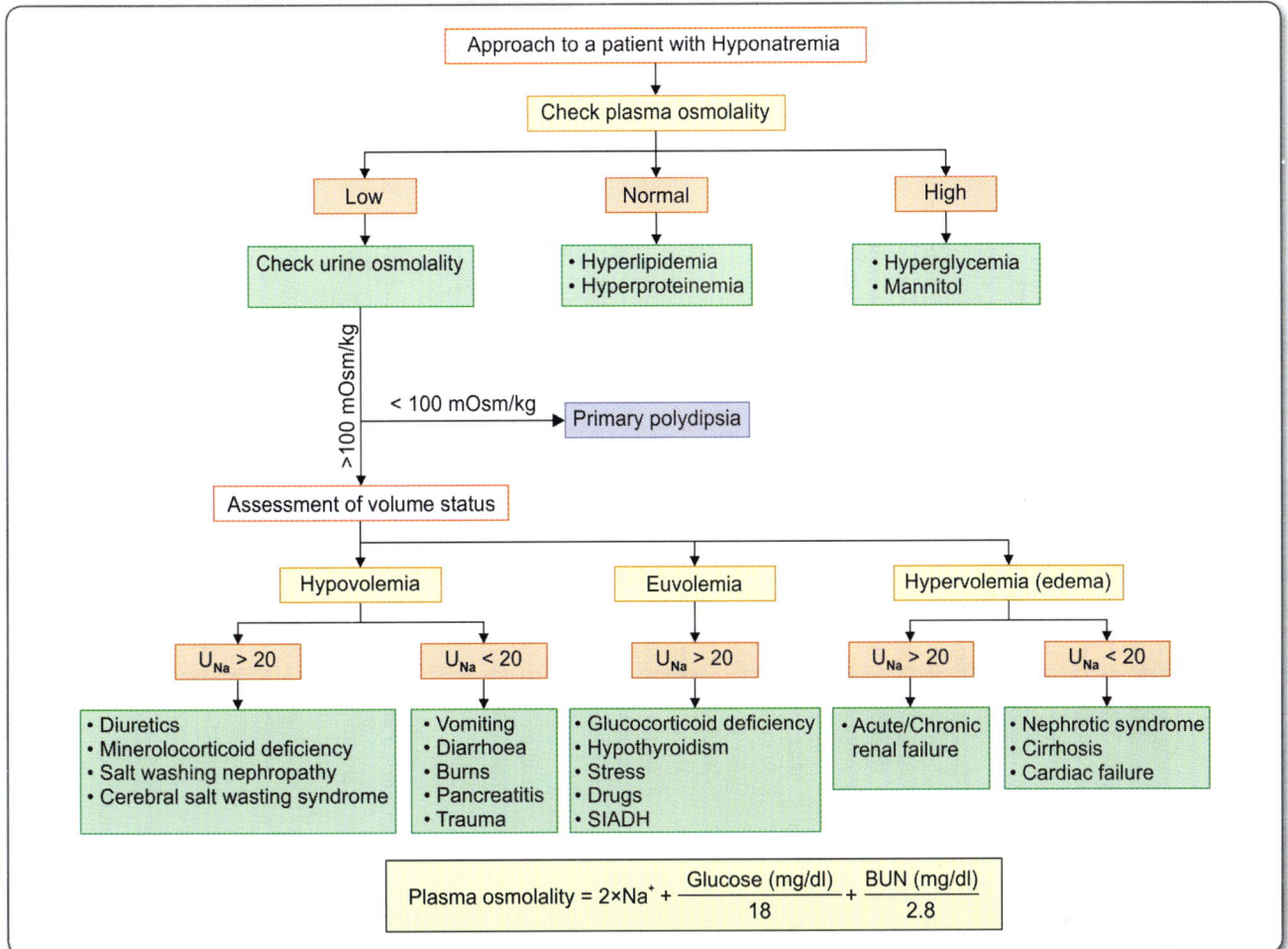

Plasma osmolality diagram content:

- Approach to a patient with Hyponatremia
- Check plasma osmolality
  - Low → Check urine osmolality
  - Normal → • Hyperlipidemia • Hyperproteinemia
  - High → • Hyperglycemia • Mannitol
- Check urine osmolality
  - >100 mOsm/kg → Assessment of volume status
  - < 100 mOsm/kg → Primary polydipsia
- Assessment of volume status
  - Hypovolemia
    - $U_{Na} > 20$: • Diuretics • Minerolocorticoid deficiency • Salt washing nephropathy • Cerebral salt wasting syndrome
    - $U_{Na} < 20$: • Vomiting • Diarrhoea • Burns • Pancreatitis • Trauma
  - Euvolemia
    - $U_{Na} > 20$: • Glucocorticoid deficiency • Hypothyroidism • Stress • Drugs • SIADH
  - Hypervolemia (edema)
    - $U_{Na} > 20$: • Acute/Chronic renal failure
    - $U_{Na} < 20$: • Nephrotic syndrome • Cirrhosis • Cardiac failure

$$\text{Plasma osmolality} = 2 \times Na^+ + \frac{\text{Glucose (mg/dl)}}{18} + \frac{\text{BUN (mg/dl)}}{2.8}$$

Volume Status	Total Body Water	Total Body Sodium
Hypovolemia	↓	↓↓
Euvolemia	↑	↔
Hypervolemia	↑↑	↑

Lab Parameters	SIADH*	CSW**	Central DI	Nephrogenic DI	Primary Polydipsia
ADH levels	↑	N/↓	↓	↑	↓
Urine output	↓/N	↑	↑ (>3 L/Day)	↑	↑
Serum sodium	↓	↓	↑	↑	↓
Serum osmolality	↓↓	↓	↑	↑	↓
Urine sodium	↑	↑↑	↓		↓
Urine osmolality	↑	↑	↓ (<200)	↓ (<200)	↑
Urine osmolality after water deprivation			No change	No change	↑
Urine osmolality after AVP			↑	No change	↑
Hydration	Euvolemia	Dehydration	Dehydrated	Dehydrated	Over hydration
Treatment	Fluid restriction – TOC Loop diuretics, Demeclocycline	IV hypertonic saline Fludrocortisone	Desmopressin	Thiazide diuretics Amiloride	Fluid restriction

* Syndrome of Inappropriate ADH Release | ** Cerebral Salt Wasting Syndrome |

POTASSIUM IMBALANCE

	Hypokalemia	Hyperkalemia
Definition	▪ Hypokalemia is defined as a potassium level <3.5 mEq/L ▪ Moderate hypokalemia is a serum level of <3.0 mEq/L ▪ Severe hypokalemia is defined as a level <2.5 mEq/L	▪ Hyperkalemia is defined as a potassium level >5.5 mEq/L ▪ Moderate hyperkalemia is a serum potassium >6.0 mEq/L ▪ Severe hyperkalemia is a serum potassium >7.0 mEq/L

Etiology	▪ **Low dietary intake**
	▪ **Redistribution into cells:**
	  ○ Metabolic alkalosis
	  ○ Insulin
	  ○ β₂ agonist (salbutamol)
	  ○ Hypokalemic periodic paralysis
	  ○ Thyrotoxic periodic paralysis
	▪ **Non renal loss:**
	  ○ Vomiting
	  ○ Diarrhoea
	  ○ Sweating
		▪ **Renal loss:**
		  ○ **Cushing's syndrome**
		  ○ **Bartter's syndrome**
		  ○ **Gitelman's syndrome**
		  ○ **Liddle's syndrome**
		  ○ Diuretics/Osmotic diuresis
		  ○ Magnesium deficiency
		  ○ Hyperaldosteronism
		  ○ Proximal & distal RTA
		  ○ DKA
		  ○ **Amphotericin B**
		  ○ Salt wasting nephropathies
			▪ **Increased dietary intake/ iatrogenic**
			▪ **Tissue breakdown:**
			  ○ Severe exercise
			  ○ Bleeding, Hemolysis
			  ○ Rhabdomyolysis
			▪ **Impaired excretion:**
			  ○ Potassium sparing diuretics
			  ○ **ACE inhibitors/ARBs**
			  ○ Renin inhibitors
			  ○ Acute or chronic renal failure
			  ○ **Addison's disease**
			  ○ Hypoaldosteronism
			  ○ **Congenital adrenal hypoplasia** (21-α hydroxylase deficiency)
				▪ **Extracellular shift:**
				  ▪ **Metabolic acidosis**
				  ○ Digoxin
				  ○ Uncontrolled diabetes
				  ○ Hyperkalemic periodic paralysis
				  ▪ **Pseudohyperkalemia**
				  ○ Thrombocytosis
				  ○ Leukocytosis
				  ○ Erythrocytosis

Clinical features	▪ Fatigue, Myalgia, Muscular weakness ▪ Constipation, Ileus, Urinary retention ▪ Polyuria ▪ Hypoventilation ▪ Hyporeflexia and Complete paralysis ▪ Increased risk of arrhythmias	▪ Fatigue, Myalgia, Muscular weakness ▪ Tingling around lips ▪ Hyporeflexia and Complete paralysis ▪ Fatal cardiac arrhythmias
Treatment	▪ Supplementation with Potassium chloride >Potassium bicarbonate either oral or IV. ▪ Potassium rich food like fruit juices, banana, coconut, dry fruits etc.	▪ Calcium gluconate or CaCl₂ – Stabilize the cardiac cell membrane ▪ First line treatment of severe hyperkalemia ▪ Insulin and dextrose infusion – increase cellular uptake of K⁺ ▪ Sodium bicarbonate infusion – intracellular shifting ▪ β₂ agonist (salbutamol) nebulisation ▪ Loop/Thiazide diuretics ▪ Cation exchange resins ▪ Dialysis

Contd...

Hypokalemia

ECG Changes

Features include:
- Increased amplitude and width of the P wave
- Prolongation of the PR interval
- *Apparent* long QT interval due to fusion of the T and U waves (= long QU interval)
- ST depression
- T wave flattening (Earliest) and inversion
- Prominent U waves – best seen in the precordial lead
- Supraventricular arrhythmias: AF, atrial flutter, atrial tachycardia
- Ventricular arrhythmias, e.g. VT, VF and Torsades de Pointes

Tall peaked P wave may be seen in severe hypokalemia known as **Pseudo – P pulmonale.**

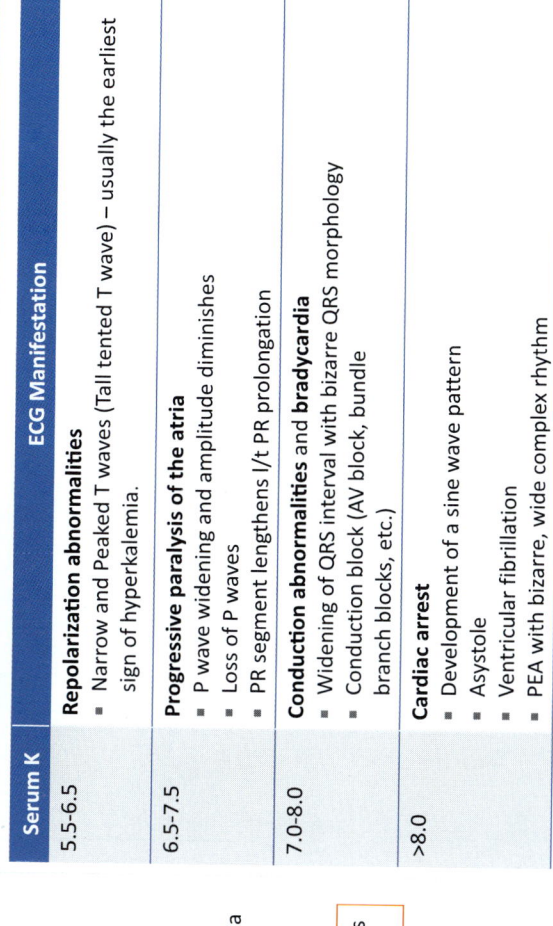

Hyperkalemia

Serum K	ECG Manifestation
5.5-6.5	**Repolarization abnormalities** - Narrow and Peaked T waves (Tall tented T wave) – usually the earliest sign of hyperkalemia.
6.5-7.5	**Progressive paralysis of the atria** - P wave widening and amplitude diminishes - Loss of P waves - PR segment lengthens l/t PR prolongation
7.0-8.0	**Conduction abnormalities** and **bradycardia** - Widening of QRS interval with bizarre QRS morphology - Conduction block (AV block, bundle branch blocks, etc.)
>8.0	**Cardiac arrest** - Development of a sine wave pattern - Asystole - Ventricular fibrillation - PEA with bizarre, wide complex rhythm

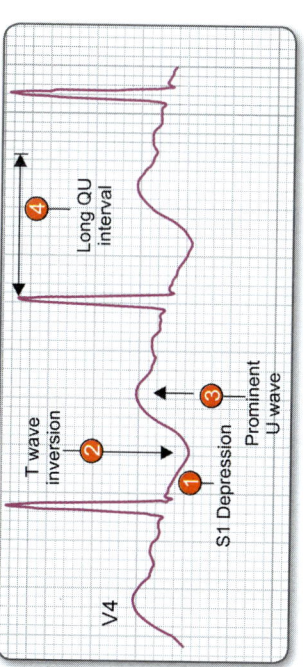

CALCIUM IMBALANCE

	Hypocalcemia	Hypercalcemia
Definition	Serum Calcium <8.8 mg/dL	Serum Calcium >11 mg/dL

Etiology	• Hypoalbuminemia
	• **Hypoparathyroidism:**
	  ○ Di George syndrome
	  ○ Hypomagnesemia
	• Vitamin D deficiency
	• Chronic renal failure
	• **Severe hyperphosphatemia:**
	  ○ Tumor lysis syndrome
	  ○ Acute renal failure
	  ○ Rhabdomyolysis
	• **Miscellaneous:**
	  ○ Metabolic or respiratory alkalosis
	  ○ Acute pancreatitis
	  ○ Massive transfusion of citrated blood
	  ○ Hungry bone syndrome
	  ○ Osteoblastic metastasis (CA prostate)
	  ○ Loop diuretics
		• **Excessive PTH production:**
		  ○ Primary hyperparathyroidism
		  ○ Tertiary hyperparathyroidism
		  ○ Lithium therapy
		• **Hypercalcemia of Malignancy:**
		  ○ Multiple Myeloma, CA Breast, CA lung
		• **Increase in bone resorption:**
		  ○ Hyperthyroidism
		  ○ Immobilization
		• **Excessive Vitamin D production:**
		  ○ Vitamin D intoxication
		  ○ Granulomatous diseases like sarcoidosis, tuberculosis
		• **Milk alkali syndrome**
		• **Decreased renal excretion:**
		  ○ Thiazide diuretics
		  ○ Acute adrenal insufficiency
		  ○ Familial hypocalciuric hypercalcemia

Clinical features	• Weakness, Paresthesia • Muscle spasm, Carpopedal spasm, Laryngeal spasm, Tetany • Lethargy, Confusion, Seizure • **Chvostek's sign** → contraction of facial muscle on tapping facial nerve • **Trousseau's sign** → Inflation of BP cuff leads to carpal spasm	• Weakness, Fatigue • Depression, Confusion, Coma • Constipation, Anorexia, Pain abdomen • Polyuria, Nocturia, Nephrolithiasis
Treatment	• 10% calcium gluconate in acute symptomatic patients • Vitamin D supplementation • Magnesium correction	• Hydration with normal saline – treatment of choice • Forced diuresis with loop diuretics – Loop loose calcium • Hemodialysis • Bisphosphonates, Calcitonin, Glucocorticoids
ECG Changes	• **Prolongation** of QTc primarily by prolonging the ST segment. • **Torsades de pointes** (less common)	• The main ECG abnormality is **shortening** of the QT interval • Bradycardia, AV Block • In severe hypercalcaemia, Osborn waves (J waves) may be seen

Short QT ECG (Hypercalcemia) and ECG strip (Hypocalcemia).

APPROACH TO AN ACID-BASE DISORDERS

- Four primary acid-base disorders are defined depending upon the primary disturbance. If the initial disturbance affects bicarbonates:
  - Rise in bicarbonate →Metabolic alkalosis
  - Fall in bicarbonate →Metabolic acidosis

- If the initial disturbance affects $PaCO_2$:
  - Rise in $PaCO_2$ → Respiratory acidosis
  - Fall in $PaCO_2$ → Respiratory alkalosis

Acid-Base Disorders	pH	Primary Change	Compensatory Change
Metabolic acidosis	↓	HCO_3 ↓	$PaCO_2$ ↓
Respiratory acidosis	↓	$PaCO_2$ ↑	HCO_3 ↑
Metabolic alkalosis	↑	HCO_3 ↑	$PaCO_2$ ↑
Respiratory alkalosis	↑	$PaCO_2$ ↓	HCO_3 ↓

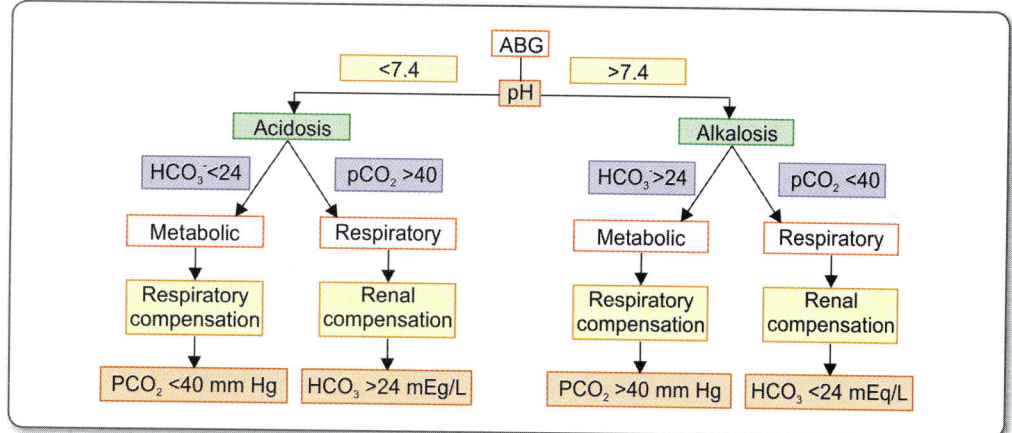

- The body tries to neutralize the effect of the primary change on pH by a process called compensation. For example, metabolic acidosis due to fall in bicarbonate produces low pH which stimulate the respiratory centre causing hyperventilation and CO_2 washout resulting in fall in $PaCO_2$. Thus, metabolic acidosis leads to compensatory respiratory alkalosis. Note that in each case, the compensatory changes take place in the same direction as the primary change. This is known as "Same Direction Rule" of compensation.

Anion Gap (AG)

- The difference between unmeasured cation and anion is termed as Anion Gap.
- AG is most useful to establish etiological diagnosis of metabolic acidosis.

$$AG = Na - (Cl + HCO_3) = 12 \pm 2 \text{ mEq/L}$$

- Anion gap reflects unmeasured anions in plasma.

- A fall in the serum albumin by 1 g/dl decreases AG by 2 mEq/L.
- A decreased anion gap (<6 mEq/L) may suggest:
  - Hypoalbuminemia as in Nephrotic syndrome
  - **Plasma cell dyscrasia** (multiple myeloma)
  - Bromide intoxication

Metabolic Acidosis

- On the basis of AG, causes of metabolic acidosis can be divided into two groups:

Normal AG Metabolic Acidosis (NAGMA)	Increase AG Metabolic Acidosis
▪ **GI loss of HCO$_3$:** 　○ Diarrhea, Cholera, Fistula ▪ **Renal loss of HCO$_3$:** 　○ Proximal RTA (Type 2) 　○ Carbonic anhydrase inhibitor ▪ Failure of renal H$^+$ ion excretion: 　○ Distal RTA (Type 1) ▪ Addition of H$^+$ ion: 　○ NH$_4$Cl infusion ▪ Pancreatitis ▪ Ureterosigmoidostomy ▪ Ileostomy fluid loss	▪ **Metabolic disorders:** 　○ Lactic acidosis 　○ DKA 　○ Alcoholic ketoacidosis ▪ **Addition of exogenous acid:** 　○ **S**alicylate poisoning 　○ **M**ethanol poisoning 　○ **E**thylene glycol poisoning 　○ **P**araldehyde 　○ **M**etformin ▪ Failure of renal H$^+$ ion excretion: 　○ **R**enal failure

* NAGMA is aka Hyperchloremic Metabolic Acidosis

Mnemonic for Increase AG Metabolic acidosis: DR MAPLES

Urinary Anion Gap

- UAG is the reflection of kidney's ability to excrete NH$_4$Cl.
- Normally it is either 0 or a positive value.
- It is useful to differentiate between the renal and GI causes of acidosis.
- UAG is negative in case of metabolic acidosis secondary to GI causes (diarrhea) as NH$_4$Cl excretion via kidneys is intact.

- In metabolic acidosis due to RTA/ Renal failure where NH$_4$Cl excretion is impaired, UAG is positive.

$$UAG = Urinary (Na + K - Cl) = 80 - NH_4$$

Other Acid-Base Disorders

Metabolic Alkalosis	Respiratory Acidosis	Respiratory Alkalosis
▪ **Vomiting/gastric suction** ▪ **Cushing syndrome** ▪ **Hypokalemia** ▪ **Multiple blood transfusion** ▪ Pyloric stenosis ▪ Diuretics ▪ Hyperaldosteronism/ Conn's syndrome ▪ Bartter syndrome	▪ **Asthma** ▪ **COPD** ▪ **ARDS** ▪ **Hypoventilation** ▪ Obesity ▪ Myasthenia ▪ Pneumothorax ▪ Pulmonary edema	▪ **Normal pregnancy** ▪ **High altitude residence** ▪ **Hyperventilation syndrome** ▪ CHF ▪ Hepatic failure ▪ Salicylate intoxication

Treatment

Metabolic Alkalosis	Respiratory Acidosis	Respiratory Alkalosis
▪ Correction of hydration and electrolytes ▪ Isotonic saline (avoid Ringer lactate) ▪ H$_2$ blocker/PPI	▪ Patent airway and adequate oxygenation ▪ Mechanical ventilation ▪ Alkali therapy	▪ Oxygen supplementation ▪ **Rebreathing in paper bag** ▪ Pre-treatment with acetazolamide

IMPORTANT FEVERS

	Fever Type	Caused by
Quotidian fever	Fever with a periodicity of 24 hours (occurs daily)	Typical of *Plasmodium falciparum* or *Plasmodium knowlesi* malaria
Tertian fever	Fever with a periodicity of 48 hours (Every 3rd day)	Typical of *Plasmodium vivax* or *Plasmodium ovale* malaria
Quartan fevers	Fever with a periodicity of 72 hours	Typical of *Plasmodium malariae* malaria
Viral Hemorrhagic fevers	Hemorrhagic fevers	Ebola virus, Chikungunya Dengue viruses type 1-4 (Flaviviruses) Yellow fever (Flaviviruses) KFD (Flaviviruses) Crimean Congo HF (Norovirus)
	Hemorrhagic fever with renal syndrome	Hantan virus
	African hemorrhagic fever	Marburg & Ebola viruses
Miscellaneous	Brazilian purpuric fever	*H. influenzae biogroup aegyptius*
	Query fever/Q fever	*Coxiella burnetii*
	Oroya fever	*Bartonella bacilliformis*
	Glandular fever/Kissing disease	*Epstein-Barr virus*
	Undulant/Malta/Mediterranean fever	Brucellosis
	Pontiac fever	*Legionella*
	Boutonneuse fever/ Mediterranean spotted fever/ Indian tick typhus	*Rickettsii conorri*
	Familial Mediterranean fever	Inherited disease (Mutation in the gene MEFV, XLR)
	Pel-Ebstein fever	Hodgkin's lymphoma
	Picket fence fever	Lateral Sinus thrombosis
	Step Ladder Fever	Typhoid
	Remittent fever	Infective endocarditis
	Saddle back fever	Dengue fever
	Relapsing fever	*Borrelia*
	Trench fever	*Bartonella quintana*

- Pel-Ebstein fever is a type of fever lasting for 3–10 days followed by an afebrile period of 3–10 days.
- Remittent fever – Fever with temperature fluctuation >1° F but do not touch baseline.

AUTOIMMUNE DISEASES

Autoantibodies	Conditions
Anti-Centromere Antibodies	Limited Cutaneous Systemic Sclerosis (Crest Syndrome)
Anti Topoisomerase I (Anti Scl-70)	Systemic Sclerosis/Scleroderma
Anti-dsDNA Antibody Anti-Smith Antibody (Most Specific)	SLE
Anti-Histone Antibodies (Mn: His Stone Dil)	SLE Drug-Induced Lupus Erythematosus
Anti-Jo1	Polymyositis Dermatomyositis
Anti SS-A/Anti-Ro Antibodies Anti SS-B/Anti La Antibodies	Primary Sjögren Syndrome
Anti-CCP Antibodies	Rheumatoid Arthritis
Anti U-1 RNP Antibodies	Mixed Connective Tissue Disease
C-ANCA	Wegener Granulomatosis
P-ANCA	Microscopic Polyangiitis Churg Strauss Syndrome
Anti-Transglutaminase Antibodies	Celiac Disease Dermatitis Herpetiformis
Anti Gliadin Antibodies	Celiac Sprue
Anti Parietal Cell Antibodies	Pernicious Anemia
Anti GAD Antibodies	Type I DM
Anti Basement Membrane Antibodies	Goodpasture Syndrome
Anti Thyroglobulin Antibodies Anti Peroxidase Antibodies	Hashimoto thyroiditis
Anti-Thyroid Autoantibodies	Hashimoto Thyroiditis Graves Disease
Anti-Smooth Muscle Antibody	Chronic Autoimmune Hepatitis
Anti-Mitochondrial Antibody	Primary Biliary Cirrhosis
Anti MI 2 Antibodies	Dermatomyositis

Emergency Medicine

TYPES OF SHOCKS

Types	Causes	Pathophysiology	Clinical Feature	Treatment
Hypovolemic	▪ Hemorrhage ▪ Dehydration	▪ Preload ↓ ▪ Contractility normal or ↑ ▪ Afterlod (SVR) ↑	▪ HR ↑ ▪ BP ↓ ▪ Cardiac output ↓ ▪ CRT Delayed ▪ Extremities cool & pale ▪ Weak thready pulse	▪ Prevent losses ▪ Secure large bore IV access ▪ Fluid resuscitation with crystalloids
Cardiogenic	▪ Myocarditis ▪ Dysrhythmia	▪ Preload ↓ ▪ Contractility ↓ ▪ Afterlod (SVR) ○ ↑ (Rt ventricular) ○ ↓ (Left ventricular)	▪ HR ↑ ▪ BP ↓ ▪ Cardiac output ↓ ▪ CRT delayed	▪ Inotropes ▪ Cautious use of fluids, ECMO ▪ DOC: Noradrenaline
Obstructive	▪ Tamponade ▪ Tension pneumothorax ▪ Pulmonary embolus ▪ Chest trauma	▪ Preload ↓ ▪ Contractility normal ▪ Afterlod (SVR) ↑	▪ HR ↑ ▪ BP ↓ ▪ Cardiac output ↓ ▪ CRT Delayed ▪ Extremities cool	▪ Pericardiocentasis ▪ Chest tube
Dissociative	▪ CO poisoning ▪ Cyanide	▪ Variable	▪ HR ↑ ▪ BP Normal or ↑ ▪ Cardiac output ↑ ▪ CRT normal ▪ Extremities normal	▪ Antidotes ▪ Hyperbaric oxygen therapy
Distributive				
1. Septic	▪ Infections ▪ Sepsis	▪ Preload ↓ ▪ Contractility normal or ↓ Afterload ↓	▪ HR ↑ ▪ BP ↓ ▪ Cardiac output ↓ ▪ CRT Flash/delayed ▪ Extremities warm & pink	▪ IV Antibiotics, Fluids ▪ IV Noradrenaline → drug of choice
2. Anaphylactic	▪ Anaphylaxis	▪ Preload ↓ ▪ Contractility variable ▪ Afterlod ↑↓	▪ HR ↑ ▪ BP ↓ ▪ Cardiac output ↓ ▪ CRT Flash/delayed ▪ Extremities warm	▪ IV Epinephrine ▪ Fluids
3. Neurogenic	▪ Spinal cord injury ▪ Traumatic brain injury (TBI)	▪ Preload ↓ ▪ Contractility normal ▪ Afterload (SVR) ↓ ▪ Loss of sympathetic tone	▪ HR ↓ ▪ BP ↓ ▪ Cardiac output ↓ ▪ CRT Flash/normal ▪ Extremities warm	▪ High flow O_2 ▪ Fluid resuscitation ▪ Vasopressors

2015 ACLS GUIDELINES

- Chest compression rate should be at the rate of 100-120/min instead of at least 100/min.
- Depth of compression should be 2 inch but not more than 2.4".
- Deliver 1 breath every 6 seconds (i.e. 10 breaths/min.) while advanced airway in place (instead of 1 breath every 6 to 8 seconds previously).
- Vasopressin in high dose was used in place of adrenaline in past. However it is removed from algorithm in latest 2015 ACLS guidelines.
- Extracorporeal CPR may be considered as an alternative to conventional CPR.

Other Drugs used in ACLS

Drug	Indication
Adenosine	SVT/PSVT
Amiodarone	Pulseless VT
Atropine	Symptomatic Bradycardia
Dopamine	Bradycardia
Epinephrine (Adrenaline)	Cardiac Arrest (Vasopressin in high dose can also be used)
Lignocaine	VT
MgSO$_4$	Torsades de pointes, Severe Asthma

ADULT BLS ALGORITHM 2016 (C → A → B)

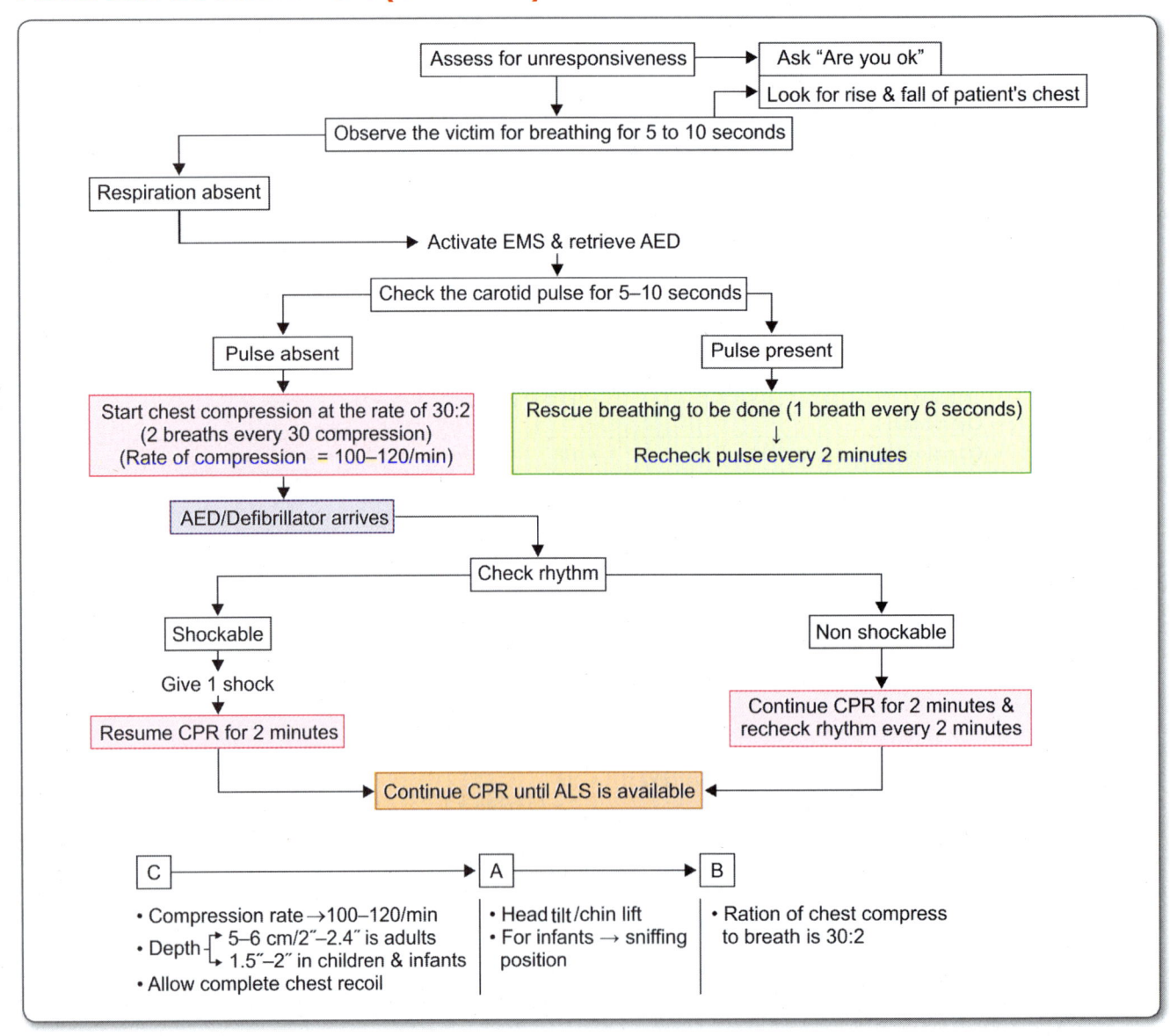

SUMMARY OF STEPS OF CPR (COURTESY: BLS ALGORITHM AND IAP-ALS GROUP)

Component	Recommendations		
	Adults & Adolescents	Children (1 year to puberty)	Infants
Assessment	▪ Unresponsive (for all ages)		
	▪ No breathing or no normal breathing (i.e. only gasping)	▪ No breathing or only gasping	
	▪ No pulse felt within 10 seconds		
Activate ERS	▪ If you are alone, activate ERS and get an AED	▪ If you are alone and did not witness arrest, provide 2 mins. CPR, then activate ERS and get an AED	
CPR sequence	▪ Chest compressions, Airway, Breathing (C-A-B)		
Compression rate	▪ 100-120/min		
Compression depth	▪ At least 2 inches (5 cm)	▪ At least 1/3 AP diameter About 2 inches (5 cm)	▪ At least 1/3 AP diameter About 2 inches ▪ About 1½ inches (4)
Chest wall recoil	▪ Allow complete recoil between compressions ▪ Rotate compressors every 2 minutes		
Compression interruptions	▪ Minimize interruptions in chest compressions ▪ Attempt to limit interruptions to <10 seconds		
Airway	▪ Head tilt-chin lift (suspected trauma → jaw thrust)		
Ventilation	▪ Mouth-to-mouth breathing/Mouth-to-mouth mask breathing	▪ Mouth-to-Nose and mouth breathing	
Compression ventilation ratio (until advanced airway placed)	▪ 30:2 (1 or 2 rescuers)	▪ 30:2 (Single rescuer) ▪ 15:2 (2 rescuers)	
Ventilations with advanced airway	▪ 1 breath every 6–8 seconds (8-10 breaths/min) ▪ Asynchronous with chest compressions ▪ About 1 second per breath ▪ Visible chest rise		
Defibrillation	▪ Attach and use AED as soon as available. ▪ Minimize interruptions in chest compression before and after shock; ▪ Resume CPR beginning with compressions immediately after each shock.		

Abbreviations: AED, automated external defibrillator, AP, anterior-posterior; CPR, cardiopulmonary resuscitation

ADULT ACLS CARDIAC ARREST ALGORITHM

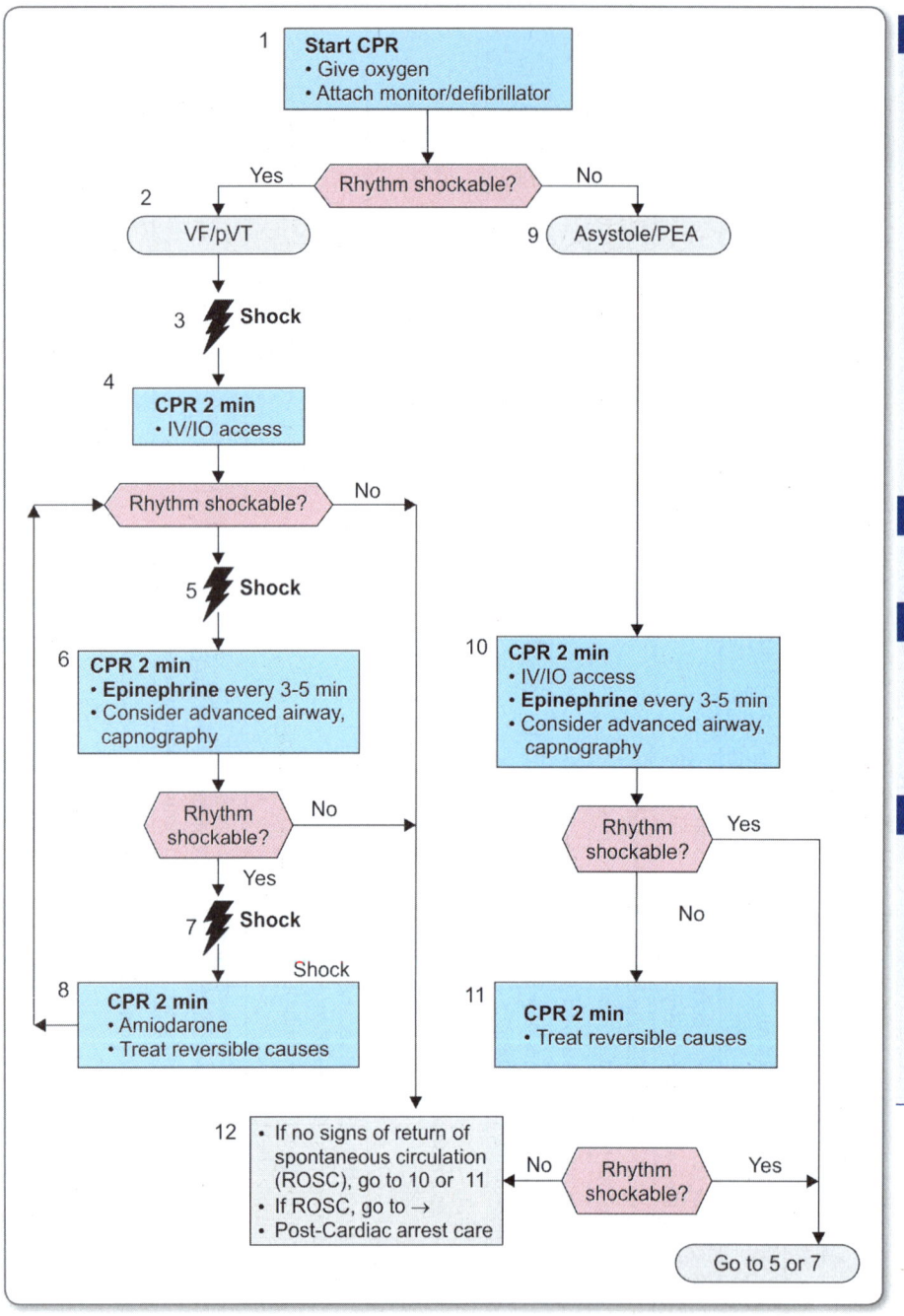

CPR Quality

- Push hard (at least 5 cm) and fast (100-120/min) and allow complete chest recoil
- Rotate compressor every 2 minutes or sooner if fatigued
- If no advanced airway→ 30:2 compression: ventilation ratio
- Quantitative waveform capnography
  - If PETCO$_2$ <10 mm Hg, attempt to improve CPR quality
- Intra-arterial pressure
  - If relaxation phase (diastolic) pressure <20 mm Hg, attempt to improve CPR quality

Shock Energy for Defibrillation

- Biphasic = 120-200 J
- Monopolistic = 360 J

Drug Therapy

- **Epinephrine** IV/IO dose: 1 mg every 3-5 minutes
- **Amiodarone** IV/IO dose:
  - First dose: 300 mg bolus
  - Second dose: 150 mg.

Advanced Airway

- Endotracheal intubation or supraglottic advanced airway
- Waveform capnography or capnometry to confirm and monitor ET tube placement
- Once advanced airway in place, give 1 breath every 6 seconds (10 breaths/min) with continuous chest compressions

ECG RHYTHMS IN CARDIAC ARREST

ECG Rhythms in Cardiac Arrest	
Shockable	**Nonshockable**
▪ Ventricular fibrillation	▪ Bradyarrhythmia
▪ Ventricular tachycardia	▪ Asystole
▪ Atrial flutter and fibrillation	▪ Pulseless electrical activity

TRAUMA MANAGEMENT

- A patient with blunt abdominal trauma presented to casualty with hypotension and tachycardia. The investigation to be done in this patient is → FAST sonogram.
- A patient presents with internal bleeding after blunt trauma abdomen. Next management in unstable patient → FAST.
- Tripod fracture is seen in → Zygomatic bone.
- What is the treatment for blunt trauma of kidney → Conservative.
- Perineal hematoma after trauma is due to → Rupture of bulbar urethra.
- Most common organ injury in sharp penetrating trauma → Liver.
- Best investigation to be done immediately when a patient comes with blunt abdominal trauma is → USG.
- A Child presented with blunt trauma abdomen, the first investigation to be done is → USG.
- The Mangled Extremity Severity Score (MESS score) used to predict necessity of amputation after lower extremity trauma. It contains:-
  ◦ Mechanism (Skeletal/soft tissue) of injury
  ◦ Limb ischemia
  ◦ Age
  ◦ Shock
- In Acute trauma → T_3 T_4 decreases, insulin decreases, cortisol & glucagon increases.
- ***TRISS calculator*** determines the probability of survival of a patient in blunt or penetrating trauma from the ISS (Injury severity score), RTS (revised trauma score) and patient's age.
- ***The revised trauma score (RTS)*** is made up of a combination of results from three categories; Glasgow Coma Scale, Systolic blood pressure, and respiratory rate.
- ***The ISS (Injury severity score)*** is defined as the sum of squares of the highest AIS grade in the 3 most severely injured body regions. Six body regions are defined, as follows: The thorax, abdomen and visceral pelvis, head and neck, face, bony pelvis and extremities,
- A 25-year-old male presents with road traffic accidents with a BP of 100/80 mm Hg and a pulse of 84/min. Best fluid for resuscitation is → Crystalloid.
- A 30-year-old male is hit by an iron rod resulting in a Gr IIIA open fracture of the tibia. The protocol for tetanus immunization in this patient who had last taken tetanus toxoid 12 years back is → TT one dose + Ig.
- In case of polytrauma with multiple injuries to the chest, neck and abdomen, highest priority is given to → Stabilizing of cervical spine.
- Organ most damaged in bomb explosion → Ear.
- The least common organ injured by blast injury is → Spleen.

IMPORTANT TRAUMA SCORE

Physiologic	Anatomic	Combined
Revised Trauma Score	Abbreviated Injury Score	TRISS
APACHE	Injury Severity Score	ASCOT
SOFA	New Injury Severity Score	ICISS
Emergency Trauma Score	PATI	
	ICISS	
	TMPM-ICD9	

SCORES & THEIR VARIABLES

Glasgow Coma Score	Revised Trauma Score	Mangled Extremity Score	SIRS (≥2 of the following)
Best Motor Response	GCS Score	Skeletal and Soft Tissue Injury	Heart Rate >90 bpm
Best Verbal Response	Systolic Blood Pressure	Limb ischemia	WBC Count >12,000 or <4000
Eye Opening	Respiratory Rate	Shock	Respiratory Rate >20/min
		Age	Temperature >100.4°F or <96.8°F

28. All are included in diagnostic criteria for SIADH in children except? *(PGMEE 2014-15)*
a. Urine sodium < 20 mEq/dl
b. Urine osmolality > 100 mEq/dl
c. Serum osmolality < 280 mosm
d. Normal creatinine clearance

[Ref: Nelson 18th /ed. table 52.3, Harrison's 19th/e pg. 301]

POTASSIUM IMBALANCE

29. Which of the following is not true about treatment of severe hyperkalemia? *(NEET Pattern 2019)*
a. Most effective and rapid way of lowering potassium is by hemodialysis
b. Calcium gluconate causes transcellular shift of potassium
c. Calcium gluconate is the fastest acting agent
d. Calcium gluconate onset of action is within 5 mins of administration

30. Hypokalemia is seen in all except? *(PGMEE 2014-15)*
a. Bartter syndrome
b. Reninoma (JG cell tumour]
c. Hypokalemic periodic paralysis
d. 21 hydroxylase deficiency

[Ref: Harrison's 19th/e pg. 307]

31. Sine wave pattern on ECG is done when serum potassium exceeds_____ mEq/dl? *(PGMEE 2014-15)*
a. >6 mEq/dl
b. >7 mEq/dl
c. >8 mEq/dl
d. >10 mEq>dl

[Ref: Harrison's 19th/e pg. 310]

32. Decreased dietary intake of potassium is incriminated in leading to all except? *(PGMEE 2014-15)*
a. CHF
b. Stroke
c. Diabetes mellitus
d. Hypertension

[Ref: Harrison's 19th/e pg. 304]

Explanation

- Hypokalemia is associated with increase mortality due to adverse effect on blood pressure, cardiac rhythm and increase cardiovascular morbidity.

33. Which of the following genetic abnormalities is associated with the development of hyperkalemia:
a. Autosomal dominant polycystic kidney disease
b. Liddle's syndrome
c. 11b - hydroxylase deficiency
d. Gitelman's syndrome

[Ref: Harrison's 19th/e Table 63-5, pg. 309]

34. Most rapid way of lowering potassium is *(PGMEE 2014-15)*
a. Albuterol
b. Sodium bicarbonate
c. Insulin drip
d. Calcium gluconate

[Ref: Harrison's 19th/e pg. 312]

35. Hyperkalemia is caused due to all of the following EXCEPT: *(PGMEE 2014-15)*
a. Addisons's disease
b. Acute renal failure
c. Excess hemolysis
d. Alkalosis

[Ref: Harrison's 19th/e pg. 309-310]

28.	a
29.	b
30.	d
31.	c
32.	c
33.	a
34.	c
35.	d
36.	c
37.	b
38.	b
39.	d

36. Hyperkalemia presents with all except? *(PGMEE 2014-15)*
a. Periodic paralysis
b. Slow idioventricular rhythms
c. Ileus
d. Hemodynamic collapse

[Ref: Harrison's 19th/e pg. 310]

37. Cardiac rhythm seen with hyperkalemia is all except? *(PGMEE 2014-15)*
a. Sinus arrest
b. Torsades de pointes
c. Ventricular fibrillation
d. Sinus bradycardia

[Ref: Harrison's 19th/e pg. 310]

Explanation

- Cardiac arrhythmias associated with hyperkalemia indude sinus bradycardias, sinus arrest, slow idioventricular rhythms, ventricular tachycardia, ventricular fibrillation & asystole.
- The electrolyte abnormalities that have been associated with Torsades include hypokalemia and hypomagnesemia

38. 1 year old male child is having a Heart Rate 40/min, BP 90/60. His serum Potassium = 6.5 what is the next best management? *(PGMEE 2015-16)*
a. Ipratropium
b. Calcium chloride
c. Sodium bicarbonate
d. Adrenaline

[Ref: Harrison's 19th/e pg. 312]

39. Which of the following is not used in the acute management of hyperkalemia? *(NEET Pattern 2017)*
a. β_2 agonist
b. Insulin
c. Calcium gluconate
d. Magnesium sulphate

[Ref: Harrison's 19th/e pg. 312]

Explanation

Management of Hyperkalemia

Immediate Antagonism of the Cardiac Effects

- Intravenous calcium serves to protect the heart, whereas other measures are taken to correct hyperkalemia. Calcium raises the action potential threshold and reduces excitability, without changing the resting membrane potential. By restoring the difference between resting and threshold potentials, calcium reverses the depolarization blockade due to hyperkalemia. Hypercalcemia potentiates the cardiac toxicity of digoxin; hence, should be used with extreme caution in patients taking this medication.

Rapid Reduction in Plasma K+ Concentration By

Redistribution into Cells

- Insulin lowers plasma K+ concentration by shifting K+ into cells. β_2 agonist, most commonly salbutamol (albuterol), are effective for the acute management of hyperkalemia. Salbutamol and insulin with glucose have an additive effect on plasma K+ concentration. Side effects include hyperglycemia and tachycardia. β_2 agonist should be used with caution in hyperkalemic patients with known cardiac disease Intravenous bicarbonate has no role in the acute treatment of hyperkalemia, but may slowly attenuate hyperkalemia with sustained administration over several hours by correcting acidosis if any.

Removal of Potassium

- This is typically accomplished in patients with moderately elevated levels and no ECG abnormalities using cation exchange resins such as sodium polystyrene sulfonate (SPS, diuretics (furosemide), and/or dialysis. Hemodialysis is the most effective and reliable method to reduce plasma K+ concentration Therapy with intravenous saline may be beneficial in hypovolemic patients with oliguria and decreased distal delivery of Na+, with the associated reductions in renal K+ excretion. Dietary restriction of potassium is also modestly helpful in chronic cases.

40. Most serious side effect with sodium polystyrene sulfonate: *(PGMEE 2014-15)*
   a. Respiratory arrest   b. Intestinal perforation
   c. Cardiac arrest   d. Rebound hyperkalemia

[Ref: Harrison's 19th/e pg. 312]

41. Which of the following presents with hypokalemia and metabolic acidosis? *(PGMEE 2015-16)*
   a. Conn's syndrome   b. Vomiting
   c. Diarrhea   d. Nasogastric suction

[Ref: Internet]

42. Hypokalemia causes death due to: *(PGMEE 2014-15)*
   a. Diastolic arrest
   b. Bidirectional Tachycardia
   c. Respiratory insufficiency
   d. Systolic arrest

[Ref: Harrison's 19th/e pg. 307]

43. In hypokalemia all ECG changes are seen EXCEPT:
   a. Decreased T wave amplitude   *(PGMEE 2014-15)*
   b. Prolonged PR interval
   c. Wide qRS complex
   d. Normal ST segment

[Ref: Harrison's 19th/e pg. 307]

44. The Maximum concentration of potassium delivered via central vein is? *(PGMEE 2014-15)*
   a. 20 mmol/hr   b. 40 mmol/hr
   c. 60 mmol/hr   d. 100 mmol/hr

[Ref: Harrison's 19th/e pg. 307]

Explanation

IV potassium therapy:

- Via peripheral vein = 20-40 mEq of KCl per litre.
- Via central vein = 10–20 mEq of KCl per hour

45. All are seen in Hypokalemia EXCEPT? *(PGMEE 2015-16)*
   a. Prolonged QU interval   b. U wave in ECG
   c. ST Depression   d. Tall T wave in ECG

[Ref: Harrison's 19th/e pg. 307, 310]

46. TTKG in hypokalemia is: *(PGMEE 2014-15)*
   a. < 3-4   b. > 6-7
   c. > 9-10   d. > 10-15

[Ref: Harrison's 19th/e pg. 311]

Explanation

- The transtubular potassium gradient (TTKG) is utilized to help determine the renal response to hyperkalemia or hypokalemia is appropriate.

$$TTKG = + \frac{[K^+]\ urine \times [OSM]\ serum}{[K^+]\ serum \times [OSM]\ urine}$$

   ○ TTKG is hyperkalemia is >7–8
   ○ TTKG is hypokalemia is <3

47. TTKG >8 is seen in all EXCEPT: *(PGMEE 2014-15)*
   a. Adrenocortical insufficiency
   b. Acute glomerulonephritis
   c. Cushing syndrome
   d. Diabetes mellitus

[Ref: Harrison's 19th/e pg. 311]

48. Hypokalemic, metabolic acidosis can occur with excess fluid loss from: *(PGMEE 2014-15)*
   a. Pancreas   b. Ileum
   c. Stomach   d. Colon

[Ref: Harrison's 19th/e pg. 305]

49. Initial ECG change in Hyperkalemia is? *(PGMEE 2015-16)*
   a. Tall tented T waves   b. PR prolongation
   c. qRS widening   d. ST segment depression

[Ref: Harrison 20th ed. pg. 310]

50. These characteristic ECG changes are seen in :- *(PGMEE 2016-17)*

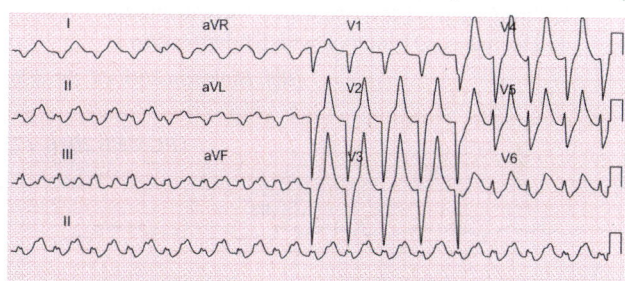

   a. Hypokalemia   b. Hyperkalemia
   c. Hypocalcemia   d. hypercalcemia

[Ref: Harrison 20th ed. pg. 310]

51. A 46 year old lady suffering from end stage renal disease broght in emergency room in altered sensorium and breathing difficulty. ECG showing following changes. Best immediate treatment for her is : *(PGMEE 2016-17)*

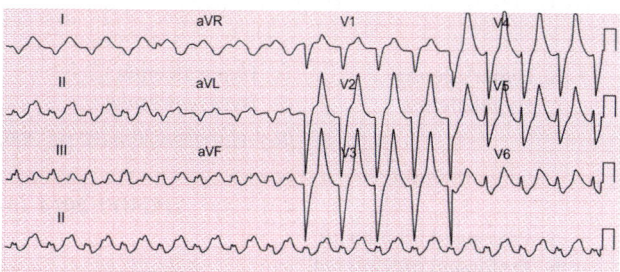

   a. Ringer lactate infusion   b. Nebulized salbutamol
   c. IV KCl injection   d. None of the above

[Ref: Harrison 20th ed. pg. 310]

40.	b
41.	c
42.	d
43.	d
44.	a
45.	d
46.	a
47.	c
48.	b
49.	a
50.	b
51.	b

52. ECG finding of Hyperkalemia: *(PGMEE 2015-16)*
- a. T wave inversion
- b. ST depression
- c. P pulmonale
- d. Wide QRS complex

[Ref: Harrison 20th ed. pg. 310]

53. All of the following are the electrocardiographic features of Hyperkalemia, EXCEPT: *(PGMEE 2014-15)*
- a. Prolonged PR interval
- b. Prolonged QT interval
- c. Sine wave patterns
- d. Loss of P waves

[Ref: Harrison 20th ed. pg. 310]

54. All are ECG changes in hypokalemia, EXCEPT: *(PGMEE 2014-15)*
- a. U wave
- b. ST segment sagging
- c. T-wave flattening or inversion
- d. QT interval shortening

[Ref: Harrison 20th ed. pg. 306]

55. All are seen in Hypokalemia except? *(All India Dec 2015 Pattern)*
- a. ST Depression
- b. Tall T wave in ECG
- c. U wave in ECG
- d. Prolonged QU internal

[Ref: Harrison 20th ed. pg. 306]

56. Pseudo P pulmonale is seen in: *(PGMEE 2018)*
- a. Hypercalcemia
- b. Hyperkalemia
- c. Hypokalemia
- d. Hypernatremia

57. The following ECG findings are seen in Hypokalemia: *(PGMEE 2014-15)*
- a. Increased PR interval with ST depression
- b. Increased PR interval with peaked T wave
- c. Prolonged QT interval with T wave inversion
- d. Decreased QT interval with ST depression

[Ref: Harrison 20th ed. pg. 306]

58. ECG strip showing which electrolyte abnormality:- *(PGMEE 2016-17)*

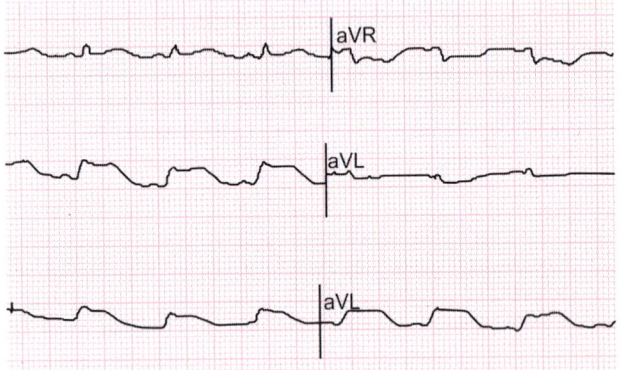

- a. Hyperkalemia
- b. Hypocalcemia
- c. Hypokalemia
- d. Hypercalcemia

[Ref: Harrison 20th ed. pg. 306]

59. Which of the following may occur due to hyperkalemia: *(PGMEE 2014-15)*
- a. Prolonged PR interval
- b. Prolonged qRS interval
- c. Ventricular fibrillation
- d. All of above

[Ref: Harrison 20th ed. pg. 310]

CALCIUM IMBALANCE

60. Chvostek's sign is elicited by: *(PGMEE 2015-16)*
- a. Tapping over extensor pollicis brevis
- b. BP cuff in arm for 5 minutes
- c. Facial nerve stimulation by tapping over the parotid
- d. Tapping over flexor retinaculum

[Ref: Harrison's 19th/e pg. 315]

61. A 55-year-old man, a chronic smoker is brought to emergency with history of polyuria, polydipsia, nausea and altered sensorium for last two days. He had been diagnosed as having squamous cell carcinoma of lung two months prior to this. On examination, he was lethargic and confused. An ECG was normal except for a narrowed QT interval. Which one of the following is the most likely metabolic abnormality? *(PGMEE 2014-15)*
- a. Hypernatremia
- b. Hyponatremia
- c. Hypokalemia
- d. Hypercalcemia

[Ref: Harrison's 19th/e pg. 2469/247]

62. Neonate is posted for Congenital Hypertrophic Pyloric Stenosis, Pre-op work up shows serum calcium = 6mg%. What should be done next? *(PGMEE 2014-15)*
- a. Serum bilirubin
- b. Serum protein
- c. USG abdomen
- d. Oxygen saturation

[Ref: Harrison's 19th/e pg. 314]

Explanation
- Measured total calcium in serum consist of about 15% bound to organic and inorganic anions, about 40% bound to albumin & the remaining as biologically active ionized calcium. Therefore, serum total calcium may under estimate biologically active calcium levels in the hypoalbuminemic patients.

63. Prolonged immobilization leads to? *(PGMEE 2014-15)*
- a. Hypercalcemia
- b. Hypocalcemia
- c. Hyperkalemia
- d. Hypokalemia

[Ref: William endocrinology 12th /e. pg. 1268, Harrison's 19th/e pg. 313]

64. Why is tetany seen with hyperventilation: *(PGMEE 2014-15)*
- a. Metabolic alkalosis
- b. Respiratory acidosis
- c. Metabolic acidosis
- d. Respiratory alkalosis

[Ref: Harrison's 19th/e pg. 323-324]

65. Tumor induced osteomalacia is caused due to? *(PGMEE 2014-15)*
- a. Calcitonin
- b. PTH
- c. FGF-23
- d. All of above

[Ref: Harrison's 19th/e pg. 2459, 2460]

Explanation
- FGF-23 is a protein belonging to the family of fibroblast growth factors. It is secreted by osteocyte and is primarily involved in regulation of phosphate metabolism as a virtue of its phosphaturetic action. Increase activity of FGF-23 is found in:-
  - Autosomal dominant Hypophosphatemic rickets
  - Tumor-induced osteomalacia
  - Chronic Kidney disease

66. Tetany may be a feature of the following EXCEPT:
(PGMEE 2014-15)
a. Thyroid surgery
b. Respiratory alkalosis
c. Hyperventilation
d. Hyponatremia

[Ref: Harrison's 19th/e pg. 314 Table 65-2]

67. Not useful for acute Hypercalcemia? *(PGMEE 2014-15)*
a. Bisphosphonates
b. Calcitonin
c. Thiazide
d. Normal saline

[Ref: William textbook of endocrinology 12th e/ pg. 1272]

68. Incorrect about hypocalcemia: *(PGMEE 2014-15)*
a. Larygospasm
b. Seizures
c. Shortening of QT interval
d. Di George syndrome

[Ref: Harrison's 19th/e pg. 314-15]

69. Hypercalcaemia is caused by all EXCEPT:
(PGMEE 2014-15)
a. Multiple myeloma
b. Hyperparathyroidism
c. Sarcoidosis
d. Hypothyroidism

[Ref: Harrison's 20th/e pg. 2924]

70. Osborn wave is seen in? *(PGMEE 2014-15)*
a. WPW syndrome type I
b. Hypercalcemia
c. Cardiac tamponade
d. Athlete

[Ref: Harrison's 19th/e pg. 1457]

Explanation

- Osborn waves or J waves or Hypothermic waves are positive deflections occuring at junction between QRS complex and ST segment. These commonly seen in hypothermia ($<32^0C$), but may also be seen in hypercalcemia, vasospastic angina or ventricular fibrillation.

ACID BASE DISORDERS

71. Blood gas parameters are in a patient of 50 kg weight is: pH-7.04, PCO_2-12, BE-29, HCO_3 -6. Dose of HCO_3 to be given in 1st hour: *(NEET 2018)*
a. 450 mEq
b. 250 mEq
c. 75 mEq
d. 150 mEq

Explanation

- Diagnosis of the patient is metabolic acidosis with respiratory compensation.
  ○ Dose of bicarbonate is calculated as
- HCO_3 deficit = [Desired HCO_3 – measured HCO_3] × 0.5 × body weight

$$= [24 – 6] × 0.5 × 50 = 450$$

72. Paracetamol poisoning produces? *(PGMEE 2009)*
a. Metabolic alkalosis
b. Metabolic acidosis
c. Coloured sweat
d. Arthralgia

[Ref: Harrison 19th/e pg320]

73. pH= 7.31 pCO2=33 mm Hg and HCO3 = 16 mEq/dl:
(PGMEE 2014-15)
a. Respiratory acidosis
b. Metabolic alkalosis
c. Metabolic acidosis
d. Respiratory alkalosis

[Ref: Harrison's 19th/e pg. 317]

74. pH = 7.55, pCO_2 = 38, HCO_3 = 33, what is the primary abnormality: *(PGMEE 2014-15)*
a. Respiratory alkalosis
b. Metabolic acidosis
c. Respiratory acidosis
d. Mixed alkalosis

[Ref: Harrison's 19th/e pg. 322]

Explanation

- Interpretation of ABG
  ○ pH = 7.55 Alkalosis (>7.4)
  ○ PCO_2 = 38 Low (<40) → Hence alkalosis
  ○ HCO_3 = 33 High (> 24) → Hence alkalosis
- Thus, this ABG shows mixed acid base disorder with both respiratory and metabolic alkalosis [Hint: Think of mixed disorder when "Same direction rule" does not follow]

75. In severe metabolic alkalosis all are seen EXCEPT:
(PGMEE'2010)
a. Pulmonary edema
b. Hypoxia
c. Tetany
d. Hypocalcaemia

[Ref: Harrison's 19th/e pg 321,322]

76. Hyperchloremic metabolic acidosis is seen in all except?
(PGMEE 2014-15)
a. Diarrhea
b. Gitelman syndrome
c. RTA 1
d. Uraemia

[Ref: Harrison's 19th/e pg. 321]

77. High anion gap acidosis is seen in all EXCEPT:
(PGMEE'2010)
a. Diabetic ketoacidosis
b. Lactic acidosis
c. Methanol poisoning
d. Renal tubular acidosis

[Ref: Harrison's 19th/e pg 318]

78. A 60 year old man is being treated for pulmonary emphysema. He is admitted with laboured breathing at rest with marked use of accessory muscles. Arterial blood gas analysis revealed: *(PGMEE 2014)*

pH	7.33
$PaCO_2$	64 mmHg
PaO_2	50 mmHg
HCO_3	34 mEq/L

Possible diagnosis
a. Compensated metabolic alkalosis
b. Chronic compensated respiratory acidosis
c. Acute respiratory acidosis
d. Hyperventilation is the main factor

[Ref: Harrison 19th p 322-323]

79. A factory worker was found unresponsive in his workplace. He is afebrile anicteric, tachypneic drowsy pale discoloration with clear lung field and hyperdynamic cardiovascular findings. His ABG with 100% oxygen after intubation was *(PGMEE 2014-15)*

pH	=	7.45
pO2	=	80 mm Hg
pCO_2	=	30 mm Hg
SaO_2	=	95%

What is the most likely diagnosis?
a. Adult Respiratory distress syndrome
b. Carbon monoxide poisoning
c. Organo-phosphorus poisoning
d. Cyanide poisoning

[Ref: Harrison 19th p 248]

66.	d
67.	c
68.	c
69.	d
70.	b
71.	a
72.	b
73.	c
74.	d
75.	a
76.	b
77.	d
78.	b
79.	b

80. Best for management of respiratory alkalosis?
(PGMEE 2014-15)

a. Acetazolamide
b. IPPV
c. Normal saline
d. Rebreathing in paper bag

[Ref: Harrison's 19th/e pg. 324]

81. A patient with blood chemistry of pH 7.3, CO2 of 60 and HCO₃ of 28 mEq/dl are indicative of: *(PGMEE 2014-15)*

a. Partially compensated respiratory acidosis
b. Uncompensated respiratory acidosis
c. Fully compensated respiratory alkalosis
d. Metabolic alkalosis with respiratory alkalosis

[Ref: Harrison 19th p 322-23]

82. A 70 year old man with history of CHF presents with increased shortness of breath and leg swelling. ABG: pH 7.24, pCO2 = 60 mmHg, PO2 = 52, HCO3– =27 *(PGMEE 2014-15)*

a. Respiratory alkalosis
b. Metabolic alkalosis
c. Metabolic acidosis
d. Respiratory acidosis

[Ref: Harrison's 19th/e pg. 323]

83. A plasma HCO_3^- concentration of 15 mEq/L and a plasma pCO_2 of 30 mmHg with a pH of 7.5 represents: *(PGMEE 2014-15)*

a. Simple metabolic acidosis
b. Compensated respiratory alkalosis
c. Simple respiratory alkalosis
d. Compensated metabolic acidosis

[Ref: Harrison's 19th/e pg. 323]

84. Type B lactic acidosis occurs due to? *(PGMEE 2014-15)*

a. Cyanide poisoning
b. Diabetes mellitus
c. CHF
d. Short gut syndrome

[Ref: Harrison's 19th/e pg. 318]

Explanation

Types of Lactic Acidosis

Type - A	Type - B
Occurs in associated with poor oxygenation of blood or tissue perfusion	May be associated with occult tissue hypoperfusion (usually no clinical evidence of poor oxygenation or hypoperfusion)
Eg:- ▪ Cardiac failure ▪ Shock ▪ Severe anemia ▪ Cyanide poisoning ▪ CO poisoning	Eg:- ▪ Renal failure ▪ Hepatic failure ▪ Diabetes mellitus ▪ Malignancy ▪ Drugs (isoniazid, biguanides, alcohol, Salicylates) ▪ Severe Infection (Malaria, Cholera)

85. Fomepizole is used for: *(PGMEE 2014-15)*

a. Type A Lactic acidosis
b. Ethyl alcohol poisoning
c. Ether poisoning
d. Ethylene glycol poisoning

[Ref: Harrison's 19th/e pg. 319]

Explanation

▪ Indications:
 ○ Methanol poisoning
 ○ Ethylene glycol poisoning
▪ MOA: Inhibits alcohol dehydrogenase enzyme

86. Most common acid base disturbance in critically ill patients? *(PGMEE 2014-15)*

a. Chronic respiratory alkalosis
b. Chronic respiratory acidosis
c. Metabolic acidosis
d. Metabolic alkalosis

[Ref: Harrison's 19th/e pg. 323]

87. pH = 7.27, HCO_3^- = 10 mEq/dl pCO_2 = 23 mm Hg: *(PGMEE 2014-15)*

a. Respiratory alkalosis
b. Metabolic alkalosis
c. Respiratory acidosis
d. Metabolic acidosis

[Ref: Harrison's 19th/e pg. 317]

88. In metabolic acidosis caused by diabetic ketoacidosis, which of the following would be greater than normal:

a. Anion gap *(PGMEE 2014-15)*
b. Arterial pCO_2
c. Concentration of plasma HCO3–
d. All of the above

[Ref: Harrison's 19th/e pg. 317]

89. pH = 7.46 , pCO_2 = 57 mm Hg and HCO_3 = 42 mEq: *(PGMEE 2014-15)*

a. Metabolic alkalosis with compensatory respiratory acidosis
b. Metabolic acidosis with compensatory respiratory alkalosis
c. Respiratory acidosis with compensatory metabolic alkalosis
d. Respiratory alkalosis with compensatory metabolic acidosis

[Ref: Harrison's 19th/e pg. 316, Table 66-2]

90. 29 year old female with history of Sjogren's syndrome presents with a 2 day episode of watery diarrhea 2 days ago. Physical examination is unremarkable. Because of her history, the physician decides to check her urine electrolytes. Urine chemistry: K=31, Na=100, Cl=105. Her current diagnosis is? *(PGMEE 2014-15)*

a. Hypochloremic Metabolic alkalosis
b. Respiratory alkalosis
c. Malignant hypertension
d. Renal tubular acidosis

[Ref: Harrison's 19th/e pg. 323, 320, 64e-6]

Explanation

▪ **UAG** = Urinary (Na + K - Cl) = 100 + 31 - 105 = 26 (positive value)
▪ **In** metabolic acidosis d/t Renal tubular acidosis or renal failure the UAG is positive.
▪ [Note: UAG is useful for differentiation between GI & renal causes of hyperchloremic acidosis. Hence we can presume that patient is in metabolic acidosis]

80.	d
81.	a
82.	d
83.	b
84.	b
85.	d
86.	a
87.	d
88.	a
89.	a
90.	d

91. All are useful for treatment of metabolic alkalosis except? *(PGMEE 2014-15)*
a. Sodium chloride
b. Potassium chloride
c. Hydrochloric acid
d. Ammonium chloride

[Ref: Harrison's 19th/e pg. 322]

92. In which of the following vomiting is not associated? *(PGMEE 2014/15)*
a. Hypercapnia
b. Hyponatremia
c. Diabetes Mellitus
d. Hypocalcemia

[Ref: Harrison's 19th/e pg. 300, 2422, 2559]

93. Hypertension, hypokalemia and hypernatremia with metabolic alkalosis is seen in:- *(PGMEE 2016-17)*
a. 1° aldosteronism
b. Liddle's syndrome
c. Barther's syndrome
d. Gitelman syndrome

[Ref: Harrison's 20th/e pg. 2729]

ANION GAP

94. Increased anion gap is seen in all except?
a. Starvation *(PGMEE 2014-15)*
b. Phenformin
c. Ethylene glycol poisoning
d. Fistula

[Ref: Harrison's 19th/e pg. 317]

95. All of the following are cause of metabolic acidosis with normal anion Gap Except: *(NEET Pattern 2017)*
a. Proximal renal tubular acidosis
b. Salicylate poisoning
c. Diarrhea
d. Pancreatitis *[Ref: S Pandya 2/e, P. 215]*

96. Anion gap is defined as:- *(PGMEE 2016-17)*
a. Difference between unmeasured anions and all measured cations
b. Difference between measured anions and cations
c. Difference between unmeasured anion and cations
d. Difference between all measured anions and unmeasured cations

97. Normal anion gap is seen in: *(PGMEE 2015-16)*
a. Diabetic ketoacidosis
b. Renal tubular acidosis
c. Starvation ketoacidosis
d. Lactic acidosis

98. Metabolic acidosis with a normal anion gap is found in a patient with: *(PGMEE 2014-15)*
a. Alcohol intoxication
b. Small bowel fistula
c. Shock
d. Aspirin ingestion

[Ref: Harrison's 19th/e pg. 317]

99. Normal anion gap is seen in: *(PGMEE 2015-16)*
a. Diabetic ketoacidosis
b. Methanol toxicity
c. Chronic renal failure
d. Renal tubular acidosis

[Ref: Harrison's 19th/e pg.320]

100. Normal anion gap acidosis seen in? *(PGMEE 2011)*
a. Methanol poisoning
b. Keto acidosis
c. Lactic acidosis
d. Hyperchloremic acidosis

[Ref: Harrison's 19th/e pg 316]

101. Widened anion gap is caused by all EXCEPT:
a. Lactic acidosis
b. Methanol poisoning
c. Diabetic keto-acidosis
d. Diarrhea

[Ref: Harrison's 19th/e pg 316]

102. All are causes of increased anion gap except? *(PGMEE 2014-15)*
a. Starvation
b. Diabetic ketoacidosis
c. Diabetic nephropathy
d. Renal tubular acidosis

[Ref: Harrison's 19th/e pg. 317]

103. Reduced anion gap is seen in? *(PGMEE 2014-15)*
a. Fanconi syndrome
b. Fistula
c. Renal tubular acidosis Type 4
d. Nephrotic syndrome

[Ref: Harrison's 19th/e pg. 317]

104. Urinary anion gap is increased in: *(PGMEE 2014-15)*
a. Diarrhea
b. Water intoxication
c. Ureterosigmoidostomy
d. Renal tubular acidosis

[Ref: Oski essential pediatrics, 2nd/e pg. 504]

MISCELLANEOUS

105. Fever increases water losses by _____ml/day per degree Celsius: *(PGMEE 2014-15)*
a. 100
b. 200
c. 400
d. 800

[Ref: Internet]

Explanation
- With fever, each degree rise in temperature above 98.6^0F (37^0C) adds 2.5 mL/kg/day to normal insensible water loss. Normal daily insensible water loss is nearly 600-900 mL.

106. Man working in hot environment and drinking lots of water without intake of salts is liable to develop? *(PGMEE 2015-16)*
a. Heat hyperpyrexia
b. Heat encephalopathy
c. Heat stroke
d. Heat cramps

[Ref: Harrison's 19th/e pg. 479e-2]

107. Insensible losses of water per day are: *(PGMEE 2014-15)*
a. 400 ml per day
b. 1200 ml per day
c. 800 ml per day
d. 1500 ml per day

[Ref: Harrison's 19th/e pg. 298]

108. Extracellular bicarbonate ions serve as an effective buffer for all of the following EXCEPT: *(PGMEE 2014-15)*
a. Sulphuric acid
b. Carbonic acid
c. Lactic acid
d. Phosphoric acid

[Ref: Guyton, 9th /e pg. 387-389]

109. The enteric fluid with an electrolyte (Na+, K+, Cl) content similar to that of Ringer's lactate is: *(PGMEE 2014-15)*
a. Contents of small intestine
b. Pancreatic secretions
c. Contents of right colon
d. Saliva *[Ref: Harrison's 19th/e pg. 305]*

110. High urinary chloride is seen in all except? *(PGMEE 2014-15)*
a. Thiazide
b. Gitelman syndrome
c. Barter syndrome
d. Vomiting

[Ref: Harrison's 19th/e pg. 306, 307]

111. Shohl's solution is: *(PGMEE 2014-15)*
a. Sodium citrate
b. Radio-iodine
c. Lugol iodine
d. Potassium binding resin

[Ref: Harrison's 19th/e pg. 318, 320]

91.	d
92.	a
93.	a,b
94.	d
95.	b
96.	c
97.	b
98.	b
99.	d
100.	d
101.	d
102.	d
103.	d
104.	d
105.	b
106.	d
107.	c
108.	b
109.	a
110.	d
111.	a

21. What is the sequence of events according to BLS
(NEET Pattern 2017)
   a. Start CPR, give 2 rescue breath, assess pulse
   b. Give rescue breath, see pulse, start CPR
   c. Assess patient, activate emergency response team, and call for defibrillator, start CPR
   d. Assess pulse, Defibrillator, start CPR

Ref: Ajay Yadav Short book of Anaesthesia 5th edition pg 254

Explanation

Basic steps in Adult BLS

- Assesment and scene saftey are first priority. If you are roadside first ensure a safe place. Then check the victim for response.
- Activate ERS (Emergency response system) and get AED (automated defibrillator).
- Pulse check : Carotid in adults, brachial artery in infants
- If no pulse felt in 10 seconds → Begin CPR using CAB sequence: Give 30 Chest compressions and 2 breaths (compression:ventilation ratio of 30:2)
- C = Chest compressions to start circulation
- A = Airway opening for breaths
- Use head tilt-chin lift & jaw thrust maneuver
- Only jaw thrust if cervical spine injury is suspected.
- B = Breathing (Deliver effective breaths, look for chest rise)
- Compression rate at least 100/min
- Give rescue breaths every 5-6 seconds (~10-12 breaths/min)
- Check the pulse every 2 min or 5 cycles of CPR.

21.	c
22.	b
23.	c
24.	c
25.	d
26.	d
27.	c
28.	c

22. The ideal parameters for cardiac massage in cardiopulmonary resuscitation are all except – *(PGMEE 2015)*
   a. Compression to be given over lower third of sternum
   b. Ratio of compression to ventilation should be 15:2
   c. Force should depress sternum approximately 1/3 of chest wall diameter
   d. Force should depress sternum by 1½ inches

[Ref: Morgan 5th/e p. 1240]

23. During cardiopulmonary resuscitation, cardiac massage is given – *(PGMEE 2014)*
   a. Upper third of sternum   b. Mid third of sternum
   c. Lower third of sternum   d. Precordium

[Ref: Morgan 5th/e p. 1240]

24. Machine used noninvasively to monitor an external chest compression during cardiopulmonary resuscitation is –
   a. Zoll pA02 monitor   *(PGMEE 2015)*
   b. Zoll depth synchronizer
   c. Zoll AED- plus automatic external defibrillator
   d. Zoll strength sensor

MECHANICAL VENTILATION

25. The following modes of ventilation may be used for weaning off patients from mechanical ventilation except–
   a. Pressure support ventilation (PSV)   *(PGMEE 2015)*
   b. Synchronized intermittent mandatory ventilation (SIMV)
   c. Assist - control ventilation (ACV)
   d. Controlled mechanical ventilation [CMV]

[Ref: Morgan 5th/e p. 1291]

26. Which of the following system can be used to produce PEEP? *(PGMEE 2015)*
   a. Pneumatic system   b. Spring system
   c. Ball valve system   d. All of the above

27. A ventilator pressure relief valve stuck in closed position can result in – *(DNB pattern 2008)*
   a. Volutrauma   b. Hypoventilation
   c. Barotrauma   d. Hyperventilation

[Ref: Morgan's 5th/e pg.71]

Explanation

- The ventilator pressure-relief valve (**pop off valve**) is pressure controlled via pilot tubing that communicates with the ventilator bellows chamber. During the expiratory phase of the mechanical ventilation cycle the spill valve vents excess gas; during inspiration it closes.
- If the ventilator pressure relief valve were to stuck in the closed position, there would be a rapid buildup of pressure within the circle system that would be readily transmitted to the patient. Barotrauma to the patient's lungs would result if this situation were to continue unrecognized.

28. All of the following are recognised strategies in the prevention of ventilator-associated pneumonia (VAP) except – *(PGMEE 2018)*
   a. Daily sedation holds
   b. Head-up positioning of 30 to 45°
   c. Daily ventilator tubing changes
   d. Chlorhexidine mouthcare

[Ref: Morgan's 5th/e p.-]

Explanation

- Daily sedation holds have been demonstrated to reduce patient time spent on the ventilator, and thus decreases the incidence of VAP
- Head-up positioning of 30 to 45° reduces micro-aspiration, and thus the incidence of VAP
- Prone positioning improves mortality in severe ARDS, but its impact on VAP rates per se is as yet unclear.
- Chlorhexidine mouthwashes has been demonstrated to reduce the incidence of VAP
- Daily changes of ventilator tubing may increase the VAP risk due to cross-contamination from excess handling of equipment.

Neurosciences

FACTS

- Neural tube defects occurs in 3rd - 4th week of IUL
- In NTD, following markers increases in the amniotic fluid:
  - Alpha fetoprotein
  - Acetylcholine esterase
- Periconceptional use of folic acid decreases the incidence of NTD by: 50-70%
- **Dose of folic acid for:**
  - Primary prevention of NTD: 0.4 mg/day
  - Secondary prevention of NTD: 5 mg/day
- Vitamin deficiency responsible for Neonatal seizure: Pyridoxine (Vitamin B$_6$)
- Type of cerebral palsy commonly associated with scoliosis and other orthopedic problem: Spastic quadriplegia
- Kernicterus (bilirubin deposition in Basal Ganglia) can leads to: Choreoathetoid/ Dystonic Cerebral palsy
- Ideal interspace for lumbar puncture in pediatric age group: L$_{3-4}$/L$_{4-5}$
- Peak age of onset of Juvenile Myoclonic Epilepsy: 12-16 years
- To label as Mental retardation, IQ should be less than: 70
- Vitamin K prevent intraventricular hemorrhage in premature infant
- Banana sign in fetal brain is seen in: Spina bifida
- Scarf sign is seen in: Floppy infant
- Neurons most sensitive to hypoxic damage: CA1 neurons in hippocampus and entorhinal cortex.
- Basal exudates in CT is a feature of TB meningitis
- Causative agent of Progressive multifocal leukoencephalopathy (PML): JC virus
- Intrauterine infection which can cause aqueductal stenosis: Mumps
- Eosinophilic meningitis is caused by:
  - Angiostrongylus – MCC
  - Coccidioides immitis
  - Neurocysticercosis
  - Neoplastic diseases
- Water shade infarcts are seen in: Diffuse axonal injury (Global hypoxic damage to brain)
- Berry aneurysm is due to: Congenital defect in tunica media
- Subdural hematoma is due to rupture of → Communicating veins to superior sagittal sinus.
- Common site for extradural hematoma is → Temporoparietal
- Lucid interval is seen in → Extradural hemorrhage
- Which of the following requires emergency operation in setting without tertiary care facilities → Extradural hemorrhage.
- Traumatic optic neuropathy due to closed head trauma commonly affects which part of optic nerve → Optic canal.
- In treatment of head-injuries one of the following is contraindicated → Narcotics.
- Puff of smoke appearance in angiogram: Moya-Moya disease
- Devic's disease or Neuromyelitis optica is characterized by: Spinal cord demyelination + B/L optic neuritis.
- Early onset AD (Alzheimer's dementia) is related to: Mutations in Presenilin genes (Presenilin 1 gene at chromosome 14 & Presenilin 2 at chromosome 1)
- **Degeneration in nucleus basalis of Meynert occurs in:**
  - Parkinson' disease
  - Alzheimer's disease
- SOD1 mutations are seen in: ALS (amyotrophic lateral sclerosis).
- Myotonic dystrophy is inherited as autosomal dominant disorder
- Most important histological indicator of brain injury: Gliosis
- **SCN4A gene** mutation is present in hyperkalemic periodic paralysis
- Lead and Mercury mainly causes motor neuropathy
- Arsenic causes sensorimotor neuropathy
- DOC for Neonatal seizure: Phenobarbitone
- DOC for Infantile spasm (West Syndrome): ACTH
- DOC for Infantile spasm associated with Tuberous sclerosis: Vigabatrin

REMEMBER

Subdural effusion is seen in meningitis due to: [Mn: SHiP]
- *H. influenza*
- *Pneumococcus*

Triad of Normal pressure hydrocephalus: [Mn: DUA]
- **D**ementia
- **U**rinary incontinence
- **A**bnormal gait

Bacterial meningitis where steroids are indicated:
- TB Meningitis
- *H. influenza* type B
- Pneumococcal meningitis

Descending Motor Paralysis is seen in:
- **D**iphtheria
- **P**olio
- Botulinum

Neuroglial Cells

Neuroglial Cells	Location	Function
Astrocytes	CNS	▪ Maintain blood brain barrier ▪ Repair and form scar
Ependymal cells	CNS	▪ CSF production
Microglia & Gitter cells	CNS	▪ Phagocytic function
Oligodendrocytes	CNS	▪ Myelination of CNS neurons
Schwann cells	PNS	▪ Myelination of peripheral neurons

Neurodegenerative Disorders

Neurodegenerative Diseases	Lesion	Composition	Location	Affected Part of Brain
Alzheimer disease	Neurofibrillary tangles Senile plaques	Tau protein/Aβ	Intracytoplasmic Extracellular	Hippocampus
Frontotemporal dementia	Neurofibrillary tangles	Tau protein/Aβ	Intracytoplasmic	Frontal and Temporal lobe
Parkinson disease	Lewy body	α synuclein	Intracytoplasmic	Substantia Nigra and Locus Ceruleus
Multiple System Atrophy	Glial inclusions	α synuclein	Intracytoplasmic	Basal ganglia and Cerebellum
Rabies	Negri bodies	Viral RNA	Intracytoplasmic	Brain, Spinal cord and Neurons

MOST COMMON

- MC site of NTD: Lumbosacral region
- MC location of Myelomeningocele: Lumbosacral region
- MC genetic cause of Mental Retardation: Down's syndrome
- MC seizure disorder during childhood: Febrile seizure
- MCC of neonatal seizure: Hypoxia
- MC presentation of neonatal seizure: subtle type
- MC consequence of periventricular leukomalacia: Spastic diplegia
- MCC of neonatal meningitis: Group B Streptococci (*S. agalactiae*)
- MCC of meningitis in adults: *S. pneumoniae*
- MCC of viral meningoencephalitis: Enterovirus
- MCC of meningitis in patient with VP shunt: *S. epidermidis*
- MC neurological sequelae of meningitis: SNHL
- MCC of meningoencephalitis: Enterovirus

- MCC of acquired aqueductal stenosis: Mumps
- MCC of suprasellar midline calcification: Craniopharyngioma
- MC form of intracranial hemorrhage in a preterm neonate is: subependymal hemorrhage
- MCC of cerebrovascular diseases/stroke: ischemic stroke
- MCC of ischemic stroke is embolism
- MCC of hemorrhagic stroke: Hypertension
- MC site of hypertensive bleed: Basal ganglia/ Putamen
- MC type of intracranial hemorrhage: Intracerebral hemorrhage
- MCC of SAH: Berry aneurysm
- MC location of berry aneurysm: Anterior circulation on circle of Willis
- MC demyelinating disease: Multiple sclerosis
- MC site of Syringomyelia: Cervical region
- MCC of Motor Neuron Disease: Amyotrophic Lateral Sclerosis

- MC cause of peripheral neuropathy → DM
- MC type of neuropathy in diabetes → DSPN (Distal Symmetrical Sensory and Sensorimotor Polyneuropathy).

- MC cause of small fiber neuropathy – Idiopathic
- MC systemic cause of small fiber neuropathy – DM

SYNDROMES

❶ Kluver Bucy syndrome
- Due to bilateral lesion of medial temporal lobe, especially amygdala. Feature–
  - Amnesia
  - Diminished fear response/placidity/ tameness
  - Hyperphagia
  - Hyper sexuality
  - Hyperorality
  - Visual agnosia (Can see but can't recognize)

❷ Horner's syndrome [Mn: SAMPLE]
- Damage of **S**ympathetic trunk leads to –
  - **A**nhidrosis
  - **M**iosis
  - **P**artial ptosis – Ipsilateral
  - **L**oss of ciliospinal reflex
  - Pseudo **E**nophthalmos
  - Anisocoria & Pupillary dilation lag
  - Heterochromia iridum → In congenital Horner syndrome

❸ Melkersson Rosenthal syndrome
- Inheritance : AD
- Recurrent facial paralysis
- Swelling of the face and lips
- Fissured tongue

❹ Moebius syndrome
- VI & VII CN palsy

❺ Frey's syndrome
- Redness & sweating in the cutaneous distribution of auriculotemporal nerve

❻ Steel Richardson syndrome/Progressive supranuclear palsy
- Postural instability and falls
- Supranuclear ophthalmoplegia
- Resting tremor is unusual
- MRI – Hummingbird sign

❼ Bruns-Garland syndrome
- Proximal neuropathy in Diabetes mellitus
- Aka Diabetic amyotrophy

❽ Locked-in syndrome
- Complete paralysis of all voluntary muscles except vertical eye movements or blinking
- Patient is conscious and awake but cannot move
- Due to infarct or bleeding in pons

❾ Tourette's syndrome
- C/b multiple motor and vocal tics
- Usual age of presentation is < 18 years
- Associated behavioral disorders are OCD, ADHD, anxiety, depression etc
- DOC – Neuroleptics/Antipsychotics

Parkinsonism-plus Syndrome

- **Multiple System Atrophy – C**
  - Prominent **c**erebellar sign
  - Hot cross bun sign
- **MSA-P:** Prominent orthostatic hypotension
- **Progressive supranuclear palsy**
  - Diplopia, Impaired down gaze

- MRI-Hummingbird/Penguin sign
- Morning glory sign
- **Dementia with Lewy Bodies**
  - Dementia is an early feature
  - Early hallucination
  - Late development of PD features

Stroke Syndromes

Affected Artery	Syndromes Associated
Middle Cerebral Artery	Gerstmann syndrome, Broca's Aphasia, Wernicke's Aphasia
Posterior Cerebral Artery P1 segment	Weber syndrome, Claude syndrome, Dejerine Roussy syndrome
Posterior Cerebral Artery P2 segment	Anton syndrome, Balint syndrome
Vertebral Artery & PICA	Medullary syndrome

Anton Syndrome
- Due to bilateral infarction in the distal PCA territory
- Cortical blindness – blindness with preserved pupillary light reaction
- Patient unaware of blindness or deny it

Bálint's Syndrome
- Due to bilateral parieto-occipital infarction
- Characterized by triad of:
  - Oculomotor apraxia – difficulty in fixating the eyes
  - Optic ataxia - loss of hand eye movement
  - Simultanagnosia – inability to examine an entire picture

Gerstmann Syndrome

- Due to involvement of parietal lobe in the dominant hemisphere
- Characterized by Acalculia, Agraphia, Finger agnosia & right left confusion

Dejerine Roussy Syndrome

- Aka Thalamic pain syndrome
- Due to stroke causing lesion in thalamus
- Manifestation: chronic pain present on C/L side of body
- Sensory loss of all modalities on C/L side of body

GLASGOW COMA SCALE

Eye Opening	Score	Verbal Response	Score	Motor Response	Score
Spontaneous	4	Oriented	5	Obeys command	6
To speech	3	Confused	4	Localizing to pain	5
To pain	2	Inappropriate words	3	Withdrawal to pain	4
None	1	Incomprehensible sounds	2	Flexion to pain	3
		None	1	Extension to pain	2
				None	1

- Minimum score – 3
- Maximum score – 15
- Mnemonic for Motor response: Old Local Wine For my Ex

UMN & LMN LESIONS

Features	Upper Motor Neuron	Lower Motor Neuron
Site of lesion	Pyramidal & Extrapyramidal tracts	Spinal motor neuron
Weakness	Spastic paresis	Flaccid paralysis
Wasting	+/– (Disuse atrophy)	++
Tone	Hypertonia (Clasp knife spasticity)	Hypotonia
Power	Decreased	Decreased (Profound)
Fasciculations	Absent	May be present
Reflexes		
Superficial reflex	Absent	Present
Deep reflex	Exaggerated	Absent
Planter reflex	Extensor (Babinski positive)	Flexor (Babinski negative)
Clonus	Present	Absent
Hoffmann's reflex*	Present	Absent

*Flicking of terminal phalanx of middle/ring finger causes reflex flexion of distal phalanx of thumb

COMMON EEG FINDINGS

EEG Findings	Diagnosis
3 Hz spike/spike & wave/spike & dome pattern	**Absence seizure**
4-6 Hz irregular spike & wave pattern	**Juvenile Myoclonic Epilepsy (Janz syndrome)**
Hypsarrhythmic pattern	**Infantile spasm/West syndrome**
Periodic Lateralized Epileptic Discharges (PLEDS)	**HSV encephalitis**
Periodic sharp wave pattern	**Creutzfeldt Jakob Disease**
<3 Hz Spike and wave	**Lennox Gastaut syndrome**
Rademecker complex	**SSPE**
Triphasic wave	**Hepatic encephalopathy**
Spikes in the centrotemporal region	**Benign Rolandic Epilepsy/BECTS**

COMMON EMG FINDINGS

EMG Finding	Site of Pathology	Disease
Fasciculation and Fibrillation	Anterior Horn Cell	Motor neuron disease/ ALS, Polio
Decremental response	Neuromuscular junction	Myasthenia

HEADACHE

Diagnosis	Symptom	Patient Characteristic	Relief of Symptom	Associated Features
Migraine	▪ Unilateral ; Throbbing or pulsatile ▪ Lasts 4 – 72 hours	▪ 5 – 40 years ▪ More common in women	▪ Dark room, sleep ▪ NSAIDs, Triptans	▪ Sensitivity to light & sound ▪ Nausea, aura, photophobia
Tension type	▪ Bilateral and nonpulsatile ▪ Tight band like sensation	▪ 10 – 50 years ▪ More common in women	▪ Physical activity	▪ Stressful events
Cluster headache	▪ Unilateral, Orbital, supraorbital or temporal ▪ Last 15 – 180 minutes	▪ 25 – 40 years ▪ More common in men	▪ With oxygen	▪ Rhinorrhea, lacrimation ▪ Occurs in grouped attacks/ Clusters
Trigeminal neuralgia	▪ Brief, paroxysmal, unilateral, stabbing pain in the distribution of V CN	▪ >50 years	▪ Carbamazepine	▪ Presence of trigger zone
Paroxysmal hemicrania	▪ Unilateral headache lasting 2 – 30 min	▪ Mean age of onset 34 years	▪ Indomethacin	

APHASIA

- *Aphasia* is an impairment of language, affecting the production or comprehension of speech and the ability to read or write.
- The areas that are critical for language make up a distributed network located along the perisylvian region of the *left* hemisphere.
- One hub, located in the inferior frontal gyrus, is known as Broca's area. Damage to this region impairs phonology, fluency, and the grammatical structure of sentences.
- The location of a second hub, known as *Wernicke's area*, is less clearly settled but is traditionally thought to include the posterior parts of the temporal lobe.

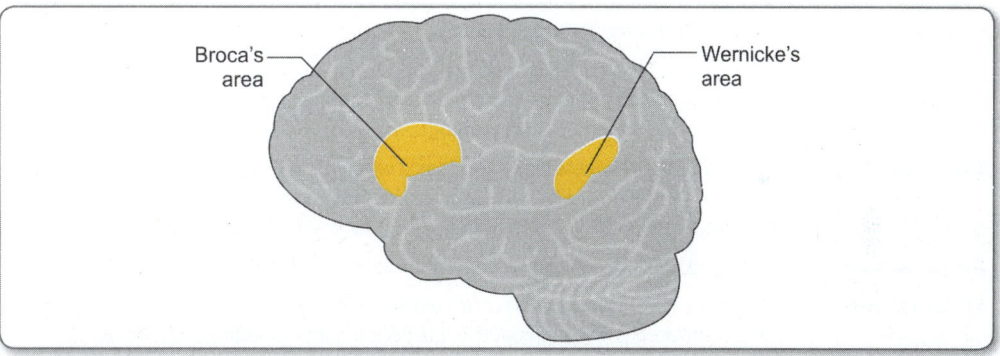

Types

	Wernicke's Aphasia	Broca's Aphasia
Aka	Jargon aphasia	Expressive aphasia/Motor aphasia
Site of lesion	Posterior part of superior temporal gyrus	Inferior frontal gyrus
Brodmann's area	22	44 and 45
MC cause	Occlusion of inferior division of MCA	Occlusion of superior division of MCA
Comprehension	Impaired	Preserved except grammar
Fluency	Preserved/Increased	Decreased/Non-fluent
Naming	Impaired	Impaired
Repetition	Impaired	Impaired
Reading	Impaired	Preserved
Writing	Impaired	Impaired
Insight	Absent	Preserved
Associated findings	Paraphasic speech Strings of neologism Right hemianopia Superior quadrantanopia	Telegraphic speech Word finding pauses Agrammatism Syntax error

AGNOSIA

- It is the inability to process sensory information.
- Often there is a loss of ability to recognize objects, persons, sounds, shapes, or smells while the specific sense is not defective nor is there any significant memory loss.

Types	Description
Anosognosia	▪ This is the inability to gain feedback about one's own condition or loss of appreciation that something is wrong. ▪ It is most commonly referred to in cases of paralysis following stroke.
Associative visual agnosia	▪ Patients can describe visual scenes and classes of objects but still fail to recognize them. They may, for example, know that a fork is something you eat with but may mistake it for a spoon. It results from inferior temporal lobe lesion.
Astereognosis	▪ Also known as somatosensory agnosia. Patient finds it difficult to recognize objects by touch based on its texture, size and weight. However, they may be able to describe it verbally or recognize same kind of objects from pictures or draw pictures of them. Can result from lesions or damage in somatosensory cortex.
Auditory agnosia	▪ Auditory agnosia is defined as impairment in identification and perception of sounds despite having normal hearing.
Auditory verbal agnosia	▪ Also known as pure word deafness (PWD). This presents as a form of meaning 'deafness' in which hearing is intact but there is significant difficulty recognising spoken words as semantically meaningful.
Cerebral achromatopsia	▪ Cerebral achromatopsia (coloragnosia): It is a type of color blindness caused by damage to the occipital or temporal cortex. ▪ Here the subject finds difficulty in identifying or differentiating colors.
Cortical deafness	▪ Cortical deafness means people do not perceive any auditory information despite having normal hearing.
Finger agnosia	▪ Is the inability to distinguish the fingers on the hand? It is present in lesions of the dominant parietal lobe, and is a component of **Gerstmann** syndrome.
Prosopagnosia	▪ Aka face blindness and facial agnosia: Patients cannot recognize familiar faces, including, sometimes even their own.
Pure alexia	▪ Pure alexia is inability to read words.
Semantic agnosia	▪ Those with this form of agnosia are effectively 'object blind' until they use non-visual sensory systems to recognise the object. For example, feeling, tapping, smelling, rocking or flicking the object, may trigger realisation of its semantics (meaning).
Simultagnosia	▪ The inability to process visual input as a whole. The person instead processes sensory inputs in a bit-by-bit fashion. When looking at a picture they can describe the parts of the picture but struggle to comprehend the picture as a whole. It is seen in **Bálint's** syndrome
Tactile agnosia	▪ Impaired ability to recognize or identify objects by touch alone.
Visual agnosia	▪ A patient with visual agnosia is unable either to name a visually presented object or to describe its use. ▪ It is associated with lesions of the left occipital lobe and temporal lobes.

HEMORRHAGES IN RELATION TO SKULL & BRAIN

Hemorrhage	Location	Cause	Diagnosis
Caput Succedaneum	Diffuse ecchymotic swelling of **S**oft tissues of scalp	Prolonged labor	Clinical
Cephalohematoma	Subperiosteal hematoma over parietal bone	Difficult extraction of baby (Vacuum/forceps assisted)	Clinical
Extra Dural or Epidural Hemorrhage (EDH)	Hemorrhage b/w Periosteum and Dura mater	Injury to Middle Meningeal Artery	NCCT – Biconvex or lentiform shape hematoma
Sub Dural Hemorrhage (SDH)	Hemorrhage b/w Dura mater and arachnoid mater	Injury to cortical bridging veins usually 2° to trauma	NCCT – Concavo-convex hematoma
Sub Arachnoid Hemorrhage (SAH)	Hemorrhage in subarachnoid space i.e. b/w arachnoid mater and Pia mater	Spontaneous rupture of aneurysm	NCCT – Blood in sylvian fissure
Intraventricular Hemorrhage (IVH)	Hemorrhage in ventricular spaces	Secondary to expansion of SAH or ICH	Blood in CSF
Intracerebral/ parenchymal Hemorrhage (ICH)	Hemorrhage in brain parenchyma MC site – Putamen	MC cause – Hypertension	NCCT head

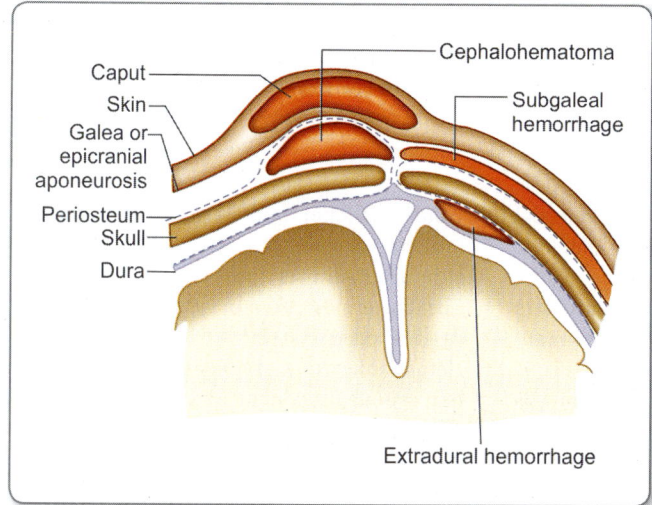

Hemorrhages in relation to skull

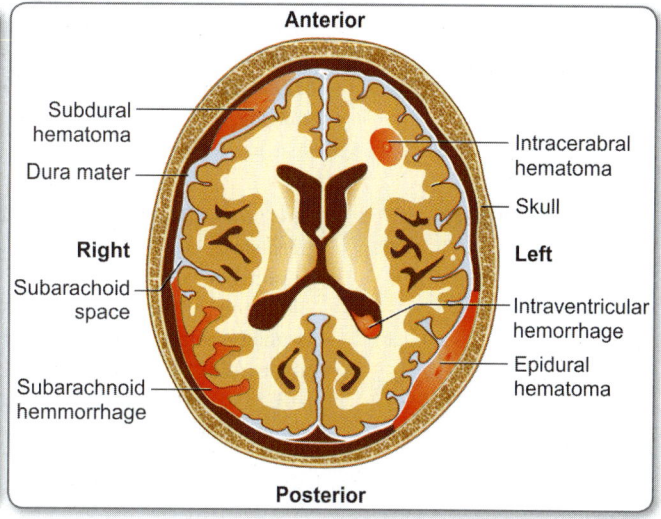

Hemorrhages in relation to brain

SUB ARACHNOID HEMORRHAGE

- The MC cause of SAH is rupture of a *Saccular (berry) aneurysm,* found near major arterial branch points in the anterior circulation.
- Severe headache associated with exertion is the presenting complaint. The patient often describes the headache as "the worst headache of my life".
- Thunderclap headache is a variant of migraine that simulates an SAH.
- The clinical manifestations of SAH can be graded using the Hunt-Hess or World Federation of Neurosurgical Societies classification Schemes.
- The hallmark of SAH is blood in the CSF.
- Initial investigation of choice remains NCCT head as soon as possible.
- If the CT scan is inconclusive of SAH and no SOL or hydrocephalus noted, then a CSF study (lumbar puncture) must be done to look for blood in subarachnoid space.
- Grossly, CSF may have xanthochromic appearance due to lysis of RBCs and conversion of hemoglobin to bilirubin.
- Once the diagnosis of SAH from a ruptured saccular aneurysm is suspected, four-vessel conventional x-ray angiography (both carotids and both vertebral) is performed to localize and define the anatomy of the aneurysm.
- CT angiography is an alternative method for locating the aneurysm and may be sufficient to plan definitive therapy.
- The ECG frequently shows ST-segment and T-wave changes like prolonged QRS complex, increased QT interval, and prominent "peaked" or deeply inverted symmetric T waves.

Site of aneurysm	Clinical presentation
▪ Junction of PCoA and ICA	Ophthalmoplegia due to III CN palsy, Ptosis
▪ Cavernous sinus	VI CN palsy
▪ MCA aneurysm	Pain in or behind the eye

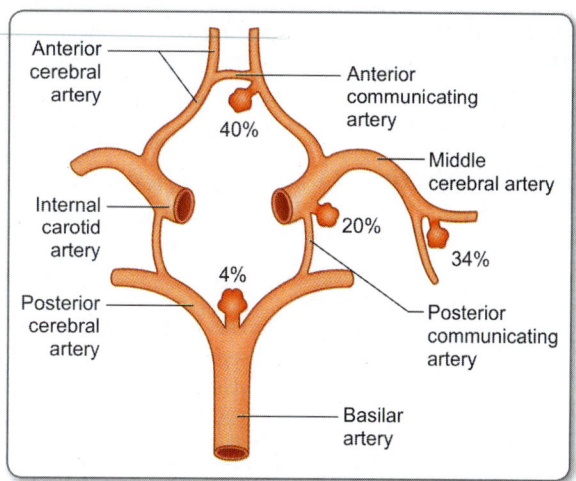

MANAGEMENT OF ISCHEMIC STROKE

- NCCT brain remains the investigation of choice in acute stroke.
- MRI is more sensitive than CT for acute stroke imaging.

- Perform an emergency NCCT scan to differentiate between ischemic stroke and hemorrhagic stroke.

Medical Support

- The immediate goal is to optimize cerebral perfusion in the surrounding ischemic penumbra.
- Blood pressure should be lowered only if there is malignant hypertension or concomitant myocardial ischemia, or if blood pressure is >185/110 mm Hg and thrombolytic therapy is anticipated.

- Water restriction and IV mannitol to reduce intracranial pressure (ICP) may be used, although their usefulness is unknown.
- Corticosteroids are not useful to decrease cerebral edema
- Hemicraniectomy reduces the mortality but overall functional outcome of patients' undergone surgery is no better than one on medical management.

Intravenous Thrombolysis

- The only fibrinolytic agent that has been shown to benefit selected patients with acute ischemic stroke is alteplase (rtPA).
- Despite an increased incidence of symptomatic intracranial hemorrhage, treatment with IV rtPA within 3 to 4.5 h of the onset of ischemic stroke improved clinical outcome.

- IV rtPA is administered by calculating total dose (0.9 mg/kg to a 90 mg maximum) and administering 10% as a bolus, then the remainder over 60 min.
- NIH stroke scale/score (NIHSS) is done to ascertain the need of thrombolysis

Administration of rtPA for Acute Ischemic Stroke (AIS)

Indication	Contraindication
▪ Clinical diagnosis of stroke ▪ Onset of symptoms to time of drug administration ≤4.5 h ▪ CT scan showing no hemorrhage or edema of >1/3 of the MCA territory ▪ Age ≥18 years ▪ SBP <185 mmHg; DBP <110 mmHg ▪ Blood glucose >50 mg/dL ▪ Consent by patient or surrogate	▪ Prior stroke or head injury within 3 months; prior intracranial hemorrhage ▪ Rapidly improving symptoms ▪ Minor stroke symptoms ▪ Use of heparin within 48 h and prolonged PTT, or elevated INR ▪ Sustained BP >185/110 mmHg despite treatment ▪ Platelets <100,000; glucose <50 or >400 mg/dL ▪ Major surgery in preceding 14 days ▪ Gastrointestinal bleeding in preceding 21 days ▪ Recent myocardial infarction

Mechanical Thrombectomy

- Mechanical clot disruption is an alternative for patients in whom fibrinolysis is ineffective or contraindicated.

- Can be performed up to 24 hours in select patients.

Antithrombotic Treatment

- Aspirin is the only antiplatelet agent that has been proven effective for the acute treatment of ischemic stroke.

- Use of aspirin within 48 h of stroke onset reduced both stroke recurrence risk and mortality minimally.

Imaging in a Patient of Stroke

- The earliest CT sign visible is a hyperdense segment of a vessel, representing direct visualisation of the intravascular thrombus/

embolus. It is most often observed in the middle cerebral artery and k/a **hyperdense MCA sign or MCA dot sign.**

BRAIN STEM STROKE SYNDROMES

Midbrain Syndromes

Syndromes	Site of Lesion	CN Involved	Tracts Involved	Features
Weber's syndrome	Ventromedial midbrain	CN III	▪ Corticospinal & Corticobulbar tract (cerebral peduncle) ▪ Substantia Nigra	▪ I/L Oculomotor palsy ▪ C/L or Crossed Hemiplegia/hemiparesis ▪ C/L lower facial weakness (UMN type) ▪ C/L parkinsonian rigidity
Benedikt syndrome	Tegmentum	CN III	▪ **R**ed nucleus ▪ Superior cerebellar peduncle ▪ Corticospinal & Corticobulbar tract	▪ I/L Oculomotor palsy ▪ C/L Hemiparesis ▪ C/L Cerebellar ataxia, Tremor
Claude's syndrome	Tegmentum	CN III	▪ Red nucleus ▪ Superior cerebellar peduncle ▪ Brachium conjunctivum	▪ I/L Oculomotor palsy ▪ C/L Cerebellar ataxia, Tremor
Nothnagel's syndrome	Tectum	CN III (U/L or B/L)	▪ Superior cerebellar peduncle ▪ Brachium conjunctivum	▪ I/L Oculomotor palsy ▪ C/L Cerebellar ataxia
Parinaud's syndrome	Dorsal midbrain	None	▪ Rostral midbrain and pretectum near the level of superior colliculus	▪ Limited upward gaze (Vertical gaze palsy) ▪ Downgaze at rest (sunsetting sign) ▪ Eyelid retraction (collier's sign) ▪ Pseudo Argil Robertson pupil

Mnemonic: for Red nucleus involvement – RBC |

Pontine Syndromes

Syndromes	Structures Involved	Ipsilateral	Contralateral
Millard Gubler syndrome	▪ CN VI & VII* ▪ Corticospinal tract	▪ Diplopia + LR palsy ▪ LMN type of facial palsy	▪ Hemiplegia
Foville's syndrome	▪ Nucleus of CN VI & VII ▪ Corticospinal tract	▪ Horizontal gaze palsy ▪ LMN type of facial palsy	▪ Hemiparesis ▪ Internuclear ophthalmoplegia

*****Mnemonic** – CN involved in both the syndromes corresponds to the letter in the name |

Medullary Syndromes

	Lateral Medullary Syndrome/Wallenberg Syndrome		Medial Medullary Syndrome/ Dejerine Syndrome
Vascular involvement	▪ Vertebral artery → MC ▪ Posterior Inferior Cerebellar Artery (PICA)		▪ Anterior spinal artery ▪ Vertebral artery
Structures involved	▪ Trigeminal nucleus (V) ▪ Vestibular nucleus (VIII) ▪ Nucleus Ambiguus (motor IX & X)	▪ Sympathetic tract ▪ Lateral spinothalamic tract ▪ Spinocerebellar tract	▪ XII CN and nucleus ▪ Pyramid ▪ Medial lemniscus
Ipsilateral (Clinical Features)	▪ Pain, Numbness, Impaired sensation over ½ of face (V) ▪ Vertigo , Nystagmus, Diplopia (VIII) ▪ Dysphagia, Hoarseness, palatal paralysis, decreased gag reflex (IX & X) ▪ Loss of taste & weakness of lower face ▪ Horner's syndrome – sympathetic tract involvement		▪ LMN paralysis of ½ of tongue with atrophy (XII)
Contralateral (Clinical Features)	▪ Impaired pain and temperature – spinothalamic involvement		▪ Spastic paralysis of arms and legs ▪ Loss of tactile, vibration & proprioception over ½ of body

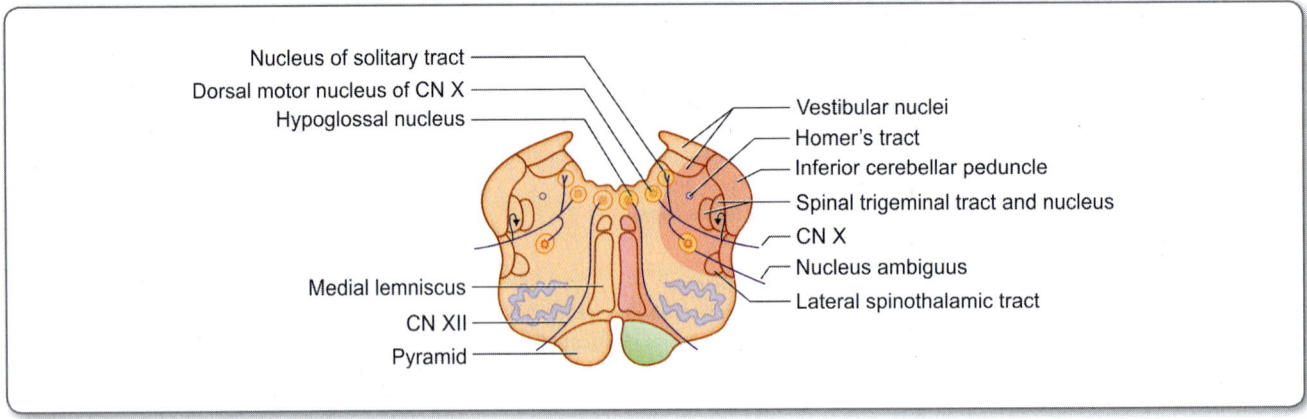

Cross section of Medulla

DIFFERENTIAL DIAGNOSIS OF ATAXIC DISORDERS

	Friedreich's Ataxia	Ataxia Telangiectasia	SACD	Tabes Dorsalis	Cerebellar Ataxia

General	▪ AR demyelinating disorder
	▪ MC form of inherited ataxia
	▪ Due to mutation in gene *Frataxin* located on chromosome 9
		▪ AR multisystem disorder
		▪ Due to mutation in the *ATM* gene located on chromosome 11
		▪ Patient present in 1st decade of life
			▪ Demyelination disorder
			▪ Due to deficiency of Vitamin B$_{12}$
				▪ Demyelination & degenerative disease
				▪ Involve the posterior columns and posterior roots
					▪ **Etiology:**
					  ○ Alcohol
					  ○ Multiple sclerosis
					  ○ Multiple system atrophy
					  ○ Ataxia Telangiectasia

Pyramidal tract	▪ Involved	▪ Less involved	▪ Involved	▪ Not involved	▪ Not involved
Posterior column	▪ Involved	▪ Involved	▪ Involved	▪ Involved	▪ Not involved
Clinical features	▪ Progressive Ataxia – MC feature ▪ Paresthesia ▪ Loss of pain sensation, vibration & joint position ▪ Dysarthria, Dysphagia ▪ Cardiomyopathy, Diabetes	▪ Cerebellar ataxia ▪ Oculomotor apraxia ▪ Sensation usually intact ▪ High incidence of recurrent pulmonary infection & neoplasms ▪ Telangiectasia	▪ Sensory ataxia ▪ Narrow base ataxic gait ▪ Paresthesia ▪ Loss of pain sensation, vibration & joint position ▪ Dementia ▪ Optic atrophy	▪ Sensory ataxia ▪ Narrow base ataxic gait ▪ Paresthesia ▪ Loss of pain sensation, vibration & joint position ▪ Atonic bladder ▪ Charcot's joint	▪ Truncal ataxia ▪ Wide based gait ▪ Sensation intact ▪ Dysmetria ▪ Dysarthria ▪ Scanning speech ▪ Intentional tremor
On examination	▪ Normal tone ▪ Nystagmus ▪ Positive Romberg sign	▪ Hypotonia ▪ Nystagmus ▪ Negative Romberg sign	▪ Motor deficit & spasticity (UMN type) ▪ Positive Romberg sign	▪ Hypotonia ▪ Argyll Robertson pupil ▪ Positive Romberg sign	▪ Hypotonic ▪ Dysdiadochokinesia ▪ Negative Romberg sign
Reflex	▪ Areflexia	▪ Areflexia	▪ Areflexia	▪ Areflexia	▪ Pendular knee jerk
Planter	▪ Extensor	▪ Extensor/Equivocal	▪ Extensor	▪ Absent	▪ Flexor

IMPORTANT NEURO DEGENERATIVE DISORDERS

	Alzheimer's Disease	Parkinson's Disease	Huntington's Disease
General feature	▪ MC cause of cortical dementia ▪ Involvement – Medial Temporal lobe (entorhinal cortex and hippocampus) & nucleus basalis of Meynert	▪ Neurodegenerative disease of basal ganglia	▪ Degenerative disorder of basal ganglia and cerebral cortex ▪ Autosomal dominant inheritance
Risk factors/ Etiology/ Pathogenesis	▪ **Mutations associated with early onset AD:** ○ The Amyloid precursor protein (**APP**) gene on chromosome 21 ○ The presenilin – 1 (**PS 1**) gene on chromosome 14 ○ The presenilin – 2 (**PS 2**) gene on chromosome 1 ○ Trisomy 21 (Downs) ▪ Advancing age ▪ Positive family history ▪ Down syndrome ▪ APOE 4 genotype ▪ Hypertension ▪ Female gender ▪ Lower education ▪ Clusterin	▪ MC genetic cause of PD – mutation in gene coding LRRK2 ▪ Mutation in GTP-1 gene ▪ Loss of dopaminergic neurons of the Substantia nigra pars compacta (SNpc) ▪ Hyperactivity of cholinergic neurons ▪ Presence of intracytoplasmic eosinophilic Lewy bodies made up of α-synuclein	▪ Loss of striatal neurons & atrophy of caudate nucleus and putamen ▪ Triple nucleotide expansion disorder ▪ CAG repeats in huntingtin gene located on chromosome 4 ▪ Exhibit Anticipation phenomenon – Symptoms appear earlier in next generation
Clinical features	▪ Episodic memory loss and difficulty in recalling events or people due to Hippocampal involvement ▪ Cognitive and behavior abnormality ▪ Language disorder as anomic aphasia or anomia ▪ Apraxia and sundowning ▪ Extrapyramidal symptoms in later stages	▪ Asymmetric resting tremors (pin rolling tremor) – MC initial symptom ▪ Bradykinesia ▪ Rigidity – Lead pipe & cog wheel rigidity ▪ Gait disturbance – Festinant gait ▪ Postural instability; Decreased arm swing ▪ Masked expressionless facies ▪ Dementia & cognitive impairment	▪ Age of onset – between 25 and 45 years ▪ Age of onset depends on the number of CAG repeats ▪ Movement disorder (MC is Chorea) ▪ Dementia ▪ Behavioral changes
Diagnosis 	▪ Degeneration in nucleus basalis of Meynert occurs → Cholinergic deficiency ▪ Decrease in Ach, Norepinephrine & Serotonin levels ▪ Brain biopsy reveals: ○ **Neurofibrillary tangles** (ghost tangles) – Intracellular accumulation of tau proteins, mostly in Hippocampus ○ Amyloid angiopathy; **Hirano bodies** ○ **Senile plaque/Neuritic plaques** – Extracellular accumulation of β amyloid protein (derived from APP) in Hippocampus ▪ MRI – Diffuse Cortical & Hippocampal atrophy; Hydrocephalus ex vacuo	▪ Clinical diagnosis ▪ 2 out of the following 3 cardinal signs are required to make the diagnosis ○ Resting tremor ○ Rigidity ○ Bradykinesia ▪ H/P – eosinophilic intracytoplasmic inclusion bodies k/a Lewy bodies	▪ Genetic testing for CAG repeats ▪ Family history
Treatments	▪ Centrally acting Acetylcholinesterase inhibitors (AChEIs) like Donepezil, Rivastigmine & Galantamine ▪ NMDA antagonist Memantine	▪ Levodopa/Carbidopa ▪ MAO B inhibitors – Selegiline, Rasagiline ▪ Dopamine agonist – Ropinirole, Pramipexole ▪ Anticholinergic agents like Trihexyphenidyl & Benztropine ▪ Amantadine ▪ Deep brain stimulation targeting Globus Pallidum and subthalamic nucleus	▪ Tetrabenazine & Deutetrabenazine – Vesicular Monoamine Transporter 2 (VMAT 2) inhibitors

HYPERKINETIC MOVEMENT DISORDERS

Disorders	Characteristic	Site of Lesion	Seen in
Tremor	▪ Rhythmic oscillation of a body part due to intermittent muscle contractions. ▪ It can be resting, postural or kinetic (action/ intentional).	▪ Substantia nigra in Parkinson disease	▪ Physiological tremor ▪ Essential tremor ▪ Parkinson disease – resting tremor ▪ Cerebellar disease – intentional tremor
Dystonia	▪ Involuntary, patterned, sustained or repeated muscle contractions often associated with twisting movements and abnormal posture	▪ Striatum ▪ Cerebellum	▪ Huntington's disease ▪ Parkinson disease ▪ Wilson disease ▪ Neuroleptic/Antipsychotics
Athetosis	▪ Slow, distal, writhing, involuntary movements with a propensity to affect the arms and hands	▪ Striatum ▪ Thalamus	▪ Cerebral palsy
Chorea	▪ Rapid, semi-purposeful, graceful, dance-like nonpatterned involuntary movements involving distal or proximal muscle groups.	▪ Caudate nucleus in Huntington ▪ Striatum	▪ Huntington's disease ▪ Rheumatic fever (Sydenham's chorea)
Myoclonus	▪ Sudden, brief (<100 ms), jerk-like, arrhythmic muscle twitches		▪ Asterixis (Negative myoclonus) ▪ Juvenile Myoclonic epilepsy
Tic	▪ Brief, rapid, recurrent, and purposeless stereotyped motor contractions that can often be suppressed for a short time. It can be motor or phonetic. Examples are eye blinking and throat clearing.		▪ Tourette's syndrome
Ballism/ Hemiballismus	▪ Large amplitude, wild, flinging movement mostly affecting the proximal muscles	▪ Contralateral Subthalamic nucleus	

Type of Tremor	Characteristics	Seen in
Enhanced Physiologic tremor	▪ High-frequency (10–12 Hz) ▪ Postural or kinetic tremor	▪ Anxiety, Hyperthyroidism ▪ Lithium, Alcohol
Essential tremor *(MC movement disorder)*	▪ High-frequency (6–10 Hz) ▪ Postural or kinetic tremor ▪ Bilateral and symmetrical ▪ Improved by alcohol and worsened by stress	▪ Approximately 50% of cases have a positive family history with an autosomal dominant pattern of inheritance
Resting/static tremor	▪ Low frequency (4 – 6 Hz) ▪ Pill – rolling tremor	▪ Parkinson disease
Intentional tremor	▪ Low frequency (<5 Hz)	▪ Cerebellar lesions
Flapping tremor/ Asterixis/Liver flap	▪ Brief interruptions of sustained voluntary muscle contraction causing brief lapses of posture	▪ Hepatic encephalopathy ▪ Metabolic encephalopathy Azotemia ▪ Respiratory failure
Perioral tremor	▪ Involuntary, fine, rhythmic motions of the mouth along a vertical plane	▪ Rabbit syndrome
Wing beating tremor		▪ Wilson disease

Hallervorden Spatz Disease
- Aka Pantothenate kinase associated neurodegeneration (PKAN)
- Caused by mutation in the PANK 2 gene
- Characterized by accumulation of iron in the basal ganglia
- MRI – Eye of tiger sign

Drug Induced Movement Disorders
- Primarily associated with drugs that block dopamine receptors (neuroleptics) or central dopaminergic transmission.
- These drugs are widely used in psychiatric illness.

Dystonia	Akathisia	Tardive Dyskinesia
▪ Develop within minutes of exposure – Acute onset ▪ Most common acute hyperkinetic drug reaction ▪ It is an involuntary, patterned, sustained or repeated muscle contractions often associated with twisting movements and abnormal posture. E.g. blepharospasm, torticollis, or oromandibular dystonia ▪ Rx: anticholinergics (benztropine or diphenhydramine), benzodiazepines (lorazepam, clonazepam, or diazepam), or dopamine agonists.	▪ Subacute onset ▪ It consists of motor restlessness with a need to move that is alleviated by movement. ▪ Therapy consists of removing the offending agent. ▪ Rx: Benzodiazepines, anticholinergics, beta blockers, or dopamine agonists.	▪ Develop months to years after initiation of neuroleptic treatment. ▪ Most common and typically presents with Choreiform movements involving the mouth, lips, and tongue. ▪ Trunk and limbs are involved in severe cases.

MULTIPLE SCLEROSIS

- It is a chronic inflammatory demyelinating disorder of CNS.
- Sine qua non of MS is that symptomatic episodes are separated in time and space i.e. episodes are separated by gap of months or years and involvement of different anatomic locations.

Clinical Features

- Sensory loss (paresthesia) – MC initial symptom
- Muscle weakness, spasticity
- Bladder, bowel & sexual dysfunction
- Cerebellar symptoms – Nystagmus, Intentional tremor & Scanning speech → **Charcot neurological triad**
- Optic neuritis, diplopia (may result from internuclear ophthalmoplegia)
- Heat intolerance

- Useless hand syndrome of Oppenheimer
- **Uhthoff phenomenon** – heat intolerance leading to blurring of vision or exacerbation of symptoms induced by exercise, a hot meal or a hot bath
- **Pulfrich effect** – sense of disorientation in moving traffic
- **Lhermitte's symptom** – electric shock like sensation induced by neck flexion
- Hyper reactive reflexes, Babinski +ve

Types

- **Relapsing MS (RMS)/Bout onset MS:**
  - MC type – 90%
  - Recurrent attacks in different parts of nervous system which resolve completely with little or no residual effects

- Secondary progressive MS (SPMS)
- Primary progressive MS (PPMS)

Diagnosis

- By **McDonald criteria**
- MRI – **Dawson finger** appearance

- CSF – Oligoclonal bands
- Expanded Disability Status Score (EDSS) – measures neurological impairment in MS

Treatment

- Acute exacerbation – Methylprednisolone/Plasmapheresis
- Disease modifying therapies:
  - Interferon β1a & 1b; Peg IFN β1a
  - Glatiramer – immunomodulator
  - Mitoxantrone – immunosuppressant
  - Dimethyl fumerate – Nrf 2 pathway activator
  - Teriflunomide – inhibit dihydro-orotate dehydrogenase

- Natalizumab – Recombinant antibody against α_4 subunit of $\alpha_4\beta_1$ and $\alpha_4\beta_7$
  - ▪ Associated with the risk of PML
- Alemtuzumab – Recombinant antibody against CD52
- Ocrelizumab – Monoclonal Ab against CD 20
- Fingolimod; Amantadine

NEUROMYELITIS OPTICA (DEVIC'S DISEASE)

- NMO is an autoimmune, inflammatory disorder characterized by recurrent attacks of optic neuritis (ON) and myelitis

- More frequent in females M:F = 1: 3
- Usually seen in adulthood

MULTIPLE CHOICE QUESTIONS

CHAPTER 1: NEUROSCIENCES

NEUROPHYSIOLOGY

CELLS OF CNS & NEURONAL INJURY

1. Cell most sensitive to hypoxia is ?　　*(PGMEE 2016)*
- a. Neuron
- b. Liver cell
- c. Stem cell
- d. Muscle

[Ref: Robbins 9th/e pg. 130]

2. Damage to nervous tissue is repaired by which cells of CNS　　*(PGMEE 2016)*
- a. Neuroglia
- b. Axons
- c. Microglia
- d. Fibroblasts

[Ref: Robbins 9th/e pg. 1282]

3. Cells which do NOT participate in repair after damage to nervous tissue after brain infarction
　　(PGMEE 2013-14, 2012-13)
- a. Astrocytes
- b. Microglia
- c. Endothelial cells
- d. Fibroblasts

[Ref: Robbins 9th/e pg. 1253]

4. Phagocytosis in brain is caused by　　*(PGMEE 2013-14)*
- a. Astrocytes
- b. Oligodendrocytes
- c. Microglia
- d. Fibroblasts

[Ref: Harrison's 20th/e pg. 3040]

5. Modified macrophages in the brain are:-
　　(PGMEE 2013-14, 2012-13)
- a. Astrocytes
- b. Oligodendrocytes
- c. Microglia
- d. Macroglia

[Ref: Harrison's 20th/e pg. 3040]

6. Cells which are NOT of reticuloendothelial system origin　　*(PGMEE 2016-17)*
- a. Astrocytes
- b. Oligodendrocytes
- c. Microglia
- d. Macroglia

[Ref: Robbins 9th/e pg. 1282]

7. Negri bodies are intracytoplasmic eosinophilic inclusion bodies seen in Rabies. Negri bodies are found in:-
- a. Affected neurons in CNS　　*(PGMEE 2013-14)*
- b. Oligodendrocytes
- c. Remaining neurons in CNS
- d. Astrocytes

[Ref: Robbins 9th/e pg. 1277]

8. Rosenthal fibres are:　　*(PGMEE 2016-17, 2015, 2012-13)*
- a. Intranuclear inclusions
- b. Intracytoplasmic inclusions
- c. Present extracellularly
- d. Part of cell membrane

[Ref: Robbins 9th/e pg. 1253]

Explanation

Rosenthal fibres

- Rosenthal fibres are corkscrew eosinophilic (pink) bundle which are associated with either pilocytic astrocytoma or Alexander's Disease.
- These are intracytoplasmic eosinophil inclusions; composed of Glial Fibrillary Acid Protein (GFAP).

9. Rosenthal fibres are seen in:　　*(PGMEE 2015-16)*
- a. Medulloblastoma
- b. Pilocytic astrocytoma
- c. Glioblastoma
- d. Ependymoma

[Ref: Robbins 9th/e pg. 1309]

10. Rosenthal fibres in astrocytoma are composed of:
　　(PGMEE 2015, 2012-13)
- a. Heat shock proteins
- b. Fibrillar proteins
- c. GFAP
- d. Globulins

[Ref: Robbins 9th/e pg. 1253]

11. What are nitrergic neurons:　　*(PGMEE 2015-16)*
- a. 1st order neurons releasing calcitonin Gene related peptide
- b. 1st order neurons releasing nitric oxide
- c. Post ganglionic neurons releasing nitric oxide
- d. Post ganglionic neurons releasing substance P

[Ref: Vascular medicine 3rd ed. / 84]

HIGHER FUNCTIONS

12. Right hand dominant patient presents with normal comprehension but speaks with short utterances of a few words at a time, comprised mostly of nouns. What is the most probable location of the lesion?
- a. Right inferior frontal gyrus　　*(NEET Pattern 2019)*
- b. Left inferior frontal gyrus
- c. Right superior temporal gyrus
- d. Left superior temporal gyrus

13. Pure word deafness is associated with:
- a. Posterior cerebral artery stroke　　*(NEET Pattern 2019)*
- b. Vertebral artery aneurysm
- c. Basilar artery aneurysm
- d. Middle cerebral artery stroke

14. Global aphasia is seen due to:　　*(NEET Pattern 2019)*
- a. Strokes involving entire middle cerebral artery distribution in left hemisphere
- b. Strokes involving entire middle cerebral artery distribution in right hemisphere
- c. Strokes involving entire posterior cerebral artery distribution in left hemisphere
- d. Strokes involving entire posterior cerebral artery distribution in right hemisphere

1.	a
2.	a
3.	d
4.	c
5.	c
6.	c
7.	c
8.	b
9.	b
10.	c
11.	b
12.	b
13.	d
14.	a

15. Motor aphasia refers to defect in: *(NEET 2018)*
   a. Peripheral speech apparatus
   b. Verbal expression
   c. Auditory comprehension
   d. Verbal comprehension

Explanation

- Motor aphasia also known as expressive aphasia is a disorder of thought and word finding resulting in inadequate verbal expression.

Defect in understanding:	Receptive aphasia / Sensory aphasia
Defect in thought and word finding:	Motor / Expressive aphasia
Defect in voice production:	Dysphonia
Defect in articulation:	Dysarthric

16. Prosopagnosia is inability to recognize:- *(PGMEE 2018)*
   a. Faces   b. Objects
   c. Taste   d. Language

17. Prospagnosia is caused by lesion of: *(NEET 2016)*
   a. Parieto-occipital   b. Occipito-termporal
   c. Frontal lobe   d. Parietal lobe

18. Frontal lobe syndrome consists of: *(NEET Pattern 2019)*
   a. Irritability   b. Euphoria
   c. Indifference   d. All of the above

19. Which of the following Broadman's area is involved in Broca's motor aphasia: *(NEET 2018)*
   a. 44,45   b. 22
   c. 17,18,19   d. 4,6

20. Broca's area is located in :- *(PGMEE 2018)*
   a. Superior frontal gyrus   b. Inferior frontal gyrus
   c. Superior temporal gyrus d. Occipital gyrus

21. Which part of brain is involved in narcolepsy? *(DNB December 2011)*
   a. Neo cortex   b. Medulla
   c. Pons   d. Hypothalamus

[Ref: Harrison's 20th/e pg. 172]

Explanation

- Hypocretin producing neurons in the brain are markedly reduced in Narcolepsy. Narcolepsy is due to hypothalamic dysfunction in relation to lack of hypocretin production.

22. A patient is unable to solve mathematical calculations, which part of his brain is damaged? *(PGMEE 2015-16)*
   a. Temporal lobe   b. Frontal lobe
   c. Occipital lobe   d. Parietal lobe

[Ref: Harrison's 20th/e pg. 3070]

CSF

23. CSF is absorbed by :- *(PGMEE 2015-16)*
   a. Choroid plexus
   b. Dura matter
   c. Sub-arachnoid granulations
   d. Pia matter

[Ref: Harrison's 19th/e pg. 443e-4]

24. CSF glucose level is: *(PGMEE 2014/15)*
   a. Half the plasma glucose
   b. 1/3 plasma glucose
   c. 2/3 plasma glucose
   d. Same as plasma glucose

[Ref: Harrison's 20th/e pg. 864]

25. Specific gravity of CSF is? *(DNB June 2009)*
   a. 1.003 – 1.008   b. 1.005 – 1.009
   c. 1.001 – 1.003   d. 1.010 – 1.013

[Ref: Ganong's 25th /e pg. 603]

INTRACRANIAL PRESSURE (ICP/ICT)

26. Pseudotumour cerebri is caused by all EXCEPT:
   a. Vitamin A toxicity   *(PGMEE 2014/15)*
   b. Obesity
   c. Sudden stoppage of steroids
   d. PCM toxicity

27. Increased ICT is shown by? *(PGMEE 2015-16)*
   a. Miosis   b. Reduction in GCS
   c. Tachycardia   d. Systemic hypotension

[Ref: Harrison's 20th/e pg. 2077]

Explanation

- Signs & symptoms of raised ICT:
  - Headache
  - Nausea, Vomiting
  - Blurring Vision
  - Papilledema
  - 6th CN palsy → False localizing sign
  - Pupillary dilatation
  - Diminished level of consciousness
  - Cushing's triad (Bradycardia, hypertension, Irregular respiration)

28. All are seen in Benign Intracranial Hypertension except? *(NEET Pattern 2015)*
   a. Normal ventricles   b. Lateral rectus palsy
   c. Papilledema   d. Proptosis

29. DOC for idiopathic intra-cranial hypertension: (I.I.H) *(PGMEE 2014/15)*
   a. Glycerol   b. Dexamethasone
   c. Mannitol   d. Acetazolamide

30. Increased intra-cranial tension is related to: *(PGMEE 2015-16)*
   a. Hypotension and tachycardia
   b. Hypertension and bradycardia
   c. Hypertension and tachycardia
   d. Hypotension and bradycardia

31. Dilated ventricles with normal CSF pressure is seen in: *(PGMEE 2014/15)*
   a. Hydrocephalus   b. Pseudotumour cerebri
   c. Normal variant   d. Hydrocephalus ex-vacuo

32. Most common false neurological sign is:- *(DNB Dec'2010)*
   a. Wasting of hands   b. Unilateral papilledema
   c. Diplopia   d. Abnormal unilateral pupil

[Ref: Journal of Neurology, Neurosurgery Psychiatry 2003; 74:415-418 Doi:10.1136/jnnp.74.4.415]

15.	b
16.	a
17.	b
18.	d
19.	a
20.	b
21.	d
22.	d
23.	c
24.	c
25.	b
26.	d
27.	b
28.	d
29.	d
30.	b
31.	d
32.	c

Explanation

SAH

- Sudden onset headache in the absence of focal neurologic symptoms is the hallmark of aneurysmal rupture; however, focal neurologic deficits may occur. *Saccular aneurysm* is the most common type of intracranial aneurysm. Other aneurysm types include atherosclerotic (fusiform; mostly of the basilar artery), mycotic, traumatic, and dissecting. These latter three, like saccular aneurysms, are most often found in the anterior circulation.
- About 90% of saccular aneurysms are found near major arterial branch points in the anterior circulation.
- The most frequent cause of clinically significant subarachnoid hemorrhage is rupture of a *Saccular (berry) aneurysm.*
- In ~45% of cases of SAH, severe headache associated with exertion is the presenting complaint. The patient often describes the headache as "the worst headache of my life". Thunderclap headache is a variant of migraine that simulates an SAH. Before concluding that a patient with sudden, severe headache has thunderclap migraine, a definitive workup for aneurysm or other intracranial pathology is required.
- The initial clinical manifestations of SAH can be graded using the Hunt-Hess or World Federation of Neurosurgical Societies classification Schemes.
- The hallmark of aneurysmal rupture is blood in the CSF. Initial investigation of choice remains NCCT head as soon as possible.
- If the CT scan is inconclusive of SAH and no SOL or hydrocephalus noted, then a CSF study (lumbar puncture) must be done to look for blood in subarachnoid space.
- Grossly, CSF may have xanthochromic appearance due to lysis of RBCs and conversion of hemoglobin to bilirubin.
- Once the diagnosis of SAH from a ruptured saccular aneurysm is suspected, four-vessel conventional x-ray angiography (both carotids and both vertebrals) is performed to localize and define the anatomy of the aneurysm and to determine if other unruptured aneurysms exist. CT angiography is an alternative method for locating the aneurysm and may be sufficient to plan definitive therapy.
- The electrocardiogram (ECG) frequently shows ST-segment and T-wave changes like prolonged QRS complex, increased QT interval, and prominent "peaked" or deeply inverted symmetric T waves.

91. The investigation to be performed in patient of SAH with normal CT scan? *(PGMEE 2014/15)*
a. Contrast enhanced CT
b. Gadolinium enhanced MRI
c. MRI
d. Three tube test

[Ref: Page 983, CMDT 2016]

91.	d
92.	a
93.	d
94.	a
95.	d
96.	a
97.	c

Explanation

- In this test, LP is done, CSF in collected in three test tube RBC are counted in each tube. SAH will have constant number of RBC in each tube.

92. In relation to Traumatic brain injury (TBI), which of the following is NOT true:- *(PGMEE 2018)*
a. MRI is diagnostic modality and should be done urgently
b. Useful in depressed fracture
c. Midline shift with intracranial bleed requires surgery
d. Motor response is prognostic indicator

[Ref: Sabiston's 19th/e pg. 440]

Explanation

- Computed tomography (CT) of the head without IV contrast is the most important diagnostic study during the initial evaluation of TBI because it provides a highly sensitive determination of acute intracranial pathology. Imaging of the cranium with magnetic resonance imaging (MRI) may be able to provide better anatomic detail, especially in the setting of ischemia, but has no role in the initial evaluation of the brain injured patient.

93. A patient was brought in casualty after a road traffic accident. He is comatose with unilaterally dilated pupil. The NCCT of the patient shows a lesion peripherally present with concavo-convex border. What is the probable diagnosis? *(PGMEE 2015-16)*
a. Sub-arachnoid hemorrhage
b. Epi-dural hematoma,
c. Intra-parenchymal bleeding
d. Sub-dural hematoma

[Ref: Harrison's 19th/e pg.1772, 442e]

94. Lucid interval is seen in:- *(PGMEE 2016-17)*
a. EDH   b. SDH
c. SAH   d. Parenchymal bleed

[Ref: Harrison's 19th/e pg. 2576-77]

95. Acute extradural hemorrhage (EDH) is seen as: *(PGMEE 2015-16)*
a. Hypodense biconvex
b. Hypodense biconcave
c. Hyperdense biconcave
d. Hyperdense biconvex

[Ref: Internet]

96. Which can be safely given in hemorrhagic stroke? *(PGMEE 2015)*
a. Normal Saline   b. Hypertonic fluids
c. Colloids   d. Blood transfusion

[Ref: Harrison's 19th/e p. 1779]

97. Subdural haemorrhage is due to injury to:- *(PGMEE 2016-17)*
a. Middle meningeal artery
b. Middle meningeal vein
c. Cortical bridging veins
d. Middle cerebral vein

[Ref: Harrison's 19th/e pg.1772, 442e]

98. Which of the following nerve is first affected in berry aneurysm: *(PGMEE 2015-16)*
a. 3rd nerve
b. 4th nerve
c. 5th nerve
d. 6th nerve

[Ref: Harrison's 19th/e pg. 1784-85]

99. Least common site for Berry Aneurysm: *(PGMEE 2014/15)*
a. Junction of anterior cerebral artery and internal carotid artery
b. Posterior cerebral artery
c. Vertebral artery
d. Basilar artery

[Ref: Neuro-Imaging, Roy Riascos, Pg 1061]

100. Most common vessel involved in rupture of Berry aneurysm :- *(PGMEE 2016-17)*
a. ACA
b. Anterior communicating artery
c. MCA
d. PCA

101. Death after rupture of Berry aneurysm is due to:
a. Re-bleeding *(PGMEE 2014/15)*
b. Myocardial infarction
c. Intra-ventricular hemorrhage
d. Cerebral ischemia

[Ref: Harrison's 19th/e pg. 1785]

102. Which vessel DOESN'T form circle of willis: *(PGMEE 2015-16)*
a. Internal carotid artery
b. Anterior cerebral artery
c. Posterior cerebral artery
d. Middle cerebral artery

[Ref: Gray's Anatomy 40th ed. / 246]

103. Anterior inferior cerebellar arterial occlusion can cause: *(PGMEE 2014/15)*
a. Contralateral lower leg weakness
b. Hemianaesthesia of opposite half of the face
c. Hemianopia
d. Urinary retention

[Ref: Harrison's 19th/e pg. 2576]

104. Hemiparesis is *not* seen with: *(PGMEE 2014/15)*
a. Weber syndrome
b. Middle cerebral artery stroke
c. Posterior cerebral artery stroke
d. Vertebral artery stroke

[Ref: Harrison's 19th/e pg. 2576-77]

105. Elderly man complains of three episodes of visual loss in right eye over 20 minutes. Blood vessel involved is: *(PGMEE 2014/15)*
a. Anterior cerebral artery
b. Basilar artery
c. Internal carotid artery
d. Middle cerebral artery

[Ref: Harrison's 19th/e pg.2568]

106. Which is true about CADASIL? *(PGMEE 2014/15)*
a. Onset is usually in the fourth or fifth decade of life
b. White matter changes
c. Monogenic stroke syndrome
d. All of the above

[Ref: Harrison's 19th/e pg. 2568]

Explanation

- CADASIL stands for cerebral autosomal dominant arteriopathy with subcortical infarcts and leuko encephalopathy.
- Caused by mutation in NOTCH3
- **Age of onset:** 45–50 years
- **Feature:** Dementia, migraine, recurrent strokes
- **MRI:** Deep white mater changes predominantly involving temporal lobe

107. Features of posterior inferior cerebellar artery thrombosis include all of the following EXCEPT:
a. Sudden onset of severe vertigo *(PGMEE 2014/15)*
b. Horner's syndrome
c. Acute cerebellar symptoms with nystagmus to the side of lesion the involvement
d. Palsy of 10,11,12 nerves

[Ref: Harrison's 19th/e pg. 2576]

108. Following are features of ischemia in anterior choroidal artery territory EXCEPT: *(PGMEE 2014/15)*
a. Hemiparesis
b. Predominant involvement of the anterior limb of internal capsule
c. Homonymous hemianopia
d. Hemisensory loss

[Ref: Harrison's 19th/e pg. 2573-74]

109. A 80 year diabetic patient presents with right sided weakness of face, arm and leg. Sensation, speech and comprehension are intact. Blood vessel involved is: *(PGMEE 2014/15)*
a. Anterior cerebral artery
b. Anterior choroidal artery
c. Internal carotid artery
d. Lenticulostriate artery

[Ref: Harrison's 19th/e pg. 2572]

110. Pin point pupils are due to damage to: *(PGMEE 2014/15)*
a. Edinger Westphal nucleus
b. Descending sympathetic pathways
c. Superior colliculus
d. Lateral geniculate body

[Ref: Harrison's 19th/e pg. 1774]

111. History of transient ischemic attack, excludes:
a. Amaurosis fugax *(PGMEE 2014/15)*
b. Seizures
c. Weak shoulder shrugging
d. Asymmetrical mouth retraction

[Ref: Harrison's 19th/e pg. 2568]

98.	a
99.	c
100.	b
101.	d
102.	d
103.	b
104.	d
105.	c
106.	d
107.	d
108.	b
109.	d
110.	b
111.	b

112. Pontine Stroke is associated with all EXCEPT:
(PGMEE 2014/15)
a. Vagal palsy   b. Pyrexia
c. Quadriparesis   d. Bilateral pin point pupil

[Ref: Harrison's 19th/e pg. 2579f]

113. Posterior cerebral artery occlusion leads to loss of memory due to involvement of: *(PGMEE 2014/15)*
a. Superior temporal gyrus
b. Supra marginal gyrus
c. Hippocampus
d. Angular gyrus

[Ref: Harrison's 19th/e pg. 2575]

114. In a patient with ruptured cerebral aneurysm, cause of delayed neurological symptoms are, all EXCEPT:
a. Hydrocephalus   *(PGMEE 2014/15)*
b. Rebleed
c. Enlargement of aneurysm
d. Spasm

[Ref: Harrison's 19th/e pg. 1785]

115. Thrombosis of Anterior cerebral artery, distal to the communicating branch leads to: *(PGMEE 2014/15)*
a. Seizures
b. Ipsilateral hemiparesis
c. Contralateral Hemiparesis
d. Incontinence

[Ref: Harrison's 19th/e pg. 2573]

116. Retrograde amnesia in injury to which lobe:-
(PGMEE 2016-17)
a. Frontal lobe
b. Temporal lobe
c. Parietal lobe
d. Occipital lobe

117. A patient came with symptoms of stroke and the following was seen on the NCCT. What should be next step? *(NEET Pattern 2017)*

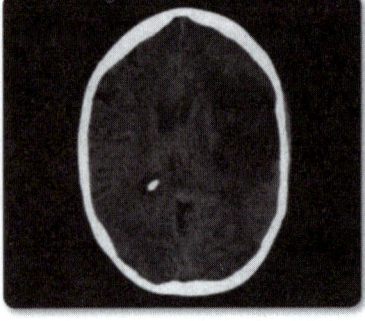

a. IV mannitol
b. Decompressive craniotomy
c. Thrombectomy
d. Aspirin and clopidogrel

Explanation

- Image shown here is a NCCT head showing wedge shaped hypodense area in left frontal region suggestive of ischemic stroke in the left MCA territory with compression of the left anterior horn and slight midline

shift. Right lateral ventricle shows calcification of the choroid plexus.

Now let's discuss each option

- Trials have shown neither beneficial nor harmful effects of mannitol in patients with stroke to reduce swelling. There is not enough of evidence to decide if mannitol improves survival or prevent disability after stroke. Hence, use of mannitol is not a part of standard of care in stroke and may be judiciously used depending on clinical status of patient (which is not provided in the question).
- Decompressive hemicranioctomy for space occupying MCA infarction results in large reductions in mortality; the level of function in the survivors, and implications, remain controversial. It is a reserve modality in current practice for cases of malignant MCA infarct as a life saving measure.
- Thrombectomy cannot be considered in this case as time frame of presentation is not specified.
- Aspirin is the only antiplatelet agent that has been proven effective for the acute treatment of ischemic stroke. Combination of aspirin and clopidogrel has shown no added advantage and data on clinical safety is limited in this regard.
- Thus the correct answer to this question should be none; but to mark one, IV mannitol seems the most appropriate answer.

118. Thrombosis of the Superior branch of middle cerebral artery leads to: *(PGMEE 2014/15)*
a. Urinary retention
b. Grasp reflex
c. Bitemporal hemianopia
d. Motor aphasia

[Ref: Harrison's 19th/e pg. 2573]

119. All are true about Broca's aphasia EXCEPT:
a. Repetition is impaired   *(PGMEE 2014/15)*
b. Damage to posterior part of inferior frontal Gyrus
c. Syntax is preserved
d. Non fluent aphasia

[Ref: Harrison's 19th/e pg. 177T, 178]

120. Which of the following is not a usual feature of right middle cerebral artery territory infarct?
(PGMEE 2014/15)
a. Dysarthria   b. Hemiparesis
c. Facial weakness d. Aphasia

[Ref: Harrison's 19th/e pg. 2573]

121. A lady can't speak but can tell by writing. Which of the following brain areas is affected? *(PGMEE 2015-16)*
a. Broca's area   b. Insula
c. Paracentral lobule d. Wernicke's area

[Ref: Harrison's 19th/e pg. 177]

122. Left lobe of the brain is responsible for:
(PGMEE 2014/15)
a. Enjoying music   b. Processing of speech
c. Spatial orientation d. Fine motor movement

[Ref: Harrison's 18th ed. P-202]

123. Duration of TIA is less than? *(PGMEE 2015-16)*
a. 12 hours
b. 24 hours
c. 48 hours
d. 36 hours

[Ref: Harrison's 19th/e pg. 2568]

124. A patient presents with subarachnoid haemorrhage. NCCT reveals blood in the fourth ventricle. The bleeding is most likely to occur from an aneurysm of which of the following arteries? *(PGMEE 2012)*
a. AICA
b. PICA
c. Basilar top region
d. Anterior communicating artery

[Ref: Handbook of Neurosurgery, Greenberg, Pg. 2601]

125. The most common cause of embolic stroke:
a. Paradoxical embolism
b. Carotid artery atherosclerosis
c. Non rheumatic atrial fibrillation
d. LV aneurysm

[Ref: Harrison's 19th/e pg. 2565]

126. What is true about Lacunar stroke: *(PGMEE 2014/15)*
a. Young male with mycotic aneurysm
b. Male with HTN
c. Female on OCP
d. Young male with AV malformation

[Ref: Harrison's 19th/e pg. 2565]

127. Most common site of cerebral infarction is in the territory of: *(PGMEE 2014/15)*
a. Posterior cerebral artery
b. Anterior cerebral artery
c. Middle cerebral artery
d. Posterior inferior cerebellar artery

[Ref: Harrison's 19th/e pg. 2572]

128. Hemiplegia is most often caused by thrombosis of:
a. Anterior cerebral artery *(PGMEE 2014/15)*
b. Basilar artery
c. Posterior cerebral artery
d. Middle cerebral artery

[Ref: Harrison's 19th/e pg. 2572-73]

129. Presence of hemiplegia with homonymous hemianopia with gaze to same side is seen with occlusion of which brain vessel? *(PGMEE 2014/15)*
a. Basilar artery
b. Internal carotid artery
c. Anterior cerebral artery
d. Middle cerebral artery

[Ref: Harrison's 19th/e pg. 2573]

130. Cerebral infarct is earliest detected by:
(PGMEE 2014/15)
a. CT scan
b. PET scan
c. MRI scan
d. Diffusion weighted MRI

[Ref: Harrison's 19th/e pg. 2580]

131. A hypertensive patient presents with severe headache and vomiting. He has got neck stiffness but no Focal Neurological Deficit. What is the most probable diagnosis? *(PGMEE 2014/15)*
a. SAH
b. Meningo-encephalitis
c. Meningitis
d. Intra-cerebral bleed

[Ref: Harrison's 19th/e pg. 1785]

132. Hemianopia, cortical blindness, amnesia and thalamic pain are associated with the occlusion of: *(PGMEE 2014/15)*
a. Anterior cerebral artery
b. Basilar artery
c. Middle cerebral artery
d. Posterior cerebral artery

[Ref: Harrison's 20th/e pg. 3073, 74]

133. A diabetes patient with BP of 220/130 mm Hg is brought to the casualty in comatose state. CT scan shows a large infarct. What is the target BP of this patient to initiate thrombolysis? *(PGMEE 2014/15)*
a. Less than 200/130
b. Less than 185/110
c. Less than 160/100
d. Less than 140/90

[Ref: Harrison's 20th/e pg. 3081]

134. Hypertensive patient presents with one day history of headache, nausea, vomiting and difficulty in walking. Diagnosis is? *(PGMEE 2014/15)*
a. Extradural haemorrhage
b. Sub-arachnoid haemorrhage
c. Sub-dural haemorrhage
d. Intra-parenchymal haemorrhage

[Ref: Harrison's 19th/e pg. 2582]

135. A 26 year old healthy female got pregnant for the first time and a LSCS was done for fetal distress. Mild hypertension was present during pregnancy. 2 days after delivery she had headache and seizures. CT shows 2X3 cm para-sagittal lesion. Urinalysis shows no proteinuria. Diagnosis is: *(NEET Pattern 2013)*
a. Hypertensive I.C.H.
b. Sagittal sinus thrombosis
c. Pituitary apoplexy
d. Eclampsia

136. A road traffic accident patient in the casualty is comatose with unilaterally dilated pupil. The NCCT of the patient shows a lesion peripherally present with concavo-convex border. What is the probable diagnosis?
a. Sub-dural hematoma *(PGMEE 2015)*
b. Intra-parenchymal bleeding
c. Epi-dural hematoma
d. Sub-arachnoid hemorrhage

[Ref: Harrison 19th/e p. 1772]

137. Commonest cause of cerebrovascular accident: *(PGMEE 2015-16)*
a. Hemorrhage
b. Aortic dissection
c. Embolism
d. Thrombosis

[Ref: Harrison's 20th/e pg. 3069]

138. Target BP before thrombolysis in ischemic stroke is below:- *(PGMEE 2015-16)*
a. 185/110 mm Hg
b. 165/100mm Hg
c. 145/100 Hg
d. 120/80mmHg

[Ref: Harrison 20th ed. pg. 3081]

139. A hypertensive patient is brought with a BP of 220/130 mmHg to the casualty. CT scan shows an infarct. What should be the primary BP of the patient to start thrombolysis? *(PGMEE 2014-15)*
a. <200/150
b. <180/110
c. <165/120
d. <140/90

[Ref: Harrison 20th ed. pg. 3081]

123.	b
124.	b
125.	c
126.	b
127.	c
128.	d
129.	d
130.	d
131.	a
132.	d
133.	b
134.	d
135.	b
136.	a
137.	d
138.	a
139.	b

140. After an attack of TIA (Transient Ischemic attack), maximum risk of stroke is seen at: *(NEET 2018)*
a. Within 48 hr
b. within 1 month
c. 1 wk
d. 1 year

[Ref:Harrison's 19th/e pg. 2559]

Explanation

- The risk of stroke following a TIA episode is ~10–15% in the first 3 months, with most events occurring in the first 2 days.
- The risk of stroke following a TIA can be estimated using the ABCD₂ score.It scores things such as your **a**ge, **b**lood pressure and whether you have **d**iabetes. It also looks at the **c**omplaints (symptoms) you had and how long they lasted for.

BRAIN STEM SYNDROMES

141. Lateral medullary syndrome or Wallenberg syndrome involves all EXCEPT: *(DNB Dec 2009)*
a. 5th cranial nerve
b. 9the cranial nerve
c. 10th cranial nerve
d. 12th cranial nerve

[Ref: Harrison's 20th/e pg. 3073]

142. Which of the following is not involved in lateral medullary syndrome? *(PGMEE 2014/15)*
a. Sympathetic tract
b. IX, X, XI cranial nerves
c. XIIth cranial nerve
d. Spinothalamic tract

[Ref: Harrison's 20th/e pg. 3073]

143. Most common cause of lateral medullary syndrome is occlusion of: *(PGMEE 2014/15, 2009)*
a. Superior cerebellar artery
b. Anterior inferior cerebellar artery
c. Posterior inferior cerebellar artery
d. Intracranial portion of the vertebral artery

[Ref: Harrison's 20th/e pg. 3073]

144. Embolism of PICA causes: *(NEET Pattern 2019)*
a. Wallenberg syndrome
b. Weber syndrome
c. Horner syndrome
d. Medial medullary syndrome

[Ref: Harrison's 20th/e pg. 3073]

145. Thrombosis of PICA leads to *(PGMEE 2019)*
a. Weber syndrome
b. Medial medullary syndrome
c. Wallenberg syndrome
d. Millard Gubler syndrome

[Ref: Harrison's 20th/e pg. 3073]

146. Lateral medullary syndrome is associated with:
a. Dense hemianesthesia *(PGMEE 2014/15)*
b. No sensory deficit is seen
c. Crossed hemianesthesia
d. Dissociative anesthesia

[Ref: Harrison's 20th/e pg. 3073]

147. Characteristic features of a lesion in the lateral part of the medulla include all EXCEPT: *(PGMEE 2014/15)*
a. Contralateral loss of proprioception to the body and limbs
b. Dysphagia
c. Nystagmus
d. Ipsilateral Horner's syndrome

[Ref: Harrison's 20th/e pg. 3073]

148. Ipsilateral 3rd nerve palsy with contralateral hemiplegia is known as: *(PGMEE 2014/15)*
a. Millard Gubler syndrome
b. Benedicts syndrome
c. Foville syndrome
d. Weber's syndrome

[Ref: Harrison's 20th/e pg. 3072]

149. True about Weber's syndrome are all EXCEPT:
a. Diplopia *(DNB Dec 2009)*
b. Opthalmoplegia
c. Contralateral hemiplegia
d. Contralateral facial nerve palsy

[Ref: Harrison's 20th/e pg. 3073]

150. Weber syndrome is characterized by: *(PGMEE 2018)*
a. Ipsilateral 3rd nerve palsy
b. Contralateral hemiplegia
c. Involvement of dorsal midbrain
d. Involvement of cerebral peduncle

151. Thrombotic occlusion of Posterior inferior cerebellar artery is associated with: *(PGMEE 2018)*
a. Benedict syndrome
b. Wallenberg syndrome
c. Medial medullary syndrome
d. Schmidt's syndrome?

152. In Balint syndrome all are seen except? *(PGMEE 2015)*
a. Optic ataxia
b. Ocular apraxia
c. Opsoclonus
d. Simultagnosia

[Ref: Harrison's 20th/e pg. 162]

Explanation

- Balint's Syndrome is an uncommon triad of **Simultagnosia** (Inability to perceive the visual field as a whole), **Oculomotor apraxia** (Difficulty in fixating the eyes) and **Optic ataxia** (Inability to move the hand to a specific object by using vision).
- It is seen in parietal lobe lesions.

NEURODEGENERATIVE DISORDER

DEMENTIA

153. Reversible dementia is seen in *(PGMEE 2014/15)*
a. Wilson
b. Myxedema
c. Alzheimer's
d. Huntington disease

[Ref: Harrison's 20th/e pg. 154]

Explanation

- Reversible causes of dementia:
  - D - Drug intoxication; Depression (pseudodementia)
  - E - Endocrine (Hypothyroidism)

140.	a
141.	d
142.	c
143.	d
144.	a
145.	c
146.	c
147.	a
148.	d
149.	d
150.	c
151.	b
152.	c
153.	b

- ○ M - Metabolic Autoimmune causes
- ○ E - Electrolyte imbalance (Hyponatremia)
- ○ N - Nutritional (Vit B_{12} deficiency, Thiamine deficiency) & NDH
- ○ T - Brain tumor
- ○ I - Infectious causes
- ○ A - Alcohol intoxication/withdrawal

154. Incorrect about Dementia pugilistica:
(PGMEE 2015-16)
a. Decreased cognition   b. Difficulty in gait
c. Seen in boxers   d. Nystagmus

[Ref: Harrison's 20th/e pg. 3114]

Explanation

- ■ Dementia pugilistica
  - ○ Aka punch - drunk syndrome; Chronic traumatic encephalopathy
  - ○ Seen in boxers & contact sport athletes
  - ○ CF : Decline in cognition, gait difficulty, intentional tremors, memory loss & dementia

155. Which of the following sites is responsible for the amnestic defect in Wernicke's Korsakoff- syndrome -
(PGMEE 2015)
a. Mamillary body & Thalamus
b. Putamen
c. Medial fore brain bundle
d. Subthalmic nucleus

[Ref: Harrison's 20th/e pg. 3112]

156. Wernicke's Encephalopathy seen in which deficiency:-
(PGMEE 2016-17)
a. Thiamine   b. Niacin
c. Riboflavin   d. Pyridoxine

[Ref: Harrison's 20th/e pg. 3112]

157. Wernicke's encephalopathy develops secondary to accumulation of which substrate? *(NEET Pattern 2019)*
a. Glutamate
b. Lactate
c. Acetate
d. Aspartate

158. A chronic alcoholic developed ataxia, nausea, vomiting, and ophthalmolegia. Diagnosis is :- *(PGMEE 2016-17)*
a. Korsakoff psychosis
b. Wernickes encephalopathy
c. Cerebellar infarction
d. Alcohol Intoxication

[Ref: Harrison's 20th/e pg. 3112]

159. Which of the following is not involved in Wernicke's Korsakoff psychosis- *(PGMEE 2015)*
a. Mamillary body
b. Periventricular Grey matter
c. Thalamus
d. Hippocampus

[Ref: Harrison's 20th/e pg. 3112]

ALZHEIMER'S DISEASE (AD)

160. Which Apo E protein is associated with Alzheimer disease *(PGMEE 2019)*
a. APO EI   b. APO EII
c. APO EIII   d. APO EIV

[Ref: Harrison's 20th/e pg. 3108]

161. Which of the following disease occurs in increased frequency in patient with Downs syndrome
(PGMEE 2019)
a. Alzheimer disease   b. Lewy body dementia
c. Parkinson disease   d. None of the above

162. Risk factors for Alzheimer's disease include?
(PGMEE 2019)
a. Klinefelter syndrome   b. Noonan syndrome
c. Down's syndrome   d. None

[Ref: Harrison's 20th/e pg. 3108]

163. Which lobe is affected in the early course of Alzheimer's disease? *(NEET Pattern 2019)*
a. Medial temporal lobe   b. Lateral temporal lobe
c. Parietal lobe   d. Frontal lobe

164. True about Alzheimer disease are all except
(PGMEE 2018)
a. Neurofibrillary tangles are intracellular inclusions
b. Amyloid plaques are extracellular deposits
c. Destruction of cholinergic neuron in Nucleus basilis of Meynert
d. Short term memory loss is seen

[Ref: Harrison's 20th/e pg. 3108, 09]

165. Neurofibrillary tangles are seen in? *(DNB June 2010)*
a. Alzheimer's disease   b. Lewy body disease
c. Shy dragger syndrome   d. Neurosyphilis

[Ref: Harrison's 20th/e pg. 3108]

166. Alzheimer type II astrocytes are not seen in?
(PGMEE 2015-16)
a. Alzheimer's disease   b. Chronic liver disease
c. Hyperammonemia   d. Wilson's disease

[Ref: Robbins 9th/e pg. 1253]

167. Rapidly progressive dementia is seen in?
(PGMEE 2016-17)
a. Alzheimer's disease   b. Vascular dementia
c. HIV Dementia   d. Parkinson's disease

[Ref: Robbins 9th/e pg. 1287]

168. Alzheimer's disease is associated with all EXCEPT?
(PGMEE 2016-17)
a. Chromosome 1   b. Chromosome 21
c. Chromosome 19   d. Chromosome 22

[Ref: Harrison's 20th/e pg. 3110]

169. All of the following inclusions are seen in Alzheimer's disease EXCEPT? *(PGMEE 2016-17)*
a. Senile plaques
b. Neurofibrillary tangles
c. Cerebral amyloid angiopathy
d. Lafora bodies

[Ref: Harrison's 20th/e pg. 3108]

154.	d
155.	a
156.	a
157.	a
158.	b
159.	d
160.	d
161.	a
162.	c
163.	a
164.	d
165.	a
166.	a
167.	c
168.	d
169.	d

202. Which of the following is not a test for integrity of 7th and 9th nerve: *(PGMEE 2015-16)*
- a. Taste
- b. Palate symmetry
- c. Tongue protrusion
- d. Position of uvula

[Ref: Harrison's 20th/e pg. 3028]

203. Right 12th nerve damage leads to ? *(PGMEE 2015-16)*
- a. Tongue deviation to left on protrusion
- b. Tongue deviation to right on protrusion
- c. Nasal twang to voice
- d. Scanning speech defects

[Ref: Harrison's 19th/e Ch 367]

Explanation

CN lesion	Side of deviation	Structure affected
5th CN	I/L OR Paralysed site	Jaw deviation
7th CN	C/L or opposite side	Angle of mouth
10th CN	Dviates away from sili of lesia - cl	Uvcula
12th CN	Towards affected site	Tongue

204. Cranial Nerve 8 palsy causes all EXCEPT: *(PGMEE 2015-16)*
- a. Motion sickness
- b. Vertigo
- c. Gag reflex
- d. Tinnitus

[Ref: Harrison's 20th/e pg. 3028]

205. The triad of strabismus, diplopia and ptosis are caused due to damage of which nerves: *(PGMEE 2014/15)*
- a. Oculomotor
- b. Cervical sympathetic truk
- c. Abducent
- d. Trochlear

[Ref: Harrison's 19th/e pg. 2537]

206. Facial nerve involvement in herpes zoster is known as?
- a. Ramsay hunt syndrome *(DNB Dec 2009)*
- b. Melkersson Rosenthal syndrome
- c. Jaw wrinkling syndrome
- d. Frey's syndrome

[Ref: Harrison's 20th/e pg. 3155]

MULTIPLE SCLEROSIS

207. Which of the following is the most common initial presenting feature of multiple sclerosis-
- a. Optic neuritis *(PGMEE 2015 , 2011)*
- b. Diplopia
- c. Cerebellar ataxia
- d. Internuclear ophthalmoplegia

[Ref: Harrison's 20th/e pg. 3188]

208. 30 year old female presents with complaints of gradual onset weakness of legs for >1 month with reduction in visual acuity and urinary incontinence for past few days. Contrast MRI shows periventricular lesions. Which of the following drugs is not used in these patients? *(PGMEE 2014/15)*
- a. Glatiramer acetate
- b. Beta interferon
- c. Mitotane
- d. Fingolimod

[Ref: Harrison's 19th/e pg. 2669]

209. Multiple sclerosis is not associated with? *(DNB June 2011)*
- a. Hydrocephalus
- b. Amiodarone
- c. Optic neuritis
- d. Spinal cord involvement

[Ref: Robbin's 7th/e pg. 1384; Harrison's 19th/e pg. 2663]

210. Most common type of multiple sclerosis? *(PGMEE 2015)*
- a. Progressive relapsing multiple sclerosis
- b. Relapsing remitting type
- c. Primary progressive multiple sclerosis
- d. Secondary progressive multiple sclerosis

[Ref: Harrison's 20th/e pg. 3189]

211. Drug that causes maximum reduction in appearance of new lesions and change in disease severity in multiple sclerosis is: *(PGMEE 2014/15)*
- a. Glatiramer
- b. Natalizumab
- c. Interferon beta 1a
- d. Interferon beta 1b

[Ref: Harrison's 20th/e pg. 3196]

212. Pulfrich effect is seen in: *(PGMEE 2014/15)*
- a. Red green color blindness
- b. C.I.D.P
- c. C.R.P.S
- d. Multiple sclerosis

SPINAL CORD SYNDROMES

213. Most common part of spine involved in malignant spinal cord compression: *(PGMEE 2014-15)*
- a. Cervical
- b. Sacral
- c. Lumbar
- d. Thoracic

[Ref: Harrison's 20th/e pg. 3175]

Explanation

- Malignant/ metastatic spinal cord syndrome is a oncological emergency and may be the first presentation of cancer.
- Most common route of spread is hematogenous.
- Most common site of compression is the lower thoracic vertebrae followed by lumbar spine.
- Most common malignancy associated are: Breast > Lung > Prostate > Multiple myeloma

214. Clinical features of conus medullaris are all EXCEPT:
- a. Late bladder involvement *(DNB June 2011)*
- b. Lower sacral and coccygeal involvement
- c. Sacral anesthesia
- d. Extensor plantar

[Ref: Harrison's 20th/e pg. 3173]

215. Which is not true of Tables dorsalis? *(DNB June 2010)*
- a. Seen in neuro syphilis
- b. Abdominal pain and visceral symptoms occur
- c. Deep tendon reflexes are retained
- d. Paresthesia is seen

[Ref: Harrison's 20th/e pg. 3181]

202. c
203. b
204. c
205. a
206. a
207. a
208. c
209. a
210. b
211. b
212. d
213. d
214. a
215. c

216. Dissociative sensory loss is seen in all EXCEPT:
a. Anterior spinal artery occlusion **(PGMEE 2014/15)**
b. Leprosy
c. Hydromyelia
d. Multiple system atrophy

[Ref: 250 cases in clinical medicine pg. 70-71]

Explanation

- Dissociative sensory loss refers to the selective loss of fine touch and proprioception without loss of pain and temperature sensation, OR vice versa.
- Pain and temperature is carried by Lateral Spinothalamic tract whereas touch and proprioception by dorsal column.
- Causes:
  ○ Syringomyelia
  ○ Diabetes
  ○ Brown sequard syndrome
  ○ Anterior spinal artery thrombosis
  ○ SACD
  ○ MS
  ○ Tabes dorsalis

217. Dose of methylprednisolone following spine injury:
  (PGMEE 2014/15)
a. 30 mg/kg within 3 hrs of injury
b. 45 mg/kg within 6 hrs of injury
c. 50 mg/kg within 9 hrs of injury
d. 60 mg/kg within 12 hrs of injury

218. Dissociative sensory loss is not seen in:
  (PGMEE 2014/15)
a. Syringomyelia
b. Damage to spino-thalamic pathways
c. Diabetes mellitus
d. Cauda equina syndrome

[Ref: Harrison's 19th/e pg. 2651]

219. Hypotension in acute spinal cord injury is due to:
  (PGMEE 2014/15)
a. Vasovagal Attack
b. Loss of Parasympathetic tone
c. Orthostatic Hypotension
d. Loss of sympathetic tone

[Ref: CMDT 2013, Pg 1018]

BROWN SEQUARD SYNDROME

220. In Brown Sequard syndrome all are seen except-
a. C/L spinothalamic tract involvement
b. Ipsilateral extensor plantar response
c. Ipsilateral pyramidal tract involvement
d. C/L posterior column involvement

[Ref: Harrison 18th/e p. 3361, 191]

221. Brown sequered syndrome is characterized by all EXCEPT:- **(PGMEE 2018)**
a. Contralateral loss of pain
b. Contralateral loss of temperature
c. Ipsilateral loss of vibration sense
d. Ipsilateral loss of joint and position

222. True regarding brown Sequard syndrome on the side of lesion **(PGMEE 2019)**
a. Loss of pain and temperature
b. Loss of stereognosis
c. Hyperaesthesia
d. Loss of vibration and proprioception

SACD

223. Sub-acute combined degeneration of spinal cord is seen in: **(PGMEE 2014/15)**
a. Thiamin deficiency
b. Industrial toxin damage to spinal cord
c. Tuberculosis of spine
d. Pernicious anemia

[Ref: Harrison's 20th/e pg. 3181]

224. Subacute combined degeneration of spinal cord is caused by deficiency of? **(PGMEE 2012)**
a. Vitamin B_1 b. Vitamin B_5
c. Vitamin B_6 d. Vitamin B_{12}

[Ref: Harrison's 20th/e pg. 3181]

SYRINGOMYELIA

225. Onion skin pattern of sensory loss in face is seen:
a. Amyloidotic polyneuropathy **(PGMEE 2014/15)**
b. Diabetes mellitus
c. Syringomyelia
d. Leprosy

[Ref: Harrison's 19th/e pg. 2658]

Explanation

- Onion skin pattern of facial sensory loss refers to graded sensory loss with perioral sparing (Dejerine pattern). It is seen in intramedullary or cervicomedullary lesion due to involvement of the trigeminal nucleus which extends into the entire brainstem.

GULLAIN-BARRE SYNDROME

226. Ascending motor weakness without bowel or bladder involvement **(PGMEE 2019)**
a. Transverse myelitis
b. GBS
c. Polio myelitis
d. Inflammatory myopathy

[Ref: Harrison's 20th/e pg. 3225]

227. True about Gullain-Barre syndrome is all EXCEPT:
a. Inflammatory **(DNB December 2011)**
b. Plasmapheresis can be done
c. Descending paralysis
d. Demyelinating

[Ref: Harrison's 20th/e pg. 3225]

Explanation

- In GBS ascending paralysis (distal to proximal) is seen.

216. d
217. a
218. d
219. d
220. d
221. None
222. d
223. d
224. d
225. c
226. b
227. c

228. CSF finding in Gullian Barre syndrome is?
(PGMEE 2015-16)
a. Normal cells with increased protein
b. Normal cells and normal protein
c. Increased cells with low sugar
d. Increased protein with increased cells
[Ref: Harrison's 20th/e pg. 3227]

229. All are true regarding treatment of Guillain-barre syndrome EXCEPT: *(DNB June 2011)*
a. Corticosteroid used for early recovery and prevent long stay
b. High-dose intravenous immune globulin (IVIg) and plasmapheresis are equally effective
c. Plasmapheresis can be done
d. High-dose intravenous immune globulin (IVIg) can be initiated
[Ref: Harrison's 20th/e pg. 3229]

230. A man has acute onset of paraplegia with symmetrical bilateral areflexia. Diagnosis is: *(PGMEE 2015-16)*
a. Poliomyelitis
b. Acute transverse myelitis
c. Guillian Barre syndrome
d. Subacute combined degenerative disorder
[Ref: Harrison's 20th/e pg. 3225]

231. Which is not seen in Miller Fisher syndrome:
a. Anti-GQ1 antibodies *(PGMEE 2014/15)*
b. Postural hypotension
c. Cranial nerve palsy
d. Ataxia
[Ref: Harrison's 20th/e pg. 3226]

Explanation
- Subtypes of GBS include AMAN, AMSAN and Miller-Fisher syndrome.
- Miller-Fisher syndrome presents as a triad of Areflexia, Ataxia and Ophthalmoplegia.
- Anti-GQ1b antibodies are seen in Miller Fisher syndrome

232. Miller Fisher test is used for: *(PGMEE 2014/15)*
a. Grading muscle involvement in ALS
b. Severity of paralysis in Gullian Barre syndrome
c. Measuring disability in multiple sclerosis
d. Evaluating cognition in normal pressure hydrocephalus
[Ref: Page 625, Neurology Review, Andrew Tarulli, 2011]

PERIPHERAL NEUROPATHY

233. Palpable nerves are seen in: *(PGMEE 2014/15)*
a. Myotonic dystrophy
b. Diabetes mellitus
c. Charcot Marie Tooth disease
d. Neurosyphilis
[Ref: Harrison's 18th ed., ch:384]

Explanation
- Causes:
  ○ Leprosy
  ○ Amyloidosis
  ○ Diabetes
  ○ Neurofibromatosis
  ○ Charcot-Marie-Tooth disease

234. Isaac syndrome is characterised by? *(PGMEE 2015)*
a. Limbic encephalitis
b. Opsoclonus
c. Encephalomyelitis
d. Peripheral nerve excitability
[Ref: Harrison 19th/e p. 619]

Explanation
- Isaac syndrome is a form of peripheral nerve hyperexcitability resulting in spontaneous muscular activity.

235. A patient after alcoholic drink fell asleep in chair overnight with hanging arm and develops Saturday Night Palsy. Which of the following best describes the clinical manifestations? *(PGMEE 2015-16)*
a. Neuropraxia b. Necroptosis
c. Neurotmesis d. Axonotmesis
[Ref: Maheshwari 5th ed. /69]

236. Arsenic poisoning causes? *(PGMEE 2015-16)*
a. Mononeuritis multiplex b. Myelopathy
c. Radiculopathy d. Polyneuritis
[Ref: Harrison's 20th/e pg. 3298]

237. High Steppage Gait is seen in? *(PGMEE 2015-16)*
a. Foot drop b. Leprosy
c. Frontal lobe stroke d. Tabes dorsalis
[Ref: Harrison's 20th/e pg. 145]

DISORDERS OF N-M JUNCTION

238. About myasthenia gravis pathogenesis, true is: *(NEET Pattern 2019)*
a. Antibody against Ca receptor
b. Blockage of nerve conduction through myoneural junction
c. Antibody against Ach receptor
d. Ach is not secreted

239. Lambert-Eaton syndrome true is: *(NEET Pattern 2019)*
a. It is a paraneoplastic syndrome associated with squamous cell carcinoma of lung
b. With continuous stimulation there is marked increase in amplitude of action potentials
c. IgM antibodies against ligand gated calcium channels
d. There is increase in release of presynaptic acetylcholine

240. A patient had proptosis and ptosis, which was relieved within 5 mins of administering IV drug. What is the diagnosis?
a. Myasthenia gravis
b. 3rd nerve palsy
c. Grave's ophthalmopathy
d. 6th nerve palsy
[Ref: Harrison's 20th/e pg. 3234]

Answers
228. a
229. a
230. c
231. b
232. d
233. b,c
234. d
235. a
236. d
237. a
238. c
239. b
240. a

Explanation

- Reversibility of clinical feature is a characteristic feature of Myasthenic weakness.
- The drug administered iv is Edrophonium (tensilon) which is a short-acting AChE inhibitor that improves muscle weakness in patients with MG. Pharmacologic inhibition of AChE increases ACh concentration at the NMJ, improving the chance for interactions between ACh and its receptor. This test evaluates weakness (eg, ptosis, partial or complete ophthalmoplegia, and forced hand grip) in an involved group of muscles before and after intravenous (IV) administration of edrophonium. Edrophonium is used most commonly for diagnostic testing because of the rapid onset (30 s) and short duration (~5 min) of its effect.

241. Most common manifestation of myasthenia gravis
(PGMEE 2019)
a. Proptosis   b. Anhidrosis
c. Ptosis   d. Enophthalmos

242. Myasthenia gravis is associated with- *(PGMEE 2012-13)*
a. Thymoma   b. Lymphoma
c. Thymic carcinoma d. Thymic hyperplasia
[Ref: Harrison's 20th/e pg. 3232]

243. Pathogenesis of Myasthenia gravis:- *(PGMEE 2018)*
a. Auto- antibodies against acetylcholine receptors
b. Mutations in raynodine receptors
c. Autoantigens synaptotagmin
d. Antibodies against acetylcholine esterase
[Ref: Harrison's 20th/e pg. 3232]

244. Not associated with thymoma?
a. Red cell aplasia *(PGMEE 2014-15, DNB June 2010)*
b. Myasthenia gravis
c. Hypergammaglobulinemia
d. Ulcerative colitis
[Ref: Harrison's 20th/e pg. 553]

Explanation

- Paraneoplastic syndromes associated with thymic tumors:
  ○ Myasthenia gravis
  ○ Rheumatoid arthritis
  ○ Pure red cell aplasia
  ○ Ulcerative colitis
  ○ Hypogammaglobulinemia

245. Good's syndrome is: *(PGMEE 2014-15)*
a. Thymic hyperplasia with myasthenia gravis
b. Thymic hypoplasia
c. Thymoma with hypo-gammaglobulinemia
d. Thymoma with anti-basement membrane antibodies
[Ref: Harrison's 19th/e pg. 1839]

246. True about Myasthenia gravis are all EXCEPT:-
a. Lactase ↓ *(PGMEE 2016-17)*
b. Glucose levels are normal
c. As the activity increases fatigability increases
d. Thymectomy is required in all cases
[Ref: Harrison's 20th/e pg. 3237]

247. Eaten Lambert syndrome is associated with ?
(PGMEE 2014-15)
a. Anti – HU antibodies   b. Anti GQ1B antiboy
c. Anti – Jo-1 antibody   d. Anti P/Q antibodies
[Ref: Harrison's 20th/e pg. 3235]

248. Which one of the following is correct regarding Eaton-Lambert syndrome- *(PGMEE 2015)*
a. It is commonly associated with adenocarcinoma of lung
b. It commonly affects the ocular muscle
c. Repeated electrical stimulation enhances muscle power in it
d. Neostigmine is the drug of choice for this syndrome
[Ref: Harrison's 20th/e pg. 3235]

249. Episodic weakness is seen in all of the following EXCEPT:
(DNB December 2011)
a. Hypercalcemia   b. Hypokalemia
c. Hyperglycemia   d. Eaton lambert syndrome
[Ref: Harrison's 19th/e pg.462e-16, 462e-17]

250. Which drug is used for Myaesthenia Gravis testing-
(PGMEE 2015)
a. Edrophonium   b. Adrenaline
c. Phycostigmine d. Acetylcholine
[Ref: Harrison's 20th/e pg. 3234]

251. Ice pack test is done for: *(PGMEE 2014/15)*
a. Myasthenia Gravis
b. Hypokalemic periodic paralysis
c. Hyperparathyroidism
d. Multiple system atrophy
[Ref: Harrison's 20th/e pg. 3233]

MUSCULAR DYSTROPHIES AND MYOPATHIES

252. Duchenne muscular dystrophy is inherited as?
(PGMEE 2012)
a. Autosomal recessive   b. Autosomal recessive
c. X- linked recessive   d. X-linked dominant
[Ref: Harrison's 20th/e pg. 3244]

Explanation

Duchenne muscular dystrophy

- DMD involves proximal muscles. missing structural protein dystrophin → muscle fibre fragility → fibre breakdown → necrosis and regeneration.
  ○ Clinical features
  ○ Proximal muscle weakness by age 3, positive Gower's sign (i.e. child uses hands to "climb up" the legs to move from a sitting to a standing position), waddling gait, toe walking. hypertrophy of calf muscles and wasting of thigh muscles, decreased reflexes dystrophin is expressed in the brain, and boys with DMD may have delayed motor and cognitive development; this is not progressive cardiomyopathy moderate intellectual compromise
- Diagnosis
  ○ Family history (pedigree analysis)
  ○ Increased CK (50-100x normal) and lactate dehydrogenase

- Muscle biopsy, electromyography (EMG)
  - Complications
    - Patient usually wheelchair-bound by 12 years of age
    - Early flexion contractures, scoliosis, develop osteopenia of immobility, increased risk of fracture
    - Death occurs due to pneumonia/respiratory failure or CHF in 2nd-3rd decade
  - Treatment
    - Supportive (e.g. physiotherapy, wheelchairs, braces), prevent obesity,surgical (for scoliosis) use of steroids (e.g. prednisone or deflazacort)
    - Gene therapy trials underway

253. Which of the following is not X linked condition - *(PGMEE 2012-13)*
a. Duchenne muscular dystrophy
b. Emery- Dreifuss muscular dystrophy
c. Facioscapulohumeral muscular dystrophy
d. Becker muscular dystrophy

[Ref: Harrison's 20th/e pg. 3249]

Explanation

	X-linked muscular dystrophies	Autosomal

Herediatry Myopathies	■ Duchenne muscular dystrophy
	■ Becker muscular dystrophy
	■ Emery - Dreifuss muscular dystrophy (EDMD1) ass with EMD gene
		■ Limb - Girdle muscular dystrophies
		  ○ LGMD1 - AD
		  ○ LGMD2 - AR
		■ E DMD 2 (AD) & EDMD 3 (AR)
		■ Myotonic dystrophy - AD
		■ Facios capuohumeral muscular dystrophy - AD
		■ Oculopharyngeal dystrophy - AD

Protein defect	M/s disorder
Dystrophin	DMD (absent); BMD (reduced)
Sarcoglycans	UG MD2
Lamionin - α2	Merosin deficient cong. - m/s dystrophy
Emerin	EDMD
SERCA-1	Brody diseases
8	

254. Dystrophin is lacking in- *(PGMEE 2012-13)*
a. Peroneal muscular atrophy
b. Duchenne's muscular dystrophy
c. Polio
d. None of the above

[Ref: Harrison's 20th/e pg. 3244]

255. Not a common feature of Duchenine muscular dystrophy is? *(DNB June 2011; PGMEE 2012-13)*
a. X- linked recessive
b. Gower sigh positive
c. Distal muscle involvement
d. Pseudo hypertrophy

[Ref: Harrison's 20th/e pg. 3244]

256. Protein defective in congenital muscular dystrophy: *(PGMEE 2014/15)*
a. Merosin
b. Sarcoglycan
c. Laminin
d. Dystrophin

Explanation

- Merosin is deficient in congenital muscular dystrophy.
- Mutation in Sarcoglycan gene causes Limb girdle muscular dystrophy.
- Dystrophin protein is defective in Duchenne muscular dystrophy.

257. All of following are examples of proximal myopathy (weakness) EXCEPT? *(PGMEE 2015-16)*
a. Thyroid myopathy
b. Duchenne's muscular dystrophy
c. Drug induced myopathy
d. Myasthenia gravis

[Ref: Harrison's 20th/e pg. 3240]

258. Parking lot inclusions are seen in: *(PGMEE 2015)*
a. Mitochondrial myopathy
b. Nemaline myopathy
c. Central myopathy
d. Lipid Myopathies

[Ref: Robbins 9th/pg 1274]

259. The term 'ragged red fibers' is applied to describe the skeletal muscle fibers in:- *(PGMEE 2015-16)*
a. Duchenne Muscular Dystrophy
b. Myotonic dystrophy
c. Amyotrophic Lateral Sclerosis
d. Mitochondrial myopathy

[Ref: Harrison's 20th/e pg. 3251]

PERIODIC PARALYSIS

260. SCN4A defect is seen in: *(PGMEE 2014/15)*
a. Brugada syndrome
b. Para-myotonia congenital
c. Lambert Eaton syndrome
d. Hyperkalemic periodic paralysis

[Ref: CMDT 2013, Pg 1036; Harrison 19th p 444e]

261. Which is true about Thyrotoxic Periodic paralysis.
a. Sodium channel defect *(PGMEE 2014-15)*
b. Hypokalemic periodic paralysis
c. Precipitated by fasting
d. Associated with myxedema coma

Explanation

Thyrotoxic Periodic Paralysis: (TPP)

- **MC** secondary hypokalemic PP.
- Thyrotoxic PP is a genetic disorder unmasked by thyrotoxicosis.
- Due to mutation in the KCNJ18 gene that encodes for the inwardly rectifying potassium channel (Kir 2.6)
- Clinical feature: Episodic weakness (proximal)
- Precipitated by hyperinsulinemia, carbohydrate load, exercise
- Associated with Myasthenia gravis.

253. c
254. b
255. c
256. a
257. d
258. a
259. d
260. d
261. b

262. Drug of choice for an attack of periodic paralysis with calcium channel defect is: *(PGMEE 2014-15)*
   a. ACTH
   b. Potassium chloride
   c. Calcium chloride
   d. Adrenaline

[Ref: Harrison's 19th/e pg. 444e]

INFECTIONS OF THE CNS

MENINGITIS

263. Latex agglutination test in CSF is done for detection of: *(PGMEE 2014-15)*
   a. Cryptococcus   b. E.coli
   c. Tuberculosis   d. Coxsackie

[Ref: Pubmed]

264. Aseptic meningitis is caused by? *(PGMEE 2015-16)*
   a. Indomethacin
   b. Icatibant
   c. Aspirin
   d. Ibuprofen

265. In tubercular meningitis what is not seen?
(DNB June 2011)
   a. Low sugar   b. Opening pressure is low
   c. High protein   d. Lymphocytic

[Ref: Harrison's 20th/e pg. 1000]

266. Most common cause of Carcinomatous meningitis:
(PGMEE 2014-15; PG 2015)
   a. Malignant melanoma   b. Carcinoma lung
   c. Carcinoma gut   d. Carcinoma breast

[Ref: Harrison's 20th/e pg. 650]

267. Which of the following statements about Mollaret's meningitis is true:- *(PGMEE 2015-16)*
   a. Is a recurrent, benign septic meningitis,
   b. Caused by Herpes simplex 2 in most of the cases.
   c. Does not resolve without treatment
   d. Is also referred to as "Benign Recurrent" Neutrophilic Meningitis

Explanation

- AKA benign recurrent aseptic meningitis, benign recurrent lymphocytic meningitis.
- Caused by HSV-2 > HSV-1
- Management is supportive.

268. A 32 years old HIV +ve female presented with headache and nuchal stiffness. On lumbar puncture examination clear CSF was obtained with leucocytes >100/cu.mm. India ink staining was positive. The most probable diagnosis is? *(PGMEE 2015-16)*
   a. Candida Meningitis
   b. Cryptococcus meningitis
   c. Cryptosporidium
   d. Tubercular Meningitis

[Ref: Harrison's 20th/e pg. 864, 1009]

269. Which of the following is not seen in tubercular meningitis: *(PGMEE 2015-16)*
   a. It is seen most often in young children but also develops in adults.
   b. Culture of CSF is diagnostic in majority of cases and remains the gold standard.
   c. Cerebrospinal fluid reveals a low leukocyte count.
   d. Evidence of old pulmonary lesions or a miliary pattern is found on chest radiography

[Ref: Harrison's 20th/e pg. 1009]

270. Steroids are used in: *(PGMEE 2014/15)*
   a. Severe typhoid
   b. H. influenzae meningitis
   c. E. coli septicemia
   d. Cerebral malaria

[Ref: Harrison's 20th/e pg. 1002]

Explanation

- Dexamethasone is given is meningitis due to H. influenza, S. pneumoniae, N. meningitidis & M. tuberculosis

271. Drug treatment is given for how many days in pneumococcal meningitis? *(PGMEE 2015-16)*
   a. 5 days   b. 7 days
   c. 14 days   d. 21 days

[Ref: Harrison's 20th/e pg. 1002]

Agent	Antibiotics	Duration
S. pneumoniae	▪ Vancomycin + ceftriaxone + steroids	10-14 days
H influenzae	▪ Ampicilin + steroids	7 days
N meningitidis	▪ Penicillin G + steroids	7 days
Listeria monocytogenes	▪ Ampicillin/Penicillin G	14-21 days
S agalactiae	▪ Ampicillin/Penicillin G	14-21 days
Pseudomonas	▪ Ceftazidime/Cefepime	21 days
S epidermidis	▪ Vancomycin	21 days

272. Neisseria meningitides infection is characteristic of deficiency of: *(PGMEE 2014-15)*
   a. C2   b. C3
   c. C4   d. C5

[Ref: Harrison's 20th/e pg. 116]

273. A Patient presents with headache and Nuchal rigidity. Lumbar Puncture was performed and CSF shows normal protein and normal glucose with clear CSF. Microscopic examination of CSF showed 50 lymphocytes/cu.mm with lymphocytic pleocytosis. What is the diagnosis? *(PGMEE 2015-16)*
   a. Viral meningitis
   b. Bacterial meningitis
   c. Neoplastic meningitis
   d. Fungal meningitis

[Ref: Harrison's 20th/e pg. 864]

262. b
263. a
264. d
265. b
266. d
267. b
268. b
269. c
270. b
271. c
272. d
273. a

301. Bilateral proptosis in children is seen in:
 a. Cavernous hemangioma   *(NEET Pattern 2012)*
 b. Leukemia
 c. Malignant fibrous Histiocytoma
 d. Neurofibromatosis

[Ref: Nelson ch. 632/Tumors of the Orbit]

302. Neurological manifestation of Whipple's disease is:
 a. Encephalopathy   *(PGMEE 2014-15)*
 b. Cerebellar ataxia
 c. Focal neurological deficits
 d. Seizures

[Ref: Harrison's 19th/e pg. 1945]

303. Acute onset areflexia quadriparesis with blurred vision and absent pupillary response in a 20 years old male, the most probable diagnosis is?   *(DNB June 2011)*
 a. Diphtheria
 b. Botulism
 c. Polio
 d. Porphyria

[Ref: Harrison's 20th/e pg. 1107]

301. b
302. b,d
303. b

Ophthalmology

ANATOMY

- The eye of a newborn is usually: Hypermetropic
- Normal visual acuity is attained by the age of: 6 years
- Visual axis is the line joining the object and the fovea
- *Goblet cells* → Mucin secreting cells present in conjunctiva
- *Muller cells* → Glial cells in the retina
- *Amacrine cells* → interneurons that produce pure depolarizing potential
- Inferior stability to the eyeball is provided by: suspensory ligament of lock wood

Refractive Index

Medium	Index
Air	1
Cornea	1.376
Lens	1.386 – 1.406
Lens nucleus	1.46
Aqueous humor Vitreous humor	1.336

- Sclera is thinnest at: Posterior to insertion of rectus muscle
- Predominant type of collagen in the sclera: Type I
- Pars plana is between choroid and ciliary body

Glands involved in:

Hordeolum externum (stye)	Gland of Zeis/Gland of Moll
Hordeolum internum	Meibomian gland (Sebaceous gland)
Chalazion	

Visual Pathway

1st order neurons → **Photoreceptors**
2nd order neurons → **Bipolar cells**
3rd order neurons → **Optic nerve**
4th order neurons → **Optic radiation**

Dimensions

- AP diameter of eyeball: 24 mm
- Direct distant ophthalmoscopy is done at distance of: 22- 25 cm
- Diameter of thee Corneal: 10.5 mm vertical ´× 11.5 horizontal

- Diameter of macula: 5 mm
- Diameter of optic disc: 1.5 mm
- Distance between optic disc & centre of macula (fovea): 3 mm or 2 disc diameter
- Normal IOP: 11-21 mmHg

Derivatives

Surface Ectoderm	Neuroectoderm	Neural Crest	Mesoderm
▪ Skin of eyelid ▪ Corneal epithelium ▪ **Lens**	▪ Epithelial lining of Ciliary body & Iris ▪ Retina & RPE ▪ Optic nerve ▪ 2° & 3° vitreous	▪ Descemet membrane ▪ Sclera ▪ Ciliary muscles ▪ Melanocytes	▪ Extraocular muscles ▪ Sclera ▪ Choroid ▪ 1° Vitreous ▪ Corneal stroma & Bowman's membrane

OPTOMETRY

- Total dioptric power of schematic eye is: + 58 D
  - Cornea→ 43 D
  - Lens → 15 D
- Total dioptric power of reduced eye is: + 60 D
  - Cornea → 44 D
  - Lens → 16 D

- Power is inversely related to focal length.
- Refractive Power (D) = 1/Focal length (in meters)
- 1 mm change in the axial length leads to change of __ diopter in refractive power: 3D
- 1 mm change in corneal curvature leads to change of __ diopter refractive power: 6D

- Ishihara cards detect: Red & Green color Vision
- The colors best appreciated by the central cones of fovea-macular area are: Red and green (remember it with traffic signal color that we follow)
- Ethambutol causes impairment of which color vision: Red - Green

CORNEA

- Neurotrophic keratopathy is caused by: Trigeminal nerve palsy
- Exposure keratopathy is caused by: Facial nerve palsy
- Vortex keratopathy/Cornea verticillate is caused by: Amiodarone
- Photophthalmia is caused by exposure to: UV rays
- Thickness of cornea is measured by: Pachymeter

- Most sensitive method for detecting Keratoconus: Corneal topography
- Specular microscopy is used to analyze: Corneal endothelium → cell size, shape & count

Fuch's Endothelial Dystrophy:
- Slowly progressive bilateral condition
- Common in middle age females
- Beaten metal appearance of the endothelium

Layers of Cornea

Epithelium	- Stratified non-keratinized squamous epithelium
Bowman's layer	- Do not regenerate - Involved in Reis-Buckler dystrophy
Dua's layer	- Toughest layer
Endothelium	- Maintains corneal transparency

Corneal Preservation

Short Term	Intermediate Term	Long Term
- In McCarey Kaufman (MK) media - Shelf life: 2-3 days	- In chondroitin sulfate media - Shelf life: 7-14 days	- Cryopreservation in liquid nitrogen - Shelf life: up to 1 year

CONJUNCTIVA

- Epithelial lining of conjunctiva is: Stratified squamous non-keratinized
- Maximum density of goblet cells is seen in: Nasal conjunctiva
- Intracytoplasmic inclusion bodies know as HP bodies are produced by: **C**hlamydia *trachomatis*
- *Ophthalmia neonatorum/Neonatal conjunctivitis is caused by:*
  - *Chlamydia* → MCC in developed countries
  - *N. gonorrhea*
  - *S. aureus*
  - Chemical conjunctivitis → 1% $AsNO_3$

- Late onset endophthalmitis after cataract surgery is caused by: *Propionibacterium acne*

Conditions	Etiology
Angular conjunctivitis	- *Moraxella lacunata*
Mucopurulent conjunctivitis	- *S. aureus*
Hemorrhagic conjunctivitis	- Enterovirus 70* - Coxsackie virus 24 - Echo virus - Adenovirus
Inclusion conjunctivitis	- C. trachomatis D-K

Pterygium

- Degenerative and hyperplastic condition of conjunctiva
- Subconjunctival fibrovascular tissue encroaching the cornea
- *Etiology*: Exposure to UV-B rays
- *Clinical features:*
  - It presents as a triangular fold of conjunctiva
  - Usually present on nasal side
  - Always situated in palpebral aperture
  - Stocker's line – deposition of iron on its leading edge

- *Complication*: corneal astigmatism
- Rx: Excision, PERFECT surgery

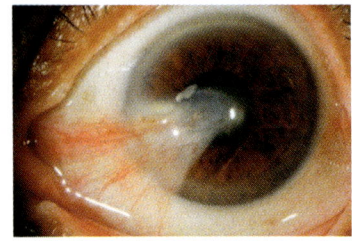

LENS

- Lens capsule is thinnest at the: posterior pole
- Which type of cataract is visually most handicapping: Post subcapsular cataract
- Best irrigation fluid for cataract surgery: Balanced Salt solution + Glutathione
- Ideal age for cataract surgery in children: 4 – 6 weeks
- MC late complication following cataract surgery: Posterior capsular opacification
- Biometry → Procedure of calculation of power of IOL
- IOL calculation is done by: SRK II formula → Power = A – (2.5 L + 0.9 K)
  - A = constant
  - L = axial length measured by A scan
  - K = corneal curvature measured by keratometry

Cataract

Symptoms/Sign	Type
▪ Second sight or myopic shift ▪ Frequent changes of glasses ▪ Colour shift; Index myopia	Nuclear cataract
▪ Index hypermetropia	Cortical cataract
▪ Difficulty seeing objects in bright light/ Headlight of coming cars	Posterior subcapsular cataract Nuclear cataract
▪ Fluctuating refractive error	Diabetic cataract
▪ Polychromatic lustre	Complicated cataract (Posterior subcapsular cataract)
▪ Bread crumb appearance	

Conditions	Cataract
▪ Diabetes	Snow flake cataract
▪ GalactOsemia	Oil droplet cataract
▪ Wilson disease	Sunflower cataract /Pseudo cataract (Mn: WILSUN)
▪ Myotonic dystrophy	ChristMas tree cataract
▪ Blunt Trauma	RoseTTe Cataract
▪ Steroid therapy	Posterior subcapsular cataract
▪ Congenital Rubella Syndrome	Nuclear cataract

Procedure	Conventional ECCE	Manual SICS	Phacoemulsification	FLACS*
Incision	10 to 2 o'clock	4-6 mm	1.5-2.4 mm	< 2 mm
Comment	Anterior capsulotomy done	Self-sealing sclerocorneal incision	Self-sealing sclerocorneal incision	It is a microincision cataract surgery
* Femtosecond Laser Assisted Cataract Surgery					

Intraocular Lens

Types	Material	Remarks
Soft IOLs	HEMA	Allergic conjunctivitis
Rigid IOLs	PMMA	use to treat astigmatism &Keratoconus
Rollable IOLs	Acrylic	Used in microincision cataract surgery
Foldable IOLs	Silicone, Acrylic, Hydrogel	After Phacoemulsification

Ectopia Lentis/ Subluxated Lens

Conditions	Features
Marfan syndrome	▪ Autosomal Dominant condition ▪ Bilateral symmetrical supero-temporal subluxation
Weill – Marchesani syndrome	▪ Microspherophakia ▪ Downward and forward subluxation
Homocystinuria	▪ AR inheritance ▪ Mental retardation; Marfanoid features ▪ Bilateral infero-nasal subluxation

RETINA

- Aniseikonia: **significant difference in the perceived size of images from both the retina**
- Macula is on temporal side while optic disc is on nasal side in fundus.
- The gene for rhodopsin is located on: Chromosome 3q
- Maximum cones are present at: Fovea
- Rods are absent at: Foveola /Fovea
- Thinnest part of retina: Foveola
- Waxy exudates and pale disc with pigmentation around retinal vessel: Retinitis Pigmentosa
- Earliest manifestation of Diabetic retinopathy: Microaneurysms
- MI factor for development of diabetic retinopathy: Duration of diabetes
- ETDRS (Early Treatment for Diabetic Retinopathy Study) chart is used for visual evaluation in diabetics
- Arden ratio of flat electrooculogram: < 1.25
- Earliest indication of optic nerve disease: RAPD/Marcus Gunn pupil
- Relative Afferent Pupillary Defect (RAPD) → Pupil dilates on exposure to light in affected eye.
- Nerve fibers of the optic nerve originate in the: Retinal ganglion cells (2nd order neuron)
- Loss of light reflex with normal near reflex is seen in: ARP (Light – Near dissociation)

- Only disease in which ERG is normal but EOG is abnormal: Best's disease (AD inheritance)
- Amsler grid is used to detect: maculopathy
- Fluid accumulation in CSR occurs in the: subretinal space
- Eale's disease is characterized by recurrent vitreous hemorrhage
- *Ring scotoma/tubular vision is seen in:*
  - Glaucoma
  - Retinitis Pigmentosa
- *Dysfunction of retinal pigment epithelium (RPE) can lead to:*
  - Age Related Macular Degeneration (ARMD)
  - Central Serous Retinopathy (CSR)
  - Exudative Retinal Detachment
- *Waves in electroretinogram (ERG):*
  - a wave → from photoreceptors (rods & cones)
  - **b** wave → from **b**ipolar & Muller cells
  - c wave → from retinal pigmented epithelium

Retinopathy of Prematurity (ROP)/Retrolental fibroplasia:

- MI risk factor: Prematurity
- Screening of ROP:
  - 28-34 weeks of GA → 4 weeks of post natal age
  - < 28 weeks of GA → 3 weeks of post natal age

Retinitis Pigmentosa

- It is the MC hereditary fundus dystrophy
- Genetic defect causes apoptosis of rods >> cones
- *Symptoms*:
  - Night blindness – earliest symptom
  - Peripheral vision loss
- *Fundoscopic* findings:
  - Bone spicules – retinal hyperpigmentation
  - Waxy disc pallor
  - Arteriolar attenuation
- *Syndromes* associated with RP:
  - Usher syndrome – MC
  - Kearn-Sayre syndrome
  - Bardet-Biedl syndrome

  - Refsum syndrome
  - Neuropathy, Ataxia & Retinitis Pigmentosa
- Perimetry → Ring scotoma which progresses to tunnel vision
- Electroretinogram → decreased amplitude of 'a' and 'b' waves

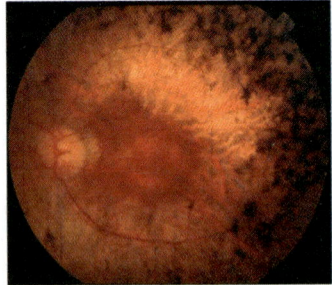

Signs of Hypertensive Retinopathy

▪ Salus's sign – deflection of retinal vein as it crosses the arteriole	Grade 2
▪ Bonnet sign – banking of the retinal vein distal to the AV crossing ▪ Gunn's sign – tapering of the retinal vein on either side of the AV crossing ▪ Copper wiring appearance	Grade 3
▪ Optic disc swelling/Papilledema ▪ Silver wiring appearance of arterioles	Grade 4

Diabetic Retinopathy

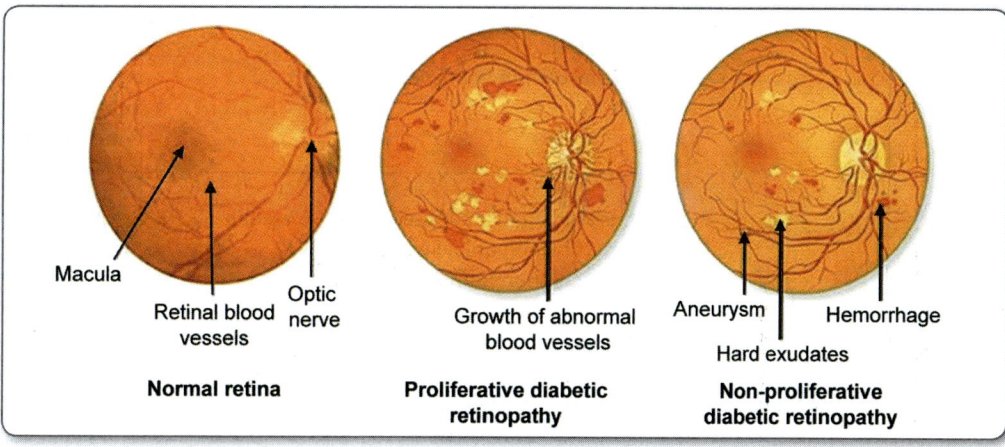

GLAUCOMA

- Most important mechanism of aqueous humor secretion: Active secretion by Na-K-ATPase
- Rate of formation of aqueous humor: 2-3 μl/min

- Colored halos of glaucoma and cataract are differentiated by: Fincham's test
- Glaukomflecken → Anterior subcapsular lens opacity following an attack of glaucoma
- 100-day glaucoma is seen in: CRVO

Disc changes:
- Notching of Neuroretinal rim
- Vertical oval cup
- Splinter hemorrhage on disc margin
- Thinning of Neuroretinal rim
- Nasal shifting of disc vessels
- Bayoneting sign – Angulation of vessel at margin
- Laminar dot sign
- Marked cupping of disc

Visual field changes:
- Isopter contraction – earliest visual field defect
- Baring of Blind spot
- Paracentral scotoma
- Seidel's scotoma – Extension of blind spot
- Arcuate or Bjerrum scotoma
- Ring scotoma or double Arcuate scotoma
- Nasal step of Roenne
- Tubular vision
- Temporal field defect – last change

Management	Primary Open Angle Glaucoma	Primary Angle Closure Glaucoma
Pharmacotherapy	▪ Prostaglandin analogues – Latanoprost, Bimatoprost, Travoprost = 1st line ▪ Alpha 2 adrenergic agonists – Brimonidine ▪ Beta blockers – Timolol, Betaxolol ▪ CA inhibitors – Acetazolamide, Brinzolamide	▪ IV mannitol ▪ IV acetazolamide ▪ Alpha 2 adrenergic agonists – Brimonidine ▪ Topical beta blockers ▪ Prostaglandin analogues
Laser therapy	▪ Laser trabeculoplasty	▪ Laser iridotomy – TOC
Surgery	▪ Trabeculectomy	▪ Trabeculectomy → Filtration surgery

MISCELLANEOUS

- Xerophthalmia – Deficiency of Vitamin A
- Acute retrobulbar neuritis – Deficiency of Vitamin B1
- All dystrophies are inherited as AD except: Macular dystrophy (AR)
- Only mydriatic drug with no cycloplegia: Phenylephrine
- Malignancy caused by chalazion is: Meibomian gland adenocarcinoma

- Persistent Hyperplasia Primary Vitreous (**P**HPV) is associated with: **P**atau syndrome
- **A**nterior Lenticonus – **A**lport's syndrome
- Posterior Lenticonus – Lowe's syndrome
- Band-shaped **K**eratopathy is due to deposition of: Calcium (**K**alcium)
  - Associated condition: JRA, Sarcoidosis
- *Complications:*
  - Hypermetropia: PACG (due to shallow AC)

- ○ Myopia: Macular degeneration (MC) & Retinal Detachment
- ○ Bacterial conjunctivitis: Marginal corneal ulcer

- • *Juvenile Rheumatoid Arthritis:*
  - ○ JRA is a contraindication to put IOL after cataract surgery
  - ○ Subtype of JRA associated with Uveitis: Pauciarticular JRA

MOST COMMON

- • MC cause for angular conjunctivitis: Moraxella
- • MC cause of amblyopia: Squint
- • MC site of coloboma: Inferonasal quadrant
- • MC cause of cataract: Senile/age related
- • MC congenital cataract: Punctate cataract/ Blue dot cataract
- • MC cataract in diabetics: Posterior subcapsular cataract
- • MC type of cataract following radiation: Posterior subcapsular cataract
- • MC degeneration seen in myopia: Lattice type
- • MC stromal dystrophy: Lattice dystrophy
- • Least common corneal dystrophy: Macular dystrophy
- • MC cause of vitreous hemorrhage in adult: Proliferative diabetic retinopathy
- • MC cause of vitreous hemorrhage in young male: Eale's disease
- • MC ocular manifestation of Sturge Weber syndrome: Glaucoma

- • MC type of scleritis: non necrotizing anterior scleritis
- • MC systemic illness associated with scleritis: Rheumatoid arthritis
- • MC systemic condition associated with uveitis: Ankylosing spondylitis
- • MC cause of Chorioretinitis: Toxoplasmosis
- • MC ocular opportunistic infection in AIDS: CMV retinitis
- • MC ocular manifestation of Congenital Rubella Syndrome: Salt and pepper retinopathy
- • MC Primary intraocular tumor in adults: Choroidal melanoma
- • MC malignant orbital tumor in children: Rhabdomyosarcoma
- • MC primary malignant intraocular tumor of childhood: Retinoblastoma
- • MC presentation of Retinoblastoma: Leukocoria

SYNDROMES

❶ *Reiter's syndrome:*
  - ○ Uveitis
  - ○ Arthritis
  - ○ Urethritis

❷ *Behcet's disease:*
  - ○ *HLA B 51 +ve*
  - ○ Recurrent oral ulceration/Aphthous ulcer
  - ○ Genital ulceration
  - ○ Erythema nodosum
  - ○ Bilateral recurrent non granulomatous iridocyclitis with transient hypopyon

❸ *VKH syndrome:* [**Mn**: *VAPER*]
  - ○ **V**itiligo
  - ○ **A**lopecia
  - ○ **P**an uveitis (Granulomatous)
  - ○ **E**xudative **R**etinal detachment

❹ *Leber Hereditary Optic Neuropathy:*
  - ○ Mitochondrial inheritance
  - ○ Bilateral but asymmetrical condition
  - ○ Central/ Centrocaecal scotoma
  - ○ Pupillary response is normal
  - ○ Circumpapillary telangiectasia

❺ *Wolfram syndrome:* [**Mn**: *DIDMOAD*]
  - ○ **D**iabetes **I**nsipidus
  - ○ **D**iabetes **M**ellitus

  - ○ **O**ptic Atrophy
  - ○ **D**eafness

❻ *Foster – Kennedy syndrome:*
  - ○ Ipsilateral Optic atrophy
  - ○ Contralateral papilledema
  - ○ Central scotoma
  - ○ Anosmia
  - ○ MC cause – frontal lobe tumors

❼ *Horner's syndrome:*
  - ○ Sympathetic pathway damage
  - ○ MC cause – Pan coast tumor
  - ○ Miosis
  - ○ Partial Ptosis
  - ○ Enopthalmosis – sinking of the eyeball
  - ○ Hemifacial anhidrosis
  - ○ Heterochromia iridis – in congenital Horner syndrome

❽ *Vogt's triad:*
  - ○ Postcongestive triad of angle closure glaucoma
  - ○ Characterized by:
    - ▪ Glaucomflecken (anterior subcapsular lens opacity)
    - ▪ Segmental iris atrophy
    - ▪ Slightly dilated non-reacting pupil

EYE FINDINGS

Signs

- Cattle track sign – slugging and segmentation of blood column in retinal vein → CRAO
- Candle wax dripping → Sarcoidosis
- Lander's sign → Sarcoidosis
- Amsler's sign → Fuch's heterochromic iritis
- Snow banking & snow ball sign→ Pars planitis
- Laminar dot sign → Glaucoma

Cherry red spots are seen in:

- Central Retinal Artery Occlusion
- Tay-Sachs disease
- GM1 Gangliosidosis
- Gaucher's disease
- Niemann-Pick disease
- Metachromatic leukodystrophy
- Commotio retinae/Blunt trauma

Fluorescein Angiography

- Window defect → Age-Related Macular Degeneration (ARMD)

- Smokestack appearance/Ink blot appearance/ Enlarging dot sign: Central Serous Retinopathy (CSR)

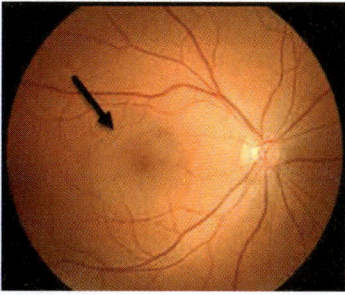

Ophthalmoscopy

	Direct	Indirect
Image	Erect & virtual	Inverted & real
Magnification	15 times	4-5 times

Roth's Spots

- Roth's Spots are retinal hemorrhages with white or pale center
- Seen in various illness like:
  - Subacute bacterial endocarditis – pathognomonic
  - Leukemia
  - Diabetes retinopathy
  - Carbon monoxide poisoning
  - Hypertensive retinopathy
  - Pernicious anemia
  - HIV retinopathy

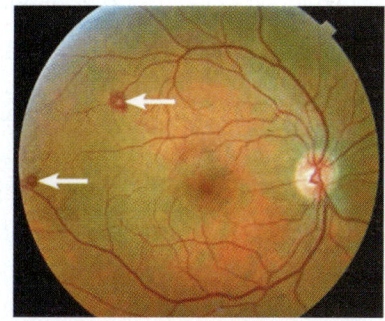

MANAGEMENT

Conditions	Management
TOC for high myopia	Contact lens
Posterior Capsule opacification/After cataract	**Nd: Yag Laser posterior capsulotomy** (wavelength = 1064 nm) Principle – photodisruption
Anterior uveitis	Topical steroids
DOC for POAG	Prostaglandin analogues
Background diabetic retinopathy (DR)	Strict metabolic control
Non-proliferative DR	Strict metabolic control
Proliferative DR	Pan retinal photocoagulation (PRP)
Clinically significant macular edema (CSME)	Focal: **Focal laser;** Diffuse: **Grid laser**
Retinopathy of prematurity	**Laser photocoagulation**
Coat's disease	**Laser photocoagulation**
Wet ARMD	Photodynamic therapy; **Intravitreal anti VEGF injection**
Central serous retinopathy (CSR)	**Wait and watch (Spontaneous resolution)**
Endophthalmitis	**Intravitreal antibiotics**

NAMED FEATURES

Features	Disease
▪ Foster's Fuch spot ▪ Myopic crescents ▪ Weis ring	Myopia
▪ Pseudopapillitis ▪ Shot silk appearance	Hypermetropia
▪ Elschnig pearls ▪ Sommering ring	After cataract/ Posterior capsular opacification
▪ Spoke of wheel appearance	Zonular cataract/Lamellar cataract
▪ Pin cushion distortion ▪ Roving ring scotoma (Jack in box phenomenon)	Aphakia
▪ Snow ball opacity in vitreous	Pars planitis
▪ Krachmer spots; Khodadoust line	Features of graft rejection
▪ Keratic precipitate (KP) ▪ Mutton fat KP ▪ Iris nodule (Koeppe and Busacca)	Pathognomic sign of anterior uveitis Granulomatous anterior uveitis Granulomatous anterior uveitis
▪ **S**alt and **P**epper fundus ▪ Sauce and **C**heese retinopathy ▪ Iris Pear**L** ▪ Lisch **N**odule	**Syp**hilis & Rubella **C**MV **L**eprosy **N**eurofibromatosis 1
▪ **S**almon patch appearance of cornea ▪ Iris ro**S**eola	Syphilis
▪ Sago grain appearance of conjunctiva	Trachoma
▪ Uyemura spots	Xerophthalmia fundus /Night blindness
▪ Brush field spots	Down's syndrome
▪ **B**ulls eye retinopathy	Chloroquine
▪ Cornea verticillata (corneal epithelial deposits)	Chloroquine and Amiodarone
▪ Bread crumb like deposits in anterior cornea	Granular corneal dystrophy
▪ Krukenberg spindles	Pigmentary glaucoma
▪ Haab's striae	Congenital glaucoma/Buphthalmos
▪ Drusen – yellow deposits in the retina	Non exudative ARMD
▪ Hollenhorst plaques	CRAO
▪ Splashed tomato fundus/Tomato ketchup fundus	CRVO
▪ Vossius ring	Concussion injuries

IMPORTANT DISEASES

	Trachoma	Vernal Keratoconjunctivitis/Spring Catarrh	Phlyctenular Keratoconjunctivitis
Etiology	■ *C. trachomatis* serotype A, B, Ba, C ■ MCC in India – Type C ■ Causes mixed follicular and papillary conjunctivitis ■ Involves both cornea and conjunctiva	■ Type I HSR/Allergic inflammatory response to *exogenous* allergen ■ Seen during spring and summer ■ Primarily affect boys	■ Type IV HSR/Allergic inflammatory response to *endogenous* allergen ■ Triggers → *S. aureus* & *M. tuberculosis* protein

Clinical features	■ Age group: 3-5 years
	Conjunctival signs:
	■ Papillary hyperplasia; Concretions
	■ Follicles: Common on **upper** tarsal conjunctiva
	■ Arlt's line: linear scar present in sulcus subtarsalis
	■ Presence of follicles on **bulbar** conjunctiva is the pathognomonic sign
	Corneal signs:
	■ Herbert follicles around limbus
	■ Herbert pits, Pannus
	■ Corneal ulcer and opacity
	Complication:
	■ Entropion, Trichiasis, Xerosis
		■ Age group: 5-20 years
		■ Recurrent, bilateral, self-limiting condition
		■ Marked itching, burning with ropy discharge
		■ Palpebral form: Most Common
		  ○ Upper palpebrae shows papillary hypertrophy with cobblestone appearance
		■ Bulbar form:
		  ○ Horner Trantas spot along the limbus
		Corneal signs:
		■ Shallow transverse (shield) ulcer
		■ Pseudogerontoxon: characterized by classical 'Cupid's Bow' outline
			■ Age group: 5-15 years
			■ Unilateral condition
			■ Itching is a less prominent feature
			■ Characteristic phlyctens (white pinkish nodule) are present near limbus
			■ Scrofulous ulcer
			■ Fascicular ulcer

Treatment	■ SAFE strategy – if prevalence > 10%
	  ○ **S**urgery for trichiasis & entropion
	  ○ **A**ntibiotics – DOC: Azithromycin
	  ○ **F**acial hygiene
	  ○ **E**nvironmental cleanliness
		■ Sodium cromoglycate → Mast cell stabilizers
		■ Topical antihistaminic
			■ DOC – Topical steroids

	Bacterial Corneal Ulcer	Fungal Keratitis	Acanthamoeba Keratitis

Etiology	■ Bacteria that can invade normal corneal epithelium:
	  ○ *N. meningitis* (Men)
	  ○ *Listeria monocytogenes* (Like)
	  ○ *C. diphtheria* (Dipti)
	  ○ *Shigella* (Sheila)
	  ○ *N. gonorrhoea* (Go)
	  ○ *H. influenza* (Home)
		■ *A. fumigatus* (filamentous fungi) – Most common cause
		■ *Candida* (Non filamentous fungi)
		■ Risk factor: History of ocular trauma by vegetable or organic matter
			■ Free living amoeba
			■ Fresh water protozoan
			■ It can also cause Granulomatous Amoebic Encephalitis
			■ **Risk factors:**
			  ○ Contaminated water
			  ○ Soft contact lens users*
			  ○ Trauma

Clinical features	■ Symptoms = Signs
	■ Hypopyon – **P**seudomonas & **P**neumococcal infection
	  ○ Sterile in nature
	  ○ Mobile
	■ Ulcus serpens in Pneumococcal infection
	
	Complications:
	■ Corneal opacity
	■ Descemetocele
	■ Perforation
		■ Signs >>> Symptoms
		■ Hypopyon – known as pseudo hypopyon as it is:
		  ○ Non-sterile/Infected
		  ○ Immobile/non shifting
		■ Greyish white dry-looking ulcer
		■ Pigmented ulcer
		■ Elevated rolled out feathery margin
		■ Multiple small satellite lesion
		■ Immune ring of Wessley
		■ Perforation is rare
			■ Severe pain (Symptoms >>> Signs)
			■ Ring-shaped infiltrate
			■ Pseudo dendritic epithelial lesion which resemble herpes simplex keratitis
			
			*MC organism responsible for corneal ulcer in contact lens user → *Pseudomonas*

Treatment	■ Fortified Gentamycin/Tobramycin ■ Fortified Cephazolin (5%) ■ Atropine ↓ posterior synechiae formation & pain due to ciliary spasm	■ For filamentous fungal keratitis: ○ DOC – Natamycin ■ Candida: DOC – Amp B ■ Topical steroids – Contraindicated	■ Diagnosed by Calcofluor stain & culture on non-nutrient *E. coli* enriched agar ■ DOC – Polyhexamethyl biguanide

	Herpes Simplex Keratitis	Herpes Zoster Ophthalmicus	Keratoconus
Etiology	• Herpes Simplex virus 1 (MC) • Herpes Simplex virus 2	• By Varicella Zoster virus • Due to reactivation of latent infection • Involves Ophthalmic division of V CN/Frontal nerve/Gasserian ganglion	• B/L progressive corneal disease • Characterized by paraxial stromal thinning • Apical protrusion of anterior cornea • Associated syndromes: EDS, Marfan, Down

Clinical features	• Pain ++
	• Follicular conjunctivitis
	• Superficial Punctate keratitis
	• Dendritic ulcer→ typical lesion of herpes keratitis
	• Marked diminution of corneal sensation
	• Geographical ulcer
	• Stromal keratitis
	• Disciform keratitis
	• Metaherpetic keratitis
	• Recurrence is common
		• Elderly & immunocompromised are particularly prone
		• Limited to one side of face
		• Severe neuralgic pain along the course of the involved nerve
		• Conjunctivitis
		• Zoster keratitis → Nummular keratitis, Disciform keratitis
		• Pseudo dendritic ulcer
		• Motor nerve palsies (3rd, 4th, 6th, 7th)
		• **Hutchinson's rule:**
		  ○ Interstitial keratitis
		  ○ VIII nerve deafness
		  ○ Notched incisor teeth
			• Vision becomes blurred & distorted with glare & halos around light
			• Myopia, astigmatism
			• Distorted window reflex/corneal reflex
			• Retinoscopy – Yawning/Scissoring reflex
			• Direct Ophthalmoscopy – Oil drop reflex
			• Munson's sign
			• **Slit lamp:**
			  ○ Fleischer's ring – due to iron deposition
			  ○ Vogt's striae – break in the Descemet membrane
			• Fe deposits at the base of Fleisher's ring
			• Rizzuti's sign

Treatments	• **Epithelial keratitis:**
	  ○ Topical antiviral
	  ○ Topical steroids – Contraindicated
	• **Stromal Keratitis:**
	  ○ Topical steroids
	  ○ Topical/Oral antiviral
	• **Metaherpetic keratitis:**
	  ○ Drugs not effective
		• DOC – Acyclovir	• Spectacles for astigmatism
			• Semi soft contact lens
			• Definitive Rx → Penetrating Keratoplasty
			• TOC → Corneal collagen cross linking

	Optic Neuritis	Papilledema
General	• Inflammatory/Demyelinating disease of optic nerve	• Non-inflammatory edema of the optic disc due to ↑ ICT

Pathology	• **Etiology:**
	  ○ Diabetes, Tobacco, vitamin B_{12} deficiency, Multiple Sclerosis, Ethambutol, Methyl alcohol
	• **Types:**
	  ○ Papillitis – MC in children
	  ○ Retrobulbar neuritis – MC in adult
		• ↑ Intracranial tension → impairment of axonal flow → edema of optic nerve head
		
		• **Foster Kennedy syndrome:**
		  ○ Ipsilateral Optic atrophy, central scotoma with contralateral Papilledema

Symptoms	• More common in young females • Sudden, progressive, unilateral loss of vision • Painful ocular movements in retrobulbar type	• Vision is initially normal → Transient obscuration of vision → Gradual progress painless loss of vision • Headache, Vomiting, LOC due to ↑ ICT
Signs	• ↓ Visual acuity (V/A) with gradual recovery • RAPD or Marcus Gunn pupil (Pupillary reflex is lost) • Field defect – Central/Centrocaecal Scotoma • Papillitis – Swelling of the optic nerve Head • In Retrobulbar, fundus is normal • Uhthoff phenomenon – vision loss is exacerbated by heat or exercise • Pulfrich phenomenon • Visual evoked potentials (VEP) – abnormal	• V/A is preserved till late stage • Visual field –initially normal f/b progressive contraction • Blurring of disc margin – 1st sign • Disc margins gets elevated • Hyperemia of disc • Enlargement of blind spot • Physiological cup – Obliterated • Secondary optic atrophy • Optic disc – dirty yellow appearance
Treatment	• High dose IV methylprednisolone	• Treat the underlying cause

MULTIPLE CHOICE QUESTIONS

CHAPTER 1A: ANATOMY AND DEVELOPMENT

DEVELOPMENT OF EYE

1. Secondary vitreous develops from? *(PGMEE 2009)*
   a. Neural ectoderm
   b. Endoderm
   c. Mesoderm
   d. All

   [Ref: Parsons' 23rd/e pg. 4]

2. Which of the following is neuro ectodermal in origin?
   a. Choroidal plexus *(PGMEE 2010)*
   b. Trabecular
   c. Primary vitreous humor
   d. Iris epithelium

   [Ref: Parsons' 23rd/e pg. 4]

3. Corneal stroma is derived from: *(PGMEE 2013)*
   a. Intermediate mesoderm
   b. Paraxial mesoderm
   c. Lateral plate mesoderm
   d. Ectoderm

   [Ref: Parsons' 23rd/e pg. 4]

4. True about newborn eye are all EXCEPT?
   a. Hypermetropic eye of +2 to+3 D *(PGMEE 2017)*
   b. Optic nerve is myelinated only upto lamina cribrosa
   c. Axial length at birth is 16.5 mm
   d. 6/6 vision comes by 6 month

   [Ref: Parsons' 23rd/e pg. 63]

Explanation

Newborn eye

- At birth, the average axial length is 18 mm, the cornea is more curved and anterior chamber is slightly shallow. Overall, the eye of the newborn is hypermetropic
- Newborn eye is hypermetropic eye of +2 to+3 D.
- Maximum growth occurs within 2 years.
- Foveal reflex develops at 5-6 (five) months of age
- Optic nerve is myelinated only upto lamina cribrosa.
- **6/6 vision comes by 6 year.**

5. 6/6 visual acuity is attained by the age of:
   (Recent Pattern June 2018)
   a. 6 months   b. 1 year
   c. 6 years   d. 18 years

   [Ref: Parsons' 23rd/e pg. 25]

Explanation

Eye in postnatal period

- The most common visual acuity test in infants is an assessment of their ability to fixate and follow a target.
- Fixation starts developing by 4-6 weeks. Critical period for development of fixation reflex is 2-4 months.

- Development of fixation is completed by 6 months. So there are three points to remember:
  ○ Fixation starts developing → 4-6 weeks (1-11/2 months).
  ○ Critical period for development → 2-4 months.
  ○ Binocular vision and eye coordination are established → 3 months
  ○ Fixation development is completed → 6 months.
  ○ Macula is fully developed by 4-6 months.
  ○ Fusional reflex, stereopsis and accommodation is well developed by 4-6 months.
  ○ Cornea attains normal adult diameter by 2 years of age.
  ○ Lens grows throughout life.
  ○ Full visual acuity (6/6) or (20/20) is attained by 5-6 years of life.

ANATOMY OF EYEBALL

6. Whitnall's ligament refers to: *(PGMEE 2015-16)*
   a. Suspensory ligament of lens
   b. Superior oblique tendon
   c. Superior transverse ligament to the eye
   d. None of the above

   [Ref: BDC 7th/e vol. 3 pg. 27]

Explanation

Ligaments in relation to eye

- *Whitnall's ligament*: Superior transverse ligament to the eye. Primarily a support for the upper eyelid and superior orbit.
- *Suspensory ligament of Lockwood*: Thickened part of tenon's capsule found in orbit.
- *Weigert's ligament*: Hypocapsular ligament.
- *Suspensory ligament or Zonule of Zinn*: The lens is held in place by this ligament
- *Annulus of Zinn*: A common tendinous ring from which the rectus muscle origin

7. Lacrimal gland receives post ganglionic innervation through? *(PGMEE Aug 13 Pattern)*
   a. Submandibular ganglion
   b. Pterygopalatine ganglion
   c. Ciliary ganglion
   d. Otic ganglion

   [Ref: BDC 7th/e vol. 3 pg. 76]

8. Parasympathetic fibres to eye come via:
   a. Ciliary ganglion *(PGMEE June 14)*
   b. Geniculate ganglion
   c. Superior cervical ganglion
   d. Sphenopalatine ganglion

   [Ref: BDC 7th/e vol. 3 pg. 220]

1.	a
2.	d
3.	c
4.	d
5.	c
6.	c
7.	b
8.	a

BASIC PRINCIPLES IN REFRACTION OF EYE

1. Diopteric power of a normal eye is   *(PGMEE 2014)*
   a.   + 6D
   b.   + 43D
   c.   + 60D
   d.   + 17D

   [Ref: Parsons' 23rd/e pg. 45]

Explanation

- Diopteric power of reduced eye → 60 D (Cornea 43 D and lens 17 D).
- Total optical power of the relaxed eye is approximately 60 dioptres.
- The cornea anterior surface has highest refractive power in the human eye, about 48 D.

2. Most important factor determining convergence of light rays on retina is -   *(PGMEE 2014)*
   a.   Dioptric power of lens
   b.   Physical state of the vitreous
   c.   Length of the eyeball
   d.   Refractive index of cornea (curvature of cornea)

   [Ref: Parsons' 23rd/e pg. 50]

3. Which component of the eye has maximum refractive index -   *(PGMEE 2012; NEET Pattern 10, 09, 08)*
   a.   Posterior surface of the lens
   b.   Cornea
   c.   Centre of the lens
   d.   Anterior surface of the lens

   [Ref: Parsons' 23rd/e pg. 44]

Explanation

- Centre (core) of the lens or nucleus has maximum refractive index → 1.406.

Refractive Index and Refractive Power

	Vitreous, aqueous	Cornea	Lens Cortex	Lens core/ Nucleus	Lens Average
R.I.	1.336	1.376	1.386	1.406 (Max^m RI)	1.39
Power		+43–45 D			+ 17 D

4. When water enters eyes, blurring of vision due to?
   a.   Impurities of water   *(DNB Jun'2009)*
   b.   Extra refraction through water
   c.   Elimination of refraction through cornea
   d.   Speed of light is more through water

   (Ref: Parsons' 23rd/e pg. 50)

5. Shortening of 2 mm of axial length of eye ball causes-   *(PGMEE 2013)*
   a.   3D myopia
   b.   6D myopia
   c.   3D hypermetropia
   d.   6D hypermetropia

   [Ref: Parsons' 23rd/e pg. 63]

Answers

1. c
2. d
3. c
4. c
5. d
6. d
7. a
8. b
9. a
10. c

Explanation

- Axial ametropia:
  o Abnormal length of the globe - too long in myopia, too short in hypermetropia.
  o A 1 mm elongation produces approximately 3 D of myopia and 1 mm shortening 3 D of hypermetropia.

6. If a person has 6/6 vision & he can read the line 6/24. At what distance is he reading the chart: *(Recent Pattern June 2018)*
   a.   24 meter
   b.   6 m
   c.   6 feet
   d.   24 feet

   [Ref: Parsons' 23rd/e pg. 89]

7. If a person is reading from 6/24 to 6/6, which of the following change is occurring in the eye of the person reading :   *(Recent Pattern June 2018)*
   a.   Change in the axial length of eye
   b.   Altering the thickness of lens
   c.   Removal of vitreous
   d.   Change in the depth of AC

   [Ref: Parsons' 23rd/e pg. 48]

8. Maximum refraction takes place between?   *(DNB JUNE 2011)*
   a.   Tear film and cornea
   b.   Air and tear film
   c.   Cornea and aqueous
   d.   Aqueous and lens

   [Ref. Parsons' 23rd/e pg. 45]

9. Visual axis is -   *(PGMEE 2012)*
   a.   Object to fovea
   b.   Centre of cornea toCentre of rotation
   c.   Centre of lens to cornea
   d.   None

   [Ref: Parsons' 22nd/e pg. 416]

Explanation

- *Visual axis:*
  o A straight line that passes through both the centre of the pupil and the centre of the fovea. I.e. it passed from object to fovea
  o Passes through the nodal point and the fovea centralis thus crossing the optical axis and making small angle with it (gamma angle).
- *The optical axis:*
  o A straight line passing through the centre of cornea and posterior surface of lens to meet retina.

10. Focal length of 0.25 m power of lens is   *(PGMEE 2015)*
   a.   40 D
   b.   1/4 D
   c.   4 D
   d.   25 D

   [Ref: Parsons' 23rd/e pg. 51]

Explanation

- D = 1/f where D is power in diopters and f is focal length in metres

11. Pin hole can reduce refractive error upto-

(PGMEE 2014)

a. 1 D
b. 3D
c. 3 D
d. 10 D

[Ref: Parsons' 22ⁿᵈ/e pg. 77]

12. Accommodation is due to - *(PGMEE 2012)*
   a. Relaxation of ciliary muscles
   b. Contraction of dilator pupillae
   c. Contraction of ciliary muscles
   d. None *[Ref: Parsons' 23ʳᵈ/e pg. 50]*

13. If you look at a near object than what will happen:

(Recent Pattern June 2018)

a. Lens becomes thin and more curved and dioptric power of lens increases
b. Suspensory ligaments of the eye are stretched
c. Cilliary muscles contracted
d. ↑ in muscle tension on the lens

[Ref: Parsons' 23ʳᵈ/e pg. 50]

Explanation

Accommodation power

- The ability of eye to change the shape of its lens is called accommodation.
- Accommodation is achieved by contraction or relaxation of cilliary muscles, which slacken or stretch the suspensory ligaments.
- When we focus a near object, following changes occur in lens:-
  ○ Lens becomes more rounded at the centre. The lens thickens along AP axis by 3.5 to 4 mm
  ○ The horizontal lens diameter decreases from 10 mm to 9.6 mm
  ○ Anterior radius of curvature of lens decreases so that 3rd purkinje image moves forward & decreases in size.

Accommodation changes to near and distant object

Object	Near	Far (distant)
Ciliary muscles	Contracts	Relaxed
Suspensory ligament	Slackened	Stretched
Muscle tension on the lens	Low	High
Shape of lens	Rounded, more curved	Thin, less curved

14. For refraction in a hypermetropic child, which is the best drug? - *(PGMEE 2014)*
   a. Atropine ointment
   b. Homatropine
   c. Atropine drops
   d. Phenylephrine

[Ref: Parsons' 23ʳᵈ/e pg. 59]

ERRORS OF REFRACTION

MYOPIA

15. Identify the refractive error *(NEET Pattern 2017)*
   a. Myopia
   b. Hypermetropia
   c. Presbyopia
   d. Astigmatism

[Ref: Parsons' 23ʳᵈ/e pg. 46]

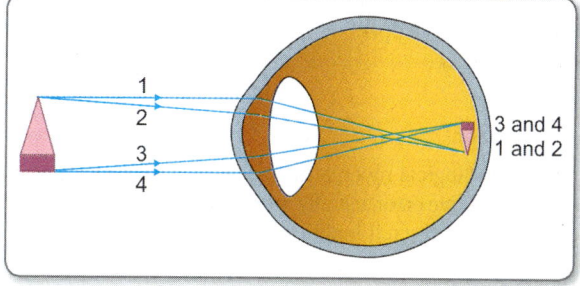

Explanation

- Myopia (aka Near-sightedness/ short-sightedness), is a dioptric condition of the eye where light focuses in front of, instead of on, the retina.
- Myopia can be classified low , moderate and high depending upon the extent of refractive error:-
  ○ Low myopia (< 4D)
  ○ Moderate myopia (4-6D), and
  ○ High myopia (> 6D)
- *Simple Myopia* when only associated with high refractive error
- *Pathological myopia*, where certain progressive degenerative changes may be observed.

16. True about amplitude of accommodation?

(PGMEE 2009)

a. Is the difference between near point and far point
b. Changes with spherical aberration
c. Increases as age advances
d. Is about 10 diopters in emmetropic eye

[Ref: Khurana 4ᵗʰ/e pg 41; Parsons' 23ʳᵈ/e pg. 51]

Explanation

- The amount or *amplitude of accommodation* can be calculated, not only of emmetropic but also of hypermetropic or myopic eyes. This is given by the formula A = P- R, which states that the amplitude of accommodation (A) is equal to the refractive power of the eye when fully accommodated
- (P) (i.e. the reciprocal of the distance of the near point in metres) less the refractive power of the eye at rest (R) (i.e. the reciprocal of the distance of the far point in metres).
- Thus, the emmetropic child of 10 has an amplitude of accommodation (A) of 100/7 2 1/` 5 14 2 0 5 14 D.
- The amplitude of accommodation decreases as age advances.
- The *range of accommodation*, i.e. the distance between the far point and the near point, is not always the same for a given amplitude.

17. The most common cause of myopia is: *(PGMEE 2014)*
   a. The viscosity of aqueous humour is increased
   b. The thickness of lens is increased
   c. The viscosity of vitreous humour is increased
   d. Antero-posterior diameter is increased

[Ref: Parsons' 23ʳᵈ/e pg. 63]

18. Choroidal vascularization is seen in: *(PGMEE 2013)*
   a. Hypermetropia
   b. Astigmatism
   c. Presbyopia
   d. Myopia

[Ref: Yanoff & Ducker 2nd/e p. 919-920]

11.	b
12.	c
13.	c
14.	a
15.	a
16.	d
17.	d
18.	d

19. Forster - Fuchs spots are seen in - *(PGMEE 2012)*
   a. Hypermetropia
   b. Astigmatism
   c. Myopia
   d. None

   [Ref: Parsons' 23rd/e pg. 225-226]

Explanation

- Pathological myopia is associated with a highly myopic refractive error, usually more than 6 D of myopia, with an elongated axial length and chorioretinal degeneration. Peripapillary atrophy, temporal crescent, macular atrophy, Forster-Fuchs spot, lacquer cracks, lattice degeneration and diffuse chorioretinal atrophy are seen in various degrees and combinations in these cases.

20. Refractive surgery most commonly performed for myopia: *(PGMEE 2013)*
   a. Photorefractive keratectomy
   b. LASIK
   c. Lensectomy
   d. Radial keratotomy

   [Ref: Parsons' 23rd/e pg. 65]

21. Maximum correction of myopia can be done by -
   a. Photorefractive keratotomy *(PGMEE 2013)*
   b. LASIK
   c. Clear lens extraction
   d. Radial keratotomy

   [Ref: Parsons' 22nd/e pg.74]

22. In senile nuclear cataract what type of myopia is seen- *(PGMEE 2013)*
   a. Index myopia
   b. Positional myopia
   c. Axial myopia
   d. Curvature myopia

   [Ref: Parsons' 23rd/e pg. 64]

19.	c
20.	b
21.	c
22.	a
23.	b
24.	c
25.	c

Explanation

- *Pathological curvature* myopia is seen typically in keratoconus.
- *Index myopia accounts* for myopia as a premonitory symptom of senile cataract

23. A patient with open angle glaucoma with myopia of 7 dioptre complains of blurring of vision on administration of pilocarpine drops. The reason for blurring of vision is? *(PGMEE 2015)*
   a. ↑hypermetropic asymmetry
   b. ↑myopic asymmetry
   c. ↑astigmatism
   d. Small pupil

   [Ref: Parsons' 22nd/e pg. 57]

Explanation

- There is frequent complaints of myopia after pilocarpine instillation esp in young glaucoma patients. According to literature this myopia can go as far as 17 diopter. The average myopization after 2% pilocarpine is 5 diopter for persons between 21 and 35 years of age.

24. A 50-year-old myopic patient with astigmatism with the rule comes to eye OPD. Which of the following prescription will best suit him:- *(PGMEE 2018)*
   a. +3 spherical, -1 cylindrical with 90 degree axis
   b. +2 Spherical only
   c. -2 spherical / +1 cylindrical, 180 degree
   d. –2 spherical / +1 cylindrical, 90 degree

   [Ref. Parsons' Diseases of the Eye 22nd /e pg. 73, 53]

Explanation

- There are 2 major types of eye glasses/lenses: spherical and cylindrical.
  - **Spherical glasses** have a single dioptric power and create a single point of focus. Their power is same in all meridians and curvature is of a single radius.
  - **Cylindrical glasses** are used for myopia and hyperopia not useful in astigmatism.
- Prescriptions used for correction of astigmatism include: spherical power, cylindrical power, and axis. The axis designates the meridian of the lens that only has the sphere power from 1 to 180; the full cylinder power is located 90° away from the axis.
- A sample prescription for astigmatism is given below:
  - OD-.50 –1.00 × 180
  - OS-.50 –2.00 × 175
- Here the OD or spherical component of the right lens is −.50, means that the patient is slightly myopic. The cylindrical power is −1.00, means the patient has astigmatism in the right eye. To determine the full power of cylindrical glass, which is present 90° away from the axis, it is necessary to combine the powers of sphere & and cylinder using formula: −.50 · (−1.00) + −1.50
- There are seven major categories of refractive errors to which prescriptions can fall:

Eye condition	Basis	Prescription
Simple myopic astigmatism	–	(−) minus plane glass
Simple myopia	–	(−) minus Sphere
Compound myopic astigmatism	–	major meridian will be (−) (−) on both 90° and 180° axis
Simple hyperopia	–	(+) Sphere
Simple hyperopic astigmatism	–	(+) Sphere
Compound hyperopic astigmatism	–	major meridian will be (+) (+) on both 90° and 180° axis Sphere
Mixed astigmatism	–	major meridian will be opposite i.e. (−)(+)(+)(−) on both 90° and 180° axis Sphere

HYPERMETROPIA

25. Pseudopapillitis is seen in *(PGMEE 2014)*
   a. Squint
   b. Presbyopia
   c. Hypermetropia
   d. Myopia

   [Ref: Parsons' 23rd/e pg. 67]

Explanation

- A bright reflex, suggesting the appearance of watered silk, is commoner in hypermetropic than in emmetropic or myopic eyes; in some cases due to a small optic nerve head with densely packed nerves, the appearance resembles optic neuritis - a condition known as pseudopapillitis.

26. All are true about hypermetropia except-
  a. Accommodative squint   **(PGMEE 2013)**
  b. Pseudopapillitis
  c. Near point comes closer
  d. Long-sightedness

  [Ref: Parsons' 23rd/e pg. 66]

27. Esotropia is commonly seen in which type of refractive error ?   **(PGMEE 2019)**
  a. Myopia   b. Hypermetropia
  c. Astigmatism   d. Presbyopia

  [Ref: Parsons' Diseases of the eye 22nd/e pg. 246]

ASTIGMATISM

28. Astigmatism is due to -   **(PGMEE 2014)**
  a. Forward displacement of the lens
  b. Irregularity of curvature of lens
  c. Backward displacement of lens
  d. Irregularity of curvature of cornea

  [Ref: Parsons' 23rd/e pg. 67]

29. Which one is "against the rule" astigmatism ?   **(PGMEE 2019)**
  a. $+2.00 \times 90*$
  b. $-2.00 \times 90*$
  c. $+1.50 \times 180*$
  d. $-1.50 \times 180*$

  [Ref: Parsons' Diseases of the eye 22nd/e pg. 53, 76]

APHAKIA & ANISEIKONIA

30. Which of the following is a sign of Aphakia:
  a. Absent 1st & 2nd Purkinje images   **(PGMEE 2015)**
  b. Iridodonesis
  c. Shallow anterior chamber
  d. White pupillary reflex

  [Ref: Parsons' 22nd/e pg.76]

Explanation

  ■ Iridodonesis → Vibration of iris with eye movement.

31. In aphakia purkinje images absent are   **(PGMEE 2013)**
  a. 1st & 3rd   b. 2nd & 4th
  c. 2nd & 3rd   d. 3rd & 4th

  [Ref: Parsons' 22nd/e pg.76]

32. Jack in box scotoma is seen after correction of Aphakia by: **(PGMEE 2012)**
  a. Contact lens   b. Spectacles
  c. IOL   d. None

  [Ref: Parsons' 23rd/e pg. 68]

Explanation

  ■ The difficulties of aphakia and its correction by spectacles include
    ○ An image magnification of about 25%–30%
    ○ Spherical aberrations producing a 'pin cushion effect'
    ○ Lack of physical coordination.
    ○ A **'jack-in-the-box' ring scotoma** from prismatic effects at the edge of the lens.
    ○ Prismatic errors resulting from displaced optical centres of the lenses.
    ○ Reduced visual fields and poor eccentric acuity.

  ○ Inaccurate correction because of erroneous vertex distances.
  ○ Physical inconvenience and cosmetic deficiency of heavy spectacle lenses.

33. Treatment of choice for aniseikonia   **(PGMEE 2013)**
  a. Spectacles
  b. Contact lens
  c. Surgery
  d. Orthoptic exercise

  [Ref: Parsons' 23rd/e pg. 69]

34. Treatment of presbyopia   **(PGMEE 2015)**
  a. Radial Keratotomy
  b. LASIK
  c. Convex lens
  d. Both b & c

  [Ref: Parsons' 23rd/e pg. 74]

Explanation

  ■ Both presbyopic lasik and convex lens are used for correction of presbyopia.
  ■ Apart from this multifocal IOL implant, multifocal contact lens and surgically implanted corneal inlays can be used to correct presbyopia.

35. A 50-year-old emmetropic elderly male presents with presbyopia. What power of the lens commonly prescribed to this patient:-   **(PGMEE 2018)**
  a. +2D   b. +3D
  c. +5D   d. +1D

Explanation

Rule of Thumb for Prescribing Presbyopic Glasses

  ■ Presbyopia is physiological weakness of accommodation due to advancing age leading to progressive diminution in near vision.
  ■ A rough guide to prescribe presbyopic lenses is given below. Start with +1D presbyopic lens at the age of 40 and increase by 0.5 D at every 5 years.

Age	Required lens
35	0.5 D
40	+1 D
45	+1.5 D
50	+2D
55	+2.5D
60	+3D
65	+3.5D

  ■ Laser vision enhancement is presbyopia correcting IOL(Intra ocular lens) surgery in a patient with a high level of pre-existing astigmatism (i.e. >3 D), a bioptics approach (i.e., IOL followed by laser vision enhancement) may be needed.

    ○ For minor astigmatism → Limbal Relaxing Incisions (LRI) are useful.
    ○ Presbyopia-correcting IOL surgery followed by LASIK or PRK is also used.

26.	c
27.	b
28.	d
29.	a
30.	b
31.	d
32.	b
33.	b
34.	d
35.	a

CONTACT LENS

36. Soft contact lens are made up of - *(PGMEE 2015)*
   a. Silicone
   b. HEMA
   c. PMMA
   d. Glass

[Ref: Parsons' 23ʳᵈ/e pg. 72]

37. Most common infection in contact lens users is-
(PGMEE 2013)
   a. Streptococcus   b. Neisseria
   c. Pseudomonas   d. Staphylococcus

[Ref: Parsons' 22ⁿᵈ/e pg.82]

38. Contraindication of LASIK *(PGMEE 2013)*
   a. Keratoconus   b. Myopia of 8D
   c. Normal cornea   d. >20 years

[Ref: Parsons' 23ʳᵈ/e pg. 65]

36. b
37. c
38. a

1. **Conjunctival epithelium is -** *(PGMEE 2014)*
   a. Stratified columnar
   b. Transitional
   c. Stratified non keratinized squamous coloum
   d. Pseudostratified

   [Ref: Parsons' 23rd/e pg. 139]

2. **Normal conjunctival flora is -** *(PGMEE 2014)*
   a. Coagulase negative staphylococci
   b. Pseudomonas
   c. Lactobacillus
   d. E. coli

   [Ref: Parsons' 23rd/e pg. 140]

INFECTIVE CONJUNCTIVITIS

OPHTHALMIA NEONATORUM (NEONATORUM CONJUNCTIVITIS)

3. **Neonatal conjunctivitis is caused by all except -**
   (PGMEE 2012; 2016-17)
   a. Gonococcus   b. Pseudomonas
   c. Chlamydia   d. Aspergillus

   [Ref: Parsons' 23rd/e pg. 152-153]

4. **Most dangerous eye infection in newborn which can lead to blindness:-** *(PGMEE 2018)*
   a. Chlamydia
   b. Gonococcus
   c. Chemical conjunctivitis
   d. Trachoma

   [Ref: Parsons' 23rd/e pg. 152-153]

5. **Most common form of conjunctivitis in newborn within few hours of birth is:-** *(PGMEE 2018)*
   a. Chlamydia
   b. Nisseria
   c. Trachoma
   d. Chemical conjunctivitis

   [Ref: Parsons' 23rd/e pg. 154]

Explanation

Ophthalmia Neonatorum

- Ophthalmia neonatorum is a purulent conjunctivitis occurring during the first four weeks of life.
- Also called neonatal conjunctivitis.
- Etiology:-
  ○ The two MC causative agents are **Neisseria gonorrhoeae** and **Chlamydia trachomatis**, the former being of more concern here because of its propensity to cause blindness. Infection is acquired from infected mothers during passage through the birth canal.
  ○ Chlamydial ophthalmia (caused by **Chlamydia trachomatis**) is the most common bacterial cause; it accounts for up to 40% of conjunctivitis in neonates < 4 wk of age.
  ○ Hyperacute cases are usually caused by Neisseria gonorrhoeae or N. meningitidis.
  ○ Acute bacterial conjunctivitis caused by Staphylococcus aureus, Streptococcus pneumoniae, and Haemophilus influenzae.
  ○ Chronic cases of bacterial conjunctivitis are those lasting longer than 3 weeks, and are typically caused by Staphylococcus aureus, Moraxella lacunata, or gram-negative enteric flora.
  ○ Neisseria gonorrhoeae causes gonococcal conjunctivitis, s is a **potentially devastating ocular infection**, because N. gonorrhoeae can cause severe ulcerative keratitis, which may **rapidly progress to corneal perforation → Resulting in blindness**.
- Crede's method is use of 1% AgNO3 (Silver nitrate)
- Time of presentation
  ○ 24 hrs → Chemical conjunctivitis
  ○ 2-4 days → Neisseria gonorrhoeae (hyperacute conjunctivitis)
  ○ 4-10 days → Chlamydia trachomatis

Ophthalmia Neonatorum: Mode of Presentation, Differential Diagnosis and Treatment

Time of Onset After Birth	Differential Diagnosis	Treatment
Within the first 48 hours	Neisseria gonorrhoeae	Ceftriaxone injection i.m., gentamicin drops, bacitracin eye ointment
	Chemical	Wash eyes, apply erythromycin ointment and observe, usually improves in 24 hours
48-72 hours	Other bacteria	Neomycin-bacitracin eye ointment, gentamicin or tobramycin drops
5-7 days	Herpes simplex virus (HSV II)	Acyclovir 3% eye ointment, systemic acyclovir for systemic involvement in consultation with a paediatrician
>1 week	Chlamydia trachomatis (D-K)	Erythromycin or chlortetracycline eye ointment, oral erythromycin for systemic infection

6. **All of the following are true regarding inclusion body conjunctivitis EXCEPT:-** *(PGMEE 2012)*
   a. Acquired while passage from birth canal
   b. Caused by chlamydia
   c. Self limiting
   d. Present only in infants

   [Ref: Neena pg. 125; Parsons' 23rd/e pg. 153]

BACTERIAL CONJUNCTIVITIS

7. **Angular conjunctivitis is caused by:**
   (PGMEE 2013; 2016-17)
   a. Morax-Axenfeld diplobacilli
   b. Adenovirus type 32
   c. Brahnamella
   d. H. influenza

   [Ref: Parsons' 23rd/e pg. 145]

Explanation

Angular (Diplobacillary) Conjunctivitis

- Caused by **Moraxella axenfield** & Moraxella lacunata bacilli.
- T/t includes → Antibiotics + Zinc containing ophthalmic drops.

8. **All are true about Membranous conjunctivitis EXCEPT:**
   (DNB JUNE 2011)
   a. Easy to peel
   b. Caused by corynebacterium
   c. May lead to loss of central vision
   d. None of above

   [Ref: Parsons' 23rd/e pg. 145]

VIRAL CONJUNCTIVITIS

9. **Most of the viral infections of eye present as -**
   (PGMEE 2013)
   a. Keratoconjunctivitis   b. Keratitis
   c. Conjunctivitis   d. None

   [Ref: Parsons' 23rd/e pg. 147]

10. **Epidemo keratoconjuctivitis is caused by:**
    (DNB December 2011; PGMEE 2016-17)
    a. HSV   b. Adenovirus
    c. Chlamydia   d. HIV

    [Ref: Parsons' 23rd/e pg. 148]

11. **Haemorrhagic conjunctivitis is caused by?**
    (DNB Jun'2009; PGMEE 2016-17)
    a. Enterovirus 70   b. Coxsackie B virus
    c. Enterovirus 72   d. Calicivirus

    [Ref: Parsons' 22nd/e pg.172]

Explanation

Acute hemorrhagic conjunctivitis

- Also called "Apollo 11 disease" or "Epidemic haemorrhagic conjunctivitis".
- **Caused by:**
  ○ Bacteria → Hemophillous , pneumococcus

○ Viruses → **Enterovirus –70** (Most common), entero virus 71, Adenovirus 11, Coxsackie A 24, Echo virus 34.
- CF: Symptoms of conjunctivitis + sub conjunctival hemorrhages . Punctate keratopathy may be present.

12. **Subtype of enteroviruses involved in hemorrhagic conjunctivitis:** *(Recent Pattern June 2018)*
    a. Enterovirus 70   b. Enterovirus 71
    c. Enterovirus 72   d. Enterovirus 69

    [Ref: Parsons' 23rd/e pg. 148]

Explanation

- Acute hemorrhagic conjunctivitis (AHC) is a highly contagious conjunctivitis caused by two main virus types: Enterovirus and Coxsackievirus
- Also known as pink eye. Symptoms include excessively red, swollen eyes as well as subconjunctival Hemorrhages (aka pink eye).
- This disease is transmitted person-to-person usually through contact with contaminated hands or through sharing of contaminated personal-care items.

ALLERGIC CONJUNCTIVITIS

VERNAL KERATO-CONJUNCTIVITIS (SPRING CATARRH)

13. **Spring catarrh is:** *(PGMEE 2012)*
    a. Type I hypersensitivity reaction
    b. Type II hypersensitivity reaction
    c. Type III hypersensitivity reaction
    d. Type IV hypersensitivity reaction

    [Ref: Parsons' 23rd/e pg. 155]

Explanation

- Type I hypersensitivity reactions to pollen and other atmospheric exogenous allergens mediated by IgE play an important role in spring catarrh.

14. **"Ropy discharge" from the eye is seen in -**
    a. Spring catarrh   *(PGMEE 2012, Al 91)*
    b. Swimming pool conjunctivitis
    c. Phlyctenular conjunctivitis
    d. Epidemic keratoconjunctivitis

    [Ref: Parsons' 23rd/e pg. 141]

Explanation

- Mucoid (stringy or ropy) discharge is highly characteristic of allergy or dry eyes. A muco-purulent or purulent discharge, often associated with morning crusting and difficulty opening the eyelids, strongly suggests a bacterial infection

15. **Pseudogerontoxon is seen in :-** *(PGMEE 2016)*
    a. Spring catarrh   b. Chlamydia
    c. Trachoma   d. Fungal ulcer

    [Ref: Nenna 6th/e pg. 135]

16. **Maxwell Lyon sign is seen in :** *(DNB 2007)*
    a. Spring catarrh
    b. Dendritic ulcerative keratitis
    c. Symphathetic ophthalmitis
    d. Angular conjunctivitis

    [Ref: Neena 6th/e pg. 134]

6.	d
7.	a
8.	a
9.	a
10.	b
11.	a
12.	a
13.	a
14.	a
15.	a
16.	a

17. Cobble stone appearance of palpebral conjunctiva is seen in *(PGMEE 2016)*
a. Vernal keratoconjunctivitis
b. Bacterial conjunctivitis
c. Fungal keratitis
d. Trachoma

[Ref: Parsons' 23rd/e pg. 155]

18. Content of cobblestone in vernal conjunctivitis is? *(DNB Jun'2009)*
a. Eosinophils
b. Basophils
c. Lymphocytes
d. Histiocytes

[Ref: Parsons' 23rd/e pg. 155]

19. Complication of vernal kerato conjunctivitis - *(PGMEE 2012)*
a. Keratoconus
b. Vitreous hemorrhage
c. Cataract
d. Retinal detachment

[Ref: Parsons' 23rd/e pg. 156]

20. Treatment of vernal keratoconjunctivitis includes all except - *(PGMEE 2012)*
a. Cromoglycate
b. Steroids
c. Olopatadine
d. Antibiotics

[Ref: Parsons' 23rd/e pg. 155]

21. Horner trantas spot is seen in? *(DNB Dec'2010)*
a. Trachoma
b. Giant Papillary conjunctivitis
c. Vernal keratoconjunctivitis
d. Phlyctenular keratoconjunctivitis

[Ref: Parsons' 23rd/e pg. 155]

PHLYCTENULAR CONJUNCTIVITIS

22. Phlycten is due to- *(PGMEE 2014; 2016-17)*
a. Endogenous allergy
b. Fungal keratitis
c. Viral keratitis
d. Exogenous allergy

[Ref: Parsons' 23rd/e pg. 157]

Explanation

■ There is considerable evidence that phlyctenular conjunctivitis is an allergic condition caused by endogenous bacterial proteins, which in most cases are tuberculous but in other cases may be derived from mild, long-standing infections such as those of the tonsils or adenoids.

23. Phlyctenular conjunctivitis is caused by: *(PGMEE 2013)*
a. Pneumococcus
b. Chlamydia
c. Aspergillus
d. Tuberculous proteins

[Ref: Parsons' 23rd/e pg. 157]

Explanation

Phlyctenular conjunctivitis

■ Occurs due to allergy towards endogenous antigen of Staph aureus or TB (type IV hypersensitivity reaction).
■ **C/F:** Itching & Watering
■ **O/E:** Small nodules of phlycten at limbus, conjunctival congestion

■ Can involve cornea to form fascicular ulcer → Ring ulcer.
■ Axillary or cervical lymphadenopathy may be seen.
■ Rx:-
   ○ Olopatadine & Epinastine (Antihistaminics)
   ○ Na+ chromoglycate (mast cell Stabilizer
   ○ Mild steroids – Fluromethalone

24. Treatment of phylctenular conjunctivitis is?
a. Systemic steroids *(PGMEE 2011)*
b. Miotics
c. Antibiotics
d. Topical steroids

[Ref: Parsons' 23rd/e pg. 157]

PTERYGIUM

25. Conjunctival mucosal overgrowth over cornea is seen in: *(PGMEE 2013)*
a. Vernal keratoconjunctivitis
b. Pinguecula
c. Pterygium
d. Herbert's pit

[Ref: Parsons' 23rd/e pg. 159]

26. Pterygium is an growth extending from the medial canthus of eye. Which of the following statement does not holds true for it: *(Recent Pattern June 2018)*
a. Arises from descemet's membrane
b. Non-neoplastic growth
b. Elastotic degeneration
d. Associated with Vit. A deficiency

[Ref: Parsons' 23rd/e pg. 159]

Explanation

Pterygium

■ Pterygium is a non-neoplastic wing-shaped growth of conjunctiva upon the cornea from either side within the interpalpebral fissure.
■ Always situated in the palpebral aperture.
■ Pathologically pterygium is a degenerative & hyperplastic condition of conjunctiva. The subconjunctival tissue undergoes elastotic degeneration & proliferates as vascularised granulation tissue under the epithelium, which ultimately encroaches the cornea.
■ **The corneal epithelium, Bowman's layer & stroma are destroyed.**
■ Etio: more common in people with excess outdoor exposure to sunlight (UV rays) dry, heat, high wind & abundance of dust.
■ CF:
   ○ It presents as a triangular fold of conjunctiva encroaching the cornea in the area of palpebral aperture, **usually on the nasal side**.
   ○ Other findings are **stocker's line** (deposition of **iron**).
   ○ Asymptomatic in the early stages, except for cosmetic intolerance. In prolonged cases visual disturbance (due to encroachment of pterygium on pupillary area and corneal astigmatism) may occur late.
   ○ Occasionally diplopia may occur due to limitation of ocular movements.

17.	a
18.	a
19.	a
20.	d
21.	c
22.	a
23.	d
24.	d
25.	c
26.	a

27. Stocker's line is seen in *(PGMEE 2013, NEET Pattern 10)*
   a. Congenital Ocular Melanosis
   b. Pterygium
   c. Conjunctival epithelial melanosis
   d. Pinguecula

[Ref: Parsons' 22nd/e pg.184; Nema pg. 139]

28. Visual impairment in pterygium is due to
   (PGMEE 2015; 2016-17)
   a. Myopia   b. Hazy cornea
   c. Astigmatism   d. Hypermetropia

[Ref: Parsons' 23rd/e pg. 159]

29. What is the most common problem following surgical excision of pterygium? *(PGMEE 2016-17)*
   a. Scleral scarring   b. Recurrence
   c. Corneal ulceration   d. Astigmatism

[Ref: Parsons' 23rd/e pg. 160]

30. A 20 years female is diagnosed to have pterygium. She does not have any clinical symptoms except for cosmetic concern. Treatment should be - *(PGMEE 2014)*
   a. Antihistaminics   b. Left alone
   c. Antibiotics   d. Surgical excision

[Ref: Parsons' 23rd/e pg. 159]

Explanation

Pterygium

- Degenerative connective tissue disorder of subconjunctival fibrovascular tissue, which encroaches cornea.
- There is wing shaped fibrovascular fold of conjunctiva encroaching upon the cornea from either side. **MC nasally**.
- Gross:- Islets of Vogt, stocker's line (d/to deposition of **iron)** and Fuch's patches (minute dispersed grey blemishes) are seen on head end.
- More common in hot climate, in elderly males. Relation with UV-B exposure.
- Histo: Elastotic degeneration with hyalinization of conjunctival stroma is seen. Bowman's membrane is destroyed.
- A pterygium is best left alone unless it is progressing towards the pupillary area, causes excessive astigmatism, a restriction of ocular motility or is disfiguring.
- Recurrence after surgery is common. It is prevented by Mitomycin C, autoconjunctival graft, amniotic membrane graft, PERFECT surgery (pterygium extended resection followed by extended conjunctival transplantation).

31. Identify the condition shown in the given image:

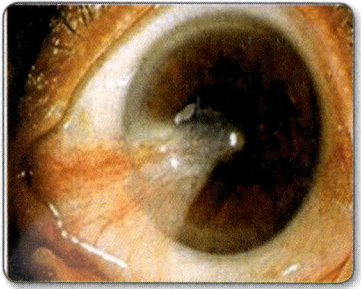

27. b
28. c
29. b
30. d
31. c
32. a
33. d
34. a
35. a

   a. Pinguecula   *(NEET Pattern 2017)*
   b. Ocular surface squamous neoplasia
   c. Pterygium
   d. Ocular dermoid

[Ref. Parsons' 23rd/e pg. 160]

Explanation

- *Pterygium* is a triangular /wing like encroachment of the conjunctiva onto the cornea in the interpalpebral region, due to fibrovascular proliferation of the subconjuctival tissues. It occurs at the nasal or temporal limbus. Nasal pterygium is more common.
- Surgical excision of pterygium is indicated if there is:
  ○ Encroachment upon the excision surgery include:
  ○ Significant astigmatism
  ○ Cosmetic concerns.
- *Pinguecula* is a growth that looks like a yellow spot or bump on the conjunctiva. It often appears on the side of the eye near your nose. A pinguecula is a deposit of protein, fat, or calcium

32. In the given condition, cause of defective vision is
   (PGMEE 2019)

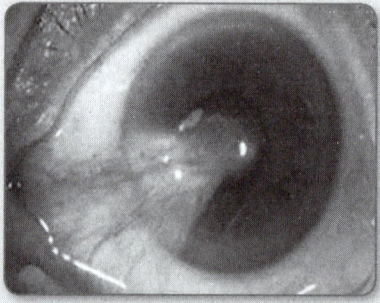

   a. Visual axis is obscured
   b. Astigmatism
   c. Hypermetropia
   d. Diplopia

[Ref: Parsons' 22nd/e pg. 184]

TRACHOMA

33. All are corneal signs of Trachoma except –
   (PGMEE 2013; 2016-17)

   a. Herbert follicles
   b. Pannus
   c. Opacity
   d. Arlt's line

[Ref: Parsons' 23rd/e pg. 150-151]

34. Arlt's line is seen in? *(DNB Jun'2009)*
   a. Trachoma
   b. Vernal catarrh
   c. Angular conjunctivitis
   d. Spring catarrh

[Ref: Nema 6th/e pg. 127]

35. Herbert pits are seen in : *(DNB 2007; PGMEE 2016-17)*
   a. Trachoma   b. Psoriasis
   c. Spring catarrh   d. Fungal keratitis

[Ref: Parsons' 23rd/e pg. 150]

36. Cicatrising trachoma is seen in - *(PGMEE 2013)*
a. Stage-1
b. Stage-2
c. Stage-3
d. Stage-4

[Ref: Parsons' 22nd/e pg.174]

Explanation

- *Mac Callan Classification (1908) is based on conjunctival findings alone:*
  - Stage I: Incipient trachoma or stage of infiltration: It is characterized by hyperaemia of palpebral conjunctiva and immature follicles.
  - Stage II: Established trachoma: It is characterized by appearance of mature follicles, papillae and progressive corneal pannus.
    II A: Follicular hypertrophy
    II B: Papillary hypertrophy
  - Stage III: Cicatrizing trachoma: It includes obvious scarring of palpebral conjunctiva.
  - Stage IV: Healed trachoma: The disease is quite and cured but sequelae due to cicatrisation give rise to symptoms.

37. Which of the following is not a sequelae of trachoma? *(DNB Jun'2009)*
a. Dacrocystitis
b. Tylosis
c. Pseudocyst
d. Proptosis

[Ref: Parsons' 23rd/e pg. 150; Nema 6th/e pg. 129]

38. Cause of blindness in trachoma:- *(PGMEE 2015)*
a. Scarring
b. Entropion
c. Pannus
d. Chronic dacrocystitis

[Ref: Parsons' 22nd/e pg. 174; Nema 6th/e pg. 129]

39. In the grading of trachoma, trachomatous inflammation follicular is defined as the presence of:- *(PGMEE 2015)*
a. ⩾3 follicles in the upper tarsal conjunctiva
b. ⩾3 follicles in the lower tarsal conjunctiva
c. ⩾5 follicles in the lower tarsal conunctiva
d. ⩾5 follicles in the upper tarsal conjunctiva

[Ref: Parsons' 23rd/e pg. 151]

40. Drug of choice for mass treatment of trachoma in India- *(PGMEE 2014 & 2015)*
a. Sulfonamide
b. Chloramphenicol
c. Oral Azithromycin
d. Penicillin

[Ref: Parsons' 23rd/e pg. 150; Nema 6th/e pg. 130]

41. Tetracycline ointment for mass prophylaxis *(PGMEE 2012)*
a. 0.1%　　　　b. 0.5%
c. 1%　　　　　d. 5%

[Ref: Parsons' 23rd/e pg. 150]

MISCELLANEOUS

42. Subconjunctival hemorrhage occurs in all conditions except - *(PGMEE 2015)*
a. Passive venous congestion
b. High intraocular tension
c. Trauma
d. Pertusis

[Ref: Parsons' 23rd/e pg. 142]

Explanation

- Systolic hypertension (not high IOT) can cause subconjunctival h'age.
- Other causes of subconjunctival h'age are
  - Spontaneous h'age in elderly people with fragile vessels or those with systolic hypertension or after local ocular trauma or eye surgery
  - In children with whooping cough and in scurvy, in blood diseases such as purpura or in malaria.
  - Bleeding diatheses or leukaemia
  - Secondary to a fracture of the base of the skull.
  - Severe or prolonged pressure on the thorax.

43. Subconjunctival cyst is seen in- *(PGMEE 2015)*
a. Chagas disease　　b. Leishmaniasis
c. Cysticercosis　　　d. Toxoplasmosis

[Ref: Parsons' 23rd/e pg. 161; Nema 6th/e pg. 140]

44. Epithelial xerosis of conjunctiva is caused by - *(PGMEE 2013)*
a. Xerophthalmia　　b. Diphtheria
c. Pemphigus　　　　d. Trachoma

[Ref: Parsons' 23rd/e pg. 163]

45. Circumcorneal congestion is not seen is?
a. Acute bacterial conjunctivitis　*(DNB June 2011)*
b. Scleritis
c. Acute glaucoma
d. Acute iritis

[Ref: Parsons' 23rd/e pg. 143]

Explanation

- In acute bacterial conjunctivitis the whole conjunctiva is fiery red (pink eye). All conjunctival vessels are congested a phenomenon less marked in the circumcorneal zone.
- *Circumcorneal congestion (ciliary flush)* may be seen due to enlargement of the episcleral vessels in the region of the ciliary body. It is seen in scleritis, acute glaucoma and acute iritis.
- Keratic precipitates (KPs) are cellular deposits on the corneal endothelium.

36.	c
37.	d
38.	a
39.	d
40.	c
41.	c
42.	b
43.	c
44.	a
45.	a

ANATOMY & PHYSIOLOGY

1. Corneal epithelium is composed of: *(PGMEE 2014)*
   a. Columnar epithelium
   b. Stratified keratinized epithelium
   c. Psudostratified epithelium
   d. Stratified non- keratinized squamous epithelium

   [Ref: Parsons' 23rd/e pg. 168]

2. Mucus in tear film secreted by?

(PGMEE June 14 Pattern)

   a. Conjunctival goblet cells
   b. Lacrimal glands
   c. Zeis gland
   d. Moll glands

   [Ref: Parsons' 23rd/e pg. 423]

3. Cornea is supplied by: *(PGMEE June 14 Pattern)*
   a. Lacrimal branch of trigeminal nerve
   b. Frontal branch of trigeminal nerve
   c. Nasociliary branch of ophthalmic nerve
   d. Trochlear nerve

   [Ref: BDC 7th/e vol. 3 pg. 300; Parsons' 23rd/e pg. 168]

4. Afferent component in corneal reflex is mediated by:

(PGMEE 2012-13)

   a. Optic nerve
   b. Ophthalmic nerve
   c. Oculomotor nerve
   d. Facial nerve

   [Ref: BDC 7th/e vol. 4 pg. 69; Parsons' 23rd/e pg. 173]

5. Schwable's line is seen in which layer of cornea-

(PGMEE 2015)

   a. Descemet's membrane
   b. Stroma
   c. Bowmann's membrane
   d. Substantia propria

   [Ref: Parsons' 22nd/e pg.194; Nema 6th/e pg. 249, 146]

6. Avascular coat, in eye is - *(PGMEE 2014)*
   a. Choroid   b. Sclera
   c. Retina   d. Cornea

   [Ref: Parsons' 23rd/e pg. 169]

7. Anisocornia in dim light is maximally seen in –
   a. Pharmacological mydriasis   *(PGMEE 2012)*
   b. Horner syndrome
   c. Parasymapathetic paralysis
   d. 3rd nerve palsy   *[Ref: Parsons' 22nd/e pg. 367]*

8. Corneal deturgescence is maintained by:

(PGMEE 2016-17)

   a. Endothelium
   b. Descemet's membrane
   c. Stroma
   d. Epithelium

   [Ref: Parsons' 22nd/e pg. 194]

Answers:

1.	d
2.	a
3.	c
4.	b
5.	a
6.	d
7.	b
8.	a
9.	b
10.	c
11.	b

Explanation

- Corneal deturgescence is part of a process in which the water content of the cornea is controlled by a dynamic process of pumping and leaking. The enzymes associated with pumping (corneal deturgescence) in fresh tissue and tissue cultures have been only partially defined and characterized.

9. Density of cells in adult corneal endothelium:

(PGMEE 2016-17)

   a. 2000 cells/mm²
   b. 2800 cells/mm²
   c. 4000 cells/mm²
   d. 5000 cells/rnth²

   [Ref: Parsons' 23rd/e pg. 118]

10. The refractive power of cornea is : *(DNB 2007)*
   a. 15   b. 30
   c. 44   d. 60

   [Ref: Parsons' 22nd/e pg192]

11. What happens to corneal endothelium after injury-

(PGMEE 2015)

   a. Regenerates rapidly   b. Never regenerates
   c. Forms a scar   d. Slowly regenerates

   [Ref: Parsons' 23rd/e pg. 168]

Explanation

- Epithelium regenerates while endothelium never regenerate
- In case the cornea sustains injury due to any cause such as trauma, infection or surgery, and if the injury is superficial involving only the epithelium, the stratified squamous epithelium covering the anterior surface of the cornea rapidly regenerates.
- This regeneration of corneal epithelial cells is mainly from stem cells, palisades of Vogt at the limbus.
- The corneal endothelium does not regenerate
- The corneal epithelium and endothelium maintain a steady fluid content of the corneal stroma.

Cornea anatomy & physiology

- Develops from:-
  ○ Surface ectoderm → epithelium
  ○ Neural crest → endothelium, and stroma of cornea
- Corneal transparency is the result of avascularity, relative dehydration, peculiar arrangement of corneal lamellae (Lattice theory of Maurice).
- Cornea attains adult size by 2 years of age.
- Cornea gets its nourishment from atmospheric oxygen and from the superficial plexus formed by episcleral branches of anterior ciliary arteries (annular plexus). Cornea has no blood vessels of its own. it is nourished by aqueous humor.

- Endothelial ionic pump of the cornea c/b blocked by inhibition of anaerobic glycolysis. Corneal edema occurs due to accumulation of lactate.
- Corneal epithelium: Stratified SqE.
- Refractive power of cornea is → 45D.
- Bowman's membrane once destroyed it can not regenerate.
- Endothelial cell layer is most **metabolically active** layer. Normal number of endothelial cells are 2500 cells/mm^2. Plexus in corneal endothelium – annular plexus.
- Stains used for corneal staining → Fluoriscein, alcian blue and Rose Bengal.

INVESTIGATIONS

12. Placido disk is used to examine- *(PGMEE 2016-17)*
a. Anterior corneal surface
b. Lens surface
c. Retina
d. Optic nerve
[Ref: Parsons' 23rd/e pg. 99]

13. Keratometer is used for: *(Recent Pattern June 2018)*
a. Corneal thickness
b. Corneal diameter
c. Corneal curvature
d. Distance between cornea and pupil
[Ref: Parsons' 23rd/e pg. 170]

Explanation

- A keratometer (aka ophthalmometer), is a diagnostic instrument for measuring the **curvature of the anterior surface of the cornea**, particularly for assessing the extent and axis of astigmatism.

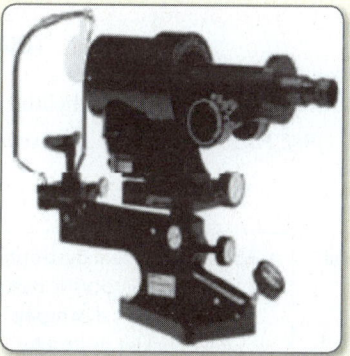

CORNEAL ULCERS

14. Organism which does NOT invade intact cornea- *(PGMEE 2014)*
a. C. diphtheriae
b. Pseudomonas
c. Meningococci
d. Gonococci
[Ref: Parsons' 23rd/e pg. 174]

Explanation

Organism invading intact cornea
- Meningococcus
- Gonococus
- Hemophillus
- Listeria
- Shigella
- Diphtheria

15. Which organism can penetrate the intact cornea? *(DNB Dec'2010)*
a. Gonococcus
b. Pseudomonas
c. Staphylococcus
d. Klebsiella
[Ref: Parsons' 23rd/e pg. 175]

16. Ulcer serpens is caused by- *(PGMEE 2016-17)*
a. Gonorrhoea niesseria
b. Pseudomonas pyocynaeceous
c. Corynebacteria
d. Pneumococcus
[Ref: Nema 6th/e pg. 149]

FUNGAL CORNEAL ULCER

17. Hypopyon in a fungal corneal ulcer contains
a. Fungal spores *(PGMEE 2015)*
b. Sterile material
c. Purulent material
d. Fungal filaments
[Ref: Parsons' 23rd/e pg. 172, 176; Nema 6th/e pg. 153]

Explanation

- The hypopyon, if present, is thick and immobile and is due to direct invasion into the anterior chamber of fungal hyphae enmeshed in thick exudates

18. Immune ring is a feature of: *(PGMEE 2013)*
a. Fungal corneal ulcer
b. Herpes simplex keratitis
c. Interstitial keratitis
d. Bacterial corneal ulcer
[Ref: Parsons' 23rd/e pg. 176]

Explanation

- Immune rings are seen in acanthamoeba, herpes, pseudomonas and fungus infections.
- An immune ring *(of Wessely)* may be visible due to deposition of immune complexes and inflammatory cells around the ulcer. **Acanthamoeba** is the most common cause of Wessely immune ring in cornea.
- Satellite lesions.

19. Steroid is contraindicated in: *(PGMEE 2015)*
a. Fungal corneal ulcer
b. Atopic dermatitis
c. Exposure keratitis
d. Herpetic keratitis
[Ref: Parsons' 23rd/e pg. 178]

20. Non-sterile hypopyon is seen in: *(PGMEE 2013)*
a. Pneumococcus infection
b. Fungal infection
c. Gonococcal infection
d. Pseudomonas infection
[Ref: Parsons' 23rd/e pg. 176; Nema 6th/e pg. 153]

21. Satellite lesion is seen which corneal ulcer? *(DNB Dec'2009; PGMEE 2016-17)*
a. Trachoma
b. Fungal
c. Angular
d. Herpes
[Ref: Parsons' 22nd/e pg. 205]

12.	a
13.	c
14.	b
15.	a
16.	d
17.	b
18.	a
19.	a
20.	b
21.	b

HERPES KERATITIS

22. All of the following are true about findings in herpetic keratitis EXCEPT:- *(PGMEE 2012)*
- a. Dendritic ulcers
- b. Disciform Keratitis
- c. Stromal Keratitis
- d. Cornea guttata

[Ref: Parsons' 23rd/e pg. 180]

Explanation
- Dendritic ulcers may be seen in severe cases.

23. Ameboid ulcer is a feature of- *(PGMEE 2013)*
- a. Herpetic corneal ulcer
- b. Mycotic corneal ulcer
- c. Bacterial corneal ulcer
- d. Parasitic corneal ulcer

[Ref: Nema 6th/e pg. 159]

Explanation
- The dendritic ulcer can spread in many directions and lead to an amoeboid configuration commonly known as geographical ulcer.
- The geographical lesion is a result of rapid viral replication owing to reduced tissue resistance particularly after the indiscriminate use of topical corticosteroids

24. Treatment of mooren's ulcer is? *(DNB Jun'2009; PGMEE 2016-17)*
- a. Corneal graft
- b. Immunosuppressive
- c. Topical steroids
- d. All of the above

[Ref. Parsons' 23rd/e pg. 184; Nema 6th/e pg. 155]

25. Disciform keratitis is seen - *(PGMEE 2016-17)*
- a. HSV
- b. Rubella
- c. HBV
- d. HIV

[Ref: Parsons' 23rd/e pg. 180]

HERPES ZOSTER OPHTHALMICUS

26. Corneal sensation is lost in- *(PGMEE 2014)*
- a. Trachoma
- b. Conjunctivitis
- c. Fungal infection
- d. Herpes simplex

[Ref: Parsons' 23rd/e pg. 173]

Explanation
- *Loss of corneal sensations* is typically seen in diseases associated with damage to the corneal nerves as seen in herpes simplex or herpes zoster infections or lesions affecting the ophthalmic division of the trigemina nerve.
- This is tested by touching it with a wisp of cotton wool or a Cochet-Bonnet aesthesiometer

27. In herpes zoster ophthalmicus least involved nerve is? *(DNB June 2011)*
- a. Facial
- b. Infraorbital
- c. Nasociliary
- d. Lacrimal

[Ref: Parsons' 23rd/e pg. 181, 182]

Explanation
- The supraorbital, supratrochlear and infratrochlear branches are nearly always involved; frequently, the nasal branch and only rarely the infraorbital branch.

- In some cases, there is associated paralysis of the motor cranial nerves, especially the oculomotor, abducens and facial, which usually passes off within 6 weeks. Facial palsy is dangerous, as it causes exposure of the cornea.

28. Hutchinson's rule is related to – *(PGMEE 2013)*
- a. Mycotic keratitis
- b. Herpes simplex keratitis
- c. Herpes zoster ophthalmicus
- d. None

[Ref: Parsons' 23rd/e pg. 182]

29. False regarding herpes zoster ophthalmicus:
- a. Vesicles appear before pain *(DNB Dec'2010)*
- b. Lesion doesn't cross the midline
- c. Ophthalmic division is commonly involved
- d. Involvement of tip of nose denotes eye involvement

[Ref. Parsons' 23rd/e pg. 181 & H. V nema 161]

30. Ocular symptom NOT seen in Herpes zoster ophthalmicus: *(PGMEE 2014; DNB 2007)*
- a. Cranial nerve palsies
- b. Nummular & Disciform keratitis
- c. Anterior uveitis
- d. Glaucoma *[Ref: Parsons' 23rd/e pg. 182]*

31. Neurotrophic keratopathy is caused by - *(DNB Jun'2010, PGMEE 2014; 2016-17)*
- a. Trigeminal nerve palsy
- b. Bell's palsy
- c. Facial and trigeminal nerve palsy both
- d. Oculomotor palsy

[Ref: Parsons' 23rd/e pg. 192; Nema 6th/e pg. 164]

CORNEAL DYSTROPHY

32. Reis-Buckler dystrophy affects which layer of cornea- *(PGMEE 2016-17)*
- a. Bowman's membrane
- b. Stroma
- c. Endothelium
- d. Epithelium

[Ref: Parsons' 23rd/e pg. 186; Nema 6th/e pg. 168]

Explanation

Anterior corneal dystrophies	Epithelial corneal dystrophies ○ Cogan's microcystic dystrophy ○ Meesmann's dystrophy ○ Reis-Buckler dystrophy ○ Thiel-Behnke dystrophy
	Stromal corneal dystrophies ○ Granular ○ Macular ○ Lattice
Posterior corneal dystrophies	Endothelial corneal dystrophy (Fuchs) Posterior polymorphous dystrophy
Ectatic corneal dystrophies	Keratoconus Keratoglobus Pellucid marginal degeneration

33. Recurrent corneal erosion seen in- *(PGMEE 2012)*
- a. Keratoconus
- b. Keratoglobus
- c. Peutz- anomalies
- d. Corneal dystrophy

[Ref: Parsons' 23rd/e pg. 186]

22.	d
23.	a
24.	d
25.	a
26.	d
27.	b
28.	c
29.	a
30.	c
31.	a
32.	a
33.	d

34. Not true about Fuch's corneal dystrophy: *(PGMEE 2013)*
a. Endothelial dystrophy
b. Occurs in old age
c. Posterior dystrophy
d. Unilateral condition

[Ref: Parsons' 23rd/e pg. 188]

35. Which one of the following stromal dystrophy is a recessive condition? *(PGMEE 06)*
a. Granular dystrophy
b. Fleck dystrophy
c. Macular dystrophy
d. Lattice dystrophy

[Ref: Parsons' 23rd/e pg. 187]

36. All are true about Bullous keratopathy except- *(PGMEE 2015)*
a. Lenses can be prescribed for such patients
b. Treatment is kertoplasty
c. Seen in Fuchs dystrophy
d. Seen in Macular dystrophy

[Ref: Parsons' 23rd/e pg. 188; Nema 6th/e pg. 171]

KERATOCONUS

37. Thinning of cornea occurs in *(PGMEE 2014)*
a. Megalocornea
b. Keratoconus
c. Endothelial dystrophy
d. Bullous keratopathy

[Ref: Parsons' 22nd/e pg.216]

38. All are seen in keratoconus except: *(DNB Dec'2010*
a. Munson sign
b. Keyser Fleischer ring
c. Scissoring reflex in retinoscopy
d. Progressive vision loss due to increasing myopia and irregular astigmatism

[Ref. Parsons' 23rd/e pg. 191; Nema 6th/e pg. 171]

39. Scissore reflex is seen in: *(PGMEE 2016-17; 13)*
a. Interstitial keratitis
b. Open angle glaucoma
c. Keratoconus
d. Phlyctenular conjunctivitis

[Ref: Parsons' 23rd/e pg. 191; Nema 6th/e pg. 171]

40. Munson's sign is seen in- *(PGMEE 2015)*
a. Keratomalacia
b. Keratoconus
c. Keratoglobus
d. All of these

[Ref: Parsons' 23rd/e pg. 190]

41. To prevent keratoconus what is used *(PGMEE 2012)*
a. Glasses
b. Cycloplegics
c. Antibiotics
d. None

[Ref: Parsons' 22nd/e pg.216]

PHOTOPHTHALMIA

42. Photophthalmia involves which part of eye: *(PGMEE 2013)*
a. Cornea
b. Retina
c. Iris
d. Vitreous

[Ref: Parsons' 23rd/e pg. 193]

43. Snow blindness is caused by: *(PGMEE 2016-17)*
a. Ultra-voilet rays
b. Infrared rays
c. Microwaves
d. Defect in mirror

[Ref: Parsons' 23rd/e pg. 193]

CORNEAL TRANSPLANTATION

44. Safe size of corneal graft with less chances of failure is: *(PGMEE 2015)*
a. 75 mm
b. 65 mm
c. 55 mm
d. 45 mm

[Ref: Parsons' 22nd/e pg.221]

45. Golden period of eye donation: *(PGMEE 2015)*
a. 6 hours
b. 12 hours
c. 18 hours
d. 24 hours

[Ref: Parsons' 23rd/e pg. 194]

46. Following corneal transplantation, most common infection to occur: *(PGMEE 2012)*
a. Staph epidermidis
b. Pseudomonas
c. Streptococcus
d. Klebsiella

[Ref: internet]

OTHER CORNEAL DISEASES

47. Prominent corneal nerves are seen in all except: *(PGMEE 2014)*
a. Ichythyosis
b. Macular dystrophy
c. Refsum's syndrome
d. Ectodermal dysplasia

[Ref: Parsons' 23rd/e pg. 172]

Explanation

Prominent or enlarged corneal nerves are seen in

- Keratoconus
- MEN IIb syndrome
- Neurofibromatosis and
- Refsum syndrome

48. Cornea verticillate is caused by: *(PGMEE 2016-17)*
a. Amiodarone
b. Tetracycline
c. Timolol
d. Erythromycin

[Ref: Parsons' 23rd/e pg. 193]

Explanation

Cornea Verticillata

- Whorl-like opacity in the corneal epithelium seen in patients on long-term treatment with medication such as amiodarone, chloroquine, phenothiazines and indomethacin. It is also seen in patients with Fabry disease and its carrier state

49. Decreased corneal sensations can be seen in: *(PGMEE 2013)*
a. Bacterial corneal ulcer
b. Leprosy
c. Interstitial keratitis
d. Mycotic corneal ulcer

[Ref: Parsons' 23rd/e pg. 173; Nema 6th/e pg. 495]

34.	d
35.	c
36.	d
37.	b
38.	b
39.	c
40.	b
41.	d
42.	a
43.	a
44.	a
45.	a
46.	a
47.	b
48.	a
49.	b

50. Interstitial keratitis is caused by all excepts-

a. TB **(PGMEE 2013)**
b. Pertussis
c. Typhoid
d. Lyme disease

[Ref: Parsons' 23rd/e pg. 185]

Explanation

- *Possible causes*: These may be measles, typhoid, syphilis, tuberculosis and idiopathic.
- *Cogan syndrome*: Interstitial keratitis and deafness (Cogan syndrome) is a rare disease affecting young adults.

51. Superficial corneal vascularisation is caused by-

(PGMEE 2016-17)

a. Chemical burn b. Graft rejection
c. Contact lens d. Interstitial keratitis

[Ref: Nema 6th/e pg. 175]

Explanation

- The superficial vascularization of cornea is common and it is seen in the following conditions
  - Trachoma
  - Superficial corneal ulcers
  - Phlyctenular keratoconjunctivitis
  - Rosacea keratitis, and
  - Contact lens wearers
- The deep vascularization of cornea is seen in the following diseases:
  - Interstitial keratitis
  - Deep corneal ulcers
  - Sclerosing keratitis
  - Disciform keratitis, and
  - Chemical burns

SCLERA

ANATOMY

52. Thickest portion of sclera is: **(PGMEE 2016-17)**

a. Anterior to rectus muscle insertion
b. Posterior pole
c. Limbus
d. Posterior to rectus muscle insertion

[Ref: Parsons' 23rd/e pg. 198]

Explanation

- It is 1 mm thick posteriorly, 0.66 mm at the insertions of the rectus muscles, 0.33 mm beneath the rectus muscles and thinnest just behind their insertions.

53. Sclera is thinnest at:

a. Equator **(PGMEE 2012-13, 2014; DNB Jun'2009)**
b. Limbus
c. Anterior to attachment of superior rectus
d. Posterior to attachment of superior rectus

[Ref: BDC 7th/e vol. 3 pg. 299; Parsons' 23rd/e pg. 198]

54. Blue sclera is characteristic of? **(PGMEE June' 2012)**

a. Tetracyline hypoplasia
b. Osteogenesis imperfecta
c. Amelogenesis Imperfecta
d. Fluorosis

[Ref. Parsons' 23rd/e pg. 203]

Explanation

- Osteogenesis imperfecta
- Other systemic diseases that may be associated with blue sclera are Ehlers-Danlos syndrome, Marfan syndrome and pseudoxanthoma elasticum.
- Keratoconus and Keratoglobus

STAPHYLOMA

55. Staphlyoma involves: **(PGMEE 2012)**

a. Conjunctiva with cornea
b. Iris with conjunctiva
c. Choroid with retina
d. Iris with cornea

[Ref: Parsons' 23rd/e pg. 202; Nema 6th/e pg. 184]

56. Most common cause of anterior staphyloma -

(PGMEE 2013)

a. Scleritis b. High myopia
c. Trauma d. Corneal ulcer

[Ref: Parsons' 23rd/e pg. 202]

57. Most common cause of posterior staphyloma:

(PGMEE 2012)

a. Glaucoma b. Myopia
c. Trauma d. Scleritis

[Ref: Parsons' 23rd/e pg. 203]

58. Posterior styphayloma is a feature of:

(PGMEE 2015, DNB December 2011)

a. Congenital myopia b. Simple myopia
c. Pathological myopia d. Hypermetropia

[Ref: Parsons' 23rd/e pg. 203]

59. Post trauma/infection, iris gets attached to the cornea, becomes adherent to it and leads to opacity. The condition is: **(PGMEE 2017)**

a. Posterior staphyloma b. Anterior staphyloma
c. Adherent leucoma d. Adherent staphyloma

[Ref: Khurana 5th /e pg128; Nema 6th/e pg. 61]

SCLERITIS

60. Most common type of scleritis: **(PGMEE 2013)**

a. Necrotizing b. Posterior
c. Non-necrotizing d. None

[Ref: Parsons' 22nd/e pg. 227; Nema 6th/e pg. 182]

Explanation

Anterior scleritis	■ Non-necrotizing scleritis
	○ Nodular (is more frequent 95%)
	○ Diffuse
	■ Necrotizing scleritis
	○ With inflammation (seen in ant. uveitis)
	○ Without inflammation (scleromalacia perforans): Seen in RA
Posterior scleritis	

50.	b
51.	c
52.	b
53.	d
54.	b
55.	d
56.	d
57.	b
58.	c
59.	c
60.	c

1.   c
2.   c
3.   b
4.   d
5.   b
6.   c
7.   a

ANATOMY

1. Continuation of inner layer of choroid is:
   a. Sclera   **(PGMEE 2012-13)**
   b. Nonpigmented layer of retina
   c. Pigmented layer of retina
   d. None
      [Ref: BDC 7th/e vol. 3 pg. 302-303; Parsons' 23ʳᵈ/e pg. 9]

2. Intermediate layer of uvea is: **(PGMEE 2017)**
   a. Sclera   b. Iris
   c. Pars plana   d. Choroid
   [Ref: BDC 7th/e vol. 3 pg. 302-303; Parsons' 23ʳᵈ/e pg. 211]

UVEITIS

3. All are cause of chronic granulomatous uveitis except –
   a. Sarcoidosis   **(PGMEE 2014)**
   b. Fuchs heterochromic iridocyclitis
   c. Brucellosis
   d. Tuberculosis

      [Ref: Parsons' 23ʳᵈ/e pg. 211]

Explanation

Causes of granulomatous and non-granulomatous uveitis

Granulomatous uveitis	Non-Granulomatous uveitis	Both G/NG uveitis
Sarcoidosis	Behcet's syndrome	Toxoplasmosis
Tuberculosis	Psoriasis	Syphilis
Vogt Koyanagi Harada (VKH) syndrome	Ankylosing spondylitis	
Sympathetic ophthalmitis	Early onset & pauciarticular JRA	
[Mn] : TVSS Grand]	Reiter's disease	

   ■ Both granulomatous/non granulomatous & anterior and posterior uveitis are seen in Syphilis and toxoplasmosis.

4. Most common cause of anterior uveitis associated with arthritis -   **(PGMEE 2012, 2016-17)**
   a. Rheumatoid arthritis
   b. Tuberculosis
   c. Syphilis
   d. Ankylosing spondylitis

      [Ref: Parsons' 23ʳᵈ/e pg. 220]

5. All of the following has HLA B-27 associated with uveitis except -   **(PGMEE 2015)**
   a. Reiters syndrome   b. Behcets syndrome
   c. Ankylosing spondylitis   d. None of the above

      [Ref: Parsons' 23ʳᵈ/e pg. 221]

Explanation

   ■ HLA B-27 → In Reiters syndrome and Ankylosing spondylitis.
   ■ Human leukocyte antigen B-6 → In Behcets syndrome

6. In acute anterior uveitis, size of pupil is –   **(PGMEE 2013)**
   a. Oval   b. Circular
   c. Small, irregular   d. Any of the above

      [Ref: Parsons' 23ʳᵈ/e pg. 104]

Explanation

Papillary findings in various diseases

   ■ 'Muddy' iris with a small, irregular pupil and sluggish reaction to light are indicative of uveitis
   ■ Dilatation of the pupils with retained mobility found sometimes in myopia
   ■ Pupils are small in babies
   ■ Very large, nonreactive pupils suggest that a mydriatic has been used.
   ■ The pupils are also large and immobile in bilateral lesions affecting the retina and the optic nerve (as in optic nerve atrophy).
   ■ Bilateral dilated pupils, in bilateral blindness, can be distinguished

Pupilloplegia

   ■ Dilated and immobile pupils also result from third nerve palsies *(absolute paralysis of the pupil)*
   ■ Small, immobile pupils suggest the use of drugs, either locally (miotics) or systemically (morphine). A small, sluggish pupil with 'muddiness' of the iris is associated with an active iritis.
   ■ A small, immobile pupil suggests old iritis with bilateral, small pupils may be due to irritation of the third nerves.
   ■ In acute angle-closure glaucoma, the pupil is usually large, immobile and oval, with the long axis vertical.

7. Iris bombe is due to –   **(PGMEE 2014, 2016-17)**
   a. Ring synechiae
   b. Total posterior synechiae
   c. Anterior synechiae
   d. Segmental posterior synechiae

      [Ref: Parsons' 23ʳᵈ/e pg. 209]

Explanation

   ■ In severe cases of plastic iritis or after recurrent attacks, the whole pupillary margin may become tied down to the lens capsule, called **annular** or **ring synechiae** or **seclusio pupillae**.
   ■ If unrelieved, it inevitably leads to a secondary angle-closure glaucoma.

- The aqueous, unable to pass forwards into the anterior chamber, collects behind the iris, which becomes bowed forwards like a sail - a condition which is called *iris bombe*.

KERATIC PRECIPITATES (KP'S)

8. Granular keratic precipitates are made of:
(PGMEE 2015)
- a. Epitheloid cells
- b. Lymphocytes
- c. Macrophages
- d. RBC

[Ref: Parsons' 23rd/e pg. 206]

9. Red keratic precipitates are seen in - *(PGMEE 2013)*
- a. Old healed uveitis
- b. Hemorrhagic uveitis
- c. Granulomatous uveitis
- d. Acute anterior uveitis

[Ref: Parsons' 23rd/e pg. 101]

10. 1st sign of anterior uveitis- *(PGMEE 2014)*
- a. Keratic precipitate
- b. Miosis
- c. Hypopyon
- d. Aqueous flare

[Ref: Parsons' 22nd/e pg. 235]

11. Keratic precipitates are on which layer of cornea-
(PGMEE 2012)
- a. Epithelium
- b. Endothelium
- c. Stroma
- d. Bowman's membrane

[Ref: Parsons' 23rd/e pg. 209, 101]

12. Mutton fat keratic precipitate and Busacca's nodules is seen in - *(PGMEE 2012, 2016-17)*
- a. Non-granulomatous uveitis
- b. Choroiditis
- c. Posterior uveitis
- d. Granulomatous uveitis

[Ref: Parsons' 23rd/e pg. 101]

Explanation

Keratic precipitates

- These are deposits of leukocytes and other inflammatory cells and debris on the back (endothelium) of cornea.
- Seen in cyclitis, iridocyclitis & choroiditis
- Types of KP's

Type	Found in
Fine and grey	Non granulomatous uveitis
Mutton fat KPs (large, greasy, granular mainly lymphocytic)	Granulomatous uveitis

- Types of nodules seen in granulomatous uveitis
  - *Koeppe's nodules* are smaller in size and are seen at the pupillary border.
  - *Bussaca's nodules* are larger in size and are seen in the surface of iris away from pupil (near the collarete).

OTHER FINDINGS IN UVEITIS

13. Which of the following indicates activity of anterior uveitis- *(PGMEE 2015)*
- a. Cells in anterior chamber
- b. Corneal edema
- c. Keratic precipitate
- d. Circumcorneal congestion

[Ref: Parsons' 23rd/e pg. 103]

14. A patient having posterior synechiae was treated with topical mydriatic and developed irregular pupil. Most likely cause is? *(PGMEE 2015)*
- a. Festooned pupil
- b. Chalcosis
- c. Occlusio pupillae
- d. Aniridia

[Ref: Parsons' 23rd/e pg. 209]

15. Most common symptom of posterior uveitis -
(PGMEE 2015)
- a. Pain
- b. Diminished vision
- c. Photophobia
- d. Lacrimation

[Ref: Parsons' 23rd/e pg. 211]

16. Phthisis bulbi means *(PGMEE 2015)*
- a. Final end stage of chronic scleritis
- b. Final end stage of chronic uveitis
- c. Developmental hypoplasia of optic cup
- d. All of the above

[Ref: Parsons' 23rd/e pg. 209]

17. Metamorphopsia is seen in- *(PGMEE 2016-17)*
- a. Anterior uveitis
- b. Glaucoma
- c. Cataract
- d. Posterior uveitis

[Ref: Parsons' 23rd/e pg. 211]

18. Koeppe's nodules are found in - *(PGMEE 2016-17)*
- a. Choroiditis
- b. Non granulomatous uveitis
- c. Granulomatous uveitis
- d. Pars planitis

[Ref: Parsons' 23rd/e pg. 206]

19. Nodules seen near the collarette are called-
(PGMEE 2015)
- a. Busacca's nodules
- b. Dalen Fuchs nodules
- c. Lisch nodules
- d. Koeppe's nodules

[Ref: Parsons' 23rd/e pg. 206]

Explanation

- Clusters of inflammatory cells forms nodules:-
  - On the pupillary border → **Koeppe nodules** or
  - On the peripheral part of the anterior surface of the iris → **Busacca nodules**.
  - **Berlin's nodules** (trabecular meshwork nodules) are seen in → the angle of anterior chamber in granulomatous uveitis.

20. Koeppe's nodules are present on - *(PGMEE 2012)*
- a. Retina
- b. Conjunctiva
- c. Iris
- d. Cornea

[Ref: Parsons' 23rd/e pg. 206]

21. Snow banking is typically seen in- *(PGMEE 2014)*
- a. Eale's disease
- b. Pars planitis
- c. Coat's disease
- d. Endophthalmitis

[Ref: Parsons' 23rd/e pg. 211]

22. Commonest complication of pars planitis
(PGMEE 2012)
- a. Vitreous hemorrhage
- b. Glaucoma
- c. Cataract
- d. Retinal detachment

[Ref: Parsons' 23rd/e pg. 211]

8.	b
9.	b
10.	d
11.	b
12.	d
13.	a
14.	a
15.	b
16.	b
17.	d
18.	c
19.	a
20.	c
21.	b
22.	c

PARS PLANITIS

23. Pars planitis is - *(PGMEE 2015)*
   a. Anterior uveitis   b. Pan uveitis
   c. Posterior uveitis   d. Intermediate uveitis

   [Ref: Parsons' 23rd/e pg. 210]

TREATMENT OF UVEITIS

24. Drug of choice for acute iridocyclitis is?
  (PGMEE 2016-17)
   a. Atropine   b. Topical Steroid
   c. Pilocarpine   d. Timolol

   [Ref: Parsons' 23rd/e pg. 212]

25. Mainstay of treatment of uveitis - *(PGMEE 2016-17)*
   a. Steroids and cycloplegics
   b. Surgery
   c. Antibiotics and steroids
   d. Antibiotics and cycloplegics

   [Ref: Parsons' 23rd/e pg. 212]

26. Uveitis with raised IOT is managed by all EXCEPT –
  (PGMEE 2013)
   a. Atropine   b. Steroid
   c. Pilocarpine   d. Timolol

   [Ref: Parsons' 23rd/e pg. 213]

Explanation

Treatment of Uveitic glaucoma (Uveitis with raised IOT)

- Secondary glaucoma (Uveitis with raised IOT) is one of the serious complications of iridocyclitis.
- The most effective treatment is to intensify atropinization and use corticosteroids
- Steroids, beta-blockers administered topically and acetazolamide given systemically
- Pilocarpine and latanoprost are contraindicated as uveitis may be exacerbated.
- Laser iridotomy is essential in all cases with annular synechiae to restore communication between the posterior and anterior chambers and thus avoid the supervention of secondary glaucoma.

27. Drug of choice for intermediate uveitis - *(PGMEE 2013)*
   a. Systemic steroids   b. Antibiotics
   c. Atropine   d. Topical steroids

   [Ref: Parsons' 23rd/e pg. 212]

Explanation

Treatment of Uveitis

- Acute anterior uveitis - Topical steroids are DOC .
- 1% Atropine eye drops give rest to the eye by relieving spasm of iris sphincter and cilliary muscle. It also prevent formation of synechiae and may break already formed synechiae. Steroids are also used.

ENDOPHTHALMITIS

28. Panophthalmitis involves - *(PGMEE 2013)*
   a. All structure of eyeball including tenon's capsule
   b. Inner and outer coat but sparing tenon's capsule
   c. Inner coat of eyeball
   d. None of the above

   [Ref: Parsons' 23rd/e pg. 214]

29. Enucleation of the eyeball is contraindicated in -
  (PGMEE 2016-17; 2013)
   a. Painful blind eye
   b. Endophthalrnitis
   c. Intraocular tumours
   d. Panophthahnitis

   [Ref: Parsons' 22nd/e pg.244]

MISCELLANEOUS

30. Iridocyclitis in a patient of MAC under treatment is due to :- *(PGMEE 2016)*
   a. Rifabutin
   b. Ethambutol
   c. Clindamycin
   d. All

   [Ref: Parsons' 22nd/e pg. 244]

31. Neovascularization of iris is frequently seen in all / except: *(Recent Pattern June 2018)*
   a. CRVO
   b. Diabetic retinopathy
   c. Fuch's heterochromic cyclitis
   d. Congenital cataract

   [Ref: Parsons' 23rd/e pg. 224]

Explanation

Rubiosis Iridis

- It is neovascularization of iris and may lead to neovascular glaucoma.
- Neovascularization develops following retinal ischemia, which is a common feature of
  - PDR (Proliferative diabetic retinopathy)
  - CRVO
  - Sickel cell retinopathy
  - Eale's disease
  - Other rare causes are Fuch's hetrochromic cyclitis, chronic intraocular inflammation, intraocular tumor, long standing retinal detachment & CRAO.

32. Iris pearl are seen in – *(PGMEE 2015; 2011; 2016-17)*
   a. Sarcoidosis
   b. Tuberculosis
   c. Leprosy
   d. Cat Scratch disease

   [Ref: Khurana Ophthalmology 4th/e p. 155; Nema 6th/e pg. 202]

33. Following is feature of Fusch's hetero chromic iridocyclitis - *(PGMEE 2015)*
   a. Posterior subcapsular cataract
   b. Keratic precipitates
   c. Heterochromia of iris
   d. All the above

   [Ref: Parsons' 23rd/e pg. 222; Nema 6th/e pg. 207]

34. Amsler sign is seen in- *(PGMEE 2013)*
   a. Uveal-effusion syndrome
   b. Fuch heterochromatic iridocyclitis
   c. Posner-schlossman syndrome
   d. None of the above

   [Ref: Parsons' 23rd/e pg. 222]

23.	d
24.	b
25.	a
26.	c
27.	d
28.	a
29.	d
30.	a
31.	d
32.	c
33.	d
34.	b

15. Identify the pathology depicted in the given image?
(PGMEE 2015)

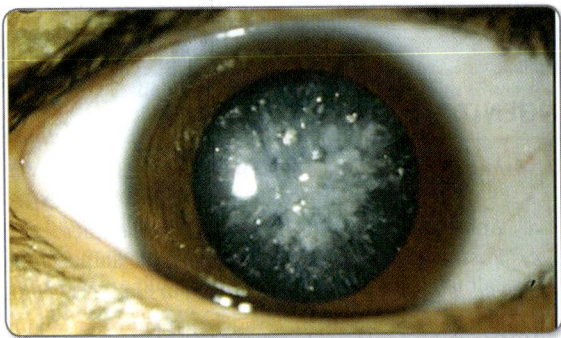

a. Blue dot cataract
b. Posterior subcapsular cataract
c. Seclusio pupillae
d. Hypopyon

[Ref: Parsons' 23rd/e pg. 241]

16. Peripheral cortical developmental cataract which is inherited as autosomal dominant and occurrs just after puberty -
(PGMEE 2015)

a. Coronary cataract
b. Total congenital cataract
c. Blue dot cataract
d. Lamellar cataract

[Ref: Parsons' 23rd/e pg. 242]

17. Pathology depicted in the slit lamp view shown image?
(PGMEE 2015)

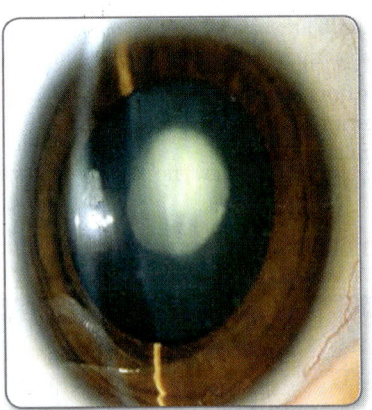

a. Zonular cataract
b. Zonular cataract
c. Blue dot cataract
d. Posterior polar cataract

[Ref: Khurana 4th /e p. 172]

18. Surgery of choice for congenital cataract -
(PGMEE 2013; 2016-17)

a. Discission
b. Needling
c. ECCE
d. ICCE

[Ref: Parsons' 22nd/e pg. 274; Internet articles]

Explanation

- *The needling operation* is described as one in which the anterior lens capsule is opened and the cortex is stirred up. Absorption is allowed for a minimum of 8 weeks after which the operation may be repeated if necessary. Some times a disscision of the posterior capsule is required at a later date.

15.	a
16.	a
17.	d
18.	b
19.	c
20.	b
21.	d

ACQUIRED CATARACT

19. Most common type of senile cataract – **(PGMEE 2013)**

a. Nuclear
b. Cupuliform cortical
c. Cunieform cortical
d. None

[Ref: Parsons' 23rd/e pg. 237]

20. Cataract brunescens results due to deposition of
(PGMEE 2013)

a. Silver
b. Melanin
c. Iron
d. Copper

[Ref: Parsons' 23rd/e pg. 238; Nema 6th/e pg. 263]

21. Second sight phenomenon is seen in – **(PGMEE 2013)**

a. Senile cataract
b. Cortical cataract
c. Tridocycitis
d. Nuclear cataract

[Ref: Parsons' 23rd/e pg. 236; Nema 6th/e pg. 264]

Explanation

Symptoms of Acquired Cataract

Symptom	Pathogenesis	Type of Cataract
Frequent change of glasses	Rapid change in refractive index of the lens	Cortical or nuclear
Reduced visual acuity usually gradual, painless, progressive	Reduction in transparency of the lens	All types
'Second sight' or myopic shift	Change in refractive index of the nucleus causes index myopia, improving near vision	Nuclear cataract
Loss of ability to see objects in bright sunlight, blinded by light of oncoming headlamps when driving at night	Loss of contrast sensitivity, which is greater at higher spatial frequencies; constriction of pupil cuts off peripheral vision from noncataractous area	Posterior subcapsular
Monocular diplopia or polyopia	Cortical spoke opacities in conjunction with water clefts that form radial wedges containing a fluid of lower refractive index than the surrounding lens	Cortical cataract (spoke or cuneiform)
Glare	Increased scattering of light	Cortical and posterior subcapsular
Coloured halos around light	Irregularity in the refractive index of different parts of the lens	Cortical cataract
Colour shift (becomes more obvious after surgery)	Blue end of the spectrum is absorbed more by the cataractous lens	Nuclear
Visual field loss	Generalized reduction in sensitivity due to loss of transparency	All types

22. Nuclear cataract can cause – *(PGMEE 2012)*
a. Hyperopia   b. Astigmatism
c. Presbyopia   d. Myopia

[Ref: Parsons' 23rd/e pg. 238]

23. Polyopia/diplopia is seen in which type of cataract:
a. Posterior subcapsular   *(PGMEE 2013)*
b. Cortical
c. Anterior polar
d. Nuclear

[Ref: Parsons' 23rd/e pg. 236]

24. Lens proteins become liquid in? *(PGMEE 2015)*
a. Hypermature cataract
b. Mature cataract
c. Immature cataract
d. None of the above

[Ref: Parsons' 23rd/e pg. 238]

25. Chronic systemic steroid use causes?
(DNB December 2011; PGMEE 2016-17)
a. Open angle glaucoma
b. Conjuctival and lid papillomatis
c. Uveitis
d. Cataract

[Ref: Parsons' 22nd/e pg 261]

CATARACT ASSOCIATED WITH SYSTEMICS DISEASES

26. Diabetic cataract occurs to accumulation of:
(PGMEE 2015; 2016-17)
a. Fructose   b. Galactitol
c. Glucose   d. Sorbitol & Fructose

[Ref: Parsons' 22nd/e pg. 268; Nema 6th/e pg. 265]

27. Typical appearance of true diabetic cataract is:
(DNB Dec'2010; 2016-17)
a. Sunflower type
b. Polychromatic lusture
c. Breadcrumb type
d. Snow flake appearance

[Ref: Parsons' 23rd/e pg. 239]

28. Cataract in case of diabetes mellitus is due to accumulation of: *(PGMEE 2015)*
a. Calcified crystallins   b. Calcified fibrillins
c. Glycated fibrillins   d. Glycated crystallins

[Ref: Parsons' 23rd/e pg. 239]

29. "Bread-crumb" appearance and polychromatic lustre is seen in: *(PGMEE 2016, 17, 13, 12)*
a. Congenital cataract
b. Diabetes mellitus
c. Complicated cataract
d. Post radiation cataract

[Ref: Parsons' 23rd/e pg. 239]

Explanation
- In the beam of the slit lamp, the opacities have an appearance like breadcrumbs and a characteristic rainbow display of colours often replaces the normal achromatic sheen *(polychromatic lustre)*

30. Oil drop cataract is characteristic of –
(PGMEE 2013; 2016-17)
a. Diabetes   b. Chalcosis
c. Galactossemia   d. Wilson's disease

[Ref: Nema 6th/e pg. 266]

Explanation
- The dust-like lenticular opacities manifest soon after birth (within 2 months) and the nucleus and deep cortex become opaque causing a classical "oil droplet" appearance on retroillumination.

31. Sunflower type cataract is characteristically seen in –
(PGMEE 2016-17, 2012)
a. Congenital syphilis
b. Diabetes
c. Stragardt's disease
d. Chalcosis/(Wilson's disease)

[Ref: Parsons' 23rd/e pg. 235; Nema 6th/e pg. 266]

32. Christmas tree cataract is seen in – *(PGMEE 2012)*
a. Down's syndrome   b. Rubella
c. Diabetes   d. Myotonic dystrophy

[Ref: Parsons' 23rd/e pg. 240]

33. Christmas tree cataract is seen in:
(Recent Pattern June 2018)
a. Down's syndrome   b. Trauma
c. Diabetes mellitus   d. Myotonic dystrophy

[Ref: Parsons' 23rd/e pg. 240]

Explanation
- Christmas tree cataract is seen in dystrophia myotonica.
- There are fine dust like opacities interspersed with tiny iridescent spots in the cortex underneath the capsule in 90% of cases.
- These opacities may or may not be a/w with posterior subcapsular stellate opacities.
- Sunflower cataract is seen in Wilson's disease, chalcosis & penetrating trauma
- Snowflake cataract is seen in diabetes mellitus

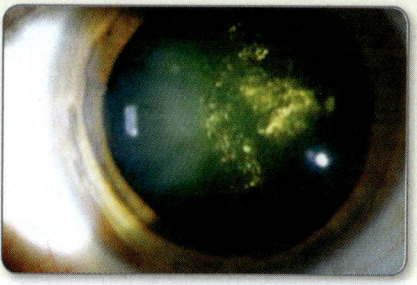

34. Rosette cataract seen in? *(PGMEE 2014)*
a. Ocular trauma   b. Diabetes
c. Wilson's d/s   d. None

[Ref: Parsons' 23rd/e pg. 499]

AFTER CATARACT

35. Elsching's pearls are seen in: *(PGMEE 2016-17)*
a. Secondary cataract   b. Congenital cataract
c. Complicated cataract   d. Wilson's disease

[Ref: Parsons' 23rd/e pg. 258; Nema 6th/e pg. 288]

22.	d
23.	b
24.	a
25.	d
26.	d
27.	d
28.	d
29.	c
30.	c
31.	d
32.	d
33.	d
34.	a
35.	a

36. Ring of Sommering is seen in - *(PGMEE 2014)*
a. After cataract
b. Galactosemia
c. Dislocation of lens
d. Acute congestive glaucoma

[Ref: Parsons' 23rd/e pg. 258]

37. Which laser is used in the management of after cataract - *(PGMEE 2015; 2016-17)*
a. Krypton
b. Excimer
c. Nd- YAG
d. Argon

[Ref: Parsons' 23rd/e pg. 259]

MANAGEMENT OF CATARACT

38. Best way to prevent infection after cataract surgery is-
a. Thorough irrigation *(PGMEE 2013)*
b. Eyebrows shaving
c. Antibiotics
d. Mydriatics

[Ref: Parsons' 22nd/e pg. 276]

39. Site of bleeding after cataract surgery is:
a. Anterior choroidal vessels *(DNB Dec'2010)*
b. Anterior ciliary vessels
c. Posterior choroidal vessels
d. Posterior ciliary vessels

[Ref: Parsons' 22nd/e pg.278]

40. Recovery in cataract surgery is fastest with which of the following- *(PGMEE 2014)*
a. Phacoemulsification
b. ECCE
c. ICCE
d. ECCE with ICI

[Ref: Parsons' 23rd/e pg. 253]

36.	a
37.	c
38.	c
39.	d
40.	a
41.	b
42.	b
43.	d
44.	c
45.	a

Explanation

Summary of Postoperative Medication and Care

	Extracapsular	Phacoemulsification
	Cataract extraction	
Topical steroidantibiotic eye drops[a]	6-8 weeks	3-4 weeks
Mydriaticcycloplegic	1-2 weeks	1-2 weeks
Medication to reduce the intraocular pressure	1-2 weeks	1-2 weeks
Refraction and prescription of glasses[b]	6-8 weeks	1-2 weeks
General precautions, restriction of physical activity	6-8 weeks	1-2 weeks

[a]Some surgeons use nonsteroidal anti-inflammatory agents.

[b]Following ICCE and ECCE, sutures are removed at this stage.

41. Phacoemulsification incision is at *(PGMEE 2015; 2016-17)*
a. Sclera
b. Sclero-corneal junction
c. Cornea
d. None of the above

[Ref: Parsons' 23rd/e pg. 251]

Explanation
- The site of incision can be superior or temporal.
- The incision could be at the limbus after cutting the conjunctiva and cauterizing bleeding vessels, or 'clear cortneal' just anterior to the limbus

42. Which is not a cataract surgery- *(PGMEE 2012)*
a. IOL
b. Goniotomy
c. Lensectomy
d. Phacoemulsification

[Ref: Parsons' 23rd/e pg. 247-48]

Explanation
- The different methods are as follows:
  - Conventional ECCE
  - ECCE by small-incision cataract surgery (SICS) or small-incision manual nucleus fragmentation
  - Lensectomy
  - Phacoemulsification
  - Femtosecond laser-assisted cataract surgery

43. Treatment of traumatic cataract in children- *(PGMEE 2012)*
a. Contact lens
b. Lensectomy
c. Glasses
d. ECCE + IOL

[Ref: Parsons' 22nd/e pg. 277]

44. Most common complication of extracapsular cataract surgery is - *(PGMEE 2015)*
a. Vitreous haemorrhage
b. Retinal detachment
c. Opacification of posterior capsule
d. None *[Ref: Parsons' 22nd/e pg. 285]*

45. A diabetic patient who underwent cataract surgery few days back comes back with complaints of red, painful eye with hypopyon as shown in image. Best treatment for him is: *(PGMEE 2018)*

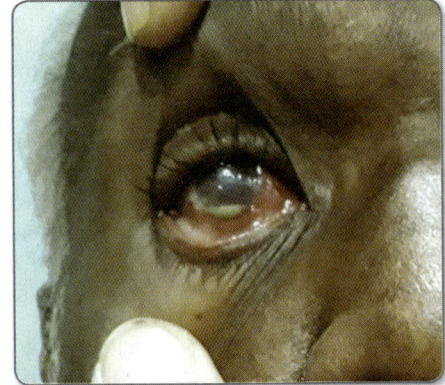

a. Tapping of fluid + Intravitreal antibiotics
b. Steroids
c. IV Mannitol
d. Pad and bandages

[Ref: Nema 6th/e pg. 279]

Explanation

Post Cataract Endophthalmitis

- Delayed onset exogenous endophthalmitis can occur after cataract surgery or Glaucoma filtration operation.
- The cardinal features of endophthalmitis are pain, swelling of lids and decreased vision (here due to hypopyon).
- A high index of suspicion arises in post operative cases (here the patient is presenting few weeks post cataract surgery).
- M/c causative organism includes Staphylococcus epidermidis. *Propionibacterium acne* is also common. Prolonged surgery > 60 minutes, vitreous loss and diabetes mellitus are risk factors for development of endophthalmitis.
- Treatment:
  - **Intravitreal antibiotics are TOC** and are injected after taking samples for cultures.
  - If there is no improvement after 48 hrs - Repeat vitreous tap
  - If no response after 2 intravitreal injections i.e. patient not responding to medical therapy→ procede for vitrectomy which is used to remove the infected vitreous and facilitate better penetration of the antibiotics..
  - Steroid therapy may be used concurrently with caution.

46. A patient developed endopthalmitis after 5 days of cataract surgery. All can be used in the management except? *(NEET Pattern 2017)*

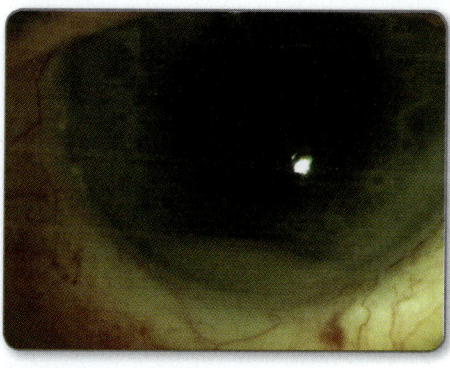

a. Intravitreal antibiotic injection
b. Intravitreal steroids
c. Pars plana vitrectomy
d. Topical antibiotics

[Ref: Nema 6th/e pg. 279]

Explanation

- Endophthalmitis is the infection of the eye involving the viterous. This can occur at any time following cataract surgery ranging from within 2 days to few months after surgery.
- Post operative endophthalmitis is treated by intravitreal antibiotics after obtaining viterous tap or vitrectomy. Topical antibiotics are being used by some ophthalmologists.

47. Best site for IOL implantation- *(PGMEE 2013)*
a. Anterior chamber
b. Ciliary sulcus
c. Capsular bag in posterior chamber
d. Iris

[Ref: Parsons' 23rd/e pg. 254]

Explanation

- Intraocular lenses are specifically designed according to the intended location (posterior chamber, anterior chamber and scleral fixated)
- The lens is best placed in the posterior chamber in the capsular bag.

48. Foldable lens is made up of: *(PGMEE 2013)*
a. Hydrogel
b. Silicon
c. PMMA
d. None

[Ref: Parsons' 23rd/e pg. 257]

ECTOPIA LENTIS

49. Dislocation of lens is seen in all the following conditions EXCEPT:- *(PGMEE 2012, 2000)*
a. Homocystinuria
b. Congenital Rubella
c. Marfan's Syndrome
d. Weill Marchesani's Syndrome

[Ref: Parsons' 23rd/e pg. 245]

50. Causes of ectopia lentis are all except *(DNB Dec'2010)*
a. Homocystinuria
b. Sulphite oxidase deficiency
c. Cogon Reese syndrome
d. Marfan's syndrome

[Ref: Parsons' 23rd/e pg. 245]

51. Typically bilateral inferior subluxations of the lens is seen in - *(PGMEE 2015)*
a. Homocystinuria
b. Ocular trauma
c. Hyperinsulinemia
d. Marfan's syndrome

[Ref: Parsons' 23rd/e pg. 245]

52. In Marfan's syndrome lens dislocation is commonly seen: *(PGMEE 2014; 2016-17)*
a. Supero-temporally
b. Downwards
c. Upwards
d. Nasally

[Ref: Parsons' 23rd/e pg. 245]

53. Marfan's syndrome associated with? *(DNB Jun'2010)*
a. Retinal detachment
b. Vitreous hemorrhage
c. Roth spots
d. Ectopia lentis

[Ref: Parsons' 23rd/e pg. 245]

46.	b
47.	c
48.	b
49.	b
50.	c
51.	a
52.	a
53.	d

54. Identify the pathology depicted below *(PGMEE 2015)*

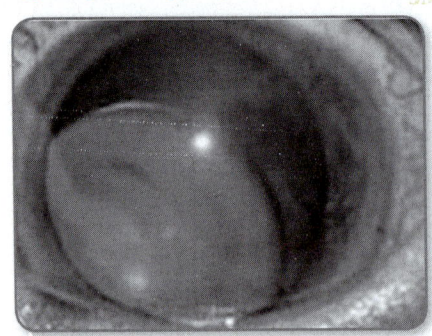

a. Corneal dehiscence
b. Lens subluxation
c. Iris subluxation
d. Vitreous haemorrhage

[Ref: Parsons' 23rd/e pg. 245]

LENTICONUS

55. Posterior lenticonus is seen in – *(PGMEE 2013; 2016-17)*

a. Lowe's syndrome
b. Homocystinuria
c. Marfan syndrome
d. Alport's syndrome

[Ref: Parsons' 23rd/e pg. 245]

56. Anterior lenticonus is found in:

(DNB 2007, PGMEE 2014)

a. Down's syndrome
b. Lowe's syndrome
c. Alport's syndrome
d. Alstrom's syndrome

[Ref: Parsons' 23rd/e pg. 245]

Explanation

- Anterior lenticonus : seen in Alport syndrome, Waardenbenburg syndrome
- Posterior Leniconus:
  ○ More common
  ○ Seen in Alport syndrome & Lowe syndrome

57. Which type of lenticonous is more common in males?
(DNB Jun'2009)

a. Posterior
b. Anterior
c. Both are equally common
d. Inferior

[Ref: Parsons' 23rd/e pg. 245]

54. b
55. a
56. c
57. a

PHYSIOLOGY

1. Normal rate of aqueous production: *(PGMEE 2013)*
- a. 2 ml/min
- b. 5 ml/min
- c. 2 μL/min
- d. 5 μL/min

[Ref: Parsons' 22nd/e pg. 289]

2. Von Herick's angle grade '3' of anterior chamber denotes— *(PGMEE 2013)*
- a. Closed angle
- b. Wide open angle
- c. Moderately narrow angle
- d. Open angle

[Ref: Parsons' 22nd/e pg. 296; Nema 6th/e pg. 217 table]

Explanation

Shaffer's grading of the angle of the anterior chamber

Grade	AC angle	Angle width in degrees	Structure visible	Chances of closure
IV	Wide open	45	Schwalbe's line to ciliary body	Nil
III	Open	20 to <45	Schwalbe's line to scleral spur	Nil
II	Moderately	10 to 20	Schwalbe's line to trabeculum	Possible
I	Very narrow	10	Schwalbe's line only	High
0	Closed	0	None	Already closed

3. The normal cup disc ratio is - *(PGMEE 2015)*
- a. 0.3
- b. 0.6
- c. 1.2
- d. 2.4

[Ref: Parsons' 23rd/e pg. 263]

4. Normal intraocular pressure is – *(PGMEE 2015)*
- a. 7 - 14 mm Hg
- b. 2.1 -6 mm Hg
- c. 15 - 17 mm Hg
- d. 16-32 mm Hg

[Ref: Parsons' 23rd/e pg. 108]

OPEN ANGLE GLAUCOMA

5. Rapid change of presbyopic glass is a feature of - *(PGMEE 2014; 2016-17)*
- a. Intumescent cataract
- b. Retinal detachment
- c. Open angle glaucàma
- d. Senile cataract

[Ref: Parsons' 23rd/e pg. 267]

6. Which of the following drug is not used topically for treatment of open angle glaucoma – *(PGMEE 2014)*
- a. Acetazolamide
- b. Brimonidine
- c. Latanoprost
- d. Dorzolamide

[Ref: Parsons' 23rd/e pg. 279]

Explanation
- Acetazolamide is used orally. Oral acetazolamide or glycerol takes about 0.5-1 hour to control moderately high intraocular pressures
- Miotics are essential for the treatment of PACG until an iridotomy is preformed.

7. Drug used in refractory glaucoma:- *(PGMEE 2015)*
- a. ACE inhibitor
- b. Systemic glucocorticoid
- c. Alpha agonist
- d. Beta blocker

[Ref: Parsons' 23rd/e pg. 267, 279]

8. The first line treatment of open angle glaucoma is:-
- a. Pilocarpine *(PGMEE 2012)*
- b. Carbonic anhydrase inhibitor
- c. Timolol
- d. Epinephrine

[Ref: Parsons' 23rd/e pg. 267]

9. Drug kept as a last resort in the management of primary open angle glaucoma is - *(PGMEE 2015)*
- a. Topical beta blocker
- b. Oral acetazolamide
- c. Latanoprost
- d. Brimonidine

[Ref: Parsons' 22nd/e pg. 307]

10. Argon Laser Trabeculoplasty is done in: *(DNB 2008)*
- a. Open angle glaucoma
- b. Secondary glaucoma
- c. Angle recession glaucoma
- d. Angle closure glaucoma

[Ref. Parsons' 23rd/e pg. 269]

ANGLE CLOSURE GLAUCOMA

11. In acute angle closure glaucoma all are seen EXCEPT: *(DNB Jun'2010)*
- a. Cupping of disc
- b. Oval cup
- c. Snow banking
- d. Bayoneting sign

[Ref. Parsons' 22nd/e pg.297]

12. Painless loss of vision is seen in all except: *(PGMEE 2011)*
- a. Papilloedema
- b. Papillitis
- c. CRAO
- d. Angle closure glaucoma

[Ref: Parsons' 23rd/e pg. 511]

Explanation

Painless loss of vision is commonly due to:
- Retinal vascular occlusion
- Arteritic is ischaemic optic neuropathy (no pain in the eye per se, but headache)
- Nonarteritic anterior ischaemic optic neuropathy (NAION)
- Retinal detachment

1.	c
2.	d
3.	a
4.	c
5.	c
6.	a
7.	c
8.	c
9.	b
10.	a
11.	c
12.	d

13. All EXCEPT one predisposes to angle closure glaucoma:-
(PGMEE 2012; NEET Pattern 00)
- a. Small cornea
- b. Short axial length of eye ball
- c. Shallow AC
- d. Flat cornea

[Ref: Parsons' 23rd/e pg. 270]

14. Secondary angle closure glaucoma is caused by:-
- a. Corticosteroid induced   **(PGMEE 2015)**
- b. Congenital glaucoma
- c. Subluxation of lens
- d. Angle recession glaucoma

[Ref: Parsons' 23rd/e pg. 274]

Explanation
- *Secondary angle closure glaucoma* occurs due to changes in the lens
  - **Phacomorphic glaucoma**:- The lens becomes intumescent, either by the rapid development of Cataractous changes or after a traumatic rupture of its capsule.
  - **Phacotopic glaucoma**:- An anterior subluxation or dislocation of the lens.
- *Secondary open angle glaucoma* occurs may develop if the lens has been damaged or if lens proteins from a hypermature senile cataract escape into the aqueous. This is called **phacolytic glaucoma**.
- **Pseudophakic and aphakic glaucomas** are among the common secondary glaucomas, due to the larger number of cataract surgeries especially after pediatric cataract surgeries.

15. Not a symptom of angle closure glaucoma -
(PGMEE 2012; 2016-17)
- a. Headache
- b. Coloured Halos
- c. Blurring of vision
- d. Metamorphosia

[Ref: Parsons' 23rd/e pg. 272; Nema 6th/e pg. 241]

Explanation
- Severe ocular pain, headache, blurred vision, rainbow-colored halos around the light, nausea and vomiting.

16. In acute congestive glaucoma, pupil is - **(PGMEE 2012)**
- a. Oval and horizontal
- b. Slit like
- c. Oval and vertical
- d. Circular

[Ref: Parsons' 23rd/e pg. 272]

17. Mild dilated fixed pupil seen in - **(PGMEE 2014)**
- a. Chronic congestive glaucoma
- b. Iridocyclitis
- c. Open angle glaucoma
- d. Acute congestive glaucoma

[Ref: Parsons' 23rd/e pg. 272]

18. Fincham's test differentiates cataract from -
- a. Open angle Glaucoma   **(PGMEE 2016-17)**
- b. Conjunctivitis
- c. Iridocyditis
- d. Acute primary angle closure glaucoma

[Ref: Parsons' 23rd/e pg. 271; Nema 6th/e pg. 241]

CONGENITAL GLAUCOMA

19. Most common symptom in buphthalmos is-
- a. Photophobia   **(PGMEE 2013)**
- b. Pain
- c. Itching
- d. Lacrimation

[Ref: Parsons' 22nd/e pg. 304]

Explanation
- Three symptoms typically characterize primary congenital glaucoma:
  - Excessive tearing (epiphora)
  - Sensitivity to light (photophobia)
  - Spasms or squeezing of the eyelid (blepharospasm)

20. Habbe striae are seen in- **(PGMEE 2013; 2016-17)**
- a. Trachoma
- b. Buphthalmos
- c. Keratoconus
- d. Keratoglobus

[Ref: Parsons' 23rd/e pg. 277]

21. A child presents with lid lag and an enlarged cornea having a diameter of 13mm. Examination of the eye reveals double contoured opacities concentric to the limbus. Which of the following is the most likely diagnosis- **(PGMEE 12)**
- a. Thyroid Endocrinopathy
- b. Deep keratitis
- c. Superficial keratitis
- d. Congenital Glaucoma

[Ref: Parsons' 23rd/e pg. 277]

22. Initial treatment of buphthalmos is – **(PGMEE 2015)**
- a. Goniotomy
- b. Carbonic anhydrase inhibitors
- c. Topical piocarpine
- d. Laser trabeculolasty

[Ref: Parsons' 23rd/e pg. 278]

Explanation
- Medications are not very effective.
- The most effective surgery is goniotomy or trabeculotomy in which the anomalous architecture of the angle is cut through to allow the entry of aqueous into the canal of Schlemm.

OTHER GLAUCOMAS

23. False about phacolytic glaucoma
(PGMEE 2012; 2016-17)
- a. Due to contact of iris to lens
- b. Open angle glaucoma
- c. Seen in hypermature stage of cataract
- d. Lens induced glaucoma

[Ref: Parsons' 23rd/e pg. 274]

24. A 40 years male with spherophakia is at risk for developing- **(PGMEE 2015)**
- a. Phacomorphic glaucoma
- b. Phacoanaphylactic glaucoma
- c. Phacolytic glaucoma
- d. None of the above

[Ref: Parsons' 23rd/e pg. 274]

13.	d
14.	c
15.	d
16.	c
17.	d
18.	d
19.	d
20.	b
21.	d
22.	a
23.	a
24.	a

25. Mechanism of steroid induced glaucoma is:
(*PGMEE 2014*)
a. Deposition of hemosiderine
b. Neovascularization of Iris
c. Narrowing of angle of anterior chamber
d. Inhibition of PGE & PGF

[Ref: Parsons' 23rd/e pg. 276]

26. Which one of the procedure involves using glaucoma drainage device? (*PGMEE 2019*)
a. Seton operation
b. Deep sclerectomy
c. Viscocanalostomy
d. Trabeculectomy

[Ref: A K Khurana Comprehensive Ophthalmology 7th/e pg. 263]

27. Arcuate field defect akin to glaucoma is seen in all except- (*PGMEE 2013*)
a. Occipital lobe infarct
b. Optic nerve lesion
c. Pituitary tumor
d. None of the above

[Ref: Parsons' 23rd/e pg. 262; Nema 6th/e pg. 228]

Explanation
- Arcuate or Bjerrum's scotomas are usually associated with glaucoma.
- They can also be found in other conditions such as sudden drop of blood pressure, coronary thrombosis, opticochiasmatic arachnoiditis, pituitary adenoma and drusen of the optic nerve head.

28. In glaucoma which field of vision is lost in the last:-
(*PGMEE 2018*)
a. Nasal
b. Temporal
c. Superior
d. Central

Explanation

Visual Field Changes in Glaucoma
- Temporal island is the most resistant in advanced changes. Temporal vision remains till last.

Changes	Findings
Early non-specific changes	Isopter contraction Baring of blind spot
Early significant changes	Peripheral nasal step, Small wing shaped paracentral scotoma, Siedel's sickle-shaped scotoma
Late changes	Arcuate (Bjerrum) scotoma, Ring/double arcuate scotoma
Advanced glaucomatous changes	Tubular vision: Only a small island of central vision accompanied by temporal island No light perception: Complete visual field defect (**temporal island is the most resistant i.e. lost in last**)

29. Krukenberg spindles - (*PGMEE 2013*)
a. Involves posterior surface of lens
b. Involves anterior surface of cornea
c. Involves posterior surface of cornea
d. Involves anterior lens surface

[Ref: Parsons' 23rd/e pg. 276]

30. Pigmentary glaucoma- findings seen is -
a. Flesscher's line (*PGMEE 2012; 2016-17*)
b. Krukenberg's spindles
c. Hadson hauti line
d. Fevy line

[Ref: Parsons' 23rd/e pg. 276; Nema 6th/e pg. 249]

31. Hypersecretory glaucoma is seen in - (*PGMEE 2014*)
a. Diabetes
b. Epidemic dropsy
c. Hypertension
d. Marfan's syndrome

[Ref: Nema 6th/e pg. 250]

ANTIGLAUCOMA MEDICATIONS

32. Which antiglaucoma drug decreases aqueous formation- (*PGMEE 2015; 2016-17*)
a. Clonidine
b. Piocarpine
c. Mannitol
d. Prostaglandins

[Ref: Parsons' 22nd/e pg. 306; Nema 6th/e pg. 105]

33. Drug of choice for acute congestive glaucoma is -
(*NEET Pattern 99, 94; PGMEE 2012*)
a. Atropine
b. Timolol
c. Levobunanol
d. IV Acetazolamide

[Ref: Parsons' 23rd/e pg. 272]

Explanation
- Eyes with acute PACG generally have an intraocular pressure of over 50 mm Hg.
- This needs to be controlled immediately with intravenous acetazolamide 500 mg, and/or intravenous mannitol
- After the control of intraocular pressure, a laser iridotomy is mandatory in all eyes with any form of PACG and also prophylactically in the unaffected (fellow), eyes.

34. Intravenous Mannitol is indicated in (*PGMEE 2019*)
a. Primary Open angle glaucoma
b. Acute angle closure attack
c. Normal tension glaucoma
d. Sympathetic ophthalmitis

[Ref: Parsons' Diseases of the eye, 22nd/e pg. 53, 76; A K Khurana Comprehensive Ophthalmology, 7th/e pg. 472]

35. The ocular hypotensive agent causing apnoea in infants is: (*PGMEE 2019*)
a. Latanoprost
b. Timolol
c. Betaxolol
d. Brimonidine

[Ref: A K Khurana Comprehensive Ophthalmology, 7th/e pg. 469]

36. Anticholinergic used in all except:
a. Uvietis (*DNB Dec'2010; 2016-17*)
b. OPC poisoning
c. Fundus examination
d. Glaucoma

[Ref. Parsons' 23rd/e pg. 134]

37. Main MOA brimonidine in glaucoma- (*PGMEE 2015*)
a. Reduce vitreous volume
b. Increased aqueous production
c. Increased uveoscleral outflow
d. Increased trabecular outflow

[Ref: Nema 6th/e pg. 105]

25.	d
26.	a
27.	d
28.	b
29.	c
30.	b
31.	b
32.	a
33.	d
34.	b
35.	d
36.	d
37.	c

38. Selective alpha 2 against used in glaucoma:
(PGMEE 2015)

a. Timolol
b. Brimonidine
c. Dipivefrine
d. Epinephrine

[Ref: Nema 6th/e pg. 105]

Explanation
- It decreases the aqueous production and episcleral venous pressure and improves the aqueous humor outflow.

39. Which of the following antiglaucoma medications can cause drowsiness? *(PGMEE 2013; 2016-17)*

a. Brimonidine
b. Timolol
c. Dorzolamide
d. Latanoprost

[Ref: Nema 6th/e pg. 105]

40. Following are the side effects of apraclonidine except-
(PGMEE 2015)

a. Eye lid retraction
b. Follicular conjunctivitis
c. Watering of mouth
d. Lid dermatitis

Explanation
- Apraclonidine causes dryness of mouth.

38. b
39. a
40. c

1. Attachment of vitreous is strongest at?

   a. Foveal region   **(PGMEE 2013; 2016-17)**

   b. Margin of optic disc

   c. Across ora serrata

   d. Back of lens

[Ref: Parsons' 23rd/e pg. 286]

Explanation

- The ora serrata marks the end of the choroid and retina and is grey to brownish-black in colour.
- The viterous base straddles the ora serrata and is firmly attached here.

2. Space of cloquet is phylogenetically related to -

   a. Central retinal vein   **(PGMEE 2015)**

   b. Central Retinal artery

   c. Hyaloid artery

   d. Iris

[Ref: Parsons' 23rd/e pg. 9]

3. Muscae volitantes are seen in -   **(PGMEE 2014)**

   a. Remains of primitive hyloid vasculature

   b. Vitreous hemorrhage

   c. Eale's disease

   d. Vitreous detachment

[Ref: Nema 6th/e pg. 315]

VITREOUS HEMORRHAGE

4. The most common cause of vitreous hemorrhage in young—   **(PGMEE 2013 2016-17)**

   a. Hypertension   b. Trauma

   c. Diabetes   d. Retinal hole

[Ref: Parsons' 23rd/e pg. 317]

Explanation

- The common causes of vitreous haemorrhage are proliferative diabetic retinopathy, retinal tears, BRVO, retinal vasculitis and peripheral retinal neovascularization.
- Trauma is the commonest cause in the young.

5. M/c cause of vitreous hemorrhage in adults—   **(PGMEE 2019)**

   a. Hypertension   b. Trauma

   c. Diabetes   d. Retinal hole

[Ref: Parsons' 23rd/e pg. 292]

6. Immediate management of vitreous hemorrhage in eye -   **(PGMEE 2015)**

   a. Conservative   b. Steroids

   c. Antibiotics   d. Vitrectomy

[Ref: Parsons' 23rd/e pg. 317]

7. Recurrent periphlebitis retinae with vitreous hemorrhage is seen in:-   **(PGMEE 2013; 2016-17)**

   a. Coat's d/s   b. Best d/s

   c. Retinitis pigmentosa   d. Eale's d/s

[Ref: Parsons' 23rd/e pg. 301]

8. Eale' disease is:-   **(PGMEE 2012, DNB June'2011)**

   a. Recurrent anterior uveitis

   b. Recurrent vitreous hemorrhage

   c. Recurrent sub-conjunctival hemorrhage

   d. Recurrent macular hemorrhage

[Ref: Parsons' 23rd/e pg. 301]

9. Treatment of choice for Eale's disease -   **(PGMEE 2013)**

   a. Surgery   b. Corticosteroids

   c. Antibiotics   d. Antihistaminics

[Ref: Parsons' 23rd/e pg. 301; Nema 6th/e pg. 312]

10. A 65 years old diabetic & hypertensive male presents with sudden loss of vision. His fundus image is shown below. diagnosis: **(Recent Pattern June 2018)**

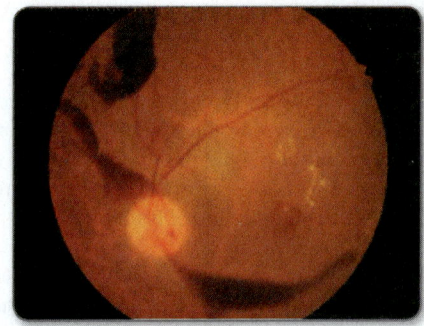

   a. Central serous retinopathy

   b. Central retinal arterial occlusion

   c. Background retinopathy

   d. Vitreous haemorrhage

[Ref: Parsons' 23rd/e pg. 317]

Explanation

- There is sub hyaloid h'ge visible in photograph which is seen in proliferative stage of diabetic retinopathy. Vitreous h'ge also occurs in PDR which is the cause of sudden loss of vision. background retinopathy does not cause sudden loss of vision or even significant loss of vision.
- Diabetes can affect the small vessels at the retina leading to diabetic retinopathy.
- Findings seen in diabetic retinopathy:-
  ○ Background retinopathy: seen as tiny red dots due to changes in blood vessels (**microaneurysms**) and **dot & blot haemorrhages** (similar to bruises on the skin).

1.	c
2.	c
3.	a
4.	b
5.	c
6.	a
7.	d
8.	b
9.	b
10.	d

DISEASES OF RETINA

11. The junction between Retina & Ciliary body is known as? *(PGMEE 2013; 2016-17)*
a. Pars plana
b. Pars plicata
c. Equator
d. Ora serrata

[Ref: Parsons' 23rd/e pg. 8]

Explanation

- The inner surface of the ciliary body is divided into two regions - the anterior part is corrugated with a number of folds called the **pars plicata;** the posterior is called the **pars plana.**
- The ciliary body extends backward as far as the **ora serrata**, at which point the retina proper begins abruptly.

12. The pigmented neurosensory epithelium of retina is continuation of? *(PGMEE 2016-17, DNB JUNE 2011)*
a. Pigmentary retinal epithelum
b. Bruch's membrane of choroid
c. Ora serrata
d. Non-pigmented epithelium of choroid (anterior layer of iris)

[Ref: Parsons' 23rd/e pg. 9]

Explanation

- The anterior layer in the iris is found to be continuous with the outer layer in the ciliary body, and this again is continued into the pigment epithelium of the retina as a single layer of hexagonal cells lying immediately adjacent to the membrane of Bruch.

13. Extra retinal fibrovascular proliferation at ridge between normal avascular retina is which grade of ROP? *(DNB June 2011)*
a. ROP 1
b. ROP 2
c. ROP 3
d. ROP 4

[Ref: Parsons' 23rd/e pg. 294]

14. Photosensitive layer of retina: *(PGMEE 2015)*
a. External limiting membrane
b. Layers of rods and cones
c. Internal limiting membrane
d. Pigment layer

[Ref: Parsons' 23rd/e pg. 10]

15. Blind spot of Mariotte is found at: *(PGMEE 2013)*
a. Macula lutea
b. Ora serrata
c. Optic disc
d. Fovea centralis

[Ref: Parsons' 23rd/e pg. 20]

16. Broadest neuroretinal rim is seen in – *(PGMEE 2016-17)*
a. Inferior pole
b. Temoral lobe
c. Nasal pole
d. Superior pole

[Ref: Parsons' 22nd/e pg. 289]

17. All are seen in CMV retinitis except: *(PGMEE 2013)*
a. Vitreous hemorrhage
b. Brush-fire appearance
c. Perivasculitis
d. Immunosuppression

[Ref: Parsons' 23rd/e pg. 300]

RETINAL FINDINGS

18. Cotton wool spots are commonly seen in All except:
a. Hypertension
b. DM *(PGMEE 2014)*
c. CMV
d. HIV

[Ref: Parsons' 23rd/e pg. 288]

19. Both soft and hard exudates are seen in:- *(PGMEE 2013; 2016-17)*
a. Eale's disease
b. DM
c. Hypertension
d. All of the above

[Ref: Parsons' 22nd/e pg. 311,315]

20. Cherry red spot is seen in all EXCEPT: *(PGMEE 2016-17)*
a. CMI gangliosidosis
b. Niemann pick disease
c. Tay sach' disease
d. None

[Ref: Parsons' 22nd/e pg. 321]

21. Cherry red spot is seen in:- *(PGMEE 2012)*
a. Central retinal artery thrombosis
b. Retinitis pigmentosa
c. Eale's disease
d. Central retinal vein occlusion

[Ref: Parsons' 23rd/e pg. 297]

HYPERTENSIVE RETINOPATHY

22. Characteristic finding in long standing hypertensive retinopathy : *(PGMEE 2013)*
a. Micro aneurysms
b. Increased light reflex
c. Tortuous arteries
d. AV nicking

[Ref: Parsons' 23rd/e pg. 288]

23. Marcus-Gunn sign is seen in - *(PGMEE 2014; 2016-17)*
a. Diabetic retinopathy
b. Hypertensive retinopathy
c. Retinal detachment
d. Retinitis pigmentosa

[Ref: Parsons' 22nd/e pg. 312]

DIABETIC RETINOPATHY

24. Degree of diabetic retinopathy depends on *(PGMEE 2015)*
a. Retinal involvement
b. Type of disease
c. Duration of disease
d. Severity of disease

[Ref: Parsons' 23rd/e pg. 289]

25. Identify the fluorescein angiography picture *(NEET Pattern 2017)*

a. Non proliferative diabetic retinopathy (NPDR)
b. Proliferative diabetic retinopathy (PDR)
c. Familial dominant drusen
d. Birdshot choroidopathy

11.	d
12.	d
13.	c
14.	b
15.	c
16.	a
17.	a
18.	c
19.	d
20.	d
21.	a
22.	d
23.	c
24.	c
25.	a

Explanation

- Above shown is the classical fluorescein angiography picture of Non proliferative diabetic retinopathy (NPDR).
- Fluorescein Angiography helps in the differentiation of retinal disease and is used to determine if laser treatment of the retina is warranted.
  - Sodium Fluorescein contrast agent is injected into antecubital (forearm) veins.
  - The dye travels quickly in circulation, and is photographed in black and white as it travels through the eye.
  - Fundus photograph and angiogram of patient with mild non-proliferative diabetic retinopathy (NDPR) shown in the above image.
- Proliferative DR looks like as given below

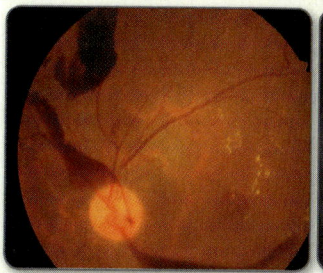 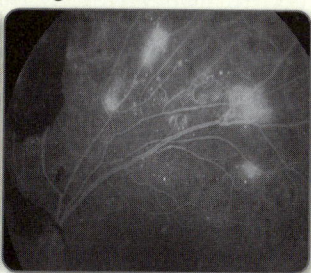

26. All are seen in non-proliferative diabetic retinopathy except: *(PGMEE 2013)*

a. Hard exudates
b. Neovascularization
c. Macular edema
d. Microaneurysm

[Ref: Parsons' 23rd/e pg. 289]

27. Earliest feature of diabetic retinopathy is?
a. Microaneurysms *(DNB Jun'2009; 2016-17)*
b. Cotton wool spots
c. Dot-&-blot haemorrhages
d. Hard exudates

[Ref: Parsons' 23rd/e pg. 290 table]

28. One of the following is NOT a sign of diabetic retinopathy
a. Choroidal neovascularization *(PGMEE 2014)*
b. Micro aneurysms
c. Hard exudates 4
d. Cotton wool spots

[Ref: Parsons' 23rd/e pg. 292]

29. Vitreous hemorrhage in diabetic retinopathy are seen in: *(PGMEE 2012; 2016-17)*
a. Proliferative diabetic retinopathy
b. Non-proliferative diabetic retinopathy
c. Both
d. None *[Ref: Parsons' 23rd/e pg. 292]*

30. Diabetic ischemic maculopathy is characterized by all except - *(PGMEE 2015)*
a. Areas of non perfusion are evident on fluorescein angiography
b. Microaneurysms and hemorrhagcs are seen
c. Mild visual loss
d. It occurs due to microvascular blockage

[Ref: Parsons' 23rd/e pg. 289]

Explanation

- Macular oedema occurs in a large number of eyes and, with central hard exudates, is the commonest cause of diminution of vision in diabetic retinopathy.
- Caused by leakage from dilated capillaries
- A mixed histological picture of oedema and ischaemia at the macular area is fairly common.

31. Panretinal photocoagulation is indicated in *(PGMEE 2014)*

a. Macular edema
b. Retinal breaks
c. Proliferative diabetic retinopathy
d. Tractional retinal detachment

[Ref: Parsons' 23rd/e pg. 291]

Explanation

Type of Retinopathy	Therapy	Indications
Mild nonproliferative	Control of diabetes; regular review	All
Maculopathy		
▪ CSME	Focal photocoagulation	Discrete areas of leakage on fluorescein angiography
Diffuse leak around macula	Grid laser/IVTA/anti-VEGF	
▪ Circinate	Focal photocoagulation	
Severe nonproliferative retinopathy	Frequent review	
Proliferative retinopathy	Panretinal photocoagulation	NVE/NVD
Advanced diabetic eye disease	Vitreoretinal surgery with photocoagulation	▪ Persistent vitreous haemorrhage ▪ Tractional retinal detachment

CSME, clinically significant macular oedema; NVD, neovascularization of the disc; NVE, neovascularization elsewhere.

32. Which of the following agents is not used in the treatment of Diabetic Macular Edema/ Retinopathy: *(PGMEE 11)*

a. Benfotiamine
b. Tamoxifen
c. Ruboxistaurim
d. Pyridazinones

[Ref: Parsons' 22nd/e pg. 315]

Explanation

- Drugs used in the treatment of diabetic macular edema/ retinopathy are:
  - Intravitreal fluocinolone acetonide
  - Intravitreal dexamethasone
  - Thiozolidinediones
  - Anti-VEGF agents.

26.	b
27.	a
28.	a
29.	a
30.	c
31.	c
32.	b

33. Cotton wool spots in diabetic retinopathy are due to:
(DNB 2007)

a. Retinal edema
b. Retinal holes
c. Retinal haemorrhage
d. Macular degeneration

[Ref: Parsons' 23rd/e pg. 292]

CRAO & CRVO

34. Cattle track appearance (PGMEE 2016-17)

a. CRVO
b. CRAO
c. Diabetic retinopathy
d. Syphilitic retinopathy

[Ref: Parsons' 23rd/e pg. 297]

35. Cherry red spot is seen in all, except : (DNB 2007)

a. CRAO
b. Tay Sach' s disease
c. Niemman pick's disease
d. Central retinal vein occlusion

[Ref: Parsons' 23rd/e pg. 297]

36. Differences between CRVO and Carotid artery occlusion are all, except: (DNB 2008)

a. Retinal vein dilation
b. Tortuosity in retinal veins
c. Pressure in retinal artery
d. None of the above

37. Central Retinal artery occlusion is known to be associated with - (PGMEE 12)

a. Diabetic Retinopathy
b. CMV retinitis
c. Panophthalmitis
d. Orbital mucormycosis

[Ref: Parsons' 22nd/e pg. 320]

CENTRAL SEROUS RETINOPATHY

38. Umbrella configuration on fluoroscein angiogrphy is seen in:- (PGMEE 2013)

a. Eale's disease
b. Retinitis pigmentosa
c. Central serous retinopathy
d. Rhegmatogenous retinal detachment

[Ref: Nema 6th/e pg. 312]

39. Enlarging dot sign in fundus fluorescein scanning is seen in:- (PGMEE 2014; 2016-17)

a. Central serous retinopathy
b. Coat's disease
c. Cystoid macular edema
d. Significant macular edema

[Ref: Parsons' 23rd/e pg. 223; Nema 6th/e pg. 312]

RETINAL DETACHMENT

40. In retinal detachment - (PGMEE 2012, 07)

a. Effusion of fluid into the suprachoroidal space
b. Retinoschisis
c. Separation of sensory retina from pigment epithelium
d. None of the above

[Ref: Parsons' 23rd/e pg. 306]

33.	a
34.	b
35.	d
36.	a
37.	d
38.	c
39.	a
40.	c
41.	b
42.	d
43.	a
44.	b
45.	c
46.	b
47.	b
48.	d

41. Retinal detachment occurs between -
(PGMEE 2013; 2016-17, DNB Jun'2010)

a. Layers of neurosensory retina
b. Neurosensory retina and pigment epithelium
c. Pigment epithelium and choroid
d. None of the above

[Ref: Parsons' 23rd/e pg. 306]

42. Retinal tears seen most commonly seen in:

a. Tractional retinal detachment (PGMEE 2015)
b. Secondary retinal detachment
c. Exudative retinal detachment
d. Primary retinal detachment

[Ref: Parsons' 23rd/e pg. 306]

43. Causes of exudative retinal detachment are all except:

a. High myopia (PGMEE 2013)
b. Scleritis
c. Central serous retinopathy
d. Toxemia of pregnancy

[Ref: Parsons' 23rd/e pg. 306]

44. Retinal detachment is not seen in:

a. Aphakia (PGMEE 2014; 2016-17)
b. Hypermetropia
c. Choroiditis
d. High myopia

[Ref: Parsons' 23rd/e pg. 306; Nema 6th/e pg. 322]

45. Shaffer's sign is seen in - (PGMEE 2016-17)

a. Tractional retinal detachment
b. Exudative retinal detachment
c. Rhegmatogenous retinal detachment
d. Vitreous haemorrhage

[Ref: Parsons' 23rd/e pg. 307]

46. Scleral buckling is used for treatment of –
(PGMEE 2013)

a. Scleritis
b. Retinal detachment
c. Cataract
d. Vitreous hemorrhage

[Ref: Parsons' 23rd/e pg. 310]

47. In retinal sealing /retinopexy, what is used?
(PGMEE 2015, NEET Pattern14)

a. Nitrous oxide
b. Sulphur hexafluoride
c. Carbon monooxide
d. SO_2

[Ref: Parsons' 23rd/e pg. 311]

Explanation

- The gases commonly employed for tamponading the retina are sulphur hexafluoride (SF6) or perfluoropropane.
- Sulphur hexafluoride is an inert gas

48. A patient presented with sudden onset of floater & perception of falling of a curtain {veil} in front of the eye which one of thefollowingis the most appropriate diagnosis- (PGMEE 2011)

a. Vitreous hemorrhage
b. Glaucoma
c. Eale's disease
d. Retinal detachment

[Ref: Parsons' 23rd/e pg. 307]

RETINITIS PIGMENTOSA

49. Which of the following parameter is decreased in Retinitis pigmentosa ? *(PGMEE 2019)*
a. Docosahexanoic acid
b. Arachidonic acid
c. Trielonic acid
d. Thromboxane

[Ref: https://iovs.arvojournals.org/data/journals/ iovs/933393/2596.pdf by J Gong - 1992]

50. Fundus in retinitis pigmentosa is - *(PGMEE 2012)*
a. No pigmentation
b. White spots with red disc
c. Jet- black spots with pale-waxy disc
d. Dilatation of arterioles

[Ref: Parsons' 23rd/e pg. 303-304]

51. About retinitis pigmentosa all are true EXCEPT: *(DNB JUNE 2011)*
a. Night bliness
b. Attenuation of retinal vessels
c. Early loss of central vision
d. Waxy disc

[Ref: Parsons' 23rd/e pg. 303]

52. In Retinitis pigmentosa there is defect in which gene - *(PGMEE 2016-17)*
a. Pigmented epithelium   b. Scotopsin
c. Rhodopsin   d. Periferin

[Ref: Parsons' 22nd/e pg. 327]

53. Earliest symptom of retinitis pigmentosa - *(PGMEE 2013)*
a. Tubular vision   b. Ring scotoma
c. Night blindness   d. None

[Ref: Parsons' 23rd/e pg. 303]

54. A23-year-old male presents with night blindness and tubular vision. On examination, IOP was observed to be 18mm and the anterior segment was unremarkable. Fundoscopy revealed attenuation of arterioles and waxy pallor of the optic disc with bony corpuscles like spicules of pigmentation in mid peripheral retina. On perimetry, ring scotomas were observed. Which of the following is the most likely diagnosis. *(PGMEE 2012)*
a. Primary open angle glaucoma
b. Pigmentary retinal dystrophy
c. Diabetic retinopathy
d. Lattice degeneration of retina

[Ref: Parsons' 23rd/e pg. 303]

MISCELLANEOUS

55. Photoretinitis is due to- *(PGMEE 2013; 2016-17)*
a. Blunt trauma   b. Snow reflection
c. Solar eclipse   d. None of the above

[Ref: Parsons' 23rd/e pg. 301]

56. Macular edema most common cause is - *(PGMEE 2014)*
a. Uveitis   b. Secondary glaucoma
c. Retinitis pigmentosa d. Cataract surgery

[Ref: Parsons' 22nd/e pg. 285; Nema 6th/e pg. 299]

57. Treatment of choice for clinically significant macular edema in a diabetic is? *(DNB Dec'2010; 2016-17)*
a. Control of diabetes
b. Focal photocoagulation
c. Panretinal photocoagulation
d. Vitreoretinal surgery

[Ref: Parsons' 23rd/e pg. 291]

58. Purtscher retinopathy is seen in patients with -
a. Diabetes mellitus   *(PGMEE 2015; 2016-17)*
b. Chronic pancreatitis
c. Occlusion of anterior retinal artery
d. Head trauma

[Ref: Parsons' 22nd/e pg. 324]

59. Purtschner's retinopathy is seen in all EXCEPT: *(PGMEE 2014-15)*
a. Fat embolism
b. Pancreatitis
c. Chest trauma
d. Unilateral carotid artery occlusion

[Ref: Harrison's 19th/e pg. 40e-4]

60. Sea fan retinopathy is seen in:
a. Diabetes   *(Recent Pattern June 2018)*
b. Sickle cell anemia retinopathy
c. Hypertension
d. Central retinal vein occlusion

[Ref: Parsons' 23rd/e pg. 296]

Explanation

Proliferative Sickle Retinopathy (PSR):
- Goldberg classification of PSR

Stage I	Peripheral arterial occlusion.
Stage II	Peripheral arteriovenous anastomoses, representing dilated pre-existing capillaries (hairpin loop)
Stage III	Neovascular and fibrous proliferation (sea fan) occurring at the posterior border of nonperfusion. A subsequent white sea fan appearance is due to auto-infarction of the neovasculature.
Stage IV	Vitreous hemorrhage
Stage V	Tractional retinal detachment

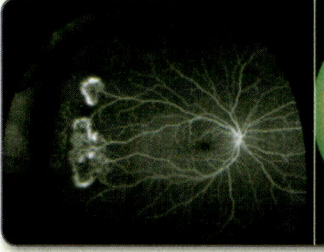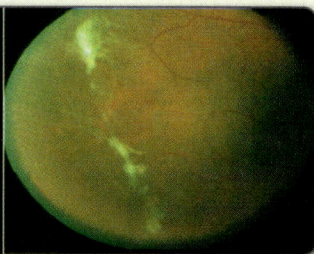

61. "Brush-fire" pattern is seen in - *(PGMEE 2013; 2016-17)*
a. Congenital rubella
b. Toxoplasmosis
c. Syphilis
d. CMV retinitis

[Ref: Parsons' 22nd/e pg. 324]

49.	a
50.	c
51.	c
52.	d
53.	c
54.	b
55.	c
56.	d
57.	b
58.	d
59.	d
60.	b
61.	d

62. Salt & pepper fundus - *(PGMEE 2016-17)*
a. Congenital syphilis
b. Cong histoplasmosis
c. Cong toxoplasmosis
d. Sarcoidosis

[Ref: Parsons' 23rd/e pg. 300]

63. Pizza pie appearance is seen in - *(PGMEE 2015)*
a. CMV retinitis
b. Toxoplasmosis
c. Drug toxicity
d. Congenital rubella

[Ref: Parsons' 22nd/e pg. 324]

64. Head light in fog appearance is seen in - *(PGMEE 2012)*
a. Herpes
b. Toxocara
c. Syphilis
d. Toxoplasmosis

[Ref: Parsons' 22nd/e pg. 325]

65. Roth spots are seen in - *(PGMEE 2012; 2016-17)*
a. DM retinopathy
b. Bacterial endocarditis
c. HTN retinopathy
d. None

[Ref: Parsons' 23rd/e pg. 300; Nema 6th/e pg. 310]

66. Roth's spots are seen in *(PGMEE 2018)*
a. Vitreoretinal hemorrhage
b. Acute leukemia
c. Lymphoma
d. None of the above

[Ref: Parsons' 23rd/e pg. 300]

Explanation
- Roth's spots (named after Moritz Roth) are retinal hemorrhages with white or pale centers.

- Composed of coagulated fibrin including platelets, focal ischemia, inflammatory infiltrate, infectious organisms, or neoplastic cells.
- Roth's spots may be seen in:
  - Leukemia,
  - Diabetes,
  - SABE (Subacute bacterial endocarditis)
  - Pernicious anemia,
  - Ischemic events, hypertensive retinopathy and
  - Rarely in HIV retinopathy.

67. Drugs causing macular toxicity when given intra-vitreally- *(PGMEE 2013)*
a. Dexamethasone
b. Gentamycin
c. Ceftazidime
d. Vancomycin

[Ref: Nema 6th/e pg. 313]

68. Parachute lesions are seen in- *(PGMEE 2013)*
a. Sickle cell anemia
b. Eale's disease
c. Diabetes
d. All of the above

[Ref: yanoff & Duker 3rd / e p. 628]

69. Birdshot retinopathy is characterized by all except-
a. Creamy yellow spots *(PGMEE 2013)*
b. Common in females
c. HLA-A29 positive
d. Unilateral

[Ref: Khurana 5th /e pg. 161]

Explanation
- Birdshot chorioretinopathy, also known as birdshot uveitis, birdshot retinopathy, or HLA-A29 uveitis, is an uncommon chronic posterior uveitis characterized by vitritis and multiple ovoid spots, which are orange to cream in color and hypopigmented.

62.	a
63.	a
64.	d
65.	b
66.	b
67.	b
68.	d
69.	d

VISUAL PATHWAY

1. Longest part of optic nerve - *(PGMEE 2013; 2016-17)*
a. Intraorbital
b. Intra-cranial
c. Intra-ocular
d. Extra-cranial

[Ref: Parsons' 23rd/e pg. 321]

Explanation

- The optic nerve has four parts
  - Intraocular portion (1 mm); Intraorbital portion (25-30 mm); Intracanalicular portion (5-9 mm); Intracranial portion (10-16 mm), which goes up to the optic chiasma. The axons are second-order neurones

2. Optic nerve is: *(PGMEE 2016-17)*
a. First order neuron
b. Second order neuron
c. Third order neuron
d. Fourth order neuron

[Ref: Parsons' 23rd/e pg. 321]

3. End organ for vision: *(PGMEE 2014)*
a. Rods and cones
b. Ganglion cell
c. Lateral geniculate body
d. Bipolar cell

[Ref: Parsons' 23rd/e pg. 10 & 27]

Explanation

Photoreceptors (rods and cones):

- Most externally; in contact with the pigment epithelium is neural epithelium, which are the end-organ of vision

4. Methanol damages: *(PGMEE 2016-17)*
a. Cones
b. Ganglion cells of retina
c. Germinal cell layer
d. Rods

[Ref: Parsons' 23rd/e pg. 338]

5. Methyl alcohol causes blindness by acting on?

(DNB JUNE 2011)
a. Ganglion cells
b. Rods only
c. Rods & Cones
d. Nerve fibers

[Ref: Parsons' 23rd/e pg. 338]

Explanation

- Methanol causes circumscribed swelling of myelin behind the lamina cribrosa of optic nerve head and OCT findings show ganglion cell layer loss, selective loss of nasal fibre layers and inner nclear layer microcysts in corresponding area of GCL loss.
- Ophthalmoscopically, there may be blurring of the edges of the discs.
- Later there are signs of optic atrophy, usually of the primary type.

- Pathologically, there is widespread degeneration of the ganglion cells of the retina probably caused by histotoxic anoxia and relative axonal preservation in the retrolaminar portion of the optic nerve

6. First order neuron in optic pathway:- *(PGMEE 2013)*
a. Cells of lateral geniculate body
b. Photoreceptors
c. Bipolar cells of inner nuclear layear
d. Astrocytes

[Ref: Ganong's 23rd /e pg.194; Parsons' 23rd/e pg. 27]

7. Superior colliculus is concerned with:

(DNB 2008; PGMEE 2016-17)
a. Olfaction
b. Hearing
c. Vision
d. Pain sensation

[Ref. Parsons' 22nd/e pg32]

8. Ocular bobbing is related to lesions of:-

(PGMEE 2016-17)
a. Medulla
b. Pons
c. Cortex
d. Midbrain

[Ref: Parsons' 23rd/e pg. 460]

PUPILLARY REFLEXES

9. Nerve carrying motor component of light reflex-

(PGMEE 2013)
a. 1st nerve
b. 2nd nerve
c. 3rd nerve
d. 4th nerve.

[Ref: Parsons' 23rd/e pg. 32]

10. A patient presented with normal eyesight and absence of direct and consensual light reflexes. Which of the following cranial nerves is suspected to be lesioned?

(PGMEE 2013)
a. Trochlear
b. Abducent
c. Optic
d. Occulomotor

[Ref: Parsons' 22nd/e pg. 412]

11. Swinging light test is positive in – *(PGMEE 2016-17)*
a. Glaucoma
b. Keratoconus
c. Retrobulbar neuritis
d. Conjunctivitis

[Ref: Parsons' 23rd/e pg. 105]

12. Marcus Gunn pupil is due to - *(PGMEE 2013)*
a. Cerebral lesion a
b. Total afferent pupillary defect
c. Efferent pathway defect
d. Relative afferent pupillary defect

[Ref: Parsons' 23rd/e pg. 333]

1.	a
2.	b
3.	a
4.	b
5.	a
6.	c
7.	c
8.	b
9.	c
10.	d
11.	c
12.	d

13. **50-years-old male presents with history of a sexually transmitted disease 20 years back now presents with visual abnormality. Which of the following statement is true about pupillary and accommodation reflex in this patient:-** *(PGMEE 2018)*
    a. Normal pupillary and accommodation reflex
    b. Abnormal pupillary reflex with abnormal accommodation
    c. Absent pupillary reflex with normal accommodation
    d. Normal papillary reflex with absent accomodation

[Ref: Parsons' 23rd/e pg. 472]

Explanation
- The patient in above question was most likely suffering from syphilis. Neurosyphilis takes 20-30 years of incubation period to develop. Argyl robertson pupil is characteristic pupillary changes seen in neurosyphilis.
- Argyl robertson pupil is characterized by :-
  ○ Presence of Accomodation reflex
  ○ Absence of light reflex

14. **Relative afferent pupillary defect [RAN)] is characteristically seen in damage to:-** *(PGMEE 2016-17)*
    a. Lateral geniculate body
    b. Optic tract
    c. Occulomotor nerve
    d. Optic nerve

[Ref: Parsons' 23rd/e pg. 333]

15. **Wernicke's hemianopic pupillary response is seen in lesions at** *(PGMEE 2016-17)*
    a. Optic tract
    b. Optic chiasma
    c. Optic radiation
    d. Lateral geniculate body

[Ref: Parsons' 23rd/e pg. 105; Nema 6th/e pg. 342]

16. **Light reflex absent but accommodation reflex present is seen in -** *(PGMEE 2016-17)*
    a. Adies pupil
    b. Hutchisons pupil
    c. Argyl Robertson pupil
    d. Honer's syndrome

[Ref: Parsons' 23rd/e pg. 34]

17. **3rd cranial nerve palsy in diabetes mellitus is characterized by:** *(PGMEE 2018)*
    a. Pseudoptosis
    b. Proptosis
    c. Decrease pupillary reflex
    d. Normal pupillary reflex

[Ref: Harrison 20th/e]

Explanation

3rd CN/ Oculomotor Palsy in DM
- 3rd CN palsy is most frequent in elderly >60 years and in those with prominent or long-standing atherosclerotic risk factors, such as diabetes or hypertension. The key finding in these patients are:-
  ○ Relative sparing of the pupillary sphincter
  ○ Complete or near-complete palsy of the extraocular muscles innervated by the 3rd CN, including levator palpebrae.
  ○ These patients may have very severe pain in the eye or orbit on the same side.

13.	c
14.	d
15.	a
16.	a,c
17.	d
18.	d
19.	d
20.	a
21.	b
22.	a

18. **Neutral density filter –** *(PGMEE 2014)*
    a. Malingering
    b. Efferent pupillary defect
    c. Amblyopia
    d. Afferent pupillary defect

[Ref: Parsons' 22nd/e pg. 413]

LESION OF VISUAL PATHWAY

19. **Homonymous hemianopia is seen in all EXCEPT: -**
    a. Lesions of lateral geniculate body *(PGMEE 2015)*
    b. Visual cortex lesion
    c. Optic tract lesion
    d. Lesions of optic nerve

[Ref: Parsons' 23rd/e pg. 455]

20. **A patient presents with Right homonymous hemianopia. Most likely site of lesion is:** *(Recent Pattern June 2018)*
    a. Left optic radiation
    b. Right geniculate body
    c. Right optic nerve
    d. Right optic radiation

[Ref: Parsons' 23rd/e pg. 455]

Explanation
- Lesions from the optic tract to visual cortex can cause contralateral homonymous hemianopsia. A left homonymous hemianopsia can be caused by a lesion in the right optic tract or the right side of the brain.
- It is caused by lesions of the retrochiasmal visual pathways, i.e.
  ○ lesions of the right optic tract
  ○ the lateral geniculate body
  ○ optic radiation
  ○ cerebral visual (occipital) cortex
- Transient homonymous hemianopsia may occur with migraine.
- Visual field defects
  ○ Homonymous hemianopia: Lesions of optic tract (incongruous defects)
  ○ Homonymous quadrantanopia: Lesion of temporal lobe (superior)
  ○ Bitemporal hemianopia: Lesions of optic chiasm

REMEMBER

- Lesions anterior to chiasma → Scotoma, monoocular blindness.
- Lesions at chiasma → Heteronymous hemianopsia
- Lesions in the optic radiation → Quadrantanopsia

21. **Homonymous hemianopia is caused by lesion of?** *(DNB December 2011)*
    a. Occipital lobe
    b. Optic tract
    c. Optic nerve
    d. Chiasma

[Ref: Parsons' 23rd/e pg. 455]

22. **Lesion of right optic tract will leads to:** *(PGMEE 2016-17)*
    a. Left homonymous hemianopia
    b. Bitemporal hemianopia
    c. Binasal hemianopia
    d. Right homonymus hemianopia

[Ref: Parsons' 23rd/e pg. 455]

23. **Site of lesion in Bitemporal hemianopia is -**
    (PGMEE 2016-17; NEET Pattern 93)
    a. Optic tract
    b. Optic radiation
    c. Optic chiasma
    d. Optic nerve

    [Ref: Parsons' 23rd/e pg. 455]

24. **Visual field defect in pituitary stalk tumour with suprasellar extension is -** **(PGMEE 2015)**
    a. Homonymous hemianopia
    b. Binasal hemianopia
    c. Pie in the sky vision
    d. Bitemporal hemianopia

    [Ref: Parsons' 23rd/e pg. 456; Nema 6th/e pg. 342]

25. **Altitudinal visual field defect is seen in**
    a. Anterior ischemic neuropathy **(PGMEE 2016-17)**
    b. Retinitis pigmentosa
    c. Buphathalmos
    d. Papilloedema

    [Ref: Parsons' 23rd/e pg. 328]

26. **Macular sparing is seen in the affection of -**
    (PGMEE 2016-17)
    a. Optic chiasma
    b. Optic tract
    c. Occipital lobe
    d. Opric nerve

    [Ref: Parsons' 23rd/e pg. 455]

PAPILLOEDEMA

27. **Earliest sign of papilloedema-** **(PGMEE 2016-17)**
    a. Blurring of disc margin
    b. Cotton-wool spots
    c. Obliteration of cup
    d. Less of pulsation

    [Ref: Parsons' 23rd/e pg. 325]

28. **All are causes of papilloedema except:**
    a. Cerebral tumors **(DNB 2008; PGMEE2016-17)**
    b. Friedreich's ataxia
    c. Cavernous sinus thrombosis
    d. Cerebral abscess

    [Ref: Parsons' 23rd/e pg. 324]

29. **Fundoscopic features of papilledema include all the following except -** **(PGMEE 2014)**
    a. Bending of blood vessels
    b. Ill- defined disc margin
    c. Absent venous pulsation
    d. Deep physiological cup

    [Ref: Parsons' 23rd/e pg. 325]

OPTIC NEURITIS

30. **Vitamin B12 deficiency is likely to cause -**
    a. Bitemporal herninanopia **(PGMEE 2012)**
    b. Centrocecal scotoma
    c. Heteronymous hemianopia
    d. Binasal hemianopia

    [Ref: Parsons' 22nd/e pg. 359]

31. **Optic neuritis causes –** **(PGMEE 2016-17)**
    a. Sudden painless loss of vision
    b. Sudden painful loss of vision
    c. Gradual painful loss of vision
    d. Gradual painless loss of vision

    [Ref: Parsons' 23rd/e pg. 513]

OPTIC ATROPHY

32. **Consecutive optic atrophy is seen in:** **(PGMEE 2012)**
    a. Papilitis
    b. Retinitis-pigmentosa
    c. Retinal detachment
    d. Papilloedema

    [Ref: Parsons' 23rd/e pg. 335]

Explanation

- Optic atrophy follows extensive disease of the retina from destruction of the ganglion cells, as in pigmentary retinal dystrophy or occlusion of the central artery; these cases are sometimes called *consecutive optic atrophy*.

33. **Which of the following is seen in Giant cell arteritis:**
    a. Small optic disc **(Recent Pattern June 2018)**
    b. AION
    c. NAION
    d. palpable temporal artery pulsation

    [Ref: Parsons' 23rd/e pg. 328]

Explanation

- GCA is associated with Arteritic anterior ischaemic optic neuropathy (AION)

34. **Fundoscopy of a patient shows chalky white optic disc with well defined margins. Retinal vessels and surrounding Retina appears normal. Which of the following is the most likely diagnosis -** **(PGMEE 2012)**
    a. Glaucomatous optic atrophy
    b. Consecutive optic atrophy
    c. Post-neuritic secondary optic atrophy
    d. Primary Optic Atrophy

    [Ref: Parsons' 23rd/e pg. 336]

35. **In optic atrophy, the optic disc appears to pale is index of-** **(PGMEE 2014)**
    a. Gliosis
    b. Atrophy of the nerve fibre
    c. Los of vasculature
    d. All of the above

    [Ref: Parsons' 23rd/e pg. 336]

MISCELLANEOUS

36. **Following are the clinical features of Leber optic neuropathy EXCEPT:–** **(PGMEE 2015)**
    a. Males can transmit the disease
    b. It is a example of gradual painless visual loss
    c. No leak of dye is observed in fluorescein angiography
    d. Seen in the 2nd or 3rd decade of life

    [Ref: Parsons' 23rd/e pg. 340]

Explanation

- Usually commences at about the 20th year of life.
- A genetic aetiology has now been established. Transmission of the disease is generally through an unaffected female to all offspring, but the disease manifests mostly in males.
- Herediatry transmission is by mitochondrial
- Vision generally falls rapidly at first; the loss is gradural thereafter
- In two-third of the cases, there is a central or centrocaecal scotoma.

23.	c
24.	d
25.	a
26.	c
27.	a
28.	b
29.	d
30.	b
31.	b
32.	b
33.	b
34.	d
35.	c
36.	a

37. A person has defective blue colour appreciation. His condition is better named as – *(PGMEE 2013)*
a. Deuteranomalous
b. Tritanomalous
c. Deuteranopia
d. Tritanopia

[Ref: Parsons' 23rd/e pg. 80; Nema 6th/e pg. 347]

Explanation

Protanopes	Are insensitive to red light (defective red sensation)
Deuteranopes	Have a defective green sensation
Tritanopes	Are rare. They have some insensitivity to blue light

38. Amaurosis fugax is due to – *(PGMEE 2012)*
a. Tobacco
b. Papilloedema
c. Optic neuritis
d. TIA

[Ref: Parsons' 23rd/e pg. 79]

39. Down-beat nystagmus is seen in lesion of:
a. Hippocampus *(PGMEE 2013)*
b. Brainstem
c. Basal ganglia
d. Cervicomedullary junction

[Ref: Parsons' 23rd/e pg. 460]

40. Illuminated frenzel glasses are used in detecting-
a. Heterophoria *(PGMEE 2015)*
b. Astigmatism
c. Esotropia
d. Nystagmus

[Ref: Common neuro-ophthalmic pitfalls case based teaching by Purvin pg. 110]

Explanation

- Frenzel goggles are a diagnostic tool used in ophthalmology, otolaryngology and audiovestibular medicine for the medical evaluation of involuntary eye movement (nystagmus). They are named after Frenzel, a German physician.

37.	b
38.	d
39.	d
40.	d

FRACTURE OF ORBIT

1. Enophthalmos caused by fracture of: *(PGMEE 2016-17)*
a. Floor of orbit
b. Medial wall of orbit
c. Lateral wall of orbit
d. Roof of orbit

[Ref: Parsons' 23rd/e pg. 436]

2. Blow out fracture of orbit most commonly affects:-
(PGMEE 2018 & 2013)
a. Medial wall
b. Lateral wall
c. Floor
d. Roof

[Ref. Parsons' 23rd/e pg. 450]

Explanation

Blow out Fracture of Orbit

- Orbital floor fracture is also known as "blowout" fracture of the orbit.
- Typically caused by sudden increase in orbital pressure from external impact by an object of larger diameter than orbit. e.g. a fist/ a cricket ball or a tennis ball
- Blow out fracture of orbit occurs when there is a fracture of one of the walls of orbit but the **orbital rim remains intact**.
- The anatomy of the orbital floor predisposes it to fracture.
  - Bones of lateral wall & roof are usually withstand trauma d/to thick wall.
  - By contrast, the bone of the orbital floor overlying the neurovascular bundle (thin bone covering infraorbital canal) is predisposed where isolated orbital floor fractures invariably occur.
- It is estimated that about 10% of all facial fractures are isolated orbital wall fractures (**the majority of these being the orbital floor**), and that 30-40% of all facial fractures involve the orbit.
- The inferior orbital neurovascular bundle comprising the infraorbital nerve and artery) courses within the bony floor of the orbit.
- *Signs of blow out #*
  - **Diplopia on looking upward and laterally** (d/ to trapping of inferior rectus m/s and traumatic enophthalmos).
  - Proptosis
  - Periorbital edema
  - Emphysema of eyelids involving medial wall
  - Anaesthesia in the distribution of infraorbital nerve (cheek, lower lid, upper lip & teeth).
- *Investigations in a case of blowout #*
  - **Hanging drop sign** on Water's view X-ray/ 30⁰ Occipito-mental view.
  - **Tear drop sign** on antral CT Scan

- **T/t:** Reconstruction of floor by elevation + Fixation. Orbital floor exploration, if there is trapping of inferior rectus.

🔲 *Important negative points: Orbital #*
- NOT seen in blow out # → Ptosis, Exopthalmos
- NOT involved in blow out # of orbit → # of orbital Rim.

3. A 25 year old young male met with a road traffic accident now he complaints of restricted eye movements. A clinical image and CT image is shown below. What will be the diagnosis? *(PGMEE June 2019)*

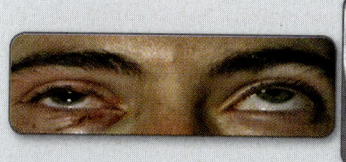 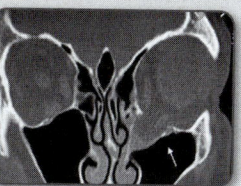

a. Le- fort fracture
b. Fracture maxilla
c. Fracture zygomatic
d. Blow out fracture

[Ref: Parsons' 23rd/e pg. 436]

4. Unilateral lacrimal gland destruction may be caused by
a. Fracture of sphenoid *(PGMEE 2012)*
b. Fracture of roof of orbit
c. Fracture of lateral wall
d. Inferior orbital fissure fracture

[Ref: Parsons' 22nd/e pg. 499]

DISEASES OF ORBIT

PROPTOSIS

5. Commonest cause for bilateral proptosis in children is -
(PGMEE 11)
a. Fibrous histiocytoma
b. Chloroma
c. Rhabdomyosarcoma
d. Cavernous hamangioma

[Ref: Parsons' 23rd/e pg. 435]

6. Most common cause of intermittent proptosis
a. Trauma *(PGMEE 2012)*
b. Retinoblastoma
c. Cavernous sinus thrombosis
d. Orbital varices

[Ref: Parsons' 23rd/e pg. 436]

7. Pulsatile proptosis is a feature of -
a. Retinoblastoma *(PGMEE 2013; 2016-17)*
b. Carotid-cavernous fistula
c. Covernous sinus thrombosis
d. Orbital varix

[Ref: Parsons' 23rd/e pg. 436]

1.	a
2.	c
3.	d
4.	b
5.	d
6.	d
7.	b

8. A hectic bout of fever with bilateral proptosis in a 25 years old diabetic following an injury to face is most diagnostic of? **(DNB June 2011)**
   a. Cavernous sinus thrombosis
   b. Thyrotoxicosis
   c. Orbital tumor
   d. Intracranial neoplasm

   [Ref: Parsons' 23rd/e pg. 439]

9. **Most common cause of unilateral proptosis is -**
   a. Retinoblastoma **(PGMEE 2013)**
   b. Raised intracranial tension
   c. Intraocular haemorrhage
   d. Orbital cellulitis

   [Ref: Parsons' 23rd/e pg. 435]

10. **The most common cause of proptosis in adults is:**
    a. Orbital cellulitis **(PGMEE 2019)**
    b. Preseptal cellulitis
    c. Thyroid eye disease
    d. Capillary hemangioma

    [Ref: A K Khurana Comprehensive Ophthalmology 7th/e pg. 398]

11. **Axial proptosis is produced by tumors lying in -**
    a. Subperiosteal space **(PGMEE 2015)**
    b. Peripheral space
    c. Tenon space
    d. Retrobulbar space

    [Ref: Parsons' 23rd/e pg. 435]

Explanation

- The proptosis can be axial.
- The causative lesion will commonly be found to originate in the intraconal space (or retrobulbar space), E.g. optic nerve gliomas, meningiomas and cavernous haemangiomas.

12. **Intermittent proptosis is seen in?** **(PGMEE 2009)**
    a. Orbital tumor
    b. Orbital cellulitis
    c. Orbital varices
    d. Cavernous sinus thrombosis

    [Ref: Parsons' 23rd/e pg 449]

THYROID OPHTHALMOPATHY

13. **Earliest symptom of thyroid ophthalmopathy –**
    a. Ophthalmoplegia **(PGMEE 2016-17)**
    b. Lid rectraction
    c. Diplopia
    d. Proptosis

    [Ref: Parsons' 23rd/e pg. 447]

14. **Dysthyroid ophthalmopathy all are true except -**
    (PGMEE 2014)
    a. Proptosis
    b. Optic neuritis
    c. Exophthalmos
    d. Myopathy

    [Ref: Parsons' 23rd/e pg. 447]

15. **The most common ocular motility problem in thyroid myopathy is due to involvement of**
    a. Inferior oblique **(PGMEE 2012; 2016-17)**
    b. Medial rectus
    c. Inferior rectus
    d. Sueprior rectus

    [Ref: Name 6th/e pg. 456]

Explanation

- The inferior rectus muscle is most frequently involved followed by medial rectus and superior rectus.

16. **Last ocular muscle to be involved in Grave's disease-**
    (PGMEE 2015)
    a. Superior rectus   b. Lateral rectus
    c. Inferior oblique   d. Inferior rectus

    [Ref: Name 6th/e pg. 456]

17. **Most common ocular movement affected in thyroid ophthalmopathy-** **(PGMEE 2013)**
    a. Depression   b. Adduction
    c. Elevation   d. Abduction

    [Ref: Name 6th/e pg. 456]

MISCELLANEOUS

18. **Paralysis of 3rd, 4th, 6th nerves with involvement of ophthalmic division of 5th nerve, localizes the lesion to:**
    (PGMEE 2013)
    a. Brainstem   b. Apex of orbit
    c. Base of skull   d. Cavernous sinus

    [Ref: Parsons' 23rd/e pg. 439]

19. **A 19 year-old-young girl with previous history of repeated pain over medial canthus and chronic use of nasal decongestants, presented with abrupt on set of fever with chills & rigor, diplopia on lateral gaze, moderate proptosis & chemosis. On examination optic disc is congested. Most likely diagnosis is:**
    a. Acute Ethmoidal sinusitis **(NEET Pattern 09)**
    b. Orbital cellulitis
    c. Orbital apex syndrome
    d. Cavernous sinus thrombosis

    [Ref: Parsons' 23rd/e pg. 440]

20. **Most common orbital cyst in children-** **(PGMEE 2015)**
    a. Dermoid cyst
    b. Clobomatous cyst
    c. Lymphoma
    d. Neuroenteric cyst

    [Ref: Parsons' 23rd/e pg. 442]

21. **Orbital apex syndrome constitutes all except -**
    a. Pain over distribution of optic nerve **(PGMEE 2014)**
    b. Proptosis
    c. Ophthalmoplegia
    d. CSF rhinorrhea

    [Ref: Dhingra 5th /e p. 213; Parsons' 23rd/e pg. 437]

22. **All nerve are involved in superior orbital fissure syndrome except -** **(PGMEE 2013)**
    a. 1st   b. 3rd
    c. 4th   d. 6th

    [Ref: Clinical ophthalmology 5th /e p. 670]

8.	a
9.	d
10.	c
11.	d
12.	c
13.	b
14.	b
15.	c
16.	c
17.	c
18.	d
19.	d
20.	a
21.	d
22.	a

LIDS

23. Muller's muscle is found in: *(PGMEE 2013)*
a. Middle ear
b. Pharynx
c. Eye lid
d. Tongue

[Ref: Parsons' 23rd/e pg. 401]

Explanation

- Besides striped muscles, there are layers of unstriped muscle in each lid, Muller's muscle in the upper lid and inferior tarsal muscle of lower lid.

24. Gland of Moll opens in/on the – *(PGMEE 2016-17)*
a. Hair follicle
b. Tarsal plate
c. Ducts of Meibomian glands
d. Skin

[Ref: Parsons' 23rd/e pg. 400]

Explanation

- The sweat glands near the edge of the lid are also unusually large and known as Moll glands. They are situated immediately behind the hair follciles, and their ducts open into the ducts of the Zeis glands or hair follicles.

25. Infection of which structure is called stye:
a. Conjunctiva *(PGMEE 2012)*
b. Zeis glands
c. Tarsal glands
d. skin

[Ref: Parsons' 23rd/e pg. 403]

26. Hardeolum internum is - *(PGMEE 2013; 2016-17)*
a. Chronic infection of Zeis gland
b. Acute infection of Moll gland
c. Acute infection of Zeis gland
d. Acute infection of Meibomian gland

[Ref: Parsons' 23rd/e pg. 404]

Explanation

- *Hardeolum externum (stye)* is acute inflamma[n] of glands of Zeiss and Moll.
- *Hardeolum internum* is acute suppurative inflamma[n] of meibomian glands.
- *Chalazion* is chronic lipogranulomatous, painless inflamma[n] of meibomian glands.
- *Blepharitis* is inflammation of the eyelid. It is a/w acne rosacea or seborrheic dermatitis.

27. Fusion of palpebral and bulbar conjunctiva is -
a. Symblepharon *(PGMEE 2012)*
b. Tylosis
c. Ectropion
d. Trichiasis

[Ref: Parsons' 23rd/e pg. 410]

CHALAZION

28. All of the following are true regarding chalazion EXCEPT: *(DNB Dec'2009)*
a. Vertical incision given to squeeze out contents
b. It's a granulomatous condition
c. Incision and curettage done
d. Horizontal incision to be made to squeeze out contents

[Ref: Parsons' 23rd/e pg. 404]

29. Chalazion of lid is - *(PGMEE 2012, NEET Pattern 08.1)*
a. Chronic lipogranulomatous inflammation
b. Chronic nonspecific inflammation
c. Liposarcoma
d. Caseous necrosis

[Ref: Parsons' 23rd/e pg. 404]

30. A recurrent chalazion should be subjected to histopathologic evalution to exclude the possibility of-
a. Malignant melanoma *(NEET 06, PGMEE 2012)*
b. Meibomian cell carcinoma
c. Basal cell carcinoma
d. Squamous cell carcinoma

[Ref: Parsons' 23rd/e pg. 404]

PTOSIS

31. Upper lid retractors include? *(PGMEE 2013)*
a. Superior oblique and superior rectus
b. Levator palpabrae superioris and superior oblique
c. Levator palpabrae superioris & muller muscle
d. Muller muscle and superior rectus

[Ref: Parsons' 23rd/e pg. 411]

32. Ptosis results from trauma to which nerve?
a. III   b. VI *(PGMEE 2016-17)*
c. VII   d. VIII

[Ref: Parsons' 23rd/e pg. 415]

33. Most common cause of ptosis - *(PGMEE 2013)*
a. Idiopathic   b. Paralysis of 3rd nerve
c. Congenital   d. Myasthenia gravis

[Ref: Parsons' 23rd/e pg. 412]

34. A 3 year old child is presenting with drooping of upper lid since birth. On examination , the palpebral aperture height is 6 mm and with poor levator palpebrae superioris function. What is the procedure recommended? *(PGMEE 2019)*
a. Observation
b. Fasanella Servat operation
c. Frontalis Sling surgery
d. Mullerectomy

[Ref: A K Khurana Comprehensive Ophthalmology 7th/e. pg. 395]

35. Marcus Gunn jaw winking phenomenon is due to relation between which cranial nerves: *(PGMEE 2016-17)*
a. VII + VIII   b. III + V
c. V + VII   d. III + VI

[Ref: Merritts neurology p. 603; Parsons' 23rd/e pg. 412]

23.	c
24.	a
25.	b
26.	d
27.	a
28.	d
29.	a
30.	b
31.	c
32.	a
33.	c
34.	c
35.	b

36. Ocular muscle involved in Marcus Gun jaw winking phenomenon is - *(PGMEE 2015)*
a. Medial rectus
b. Levator palpebrae
c. Lateral rectus
d. Orbicularis oculi

[Ref: Parsons' 23rd/e pg. 412]

37. A patient with ptosis presents with retraction of the ptotic eye lid on chewing. This represents: *(PGMEE 10)*
a. Third nerve misdirection syndrome
b. Occulomotor palsy
c. Abducent palsy
d. Marcus Gunn Jaw winking sydrome

[Ref: Parsons' 23rd/e pg. 412]

38. Treatment of congenital ptosis with poor elevation is- *(PGMEE 2013)*
a. FS operation
b. Frontalis sling
c. Levator resection
d. None of the above

[Ref: Parsons' 23rd/e pg. 412, 413]

Explanation

- The *Fasanella-Servat operation* is indicated for cases of minimal ptosis of 15.2 mm with good function of the levator and a good lid fold.

Ptosis Surgery	Requisite Levator Action	Amounty of Ptosis That Can Be Treated	Indications
Fasanella-Servat	Good	≤ 2 mm	Horner syndrome, mild congenital ptosis
Levator resection - anterior approach	Good/moderate/poor	Any	Congenital or acquired ptosis
Levator resection - conjunctival approach	Good/moderate	Any	Congenital or acquired ptosis
Levator resection with aponeurotic reinsertion	Good/moderate	Any	Acquired aponeurotic ptosis
Frontalis suspension	Poor	Severe	Congenital-especially Marcus Gunn ptosis or for temporary relief

- For mild ptosis having a positive phenylephrine test, internal conjunctival Muller muscle resection is preferred.
- In moderate-to-severe ptosis with a moderate levator action, levator resection can be carried out.

39. Treatment for mild ptosis is - *(PGMEE 2016-17)*
a. Frontalis sling operation
b. Everbusch's operation
c. Levator resection
d. Fasanella servat operation

[Ref: Parsons' 23rd/e pg. 412]

40. A patient with ptosis, upper 4 mm of cornea is covered by upper eyelid. Grade of Ptosis is: *(PGMEE 2013)*
a. Moderate
b. Profound
c. Severe
d. Mild

[Ref: Parsons' 23rd/e pg. 411]

Explanation

- *Callahan and Beard classification of ptosis is as follows:*
  ○ Mild: ≥2 mm
  ○ Moderate: ≥3 mm
  ○ Severe: ≥4 mm

MISCELLANEOUS

41. Distichiasis is *(PGMEE 2016-17)*
a. Abnormal extra row of cilia
b. Abnormal eversion of eyelashes
c. Misdirected cilia
d. Abnormal inversion of eyelashes

[Ref: Parsons' 23rd/e pg. 420]

42. Blephritis acarica is caused by- *(PGMEE 2014)*
a. Ascaricus
b. Demodex folliculorum
c. Streptococcus
d. Propionibacterium

[Ref: Parsons' 23rd/e pg. 402]

Explanation

- Occasionally, parasites cause blepharitis - *blepbaritis acarica*, due to *Demodex folliculorum*, and *phthiriasis palpebrarum*, due to the crab louse, very rarely due to the head louse.

43. Loss of eyelashes is - *(PGMEE 2012)*
a. Madarosis
b. Ectropion
c. Tylosis
d. Trichiasis

[Ref: Parsons' 23rd/e pg. 402]

44. Most common cause of trichiasis is – *(PGMEE 2014)*
a. Trachoma
b. Congenital
c. Blephritis
d. Stye

[Ref: Parsons' 23rd/e pg. 405]

45. Trichiasis is characterised by:- *(PGMEE 2016)*
a. Thickening of eyelids
b. Inward misdirection of cilia
c. Inward misdirection of lid
d. Extra row of lashes

[Ref: Parsons' 23rd/e pg. 405]

46. Most common malignant tumour of eyelid is - *(NEET Pattern 09, Nov 93, June 92; PGMEE 2012)*
a. Sebaceous gland carcinoma
b. Malignant melanoma
c. Basal cell carcinoma
d. Squamous cell carcinoma

[Ref: Parsons' 23rd/e pg. 418]

36.	b
37.	d
38.	b
39.	d
40.	d
41.	a
42.	b
43.	a
44.	a
45.	b
46.	c

47. MC tumor of lacrimal gland. *(NEET Pattern 2017)*
a. Adenoid cystic carcinoma
b. Non Hodgkin lymphoma
c. Mucoepidermoid cancer
d. Pleomorphic adenoma

[Ref. Parsons' 23ʳᵈ/e pg. 424]

Explanation

- Tumors of the lacrimal glands show marked resemblance to those of the parotids. Pleomorphic adenocarcinoma (mixed tumour) is commonest.
- Non epithelial tumors comprise 70-80% of solid lacrimal masses whereas only 20-25% are epithelial.
- Pleomorphic adenoma is the most common benign epithelial lacrimal tumor, whereas adenoid cystic carcinoma is the most common malignant epithelial lesion.
- Radical excision is TOC for malignant lesions.

48. Basal cell carcinoma is seen in most commonly in which eyelid- *(PGMEE 2016-17; 2013)*
a. Upper medial
b. Upper lateral
c. Lower medial
d. Lower lateral

[Ref: PParsons' 23ʳᵈ/e pg. 417]

49. Lower lid surgery in which plication of the lower lid retractors is done is called - *(PGMEE 2015)*
a. Modified wheelers
b. Jones
c. Quickert
d. Weiss

[Ref: Parsons' 23ʳᵈ/e pg. 406; Nema 6ᵗʰ/e pg. 421]

Explanation

- *Tucking of inferior lid retractors (Jones, Reeb and Wobig):* In cases of severe entropion, tucking of the inferior.

50. The operation for plication of lower lid retractors is done for? *(DNB June 2011)*
a. Senile Ectropion
b. Paralytic entropion
c. Cicatrical entropion
d. Senile entropion

[Ref: Parsons' 23ʳᵈ/e pg. 406]

51. Identify the pathology depicted in the image? *(PGMEE 2015)*

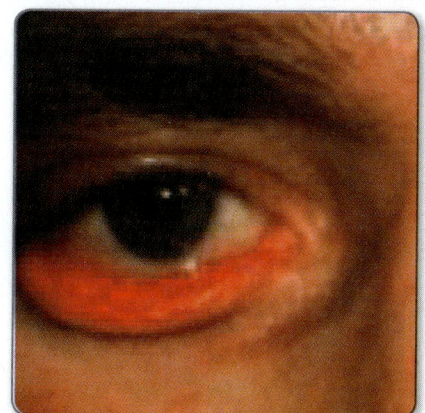

a. Esotropia
b. Entropion
c. Districhiasis
d. Ectropion

[Ref: Khurana 4th /e p. 351; Parsons' 23ʳᵈ/e pg. 409]

52. Horner's syndrome, all are true except: *(PGMEE 2016-17)*
a. Enophthalmos
b. Mydriasis
c. Ptosis
d. Unilateral loss of sweating

[Ref: Parsons' 23ʳᵈ/e pg. 104, 415]

53. Madarosis is seen in - *(PGMEE 2012)*
a. Acromegaly
b. Addison's disease
c. Hypothyroidism
d. Vitiligo

[Ref: Nema 6ᵗʰ/e pg. 415]

LACRIMAL APPARATUS

54. Meibomian glands secrete which component of tear- *(PGMEE 2016-17)*
a. Protein
b. Mucin
c. Lipid
d. Water {aqueous}

[Ref: Parsons' 23ʳᵈ/e pg. 423]

55. Congenital dacrocystitis, the block is at- *(PGMEE 2012)*
a. Nasolacrimal duct
b. Lacrimal calnaliculi
c. Punctum
d. None

[Ref: Parsons' 23ʳᵈ/e pg. 426]

56. Treatment of dacryocystitis in three months old child — *(PGMEE 2015)*
a. Massaging
b. Weekly probing
c. Syringing
d. Daily probing

[Ref: Parsons' 23ʳᵈ/e pg. 426]

Explanation

Dacrocystitis

- Inflammation/infection of lacrimal sac, secondary to obstruction of the nasolacrimal duct at the junction of lacrimal sac.
- MC organism implicated → Staph. aureus.
- Acute dacrocystitis with orbital cellulitis necessitates hospitalization with i/v antibiotics.
- T/t:-
  ○ < 6 month → Antibiotic eye drops + massaging
  ○ 6-18 month → Probing
  ○ > 18 months → DCR (dacrocystorhinostomy) opening of which is made in middle meatus.

57. Primary treatment of dacrocystitis – *(PGMEE 2016-17)*
a. Massage
b. Antibiotic drops
c. Surgery
d. Probing

[Ref: Parsons' 23ʳᵈ/e pg. 426]

58. Immediate treatment of acute dacryocystitis is-
a. Nasal decongestants *(PGMEE 2015)*
b. Antibiotics and drainage of abscess if present
c. Dacryocystectomy
d. Dacrycystorhinostomy

[Ref: Orbit, Eyelids and Lacrimal System, section 7. Basic and Clinical Science Course, AAO, 2011-2012]

59. Treatment of acute dacrocystitis in stage of cellulitis is – *(PGMEE 2015)*
a. Abscess drainage
b. DCR
c. DCT
d. IV Antibiotics

[Ref: Parsons' 23ʳᵈ/e pg. 427]

47.	d
48.	c
49.	b
50.	d
51.	d
52.	b
53.	d
54.	c
55.	a
56.	a
57.	a
58.	b
59.	d

60. Surgery of choice in dacrocystitis
a. Dacryocystectomy
b. Conjunctivo-cystorhinostomy
c. Dacryocystorhinostomy
d. None   [Ref: Parsons' 23rd/e pg. 426]

61. Dacrocytorhinostomy involves- **(PGMEE 2013)**
a. Complete excision of lacrimal
b. Connecting the lacrimal sac to nose by breaking the medial wall
c. Insertion of drainage tube in the lacrimal sac
d. Opening up the terminal blocked end of nasolacrimal duct

[Ref: Parsons' 23rd/e pg. 426]

62. During DCR surgery an osteotomy was done in the anterior and superior region. Which area does it accidentally open into? **(DNB Jun'2010)**
a. Superior Meatus
b. Maxillary Antrum
c. Anterior ethomoidal Sinus
d. Middle Meatus

[Ref: Parsons' 22nd/e pg.431]

63. Dacrocystorhinostomy, where the duct is opened - **(PGMEE 2016-17)**
a. Inferior meatus
b. Sphenoethmoidal recess
c. Middle meatus
d. Superior meatus

[Ref: Parsons' 23rd/e pg. 426]

64. For congenital obstruction of nasolacrimal duct, probing is done at what age? **(PGMEE 2015)**
a. 2 months
b. 6 months
c. 9 months
d. 14 months

[Ref: Parsons' 23rd/e pg. 426]

65. Probing and irrigation is not done in - **(PGMEE 2015)**
a. Acute dacryocystitis
b. Trauma to eye
c. Congenital dacryocystitis
d. Lacrimal fistula

[Ref: Parsons' 23rd/e pg. 427]

66. Schirmer's test detects abnorniality of which nerve- **(PGMEE 2016-17)**
a. Glossopharyngeal
b. Oculomotor
c. Hypoglossal
d. Facial

[Ref: Parsons' 23rd/e pg. 425]

67. Identify the pathology depicted in the image? **(PGMEE 2015)**

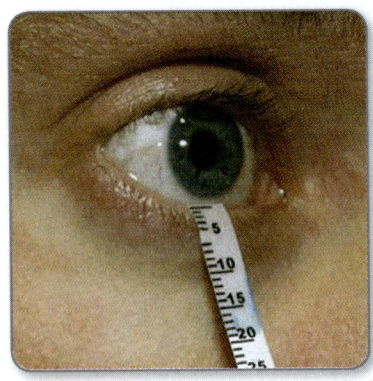

a. Schirmer's test
b. Enophthalmos
c. Proptosis
d. Exophthalmos

68. Pleomorphic adenoma of the lacrimal gland moves the eyeball - **(PGMEE 2015)**
a. Upwards and outards
b. Downwards and inwards
c. Downwards and outwards
d. Upwards and inwards

[Ref: Parsons' 23rd/e pg. 424]

Explanation
■ Impairment of eye movements. The globe is pushed downwards and inwards (Fig. 24.2). Ocular movement outwards, and especially outwards and upwards, is limited. There may be some proptosis.

69. Beaded margin of eyelid is seen in: **(DNB Dec'2010)**
a. Erythema granuloma annulare
b. Granuloma annulare
c. Leprosy
d. Lipoid proteinosis

[Ref: Internet]

70. Ankyloblepharon is – **(PGMEE 2016)**
a. Adhesion b/w bulbar & palpebral conjunctiva
b. Thickening of lid margin
c. Anterior scleral perforation
d. Adhesion of both lid margins together

[Ref: Parsons' 23rd/e pg. 410]

60.	c
61.	b
62.	c
63.	c
64.	c
65.	a
66.	d
67.	a
68.	b
69.	d
70.	d

OPHTHALMOSCOPY

1. Area of fundus seen with direct ophthalmoscope is: *(PGMEE 2012)*

a. 1 DD　　　　　　b. 2 DD
c. 3 DD　　　　　　d. 4 DD

[Ref: Parsons' 22nd/e pg. 137]

2. The magnification obtained with a direct ophthalmoscope is: *(PGMEE 2016-17)*

a. 5 times
b. 2DD
c. 15 times
d. 4 DD

[Ref: Parsons' 23rd/e pg. 117]

3. Image formed in direct opthalmoscopy is:

a. Real and erect　　　*(PGMEE 2014)*
b. Virtual and inverted
c. Virtual and erect
d. Real and inverted

[Ref: Parsons' 23rd/e pg. 117]

4. Which of the following is false about indirect ophthalmoscopy? *(NEET 13; PGMEE 2016-17)*

a. Convex lens is used
b. It is so bright that regular haziness in penetrated.
c. Magnification is 4-5 times
d. Image is virtual and erect

[Ref: Parsons' 23rd/e pg. 113]

5. Indirect ophthalmoscopy is done for: *(PGMEE 2014)*

a. Angle of ant. chamber
b. Central retina
c. Sclera
d. Periphery of retina

[Ref: Parsons' 23rd/e pg. 113]

FLUOROSC IN ANGIOGRAPHY

6. Fluorescent dye for ophthalmological diagnosis is injected in: *(PGMEE 2016-17, 15)*

a. Popliteal vein
b. Subclavian vein
c. Femoral vein
d. Antecubital vein

[Ref: Nema 6th/e pg. 83]

7. Fluoroscein dye study is done to detect - *(PGMEE 2015)*

a. Assess retinal function of babies
b. Posterior segment of eye
c. Macular pathology
d. Retinal vascular pathology

[Ref: Parsons' 23rd/e pg. 119]

8. Indocyanine Green Angiography [ICG Angiography] is most useful in detecting: *(PGMEE 2014)*

a. Angioid streakswith choroidal Neovascularization (GNV)
b. Classic choroidal Neovascularization (Classic GNV)
c. Occult Choroidal Neovascularization (Occult GNV)
d. Polypoidal choroidal vasculopathy

[Ref: Parsons' 23rd/e pg. 119]

ERG

9. Waves present in electroretinogram are all EXCEPT: *(DNB Jun'2010)*

a. a wave　　　　　　b. b wave
c. c wave　　　　　　d. d wave

[Ref: Parsons' 23rd/e pg. 123]

10. True about electroretinogram (ERG):- *(PGMEE 2013)*

a. 'a' wave is positive wave
b. 'a' wave arises from pigmented epithelium
c. 'b' wave arises from rods and cones
d. 'c' wave is positive wave

[Ref: Parsons' 23rd/e pg. 123]

11. A wave in ERG is due to activity of:- *(PGMEE 2016-17)*

a. Pigmented epithelium
b. Bipolar cell
c. Ganglion cells
d. Rods and cones

[Ref: Parsons' 23rd/e pg. 123]

CLINICAL EXAMINATION & EYE TESTING

12. Amaurosis fugax refers to occlusion of : *(DNB 2008; PGMEE 2016-17)*

a. Middle cerebral artery
b. Retinal arteriole
c. Renal vessels
d. Mesenteric vessels

[Ref: Parsons' 23rd/e pg. 463]

13. Abnormally eccentric placed pupil is called- *(PGMEE 2012)*

a. Corectopia
b. Anisocoria
c. Ectopia lentis
d. Polycoria

[Ref: Parsons' 23rd/e pg. 229; Nema 6th/e pg. 66]

Explanation

- Rarely, there can be more than one pupillary aperture called polycoria.
- Occasionally, the location of pupil may be eccentric (corectopia).

1.	b
2.	c
3.	c
4.	d
5.	d
6.	d
7.	d
8.	c
9.	d
10.	d
11.	d
12.	a
13.	a

14. Specific for albinism – *(PGMEE 2013)*
a. Decreased visual activity
b. Nystagmus
c. Photophobia
d. Red reflex

[Ref: Pasricha p.221; Parsons' 23rd/e pg. 230]

15. Brushfield spots in iris are seen in:
(PGMEE 2015, 2016-17)
a. Down syndrome
b. Toxoplasmosis
c. Tuberous sclerosis
d. Neurofibromatosis

[Ref: Parsons' 23rd/e pg. 103; Nema 6th/e pg. 268]

Explanation

- Multiple punctate and flake-like opacities are found early in life in the lens cortex. Congenital cataract involving the fetal nucleus, Brushfield spots, white or gray thickening of the midperipheral iris arranged in a ring concentric with the pupil are found in 85% patients.
- Brushfield spots are seen in Down syndrome
- Pedunculated nodules (Lisch) are seen in neurofibromatosis.

16. Lisch nodule seen in – *(PGMEE 2015)*
a. Chronic iridocyclitis
b. Trachoma
c. Neurofibromatosis
d. Sympathetic ophthalmitis

[Ref: Parsons' 23rd/e pg. 103]

17. All of the following are causes of night blindness Except:
(PGMEE 2011)
a. High myopia
b. Vitamin A deficiency
c. Oguchi disease
d. Devics disease

[Ref: Parsons' 23rd/e pg. 79]

18. Curvature of cornea can be measured by -
(PGMEE 2016-17)
a. Direct ophthalmoscopy
b. Perimetry
c. Retinoscopy
d. Keratometry

[Ref: Parsons' 23rd/e pg. 170]

19. Increased intraocular tension can be diagnosed by-
(PGMEE 2015)
a. Placido's disc
b. Pachymeter
c. Keratometer
d. Tonometer

[Ref: Parsons' 23rd/e pg. 108]

20. Inverted Purkinje image is seen on- *(PGMEE 2013)*
a. Posterior surface of cornea
b. Anterior surface of lens
c. Anterior surface of cornea
d. Posterior surface of lens

[Ref: Nema 6th/e pg. 68]

21. Fluorescence stain is used in the eye to stain -
(PGMEE 2016-17)
a. Choroid
b. Retina
c. Cornea
d. Iris

[Ref: Parsons' 23rd/e pg. 101]

22. Which of the following are contrast sensitivity testing charts? *(PGMEE 2015)*
a. Pelli Robson charts
b. Snellen type chart
c. Regan charts
d. Both a & c are correct

[Ref: Parsons' 23rd/e pg. 95]

14.	d
15.	a
16.	c
17.	d
18.	d
19.	d
20.	d
21.	c
22.	d
23.	d
24.	d
25.	a
26.	c
27.	d
28.	a
29.	d
30.	b
31.	b

23. Slit lamp examination helps in examination of-
a. Posterior 1/3rd of choroid *(PGMEE 2013)*
b. Anterior 1/3rd of choroid
c. Anterior 2/3rd of choroid
d. Posterior capsule

[Ref: Parsons' 23rd/e pg. 106]

24. Slit-lamp bimicroscopy is indicated in: *(PGMEE 2014)*
a. Disease of anterior chamber
b. Lens opacities
c. Corneal opacities
d. All of the above

[Ref: Parsons' 23rd/e pg. 107]

25. Imbert-Fick law is associated with:-
a. Applanation tonometry *(PGMEE 2015; 2016-17)*
b. Keratometry
c. Schiotz tonometry
d. Pachymetry

[Ref: Parsons' 23rd/e pg. 108]

26. Corneal thickness is measured by all except:
(PGMEE 2014)
a. Orbscan
b. OCT
c. Javal Schiotz method
d. Utrasonography

[Ref: Parsons' 23rd/e pg. 170]

Explanation

- The corneal thickness can be measured manually by an optical pachymeter attached to slit lamp, with an ultrasonic pachymeter or a slit-scanning topography system.
- The corneal endothelium can be viewed with the slit lamp in the zone of specular reflection and the cells are counted using a specular microscope.

27. Corneal endothelial cell count is done by:
(PGMEE 2012)
a. Gonioscopy
b. Slit lamp
c. Keratometry
d. Specular microscopy

[Ref: Parsons' 23rd/e pg. 170]

28. In specular microscopy endothelial density is measured by- *(PGMEE 2013)*
a. Fixed frame analysis
b. Optical focusing
c. Optical doubling
d. None

[Ref: Parsons' 23rd/e pg. 170]

29. Corneal sensation is tested by - *(PGMEE 2016-17)*
a. Keratometry
b. Specular microscopy
c. Pachymeter
d. Aesthesiometer

[Ref: Parsons' 23rd/e pg. 101]

30. Swinging flash light test is used to examine: *(DNB 2008)*
a. Cornea
b. Pupil
c. Lens
d. Conjunctiva

[Ref: Parsons' 23rd/e pg. 105]

31. Argyll Robertson pupil is seen in? *(DNB June' 2012)*
a. Multiple sclerosis
b. Neurosyphilis
c. Mid brain tumor
d. All

[Ref: Parsons' 23rd/e pg. 106]

32. Campimetry is used to measure:
                    (DNB 2007; PGMEE 2016-17)
  a. Squint
  b. Malignant melanoma
  c. Pattern of retina
  d. Field charting

[Ref: Parsons' 23rd/e pg. 90; Nema 6th/e pg. 80]

Explanation

Campimetry (scotometry)

- It is a type of kinetic perimetry, which enables the examiner to explore the central and paracentral areas (30°) of the visual field. Bjerrum's screen (at 1 or 2 meters distance) is used to chart the field.

33. Photostress test is useful in disease of:-   **(DNB 2007)**
  a. Macula   b. Optic nerve
  c. Refractive error   d. Optic tract

[Ref: Parsons' 23rd/e pg. 90]

34. Amsler grid test is for   **(PGMEE 2016-17)**
  a. Visual field charting
  b. Corneal thickness
  c. Calculation of squint angle
  d. Macular function   *[Ref: Parsons' 23rd/e pg. 83]*

Explanation

Metamorphopsia

- This can be reviewed for any changes over time using an Amsler grid, which tests the central 10° of vision. It is associated with diseases affecting the macula such as central serous choroidopathy, age-related macular degeneration, diabetic macular oedema and macular hole.

35. This test is used in: **(PGMEE 2019)**

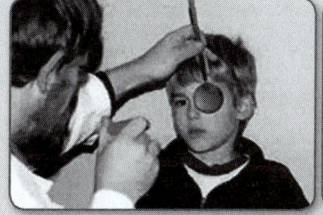 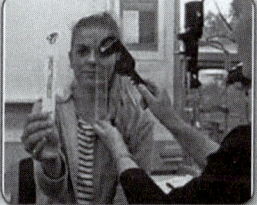

  a. Squint   b. Heterophoria
  c. Esotropia   d. All the above

[Ref: Parsons' Diseases of the eye, 22nd/e pg. 184; A K Khurana Comprehensive Ophthalmology 7th/e pg. 365]

36. Identify the instrument: **(PGMEE 2019)**

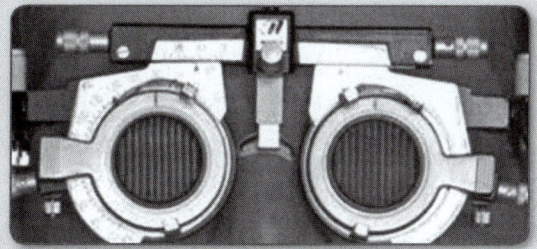

  a. Maddox rod   b. Maddox wing
  c. Maddox glass   d. Red glass

[Ref: A K Khurana Comprehensive Ophthalmology 7th/e pg. 203, 360]

37. Amsler's grid is used to evaluate -   **(PGMEE 2015)**
  a. Central 20 degrees of vision
  b. Peripheral vision
  c. Central 10 degress of vision
  d. Lens opacity   *[Ref: Parsons' 23rd/e pg. 83]*

38. Floaters can be seen in following except- **(PGMEE 2015)**
  a. Acute congestive Glaucoma
  b. Retinal detachment
  c. Uveitis
  d. Vitreous haemorrhage   *[Ref: Parsons' 23rd/e pg. 83]*

39. Following are the causes of sudden loss of vision except:
                    (PGMEE 2016-17)
  a. Central serous retinopathy
  b. Endophthalmitis
  c. Corneal ulceration
  d. Angle closure glaucoma

[Ref: Parsons' 23rd/e pg. 511]

40. Shadow test is used in-   **(PGMEE 2015)**
  a. Retinoscopy   b. Keratometry
  c. Gonioscopy   d. Ophthalmoscopy

[Ref: Parsons' 23rd/e pg. 57]

41. No movement of Red reflex in retinoscopy:
                    (PGMEE 2015)
  a. Myopia of 3D   b. Hypermetropia
  c. Myopia of 1D   d. No refractive error

[Ref: Parsons' 23rd/e pg. 57]

42. Objective assessment of the refractive state of the eye is done by –   **(PGMEE 2012)**
  a. Gonioscopy   b. Ophthalmoscopy
  c. Keratoscopy   d. Retinoscopy

[Ref: Parsons' 23rd/e pg. 54]

43. Methods to measure error of refraction are all except -
                    (PGMEE 2013)
  a. Retinoscopy   b. Binocular balancing
  c. Keratometry   d. Refractometry

[Ref: Parsons' 23rd/e pg. 54, 59]

44. Jackson's cross cylinder test is used for?- **(PGMEE 2015)**
  a. Objective refining   b. Subjective balancing
  c. Subjective verification d. Subjective refraction

(Ref: Internet]

45. Duochrome test is for   **(PGMEE 2012)**
  a. Subjective verification of refraction
  b. Subjective refinement of refraction
  c. Subjective binocular balancing
  d. None

[Ref:- Khurana 5th/e pg 588]

46. Binocular single vision is tested by –
  a. Amsler grid   b. Cardboard test
  c. Synoptophore   d. Maddox rod

[Ref: Parsons' 23rd/e pg. 373]

Explanation

- **Synoptophore:** Binocular viewing device that can be used to determine fusion ability of individuals with diplopia who have had long-standing severe monocular visual loss in which the vision has been restored.

32.	**d**
33.	**a**
34.	**d**
35.	**d**
36.	**a**
37.	**c**
38.	**a**
39.	**c**
40.	**a**
41.	**c**
42.	**d**
43.	**b**
44.	**d**
45.	**b**
46.	**c**

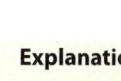

47. Identify the instrument depicted in the image?
(PGMEE 2015)

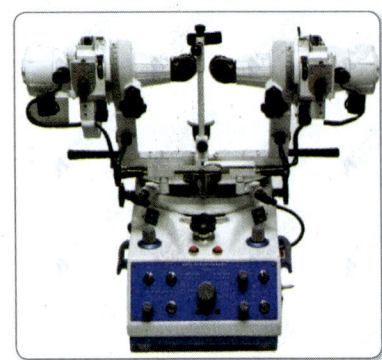

a. Tonometer   b. Perimeter
c. Operating microscope   d. Synoptophore

[Ref: Parsons' 23rd/e pg. 373]

48. Identify the instrument given in the image?
(PGMEE 2015)

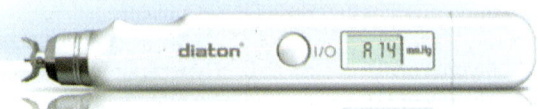

a. Tonometer   b. Pachymeter
c. Keratometer   d. Buphthalmometer

[Ref: Khurana 5th /e p. 479]

MISCELLANEOUS

49. To assess stereopsis , test done is :-   *(PGMEE 2016)*
a. Titmus fly test
b. Amsler grid
c. Fincham test
d. Worth test

[Ref: Parsons' 23rd/e pg. 96]

Explanation

- Tests to further quantify the extent of stereopsis, i.e. measure stereoacuity, included various means of dissociating the images presented to the right and left eyes by using different coloured glasses or polarized lenses and appropriately designed pictures such as the Titmus fly test, TNO test and Randot stereoacuity test

50. Worth -4-dot Test in a normal person is: *(PGMEE 2016)*
a. 2 green, 4 red, 1 white
b. 2 green, 2 red, 1white
c. 2 green, 1 red, 1 white
d. 2 green, 1 red, 2 white

[Ref: Parsons' 23rd/e pg. 372]

51. Image seen through prism?   *(PGMEE 2014)*
a. Titled
b. Near the apex
c. Near the base
d. Inverted

[Ref: Parsons' 23rd/e pg. 373]

47. d
48. a
49. a
50. c,d
51. b

PREVENTIVE OPHTHALMOLOGY

1. Most common cause of blindness in India is?

    (DNB Jun'2009)

a. Glaucoma

b. Cataract

c. Trachoma

d. Refractory errors

[Ref: Parsons' 23rd/e pg. 532]

2. Vitamin A supplementation in a 10 month old child with xerophthalmia is?

    (DNB December 2011; PGMEE 2016-17)

a. One dose of 1 lakh units i/m

b. Two doses of 1 lakh units i/m 1week apart

c. Three doses of 1 lakh units orally on 3 successive days

d. Two doses of 2 lakh units orally on 2 successive days

[Ref: Parsons' 23rd/e pg. 163]

3. In xerophthalmia classification X 2 stage is:

    (PGMEE 2015)

a. Corneal xerosis

b. Corneal scar

c. Bitots spots

d. Corneal ulceration

[Ref: Park's 24th/e pg. 654]

4. What is the correct sequence of xerophthalmia

    (PGMEE 2015)

a. Corneal ulcer → Nightblindness → Conjunctival xerosis → corneal xerosis

b. Conjunctival xerosis → corneal xerosis → corneal ulcer → Nightblindness

c. Nightblindness → Conjunctival xerosis → corneal xerosis → corneal ulcer

d. Corneal xerosis → corneal ulcer → Nightblindness → Conjunctival xerosis

[Ref: Parsons' 22nd/e pg. 188]

5. The dosage of Vitamin A in keratomalacia in a 2 year old boy who is 12 kg weight is   *(PGMEE 2019)*

a. Vitamin A: 2 lakh I U, oral, 1st, 2nd and 14th day

b. Vitamin A: 1 lakh I U, oral, 1st, 2nd and 14th day

c. Vitamin A: 2 lakh I U, oral , 1st, 2nd and 3rd day

d. Vitamin A: 1 lakh I U, oral, 1st, 2nd and 3rd day

[Ref: Parsons' Diseases of the eye 22nd/e pg. 218; A K Khurana Comprehensive Ophthalmology 7th/e pg. 488]

6. Identify the pathology depicted in the image?

    (PGMEE 2015)

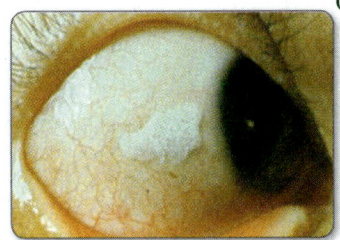

a. Foreign body

b. Anterior staphyloma

c. Bitot's spots

d. Normal anatomical variant

[Ref: Parsons' 22nd/e pg. 188]

7. Which is not done in vision centre?

a. Eye check-up

b. Cataract surgery

c. Prescription of glasses

d. School health programme

[Ref: Park 23rd/e pg. 403]

SYSTEMIC OPHTHALMOLOGY

8. Which of the following is seen in Horner's syndrome?

    (DNB Jun'2009; PGMEE 2016-17)

a. Anhidrosis   b. Cheilitis

c. Optic neuritis   d. Blepharitis

[Ref: Parsons' 23rd/e pg. 104 & 415]

9. Horner's syndrome causes all, except: *(DNB 2007)*

a. Enophthalmos

b. Mydriasis

c. Anhidrosis

d. Narrowed palpebral fissure

[Ref: Parsons' 23rd/e pg. 104 & 415]

10. Uveoparotitis is seen in?   *(DNB Dec'2009)*

a. Mumps   b. SLE

c. Scleroderma   d. Sarcoidosis

[Ref: Parsons' 23rd/e pg. 221]

Explanation

- *Uveoparotid fever* or *Heerfordt disease*, which is bilateral and characterized by a simultaneous involvement of the entire uveal tract, parotid gland and frequently the cranial nerves.
- Half the cases with a granulomatous iridocyclitis
- Half with a painful swelling of the parotid resembling that due to mumps.

1.	b
2.	c
3.	a
4.	c
5.	a
6.	c
7.	b
8.	a
9.	b
10.	d

11. Behcet's disease is characterized by:
a. Hypoyon   **(DNB Jun 2010; 2016-17)**
b. Hyphema
c. Subconjuctival hemorrhage
d. Scleritis

[Ref: Parsons' 23rd/e pg. 221]

12. Spontaneous absorption of lenticular material is seen in: **(DNB 2008)**
a. Myotonic dystrophy
b. Hallermann Streiff syndrome
c. Aniridia
d. Persistent hyperplastic primary vitreous

[Ref: Internet]

13. Kayser Fleisher ring is characteristic of?
      (PGMEE June 2012; 2016-17)
a. Hemosiderosis   b. Wilson disease
c. Tyrosinemia   d. Hereditary cataract

[Ref: Parsons' 23rd/e pg. 488]

14. Eye involvement is seen in?   **(DNB Jun'2009)**
a. Seronegative JRA   b. Seropositive JRA
c. Osteoarthritis   d. All

[Ref: Parsons' 23rd/e pg. 221]

Explanation
- The pauciarticular subset of JCA involves mainly girls 2-6 years of age, who are positive for ANA and negative for RF, Ocular involvement is common (50% of patients), predominantly manifesting as a bilateral chronic uveitis of insidious onset, often with minimal signs such as mild pain and redness
- Spondyloarthropathy affecting males older than 12 years who are positive for the HLA-B27 antigen. This group is affected by an acute unilateral iritis of sudden onset.

15. After a leisure trip, a patient comes with gritty pain in eye, and joint pain. What is the most probable diagnosis?
      (DNB Dec' 2011; PGMEE 2016-17)
a. Reiter's syndrome   b. Behcet's syndrome
c. Sarcoidosis   d. SLE

[Ref: Parsons' 23rd/e pg. 220]

16. Macula involvement is common in –   **(PGMEE 2014)**
a. Syphilis   b. Malaria
c. CMV   d. Toxoplasma

[Ref: Parsons' 23rd/e pg. 488]

MISCELLANEOUS

17. All are ophthalmological emergencies except -
a. CRAO   **(PGMEE 2016-17)**
b. Acute congestive glaucoma
c. Endophthalmitis
d. CRVO

[Ref: Parsons' 23rd/e pg. 513]

Explanation

Common Eye Emergencies and Key Steps in Management

Ischaemic optic neuropathy	Must rule out giant cell arteritis (GCA)
Central retina artery occlusion	Must rule out GCA and causes of emboli/thrombus
Macula-on rhegmatogenous retinal detachment	Must refer immediately to ophthalmologist
Acute third nerve palsy	Must rule out intracranial aneurysm
Corneal microbial keratitis	Must culture and treat with empirical antibiotics and follow closely
Open globe	Arrange for emergency repair
Acute angle-closure glaucoma	Must control IOP
Endophthalmitis	Must treat with antibiotics and refer
Alkali injury	Requires urgent and copious irrigation
Orbital cellulitis	Must treat with systemic antibiotics

Answers

11.	a
12.	b
13.	b
14.	a
15.	a
16.	a,d
17.	d

EXTRA EDGES

Systemic Diagnosis	Systemic Features	Extraocular Features	Intraocular Features
Homocystinuria	Mental retardation, tall, arachnodactyly, thromboembolic episodes		Subluxation of the lens
Mucopolysaccharidoses	Dysmorphia, behavioural disorders, cardiac anomalies	Corneal opacification	Pigmentary retinopathy, glaucoma, optic atrophy
Wilson disease	Extrapyramidal signs, cirrhosis	Kayser-Fleischer ring	Sunflower cataract
Diabetes mellitus	Peripheral neuropathy, glomerulosclerosis	Xanthelasma, extraocular muscle palsies, infections	Cataract, iris neovascularization, retinopathy, vitreous haemorrhage, tractional retinal detachment, optic neuropathy
Hyperthyroidism	Tachycardia, tremors of the hand	Exophthalmos, lid retraction, lid lag	Superior limbic keratitis, disc oedema
Hypoparathyroidism	Tetany, seizures	Fasciculation	Cataract, disc oedema

1. **Most common primary malignant orbital tumor in children:** *(PGMEE 2016-17)*
   a. Chloroma
   b. Melanoma
   c. Rhabdomyosarcoma
   d. Retinoblastoma

   [Ref: Parsons' 23rd/e pg. 445; Nema 6th/e pg. 445]

2. **Most common malignant intraorbital tumor in adult is -** *(PGMEE 2015)*
   a. Rhabdomyosarcoma
   b. Sarcoma
   c. Dermoid cyst
   d. Lymphoma

   [Ref: Parsons' 22nd/e pg. 379]

3. **Most common tumor to extend from intracranial to orbital portion is:** *(PGMEE 2012)*
   a. Sphenoidal wing meningioma
   b. Craniopharyngioma
   c. Pituitary adenoma
   d. Astrocytoma

   [Ref: Internet]

4. **The most common primary cause of intraocular tumor in children:** *(PGMEE 2015)*
   a. Neuroblastoma
   b. Rhabdomyosarcoma
   c. Melanoma
   d. Retinoblastoma

   [Ref: Parsons' 23rd/e pg. 349; Nema 6th/e pg. 352]

5. **The most common retrobulbar orbital mass in adults -**
   a. Cavernous haemangioma *(PGMEE 2013)*
   b. Schwanrfoma
   c. Meningioma
   d. Nerurofibroma

   [Ref: Parsons' 23rd/e pg. 443]

6. **Most common orbital tumor has its origin from -** *(PGMEE 2012; 2016-17)*
   a. Nerves
   b. Lymph node
   c. Muscle
   d. Blood vessels

   [Ref: Parsons' 23rd/e pg. 443]

7. **Most common carcinoma of conjunctiva -** *(PGMEE 2012)*
   a. Melanoma
   b. Lymphoma
   c. Squamous cell Ca
   d. Basal cell ca

   [Ref: Textbook of tumors of the eye and ocular Adexa p. 57]

RETINOBLASTOMA

8. **Retinoblastoma can occur bilaterally in how many percentage of the cases?** *(PGMEE 2015)*
   a. 10-15%
   b. 15-20%
   c. 30-35%
   d. 25%

   [Ref: Parsons' 23rd/e pg. 349]

9. **Regarding Retinoblastoma all are true EXCEPT:** *(DNB Dec'2009; PGMEE 2016-17)*
   a. 13q14 mutation
   b. Autosomal dominant
   c. 25% Bilateral
   d. 40% Heritable forms

   [Ref: Parsons' 22nd/e pg. 375]

10. **Pseudorosettes are seen in -** *(PGMEE 2014)*
    a. Phakolytic glaucoma
    b. Ophthalmic nodosa
    c. Trachoma
    d. Retinoblastoma

    [Ref: Parsons' 23rd/e pg. 349]

11. **Rees-Elsworth classification is used for:** *(DNB 2008; PGMEE 2016-17)*
    a. Neuroblastoma
    b. Nephroblastoma
    c. Retinoblastoma
    d. Hepatoblastoma

    [Ref: Parsons' 23rd/e pg. 350]

12. **Intraocular calcification in eye in child -** *(PGMEE 2015)*
    a. Malignant melanoma of choroid
    b. Retinoblastoma
    c. Toxocara
    d. Angiomatosis retinae

    [Ref: Parsons' 23rd/e pg. 350]

13. **Most common presenting feature of retinoblastoma –** *(PGMEE 2013)*
    a. Proptosis
    b. Pain
    c. White reflex
    d. Photophobia

    [Ref: Parsons' 23rd/e pg. 349]

14. **All are presentation of retinoblastoma except -** *(PGMEE 2013)*
    a. Cataract
    b. Squint
    c. Glaucoma
    d. Leucocoria

    [Ref: Parsons' 23rd/e pg. 349]

Explanation
- The child is usually brought to the surgeon on account of a peculiar yellow reflex from the pupil, leucocoria or 'amaurotic cat's 'eye' divergent squint, cataract, buphthalmos, a hypopyon or proptosis.

15. **The most common mode of spread of Retinoblstoma is -** *(PGMEE 2012)*
    a. Trans-scleral
    b. Hematogenous
    c. Optic nerve
    d. Lymphatogenous

    [Ref: Parsons' 23rd/e pg. 350]

16. **Leucokoria can be seen in all except –** *(PGMEE 2014)*
    a. Congenital glaucoma
    b. Retinoblastoma
    c. Fungal endopthalmitis
    d. Persistant hyperplastic primary vitreous

    [Ref: Nema 6th/e pg. 68]

Explanation

The common causes of leukocoria are

- Retinoblastoma
- Total retinal detachment
- Endophthalmitis
- Retinopathy of prematurity
- Toxocariasis
- Coat's disease
- Persistent hyperplastic primary vitreous (PHPV)

1.	c
2.	d
3.	a
4.	d
5.	a
6.	d
7.	c
8.	d
9.	d
10.	d
11.	c
12.	b
13.	c
14.	None
15.	c
16.	a

17. Pseudoglioma differs from Retinoblastoma in that pseudoglioma is associated with - *(PGMEE 95)*
a. Blurring of vision
b. Enlargement of the optic foramen
c. Decreased intraocular pressure
d. All of the above

[Ref: Parsons' 23rd/e pg. 351]

18. Treatment of metastatic disease in retinoblastoma is —
a. Cryo *(PGMEE 2014)*
b. Chemotherapy
c. Enucleation
d. Radiotherapy

[Ref: Parsons' 23rd/e pg. 352]

19. A 5 yr old boy presented with leukocoria in right eyeball diagnosed to be retinoblastoma involving full eyeball, while other eye had 2-3 small lesions in the periphery. What will be the ideal management for this patient? *(PGMEE 2011)*
a. 6 cycles of chemotherapy
b. Enucleation of right eye & conservative management of the other eye
c. Enucleation of right eye and focal therapy of the other eye
d. Enucleation of both eyes

[Ref: Parsons' 23rd/e pg. 352]

MISCELLANEOUS

20. Most common site of distant metastasis in intraorbital malignant melanoma is *(PGMEE 2013)*
a. Brain
b. Lymph nodes
c. Lung
d. Liver

[Ref: Clinical oncology p. 786]

21. Most common type of optic nerve glioma is: *(PGMEE 2013)*
a. Protoplasmic
b. Fibrous
c. Pilocytic
d. Gemistocytic

[Ref: Sunita Agrawal Vol 2 p. 385]

22. Retinal astrocytoma is seen in: *(PGMEE 2012)*
a. Tuberous sclerosis
b. Von Hippel-Lindau syndrome
c. Sturge weber syndrome
d. None

[Ref: Textbook of ocular pathology pg. 53]

23. Most common intracranial tumor encroaching the orbit is? *(DNB JUNE'2011)*
a. Sphenoid wing meningioma
b. Glioblastoma multiforme
c. Astrocytoma
d. Medulloblastoma

[Ref: Parsons' 22nd/e pg.380]

24. Second common malignancy in patients of retinoblastoma is? *(DNB December 2011)*
a. Osteosarcoma
b. Osteoblastoma
c. Medulloblastoma
d. Ewing's sarcoma

[Ref: Parsons' 22nd/e pg.380]

25. Most common intraocular malignancy in adults is: *(DNB Dec'2010)*
a. Rhabdomyosarcoma
b. Melanoma of uvea
c. Retinoblastoma
d. Melanoma of choroid

[Ref: Parsons' 23rd/e pg. 346]

17. c
18. b
19. c
20. d
21. c
22. a
23. d
24. a
25. d

1. Bett's classification deals with *(PGMEE 2015)*
- a. Ocular foreign body
- b. Maculopathy
- c. Squint
- d. Ocular trauma

[Ref: Parsons' 23rd/e pg. 494]

Explanation

Mechanical eye injury	Closed-globe injuries	Contusion	
		Lamellar laceration	
		Superficial foreign body	
	Open-globe injuries	Laceration*	Penetrating‡ injury
			Perforating injury¥
			Intraocular foreign body
		Rupture†	

- BETTS classification of ocular trauma. *Outside-in injury; †inside-out injury; ‡single break in eye wall; ¥through-and-through injury of globe, dual breaks or double perforation. (Adapted from Kuhn et al. Ophthalmology 1996; 103:240-243.)

2. All can occur due to blunt trauma of eye except -
- a. Berlin's edema *(PGMEE 2016-17)*
- b. Rosette cataract
- c. Sympathetic ophthalmitis
- d. Angle recession

[Ref: Parsons' 23rd/e pg. 496-500]

Explanation

Blunt trauma to eye causes
- Blunt trauma to the eye occurs as a result of injury by tennis ball, fist, stick, stone etc.
- Contusion injuries may vary from a simple corneal abrasion to an extensive intraocular damage.
- Effects:-
  ○ Traumatic hyphaema
  ○ *Berlin's edema* (COMMOTIO RETINAE) following a blow on the eye. It manifests as milky white cloudiness involving a considerable area of **posterior pole** with a cherry- red spot in the foveal region
  ○ Angle recession
  ○ Iridodialysis, iridoplegia
  ○ VOSSIUS RING is a circular ring of brown pigment seen on the anterior capsule of lens.It occurs due to striking of contracted pupillary margin against the lens

3. Vossius ring is seen in the - *(PGMEE 2014)*
- a. Posterior capsule of the lens
- b. Anterior capsule of the lens
- c. Iris
- d. Cornea

[Ref: Parsons' 23rd/e pg. 498]

4. Ophthalmologic examination of a patient shows 'vossius ring' which is characteristic of the following condition: *(Recent Pattern June 2018)*
- a. Penetrating injury
- b. Concussion injury
- c. Lens dislocation
- d. Extracapsular extraction

[Ref: Parsons' 23rd/e pg. 498]

Explanation
- Vossius Ring is a circular deposit of dark brown iris pigments as a complete or incomplete ring on the **anterior lens capsule** d/to blunt trauma to the eye.
- Seen in traumatic iritis which frequently develops after closed globe concussion injury.
- Symptoms include pain, especially in bright light, blurred vision, and tenderness of the globe.
- Slit Lamp examination reveals inflammatory cells and flare in the AC, and finely dispersed cellular keratic precipitates on the corneal endothelium.

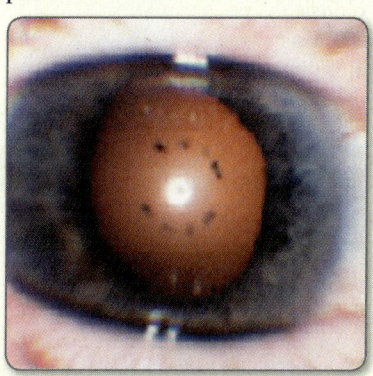

5. Secondary glaucoma associated with angle recession is seen in – *(PGMEE 2014; 2016-17)*
- a. Penetrating injury
- b. Penetrating injury
- c. Chemical injury
- d. Concussion injury

[Ref: Parsons' 23rd/e pg. 501]

Explanation
- Angle recession is associated with traumatic effects on the outflow channels leading to an insidious glaucoma. *Ghost cell* obstruction of the trabeculae in long-standing vitreous haemorrhages may also induce a secondary glaucoma.

6. Commotio retinae affects which part of retina - *(PGMEE 2013)*
- a. Peripheral retina
- b. Superior-nasal part
- c. Inferior-nasal part
- d. Posterior pole

[Ref: Parsons' 23rd/e pg. 500]

1.	d
2.	c
3.	b
4.	b
5.	d
6.	d

7. A boy gets hit by a tennis ball in the eye following which he has complaints of decreased vision. Which of the following indicates that blunt injury is due to the ball?

(PGMEE 11)

a. Pars planitis
b. Equatorial edema
c. Vitreous base detachment
d. Optic neuritis

[Ref: Parsons' 23rd/e pg. 500]

SYMPATHETIC OPHTHALMITIS

8. Sympathetic ophthalmitis results due to

(PGMEE 2016-17)

a. Glaucoma
b. Uveitis
c. Penetrating injury of ciliary body
d. Trachoma

[Ref: Parsons' 23rd/e pg. 506]

9. Dalen fuchs nodule is pathognomc of?

(PGMEE 2016-17; 2011)

a. Sympathetic opthalmitis
b. Sarcoidosis
c. Tuberculosis
d. Retinitis pigmentosa

[Ref: Parsons' 23rd/e pg. 506]

FOREIGN BODY

10. MC retained foreign body intraocularly:

(PGMEE 14)

a. Silver
b. Airgun pellets
c. Iron
d. Glass

[Ref: Parsons' 23rd/e pg. 504]

11. Inert foreign body in the eye -

(PGMEE 2013)

a. Silver
b. Nickel
c. Iron
d. Copper

[Ref: Parsons' 23rd/e pg. 503]

Explanation

- *Glass, plastics* and *porcelain* and inert. *Stone* may occasionally give rise to chemical changes, depending on its composition. Of the metals, *gold, silver, platinum* and *titanium* are inert. *Lead*, excites little reaction. *Aluminium* frequently becomes powdered and excites a local reaction, *Iron* and *copper*; the two most common materials found, undergo electrolytic dissociation.

12. What is deposited in Kyser-Fleischer ring:

a. Heme
b. Copper *(PGMEE 2012)*
c. Mercury
d. Lead

[Ref: Parsons' 23rd/e pg. 504]

13. Copper deposition in cornea leads to: *(PGMEE 2013)*

a. Keratoglobus
b. Siderosis
c. KF ring
d. Keratoconus

[Ref: Parsons' 23rd/e pg. 504]

Explanation

- The typical sites for deposition are in the deeper parts of the cornea level of Descemet's membrane.
- Mostly at the periphery causing the appearance of golden-brown ring, which resembles the Kayser-Fleischer ring

14. Kayser flescher ring is seen in: *(PGMEE 2015; 2016-17)*

a. Chalcosis
b. Chemical injuries
c. Open angle glaucoma
d. Siderosis

[Ref: Parsons' 23rd/e pg. 504]

15. Identify the pathology depicted in the given Image?

(PGMEE 2015)

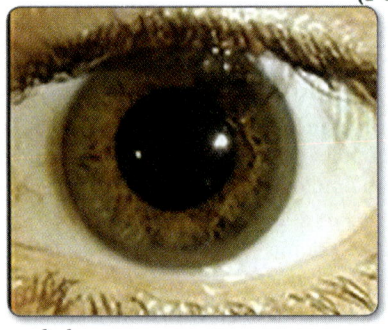

a. Corneal ulcer
b. Aniridia
c. Circumcorneal congestion
d. Kayser-Fleischer ring

[Ref: Parsons' 22nd/e pg. 433]

ALKALI BURNS

16. Alkali causes – *(PGMEE 2016-17)*

a. Retinal detachment
b. Symblepharon
c. Optic neuritis
d. Papilloedema

[Ref: Parsons' 23rd/e pg. 164 & 492]

Explanation

- Chemical and thermal burns, cicatrizing conjunctival diseases such as Stevens-Johnson syndrome and pemphigoid are co0mmon causes.
- This leads to a diminished vascularity of the anterior segment, corneal opacification and melting, cataract and symblepharon. Ammonia and sodium causes necrosis of the cornea.

17. 'Ischemic necrosis' in alkali burn is: *(PGMEE 2015)*

a. Stage I
b. Stage II
c. Stage III
d. Stage IV

[Ref: Parsons' 23rd/e pg. 493]

18. Alkali injury to eye causes? *(DNB JUNE 2011)*

a. Globe perforation
b. Optic neuritus
c. Thyrotoxicosis
d. Symblepharon

[Ref: Parsons' 23rd/e pg. 492]

7.	c
8.	c
9.	a
10.	c
11.	a
12.	b
13.	c
14.	a
15.	d
16.	b
17.	a
18.	d

EXTRAOCULAR MUSCLES

1. Primary action of superior oblique is:
                                                                    (PGMEE 2012-13)
a. Intorsion   b. Depression
c. Abduction   d. Adduction
    [Ref: BDC 7th/e vol. 3 pg. 216; Parsons' 23rd/e pg. 357]

2. Yoke muscle pair: *(PGMEE 2012-13)*
a. Rt LR + Rt MR   b. Rt IR + Rt SR
c. Rt LR + Lt MR   d. Lt LR + Lt MR
    [Ref: BDC 7th/e vol. 3 pg. ..... ; Parsons' 23rd/e pg. 359]

3. All extra-ocular muscles are supplied by the oculomotor nerve except: *(PGMEE 2012-13)*
a. Inferior oblique
b. Superior rectus
c. Lateral rectus
d. Medial rectus
    [Ref: BDC 7th/e pg. 215; Parsons' 23rd/e pg. 360]

4. Main action of superior rectus: *(PGMEE 2012-13)*
a. Intorsion
b. Extorsion
c. Elevation
d. Depression
    [Ref: BDC 7th/e vol. 3 pg. 216; Parsons' 23rd/e pg. 357]

5. Distance of medial rectus from limbus -   *(PGMEE 2012)*
a. 4.5 mm   b. 5.5 mm
c. 7.0 mm   d. 10 mm

    [Ref: Parsons' 23rd/e pg. 356]

Explanation

- The medial rectus is inserted into the sclera about 5.5 mm to the nasal side of the corneoscleral margin, the inferior rectus 6.6 mm below, the lateral rectus 7 mm to the temporal side and the superior rectus 7.75 mm above.

6. Longest and thinnest extrocular muscle -
                                                                    (PGMEE 2014; 2016-17))
a. SR   b. IR
c. SO   d. IO

    [Ref: Parsons' 22nd/e pg. 404]

7. Downward and lateral gaze is action of -
                                                                    (PGMEE 2012; A1IMS Dec 92.)
a. Inferior oblique   b. Lateral rectus
c. Medial rectus   d. Superior oblique

    [Ref: Parsons' 23rd/e pg. 356]

8. Secondary action of Superior Rectus Muscle is?
                                                                    (PGMEE 2013)
a. Abduction & intorsion   b. Abduction & extorsion
c. Adduction & extorsion   d. Adduction & intorsion

    [Ref: Parsons' 23rd/e pg. 357]

Explanation

Actions of the Extraocular Muscles

Muscle	Primary Action	Subsidiary Actions
Medial rectus (MR)	Adduction	None
Lateral rectus (LR)	Abduction	None
Superior rectus (SR)	Elevation (best when eye in abducted position)	Incycloduction (intorsion) and adduction
Inferior rectus (IR)	Depression (best when eye is in abducted position)	Excycloduction (extortion) and adduction
Superior oblique (SO)	Incycloduction (intorsion)	Depression (best when eye is in adducted position) and abduction
Inferior oblique (IO)	Excycloduction (extortion)	Elevation (best when eye is in adducted position) and abduction

9. Superior oblique testing for 4th nerve is done by checking its intorsion while asking the subject to look –
                                                                    (PGMEE 2016-17))
a. Straight down   b. Straight up
c. Down and in   d. Down and out

    [Ref: Parsons' 23rd/e pg. 359]

10. Yolk muscle for left superior rectus is –   *(PGMEE 2013)*
a. Right superior rectus   b. Left inferior rectus
c. Right inferior oblique   d. Right superior oblique

    [Ref: Parsons' 23rd/e pg. 359]

11. Yoke muscle for left inferior rectus is –
                                                                    (PGMEE 2013; 2016-17)
a. Right superior rectus   b. Left inferior rectus
c. Right inferior oblique   d. Right superior oblique

    [Ref: Parsons' 23rd/e pg. 359]

OPHTHALMOPLEGIA & SQUINT

12. All are feature of 3rd nerve palsy except - *(PGMEE 2013)*
a. Loss of light reflex   b. Mydriasis
c. Adducted eye   d. Ptosis

    [Ref: Parsons' 23rd/e pg. 393]

Explanation

- There is ptosis, eye is seen to be deflected outwards (divergent squint or exotropia) and rotated internally (intorted). The pupil is semidilated and immobile, and accommodation is paralysed. Slight degree of proptosis. There is limitation of movements upwards and inwards.

1.	a
2.	c
3.	c
4.	c
5.	b
6.	c
7.	d
8.	d
9.	c
10.	c
11.	d
12.	c

13. A patient is unable to move eye outward beyond midline. The lesion is in *(PGMEE 2012-13)*

a. Obturator nerve
b. Trochlear nerve
c. Abducent nerve
d. None

[Ref: BDC 7th/e vol. 3 pg. 220; Parsons' 23rd/e pg. 392]

14. The following picture exhibit which cranial nerve palsy.? *(NEET Pattern 2017)*

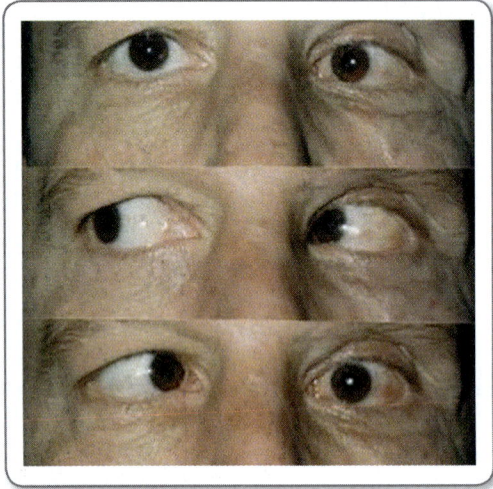

a. Oculomotor nerve
b. Trochlear nerve
c. Abducent nerve
d. Vestibulocochlear nerve

[Ref: Parsons' 23rd/e pg. 392]

13. c
14. c
15. b
16. d
17. b

Explanation

- 6th cranial nerve (abducent nerve) palsy leads to abduction of the eyeball as it supplies LR muscle. If the patient is asked to look at the left side, concomitant palsy of the left lateral rectus leads to inability to move the left eyeball to the left side (abduction of left eye), whereas the right eyeball moves normally.

To Summarize

- 6th nerve palsy – failure of lateral gaze
- 3rd nerve palsy – eyeball down and out, dialted pupil, Ptosis
- 4th nerve palsy – vertical diplopia on looking down – difficulty in going downstairs, reading book

Oculomotor Palsy

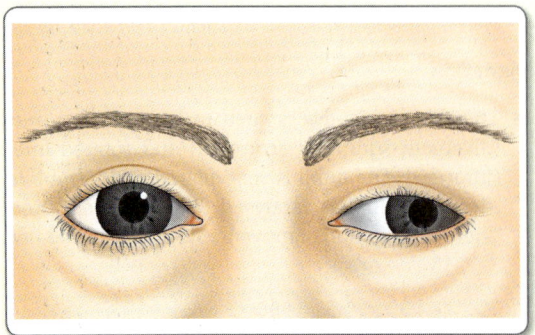

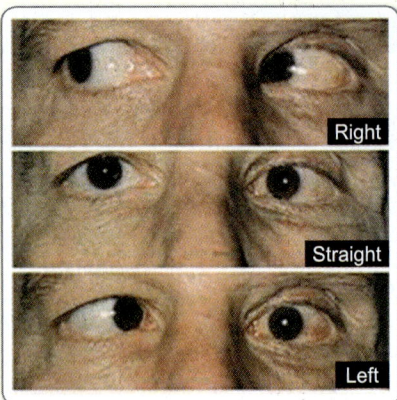

Superior Oblique Palsy

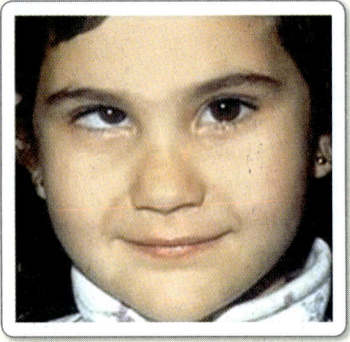

15. Treatment of choice for amblyopia is *(PGMEE 2012; PGMEE 94)*

a. Spectacles
b. Conventional occlusion
c. Surgery
d. Convergent exercises

[Ref: Parsons' 23rd/e pg. 374]

MISCELLANEOUS

16. Duanne syndrome involves- *(PGMEE 2013; 2016-17)*

a. Inferior oblique
b. Superior rectus
c. Superior oblique
d. Lateral rectus

[Ref: Parsons' 22nd/e pg. 406]

17. Fusion of visual reflexes in binocular vision is *(PGMEE 2014)*

a. Grade 1
b. Grade 2
c. Grade 3
d. Grade 4

[Ref: Parsons' 22nd/e pg. 411; Nema 6th/e pg. 389]

Explanation

Grades of Binocular Vision

- Binocular vision is precisely measured on a synopto-phore. It is of three grades
- *Grade I: Simultaneous Macular Perception*
  ○ It is the ability of eyes to perceive two dissimilar objects simultaneously. When dissimilar test targets are presented, a lion on one side and a cage on the other, the subject sees the lion as being in the cage. If one object is not seen, the eye on the corresponding side is suppressed.
- *Grade II: Fusion*
  ○ Fusion is the cortical unification of visual objects. It is only possible by the simultaneous stimulation

of corresponding areas on the retina. Two similar targets, which individually lack some detail but when super.imposed form a complete image, are used for the assessment of fusion. If a complete image is perceived and maintained, despite the targets being moved on either side from 5^0 to 10^0 while testing on a synoptophore, fusion is present.

- *Grade III: Stereopsis*
  - The third grade of binocular vision is stereopsis or three-dimensional vision: It is the ability to obtain an impression of the depth byb the sup[erimposition of two images of the same object taken from slightly different angles. The stereopsis can be measured by stereopsis slides on a synoptophore.

18. Ophthalmoplegic migraine means: *(NEET Pattern 03)*
- a. Headache associated with 3rd, 4th & 6th nerve palsy
- b. Recurrent transient 3 nerve palsy associated with headache
- c. Headache associated with optic neuritis
- d. Headache with irreversible loss of ophthalmic nerve function

[Ref: Parsons' 23rd/e pg. 468]

19. Ataxia, nystagmus and ophthalmoplegia is seen in- *(PGMEE 2012)*
- a. Chronic progressive external ophthalmoplegia
- b. 3rd nerve palsy
- c. Mysthenia gravis
- d. Demylination in MLF

[Ref: Parsons' 23rd/e pg. 474]

Explanation

- Unilateral internuclear ophthalmoplegia with ataxic nystagmus indicates demyelination in the medial longitudinal fasciculus. Sixth is more often affected (than the third, and total third nerve paralysis is never seen.)

20. Which of the following best defines the "Saccade"
- a. Involuntary slow eye movement
- b. Abrupt, involuntary rapid eye movements
- c. Abrupt, involuntary slow eye movements
- d. Voluntary slow eye movements

[Ref: Parsons' 22nd/e pg. 409]

21. Structure associated with horizontal movement of eye is? *(DNB Jun'2010)*
- a. Thalamus
- b. Pons
- c. Medulla
- d. Midbrain

[Ref: Parsons' 23rd/e pg. 360]

22. Left sided lateral gaze is affected in lesion of - *(PGMEE 2014)*
- a. Right frontal lobe
- b. Right occipital lobe
- c. Left occipital lobe
- d. Left frontal lobe

[Ref: Parsons' 23rd/e pg. 361]

23. BSGT stands for: *(PGMEE 2015)*
- a. Bagolini striated glasses test
- b. Bagolini smooth glasses test
- c. Bagolini shiny glasses test
- d. Bagolini second glue test

[Ref: Wikipedia]

24. A patient comes with recent onset paralytic squint. Which of this is true of paralytic squint?
- a. Congenital   *(PGMEE 2016-17)*
- b. Ambylopia is present
- c. Diplopia
- d. Secondary deviation is equal to primary deviation

[Ref: Parsons' 23rd/e pg. 386]

Explanation

- The signs and symptoms of paralysis of any extraocular muscle are as follows:
  - Squint
  - Limitation of ocular movements
  - Diplopia
  - False orientation
  - Abnormal position of the head
  - Vertigo

25. A patient was suffering from ptosis and hypotropia. After giving an IV drug to the patient, in 6 mins his ptosis & hypotropia improved. What is the probable diagnosis? *(NEET Pattern 2017)*
- a. 6th nerve palsy
- b. Tolosa Hunt syndrome
- c. Third nerve palsy
- d. Myasthenia gravis

[Ref. Parsons' Diseases of the Eye 22nd/e pg. 474]

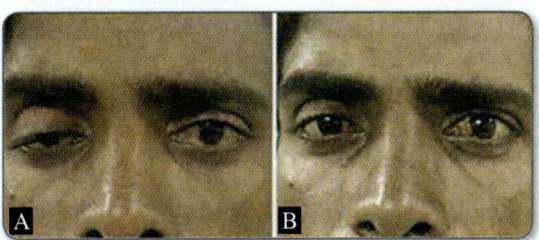

Explanation

- The term hypertropia and hypotropia are used to in relation to vertical strabismus /misalignment.
  - Hypertropia is an abnormal eye higher than the normal eye.
  - Hypotropia is when the abnormal eye is lower than the normal eye.
- Esotropia is inward turning of the eyes (aka "crossed eyes").
- Exotropia is the term used to describe outward turning of the eyes (aka "wall-eyed")
- *Myasthenia gravis* is characterised by triad of ptosis, diplopia, weakness of eye muscles. MG is a disorder of N-M junction caused by autoantibodies to post synaptic acetylcholine receptors. Use of acetyl-cholinesterase inhibitors (e.g. pyridostigmine/edrophonium) reverses the myasthenic symptoms. Improvement after giving IV edrophonium is known as **tensilon test**. It is mainly used as diagnostic test for MG. It is also used to distinguish a myasthenic crisis from a cholinergic crisis in individuals undergoing t/t for myasthenia gravis.
- *Tolosa-Hunt syndrome* is a rare disorder char/ by severe periorbital headaches, along with decreased and painful eye movements (ophthalmoplegia).

18.	a
19.	d
20.	b
21.	b
22.	a
23.	a
24.	c
25.	d

LASERS IN OPHTHALMOLOGY

1. Type of laser used for iridotomy: *(PGMEE 2013)*
   a. Nd: YAG
   b. Krypton red
   c. Diode
   d. Excimer

[Ref: Parsons' 23rd/e pg. 137]

Explanation

Lasers Used in Ophthalmology

Laser	Wave-length (nm)	Clinical Applications
Nd: YAG (Neodymium-Yttrium-Aluminium-Garnet)	1064	Posterior capsulotomy, iridotomy, vitreolysis
Frequency-doubled Nd:YAG	532	Retinal photocoagulation, cyclophotocoagulation
Argon green	514	Trabeculoplasty, iridoplasty, pupillomydriasis, retinal photocoagulation[a]
Diode laser	800	Retinal photocoagulation
Krypton red	714	Retinal photocoagulation
Excimer (argon fluoride)	193	Photorefractive keratectomy (PRK), photorefractive keratectomy (PTK), LASIK, LASEK
Femtosecond laser (neodymium-glass)	1053	Femtosecond laser-assisted refractive surgery, lamellar and fullthickness corneal transplants

[a]Retinal photocoagulation includes treatment for diabetic retinopathy, other causes of retinal neovascularization or retinal oedema, retinal breaks, central serous retinochoroidopathy, subretinal neovascular membranes, small retinal tumours and angiomas. Argon green laser is the most widely used, but other lasers are increasingly being used as substitutes in certain situations.

2. YAG laser capsulotomy is used in *(PGMEE 2016-17)*

   a. Diabetes   b. Refractive errors
   c. After-cataract   d. Retinal detachment

[Ref: Parsons' 23rd/e pg. 259]

Explanation

- 'After' cataracts, if thin, can be cleared centrally by a YAG laser capsulotomy.

3. Laser used in LASIK surgery *(PGMEE 2016-17)*
   a. Argon
   b. Nd-yag
   c. Holmium
   d. Excimer *(Argon fluoride)*

[Ref: Parsons' 23rd/e pg. 137]

4. The wavelength of laser {in nanometers) for shaping cornea in refractive surgery is: *(PGMEE 12)*
   a. 45mm   b. 193 nm
   c. 532 nm   d. 1064 mn

[Ref: Parsons' 23rd/e pg. 196]

Explanation

Phototherapeutic Keratectomy

- The excimer laser (198 nm) can be used to ablate the superficial layers of the cornea to remove superficial opacities in conditions such as band-shaped keratopathy, superficial scars, oil droplet keratopathy, Reis-Buckler dystrophy and Salzmann nodular degeneration. Only superficial lesions (100 mm depth) can be thus treated.

5. Confocal scanning laser ophthalmoscope uses:
   a. Excimerlaser *(PGMEE 2015; 2016-17)*
   b. Diode laser
   c. YAG laser
   d. Infrared laser

[Ref: Parsons' 22nd/e pg. 608]

6. Which of the following is/are the side effect/s of using argon laser - *(PGMEE 2015)*
   a. Crusting
   b. Keloid formation
   c. Hypopigmentation
   d. All the above

7. How many incisions are used in the divided system approach of pars planavitrectomy? *(PGMEE 2015)*
   a. 1
   b. 2
   c. 3
   d. 4

[Ref: Parsons' 22nd/e pg. 404]

ANAESTHESIA IN OPHTHALMOLOGY

8. Peribulbar injection is given in:- *(PGMEE 2014)*
   a. Periorbital space
   b. Outside muscle
   c. Subtenon space
   d. Subperiorbital space

[Ref: Parsons' 23rd/e pg. 567]

1.	a
2.	c
3.	d
4.	b
5.	b
6.	d
7.	c
8.	b

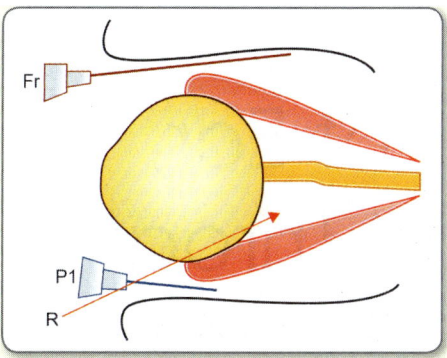

Fig.: Sagittal section of the orbit showing the sites of insertion of the needles for retrobulbar (blue, R), peribulbar (red, P1) and frontal (green, Fr) blocks.

9. Retrobulbar injection is given in:　　　(PGMEE 2013)
a. Inside muscle cone
b. Outside muscle cone
c. Subtenon space
d. Subperiosteum

[Ref: Parsons' 23ʳᵈ/e pg. 567]

10. Shortest acting mydriatic is?
a. Tropicamide　　　(DNB JUNE 2011; PGMEE 2016-17)
b. Atropine
c. Phenylephrine
d. Hyoscine

[Ref: Parsons' 23ʳᵈ/e pg. 134]

11. Shortest acting mydriatic agent is:
a. Tropicamide　　　(Recent Pattern June 2018)
b. Atropine
c. Cyclopentolate
d. Homatropine

[Ref: Parsons' 23ʳᵈ/e pg. 134]

Explanation

- Tropicamide is an antimuscarinic drug that produces short acting mydriasis (dilation of the pupil) and cycloplegia when applied as eye drops.
- It is used to allow better examination of the lens, vitreous humor, and retina.

CHAPTER-15 ● LASERS, ANAESTHESIA AND DRUGS

9.　a
10.　c
11.　a

4

Diseases of Ear, Nose and Throat

ANATOMY AND EMBRYOLOGY OF EAR

- Mastoid antrum and inner ear are situated in ____ part of temporal bone: Petrous.
- Korner's septum: persistent petrosquamous suture
- Collaural fistula → anomaly of the 1st brachial cleft

- Type of joint between the ossicles: Synovial joint
  - Between **M**alleus and **I**ncus → **S**addle joint
  - Between incus and stapes → Ball and socket

Structures	Origin
▪ Tragus	1st brachial arch
▪ Pinna except tragus	2nd pharyngeal arch
▪ External Auditory Canal (EA**C**)	1st ectodermal <u>c</u>left
▪ Tympanic cavity, Eustachian tube and Middle ear	1st endodermal pouch
▪ Malleus and Incus	1st brachial arch
▪ Stapes suprastructure	2nd brachial arch
▪ Stapes footplate	Otic capsule / Neuroectoderm
▪ Bony labyrinth	Otic capsule
▪ Membranous labyrinth	Otic vesicle
▪ Tympanic Membrane (TM)	All 3 germ layers

External Ear and Tympanic Membrane

- 1st part of the EAC to develop: Bony part.
- Pinna and EAC is made up of: Auricular cartilage (yellow elastic cartilage)
- Length of External Auditory Canal – 24 mm
  - Outer 1/3rd / Cartilaginous part – 8 mm
  - Inner 2/3rd / Bony part – 16 mm
- Narrowest part of EAC → Isthmus

- Present 6 mm lateral to TM
- Cone of light is seen in → Anteroinferior quadrant of TM.
- Movement of TM is more at periphery
- Color of normal TM – Pearly white
- Pars flaccid is aka Shrapnell's membrane
- Ceruminous glands are → Apocrine sweat glands.

Middle Ear

- *Prussak's Space:*
  - Communicates with Epitympanum.
  - Present between pars flaccida and neck of Malleus
  - MC site for primary cholesteatoma.
- Deepest part of middle ear: Epitympanum – 6 mm wide
- Narrowest part of middle ear: Mesotympanum – 2 mm wide
- Distance between TM and promontory: 2 mm
- Promontory is formed by: Basal turns of cochlea.
- *Oval window:*
  - Covered by foot plate of stapes
  - Overlies the opening of Scala vestibule
- *Round window:*

- Covered by secondary TM
- Overlies the opening of Scala tympani
- Oval and round windows are separated by → Subiculum.
- Tendon of tensor tympani takes a turn at: Processus cochleariformis
- Largest/Most constant mastoid air cell – Antrum
- Protympanum – part of middle ear around the opening of Eustachian tube
- ET opens in ____ wall of middle ear: Anterior.
- Roof of middle ear is formed by: Tegmen tympani

Muscle involved in opening and closing of Eustachian tube (ET):
- Tensor palatini
- Tensor tympani

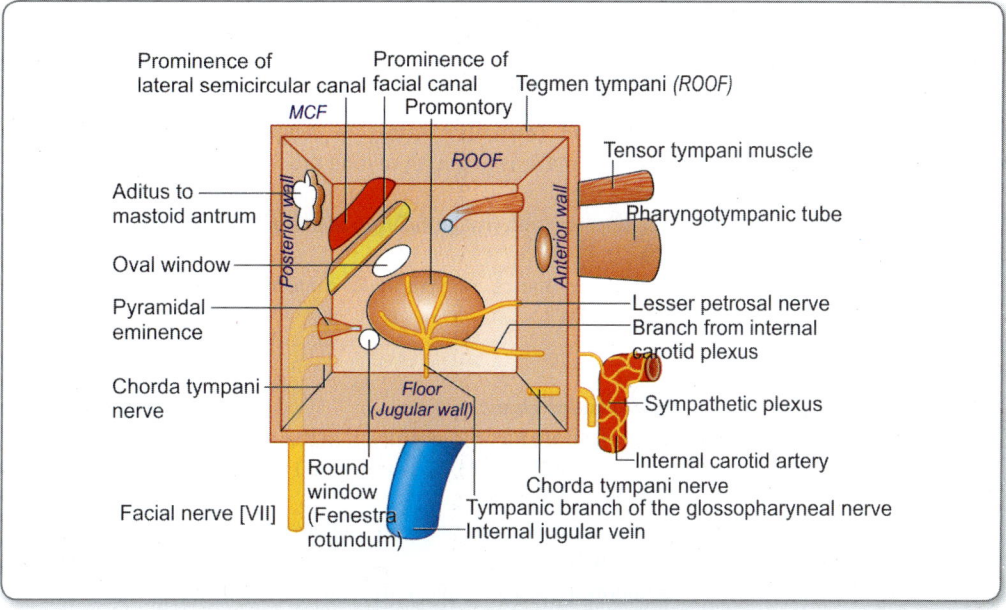

Boundaries and Contents of Middle Ear Cavity

Inner Ear

- Otoacoustic Emission (**O**AE) is generated from → **O**uter hair cells.
- **Organ of corti:**
  - Sense organ of hearing
  - Present over basilar membrane in scala media
  - Supporting cell of Organ of Corti – Deiter cell.
- Stria vascularis secretes endolymph which fills the membranous labyrinth/Scala media
- Helicotrema connects scala vestibule and scala tympani

- Perilymph is present in scala vestibule and scala tympani
- Cochlear aqueduct connects scala tympani with subarachnoid space–infection of inner ear can spread to CNS via this route
- Semicircular canals respond to angular acceleration and deceleration
- Endolymphatic duct connects utriculosaccular duct to endolymphatic sac

	Perilymph	Endolymph
Location	▪ Between bony and membranous labyrinth	▪ Inside membranous labyrinth
Composition	▪ Similar to ECF (High Na⁺ low K⁺)	▪ Similar to ICF (High K⁺ low Na⁺)
Synthesis	▪ Ultra filtrate of plasma	▪ Striae vascularis
Drainage	▪ Into the CSF via aqueduct of cochlea	▪ Absorbed via endolymphatic sac

Landmarks

- ***Incisura terminalis:***
  - Part of pinna between tragus and crus of helix
  - Devoid of cartilage
  - Site of incision for endaural surgery
- Citelli's angle – angle between sigmoid sinus and tegmen
- Surgical landmark for endolymphatic sac: Donaldson's line
- Trautmann's triangle: Landmark to approach posterior cranial fossa

Landmark for mastoid antrum:

- MC Evan's triangle (Spine of Henle).
- Simba choncha.

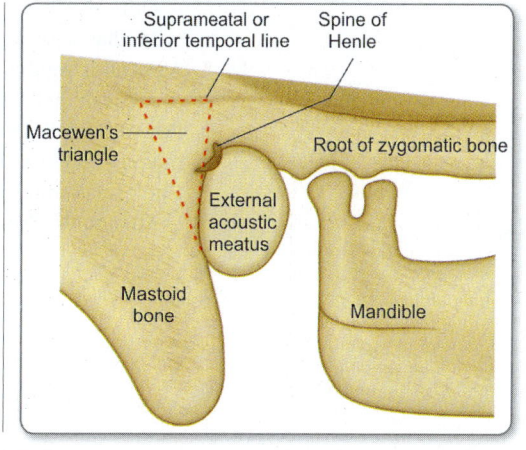

PHYSIOLOGY OF HEARING

- Surface area of TM → 90 mm^2.
- Working surface area of TM → 45-55 mm^2.
- Areal Ratio [55/ surface area of stapes footplate] = 17:1.
- *Lever ratio (ossicular ratio)* → length of Handle of malleus to length of long process of incus = 1.3:1.
- Transformer ratio (magnification of sound) → 22:1
- Natural resonance of tympanic membrane: 800-1600 Hz

- Endocochlear potential is: + 80 mV
- Impendence matching mechanism OR Transformer action is carried out by → Ossicles.
- *Direction of nystagmus in Caloric test:*
  - **C**old water → **O**pposite side
  - **W**arm water → **S**ame side
- Most important wave in BERA → Wave V
  - Produced by – Lateral lemniscus

EXTERNAL EAR

- *Preauricular sinus:*
  - Results from incomplete fusion of the hillocks of His which arise from the 1st and 2nd brachial arches.
  - Commonly located between tragus and crux of helix
- Cauliflower/Boxer's ear is due to repeated blunt trauma
- Bat ear → absent antihelix
- Mozart ear → fusion of helix and antihelix
- Exostosis of EAC is seen in *swimmer* ∴ also known as Surfer's ear.
- Syringing to remove wax is done in Posterosuperior direction.

- Myringitis bullosa is caused due to → Viral infection.
- *Keratosis obturans:*
  - Accumulation of pearly white, desquamated keratinous material in the bony part of EAC
  - Can cause erosion and widening of meatus
  - May lead to palsy of VII cranial nerve
  - May be associated with bronchiectasis and sinusitis
- *Malignant/Necrotizing Otitis Externa:*
  - MC cause – P. aeruginosa
  - Common in elderly with h/o diabetes or immunosuppression
  - Multiple CN can be involved

MIDDLE EAR

- Acute necrotizing otitis media is caused by: β hemolytic streptococci
- Cartwheel appearance of TM is seen in → ASOM.
- 1st sign of acute mastoiditis → Ironing out of its surface.
- In case of ASOM with bulging TM, to prevent perforation myringotomy is done in → Posteroinferior quadrant.
- *Myringotomy*
  - In ASOM → Posterior inferior quadrant.
  - Otitis media with effusion/Serous Otitis Media → Anterior inferior quadrant.
- Aero otitis media (Barotrauma) occur during descend of flight, SCUBA diving etc.
- Pressure gradient required to cause aero-otitis media → 90 mm Hg.
- Cholesteatoma/Epidermosis/Keratoma:
  - Misnomer – No cholesterol; Not a tumor

- Presence of stratified squamous epithelium in middle ear
- Levenson criteria is used for diagnosis of congenital cholesteatoma
- Secondary acquired cholesteatoma is seen in → Marginal Perforation.
- MC site for residual cholesteatoma after surgery: Sinus tympani
- In intact canal wall surgeries, the middle ear is approached through the suprapyramidal recess

Complications of Acute Mastoiditis/ASOM:

- Bezold's abscess → Occurs deep to Sternocleidomastoid muscle along with mastoid tip.
- Citelli's abscess → Along posterior belly of digastric.
- Luc's abscess → Along posterior wall of EAC.

	Otitis Media with Effusion (Glue Ear)	Acute Suppurative Otitis Media	Chronic Suppurative Otitis Media
Etiology	■ Adenoid hyperplasia ■ Tumors of nasopharynx	■ *S. pneumoniae* – MCC ■ *H. influenzae* ■ *M. catarrhalis*	■ *P. aeruginosa* – MCC ■ *S. aureus* ■ *Proteus*
Features	■ Nonpurulent sterile effusion of the ME	■ Pyogenic inflammation of ME	■ Perforation of TM + discharge from ME
Manifestations	■ Hearing loss, aural fullness	■ Fever, Otalgia, Hearing loss	■ Hearing loss without Otalgia
Complications	■ Tympanosclerosis ■ Atelectasis of middle ear ■ Cholesteatoma ■ Retraction pockets in TM	■ Development of chronic otitis media ■ Acute mastoiditis or labyrinthitis ■ Meningitis, Encephalitis, Brain abscess ■ Facial nerve palsy	■ Intracranial abscess ■ Lateral sinus thrombophlebitis ■ Meningitis, Intracranial abscess ■ Facial paralysis
On Examination	■ Fluid level and air bubbles ■ TM – dull, lustreless, loss of light reflex ■ Type B tympanogram	■ Inflammation of TM ± Bulging ■ Perforation in posteroinferior quadrant ■ Pulsatile otorrhea	■ Granulation tissue in ME ■ Conductive hearing loss
Management	■ Antimicrobials, Steroids, Antihistaminic ■ Surgery – Myringotomy	■ Antibiotics – initial therapy of choice ■ Myringotomy – for impending rupture	■ Antibiotics ± steroids ■ Surgery – Tympanoplasty

Types of CSOM

	Tubotympanic or Safe Type	Attico-antral or Unsafe Type
Perforation	■ Central	■ Attic or marginal
Cholesteatoma	■ Absent	■ Present
Granulation	■ Uncommon	■ Common
Otorrhea	■ Profuse, Mucoid ■ Odorless, No blood stained	■ Scanty, Purulent ■ Foul smelling, Blood stained
Complication	■ Rare (hence k/a safe type)	■ Common
Management	■ Medical ■ Surgical – Tympanoplasty	■ Only surgical – Mastoidectomy

INNER EAR

- Part of cochlea damaged in drug toxicity → Basal turns.
- Blood supply of labyrinth → Labyrinthine artery – branch of Anterior Inferior Cerebellar Artery.
- $CaCO_3$ crystals present in Macula → Otoconia – can lead to BPPV
- **O**totoxicity is due to damage to → **O**uter hair cells of cochlea.
- Drug induced ototoxicity leads to: High frequency hearing loss.

- Pathology of Basal turns causes high frequency hearing loss as seen in:
  - Ototoxicity
  - Presbycusis
- Pathology of Apical turns causes low frequency hearing loss as seen in early Meniere disease.
- 1st cranial nerve to be involved in acoustic neuroma: 5th CN → manifest as absent corneal reflex

MISCELLANEOUS

- Viral infections a/w hearing loss → MMR.
- Impedance audiometry is an objective test for pathology of Middle ear.
- Vertical nystagmus is seen in lesion of → Brain stem.
- Myringoplasty = repair of perforation of TM
- Tympanoplasty = Myringoplasty + ossicular reconstruction

- In cochlear implant, electrodes are placed in scala tympani.
- Narrowest segment of Facial nerve → Labyrinthine segment (aka physiological bottle neck of facial nerve).
- Permissible level of noise in industries in India → 90 dB for 8 hours a day × 5 days a week.

REMEMBER

Pneumatic bones:
- Maxilla
- Ethmoid
- Sphenoid
- Frontal bone

Tubercular Otitis Media:
- Painless condition
- Foul smelling discharge
- Multiple TM perforation
- Pale granulation tissue present
- Fails to responds to usual antimicrobial.

Ear structures which are fully developed at birth:
- Tympanic membrane
- Middle ear

- Ossicles
- Mastoid antrum
- Cochlea and Labyrinth

EAC has two deficiencies through which parotid infection can appear in EAC and vice versa:
- Fissure of Santorini in cartilaginous part [**Mn.** Santro Car]
- Foramen of **H**uschke in **BO**ny part [**Mn.** HBO]

Components of Auditory Pathway:
- **E** → 8th CN
- **C** → Cochlear nucleus
- **O** → Olivary complex
- **L** → Lateral lemniscus
- **I** → Inferior colliculus

NERVE SUPPLY

Pinna

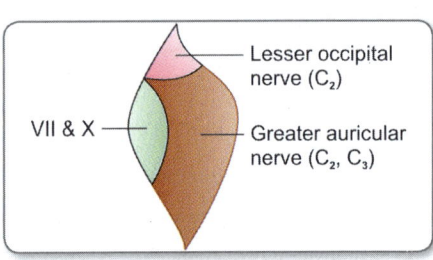

Medial surface

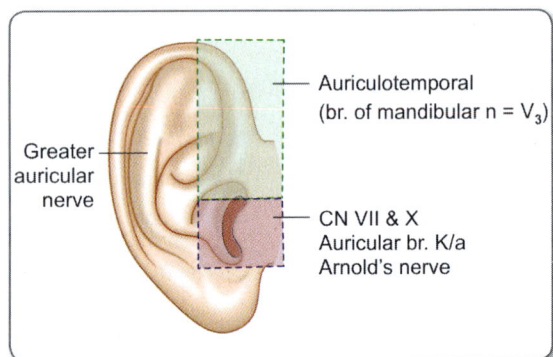

Lateral surface

External Auditory Canal

- **Roof and Anterior wall:**
  - Auriculotemporal nerve (branch of mandibular nerve)
- **Floor and Posterior wall:**
  - Auricular branch of Vagus
  - Aka Arnold's nerve or Alderman's nerve
- Posterior wall is also supplied by sensory division of facial nerve

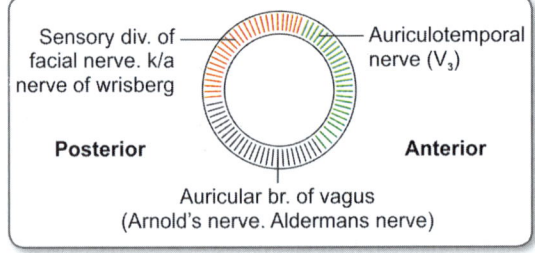

Tympanic Membrane

- **Lateral surface:**
  - Anterior ½ → Auriculotemporal nerve
  - Posterior ½ → Auricular branch of Vagus

- **Medial surface:**
  - Tympanic branch of Glossopharyngeal nerve
  - Also known as **Jacobson's nerve**.

- Sensory supply of middle ear is from → Tympanic branch of Glossopharyngeal nerve
- **Corda tympani:**
  - Taste sensation from anterior 2/3rd of tongue
  - Located in posterior wall of middle ear
  - Runs between malleus and incus
- Tensor tympani (derivative of 1st arch) is supplied by branch from medial pterygoid nerve – which is a branch of mandibular division of CN V
- Stapedius is supplied by facial nerve
- Nerve of Pterygoid canal → **Vidian nerve.**
- **Singular nerve:**
  - Branch of inferior vestibular nerve.
  - Supplies posterior Semicircular canal
- **Jacobson's nerve:** Leads to referred otalgia from tonsillitis
- **Arnold's nerve:** Leads to cough on stimulation.
- **Wrisberg nerve:** related to Hitzelberger's sign seen in Acoustic neuroma

REFERRED OTALGIA

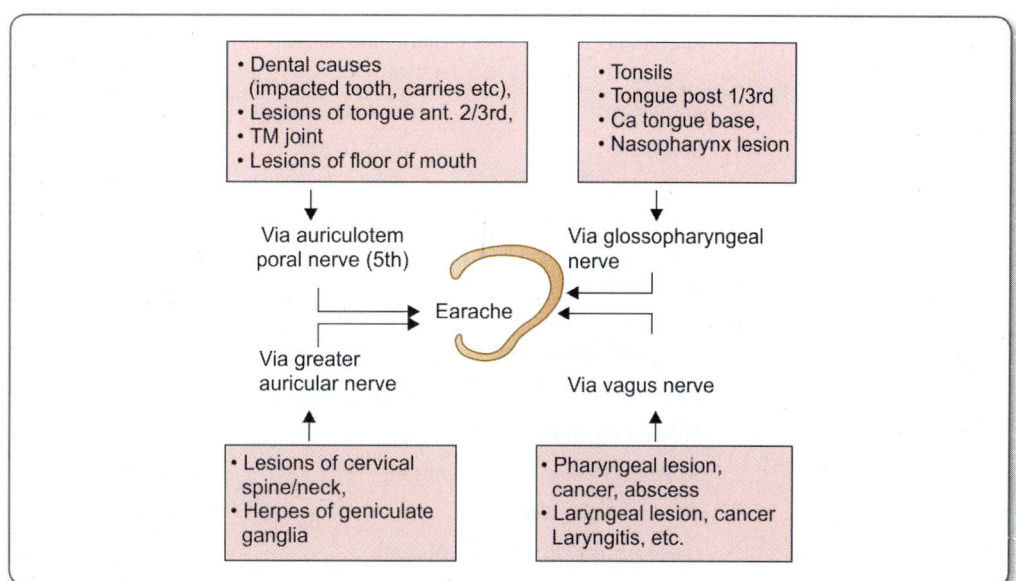

HEARING LOSS

- Normal conversation sound level → 60 dB.
- Pain in ear is experienced at 130 dB

Condition	Hearing Loss
Perforation of TM	10-40 dB
Wax/Complete obstruction of ear canal	30 dB
Ossicular dislocation with perforated TM	38 dB
Ossicular dislocation with intact TM	54 dB

Assessment of Hearing Loss

- Minimum hearing loss required for Weber test to lateralize: 5 dB.
- Minimum hearing loss for Rinne test to be negative: 15 dB
- Best tuning fork test → Weber's.
- False negative Rinne test is seen in → severe unilateral SNHL.
- **Bing test** → test of bone conduction
  - Examine the effect of occlusion of ear canal (by pressing the tragus inwards) on hearing
- **Gelle's test** → On ↑ air pressure in the EAC, hearing by BC is decreased.
  - Negative in otosclerosis due to fixity.

Fistula Test	Diagnosis
Negative	▪ Normal person
Positive	▪ Stapedectomy ▪ Fenestration surgery ▪ Erosion of horizontal SCC
False positive Hennebert sign	▪ Congenital Syphilis ▪ Meniere's disease
False negative	▪ Dead inner ear ▪ Cholesteatoma

Hearing Loss	Rinne Test	Weber Test	Bing Test	Gelle Test	ABC Test
None/Normal ear	AC > BC (+ve)	Midline	Hears louder when ear canal is occluded	Positive	Equal to examiner
Sensorineural HL	AC > BC (+ve)	Lateralization to normal ear			Decreased
Conductive HL	BC > AC (-ve)	Lateralization to diseased ear	No change on occlusion	Negative in otosclerosis	Equal to examiner

Types of Hearing Loss

	Conductive Hearing Loss	Sensorineural Hearing Loss	
		Cochlear	Retrocochlear
Pathology	▪ Up to foot plate of stapes	▪ Damage to cochlear hair cells	▪ 8th CN / Central connection
Audiometry	▪ Air Bone gap present	▪ No Air Bone gap	▪ No Air Bone gap
Hearing loss	▪ Up to 50-60 db	▪ >60 db	▪ >60 db
Speech Discrimination Score	▪ 95-100%	▪ Low (<90%)	▪ Very low (<40%)
Recruitment Phenomenon	▪ Absent	▪ Present (diagnostic)	▪ Absent
Short Increment Sensitivity Index (SISI)	▪ 15%	▪ Better than N (>60 %)	▪ Low (<20%)
Tone Decay	▪ Absent/not significant	▪ Not significant	▪ Significant
Rollover Phenomenon	▪ Absent	▪ Absent	▪ Present
Stapedial Reflex	▪ Absent	▪ Present	▪ Absent
Acoustic Reflex Decay		▪ Absent	▪ Present
Otoacoustic Emissions	▪ Absent	▪ Absent	▪ Present
Examples	▪ Wax impaction ▪ Otosclerosis ▪ CSOM ▪ Serous Otitis Media	▪ Meniere disease ▪ Noise induced hearing loss ▪ Alport syndrome, Ototoxicity, ▪ Distal RTA, Batter syndrome	▪ Acoustic neuroma

TYMPANOMETRY

Type	Pathology	Etiology
Type A	Normal middle ear status	Normal ear
Type B (Flat curve)	Fluid in middle ear	Glue ear
Type A$_s$	Decrease compliance of middle ear	Otosclerosis
Type A$_D$	Increase compliance of middle ear	Ossicular **d**isruption
Type C	Negative pressure in middle ear	Eustachian tube obstruction with retraction of tympanic membrane
Type U (Trough shaped)		Congenital deafness

NOSE

- *Nasal septum is formed by:*
  - Septal cartilage – Quadrangular shaped
  - Perpendicular plate of Ethmoid bone
  - Vomer
  - Crest of nasal bone
- Nasolacrimal duct is guarded by valve of Hasner
- Largest paranasal sinus: Maxillary sinus (aka antrum of Highmore)
- Choanal atresia may be associated with CHARGE syndrome
- Mulberry mucosa is seen in → Hypertrophic rhinitis.
- Strawberry like appearance of nose → Sarcoidosis.
- Vidian neurectomy is done in vasomotor rhinitis
- Rhinitis medicamentosa is due to excessive use of nasal decongestants
- Rhinophyma/Potato nose is due to benign hypertrophy of sebaceous gland

- Rhinosporidium seeberi is an aquatic parasite of the class Mesomycetozoea
- Best view for maxillary sinus: Waters' view
- Best view for frontal sinus: Caldwell view
- Caldwell-Luc operation is done to approach: Maxillary sinus
- First step in FESS: Uncinectomy
- Killian's incision is used for submucosal resection of nasal septum

Meatus	Opening Structure
Sphenoethmoidal recess	▪ Sphenoid air sinus
Superior meatus	▪ Posterior ethmoidal sinus
Middle meatus	▪ Maxillary, Frontal and Anterior ethmoidal sinus ▪ Also contains Bulla ethmoidalis and Hiatus semilunaris
Inferior meatus	▪ Nasolacrimal duct

	Rhinolalia Clausa	Rhinolalia Aperta
Definition	▪ Hyponasality of tone	▪ Hypernasality of tone
Pathology	▪ Lack of nasal resonance due to blockage of nose or nasopharynx	▪ Excess of nasal resonance due to abnormal communication between oral and nasal cavities
Etiology	▪ Rhinosinusitis ▪ Allergic rhinitis ▪ Nasal polyps or mass ▪ Hypertrophy of Adenoids	▪ Cleft of soft palate ▪ Short soft palate ▪ Soft palate paralysis

	Rhinoscleroma	Rhinosporidiosis
Definition	▪ Chronic granulomatous condition of the nose and upper respiratory tract	▪ Chronic granulomatous infection of the mucous membrane
Etiology	▪ *Klebsiella rhinoscleromatis*	▪ *Rhinosporidium seeberi*
Epidemiology	▪ More common in northern India	▪ More common in south India
Transmission	▪ Direct inhalation	▪ Water borne (bathing in ponds)
Features	▪ Crusting and foul smelling nasal discharge ▪ Woody hard nose	▪ Strawberry like polypoidal mass which is highly vascular and bleeds easily upon manipulation
Diagnosis	▪ Biopsy – Mikulicz and Russell bodies ▪ Culture – MacConkey agar	▪ Biopsy – Sporangia containing endospores
Management	▪ Antibiotics – Tetracycline (DOC) ▪ Surgery to relieve any obstruction	▪ Complete surgical excision with cauterization of base

	Antrochoanal Polyp	Ethmoidal Polyp [Mn: Adult BMR]
Origin	▪ Maxillary Sinus	▪ Ethmoidal sinus
Etiology	▪ Infection	▪ Allergy
Age group	▪ Common in children	▪ Common in **a**dults
Laterality	▪ Unilateral	▪ **B**ilateral
Number	▪ Single	▪ **M**ultiple
Recurrence	▪ Less common	▪ **R**ecurrence rate high
Growth	▪ Posteriorly towards choana	▪ Anteriorly towards nares
Investigation	▪ Posterior rhinoscopy	▪ Anterior rhinoscopy
Treatments	▪ TOC: FESS/Polypectomy ▪ Recurrence → TOC is FESS ▪ Caldwell Luc operation is done if FESS is not available.	▪ TOC: FESS/Polypectomy ▪ Recurrence → TOC is FESS ▪ Topical steroids spray (Fluticasone, Budesonide) ▪ Oral steroids

	Allergic Rhinitis	Atrophic Rhinitis/Ozaena
General feature	▪ Inflammation of nasal mucosa	▪ Progressive atrophy of mucosa & bone.
Etiology	▪ Genetic, Environmental allergens	▪ *Klebsiella ozaenae*
Clinical features	▪ Rhinorrhea, Postnasal drip ▪ Common in childhood and adolescent age ▪ Eustachian tube dysfunction leading to serous otitis media ▪ Hypertrophy of turbinates ▪ **Allergic shiners** – dark circle around the eye ▪ **Dennie Morgan lines** – prominent crease below inferior eyelid ▪ **Allergic salute** – horizontal nasal crease	▪ More common in females ▪ Pubertal age group ▪ Always bilateral ▪ Nasal blockage due to excessive crust formation ▪ Epistaxis on removal of crust ▪ Merciful anosmia (Bad smell from patient but patient is unaware) ▪ Roomy nasal cavities due to atrophy of turbinates ▪ Atrophic pharyngitis +/-.
Treatments	▪ Avoidance of allergen ▪ Antihistaminics and decongestants ▪ Intranasal steroid spray	▪ *Alkaline nasal douching* → composition = $NaHCO_3$, NaCl, Sodium biborate ▪ Surgery → Young's operation

PHARYNX

- Pharynx extends from base of skull to lower border of cricoids cartilage
- Eustachian tube opens about 1.25 cm behind the posterior end of inferior turbinate
- Passavant's ridge is formed by palatopharyngeal muscle
- Nodes of Rouvier are present in retropharyngeal space/space of Gillette
- Lymphatics from tonsils drain into the jugulo-digastric lymph node
- MC infective cause of acute tonsillitis: beta hemolytic streptococcus

Thornwaldt cyst:
- Benign mucosal cyst of the posterior nasopharynx
- Rx: Antibiotics + Marsupialization

	Retropharyngeal Abscess	Parapharyngeal Abscess	Peritonsillar Abscess/ Quinsy	Ludwig's Angina
Description	▪ Acute – suppuration of retropharyngeal LN ▪ Chronic – caries of cervical spine	▪ Collection of pus between the superior constrictor and Pterygoid muscle	▪ Collection of pus between the tonsillar capsule and the superior constrictor muscle	▪ Infection of Submandibular space (= sublingual + submaxillary) ▪ MCC – Dental infection
Manifestations	▪ Neck stiffness, Torticollis ▪ Odynophagia ▪ Neck swelling ▪ Aspiration pneumonia	▪ Trismus ▪ Tonsils are pushed medially ▪ Neck swelling at upper 1/3rd of SCM	▪ Odynophagia ▪ Dribbling of saliva from angle of mouth ▪ Hot potato voice	▪ Odynophagia, Trismus ▪ Woody hard swelling in the floor of mouth
Management	▪ Intraoral or external neck incision and drainage ▪ Broad spectrum antibiotics	▪ External neck incision and drainage of pus ▪ Broad spectrum antibiotics	▪ Intraoral incision and drainage + Antibiotics ▪ Tonsillectomy is done 4-6 weeks later	▪ External neck incision and drainage of pus ▪ Broad spectrum antibiotics

ANATOMY OF LARYNX

- *Cartilages of larynx:*
  - Paired – **A**rytenoid, **C**orniculate, **C**uneiform
  - Unpaired – **C**ricoid, **E**piglottis, **T**hyroid
  - Epiglottis is made up of: Elastic cartilage
- Corniculate cartilage is aka → Cartilage of Santorini.
- Cuneiform cartilage is aka → Cartilage of Wrisberg.
- Average length of male vocal cord → 18-23 mm.
- Average length of female vocal cord (VC) → 16-17 mm.
- False VC is formed by → Quadrangular fold.
- True VC is formed by → Cricovocal membrane.
- Weakness of Thyroarytenoid leads to → Elliptical defect of vocal cord.
- Weakness of Interarytenoids leads to → Posterior triangle defect of vocal cord.
- Weakness of both muscle leads to → Key hole defect of VC

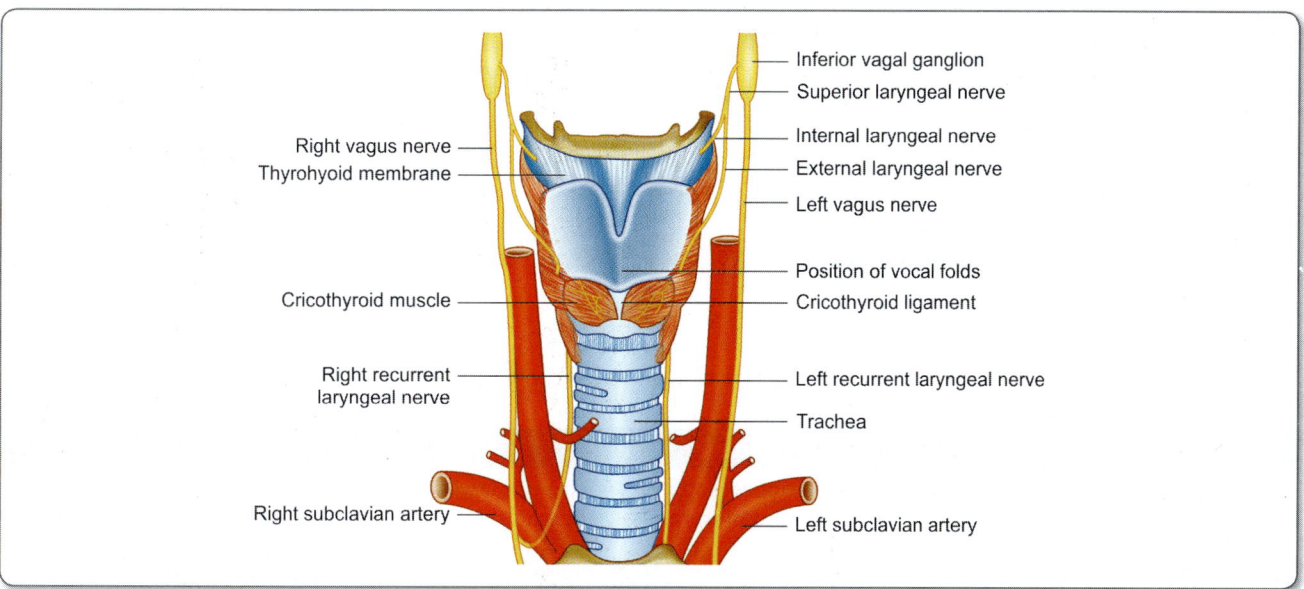

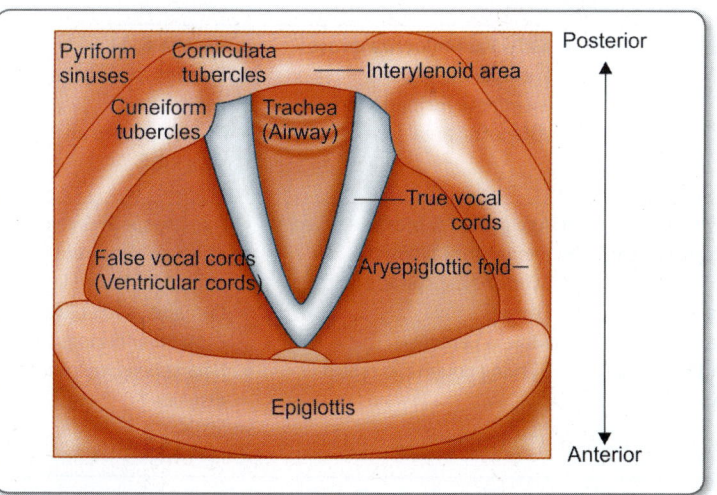

- Thyrohyoid membrane is pierced by → Internal branch of SLN.
- Laryngeal saccule arises from the roof of ventricles of larynx
- Only abductor of VC → Posterior Cricoarytenoid.

Tensor muscle of Vocal Cords:
- Internal part of Thyroarytenoid aka Vocalis.
- Cricothyroid muscle (lies outside larynx).

Motor Supply of Larynx:
- All muscles of larynx are supplied by → Recurrent Laryngeal Nerve (**RLN**)
- **Exception:** Cricothyroid—supplied by → External division of Superior Laryngeal Nerve.

Sensory supply of Larynx:
- Till VC → Internal branch of SLN
- Below VC → Recurrent laryngeal nerve

PATHOLOGY OF LARYNX

- Ω-Shaped epiglottis → Laryngomalacia.
- Turban epiglottis → TB larynx.
- External laryngocele pierces → Thyrohyoid membrane.
- Laryngocele → Congenital anomalous dilatation of laryngeal saccule
- Inspiratory stridor is produced in obstructive lesions of: Supraglottis
- Cadaveric/Intermediate position of vocal cords is seen in complete paralysis of cords.
- Site of vocal cord nodules is at the junction of → Anterior 1/3rd and Posterior 2/3rd of VC.
- Intubation granuloma is seen at the junction of → Anterior 2/3rd and Posterior 1/3rd of VC.
- *Dysphonia plica ventricularis* → low pitched voice produced from false vocal cord

- Pseudosulcus in larynx is due to: Pharyngolaryngeal reflex
- Functional aphonia is MC seen in emotionally insecure young females
- *Phonasthesia* = Weakness of voice due to fatigue
- Myers-Cotton grading system is used for: Subglottic stenosis

Puberphonia:
- Functional disorder characterized by persistence of high-pitched voice after puberty
- Common in emotionally distressed adolescent males
- Rx: Voice therapy k/a Gutzman's pressure test

	TB Larynx	Atrophic Laryngitis
General features	▪ Secondary to pulmonary TB ▪ Lesion begins from posterior part of larynx	▪ Also known as Laryngitis Sicca ▪ Due to *Klebsiella ozaenae* ▪ Loss of mucus-producing glands ▪ Chronic dry cough
Clinical features	▪ Painful phonation ▪ Odynophagia ▪ **Mouse bitten appearance** of VC ▪ **Turban epiglottis**	▪ F>>M ▪ Excess crust formation which may be hemorrhagic ▪ MC site: False VC, subglottic region
Diagnosis	▪ Biopsy	▪ Laryngoscopy
Treatment	▪ ATT	▪ MLS removal of crust

	Laryngomalacia	Acute Epiglottitis	Croup	Juvenile Papillomatosis
General	▪ MC congenital anomaly of Larynx ▪ **MCC of stridor** in infants ▪ Also known as congenital laryngeal stridor	▪ Inflammation of epiglottis and other supraglottic structures	▪ Aka acute laryngotracheo-bronchitis	▪ Formation of warts in the larynx ▪ Also known as "Recurrent Respiratory Papillomatosis" ▪ Premalignant condition for CA larynx
Etiopathology	▪ Weakness of supraglottis leading to collapse of supraglottis	▪ *H. influenza* type B	▪ MC – Parainfluenza viruses ▪ Pathogenesis → edema formation in subglottic area	▪ **HPV → 6, 11** ▪ Transmission: Maternal genital tract ▪ Involves supra and subglottis

Clinical features	▪ Inspiratory stridor
	  ○ Seen after 7 days of life
	  ○ ↓ in prone position
	  ○ ↑ on crying, supine position and feeding
	▪ Cry of the baby → Normal
	▪ Cyanosis ±
		▪ Age group → 2–7 years
		▪ Respiratory distress, stridor, fever, dysphagia
		▪ Drooling of salvia
		▪ **Tripod sign** → patient prefers sitting and bending forward position
			▪ Age group: 3 month – 3 years
			▪ Respiratory distress
			▪ Stridor on inspiration
			▪ Fever
			▪ Male > Female
			▪ Barking cough f/b croup
				▪ Age group: 2–5 years
				▪ Multiple recurrent papilloma in the larynx
				▪ Can also involve trachea, Bronchi and lungs
				▪ Hoarseness, respiratory distress
				▪ Stridor
				▪ Recurrence – Common

Investigations	▪ Laryngoscopy → collapse of supraglottis leading to Ω shaped epiglottis (elongated and curled on itself)	▪ X-ray → Thumb sign (thick epiglottis) and Vallecula sign ▪ Indirect laryngoscopy is preferred	▪ X-ray: Steeple sign /Pencil tip sign → Narrowing of subglottic region ▪ Widening/distension of hypopharynx	▪ Direct laryngoscopy and biopsy
Management	▪ Conservative ▪ Resolves spontaneously within 2 years ▪ Excellent prognosis	▪ It is an airway emergency ▪ Establish airway → intubation/Tracheostomy ▪ IV Ab and IV steroids ▪ DOC: Ceftriaxone	▪ Airway emergency ▪ Bronchodilator ▪ Antibiotics if secondary bacterial infection present ▪ Excellent prognosis	▪ TOC: CO_2 laser/MLS ▪ If patient present with respiratory distress and stridor → TOC → Tracheostomy ▪ Intubation can spread the disease further into lungs ▪ May resolve spontaneously ▪ Caesarean section is done in pregnant women with active genital warts

THYROPLASTY

Types	Surgery Procedure	Indication
Type - I	▪ Medialization of Vocal cords	Bilateral Adductor palsy
Type - II	▪ Lateralization of Vocal cords	Bilateral Abductor palsy
Type - III	▪ Shortening/Loosening of cords	Puberphonia
Type - IV	▪ Lengthening/tightening of cords	Androphonia

REMEMBER

Variation of Ethmoid bone anatomy:
- Haller cell (Variation of anterior ethmoid cells) lies in Orbital floor. [**Mn:** hall and floor]
- **On**odi cells (Variation of posterior ethmoid cells) lie in relation to <u>o</u>ptic <u>n</u>erve.

Ethmoidal Poly is associated with:
- Asthma
- Kartagener syndrome
- Young syndrome
- Cystic fibrosis

Samter triad:
- Aspirin intolerance + Nasal Polyp + Asthma

Indications of FESS:
- Chronic sinusitis not responding to medical management
- Nasal Polyps
- Epistaxis

Precancerous conditions of Larynx:
- Keratosis larynx
- Juvenile papilloma of larynx
- Leukoplakia and Erythroplakia

Carcinoma Larynx:
- More common in males
- Risk factors:
  - ◆ Tobacco smoking – MI
  - ◆ Alcohol
  - ◆ Asbestosis
  - ◆ Radiation
  - ◆ Gas (mustard)
- MC histological type: Squamous cell carcinoma
- MC site: Glottis > Supraglottis > Subglottis
- **Glottis** –Good prognosis
- **Supraglottis** – Poor prognosis
- **Subglottic** – Worst prognosis
- Hoarseness of voice – earliest in glottis carcinoma
- Lymph node enlargement – max with supraglottic CA
- Nodal metastases – early in supraglottic

Sinus of Morgagni:
- Space between the base of skull and upper border of superior constrictor muscle
- Structures passing through it –
  - ◆ Eustachian tube
  - ◆ Levator veli palatini
  - ◆ Tensor veli palatini
  - ◆ Ascending palatine artery

Predisposing Factors:
- **Keratosis Larynx** – Smoking
- **Rienke's edema** (Swelling of vocal cords) – Vocal abuse, Smoking
- **Dysphonia plica ventricularis** – In people who mimic others
- **Juvenile papilloma of larynx** – Vaginal delivery by infected mother.

SYNDROMES

Syndrome	Features	Seen in	Comment
Gradenigo Syndrome	▪ Ear discharge (Otorrhea). ▪ Retro orbital pain due to V CN. ▪ Diplopia due to VI CN.	▪ Petrositis (complication of ASOM/CSOM)	▪ Treatment → surgery
Melkersson Rosenthal syndrome	▪ Fissured tongue ▪ Swollen lips ▪ Recurrent facial nerve paralysis		
Vander Hove syndrome	▪ Otosclerosis ▪ Osteogenesis imperfecta ▪ Blue sclera		▪ As tympanogram

MOST COMMON

- MC Tuning fork used in ENT → 512 Hz.
- MC cause of chondritis of aural cartilage → Pseudomonas.
- MC SCC involved in BPPV → Posterior SCC.
- MC cause of hearing loss → Impacted wax.
- MC cause of hearing loss in children → Secretory otitis media/Otitis media with effusion
- MC fungus causing Otomycosis → Aspergillus niger
- MC organism causing ASOM → *S. pneumoniae* > *H. influenzae* > *Moraxella*.
- MC complication of ASOM → Acute mastoiditis.
- MC intracranial complication of ASOM → Meningitis.
- MC site of perforation of TM in ASOM → Anteroinferior quadrant
- MC site of unsafe CSOM → Marginal perforation of TM in Posterosuperior quadrant.
- MC ossicle to be eroded in CSOM → Long process of Incus.
- MC complication of CSOM → Mastoiditis.
- MC intracranial complication of CSOM → Brain abscess.
- MC graft material used in Tympanoplasty → Temporalis fascia
- MC # of Temporal bone → Longitudinal
- MCC of Iatrogenic traumatic facial nerve palsy → Mastoidectomy. MC injured part → 2nd Genu.
- MC site of origin of otosclerosis → Anterior to oval window and that point is known as *Fissula ante fenestrum*.
- MC site of cochlear otosclerosis → Round window.
- MC site of origin of Acoustic neuroma/ Vestibular schwannoma→ Inferior vestibular division of 8th CN.
- MC variety of CP angle tumor → Vestibular Schwannoma.
- MC tumor of middle ear → Glomus tumor.
- MC site of origin of laryngeal **c**hrondroma/ **C**hondrosarcoma→ **C**ricoid.
- MC cause of VC paralysis → Thyroidectomy (Iatrogenic).
- MC cause of B/L RLN palsy → Neck surgery
- MC cause of stridor/Noisy breathing in infants → Laryngomalacia/Congenital laryngeal stridor.
- MC congenital anomaly of larynx → Laryngomalacia
- MC histological variant of CA larynx → Squamous cell carcinoma.
- MC site of distant metastasis in CA larynx → Lung.
- MC cause of septal perforation → Trauma
- MC cause of chronic fungal sinusitis → Aspergillus fumigatus.
- MC sinus to form aspergilloma → Maxillary sinus.
- MC sinus to develop **M**alignancy and to form **A**spergilloma → **Ma**xillary sinus
- MC sinus to develop Osteoma and Mucocoele → Frontal Sinus [**Mn**: FROM]
- MC sinusitis in children → Ethmoid.
- MC sinusitis in Adult → Maxillary.
- MC benign tumor of sinus → Osteoma.
- MC # bone of face → Nasal bone.
- MC site of Traumatic CSF leak → Fovea ethmoidalis (Roof of ethmoid bone).

INVESTIGATION

- Diagnostic test for BPPV → Dix Hallpike maneuver.
- Caloric test → Checks only lateral SCC.
- Gold standard investigation for hearing loss → BERA.
- Otoacoustic Emissions (OAE):
  - Produced by **O**uter Hair cells of cochlea
  - IOC for screening of hearing in neonates
- IOC for **O**totoxicity → **O**AE.
- Tobey ayer test (based on lumbar puncture) and Crowback test (based on fundus examination) is done in → Sigmoid sinus thrombosis.
- Increase latency of 5th wave in BERA is seen in → Acoustic neuroma.
- Gold standard investigation for acoustic neuroma → Gadolinium enhanced MRI.
- Low frequency hearing loss/Rising curve in audiometry is seen in → Meniere's disease.
- Glycerol test:
  - Glycerol causes improvement in hearing
  - Seen in patient with Meniere's disease.
- VEMP → This test checks inferior vestibular division of 8th CN. Indications are:
  - Superior SCC dehiscence syndrome
  - Acoustic neuroma
  - BPPV
- Best investigation to study movements and lesions of VC → Videostroboscopy.
- Diagnostic test for laryngopharyngeal reflux (LPR) → 24 hours double probe pH monitoring.
- IOC for sinus imaging → CT scan.
- Confirmatory test for CSF Rhinorrhea → β_2 transferrin estimation.
- Best radiological test to detect site of leakage in CSF Rhinorrhea → HRCT of skull bone

MANAGEMENT

- Ideal age for otoplasty (plastic reconstruction of ear) → >6 years.
- *Epley maneuver* (Particle repositioning maneuver) is done for → BPPV.
- *Microwick* is used for Transtympanic delivery of drugs in case of → Sudden SNHL.
- Carbogen is beneficial in case of → Sudden SNHL.
- Icthammol Glycerin packing is used for → Otitis Externa.
- Icthammol is an antiseptic while glycerin decreases edema.
- TOC in safe CSOM → Myringoplasty.
- TOC in unsafe CSOM → MRM.
- *Management of Otosclerosis*
  - Surgery → Stapedectomy / Stapedotomy.
  - If patient refuse to Surgery → Hearing aid
  - In patient with Schwartz sign positive → NaF is TOC
- If patient of Acoustic neuroma refuses for Surgery, then TOC → γ knife.
- Surgical site for cochlear implant → Facial recess.

- *TOC in:*
  - Puberphonia → Speech therapy – Gutzmann's maneuver.
  - Androphonia (Masculinization of female voice) → Speech therapy
- *Keratosis larynx:*
  - Stop smoking.
  - Decortication of vocal cord
- Rienke's edema: Decortication of vocal cord (Type I cordectomy)
- TOC for Juvenile papillomatosis→ CO_2 laser.
- TOC for vocal nodule → Speech therapy → if fails → MLS (Microlaryngeal surgery).
- In functional aphonia, speech therapy is → Ineffective.
- DOC for treatment of laryngotracheal stenosis → Topical mitomycin C.
- Vasomotor rhinitis → Vidian neurectomy.
- CA Maxilla → Total maxillectomy f/b Radiotherapy.
- CSF Rhinorrhea → Antibiotics + Wait and Watch.

TRACHEOSTOMY

Type	Procedure	Indications	Remark
Cricothyrotomy/ Laryngotomy	▪ Emergency surgery to open airway through Cricothyroid membrane	▪ Acute respiratory obstruction where there is no time for tracheostomy/ no competent surgeon is available to do the operation or no facility for ET intubation.	▪ Done in emergency situations.
High tracheostomy	▪ Tracheostoma made above the level of thyroid isthmus (isthmus lies against 2nd-4th tracheal rings)	▪ Only indication is carcinoma of larynx.	▪ Risk of perichondritis of the cricoid cartilage and subglottic stenosis.
Mid tracheostomy	▪ A mid tracheostomy is the preferred one ▪ It is done at the level of isthmus through the 2nd or 3rd tracheal rings and would entail division of the thyroid isthmus	▪ Elective indications	▪ Less chance of perichondritis, stenosis and pneumothorax
Low tracheostomy	▪ Tracheostoma made below the level of thyroid isthmus	▪ To create permanent tracheostoma	▪ Pneumothorax is an important complication

- Permanent tracheostomy → This may be required for cases of bilateral abductor paralysis or laryngeal stenosis.

	Acoustic Neuroma	Glomus Jugulare	Meniere's Disease
General features	▪ Also known as vestibular schwannoma ▪ MC variety of CP angle tumor ▪ Benign tumor of 8th cranial nerve ▪ MC site of origin → inferior vestibular division of 8th cranial nerve ▪ It is a slow growing tumor	▪ Also known as non-chromaffin paraganglioma ▪ MC tumor of middle ear ▪ Benign tumor ▪ Multicentric and locally invasive in nature ▪ Non capsulated and Highly vascular tumor ▪ Slow growing tumor	▪ Also known as endolymphatic hydrops ▪ It is an episodic disease which lasts for < 24 hours ▪ Due to ↑ in endolymph due to ↑ production or faulty absorption of it ▪ Site of pathology → Cochlea
Clinical features	▪ Equal incidence in male and female ▪ Age group → 40-60 years ▪ Earliest feature: U/L gradually progress SNHL ▪ Earliest sign: Absence of corneal reflex due to 5th CN involvement ▪ Tinnitus, Nystagmus ▪ Hitzelberger's sign due to 7th CN involvement ▪ Mostly unilateral but in NF 2, it is B/L	▪ Female > Male ▪ Age group → 40-60 years ▪ Earliest feature – Pulsatile/Fluctuating tinnitus ▪ Mass in middle ear with bleeds on touching ▪ Can erode TM and grows in to EAC ▪ Brown sign → Tumor blanches on seigalization	▪ Male > Female ▪ Age group → 30-40 years ▪ Each episode consists of Tinnitus, Vertigo, SNHL ▪ Tinnitus persist between two episodes ▪ Vertigo on hearing loud sound → Tullio's phenomenon ▪ Fluctuating deafness which improves after attack ▪ Aural fullness ▪ Unilateral condition
Investigation	▪ Audiometry → SNHL (Retrocochlear type) ▪ Recruitment phenomenon → negative ▪ Rollover phenomenon → positive ▪ Stapedial reflex → absent ▪ BERA →↑ 5th wave latency ▪ Gold standard: Gadolinium enhanced MRI	▪ Audiometry → Conductive hearing loss ▪ Otoscopy → Rising sun appearance ▪ CT → Phelp sign i.e. erosion of bony canal between carotid canal and jugular foramen ▪ Biopsy → Contraindicated	▪ Audiometry → Low frequency SNHL ▪ Rising curve in audiogram ▪ Recruitment phenomenon → positive ▪ Electrocochleography → Diagnostic test ▪ Summating potential ↑, Summating potential to Action potential (SP/AP)> 30%
Complications	▪ Dead ear ▪ Facial paralysis	▪ CN involvement: 7, 9, 10, 11 and 12	

Management	▪ Treatment of choice → Surgery
	▪ If patient refuses surgery → Stereotactic Radiotherapy with:
	  ○ Gamma knife using Cobalt 60
	  ○ Cyber knife
	▪ For patient with bilateral schwannoma as in NF-2 → auditory Brainstem implant → placed on lateral recess of 4th ventricle
		▪ Treatment of choice → Surgical removal after preoperative embolization
		▪ Stereotactic Radiotherapy
			▪ Medical Management: for vertigo
			  ○ Antihistaminics – Prochlorperazine
			  ○ Anxiolytics → Diazepam
			  ○ Vasodialators→ Betahistine
			  ○ Inhaled Carbogen – 5 % CO_2
			  ○ Acetazolamide
			  ○ Refractory cases:
			  ○ Transtymapnic injection of Gentamycin using microwick – chemical labyrinthectomy
			  ○ Endolymphatic sac decompression
			  ○ Meniett device – shock wave therapy

Extra edge	▪ Arises from Schwann cell sheath present around the nerve	▪ Arises from glomus cells present around jugular bulb ▪ Cell of origin - sympathetic neurons	▪ **Hennebert sign:** false +ve fistula test may be + ▪ Patient with recruitment phenomena are poor candidate for hearing aid ▪ **Lermoyez syndrome:** improvement in hearing and tinnitus during attack

MULTIPLE CHOICE QUESTIONS

CHAPTER 1: EAR

DEVELOPMENT OF EAR

1. Ear pinna develops from? *(DNB pattern 2007)*
a. Ectoderm
b. Endoderm
c. Mesoderm
d. All

[Ref: Dhingra's 7th/e pg. 12; S.K. De 9th/e pg. 13]

Explanation

Development of ear

- Developmentally, the internal ear appears first from an ectodermal vesicle, the otocyst. The middle ear develops next from the endoderm of the tubotymanic recess. The external ear appears last from the ectodermal first branchial cleft.
- Around 6th week of intrauterine life six 'hillocks or tubercles of His' appear around the 1st brachial cleft
- The 1st tubercle is derived from the first brachial arch and rest from the 2nd brachial arch (some authors believe that the 1st three tubercle develops from the first arch and rest from 2nd arch)
- Structure derived from various hillocks
  - 1st hillock → tragus
  - Second → crus of halix
  - Third → helix
  - Fourth → antihelix
  - Fifth → anti tragus and scapha
  - Sixth → ear lobule
- Defective fusion of hillocks gives rise to Preauricular sinus
- Failure of development of hillocks cause anotia
- Defective development of 4th tubercle can cause absence of of antihelix leading to 'Bat ear'

2. Ear structure fully developed at birth?
(DNB pattern 2009)
a. Mastoid air cells
b. Orbit
c. cornea
d. Ear ossicles

[Ref: Dhingra's 7th/e pg. 12; S.K. De 9th/e pg. 13]

3. Which of the following attains adult size before birth?
(DNB pattern 2007, 2009)
a. Parietal bone
b. Mastoid
c. Maxilla
d. Ear ossicles

[Ref: Scott Brown Otorhinolaryngology, 7th/e pg. 815]

Explanation

- The mastoid antrum is an air-filled sinus within the petrous part of the temporal bone.
- It communicates with the middle ear by way of the aditus and has mastoid air cells arising from its walls.

- The antrum, but not the air cells, is well developed and almost adult size at birth and has a volume of about 2mL.
- In most of the population, the mastoid air cell system is fairly extensive with air cells extending into the mastoid tip, the retrofacial region, the sinodural angle and anteriorly into the petrous apex and arch of the zygoma.
- Alternatively, the mastoid antrum may be the only airfilled space in the mastoid process when the name acellular or sclerotic is applied.
- Cornea- at birth a normal human cornea measures about 9.5 to 10mm while adult cornea measures around 12mm - 12.5 mm. adult corneal diameter is reached at 2 years of age.
- Adult orbit size reached at 15 -16 years of age.

4. Which of the following is not a derivative of the middle ear cleft - *(PGMEE 2015)*
a. Mastoid air cell
b. Eustachian tube
c. Tympanic cavity
d. Semicircular canal

[Ref: Dhingra's 7th/e pg.12]

5. When does the cochlea fully develops in the developing fetus? *(PGMEE 2015)*
a. 3rd to 8th week
b. 8th to 12th week
c. By the end of 20th week
d. First week

[Ref: Dhingra's 7th/e pg.14]

6. The following structure represents all the 3 components of the embryonic disc - *(PGMEE 2014)*
a. Meninges
b. Retina
c. Tympanic membrane
d. None of the above

[Ref: Dhingra's 7th/e pg.12]

7. Collaural fistula is an abnormality of - *(PGMEE 2015)*
a. 1st branchial arch
b. 1st branchial cleft
c. 2nd branchial arch
d. 2nd branchial cleft

[Ref: Dhingra's 7th/e pg.53]

8. Korner's septum arises from:- *(PGMEE 2016-17)*
a. Petro occipital suture
b. Petro squamous suture
c. Temporo parietal suture
d. Fronto-temporal suture

[Ref: Dhingra's 7th/e pg. 8]

9. Trautmann's triangle is bounded by all except: *(PGMEE 2012-13)*
a. Posterior margin of external meatus
b. Sigmoid sinus
c. Bony labyrinth
d. Superior petrosal sinus and dura

[Ref: Dhingra's 7th/e pg. 457]

1.	a
2.	d
3.	d
4.	d
5.	c
6.	c
7.	b
8.	b
9.	a

OTALGIA

10. All of the following nerves are involved in referred ear pain (Otalgia) EXCEPT: – *(PGMEE 2013)*

a. Abducens nerve
b. Glossopharyngeal nerve
c. Trigeminal nerve
d. Vagus nerve

[Ref: Dhingra's 7th/e pg. 5 & 143]

11. Which nerve is responsible for referred pain in ear: *(PGMEE 2012-13)*

a. Olfactory
b. Trochlear
c. Glossopharyngeal
d. Abducent

[Ref: BDC 7th/e vol. 3 pg. 292; Dhingra's 7th/e pg. 143]

12. Referred otalgia can be due to?

a. Carcinoma larynx
b. Carcinoma oral cavity
c. Carcinoma tongue
d. All of the above

[Ref: Dhingra's 7th/e pg. 143]

13. Referred pain in ear is due to all except:

a. Furunculosis
b. Oral cavity tumors
c. TM joint problems
d. Teething

[Ref: Dhingra's 7th/e pg. 143]

Explanation

- Ear receives nerve supply from
  - Vth (auriculotemporal br.)
  - IXth (tympanic br.) and Xth (auricular br.)
  - Cranial nerves; and from C2 (lesser occipital) and C2 and C3 (greater auricular), pain may be referred from remote areas supplied by these nerve
- Via Vth cranial nerve
  - Dental - Caries tooth, apical abscess, impacted molar, malocclusio.
  - Oral cavity- Benign or malignant ulcerative lesions of oral cavity
  - Temporomandibular joint disorders. Bruxism, osteoarthritis , recurrent dislocation.
  - Sphenopalatine neuralgia.
- Via IXth cranial nerve
  - Oropharynx - Acute tonsillitis, peritonsillar abscess, tonsillectomy, Benign or malignant ulcers of soft palate, tonsil and its pillars.
  - Base of tongue. Tuberculosis or malignancy.
  - Elongated styloid process.
- Via Xth cranial nerve Malignancy or ulcerative lesion of: vallecula, epiglottis, larynx or laryngopharynx, oesophagus.
- Via C2 and C3 spinal nerves Cervical spondylosis, caries spine.

EXTERNAL EAR

SURGICAL ANATOMY

14. Incisura terminalis is between:- *(PGMEE 2015)*

a. Tragus and crux of helix
b. Ear lobule and antihelix
c. Antihelix and external auditory meatus
d. Tragus and ear lobule

[Ref: Dhingra's 7th/e pg. 3]

15. The most common site of Darwin tubercle is:-

a. Near tragus *(PGMEE 2016-17)*
b. Over posterior aspect of helix
c. Over apex of helix
d. Upper crus of antihelix

[Ref: Dhingra's 7th/e pg. 51]

EXTERNAL AUDITORY CANAL

16. Posterior wall and floor of external auditory canal is supplied by- *(PGMEE 2015)*

a. Lesser petrosal nerve
b. Arnold nerve
c. Facial nerve
d. Vidian nerve

[Ref: Dhingra's 7th/e pg. 5]

Explanation

Part of EAC	Nerve supply
Ant. wall & roof	Auriculotemporal nerve.
Post. wall & floor	Auricular br. of vagus (Arnold nerve).
Post. wall	Auricular br. of vagus, sensory fibers of VIIth CN.

17. Length of external auditory canal is:- *(PGMEE 2016-17; PGMEE 2012)*

a. 2.4 cm
b. 4.2 cm
c. 2.4 mm
d. 42 cm

[Ref: Dhingra's 7th/e pg.3]

Explanation

- The external auditory canal extends from the concha of the auricle to the tympanic membrane and is approximately 2.4 cm (or 24 mm).
- In the adult, the lateral cartilaginous portion is about 8mm long and is continuous with the auricular cartilage.
- The bony canal wall, about 16mm long, is narrower than the cartilaginous portion.
- In adults, the cartilaginous portion runs inwards slightly downwards and forwards.
- In the neonate, there is virtually no bony external meatus as the tympanic bone is not yet developed, and the tympanic membrane is more horizontally.

18. Cartilagenous part of external auditory canal is- *(PGMEE 2014)*

a. Medial 1/3
b. Lateral 1/3
c. Medial 2/3
d. Lateral 2/3

[Ref: Dhingra's 7th/e pg. 3]

19. Most common benign tumor of external auditory meatus:- *(PGMEE 2016-17)*

a. Osteoma
b. Exostoses
c. Ceruminoma
d. Cholestatoma

[Ref: Dhingra's 7th/e pg. 118]

Explanation

- **Exostoses are** m/c benign tumors of external auditory meatus.
- SqCC is m/c malignant tumor of external auditory meatus.

10.	a
11.	c
12.	d
13.	a
14.	a
15.	c
16.	b
17.	a
18.	b
19.	b

20. Exostosis due to repetitive exposure to cold water is common in which part of the temporal bone?
   (PGMEE 2015)
   a. Squamous part
   b. Mastoid part
   c. Tympanic part
   d. Meatal part of tympanic ring

   [Ref: Dhingra's 7th/e pg. 118]

21. External auditory canal exostosis occurs due to-
   (PGMEE 2015)
   a. Repeated instrumentation
   b. Recurrent otitis externa
   c. Wide external auditory meatus
   d. Recurrent prolonged cold water exposure

   [Ref: Dhingra's 6th/e pg.107,447]

Explanation

- Chronic aural suppuration seen in the preantibiotic era was soon followed by exostoses.
- Today, prolonged contact of the external ear canal with cold sea water is the most prevalent cause (aquatic theory).

22. Identify the condition of the given image:
   (PGMEE 2019)

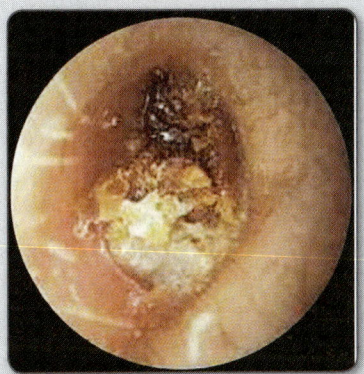

   a. Acquired cholesteatoma
   b. Congenital cholesteatoma
   c. Rupture of tympanic membrane
   d. Keratosis obturans

   [Ref: PL Dhingra 7th/e chap 8, diseases of external ear, pg. 58]

23. Keratosis obturans is -
   (PGMEE 2012)
   a. Cholesterol crystals surrounded by calcium
   b. Desquamated epithelial cell + Cholesterol
   c. Foreign body in external auditory canal
   d. Wax in external auditory canal

   [Ref: Dhingra's 7th/e pg. 58; Hazarika 2nd edition page 124]

Explanation

Karatosis obturans

- Firm mass consisting of wax, desquamated keratinizing epithelium and cholesterol in EAC simulating a cholesteatoma mass.
- A/w osteitis, granulation tissues in deep bony canal, cause widening of bony meatus.
- CF: Severe pain, CD/Hearing loss, tinnitis, discharge from ear, facial palsy of LMN type may occasionally occur.
- Removal after using waxolytic agent. Sometimes it is removed under general anaesthesia.

24. Cauliflower ear is due to:-
   (PGMEE 2014)
   a. Haematoma
   b. Carcinoma
   c. Fungal infection
   d. Herpetic infection

   [Ref: Dhingra's 7th/e pg. 52]

25. Ceruminous glands are modified
   (PGMEE 2015)
   a. Sweat glands
   b. Sebaceous glands
   c. Eccrine glands
   d. None of the above

   [Ref: Dhingra's 7th/e pg. 56]

TYMPANIC MEMBRANE

26. Resonance of tympanic membrane –
   (PGMEE 2012)
   a. 800 Hz
   b. 800-1600 Hz
   c. 3000 KHz
   d. 3000 Hz

   [Ref: Dhingra's 7th/e pg. 17]

Explanation

Natural Resonance and Efficiency of Auditory Apparatus

External auditory canal	3000 Hz
Tympanic membrane	800-1600 Hz
Middle ear	800 Hz
Ossicular chain	500-200 Hz

27. Ratio of tympanic membrane to oval window is -
   a. 17:1   *(PGMEE 2012)*
   b. 22:1
   c. 25:1
   d. 50:1

   [Ref:Dhingra's 7th/e pg. 17]

28. The angle made by the tymphanic membrane with the floor of external auditory canal:- *(PGMEE 2016-17)*
   a. 15°
   b. 30°
   c. 45°
   d. 90°

   [Ref: Internet, semanticscholar.org]

29. Impedance matching occurs at:
   (Recent Pattern June 2018)
   a. Difference of surface area of tympanic membrane and foot plate
   b. Semicircular canal fluid
   c. Utricle and Saccule
   d. None

   [Ref: Dhingra's 7th/e pg. 16]

Explanation

- The area of tympanic membrane is much larger than area of stapes footplate, the average ratio being 21:1.
- As the effective vibratory area of tympanic membrane is only two thirds, the effective areal ratio is reduced to 14:1 which helps in impedance matching/ transformer action.

20.	d
21.	d
22.	d
23.	b
24.	a
25.	a
26.	b
27.	a
28.	c
29.	a

30. The angle that tympanic membrane makes with the horizontal plane is: *(PGMEE 2013)*

a. 25°
b. 15°
c. 45° - 55°
d. 55° - 65°

[Ref: BDC 7th/e vol. 3 pg. 285]

Explanation

- It is oval in shape, measuring 9 × 10 mm. It is placed obliquely at an angle of 55⁰ with the floor of the meatus. It face downwards, forwards and laterally *(Ref: BDC 3rd/e pg. 311)*.
- Tympanic membrane is almost horizontal infants. In adults it forms 40°-45° angle with the floor of the external auditary canal *(Ref: S.K. De 9th/e pg. 15)*.

31. Pars flaccida of the tympanic membrane is also called - *(PGMEE 2014)*

a. Reissner's membrane
b. Secondary tympanic membrane
c. Basilar membrane
d. Shrapnells membrane

[Ref: Dhingra's 7th/e pg. 3]

32. Nerve supply of the tympanic membrane is by – *(PGMEE 2012)*

a. Lesser occipital
b. Parasympathetic ganglion
c. Auriculotemporal
d. Greater occipital

[Ref: Dhingra's 7th/e pg. 5]

33. Retraction of tympanic membrane touching the promontory is called- *(PGMEE 2013)*

a. Mild retraction
b. Adhesive otitis
c. Atelectasis
d. Severe retraction

[Ref: Dhingra's 7th/e pg. 59; Color atlas of otoscopy p.53]

34. Blue ear drum is seen in- *(PGMEE 2012)*

a. Serous otitis media
b. CSOM
c. Perforation
d. ASOM

[Ref: Dhingra's 7th/e pg. 69]

35. Retraction of tympanic membrane touching promontory. What is sade's grade- *(PGMEE 2013)*

a. 1
b. 2
c. 3
d. 4

[Ref: Color atlas of otoscopy p.53; Hazarika 2ⁿᵈ e/pg 163]

30.	c
31.	d
32.	c
33.	c
34.	a
35.	c
36.	d
37.	c
38.	d
39.	b
40.	d

Explanation

Sade's classification

- Sade's classification is based on retraction of pars tensa of TM
  - Grade I - Mild retraction not touching the long Process of incus.
  - Grade II - Retracted drum touching the long process of incus.
  - Grade III - Retracted drum/TM touching the promontory (Atelectasis)
  - Grade IV - Drum adherent to the promontory (Adhesive otitis media)

Toss classification

- Toss classification is for retraction of pars flaccida
  - Grade I - Mild attic retraction, not touching neck of malleus
  - Grade II - Attic retraction touching neck of malleus

- Grade III - Limited outer attic wall erosion
- Grade IV - Severe outer attic wall erosion

36. Most common perforation site in tympanic membrane - *(PGMEE 2014)*

a. Posterosuperior
b. Posteroinferior
c. Anterosuperior
d. Anterinferior

[Ref: Dhingra's 7th/e pg. 76-77]

Explanation

- Traumatic perforations are m/c
- Traumatic TM perforations are common in young males
- Slap is the m/c cause of perforation & involves antero-inferior quadrant.
- Marginal perforation m/c involve postero-superior quadrant.

37. Otoscopic finding shown below is of: *(PGMEE 2016-17)*

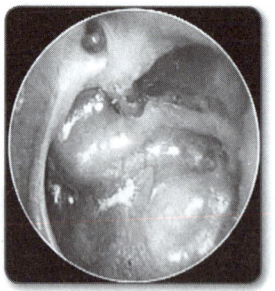

a. Normal tympanic membrane
b. Perforated tympanic membrane
c. Retracted and atelactatic tympanic membrane
d. Bulging tympanic membrane

[Ref: Dhingra's 7th/e pg. 75]

38. Organism responsible for multiple perforations of tympanic membrane:- *(PGMEE 2016-17)*

a. Moraxella catarrhalis
b. Mycobacterium Leprae
c. Staph. aureus
d. Mycobacterium tuberculosis

[Ref: Dhingra's 7th/e pg. 81]

39. Cause of myringosclerosis – *(PGMEE 2013)*

a. Otosclerosis
b. Grommet insertion
c. Genetic
d. None

[Ref: Dhingra's 7ᵗʰ/e pg. 59]

MIDDLE EAR

MIDDLE EAR ANATOMY

40. Which structure prevents spread of infection form middle ear to brain- *(PGMEE 2013)*

a. Petrous apex
b. Cribriform plate
c. Fundus tympani
d. Tegmen tympani

[Ref: Dhingra's 7th/e pg.5]

Explanation

- The **roof** is formed by a thin plate of bone called tegmen tympani.
- It also extends posteriorly to form the roof of the aditus and antrum.
- It separates tympanic cavity from the middle cranial fossa.

41. What overlies the lateral wall of the mastoid antrum? (PGMEE 2012-13)
   a. Mastoid process
   b. Tegmen tympani
   c. Tympanic plate
   d. Suprameatal triangle
   [Ref: BDC 7th/e vol. 3 pg. 292; Dhingra's 7th/e pg. 7]

42. Scutum is - (PGMEE 2015)
   a. Cartilaginous part of outer attic wall
   b. Bony part of inner attic wall
   c. Cartilagenous part of inner attic wall
   d. Bony part of outer attic wall
   [Ref: Dhingra's 7th/e pg.7]

Explanation

- The lateral wall of middle ear formed largely by the tympanic membrane and to a lesser extent by the bony outer attic wall called *scutum*.

43. All of the following are true about the middle ear cavity except: (PGMEE 2012-13)
   a. Anterior wall has opening of two canals
   b. Roof is formed by tegmen tympani
   c. Medial wall is formed by tympanic membrane
   d. Floor has bulb of internal jugular vein
   [Ref: BDC 7th/e vol. 3 pg. 288 and Dhingra's 7th/e pg. 6]

44. Tympanic branch of the middle ear is derived from: (PGMEE 2012-13)
   a. Facial nerve
   b. Glossopharyngeal nerve
   c. Chorda tympani
   d. Nerve to stapedius
   [Ref: BDC 7th/e vol. 3 pg. 292 and Dhingra's 7th/e pg. 5]

45. Chorda tympani is a part of: (PGMEE 2013)
   a. Middle ear
   b. External auditory canal
   c. Inner ear
   d. None of the above
   [Ref: BDC-III 7th/e pg. 290]

46. Sensory nerve supply of middle ear cavity is provided by - (PGMEE 2012, AI 95)
   a. Facial
   b. Vagus
   c. Trigeminal
   d. Glossopharyngeal
   [Ref: Dhingra's 6th/e pg.7]

47. Middle superior alveolar nerve is a branch of:
   a. Nasal branch of maxillary nerve (DNB pattern 2009)
   b. Mandibular branch of trigeminal nerve
   c. Inferior alveolar
   d. Infraorbital branch of maxillary nerve
   [Ref: BD Chaurasia, 4th/e pg. 118]

48. All of the following are a part of medial wall of the middle ear except- (PGMEE 2015)
   a. Subiculum
   b. Promontory
   c. Pyramid
   d. None of the above
   [Ref: Dhingra's 7th/e pg. 7; BDC vol-3 8th/e pg. 318 color plate]

Explanation

Structure	Formed by	Imp. structures in relation to it
Ant. wall (carotid wall)	Thin bony plate	2 openings: 1 (upper) for canal for tensor tympani & 1 (lower) for ET
Post wall (mastoid wall)	Mastoid	Pyramid, Auditus, fossa incudis

Structure	Formed by	Imp. structures in relation to it
Roof	Tegmen tympani	Cholesteatoma covers site of fistula
Floor (jugular wall)	Thin bony plate	Has bulb of IJV
Medial wall (labyrinthine wall)	Bony labyrinth	Has promontary (due to basal coil of chochlea) Has Round window covered by 2⁰ TM
Lateral wall	TM & scutum	Petrotympanic fissure, canaliculus for the chorda tympani nerve

49. Superior wall of middle ear is formed by: (PGMEE 2013)
   a. Jugular bulb
   b. Tympanic membrane
   c. Tegmen tympani
   d. None
   [Ref: BDC 7th/e vol. 3 pg. 288; Dhingra's 7th/e pg. 5]

50. Middle ear is separated from cerebrum by: (PGMEE 2013)
   a. Tegmen tympani
   b. Sphenoid bone
   c. Carotid wall
   d. Jugular wall
   [Ref: BDC 7th/e vol. 3 pg. 288; Dhingra's 7th/e pg. 5]

51. Which of the following is related to floor of middle ear: (PGMEE 2012-13)
   a. Internal carotid artery
   b. Round window
   c. Internal jugular vein
   d. Tegmen tympani
   [Ref: BDC 7th/e vol. 3 pg. 289; Dhingra's 7th/e pg. 5]

52. Secondary tympanic membrane is present over-
   a. Lateral wall of middle ear (PGMEE 2014)
   b. Oval window
   c. Round window
   d. Scala media
   [Ref: Dhingra 5th/e pg.9]

MIDDLE EAR (INTRATYMPANIC) MUSCLES

53. Number of muscles in middle ear: (PGMEE 2013)
   a. 1
   b. 2
   c. 4
   d. 3
   [Ref: BDC-III 6th/e pg. 280; Dhingra's 7th/e pg. 9]

54. Muscle entering middle ear from pyramid apex is: (PGMEE 2012-13)
   a. Stapedius
   b. Tensor tympani
   c. Auricularis
   d. Tensor palatine
   [Ref: BDC 7th/e vol. 3 pg. 291; Dhingra's 7th/e pg. 6]

55. Tensor tympani muscle is attached to:- (PGMEE 2016-17)
   a. Tympanic membrane
   b. Handle of malleus
   c. Stapes
   d. Incus
   [Ref: Dhingra's 7th/e pg. 9]

56. Pyramid of ear gives attachment to: (PGMEE 2012-13 & 16-17)
   a. Tensor tympani
   b. Stapedius
   c. Levator palati
   d. Tensor palati
   [Ref: Dhingra's 7th/e pg. 6]

41.	d
42.	d
43.	c
44.	b
45.	a
46.	d
47.	d
48.	d
49.	c
50.	a
51.	c
52.	c
53.	b
54.	a
55.	b
56.	b

57. Stapedius muscle is attached to:- *(PGMEE 2016-17)*
   a. Pyramids
   b. Precessus cochliformis
   c. Neck of malleus
   d. Neck of stapes

   [Ref: Dhingra's 7th/e pg. 6]

58. Attenuation reflex is lost in case of?
   a. Stapedial palsy
   b. Glomus tumor
   c. Internal ear pathology
   d. Malingerers

Explanation

- **The acoustic reflex** threshold test determines the softest level of sound that elicits stapedial muscle contraction.
- This normally occurs bilaterally after either ipsilateral or contralateral stimulation when a pure tone or noise is presented to a normal-hearing ear at levels of 70 to 100 dB HL.
- The middle ear muscle reflex has various functions..
  - First, the reflex provides protection from noise damage. Although the reflex is too slow to protect the ear from sudden impulsive noise, it may have an effect with longer lasting noises.
  - Patients with Bell's palsy and paralysis of the stapedius muscle had greater temporary threshold shifts in response to intense frequency noises in the affected than in the unaffected ear.
  - Second, **the reflex may provide selective attenuation of low frequency stimulus components**.
  - Third, the reflex may also have a beneficial effect in reducing the influence of some of the resonances in the middle ear
  - stapedial reflex measures include the acoustic reflex threshold and acoustic reflex decay. Both of these tests measure changes in tympanic membrane compliance caused by contraction of the stapedius muscle and are particularly useful for differentiation of cochlear and retrocochlear lesion sites
  - The stapedius reflex also provides valuable clinical information regarding the level of a facial nerve lesion in patients with facial nerve paralysis. If the lesion is proximal, an absent stapedius reflex may be expected. If the lesion is distal to the stapedius branch, an intact reflex may be expected.

EAR OSSICLES

59. Type of joint between the ear ossicles :-
   a. Primary cartilaginous
   b. Synovial joint
   c. Secondary cartilaginous
   d. Fibrous joint

   [Ref: Gray's Anatomy 38th/e pg. 10]

60. Ear ossicles articulate with each other through which type of joints? *(PGMEE 2012-13)*
   a. Synostosis
   b. Synovial
   d. Syndesmosis
   c. Synchondrosis

   [Ref: BDC 7th/e vol. 3 pg. 290 and 6th/e pg. 280]

61. Trauma to ear causes:- *(PGMEE 2016-17)*
   a. Malleus dislocation
   b. # of stapes
   c. Dislocation of stapes
   d. Dislocation of incus

   [Ref: Internet]

62. All of the following are true about ear ossicles except: *(PGMEE 2012-13)*
   a. Transmit vibrations from tympanic membrane to inner ear
   b. Give the eardrum mechanical advantage via lever action
   c. The muscles are highly developed like in bats for echo location.
   d. Are controlled by muscles as part of the accoustic Reflex

   [Ref: BDC 8th/e vol. 3 pg. 317; Dhingra's 7th/e pg. 17]

Explanation

- Movements of the stapes footplate, transmitted to the cochlear fluids, move the basilar membrane and set up shearing force between the tectorial membrane and the hair cells.

63. Stapes foot plate covers: *(DNB pattern 2009)*
   a. Inferior sinus tympani
   b. Round window
   c. Oval window
   d. Pyramid

   [Ref: Dhingra's 7th/e pg. 9]

EUSTACHIAN TUBE

64. The length of Eustachian tube is *(PGMEE 2015)*
   a. 16 mm
   b. 24 mm
   c. 36 mm
   d. 40 mm

   [Ref: Dhingra's 7th/e pg. 61]

65. Which of the following causes opening of Eustàchian tube? *(PGMEE 2014)*
   a. Tensor veli palatini (main)
   b. Salpingopharyngeus
   c. Levator veli palatini (Assist)
   d. Tensor veli palatini & Levator veli palatini

   [Ref: Dhingra's 7th/e pg. 61]

Explanation

- Muscles which help in opening of eustachian tube:-
  - Main muscle → Tensor veli palatini
  - Assisting muscle → Levator veli palatini

66. Eustachian tube opens into: *(PGMEE 2016-17; 2014, 2013)*
   a. Anterior wall of middle ear
   b. Medial wall of middle ear
   c. Lateral wall of nose
   d. Nasopharynx

   [Ref: Dhingra's 7th/e pg. 61]

67. Eustachian tube passes: *(PGMEE 2012-13)*
   a. Between superior and middle constrictors
   b. Above superior constrictor
   c. Below inferior constrictor
   d. Between middle and inferior constrictor

   [Ref: BDC 8th/e vol. 3 pg. 264]

Explanation

- Eustachian tube (pharyngotympanic tube or auditory tube) passes through the space between superior constrictor muscle and base of skull (**sinus of Morgagni**).

57.	d
58.	a
59.	b
60.	b
61.	d
62.	c
63.	c
64.	c
65.	d
66.	a
67.	b

68. Blood supply of the Eustachian tube is by all except:
   a. Ascending pharyngeal artery   *(PGMEE 2012-13)*
   b. Artery of pterygoid canal
   c. Middle meningeal artery
   d. Facial artery

[Ref: BDC 7th/e vol. 3 pg. 245]

Explanation

- Blood supply of the Eustachian tube is provided by branches of external carotid artery including:-
   ○ Ascending pharyngeal artery.
   ○ Maxillary artery
   ○ Middle menengeal artery
   ○ Artery to pterygoid canal.

69. Patulous eustachian tube is seen in?   *(PGMEE 2012-13)*
   a. CSOM   b. Cleft palate
   c. Pregnancy   d. Down's syndrome

[Ref: Dhingra 6th/e pg. 61]

Explanation

Patulous Eustachian Tube is seen in

- Most of the time it is idiopathic
- Pregnancy especially third trimester.
- Multiple sclerosis

70. All are tests to check eustachian tube patency except-
   a. Tonybee's and Frenzel maneuver   *(PGMEE 2015)*
   b. Fistulas test and Calorie test
   c. Politzer test
   d. Valsalva maneuver

[Ref: Dhingra's 7th/e pg. 62-63]

71. Ostmann fat pad is related to -   *(PGMEE 2015)*
   a. Eustachian tube   b. Buccal mucosa
   c. Tip of nose   d. Ear lobule

[Ref: Dhingra's 6th/e pg. 59]

PHYSIOLOGY OF HEARING

72. Semicircular canal perceives?
   a. Linear acceleration   b. Angluar acceleration
   c. Both   d. None

[Ref: Dhingra's 7th/e pg. 19]

Explanation

Semicircular canal

- They respond to **angular acceleration and deceleration**.
- The three canals l ie at right angles to each other but the one which lies at right angles to the axis of rotation is stimulated the most.
- Thus horizontal canal will respond maximum to rotation on the vertical axis and so on .
- Due to this arrangement of the three canals in three different planes, any change in position of head can be detected.
- Stimulation of semicircular canals produces nystagmus and the direction of nystagmus is determined by the plane of the canal being stimulated.
- Thus, nystagmus is horizontal from horizontal canal, rotatory from the superior canal, and vertical from the posterior canal.
- The stimulus to semicircular canal is flow of endolymph which displaces the cupula. The flow may be towards the cupula (ampullopetal) or away from it (ampuHofugal).

- Ampullopetal flow is more effective than ampullofugal for the horizontal canal.
- The quick component of nystagmus is always opposite to the direction of flow of endolymph

73. Impedence matching occurs d/t-   *(PGMEE 2014)*
   a. Utricle & Saccule
   b. Difference of surface area of tympanic membrane and foot plate
   c. Semicircular canal fluid
   d. None

[Ref: Dhingra's 7th/e pg. 15]

74. Function of ear ossicles is -   *(PGMEE 2012)*
   a. Amplification
   b. Equilibrium
   c. Impedance matching
   d. None

[Ref: Dhingra's 7th/e pg. 16]

75. Mechanical advantage provided by lever action of malleus-   *(PGMEE 2014)*
   a. 2:1   b. 1.3:1
   c. 1.8:1   d. 1:1

[Ref: Dhingra's 7th/e pg. 16]

NEURAL TRANSMISSION

76. All are involved in auditory pathway except -
                                       (PGMEE 2013)
   a. Trapezoid body
   b. Superior olivary complex
   c. Inferior colliculus
   d. Lateral geniculate body

[Ref: Dhingra's 7th/e pg. 15]

Explanation

- Remember its medial geniculate body not the LGB.
- Pathway of hearing (auditory pathway) is depicted by the following flow diagram:

Hair cell Peripheral/Spiral ganglia central
↓
Auditory nerve
↓
Cochlear Nucleus
↓
Superior olivary Nucleus
↓
Lateral lemniscus
↓
Inferior colliculus
↓
Medial geniculate body
↓
Auditory Cortex
(**Mnemonic:** Ac SLIM)

68.	d
69.	c
70.	b
71.	a
72.	b
73.	b
74.	c
75.	b
76.	d

77. Higher auditory centre determines: *(DNB pattern 2009)*
   a. Speech discrimination   b. Sound localization
   c. Sound frequency   d. Loudness

   [Ref: Dhingra's 7th/e pg. 15]

78. Which of the following is responsible for localization of sound - *(PGMEE 2013)*
   a. Cochlear nuclei   b. Cochlea
   c. Cochlear nerve   d. Superior olivary nucleus

   [Ref: Medical physiology by Khurana p.1198]

79. Primary receptor cells of hearing-
   a. Maculae & Cristae of SCC   *(PGMEE 2012, 2014)*
   b. Supporting cells in organ of Corti
   c. Hair cells in organ of Corti
   d. Tectorial membrane

   [Ref: Dhingra's 7th/e pg. 15]

80. Otoacoustic emissions arise from: *(DNB pattern 2009)*
   a. Inner hair   b. Outer hair cells
   c. Organ of Corti   d. Both inner and outer hair cells

   [Ref: DDhingra's 7th/e pg. 29]

Explanation

Otoacoustic emissions (OAE)

- Otoacoustic emissions (OAE) are acoustic signals emitted from the cochlea to the middle ear and into the external ear canal where they are recorded.They are most probably generated by active mechanical contraction of the outer hair cells, spontaneously or in reponse to sound.
- There are four types of OAEs: spontaneous OAEs (SOAE), transient evoked OAEs (TOAE), distortion product OAEs (DPOAE), and stimulus frequency OAEs (SFOAE).
- Spontaneous OAEs: They are present in healthy normal hearing persons where hearing loss does not exceed 30dB. They may be absent in 50% of normal persons.
- Uses
  ○ OAEs are used as a screening test of hearingin neonates and to test hearingin uncooperative or mentally challenged individuals afer sedation.
  ○ They help to distinguish cochlear from retrocochlear hearing loss.OAEs are absent i n cochlear lesions.
  ○ OAEs are also useful to diagnose retrocochlear pathology, especially auditory neuropathy.
- Thus, both the saccule and the utricle sense linear accelerations caused by translational movements of the head, as well as static tilts of the head.

81. Otolith organs are concerned with function of? *(DNB December 2011)*
   a. Oculovestibular reflex   b. Rotatory nystagmus
   c. Angular acceleration   d. Linear acceleration

   [Ref: Dhingra's 7th/e pg. 19]

Explanation

Otolith organs

- On earth, the gravitational force acts permanently on us, hence gravitational acceleration needs to be detected continuously, and this function is served by the otolith organs, which detect all linear accelerations.

77.	b
78.	d
79.	c
80.	b
81.	d
82.	b
83.	d
84.	c
85.	c
86.	c

- The orientation of the otolith organs, the saccule and utricle, is relatively orthogonal to each other, with the utricle being horizontal and the saccule predominantly vertical (tangential in the head).
- Consequently, motion in the horizontal plane triggers predominantly the utricle, whereas vertical movements trigger mainly the saccule.
- Thus, both the saccule and the utricle sense linear accelerations caused by translational movements of the head, as well as static tilts of the head.

HEARING ASSESSMENT & AUDIOMETRY

TESTS OF HEARING

82. Tuning fork frequency used in ENT is? *(PGMEE 2011)*
   a. 256 Hz   b. 512 Hz
   c. 1024 Hz   d. 2048 Hz

   [Ref: Dhingra's 7th/e pg. 23]

Explanation

- Tunning fork tests are performed with tuning forks of different frequencies such as 128, 256 ,512, 1024, 2048 and 4096 Hz.
- But for routine clinical practice, tuning fork of 512 Hz is ideal.
- Forks of lower frequencies produce sense of bone vibration while those of higher frequency have a shorter decay time and are thus not routinely preferred.

83. During ear examination, cough occurs due to stimulation of:- *(PGMEE 2012)*
   a. Trigeminal nerve   b. Trochlear nerve
   c. Hypoglossal nerve   d. Vagus nerve

   [Ref: Dhingra's 7th/e pg. 5]

84. Weber's test lateralizing to the affected side means:- *(PGMEE 2015)*
   a. Mixed loss   b. Brainstem damage
   c. Conductive hearing loss   d. Sensorineural hearing loss

   [Ref: Dhingra's 7th/e pg. 24]

85. Which of the following is a cause of positive Hennebert's sign- *(PGMEE 2015)*
   a. Dead labyrinth   b. Fenestretion surgery
   c. Congenital Syphilis   d. Cholesteatoma

   [Ref: Dhingra's 7th/e pg. 49 & 508]

Explanation

Hennebert's sign	Seen in
Positive	Cholesteatoma, Fenestration operation
False Positive	Congenital syphilis
False negative	Cholesteatoma covers site of fistula

86. Fitzgerald-Hallpike test is done for: *(DNB 2007, 2008)*
   a. Tinnitus   b. Facial weakness
   c. Vestibular function   d. Vertigo

   [Ref: Dhingra's 7th/e pg. 45]

87. Which of the following tests is not used to differentiate between cochlear and retrocochear hearing loss-

(PGMEE 2015)

a. Short increment sensitivity index (SISI) test
b. Recruitment
c. Threshold tone decay test
d. None of the above

[Ref: Dhingra's 7th/e pg. 28]

88. In the right middle ear pathology, Weber's test will be -

a. Lateralised to left side   *(PGMEE 2014)*
b. Centralized
c. Lateralised to right side
d. Normal

[Ref: Dhingra's 7th/e pg. 24]

89. Positive Rinne test indicates –   *(PGMEE 2012)*

a. AC>BC   b. BC = AC
c. BC>AC   d. None

[Ref: Dhingra's 7th/e pg. 24]

90. Rinne's test negative is seen in -   *(PGMEE 2014)*

a. Menieres disese   b. CSOM
c. Presbycusis   d. Labyrinthitis

[Ref: Dhingra's 7th/e pg. 24]

91. All are tuning fork test except -

(PGMEE 2012; DNB 02)

a. Schwaback test   b. Rinne's test
c. Weber's test   d. Grants test

[Ref: Dhingra's 7th/e pg. 24]

92. Bing test is -   *(PGMEE 2013)*

a. Bone conduction test
b. Air conduction test
c. Audiometric test
d. Special test

[Ref: Dhingra's 7th/e pg. 24]

93. A 38 year old gentleman reports of decreased hearing in the right ear for the last two years. On testing with a 512 Hz tuning fork the Rinne's test without masking is negative on the right ear and positive on the left ear. With the weber's test the tone is perceived as louder in the left ear The most likely patient has - *(PGMEE 2015)*

a. Right sensorineural hearing loss
b. Left conductive hearing loss
c. Left sensorineural hearing loss
d. Right conductive hearing loss

[Ref: Dhingra's 7th/e pg. 24]

94. A 38 year old gentleman presents to ENT specialist and reports decreased hearing in the right ear for the last two years. On testing with a 512 Hz tuning fork the Rinne's test without masking is negative on the right ear and positive on the left ear. With the weber's test the tone is perceived as louder in the left ear The most likely patient ha:

(Recent Pattern June 2018)

a. Sensorineural deafness in Left ear
b. Sensorineural deafness in Right ear
c. Conductive deafness in Left ear
d. Conductive deafness in Right ear

[Ref: Dhingra's 7th/e pg. 24]

Explanation

Rinne's Test

- The Rinne test is a tuning fork test that compares hearing by air conduction and bone conduction.
- The Rinne test is based on the idea that hearing mechanism is normally more efficient by air conduction (AC) than it is by bone conduction (BC), i.e., AC > BC in normal persons.
- For this reason, a tuning fork will sound louder and longer by air conduction than by bone conduction.
- However, this air conduction advantage is lost when there is a conductive hearing loss in which case the tuning fork sounds louder by bone conduction than by air-conduction.
- Right side negative means : -
  ○ Right sided conductive deafness. or
  ○ Right sided severe sensorineural hearing loss which gives false negative results.
- Left side positive test Rinne's test means : -
  ○ Normal left ear
  ○ Left sided sensorineural hearing loss (However this is not the case in this patient as the patient is presenting with right sided hearing loss).
- Interpretation of Weber test in this patient. Weber is lateralized to right ear. That means:
  ○ Left sided sensorineural hearing loss.
  ○ Right sided conductive deafness.
  ○ Thus, this patient is suffering from severe Left side sensorineural hearing loss in which the Rinne's test is false negative and weber is lateralized to left ear.

95. All of the following are tests for vestibular dysfunction except -   *(PGMEE 2015)*

a. Electronystagmography
b. Gelle's test
c. Galvanic test
d. Optokinetic test

[Ref: Dhingra's 7th/e pg. 45]

96. Regarding electrocochelography true is:-

(PGMEE 2016-17)

a. Electrode place on promontory
b. SP is potential of outer hair cell
c. AP is potential of inner hair cell
d. Normal value is more than 0.3

[Ref: Dhingra's 7th/e pg. 28; S.K. De 9th/e pg. 34]

Explanation

- Endocochlear potential is a direct potential recorded in scalar media and generated by stria vascularis.
- Summational potential (SP) is generated predominantly by outer hair cells in organ of Corti.
- Compound action potential (AP) is an all or none response by cochlear neurones.

97. Hallpike biothermal caloric test is done at an angle of :-   *(PGMEE 2014)*

a. 15°   b. 30°
c. 45°   d. 60°

[Ref: Dhingra's 7th/e pg. 45]

87.	d
88.	c
89.	a
90.	b
91.	d
92.	a
93.	a
94.	b
95.	b
96.	a
97.	b

98. In cold caloric stimulation test, the cold water, induces nystgmus (movement of the eye ball) in the following direction : *(PGMEE 2012)*
   a. Towards the same side
   b. Towards the opposite side
   c. Upwards
   d. Downwards

   [Ref: Dhingra's 7th/e pg. 45]

99. What will happen when semicircular canal of one side is destroyed? *(PGMEE 2014)*
   a. Increased tendency to fall
   b. Sensation of Spinning of world around
   c. Increased nausea and vomiting
   d. None of the above

AUDIOMETRY

100. All are subjective tests for audiometry except -
   a. Impedance audiometry *(PGMEE 2014)*
   b. Pure tone audiometry
   c. Speech audiometry
   d. Tone decay

   [Ref: Dhingra's 7th/e pg. 26]

101. Impedance audiometry is for pathology of: *(PGMEE 2012)*

   a. Middle ear   b. Inner ear
   c. Mastoid air cell d. External ear

   [Ref: Dhingra's 7th/e pg. 27]

102. A "trough shaped curve" in audiometry is seen in -
   a. Congenital SNHL *(PGMEE 2012)*
   b. Otosclerosis
   c. Acoustic neuroma
   d. Otitis media

Explanation
   - A trough-shaped audiogram aka "ski slope" or "cookie bite" audiogram or an inverted U-shaped audiogram are seen in sudden onset SNHL and acoustic neuroma.

103. Red line in pure tone audiometry is for - *(PGMEE 2013)*
   a. Air conduction   b. Bone conduction
   c. Right ear   d. Left ear

   [Ref: Dhingra's 7th/e pg. 32]

Explanation

Symbols used in audio gram
   - Red colored symbols are used for right ear and Blue colored symbols are used for left ear

Modality	Right Ear	Left ear
Colour of graph	Red line	Blue live
AC unmasked	○	✕
AC masked	△	▢
BC unmasked	<	>
BC masked	⌐	⌐
No response	↯	↯

104. B-type tympanogram is seen in- *(PGMEE 2012)*
   a. Serous otitis media   b. Ossicular discontinuity
   c. Otosclerosis   d. All of the above

   [Ref: Dhingra's 7th/e pg. 27]

105. C-shaped curve on tympanometry is seen in:
   a. Serous otitis media *(PGMEE 2013)*
   b. Otosclerosis
   c. Eustachian tube obstruction
   d. TM perfiration

   [Ref: Dhingra's 7th/e pg. 27]

106. Stapedial reflex is mediated by- *(PGMEE 2012)*
   a. V and VII nerves   b. V and VIII nerves
   c. VII and VI nerves   d. VII and VIII nerves

   [Ref: Dhingra's 7th/e pg. 27]

107. Sound intensity of whispering is: *(PGMEE 2015)*
   a. 2 dB   b. 30 dB
   c. 90 dB   d. 120 dB

   [Ref: Dhingra's 7th/e pg. 21]

Explanation

Intensity
   - It is the strength of sound which determines its loudness. It is usually measured in decibels. At a distance of 1 m, intensity of

Whisper	30 dB
Normal conversation	60 dB
Shount	90 dB
Discomfort of the ear	120 dB
Pain in the ear	130 dB

108. During normal conversation sound heard at 1 meter distance is: *(PGMEE 2012, 2015)*
   a. 60 dB   b. 80 dB
   c. 90 dB   d. 120 dB

   [Ref: Dhingra's 7th/e pg. 21]

109. Maximum audible tolerance is?
   a. 90 db for 6 hours
   b. 90 db for 8 hours
   c. 85 db for 6 hours
   d. 85db for 8 hours

   [Ref: Dhingra's 7th/e pg. 37]

Explanation
   - Permissible exposure in cases of continuous noise or a number of short term exposures. [Government of India, Ministry of Labour, Model Rules under Factories Act 1948 (corrected up to 31.3.87)]
   - Noise level* (dBA) Permitted daily exposure (hours)

90	8.0	102	11/2
92	6.0	105	1.0
95	4.0	110	1/2
97	2.0	115	1/4
100	2.0		

   - 5 dB rule of time-intensity states that "any rise of 5 dB noise level will reduce the permitted noise exposure time to half"

98.	**b**
99.	**b**
100.	**a**
101.	**a**
102.	**c**
103.	**c**
104.	**a**
105.	**c**
106.	**d**
107.	**b**
108.	**a**
109.	**b**

110. **Pitch discrimination is best between?**
(PGMEE 2015; 2014)
   a. 1-5Hz
   b. 10-100Hz
   c. 1000-10,000 Hz
   d. 100-1000Hz
   [Ref: Dhingra's 7th/e pg. 21]

111. **What is the intensity in decibel of normal conversation in humans:** *(PGMEE 2015)*
   a. 30dB
   b. 60dB
   c. 150dB
   d. 90dB
   [Ref: Dhingra's 7th/e pg. 21]

112. **What is the continuous audible decibel without loss of hearing:-** *(PGMEE 2016-17)*
   a. 65 dB
   b. 75 dB
   c. 85 dB
   d. 45 dB
   [Ref: Dhingra's 7th/e pg. 22]

HEARING ASSESSMENT IN INFANTS

113. **In infant most sensitive audiometric screening is -**
(PGMEE 2012)
   a. BERA
   b. Tympanometry
   c. Electrocochleography
   d. Cortical evoked response
   [Ref: Dhingra's 7th/e pg. 133]

114. **Which test is used to assess Neonatal hearing loss?**
   a. SISI *(PGMEE 2015)*
   b. Calorie Test
   c. Otoacoustic emissions (OAE)
   d. Rinne's Test
   [Ref: Dhingra's 7th/e pg. 132]

115. **Best time for hearing assessment in an infant -**
(PGMEE 2015)
   a. 1st month of life
   b. 3-6 months
   c. 6-9 months
   d. 9-12 months
   [Ref: Dhingra's 7th/e pg. 132]

HEARING LOSS

116. **Viruses causing hearing loss are all except:**
(PGMEE 2013)
   a. Rota virus
   b. Mumps
   c. Rubella
   d. Measles
   [Ref: Dhingra's 7th/e pg. 129]

117. **Unilateral sensorineural hearing loss may occur in**
   a. Coronavirus
   b. Rotavirus *(PGMEE 2013)*
   c. Pertussis
   d. Mumps
   [Ref: Wiki]

118. **Recruitment phenomenon is seen in:**
   a. Otitis media with effusion *(DNB pattern 2008)*
   b. Otosclerosis
   c. Acoustic nerve schwannoma
   d. Presbyaccusis
   [Ref: Dhingra's 7th/e pg. 28]

119. **Loudness recruitment phenomenon is seen in:-**
   a. Meineire's disease *(PGMEE 2016-17)*
   b. Otosclerosis
   c. Acoustic nerve schwannoma
   d. Otitis media with effusion
   [Ref: Dhingra's 7th/e pg. 28]

120. **Stenger test and Lombard's test is used to diagnosis -**
   a. Mixed hearing loss *(PGMEE 2013)*
   b. Sensorineural hearing loss
   c. Non-organic hearing loss
   d. Conductive hearing loss
   [Ref: Dhingra's 7th/e pg. 39; Scott Brown's 7th/e p.1299]

121. **Maximum hearing loss is seen in?** *(PGMEE 2014, 13, 12)*
   a. Ossicular interruption with perforation
   b. Perforation of tympanic membrane
   c. Complete obstruction of ear canal
   d. Ossicular interruption with intact tympanic membrane
   [Ref: Dhingra's 7th/e p. 31]

Explanation

Average Hearing Loss seen in Different Lesions of Conductive Apparatus

Complete obstruction of ear canal	30 dB
Perforation of tympanic membrane (It varies and is directly proportional to the size of perforation)	10-40 dB
Ossicular interruption with intact drum	54 dB
Ossicular interruption with perforation	38 dB
Malleus fixation	10-25 dB
Closure of oval window	60 dB

- Note here that ossicular interruption with intact drum causes more loss than ossicular interuption with perforated drum.

122. **When the patient fails to understand normal speech, but can understand shouted or amplified speech the hearing loss, is termed -** *(PGMEE 2015)*
   a. Mild hearing loss
   b. Moderate hearing loss
   c. Severe hearing loss
   d. Profound hearing loss
   [Ref: Dhingra's 7th/e pg. 41]

123. **Female with stapedectomy done, has conductive hearing loss at 60 dB. Diagnosis -** *(PGMEE 2013)*
   a. Implant failure
   b. Fistula
   c. Tympanic membrane perforation
   d. Closure of oval window
   [Ref: Dhingra's 7th/e pg. 41]

124. **In noice induced hearing loss, audiogram shows a typical notch at -** *(PGMEE 2013)*
   a. 1000 Hz
   b. 2000 Hz
   c. 3000 Hz
   d. 4000 Hz
   [Ref: Dhingra's 7th/e pg. 37]

125. **If a patient gets an attack of vertigo/dizziness by loud noise, he is having -** *(PGMEE 2015)*
   a. Hyperacusis
   b. Dysplacusis
   c. Tullio phenomenon
   d. Paracusis
   [Ref: Dhingra's 7th/e pg. 511]

126. **Defective function of which of the following causes hyperacusis -** *(PGMEE 2013)*
   a. VIII nerve
   b. 7th nerve
   c. Stapedius muscles
   d. Any of the above

Explanation

- Hyperacusis is 'unusual tolerance to ordinary environmental sounds.'

110.	d
111.	b
112.	a
113.	a
114.	c
115.	a
116.	a
117.	d
118.	d
119.	a
120.	c
121.	d
122.	c
123.	d
124.	d
125.	c
126.	d

127. 65 year old person presents with hearing loss with normal speech discrimination. He is suffering from-
a. Presbycusis   *(PGMEE 2012)*
b. NOHL (Non organic hearing loss)
c. Ototoxic drug toxicity
d. Noise induced hearing loss

[Ref: Dhingra's 7th/e pg. 39]

128. If there is intolerance to loud sounds, which nerve affected:-   *(PGMEE 2012)*
a. 5th nerve   b. 7th nerve
c. 10th nerve   d. None

[Ref: Essentials of ENT p. 686]

OTITIC BAROTRAUMA

129. Otitic barotrauma results from:-   *(PGMEE 2015)*
a. Ascent in air   b. Sudden acceleration
c. Linear acceleration   d. Sudden descent in air

[Ref: Dhingra's 7th/e pg. 71]

130. All are true about otitic barotrauma EXCEPT -
                                                        (PGMEE 2013).
a. Catheterization or politerization can be used in treatment
b. Retracted tympanic membrane
c. Conductive deafness
d. Occurs during sudden ascent in aeroplane

[Ref: Dhingra's 7th/e pg. 71]

OTITIS EXTERNA

131. A clinical condition seen in a 24 year old male from New orleans characterised by a facial palsy and is often associated with facial pain and the appearance of vesicles on the ear drum, ear canal and pinna. Vertigo and sensorineural hearing loss accompanying it is suggestive of: *(PGMEE 2012-13)*
a. Turners Syndrome   b. Pendred Syndrome
c. Bells Palsy   d. Ramsay Hunt Syndrome

[Ref: Dhingra's 7th/e pg. 105]

132. Haemorrhagic otitis externa is caused by -
a. Influenza   *(PGMEE 2014)*
b. Streptococcus
c. Staphylococcus aureus
d. Proteus

[Ref: Dhingra's 7th/e pg. 55]

Explanation

Haemorrhagic otitis externa	Caused by influenza epidemics
Malignant (necrotizing) otitis externa	Caused by pseudomonas infection

133. Bullous myringitis is caused by   *(PGMEE 2013)*
a. Pseudomonas aureginosa
b. Candida
c. Pneumococcus
d. Mycoplasma pneumoniae

[Ref: Dhingra's 7th/e pg. 58]

127.	a
128.	b
129.	d
130.	d
131.	d
132.	a
133.	d
134.	c
135.	a
136.	b
137.	c

134. Sago grain appearance is seen in :   *(PGMEE 2013)*
a. Malignant otitis externa
b. Otomycosis
c. Healed myringitis bullosa
d. Keratosis obturans

[Ref: Dhingra's 6th/e pg. 55]

135. Malignant otitis externa false statement is:-
a. It is a type of malignancy   *(PGMEE 2016-17)*
b. Caused by pseudomonas
c. Seen in diabetic individual
d. IOC is Tc 99 scan

[Ref: Dhingra's 7th/e pg. 55]

136. Malignant otitis externa is caused by:
a. Staphylococcus aureus   *(PGMEE 2016-17)*
b. Pseudomonas
c. Staphylococcus epidermidis
d. Klebsiella

[Ref: Dhingra's 7th/e pg. 55]

Explanation

Malignant otitis externa

- Malignant otitis externa (MOE) is an aggressive and potentially life-threatening infection of the soft tissues of the external ear and surrounding structures, quickly spreading to involve the periostium and bone of the skull base.
- Clinicopathological classification system.
  - Stage 1: Clinical evidence of malignant otitis externa with infection of soft tissues beyond the external auditory canal, but negative Tc-99 bone scan
  - Stage 2: Soft tissue infection beyond external auditory canal with +ve Tc-99 bone scan
  - Stage 3: As above, but with cranial nerve paralysis
    - 3a Single
    - 3b Multiple
  - Stage 4: Meningitis, empyema, sinus thrombosis or brain abscess
- Pseudomonas aeruginosa is the most common pathogen and is responsible in > 95% of cases.
- The combination of pain, granulations, otorrhea and resistance to local therapy for at least eight to ten days are highly sensitive for making a diagnosis of MOE.
- Technetium (Tc-99m) radionuclide bone scans will detect bony involvement, even before HRCT scans can demonstrate bone destruction.
- The treatment of choice for MOE is systemic anti-Pseudomonas antibiotics.
- Other treatments includes; aural toilet, hyper oxygen, Surgery for the removal of sequestra, collections of pus and debridement of necrotized and granulating tissues.

137. A 60 year old diabetic patient presents with otorrhea. O/E there are extermely painful lesion in the external ear. He does not respond to antibiotics. There is evidence of granulation type tissue in the external ear and bony erosion with facial nerve palsy is noted. The most likely diagnosis is:
a. Chronic suppurative otitis media   *(PGMEE 2012)*
b. Acute suppurative otitis media
c. Malignant Otitis Externa
d. Nasopharyngeal carcinoma

[Ref: Dhingra's 7th/e pg. 55]

138. Regarding necrotizing otitis externa all are true EXCEPT:
a. Common in diabetics *(PGMEE 2012)*
b. Surgery is never indicated
c. Facial nerve involved
d. Caused by pseudomonas

[Ref: Dhingra's 7th/e pg. 55]

139. All of the following are risk factors for malignant otitis extrena except: *(PGMEE 2015)*
a. Immunodeficiency   b. Chemotherapy
c. Parotitis   d. Diabetes

[Ref: Dhingra's 7th/e pg. 55]

140. Most common cause of otomycosis:
(Recent Pattern June 2018)
a. Histoplasma   b. Rhinosporidium
c. Aspergillus   d. Actinomyces

[Ref: Dhingra's 7th/e pg. 55]

Explanation

Otomycosis (Acute fungal otitis externa)

- A fungal or yeast infection of the external auditory meatus.
- Caused by saprophytic fungi of ear canal which become pathogenic under certain conditions like warmth, humidity, DM, immunosuppression, steroids overuse.
- **Aspergillus niger** is most common cause (accounts 90%) in tropical countries.
- Other fungi which are implicated - candida albicans, phycomycetes, rhizopus, actinomyces, and penicillium.

141. Most common fungus causing otomycosis:
(PGMEE 2012)
a. Penicillin   b. Candida
c. Mucor   d. Aspergillus fumigatus

[Ref: Dhingra's 7th/e pg. 55]

Explanation

- Commonest in topical countries being aspergillus niger and occasionally candida albicans which is more common in Wester countries.

142. Ramsay hunt syndrome is caused by- *(PGMEE 2015)*
a. H. simplex   b. Adenovirus
c. Influenza   d. Varicella zoster

[Ref: Dhingra's 7th/e pg. 59, 105; S.K. De 9th/e pg. 137]

Explanation

- Caused by VZV
- Involves CN VII & VIII

OTITIS MEDIA

ACUTE SUPPURATIVE OTITIS MEDIA (ASOM)

143. Commonest cause of acute otitis media in children is -
(PGMEE 2016-17)
a. Staph aureus   b. Strepto-pneumoniae
c. H.influenzae   d. Pseudomonas

[Ref: Dhingra's 7th/e pg. 67]

144. Light house sign is a classical sign of- *(PGMEE 2015)*
a. Chronic suppurative otitis media
b. Acute supprative otitis media
c. Acoustic neuroma
d. Glomus tumour

[Ref: Dhingra's 7th/e pg. 67; S.K. De 9th/e pg. 374]

Explanation

- In stage III of suppuration in ASOM, during otoscopy the pulstating discharge may reflect the light intermittently. This is called light house sign.

145. Light house sign is seen in ASOM in which stage -
a. Stage of pre-suppuration *(PGMEE 2012)*
b. Stage of suppuration
c. Stage of resolution
d. Stage of hyperemia

[Ref: S.K. De. 9th/e pg. 74]

146. Cart-wheel appearance of tympanic membrane in ASOM is due to - *(PGMEE 2013)*
a. Perforation of tymparic membrane
b. Granulation tissue on tympanic membrane
c. Congested blood vessels along malleus
d. Edema of tympanic membrane

[Ref: Dhingra's 7th/e pg. 67]

SEROUS OTITIS MEDIA (GLUE EAR)

147. In a case of serous otitis media all are done except-
(PGMEE 2014)
a. Antibiotics are mainstay of treatment
b. Myringotomy
c. Adenoidectomy
d. Insertion of grommet

[Ref: Dhingra's 7th/e pg. 70]

148. Treatment of choice for persistent glue ear is:
(DNB pattern 2009)
a. Myringotomy with diode laser
b. Myringotomy with cold knife
c. Conservative treatment with analgesics & Antibiotics
d. Myringotomy with ventilation tube insertion

[Ref: Dhingra's 7th/e pg. 70]

149. A child has Adenoidectomy done but he has effusion in middle ear. What is done next - *(PGMEE 2012)*
a. Mastoidectomy   b. Tympanoplasty
c. Grommet insertion   d. None

[Ref: Dhingra's 7th/e pg. 70]

150. Following cause should always be excluded in case of unilateral secretory otitis media in an adult :
a. CSOM   *(PGMEE 2013)*
b. Foreign body of external ear
c. Mastoiditis
d. Nasopharyngeal carcinoma

[Ref: Dhingra's 7th/e pg. 69]

151. Glue ear - *(PGMEE 2014)*
a. Is painful
b. NaF is useful
c. Radical mastoidectomy is required
d. Is painless

[Ref: Dhingra's 7th/e pg. 69]

138. b
139. c
140. c
141. b
142. d
143. b
144. b
145. b
146. c
147. a
148. d
149. c
150. d
151. d

152. Watery otorrhoea is seen in:- *(PGMEE 2016-17)*
- a. CSOM
- b. Glomus tympanicum
- c. Otitis media with effusion
- d. # of temporal bone

CHRONIC SUPPURATIVE OTITIS MEDIA (CSOM)

153. Most common organism cultured in CSOM
- a. Staphylococcus aureus *(PGMEE 2015)*
- b. Staphylococcus epidermidis
- c. Streptococcus pneumonia
- d. Pseudomonas aeruginosa

[Ref: Dhingra's 7th/e pg. 76]

154. Commonest complication of CSOM is:
- a. Meningitis *(DNB pattern 2008)*
- b. Superiosteal abscess
- c. Brain abscess
- d. Mastoiditis

[Ref: Dhingra's 6th/e pg. 76]

155. All of the following are features of Tubotympanic CSOM except- *(PGMEE 2015)*
- a. Sometimes paradoxical improvement in hearing is seen
- b. Hearing loss
- c. Profuse discharge
- d. Extreme pain

[Ref: Dhingra's 7th/e pg. 75]

156. Treatment of choice in central safe perforation is -
- a. Conservative management *(PGMEE 2014)*
- b. Tympanoplasty
- c. Myringoplasty
- d. Modified mastoidectomy

[Ref: Dhingra's 7th/e pg. 78]

CHOLESTEATOMA

157. Central part of cholesteatoma contains – *(PGMEE 2015)*
- a. Keratinized squamous epithelium
- b. Keratin debris
- c. Coulmnar epithelium
- d. Fibrolasts

[Ref: Dhingra's 7th/e pg. 73]

158. Posterosuperior retraction pocket if allowed to progress will lead to- *(PGMEE 2013)*
- a. Tympanosclerosis
- b. Secondary cholesteatoma
- c. SNHL
- d. Primary cholesteatoma

[Ref: Dhingra's 7th/e pg. 79; S.K. De 9th/e pg. 86]

159. Which of the following is included in the Levenson criteria for congenital cholesteatoma - *(PGMEE 2015)*
- a. White mass medial to normal tympanic membrane
- b. History of prior otologic procedures
- c. Definite history of otorrhoea
- d. Atticoantral perforation of the tympanic membrane

[Ref: Dhingra's 7th/e pg. 74]

160. Which of the following structures is not at immediate risk of erosion by cholesteatoma - *(PGMEE 2015)*
- a. Long process of incus
- b. Base plate of stapes
- c. Horizontal, lateral semicircular canal
- d. Fallopian canal containing facial nerve

[Ref: Dhingra's 7th/e pg. 79]

161. Most common surgery performed for t/t of CSOM:
- a. Simple mastoidectomy *(PGMEE 2013)*
- b. Radical mastoidectomy
- c. Modified radical mastoidectomy
- d. Tympanoplasty

[Ref: S.K. De. 9th/e pg. 90]

Explanation
- Modified radical mastoidectomy → done for unsafe CSOM

162. Treatment of choice in deafness associated with attico antral perforation- *(PGMEE 2014)*
- a. Instillation of antibiotic drops
- b. Modified radical mastoidectomy
- c. Watch and wait
- d. Simple mastoidectomy

[Ref: Dhingra's 7th/e pg. 80]

163. X-ray findings in tubotympanic chronic otitis media - *(PGMEE 2013)*
- a. Clear-cut distinct bony partition between cells
- b. Sclerosis with cavity in mastoid
- c. Honeycombing of mastoid
- d. Bone destruction

[Ref: Dhingra's 7th/e pg. 78]

COMPLICATIONS OF CSOM

164. Commonest intracranial complication of CSOM is -
- a. Conductive deafness *(PGMEE 2012)*
- b. Cholesteatoma
- c. Temporal lobe abscess
- d. Meningitis

[Ref: Dhingra's 7th/e pg. 90]

165. Most common extra-cranial complication of CSOM is -
- a. Lateral sinus thrombosis *(PGMEE 2012)*
- b. Sub-periosteal (Post auricular) abscesses
- c. Facial nerve paralysis
- d. Brain abscess

[Ref: Dhingra's 7th/e pg. 86]

166. Most common nerve to be damaged in CSOM is –
- a. III *(PGMEE 2015)*
- b. VII
- c. III
- d. VI

[Ref: Dhingra's 7th/e pg. 88]

152.	d
153.	d
154.	d
155.	d
156.	a
157.	b
158.	d
159.	a
160.	b
161.	c
162.	b
163.	b
164.	d
165.	b
166.	b

167. A patient presented with the following picture of Tympanic Membrane. Most Probable diagnosis (marked with arrow): *(PGMEE 2019)*

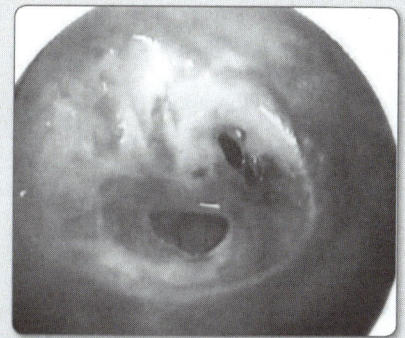

- a. Tubercular Otitis Media
- b. Syphilitic Otitis Media
- c. Pseudomonas infection
- d. Fungal Otitis Media

[Ref: PL Dhingra 7th/e chap 10, disorders of middle ear, pg. 71]

Explanation

- ■ Features of Tuberculous Otitis Media
  - ○ Multiple perforations
  - ○ Pale
  - ○ Painless
  - ○ Disproportionate hearing loss
- ■ The above picture shows multiple perforations - indicative of tuberculous otitis media.

168. True about tubercular otitis media are all except-
- a. Spreads through eustachian tube *(PGMEE 2013)*
- b. Usually affects both ears
- c. May cause multiple perforations
- d. Causes painless ear discharge

[Ref: Dhingra's 7th/e pg. 81]

169. 12 years old child presents with fever, unilateral pain behind left ear, mastoid bulging displacing the pinna forward outwards with loss of bony trabeculae. This patient has history of chronic persistent pus discharge from left ear. Treatment of choice is- *(PGMEE 2015)*
- a. Antibiotics only
- b. Mastoidectomy with incision and drainage and antibiotics
- c. Antibiotics and incision and drainage
- d. Incision and drainage only

[Ref: Dhingra's 7th/e pg. 84-86]

170. Treatment of middle ear papilloma is *(PGMEE 2015)*
- a. Myringotomy and simple excision
- b. Local infiltration with podophyllin
- c. Tympanomastoidectomy
- d. Myringotomy and simple excision

[Ref: Washington Manual of Surgical Pathology p. 86]

171. Which perforation of the tympanic membrane is most commonly seen with tubotympanic CSOM? *(PGMEE 2015)*
- a. Central
- b. Posteroinferior
- c. Anterosuperior
- d. Posterosuperior

[Ref: Dhingra's 7th/e pg. 75]

172. Commonest complication of CSOM is: *(DNB pattern 2010)*
- a. Benzold Abscess
- b. Brain abscess
- c. Meningitis
- d. Mastoiditis

[Ref: Dhingra's 7th/e pg. 84]

173. Schwartz operation is: *(DNB pattern 2007)*
- a. Radical mastoidectomy
- b. Myringotomy
- c. Cortical mastoidectomy
- d. Modified radical mastoidectomy

[Ref: Dhingra's 7th/e pg. 457]

174. An intra operative photograph of mastoidectomy. Which of the following is lateral semicircular canal *(NEET Pattern 2017)*
- a. A
- b. B
- c. C
- d. D

[Ref: Dhingra's 7th/e pg. 458]

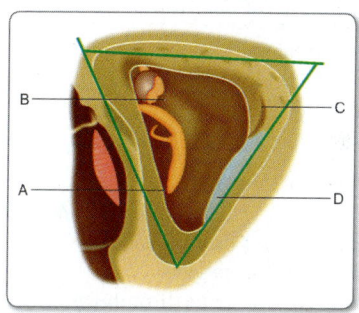

Explanation

- ■ A- Facial nerve
- ■ B-lateral semicircular canal
- ■ C- sino-dural angle
- ■ D-sigmoid sinus

ABSCESS IN RELATION TO MASTOID

175. Bezold's abscess is located deep to:- *(DNB pattern 2007; PGMEE 2015)*
- a. Submandibular region
- b. Infratemporal region
- c. Digastric triangle
- d. Sternomastoid muscle

[Ref: Dhingra's 7th/e pg. 87]

176. A young male presents with ear discharge for last 3 years; He recently developed swelling in the neck below and behind the angle of mandible. On examination there is torticollis, external auditory canal was filled with granulation tissue. What is the diagnosis? *(PGMEE 2015)*
- a. Bezold's abscess
- b. Citelli's abscess
- c. Luc's abscess
- d. Digastric abscess

[Ref: Dhingra's 7th/e pg. 87]

PETROSITIS

177. False about Gardenigo syndrome- *(PGMEE 2012)*
- a. Retrobulbar pain
- b. Petrositis
- c. Facial palsy
- d. Otitis media

[Ref: Dhingra's 7th/e pg. 88]

167.	a
168.	b
169.	b
170.	c
171.	a
172.	d
173.	c
174.	b
175.	d
176.	a
177.	c

178. All are true about Gradenigo's syndrome except -
(PGMEE 2015; 12)
a. Associated with intermittent ear discharge
b. Associated with headache
c. Causes diplopia
d. Leads to retro orbital pain

[Ref: Dhingra's 7th/e pg. 88]

Explanation

- Three classic signs of GS are: otorrhea + facial pain + horizontal diplopia (sixth nerve palsy).
- Patients may complain of earache, tenderness, fever, persistent ear discharge (not intermittent), deep unilateral facial pain, headache, diplopia, dizziness, nausea, vomiting, and confusion

LATERAL SINUS THROMBOPHLEBITIS

179. Griesinger sign is :- *(PGMEE 2016-17)*
a. Oedema of the postauricular soft tissues overlying the mastoid process
b. Retro-orbital pain
c. Periorbital ecchymosis and Raccoon's eyes
d. None of the above

[Ref: Dhingra's 7th/e pg. 93, 508]

180. Griesinger sign is seen in:
(PGMEE 2016-17, 2011)
a. Cavernous sinus thrombosis
b. Lateral sinus thrombosis
c. Superior sagittal sinus thrombosis
d. Inferior sagittal sinus thrombosis

[Ref: Dhingra's 7th/e pg. 93, 508]

178.	b
179.	a
180.	b
181.	d
182.	a
183.	d
184.	c
185.	a

Explanation

Lateral sinus thrombosis

- It is an inflammation of inner wall of lateral venous sinus with formation of a thrombus.
- The pathological process can be divided into the following stages:
  - Formation of peri-sinus abscess
  - Endophlebitis and mural thrombus formation
  - Obliteration of sinus lumen and intra sinus abscess
  - Extension of thrombus
- CF:
  - Hectic Picket-fence type of fever with rigors
  - Headache
  - Progressive anaemia and emaciation.
  - *Griesnger's sign* This is due to thrombosis of mastoid emissary vein.Oedema appears over the posterior part of mastoid.
  - Papilloedema Its presence depends on obstruction to venous return.
  - *Tobey- Ayer test* This is to record CSF pressure by manometer and t o see the effect of manual compression of one or both jugular veins. Compression of vein on the thrombosed side produces no effect while compression of vein on healthy side produces rapid rise in CSF pressure which will be equal to bilateral compression of jugular veins.

- Crowe -Beck test Pressure on jugular vein of healthy side produces engorgement of retinal veins (seen by ophthalmoscopy) and supraorbital veins. Engorgement of veins subside on release of pressure.
  - Tenderness along jugular vein
- **Treatment**
  - I/v anti bacterial therapy
  - Mastoidectomy and exposure of sinus
  - Ligation of internal jugular vein It is indicated when antibiotic and surgical treatment have failed to control embolic phenomenon
  - Anticoagulant therapy It is rarely required and used when thrombosis is extending to cavernous sinus.
- *Gradenigo's syndrome* is the classical presentation of petrositis, and consists of a triad of (a) external rectus palsy (VIth nerve palsy), (b) deep-seated ear or retro-orbital pain (Vth nerve involvement) and (c)persistent ear discharge. It is uncommon to see the full triad these days.

181. Tobey Ayer test is positive in - *(PGMEE 2013)*
a. Subarachnoid hemorrage
b. Petrositis
c. Cerebral abscess
d. Lateral sinus thrombosis

[Ref: Dhingra's 7th/e pg. 93]

182. Delta-sign is seen in- *(PGMEE 2013)*
a. Sigmoid sinus thrombosis
b. Acute mastoiditis
c. Petrositis
d. Glomus tumor

[Ref: Dhingra's 7th/e pg. 93]

INNER EAR

ANATOMY & PHYSIOLOGY

183. Site where endolymph is seen - *(PGMEE 2012)*
a. Scala vestibule   b. Organ of corti
c. Helicotrema   d. Scala media

[Ref: Dhingra 7th/e pg. 12]

184. Endolymph is secreted by: *(DNB pattern 2009)*
a. Basiliar membrane
b. Hensen cell
c. Stria vascularis   d. Cochlear duct

[Ref: Dhingra's 7th/e pg. 12]

185. A steel factory worker is suffering from noise induced hearing loss. Which of the following is most likely to be affected? *(NEET Pattern 2017)*
a. Inner hair cell   b. Macula
c. Crista ampullaris   d. Saccule

[Ref: Dhingra 5th edition, Pg-141]

Explanation

- Noise induced hearing loss cause damage to Hair cells, start in the basal turn of cochlea.
- Outer hair cells are affected before inner hair cells
- Damage depend upon the frequency of noise. 2000-3000 Hz cause more damage, intensity and duration of noise.

186. CSF is similar to – *(PGMEE 2012)*
a. Perilymph
b. Urine
c. Cortilymph
d. Endolymph

[Ref: Dhingra's 7th/e pg. 11]

187. Endolymph resembles:- *(PGMEE 2013)*
a. Plasma
b. CSF
c. ECF
d. ICF

[Ref: Dhingra's 7th/e pg. 12]

Explanation

Endolymph resembles

- It fills the entire membranous labyrinth.
- Resembles intracellular fluid, being rich in K ions.
- It is secreted by secretory cells of the stria vascularis or the cochlea and by the *dark cells.*

188. Angular movement is sensed by - *(PGMEE 2012)*
a. Cochlea
b. Semicircular canal
c. Saccule
d. Utricle

[Ref: Dhingra's 7th/e pg. 18, 19]

189. Sense of gravity is detected by - *(PGMEE 2014)*
a. Superior semicircular canal
b. Lateral semicircular canal
c. Horizontal semicircular canal
d. Utricle and saccule

[Ref: Dhingra's 7th/e pg. 18]

190. Horizontal acceleration with forward movement in the sagittal plane is detected by- *(PGMEE 2015)*
a. Lateral semicircular canal
b. Macula of saccule
c. Posterior semicircular canal
d. Macula of utricle

[Ref: Dhingra's 7th/e pg. 18]

Explanation

Maculae

- Otolith organs (i.e. utricle and saccule).
- Macula of the utricle lies in its floor in a horizontal plane.
- Macula of the saccule lies in its medial wall in a vertical plane.
- They sense position of head in response to gravity and linear acceleration.

191. Static equilibrium is due to - *(PGMEE 2012)*
a. End organ of corti
b. Cristae ampulla
c. Cupula
d. Macula

[Ref: Dhingra's 6th/e pg. 16]

192. Macula is stimulated by – *(PGMEE 2012)*
a. Gravity
b. Head position change
c. Linear acceleration
d. All of the above

[Ref: Dhingra's 7th/e pg. 19]

Explanation

- A macula consits mainly of two parts:-
  ○ A sensory neuroepithelium.
  ○ An otolithic membrane which contain the crystals of $CaCO_3$ called otoliths or otoconia.
- The cilia of hair cells project into the gelatinous layer. The linear, gravitational and head tilt movements cause displacement of otolithic membrane and thus stimulus the hair cells which lie in different planes.

193. Horizontal semicircular canal responds to-
a. Antero posterior acceleration *(PGMEE 2014)*
b. Rotational acceleration
c. Gravity
d. Horizontal acceleration

[Ref: Dhingra's 7th/e pg. 19]

194. Identify the lateral semicircular canal in the following diagram *(NEET Pattern 2017)*

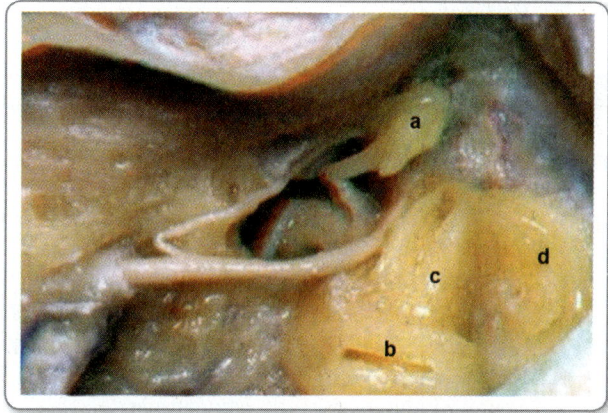

a. A
b. B
c. C
d. D

Explanation

- A – incus
- B – Posterior semicircular canal
- C – Lateral semicircular canal
- D – Superior semicircular canal

195. Endolymphatic duct connects which structure - *(PGMEE 2014)*
a. Scala vestibule to aqueduct of cochlea
b. Scala tympani to subdural space
c. Scala tympani to aqueduct of cochlea
d. Scala media to subdural space

[Ref: Dhingra 7th/e pg. 11]

Explanation

Endolymphatic duct

- Lies in bony canal
- It passes through the vestibular acqueduct
- Formed by union of ducts of saccule & utricle
- Connects scala media to subdural space
- It is exposed for drainage/shunt operation in Meniere's disease.

196. Endolymphatic duct drains into: *(DNB pattern Dec 2010)*
a. Saccule
b. Subdural space
c. Subarachnoid space
d. Epidural space

[Ref: BDC 7th/e vol. 3 pg. 296; Dhingra's 7th/e pg. 11]

Explanation

- Scala tympani is connected with the subarachnoid space through aqueduct of cochlea. The infection of labyrinth can travel along it to reach meninges
- Hyrtle's fissure is an embryonic remnant also k/as tympano-meningeal hiatus as it connects mesotympanum to the CSF of sub-arachnoid space

186.	a
187.	d
188.	b
189.	d
190.	d
191.	d
192.	d
193.	b
194.	c
195.	d
196.	a

- Endolymphatic duct is f/by union of 2 ducts, one each from the saccule & the utricle.It passes through the vestibular aqueduct. Its terminal part is dilated to form endolymphatic sac. Meniere's diaease is caused by its obstruction.

197. Infection of CNS spreads in inner ear through?
(DNB pattern Dec 2011)
- a. Cochlear Aqueduct
- b. Endolymphatic sac
- c. Hyrtle's fissure
- d. Vestibular Aqueduct

[Ref: Dhingra's 7th/e pg. 11]

DISEASES OF INNER EAR

OTOSCLEROSIS (OTOSPONGIOSIS]

198. Otosclerosis presents with? *(PGMEE 2012-13)*
- a. Fluctuating hearing loss
- b. Conductive deafness
- c. Mixed hearing loss
- d. Sensorineural deafness

[Ref: Dhingra's 7th/e pg. 96]

199. Commonest site of otosclerosis is: *(PGMEE 2015, 2007)*
- a. Utricle
- b. Ear ossicles
- c. Round window
- d. Otic capsule

[Ref: Dhingra's 7th/e pg. 95]

200. Most common site for the initiation of otosclerosis is:
- a. Fissula ante fenestrum *(PGMEE 2014)*
- b. Margins of stapes
- c. Foot plate of stapes
- d. Fissula post fenestrum

[Ref: Dhingra's 7th/e pg. 95]

201. Otosclerosis most commonly affects with race?
- a. Chinese
- b. Negros *(PGMEE 2015)*
- c. White races
- d. Japanese

[Ref: Dhingra's 7th/e pg. 95]

202. Common age for otosclerosis is – *(PGMEE 2014)*
- a. 5-10 yrs
- b. 10-20 yrs
- c. 20-30 yrs
- d. 30-45 yrs

[Ref: Dhingra's 7th/e pg. 95]

203. Autosomal Dominant disease with Carharts Notch is:
(PGMEE 2007, 2010)
- a. CSOM
- b. Acoustic neuroma
- c. Otospongiosis
- d. Meniere's disease

[Ref: Dhingra's 7th/e pg. 95]

204. Schwartze sign seen in *(PGMEE 2012)*
- a. Meniere's diseases
- b. Otosclerosis
- c. Glomus Jugulare
- d. Acoustic neuroma

[Ref: Dhingra's 7th/e pg. 96]

205. Carhartt notch appears at what frequency in otosclerotic patient: *(Recent Pattern June 2018)*
- a. 1000Hz
- b. 2000Hz
- c. 3000Hz
- d. 4000Hz

[Ref: Dhingra's 7th/e pg. 97]

Explanation

- An audiometric finding characteristic of otosclerosis is an increase in bone conduction threshold with a peak at 2,000 Hz known as Carhartt's notch. This phenomenon is attributed to "mechanical factors associated with stapedial fixation."

- Although the notch occurs at 2,000 Hz, a reduction in bone conduction sensitivity is seen from 500 to 4,000 Hz which is, on average, 5 dB at 500 Hz, 10 dB at 1000 Hz, 15 dB at 2000 Hz, and 5 dB at 4,000 Hz
- Carhartt attributed this

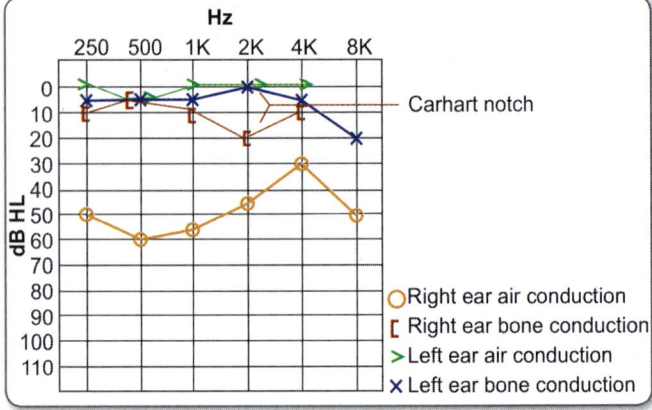

206. All of the following are true regarding otosclerosis EXCEPT:- *(PGMEE 2016-17)*
- a. Negative Gelle's test
- b. Normal bone conduction
- c. Loss of higher frequencies in air conduction
- d. Autosomal dominant inheritance

[Ref: Dhingra's 7th/e pg. 95-96]

Explanation

Gelle & Bing Tests
- Vibrating tuning fork placed over mastoid & then: External auditory canal is blocked in **Bing test** or E.A.C. pressure ↑ed by Siegalization in **Gelle test**

	Bing	Gelle
Otosclerosis	No change	No change
Normal/SNHL	Intensity ↑es	Intensity ↓es

207. In a pure tone audiogram a dip at 2000Hz (Carhart's notch) is characteristic of - *(PGMEE 2016-17; 2012)*
- a. Otosclerosis
- b. Ototoxicity
- c. Presbyacusis
- d. Noise induced hearing loss (NIHL)

[Ref: Dhingra's 7th/e pg. 96]

208. Otosclerosis treatment includes all except-
(PGMEE 2012)
- a. Stapedectomy
- b. Sodium fluoride
- c. Hearing Aids
- d. Radical mastoidectomy

[Ref: Dhingra's 7th/e pg. 97-98]

209. Role of this drug is under research in medical treatment in otosclerosis:- *(PGMEE 2016-17)*
- a. Sodium chloride
- b. Bisphosphonates
- c. Steroid
- d. Calcitonin

[Ref: Internet]

Explanation

- 3rd generation bisphosphonates (risedronate and zoledronate) are being tried for t/t of sensorineural hearing loss in otosclerosis.

210. What is the role of NaF (Sodium Fluoride) in otosclerosis?
   a. It repolarizes the cochlear cells **(PGMEE 2015)**
   b. It quickness the maturity of the active focus and reduces osteoclastic resorption
   c. It restores the electrolyte equilibrium
   d. It hastens recovery of the Overstimulated Cochlea
   [Ref: Dhingra's 7th/e pg. 97]

MENIERE'S D/S

211. Selective low frequency sensorineural hearing loss occurs in: **(PGMEE 2015)**
   a. BPPV   b. Glomus tumour
   c. Schwannoma   d. Meneire's disease
   [Ref: Dhingra's 7th/e pg. 112]

212. Fluctuating deafness is seen in: **(PGMEE 2015)**
   a. Meniere's disease   b. Otosclerosis
   c. CSOM   d. ASOM
   [Ref: Dhingra's 7th/e pg. 112; Logan Turner 10th/e pg. 335]

213. On giving glycerol, hearing defect improves . Likely condition is : **(PGMEE 2016-17, 2015)**
   a. Meniere's disease
   b. Otosclerosis
   c. Acoustic nerve schwannoma
   d. Otitis media with effusion
   [Ref: Dhingra's 7th/e pg. 113]

214. Chemical labyrinthectomy by transtympanic injections is done in Meniere's disease using which drug:- **(PGMEE 2015)**
   a. Coamoxiclav   b. Cyclosporine
   c. Gentamicin   d. Amikacin
   [Ref: Dhingra's 7th/e pg. 115]

215. Micro Wick and Microcatheter sustained release devices are used in: **(DNB pattern 2008)**
   a. Conrol of epistaxis
   b. Drooling of saliva
   c. Delivering drug to the round window
   d. Frey's syndrome
   [Ref: Dhingra's 7th/e pg. 115]

216. Fick's operation and Cody Tack's sacculotomy is done for: **(PGMEE 2015)**
   a. Benign positional paroxysmal vertigo
   b. Meniere's disease
   c. Atrophic rhinitis
   d. Otoscierosis
   [Ref: Dhingra's 7th/e pg. 115; Logan Turner 10th/e pg. 335]

ACOUSTIC NEUROMA

217. Most common tumour of CPA angle (Cerebellopontine Angle) is: **(PGMEE 2012-13; PGMEE 2015)**
   a. Cholesteatoma   b. Meningioma
   c. Acoustic neuroma   d. Neurofibroma
   [Ref: Dhingra's 7th/e pg. 125; Logan Turner 10th/e p. 341]

218. Hitzelberger's sign is seen in- **(PGMEE 2015)**
   a. Glomus Tumour
   b. Acoustic neuroma
   c. Acute suppurative otitis media
   d. Nasal angiofibroma
   [Ref: Dhingra's 7th/e pg. 125]

Explanation
- In acoustic neuroma sensory fibers of VIIth nerve are affected early.
- There is hypoaesthesia of posterior meatal wall (**Hitzelberger's sign**), loss of taste (as tested by electrogustometry) and reduced lacrimation (**+ve Schirmer test**).
- Paraesthesia of face and reduced corneal sensitivity occurs due to involvement of 5th cranial nerve. 5th CN is the earliest nerve to be involved.
- Motor fibres are more resistant and are affected late.
- Delayed blink reflex may be an early manifestation.

219. Acoustic neuroma most commonly arises from:- **(PGMEE 2007, 2009, 2010)**
   a. Cochlear division of VIIIth cranial nerve
   b. Superior division of vestibular nerve
   c. Inferior division of vestibular Nerve
   d. Facial nerve
   [Ref: Dhingra's 6th/e pg. 112; Internet NCBI]

220. Earliest nerve to be involved in acoustic neuroma:-
   a. 5   b. 7   **(PGMEE 2012)**
   c. 9   d. 10
   [Ref: Dhingra's 7th/e pg. 125]

Explanation
- Corneal reflex is lost which is related to 5th nerve

221. Earliest sign seen in Acoustic neuroma is- **(PGMEE 2014)**
   a. Loss of corneal reflex   b. Unilateral deafness
   c. Cerebellar signs   d. Facial weakness
   [Ref: Dhingra's 7th/e pg. 125]

222. Triad of Tinnitus, progressive deafness and vertigo along with facial weakness is seen in?
   a. Menier's disease   b. Lermoyez syndrome
   c. Acoustic neuroma   d. Otosclerosis

Explanation
- *Acoustic neuroma:* Symptoms caused by a acoustic neuroma depend largely on its size.
  - Hearing loss, Tinnitus, Vertigo
  - Cerebellar dysfunction
  - 5th nerve dysfunction
  - Symptoms of raised intra cranial pressure
  - Facial nerve palsy
- *Meniere's disease*, also called endolymphatic hydrops, is a disorder of the inner ear where the endolymphatic system is distended with endolymph. It is characterised by (i)vertigo, (ii) sensorineural hearing loss and (iii) tinnitus and (iv) aural fullness.
- *Lermoyez syndrome:* Here symptoms of Meniere's disease are seen in reverse order. First there is progressive deterioration of hearing, followed by an attack of vertigo, at which time the hearing recovers.

TINNITUS

223. Which of the following is a cause of objective tinnitus? **(PGMEE 2015; 2013)**
   a. Meniere's disease   b. Ototoxic drugs
   c. Impacted Wax   d. Carotid artery aneurysm
   [Ref: Dhingra's 7th/e pg. 145]

210.	**b**
211.	**d**
212.	**a**
213.	**a**
214.	**c**
215.	**c**
216.	**b**
217.	**c**
218.	**b**
219.	**c**
220.	**a**
221.	**a**
222.	**c**
223.	**d**

224. Objective tinnitus is seen in:-   *(PGMEE 2013)*
- a. Meniere's disease
- b. Glomus tumor
- c. Ear wax
- d. Acoustic neuroma

[Ref: Dhingra's 7th/e pg. 145]

VERTIGO

225. Postitional vertigo is caused by disorders of:-   *(PGMEE 2014)*
- a. Inferior SCC
- b. Superior SCC
- c. Lateral SCC
- d. Posterior SCC

[Ref: Dhingra's 7th/e pg. 47]

Explanation

Benign Paroxysmal Positional Vertigo (BPPV)

- Vertigo when the head is placed in a certain when the head is placed in a certain critical position.
- There is no hearing loss or other neurologic symptoms
- Disease is caused by a disorder of posterior semicircular

226. Name the maneuvre shown in the image: *(PGMEE 2019)*

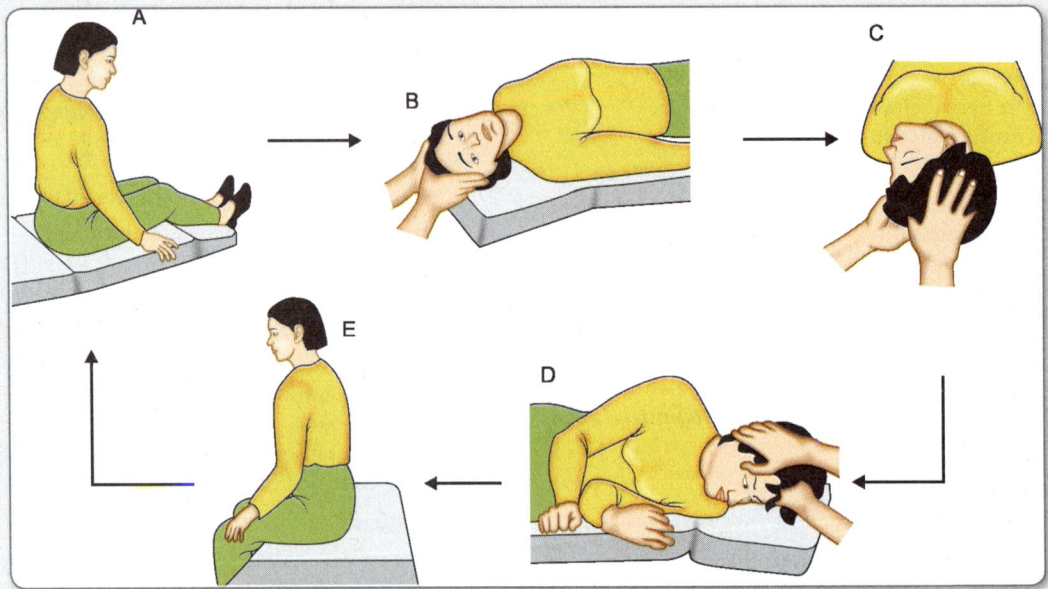

- a. Brandt daroff
- b. Epley
- c. Foster
- d. Semont

[Ref: PL Dhingra 7th/e chap 7, disorders of vestibular system, pg. 47-48]

227. Epley's test (maneuver) is used for?   *(PGMEE 2014)*
- a. Benign paroxysmal vertigo
- b. Basilar migraine
- c. Orthostatic hypotension
- d. Thoracic outlet syndrome

[Ref: Dhingra's 7th/e pg. 47]

224. b
225. d
226. b
227. a

Explanation

- First-line therapy for BPPV is organized around repositioning maneuvers that, in cases of canalithiasis, use gravity to move canalith debris out of the affected SCC and into the vestibule.
- For posterior canal BPPV, Epley maneuvers is particularly effective.
- The Epley maneuver is effective in more than 90% of cases in eliminating BPPV.
- The Semont maneuver also is effective for posterior canal BPPV but is more difficult to perform and is less effective than the simpler, more comfortable Epley maneuver.
- BPPV will be cured by respositioning maneuvers, but surgical therapy remains an option for the rare patient with disabling persistent disease ,Singular neurectomy to treat refractory BPPV was proposed by Gacek.

228. All of the following are vertigo of vestibular (peripheral) origin EXCEPT:- *(PGMEE 2012)*
a. Meniere's disease
b. Benign paroxysmal positional vertigo
c. Vertibrobasilar insufficiency
d. Vestibular neuronitis

[Ref: Dhingra's 7th/e pg. 47]

229. Bilateral past-pointing is due to defect in - *(PGMEE 2013)*
a. Vestibular system   b. Cerebellum
c. Brainstem   d. Basal ganglia

[Ref: Dhingra's 7th/e pg. 49]

230. Positive head impulse test is suggestive of- *(PGMEE 2015)*
a. Injury to peripheral vestibular nerve
b. Injury to vestibular nuclei
c. Lesion in the brain stem
d. Injury to Occulomotor nerve

[Ref: Dhingra's 6ᵗʰ/e pg. 41]

231. True about central nystagmus - *(PGMEE 2013)*
a. Not suppressed by optic fixation
b. Changing direction
c. Horizontal or vertical
d. All of the above

[Ref: Scott's Brown's 7th/e p. 3724]

GLOMUS TUMOUR

232. Earliest symptom of glomus tumor is - *(PGMEE 2015)*
a. Pulsatile tinnitus   b. Vertigo
c. Headache   d. Easache

[Ref: Dhingra's 7th/e pg. 121]

233. Positive Brown sign and a mass in ear which bleeds heavily on touching. Most likely cause is: *(DNB pattern 2008; PGMEE 2012)*
a. Ca mastoid   b. Angiofibroma
c. Glomus Jugulare   d. Acoustic neuroma

[Ref: Dhingra's 7th/e pg. 121]

234. Pulsatile Tinnitus in ear is due to:
a. Glomus jugulare tumour   *(PGMEE 2015, 2008)*
b. Mastoid reservoir phenomenon
c. Malignent otitis media
d. Osteoma

[Ref: Logan Turner 10ᵗʰ/e pg. 214; Maqbool 9ᵗʰ/e pg. 85; Dhingra's 7th/e pg. 121]

235. Glomus tumour is characterized by all of the following EXCEPT:- *(PGMEE 2013)*
a. Most common benign neoplasm of middle ear
b. "Rising sun" appearance in otoscopy
c. Cranial nerve palsy is a late feature
d. CT scan is not helpful in differentiating glomus jugulare from glomus tympanicum

[Ref: Dhingra's 7th/e pg. 121]

236. Phelps sign is seen in - *(PGMEE 2012; PGMEE 02)*
a. Glomus jugulare   b. Neurofibromatosis
c. Meniere's disease   d. Vestibular Schwannoma

237. True about Glomus jugulare are all EXCEPT:
a. Rising sun sign is seen   b. Involves cranial nerve
c. Pulsatile tinnitus is seen d. Invades epitympanum

Explanation

Glomus tumours

- Glomus tumours that originate in the temporal bone invade the jugular foramen.
- Depending on their localization, they can be divided into one of three categories – glomus jugulare, glomus jugulotympanicum and glomus tympanicum tumours.
- Only the glomus tympanicum is confined to the tympanic cavity, but this a relatively uncommon
- Glomus jugulare They arise from the dome of jugular bulb, invade the hypotympanum and jugular foramen, causing neurological signs of IXth to Xllth cranial nerve involvement.They may compress jugular vein or invade its lumen.
- Hearing loss is conductive and slowly progressive. Tinnitus is pulsatile and of swishing character, synchronous with pulse, and can be temporarily stopped by carotid pressure.
- Otoscopy shows a red reflex through intact tympanic membrane. "Rising sun" appearance is seen when tumour arises from the floor of middle ear.
- Sometimes, tympanic membrane appears bluish and may be bulging." Pulsation sign" (Brown's sign) is positive, i.e. when ear canal pressure is raised with Siegle's speculum, tumour pulsates vigorously and then blanches; reverse happens with release of pressure.
- Rule of 10s: Remember that 10% of the tumours are familial, 10% multicentric and up to 10% functional ,i.e. they secrete catecholamines
- Four –vessel angiography It is necessary when CT head shows involvement of jugular bulb, carotid artery or intradural extension.It also helps to delineate any other glomus tumour (as they may be multiple) ,find the feeding vessels or embolization of tumour if required .
- Brain perfusion and flow studies They are necessary when tumour is pressing on internal carotid artery.
- Biopsy Preoperative biopsy of the tumour for diagnosis is never done.
- Treatment: It consists of:
  ○ Surgical removal.
  ○ Radiation.
  ○ Embolisation.
  ○ Combination of the above techniques

238. According to FISCH classification, Glomus tumor invading the vertical part of carotid canal, belongs to:- *(PGMEE 2012, 2013)*
a. Type B   b. TypeC1
c. Type C2   d. Type C

[Ref: Internet]

Explanation

Fisch classification of Glomus tumor

- Type A Limited to the middle ear cavity (mesotympanum)
- Type B In the middle ear (meso- and hypotympanum) and the mastoid

228. c
229. b
230. a
231. d
232. a
233. c
234. a
235. d
236. a
237. d
238. c

- Type C Tumor invading the bone of the intralabyrinthine compartment.
  - C_1: Tumor with limited involvement of the vertical portion of carotid canal.
  - C_2: Invading vertical portion of carotid canal.
  - C_3: Invading horizontal portion of carotid canal.
- Type D Tumor with intracranial extension
  - D_1: Tumor with intracranial extension <2cm in diameter
  - D_2: Tumor with intracranial extension >2 cm in diameter.

FACIAL NERVE

239. Surgical landmark for finding the facial nerve is:-
(PGMEE 2015)
a. Cartilaginous (Tragus) pointer
b. Posterior belly of digastric
c. Tympano - mastoid suture
d. All the above

[Ref: Dhingra's 7th/e pg. 100]

240. Facial nerve exits the skull through- **(PGMEE 2015)**
a. Stylomastoid foramen
b. Foramen Lacerum
c. Foramen Rotundum
d. Internal acoustic meatus

[Ref: Dhingra's 7th/e pg. 99]

241. Shortest part of VIIth cranial nerve is in:
(DNB pattern 2007)
a. Pons
b. Stylomastoid region
c. Superior colliculus
d. Labyrinthine canal

[Ref: Dhingra's 7th/e pg. 99]

242. First branch of the facial nerve is - **(PGMEE 2012)**
a. Chorda-tympani nerve
b. Nerve to the stapedius
c. Greater superficial petrosal nerve
d. Lesser petrosal nerve

[Ref: Dhingra's 7th/e pg. 99]

LESIONS OF FACIAL NERVE

243. In facial nerve injury, loss of lacrimation is due to involvement of - **(PGMEE 2013)**
a. Greater superficial petrosal nerve
b. Buccal nerve
c. Chorda tympani nerve
d. Deep petrosal nerve

[Ref: Dhingra's 7th/e pg. 99]

244. In facial nerve injury, dryness of mouth is seen if injury occurs at:- **(PGMEE 2014)**
a. Geniculate ganglion
b. Concussion of tympanic membrane
c. Chorda tympani nerve
d. Cerebellopontine angle

[Ref: Dhingra's 7th/e pg. 99]

245. Facial nerve palsy is common in attempted removal of:-
(PGMEE 2016-17)
a. Vegetable in ear
b. Lithium battery in ear
c. Living insect in ear
d. None

[Ref: Internet, http://www.ijcmr.com]

239. d
240. a
241. d
242. c
243. a
244. c
245. b
246. b
247. b
248. a
249. d
250. a

246. Facial nerve injury with facial palsy and loss of tears, loss of taste and hyperacusis. Injury is at what level:-
a. Stylomastoid foramen **(PGMEE 2016-17)**
b. Geniculate ganglion
c. In internal acoustic meatus
d. Infrastapedial lesions

[Ref: Dhingra's 7th/e pg. 107 fig.]

247. In Ramsay Hunt syndrome, most commonly involved nerve is - **(PGMEE 2015)**
a. V
b. VII
c. VIII
d. IX

[Ref: Dhingra's 7th/e pg. 105]

248. Recurrent orofacial edema +recurrent facial palsy+fissured tongue is seen in:
(Recent Pattern June 2018)
a. Melkersson-Rosenthal Syndrome
b. Pierre Robins Syndrome
c. Ramsay Hunt syndrome
d. None

[Ref: Dhingra's 7th/e pg. 105]

Explanation

- Melkersson-Rosenthal syndrome is a rare neuro-mucocutaneous disease with a chronic intermittent course, characterized by a classic triad of:–
  - Orofacial swelling
  - Fissured tongue (lingua plicata)
  - Facial paralysis.

249. Bilateral facial nerve palsy is seen in - **(PGMEE 2012)**
a. Guillain Barre syndrome
b. Sarcoidosis
c. Sickle cell disease
d. All of the above

[Ref: Dhingra's 7th/e pg. 105]

Explanation

Recurrent facial palsy

- Recurrent facial palsy is seen in Bell palsy (3-10% cases), Melkersson syndrome, diabetes, sarcoidosis and tumours.
- Bells palsy is defined as idiopathic, peripheral facial paralysis or paresis of acute onset.
  - Any age group may be affected though incidence rises with increasing age.
  - A positive family history is present in 6-8% of patients.
  - Risk of Bell palsy is more in diabetics (angiopathy) and pregnant women (retention of fluid).
  - 80-95% patients recover fully.

Bilateral facial palsy

- Stimultaneously bilateral facial paralysis may be seen in Guillain-Barre syndrome, sarcoidosis, sickle cell disease, acute leukaemia, bulbar palsy, leprosy and some other systemic disorders.

250. Iatrogenic traumatic facial nerve palsy is most commonly caused during: **(DNB pattern 2009)**
a. Mastoidectomy
b. Stapedectomy
c. Ossiculoplasty
d. Myringoplasty

[Ref: Dhingra's 7th/e pg. 105]

251. Which of the following is not true about bell's palsy-

a. Always recurrent   **(PGMEE 2014)**

b. Increased predisposition in Diabetes Mellitus

c. Spontaneous remission

d. Acute onset

[Ref: Dhingra's 7th/e pg. 104]

Explanation

- Recurrent facial palsy is seen in Bell's palsy (3-10%) cases
- It is defined as idiopathic, peripheral facial paralysis or paresis of acute onset.
- Any age group may be affected though incidence rises with increasing age.
- A positive family history is present in 6-8% of patients.
- Risk of Bell palsy is more in diabetics (angiopathy) and pregnant women (retention of fluid)
- 80-95% patients recover fully

252. Commonest cause of facial palsy is:

(Recent Pattern June 2018)

a. Viral   b. Bacterial

c. Pressure induced   d. Idiopathic

[Ref: Dhingra's 7th/e pg. 108]

Explanation

- Bell's palsy is the most common cause of acute facial nerve paralysis.
- There is no known cause of Bell's palsy hence idiopathic (peripheral 7th cranial nerve paly), although it has been a/w herpes group (sometimes EBV) infection. About 50% of the cases of facial nerve palsy are idiopathic.
- Presumed mechanism is swelling/compression of the facial nerve due to an immune or viral disorder.
- Recent evidence suggests that herpes simplex virus infection is the MC cause and that herpes zoster may be the second MC viral cause.
- Other viruses involved in facial paralysis include coxsackievirus, CMV, adenovirus, and the EBV, mumps, rubella, and influenza B viruses.
- The swollen nerve is maximally compressed as it passes **through the labyrinthine portion of the facial canal**, resulting in ischemia and paresis.

253. Synkinesis is a sequel of -   **(PGMEE 2015)**

a. Facial nerve paralysis

b. Greater Petrosal nerve paralysis

c. Superficial temporal nerve paralysis

d. Trigeminal nerve paralysis

[Ref: Dhingra's 7th/e pg. 108]

254. True about Bell's palsy -   **(PGMEE 2012)**

a. Steroid are contraindicated

b. Antibiotics are mainstay of treatment

c. Central facial paralysis

d. Spontaneous recovery occurs in most of the cases

[Ref: Dhingra's 7th/e pg. 105]

255. All of the following are seen in Bell's palsy except -

a. Ipsilateral facial palsy   **(PGMEE 2012)**

b. Hyperacusis

c. Ipsilateral ptosis

d. Ipsilateral-loss of taste sensation

[Ref: Dhingra's 7th/e pg. 107, 108]

256. Supra nuclear lesion of facial nerve affects?

a. Lower part of face

b. Upper part of face

c. Both upper and lower face

d. Spares both upper and lower face

[Ref: Dhingra's 7th/e pg. 107]

Explanation

- It causes paralysis of only the lower half of face on the contralateral side.
- Forehead movements are retained due to bilateral innervation of frontalis muscle.
- Involuntary emotional movements and the tone of facial muscles are also retained.
- Facial nerve nucleus
  - Facial nerve is mixed nerve, motor nucleus of 7th nerve is situated in the pons
  - Upper part of the nucleus which innervates forehead muscles receive fibres from both the cerebral hemisphere so function of forehead is preserved in supranuclear lesions because of bilateral innervations.
  - Lower part of nucleus which supplies lower face gets only crossed fibres from one hemisphere
  - 7th nerve nucleus also received fibres from thalamus so emotional movements such as smiling and crying are preserved
- Course of facial nerve divided into-
  - Intracranial- brainstem to fundus of internal acoustic meatus is about 24 mm
  - Intratemporal part – from IAM to styloidmastoid foramen is about 28-30 mm. further divided into
  - Meatal segment – with in IAM, about 8-10 mm
  - Labyrinthine segment – from fundus of meatus to geniclate ganglion is about 4 mm and has narrowest diameter (.61–.68 mm)
  - Tympanic or horizontal segment – geniculate ganglion to pyramidal eminence is about 11 mm
  - Vertical or mastoid segment – pyramid to styloidmastoid foramen is about 13 mm.
  - Extracranial part: styloidmastoid foramen to termination of peripheral branch.

257. A patient presents to ENT clinic on day 3 after Bell's palsy. Best treatment for this patient is:-

(PGMEE 2015, 2012, 2013)

a. Intratympanic steroids

b. Vitamin B + vasodilators

c. Oral steroids + Acyclovir

d. Oral steroids + Vitamin B

[Ref: Dhingra's 7th/e pg. 104; IMPLANTS]

HEARING AIDS

258. Electrode of cochlear implant is placed at -

(PGMEE 2013)

a. Scala tympani

b. Scala media

c. Horizontal semicircular canal

d. Scala vestibuli

[Ref: Dhingra's 7th/e pg. 139]

251.	a
252.	d
253.	a
254.	d
255.	c
256.	a
257.	c
258.	a

259. Patient with anotia ideal hearing aid is - *(PGMEE 2015)*
   a. Vestibular
   b. Bone anchored hearing aid
   c. Pericanal device
   d. Transcutaneous

[Ref: Dhingra's 7th/e pg. 137]

Explanation

- Bone-anchored hearing aids can be used in
  - People who have chronic inflammation or infection of the ear canal and cannot wear standard "tin the ear" air-conduction hearing aids.
  - Children with malformed or absent outer ear and ear canals as in microtia or canal atresia.
  - Single-sided deafness

High-yield Points

Signs in ENT

- ✈ BATTLE SIGN- Bruising behind ear at mastoid region, due to petrous temporal bone# (middle fossa #).
- ✈ BOCCA'S SIGN - Absence of post cricoid crackle (Muir's crackle) in Carcinoma post. cricoid.
- ✈ BROWN SIGN - blanching of redness on increasing pressure more than systemic pressure see in glomus jugulare.
- ✈ BOYCE SIGN - Laryngocoele-Gurgling sound on compression of external laryngocoele with reduction of swelling.
- ✈ DODD'S SIGN/CRESCENT SIGN - X-ray finding-Crescent of air between the mass and posterior pharyngeal wall. Positive in AC ployp. Negative in Angiofibroma
- ✈ FURSTENBERGERS SIGN-This is seen when nasopharyngeal cyst is communicating intracranially,there is enlargement of the cyst on crying and upon compression of jugular vein.
- ✈ HITSELBERGER'S SIGN - In Acoustic neuroma- loss of sensation in the ear canal suppllied by Arnold's nerve (branch of Vagus nerve to ear)
- ✈ HOLMAN MILLER SIGN, ANTRAL SIGN-it is seen in angiofibroma,the tumor pushes forward on the posterior wall of the maxillary sinus..
- ✈ HONDOUSA SIGN--X-ray finding in Angiofibroma, indicating infratemporal fossa involvement characterised by widening of gap between ramus of mandible and maxillary body.
- ✈ HENNEBERT SIGN- false fistula sign(cong.syphilis, Meniere's,)
- ✈ IRWIN MOORE'S SIGN-------- positive squeeze test in chronic tonsillitis
- ✈ LIGHT HOUSE SIGN--- seeping out of secretions in acute OTITIS media
- ✈ LYRE'S SIGN - splaying of carotid vessels in carotid body tumor
- ✈ MILIAN'S EAR SIGN- Erysipelas can spread to pinna(cuticular affection), where as cellulitis cannot.
- ✈ PHELP'S SIGN - loss of crust of bone between carotid canal and jugular canal in glomus jugulare
- ✈ RACOON SIGN-Indicate subgaleal hemorrhage,and not necessarily base of skull #
- ✈ STEEPLE SIGN- X-ray finding in Acute Laryngo tracheo bronchitis
- ✈ STANKIEWICK'S SIGN - indicate orbital injury during FESS. fat protrudes into nasal cavity on compression of eye ball from ouside
- ✈ THUMB SIGN --X-ray finding A/c epiglottitis
- ✈ TRAGUS SIGN- EXTERNAL OTITIS, Pain on pressing Tragus
- ✈ TEA POT SIGN is seen in CSF rhinorrhoea.
- ✈ WOODS SIGN----- palpable jugulodigastric lymphnodes.

NOSE: ANATOMY

1. Middle superior alveolar nerve is a branch of:
(DNB pattern 2009)
a. Nasal branch of maxillary nerve
b. Mandibular branch of trigeminal nerve
c. Inferior alveolar
d. Infraorbital branch of maxillary nerve

[Ref: BD Chaurasia]

Explanation

- The middle superior alveolar nerve is a nerve that drops from the infraorbital portion of the maxillary nerve to supply the sinus mucosa, the roots of the maxillary premolars, and the mesiobuccal root of the first maxillary molar.

2. Nerve supply of tip of nose: *(PGMEE 2013)*
a. External nasal branch of ophthalmic division of trigeminal nerve
b. Buccal branch of mandibular nerve
c. Inferior orbital nerve
d. Orbital br of maxillary n
[Ref: BDC 7th/e vol. 3 pg.254 and 6th/e pg. 215]

3. Lymphatic drainage of anterior part of nose is to:
(PGMEE 2013)
a. Submandibular LN
b. Parotid
c. Retropharyngeal LN
d. Pretracheal LN
[Ref: BDC 8th/e vol. 3 pg. 277; Dhingra's 7th/e pg. 155]

4. What lies between the middle and inferior turbinate?
(PGMEE 2015)
a. Middle meatus b. Inferior meatus
c. Superior meatus d. Hiatus semilunaris
[Ref: Dhingra's 7th/e pg. 151 fig.]

5. Narrowest part of the nasal cavity is- *(PGMEE 2015)*
a. Middle turbinate
b. Choanae
c. Vestibule and internal nasal valve
d. Inferior turbinate
[Ref: Dhingra's 7th/e pg. 149]

6. Largest turbinate is: *(PGMEE 2012-13)*
a. Middle b. Inferior
c. Superior d. All are of the same size
[Ref: BDC 8th/e vol. 3 pg. 275]

Explanation

- The inferior turbinate is the largest turbinate and occupies the lower third of the lateral nasal wall. It arises from the medial wall of the maxillary sinus. Its anterior tip is located 1.5–2.0 cm inside the nasal space in adults, and the nasolacrimal duct empties into the inferior meatus

7. Which is an independent bone?
a. Superior turbinate b. Middle turbinate
c. Inferior turbinate d. All
[Ref: Dhingra's 7th/e pg. 150]

Explanation

- A series of elevations appear on the lateral wall of the nose from the sixth foetal week which will ultimately form the turbinates.
- The most inferior or maxilloturbinal forms the inferior turbinate. Inferior turbinate is a separate bone and below it ,into the inferior meatus, opens the nasolacrimal duct guarded at its terminal end by a mucosal valve called Hasner's valve.
- The middle, superior and supreme turbinates result from reduction of the complex ethmoturbinal system found in lower mammals.
- Similarly, the primitive nasoturbinal is represented by the agger nasi region and uncinate process of the ethmoid.
- The inferior concha has its own ossification centre which appears around the fifth intrauterine month.
- The turbinate possesses an impressive submucosal cavernous plexus with large sinusoids under autonomic control which provides the major contribution to nasal resistance.

8. True about external nose: *(PGMEE 2013)*
a. Upper 2/3 is bony
b. Lower 1/3 is cartilaginous
c. Single lateral cartilage
d. Bony part consist of two nasal bones
[Ref: Dhingra's 7th/e pg. 149]

9. Osteomeatal complex [OMC] connects- *(PGMEE 2015)*
a. The two nasal cavities
b. Nasal cavity with sphenoid sinus
c. Nasal cavity with maxillary, ethmoid & frontal sinus
d. Ethmoidal sinus with ethmoidal bulla
[Ref: S.K. De 9th/e pg. 161]

10. Nasal valve is formed by - *(PGMEE 2013, 2016-17)*
a. Upper lateral cartilage
b. Lower lateral cartilage
c. Upper end of lower lateral cartilage
d. Lower end of upper lateral cartilage
[Ref: Dhingra's 7th/e pg. 149]

11. Hiatus semilunaris is present in - *(PGMEE 2014)*
a. Superior meatus
b. Spenoethmoidal recess
c. Inferior meatus
d. Middle meatus

[Ref: Dhingra's 7th/e pg. 150]

1.	d
2.	a
3.	a
4.	a
5.	c
6.	b
7.	c
8.	d
9.	c
10.	d
11.	d

12. Bony nasal septum is formed by all except:
a. Sphenoid
b. Vomer *(PGMEE 2012-13)*
c. Ethmoid
d. Nasal spine of nasal bone
[Ref: BDC 8th/e vol. 3 pg. 273; Dhingra's 7th/e pg. 165]

Explanation

Septum Proper

- It consists of osteocartilaginous framework.
- The bony part is formed almost entirely by
  ○ The vomer
  ○ The perpendicular plate of ethmoid bone. However, its margins receive contribution from the crest of nasal bones, nasal spine of frontal bone, rostrum of sphenoid, crest of palatine & maxilla.
- The cartilaginous part is formed by:-
  ○ A large septal (quadrilateral) cartilage wedged between the above two bones anteriorly.
  ○ The septal processes of the inferior nasal cartilages.

13. Olfactory region in nose is: *(PGMEE 2012-13)*
a. Between middle & inferior turbinate
b. Above superior turbinate
c. Below inferior turbinate
d. None
[Ref: BDC 8th/e vol. 3 pg. 276]

14. Cribriform plate is a part which bone? *(PGMEE 2013)*
a. Ethmoid
b. Maxilla
c. Frontal
d. Nasal
[Ref: BDC 8th/e vol. 3 pg. 273; Dhingra's 7th/e pg. 153]

15. Odour receptor present in? *(PGMEE 2011)*
a. Neurons of olfactory epithelium
b. Olfactory bulbs
c. Amygdala
d. Olfactory tract

12.	d
13.	b
14.	a
15.	a
16.	b
17.	c
18.	d
19.	a
20.	b
21.	c
22.	d

Explanation

- The olfactory epithelium is a pseudostratified columnar neuroepithelium containing supporting cells, bipolar olfactory receptor neurons, and dividing basal cells located in the superior cleft between the middle and superior turbinates and the septum.
- The axons extending from the receptor neurons coalesce into bundles (cranial nerve I) that travel through the cribriform plate to make primary synapses with the olfactory bulb.
- Which individual odorant receptor types that are randomly distributed among zones within the olfactory mucosa converge to form synapses in specific glomeruli.
- The most common reasons for olfactory loss include chronic rhinosinusitis and polyps, upper respiratory infections, head trauma, and aging.
- Patient history is extremely important in determining etiology of olfactory disorders.
- Patchy replacement of olfactory mucosa with respiratory epithelium appears to be common with aging. Alzheimer's disease is closely correlated with olfactory loss independent of aging.
- Chronic rhinosinusitis can cause both a conductive loss of olfaction and a sensorineural loss.
- Nasal endoscopy is extremely useful in assessing obstruction of the olfactory cleft.

- Computed tomography scans are helpful in assessing conductive losses and chronic rhinosinusitis. Magnetic resonance imaging can be helpful if there are neurologic signs suggesting mass lesion or neurodegenerative disease.
- Patient support and counseling of hazards associated with the loss of smell are an important part of the patient visit.

16. Olfactory nerve fibres passes through? *(PGMEE 2013)*
a. Supraorbital foramen
b. Cribriform plate
c. Foramen ovale
d. Foramen rotundum
[Ref: BDC 8th/e vol. 3 pg. 273; Dhingra's 7th/e pg. 153]

Explanation

- Middle horizontal part of root is formed by the cribriform plate ethmoid through which the olfactory nerves enter the nasal cavity.

17. The maxillary sinus opens into middle meatus at the level of - *(PGMEE 2015)*
a. Infundibulum
b. Bulla ethmoidalis
c. Hiatus semilunaris
d. None of the above
[Ref: Dhingra's 7th/e pg. 151]

18. Ethmoidal sinus opens into which of the following: *(PGMEE 2012-13)*
a. Middle meatus
b. Hiatus semilunaris
c. Superior meatus
d. All of the above
[Ref: BDC 8th/e vol. 3 pg. 276]

19. Sphenoid sinus drains into which of the following: *(PGMEE 2012-13; PGMEE 2014)*
a. Spheno-ethmoidal recess
b. Superior meatus
c. Middle meatus
d. Hiatus semilunaris
[Ref: BDC 8th/e vol. 3 pg. 276; Dhingra's 7th/e pg. 151]

20. All open into middle meatus EXCEPT: *(PGMEE 2013)*
a. Frontal sinus
b. Sphenoid sinus
c. Ethmoidal sinus
d. Maxillary sinus
[Ref: BDC 7th/e vol. 3 pg. 253]

21. Paranasal sinuses are divided into anterior and posterior group in relation to: *(PGMEE 2014)*
a. Bulla ethmoidalis
b. Inferior turbinate
c. Middle turbinate
d. Superior turbinate
[Ref: Mohan Bansal p. 37; Dhingra's 7th/e pg. 209]

Explanation

- Anterior group
  ○ This includes maxillary, frontal and anterior ethmoidal.
  ○ They all open in the middle meatus and their ostia lie anterior to basal lamella of middle turbinate.
- Posterior group
  ○ This includes posterior ethmoidal sinuses which open in the superior meatus and the sphenoid sinus which opens in sphenoethmoidal recess.

22. All are part of ethmoid bone except: *(PGMEE 2014)*
a. Bulla ethmoidalis
b. Agger nasi
c. Uncinate process
d. Inferior turbinate
[Ref: Essentials of clinical anatomy p. 19]

23. Uncinate process arises from: *(PGMEE 2014)*
a. Superior meatus   b. Middle meatus
c. Maxilla   d. Nasal bone

[Ref: Dhingra's 7th/e pg. 150]

24. Nasolacrimal duct opens in-
(PGMEE 2016-17, 2014-15, 2012-13)
a. Inferior nasal meatus
b. Maxillary sinus
c. Superior nasal meatus
d. Middle nasal meatus

[Ref: Dhingra's 7th/e pg. 150]

25. Valve of Hasner is found at/gaurds: *(PGMEE 2013)*
a. Opening of nasolacrimal duct
b. Frontal sinus opening
c. Sphenoidal sinus opening
d. Ethmoidal sinus opening

[Ref: Dhingra's 7th/e pg. 150]

26. Valve of Rosenmuller is located at:
(PGMEE 2014)
a. Opening of nasolacrimal duct
b. Cystic duct
c. Junction of lacrimal sac and canaliculus
d. None

[Ref: Internet]

Explanation

Valve of Rosenmuller.
- A fold of mucous membrane found at the junction between the common canaliculus and the lacrimal sac. It is not strictly a valve because fluids can be blown back to emerge at the puncta.

27. In DCR (dacrocystorhinostomy) opening of NLD is made in:- *(PGMEE 2016-17)*
a. Inferior meatus
b. Middle meatus
c. Superior meatus
d. Posterior to inferior meatus

[Ref: Parson's Diseases of the Eye 22nd/e pg.477]

28. Concha bullosa is :- *(PGMEE 2016-17)*
a. Aerated middle turbinate
b. Aerated superior turbinate
c. Infection of nasal bulla
d. Middle ear streptococcus infection

[Ref: Dhingra's 7th/e pg. 153]

29. Ethmoidal infundibulum lies between - *(PGMEE 2015)*
a. Bulla ethmoidalis and uncinate process of ethmoid
b. Wing of sphenoid and maxillary antrum
c. Hiatus semilunaris and Inferior meatus
d. Middle and inferior turbinate

[Ref: Dhingra's 7th/e pg. 151]

30. Ethmoidal Bullae are seen in- *(PGMEE 2015)*
a. Middle ethmoid air cells
b. Superior ethmoidal air cells
c. Posterior ethmoidal air cels
d. Inferior ethmoidal air cells

[Ref: Dhingra's 7th/e pg. 151]

31. All of the following structures open into hiatus semi-lunaris except: *(DNB 2008)*
a. Maxillary sinus
b. Posterior ethmoid sinus
c. Anterior ethmoid sinus
d. Frontal sinus

[Ref: Dhingra's 7th/e pg. 151]

CSF RHINORRHOEA

32. Intrathecal fluorescein with endoscopic visualization is useful in diagnosis of- *(PGMEE 2015)*
a. Rhinitis Medicamentosa
b. Multiple ethmoidal polyps
c. CSF Rhinorrhoea
d. Deviated nasal septum

[Ref: Dhingra's 7th/e pg. 183]

33. The most common site of leak in CSF rhinorrhoea is:
(DNB 2007; PGMEE 2012, AI 05)
a. Frontal sinus   b. Sphenoid sinus
c. Cribriform plate   d. Tegmen tympani

[Ref: Dhingra's 7th/e pg. 183]

34. Most common cause of leakage of CSF through nose-
(PGMEE 2014)
a. Intracranial infection   b. Itrogenic trauma
c. Accidental trauma   d. Congenital defects

[Ref: Dhingra's 7th/e pg. 183]

35. Queckensted test in done for – *(PGMEE 2013)*
a. Beta 2 microglobulin   b. Acoustic neuroma
c. Otosclerosis   d. CSF spinal block

[Ref: Dhingra 6th/e pg.165]

36. Target sign is seen in a blot test from nasal discharge in which of these condition? *(NEET Pattern 2017)*
a. Traumatic CSF leak   b. Fracture mastoid
c. Spontaneous CSF leak   d. Meningoencephalocele

[Ref: Dhingra's 7th/e pg. 184]

Explanation
- In traumatic CSF leak, when CSF is mixed with blood Target sign (or Double ring sign) is helpful in differentiation of CSF from nasal discharge
- In this sign discharge collected on a piece of filter paper shows a central spot of blood while CSF spread out like a halo around it.

37. CSF rhinorrhoea is diagnosed by *(PGMEE 2015)*
a. Thyroglobulin
b. Beta 2 transferrin
c. Beta 2 microglobulin
d. Transthyretin

[Ref: Dhingra's 7th/e pg. 184]

38. In evaluation of a case of immotile nasal cilia, which of the following investigation should prove useful?
a. Sweat sodium levels   *(PGMEE 2015)*
b. Nitric oxide test
c. Xray nasal and paranasal sinuses
d. Rhinogram

[Ref: Dhingra 6th/e pg.164]

23.	b
24.	a
25.	a
26.	c
27.	b
28.	a
29.	a
30.	a
31.	b
32.	c
33.	c
34.	c
35.	d
36.	a
37.	b
38.	b

39. Management for CSF rhinorrhoea is *(PGMEE 2015)*
   a. Immediate surgery
   b. Plain X-ray and packing of nose
   c. Nasal packing only
   d. Antibiotics and observation

[Ref: Dhingra 7th /e pg. 185]

EXTERNAL NOSE AND NASAL DEFORMITIES

40. All are true about nasolabial cyst except: *(DNB 2009)*
   a. Bilateral
   b. Usually seen in adults
   c. Presents submucosally in anterior nasal floor
   d. Arises from odontoid epithelium

[Ref: Cummins Oto laryngology, 4th/e pg. 1527]

41. Potato tumor is – *(PGMEE 2013)*
   a. Rhinosporidiosis
   b. Tubercular infection
   c. Nosopharyngeal angiofibroma
   d. Hypertrophied sebaceous gland

[Ref: Dhingra's 7th/e pg. 162]

Explanation

  ▪ Rhinophyma or potato tumour is a slow-growing benign tumour due to hypertrophy of the sebaceous glands of the top of nose often seen in cases of long-standing acne rosacea.
  ▪ It presents as a pink, lobulated mass over the nose.

42. Crooked nose is due to? *(PGMEE 2012-13)*
   a. Deviated dorsum and septum
   b. Deviated Ala
   c. Hump in nasal septum
   d. Deviated septum

[Ref: Dhingra's 7th/e pg. 161]

43. Saddle nose is – *(PGMEE 2013)*
   a. Deviated nose   b. Crooked nose
   c. Depressed nose   d. C-shaped

[Ref: Dhingra's 7th/e pg. 161]

44. All of the following are causes of saddle nose deformity except – *(PGMEE 2015)*
   a. Sarcoidosis   b. Hematoma
   c. Leprosy   d. Trauma

[Ref: Dhingra's 7th/e pg. 161]

45. Most common cause of saddle nose deformity is - *(PGMEE 2015)*
   a. Lupus Vulgaris   b. Secondary syphilis
   c. Tertiary syphilis d. Trauma to the nose

[Ref: Dhingra's 7th/e pg. 161]

Explanation

  ▪ Depressed nasal dorsum may involve bony, cartilaginous or both
  ▪ Nasal trauma causing depressed fractures is the most common aetiology.
  ▪ Excessive removal of septum
  ▪ Destruction of septal cartilage by haematoma or abscess, sometimes by leprosy, tuberculosis or syphilis.

39.	d
40.	d
41.	d
42.	a
43.	c
44.	a
45.	d
46.	c
47.	d
48.	a
49.	b
50.	a

46. A 55 year old diabetic patient presents with blackish nasal discharge and a blackish mass is the nose which is rapidly destructive, most likely diagnosis is: *(PGMEE 2012-13; DNB 2010)*
   a. Sporotrichosis   b. Actinomycosis
   c. Mucormycosis   d. Rhinosporiodosis

[Ref: Dhingra's 7th/e pg. 178]

CHOANAL ATRESIA

47. Choanal atresia is most commonly due to-
   a. Presence of gingivonasal covering *(PGMEE 2015)*
   b. Due to respiratory distress at birth
   c. Presence of nasal synechiae
   d. Persistence of bucconasal membrane

[Ref: Dhingra's 7th/e pg. 183]

Explanation

Choanal Atresia

  ▪ Choanal Atresia is due to persistence of bucconasal membrane
  ▪ May U/L or B/L, unilateral is most common
  ▪ Bony (90%) or membranous (10%)
  ▪ B/L atresia presents with respiratory obstruction and surgical emergency as newborn is natural nose breather.
  ▪ D/g by
    ○ Failure to pass a catheler from nose to pharynx
    ○ Putting a few drop of dye (methylene blue) into nose & seeing its passage into pharynx.
    ○ Putting radio opaque dye into the nose & taking a lateral film.
  ▪ Treatment
    ○ A feeding nipple with a large hole provides a good oral airway (*Mc Govern's technique*)
    ○ Definitive treatment by Transnasal or transpalatal approach usually at 1.5 yrs of age. It is corrected by nasal endoscope and drill.

48. Which of the following is a surgical emergency? *(PGMEE 2012-13)*
   a. Bilateral choanal atresia
   b. Laryngocele
   c. Laryngomalacia
   d. Unilateral choanal atresia

[Ref: Dhingra's 7th/e pg. 183]

DISEASES OF NASAL SEPTUM

49. Shape of nasal septum is :- *(PGMEE 2016-17)*
   a. Triangular   b. Quadrilateral
   c. Square   d. Rectangular

[Ref: Dhingra's 7th/e pg. 166 fig.]

50. Septal perforation is not seen in: *(DNB 2010)*
   a. Rhinophyma   b. Septal abscess
   c. Trauma   d. Leprosy

[Ref: Dhingra's 7th/e pg. 168]

51. Nasal septum perforation occurs in all the following except - *(PGMEE 2012)*
 a. Syphilis b. Nasal surgery
 c. Tuberculosis d. Rhinosporidiosis

[Ref: Dhingra's 7th/e pg. 168]

52. Cottle's test is used to test patency of nares in :
 a. Atrophic rhinitis *(PGMEE 2014, 2015)*
 b. Rhinosporidosis
 c. Antrochoanal polyp
 d. Deviated nasal septum

[Ref: Dhingra's 7th/e pg. 167]

53. Submucosal resection is the treatment of choice of:-
 a. Nasal polyp *(PGMEE 2015)*
 b. DNS in adults
 c. Sluder's Neuralgia
 d. DNS in children

[Ref: Dhingra's 7th/e pg. 168]

54. After DNS operation pig snout deformity is caused by:- *(PGMEE 2016-17)*
 a. Excessive removal of dorsal strut of the septum
 b. Removal of columella cartilage
 c. Septal perforation
 d. All of the above

[Ref: Internet link http://www.drtbalu.com]

55. All of the following are features of nasal foreign body except- *(PGMEE 2015)*
 a. Septal perforation b. Nasal obstruction
 c. Epistaxis d. Foul smelling discharge

[Ref: Dhingra's 7th/e pg. 181]

56. All of the following are causes of perforation of cartilaginous part of nasal septum except- *(PGMEE 2015)*
 a. Leprosy b. Lupus
 c. Tuberculosis d. Syphilis

[Ref: Dhingra's 7th/e pg. 169]

Explanation
- Chronic granulomatous conditions like lupus, tuberculosis and leprosy cause perforation in the cartilaginous part while syphilis involves the bony part

57. Nose is commonly involved in:- *(PGMEE 2013)*
 a. Primary stage of syphilis
 b. Secondary stage of syphilis
 c. Tertiary stage of syphilis
 d. Equally involved in all stages

[Ref: Dhingra's 7th/e pg. 168]

58. Apple jelly nodules on the nasal septum are found in cases of - *(PGMEE 2014)*
 a. Tuberculosis b. Syphilis
 c. Lupus Vulgaris d. Rhinoscleroma

[Ref: Dhingra's 7th/e pg. 176]

59. Treatment of septal hematoma is? *(DNB Dec'2011, PGMEE 2014)*
 a. Incision and drainage b. Nasal packing
 c. Antibiotics d. Nasal decongestants

[Ref: Dhingra's 7th/e pg. 168]

Explanation

Septal Hematoma
- It is collection of blood under the pericondrium or periosteum of the nasal septum. It often results from nasal trauma or septal surgery. In bleeding disorders, it may occur spontaneously.
- Small haematomas can be aspirated with a wide bore sterile needle.
- Larger haematomas are incised and drained by a small antero-posterior incision parallel to the nasal floor. Excision of a small piece of mucosa from the edge of incision gives better drainage.
- Following drainage, nose is packed on both sides to prevent re accumulation .Systemic antibiotics should be given, to prevent septal abscess

60. Nasal bone fracture is corrected by? *(PGMEE 2016-17)*
 a. Citelli's forceps b. Luc's forceps
 c. Tilly's forceps d. Walsham's forceps

[Ref: Dhingra's 7th/e pg. 517]

Explanation
- Walsham's forceps used for the disimpacting and reducing fracture of nasal bone.
- Asch's forceps for reducing fractures of nasal septum.
- Tilley's forcep used for nasal packing, ear dressing.
- Luc's forceps used in Caldwell-luc operation, septoplasty, polypectomy, to take biopsy.

OTHER DISEASES OF NOSE

61. A roomy nasal cavity with thick crust formation and woody hard external nose is seen in? *(DNB Dec'2011)*
 a. Rhinoscleroma b. Vasomotor rhinitis
 c. Atrophic rhinitis d. Rhinosporidiosis

[Ref: Dhingra's 7th/e pg. 175]

Explanation
- Rhinoscleroma resembles atrophic rhinitis in clinical features in early stage with woody nose an additional feature.
- **ATROPHIC RHINITIS (OZAENA)**
  - It is a chronic inflammation of nose characterised by atrophy of nasal mucosa and turbinate bones. The nasal cavities are roomy and full of foul-smelling crusts.
  - Atrophic rhinitis is of two types:primary and secondary.
  - Atrophic rhinitis has been attributed to infection from bacteria, such as Klebsiella ozaenae.
  - secondary atrophic rhinitis, which may result from chronic granulomatous infections, infectious rhinosinusitis, irradiation, radical nasal surgery and trauma.
  - Pathology-
    - Ciliated columnar epithelium is lost and is replaced by stratified squamous type.
    - There is a trophy of seromucinous glands, venous blood sinusoids and nerve elements.

51.	d
52.	d
53.	b
54.	a
55.	a
56.	d
57.	c
58.	c
59.	a
60.	d
61.	a

81. Lines of Sebileau pass through- *(PGMEE 2015)*
a. Floor of orbit and nasal cavity
b. Floor of nasal cavity and maxillary antrum
c. Floor of orbit and floor of maxillary antrum
d. Floor of orbit and roof of mouth

[Ref: Dhingra 7th/e pg. 233]

Explanation

- Lederman's classification
  - It uses two horizontal lines of Sebileau; one passing through the floors of orbits and the other through floors of antra.

82. Which sinus is absent at birth: *(PGMEE 2014)*
a. Frontal
b. Maxillary
c. Ethmioid
d. None of the above

[Ref: Dhingra's 7th/e pg. 211]

83. Paranasal sinuses present at birth - *(PGMEE 2013)*
a. Frontal and ethmoid
b. Ethmoid and maxillary
c. Frontal and maxillary
d. Sphenoid and ethmoid

[Ref: Dhingra's 7th/e pg. 211; Textbook of human embryology p. 819]

84. First paranasal sinus to develop at birth is *(PGMEE 2012; 98)*
a. Maxillary
b. Sphenoidal
c. Frontal
d. Ethmoidai

[Ref: Dhingra's 7th/e pg. 211]

85. Which of the following sinus grow till early adulthood? *(NEET Pattern 2017)*
a. Frontal
b. Ethmoid
c. Sphenoid
d. Maxillary

[Ref: B D Chaurasia vol.3 7th/e pg. 255]

81.	c
82.	a
83.	b
84.	a
85.	a
86.	d
87.	d
88.	c
89.	d

Explanation

The Development of the Sinuses

Sinus	Gestational month when development starts	Present in clinically significant size	Fullly developed
Maxillary	2	Birth	12 years
Ethmoid	3	Birth	12 years
Frontal	4	3 years	18-20 years
Sphenoid	3	8 years	12-15 years

- Maxillary sinus –
  - begin to develop during late fetal life.
  - Small at birth
  - Grow slowly until ouberty and are not fully developed until all of the permenant teeth have erupted in early adulthood
- Frontal or sphenoid – not seen at birth.
- Ethmoidal sinuses – small before 2 years and they do not grow rapidly until 6 to 8 years of age
- Frontal sinuses visible on the radiograph by radiograph by 7 years

86. Maxillary sinus fully develops at the age of:- *(PGMEE 2016-17)*
a. 2 months
b. 6 months
c. 2 years
d. 15 years

[Ref: Dhingra's 7th/e pg. 211]

87. Which facial sinus continues to grow even in adulthood? *(NEET Pattern 2017)*
a. Frontal
b. Maxillary
c. Ethmoid
d. Sphenoid

[Ref: Dhingra's 7th/e pg. 211]

Explanation

Maxillary Sinus
- Present at birth
- Rapidly grows from birth to 3 yrs and from 7 to 12 yrs
- Adult size at 15 years of age

Ethmoid Sinus
- Present at birth

Frontal Sinus
- Not present at birth
- Invade frontal bone at age of 4 yrs
- Size increase until teens

Sphenoid Sinus
- Not present at birth
- Reach sella turcica by age of 7yrs
- Dorsum sella by late teens
- Reaches full size b/w 15 yrs to adulthood.

88. Which among the following sinuses is most commonly affected in a child - *(PGMEE 2014)*
a. Sphenoid
b. Maxillary
c. Ethmoid
d. Frontal

[Ref: Dhingra's 7th/e pg. 216]

89. Water's view is done to visualize which of the following sinus? *(PGMEE 2018)*
a. Frontal
b. Ethmoidal
c. Sphenoidal
d. Maxillary

[Ref: Dhingra's 7th/e pg. 493]

Explanation

- *Water's view* is used to visualize Maxillary sinuses.
  - Also called occipitomental view
  - Nose and chin of the patient touches the film while x-ray beam is projected 45 degree to the orbitomeatal line
  - Sphenoid sinus also seen if film is taken with open mouth
- *Caldwell's view* (or Occipitofrontal view) is a radiographic view of skull, where
  - X-ray plate is angled at 20° to orbitomeatal line.
  - The rays pass from behind the head and are perpendicular to radiographic plate.
  - It is commonly used to get better view of frontal and ethmoid sinuses.
- Submentovertical/Basal view **(Hirtz view)** is best for sphenoid sinus.

View	Used for
Occipitofrontal view	Superior orbital fissure
Periorbital view	Internal auditory meatus
Occipitofrontal (Caldwell's view)	Pterygoid canal
Submentovertical view (Hirtz view)	Best for sphenoid sinus, also used for Carotid canal, Foramen ovale, Foramen Spinosum, Foramen Magnum, Jugular Foramen
Rheese view	Optic foramen
Reversed stenver's view	Hypoglossal canal

90. Onodi cells and Haller cells are seen in relation to following respectively - *(PGMEE 2011; 09)*

a. Optic nerve and nasolacrimal duct
b. Optic nerve and internal carotid artery
c. Optic nerve and floor of the orbit
d. Orbital floor and nasolacrimal duct

[Ref: Dhingra's 7th/e pg. 210]

91. Maxillary sinus epithelium is - *(PGMEE 2014)*

a. Keratinized squamous
b. Non ciliated columnar
c. Squamous
d. Ciliated columnar

[Ref: Dhingra's 7th/e pg. 211]

92. Antrum of Highmore is – *(PGMEE 2012)*

a. Maxillary
b. Frontal
c. Sphenoid
d. Ethmoid

[Ref: Dhingra's 7th/e pg. 209]

SINUSITIS

93. Sinus which is least involved in isolated sinusitis :- *(PGMEE 2012)*

a. Sphenoid
b. Maxillary
c. Frontal
d. Ethmoid

[Ref: Dhingra's 7th/e pg. 216]

94. Most common sinus to be involved in acute sinusitis- *(PGMEE 2013)*

a. Frontal
b. Maxillary
c. Sphenoid
d. Ethmoid

[Ref: Dhingra 7th/e pg. 214; S.K. De 9th/e pg. 220]

Explanation

- It is the commonest of all sinus infection.
- Source of infection is usually from nose or dental sepsis from upper jaw as the roots of premolar and molar teeth lie close to the floor of the maxillary antrum.

95. Symptoms of sinusitis are all EXCEPT: - *(PGMEE 2013)*

a. Nasal blockage
b. Facial congestion
c. Halitosis
d. Nasal congestion

[Ref: Dhingra's 7th/e pg. 213]

96. Patient with toothache and sinusitis. Which sinus is involved- *(PGMEE 2013)*

a. Frontal
b. Ethmoid
c. Maxillary
d. Sphenoid

[Ref: Dhingra's 7th/e pg. 214]

97. Which of the following is false regarding frontal sinusitis- *(PGMEE 2015)*

a. Pain shows periodicity
b. Tenderness is present just above the medial canthus of eye
c. Pain is referred to as office headache
d. Most common sinus involved in infants and children

[Ref: Dhingra's 7th/e pg. 215]

Explanation

Headache/Pain in sinusitis

- Maxillary sinusitis
  - Headache usually confined to forehead and may thus confused with frontal sinusitis.
- Fronal sinusitis
  - It show characteristic periodicity - come on waking gradually increases and reaches its peak by about mid day and start subsiding so called 'office-headache' because of presence during office hours.
- Ethmoid sinusitis
  - It localised over bridge of the nose, medial & deep to the eye, aggravated by movement of eye ball.
- Sphenoid sinusitis
  - Usually localised to the occiput or vertex region.

98. A 55 year old patient presents with seeing double, periorbital edema and headache. He has BP 130/80 mmHg. On evaluation he was found to have fever. Opthalmologist finds gaze palsy with ptosis and dilated pupil. Most likely cause is: *(PGMEE 2012-13)*

a. Infection within venous sinuses
b. Mandibular nerve palsy
c. Immunological disease
d. Infection of orbit

[Ref: Dhingra's 7th/e pg. 226]

99. Orbital cellulitis most commonly occurs after infection of which sinus: *(DNB 2011)*

a. Maxillary sinus
b. Sphenoid sinus
c. Frontal sinus
d. Ethmoid sinus

[Ref: Dhingra's 7th/e pg. 226]

90.	c
91.	d
92.	a
93.	a
94.	b
95.	c
96.	c
97.	d
98.	a
99.	d

Explanation

- Most important and frequent acute complication of ethmoid rhinosinusitis is orbital cellulitis

Complications of rhinosinusitis-

- Orbital: Orital cellulitis is clinically classified into five stages:
- Preseptal cellulitis- Inflammation does not extend beyond the orbital septum (the site at which the medial orbital periosteal reflection attaches to the medial eyelid at the tarsal plate).
- Postseptal cellulitis or orbital cellulitis without abscess. Inflammation extends into the tissues of the orbit.
- Subperiosteal abscess-There is abscess formation deep to the periosteum of the orbital bones, usually the lamina papyracea.
- Orbital abscess-There is abscess formation within the orbit which has breached the periosteum.

- Cavernous sinus thrombosis/abscess- The inflammatory process has extended through the optic foramen into the cavernous sinus which thromboses and possibly progresses to abscess formation
- Sphenoid rhinosinusitis can result in cavernous sinus thrombosis by direct spread
  ○ Intracranial:
    - Meningitis
    - Epidural abscess
    - Subdural abscess
    - Intracerebral abscess
    - Cavernous or sagittal sinus thrombosis
  ○ Bony: osteomyelitis (pott's puffy tumor)
  ○ Mucocoele/pyocoele

100. All of the following are complication of maxillary sinus lavage and insufflations except- *(PGMEE 2015)*
a. Facial nerve injury
b. Orbital injury
c. Epistaxis
d. Air embolism

[Ref: Dhingra's 6th/e pg. 465]

101. Most definitive diagnosis of sinusitis is: *(PGMEE 2013)*
a. Sinuscopy
b. Proof puncture
c. X- ray PNS
d. Transillumination test

[Ref: Dhingra 6th/e p. 187]

102. Endoscopic sinus surgery prerequisite- *(PGMEE 2013)*
a. Mucocilliary clearing testing
b. CT of PNS
c. MRI of paranasal sinus
d. Acoustic tests

[Ref: Dhingra's 7th/e pg. 477]

103. Most common complication of Sinusitis is: *(PGMEE 2012)*
a. Meningitis
b. Septicemia
c. Brain abscess
d. Orbital cellulitis

[Ref: Dhingra's 7th/e pg. 216, 225]

104. Most common cause of fungal sinusits - *(PGMEE 2013)*
a. Candida
b. Aspergillus niger
c. Aspergillus flavus
d. Aspergillus fumigatus

[Ref: Dhingra 6th/e p. 196; S.K. De 9th/e pg. 229]

105. Pneumatocele is seen in fracture of – *(PGMEE 2014)*
a. Maxillary sinus
b. Sphenoid sinus
c. Ethmoid sinus
d. Frontal sinus

106. Mucocele is commonly seen in which sinus. *(DNB 2007)*
a. Frontal
b. Sphenoid
c. Maxillary
d. Ethmoid

[Ref: Dhingra's 7th/e pg. 223]

100.	a
101.	a
102.	b
103.	d
104.	d
105.	d
106.	a
107.	b
108.	c
109.	c
110.	a
111.	a

107. Pott's puffy tumour is:
(Recent Pattern June 2018, PGMEE 2019)
a. Subperiosteal abscess of ethmoid bone
b. Subperiosteal abscess of frontal bone
c. Mucocele of frontal bone
d. Mucocoele of ethmoid bone

[Ref: Dhingra's 7th/e pg. 224]

Explanation

- Pott's Puffy tumor occurs if infection of frontal sinusitis spreads to the marrow of the frontal bone, causing localized osteomyelitis with bone destruction that can result in collection of pus under periosteum and doughy swelling of the forehead.
- Surgical drainage and débridement must be undertaken

108. Most common site for osteoma among PNS -
(DNB Dec'2011; PGMEE 2013)
a. Maxillary sinus
b. Sphenoid sinus
c. Frontal sinus
d. Ethmoid sinus

[Ref: Dhingra's 7th/e pg. 231; S.K. De 9th/e pg. 235]

Explanation

Osteoma

- Localised ivory osteoma
  ○ Occurs commonly in the frontal sinus.
  ○ It is ivory hard in consistency
- Cancellous osteoma
  ○ Occurs commonly in the maxillary and the ethmoid sinuses.
  ○ It can grow rapidly in younger patients.

MALIGNANCY OF PARANASAL SINUS

109. Sinonasal neoplasm is commonly seen in which industry- *(PGMEE 2014)*
a. Fishing
b. Building
c. Hard wood
d. Iron steel

[Ref: Dhingra's 7th/e pg. 231]

Explanation

- People working in hardwood furniture industry, nickel refining, leather work and manufacture of mustard gas have shown higher incidence of sinunasal cancer.

110. Wood workers are associated sinus Ca-
(PGMEE 2012, 06)
a. Adeno Ca
b. Sq. cell Ca
c. Anaplastic Ca
d. Melanoma

[Ref: Dhingra 7th/e pg. 231]

Explanation

- Worker of furniture industry develop adenocarcinoma of the ethmoids and upper nasal cavity, while those engaged in nickel refining get squamous cell and anaplastic carcinoma.

111. Ohngren's line passes from - *(PGMEE 2015)*
a. Medial canthus to angle of mandible
b. Lateral canthus to mastoid process
c. Medial canthus to mastoid process
d. Lateral canthus to angle of mandible

[Ref: Dhingra 7th/e pg. 233]

Explanation

- Ohngren's line extends from medial canthus of eye to the angle of mandible.
- Growths anteroinferior to this plane (infrastructural) have a better prognosis than those posterosuperior to it (suprastructural)

112. Maxillary carcinoma in a 60 year old male involving anterolateral part of maxilla preferred treatment is - *(PGMEE 2015)*

a. Radiotherapy followed by total/extended maxillectomy
b. Total/extended Maxillectomy followed by radiotherapy
c. Radiotherapy only
d. Total/extended maxillectomy alone

[Ref: S.K. De 9th/e pg.239]

EPISTAXIS

113. Epistaxis in elderly person is commonly due to: *(PGMEE 2012-13 & 2014-15)*

a. Allergic rhinitis
b. Foregin body
c. Hypertension
d. Nasopharyngeal carcinoma

[Ref: Dhingra 7ᵗʰ/e pg. 158; S.K. De 9th/e pg. 214]

Explanation

Age group

- Epistaxis can occur in any age group, but aetiology varies:
  - **Children:** Commonest cause is anterior *epistaxis from Little's area* either spontaneous or due to nose picking; other causes are injury nose, exanthematous fevers, foreign body nose, diphtheretic rhinitis, enlarged adenoids, etc.
  - **Adolescents and young adult:** *Juvenile nasopharyngeal angio-fibroma* (in male) *should be suspected first* ; other causes are trauma, sinusitis, etc.
  - **Adult:** Acute and chronic sinusitis, injury nose (playing, boxing, etc.) head injury, specific rhinitis, etc.
  - **Elderly : Hypertension is the commonest cause**

114. Which artery is responsible for epistaxis after ligating of external carotid artery? *(PGMEE Dec'2011)*

a. Ethmoidal artery
b. Ascending pharyngeal.
c. Superior labial artery
d. Greater palatine artery

[Ref: Dhingra 7ᵗʰ/e pg. 198]

Explanation

Ethmoidal artery is the branch of internal carotid artery so it is responsible for epistaxis after ligation of external carotid artery

- Blood supply of Nasal Septum
  - Internal Carotid System
    - Anterior ethmoidal artery &Posterior ethmoidal artery
      branches of ophthalmic
  - External Carotid System

- Sphenopalatine artery (branch of maxillary artery) gives nasopalatine and posterior medial nasal branches.
- Septal branch of greater palatine artery (Br.of maxillary artery).
- Septal branch of superior labial artery (Br. of facial artery).
- Lateral Wall
  - Internal Carotid System
  - Anterior ethmoidal & Posterior ethmoidal branches of ophthalmic artery
  - External Carotid System
    - Posterior lateral nasal branches → From sphenopalatine artery
    - Greater palatine artery → From maxillary artery
    - Nasal branch of anterior superior dental → From infraorbital branch of maxillary A.
    - Branches of facial artery to nasal vestibule.

115. All of the following blood vessels are a part of Kiesselbach's plexus except- *(PGMEE 2015; DNB 2011)*

a. Posterior ethmoidal artery
b. Superior labial artery
c. Anterior Enthmoidal artery
d. Greater palatine artery

[Ref: Dhingra's 7th/e pg. 198]

116. The artery which leads to bleeding in Woodruff's area is-

a. Greater palatine artery *(PGMEE 2015; 2016)*
b. Sphenopalatine artery
c. Anterior ethmoidal artery
d. Superior labial artery

[Ref: Dhingra's 7th/e pg. 197 fig.]

117. Woodruff's plexus is situated in-

a. Below superior turbinate *(PGMEE 2015, 2016-17)*
b. Posterior end of inferior turbinate
c. Near hiatus semilunatis
d. Anterior end of middle turbinate

[Ref: Dhingra's 7th/e pg. 197]

118. Kiesselbach's plexus is present at: *(PGMEE 2015, 2013)*

a. Medial wall of nasopharynx
b. Posterior part of the nasal cavity
c. Anteroinferior part of nasal septum
d. Lateral wall of nasal cavity

[Ref: Dhingra's 7th/e pg. 197]

119. Which of the following arteries in kiesselbach's plexus is not the branch of ECA (External carotid artery) ?

a. Sphenopalatine artery *(NEET Pattern 2017)*
b. Greater palatine artery
c. Anterior, middle and posterior ethmoidal artery
d. Septal branch of superior labial artery

[Ref: Dhingra's 7th/e pg. 198; BDC vol.III 253]

Explanation

- Little's area is situated in the antero-inferior part of nasal septum just above the vestibule. 4 arteries here to form a vascular plexus called kiesselbach's plexus
- All arteries are the branch of ECA except anterior, middle and posterior ethmoidal arteries which is the branch of ICA.

112.	**a**
113.	**c**
114.	**a**
115.	**a**
116.	**b**
117.	**b**
118.	**c**
119.	**c**

- Commom site for epistaxis in children's and young adults
- Little's area – Kiesselbach's area – anteroinferior part of nasal septum is highly vascular and it is formed by
  - Sphenopalatine artery – branch of maxillary which in turn branch of external carotid
  - Greater palatine artery - branch of maxillary which in turn branch of external carotid
  - Anterior ethmoidal artery – branch of ophthalmic artery – branch of internal carotid
  - Septal branch of superior labial artery – branch of facial which in turn branch of external carotid

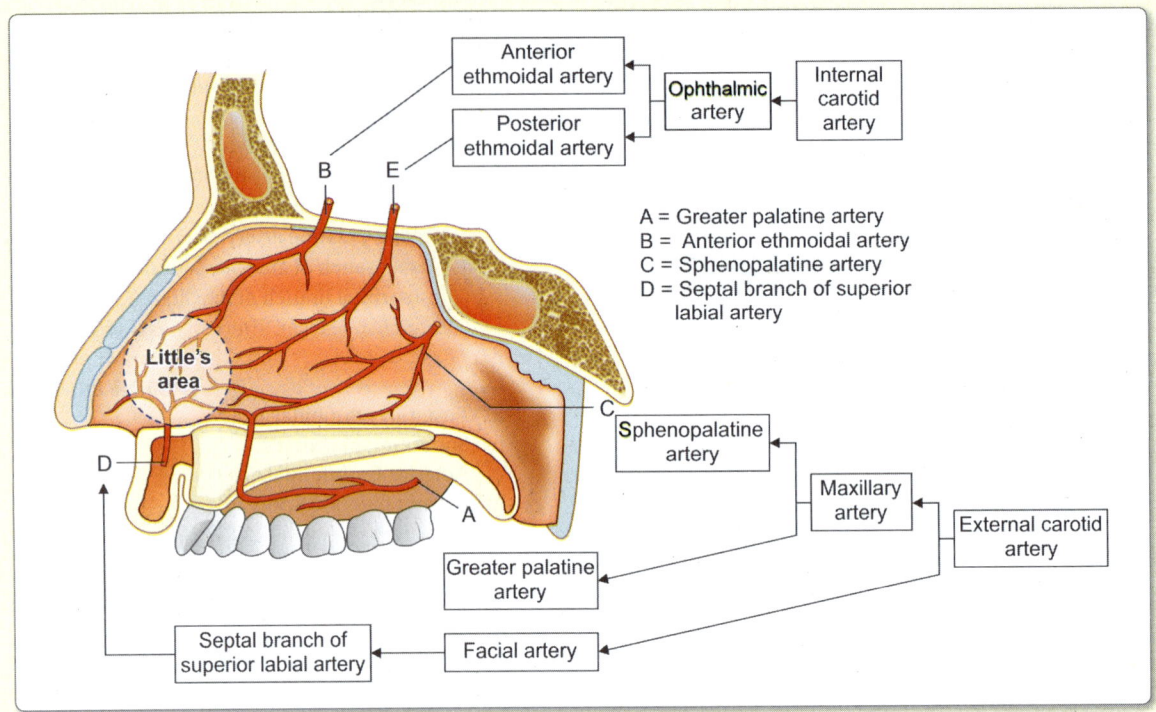

A = Greater palatine artery
B = Anterior ethmoidal artery
C = Sphenopalatine artery
D = Septal branch of superior labial artery

120. d
121. a
122. c

120. Main vascular supply of Little's area are all, except: *(PGMEE 2013)*
   a. Septal branch of superior labial artery
   b. Anterior ethmoidal artery
   c. Nasal branch of sphenopalatine artery
   d. Palatal branch of sphenopalatine
                 [Ref: Dhingra's 7th/e pg. 198 fig]

121. Cause of epistaxis are all except- *(PGMEE 2012)*
   a. Allergic rhinitis   b. Hypertension
   c. Foreign body   d. Tumor
              [Ref: Dhingra's 7th/e pg. 197-198]

Explanation

Local Causes

- Idiopathic—spontaneous
- Trauma:
  - Nose picking
  - Foreign body
  - Nasal oxygen and continuous positive airway pressure
  - Nasal fracture
- Inflammatory/infectious:
  - Common cold, viral rhinosinusitis
  - Allergic rhinosinusitis
  - Bacterial rhinosinusitis
  - Granulomatous diseases

  - Environmental irritants (cigarette smoking, chemicals, pollution, altitude)
- Postoperative—iatrogenic
  - Nasal surgery
- Primary neoplasm:
  - Hemangioma of the septum, turbinates
  - Hemangiopericytoma
  - Nasal papilloma
  - Pyogenic granuloma
  - Angiofibroma
  - Carcinoma and other nasal malignancies
- General Disorders, Systemic Causes
  - Hypertension (not more common, but more troublesome)
  - Arteriosclerosis
  - Platelet deficiencies, dysfunction; coagulopathies (e.g., warfarin, liver disease)
  - Leukemia, von Willebrand's disease
  - Hereditary hemorrhagic telangiectasia

122. Recurrent epistaxis in a 15 year old male the most common cause is - *(PGMEE 2012)*
   a. Foreign body
   b. Rhinosporiodiosis
   c. Juvenile nasopharyngeal fibroma
   d. Hematological disorder
                [Ref: Dhingra's 7th/e pg. 198]

123. Commonest cause of epistaxis in children is:
a. Enlarged adenosis   **(PGMEE 2014)**
b. Foreign body
c. Nasal diphtheria
d. Trauma

[Ref: Atlas of pediatric emergency 5th/e p. 417; Dhingra's 7th/e pg. 197; S.K. De 9th/e pg. 214]

124. Most common site of nose bleed in a child-
    (PGMEE 2012)
a. Little's area   b. Woodruff area
c. Brown area   d. None

[Ref: Atlas of pediatric emergency 5th/e p. 417; Dhingra's 7th/e pg. 197]

125. Most common cause of bleeding in children
a. Tumor   **(PGMEE 2012)**
b. Nose picking
c. Hypertension
d. None

[Ref: Dhingra's 7th/e pg. 197]

126. Posterior epistaxis is commonly seen in -(PGMEE 2014)
a. Foreign bodies of the nose
b. Children with ethmoidal polyps
c. Hypertension
d. Nose picking

[Ref: Dhingra's 7th/e pg. 199]

Explanation

Differences between Anterior and Posterior Epistaxis

	Anterior epistaxis	Posterior epistaxis
Incidence Site	▪ More common ▪ Mostly from Little's area of anterior part of lateral wall	▪ Less common ▪ Mostly from posterosuperior part of nasal cavity; often difficult to localize the bleeding point ▪ After 40 years of age
Age	▪ Mostly occurs in children or young adults	▪ After 40 years of age
Cause	▪ Mostly trauma	▪ Spontaneous; often due to hypertension or arteriosclerosis (uncommon d/to trauma)
Bleeding	▪ Usually mild, can be easily controlled by local pressure or anterior pack	▪ Bleeding is severe, requires hospitalization; postnasal pack often required

127. Traumatic epistaxis is not a cause in -   **(PGMEE 2014)**
a. Anterior epistaxis
b. Posterior epistaxis
c. Childhood
d. Adulthood

[Ref: Dhingra's 7th/e pg. 199]

128. A boy has developed epistaxis. What is the treatment of choice -   **(PGMEE 2013)**
a. Digital pressure
b. Surgical ligation
c. Cauterization of vessels
d. Nasal packing

[Ref: Dhingra's 7th/e pg. 199]

129. Young's surgery is used in the treatment of-
a. Nasal polyp   **(PGMEE 2015)**
b. Epistaxis
c. Maxillary sinus carcinoma
d. Deviated nasal septum

[Ref: Dhingra 6th/e pg. 179]

NASAL POLYPOID MASSES

130. Ethmoidal polyp is associated most commonly with -
a. Superior meatus   **(PGMEE 2015)**
b. Sphenoethmoidal recess
c. Middle meatus
d. Inferior meatus

[Ref: Dhingra's 7th/e pg. 193]

131. True about Antrochoanal polyp is?   **(PGMEE 2014)**
a. Bleeding is common
b. Multiple
c. Single and grows posteriorly
d. None

[Ref: Dhingra's 7th/e pg. 195]

132. All are true about antrochoanal polyp except:
a. Unilateral and single
b. Grows backwards to the choana
c. Avulsion is the treatment of choice
d. Common in children

Explanation

▪ *Differences between antrochoanal and ethmoidal polypi*

	Antrochoanal polypi	Ethmoidal polypi
Age	Common in children	Common in adults
Aetiology	Infection	Allergy or multifactorial
Number	Solitary	Multiple
Laterality	Unilateral	Bilateral
Origin	Maxillary sinus near the ostium	Ethmoidal sinuses, uncinate process middle turbinate and middle meatus

contd...

123.	d
124.	a
125.	b
126.	c
127.	b
128.	a
129.	b
130.	c
131.	c
132.	c

	Antrochoanal polypi	Ethmoidal polypi
Growth	Grows backwards to the choana; may hangdown behind the soft palate	Mostly grow anteriorly and may present at the nares
Size & shape	Trilobed with antral, nasal and choanal parts.	Usually small & grape like masses
Treatment	Polypectomy; endoscopic removal or Caldwell-Luc	Polypectomy Endoscopic surgery or ethmoidectomy (which may be in tranasal, extra nasal or transantral)

133. **The most appropriate management for Antrochoanal polyp in children is:** *(DNB 2009)*
   a. Wait and watch
   b. Corticosteroids
   c. Intranasal polypectomy
   d. Caldwell Luc operation

   [Ref: Dhingra's 7th/e pg. 193]

134. **X-ray showing air column between soft tissue mass and posterior wall of nasopharynx is suggestive of-** *(PGMEE 2015)*
   a. Nasal myiasis   b. Antrochoanal polyp
   c. Ethmoidal polyp   d. None of the above

   [Ref: Dhingra's 7th/e pg. 193]

Explanation

- X-ray (lateral view), soft tissue nasopharynx, reveals a globular swelling in the postnasal space by the presence of a column of air behind the polyp.

135. **What is the treatment of choice for ethmoidal polyps?** *(PGMEE 2015)*
   a. Functional Endoscopic sinus surgery with polypectomy
   b. Transantral ethmoidectomy
   c. Extranasl ethmoidectomy
   d. Intranasal ethmoidectomy

   [Ref: Dhingra 7th/e pg. 196]

Explanation

Endoscopic sinus surgery	These days, ethmoidal polypi are removed by *functional endoscopic sinus surgery* (FESS).
Simple polypectomy	One or two pedunculated polyps can be removed with snare.
Intranasal ethmoidectomy	When polypi are multiple and sessile
Extranasal ethmoidectomy	This is indicated when polypi recur after intranasal procedures
Transantral ethmoidectomy	This is indicated when infection and polypoidal changes are also seen in the maxillary antrum.

136. **Recurrent polyp are seen in:-** *(PGMEE 2013)*
   a. Antrochoanal polyp   b. Hypertrophic turbinate
   c. Nasal polyp   d. Ethmoidal polyp

   [Ref: Dhingra's 7th/e pg. 195]

137. **Samters triad is:-** *(PGMEE 2016-17)*
   a. Asthma, aspirin hypersensitivity, nasal mass
   b. Asthma, Brufen hypersensitivity, nasal allergy
   c. Asthma, aspirin hypersensitivity, nasal polyps
   d. COPD, aspirin hypersensitivity, nasal polyps

   [Ref: Dhingra's 7th/e pg. 194]

138. **All of the following are features of ethmoidal polyp except-** *(PGMEE 2015)*
   a. Commonly Singular   b. Commonly bilateral
   c. Common in adults   d. Is usually allergic

   [Ref: Dhingra's 7th/e pg. 195]

139. **What is not true about use of intranasal steroids in nasal polyposis-** *(PGMEE 2013)*
   a. Effective in eosinophilically predominant polyp only
   b. Reduce obstruction
   c. Reduce recurrence
   d. May cause epistaxis

   [Ref: Dhingra's 7th/e pg. 196]

140. **Treatment modalities of multiple bilateral ethmoidal polyps are all except:** *(PGMEE 2015)*
   a. Caldwall Luc operation
   b. Intranasal ethmoidectomy
   c. Functional endoscopic sinus surgery
   d. Extranasal ethmoidectomy

   [Ref: Dhingra's 7th/e pg. 196]

141. **In Cadwell Luc operation, the approach is through the-** *(PGMEE 2015)*
   a. Superior meatus
   b. Through the sphenopalatine recess
   c. Sublabial Approach leading to opening of mandibular antrum
   d. Opening of maxillary antrum through gingivolabial approach

   [Ref: Dhingra's 7th/e pg. 196]

TUMOURS OF NOSE AND PNS

142. **Most common malignant tumor of nose -** *(PGMEE 2013)*
   a. Squamous cell carcinoma
   b. Basal cell carcinoma
   c. Malignant melanoma
   d. None of the above

   [Ref: Dhingra's 7th/e pg. 229]

143. **Most common tumor of nasal cavity -** *(PGMEE 2014)*
   a. Adenoma   b. Admantinoma
   c. Myxoma   d. Papilloma

   [Ref: Neuroradiology : Differential diagnosis p. 355]

144. **Inverted papilloma of nose arise from -** *(PGMEE 2013)*
   a. Tip of the nose   b. Roof of the nose
   c. Nasal septum   d. Lateral wall of the nose

   [Ref: Dhingra's 7th/e pg. 227]

133.	c
134.	b
135.	a
136.	d
137.	c
138.	a
139.	a
140.	a
141.	d
142.	a
143.	d
144.	d

145. Which of the following is not true about inverted papiloma: *(PGMEE 2015)*

a. 10-15 % of the cases may be associated with squamous cell carcinoma

b. It is more common in females

c. It is almost always unilateral

d. It is also called Ringertz tumor

[Ref: Dhingra's 7th/e pg. 227]

146. Osteoma of PNS is commonest in: *(DNB 2011)*

a. Ethmoidal   b. Frontal

c. Sphenoid   d. Maxillary

[Ref: Dhingra 6th/e pg. 205]

147. Ohngren's classification of maxillary sinus carcinoma is based on: *(DNB 2010)*

a. Imaginary plane between medial canthus of eye and angle of mandible.

b. Two horizontal lines, one passing through floor of orbit and other through floor of antrum

c. Imaginary plane between lateral canthus of eye and angle of mandible.

d. None

[Ref: Dhingra's 7th/e pg. 233]

148. Ohngren's line that divides maxillary sinus into superolateral and inferomedial zone is related to? *(PGMEE 2011)*

a. Infratemporal carcinoma

b. Maxillary carcinoma

c. Maxillary osteoma

d. Maxillary sinusitis

[Ref: Dhingra's 7th/e pg. 233]

Explanation

Classification of maxillary sinus carcinoma

- Ohngren's classification-
  - An imaginary plane is drawn, extending between medial canthus of eye and the angle of mandible.
  - Growths situated above this plane (suprastructural) have a poorer prognosis than those below it (intrastructural).
- AJCC (American Joint Committee on Cancer) classification:
  - AJCC classification is only for squamous cell carcinoma. SCC graded into
    - Well differentiated
    - Moderately differentiated and
    - Poorly differentiaed
    - Figure 40.5
    - Lederman's classification-
  - It uses two horizontal lines of Sebileau; one passing through the floors of orbits and the other through floors of antra, thus dividing the area into:
    - Suprastructure: Ethmoid ,sphenoid and frontal sinuses and the olfactory area of nose.
    - Mesostructure: Maxillary sinus and the respiratory part of nose.
    - Infrastructure: Containing alveolar process.

- This classification further uses vertical lines, extending down the medial walls of orbit to separate ethmoid sinuses and nasal fossa from the maxillary sinuses.

TNM classification-

- Maxillary sinus
  - T1 Tumour limited to the antral mucosa with no erosion of bone
  - T2 Tumour causing bone erosion or destruction, except for the posterior antral wall, including extension into the hard palate and/or middle
  - Meatus
  - T3 Tumour invades any of the following: bone of the posterior wall of the maxillary sinus, subcutaneous tissues, skin, floor or medial wall of the
  - Orbit, infratemporal fossa, pterygoid plates, ethmoid sinus
  - T4a Tumour invades any of the following: anterior orbital contents, skin of cheek, pterygoid plates, infratemporal fossa, cribriform plate,
  - Sphenoid or frontal sinuses
  - T4b Tumour invades any of the following: orbital apex, dura, brain, middle cranial fossa, cranial nerves other than the maxillary division of V2,
  - nasopharynx or clivus.
- Ethmoid sinus
  - T1 Tumour confined to ethmoid with or without bone erosion
  - T2 Tumour extends into the nasal cavity
  - T3 Tumour extends into the anterior orbit and/or maxillary sinus
  - T4a Tumour invades any of the following: anterior orbital contents, skin of the nose or cheek, minimal anterior intracranial extension, pterygoid
  - plates, sphenoid or frontal sinuses
  - T4b Tumour invades any of the following: orbital apex, dura, brain, middle cranial fossa, cranial nerves other than V2, nasopharynx or clivus.
- Nasal cavity
- T1 Tumour involves one subsite
  - T2 Tumour involves two subsites or ethmoid
  - T3 Tumour extends into the anterior orbit and/or maxillary sinus
  - T4a Tumour invades any of the following: anterior orbital contents, skin of the nose or cheek, minimal anterior intracranial extension, pterygoid
  - plates, sphenoid or frontal sinuses
  - T4b Tumour invades any of the following: orbital apex, dura, brain, middle cranial fossa, cranial nerves other than V2, nasopharynx or clivus.
- Within the nose, four subsites are recognized, namely septum, floor, lateral wall and vestibule.

149. Treatment of choice for Maxillary sinus carcinoma Stage T3 N0 M0: *(DNB 2007)*

a. Radiotherapy

b. Surgery + Radiotherapy

c. Chemotherapy

d. Radiotherapy + Chemotherapy

[Ref: Dhingra's 7th/e pg. 234]

145.	b
146.	b
147.	a
148.	b
149.	b

Explanation

- T3 and T4 lesions are treated by combined modalities of radiation and surgery.
- Radiation in such cases may be given preoperatively or postoperatively.

150. **What is the cause of sudden death in a patient who recently underwent maxillary sinus irrigation ?**
   a. Air embolism
   b. Meningitis
   c. Septicemia
   d. Maxillary artery thrombosis

[Ref: Dhingra's 7th/e pg. 466]

Explanation

Maxillary sinus irrigation

- Maxillary sinus irrigation
  ○ This procedure involves puncturing the medial wall of maxillary sinus in the region of inferior meatus and irrigating the sinus.
  ○ Indicatoins: Chronic and subacute maxillary sinusitis with dual purpose of: (a) confirming the diagnosis and (b) washing out the pus.
  ○ Contraindication : Acute maxillary sinusitisf or fear of osteomyelitis.
- Complications
  ○ Swelling of check. This is due to faulty technique.
  ○ Orbital injury and cellulites
  ○ Puncture of the posterior antral wall.
  ○ Bleeding due to injury to nasal mucosa.
  ○ Air embolism: It is rare but may prove fatal. This complication can be prevented by avoiding insufflation of air into the antrum after lavage

151. **People working in wood industry are exposed to increased risk of?** *(PGMEE 2011)*
   a. Sarcoma of PNS
   b. Osteomas of PNS
   c. SCC of paranasal sinuses
   d. Adenocarcinoma of PNS

[Ref: Dhingra's 7th/e pg. 231]

Explanation

- Workers exposed to hard wood have a 70 times increased incidenc of sinonasal adenocarcinoma, particularly in the ethmoid sinuses.
- The type of wood is a significant factor, with African mahogany being the most dangerous. It is thought that biologically active compounds in wood dust impair mucociliary clearance and predispose to carcinogenesis
- While hardwood exposure increases the risk of developing adenocarcinoma, soft wood exposure increases the risk of developing squamous cell carcinoma.
- Exposure to nickel increases the risk of developing sinonasal squamous cell carcinoma 250 times.
- Other chemicals linked to sinonasal malignancy include chromium, polycyclic hydrocarbons, aflatoxin (found in certain foods and dust), mustard gas and thorotrast (thorium dioxide used in paints for watch dials)
- Maxillary sinus tumours are the most common (55 percent) followed by the nasal cavity (35 percent),

ethmoid sinuses (9 percent) and rarely frontal and sphenoid sinuses (1 percent).
- They have a slow growth rate and rarely metastasize. Several histological subtypes of sinonasal adenocarcinoma are recognized,namely papillary, sessile, mucoid, neuroendocrine, intestinal and undifferentiated.
- Papillary adenocarcinomas tend to be locally malignant only and are the least aggressive form.
- Sessile and mucoid adenocarcinomas have the worst prognosis.

152. **Dangerous area of face is so called because?**
   a. Its infection can lead to cavernous sinus thrombobosis and can be life threatening
   b. It's easily hurt in injuries
   c. It is easily scarred
   d. Trauma here leads to massive bleeding and Death

Explanation

- The danger triangle of the face consists of the area from the corners of the mouth to the bridge of the nose, including the nose andmaxilla.
- Due to the special nature of the blood supply to the human nose and surrounding area, it is possible for retrograde infections from the nasal area to spread to the brain.
- This is possible because of venous communication (via the ophthalmic veins) between the facial vein and the cavernous sinus. The cavernous sinus lies within the cranial cavity, between layers of the meninges and is a major conduit of venous drainage from the brain.
- It is a common misconception that the veins of the head do not contain one-way valves like other veins of the circulatory system. In fact, it is not the absence of venous valves but the existence of communications between the facial vein and cavernous sinus and the direction of blood flow that is important in the spread of infection from the face. Most people, but not all, have valves in the veins of the face.[

Cavernous Sinus Thrombosis

- Cavernous sinus thrombosis results from septic phlebitis of the ophthalmic veins and involvement of the cavernous sinus.
- Initially, the orbital signs are unilateral but these become progressively bilateral causing proptosis with third, fourth and sixth cranial nerve palsies.
- It can prove to be fatal with quoted mortality rates of 30 percent.
- CT scanning of the head with contrast will confirm the diagnosis.
- Intravenous broad-spectrum antibiotics should be started immediately, together with heparin anticoagulation.
- Staphylococcus aureus, Streptococcus and Pneumococcus are the most likely organisms.

MISCELLANEOUS

153. **Weber ferguson approach is used for?**
   a. Mastoidectomy   b. Maxillectomy
   c. Myringoplasty   d. Mandibulectomy

[Ref: Dhingra's 7th/e pg. 455]

150. a
151. d
152. a
153. b

Explanation

Surgical Approaches to the Ear Surgeries

1. Endo meatal or transcanal approach
   - It is used to raise a tympano meatalflap in order to expose the middle ear .most commonly used for stapedectomy and inlay Myringoplasty.
   - Also used commonly for exploratory tympanotomy to find cause for conductive hearing loss, ossicular reconstruction.

2. Endaural approach It is used for:
   - Excision of osteomasor exostosis of ear canal.
   - Large tympanic membrane perforations.
   - Attic cholesteatomas with limited extension into the antrum.
     - Modified radical mastoidectomy where disease is limited to attic, antrum ,and part of mastoid.

3. Postaural (or Wilde's) approach used for:
   - Cortical mastoidectomy.
   - Modified radical and radical mastoidectomy.
   - Tympanoplasty :when perforation extends anterior to handle of malleus.
   - Exposure of CN VII in vertical segment.
   - Surgery of endolymphatic sac.
   - **Surgical approaches for Maxillectomy Three different soft tissue approaches are used.**

- Lateral rhinotomy: It gives excellent exposure of both the nasal cavities and medial maxilla with a cosmetically acceptable incision in the lateral nasal crease.
- Weber–Fergusson: It is rarely used unless there is need for an orbital exenteration.
- Midfacial degloving: more cosmetic alternative to both. This technique combines a bilateral sublabial approach to the anterior wall of the maxilla with a midline.

154. Which of following is seen in Young's syndrome?
   a. Azoospermia   b. Bronchiectasis
   c. Infertility   d. All above

Explanation

- Young's syndrome.
  - It consists of recurrent respiratory disease with chronic rhinosinusitis, nasal polyps, bronchiectasis and azoospermia.
- Kartagener's syndrome (Primary ciliary dyskinesia)
  - This consists of bronchiectasis sinusitis, situs inversus and ciliary dyskinesis.
  - Absent mucociliary clearance and recurrent bacterial infections result in nasal polyposis.
- Churg-Strauss syndrome. Consists of asthma, fever, eosinophilia, vasculitis and granuloma.

154. d

ANATOMICAL AND PHYSIOLOGICAL ASPECT

1. All of the following are true about the larynx except:
(PGMEE 2012-13)
a. All intrinsic muscles are supplied by the recurrent laryngeal nerve
b. Posterior cricoarytenoids abduct the vocal cords
c. Cricothyroid is supplied by the external laryngeal nerve
d. Lymphatic draining of the larynx is to the deep cervical nodes.
[Ref: BDC 8th/e vol. 3 pg. 293; Dhingra 7th/e pg. 320, 337]

Explanation

- *Motor supply of larynx:* All the intrinsic muscles of the larynx are supplied by the recurrent laryngeal nerve except the cricothyroid, which is supplied by the external branch (ELN) of the superior laryngeal nerve.
- *Sensory supply of larynx:* The internal laryngeal nerve supplies the mucous membrane above the vocal cord. The recurrent laryngeal nerve supplies it below the vocal cord.

2. Function of larynx: (PGMEE 2013)
a. Protection of airway
b. Speech
c. Conduit of air
d. All
[Ref: BDC 8th/e vol. 3 pg. 294; Dhingra 7th/e pg. 323]

3. Side walls of inlet of larynx are formed by:
a. True vocal cord (PGMEE 2013)
b. Aryepiglotic folds
c. Vocal folds
d. False vocal cord
[Ref: Dhingra 7th/e pg. 321]

1.	a
2.	d
3.	b
4.	a
5.	a
6.	d
7.	d
8.	a

Explanation

- Inlet of larynx is an oblique opening bounded:-
  ○ Anteriorly by free margin of epiglottis
  ○ On the sides, by aryepiglottic fold and
  ○ Posteriorly by interarytenoid fold.

4. Part of larynx above the vocal cord is known as
a. Supraglottis (PGMEE 2016-17)
b. Infraglottis
c. Rima vestibuli
d. Saccule of larynx
[Ref: BDC 7th/e vol. 3 pg. 266; Dhingra 7th/e pg. 321]

Explanation

- **Vestibule and vocal cords (vocal folds) divide the cavity of larynx into 3 parts:-**
  ○ **Supraglottis(Vestibule):** Part above the vestibular fold

○ **Glottis:** Part between the vestibular and vocal folds. contain Ventricle (sinus) of larynx
○ **Infraglottis:** The part below the vocal folds

5. Inspiratory stridor is found in what kind of lesions:
(PGMEE 2019)
a. Supraglottic
b. Subglottic
c. Tracheal
d. Bronchus
[Ref: PL Dhingra 7th/e chap 59 - congenital lesions of larynx and stridor, pg. 333-334]

6. Laryngocele arises from- (DNB 2009)
a. True cords
b. Subglottis
c. Anterior commissure
d. Saccule of the ventricle
[Ref: Dhingra 7th/e pg. 333]

7. External laryngocele arises from herniation through?
a. Cricovocal membrane (DNB Dec'2010)
b. Cricoepiglottic membrane
c. Thyroid membrane
d. Thyrohyoid membrane
[Ref: Dhingra 7th/e pg. 345]

Explanation

Laryngocoele:

- It is an air or mucus filled dilation of saccule or appendix of laryngeal ventricle.
- Common in glass blowers, weight lifters and Trumpet players due to raised intralaryngeal pressure.
- 3 types
  ○ External: distended saccule **herniates through thyrohyoid membrane** and presents as a cystic mass in neck.
  ○ Internal: air containing sac confined to area of false vocal fold and aryepiglottic fold.
  ○ Mixed
- Bryce's sign: Gurgling and hissing sound in throat on compressing the external neck mass.
- Treatment: Excision or marsupialisation.

8. All of the following are extrinsic laryngeal membranes except- (PGMEE 2015)
a. Quadrangular membrane
b. Cricotracheal membrane
c. Thyrohyoid membrane
d. Hyoepiglottic ligament
[Ref: Dhingra 7th/e pg. 320]

Explanation

Extrinsic	**Intrinsic**
▪ Thyrohyoid membrane	▪ Cricovocal membrane
▪ Cricotracheal membrane	▪ Quadrangular membrane
▪ Hyoepiglottic ligament	

9. **Direct bronchoscopy can visualize all, except:**
   a. Subcarinal lymph nodes   *(DNB 2009)*
   b. Vocal cords
   c. First segmental subdivision of branch
   d. Trachea

   [Ref: Logan Turner 10th/e pg. 391, 392, Cummins ENT, Sabiston Surgery; Dhingra 7th/e pg. 484]

10. **Supraglottic part of larynx is drained by**
    (PGMEE 2016-17)
    a. Anterosuperior part of deep cervical LN
    b. Posterosuperior part of deep cervical LN
    c. Superficial cervical group of LN
    d. Juguloomohyoid LN

    [Ref: Dhingra 7th/e pg. 322]

11. **Which of the following is the only intrinsic muscle of larynx that lies outside the laryngeal framework-**
    (PGMEE 2012)
    a. Lateral cricothyroid   b. Superior constrictor
    c. Cricothyroid   d. Cricopharyngeus

    [Ref: Scott-Brown's pg. 637]

12. **X-ray of lateral view of neck is shown below. The arrow mark indicates :-** *(PGMEE 2016-17)*

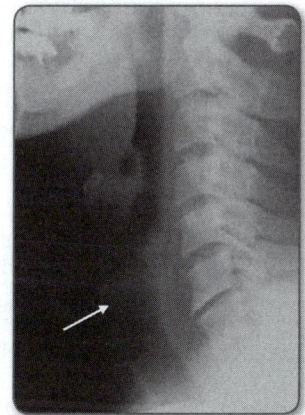

    a. Cricoid cartilage   b. Thyroid cartilage
    c. Arytenoid cartilage   d. Epiglottis

13. **Which of the following doesn't elevate the larynx:**
    (PGMEE 2012-13)
    a. Sternohyoid   c. Mylohyoid
    b. Thyrohyoid   d. None
    [Ref: BDC 8th/e vol. 3 pg. 292; Dhingra 7th/e pg. 321]

Explanation

Extrinsic muscles

- Elevators
  - *Primary elevators* act directly as they are attached to the thyroid cartilage and include stylopharyngeus, salpingopharyngeus, palatopharyngeus and thyrohyoid.
  - *Secondary elevators* act indirectly as they are attached to the hyoid bone and include mylohyoid (main), digastric, stylohyoid and geniohyoid.
- Depressors
  - They include sternohyoid, sternothyoid and omohyoid.

LARYNGEAL NERVES

14. **Recurrent laryngeal nerve lies in relation to?**
    (PGMEE 2012)
    a. Superior thyroid artery   b. Inferior thyroid artery
    c. Superior thyroid vein   d. Inferior thyroid vein
    [Ref: BDC 7th/e vol. 3 pg. 147; Dhingra 7th/e pg. 337]

15. **Internal laryngeal nerve runs along which border of pharyngeal muscle:** *(PGMEE 2013)*
    a. Lateral   b. Medial
    c. Superior   d. Inferior
    [Ref: BDC 7th/e vol. 3 pg. 100-101; Dhingra 7th/e pg. 337 fig.]

16. **Nerve supply of cricothyroid:** *(PGMEE 2014)*
    a. Recurrent laryngeal nerve
    b. Internal laryngeal nerve
    c. External laryngeal nerve
    d. None of the above

    [Ref: BDC 7th/e vol. 3 pg. 267]

17. **Which muscle of larynx is not supplied by recurrent laryngeal nerve:** *(PGMEE 2013)*
    a. Thyroarytenoid   b. Vocalis
    c. Cricothyroid   d. Interarytenoid
    [Ref: BDC 7th/e vol. 3 pg.267]

18. **Galen's anastomosis is between:** *(PGMEE 2013)*
    a. Internal laryngeal nerve and external laryngeal nerve
    b. Recurrent laryngeal and internal laryngeal nerve
    c. Recurrent laryngeal nerve and external laryngeal nerve
    d. None of the above

    [Ref: Essentials of clinical anatomy p. 1212]

19. **Sensory supply of larynx, below the vocal cord:**
    (PGMEE 2012-13)
    a. Superior laryngeal nerve
    b. Internal laryngeal nerve
    c. Recurrent laryngeal nerve
    d. Inferior laryngeal nerve
    [Ref: BDC 7th/e vol. 3 pg. 271; Dhingra 7th/e pg. 337]

20. **Nerve supply of larynx above level of vocal cord:**
    a. Superior laryngeal   *(PGMEE 2013)*
    b. Recurrent laryngeal
    c. External laryngeal
    d. Glossopharyngeal
    [Ref: BDC 7th/e vol. 3 pg. 271; Dhingra 7th/e pg. 337]

LARYNGEAL CARTILAGES

21. **X-ray neck. (Lateral view). structure marked by the arrow arrow is:** *(PGMEE 2016-17)*

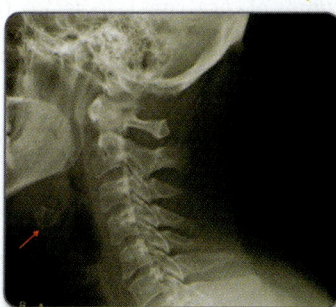

    a. Cricoid   b. Thyroid
    c. Hyoid   d. Epiglottis

9.	a
10.	a
11.	c
12.	a
13.	a
14.	b
15.	c
16.	c
17.	c
18.	b
19.	c
20.	a
21.	c

22. The distance between the upper incisor to hyoid bone:-
(PGMEE 2016-17)

a. 12 cm   b. 15 cm
c. 20 cm   d. 18 cm

[Ref: Internet]

23. Laryngeal cartilage forming complete circle:

a. Thyroid
b. Cricoid   *(PGMEE 2013)*
c. Arytenoid
d. Corniculate

[Ref: BDC 7th/e vol. 3 pg. 264; Dhingra 7th/e pg. 319]

24. Which laryngeal cartilage is not elastic:
(PGMEE 2012-13)

a. Epiglottis
b. Corniculate
c. Thyroid
d. Cuneiform

[Ref: BDC 7th/e vol. 3 pg. 265; Dhingra 7th/e pg. 319]

Explanation

- Thyroid, cricoid and most of the arytenoid cartilages are hyaline cartilages whereas epiglottis, corniculate, cuneiform and tip of arytenoid near the corniculate cartilage are elastic fibrocartilage.

25. Which of the following cartilage has signet ring shape -
(PGMEE 2013)

a. Thyroid   b. Arytenoid
c. Cuneiform   d. Cricoid

[Ref: Dhingra 7th/e pg. 319]

26. Elastic cartilage is present in –   *(PGMEE 2014)*

a. Thyroid cartilage
b. Epiglottis
c. Cricoid
d. Aretynoid cartilage

[Ref: Dhingra 7th/e pg. 319]

VOCAL CORDS (VOCAL FOLDS)

27. Anterior posterior diameter of vocal cords in males & females respectively is: *(PGMEE 2013)*

a. 36 & 48 mm
b. 24 & 36 mm
c. 23 & 17 mm
d. 48 & 36mm

[Ref: Textbook of clinical anatomy p. 442; Dhingra 7th/e pg. 321]

28. Sensory supply of vocal cord is from: *(PGMEE 2013)*

a. Recurrent laryngeal nerve
b. Internal laryngeal nerve
c. Superior laryngeal nerve
d. All of the above

[Ref: BDC 8th/e vol. 3 pg. 293; Dhingra 7th/e pg. 337]

29. Abductor of vocal cord is:
(DNB Dec' 2011, 2007, PGMEE 2012, 2016-17)

a. Lateral cricoarytenoid
b. Cricothyroid
c. Posterior cricoarytenoid
d. Interarytenoid

[Ref: BDC 8th/e vol. 3 pg. 292; Dhingra 7th/e pg. 320]

22.	b
23.	b
24.	c
25.	d
26.	b,d
27.	c
28.	d
29.	c
30.	a

Explanation

Laryngeal Muscles` There are two groups of laryngeal muscles	
Intrinsic muscles	Extrinsic muscles
moves the cartilage in the larynx,control the position and shape of vocal fold and control the elasticity and viscosity of each layer of vocal cord	they attach the to neighbouring structures and mailntain the position of the larynx in the neck
Functions of the intrinsic muscles	
Control the tension of the vocal folds (Tensors)	1. Cricothyroid 2. Vocalis (Internal part of thyroarytenoid) -A broad sheet of muscle which lieslateral to and above the free edge of the cricovocal ligament. The lower part of the muscle is thicker and forms a distinct bundle called the vocalis muscle.
Adductors of vocal cords	1. Lateral Cricoarytenoids 2. Transvrse arytenoids (Inter arytenoids) 3. Oblique Arytenoids (External part of Thyroarytenoids)
Abductors of vocal cords	Posterior cricoarytenoids
Opners of laryngeal inlet	Thyroepiglotticus - A continuation of the thyroarytenoid
Closures of laryngeal inlet	Aryepiglotticus - A continuation of the oblique arytenoids
Functions of the extrinsic muscles	
Elevator of larynx	Primary elevators – They are attach to thyroid cartilage and acts directly- Stylopharyngeus,Palatopharyngeus, Salpingopharyngeus Secondary elevators – Act indirectly and they are attach to hyoid bone -Diagastric,Stylohoid, Myelohyoid and Geniohyoid
Depressors of larynx	Sternohyoid, Sternothyroid and Omohyoid

- **Note:**
  - The unpaired transverse arytenoid and paired oblique arytenoid make up the interarytenoid muscle.

30. Tensor of vocal cord?   *(PGMEE 2018)*

a. Cricothyroid
b. Posterior cricoarytenoid
c. Lateral criciarytenoid
d. Thyroarytenoid

[Ref: Dhingra 7th/e pg. 320]

Explanation

- Tensors of Vocal cord: Cricothyroid and Vocalis (internal part of thyroarytenoid)
- Abductor of Vocal cord: posterior cricoarytenoid
- Adductors of vocal cord: Lateral cricoarytenoid, Interarytenoid, Thyroarytenoid.

31. Tensors of vocal cord are? *(DNB Dec' 2010)*

a. Posterior cricothyroid, internal interarytenoid
b. Cricothyroid and internal thyroarytenoid
c. Thyroarytenoid, internal interaryenoid
d. Lateral Cricothyroid, internal interarytenoid

[Ref: Dhingra 7th/e pg. 320]

32. Cadaveric position of vacal cords in seen in?

a. Bilateral recurrent and superior laryngeal nerve palsy
b. Bilateral recurrent laryngeal nerve palsy
c. Unilateral superior laryngeal nerve palsy
d. Bilateral superior laryngeal nerve palsy

[Ref: Dhingra 7th/e pg. 338]

Explanation

Vocal cord paralysis

- It may be unilateral or bilateral and complete or incomplete. Thus it can have four possible combinations.
- Unilateral complete Paralysis (Unilateral adductor Paralysis)
  - Both recurrent and the superior laryngeal nerves are paralysed
  - The cord will be in cadaveric position
  - The patient will be aphonic at the onset of paralysis but after 1-2 week, the opposite cord will cross the midline on phonation and voice will begin to return
  - Diplophonia; the quality of voice is harsh, warbling and breathy which is produced by two different level of vocal cord (paralysed cord falls downwards and medially)
  - Treatment includes medialization of vocal cord, injection of Teflon and crico-arytenoid arthrodesis.
- Bilateral complete paralysis (Bilateral adductor paralysis)
  - Both the vocal cord are in cadaveric position
  - Patient has aphonia and it does not recover
  - Patient has difficulty in swallowing so all patient sooner or later develop bronchopneumonia and traceostomy.
- Unilateral incomplete Paralysis (unilateral abductor paralysis)
  - The vocal cord is fixed in the paramedian position.
- Bilateral incomplete paralysis (Bilateral abductor paralysis)
  - Both the vocal cord are in the paramedian position and sooner or later every patient will have stridor.
- Note:-
  - Semons's law: In all progressive organic lesions of motor laryngeal nerve, the abductor of the vocal cords are paralysed much earlier than adductors. The reason are
  - Adductors are first to develop so last to go.
  - Bulk of abductor muscles is less
  - Chronaxy (response to the electric stimulation) is more in abductor.
  - Exception of semon's law: Tuberculosis and Malignancy
  - All the muscles of larynx are supplied by recurrent laryngeal laryngeal nerve except cricothyroid, which is supplied by external branch of superior laryngeal nerve.
- Loop of Galen is formed by superior laryngeal nerve with ascendind branch of recurrent laryngeal nerve.

33. Cadaveric position of vocal cords – *(PGMEE 2013)*

a. Midline
b. 1.5 mm from midline
c. 3.5 mm from midline
d. 7.5 mm from midline

[Ref: Dhingra 7th/e pg. 338]

CONGENITAL ANOMALIES OF LARYNX

LARYNGOMALACIA

34. Most common congenital anomaly of larynx- *(PGMEE 2014)*

a. Laryngeal web
b. Laryngomalacia
c. Vocal and palsy
d. Laryngeal stenosis

[Ref: Dhingra 7th/e pg. 333]

35. All of the following are true about laryngomalacia EXCEPT: *(PGMEE 2015)*

a. Usually noticed in the first few weeks of life
b. Reassurance of the patient is the treatment of choice
c. Omega shaped epiglottis is seen on direct laryngoscopy
d. Expiratory stridor is characteristic

[Ref: Dhingra 7th/e pg. 333]

36. All of the following statements about Laryngomalacia are true, Except: *(PGMEE 2012)*

a. Stridor is increased on crying and relieved on lying prone
b. Surgical Tracheostomy is the treatment of choice
c. It is the most common congenital anomaly of the larynx
d. It is associated with an omega shaped epiglottis

[Ref: Dhingra 7th/e pg. 333]

37. Inspiratory stridor is clinical finding when the pathology lies in: *(Recent Pattern June 2018)*

a. Supraglottis
b. Subglottis
c. Trachea
d. Bronchus

[Ref: Dhingra's 7th/e pg. 334]

Explanation

- The stridor is a physical sign which is caused by a narrowed or obstructed airway. It can be inspiratory, expiratory or biphasic, although it is usually heard during inspiration.
- Inspiratory stridor often occurs in children with croup.
- Pathology lies in pharynx and supraglottis.
- DIAGRAM

31.	b
32.	a
33.	c
34.	b
35.	d
36.	b
37.	a

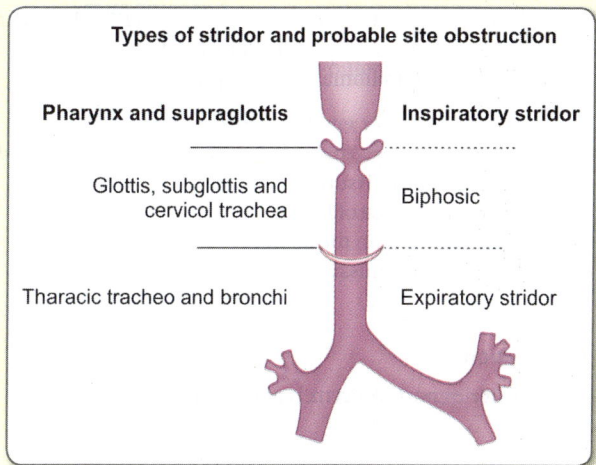

Types of stridor and probable site obstruction

Pharynx and supraglottis	Inspiratory stridor
Glottis, subglottis and cervicol trachea	Biphosic
Tharacic tracheo and bronchi	Expiratory stridor

MALIGNANCIES

SQUAMOUS PAPILLOMA OF LARYNX

63. Identify the lesion of vocal cord in the image given below: *(PGMEE 2019)*

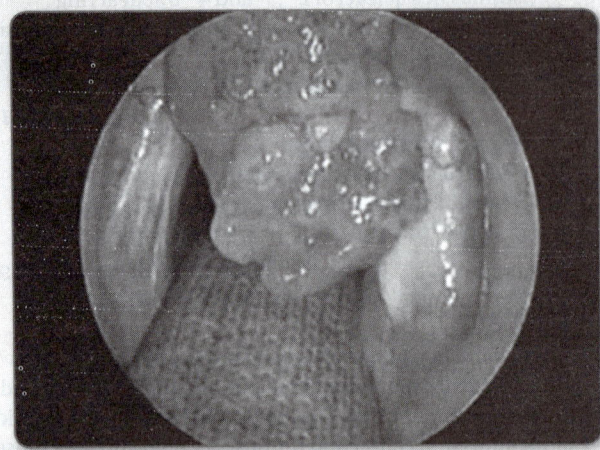

   a. Reinke's edema
   b. Laryngeal Papilloma
   c. Malignancy
   d. Tracheomalacia

[Ref: PL Dhingra 7th/e chap 61 - benign tumours of larynx, pg. 344-345]

64. Juvenile papillomatoses is caused by *(PGMEE 2012)*
   a. HPV
   b. HSV
   c. CMV
   d. EBV

[Ref: Dhingra 7th/e pg. 345]

65. HPV serotypes associated in laryngeal papillomatosis: *(Recent Pattern June 2018)*
   a. 16, 18   b. 31, 35
   c. 6, 11   d. 13, 16

[Ref: Dhingra's 7th/e pg. 345]

Explanation

Conditions associated	HPV serotypes
Respiratory papillomatosis	6, 11
Laryngeal papillomatosis	2, 6, 11, 16
Laryngeal Carcinoma	6, 11
Squamous cell carcinoma of esophagus	16, 18
Bowen disease	16, 18, 31, 34
Carcinoma of cervix	16, 18, 31, 33
Carcinoma of vulva	6, 11, 16, 18
Carcinoma in situ of penis (Erythroplasia of Queyrat)	16
Carcinoma of penis	16, 18

- Laryngeal papillomas are MC benign tumor of larynx
- Single or multiple, irregular, wart like glottic masses.
- Treatment is with CO_2 laser ablation. α-IFN and indole - 3 - carbinol may also be used.

66. All of the following are true regarding Juvenile papillomatosis EXCEPT *(PGMEE 2012)*
   a. Commonly occur in children
   b. Laser surgery is the treatment of choice
   c. Stridor is common
   d. Remissions are uncommon

[Ref: Dhingra 7th/e pg. 345]

67. All are true about adult laryngeal papilloma except-
   a. More common in males *(PGMEE 2012)*
   b. Usually does not recur
   c. Posterior half of vocal cord
   d. Treatment is surgery

[Ref: Dhingra 7th/e pg. 346]

Explanation

- Usually, It is single, smaller in size, less aggressive and does not recur after surgical removal.
- It is common in males (2:1) in the age group of 30-50 years
- Usually arises from the anterior half of vocal cord or anterior commissure.
- Treatment is the same as for juvenile type.

LARYNGEAL CANCER

68. Hot potato voice is characteristic of - *(PGMEE 2013)*
   a. Subglottic carcinoma
   b. Glottic carcinoma
   c. Nasopharyngeal carcinoma
   d. Supraglottic carcinoma

[Ref: Dhingra's 6th/e pg. 306]

69. Laryngeal cancer is which type of carcinoma:- *(PGMEE 2016-17)*
   a. Transitional   b. Squamous epithelial
   c. Columnar cell   d. Mixed

[Ref: Dhingra 7th/e pg. 347]

70. TOC for glottic carcinoma with fully mobile cords:- *(PGMEE 2015)*
   a. Hemilaryngectomy   b. Radiotherapy
   c. Total laryngectomy   d. Chemotherapy

[Ref: Dhingra 7th/e pg. 351]

Explanation

- Cancer of the vocal cord without impairment of its mobility gives a 90% cure rate after irradiation and has the advantage of preservation of voice.

71. Treatment for early laryngeal tumor *(PGMEE 2016-17)*
   a. Chemotherapy
   b. Radiotherapy
   c. Total Laryngectomy
   d. Conservative laryngeal surgery

[Ref: Dhingra 7th/e pg. 351]

72. Best t/t of Ca Larynx with involvement of anterior commissure and arytenoids :- *(PGMEE 2012)*
   a. Radiotherapy followed by surgery
   b. Chemotherapy
   c. Partial Laryngectomy
   d. Total Laryngectomy

[Ref: Dhingra 7th/e pg. 351]

63.	b
64.	a
65.	c
66.	d
67.	c
68.	d
69.	b
70.	b
71.	b
72.	c

VOCAL NODULE

73. Most common cause of singers nodule is -

(PGMEE 2013)

a. Vocal abuse
b. Allergy
c. Infection
d. None

[Ref: Dhingra 7th/e pg. 343]

74. Most common location of vocal nodule - (PGMEE 2014)

a. Posterior 1/3 and anterior 2/3 junction
b. Anterior commissure
c. Anterior 1/3 and posterior 2/3 junction
d. Posterior commissure

[Ref: Dhingra 7th/e pg. 343]

MISCELLANEOUS

75. Hyponasal voice is seen in all except - (PGMEE 2013)

a. Adenoids
b. Habitual
c. Cleft palate
d. Nasal polyp

[Ref: Dhingra 7th/e pg. 357 table]

Explanation

Causes of Hyponasality and Hypernasality

Hyponasality	Hypernasality
Common cold	Velopharyngeal insufficiency
Nasal allergy	Congenitally short soft palate
Nasal polypl	Submucous palate
Nasal growth	Large nasopharynx
Adenoids	Cleft of soft palate
Nasopharyngeal mass	Paralysis of soft palate
Familial speech pattern	Postadenoidectomy
Habitual	Oronasal fistula
	Familial speech pattern
	Habitual speech pattern

76. A 5 year old boy while having dinner suddenly becomes aphonic and is brought to the casualty with complaint of respiratory distress. What should be the appropriate management? (PGMEE 11)

a. Cricothyroidotomy
b. Emergency tracheostomy
c. Humidified oxygen
d. Heimlich manoeuvre

[Ref: Dhingra 7th/e pg. 367]

77. A patient with Pancoast's tumour, develops loss of voice after radiation. It is due to:- (PGMEE 2014)

a. Irradiation to vocal cords
b. Involvement of recurrent laryngeal nerve
c. Vocal cord infiltration with secondaries
d. Radiation stenosis of larynx

[Ref: Dhingra 7th/e pg. 338]

78. Laryngotomy is done at:- (PGMEE 2016-17)

a. Thyrohyoid membrane
b. Cricothyroid membrane
c. Trachea
d. All of the above

[Ref: Dhingra 7th/e pg. 363]

Explanation

- Cricothyrotomy or Laryngotomy or Mini Tracheostomy. This is a procedure for opening the air way through the cricothyroid membrane.

79. Maintenance of airway during laryngectomy in a patient with carcinoma of larynx is best done by -

(PGMEE 2012)

a. Tracheostomy
b. Combi tube
c. Laryngeal mask airway
d. Laryngeal tube

[Ref: Dhingra 7th/e pg. 359]

80. Cotton's grading is used for? (PGMEE 2011)

a. Subglottic stenosis
b. Vocal cord misuse
c. Superior nerve palsy
d. Laryngeal carcinoma

Explanation

Subglottic stenosis:

- Most common cause of subglottic stenosis is from endotracheal intubation, either secondary to prolonged intubation, an incorrect size tube or incorrect cuff pressure
- Cotton and myer's devised a classification from 1 to 4 for grading circumferential subglottic stenosis
  - Grade 1: less than 50% luminal obstruction
  - Grade 2: 50-70% luminal obstruction
  - Grade 3: 71-99% luminal obstruction
  - Grade 4: complete luminal obstruction
- It can be managed either endoscopically or via an open procedure depend upon type of stenosis.

81. Acute laryngeal spam during indirect laryngoscopy in seen in?

a. Acute epiglottitis
b. Acute laryngo tracheo bronchitis
c. Acute tonsillitis
d. Acute laryngitis

Explanation

- Laryngitis means inflammation of the larynx. Oedema of the laryngeal lining increases the amount of pressure required to produce sound, resulting in dysphonia or aphonia. Changes to the structure of the larynx may also result in a lower register of speech.
- Mucous across the vocal cords may result in laryngeal spasm. Unless the clinician is experienced in the technique of indirect laryngoscopy, examination in the limited context of primary care is generally unhelpful.

82. All of the following are removed in vertical hemilaryngectomy except- (PGMEE 2015)

a. Half Subglottis
b. Half tongue
c. Half Supraglottis
d. Half Glottis

[Ref: Internet]

73.	a
74.	c
75.	c
76.	d
77.	b
78.	b
79.	a
80.	a
81.	d
82.	b

WALDEYER RING

ADENOIDS

1. Adenoids are lined by ? *(PGMEE 2015)*
a. Pseudostratified ciliated columnar epithelium
b. Columnar epithelium with goblet cells
c. Cuboidal epithelium
d. Non keratinized squamous epithelium

[Ref: Dhingra's 7th/e pg. 271]

2. Adenoids are also called? *(PGMEE 2012)*
a. Faucial tonsils
b. Lingual tonsils
c. Nasopharyngeal tonsils
d. Palatine tonsils

[Ref: Dhingra's 7th/e pg. 270]

Explanation

Types of tonsils	Also called
Nasopharyngeal tonsils (or pharyngeal tonsils)	■ Adenoids ■ No crypts & no capsule
Palatine tonsils	■ Simply the tonsils (Faucial tonsils) ■ Crypts + capsule
Lingual	
Tubal (Gehrlach tonsils)	■ In fossa of Rosenmuller ■ Near pharyngeal opening of ET.

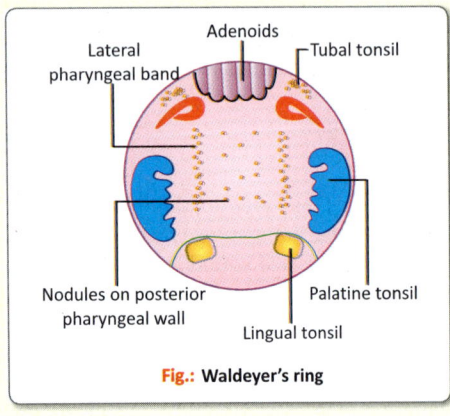

Fig.: Waldeyer's ring

3. All are true about adenoids except: *(PGMEE 2012-13)*
a. Physiological growth up to 6 years
b. Crypta magna present
c. Supplied by facial artery
d. Present in nasopharynx
[Ref: BDC 7th/e vol. 3 pg. 237; Dhingra's 7th/e pg. 269, 275]

4. All of the following are features of enlarged adenoids except:- *(PGMEE 2015)*
a. Otitis media
b. Esophagitis
c. Nasal obstruction
d. Aprosexia

[Ref: Dhingra's 7th/e pg. 275]

Explanation

- Nasal obstruction is the commonest symptom.
- Nasal discharge
- Sinusitis
- Epistaxis
- Voice change. Voice is toneless and loses nasal quality due to nasal obstruction (Hyponasality/Rhinolatia clausa)
- Tubal obstruction
- Recurrent attacks of acute otitis media
- Chronic suppurative otitis media
- Otitis media with effusion
- Adenoid facies. Chronic nasal obstruction and mouth breathing lead to characteristic facial appearance called adenoid facies.
- Pulmonary hypertension.
- Aprosexia, i.e. lack of concentration

5. Mother of a 5yr old child complaints that her child is a mouth breather and suffers recurrent cold. On examination typical facies are found. Most likely cause is - *(PGMEE 2012)*
a. Adenoids   b. Carcinoma
c. Angiofibroma   d. None

[Ref: Dhingra's 7th/e pg. 275]

6. Objective diagnosis of adenoid enlargement is made by?
a. CT scan *(PGMEE 2012-13)*
b. Lateral neck radiograph
c. Posterior rhinoscopy
d. Nasal fiberoptic endoscopy

[Ref: Dhingra's 7th/e pg. 276]

7. Treatment of hypertrophied adenoids: *(PGMEE 2012)*
a. Antibiotics
b. H_2 blockers
c. Beta-blockers
d. Nasal decongestant dropss

[Ref: Dhingra's 7th/e pg. 276]

8. Adenoidectomy with grommet insertion is treatment of choice for:- *(DNB 2010)*
a. Serous otitis media due to adenoids in children
b. Serous otitis media in adults
c. Adenoiditis in children
d. All of the above

[Ref: Dhingra's 7th/e pg. 70]

1.	a
2.	c
3.	b
4.	b
5.	a
6.	d
7.	d
8.	a

Explanation

Otitis media with effusion (OME)

- Otitis media with effusion (OME) is the chronic accumulation of mucus within the middle ear and sometimes the mastoid air cell system.
- In children, the prevalence is bimodal with the first and largest peak of 20 percent at two years of age and a second peak of percent at around five years of age
- In the majority of children their OME causes only a mild hearing impairment that is unlikely to be disabling.
- Any effect of this hearing impairment on speech and language and cognition is small, of minor significance and likely to spontaneously correct with age.
- Attic retractions are an OME disease effect with an incidence of 14 percent in the most severely affected children. What proportion of these retractions progress to cholesteatoma is not known.
- The arbitrary cut-off in hearing thresholds that is taken to indicate a potentially disabling effect that could be improved by ventilation tubes is now taken as 25 dB HL or poorer in both ears.
- Children who persist with OME and a bilateral 25 dB HL over a 12-week-period can benefit from the beneficial effects of ventilation tubes on the hearing over the next nine months.
- Even when a ventilation tube is functioning, there is still a residual conductive impairment of around 13 dB.
- If ventilation tubes are to be inserted there is a strong argument that adenoidectomy should be performed at the same time, particularly if there is concern regarding the general health of the upper respiratory tract.
- Adenoidectomy extends the period of benefit to the hearing of short-term ventilation tubes up to two years by a magnitude of around 2 to 3 dB.
- It also reduces the proportion of children eligible for reinsertion of short term tubes from around 50 to 25 percent.

TONSILS

9. **Bed of tonsil is formed by -**   *(PGMEE 2013)*
   a. Inferior constrictor & styloglossus m/s
   b. Middle constrictor & styloglossus m/s
   c. Superior constrictor & styloglossus m/s
   d. Platysma & stylopharyngeus m/s
   [Ref: BDC 7th/e vol. 3 pg. 237; Dhingra's 7th/e pg. 291]

10. **Anterior tonsillar pillar is formed by-**
        (PGMEE 2015, 2013)
    a. Valleculae   b. Palatopharyngeal fold
    c. Pterygopalatine arch   d. Palatoglossal fold
    [Ref: Gray's Anatomy 20th/e]

Explanation

- Ant. pillar is formed by → Palatoglossal fold/arch
- Posterior is formed by → Palatopharyngeal arch (Palatopharyngeus muscle)

11. **Blood supply of tonsil is mainly by:-**   *(PGMEE 2014)*
    a. Middle meningeal artery
    b. Maxillary artery
    c. Tonsillar branch of facial artery
    d. External carotid artery
    [Ref: Dhingra's 7th/e pg. 291]

12. **Tonsils reach their maximum size by -**   *(PGMEE 2012)*
    a. l years   b. 3 years
    c. 5 years   d. 12 years
    [Ref: Dhingra's 7th/e pg. 292]

13. **Referred ear pain (otalgia) in case of acute tonsillitis is transmitted by ?**   *(PGMEE 2018)*
    a. Auriculotemporal branch of facial nerve
    b. Glossopharyngeal nerve
    c. Trigeminal nerve
    d. Vagus nerve
    [Ref: Dhingra's 7th/e pg. 291, 143]

Explanation

- Pain from orophayrnx (acute tonsillitis, peritonsillar abscess) Base of tongue, elongated styloid process referred to ear via 9th nerve
- Palatine tonsil is supplied by Tonsillar branch of GLOSSOPHARYNGEAL NERVE and maxillary division of trigeminal nerve but glossopharyngeal is most likely to be damaged during acute tonsillitis and tonsillectomy.
- Pain from teeths, tongue, TM joints referred to ear via 5th cranial nerve
- As ears receive nerve supply from 5th, 9th and 10th cranial nerve and from C2, C3 pain may be referred from these area
- Pain from larynx, epiglottis referred via 10th nerve

14. **Sensory supply of palatine tonsil is by which cranial nerve?**   *(PGMEE 2012-13)*
    a. Lesser palatine nerve   b. Greater palatine nerve
    c. Vagus   d. Glossopharyngeal nerve
    [Ref: BDC 7th/e vol. 3 pg. 239; Dhingra's 7th/e pg. 291]

15. **Structure seen on the lateral wall of tonsillar fossa is?**   *(DNB June 2009)*
    a. Glossopharyngeal artery
    b. Facial nerve
    c. Superior constrictor muscle
    d. Palatopharyngeus muscle
    [Ref: BDC 7th/e vol. 3 pg. 238; Dhingra's 7th/e pg. 292]

Explanation

- Tonsil is related laterally to
  ○ Loose areolar tissue containing paratonsillar vein
  ○ Superior constrictor muscle
  ○ Styloglossus
  ○ Glossopharyngeal nerve
  ○ Facial artery
  ○ Medial pterygoid muscle

16. **Plica triangularis is present in:**   *(PGMEE 2012-13)*
    a. Antero-inferior part of tonsil
    b. Inlet of larynx
    c. Dorsum of tongue
    d. None
    [Ref: BDC 7th/e vol. 3 pg. 238; Dhingra's 7th/e pg. 291]

Explanation

- **Tonsil morphology:**
  ○ Plica triangularis: Triangular vestigial fold of mucosa covering **anteroinferior** part of tonsil.
  ○ Plica semilunaris: Semilunar fold which crosses upper part of the tonsillar sinus.

9.	c
10.	d
11.	c
12.	d
13.	b
14.	d
15.	c
16.	a

17. Pharyngeal tonsil is lined by? *(PGMEE 2013)*
   a. Simple cuboidal epithelium
   b. Pseudostratified columnar epithelium
   c. Non-keratinizing stratified squamous epithelium
   d. Keratinizing stratified squamous epithelium

   [Ref: Dhingra's 7th/e pg. 271]

18. Waldeyer's ring consist of all of the following except?
   a. Pharyngeal tonsils *(PGMEE 2012-13)*
   b. Palatine tonsile
   c. Tubal tonsils
   d. Posterior auricular nodes

   [Ref: BDC 7th/e vol. 3 pg. 237; Dhingra's 7th/e pg. 270]

19. Gerlach tonsil in Waldeyer's ring is - *(PGMEE 2013)*
   a. Tubal tonsil   b. Palatine tonsil
   c. Pharyngeal tonsil d. Lingual tonsil

   [Ref: Stedman's medical eponyms p. 269]

QUINSY (PERITONSILLAR ABSCESS)

20. Quinsy (Peritonsillar abscess) is caused most commonly by:- *(PGMEE 2013)*
   a. Streptococcus pneumoniae
   b. H. influenzae
   c. Mix anaerobic & aerobic infection
   d. Staphylococcus aureus

   [Ref: Dhingra's 7th/e pg. 298]

21. Trismus is seen commonly in :- *(PGMEE 2013)*
   a. Retropharyngeal abscess
   b. Quinsy
   c. Ludwig angina
   d. Parapharyngeal abscess

   [Ref: Dhingra's 7th/e pg. 298]

Explanation
   - Quinsy can cause → Hot potato voice, trismus (d/to spasm of pterygoid), ear ache & torticollis.
   - Retropharyngeal abscess produces torticollis (stiff neck), dysphagia & croupy cough.
   - Ludwig angina produces odynophagia, cellulitis and laryngeal edema.

22. Which muscle is affected in peritonsiller Abscess:- *(PGMEE 2016-17)*
   a. Sternocleidomastoid   b. Massater
   c. Medial pterygoid   d. Inferior constrictor

   [Ref: Dhingra's 7th/e pg. 298]

23. All of the following is true about quinsy EXCEPT? *(PGMEE 2012)*
   a. Does not involve floor of mouth
   b. Abscess is collected lateral to the superior constrictor
   c. Bulge in soft palate
   d. Trismus is commonly associated

   [Ref: Dhingra's 7th/e pg. 299; Longer Turner 10th/e p. 85]

24. The ideal time Tonsillectomy operation of quinsy after an attacks of quinsy - *(PGMEE 2014)*
   a. 2 weeks   b. 2-4 weeks
   c. 4-6 weeks   d. 6-12 weeks

   [Ref: Dhingra's 5th/e p. 279; Mapbool 11th /e p. 289; Logen Turner 10th/e p. 86]

PHARYNX

25. Nasopharynx is lined by which epithelium
   a. Ciliated columnar *(PGMEE 2013)*
   b. Stratified squamous keratinized
   c. Stratified squamous nonkerationized
   d. Cuboidal

   [Ref: Dhingra's 7th/e pg. 271]

26. Sinus of Morgagni is present in – *(PGMEE 2013)*
   a. Oropharynx   b. Laryngopharynx
   c. Hypophrynx   d. Nasopharynx

   [Ref: Dhingra's 7th/e pg. 271, 511]

Explanation
   - Sinus of Morgagni is a part of nasopharynx.
   - It is a space between the base of the skull and upper free border of superior constrictor muscle. Through it enters
     ○ The eustachian tube
     ○ The levator veli palatini
     ○ Tensor veli palatini and
     ○ Ascending palatine artery - branch of the facial artery
   - *Trotter (or Sinus of Morgagni) syndrome or triad* is seen in nasopharyngeal carcinoma which spreads laterally to involve the sinus of Morgagni involving mandibular nerve. It is characterized by
     ○ Conductive hearing loss (due to eustachian tube obstruction).
     ○ Ipsilateral immobility of soft palate.
     ○ Neuralgic pain in the distribution of V3.
     ○ Trismus and preauricular fullness may be associated with the above.

27. Sinus of Morgagni lies between: *(PGMEE 2014)*
   b. Middle constrictor and superior constrictor
   a. Middle constrictor and inferior constrictor
   c. Superior constrictor and skull
   d. None of the above

   [Ref: BDC 8th/e vol. 3 pg. 264; Dhingra's 7th/e pg. 271]

28. Which of the following structure passes through sinus of Morgagni:- *(PGMEE 2016-17)*
   a. Palatoglossus
   b. Palatopharyngeus
   c. Tensor tympani
   d. Levator veli palatini muscle

   [Ref: BDC 7th/e vol. 3 pg. 242; Dhingra's 7th/e pg. 271]

29. Trotter's triad consists of following, except:
   a. Ipsilateral soft plate immobility *(DNB pattern 2008)*
   b. Conduction deafness
   c. VII nerve palsy
   d. Trigeminal neuralgia

   [Ref: Dhingra's 7th/e pg. 511]

30. Trotter's triad includes all except – *(PGMEE 2012)*
   a. Conductive deafness
   b. Diplopia
   c. Palatal palsy
   d. Sensory disturbance over distribution of 5th cranial nerve

   [Ref: Dhingra's 7th/e pg. 511]

17.	b
18.	d
19.	a
20.	c
21.	b
22.	c
23.	b
24.	c
25.	a
26.	d
27.	c
28.	d
29.	c
30.	b

31. **Passavant ridge is formed by:** *(PGMEE 2012-13, 2015)*
   a. Tensor veli palati and superior constrictor
   b. Palatopharyngeous and superior constrictor
   c. Palatoglossus and superior constrictor
   d. Palatopharyngeous and inferior constrictor

   [Ref: BDC 8th/e vol. 3 pg. 266; Dhingra's 7th/e pg. 271]

Explanation

- *Passvant's ridge* is a small cushion in posterior pharynx formed by contraction of superior pharyngeal constrictor.
- It is a mucosal ridge raised by fibres of palatopharyngeus.

32. **Passavant ridges is due to contraction of?**
   (PGMEE 2013)
   a. Palatoglossus   b. Superior constrictor
   c. Inferior constrictor   d. Middle constrictor

   [Ref: BDC 7th/e vol. 3 pg. 234]

33. **Killian dehiscence is found in:** *(PGMEE 2012-13)*
   a. Middle constrictor   b. Inferior constrictor
   c. Superior constrictor   d. None

   [Ref: BDC 8th/e vol. 3 pg. 265; Dhingra's 7th/e pg. 269]

Explanation

Killian's Dehiscene

- Inferior constrictor muscle has two parts; thyropharyngeus with oblique fibres and cricopharyngeus with transverse fibres.
- Between these two parts exists a potential gap called *Killian's dehiscence*.
- It is also called "gateway of tears" as perforation can occur at this site during oesophagoscopy.
- This is also the site for herniation of pharyngeal mucosa in cases of pharyngeal pouch.

34. **Location of Piriform fossa:** *(PGMEE 2012-13)*
   a. Oropharynx
   b. Nasopharynx
   c. Laryngeal part of pharynx
   d. Centre of Larynx

   [Ref: BDC 8th/e vol. 3 pg. 291; Dhingra's 7th/e pg. 272]

35. **Lymphatic drainage of oropharynx is mainly through-**
   (PGMEE 2013)
   a. Superficial cervical lymph nodes
   b. Submandibular nodes
   c. Jugulodigastric nodes of upper jugular chain
   d. Jugulo-omohyoid nodes

   [Ref: Dhingra's 7th/e pg. 271]

36. **Which of the following mobile painless swelling produces lump in throat but does not interfere with swallowing:** *(Recent Pattern June 2018)*
   a. Thyroglossal cyst   b. Globus pharyngeus
   c. Retrosternal goitre   d. Subhyoid bursitis

   [Ref: Dhingra's 7th/e pg. 389]

Explanation

- The sensation of difficulty in swallowing (dysphagia) in the absence of any apparent physical abnormality is often commonly described as having "lump in the throat".

- The MC cause of lump in throat is tightening of the cricopharyngeal muscle surrounding the esophagus, it is called **globus pharyngeus or globus hystericus**.
- The majority of patients complaining of the sensation of a lump in the throat suffer from this condition.
- Clinical examination of the pharynx, larynx and base of tongue is normal.
- T/t: Reassurance to the patient

ANGIOFIBROMA

37. **A 15 year old male presents with a mass in the posterior nasopharynx near inferior meatus. It suddenly starts bleeding heavily when biopsy was attempted. Investigation of choice for this condition-**
   a. MRI   *(PGMEE 2015)*
   b. CT head with contrast
   c. Carotid Angiography
   d. Xray paranasal sinuses

   [Ref: Dhingra's 7th/e pg. 280]

38. **Nasal angiofibroma is common in:-** *(PGMEE 2013)*
   a. Adolescent male   b. Elderly female
   c. Elderly male   d. Adult male

   [Ref: Dhingra's 7th/e pg. 279]

39. **Juvenile Nasopharyngeal angiofibroma is:** *(DNB 2010)*
   a. Is malignant neoplasm common in females
   b. Is benign neoplasm common in adolescents males
   c. Is malignant neoplasm in males
   d. Is benign neoplasm in females

   [Ref: Dhingra's 7th/e pg. 279]

40. **Frog face deformity of nose caused by-** *(PGMEE 2014)*
   a. Antral polyp   b. Angiofibroma
   c. Rhinoscleroma   d. Ethmoidal polyp

   [Ref: Dhingra's 7th/e pg. 279]

Explanation

- Extension of nasopharyngeal angiofibroma into orbits giving rise to proptosis and "frog-face deformity".
- Nasopharyngeal angiofibroma enters through the inferior orbital fissure and also destroys apex of the orbit.

41. **Antral sign or Holman Miller sign in contrast CT head is seen in -** *(PGMEE 2012)*
   a. Laryngeal carcinoma
   b. Cranipharyngioma
   c. Nasopharyngeal carcinoma
   d. Nasopharyngeal angiofibroma

   [Ref: Dhingra's 7th/e pg. 281]

42. **Which of the following is not true for juvenile angiofibroma**
   a. Surgical excision is TOC   *(PGMEE 2012)*
   b. Presentation is commonly in second decade
   c. Biopsy for diagnosis
   d. Benign tumor

   [Ref: Dhingra's 7th/e pg. 279, 281]

43. **Investigation of choice for nasopharyngeal angiofibroma -** *(PGMEE 2013)*
   a. X-ray   b. CT- contrast
   c. Plane-CT   d. MRI

   [Ref: Dhingra's 7th/e pg. 280]

31.	b
32.	b
33.	b
34.	c
35.	c
36.	b
37.	b
38.	a
39.	b
40.	b
41.	d
42.	c
43.	b

44. Young patient with headache, epiphora, bilateral nasal obstruction, no fever. Diagnosis- *(PGMEE 2013)*
- a. Nasal polyp
- b. Rhinoscleroma
- c. Nasal carcinoma
- d. Juvenile angiofibroma

[Ref: Dhingra's 7th/e pg. 279]

45. A 13 year old boy presents with swelling in the cheek with recurrent epistaxis. Most likely cause is - *(PGMEE 2012, UP 08)*
- a. Rhabdomyosarcoma
- b. Ca Nasopharynx
- c. Angiofibroma
- d. None

[Ref: Dhingra's 6th/e pg. 246]

NASOPHARYNGEAL CA

46. 70 year old man presents with cervical lymphadenopathy. What can be the cause - *(PGMEE 2012)*
- a. Nasopharyngeal carcinoma
- b. Angiofibroma
- c. Acoustic neuroma
- d. Otosclerosis

[Ref: Dhingra's 7th/e pg. 283]

47. Which of the following is an important etiological factor for nasopharyngeal carcinoma? *(PGMEE 2015)*
- a. Epstein Barr virus
- b. Cytomegalovirus
- c. Human Herpes Virus
- d. Varicella

[Ref: Dhingra's 7th/e pg. 283]

48. Nasopharyngeal carcinoma affects which age group :- *(PGMEE 2014)*
- a. 3rd decade
- b. Adolescents
- c. Children
- d. 5th to 7th decade

[Ref: Dhingra's 7th/e pg. 284]

49. Most common presentation in nasopharyngeal carcinoma is with - *(PGMEE 2012)*
- a. Epistaxis
- b. Cervical lymphadenopathy
- c. Nasal stuffiness
- d. Hoarseness of voice

[Ref: Dhingra's 7th/e pg. 285]

Explanation

Cervical Nodal Metastases
- This may be the only manifestation of nasopharyngeal cancer.
- Nodal metastases are seen in 75% of the patients, when first seen, about half of them with bilateral nodes.

50. A person with neck nodes and B type tympanogram - *(PGMEE 2012)*
- a. Nasopharyngeal CA
- b. Angiofibroma
- c. Acoustic neuroma
- d. None

[Ref: Logan Turner 10th/e p. 109; Dhingra's 7th/e pg. 285, 284]

51. Investigation of choice for nasopharyngeal carcinoma :- *(PGMEE 2016-17)*
- a. MRI
- b. Plain CT scan
- c. Ultrasound
- d. X-ray PNS

[Ref: Dhingra's 7th/e pg. 285]

52. Trotter's triad is seen in: *(PGMEE 2016-2017; 12)*
- a. Maxillary ca
- b. Maxillary sinusitis
- c. Nasopharyngeal ca
- d. Angiofibroma

[Ref.:Dhingra's 7th/e pg. 511]

53. Most common site of origin of nasopharyngeal carcinoma is: *(PGMEE 2012 & 2015)*
- a. Antrochonal region
- b. Valleculae
- c. Palatine tonsils
- d. Fossa of Rosenmuller

[Ref: Dhingra's 7th/e pg. 284]

54. Radiotherapy is the treatment of choice for: *(DNB 2008)*
- a. Subglottic CA T3NO
- b. Glottic CA T3NI
- c. Nasopharyngeal carcinoma T3N1M0
- d. Supraglottic CA T3NO

[Ref: Dhingra's 7th/e pg. 285]

55. All of the following statements about Nasopharyngeal carcinoma are true, except: *(PGMEE 10)*
- a. Bimodal age distribution
- b. Nasopharyngectomy with radical Neck dissection is the treatment of choice
- c. IgA antibody to EBV is observed
- d. Squammous cell carcinoma is the most common histological subtype

[Ref: Dhingra's 6th/e pg. 253]

Explanation
- Nasopharyngeal carcinoma has 2 peaks.. 15-25 yrs and 55-65yrs

PARAPHARYNGEAL ABSCESS

56. Most common cause of parapharyngeal abscess: *(PGMEE 2014)*
- a. Penetrating trauma
- b. Haematogenous spread
- c. Removal of tonsil
- d. Blunt trauma

[Ref: Dhingra's 7th/e pg. 301; Logan Turner 10th/e p. 106]

57. A middle aged diabetic patient 1 week after the extraction of Lower 3rd molar, presents with swelling in posterior one third of the neck and sternocleidomastoid pushed medially. Most likely diagnosis is: *(PGMEE 2012-13)*
- a. Cold abscess
- b. Peritonsillar abscess
- c. Retropharngeal abscess
- d. Parapharyngeal abscess

[Ref: Dhingra's 7th/e pg. 301]

58. Most common cause of parapharyngeal abscess in adults - *(PGMEE 2013)*
- a. TB
- b. Lymphadenitis
- c. Tonsillitis
- d. Tooth extraction

[Ref: Logan Turner 10th/e p. 106]

59. All of the following are true regarding parapharyngeal abscess EXCEPT:- *(PGMEE 2012)*
- a. Midline swelling
- b. Abscess in pharyngo maxillary space
- c. Trismus may be seen
- d. Torticollis is due to spasm of prevertebral muscles

[Ref: Logan Turner 10th/e p. 106; Dhingra's 7th/e pg. 303]

44.	d
45.	c
46.	a
47.	a
48.	d
49.	b
50.	a
51.	a
52.	c
53.	d
54.	c
55.	b
56.	c
57.	d
58.	d
59.	a

RETROPHARYNGEAL ABSCESS

60. What is present in the retropharyngeal space:
   a. Platysma   **(PGMEE 2012-13)**
   b. Loose areolar tissue & lymph nodes
   c. Hypoglossal nerve
   d. Vertebrae

   [Ref: BDC 7th/e vol. 3 pg. 232]

61. Gillete's space indicates which of the following?
                                  (PGMEE 2012-13)
   a. Paravertebral space
   b. Prevertebral space
   c. Retropharyngeal space
   d. Perotinsillar space

   [Ref: Dhingra's 7th/e pg. 299]

62. Gillette's space is –   **(PGMEE 2012)**
   a. Parapharyngeal space
   b. Peritonsilar space
   c. Retropharyngeal space
   d. Paratracheal space

   [Ref: Dhingra's 7th/e pg. 299]

63. Most common cause of chronic retropharyngeal abscess:-   **(PGMEE 2016-17)**
   a. Dental caries
   b. Caries of cervical spine
   c. Torticollis
   d. Foreign body

   [Ref: Dhingra's 7th/e pg. 299]

64. Which of the following is not true about acute retropharyngeal abscess -   **(PGMEE 2012)**
   a. Dysphagia
   b. Swelling on posterolateral wall of pharynx
   c. Torticollis
   d. Caries of cervical spine is usually a common cause

   [Ref: Dhingra's 6th/e pg. 300]

65. Nodes of Rouviere are: –   **(PGMEE 2012)**
   a. Pretracheal node
   b. Retropharyngeal nodes
   c. Adenoids
   d. Parapharyngeal node

   [Ref: Dhingra's 7th/e pg. 510]

Explanation
- Node of Rouviere is the most superior node of the lateral group of retropharyngeal nodes.

LUDWIG'S ANGINA

66. Most common cause of Ludwig's angina is
   a. Retropharyngeal abscess   **(PGMEE 2013)**
   b. Parotid infection
   c. Tooth infection
   d. None

   [Ref: Dhingra's 7th/e pg. 297; Logan Turner 10th/e p. 107, 108]

67. Ludwig's angina is infection of: -   **(PGMEE 2012)**
   a. Sublingual space
   b. Peritonsilar space
   c. Submandibular space
   d. Parapharyngeal space

   [Ref: Dhingra's 7th/e pg. 297]

Explanation

Vincent's Angina Vs. Ludwig's Angina

Vincent's angina	Ludwig's angina
▪ Also k/as *acute necrotizing ulcerative gingivitis/Trench Mouth*	▪ Usually starts in infected Lower Molar 2nd and 3rd. (Cellulitis of floor of mouth)
▪ Halitosis and ulceration of the interdental papillae.	▪ Rapidly spreading, Life-threatening cellulitis of sublingual/submand spaces.
▪ Causative organism: Fusiform bacillus and Borellia vincenti	▪ Causative organism: Polymicrobial infection
▪ Patch (grayish-white pseudomembrane) in mouth Tracheostomy in case of glottic edema penicillin (high doses) + **IV metronidazole** therapy.	▪ T/t: Intubation/emergency

68. Ludwig's angina begins in: **(Recent Pattern June 2018)**
   a. Submandibular space   b. Sublingual space
   c. Parotid space   d. Retropharyngeal space

   [Ref: Dhingra's 7th/e pg. 297]

Explanation
- Ludwig's angina is a rapidly spreading bilateral cellulitis that involves the floor of mouth beneath the tongue (sublingual space, submandibular space and submental space).
- Ludwig's angina usually begins in the submandibular space, and then rapidly spreads to involve the sublingual space, usually on a bilateral basis.
- MC cause is infection of the root of the teeth (Dental infection), especially 2nd and 3rd mandibular molar.
- Other causes are mouth injury, mandibular fracture, and submandibular sialadenitis.

60.	b
61.	c
62.	c
63.	b
64.	d
65.	b
66.	c
67.	c
68.	a

MAXILLOFACIAL TRAUMA

MAXILLA

1. Lefort classification involves which bone fracture?
(PGMEE 2012)
a. Nasal bone
b. Zygomatic arch
c. Mandible
d. Maxilla

[Ref: Dhingra's 7th/e pg. 204; Bailey & Love 27th/e pg. 360]

Explanation

- # Middle third of face
  ○ Nasal bones and septum Naso-orbital area
- # Maxilla
  ○ Le Fort I (transverse)
  ○ Le Fort II (pyramidal)
  ○ Le Fort III (craniofacial dysjunction)

2. In Jarjavay fracture of nasal bone, the fracture line is-
(PGMEE 2012)
a. Oblique
b. Comminuted
c. Vertical
d. Horizontal

[Ref: Logan Turner 10th/e p. 21]

Explanation

- A priority is to distinguish simple fractures limited to the nasal bones (Type 1) from fractures that also involve other facial bones and/or the nasal septum (Types 2 and 3). ... A fracture that runs horizontally across the septum is sometimes called a "Jarjavay fracture", and a vertical one, a "Chevallet fracture".

3. Transverse fracture of maxilla is – *(PGMEE 2013)*
a. Le Fort-1
b. Let Fort- 2
c. Le Fort-3
d. Craniofacial disjunction

[Ref: Dhingra's 7th/e pg. 204]

4. Pyramidal fracture of maxilla is – *(PGMEE 2015)*
a. Le Fort-1
b. Le Fort-2
c. Le Fort-3
d. Craniofacial disruption

[Ref: Dhingra 6th/e p. 185]

5. Fracture of middle 1/3ʳᵈ of face does not lead to:-
(PGMEE 2014)
a. Malocclusion of teeth
b. Lengthening of face
c. Proptosis
d. Anaesthesia of upper lip

[Ref: Dhingra's 7th/e pg. 207]

Explanation

- Fractures of Maxilla can lead to:-
  ○ Malocclusion of teeth with anterior open bite
  ○ Elongation of midface
  ○ Mobility in the maxilla
  ○ CSF rhinorrhoea. Cribriform plate is injured in Le Fort II and Le Fort III fractures.

ZYGOMA

6. Tripod fracture is seen in- *(PGMEE 2015)*
a. Nasal bone
b. Maxilla
c. Mandible
d. Zygoma

[Ref: Dhingra's 7th/e pg. 205]

7. Nerve most commonly injured in fracture zygoma is:
a. Inferior alveolar nerve *(PGMEE 2011)*
b. Supraorbital nerve
c. Zygomaticotemporal nerve
d. Infraorbital nerve

[Ref: Dhingra's 7th/e pg. 205]

ORBITAL FLOOR

8. Blow out fracture refers to- *(PGMEE 2012)*
a. Fracture of roof of orbit
b. Fracture of zygoma
c. Fracture base of skull
d. Fracture of floor of orbit

[Ref: Dhingra's 7th/e pg. 206]

9. Tear drop opacity in Water's view is seen in:
a. Fracture mandible *(PGMEE 2013)*
b. Fracture maxilla
c. Fracture zygomatic arch
d. Blow out fracture of orbital floor

[Ref: Dhingra's 7th/e pg. 206]

10. A patient presents with enophthalmos after a trauma to face by blunt object. There is no fever or extraocular muscle palsy. Diagnosis is – *(PGMEE 2014)*
a. Fracture maxilla
b. Fracture ethmoid
c. Blowout fracture
d. Fracture zygoma

[Ref: Dhingra's 7th/e pg. 206]

PAROTID SURGERY

Given in Surgery

MISCELLANEOUS

11. Delphian nodes are:
a. Pretracheal
b. Prelaryngeal nodes
c. Supraclavicular
d. Paratracheal

[Ref: Dhingra's 7th/e pg. 440]

Explanation

Enlarged Nodes	Also known as
Transverse cervical chain (supraclavicular nodes)	Scalene Node
Prelaryngeal node (Delphian node)	Lies on cricothyroid membrane and drains subglottic region of larynx and pyriform sinuses
Retropharyngeal nodes	Most superior node of the lateral group is called node of Rouviere

12. Which of the following cancers do not present with cervical lymphnode involvement: *(PGMEE 2015)*
a. Oral cancer
b. Papillary thyroid cancer
c. Subglottic Cancer
d. Glottic Cancer

[Ref: Dhingra's 7th/e pg. 450]

1.	d
2.	d
3.	a
4.	b
5.	c
6.	d
7.	d
8.	d
9.	d
10.	c
11.	b
12.	d

Endocrinology

FACTS

- Gonads to testis differentiation is done by: SRY gene
- Testis starts producing testosterone under the influence of: Placental hCG
- 1st sign of pubertal changes in boys: Enlargement of testis
- 1st sign of pubertal changes in girls: Thelarche
- *Normal consonance of puberty is*
  - Girls: Thelarche → Pubarche → Menarche
  - Boys: **G**onadarche → **P**ubarche → **S**permarche
- Maximum level of ACTH and cortisol is at the time of early morning
- In secondary adrenal insufficiency: Aldosterone secretion is not affected therefore electrolytes are usually normal
- Midline facial defect, Single central incisor Micro penis, Hypoglycemia are the features seen in the deficiency of: Growth hormone
- Most of the affected children of Hashimoto's disease are clinically: Euthyroid i.e. TSH levels are raised but T$_4$ is normal, with Anti TPO & Anti Tg Ab positive.
- Earliest sign of congenital hypothyroidism: prolongation of physiological jaundice
- Earliest manifestation of Cushing's syndrome: Loss of diurnal variation in serum cortisol
- Major source of circulating IGF-I: Liver
- Weak giants are the consequence of pituitary adenoma
- *Whipple's triad:* Seen in Insulinoma and other conditions causing hypoglycemia.
  - Symptoms of hypoglycemia
  - Low plasma glucose levels
  - Relief of symptoms after plasma glucose is raised
- *Pemberton sign:*
  - Development of facial plethora on elevation of both the arms
  - Seen in Retrosternal goiter & mediastinal tumor

Hypothalamic Peptides

Hormones	Effect on Pituitary
Ghrelin	GH Release
Gonadotropin Hormone (GnRH)	LH & FSH Release
Thyrotropin Hormone (TRH)	TSH, **PRL**, GH, CRH Release
Corticotropin Releasing Hormone (CRH)	ACTH Release
Arginine Vasopressin (AVP)	ACTH Release
Somatostatin	Inhibits GH Release and TSH Release
Prolactin Inhibiting Hormone	Inhibits PRL, TSH, GH, LH, FSH Release

MOST COMMON

- MC hyperfunctioning pituitary adenoma: Prolactinoma
- MC pituitary hormone hypersecretion syndrome: Hyperprolactinemia
- MCC of Acromegaly: Growth hormone secreting pituitary adenoma
- MCC of death in children with DKA: Cerebral edema
- MC mononeuropathy in DM: 3rd CN palsy
- MC gland involved in MEN 1: Parathyroid

SYNDROMES

❶ Nelson syndrome:
- Due to rapid enlargement of an ACTH secreting pituitary adenoma
- Seen in patients with Cushing's syndrome after bilateral adrenalectomy
- B/L adrenalectomy → Loss of hypothalamic suppression → ↑ CRH → Growth of adenoma

❷ Kallman syndrome:
- X-linked inheritance
- KAL gene mutation
- Defect in GnRH synthesis in hypothalamus
- Associated with hypogonadotropic hypogonadism
- Olfactory bulb agenesis leads to anosmia or hyposmia

❸ McCune Albright syndrome:
- Cafe au -lait spots
- Polyostotic fibrous dysplasia
- Precocious puberty

❹ Laron's Syndrome/dwarfism:
- Defect of GH receptor structure/signaling.
- Growth failure results due to GH resistance/insensitivity.

❺ Jansen's disease:
- Constitutively active PTH/PTHrP receptor in target tissues

❻ Pendred syndrome:
- AR disorder of defective organification of Iodine
- Caused by mutation in the *pendrin* gene
- Manifestations include SNHL & Goiter

❼ Complete Androgen insensitivity syndrome:
- Genotype: XY
- Phenotype: female

❽ Sheehan syndrome/Postpartum hypopituitarism:
- Necrosis of pituitary gland as a result of severe hypotension or shock caused by massive hemorrhage (e.g. PPH) during or after delivery
- Leads to anterior pituitary hormone deficiency

❾ Wolman Disease:
- It is an example of Lysosomal storage disorders.
- AR disorder characterized by complete absence of an enzyme – Lysosomal Acid Lipase.
- Newborn becomes symptomatic during first week of life.
- Characterized by abdominal distension, Hepatosplenomegaly, **adrenal calcification** etc.

MICRODELETION SYNDROMES

Syndrome	Deletion	Clinical Features	Endocrine Features
Prader Willi Syndrome	15q11-13	▪ Muscular Hypotonia ▪ Excess appetite, Mental retardation ▪ Sleep apnea, Dysmorphim	▪ Short stature ▪ Hypogonadism ▪ Progressive obesity
Williams Syndrome	7q 11	▪ Supravalvular Aortic Stenosis ▪ Peripheral pulmonary artery stenosis ▪ Elfin facies; Mental retardation	▪ Infantile Hypercalcemia
CATCH-22/ DiGeorge Syndrome	22q 11	▪ **C**ardiac abnormalities ▪ **A**bnormal facies ▪ **T**hymic hypoplasia/absence ▪ **C**left palate	▪ **H**ypocalcemia ▪ Hypoparathyroidism ▪ Short stature
WAGR Syndrome	11p 13	▪ **W**ilm's tumor ▪ **A**niridia ▪ Mental **R**etardation ▪ Hemihypertrophy	▪ **G**enitourinary abnormality like undescended testes

PITUITARY ADENOMAS

Functions of prolactin
- Induces and maintains lactation
- Suppress sexual drive

- ↓ GnRH, LH & FSH
- ↓ estrogen l/t anovulation

Etiology for Hyperprolactinemia

- Pregnancy
- Lactation
- Hypothyroidism
- Prolactinoma
- Acromegaly
- Tumors

- Atypical antipsychotics
- Haloperidol
- Metoclopramide
- α-Methyl-dopa
- Phenothiazines

	Prolactinoma	Acromegaly
Pathology	▪ Most common hormone secreting pituitary tumor. ▪ Depending on size, it can be classified as Microadenoma (<1 cm) or Macroadenoma (>1 cm).	▪ Disorder of GH hypersecretion in adulthood ▪ Characterized by excess of IGF-I (aka **Somatomedin C**) ▪ MC Cause – GH secreting pituitary adenoma.

Clinical features	▪ Headache
	▪ **Visual problems**:
	  ○ Superior temporal quadrantanopia in asymmetric lesion
	  ○ Bitemporal hemianopsia (compression of optic chiasm) to total vision loss.
	  ○ Ophthalmoplegia (from compression of CN III, IV, or VI).
	
	In Women
	▪ Infertility
	▪ Menstrual disturbance – Oligo/Amenorrhea
	▪ Galactorrhea
	▪ Osteoporosis
	
	In Men
	▪ Decreased libido
	▪ Erectile dysfunction
	▪ ↓ spermatogenesis & Infertility
		▪ Coarse facial features and a large fleshy nose.
		▪ Acral bony overgrowth results in frontal bossing, mandibular enlargement with **prognathism**, and widened space between the lower incisor teeth.
		▪ Soft tissue swelling results in **increased heel pad thickness, increased shoe or glove size**, ring tightening
		▪ Galactorrhea, Hypogonadism
		▪ **High blood pressure**
		▪ **Diabetes mellitus** + intolerance of a glucose
		▪ Generalized visceromegaly
		▪ Increased risk for colorectal cancer and premalignant adenomatous polyps.

Lab Investigations	▪ Basal, fasting morning PRL levels are increased ▪ Serum TSH – to exclude the possibility of an elevated PRL level occurring secondary to an elevated TRH level. ▪ ↓Serum testosterone – in males presenting with symptoms of hypogonadism	▪ Serum IGF-I levels are elevated ▪ The diagnosis of acromegaly is confirmed by demonstrating the **failure of GH suppression** within 1–2 h of an oral glucose load. ▪ PRL should be measured (elevated in ~25% of patients).
Imaging	▪ Gadolinium enhanced MRI >> CECT	▪ MRI

Treatment	▪ Microadenomas rarely progress to become Macroadenoma→ no treatment required in asymptomatic patients and if fertility is not desired.
	▪ **DOC/1ˢᵗ line** for symptomatic Microadenoma OR Macroadenoma : *Dopamine agonist* – Cabergoline and Bromocriptine
	▪ **Preferred surgical treatment**: Transsphenoidal pituitary adenomectomy. Indications for debulking surgery include:
	  ○ Dopamine resistance or intolerance
	  ○ Presence of an invasive Macroadenoma with compromised vision that fails to improve after drug treatment.
		▪ *Surgical:* Transsphenoidal resection
		  ○ Preferred primary treatment for both Microadenomas and macroadenomas.
		▪ *Pharmacotherapy:* Used as adjuvant treatment
		  ○ *Somatostatin analogues:* Octreotide and Lanreotide are the preferred medical treatment
		  ○ *Dopamine agonist:* Bromocriptine and cabergoline
		  ○ *GH Receptor Antagonist:* Pegvisomant

SYNDROME OF INAPPROPRIATE ADH SECRETION

Physiology of ADH/AVP Release	■ Synthesized in the neurons located in the supraoptic and paraventricular nuclei of anterior hypothalamus. ■ Secreted by posterior pituitary in response to ↑in serum osmolality & ↓ in effective circulating volume. ■ Major site of action – DCT & medullary collecting duct (via V_2 receptor)
Pathology of SIADH	■ Form of **euvolemic/ dilutional** hyponatremia resulting from inappropriate, continued secretion of the antidiuretic hormone – Arginine vasopressin (AVP). ■ Secretion is independent of serum osmolality. ■ Impaired free water excretion results in dilutionalhyponatremia. ■ Increase in Atrial Natriuretic Peptide and glomerular filtration results in natriuresis with diuresis, thus prevents development of edema.

Etiology	**Neoplasms**	**Drugs**	**Neurological**	**Pulmonary**
	■ **Lung carcinoma – Small Cell CA** ■ Duodenum CA ■ Pancreas CA ■ Bronchial adenoma ■ Carcinoid	■ **Vasopressin Desmopressin** ■ **Vincristine** ■ SSRI; MAO inhibitors ■ Carbamazepine ■ Cyclophosphamide ■ Tricyclic Antidepressants	■ **Head trauma** ■ **Encephalitis** ■ Neuropsychiatric disorders ■ Acute intermittent Porphyria ■ Cerebrovascular accidents	■ **Pneumonia** ■ **Emphysema** ■ Tuberculosis ■ Asthma ■ COPD

Clinical Feature	■ No edema , Euvolemia ■ Similar to hyponatremia
Lab	■ Hyponatremia ■ Concentrated urine with osmolality >100 mOsm/kg ■ Hypo-osmolality (<280 mosmol/L) ■ Low BUN and Uric acid ■ Urinary Na >20 mmol/L

Treatment	Depends on whether the patient is symptomatic, and whether hyponatremia is acute (<48 h) or chronic.
	Acute symptomatic: ■ First line of therapy: water restriction ■ Hypertonic (3%) saline ■ AVP receptor-2 antagonist (Tolvaptan) *Chronic and/or minimally symptomatic:* ■ Restricting total fluid intake ■ Oral vaptan ■ Tolvaptan

DIABETES INSIPIDUS (DI)

Central Diabetes Insipidus	■ Lack of ADH production & secretion ■ Sever polyuria (>8-10 L/day)
Nephrogenic Diabetes Insipidus	■ Lack of renal response to ADH
Gestational Diabetes Insipidus	■ Due to destruction of ADH by placental vasopressinase
Primary Polydipsic Diabetes Insipidus	■ Suppression of ADH release secondary to excessive fluid intake ■ Seen in conditions like dipsogenic, psychogenic or iatrogenic DI

Investigations	SIADH*	CSW**	Central DI	Nephrogenic DI	Primary Polydipsia
ADH levels	↑	N/↓	↓	↑	↓
Urine output	↓/N	↑	↑ (>3 L/Day)	↑	↑
Serum sodium	↓	↓	↑	↑	↓
Serum osmolality	↓↓	↓	↑	↑	↓
Urine sodium	↑	↑↑	↓		↓
Urine osmolality	↑	↑	↓ (<200)	↓ (<200)	↑
Urine osmolality after water deprivation			No change	No change	↑
Urine osmolality after AVP			↑	No change	↑
Hydration	Euvolemia	Dehydration	Dehydrated	Dehydrated	Over hydration
Treatment	■ Fluid restriction – TOC ■ Loop diuretics ■ Demeclocycline	■ IV hypertonic saline ■ Fludrocortisone	■ Desmopressin	■ Thiazide diuretics ■ Amiloride	■ Fluid restriction

* Syndrome of Inappropriate ADH Release | ** Cerebral Salt Wasting Syndrome |

THYROIDITIS

	Acute Suppurative Thyroiditis	Subacute Thyroiditis (aka de Quervain's Thyroiditis)	Chronic Thyroiditis

Etiology	■ Bacterial infection
	■ Fungal infection
	■ Radiation thyroiditis after I^{131}
	■ Amiodarone
		■ Viral infection
		■ Mycobacterial infection
		■ Silent thyroiditis
		■ Postpartum thyroiditis
		■ Drug induced – Amiodarone, Interferon
			■ Autoimmune
			  ○ Hashimoto's thyroiditis (MCC)
			  ○ SLE
			  ○ Rheumatoid Arthritis
			  ○ Diabetes Mellitus Type I
			  ○ Myasthenia
			■ Riedel's thyroiditis

Thyroid Function Test	■ Normal	■ Brief hyperthyroidism f/b normal function (self-limiting disease in 2 – 6 months)	■ Subclinical or permanent Hypothyroidism (↑ TSH)
Antibodies	■ Nil	■ Nil	■ Anti – TPO & Anti Tg Antibodies present
RAI uptake study	■ Normal	■ Extremely low (<5%) – d/t destruction of parenchyma	■ Not useful
Treatment	■ IV antibiotics	■ Aspirin/Prednisolone ■ Propranolol – if signs of hyperthyroidism	■ Levothyroxine

Riedel's Thyroiditis

• Chronic inflammatory disease characterized by replacement of normal thyroid parenchyma by fibrotic tissues.

• Fibrous process extends beyond the capsule to involve the adjacent structures.

CONGENITAL HYPOTHYROIDISM

Etiology	■ MC Cause: Thyroid dysgenesis (75 - 80%)
Associated with	■ **Pendred syndrome (Dyshormonogenesis)** ■ Kocher-Debre-Semelaigne Syndrome
Clinical features	■ Asymptomatic at birth due to maternal T_4 ■ Prolongation of physiological jaundice ■ Feeding deficiency ■ Oedematous facies ■ Macroglossia (Large tongue) ■ Abdominal distension ■ Hands are broad, fingers are short ■ Coarse and dry skin ■ Constipation ■ Hypothermia/Motting ■ Delayed bone age ■ Delayed puberty ■ Upper segment > lower segment ■ **Wide and open posterior fontanel** ■ **Delayed dentition** ■ Growth retardation ■ Umbilical hernia ■ Hoarse cry ■ MR within 2 years of age
Lab	■ Serum T_4 = low ■ TSH = elevated ■ Serum Prolactin = elevated
X-ray	■ Absent distal femoral epiphysis ■ Epiphyseal dysgenesis ■ Multiple epiphyseal break ■ Deformity/beaking of 12th thoracic or L_{1-2} vertebrae ■ Intersutural/wormian bone
Treatment	■ Replacement therapy with Thyroxine T_4
Screening	■ Done at postnatal age of day 2-4 → done by filter paper method ■ Can be done by assessing either TSH or T_4 ■ TSH based approach is commonly used but it does not identify central hypothyroidism
Extra Edge	■ TSH is the most sensitive marker of primary hypothyroidism ■ Blood specimen for thyroid screening is obtained from: Heel prick > Cord blood

HYPOTHYROIDISM

Types	• *Primary hypothyroidism:* Thyroid gland is unable to produce sufficient amounts of thyroid hormone. • *Secondary hypothyroidism:* Low secretion of TSH from the pituitary • *Tertiary hypothyroidism:* Inadequate secretion of TRH from the hypothalamus

Etiology	• **Primary hypothyroidism:**
	  ○ **Iodine deficiency (MCC)**
	  ○ Autoimmune : Chronic lymphocytic thyroiditis/**Hashimoto thyroiditis** (MCC in areas of adequate iodine intake)
	  ○ Drug induced : **Amiodarone, Lithium**, Phenytoin, Carbamazepine, Rifampicin, RAI[131], Radiotherapy
	  ○ **Congenital hypothyroidism**: Absent or ectopic thyroid gland, Dyshormogenesis, TSH-R mutation
	  ○ Infiltrative disorders: **Amyloidosis, Sarcoidosis, Hemochromatosis, Scleroderma**, Riedel's thyroiditis
	  ○ Subacute granulomatous thyroiditis (Also known as de Quervain's disease)
	  ○ **Pendred syndrome**, Schmidt syndrome (adrenal insufficiency and hypothyroidism)
	• **Central/Secondary hypothyroidism:**
	  ○ Hypopituitarism: Pituitary adenoma, Sheehan syndrome, Cranial irradiation
	  ○ Drugs: Dopamine, Corticosteroids

Clinical features	**Symptoms** • Decreased appetite and Weight gain • **Cold intolerance** • Constipation • Muscle pain, joint pain, weakness in the extremities • Depression, Emotional lability, Mental impairment • **Reversible dementia** • Menstrual disturbances, impaired fertility, **Galactorrhoea** • **Increase miscarriage**, Loss of libido • Paresthesia and nerve entrapment syndromes The following are symptoms more specific to Hashimoto thyroiditis: • Feeling of fullness in the throat • Painless thyroid enlargement • Exhaustion • Transient neck pain, sore throat, or both **Signs** • Coarse facial features (Puffy face, edematous eyelids) • Periorbital puffiness • Dry skin with decreased sweating • Jaundice (due to carotene accumulation),Pallor • **Alopecia** • Macroglossia • Slowed speech and movements • Goiter (simple or nodular) • Hoarseness • Bradycardia • **Pericardial effusion** • **Non-pitting pretibial edema (myxedema)** • Pitting edema of lower extremities • Hyporeflexia with delayed relaxation (**Hung up ankle reflex**), ataxia, or both
Diagnosis	• TSH assays are the most sensitive screening tool for primary hypothyroidism • **Elevated TSH with decreased T4** • Elevated TSH with normal free T4 is considered subclinical hypothyroidism • Anti – TPO antibodies are the hallmark of the Hashimoto thyroiditis • Other features: Anemia, **Dilutional hyponatremia, Hyperlipidemia, ↑ cholesterol & triglycerides** • Radioactive Iodine uptake scan and thyroid scan – Not useful
Treatment	• Monotherapy with levothyroxine (LT4) remains the treatment of choice for hypothyroidism. • The daily replacement dose of levothyroxine is usually 1.6 µg/kg body weight (typically **100–150** µg).
Wolf – Chaikoff effect	• Iodine induced hypothyroidism • Excess of iodine intake results in transient decrease in thyroid hormone synthesis
Myxedema Coma/Crisis	• Life threatening condition due to decompensation of severe hypothyroidism • Manifest with reduced level of consciousness, seizures and other features of hypothyroidism • TSH is elevated with reduced free T4 and T3 • Treatment: Levothyroxine (T4) and Liothyronine (T3), Hydrocortisone
Hashimoto's encephalopathy	• Associated with myoclonus, seizures, slow-wave activity on EEG & Anti TPO antibodies • Rx: Steroids as it is a steroid-responsive syndrome.

HYPERTHYROIDISM

Etiology	▪ Diffuse toxic goiter (Graves' disease) – MCC ▪ Toxic multinodular goiter (Plummer disease) ▪ Toxic adenoma ▪ Thyrotoxicosis factitia – excess intake of thyroid hormone ▪ TSH secreting pituitary adenoma	▪ Subacute thyroiditis ▪ Drug: Amiodarone, Iodine excess ▪ McCune Albright syndrome ▪ Struma ovarii ▪ Gestational hyperthyroidism
Clinical features	▪ Palpitations ▪ Anxiety ▪ Nervousness ▪ Heat intolerance ▪ Increased perspiration ▪ Hyperactivity ▪ Oligomenorrhea ▪ Hyperreflexia ▪ Muscle wasting ▪ Proximal myopathy without fasciculations ▪ Periodic paralysis ▪ Pretibial myxedema ▪ Chorea – rare	▪ Tachycardia, **atrial fibrillation,** Bounding pulse ▪ Systolic hypertension with wide pulse pressure ▪ Hand tremor ▪ Warm, moist, smooth skin ▪ Lid lag ▪ Ophthalmopathy ▪ Weight loss despite increased appetite

Diagnosis	▪ Suppressed TSH levels and elevated T_3 and T_4 levels
	▪ Milder thyrotoxicosis may have elevation of T_3 levels only
	▪ Subclinical hyperthyroidism features decreased TSH and normal T_3 and T_4 levels
	▪ Graves disease – Significantly elevated anti-TPO antibodies, Anti Thyroglobulin Ab, Thyroid Stimulating Immunoglobulins (TSI)
	▪ Scintigraphy:
	  ○ Graves' disease – Diffuse enlargement of thyroid lobes with uniform and elevated RAI uptake
	  ○ Toxic multinodular goiter – Irregular areas of relatively diminished and occasionally increased uptake
	  ○ Subacute thyroiditis –Very low radioactive iodine uptake	

Treatments	▪ **Methimazole:**
	  ○ It inhibits the enzyme thyroperoxidase
	  ○ More potent than propylthiouracil
	  ○ Longer duration of action
	  ○ Less protein bound
	  ○ Not recommended for use in the first trimester of pregnancy (due to risk of cutis aplasia)
	▪ **Propylthiouracil:**
	  ○ It also inhibits the enzyme thyroperoxidase
	  ○ Additionally it also inhibits **P**eripheral T_4–T_3 conversion
	  ○ DOC during the first trimester of **P**regnancy & severe thyrotoxicosis (thyroid storm)
	▪ **Potassium iodide:**
	  ○ Inhibits thyroid hormone secretion
	  ○ Primarily used for the treatment of thyroid storm or preoperative thyroidectomy (given 10–14 days before surgery)
	▪ **Nonselective beta blockers:**
	  ○ Reduce many of the symptoms of thyrotoxicosis like tachycardia, tremor, and anxiety
	  ○ Propranolol is the drug of choice for treating cardiac arrhythmias resulting from hyperthyroidism	

Jod-Basedow phenomenon	▪ Iodine induced hyperthyroidism ▪ Hyperthyroidism after intake of large amount of iodine in diet/drug/contrast	
Thyroid storm/ Thyrotoxic crisis	▪ Acute life threatening state resulting due to excessive release of thyroid hormone ▪ Rx: Propranolol, Propylthiouracil (**DOC**), Methimazole, Lugol Iodine, Potassium iodide, Glucocorticoids	

TSH Secreting Pituitary Adenoma	● Diffuse goiter with N/↑ TSH, ↑ T3 & T4 ● Confirmation: MRI/CT brain for tumor ● Rx: TNTS surgery, Sella irradiation & Octreotide	● RAI and antithyroid drugs to control hyperthyroidism
Sick Euthyroid Syndrome	● Aka low T3 syndrome ● Abnormal thyroid function test noted during acute severe non thyroidal illness	● MC abnormality is low T3, normal T4 & elevated rT3.

DISORDERS OF THE PARATHYROID GLAND

Parathyroid Hormone

- Stimulus for release – low calcium level
- Bone – releases Ca by acting on osteoblasts & osteoclasts
- Kidneys – reabsorption of Ca in collecting duct; Synthesis of 1,25 $(OH)_2$ Vit D; Excretion of phosphate
- Intestine – indirect action via Vitamin D → Ca & P absorption

	Primary Hypoparathyroidism	Primary Hyperparathyroidism	Secondary HPT	Pseudohypoparathyroidism
Pathology	▪ Decreased secretion of parathyroid hormone	▪ Excessive secretion of parathyroid hormone	▪ Excessive secretion of parathyroid hormone	▪ Defect in the biological activity of the PTH at receptor level
Causes	▪ Surgery of thyroid, laryngeal, or other neck malignancy → MCC ▪ Type I APS ▪ Neck irradiation ▪ DiGeorge syndrome	▪ Single parathyroid adenoma – MCC ▪ Parathyroid gland hyperplasia ▪ MEN 1/2A	▪ Chronic kidney disease ▪ Vitamin D deficiency	▪ PHP type 1a is characterized by the loss of Gsα function
Clinical features	▪ Hyperirritability, Seizures ▪ Paresthesias, Muscle cramps ▪ Hoarseness ▪ Chvostek sign: Facial twitching, especially around the mouth on gently tapping the facial nerve ▪ Trousseau sign: carpel spasm	▪ Osteitis fibrosa cystica (Brown tumor) ▪ Nephrocalcinosis, Renal stones ▪ Abdominal pain ▪ Peptic ulceration ▪ Acute pancreatitis ▪ Depression & other neuropsychiatric manifestation	▪ Renal failure ▪ Osteomalacia	▪ Albright hereditary osteodystrophy (AHO). ▪ Short stature ▪ Rounded face ▪ Shortened fourth metacarpals ▪ Obesity ▪ Other features of hypocalcemia

Investigations	▪ Low PTH levels
	▪ Hypocalcemia
	▪ Hyperphosphatemia
	▪ N /↓ 1,25$(OH)_2$ Vit D
	▪ Normal 25 OH vitamin D
	▪ ECG → Prolongation of the QT interval
		▪ High iPTH levels
		▪ Hypercalcemia
		▪ Hypophosphatemia
		▪ ↑ 1,25$(OH)_2$ Vit D
		▪ 24 hours urinary calcium is increased
		▪ Radiological features:
		  ○ Salt & pepper skull
		  ○ Subperiosteal bone resorption l/t tufting of the distal phalanges
			▪ High iPTH levels
			▪ Low – normal calcium
			▪ High/low phosphate
			▪ Low 25 OH Vit D
			▪ Radiological features:
			  ○ Rugger Jersey spine
				▪ High iPTH levels
				▪ PTH resistant Hypocalcemia
				▪ Hyperphosphatemia
				▪ Normal 25 OH Vit D
				▪ Failure of administered PTH to produce phosphaturia or stimulate renal production of cAMP

Treatment	▪ Recombinant PTH hormone	▪ Surgical excision of the culprit gland	▪ Medical management	▪ Calcium supplementation

Classification of Pseudohypoparathyroidism (PHP) & Pseudopseudohypoparathyroidism (PPHP)

Type	Hypocalcemia, Hyperphosphatemia	Serum PTH	Response of Urinary cAMP to PTH	Gsα Subunit Deficiency	AHO
PHP 1A	Yes	↑	↓	Yes	Yes
PHP 1B	Yes	↑	↓	No	No
PHP 2	Yes	↑	Normal	No	No
PPHP	No	Normal	Normal	Yes	Yes

Diagnostic criteria

At least one out of the four criterions must be met:
- Symptoms of diabetes + random plasma glucose concentration ≥ 200 mg/dl
- Fasting plasma glucose ≥ 126 mg/dl
- 2 hours plasma glucose ≥ 200 mg/dl during an OGTT
- HbA1C ≥ 6.5

Etiologic Classification of Diabetes Mellitus

Type I DM	Type 2 DM

- β cell dysfunction leading to absolute insulin deficiency
- Immune mediated/idiopathic
- Seen in Young lean subjects
- Associated with HLA DR 3, DR 4
- HLA DR – 2 confers protection against type 1 DM
- Lab:
  ○ Low C – peptide
  ○ Low insulin levels
  ○ Autoantibodies like GAD
	- Combination of insulin resistance with relative insulin deficiency
	- Genetic predisposition
	- Obese individual
	- Usually part of metabolic syndrome
	- Lab:
	  ○ High C – peptide levels
	  ○ High insulin levels
	  ○ No autoantibodies

	Type 1 DM	Type 2 DM	MODY
Pathophysiology	β cell destruction	Insulin resistance	β cell destruction
Genetics	HLA	Polygenic	Monogenic/AD
Family history	?	>50%	>90%
Age of onset	Childhood	Post puberty	Around 25 years
Insulin resistance	Absent	Common	Absent
Obesity	–	++	+/-
C – peptide	Low/Negative	Normal/High	Normal
Auto-antibodies	Positive	Negative	Negative

Other Specific Types Diabetes

Pancreatic disorders	Endocrinopathies	Genetic syndromes	Drug induced
Pancreatitis Cystic fibrosis **Hemochromatosis (Bronze Diabetes)** Fibrocalculous pancreatopathy Pancreatectomy Neoplasia	**Acromegaly** **Cushing's syndrome** **Pheochromocytoma** Hyperthyroidism **Glucagonoma** Somatostatinoma	**Wolfram's syndrome** Down's syndrome **Friedreich's ataxia** Laurence Moon Biedl **Myotonic dystrophy** Prader-Willi syndrome Klinefelter syndrome Turner syndrome	**Glucocorticoids** Pentamidine β- agonists Thiazides Calcineurin and mTOR inhibitors α-interferon Diazoxide

Treatment Goal
- HbA1C <7%
- Pre-prandial plasma glucose 80-130 mg/dL
- Postprandial plasma glucose <180 mg/dL
- BP <140/90 mm Hg

Spectrum

	Normal glucose tolerance	Pre-diabetes (IFG/IGT)	Diabetes
FPG	<100 mg/dl	100 – 125 mg/dl	≥126 mg/dl
2-h PP	<140 mg/dl	140 – 199 mg/dl	≥200 mg/dl
HbA1C	<5.6%	5.7 – 6.4%	≥6.5%

MODY
- Non-insulin dependent diabetes having age of onset <25 years
- Autosomal dominant inheritance
- Most common variety – MODY 3 (HNF 1 α mutation)
- MODY 1 has HNF 4 α mutation

LADA
- Type 1 DM with age of onset > 25 years of age
- Patients are usually lean and require insulin within a year of diagnosis
- GAD autoantibody positive

Dawn phenomenon
- It is an early-morning (usually between 2 a.m. and 8 a.m.) increase in blood sugar
- Occurs due to counter regulatory hormones like glucagon and cortisol which release glucose from liver or due to wearing off insulin effect
- Treated by avoiding intake of carbohydrate diet at bedtime

Somogyi phenomenon
- Rebound hyperglycemia after an episode of hypoglycemia at night around 2 am – 3 am
- Due to release of hormones like glucagon and cortisol in response to hypoglycemic episode
- Managed by decreasing the dose of insulin at night

Contd...

ENDOCRINOLOGY ● (HIGH-YIELD POINTS)

COMPLICATIONS

Microvascular complications:

Diabetic retinopathy:
- Most common Microvascular complications
- Risk of retinopathy depends on both duration and severity of hyperglycemia
- VEGF plays an important role in the development of retinopathy
- Fundoscopic examination for screening is done at the time of diagnosis in type 2 whereas after 5 years in type 1 DM
- Rx: Intravitreal triamcinolone, VEGF inhibitors (Ranibizumab, Aflibercept, Bevacizumab), Laser photocoagulation

Diabetic neuropathy:
- MC cause of peripheral neuropathy
- Manifest as Distal Symmetrical Sensorimotor Polyneuropathy (MC), Mononeuropathy, and/or Autonomic neuropathy.
- Rx: Duloxetine, Amitriptyline, Gabapentin, Pregabalin, Carbamazepine, or Opioids

Diabetic nephropathy:
- Defined by persistent albuminuria > 300 mg in 24 hours
- 1st detectable sign → Microalbuminuria
- Rx: Strict Diabetes control, Control of hypertension, ACEI/ARB
- ❖ Intensive glycemic control decreases microvascular complications.

Macrovascular:
- Coronary artery disease
- Peripheral arterial disease
- Cerebrovascular diseases
- ❖ Intensive glycemic control offers little or no benefit in reducing macrovascular events.

DKA and HHS

	DKA	HHS
S. Glucose (mg/dL)	250 – 600	600 – 1200
Ketosis	+++	+/-
Anion gap	>12 mEq/L (↑)	Near normal
Bicarbonate	<15 mEq/L	> 15 mEq/L
Osmolality (mOsm/L)	300 – 320	> 320
Sodium (mEq/L)	125 – 135	135 – 145
Arterial pH	6.8 – 7.3	> 7.3
Potassium (mEq/L)	N/↑	N
Creatinine	↑	↑↑
Manifestations	Nausea/Vomiting, Pain abdomen, Thirst/Polyuria, Dehydration, Kussmaul breathing	Confusion, Lethargy, Polyuria, Dehydration, Tachycardia
Treatment	IV fluid replacement, Low dose short acting insulin infusion	

Metabolic Syndrome
- Also known as Syndrome X or Insulin Resistance Syndrome
- Consist of central obesity, hypertriglyceridemia, low HDL, hyperglycemia & hypertension.
- 3 out of the following must be present:
  - Waist circumference: ≥ 90 cm in men; ≥ 80 cm in women
  - SBP > 130 mm Hg OR DBP > 85 mm Hg
  - Fasting Plasma Glucose ≥ 100 mg/dL or on medications
  - Fasting Triglyceride > 150 mg/dL
  - HDL <40 mg/dL in men; <50 mg/dL in women

DISORDERS OF THE ADRENAL CORTEX

	Addison Disease	Cushing's Syndrome	Primary Hyperaldosteronism
General Features	■ Addison disease is primary adrenocortical insufficiency due to the destruction or dysfunction of the entire adrenal cortex. ■ This causes deficiency of glucocorticoid, mineralocorticoid & androgens.	■ Cushing syndrome is caused by prolonged exposure to elevated levels of either endogenous glucocorticoids or exogenous (iatrogenic) glucocorticoids.	■ Primary hyperaldosteronism is excess production of aldosterone by the adrenal glands resulting in low renin activity ■ MCC of mineralocorticoid excess
Etiology	■ MCC –autoimmune destruction of the gland ■ MCC in India – Tuberculosis ■ Adrenal hemorrhage due to meningococcemia (Waterhouse – Friderichsen syndrome) ■ Metastasis especially from CA lung & breast ■ Congenital adrenal hyperplasia; APS 1 & 2 ■ Drugs like Ketoconazole, Mitotane, Aminoglutethimide	■ MCC – Exogenous steroid therapy/Iatrogenic Cushing's ■ **Endogenous Cushing's:** ○ Cushing's disease (75%) – excess ACTH secretion by pituitary adenoma ○ Ectopic ACTH production (15%) as in small cell CA of lung ○ ACTH independent Cushing's (10%) – Adrenal adenoma & carcinoma	■ MCC – Bilateral micronodular adrenal hyperplasia ■ Adrenal adenoma (Conn's syndrome)
Associated with	■ Autoimmune diseases like Hashimoto thyroiditis, Graves' disease, Vitiligo, APS-1 etc. ■ **Schmidt syndrome(APS-2):** ○ Addison disease with Hashimoto thyroiditis	■ McCune-Albright syndrome ■ MEN 1 (pituitary adenoma)	
Clinical features	■ **Hyperpigmentation of the skin** and mucous membrane (due to raised ACTH) – in 1° adrenal insufficiency only ■ Orthostatic hypotension may lead to syncope ■ Low Blood pressure ■ Salt wasting, Hyponatremia & salt craving ■ Hypoglycemia ■ Amenorrhea ■ Generalized weakness, fatigue & weight loss ■ Loss of axillary & pubic hairs ■ Acute Addison disease presents with nausea, vomiting, hyperpyrexia & shock	■ Truncal obesity, buffalo hump ■ Moon like facies & facial plethora ■ Purplish striae, easy bruising ■ Proximal muscle weakness ■ Growth impairment & short stature ■ Hirsutism, Acne ■ Hypertension, edema – d/t mineralocorticoid excess ■ Diabetes/Glucose intolerance ■ Osteoporosis & pathological fracture, Osteopenia ■ Amenorrhea, infertility & decreased libido ■ Psychiatric manifestations like depression, psychosis	■ Aldosterone causes increase sodium and water absorption at distal tubule in exchange of potassium & H^+ ion leading to: ○ Hypernatremia/Sodium retention ○ Diastolic hypertension **without** edema ○ Hypokalemia ○ Metabolic alkalosis ■ Muscle weakness and fatigue ■ Polydipsia & polyuria – due to hypokalemia induced nephrogenic Diabetes insipidus
Lab features	■ Peripheral eosinophilia ■ Hyponatremia/Hyperkalemia/Hypercalcemia ■ Increased renin levels ■ Metabolic acidosis ■ ACTH stimulation test/Cosyntropin test using synthetic ACTH in a dose of 250 mcg is diagnostic	■ Loss of diurnal variation in cortisol levels ■ Hypokalemia ■ High serum and urine cortisol levels ■ Recommended screening tests: ○ Midnight plasma or salivary cortisol (increased) ○ 24-hour urine free cortisol (> 3 times) ○ Low dose dexamethasone suppression test	■ High aldosterone ■ Low renin levels & plasma renin activity (PRA) ■ Hypokalemia, hypernatremia & metabolic alkalosis (S. Na can remain normal) ■ Screening test– Aldosterone renin ratio ■ Saline infusion test – failure of aldosterone suppression with volume expansion
Treatments	■ Glucocorticoid replacement by Hydrocortisone ■ Mineralocorticoid replacement by Fludrocortisone ■ Hydrocortisone is the drug of choice for daily maintenance in the treatment of acute adrenal crisis.	■ Surgical removal of the causal tumor ■ Transsphenoidal removal of pituitary adenoma ■ Steroid synthesis inhibitors like ketoconazole, metyrapone & etomidate	■ Pharmacologic therapy includes the following: ○ Calcium channel blockers ○ Mineralocorticoid antagonists ○ Glucocorticoids ■ Surgery is the treatment of choice

CONGENITAL ADRENAL HYPERPLASIA

- AR disorder of cortisol synthesis
- MC enzymatic defect in CAH: 21-OH deficiency (>90%)
- Diagnosed at 2 weeks of age
- ACTH levels are elevated due to loss of feedback suppression of cortisol
- Rx: hydrocortisone. If salt wasting is present add fludrocortisone
- Prenatal therapy of 21-OH deficiency: Start Dexamethasone at 6 weeks of gestation. Perform CVS to determine sex of fetus. If male-stop the treatment. If female-continue the treatment.

Enzyme Deficiency	Electrolyte Disorder	Blood Sugar Level	Male	Female
21-α-OH	$\downarrow$ Na$^+$, $\uparrow$ K$^+$ Salt wasting	Hypoglycemia	Normal with precocious puberty	Pseudo hermaphrodite (VF)
11-β-OH	$\uparrow$ Na$^+$, $\downarrow$ K$^+$ Hypertension	Normal	Normal with precocious puberty	Pseudo hermaphrodite (VF)
3-β-HSD	$\downarrow$ Na$^+$, $\uparrow$ K$^+$ Salt wasting	Hypoglycemia	Pseudo hermaphrodite (UM)	Pseudo hermaphrodite (MVF)
17-α-OH	$\uparrow$ Na$^+$, $\downarrow$ K$^+$ Hypertension	Normal	Pseudo hermaphrodite (UM)	Normal with delayed puberty
StAR/Cholesterol desmolase	$\downarrow$ Na$^+$, $\uparrow$ K$^+$ Salt wasting	Hypoglycemia	Pseudo hermaphrodite (UM)	Normal with delayed puberty

How to remember CAH:
- Learn the table in a vertical fashion, you will find a pattern
- Normal electrolyte level rules out CAH

UM - Under virilized male
MVF - Mildly virilized female
VF - Virilized female

MULTIPLE ENDOCRINE NEOPLASIA SYNDROMES

MEN	Characterized by a predilection for tumors involving two or more endocrine glands. Due to Autosomal Dominant mutations in the genes that regulate cell growth.			
MEN 1 [MC MEN] (Wermer's Syndrome)	MEN 2			MEN 4 (MENX)
	MEN 2A (Sipple Syndrome)	MEN 2B (MEN III)		
▪ Parathyroid adenoma (90%) ▪ Pancreatic islet cell tumors ▪ Pituitary adenoma *Mn: Pit Pan Par	▪ MTC (90%) ▪ Pheochromocytoma ▪ Parathyroid adenoma * MTC = Medullary Thyroid Cancer	▪ MTC (90%) ▪ Pheochromocytoma ▪ Mucosal neuromas ▪ Marfanoid habitus ▪ Medullated corneal nerve fibers		▪ Parathyroid adenoma ▪ Pituitary adenoma ▪ Reproductive organ tumor

MEN 1	Due to Loss of function mutation in the gene MENIN located on chromosome 11q13	
Parathyroid adenoma (90%)	Pancreatic islet cell tumors (30 – 70%)	Pituitary adenoma (15 – 50%)
▪ Hyperparathyroidism is the most common manifestation of type 1 MEN ▪ It results from hyperplasia of all 4 parathyroid glands	▪ Pancreatic islet cell tumors represent the second most common manifestation. Islet cell tumors encompass: ○ Gastrinoma (MC) ○ Insulinoma ○ Glucagonoma ○ Vasoactive intestinal peptide tumor (VIPoma)	▪ Prolactinoma are the most common

MEN 2	Due to Gain of function mutation in the RET proto-oncogene located on chromosome 10

MEN 4	Due to mutation of the gene encoding cyclin dependent kinase inhibitor (CDKN1B) located on chromosome 12

AUTOIMMUNE POLYGLANDULAR SYNDROMES

	APS-1 (APECED)	APS-2 (Schmidt syndrome)
Gene:	▪ AIRE	▪ HLA-DR-3, CTLA-4
Features:	▪ Autoimmune Addison disease ▪ Hypoparathyroidism ▪ Mucocutaneous candidiasis ▪ Other Autoimmune disorders ▪ Lymphoma (rare)	▪ Autoimmune Addison disease ▪ Hypothyroidism ▪ Hyperthyroidism ▪ Vitiligo ▪ Type 1 DM ▪ Pernicious anemia
Inheritance	▪ AR	▪ AD

APECED – **A**utoimmune **P**oly**E**ndocrinopathy – **C**andidiasis – **E**ctodermal **D**ystrophy |

PHEOCHROMOCYTOMA

General features	▪ Pheochromocytomas and paragangliomas are derived from the sympathetic or parasympathetic nervous system. ▪ They synthesize and store catecholamines like norepinephrine (noradrenaline), epinephrine (adrenaline), and dopamine. ▪ The classic "rule of tens" for pheochromocytomas states that ~10% are bilateral, 10% are extra- adrenal and 10% are malignant.
Etiology	▪ Either arise sporadically or be inherited as features of multiple endocrine neoplasia type 2 (MEN 2), von Hippel–Lindau (VHL) disease
Associated with	▪ MEN 2, VHL, Neurofibromatosis 1
Clinical features	▪ Classic triad – episodes of palpitation, headache, and profuse sweating ▪ Sustained or paroxysmal Hypertension ▪ Orthostatic hypotension	▪ Anxiety and panic attacks ▪ Abdominal pain, Weight loss ▪ Polyuria and polydipsia, Constipation
Lab	▪ Erythrocytosis, Elevated blood sugar, Hypercalcemia ▪ Elevated plasma and urinary levels of catecholamines and metanephrines ▪ Plasma metanephrines – highest sensitivity ▪ 24 hr urinary catecholamines & metanephrines – highest specificity ▪ Histology – characteristic "**Zellballen**" pattern ▪ Immunohistochemistry – positive for chromogranin, synaptophysin and S-100
Imaging	▪ 1st line imaging technique – CT ▪ Tumors also can be localized by ^{131}I or ^{123}I MIBG scintigraphy, ^{111}In-somatostatin scintigraphy, 18F-DOPA PET, ^{68}Ga-DOTATATE PET, or 18F-FDG PET
Treatment	▪ TOC – Complete tumor removal by partial or total adrenalectomy ▪ Oral prazosin or intravenous phentolamine can be used to manage paroxysms ▪ Pre-op BP is controlled by α blockers (oral phenoxybenzamine) – start 7-10 days prior to surgery ▪ Liberal salt & water intake to avoid severe orthostatic hypotension. ▪ Initiate β blockers only after adequate α blockade ▪ Nitroprusside infusion is useful for intraoperative hypertensive crises

MULTIPLE CHOICE QUESTIONS

CHAPTER 1: HYPOTHALAMIC AND PITUITARY HORMONES ENDOCRINOLOGY

PITUITARY GLAND

1. Which of the following is under anterior pituitary control? *(PGMEE 2014-15)*
   a. Fluid and electrolyte balance
   b. Control of blood pressure
   c. Muscle activity
   d. Gonad function

[Ref: Harrison's 20th/e pg. 2663]

2. First drug to be started in Sheehan's syndrome is? *(PGMEE 2014-15)*
   a. Gonadotropins
   b. Oestrogen
   c. Thyroxine
   d. Corticosteroids

[Ref: Harrison's 20th/e pg. 2666]

Explanation

Treatment of sheehan's syndrome

- Replacement of all deficieint hormone. Some patients mya recover TSH and even gonadotropin function after cortisol replacement alone.

3. Herring bodies are seen in? *(PGMEE 2012)*
   a. Pars tuberalis
   b. Pars intermedia
   c. Pars nervosa
   d. All of the above

Explanation

- An interesting histologic feature of the neurohypophysis (aka pars nervosa) is the presence of "Herring bodies" in the terminal portion of axon contains neurosecretory granules.

4. GNAS mutation is associated with malignancy of which cells? *(PGMEE 2015-16)*
   a. Lactotroph
   b. Somatotroph
   c. Thyrotroph
   d. None

[Ref: Robbin's 9th/e pg.]

Explanation

- Approximately 40% of somatotroph adenoma bear GNAS mutation
- GNAS mutation is also seen in pseudohypoparthyroidism and McCune-Aibright syndrome

5. Arginine vasopressin levels are increased in tumors of? *(PGMEE 2016-17)*
   a. Pituitary
   b. Hypothalamus
   c. Adrenal medulla
   d. Cerebellum

[Ref: Robbin's 9th/e pg. 1082]

6. Posterior pituitary secretes- *(PGMEE 2013-14)*
   a. FSH
   b. TSH
   c. ADH
   d. GH

[Ref: Harrison's 20th/e pg. 2684]

7. Stimulator of Growth hormone release is:- *(PGMEE 2016-17)*
   a. REM Sleep
   b. Bromocriptine
   c. **Hypoglycemia**
   d. Cortisol

[Ref: Ganong's 25th/e pg. 328,333]

Explanation

- GH release is stimulated by:
  - GHRH
  - Exercise
  - Ghrelin
  - Physical stress
  - Androgens
  - Deep sleep (mostly NREM III)
  - Hypoglycemia
  - Prolonged fasting

8. Levodopa test is used to detect: *(PGMEE 2014-15)*
   a. LH
   b. ACTH
   c. FSH
   d. GH reserve

[Ref: Pediatric endocrinology Mark A. Sparling, table 10.9, 4th ed.]

9. Hyperpigmentation is seen with excess of which hormone? *(PGMEE 2015)*
   a. FSH
   b. LH
   c. ACTH
   d. TSH

[Ref: Harrison's 20th/e pg. 2734]

10. The following are recognized features of panhypopituitarism EXCEPT: *(PGMEE 2014-15)*
   a. Increased insulin sensitivity
   b. Hyperpigmentation of the mucous membranes
   c. Low serum thyroxine and TSH levels
   d. Loss of secondary sex characters

[Ref: Harrison's 20th/e pg. 2734, 2666]

11. Short stature, secondary to growth hormone deficiency is associated with *(PGMEE 2012-13)*
   a. Height age is equal to Bone age
   b. Normal body proportion
   c. Low birth weight
   d. Normal epiphyseal development

[Ref: O.P. Ghai 8th/e pg. 511-512]

Explanation

Growth Hormone deficiency

- GHD babies are born AGA (not SGA)
- They have maintained body proportions, i.e. - proportionate short stature
- Disproportionate SS is seen in following (Upper segment: lower segment)
  - US > LS → Richets & Achondroplasia
  - US < LS → Spondylo epiphyseal dysplasia
- GHD - children have significantly delayed bone age - but which is appropriate for height age i.e., CA > HA = BA

1.	d
2.	d
3.	c
4.	b
5.	b
6.	c
7.	c
8.	d
9.	c
10.	b
11.	b

PROLACTINOMA

12. Commonest functional tumor of pituitary gland is?

a. Gonodotroponoma   b. ACTH secreting tumour

c. Prolactinoma   d. TSH secreting tumour

[Ref: Sabiston textbook of surgery, 18ᵗʰ/e chapter 72]

13. Most common cause of hypersecreting pituitary tumor is   *(DNB June' 2009)*

a. Pitutary adenoma

b. Pituitary carcinoma

c. Autoimmune disease of pituitary

d. Transection of stalk

[Ref: Sabiston textbook of surgery, 18th/e chapter 72]

14. In prolactinoma levels of serum prolactin are:

     (PGMEE 2018)-

a. >50 ng/dL   b. >100 ng/dL

c. >150 ng/dL   d. >200 ng/dL

15. In prolactinoma most common symptom other than galactorrhea is?   *(PGMEE 2015-16)*

a. Bitemporal hemianopia   b. Amennorhea

c. Thyroid dysfunction   d. Headache

[Ref: Harrison's 20th/e pg. 2676]

Explanation

Clinical manifestation of hyperprolactinemia

- Elevated prolactin inhibits GnRH secretion and consequently lowers LH and FSH secretion, manifesting as inferitilify, galactorrhea gynecomistia, impotence and amenorrhea.
- Bitemporal hemianopsia may also be present.

16. For galactorrhea and amenorrhea syndromes, additional investigation apart from serum prolactin?

     (NEET Pattern 2015)

a. TSH   b. LH

c. Urinary Ketosteroids   d. HCG

[Ref: Harrison's 20th/e pg. 2676]

17. Most common functional tumour of pituitary is:

     (PGMEE 2014-15)

a. Prolactinoma

b. GH secreting adenoma

c. ACTH secreting adenoma

d. TSH secreting adenoma

18. All of the following causes hyperprolactinemia EXCEPT:

     (PGMEE 2014-15)

a. Methyldopa   b. Phenothiazines

c. Bromocriptine   d. Metoclopramide

[Ref: Harrison's 20th/e pg. 2675]

Explanation

- Dopamine antagonists causes hyporprolactinemia.

19. Investigation to be done for hyperprolactinaemia?

     (PGMEE 2014-15)

a. Estradiol estimation   b. LH estimation

c. Diabetic status   d. Thyroid status

[Ref: Harrison's 20th/e pg. 2676]

20. Which is the first hormone to fall in the blood in Sheehan syndrome: *(PGMEE 2014-15)*

a. GH   b. ACTH

c. prolactin   d. TSH

Explanation

- Somatotrophs are most likely to be damaged by ischemic necrosis of the pituitary which is the reason behind GH deficiency in most patients with Sheehan syndrome
- The most common presenting syndrome is failure to lactate (caused by ↓prolactin levels).

21. Prolactinoma presents with: *(PGMEE 2014-15)*

a. Inferior quadrantopia

b. Superior quadrantopia

c. Priapism

d. Failure of lactation

22. A young woman comes with secondary amenorrhoea and galactorrhoea. MRI shows a tumor of <10 mm diameter in the pituitary fossa. Treatment is:

     (PGMEE 2014-15)

a. Hormonal therapy for withdrawal bleeding

b. Chemotherapy

c. Bromocriptine

d. Surgery

[Ref: Harrison's 20th/e pg. 2677]

Explanation

- Best initial therapy for hyperprolactinemia is dopamine agonists (Bromocriptine, cabergoline).

ACROMEGALY

23. Consider the following statements about acromegaly

     (PGMEE 2014-15)

i. Impaired glucose tolerance

ii. Galactorrhoea

iii. Hypertension

iv. Suppression of growth hormone with glucose

Which of these statements are correct?

a. i, ii and iv   b. ii, iii and iv

c. i, iii and iv   d. i, ii and iii

[Ref: Harrison's 20th/e pg. 2678-79]

24. A middle aged man noticed that he can no longer fit in his shoes and enlarging of jaw and phalanges. These effects are mediated by?   *(DNB Dec'2010)*

a. ACTH   b. TRH

c. Somatomedin   d. TGF beta

[Ref: Harrison's 20th/e pg. 2677]

25. All of the following are features of acromegaly except?

a. Glucose intolerance   *(PGMEE 2014-15)*

b. Non-suppression of growth hormone by glucose ingestion

c. Raised level of plasma somatomedin C

d. Low serum phosphate

[Ref: Harrison's 20th/e pg. 2679]

26. All are seen in gigantism EXCEPT: *(DNB Dec'2010)*

a. Visceromegaly   b. Mental retardation

c. Large foot   d. Cardiovascular damage

[Ref: Harrison's 20th/e pg. 2678]

12.	c
13.	a
14.	d
15.	b
16.	a
17.	a
18.	c
19.	d
20.	d
21.	b
22.	c
23.	d
24.	c
25.	d
26.	b

27. All of following are seen in GH deficiency EXCEPT:
(PGMEE 2015-16)

a. Hyperglycemia   b. Stunting
c. Delayed bone age   d. High pitched voice

[Ref: Harrison's 20th/e pg. 2667]

Explanation

- Delayed bone age + Short stature → Endocrine/Systemic disorder
- Normal bone age + Short stature → Genetic/growth plate disorder

28. Laron dwarfism is due to?   *(PGMEE 2015-16)*

a. GH deficiency
b. GHRH deficiency
c. GH receptor resistance
d. IGF-1 deficiency

[Ref: Harrison's 20th/e pg. 3417]

29. Which is NOT a side effect of GH administration?

a. Gynecomastia   *(PGMEE 2014-15)*
b. Hypoglycemia
c. Slipped capital femoral epiphysis
d. Pseudotumor cerebri

[Ref: Harrison's 20th/e pg. 2669]

30. Heel pad thickness is useful in: *(PGMEE 2014-15)*

a. Hypothyroidism
b. Acromegaly
c. PEM
d. All of the above

[Ref: Harrison's 20th/e pg. 2678]

31. Arrow headed finger on X-ray is suggestive of:

a. Acromegaly   *(PGMEE 2014-15)*
b. Hyperparathyroidism
c. Down syndrome
d. Sarcoidosis

SIADH & DIABETES INSIPIDUS

32. Which of the following are true regarding congenital nephrogenic diabetes insipidus: *(PGMEE 2014-15)*

a. ADH receptors are not sensitive
b. It is associated with SIADH
c. Serum ADH levels are normal
d. Urine is hyperosmolar

[Ref: Nelson 18th edition ch. 559, Harrison's 20th/e pg. 2687]

33. The syndrome of inappropriate ADH secretion is characterized by the following: *(PGMEE 2014-15)*

a. Hyponatremia and urine sodium excretion > 20 mEq/L
b. Hypernatremia and urine sodium excretion > 20 mEq/L
c. Hyponatremia and hyperkalemia
d. Hypernatremia and hyperkalemia

[Ref: Harrison's 20th/e pg. 298]

34. In a patient if administration of vasopressin does not increase the osmolality of urine, it indicates?

a. ADH deficiency   *(DNB June 2009)*
b. Renal hyposensitivity towards ADH
c. Psychogenic polydipsia
d. SIADH

[Ref: Harrison's 20th/e pg. 2687]

35. Inappropriate ADH secretion is seen in all EXCEPT:

a. Head injury   *(PGMEE 2014-15)*
b. Oat Cell carcinoma of Lung
c. Acute encephalitis
d. Chromophobe adenoma

[Ref: Harrison's 20th/e pg. 2690]

36. True about Nephrogenic diabetes insipidus is?
(DNB June 2011)

a. Renal tubule unresponsiveness to ADH
b. The urine osmolarity is increased after ADH administration
c. Serum Na is low
d. There is central decrease in secretion of ADH

[Ref: Harrison's 20th/e pg. 2687-87]

37. Treatment of neurogenic diabetes insipidus is?
(DNB June 2011)

a. Amiodarone   b. Desmopressin
c. Terlipressin   d. Vasopressin

[Ref: Harrison's 20th/e pg. 2687]

Explanation

Treatment of diabetes insipidus

- Central DI→Administer dDAVP (desmopressin acetate) i.v., intranasaly or orally
- Nephrogenic DI→Salt restinction, reduced water intake, hydrochlorothiazide, amiloride

38. Consider the following statements: *(PGMEE 2014-15)*
In nephrogenic diabetes insipidus the patient is likely to have:

i. High vasopressin level
ii. Poor or no response to desmopressin
iii. High plasma osmolality.
iv. Dilutional hyponatremia

Which of these statements are correct?

a. i, ii and iii
b. ii, iii and iv
c. i and iv
d. i, ii, iii and iv

[Ref: Harrison's 20th/e pg. 2686-88]

39. Mainstay of t/t of Nephrogenic Diabetes Insipidus is:
(PGMEE 2015-16)

a. Thiazide/Amiloride diureties and salt restriction
b. Desmopressin
c. Vasopressin and salt restriction
d. Desmopressin and salt restriction

[Ref: Harrison's 20th/e pg. 2688]

27.	a
28.	c
29.	b
30.	b
31.	a
32.	a
33.	a
34.	b
35.	d
36.	a
37.	b
38.	a
39.	a

40. **Polyuria with low fixed specific gravity urine is seen in?**
    a. Diabetes mellitus   *(PGMEE 2014-15)*
    b. Diabetes insipidus
    c. Chronic glomerulonephritis
    d. Potomania

    [Ref: Harrison's 19th/e pg. 2276, 1811]

41. **Urine osmolality in diabetes insipidus is:**
    (PGMEE 2014-15)

    a. <150 mosm/L   b. <300 mosm/L
    c. 600 mosm/L   d. 900 mosm/L

    [Ref: Harrison's 20th/e pg. 294]

42. **True about SIADH is all EXCEPT**   *(PGMEE 2014-15)*
    a. Hyponatraemia
    b. Urine hyposmolar
    c. Increased ADH
    d. Adequate hydration status

    [Ref: Harrison's 20th/e pg. 2690]

43. **Central diabetes insipidus is characterized by:**
    (PGMEE 2014-15)

    a. Low plasma and low urine osmolality
    b. High plasma and high urine osmolality
    c. Low plasma and high urine osmolality
    d. Low urine and high plasma osmolality

    [Ref: Harrison's 20th/e pg. 2686]

Explanation
- Central DI: ↓ urine output and ↑urine osmology
- Nephrogenic DI: No effect is seen on urine output or urine osmolarity.

44. **Syndrome of Inappropriate secretion of Anti-Diuretic hormone (SIADH) may be seen in the following EXCEPT:**
    a. Use of vincristine   *(PGMEE 2014-15)*
    b. Oat cell carcinoma of lung
    c. Porphyria-acute attack
    d. Primary pulmonary emphysema

    [Ref: Harrison's 20th/e pg. 299]

45. **Pituitary diabetes insipidus is improved by:**
    (PGMEE 2014-15)

    a. Water restriction   b. Lithium
    c. Desmopressin   d. Chlorthiazide

    [Ref: Harrison's 20th/e pg. 2688]

46. **Dilutional hyponatremia is seen in?**   *(PGMEE 2014-15)*
    a. Addison's disease
    b. Vincristine
    c. Diuretic therapy
    d. Craniphyrangioma

47. **All are true regarding ADH action except?**
    a. Postoperative secretion is more   *(PGMEE 2014-15)*
    b. ADH secretion occurs when plasma osmolality is low
    c. Acts on DCT
    d. Neuro-secretion

    [Ref: Harrison's 20th/e pg. 2684

40.	c
41.	b
42.	b
43.	d
44.	d
45.	c
46.	b
47.	b

CHAPTER-1 ᠻ HYPOTHALAMIC AND PITUITARY...

THYROID GLAND

1. Which of the following is not a feature of myxedema coma? *(NEET Pattern 2019)*
- a. Educed level of consciousness and seizures with other features of hypothyroidism is seen
- b. Hypoventilation leading to hypoxia and hypercapnea play a major role
- c. Levothyroxine can be given via intravenous and nasogastric route
- d. Levothyronine should not be used in the management

2. Thyrotoxicosis with low radioactive iodine uptake occurs in: *(NEET 2018)*
- a. Subacute thyroiditis
- b. Thyrotoxicosis
- c. Graves disease
- d. Hashimoto's

3. Long acting thyroid stimulating agent is: *(PGMEE 2014)*
- a. Antibody to thyroid cell receptors
- b. Antibody to thyroid cells
- c. Antibody to thyroid globulin
- d. Antibody to thyroxine

[Ref: Harrison's 20th/e pg. 2703]

4. Autoimmune thyroiditis is associated with all except- *(PGMEE 2013-14)*
- a. SLE
- b. DM
- c. Mysthenia gravis
- d. Psoriasis

[Ref: Robbin's 9th/e pg. 1086]

5. Which of the following is not associated with hypothyroidism:- *(PGMEE 2015-16)*
- a. Low T3
- b. Low cholesterol
- c. High TSH
- d. High Triglycerides

[Ref: Harrison's 20th/e pg. 2701]

6. The laboratory screening test which suggests normal thyroid function is: *(PGMEE 2014-15)*
- a. TSH
- b. Free T4
- c. T3
- d. Free T3

[Ref: Harrison's 20th/e pg. 2701]

7. The third generation TSH detection tests can detect TSH at a minimum level of: *(PGMEE 2014-15)*
- a. 0.4 mU/L
- b. 0.04 mU/L
- c. 0.004 mU/L
- d. 0.0004 mU/L

[Ref: Harrison's 19th/e pg. 2288]

8. Hypothyroidism in sub Himalayan is due to? *(DNB Dec'2010)*
- a. Selenium
- b. Iodine
- c. Copper
- d. Iron

9. Hypothyroidism is associated with *(PGMEE 2016-17)*
- a. Hyponatremia
- b. Hypernatremia
- c. Hypothermia
- d. Hypokalemia

10. Hypothyroidism is caused by? *(DNB June 2010)*
- a. Hemochromatosis
- b. Lithium
- c. Scleroderma
- d. All of the above

[Ref: Harrison's 20th/e pg. 2698]

11. Replacement dose of Thyroxine per day is? *(PGMEE 2014-15)*
- a. 100 mcg
- b. 200 mcg
- c. 300 mcg
- d. 400 mcg

[Ref: Harrison's 20th/e pg. 2701]

12. Presentation of hypothyroidism is? *(PGMEE 2014-15)*
- a. Pretibial myxedema
- b. Hirusutism
- c. Easily brusiable skin
- d. Galactorrhoea

[Ref: Harrison's 20th/e pg. 2699]

13. Which of the following present with hypothyroidism? *(PGMEE 2015-16)*
- a. Struma ovarii
- b. Grave's disease
- c. Myasthenia gravis
- d. Toxic multinodular goiter

[Ref: Harrison's 20th/e pg. 2699]

Explanation

- Autoimmune hypothyroidism (one of the etiology of primary hypothyroidism) may be associated with signs & symptoms of other autoimmune diseases like:

▪ Vitiligo	▪ Celiac disease
▪ Pernicious anemia	▪ Dermatitis herpetiformis
▪ Addison's disease	▪ Rheumatoid arthritis
▪ Alopecia areata	▪ SLE
▪ Type -1 DM	▪ Myasthenia gravis
	▪ Sjogren's syndrome

14. All are true about congenital Hypothyroidism EXCEPT- *(PGMEE 2013-14)*
- a. Delayed dentition
- b. Widened fontanel
- c. Distended abdomen
- d. All are true

[Ref: O.P. Ghai 8th/e/p 516-517]

15. Proptosis not seen in? *(PGMEE 2015-16)*
- a. Primary thyrotoxicosis
- b. Sarcoidosis
- c. Pituitary adenoma
- d. Hypothyroidism

[Ref: Harrison's 20th/e pg. 2699]

16. Hung up ankle jerk is seen in? *(PGMEE 2014-15)*
- a. Hypothyroidism
- b. Thyrotoxicosis
- c. Sipple syndrome
- d. Wermer syndrome

[Ref: Harrison's 20th/e pg. 2699]

1.	d
2.	a
3.	a
4.	d
5.	b
6.	a
7.	c
8.	b
9.	c>a
10.	d
11.	a
12.	a,d
13.	c
14.	d
15.	d
16.	a

17. **Which one of the following features may not be seen in hypothyroidism?** *(PGMEE 2014-15)*
   a. Cold intolerance   b. Deafness
   c. Pericardial effusion   d. Pretibial myxoedema
   [Ref: Harrison's 20th/e pg. 2700]

18. **A 17-year old girl who was evaluated for short height was found to have an enlarged pituitary gland. Her T4 was low and TSH was increased. Which of the following is the most likely diagnosis?** *(PGMEE 2014-15)*
   a. Pituitary adenoma
   b. TSH-secreting pituitary tumour
   c. Thyroid target receptor insensivity
   d. Primary hypothyroidism
   [Ref: Harrison's 20th/e pg. 2701]

Explanation

Thyroid function test in thyroid diseases

Dx	TSH	T4	T3
1° Hyperthyroidism	↓	↑	↑
2° Hyperthyroidism	Nl/↑	↑	↑
1° Hypothyroidism	↑	↓	↓
2° Hypothyroidism	↓	↓	↓

19. **Hypothyroidism is associated with the following clinical problems, EXCEPT:** *(PGMEE 2014-15)*
   a. Menorrhagia   b. Early abortions
   c. Galactorrhoea   d. Thromboembolism
   [Ref: Harrison's 20th/e pg. 2699]

20. **Reversible Dementia is a feature of?** *(PGMEE 2014-15)*
   a. Hyperparathyroidism   b. Hypothyroidism
   c. Hyperthyroidism   d. Cushing's disease
   [Ref: Harrison's 20th/e pg. 2700]

21. **TSH cannot be used for monitoring response to treatment in:** *(PGMEE 2014-15)*
   a. Primary hypothyroidism
   b. Secondary hypothyrodism
   c. Thyroprivic hypothyroidism
   d. Iodine deficiency
   [Ref: Harrison's 20th/e pg. 2701]

22. **Most common presentation of sick euthyoid state:** *(PGMEE 2014-15)*
   a. Low T3 with normal T4   b. Low T3 with low T4
   c. Low T3 with high T4   d. High T3 with high T4
   [Ref: Harrison's 20th/e pg. 2709]

23. **In myxoedema which is not correct:** *(PGMEE 2014-15)*
   a. Slow pulse   b. Hypertension
   c. Hypotension   d. Dry skin
   [Ref: Harrison's 20th/e pg. 2699]

24. **Myxoedema coma is treated with:** *(PGMEE 2014-15)*
   a. Hydrocortisone   b. Liothyronine
   c. Levothyroxine   d. All of the above
   [Ref: Harrison's 20th/e pg. 2703]

25. **Dancing carotid sign is seen in:** *(PGMEE 2014-15)*
   a. Thyrotoxicosis   b. Papillary Ca
   c. Follicular Ca   d. Hashimoto's disease
   [Ref: Bedside cardiology A. Sarkar, 1st ed. pg. 85]

26. **The most common differential diagnosis of hyperthyroidism in a young female is:** *(PGMEE 2014-15)*
   a. Hysteria   b. Essential tremor
   c. Anxiety neurosis   d. Parkinsonism
   [Ref: Harrison's 20th/e pg. 2705]

27. **Gestational hyperthyroidism occurs due to:**
   a. Beta HCG from placenta   *(PGMEE 2014-15)*
   b. Transplacental TSH transfer
   c. T.P.O antibody
   d. Anti–thyroglobulin antibody
   [Ref: Harrison's 20th/e pg. 2653]

Explanation

- Very high levels of β-HCG hormone (eg: molar pregnancy or choriocarcinoma) can activate the TSH receptor which can cause thyrotoxicosis.

28. **Which one of the following clinical signs is not seen in ophthalmic Grave's disease?** *(PGMEE 2014-15)*
   a. Lid retraction
   b. Frequent blinking
   c. Poor convergence
   d. Upper lid "lad" on down gaze

Explanation

- Thyroid associated orbitopathy (TAO) aka "Graves opthalmopathy" is associated with numerous eponymous signs:
  ○ Ballet sign → Restriction of one or more extraocular muscles
  ○ Grove sign → Resistance to pulling down the retracted upper eyelid.
  ○ Joffroy sign → absent creases in the forehead on superior gaze
  ○ Mobius sign → Poor convergence
  ○ Stellwag sign → incomplete and infrequent blinking
  ○ Vigouroux sign → Eyelid fullness.

29. **Characteristic of Graves disease are A/E:**
   a. Hyperthyroidism   *(PGMEE 2014-15)*
   b. Pretibial myxoedema
   c. Atrial fibrillation
   d. Ophthalmopathy
   [Ref: Harrison's 20th/e pg. 2704]

30. **Drugs used in thyroid crisis are A/E:** *(PGMEE 2014-15)*
   a. Propranolol   b. Carbimazole
   c. Iodine   d. Corticosteroids
   [Ref: Harrison's 20th/e pg. 2707]

31. **Cardiac manifestations of Grave's disease would include all of the following except?** *(PGMEE 2014-15)*
   a. Wide pulse pressure
   b. Atrial fibrillation
   c. Pleuropericardial scratch
   d. Aortic insufficiency
   [Ref: Harrison's 20th/e pg. 2704]

17.	None
18.	d
19.	d
20.	b
21.	b
22.	a
23.	b
24.	d
25.	a
26.	c
27.	a
28.	b
29.	c
30.	b
31.	d

32. The occurrence of hyperthyroidism following adminis-tra-tion of supplemental iodine to subjects in endemic area of iodine deficiency is due to? *(PGMEE 2014-15)*
   a. Wolf-Chaikoff effect   b. Jod-Basedow effect
   c. Pemberton effect   d. Graves' effect

[Ref: Harrison's 20th/e pg. 2703]

33. Thyroid storm is seen in: *(PGMEE 2014-15)*
   a. Thyroid surgery   b. Neonatal thyrotoxicosis
   c. Peri-operative infection d. All of the above

[Ref: Harrison's 20th/e pg. 2707]

34. Wolf Chaikoff effect is due to: *(PGMEE 2015-16)*
   a. Iodine deficiency
   b. Excessive iodine
   c. Iodine metabolism defect
   d. TPO enzyme deficiency

[Ref: Harrison's 20th/e pg. 2695]

35. Which of the following is NOT a feature of thyrotoxicosis? *(PGMEE 2015-16)*
   a. Palpitation   b. Anxiety
   c. Weight loss   d. Menorrhagia

[Ref: Harrison's 20th/e pg. 2703]

36. A young lady with tremors and diarrhea with elevated T4 and TSH levels were 8.5 mIU/L. Further examination reveals bi-temporal hemianopia. Next step of manage-ment: *(NEET Pattern 2015)*
   a. Start anti-thyroid drugs, and do urgent MRIBrain
   b. Start beta blockers
   c. Conservative management
   d. Start anti-thyroid drugs and wait for symptoms to resolve

[Ref: Harrison's 20th/e pg. 2708]

Explanation
- Elevated T_4 & TSH is suggestive of secondary hyperthy-roidism. Bitemporal hemianopia suggest underlying TSH secreting pituitary adenoma.

37. Common neurological manifestations of thyrotoxicosis include all EXCEPT: *(PGMEE 2014-15)*
   a. Hyper reflexia
   b. Muscle wasting
   c. Chorea
   d. Proximal myopathy without fasciculations

[Ref: Harrison's 20th/e pg. 2704]

38. All are true about Hashimoto encephalopathy EXCEPT:
   a. Myoclonus   *(PGMEE 2014-15)*
   b. Seizures
   c. Steroid responsive encephalopathy
   d. EEG is normal

[Ref: Harrison's 20th/e pg. 2700]

39. DOC for Hashimoto encephalopathy: *(PGMEE 2014-15)*
   a. Steroids   b. Prophythiouracil
   c. I-131   d. Liothyronine infusion

[Ref: Harrison's 20th/e pg. 2700]

32.	b
33.	d
34.	c
35.	d
36.	a
37.	c
38.	d
39.	a
40.	d
41.	c
42.	a
43.	b
44.	c
45.	a

40. Which is not seen in subacute thyroditidis:
   (PGMEE 2014-15)
   a. Raised T4 levels   b. Raised ESR
   c. Pain   d. High Radio iodine uptake

[Ref: Harrison's 20th/e pg. 2708]

41. Goitrous hypothyroidism commonly occurs in all of the following except? *(PGMEE 2014-15)*
   a. Hashimoto's thyroiditis
   b. Dyshoromonogenesis (Pendred syndrome)
   c. Thyroprivic hypothyroidism
   d. Iodine deficiency

[Ref: Harrison's 20th/e pg. 2700]

Explanation
- Goiters

Toxic Goiter	Non-Toxic Goiter
Diffuse toxic goiter (Graves disease)	Endemic goiter/Iodine deficiency
Toxic multinodular goiter	Chronic lymphocytic thyroiditis (Hashimoto disease)
Toxic adenoma (Plummer d/s)	Congenital goiter
	Pendred syndrome

  ○ Thyroprivic hypothyroidism is due to loss of parenchyma of thyroid gland.
  ○ MCC of goiter globally is iodine deficiency leading to:- Diffuse endemic goiter.

42. Pemberton sign is seen in? *(PGMEE 2014-15)*
   a. Retrosternal goiter   b. Grave opthalmopathy
   c. Thyroid crisis   d. Addisonian crisis

[Ref: Harrison's 20th/e pg. 2697]

Explanation
- Pemberton's sign:
  ○ Seen in retrosternal goiters
  ○ Positive sign is marked by the presence of facial congestion and cyanosis as well as difficulty breathing when patient raises both his arm.

43. Radioiodine uptake in endemic goitre is:
   (PGMEE 2014-15)
   a. Normal   b. Increased
   c. Decreased   d. Erratic

[Ref: Harrison's 20th/e pg. 2698]

44. Thyroid nodule in a 65 year old male who is clinically euthyroid is most likely to be- *(PGMEE 2015)*
   a. Follicular adenoma   b. Follicular carcinoma
   c. Multinodular goiter   d. Throid cyst

[Ref: Harrison's 20th/e pg. 2711, 2717]

45. Most common cause of goiter in India is *(PGMEE 2015)*
   a. Diffuse Endemic Goitre   b. Hashimoto's Thyroiditis
   c. Papillary carcinoma   d. Toxic Multinodular

[Ref: Harrison's 20th/e pg. 2698]

PARATHYROID GLAND

46. Jansen disease is?   *(PGMEE 2014-15)*
   a. Defect of PTH receptor
   b. Defect of ADH receptor
   c. Defect of GHRH receptor
   d. Defect of GH receptor

[Ref: Harrison's 19th/e pg. 2475]

47. Mechanism of action of parathyroid hormone:-
   a. ↓ Calcitriol   *(PGMEE 2016-17)*
   b. ↓ Phosphate excretion
   c. ↑ Calcium absorption
   d. Act an osteoclasts

[Ref: Harrison's 20th/e pg. 2922]

48. Parathyroid hormone will lead to:-   *(PGMEE 2016-17)*
   a. Negative feedback to calcitriol
   b. ↓ Phosphate reabsorption
   c. ↓ Calcium absorption
   d. ↑se osteoblastic activity

[Ref: Harrison's 20th/e pg. 2921]

49. Increase calcitonin levels are seen in   *(PGMEE 2019)*
   a. Hyperthyroidism
   b. Hypoparathyroidism
   c. Hyperparathyroidism
   d. Cushing Syndrome

Explanation

- Hyperparathyroidism is present in 20-30% of patients with medullary thyroid carcinoma. After successful total thyroidectomy, calcitonin is no longer detectable. Increasing concentration of calcitonin after therapy indicate relapse or metastasis.

50. Gs- alpha mutation my lead to?   *(PGMEE 2013)*
   a. Pseudopseudohhypoparathyroidism
   b. Mc cune Albright syndrome
   c. Pseudohypoparathyroidism
   d. All of the above

[Ref: Harrison's 20th/e pg. 2940]

Explanation

- G$_s$ alpha sub unit is a heterotrimeric G- protein that activates the cAMP dependent pathway by activating adenylyl cyclase.

Mutation in G$_{sa}$ subunit	
Inactivating mutations	**Activating mutation**
▪ Albright hereditary osteodystrophy	▪ Mc Cune-Albright syndrome
▪ Pseudohypoparathyroidism Ia.	
▪ Pseudo-pseudo hypoparathyroidism (PPHP)	

51. All of the following statements are true EXCEPT:
                      (PGMEE 2014-15)
   a. 25-α-hydroxylation of vitamin D occurs in the liver
   b. 1-α-hydroxylation of vitamin D occurs in the kidney
   c. In the absence of sunlight, the daily requirement of Vitamin D is 400-600 IU
   d. William's syndrome is characterized by precocious puberty, mental retardation and obesity

[Ref: Harrison's 20th/e pg. 2932]

52. Imaging of choice in parathyroid pathology is:
   a. CT scan   *(PGMEE 2014-15)*
   b. Gallium scan
   c. Thallium scan
   d. Technetium-99 sestamibi scan

[Ref: Harrison's 20th/e pg. 2928]

53. Low serum alkaline phosphatase is seen with:
   a. Hypoparathyroidism   *(PGMEE 2014-15)*
   b. Hypophosphatasia
   c. Hyperparathyroidism
   d. Pseudohypoparathyrodism

54. Hypercalcemic crisis is seen in all EXCEPT:
   a. Metastatic carcinoma breast   *(PGMEE 2014-15)*
   b. Hyperparathyroidism
   c. Pancreatitis
   d. Hodgkin's lymphoma

[Ref: Harrison's 20th/e pg. 2924]

Explanation

- Pancreatitis is associated with hypocalcemia, rescuting due to saponification of fats.

55. Hyperphosphataemia is seen in all EXCEPT:
   a. CRF   *(PGMEE 2014-15)*
   b. Prolonged phosphate intake
   c. Pseudo-pseudo-hypoparathyroidism
   d. Pseudo-hypoparathyrodism

[Ref: Harrison's 20th/e pg. 2940]

56. True about primary hyperparathyroidism is:
   a. Hypotension   *(PGMEE 2014-15)*
   b. Recurrent abortion
   c. Neuropsychiatric changes
   d. Gallstone

[Ref: Harrison's 20th/e pg. 2927]

57. Secondary hyperparathyroidism is seen in all EXCEPT:
   a. Medullary carcinoid syndrome   *(DNB June 2011)*
   b. Vitamin D deficiency
   c. Chronic renal failure
   d. Adenoma

[Ref: Harrison's 20th/e pg. 2924]

58. Tufting of distal phalanx is characteristic of:
   a. Psoriatic arthropathy   *(PGMEE 2014-15)*
   b. Sarcoidosis
   c. Hyperparathyroidism
   d. Hypoparthyroidism

[Ref: Harrison's 20th/e pg. 2927]

46.	a
47.	c,d
48.	b,d
49.	c
50.	d
51.	d
52.	d
53.	b
54.	c
55.	c
56.	c
57.	d
58.	a,c

59. Nephro-calcinosis is a feature of: *(PGMEE 2014-15)*
  a. Primary hyperparathyroidism
  b. Medullary cystic kidney
  c. Vitamin C intoxication
  d. Pseudo-hypoparathyroidism

[Ref: Harrison's 20th/e pg. 2927]

60. Brown tumor is seen in- *(PGMEE 2014)*
  a. Hyperthyroidism
  b. Hypoparathyroidism
  c. Hypothyroidism
  d. Hyperparathyroidism

[Ref: Harrison's 20th/e pg. 2115]

61. Vitamin D deficiency has all EXCEPT: *(PGMEE 2015-16)*
  a. Hypocalcemia
  b. Increased SAP
  c. Increased PTH
  d. Hyperphosphataemia

[Ref: Harrison's 20th/e pg. 2920]

Explanation

- VDD is characterized by hypocalcemia, hypophosphatemia, secondary hyperparathyroidism & ↑ ALP.

62. Which of the following finding shall be seen in patient with hyper-parathyroidism? *(PGMEE 2015-16)*
  a. Hypophosphatemia
  b. Hyperphosphatemia
  c. Hypermagnesemia
  d. Hypo magnesemia

[Ref: Harrison's 20th/e pg. 2923]

63. All are features of hyper-parathyroidism EXCEPT:
  a. Increase serum calcium *(PGMEE 2015-16)*
  b. Decreased serum phosphate
  c. Diarrhea
  d. Nephrocalcinosis

[Ref: Harrison's 20th/e pg. 2925-26]

64. Etiology of hyperparathyroidism are all except?
  a. Solitary adenoma *(PGMEE 2015-16)*
  b. Malignant
  c. Thyroid malignancy
  d. Parathyroid hyperplasia

[Ref: Harrison's 20th/e pg. 2924]

59.	a
60.	d
61.	d
62.	a
63.	c
64.	c

DIABETES MELLITUS (DM)

1. Which of the following is seen in early Type II DM: *(NEET 2018)*

a. Ketone bodies
b. Insulin resistance
c. Increase C-peptide level
d. Anti GAD antibodies

Explanation

Pathogenesis of type 2 diabetes mellitus

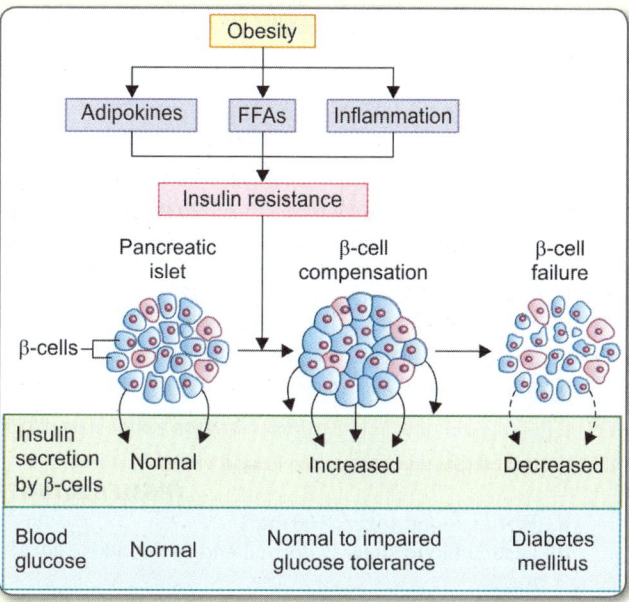

2. Hyperglycemia occurs after what % of beta cell mass is destroyed: *(PGMEE 2014-15)*

a. 20%
b. 40%
c. 60%
d. 80%

[Ref: Harrison's 18th ed. ch. 344]

3. Autonomic disturbances are seen in? *(DNB June 2009)*

a. Diabetes
b. Hyperthyroidism
c. Hyperaldosteronism
d. Hyperparathyroidism

[Ref: Harrison's 20th/e pg. 2875]

4. Incorrect about gestational diabetes mellitus?

a. Congenital malformations *(PGMEE 2014-15)*
b. Metformin is used
c. Prolonged labour
d. Large for date baby

[Ref: Harrison's 20th/e pg. 2851]

5. Not associated with diabetes mellitus: *(PGMEE 2015)*

a. Acromegaly
b. Cushing syndrome
c. Hypothyroidism
d. Phaeochromocytoma

[Ref: Harrison's 20th/e pg. 2851]

6. Mauriac's syndrome is characterized by all EXCEPT: *(PGMEE 2014-15)*

a. Diabetes
b. Obesity
c. Dwarfism
d. Cardiomegaly

Explanation

Mauriac's syndrome:

- Rare complication of Type 1 DM (poorly controlled)
- Characterized by:
  - Dwarfism
  - Obesity
  - Obesity
  - Growth failure
  - Hepatomegaly
  - Delayed puberty

7. Adrenal diabetes is caused by? *(PGMEE 2016-17)*

a. Hemochromatosis
b. Cortisol induced diabetes as seen in Cushing syndrome.
c. Addison's disease
d. Hormonal excess from adrenal medullary tumour

[Ref: Internet]

8. Term Bronze diabetes is used for? *(PGMEE 2016-17)*

a. Hemochromatosis
b. Wilson's diease.
c. Addison's disease
d. Cushing syndrome

9. Diabetes mellitus is present in all EXCEPT: *(PGMEE 2014-15)*

a. Hemochromatosis
b. Ataxia telengeictasia
c. Friedreich ataxia
d. Myotonic dystrophy

[Ref: Harrison's 20th/e pg. 2851]

10. Which one of the following statements about diabetes is not correct? *(PGMEE 2014-15)*

a. Insulin may be given i.v. in patient of diabetic ketoacidosis
b. Insulin antibodies are a hallmark for diagnosis of insulin resistance
c. During hypoglycemic episodes patient may complain of difficulty in vision
d. Positive test for ketone bodies in urine even after patients of diabetic ketosis are treated.

[Ref: Harrison's 20th/e pg. 2857]

Explanation

Insulin Resistance: (IR)

- Inadequate response of cells to a particular concentration of insulin
- Seen in
  - Obesity (MCC)
  - T_2 DM
  - Hypertension
  - Dyslipidemia
  - Type A syndrome
  - Type B syndrome
  - Leprechaunism
  - Lipodystrophy
  - Werner syndrome
  - Ataxia telangiectasia
  - Rabson-Mendenhall syndrome

1.	b
2.	d
3.	a
4.	a
5.	c
6.	d
7.	b
8.	a
9.	b
10.	b

- Diagnosis
  - Clinical
  - Lab: Plasma glucose, fasting insulin level. Lipid profile
- Rx
  - Metformin
  - Thiazolidinediones

11. Which of the following diabetes is associated with HLA?
(PGMEE 2014-15)

a. Type I
b. Type II
c. Fibro-calcific Diabetes mellitus
d. MODY

[Ref: Harrison 20th/e pg. 2486]

12. In Diabetes mellitus, most commonly implicated HLA is:- *(PGMEE 2016-17)*

a. DR 3,DR 4   b. DQ 8
c. DR 8   d. DQ 3, DR 4

[Ref: Harrison's 20th/e pg. 2855]

13. Necrobiosis lipoidica is seen in: *(PGMEE 2014-15)*

a. Diabetes insipidus   b. Lyme disease
c. Diabetes mellitus   d. Simmonds disease

[Ref: Harrison's 20th/e pg. 351]

Explanation

- It is a well circumscribed reddish brown plaque mostly located on the pretibial area. It is strongly associated to DM.

14. Secondary diabetes may be noted in all except?
(PGMEE 2014-15)

a. Acromegaly   b. Addison's disease
c. Haemosiderosis   d. Glucagonoma

[Ref: Harrison's 20th/e pg. 2851]

15. Insulin resistance is not seen in: *(PGMEE 2014-15)*

a. Type 1 DM   b. Lipodystrophy
c. Werner's syndrome   d. Ataxic telangiectasia

[Ref: Harrison's 20th/e pg. 2904]

16. Niacin is contraindicated in diabetes patient because:
(PGMEE 2018)

a. It increases insulin resistance
b. It increases metabolism of anti diabetic drugs
c. It causes scleroderma which leads to loss of injection sites
d. It causes hypoglycemia

DIAGNOSIS OF DIABETES MELLITUS

17. Patient presents with fasting plasma glucose level of 124 mg/dL and 2 hour post-prandial levels of 180 mg/dL. Which of the following is the patient diagnosis?
(NEET Pattern 2019)

a. Normal glucose tolerance
b. Impaired glucose tolerance or prediabetes
c. Diabetes mellitus
d. Diabetic ketoacidosis

18. All of the following are true about Type I DM, EXCEPT:
(PGMEE 2011)

a. Family history is present in 90% of cases
b. Antibodies against β cells
c. Prone to Diabetic Ketoacidosis (DKA)
d. Insulin is required for management of DKA

[Ref: Harrison's 20th/e pg. 2854]

19. True about type 1 diabetes mellitus *(PGMEE 2019)*

a. Increased lipolysis
b. Decreased protein catabolism
c. Decreased hepatic Glucose output
d. Increase glucose uptake

[Ref: Harrison's 20th/e pg. 2854]

20. Which is the best indicator for short term control (2-3 weeks) of blood gucose? *(PGMEE 2015)*

a. Serum fructosamine   b. Urine sugar
c. HbA 1c   d. Blood sugar

[Ref: Harrison's 20th/e pg. 2862]

21. Diabetes is diagnosed when: *(PGMEE 2014-15)*

a. The level of fasting glucose is > 100 mg/dL and that of post-prandial glucose is >140 mg/dL
b. The level of fasting glucose is > 125 mg/dL and that of postprandial glucose is > 199 mg/dL
c. The level of plasma insulin is >6 lU/dL
d. The HbA1c level is >5.5%

[Ref: Harrison's 20th/e pg. 2850]

22. Impaired glucose tolerance is said when:-
(PGMEE 2016-17)

a. Fasting blood sugar >100 mg%
b. Fasting blood sugar is normal and PP blood is 100-140 mg%
c. If Fasting blood sugar is normal and PP blood is 140-200 mg%
d. If Fasting blood sugar is 100-120 mg% and PP blood is >200 mg%

[Ref: Harrison's 20th/e pg. 2850]

23. Fasting blood sugar is 120mg/dL and 2 hr post prandial sugar after 75 gm of oral glucose administration is 180mg/dL. Diagnosis is:- *(PGMEE 2016-17)*

a. Normal individual
b. Impaired glucose tolerance
c. Pre-diabetes
d. Diabetes mellitus

[Ref: Harrison's 20th/e pg. 2850]

24. GTT post 1 hour sugar for gestational diabetes in > _____ mg%? *(PGMEE 2015)*

a. 140   b. 150
c. 180   d. 200

[Ref: ADA Guidelines 2019]

25. Post Prandial capillary glucose should be _____ mg/dl for adequate diabetes control- *(PGMEE 2015)*

a. < 100mg/dl   b. <140mg/dl
c. <180mg/dl   d. <200mg/dl

[Ref: Harrison's 20th/e pg. 2860]

11.	a
12.	a
13.	c
14.	b,c
15.	a
16.	a
17.	b
18.	a
19.	a
20.	a
21.	b
22.	c
23.	c
24.	c
25.	c

TREATMENT OF DIABETES MELLITUS

26. Oral anti-diabetic drug safe in renal failure is:
(PGMEE 2014-15)

a. Glyburide
b. Chlorpropamide
c. Repaglinide
d. Metformin

[Ref: ADA standard of care 2019]

27. The glucose lowering effect is least and delayed by several weeks with the following oral hypoglycaemic agents:

a. Insulin secretogogues
(PGMEE 2014-15)
b. DPP – IV inhibitors
c. Biguanides
d. Alpha-Glucosidase inhibitors

[Ref: Harrison's 20th/e pg. 2865]

28. Female with blood sugar of 600 mg% and sodium of 110 mEq. Insulin was given, what will happen to serum sodium levels? *(PGMEE 2015-16)*

a. Sodium increase
b. Sodium decrease
c. Sodium unaffected
d. Relative sodium deficiency

[Ref: Harrison's 20th/e pg. 301]

Explanation

- Discussed in general medicine.

29. Which of the following drugs used for Diabetes Mellitus causes lactic acidosis- *(PGMEE 2015)*

a. Metformin
b. Pioglitazone
c. Acarbose
d. Glipizide

[Ref: Harrison's 20th/e pg. 2866]

30. An obese diabetic patient was on metformin monotherapy, but his sugar levels were not well controlled. He is allergic to sulpha drugs and does not comply with injectables. He has history of pancreatitis, and family history of bladder CA. In view of the raised glucose levels, you wish to add another anti—diabetic drug. Which one would you prefer? *(NEET Pattern 2017)*

a. Liraglutide
b. Sitagliptin
c. Canagliflozin
d. Pioglitazone

Explanation

Anti-Diabetic Drugs

- *Anti-diabetes drugs which can cause weight gain :(Mn: if u SIT more, u gain weight)*
  - **S**ulfonylureas
  - **I**nsulin
  - **T**hiazolidinedione
- *Anti-diabetic drugs causing weight loss* : (Mn → u play GAMeS to lose weight)
  - G - **G**LP 1 analog (Exenatide, Liraglutide)
  - A - **A**mylin analogs (Pramlintide)
  - Me - **Me**tformin
  - S - SGLT 2 inhibitor
- As this patient is obese, so the preferred add on drug next to metformin would be a GLP 1 analog and SGLT 2 inhibitor followed by DPP 4 inhibitor. As the patient is not willing for injectables, Liraglutide is out (which in fact is the best therapy in an obese individual).

SGLT 2 inhibitors are the next consideration which is safe in this patient and would be the preferred drug. DPP 4 inhibitors are associated with increased risk of pancreatitis and Pioglitazone with bladder carcinoma.

31. Which of the following is used in management of diabetes? *(PGMEE 2014-15)*

a. Bromocriptine
b. Octreotide
c. Prednisolone
d. Pegvisomant

[Ref: Harrison's 20th/e pg. 2868]

32. Dose of insulin in diabetic nephropathy:
(PGMEE 2014-15)

a. Insulin dose should be increased in patient with ESRD
b. Insulin dose should be decreased in patients with ESRD
c. Insulin does not need change in ESRD
d. Add inhaled insulin to conventional administration

[Ref: Harrison's 20th/e pg. 2878]

33. T/t of insulin overdose *(PGMEE 2016-17)*

a. Oral or IV Glucose
b. Beta blockers
c. IV Glucagon
d. Anti-insulin antibodies

[Ref: Harrison's 20th/e pg. 2888]

34. Percentage of dose given as basal insulin in bolus-basal regimen in children is? *(PGMEE 2013)*

a. 0-25%
b. 25-50%
c. 50-75%
d. None

[Ref: Harrison's 20th/e pg. 2864]

35. Increased intracellular insulin is characterized by all EXCEPT: *(DNB Dec 2009)*

a. Increased insulin secretion
b. Hypokalemia
c. Hypoglycemia
d. Increased glucagon secretion

[Ref: Ganong's 22nd Table 19-8]

Explanation

- Inoulin reciprocally regulate glucagon secretion in humans.

36. Dawn phenonmenon is? *(PGMEE 2012)*

a. Morning hyperglycemia with midnight hyperuricemia
b. Morning hypoglycaemia due to excess insulin
c. Morning hyperglycaemia due to insufficient insulin
d. Morning hyperglycemia

[Ref: Harrison's 20th/e pg. 2864]

37. An obese patient presented in casualty with random blood sugar 400 mg%, urine sugar +++ and ketones 1+. Drug useful in management will be: *(PGMEE 2014-15)*

a. Glibenclamide
b. Troglitazsone
c. Insulin
d. Metformin

[Ref: Harrison's 20th/e pg. 2871]

38. All are short acting insulin, EXCEPT: *(PGMEE 2014-15)*

a. Lispro
b. Aspart
c. Glulisine
d. Detemir

[Ref: Harrison's 20th/e pg. 2863]

26.	c
27.	c
28.	a
29.	a
30.	c
31.	a
32.	b
33.	a
34.	b
35.	d
36.	c
37.	c
38.	d

39. Patient on insulin in CKD stage 4. What is the dose adjustment of insulin required? *(PGMEE 2015)*
   a. Add DPP-4 inhibitors   b. Decreased insulin
   c. Normal insulin   d. Increased insulin

[Ref: Harrison's 20th/e pg. 2878]

40. Mineral which potentiate action of insulin: *(PGMEE 2015)*
   a. Zinc   b. Copper
   c. Chromium   d. Selenium

[Ref: spectrum.diabetes journals.org]

COMPLICATIONS OF DIABETES MELLITUS

41. In diabetic ketoacidosis which of the following is the initial iv fluid choice: *(NEET 2018)*
   a. 0.9% sodium chloride solution
   b. Ringer's lactate solution
   c. 5-10% dextrose
   d. None

Explanation

- A crystalloid fluid is the initial fluid of choice.
- Current recommendations are to initiate restoration of volume loss with boluses of isotonic saline (0.9% NaCl) intravenously initially and thereafter, infusion of 0.45% NaCl solution.
- When blood sugar falls <180 mg/dL, isotonic NaCl is replaced with 0.45 DNS.

42. Most effective treatment in DKA is? *(PGMEE 2012)*
   a. Insulin   b. KCl
   c. Sodium bicarbonate   d. IV fluid

[Ref: Harrison's 20th/e pg. 2871]

43. The most effective correction of acidosis in diabetic ketoacidosis is by: *(PGMEE 2014-15)*
   a. I.V. bicarbonate   b. I.V. saline
   c. I.V. insulin   d. Oral bicarbonate

[Ref: Harrison's 20th/e pg. 2871]

44. Diabetes mellitus patient presents with HbA1C of 9.6%. All improve with tight glycemic control EXCEPT:
   a. Neuropathy   *(PGMEE 2014-15)*
   b. Nephropathy
   c. Retinopathy
   d. Peripheral vascular disease

[Ref: Harrison's 20th/e pg. 2876]

Explanation

- The Diabetes control and Complications Trial (DCCT) demonstrated that improvement of glycemic control reduces the risk of retinopathy, microalbuminuria, nephropathy & neuropathy. Long term follow up also demonstrated reduction in cardiovascular events (nonfatal MI, stroke or death from cardiovascular event) in individuals belonging to the intensive therapy group.

45. Which of the macrovascular complication of Diabetes occurs first :- *(PGMEE 2016-17)*
   a. Diabetic neuropathy   b. Diabetic.nephropathy
   c. Diabetic.retinopathy   d. CAD

[Ref: Harrison's 20th/e pg. 2875]

39.	b
40.	c
41.	a
42.	a
43.	c
44.	d
45.	d
46.	c
47.	c
48.	d
49.	a
50.	d
51.	b
52.	c
53.	c

46. Which of the following tests is most sensitive for detecting early diabetic nephropathy? *(PGMEE 2012)*
   a. Serum Creatinine   b. Ultra sonography
   c. Microalbuminuria   d. Creatinine clearance

[Ref: Harrison's 20th/e pg. 2878]

Explanation

- Microalbuminuria is followed by macroproteinuria.

47. The complication of diabetes which cannot be prevented by strict control of blood sugar is: *(PGMEE 2014-15)*
   a. Amyotrophy
   b. Nerve conductivity
   c. Fluorescein dye leak
   d. Microalbuminuria

48. Which drug given for painful tingling of diabetic neuropathy? *(DNB June 2011)*
   a. Gabapentin   b. Pregablin
   c. Duloxetine   d. All of them

[Ref: Harrison's 20th/e pg. 2880]

49. Mechanism of shivering in hypoglycemia:-
   a. Sympathetic overstimulation   *(PGMEE 2016-17)*
   b. Decreased peripheral circulation
   c. Hypoglycemia induced hypothermia
   d. Both B and C

[Ref: Harrison's 20th/e pg. 2884]

50. Diabetic neuropathy is a: *(DNB Dec'2010)*
   a. Autonomic neuropathy
   b. Mononeuritis
   c. Distal symmetric sensory polyneuropathy
   d. All above

[Ref: Harrison's 20th/e pg. 2879]

51. The most common form of diabetic neuropathy is:-
   (PGMEE 2015-16)
   a. Distal Motor neuropathy
   b. Distal symmetric sensory and motor neuropathy
   c. Autonomic neuropathy
   d. Distal symmetric sensory neuropathy

[Ref: Harrison's 20th/e pg. 2879]

52. Hypoglycemic unawareness is because of:
   (PGMEE 2014-15)
   a. Shifting of oral hypoglycemics to insulin
   b. Insulin resistance
   c. Autonomic neuropathy
   d. Necrobiosis lipoidica

[Ref: Harrison's 20th/e pg. 2885]

Explanation

- Hypoglycemic unawareness is defined as loss of the warning adrenergic and cholinergic symptoms (Eg. palpitation, sweating, tremors etc) that allows a patient to recognize developing hypoglycemia. It is the result of an attenuated sympathetic neural response to hypoglycemia.

53. Necrobiosis lipoidica diabeticorum is most marked on:
   (PGMEE 2014-15)
   a. Forearms   b. Face
   c. Pre-tibial   d. Sole of foot

[Ref: Harrison's 20th/e pg. 2882]

54. Retinopathy is most likely to be seen with:
(PGMEE 2014-15)
a. IDDM of 5 years duration
b. NIDDM of 8 years duration
c. Gestational diabetes
d. Juvenile diabetes started before puberty

[Ref: Harrison's 20th/e pg. 2877]

55. Diabetic ketoacidosis is associated with all EXCEPT:
(PGMEE 2014-15)
a. Utilization of glucose b. Protein catabolism
c. Positive Anion gap d. Lipolysis

[Ref: Harrison's 20th/e pg. 2870-71]

56. The following statements concerning diabetic keto-acidosis are correct EXCEPT: *(PGMEE 2014-15)*
a. Abdominal pain
b. Low BUN
c. Dehydration is out of proportion to the severity of vomiting
d. Low-dose insulin therapy is the treatment of choice:

[Ref: Harrison's 20th/e pg. 2871]

57. Which is not seen in diabetic ketoacidosis:
(PGMEE 2014-15)
a. Normal serum potassium
b. Plasma osmolality 380 mOsm
c. Urine Rothera test positive
d. Urine Benedicts test positive

[Ref: Harrison's 20th/e pg. 2870]

58. A patient with DM of 4 years duration presents with dizziness and HR 52/min, Probable cause is:
(PGMEE 2014-15)
a. Hypoglycaemia b. Inferior wall MI
c. Sick-sinus syndrome d. Autonomic dysunction

59. Early morning hyperglycemia with decreased blood glucose of 2.00 AM suggests:- *(PGMEE 2015-16)*
a. Somogyi effect
b. Insufficient Insulin
c. Dawn Phenomenon
d. None of the above

[Ref: Harrison's 20th/e pg. 3515]

60. What is correct in diabetic ketoacidosis?
(PGMEE 2014-15)
a. Low serum K⁺ b. ↑ed anion gap
c. Metabolic alkalosis d. Respiratory acidosis

[Ref: Harrison's 20th/e pg. 2870]

61. Most common oral infection in diabetes mellitus?
(PGMEE 2015)
a. Candida b. Staphylococcus
c. Streptococcus d. Aspergilius

[Ref: Harrison's 20th/e pg. 2882]

62. Aldose reductase inhibitor drugs are useful in?
(PGMEE 2015)
a. Essential fructosuria
b. Myopathy
c. Hereditary fructose intolerance
d. Diabetes neuropathy

[Ref: Harrison's 20th/e pg. 2877]

63. Foot Ulcers in diabetes are due to all except?
a. Microangiopathy *(PGMEE 2015)*
b. Neuropathy
c. Decreased immunity
d. Macroangiopathy

[Ref: Harrison's 20th/e pg. 2881]

64. Cause of death in diabetic ketoacidosis in children?
(PGMEE 2014-15)
a. Cerebral edema b. Hypokalemia
c. Infection d. Acidosis

METABOLIC SYNDROME AND OBESITY

65. Which of the following is incorrect about metabolic syndrome?
a. Obesity
b. Hyperventilation
c. Hyperlipidemia
d. Impaired Glucose tolerance test

[Ref: Harrison's 20th/e pg. 2903]

Explanation

Criteria for metabolic syndrome

- **W**aist **E**xpanded
- **I**mpired **G**lucose
- **H**ypertension
- **H**DL↓
- **T**riglycerides↑ [**Mnemonic: WEIGHT**]

66. Obesity in children is seen in: *(PGMEE 2015-16)*
a. Adrenal insufficiency
b. Pseudo-hypo-parathyroidism
c. Prader willi syndrome
d. Soto syndrome

[Ref: Harrison's 20th/e pg. 2842]

Explanation

Obesity in Children		
Genetic syndrome	*Hormonal disorders*	*Medications*
Prader-Willi syndrome	GH deficiency	Glucocorticoids
Pseudo hypoparathyroidism	GH resistance	Insulin
Laurence. Moon-Biedl syndrome	Hypothyroidism	
Cohen syndrome	Leptin deficiency	
Down syndrome	Cushing syndrome	
Turner syndrome	PCOS	

67. In morbid obesity BMI greater than? *(DNB June 2010)*
a. 30 b. 35
c. 40 d. 45

[Ref: Harrison's 20th/e pg. 2844]

54.	**a**
55.	**a**
56.	**b**
57.	**b**
58.	**d**
59.	**a**
60.	**b**
61.	**a**
62.	**d**
63.	**c**
64.	**a**
65.	**b**
66.	**b,c**
67.	**c**

68. Obesity is seen in all except: *(All India Dec 2015 Pattern)*
a. Sipple syndrome
b. Prader willi syndrome
c. Cushing syndrome
d. Pickwinian syndrome

[Ref: Harrison's 20th/e pg. 2842]

Explanation

- Obesity hypoventilation syndrome is aka Pickwickian syndrome

69. True about obesity? *(PGMEE 2015-16)*
a. More common in females
b. Prevalence decrease upto 40 years of age
c. No genetic predisposition
d. Smoking is a risk factor

[Ref: Harrison's 20th/e pg. 2838]

70. All are true about syndrome X EXCEPT:
(DNB December 2011)
a. Hypertriglyceridemia
b. Hypoinsulinemia
c. Abdominal obesity
d. Hyperglycemia

[Ref: Harrison's 19th/e pg 2405]

MISCELLANEOUS

71. Stress hormone is :- *(PGMEE 2016-17)*
a. Gonadotrophins   b. Insulin
c. Cortisol   d. Growth hormone

[Ref: Ganong's 25th/e pg. 364]

72. Pro-opiomelanocortin (POMC) is released from?
(PGMEE 2015)
a. Pituitary   b. Adrenal gland
c. Lung   d. Liver

[Ref: Harrison's 20th/e pg. 2720]

73. Zellballen pattern is seen in all of the following, except:-
(PGMEE 2015-16)
a. Acoustic neuroma   b. Carotid body tumour
c. Pheochromocytoma   d. Glomus jugulare

[Ref: Robbin's 9th/e pg. 742, 1135]

Explanation

- Zellballen pattern is seen in pheochromocytoma & paragangliomas (Glomus tumor) like glomus jugulare, carotid body tumors etc.

74. Zellballen pattern is seen in:- *(PGMEE 2016-17)*
a. Acoustic neuroma   b. Paraganglioma
c. Neurofibroma   d. Juvenile angiofibroma

[Ref: Robbin's 9th/e pg. 741-742]

68.	a
69.	a
70.	b
71.	c
72.	a
73.	a
74.	b

ADRENAL GLAND

1. **Adrenal reserve is best tested by means of infusion with:** *(PGMEE 2014-15)*
   a. Glucocorticoids
   b. ACTH
   c. Hypothyroidism
   d. Metyrapone

   [Ref: Harrison's 20th/e pg. 2720]

2. **False about Wolman disease is -** *(PGMEE 2014)*
   a. It is characterized by deficient acid lysosomal lipase
   b. It shows autosomal recessive inheritance pattern
   c. It is lysosomal storage disorder
   d. It is characterized by adrenal calcification and corneal clouding

   [Ref: Harrison's 20th/e pg. 2896]

3. **Salt losing type of adreno-genital syndromes is associated with:** *(PGMEE 2014-15)*
   a. Hypoglycemia
   b. Hypernatremia
   c. Hypertension
   d. Hypokalemia

   [Ref: Harrison's 20th/e pg. 2738]

4. **The most common cause of malignant adrenal mass is:** *(PGMEE 2015)*
   a. Lymphoma
   b. Malignant Phaeochromocytoma
   c. Adrenocortical carcinoma
   d. Metastasis from another solid tissue tumor

   [Ref: Harrison's 20th/e pg. 2731]

5. **Hypertension with hypokalemia is seen in following EXCEPT:** *(PGMEE 2014-15)*
   a. Cushing syndrome
   b. Liddle syndrome
   c. End stage renal disease
   d. Primary hyperaldosteronism

   [Ref: Pubmed]

Explanation

- Common causes of hypertension with hypokalemia:
  - Essential hypertension with diurectic use
  - Primary aldosteronism
  - Cushing's syndrome
  - Pheochromocytoma
  - Liddle syndrome
  - Renovascular disease

6. **All are features of glucocorticoid deficiency except?** *(NEET Pattern 2015)*
   a. Weight loss
   b. Fever
   c. Hyperkalemia
   d. Postural hypotension

   [Ref: Harrison's 20th/e pg. 2735]

Explanation

	Glucocorticoid deficiency	Mineralocorticoid deficiency
Low BP	+	+
Postural hypotension	+	+
Hyponatremia	+/-	+
Hyperkalemia	-	+
Constitutional symptoms	++	-
Other	■ Hypoglycemia ■ Eosinophilia ■ ↓ S. cortisol ■ ↑ ACTH	■ Salt craving ■ ↑ S. creatinine

7. **Which of the following is the most common cause of Addison's disease in India?** *(PGMEE 2015)*
   a. Autoimmune adrenal insufficiency
   b. HIV
   c. Post-partum pituitary insufficiency
   d. Tuberculosis

   [Ref: Harrison's 20th/e pg. 2733]

8. **Incorrect about Addison's disease is?** *(PGMEE 2014-15)*
   a. Hypoglycemia
   b. Hypokalemia
   c. Loss of axillary and pubic hair
   d. Salt craving

   [Ref: Harrison's 20th/e pg. 2735]

Explanation

Laboratory abnormalities in addison's disease

- Hyponatremia
- Hyperkalemia with mild to moderate acidosis
- Hypoglycemia
- Neutropenia

9. **Which of the following is not seen in Secondary Adrenal insufficiency?** *(PGMEE 2015)*
   a. Lassitude
   b. Hypoglycemia
   c. Pigmentation
   d. Postural hypotension

   [Ref: Harrison's 20th/e pg. 2735]

Explanation

- In secondary adrenal insufficiency, only deficient hormone is glucocorticoids. A distinguishing feature of primary adrenal insufficiency is hyperpigmentation caused by excess of ACTH. In secondary adrenal insufficiency the skin is pale due to lack of ACTH secretion.

1.	b
2.	d
3.	a
4.	c
5.	c
6.	c
7.	d
8.	b
9.	c

- 46,XY is seen in < 10% of patients with ovotesticular DSD
- 46,XX/46,XY mosaicism is found in 20% of patients.
- The most frequently encountered gonad in ovotesticular DSD is an **ovotestis**, which may be bilateral. If unilateral, the contralateral gonad is usually an ovary but may be a testis. The ovarian tissue is normal, but the testes is dysgenetic.
- Patients who are highly virilized and have had adequate testicular function with no uterus are usually reared as males.
- If a uterus exists, virilization is often mild and testicular function minimal; assignment of female sex may be indicated.
- Risk of developing gonadoblastomas, dysgerminomas, or seminomas is 5%.

Ovotesticular DSD
XX
XY
XX/XY chimeras

Sex Chromosome DSD
45, X (Turner syndrome and variants)
47,XXY (Klinefelter syndrome and variants)
45,X/46,XY (mixed gonadal dysgenesis, sometimes a cause of ovotesticular DSD)P
46,XX/46,XY (chimeric, sometimes a cause of ovotesticualr DSD)

42. Not a Cause of Gynaecomastia? *(PGMEE 2015-16)*
  a. Hypothyroidism
  b. Kallman syndrome
  c. Obesity
  d. Klinefelter syndrome

  [Ref: Harrison's 20th/e pg. 2780]

Explanation

Causes of gyne comastia

■ Klinefelter syndrome	■ Hyperthyroidism	■ Drugs C
■ Kallmann syndrome	■ Obesity	■ Ocp. Digitalis
■ Androgen insensitivity syndrome	■ Chronic liver disease	■ Ketoconazole
		■ Spironolactone
		■ Cimetidine

43. A patient has amenorrhea and anosmia with hypothalamic lesion. The diagnosis is? *(PGMEE 2014-15)*
  a. Kallman's syndrome
  b. Asherman's syndrome
  c. Stein Leventhal syndrome
  d. Sheehans syndrome

  [Ref: Harrison's 20th/e pg. 2797]

44. The karyotype in testicular feminization syndrome is? *(PGMEE 2013)*
  a. XX
  b. XY
  c. XXY
  d. XXXY

  [Ref: Harrison's 20th/e pg. 2765]

45. Gonadectomy is advised in: *(PGMEE 2014-15)*
  a. Kallman's syndrome
  b. Testicular feminization syndrome
  c. Hemochromatosis
  d. Sexual precocity

  [Ref: Harrison's 20th/e pg. 2765]

42.	a
43.	a
44.	b
45.	b
46.	b
47.	b
48.	c
49.	b
50.	b
51.	b
52.	d

Explanation

- Gonadectomy is advised in *testicular feminization syndrome* as the gonads are located in the abdomen. These gonads have a high incidence of malignancy.
- The sex of rearing is female. Karyotype is 46 XY.
- *Hemachromatosis* is anosmia with delayed puberty.
- GnRH Analogs are used in the Rx of precocious puberty.

46. All the following are testicular dysgenesis syndromes except: *(PGMEE 2015)*
  a. Cryptorchidism
  b. Epispadias
  c. Poor sperm quality
  d. Hypospadias

  [Ref: Harrison's 20th/e pg. 2778]

47. A child presents with ambiguous genitalia without hyperpigmentation and normal blood pressure, 2.5 cm phallus with no opening at its tip, labia developed. Gonads are not seen in inguinal region and Mullerian structures are present on USG. The most probable diagnosis is: *(PGMEE 2014-15)*
  a. AIS
  b. Maternal virilising tumor
  c. CAH
  d. 5-alpha-reductase deficiency

  [Ref: Harrison's 19th/e pg. 2362, 2366]

48. Hirsutism is seen in all EXCEPT: *(DNB June 2010)*
  a. Congenital adrenal hyperplasia
  b. Cushing syndrome
  c. Testicular feminizing syndrome
  d. Stein leventhal syndrome

  [Ref: Harrison's 17th/e ch.50, Hirsutism and vertilization Table 50-1]

49. Male pseudohermaphroditism is- *(PGMEE 2013-14)*
  a. Testis and ovary both present
  b. XY genotype, female external genitalia
  c. XX genotype, male external genitalia
  d. Male external genitalia and ovary present

  [Ref: Nelson 20th/e/p 2297]

50. Gene responsible for differentiation of gonads to testis is? *(PGMEE 2012-13)*
  a. WNT-4 gene
  b. SRY gene
  c. RSPO-1 gene mutation
  d. DAX1 gene

  [Ref: Ghai 8th/e/p 538]

51. Testes are not palpable in- *(PGMEE 2015)*
  a. WNT-4 gene mutation
  b. SRY deletion
  c. DAX 1 deletion
  d. RSPO-1 gene mutation

  [Ref: Ghai 8th/e/p 538, Nelson 20th/e/p 583]

HIRSUTISM, GYNAECOMASTIA

52. All of the following drugs causes hirsutism except: *(DNB Dec' 2011)*
  a. Flutamide
  b. Cyproterone acetate
  c. Spironolactone
  d. Mefipristone

  [Ref: Harrison's 18th/e chapter 49]

MEN

1. Which of the following are the extraintestinal manifestations of Sipple syndrome? *(NEET Pattern 2019)*
   - a. Amyloidosis
   - b. Hirschsprung disease
   - c. Cutaneous lichen
   - d. All of the above

2. Which of the following is most often involved in multiple endocrine neoplasia-I *(DNB 2007)*
   - a. Pituitary
   - b. Pancreas
   - c. Parathyroid
   - d. Thyroid

[Ref: Harrison's 20th/e pg. 2747]

3. Commonest thyroid cancer associated with neuroendocrine tumour /MEN: *(PGMEE 2016-17; 2013-14)*
   - a. Papillary
   - b. Anaplastic
   - c. Follicular
   - d. Medullary

[Ref: Harrison's 20th/e pg. 2747]

4. Wermer syndrome is- *(PGMEE 2016-17)*
   - a. MEN 1
   - b. AIP
   - c. MEN IIA
   - d. MEN IIB

[Ref: Harrison's 20th/e pg. 2747]

5. Werner syndrome is characterized by all EXCEPT: *(PGMEE 2014/15)*
   - a. Premature ageing
   - b. Pituitary adenoma
   - c. Bird like facies
   - d. Premature atherosclerosis

[Ref: Harrison's 20th/e pg. 3416]

Explanation

- Werner syndrome is a syndrome in which defective DNA helicase leads to defective gene product leading to premature aging and other mentioned features.

6. MEN type I includes tumors of all except- *(DNB June 2009, 2012-13)*
   - a. Pituitary
   - b. Pancrease
   - c. Parathyroid
   - d. Medullary carcinoma of thyroid

[Ref: Harrison's 20th/e pg. 2747]

7. A/E are involved in MEN type II A- *(PGMEE 2013-14)*
   - a. Thyroid
   - b. Parathyroid
   - c. Adernal
   - d. Pituitary

[Ref: Harrison's 20th/e pg. 2747]

8. All are associated with MEN4 except? *(PGMEE 2014-15)*
   - a. Parathyroid adenoma
   - b. Pituitary adenoma
   - c. Reproductive organ Tumors
   - d. Medullary carcinoma of thyroid

[Ref: Harrison's 20th/e pg. 2747]

9. All are features of MEN2B except? *(PGMEE 2014-15)*
   - a. Mucosal neuroma
   - b. Marfanoid Habitus
   - c. Medullated corneal nerve fibres
   - d. Meningioma

[Ref: Harrison's 20th/e pg. 2747]

10. CDKN1B gene mutation is implicated in:- *(PGMEE 2015-16)*
   - a. MEN-1
   - b. MEN-2
   - c. MEN-3
   - d. MEN-4

[Ref: Harrison's 20th/e pg. 2747]

11. Chromosome involved in MEN-II (Sipple syndrome):- *(PGMEE 2016-17)*
   - a. 17
   - b. 22
   - c. 19
   - d. 10

[Ref: Harrison's 20th/e pg. 2747]

12. MEN-2A includes :- *(PGMEE 2016-17)*
   - a. Parathyroid adenoma , pituitary tumor and phaeochromocytoma
   - b. Parathyroid adenoma, pancreatic and pituitary tumor
   - c. Parathyroid adenoma, pituitary tumor, medullary thyroid CA
   - d. Pheochromocytoma, medullary thyroid CA, parathyroid adenoma

[Ref: Harrison's 20th/e pg. 2747]

13. All of the following are seen in MEN 2b (MEN3) EXCEPT: *(DNB June 2011)*
   - a. Hyperparathyroidism
   - b. Pheochromocytoma
   - c. Medullary carcinoma
   - d. Neuromas

[Ref: Harrison's 20th/e pg. 2747]

PHEOCHROMOCYTOMA

14. Pheochromocytoma all are true except:- *(PGMEE 2016-17]*
   - a. Tumor of parasympathetic ganglion
   - b. 10% tumors are malignant
   - c. HTN with ↑VMA
   - d. MRI is not used in diagnosis

[Ref: Harrison's 20th/e pg. 2741]

15. A 40 years old lady comes with pheochromocytoma. Most characteristic symptom is? *(DNB December 2011)*
   - a. Orthostatic hypotension
   - b. Weight loss
   - c. Sweating attacks
   - d. Paroxysmal hypertension

[Ref: Harrison's 20th/e pg. 2740]

16. Which of the following is not found in pheochromocytoma? *(PGMEE 2014-15)*
   - a. Episodic hypertension
   - b. Postural hypotension
   - c. Increased hematocrit
   - d. Hypocalcemia

[Ref: Harrison's 20th/e pg. 2740]

17. Vanillyl mandelic acid (VMA) is increased in urine in? *(DNB December 2011)*
   - a. Cushing's syndrome
   - b. Pheochromocytoma
   - c. Addison's disease
   - d. Carcinoid tumour

[Ref: Harrison's 19th/e pg 2329]

1.	d
2.	c
3.	d
4.	a
5.	b
6.	d
7.	d
8.	d
9.	d
10.	d
11.	d
12.	d
13.	a
14.	d
15.	d
16.	d
17.	b

Explanation

- VMA is a meabolic by product of epinephrine and norepinephrine . It can be used to detect tumor of neural crest origin.

18. A patient with pheochromocytoma would secrete which of the following in a higher concentration?

(PGMEE 2014-15)

a. Norepinephrine   b. Epinephrine

c. Dopamine   d. VMA

[Ref: Harrison's 19th/e pg. 2329]

19. All are seen in Pheochromocytoma EXCEPT:

(DNB June 2010)

a. Weight loss   b. Headaches

c. Sweating attacks   d. Hypocalcemia

[Ref: Harrison's 20th/e pg. 2740]

20. In a patient with phenochromocytoma, all the following are seen EXCEPT: *(PGMEE 2014-15)*

a. Constipation

b. Orthostatic hypotension

c. Episodic hypertension

d. Weight gain

[Ref: Harrison's 20th/e pg. 2740]

21. The residual form of phaeochromocytoma is treated by:

(PGMEE 2014-15)

a. Strontium   b. Phosphorus

c. Cobalt-60   d. MIBG

[Ref: Harrison's 20th/e pg. 2744]

22. Pheochromocytoma is associated with- *(PGMEE 2015)*

a. Acanthosis Nigricans

b. Vitiligo

c. Ash leaf amelanotic macusles

d. Café-au-lait spots

[Ref: Harrison's 20th/e pg. 2745]

23. All are true about Pheochromocytoma EXCEPT

(DNB Dec' 2009)

a. Benign in nature

b. Malignant tumor

c. Secretes hormones

d. Hypertension is seen

[Ref: Robbin's 9th/e pg. 1133-34]

24. Pheochromocytoma secretes *(DNB Dec' 2009)*

a. Norepinephrine

b. Dopamine

c. Epinephrine

d. All of the above

[Ref: Robbin's 9th/e pg. 1133-34]

25. Mitotic figures and giant cells are seen in which tumor-

(PGMEE 2014)

a. Benign Pheochromocytoma

b. Malignant Pheochromocytoma

c. Both of the above

d. None of the above

[Ref: Robbins 9th/e pg. 1135]

26. Tumor that follows rule of 10 is- *(PGMEE 2012-13)*

a. Pheochromocytoma   b. Renal cell carcinoma

c. Oncocytoma   d. Lymphoma

[Ref: Robbin's 9th/e pg. 1134]

NEUROENDOCRINE TUMORS

27. Whipple's triad is useful for diagnosis of:

(PGMEE 2015-16)

a. Insulinoma   b. Glucagonoma

c. Somatostatinoma   d. V.I.Poma

[Ref: Harrison's 20th/e pg. 2883]

28. Migratory necrolytic erythema is a feature of :-

a. TEN   *(PGMEE 2016-17)*

b. Drug induced lupus

c. Leukocytoclastic vasculitis

d. Glucagonoma

[Ref: Harrison's 20th/e pg. 609]

29. Secretory diarrhea is caused by all except?

a. Medullary thyroid tumor   *(PGMEE 2015-16)*

b. Carcinoid Tumor

c. Somatostinoma

d. Glucagonoma

[Ref: Harrison's 20th/e pg. 263]

30. 72 hour prolonged fasting test is used for?

a. Fat absorption   *(PGMEE 2014-15)*

b. Insulinoma

c. Carbohydrate absorption

d. Amino acid absorption

[Ref: Harrison's 20th/e pg. 608]

MISCELLANEOUS

31. Prader-Willi syndrome is associated with an increase in which of the following hormones: *(PGMEE 2014-15)*

a. Ghrelin   b. GH

c. FSH   d. LH

[Ref: Prader willi syndrome: ch. 44 Nelson 18th ed.]

32. Which of these organs are not affected in autoimmune polyglandular syndrome type 2? *(PGMEE 2015)*

a. Parathyroid   b. Thyroid

c. Adrenal   d. Pancreas

[Ref: Harrison's 20th/e pg. 2734]

18.	a
19.	d
20.	d
21.	d
22.	d
23.	b
24.	d
25.	a
26.	a
27.	a
28.	d
29.	c
30.	b
31.	a
32.	a

Pulmonology

FACTS

- Chief blood supply of lungs: Pulmonary artery
- COPD and Asthma are the diseases of small airways
- Bronchiectasis involve: Medium sized airways
- TOC in Bronchiectasis: postural drainage
- Hemoptysis in bronchiectasis is due to erosion of: Bronchial arteries
- Idiopathic (Primary) PAH is associated with: **BMPR2** gene abnormality

V/Q Ratio:
- Ventilation: Best at base
- Perfusion: Best at base
- V/Q: Best at apex

Asbestosis
- **Serpentine/Chrysotile:** MC type of asbestos used in industry
- **Amphibole:** More pathogenic than chrysotile. Can cause mesothelioma

Hoover Sign:
- Paradoxical inward movement of the lower ribcage during inspiration
- Seen in advanced COPD

Hamman sign/Humman's Crunch:
- Crunching sound heard in synchrony with the heart beats
- Seen in Pneumomediastinum/Mediastinal emphysema

Hamman Rich Syndrome:
- Aka acute interstitial pneumonia
- Severe form of idiopathic ILD

Obesity Hypoventilation Syndrome:
- BMI ≥30 kg/m²
- Daytime hypoventilation ($PaCO_2$ ≥45 mm Hg)
- Sleep disordered breathing

MOST COMMON

- MC cause of drug induced asthma: Aspirin
- MC cause of pneumothorax: COPD
- MC cause of spontaneous pneumothorax: rupture of Subpleural apical blebs.
- IOC for measuring the lung volumes in COPD and bullous lesions: Body plethysmography
- MC site of bronchiectasis: Left lower lobe
- MC mutation in Cystic Fibrosis: 3 bp deletion at ΔF_{508} of *CFTR* gene
- MC infection in cystic fibrosis: *Pseudomonas*
- MC cause of CAP: *S. pneumoniae*
- MC species of Legionella causing human infection: *L. pneumophila*
- MC serotype of Legionella causing CAP: 1
- MC site of hemoptysis: Tracheobronchial tree
- MC vessels causing hemoptysis: Bronchial artery

- MC fetal response to acute hypoxia: Bradycardia
- MCC of invasive Aspergillosis: *A. fumigatus*
- MCC of chronic Aspergillosis: *A. fumigatus*
- MCC of massive exudative effusion: TB
- MC source of pulmonary emboli: Ileofemoral veins
- MC sign of pulmonary embolism: Tachypnea
- MCC of acute Cor pulmonale: Massive PTE
- MCC of Cor pulmonale: Pulmonary hypertension
- MC site of lung abscess: Posterior segments of right upper lobe or Superior segments of right lower lobe.
- MC GNB causing lung abscess: *Klebsiella*
- MC chronic occupational disease in the world: Silicosis

INVESTIGATIONS

- IOC in Bronchiectasis: HRCT → Signet ring appearance or Tram track appearance
- CXR in bronchiectasis: Tram track/Ring shadow appearance
- CXR in Klebsiella pneumonia: Bulging fissure sign

- Mainstay of diagnosis for Pneumocystis pneumonia: BAL
- IOC for Pulmonary hypertension: Cardiac catheterization
- Halo sign on CT chest: Invasive Aspergillosis
- IOC for lung CA: Bronchoscopy + Biopsy

PULMONARY FUNCTION TESTS

	OLD	IRLD	ERLD
TLC	↑	↓	↓
RV	↑	↓	N
PEFR	↓	N	↓
RV/ TLC	N	N	↑
FEV_1	↓↓	↓	↓
FVC	↓	↓↓	↓↓
FEV_1/ FVC	↓ (<70%)	N/↑	N/↑
DL_{co}	N	↓	N
Conditions	▪ Asthma ▪ Bronchiectasis ▪ Bronchiolitis ▪ COPD ▪ Cystic fibrosis	▪ Idiopathic pulmonary fibrosis/ILD ▪ Asbestosis ▪ Sarcoidosis	▪ Guillain Barre Syndrome ▪ Myasthenia gravis ▪ Ankylosing spondylosis ▪ Kyphoscoliosis ▪ Pleural effusion

OLD – Obstructive Lung Disease | IRLD – Intrinsic Restrictive Lung Disease | ERLD – Extrinsic Restrictive Lung Disease |

DL_{co} – Diffusion capacity of lung for CO |

Different respiratory volumes:
- Inspiratory Reserve Volume (IRV) = 3000 mL
- Expiratory Reserve Volume (ERV) = 1100 mL
- Residual Volume (RV) = 1200 mL
- Tidal volume (TV) = 500 mL
- Vital Capacity (VC) = TV + IRV + ERV
- Total Lung Capacity = RV + VC

Hallmark of:
- Obstructive lung disease → decrease in expiratory flow rates
- Restrictive lung disease → decrease in lung volumes

Absolute lung volume is calculated by:
- Inert gas dilution
- Body plethysmography → Most accurate

Increase in DL_{co} is seen in:
- Pulmonary hemorrhage
- Left to right shunt
- Polycythemia

Most sensitive measure of air flow obstruction:
- Large airway → Peak expiratory flow rate (PEFR)
- Small airway → MEFR /FEF_{25-75}

ILD with obstructive feature:
- Sarcoidosis
- Hypersensitivity Pneumonitis
- Lymphangioleiomyomatosis (LAM)

ASTHMA

- Single largest risk factor for Asthma: History of atopy
- Nasal polyp is seen which type of Asthma: Aspirin induced asthma/Intrinsic asthma
- GINA = Global Initiative for Asthma is a guideline for management of asthma

- NO_2 is associated with: Asthma
- **Sampter's triad** = Intrinsic asthma + Nasal polyp + Aspirin sensitivity
- Leukotriene antagonist are associated with: Churg Strauss syndrome

Types

	Allergic Asthma	Exercise Induced Asthma (EIA)	Aspirin Sensitive Asthma
Type	▪ Extrinsic asthma	▪ Intrinsic asthma	▪ Intrinsic asthma
Trigger	▪ Allergen like pollen, dust etc	▪ Aerobic exercise	▪ Aspirin and other NSAIDs
Pathology	▪ Type I Hypersensitivity	▪ Histamine release	▪ Increase production of LT and eosinophils
Manifestations	▪ Onset – Childhood ▪ Atopy/Rhinitis/Eczema ++ ▪ Family history ++ ▪ Increased serum IgE	▪ Can occur in any age ▪ More common in asthmatics and individuals with allergic rhinitis ▪ More in winter or cold weather sports	▪ Adult/late onset ▪ Non atopic individual ▪ Perennial rhinitis and nasal polyps ▪ Triad = Asthma + Aspirin sensitivity + Polyp
Treatment	▪ Controller – inhaled corticosteroids, LABA, LAMA, Theophylline, anti IgE and IL-5 Antibody ▪ Reliever – SABA, Systemic steroids	▪ Preexercise SABA like salbutamol ▪ Mast cell stabilizer – Cromolyn sodium ▪ LT receptor antagonist - Montelukast	▪ Responds well to ICS ▪ Avoid nonselective COX inhibitor
Prognosis	▪ Good	▪ Excellent	▪ Good

Monoclonal Antibodies in Asthma

- Omalizumab – inhibits binding of IgE to mast cell receptors
- Mepolizumab, Reslizumab, Benralizumab – blocks IL-5 binding to its receptor on eosinophils
- Dupilumab – blocks the action of IL-4 and IL-13

Management

- Best diagnostic test: Demonstration of reversibility of airway obstruction → ↑ in FEV_1 of ≥12% or 200 mL after administration of SABA
- DOC for chronic asthma: Inhaled corticosteroid + LABA

- Exercise induced Asthma
  - Treatment: SABA
  - Prophylaxis: Inhaled LABA/LT receptor Blocker
- Monitoring response to asthma therapy is done by measuring: PEFR

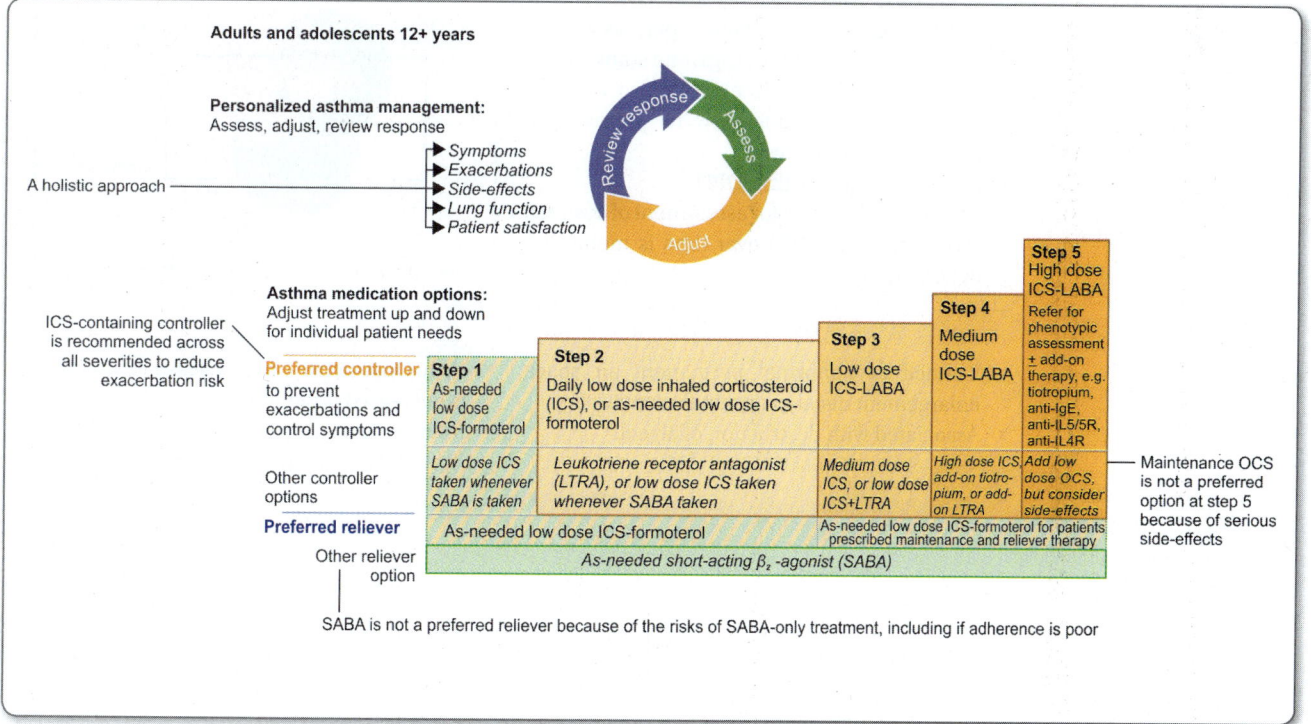

OCS-oral corticosteroids | ICS-Inhaled corticosteroids

ACUTE SEVERE ASTHMA (STATUS ASTHMATICUS)

- It is an acute exacerbation of asthma that remains unresponsive to initial treatment with bronchodilators.
- On examination – absence of wheezing (so called silent chest) indicate severe airflow obstruction.

- Pulsus paradoxus may be observed in case of severe asthma.
- DOC for acute severe asthma: Inhaled SABA + Systemic steroids

Beta 2 Agonists

- The first line of therapy is treatment with a β2-agonist, typically salbutamol.
- Most effective in the early phase of asthma.
- Acts via stimulation of cyclic adenosine monophosphate (c-AMP) mediated bronchodilation.

- Most effective route of delivery – Inhalational route
- The role of methylxanthines, such as theophylline or aminophylline, in the treatment of severe acute asthma has been diminished since the advent of potent selective beta-agonists.

Anticholinergic Agent

- Ipratropium bromide does not cross the blood-brain barrier and is the recommended agent of choice.

- Ipratropium may also be used as an alternative bronchodilator in patients who are unable to tolerate inhaled β2-agonists.

Glucocorticoids

- Glucocorticoids are the most important treatment for status asthmaticus.
- These agents can decrease bronchial hypersensitivity, mucus production, improve oxygenation, reduce theophylline or beta-agonist (by **increasing the expression of β2-receptors**) requirements, and

activate properties that may prevent late bronchoconstrictive responses.
- Corticosteroid action usually requires at least 4-6 hours to occur because protein synthesis is required before the initiation of its anti-inflammatory effects.

COPD

- Clubbing is not a feature of COPD
- ***Reid Index for Chronic Bronchitis:***
  - <0.4 is normal
  - >0.4 suggest mucus gland hyperplasia
- MI risk factor for COPD: Cigarette smoking
- Single most effective intervention to ↓ risk of developing COPD and slow its progression: Cessation of smoking
- SO_2 is associated with: COPD
- MRC grading is done for assessment of dyspnea
- Progression of COPD over time is monitored by: Change in FEV_1

- GOLD staging is done for: COPD

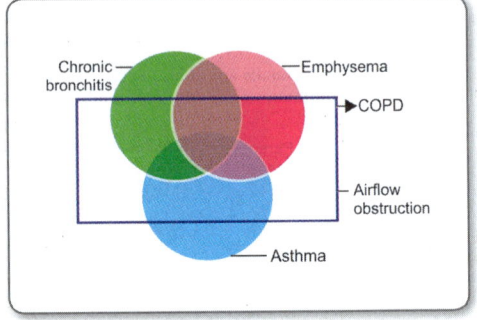

Emphysema

- Defined as abnormal permanent air space enlargement distal to terminal bronchiole
- Associated with destruction of alveoli

- Only Obstructive Lung Disease in which DL_{CO} is decreased: Emphysema
- Increase in static compliance with increase in dynamic compliance is seen in: Emphysema

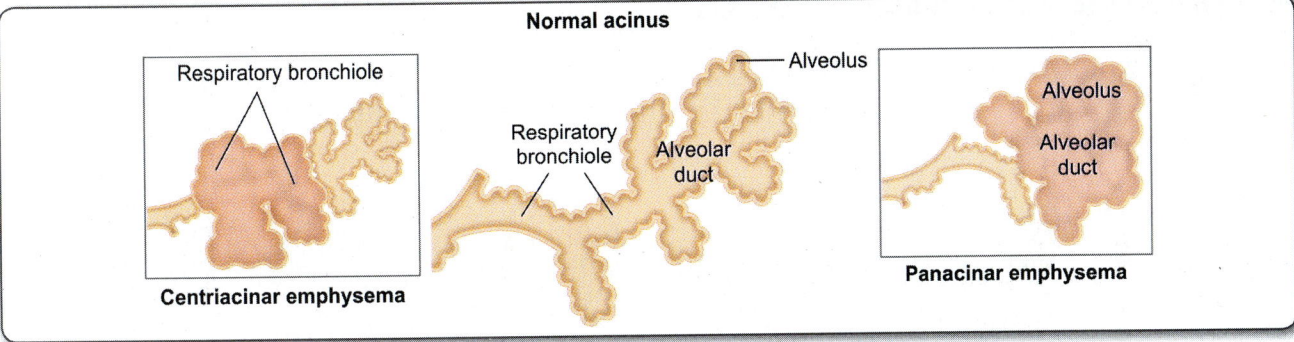

	Centriacinar/Centrilobular	Panacinar/Panlobular	Paraseptal/Distal Acinar
General	▪ MC type		▪ Subpleural location
Involves	▪ Proximal respiratory bronchioles	▪ Entire alveolus distal to terminal bronchioles	▪ Distal alveolar duct and alveolar sac
Site	▪ Upper lobes	▪ Lower lobes	▪ Upper lobe
Associated with	▪ **C**igarette smoking ▪ Dust inhalation	▪ α_1-AT deficiency (Pi ZZ) ▪ Early onset	▪ Pneumothorax ▪ Fibrosis

Diagnosis

- The formal diagnosis of COPD is made with spirometry; when the ratio of forced expiratory volume in 1 second over forced vital capacity (FEV_1/FVC) is less than 70%.
- Criteria for assessing the severity of airflow obstruction are as follows:

In patients with FEV_1/FVC <0.70		
GOLD 1	Mild	$FEV_1 \geq$ 80% of predicted
GOLD 2	Moderate	50% $\leq FEV_1$ <80% of predicted
GOLD 3	Severe	30% $\leq FEV_1$ <50% of predicted
GOLD 4	Very Severe	FEV_1 <30% of predicted

Treatment

- Bronchodilator of choice in COPD: Anticholinergics
- Only therapy that can decrease mortality in COPD patients: supplemental O_2

- Interventions shown to improve survival:
  - Smoking cessation
  - Long term oxygen therapy (LTOT)
  - Lung volume reduction surgery (LVRS)

Severity	mMRC 0–1 CAT <10	mMRC $\geq$2 CAT $\geq$10
0 or 1 moderate exacerbations (not leading to hospital admission)	**Group A** ▪ A bronchodilator	**Group B** ▪ A long-acting bronchodilator (LABA or LAMA)
$\geq$2 moderate exacerbations or $\geq$1 leading to hospitalisation	**Group C** ▪ LAMA	**Group D** ▪ LAMA or LAMA + LABA* or ▪ ICS + LABA *Consider if highly symptomatic (e.g. CAT > 20) **Cpmsoder if eos $\geq$ 300

LAMA – long-acting muscarinic receptor antagonists| LABA – long-acting beta$_2$ agonist| ICS – inhaled corticosteroids| CAT = COPD assessment test| mMRC – modified Medical Research Council dyspnoea questionnaire|

Beta 2 Agonists		Anticholinergics		Methylxanthines	PDE- 4 inhibitors
Short acting (SABA)	Long acting (LABA)	Short acting (SAMA)	Long acting (LAMA)		
▪ Salbutamol/ Albuterol ▪ Levosalbutamol ▪ Terbutaline ▪ Fenoterol	▪ Formoterol ▪ Salmeterol ▪ Indacaterol ▪ Olodaterol	▪ Ipratropium bromide ▪ Oxitropium bromide	▪ Aclidinium bromide ▪ Glycopyrronium ▪ Tiotropium ▪ Umeclidinium	▪ Aminophylline ▪ Theophylline	▪ Roflumilast

Flow Volume Loop of Major Pulmonary Pathology

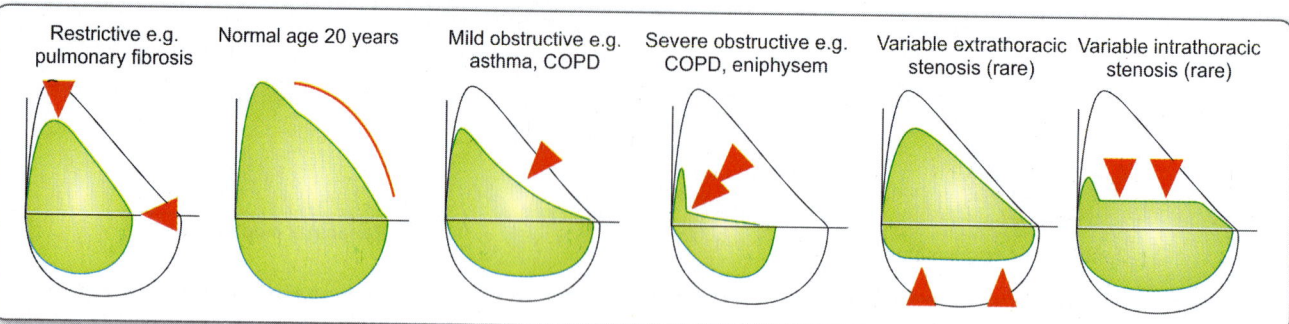

Restrictive e.g. pulmonary fibrosis | Normal age 20 years | Mild obstructive e.g. asthma, COPD | Severe obstructive e.g. COPD, eniphysem | Variable extrathoracic stenosis (rare) | Variable intrathoracic stenosis (rare)

CYSTIC FIBROSIS (MUCOVISCIDOSIS)

- CF is an AR disorder of exocrine glands.
- Locus – long arm of chromosome 7 (*CFTR* gene)
- MC mutation is ΔF 508
- MC presentation → Lung infection
- MCC of death → End stage lung disease
- *Respiratory Manifestations:*
  - Hyperviscous pulmonary secretions
  - Bronchiectasis confined to periphery and upper lobe
  - Secondary infection with *S. aureus, H influenzae, Pseudomonas* and *Burkholderia*
- *Pancreatic features:*
  - Exocrine pancreatic insufficiency leading to malabsorption, steatorrhea and failure to thrive
  - CF related Diabetes mellitus
- *Other features:*
  - Gall stone, Meconium ileus, Constipation
  - Azoospermia, Sinusitis
  - Infertility in either gender

- PFT → Obstructive airway pattern
- The Nasal Potential Difference (NPD) is a sensitive test that can be used to support or refute a diagnosis of CF.
- Newborn screening test → elevated serum trypsinogen
- Genotyping for *CFTR* gene
- Diagnostic criteria include either positive genetic testing or positive sweat chloride test (>60 mEq/L) and 1 of the following:
  - Chronic Obstructive Pulmonary Disease
  - Documented exocrine pancreatic insufficiency
  - Positive family history
- Management: Pancreatic enzyme supplements, mucolytics
- *CFTR protein potentiators:* **Ivacaftor**
- *CFTR correctors:* Elexacaftor, Lumacaftor, Tezacaftor

INTERSTITIAL LUNG DISEASE

- *Clinical manifestations:*
  - Exertional dyspnea, Non productive cough
  - Bibasilar end inspiratory crackles
- CXR in ILD: Bibasilar reticular pattern
- PFT – restrictive pattern
- HRCT: Honey combing, Ground glass opacification

- IOC for ILD: Lung biopsy > HRCT
- DOC for ILD: Steroids
- Immunosuppressants: Azathioprine, Cyclophosphamide
- Antifibrotic agent: Pirfenidone → inhibit TGF alpha and beta

Etiology

- Exposure related:
  - Asbestosis
  - Silicosis
- Associated with systemic diseases:
  - Rheumatoid arthritis
  - Scleroderma/Systemic sclerosis
  - Polymyositis/Dermatomyositis
  - Wegener's granulomatosis (GPA)
  - Churg Strauss (EGPA)
- Smoking related ILDs:
  - Desquamative interstitial pneumonia (DIP)

  - Respiratory bronchiolitis – associated (RB-ILD)
  - Pulmonary Langerhans' cell histiocytosis
- Idiopathic Interstitial Pneumonia:
  - Idiopathic pulmonary fibrosis
  - Nonspecific interstitial pneumonia
  - Cryptogenic organizing pneumonia
- Exclusively in smokers: DIP
- Non smokers > Smokers:
  - Sarcoidosis
  - Hypersensitivity pneumonitis

BAL in ILD

- Neutrophil rich: Interstitial pulmonary fibrosis (IPF)
- Eosinophil rich: Eosinophilic lung disease
- Ferruginous bodies: Asbestosis

- Lymphocyte rich:
  - CD 4: Sarcoidosis (CD4 : CD8 ratio > 3.5)
  - CD 8: Hypersensitivity pneumonitis

PNEUMONIAS

- Single most useful clinical sign of severity of pneumonia: Respiratory rate
- Friedlander's pneumonia is due to: **Klebsiella**

Color of Sputum	Agent
▪ **Rusty brown sputum**	▪ *Pneumococcus/Streptococcus*
▪ **Red currant jelly sputum**	▪ *Klebsiella*
▪ **Green sputum**	▪ *Pseudomonas*
▪ **Black sputum**	▪ ABPA

Risk Factors for MDR/Nosocomial Pneumonia:
- Hospitalization ≥2 days in past 90 days
- Use of antibiotics in past 90 days
- Hemodialysis in previous 1 month
- Immunosuppression

Causes of Community Acquired Pneumonia in Outpatients/Hospitalized Non-ICU Patients:
- *Streptococcus pneumonia* (MCC)
- *Mycoplasma pneumonia*
- *H. influenzae*
- *Chlamydia pneumoniae*
- RSV, Influenza A and B, Parainfluenza

Legionnaires Disease/Legionellosis:
- MC Cause – *L pneumophila* (Serogroup 1)
- Pontiac fever – benign, self-limited, acute febrile illness
- Disease is limited only to humans
- No man to man transmission
- No animal reservoir

Staph pneumonia is associated with:
- P → Pneumatocele (air filled cyst)
- A → Abscess formation
- C → Cavitation
- E → Empyema

Cavitation is seen in Pneumonia Caused by:
- Tuberculosis
- *Staphylococcus*
- *Klebsiella*
- *Pseudomonas, Pneumococcus*
- Anaerobic bacteria

Pneumonia Severity Index (PSI) or PORT score:
- Estimates mortality for adult patient with CAP
- Predict need for hospitalization in patient of CAP

CURB -65 Scoring:
- Predict severity and mortality of CAP
- **C** – Confusion
- **U** – Blood Urea >20 mg/dL or >7 mmol/L
- **R** – Respiratory Rate ≥30/min
- **B** – SBP <90 mm Hg; DBP ≤60 mm Hg
- **65** – Age ≥65 years

CURB Score	Recommendation
0 – 1	OPD treatment
2	Hospitalization
≥3	ICU management

Typical Vs Atypical Pneumonia

	Typical Pneumonia	Atypical Pneumonia
Pathology	▪ Presence of alveolar exudates ▪ Infiltrate is mainly neutrophilic	▪ Lacks alveolar exudates ▪ Mainly lymphocytic infiltrate
Etiology	▪ *S. pneumoniae* ▪ *H. influenzae* ▪ *M. catarrhalis* ▪ *S. aureus* ▪ *K. pneumoniae* ▪ *P. aeruginosa*	▪ *Mycoplasma* ▪ *Chlamydia* ▪ *Legionella pneumophila* ▪ *RSV, Influenza A and B, Parainfluenza* ▪ *Pneumocystis jirovecii* ▪ Fungus
Clinical Manifestations	▪ Fever, Dyspnea, Chest pain ▪ Productive cough with sputum ▪ ↑ Tactile fremitus ▪ Bronchial breath sounds	▪ Subtle pulmonary signs ▪ Extrapulmonary signs like mental confusion, diarrhea, myalgia, rash
CXR	▪ Lobar Consolidation ▪ Parapneumonic effusion	▪ Nonlobar interstitial infiltrates ▪ Ground glassing pattern
Treatment	▪ Beta lactams	▪ Resistant to beta lactams

	Pneumococcal Pneumonia	Legionnaires Disease	Mycoplasmal Pneumonia	Pneumocystis jirovecii Pneumonia
Agent	▪ Gram +ve α-hemolytic Streptococci ▪ Capsulated and Catalase –ve ▪ MCC of Community Acquired Pneumonia	▪ Legionella pneumophila – Gram -ve, non-motile ▪ Unencapsulated, Catalase +ve ▪ Transmission via aerosol inhalation	▪ Mycoplasma pneumoniae/ Eaton's agent ▪ Lack cell wall → Pleomorphic organism ▪ Not visible on Gram stain	▪ P jirovecii – a unicellular fungus
Risk factors	▪ Extreme of ages, Immunosuppression ▪ Viral infections ▪ COPD, Smoking, Malnutrition ▪ Splenectomy, Sickle cell anemia ▪ Strongest independent RF: Alcoholism	▪ Advanced age, Immunosuppression ▪ Organ transplant, Hairy cell leukemia ▪ Smoking, Alcohol ▪ Exposure to **AC** plants, stagnant water, Humidifiers	▪ Children ▪ Closed population as in military and prison population ▪ Sickle cell anemia	▪ Person receiving long-term immunosuppressive therapy ▪ HIV patient with CD4+ <200/μL ▪ Malignancies ▪ Malnutrition
Clinical Manifestations	▪ High grade fever ▪ Productive cough with Rusty brown sputum ▪ Complications: Parapneumonic effusion or Empyema	▪ High fever with chills, myalgia, headache ▪ Cough with abdominal pain, nausea, diarrhoea, confusion ▪ Nosocomial LD – patient developing symptoms ≥10 days after hospitalization	▪ Low grade fever ▪ Persistent cough	▪ Fever with chills ▪ Non productive cough ▪ Weight loss ▪ Extrapulmonary infection can involve any organ ▪ Complication: ARDS
Diagnosis	▪ Gram stain and culture of sputum ▪ Urinary Antigen detection ▪ CXR → Lobar consolidation ± Air bronchogram ± Pneumatocele ▪ Cavitation is not a feature	▪ Hyponatremia due to SIADH ▪ Urinary Ag to detect L pneumophila serogroup 1 ▪ CXR → patchy alveolar infiltrates (non diagnostic) ▪ Culture → BYCE medium ▪ PCR	▪ Hemolytic anemia, ▪ Cold agglutination +ve ▪ CXR → Bronchopneumonia, Interstitial or reticulonodular infiltrates (Non- specific) ▪ Best investigation – PCR ▪ Culture → PPLO media	▪ Elevated LDH and β 1, 3 Glucan ▪ CXR → Diffuse bilateral infiltrates ▪ HRCT → Ground glass attenuation ▪ Quantitative PCR ▪ Histopathology for definitive diagnosis using Methamine silver and Wright stain
Management	▪ DOC → β lactam or Macrolides ▪ Smoking cessation ▪ Prevention via immunization of high risk individuals with PCV 13 or PPSV 23	▪ **DOC:** Macrolide (Azithromycin) ▪ Other: Rifampicin, Levofloxacin, Doxycycline	▪ **DOC:** Macrolides (Azithromycin)	▪ **DOC:** TMP- SMX ▪ 2nd line: Pentamidine, Dapsone-Pyrimethamine, Atovaquone ▪ Corticosteroids as adjuvant ▪ Antifungals – **not** effective

HYPERSENSITIVITY PNEUMONITIS

- Acute HSP is an example of type III HSR
- Subacute and chronic HSP is an example of type IV HSR

Etiology

Disease	Source	Antigen
▪ Farmer's lung	Mouldy hay, Grains	Thermophilic actinomycetes e.g. *Saccharopolyspora*
▪ Bagassosis	Sugarcane	*Thermoactinomyces sacchari*
▪ Cheese workers lung	Cheese	*Penicillium casei*
▪ Malt worker's lung	Malt	*Aspergillus clavatus*
▪ Bird fancier's lung	Bird feathers, droppings	
▪ Hot tub lung	Contaminated water	*Cladosporium*

ALLERGIC BRONCHOPULMONARY ASPERGILLOSIS

- ABPA is a hypersensitivity disease of the lung that is virtually almost always related to *A. fumigatus*.
- Nearly all patients with ABPA have history of chronic asthma or cystic fibrosis.
- *Clinical Manifestation:*
  - Episodic wheezing, malaise, low grade fever
  - Cough with sputum, Chest pain
  - Sputum contains brownish plugs of mucus
  - Sputum and blood eosinophilia.
- Patient may have h/o recurrent pneumonia.
- As ABPA progress, central bronchiectasis becomes a dominant feature of the disease and may result in chronic bronchorrhoea and occasional hemoptysis.
- *Radiographic findings:*
  - Pulmonary infiltrates, Cavitations
  - Parallel shadow or tram line – suggestive of Bronchiectasis
  - Finger in glove sign, Ring sign

  - Diagnostic hallmark - Presence of proximal bronchiectasis
- Treatment includes systemic glucocorticoids and antifungals.

Primary/Major Diagnostic Criteria:
[**Mn: TEAR PICS**]
- Immediate type skin reactivity **T**est to Aspergillus Ag
- Peripheral blood **E**osinophilia (>1000/mm³)
- Episodic bronchial **A**sthma
- History of pulmonary infiltrates on chest **R**adiograph
- **P**recipitating serum antibodies against Aspergillus Ag
- **I**ncrease IgE levels (>1000 ng/ml)
- **C**entral Bronchiectasis on chest CT Scan
- Increase in **S**erum IgE/IgG specific to *A. fumigatus*
  - ⌃ The presence of 6 out of 8 major criteria makes the diagnosis almost certain.

REMEMBER

Light's criteria:
- Pleural Fluid/Serum protein > 0.5
- Pleural Fluid/Serum LDH > 0.6
- Pleural Fluid LDH > 2/3 of normal upper limit
- Presence of any 1 is suggestive of exudative pleural effusion

Causes of Exudative Pleural effusion:
- Parapneumonic effusion
- Tuberculous effusion
- Malignant effusion – MC CA lung or CA breast
- Rheumatoid effusion, SLE
- Pulmonary embolism
- Pancreatitis

Causes of Transudative Pleural effusion:
- Congestive heart failure
- Cirrhosis
- Nephrotic syndrome, Hypoalbuminemia
- Myxedema
- Constrictive pericarditis

Pleural effusion with High Amylase: [**Mn: POeM**]
- Pancreatic effusion
- Oesophageal rupture
- Malignacy

Pleural effusion with Low Glucose (<60 mg /dl):
[**Mn: Low MRP on Tub**]
- **M**alignant effusion
- **R**heumatoid effusion
- **P**arapneumonic effusion
- **Tub**erculous effusion

Hemorrhagic Pleural effusion:
- Trauma – MC cause
- Tubercular effusion
- Malignancy
- Pulmonary embolism
- Pancreatitis

Pleural effusion with Cholesterol Crystal:
[**Mn: My RAT Cry**]
- **My**xedema
- **R**heumatoid **A**rthritis
- **T**uberculosis

Tubercular pleural effusion:
- Exudative and hemorrhagic type
- Lymphocyte predominance with low polymorph
- Adenosine Deaminase >40 IU/L
- Mesothelial cells <5%

PNEUMOTHORAX

Primary Spontaneous Pneumothorax:
- Affects tall, thin young males
- Exclusive in smokers
- No underlying lung disease
- Associated with subpleural blebs
- Rx: Simple aspiration

Features of Tension Pneumothorax:
- ↓ Cardiac output → Hypotension
- Mediastinal and tracheal shift to opposite side
- Hyper resonance on percussion
- ↓ Vocal resonance on ipsilateral side
- No breath sounds on ipsilateral side
- Rx: Large bore needle thoracostomy f/b ICD insertion

PLEURAL EFFUSION

- Difference between Serum and Effusion protein > 3.1 g/dL → Transudative effusion
- Plasma-Pleural effusion albumin gradient (PPEAG) > 1.2 → Transudative effusion

- For blunting of the lateral CP angle on PA view, amount of effusion required: 175 mL

PULMONARY EMBOLISM

- Classical presentation: acute pleuritic type chest pain, shortness of breath and hypoxia
- Scoring system used to assess likelihood of PE/DVT: Wells' criteria
- **ECG findings in PE:**
  - Sinus tachycardia: Most common
  - RV Strain
  - $S_1 Q_3 T_3$ → McGinn sign
- **CXR in Pulmonary Embolism:**
  - Normal → Most common
  - Westermark's sign → Focal oligemia (s/o massive PE)

- Hampton's hump → Peripheral wedge shaped opacity above Diaphragm (s/o small PE)
- **Pa**lla's sign → Enlarged Right Descending **PA**
- Fleischner sign → Enlarged Pulmonary artery
- ECHO in PE: McConnell's sign (RV free wall hypokinesis with normal RV apical motion)
- IOC: CT pulmonary angiography
- Gold standard/most specific test for PE: Pulmonary angiogram
- Primary therapy: Thrombolysis

ARDS

- Also called as shock lung, wet lung etc.
- ARDS is characterized by diffuse alveolar damage and lung capillary endothelial injury.
- Type I cells, which constitute 90% of the alveolar epithelium, are injured easily.
- Neutrophils are thought to play a key role in the pathogenesis of ARDS.
- ARDS is defined radiologically by the presence of bilateral pulmonary infiltrates. While characteristic for ARDS, these radiographic findings are not specific and can be indistinguishable from cardiogenic pulmonary edema.
- According to the 2012 Berlin definition, ARDS is characterized by the following:
  - Onset – within 1 week of clinical insult or onset of respiratory symptoms

- Radiographic changes – bilateral opacities not fully explained by effusions, consolidation, or atelectasis
- Origin of edema not fully explained by cardiac failure or fluid overload; and
- Severity based on the PaO_2/FiO_2 ratio.
- *The 3 categories of severity are:*
  - *Mild* – PaO_2/FiO_2 200-300 mm Hg
  - *Moderate* – PaO_2/FiO_2 100-200 mm Hg
  - *Severe* – $PaO_2/FiO_2 \leq 100$ mm Hg
- ARDS was recognized as the most severe form of acute lung injury (ALI). ALI term is obsolete now.
- ARDS can be differentiated from cardiogenic pulmonary edema based on pulmonary capillary wedge pressure (PCWP); in cardiogenic edema, PCWP is >18; in ARDS it is <18.

Phases of ARDS

- *Features of acute/exudative phase:*
  - Lasts for first 7 days
  - Necrosis or apoptosis of Type I pneumocytes
  - Inactivated surfactants
  - Sloughing of bronchial epithelium

- Protein rich edema fluid in alveoli
- Hyaline membrane
- Interstitial edema with exudative cellular infiltrate
- Decreased lung compliance
- *Proliferative phase* lasts from day 7 to day 21.

Etiology	• Pneumonia • Sepsis • Severe trauma	• Multiple blood transfusion • Pancreatitis • Aspiration of gastric contents • Toxic gas inhalation
Management	• Mechanical ventilation with low tidal volume & high PEEP	• Prone ventilation

SLEEP APNEA

- Intermittent cessation of airflow for at least 10 seconds
- Grading of severity is done by: Apnea-Hypnea Index (AHI)
- OSA is associated with increased risk of Hypertension, Pulmonary hypertension, Diabetes, Atrial fibrillation, Heart failure and Sexual dysfunction.
- Screening tool for OSA:
  - Berlin questionnaire
  - Epworth Sleepiness scale

	Obstructive Sleep Apnea (OSA)	Central Sleep Apnea (CSA)
Definition	▪ Defined by AHI ≥5/hour	▪ Transient abolition of central drive to respiratory muscle
Mechanism	▪ Oropharyngeal occlusion	▪ Increased sensitivity to $PaCO_2$ leading to hyperventilation alternating with apnea
Risk factors	▪ Alcoholism, Hypertension ▪ Obesity	▪ Opioid medications ▪ Hypoxia
Manifestations	▪ Snoring, interrupted by apneas ▪ Excessive day time sleepiness	▪ Cheyne stokes breathing
Diagnosis	▪ Polysomnography,	▪ Polysomnography
Management	▪ TOC: Nasal CPAP ▪ CNS stimulants: Modafinil ▪ Uvulopalatopharyngoplasty	▪ Nasal CPAP

RESPIRATORY FAILURE

Parameter	Type I (MC)		Type II
Also known as	▪ Hypoxemic Respiratory failure		▪ Hypercapnic Respiratory failure
Pathology	▪ Failure of oxygenation		▪ Alveolar Hypoventilation
Alveoli	▪ Fluid filled		▪ Normal
PaO_2	▪ <60 mm Hg		▪ <60 mm Hg
$PaCO_2$	▪ Low/Normal		▪ >50 mm Hg
PA-a O_2	▪ ↑ (suggestive of parenchymal dysfunction)		▪ Normal
Causes	▪ Pneumonia ▪ ARDS ▪ Sepsis ▪ ILD ▪ Pulmonary embolism ▪ Atelectasis	▪ Pulmonary edema ▪ Pancreatitis ▪ Multiple blood transfusion	▪ Obstructive disease like COPD ▪ Myasthenia gravis ▪ Guillain Barre syndrome ▪ Amyotrophic Lateral Sclerosis ▪ ↓ Central respiratory drive ▪ Diseases of spine and chest wall

	Type III	Type IV
Definition	▪ Aka Perioperative respiratory failure ▪ Due to atelectasis	▪ Respiratory failure in patients with shock due to hypoperfusion of respiratory muscles

MULTIPLE CHOICE QUESTIONS

CHAPTER 1: PULMONOLOGY

PULMONARY FUNCTION TEST

1. The diffusion capacity of lung is decreased in all of the following conditions EXCEPT: *(PGMEE 2014-15)*
   a. Interstitial lung disease
   b. Goodpasture's syndrome
   c. Pneumocystis Jiroveci
   d. Primary pulmonary hypertension

[Ref: Harrison's 20th/e pg. 1944]

2. Which of the following does not causes hyperventilation?
   a. Anxiety   *(DNB Dec 2009)*
   b. Psychotic illness
   c. Pulmonary hypertension
   d. High altitude

[Ref: Harrison's 20th/e pg. 1935]

3. Which of the following is not true in obstructive lung disease? *(PGMEE 2014-15)*
   a. FEV1↓
   b. TLC↓
   c. FVC↓
   d. Reduced timed vital capacity

[Ref: Harrison's 20th/e pg. 1944]

4. In obstructive lung disease all are true EXCEPT:
   a. Residual volume normal
   b. FEV decrease
   c. FEV1/FVC decreases
   d. Vital capacity normal

[Ref: Harrison's 20th/e pg. 1949]

5. FeV1 of a patient is 1.5 L and FVC is 3.5 L. What is the type of lung disease *(PGMEE 2019)*
   a. Normal lung function   b. Obstructive lung disease
   c. Restrictive lung disease   d. Mixed lung disease

[Ref: Harrison's 20th/e pg. 1949]

Explanation
- $FEV_1/FEV = 1.5/3.5 = 0.43$, means obstructive lung disease.

6. Residual volume is best measured by? *(PGMEE 2014-15)*
   a. Body plethysmography   b. Helium dilution method
   c. Spirometry   d. All of above

[Ref: Harrison's 20th/e pg. 1950]

7. If FEV1 is 1.3 L, FVC is 3.1 L in an adult man, the pattern is suggestive of: *(PGMEE 2014-15)*
   a. Normal lung function
   b. Restrictive lung disease
   c. Obstructive lung disease
   d. None of the above

[Ref: Harrison's 20th/e pg. 1944]

8. All the following lung volumes can be measured by a simple spirometer EXCEPT: *(PGMEE 2014-15)*
   a. Vital capacity   b. Residual volume
   c. Tidal volume   d. Forced vital capacity

[Ref: Harrison's 20th/e pg. 1963]

9. Alveolar-arterial tension gradient increases in all EXCEPT: *(PGMEE 2014-15)*
   a. Diffusion defects   b. Hypoventilation
   c. R-L shunt
   d. Ventilation perfusion abnormality

[Ref: Harrison's 20th/e pg. 1944]

Explanation
- Alveolar gas and arterial blood oxygen tension difference is increased in conditions that cause ventilation - perfusion (V/Q) mismatch or shunt.

(A-a)O$_2$ difference	Normal (A-a)O$_2$ difference
▪ ARDS ▪ Pneumonia ▪ Obstructive lung d/s ▪ Right to left shunt ▪ Hepato pulmonary syndrome ▪ Interstitial fibrosis	▪ Hypoventilation ▪ High altitude

10. For diagnosis of obstructive airway disease, which of the following measurement is preferred: *(PGMEE 2014-15)*
   a. Vital capacity   b. Timed vital capacity
   c. Tidal volume   d. Blood gas analysis

[Ref: Harrison's 20th/e pg. 1944]

11. All show increased alveolar-arterial O2 gradient except?
   a. Bronchiectasis   *(PGMEE 2014-15)*
   b. ARDS (acute respiratory distress syndrome)
   c. Interstitial fibrosis
   d. Central hypoventilation

[Ref: Harrison's 20th/e pg. 1944]

12. The results of the pulmonary functions tests shown below, the best diagnosis is : *(PGMEE 2014-15)*

Parameters	Actual	Predicted
FEV1 (L)	1.2	3.5-4.3
FVC (L)	4.1	4.6-5.4
FEV1/FVC (%)	29	72-80
PEF (L/min)	80	440-540
DL CO	120%	100%

   a. Asthma   b. Asbestosis
   c. ARDS   d. Silicosis

[Ref: Harrison's 20th/e pg. 1949]

Answers:

1.	b
2.	c
3.	b
4.	a
5.	b
6.	a
7.	c
8.	b
9.	b
10.	b
11.	d
12.	a

13. FEVI/FVC decreased in all of the following except:
(NEET Pattern 2019)
- a. COPD
- b. COPD
- c. ARDS
- d. Bronchiectasis

14. FEV1/FVC ratio is decreased in all EXCEPT:
- a. Bronchiectasis *(PGMEE 2014-15)*
- b. Emphysema
- c. Chronic bronchitis
- d. Interstitial lung disease

[Ref: Harrison's 20th/e pg. 1944]

15. Following pulmonary changes are seen in restrictive lung disease EXCEPT: *(PGMEE 2014-15)*
- a. ↑FEV1/FVC
- b. ↓TLC
- c. ↓RV
- d. ↑VC

[Ref: Harrison's 20th/e pg. 1949]

16. Which of the following is markedly decreased in restrictive lung disease- *(PGMEE 2015)*
- a. FVC
- b. FEV1
- c. RV
- d. FEV1/FVC

[Ref: Harrison's 20th/e pg. 1949]

17. In bronchial asthma following pulmonary function abnormalities are present EXCEPT: *(PGMEE 2014-15)*
- a. Decreased FEV1
- b. Decreased maximum expiratory flow rate
- c. Increased residual volume
- d. Increased inspiratory capacity

[Ref: Harrison's 20th/e pg. 1949, 1963]

18. All are obstructive lung disease except *(PGMEE 2013-14)*
- a. Bronchitis
- b. Interstitial fibrosis
- c. Emphysema
- d. Asthma

[Ref: Harrison's 20th/e pg. 1943]

ASTHMA

19. Life threatening features of asthma are the following except: *(NEET Pattern 2019)*
- a. Silent chest
- b. Drowsy or confused patient
- c. Tachycardia
- d. Presence of pulsus paradoxus

20. Leukotriene inhibitors are used in asthma for:
(NEET Pattern 2019)
- a. Add-on therapy in patients not controlled by low dose inhaled glucocorticoids
- b. Status asthmaticus
- c. Monotherapy for acute attack
- d. None of the above

21. Commonly used route of administration for Omalizumab in asthma in: *(PGMEE 2014-15)*
- a. Subcutaneous
- b. Inhalational
- c. Intradermal
- d. Intramuscular

[Ref: Harrison's 20th/e pg. 1967]

Explanation
- Omalizumab: Humanized monoclonal antibody that binds circulating IgE Antibodies, hence used for moderate to severe allergic asthma that is poorly controlled with corticosteroids & LABA.
- Omalizumab is used as 150-300 mg injection via subcutaneous route.

22. Bronchial asthma patient on artificial ventilation requires: *(PGMEE 2014-15)*
- a. A low Inspiratory Flow
- b. An equal IE ratio of 1:1
- c. An inverse ration ventilation
- d. An IE ratio 1:2.5

[Ref: CMDT 2014 pg. 242]

23. Hyperplasia of smooth muscle of airway is seen in? *(PGMEE 2013)*
- a. Brochiectasis
- b. Asthma
- c. Emphysema
- d. Alveolar proteinosis

[Ref: Harrison's 20th/e pg. 1961]

24. Curschman's spirals are seen in *(PGMEE 2016; 2013)*
- a. Bronchial asthma
- b. Sarcoidosis
- c. Bronchiectasis
- d. Chronic bronchitis

[Ref: Robbin's 9th/e pg. 682]

25. Creola bodies are seen in- *(PGMEE 2012-13)*
- a. Bronchial asthma
- b. Bronchiectatsis
- c. Chronic bronchitis
- d. Emphysema

[Ref: Color atlas of Pulmonary Cytopathology pg. 65]

26. In a patient of bronchial asthma, silent chest signifies? *(DNB Dec'2010)*
- a. Good prognosis
- b. Not a prognostic sign
- c. Grave prognosis
- d. Bad prognosis

[Ref: GINA Guidelines 2018]

27. All are true about Aspirin sensitive asthma except? *(PGMEE 2015-16)*
- a. Nasal polyposis
- b. Treatment with inhaled corticosteroids
- c. Rhinosinusitis
- d. Increased prostaglandins

[Ref: Harrison's 20th/e pg. 1969]

28. Aspirin sensitive asthma is associated with:
- a. Extrinsic asthma *(PGMEE 2014-15)*
- b. Usually associated with urticaria
- c. Obesity
- d. Associated with nasal polyp

[Ref: Harrison's 20th/e pg. 1959]

29. Which of the following is given in the maintenance of severe persistent asthma: *(PGMEE 2015-16)*
- a. Oral Steroid
- b. Leukotriene agonist
- c. Ipratomium bromide
- d. Long acting beta2 agonist

[Ref: Harrison's 20th/e pg. 1967]

13. c
14. d
15. d
16. a
17. d
18. b
19. c
20. a
21. a
22. d
23. b
24. a
25. a
26. c
27. d
28. d
29. d

30. What is the full form of ARIA *(PGMEE 2015-16)*
a. Allergic Rhinitis Induced Asthama
b. Allergic Rhinitis and its Impact on Asthma
c. Allergy Rheumatology Immunology and Asthma
d. Acetlycholine Receptor Inducing Activity

[Ref: Pubmed. nl]

31. Which drugs are not used in severe persistent Asthma:
a. Short acting beta 2 agonist *(PGMEE 2015-16)*
b. Oral corticosteroids
c. Long acting beta 2 agonist
d. Inhaled high dose Steroids

[Ref: Harrison's 20th/e pg. 1968]

32. Drug of choice for treatment of type 2 Brittle Asthma is?
a. β-adrenergic agonist *(PGMEE 2015-16)*
b. Inhaled corticosteroids
c. Antileukotrines DM
d. Subcutaneous epinephrine

[Ref: Harrison's 20th/e pg. 1969]

33. One of the following is not an indicator of the severity of asthma: *(PGMEE 2014-15)*
a. Use of accessory muscles
b. Pulsus paradoxus
c. Cyanosis
d. Systolic BP

[Ref: GINA 2018]

34. Bronchial asthma is associated with raised levels of: *(PGMEE 2014-15)*
a. Leukotrienes   b. PGI2
c. PGE2   d. Thromboxane

[Ref: Harrison's 20th/e pg. 1962]

35. Best for treatment of Exercise induced asthma?
a. Montelukast *(PGMEE 2014-15)*
b. Salbutamol
c. Ipratropium
d. Low dose Inhaled corticosteroids

[Ref: Harrison's 20th/e pg. 1959]

36. A child of less than one year with asthma treatment:
a. MDI with Mask *(PGMEE 2013-12)*
b. MPI with mask
c. MDI with Spacer
d. MDI with Spacer with Mask

[Ref: GINA Guidelines 2018]

37. Treatment for a child having exercise induced asthma is - *(PGMEE 2012-13)*
a. Breathing exercise
b. Prophylaxis with theophylline
c. Prophylaxis with short acting Beta$_2$ agonist
d. Prophylaxis with steroids

[Ref: GINA Guidelines 2018]

38. In severe bronchial asthma, true is: *(PGMEE 2014-15)*
a. Inspiratory and expiratory rhonchi with reduced air entry
b. Hyper-resonant chest
c. Increased fremitus and absent breath sounds
d. Decreased fremitus and crackles

[Ref: Harrison's 20th/e pg. GINA Guidelines 2018]

39. A known asthmatic, presented to the emergency with severe exacerbation not relived by Salbutamol. The patient was given corticosteroids and aminophylline. What is the rationale of giving corticosteroids? *(NEET Pattern 2017)*
a. Corticosteroids facilitate the action of β agonists
b. Corticosteroids sensitize adenosine receptors to xanthines
c. Direct bronchodilator action of corticosteroids
d. Increase mucociliary clearance

[Ref: Harrison 19/e, P.1677]

40. All of the following are useful for treating acute bronchial asthma in children EXCEPT: *(PGMEE 2014-15)*
a. 100% Oxygen
b. Hydrocortisone function
c. IV aminophylline
d. Sodium Cromoglycate inhalation

[Ref: Harrison's 20th/e pg. 1968]

COPD

41. According to GOLD criteria, very severe COPD is defined as: *(PGMEE 2018)*
a. FEV1/FVC > 0.7, predicted response is < 90%
b. FEV1/FVC > 0.7, predicted response is < 80%
c. FEV1/FVC > 0.7, predicted response is < 50%
d. FEV1/FVC > 0.7, predicted response is < 30%

42. On an ABG, pH of 7.2, pO2 of 46, pCO2 of 80 are indicative of: *(PGMEE 2014-15)*
a. Acute exacerbation of COPD
b. Adult respiratory distress syndrome
c. Interstitial pneumonitis
d. Acute asthma

[Ref: Harrison's 20th/e pg. 1995]

Explanation
- ABG is suggestive of respiratory acidosis with type II respiratory failure. Among the options COPD leads to this picture severe asthma rarely cause respiratory failure.

43. In a patient with COPD, best management option is? *(PGMEE 2015-16)*
a. Quit smoking   b. Bronchodilators
c. Low flow oxygen   d. Mucolytics

[Ref: Harrison's 20th/e pg. 1997]

44. The most common type of emphysema associated with α-1 antitrypsin deficiency- *(DNB Dec 08)*
a. Centriacinar   b. Panacinar
c. Distal acinar   d. Paraseptal

[Ref: Harrison's 20th/e pg. 1992]

45. α1 Antitrysin deficiency is associated with all except *(PGMEE 2012)*
a. Fatty liver   b. Renal disease
c. Emphysema   d. Pancreatitis

[Ref: Robbin's 9th/e pg. 675]

---

30. b
31. b
32. d
33. d
34. a
35. d
36. d
37. c
38. a
39. a
40. d
41. d
42. a
43. c
44. b
45. b

46. Which of the following structures in the lung is likely to be affected the most in a patient who smoked a pack and half of cigarettes per day for 30 years and developed centrilobular emphysema:- *(PGMEE 2015)*
a. Alveolar duct
b. Terminal bronchiole
c. Alveolar sac
d. Respiratory bronchiole

[Ref: Harrison's 20th/e pg. 1992]

47. Emphysema pathologically involves beyond the:- *(PGMEE 2015)*
a. Alveolar Sac
b. Terminal bronchiole
c. Bronchi
d. Respiratory bronchiole

[Ref: Harrison's 20th/e pg. 1992]

48. Distension of distant alveoli is seen in-
a. Centriacinar emphysema *(PGMEE 2013-14)*
b. Irregular emphysema
c. Paraseptal emphysema
d. Panacinar emphysema

[Ref: Robbin's 9th/e pg. 675-676]

49. In a patient with smoking history, which is important? *(PGMEE 2015-16)*
a. Duration of smoking
b. Number of smoking
c. Brand of Cigarette
d. Filter of cigarette

[Ref: IASLC Textbook of Prevention and Early Detection of Lung Cancer: 2015 Review]

50. Emphysema presents with all EXCEPT:
a. Cyanosis *(PGMEE 2015-16)*
b. Barrel shaped chest
c. Associated with smoking
d. Type II respiratory failure

[Ref: Harrison's 20th/e pg. 1995]

Explanation
- Patients of COPD with predominant emphysema are noncyanotic at rest & hence are termed "purk puffers"

51. "Pink Puffers" are patients having which disease:- *(PGMEE 2016-17)*
a. Chronic bronchitis
b. Emphysema
c. Bronchiectasis
d. Bronchial asthma

[Ref: Harrison's 20th/e pg. 1995]

52. All are seen in emphysema EXCEPT: *(PGMEE 2014-15)*
a. Decreased vital capacity
b. Hyperinflation
c. Rhonchi
d. Reduced DLco

[Ref: Harrison's 20th/e pg. 1992, 1995]

53. Investigation of choice to distinguish between COPD and bronchial asthma is? *(PGMEE 2014-15)*
a. Allergy test to pollens
b. Non reversible airflow obstruction
c. Chest X-ray
d. Arterial blood gas analysis

[Ref: Harrison's 20th/e pg. 1949]

54. Which component of cigarette smoke is responsible for CAD? *(PGMEE 2015-16)*
a. Nicotine
b. Tar
c. Polycyclic aromatic hydrocarbons
d. Benzene

[Ref: Harrison's 20th/e pg. 3291-92]

55. The drug varenicline is used in: *(PGMEE 2014-15)*
a. Pulmonary Hemosiderosis
b. Sleep apnoea
c. Anti-trypsin deficiency
d. Nicotine dependence

[Ref: Harrison's 20th/e pg. 3294]

Explanation
- Varenicline is effective in smoking cessation as a result of its activity at the $\alpha_2\beta_2$ subtype of nicotine receptor, where it binding produces agonist activity while simultaneously preventing nicotine from binding to these receptors.

56. False about emphysema is: *(PGMEE 2014-15)*
a. Decreased FEV1
b. Decreased timed vital capacity
c. Increased residual volume
d. Increased diffusion capacity

[Ref: Harrison's 20th/e pg. 1995]

57. All are true in definition of chronic bronchitis EXCEPT: *(PGMEE 2014-15)*
a. Cough > 2 months
b. Bronchorrea
c. Hoover sign
d. Haemoptysis

[Ref: Harrison's 20th/e pg. 1995]

58. Reid's index *(PGMEE 2015, 2016; 2014; 10)*
a. Increased in bronchial asthma
b. Increased in chronic bronchitis
c. Decreased in bronchial asthma
d. Decreased in chronic bronchitis

[Ref: Robbin's 9th/e pg. 679]

59. Chronic bronchitis can be a premalignant condition, which involves:- *(PGMEE 2015)*
a. Columnar to squamous
b. Cuboidal to squamous
c. Squamous to cuboidal
d. Squamous to columnar

[Ref: Robbin's 9th/e pg. 679]

BRONCHIECTASIS

60. Imaging modality for confirming the diagnosis of bronchiectasis is? *(NEET Pattern 2019)*
a. X-ray chest
b. MRI chest
c. Chest CT scan
d. Bronchoscopy

[Ref: Harrison's 20th/e pg. 1984]

61. Bronchiectasis means:- *(PGMEE 2012-13)*
a. Inflammation of bronchi
b. Dilatation of bronchi
c. Cavitation of bronchi
d. All

[Ref: Harrison's 20th/e pg. 1984]

46. d
47. b
48. c
49. a
50. a
51. b
52. c
53. b
54. a
55. d
56. d
57. d
58. b
59. a
60. c
61. b

62. **Which of the following is most likely to be associated with bronchiectasis of the main bronchi:**
    (PGMEE 2014-15)
    a. Allergic bronchopulmonary aspergillosis
    b. Endobronchial tuberculosis
    c. Measles
    d. Chronic bronchitis

    [Ref: Harrison's 20th/e pg. 1984]

63. **Most likely precursor to bronchiectasis is:**
    a. Tuberculosis *(PGMEE 2014-15)*
    b. Carcinoma
    c. Bronchial adenoma
    d. Necrotising pneumonia

    [Ref: Harrison's 20th/e pg. 1984]

64. **Complication of Bronchiectasis:-** *(PGMEE 2016-17)*
    a. Right heart failure   b. Left ventricular failure
    c. Biventricular failure   d. Lung cancer

    [Ref: Harrison's 20th/e pg. 1985]

Explanation

- Complications of bronchiectasis are : Recurrent pneumonia, Empyema, Lung abscess, corpulmonale and pneumothorax. Massive hemoptysis, Amyloidosis & metastatic abscesses are also rarely seen.

65. **IOC for Bronchiectasis:** *(PGMEE 2015-16)*
    a. HRCT scan
    b. Spiral CT
    c. Bronchoscopy
    d. Pulmonary angiography

    [Ref: Harrison's 20th/e pg. 1984]

66. **Parents of a child with bronchiectasis may give a past history of:** *(PGMEE 2014-15)*
    a. Chickenpox   b. Mumps
    c. Whooping cough   d. Typhoid

    [Ref: Harrison's 20th/e pg. 1984]

67. **Not a CT finding in bronchiectasis:** *(PGMEE 2014-15)*
    a. Tree in bud appearance
    b. Crazy paving appearance
    c. Signet ring appearance
    d. Traction bronchiectasis with lung fibrosis

    [Ref: CMDT 2014 pg. 265, Harrison's 19th/e pg. 308e; 1694-95]

Explanation

- Crazy pauing appearance on HRCT is a feature of acute silicosis

68. **Bronchiectasis is most common in:** *(PGMEE 2014-15)*
    a. Right middle lobe
    b. Right upper lobe
    c. Left lower lobe
    d. Left upper lobe

    [Ref: http://www.ncbi.nlm.nih.gov/pmc/articles/PMC3005318]

69. **Bronchiectasis sicca is seen with:** *(PGMEE 2014-15)*
    a. TB   b. Pertussis
    c. Cystic fibrosis   d. Kartaneger syndrome

    [Ref: Pubmed]

70. **All are complications of bronchiectasis EXCEPT:**
    a. Cerebral abscess *(PGMEE 2014-15)*
    b. Lung abscess
    c. Amyloidosis
    d. Bronchogenic carnicoma

    [Ref: Harrison's 20th/e pg. 1985]

71. **Persistent coarse crepitations in the chest is diagnostic of:** *(PGMEE 2014-15)*
    a. Pulmonary TB
    b. Pulmonary oedema
    c. Cavity lesion
    d. Bronchiectasis

    [Ref: Harrison's 20th/e pg. 1944]

CYSTIC FIBROSIS

72. **All of the following clinical features are seen in a patient with cystic fibrosis, EXCEPT:** *(NEET 2018)*
    a. Pancreatic insufficiency
    b. Biliary cirrhosis
    c. Decreased Na^+ and chloride in sweat
    d. Decreased mucocilliary clearance of lungs and recurrent pneumonias

    [Ref: Harrison's 19th/e pg. 1699]

73. **Cystic fibrosis:-** *(PGMEE 2016-17)*
    a. AR
    b. AD
    c. Mitochondrial inheritance
    d. Paternal disomy

74. **Cystic fibrosis is associated with all except-**
    (PGMEE 2012-13)
    a. Nasal polyps   b. Azoospermia
    c. Infertilitiy   d. Renal failure

    [Ref: Harrison's 20th/e pg. 1986]

75. **In cystic fibrosis the most frequent pulmonary pathogen causing recurrent pneumonia is?** *(PGMEE 2014-15)*
    a. Pseudomonas
    b. Enterococci
    c. Staphylococci
    d. Klebsiella

    [Ref: Harrison's 20th/e pg. 1986]

76. **Cystic fibrosis affects all systems EXCEPT:**
    (DNB June 2010)
    a. Respiratory   b. Endocrine
    c. Genitourinary   d. Hepatobiliary

    [Ref: Harrison's 20th/e pg. 1986]

77. **The most common cause of pulmonary abscesses in cystic fibrosis is?** *(DNB Dec'2010)*
    a. Nontuberculous mycobacteria
    b. Staphylococcus aureus
    c. Burkholderia cenocepacia
    d. Pseudomonas aeruginosa

    [Ref: Mayo Clinic Internnal Medicine Board Review 9th/e pg. 845, Infectious diseases of the respiratory tract by Michael E. Ellis Page 511]

62. a	
63. d	
64. a	
65. a	
66. c	
67. b	
68. c	
69. a	
70. d	
71. d	
72. c	
73. a	
74. d	
75. a	
76. None	
77. d	

139. The following does not occur with asbestosis-
(DNB Dec 08)
- a. Methaemoglobinemia
- b. Pleural calcification
- c. Pneumoconiosis
- d. Pleural mesothelioma

[Ref: Harrison's 20th/e pg. 1977]

140. Which of the following causes malignant mesothelioma?
(PGMEE 2012)
- a. Smoking
- b. Asbestosis
- c. Pneumoconiosis
- d. Silicosis

[Ref: Harrison's 20th/e pg. 1977]

141. Asbestos causes all except?   **(PGMEE 2015-16)**
- a. Mesothelioma
- b. Pleural effusion
- c. Bronchial cancer
- d. Atelectasis

[Ref: Harrison's 20th/e pg. 1978]

142. Asbestosis causes all except?   **(PGMEE 2014-15)**
- a. Shaggy heart borders
- b. Honeycombing
- c. Hilar lymphadenopathy
- d. Basal peribronchial fibrosis

[Ref: Harrison's 20th/e pg. 1978]

143. Which is due to inorganic dust:-   **(PGMEE 2016-17)**
- a. Farmer's lung
- b. Anthracosis
- c. bagassosis
- d. Hay fever

[Ref: Harrison's 20th/e pg. 1977]

144. Which one of the following is not correct regarding silicosis?
(PGMEE 2014-15)
- a. Egg shell calcification is seen on chest X-ray
- b. It is more marked in the lower zone
- c. May lead to progressive massive fibrosis
- d. Increased timed vital capacity

[Ref: Harrison's 20th/e pg. 1979]

145. Recognized features of asbestosis do not include:
- a. Calcification of pleura   **(PGMEE 2014-15)**
- b. Egg shell calcification of hilar lymph nodes
- c. Clubbing of fingers
- d. Restrictive pattern of ventilatory defect shown by pulmonary function

[Ref: Harrison's 20th/e pg. 1978]

146. What is true regarding byssinosis: **(PGMEE 2014-15)**
- a. Dyspnea resolves after cessation of exposure
- b. Similar to chronic bronchitis and emphysema
- c. Present as mediastinal fibrosis
- d. Eosinophils are prominent in BAL

[Ref: Harrison's 20th/e pg. 1980]

147. Cotton dust is associated with: **(PGMEE 2014-15)**
- a. Byssinosis
- b. Asbestosis
- c. Bagassosis
- d. Silicosis

[Ref: Harrison's 20th/e pg. 1977]

148. The following does not occur with asbestosis:
(PGMEE 2014-15)
- a. Atelectasis
- b. Pneumoconiosis
- c. Pleural mesothelioma
- d. Pleural calcification

[Ref: Harrison's 20th/e pg. 1978]

149. A factory worker who works in cotton industry developed difficulty in breathing. Probable diagnosis is:-
(PGMEE 2016-17)
- a. Rheumatoid arthritis
- b. COPD
- c. Bronchitis
- d. Byssinosis

[Ref: Harrison's 20th/e pg. 1977]

PLEURAL EFFUSION, PNEUMOTHORAX

150. Light criteria for pleural effusion are all except?
(PGMEE 2015-16)
- a. Effusion protein/serum protein ratio greater than 0.5
- b. Effusion lactate dehydrogenase (LDH)/serum LDH ratio greater than 0.6
- c. Effusion LDH level greater than two-thirds the upper limit of the laboratory's reference range of serum LDH
- d. Effusion sugar is less than 2/3 rd of blood sugar

[Ref: Harrison's 20th/e pg. 2006]

151. Tension pneumothorex is drained by   **(PGMEE 2016-17)**
- a. Wide base needle
- b. Wide bore needle
- c. Normal needle
- d. Needle with high Gauze

[Ref: Harrison's 20th/e pg. 2009]

152. Treatment of spontaneous pneumothorax is:
- a. IPPV   **(PGMEE 2014-15)**
- b. Closed drainage
- c. Simple needle aspiration
- d. Thoractomy

[Ref: Harrison's 20th/e pg. 2009]

153. Incorrect regarding chylous pleural effusion?
- a. Most common cause is trauma   **(PGMEE 2014-15)**
- b. Milky white fluid
- c. High cholesterol
- d. Octreotide is used

[Ref: Harrison's 20th/e pg. 2008]

154. Low glucose in pleural effusion is seen in all EXCEPT:
- a. Rheumatoid arthritis   **(PGMEE 2014-15)**
- b. Empyema
- c. Malignant pleural effusion
- d. Dressler's syndrome

[Ref: Harrison's 20th/e pg. 2007]

155. Pleural fluid low in glucose is seen in all EXCEPT:
(PGMEE 2014-15)
- a. CHF
- b. Tuberculosis
- c. Mesothelioma
- d. Empyema

[Ref: Harrison's 20th/e pg. 2007]

156. Transudative type of pleural effusion is a feature of:
(PGMEE 2014-15)
- a. Variceal sclerotherapy
- b. Coronary artery bypass
- c. Peritoneal dialysis
- d. Radiation

[Ref: Harrison's 20th/e pg. 2008]

157. Which of the following conditions may lead to exudative pleural effusions: **(PGMEE 2014-15)**
- a. Cirrhosis
- b. Nephrotic syndrome
- c. Congestive heart failure
- d. Bronchogenic carcinoma

[Ref: Harrison's 20th/e pg. 2008]

139.	a
140.	b
141.	d
142.	c
143.	b
144.	b
145.	b
146.	a
147.	a
148.	a
149.	d
150.	d
151.	b
152.	c
153.	c
154.	d
155.	a
156.	c
157.	d

158. Bilateral pleural effusion is seen in *(PGMEE 2014-15)*
a. Nephrotic syndrome
b. Constrictive pericarditis
c. Congestive cardiac failure
d. All of the above

[Ref: Harrison's 20th/e pg. 2008]

159. Pleural effusion in rheumatoid arthritis is typically associated with the following features EXCEPT:
(PGMEE 2014-15)
a. Glucose > 620 mg/dl
b. Protein > 3 gm/dl
c. Pleural fluid protein to serum protein ratio of > 0.5
d. Pleural fluid LDH to serum LDH ratio of >0.6

[Ref: Harrison's 20th/e pg. 2007]

160. Pneumothorax occurs in all EXCEPT: *(PGMEE 2014-15)*
a. Langhans cell histiocytosis
b. Marfan's syndrome
c. Assisted ventilation
d. Bronchopulmonary aspergillosis

161. All of the following are causes of hemorrhagic pleural effusion EXCEPT: *(PGMEE 2014-15)*
a. Pulmonary embolism
b. Rheumatoid arthritis
c. Pancreatitis
d. TB

[Ref: Harrison's 20th/e pg. 2007-2008]

162. Which statement is true regarding pneumothorax:
a. Absent breath sounds *(PGMEE 2014-15)*
b. Decreased percussion note
c. Always needs chest tube insertion
d. Tracheal tug

[Ref: Manual of clinical medicine, 6/e]

163. Transudative pleural effusion is present in all EXCEPT:
(PGMEE 2014-15)
a. Meig's syndrome   b. CCF
c. Nephrotic syndrome d. Chronic liver disease

[Ref: Harrison's 20th/e pg. 2008]

164. A high amylase level in pleural fluid suggests a diagnosis of: *(PGMEE 2014-15)*
a. Tuberculosis
b. Malignancy
c. Rheumatoid arthritis
d. Pulmonary infarction

[Ref: Harrison's 20th/e pg. 2008]

165. Causes of haemorrhagic pleural effusion are all EXCEPT:
(PGMEE 2014-15)
a. Pulmonary infarction   b. Mesothelioma
c. Bronchial adenoma   d. Tuberculosis

[Ref: Harrison's 20th/e pg. 2007-08]

166. The most common cause of spontaneous pneumothorax is: *(PGMEE 2014-15)*
a. Tuberculosis
b. Rupture of a sub-pleural bleb
c. Bronchogenic carcinoma
d. Bronchial adenoma

[Ref: Harrison's 20th/e pg. 2009]

158. d
159. a
160. d
161. b
162. a
163. a
164. b
165. c
166. b
167. a
168. d
169. a
170. c
171. b

167. Patient presented with sudden onset difficulty in breathing with RR 28/min, normal blood pressure. X-ray was taken which is given below. What's the diagnosis?
(NEET Pattern 2017)

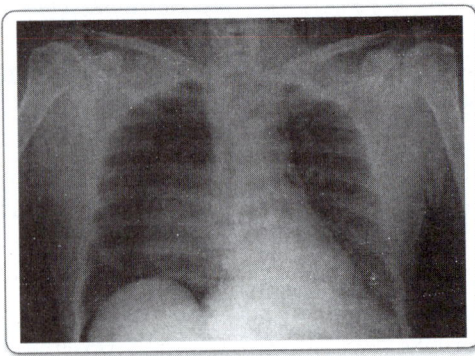

a. Massive pneumothorax
b. Hydro pneumothorax
c. Pulmonary embolism
d. Massive pleural effusion

[Ref: Harrison 19/e]

Explanation

CXR Findings in Pneumothorax

- Visceral pleural edge is visible as a very thin, sharp white line
- No lung markings are seen peripheral to this line
- The peripheral space is radiolucent compared to adjacent lung
- The lung may completely collapse
- The mediastinum may be shift away if a tension pneumothorax is present

168. Tuberculous pleural effusion is characterized by A/E:
(PGMEE 2014-15)
a. Haemorrhage
b. LDH more than 60%
c. Protein is increased
d. Mesothelial cells > 5%

[Ref: Harrison's 20th/e pg. 2008]

169. Tension pneumothorax results in all EXCEPT:
a. Respiratory alkalosis *(PGMEE 2014-15)*
b. Decreased cardiac output
c. Decreased venous return
d. Absent breath sounds

[Ref: Harrison's 20th/e pg. 2009]

170. Bilateral malignant pleural effusion is most often seen in:
a. Ca breast   b. Ca-lung
c. Mesothelioma   d. Lymphoma

[Ref: Pubmed article]

171. The antibiotic commonly used for chemical pleurodesis is: *(PGMEE 2014-15)*
a. Amoxicillin   b. Doxycycline
c. Co-trimoxazole   d. Rifabutin

Explanation
- Agents commonly used for pleurodesis : Talc (most effective), Doxycycline, Bleomycin

172. Most common cause of pleural effusion in AIDS patients?
(*PGMEE 2015*)

a. Mycoplasma
b. Pneumocystis
c. TB
d. Kaposi Sarcoma

Explanation
- MCC of pleural effusion in AIDS patient in India is Bacterial pneumonia f/b Kaposi sarcoma

PULMONARY EMBOLISM

173. Most specific finding in pulmonary embolism:-
(*PGMEE 2016-17*)

a. S1Q3T3
b. Sinus tachycardia
c. RBBB
d. Right axis deviation

[Ref: Harrison 20th ed. pg. 1912]

174. A patient of left hemiplegia with previous history of right deep vein thrombosis. Cause of hemoptysis in this patient is? (*DNB June 2010*)
a. Pulmonary thromboembolism
b. Superior Vena Cava of thyroid
c. Fat Embolism
d. Disseminated intravascular coagulation

[Ref: Harrison's 20th/e pg. 1911]

175. Most common ECG finding for pulmonary embolism?
(*PGMEE 2014-15*)

a. Sinus tachycardia
b. S1Q3T3
c. T wave inversion
d. Epsilon waves

[Ref: Harrison's 20th/e pg. 1913]

176. A patient undergoing surgery suddenly develops hypotension. The monitor shows that the end-tidal carbon dioxide has decreased abruptly by 15 mm Hg. What is the probable diagnosis? (*PGMEE 2014-15*)
a. Hypothermia
b. Pulmonary embolism
c. Massive fluid deficit
d. Myocardial depression due to anaesthetic agents

Explanation
- Rapid decrease in $ETCO_2$ implies rapid decrease in pulmonary perfusion & rapid increase in alveolar dead space, possibly due to
  - Hypotension (MC) secondary to pump failure
  - Pulmonary embolism (air or clot)
  - Cardiac arrest

177. All are seen in massive pulmonary embolism except?
a. Inter-ventricular septum deviation (*PGMEE 2014-15*)
b. Fall of SBP
c. Pulmonary plethora
d. Elevated JVP

[Ref: Harrison's 20th/e pg. 1912]

178. Most common clinical sign of pulmonary embolism is:
(*PGMEE 2014-15*)

a. Tachypnea
b. Tachycardia
c. Cyanosis
d. Sweating

[Ref: Harrison's 20th/e pg. 1911]

179. Most diagnostic of pulmonary emboli is:
(*PGMEE 2014-15*)

a. CT PA
b. V/P scan
c. HRCT
d. D- Dimer Assay

[Ref: Harrison's 20th/e pg. 1913]

180. Pulmonary embolism causes all EXCEPT:
a. Bradycardia (*PGMEE 2014-15*)
b. Decreased cardiac output
c. Arterial hypoxaemia
d. Acute right ventricular strain

[Ref: Harrison's 20th/e pg. 1912]

181. Most common source of pulmonary embolism is:
(*PGMEE 2014-15*)

a. Atherosclerosis
b. Fracture fixation
c. Pelvic surgery
d. Cardiothoracic surgery

[Ref: Harrison's 20th/e pg. 1910]

182. All of the following are true of pulmonary embolism except? (*PGMEE 2014-15*)
a. Sudden onset of pleuritic pain and haemoptysis and hypotension
b. ECG shows evidence of acute left ventricular stress
c. Blood LDH and SGOT levels are raised
d. Isotope perfusion ventilation scan is diagnostic

[Ref: Harrison's 20th/e pg. 1911]

183. Pulmonary embolism is seen in all EXCEPT:
a. Fanconi anemia (*PGMEE 2014-15*)
b. Paroxysmal nocturnal haemoglobinuria
c. Oral contraception
d. Old age

[Ref: Harrison's 20th/e pg. 1910]

184. All of the following conditions may predispose to pulmonary embolism EXCEPT: (*PGMEE 2014-15*)
a. Protein S deficiency
b. Malignancy
c. Obesity
d. Progesterone therapy

[Ref: Harrison's 20th/e pg. 1910]

185. Air embolism is diagnosed by: (*PGMEE 2014-15*)
a. ↓End tidal CO_2
b. ↓End tidal N_2
c. Doppler study
d. Ultrasound

Explanation
- Air Embolism:
  - Most sensitive investigation : Transesophageal echo
  - Most sensitive non invasive investigation : Doppler USG
  - $ETCO_2$ & ETN_2 are nonspecific diagnostic modality

186. Most common symptoms of pulmonary embolism:
(*PGMEE 2014-15*)

a. Chest pain
b. Dyspnea
c. Haemoptysis
d. Cough

[Ref: Harrison's 20th/e pg. 1911]

172.	d
173.	a
174.	a
175.	a
176.	d
177.	c
178.	a
179.	a
180.	a
181.	c
182.	b
183.	a
184.	d
185.	c
186.	b

PULMONARY INFARCTION

187. Pulmonary infraction occurs with all except-

(PGMEE 2012-13)

   a. Arterioles are blocked
   b. Blockage of 2nd and 3rd gen end arteries
   c. Saddle embolus at bifurcation
   d. None

[Ref: Robbin's 8th/e pg. 706]

188. The dome of the diaphragm is elevated in:

(PGMEE 2014-15)

   a. Typhoid fever   b. Pulmonary infarction
   c. Emphysema   d. Cirrhosis

[Ref: Harrison's 19th/e pg. 1632]

ARDS

189. A 45 years male patient who is a chronic alcoholic developed acute pancreatitis. On 4th day of admission, he developed breathlessness and bilateral basal crepitations. ABG showed pH of 7.34, pCO2 of 54 and pO2 of 55 mmHg. Chest x ray was done and is shown. What is the diagnosis

(PGMEE 2019)

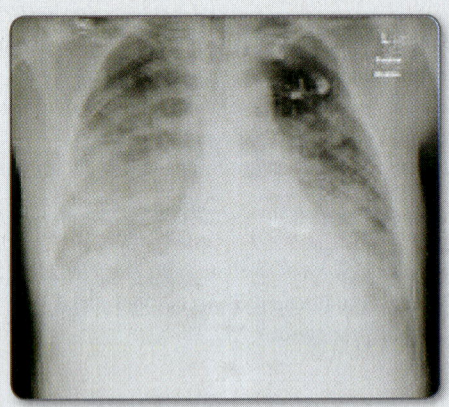

   a. Cardiogenic pulmonary edema
   b. ARDS
   c. Bilateral pneumonia
   d. Collapse

190. Drug of choice for management of acute pulmonary edema is:

(NEET Pattern 2019)

   a. Spironolactone
   b. Hydrochorthiazide
   c. Furosemide
   d. Triamterene

191. A child presents with breathlessness. Which of the following feature is not suggestive of ARDS:

   a. PCWP > 18   *(PGMEE 2018)*
   b. PaO_2/FiO_2 ratio < 100
   c. CXR suggestive of bilateral diffuse infiltrate similar in appearance to pulmonary edema
   d. Presents within 7 days

[Ref: Harrison's 20th/e pg. 2031]

Explanation

- Differentiate ARDS from cardiogenic pulmonary edema based on pulmonary capillary wedge pressure (PCWP); in cardiogenic edema PCWP >18, in ARDS <18.

192. Acute lung injury (shock lung) is characterized by which of the following: *(PGMEE 2015-16)*

   a. Diffuse pulmonary hemorrhage
   b. Alveolar proteinosis
   c. Diffuse bronchial damage
   d. Diffuse alveolar damage

[Ref: Harrison's 20th/e pg. 2031]

193. In ARDS the pathology in the lung consists of-

   a. Surfactant   *(PGMEE 2012-13)*
   b. Fibrin + necrotic epithelial cells
   c. Albumin + complement
   d. Mucus + neutrophils

[Ref: Harrison's 20th/e pg. 2031]

194. What is false about ARDS: *(PGMEE 2015)*

   a. Mucus plug in alveoli
   b. Interstitial infiltrates by cells
   c. Hyaline membrane present
   d. Interstitial edema

[Ref: Harrison's 20th/e pg. 2032]

195. Etiology of ARDS are all except: *(PGMEE 2015)*

   a. Sepsis
   b. Multiple transfusion
   c. Aspiration of gastric contents
   d. Fat embolism

[Ref: Harrison's 20th/e pg. 2031]

196. ARDS is associated with all except? *(PGMEE 2015)*

   a. Pulmonary embolism
   b. Acute pancreatitis
   c. Sepsis
   d. Aspiration

[Ref: Harrison's 20th/e pg. 2031]

197. Which is not seen in ARDS? *(PGMEE 2012)*

   a. Hypoxia
   b. Hypercapnia
   c. Pulmonary oedema
   d. Stiff lung

[Ref: Harrison's 20th/e pg. 2031-32]

198. ARDS is characterised by all except?

   a. Decreased surfactant   *(PGMEE 2015-16)*
   b. Alveolar transudate
   c. Decreased lung compliance
   d. pAO2/ FiO2 ratio <200

[Ref: Harrison's 20th/e pg. 2032]

199. ARDS includes all EXCEPT? *(PGMEE 2015-16)*

   a. Hypoxia
   b. Hypercapnia
   c. Non cardiogenic pulmonary edema
   d. Normal P.C.W.P

[Ref: Harrison's 20th/e pg. 2031]

187. d
188. b
189. b
190. c
191. a
192. d
193. b
194. a
195. d
196. a
197. b
198. b
199. b

200. The following are features of adult respiratory distress syndrome EXCEPT: *(PGMEE 2014-15)*
a. Hypoxia
b. Hypocapnia
c. Low protein Pulmonary edema
d. Stiff lungs

[Ref: Harrison's 20th/e pg. 2032]

201. Wedge pressure in ARDS is usually: *(PGMEE 2014-15)*
a. Markedly increased
b. Moderately increased
c. Normal
d. Decreased

[Ref: Harrison's 20th/e pg. 2032]

202. Correct about ARDS is: *(PGMEE 2014-15)*
a. Low tidal volume ventilation
b. High lung compliance
c. Low protein pulmonary edema
d. High pulmonary capillary pressure

[Ref: Harrison's 20th/e pg. 2034]

203. Best ventilator strategy for ARDS is? *(PGMEE 2014-15)*
a. C.P.A.P
b. High frequency jet ventilation
c. Assisted control mechanical ventilation
d. Synchronized intermittent mandatory ventilation

[Ref: Harrison's 19th/e pg. 1736-38]

204. In management of ARDS ventilator strategy is to *(PGMEE 2016-17)*
a. Increase Tidal volume   b. High PEEP
c. Decrease tidal volume   d. Increase PIP

[Ref: Harrison's 20th/e pg. 2034]

205. The point which distinguishes ARDS from cardiogenic pulmonary edema is: *(PGMEE 2014-15)*
a. Normal PO_2
b. Normal pulmonary capillary wedge pressure
c. Normal arterial alveolar gradient
d. Normal PCO_2

[Ref: Harrison's 20th/e pg. 2031]

OBSTRUCTIVE SLEEP APNEA

206. All of the following criteria are required for diagnosis of obesity hypoventilation syndrome EXCEPT
a. Hypertension   *(PGMEE 2015-16)*
b. Sleep disorder breathing
c. BMI ≥ 30 kg/m²
d. $PaCO_2$ ≥ 45 mm Hg

[Ref: Harrison's 20th/e pg. 2012]

207. 40-year-old smoker, obese, hypertension patient is having loud snoring. On sleep study patient had >5 episodes of apnea per hour of sleep at night. After control of BP and quitting smoking what is the next best management for improvement of symptoms of the patient?
a. C.P.A.P   *(PGMEE 2014-15)*
b. Uvulopalatoplasty
c. Weight reduction and diet control
d. Mandibular reposition surgery

[Ref: Harrison's 20th/e pg. 2017]

208. Not true of obstructive sleep apnoea: *(PGMEE 2014-15)*
a. Nocturnal asphyxia
b. Alcoholism is a cofactor
c. Prone to hypertension
d. Spirometry is diagnostic

[Ref: Harrison's 20th/e pg. 2015]

209. Obstructive sleep apnoea may result in all of the following EXCEPT: *(PGMEE 2014-15)*
a. Systemic hypertension   b. Pulmonary hypertension
c. Cardiac arrhythmia   d. Impotence

[Ref: Harrison's 20th/e pg. 2014-16]

210. Most common cause of obstructive sleep apnea
a. Craniofacial abnormalities   *(PGMEE 2014-15)*
b. Hypothyroidism
c. Alcoholism
d. Acromegaly

211. Duration of apnea in obstructive sleep apnea is *(PGMEE 2014-15)*
a. ≥10 sec   b. ≥20sec
c. ≥30 sec   d. ≥60 sec

[Ref: Harrison's 20th/e pg. 2013]

212. Obstructive sleep apnea is defined as _____ number of apnea events/hour? *(PGMEE 2014-15)*
a. 2   b. 3
c. 4   d. 5

[Ref: Harrison's 20th/e pg. 2013]

213. The Epworth scale is used for assessing: *(PGMEE 2014-15)*
a. Body mass index
b. Vital capacity in post-operative patients
c. Sleep apnea
d. Risk of embolism in perioperative patient

[Ref: Harrison's 20th/e pg. 2011]

RESPIRATORY FAILURE

214. Which of the following is the common cause of respiratory failure Type 2? *(PGMEE 2015-16)*
a. COPD
b. Acute attack asthma
c. ARDS
d. Pneumonia

[Ref: Harrison's 20th/e pg. 2026]

215. Type II respiratory failure is seen in:
a. Chronic bronchitis with cor-pulmonale
b. Chronic renal failure
c. Adult respiratory distress syndrome
d. Pulmonary alveolar proteinosis

[Ref: Harrison's 20th/e pg. 2026]

216. Type 3 respiratory failure occurs due to:
a. Post-operative atelectasis   *(PGMEE 2014-15)*
b. Kyphoscoliosis
c. Flail chest
d. Pulmonary fibrosis

[Ref: Harrison's 20th/e pg. 2026]

200. c
201. c
202. a
203. a
204. b
205. b
206. a
207. a
208. d
209. None
210. a
211. a
212. d
213. c
214. a
215. a
216. a

217. In type II respiratory failure there is: *(PGMEE 2014-15)*
a. Low pO_2 and Low pCO_2
b. Low pO_2 and High pCO_2
c. Normal pO_2 and High pCO_2
d. Low pO_2 and Normal pCO_2

[Ref: Harrison's 20th/e pg. 2026]

218. Respiratory failure type I consists of: *(PGMEE 2014-15)*
a. Low PaO_2, normal or low $PaCO_2$
b. Raised $PaCO_2$, low PaO_2
c. Normal PaO_2, low PO_2
d. Normal PaO_2 and $PaCO_2$ high

[Ref: Harrison's 20th/e pg. 2026]

219. All of the following are true about type I respiratory failure EXCEPT: *(PGMEE 2014-15)*
a. Decreased PaO_2
b. Decreased $PaCO_2$
c. Normal $PaCO_2$
d. Normal A-a gradient

[Ref: Harrison's 20th/e pg. 2026]

220. Acute respiratory failure does not occur with: *(PGMEE 2014-15)*
a. Porphyria
b. Myasthenia gravis
c. Polio
d. Lead poisoning

221. Alveolar hypoventilation is observed in:
a. Gulliain –Barre syndrome *(PGMEE 2014-15)*
b. Acute asthma
c. Bronchiectasis
d. CREST syndrome

[Ref: Harrison's 20th/e pg. 2026]

222. Prolonged hyperventilation may lead to all EXCEPT: *(PGMEE 2014-15)*
a. Paraesthesia
b. Alkalosis
c. Tetany
d. Somnolence

223. Which of the following is the common cause of type II respiratory failure: *(PGMEE 2015)*
a. ARDS
b. Pneumonia
c. Chronic bronchitis/COPD
d. Acute attack asthma

[Ref: Harrison's 20th/e pg. 2026]

MISCELLANEOUS

224. Brock syndrome is due to which lobe of lung? *(NEET Pattern 2019)*
a. Right lower lobe
b. Left lower lobe
c. Right middle lobe
d. Left upper lobe

225. Inspiratory squeaks are the physical examination finding of: *(NEET Pattern 2019)*
a. Pneumonia
b. Pulmonary hypertension
c. Pulmonary hypertension
d. Bronchiolitis

226. Biot breathing is seen in? *(PGMEE 2015-16)*
a. Flail chest
b. Uremia
c. High altitude
d. Lesion in the brain

[Ref: Manual of clinical medicine, 6/e]

227. Pop-corn calcification is seen with? *(PGMEE 2015-16)*
a. Pulmonary Hamartoma
b. Aspergillosis
c. Broncho-Alveolar cancer
d. Pulmonary Embolism

[Ref: Harrison's 20th/e pg. 547]

228. Partial pressure of oxygen in alveoli: *(PGMEE 2015-16)*
a. 60 mm Hg
b. 103 mm Hg
c. 136 mm Hg
d. 160 mm Hg

229. Finger in glove sign is seen in *(PGMEE 2015-16)*
a. Pulmonary alveolar proteinosis
b. Pneumocystis carinii
c. Tuberculosis
d. Bronchocele

Explanation
- Finger in glove sign is characteristically seen in bronchocele which can be secondary to ABPA, bronchogenic CA etc.

230. The following CXR shows *(PGMEE 2015-16)*

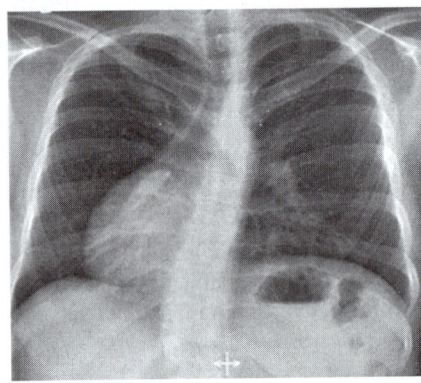

a. Dextrocardia
b. Pneumothorax
c. Pneumomediastinum
d. Pulmonary hamartoma

231. The CXR shows markings near the Costophrenic angle. Which of the following is the cause of these markings?

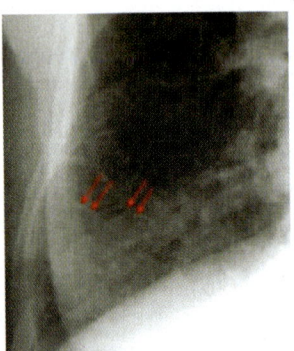

a. Lymphangitis Carcinomatosis
b. Pulmonary alveolar Proteinosis
c. Lung abscess
d. Pneumatocele

[Ref: Page 476e-3, 1552, Harrison 19th edition]

232. A patient presented with hemoptysis and persistent cough. The chest X-ray of the patient was normal. The next best investigation is? *(PGMEE 2014-15)*
a. Helical CT
b. High resolution CT
c. Bronchoscopy
d. Angiography

[Ref: Harrison's 20th ed. pg. 234]

217. b
218. a
219. d
220. d
221. a
222. d
223. c
224. c
225. d
226. d
227. a
228. b
229. d
230. a
231. a
232. b

233. Subcutaneous Emphysema may be found in the following conditions: *(PGMEE 2014-15)*
- a. Tracheostomy
- b. Hemilich maneuver
- c. Chest injury
- d. All of the above

[Ref: www.nlm.nih.gov-google, Harrison's 19th/e pg. 1703-04]

234. Bronchoalveloar lavage is beneficial in the evaluation of:
- a. Squamous cell cancer lung *(PGMEE 2014-15)*
- b. Bronchiectasis
- c. Bronchopleural fistula
- d. Pulmonary alveolar Proteinosis

[Ref: CMDT 2014 pg. 296, Harrison's 19th/e pg. 1714]

235. The most common cause of bronchiolitis is:
- a. Respiratory syncytial virus *(PGMEE 2014-15)*
- b. Adenovirus
- c. Herpes virus
- d. Influenza virus

[Ref: CMDT 2014 pg. 269, Harrison's 19th/e pg. 1205-06]

236. Most common lesion in middle mediastinum: *(PGMEE 2014-15)*
- a. Congenital cyst
- b. Lipoma
- c. Aneurysm
- d. Neurogenic tumours

[Ref: Harrison's 19th/e pg. 1664-65; 1719]

237. A patient presented with a 5 cm cavity of upper lobe of lung; choice of diagnosis will be: *(PGMEE 2014-15)*
- a. CT scan
- b. Percutaneous aspiration
- c. Bronchography
- d. Bronchoalveolar lavage and biopsy

[Ref: Pubmed article]

238. Palpatory thud, audible slap is seen in- *(PGMEE 2015)*
- a. Laryngeal foreign body
- b. Tracheal foreign body
- c. Bronchial foreign body
- d. None

239. Artery responsible for bleeding in hemoptysis is? *(PGMEE 2009)*
- a. Bronchial artery
- b. Pulmonary artery
- c. Intersegmental artery
- d. Intercostal collaterals

[Ref: Harrison's 20th/e pg. 232]

240. Blood supply of pulmonary sequestration is mainly from *(PGMEE 2015, 13-12)*
- a. Pulmonary artery
- b. Descending aorta & its branches
- c. Bronchial artery
- d. Intercostal artery

Explanation
- Pulmonary sequestration, also called accessory lung, refers to the aberrant formation of segmental lung tissue that has no connection with bronchial tree or pulmonary arteries.
- It's blood supply is mainly from descending aorta & its branches.

241. Bronchogenic sequestration is seen in which lobe- *(PGMEE 2012-13)*
- a. Right upper lobe
- b. Left upper lobe
- c. Left lower lobe
- d. Left middle lobe

[Ref: Fetal & neonatal physiology pg. 872]

Explanation
- Sequestration preferentially affects Lower Lobes. 60% of it affects Left Lower lobe & 40% affects right Lower lobe.
- Extralobar sequestrations almost always affect left lower lobe.

242. Hamartomatous lung tissue is: *(PGMEE 2015)*
- a. Hypoplasia of lung
- b. Lobar sequestration
- c. Congenital cyst
- d. Congenital cystic adenomatoid malformation

[Ref: Robbins 9th/e pg. 670]

243. Collapse of lung is called- *(PGMEE 2012-13)*
- a. Atelectasis
- b. Empysema
- c. Bronchitis
- d. Bronchiactasis

244. Most common cause for acute mediastinitis is:
- a. Esophageal perforation *(PGMEE 2014-15)*
- b. Cervical spondylitis
- c. Osteomyelitis of sternum
- d. Osteomyelitis of clavicle

[Ref: Harrison's 19th/e pg. 1719]

245. Hamman's crunch sign is seen in: *(PGMEE 2014-15)*
- a. Hamman rich syndrome
- b. Aortic aneurysm
- c. Pneumo-Mediastinum
- d. Pneumothorax

[Ref: Harrison's 19th/e pg. 1720]

246. Heart Failure cells are: *(PGMEE 2016-17, 2015)*
- a. Lipofuscin granules in cardiac cells
- b. Pigmented alveolar macrophages
- c. Pigmented pancreatic acinar cells
- d. Pigment cells seen in liver

[Ref: Robbin's 9th/e pg. 669-670]

Explanation
- Heart failure cells are hemosiderin containing macrophages present in the alveoli of patients with LV failure.

247. Heart failure cells in Lungs can be seen in:-
- a. Left heart failure *(PGMEE 2016-17)*
- b. Acute pulmonary edema
- c. Chronic pulmonary edema
- d. A and C

248. Paradoxical breathing is characteristic of: *(PGMEE 2014-15)*
- a. Pneumonia
- b. Pneumothorax
- c. Atelectasis
- d. Flail chest

233. d
234. d
235. a
236. c
237. a
238. b
239. a
240. b
241. c
242. d
243. a
244. a
245. c
246. b
247. d
248. d

CHAPTER 7

Cardiology

FACTS

- Chest pain from pericardial inflammation in pericarditis is referred by: Phrenic nerve
- Preferred site for pericardiocentesis: Sub-xiphoid
- Small /narrow cuff leads to → Falsely high BP
- Large/wide cuff leads to → Falsely lower BP
- Pathological S_3 associated with constrictive pericarditis: **Pericardial knock**
- Ω–3–FA (PUFA) has shown to ↓ total mortality and sudden death in patient with IHD.
- Cardio protective fatty acids : PUFA > MUFA
- Types of hyperlipidemia not associated with increased risk of CAD:
  - Type I → Familial hyper chylomicronemia
  - Type II → Familial mixed hypertriglyceridemia
- Bacteria which have been associated with atherosclerosis → Chlamydia pneumoniae.
- Most important modifiable risk factor for atherosclerosis → Smoking
- Most important modifiable risk factor for stroke → Hypertension
- MI risk factor for aortic aneurysm → Smoking
- *Hibernating myocardium*: ischemic myocardium with viable cells but with depressed contractile function
- *Stunned myocardium*: viable myocardium that exhibits prolonged post ischemic contractile dysfunction after coronary reperfusion is achieved.
- Reperfusion is believed to restore contractile function of → Hibernating myocardium
- Most important cause of renovascular hypertension in young female →Fibromuscular dysplasia
- Genetic abnormality associated with Pulmonary arterial hypertension → *BMPR2* mutation
- Pathognomonic feature of rheumatic fever: Aschoff's body
- Least common cause of endocarditis : ASD
- Most friable vegetations on cardiac valve: IE
- Flat verrucous lesion present in pockets of valve on either or both side of valve leaflets: Libman Sack endocarditis
- Small warty vegetations along the line of closure of valve → Rheumatic fever
- Diastolic murmur always signify structural heart diseases
- The Framingham criteria helps in diagnosis of heart failure

Electrophysiology

- Conduction of electrical impulse is fastest in purkinje system (4 m/sec).
- ECG is less sensitive in detecting ischemia over area supplied by → Left circumflex artery.
- ECG leads that is most sensitive in detecting intra operative myocardial ischemia → V5
- AV block with atrial tachycardia is seen in → Digitalis toxicity with K^+ depletion
- Fusion beats are seen in: Ventricular Tachycardia
- Idiopathic degeneration of the proximal bundle branch fibre is known as: **Lev's** disease.

Congenital Heart Diseases

- Ductus venosus is a communication between: umbilical vein and the IVC.
- In PDA, aortic attachment of ductus arteriosus is just distal to left subclavian artery
- Truncus arteriosus may be associated with: Di George syndrome
- Congenital heart diseases associated with loud S_3 → ASD, VSD, PDA [L → R Shunts]
- Most characteristic cause for wide and fixed splitting of S_2: **ASD**

Valvular Heart Diseases

Features suggestive of severe MS:
- Proximity of A_2 and Opening Snap → Time interval between A_2 and OS varies inversely with the severity of MS
- Longer duration of MDM

Features suggestive of severe MR:
- Presence of S_3 or inflow rumble at apex
- Wide Split S_2 (due to early A_2)
- Presence of MDM across MV

Valve Area

MV Pathology	Area
Normal MV	4 – 6 cm²
Mild MS	>1.5 cm²
Moderate MS	1 – 1.5 cm²
Severe MS	<1 cm²

AV Pathology	Area
Normal AV	2.5 – 3.5 cm²
Mild AS	>1.5 cm²
Moderate AS	1–1.5 cm²
Severe AS	<1 cm²

REMEMBER

- After occlusion, Umbilical **A**rteries form: **M**edial **U**mbilical **L**igament [**Mn: AMUL**]
- Umbilical vein forms: round ligament of liver (aka Ligamentum teres)
- **M**arfan syndrome is associated with: **A**ortic **R**oot dilatation [**Mn: MAR**fan]
- **Car**cinoid syndrome usually involves: **R**ight side of heart [**Mn: CaR**]

Features of HOCM:
- Pulsus bisferiens
- Reversed pulsus paradoxus
- Fusion murmur
- Double or triple apical impulse (also seen in AS)
- S_4

- Harsh diamond shaped, systolic murmur→ due to MR [Hallmark]
- Systolic anterior motion (SAM) of MV is seen
- Aggravation of symptoms of angina after taking nitrate

Classification scheme for thoracic aortic dissection:
- DeBakey classification
- Stanford classification:
  - Type A – Ascending Aorta is involved
  - Type B – Descending Aorta is involved

Conditions presenting with interarm BP difference:
- Aortic dissection
- Takayasu arteritis / Pulseless disease
- Coarctation of Aorta
- Supravalvular AS

MOST COMMON

- MC used intercostal space for pericardiocentesis: Left 5ᵗʰ ICS
- MCC of constrictive pericarditis in India → TB
- MC type of cardiomyopathy: DCM
- MC cause of DCM: Idiopathic
- MC toxin implicated in DCM: Alcohol
- MCC of sudden death in young athlete: HOCM
- MC cardiac manifestation of SLE: Pericarditis
- MC cardiac lesion in congenital rubella syndrome: PDA > PS
- MC congenital heart disease in high altitude: PDA
- MCC of LV Hypertrophy is: Systolic hypertension

- MC cause of Renovascular hypertension in:
  - Elderly: Atherosclerosis
  - Young: India – Aortoarteritis / Takayasu arteritis
    West – Fibromuscular dysplasia
- MC cause of aortic aneurysm is: Atherosclerosis
- MC cause of ascending aortic aneurysm: Marfan syndrome
- MC risk factor for aortic dissection: Hypertension
- MC Primary cardiac tumor: Myxoma
- MC site for atrial myxoma : Left atrium

Valvular Heart Diseases

- MC valvular disease associated with sudden death: AS
- MC heart valve involved in IV drug user: Tricuspid valve
- MC valve involved in carcinoid syndrome: Tricuspid valve leading to TR

- MC valvular lesion seen in MI: MR
- MC cardiac lesion complicating pregnancy: Valvular heart disease
- MC valvular lesion in pregnant women: MS

ECG & Arrhythmias

- MCC of LAD in ECG: Left anterior hemi block.
- MC type of reentrant supraventricular tachycardia: Atrioventricular nodal reentry tachycardia (AVNRT)
- MC reentrant tachycardia associated with WPW syndrome: Orthodromic AV reentrant tachycardia (AVRT).
- MC accessory pathway which leads to pre-excitation syndrome/WPW syndrome: Left sided pathways (aka Type-A WPW)

- MC mechanism of arrhythmia: Reentry
- MC arrhythmia seen after successful reperfusion of a blocked coronary vessel/ Myocardial reperfusion: Accelerated idioventricular rhythm (AIVR)
- MC arrhythmia after binge alcohol drinking: Atrial fibrillation
- MC sustained arrhythmia in older adults: Atrial fibrillation
- MCC of broad complex tachycardia : VT

SYNDROMES

❶ *Wellens Syndrome:*
- Represents critical stenosis of the proximal LAD artery
- ECG → symmetrical deep T wave inversion in precordial leads esp. V_2 and V_3

❷ *Dressler Syndrome:*
- Aka post myocardial infarction syndrome; post pericardiotomy syndrome

- Refers to pericarditis (**fibrinous** variety) developing 1 – 4 weeks after the cardiac injury
- It is an autoimmune condition due to **hypersensitivity** to myocardial antigens
- CF: Fever, Pleuritis, Chest pain, Pneumonitis, Pericardial effusion
- Treatment: NSAIDs (Aspirin, Ibuprofen), Steroids

INVESTIGATIONS

- Test of choice for detecting recurrent ischemic event in 4 to 10 day window: CK–MB
- Reversible myocardial ischemia can be detected by: Thallium scan
- PCWP closely correlates with pressure of LA.
- **Kerley 'B' lines** are invariably present if LA pressure is more than → 20 mm Hg
- Most sensitive and specific screening test for renovascular hypertension: MRA (noninvasive) > CT Angio (invasive)
- IOC for aortic aneurysm: MRI
- Best screening test to detect aortic aneurysm: USG

- Best investigation to monitor size of aortic aneurysm: CT

Pulmonary edema with:
- ↑ PCWP (>18 cm H_2O) → Cardiogenic
- Normal PCWP (<18 cm H_2O) → ARDS or Non cardiogenic pulmonary edema

Biomarkers raised in Heart failure:
- BNP/ NT-proBNP → MC and best for diagnosis of HF
- ST2
- Galectin-3

ECHO

- Early diastolic collapse of the RV free wall & late diastolic collapse of the RA → Cardiac tamponade
- Systolic Anterior Motion of MV is seen in → HOCM

- Akinesia or hypokinesia of the midsegment and apical segment of LV is characteristic of → Takotsubo Cardiomyopathy

SIGNS

- *Kussmaul's sign:* failure of JVP to fall during inspiration.
- *Ewart's sign:* dullness and bronchial breath sound below angle of left scapula in large pericardial effusion
- *Beck's triad:* Hypotension + Muffled heart sounds + Raised JVP. Seen in Tamponade

- *Broadbent's sign:* retraction of 11th & 12th ribs seen in constrictive pericarditis
- *Square root sign*/dip and plateau wave form: Constrictive pericarditis
- *Carvallo's sign:* PSM of TR becomes louder on inspiration. Helps to differentiate the PSM of MR.

Signs of Chronic AR

- **Becker sign:** systolic pulsation of the retinal arterioles.
- **Corrigan pulse (Water Hammer pulse):** forceful distention of the arterial pulse followed by quick collapse.
- **De Musset sign:** bobbing of head with each heart beat.
- **Hill sign:** Popliteal SBP > Brachial SBP by 60 mm Hg
- **Duroziez sign:** murmur over femoral artery with compression of the artery

- **Muller sign:** systolic pulsation of the uvula.
- **Quincke sign:** capillary pulsation seen on light compression of the fingernail bed
- **Traube sign (pistol shot pulse):** booming systolic and diastolic sounds over femoral artery
- **Rosenbach sign:** hepatic pulsation
- **Gerhardt sign:** splenic pulsation
- **Landolfi sign:** systolic contraction and diastolic contraction of the pupil
- **Light house sign:** alternate blanching and flushing of the forehead

MANAGEMENT

- DOC to control supraventricular tachycardia (PSVT): Adenosine
- DOC for WPW with Atrial fibrillation: Procainamide (or ibutilide)
- TOC for AF in patient with WPW syndrome who are hemodynamically unstable: DC cardioversion

- IV fluids is indicated in treatment of: Inferior wall MI
- DOC for hypertension in a patient with angina: β-blockers
- DOC for hypertension in a patient with proteinuria: ACE Inhibitors or ARB
- DOC for hypertension in a patient with diabetes: ACE Inhibitors or ARB

TYPES OF PULSES

Pulse Character	Wave	Causes
Hypokinetic Pulse - Small volume pulse with narrow pulse pressure		- CCF - Shock - Aortic sclerosis
Anacrotic Pulse/Pulsus parvus et tardus - Low amplitude (Parvus) with slow rising and late peak (tardus)		- Severe valvular **AS**
Hyperkinetic Pulse - High amplitude - Large volume with wide pulse pressure		- High cardiac output states - MR
Collapsing Pulse/Corrigan's/Water hammer pulse - Rapid upstroke due to ↑ SBP - Rapid down stroke d/t ↓ DBP		- AR, PDA, AV fistula - RSOV - Severe anemia - Beriberi - Thyrotoxicosis
Pulsus Bisferiens - Single pulse wave with 2 peaks in systole - Best felt in **B**rachial artery - Due to **B**ernouli's effect on walls of ascending aorta		- **H**OCM - Severe **AR** - AS with **AR** [**Mn:** BiHAR]
Pulsus Dicrotic - One peak in systole and other in diastole - Due to very low stroke volume		- **D**CM

Contd...

Pulse Character	Wave	Causes
Pulsus Alternans ▪ Alternate small and large volume pulse ▪ Best felt on radial or femoral artery ▪ Rhythm–regular	No compensatory pause	▪ Severe LVF ▪ MI
Pulsus Bigeminus ▪ Pulse wave with normal beat f/b premature beat and a compensatory pause (Must be distinguished from pulsus alterans) ▪ Rhythm-Irregular	Compensatory pause	▪ **V**PC ▪ **Dig**italis toxicity [**Mn:** V Dig Big]
Pulsus Paradoxus ▪ > 10 mm Hg fall in BP on inspiration ▪ *Mechanism*: On inspiration → venous return ↑ → RV enlarge → IV septum pushed to left side → LV filling ↓ → stroke volume↓ [**Mn:** AC$_2$ P$_2$ S$_2$]	Inspiration	▪ Obstructive **a**irway disease: e.g. asthma, COPD ▪ **C**ardiac tamponade ▪ **C**onstrictive pericarditis ▪ **P**ulmonary embolism ▪ **P**neumothorax ▪ **S**VC obstruction ▪ **H**emorrhagic **S**hock
Reversed Pulsus Paradoxus ▪ Inspiratory ↑ in BP		▪ HOCM ▪ IPPV

JVP

JVP		▪ Reflection of pressure changes in the RA ▪ Measured in right Internal Jugular Vein. ▪ Raised in right heart failure, volume overload states etc ▪ Raised and non-pulsatile in SVC obstruction
Waves in JVP	A wave →	Right **A**trial Contraction
	C wave →	Bulging of Tri**C**uspid valve towards the RA during RV **C**ontraction
	V wave →	**V**enous filling into the RA with closed Tricuspid valve
Descents in JVP	X descent →	RA rela**X**ation and Tricuspid valve moves downward
	Y descent →	Tricuspid valve opens and rapid empt**Y**ing of RA into RV

Clinical Abnormalities

A wave	Prominent	Tricuspid stenosis, Pulmonary stenosis, Pulmonary hypertension, RVH
	Absent	Atrial fibrillation
	Cannon	Complete heart block, Atrial flutter
C wave	Prominent	Tricuspid regurgitation
	Absent	Constrictive pericarditis
V wave	Prominent	Tricuspid regurgitation
X descent	Prominent	Constrictive **P**ericarditis, **C**ardiac **T**amponade [**Mn:** PCT]
Y descent	Prominent	**T**ricuspid **R**egurgitation, Constrictive **P**ericarditis [**Mn:** TRP]
	Slow	Tricuspid stenosis, Atrial myxoma

Kussmaul's Sign

- Defined by either a rise or a lack of fall of the JVP with inspiration
- It is absent in Cardiac Tamponade

- Seen in :
  - Constrictive Pericarditis
  - Restrictive cardiomyopathy
  - Massive Pulmonary embolism
  - Right ventricular infarction

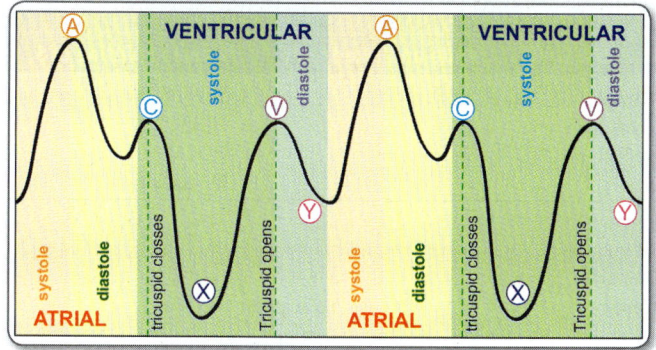

JVP waves in different phase of cardiac cycle

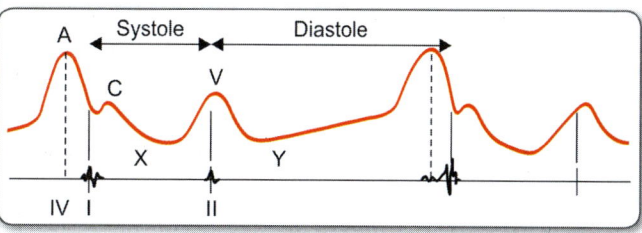

JVP waves with heart sounds

AUSCULTATION

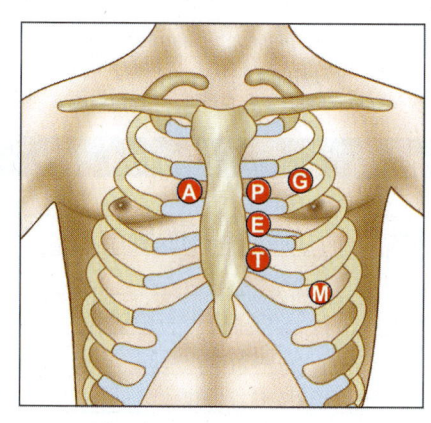

A	Aortic valve area	Second intercostal space (ICS), right sternal border
P	Pulmonic valve area	Second intercostal space (ICS), left sternal border
E	Erb's area	Third ICS, left sternal border
T	Tricuspid valve area	Fourth ICS, left sternal border
M	Mitral valve area	Fifth ICS, left mid-clavicular line
G	Gibson's area	Left 2nd intercostal space → PDA is heard here

* Erb's area or 2nd Aortic area → EDM of AR & PSM of VSD is best heard here

First Heart Sound

Soft S_1	Loud S_1	Split S_1	Reverse Split S_1	Variable

▪ MR, TR
▪ Severe or calcified MS or TS
▪ Prolonged PR interval
  ○ 1⁰ heart block
  ○ Bradycardia
	▪ Mild – moderate MS, TS
	▪ High cardiac output states
	▪ Short PR interval – WPW syndrome
		▪ RBBB
		▪ LV pacing
		▪ LV ectopics
		▪ Ebstein anomaly
		▪ ASD
			▪ LBBB
			▪ RV pacing
			▪ Severe MS
			▪ LA myxoma
				▪ Atrial fibrillation
				▪ Extrasystole
				▪ Mobitz type I Heart block

Second Heart Sound

Soft S_2	Loud S_2	Single S_2
▪ Calcified AS ▪ Calcified PS	▪ Hypertension (Loud A_2) ▪ Pulmonary hypertension (Loud P_2)	▪ Expiration ▪ Severe AS (Absent A_2) ▪ Severe PS (Absent P_2) ▪ TOF (Absent P_2)

Splitting of S$_2$			
Physiological	**Wide and Variable Split**	**Wide and Fixed Split**	**Reverse Splitting of S$_2$**
▪ Children ▪ During Inspiration	▪ MR (Early A$_2$) ▪ VSD (Early A$_2$) ▪ RBBB (Late P$_2$)	▪ ASD	▪ Severe AS ▪ LBBB ▪ HOCM ▪ RV pacing

Third and Fourth Heart Sounds

Features	S$_3$	S$_4$
Frequency	▪ **Low pitch (<20 Hz)**	▪ **Low pitch (<20 Hz)**
Auscultation	▪ Bell of stethoscope	▪ Bell of stethoscope
Heard during	▪ Early diastole/Rapid Filling phase	▪ Late Diastole due to Atrial contraction
Mechanism	▪ Sudden deceleration of blood flow in LV	▪ Increase stiffness or thickness of LV
Examples	▪ Can be physiological in patients <40 years ▪ High Cardiac Output States: Anemia, Fever, Pregnancy, Thyrotoxicosis ▪ Congestive cardiac failure, MR	▪ Hypertension ▪ LVH ▪ AS ▪ Hypertrophic cardiomyopathy
Absent in	▪ **MS**	▪ **Atrial Fibrillation**

Added Sound

Timing	Pitch	Sound	Examples
Systolic	High Pitched	Ejection Click*	AS, PS
		Mid Systolic Click	Mitral Valve Prolapse
Diastolic	High Pitched	Opening Snap	MS, TS
		Pericardial Knock	Constrictive Pericarditis
	Low Pitched	Tumor Plop	Atrial Myxoma
		S$_3$	Heart Failure
		S$_4$	LVH

*The pulmonic ejection click is the only right-sided acoustic event that decreases in intensity with inspiration.

MURMURS

Timing	Condition	Character	Radiation
Midsystolic/ Ejection systolic	Aortic stenosis	High pitch	Carotid arteries
	Pulmonary stenosis	High pitch	Towards left shoulder and neck
Holosystolic/ Pansystolic	Mitral regurgitation	High pitch	Towards left axilla
	Tricuspid regurgitation	High pitch	Towards apex
	VSD	High pitch	Across precordium
Early diastolic	Aortic regurgitation	High pitch, blowing, decrescendo	Base of heart
Mid-Late diastolic	Mitral stenosis	Low pitch, rumbling with presystolic accentuation	None
Continuous	PDA	Harsh machine like	

Named Murmur	Characteristic
Austin-Flint murmur	▪ Low pitched delayed diastolic-murmur ▪ Associated with severe **AR**
Carey-**C**oombs murmur	▪ Associated with **R**heumatic fever "RCC" ▪ Low pitched **D**DM "CCD"
Graham Steell murmur	▪ Early diastolic murmur due to functional incompetence of pulmonary valve

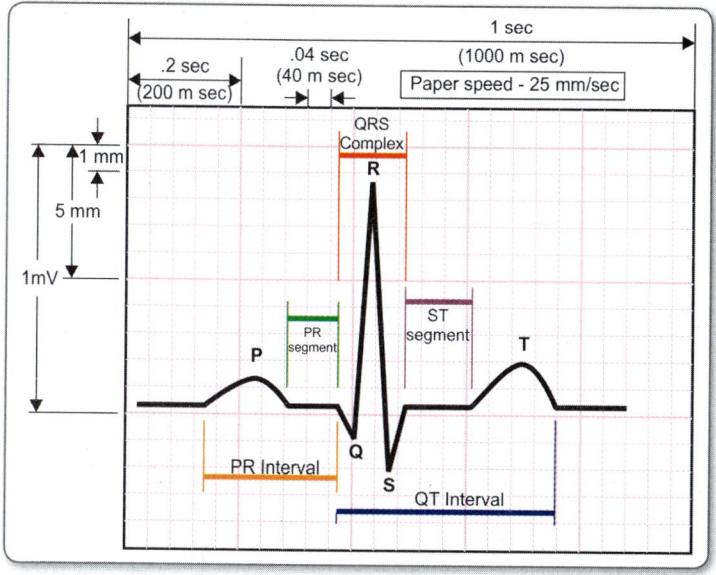

	Origin		Normal Duration	
P wave	Atrial Depolarization	*PR Interval*	120 – 200 ms
QRS	Ventricular Depolarization	*QRS complex*	80 – 120 ms
T wave	Ventricular Repolarization	*QTc Interval*	<440 ms

Rate interpretation

- Rate = 300 / No. of large square between consecutive R wave

AXIS CALCULATION

$$R < S \text{ wave} \quad \frac{\text{Lead I} \rightarrow \text{RAD}}{\text{Lead II} \rightarrow \text{LAD}}$$

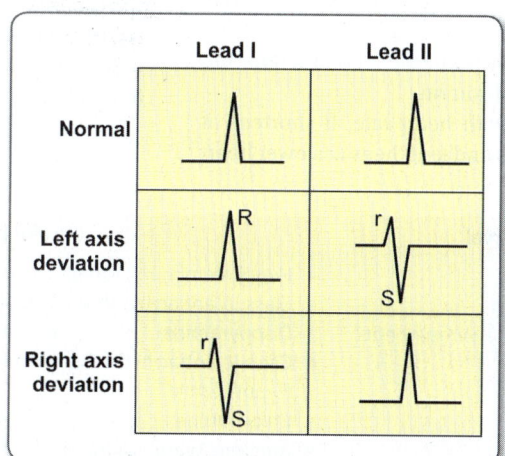

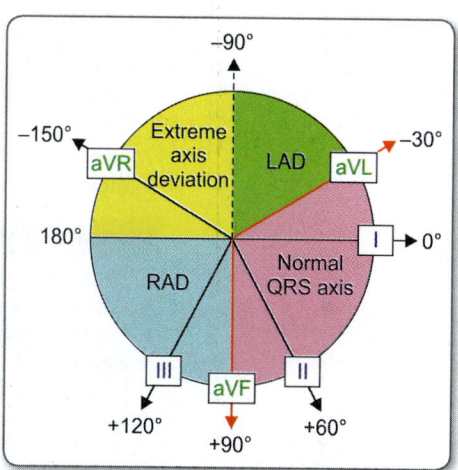

Causes of Axis Deviation

Right Axis Deviation	Left Axis Deviation
▪ RVH	▪ LVH
▪ Lateral wall MI	▪ Inferior wall MI
▪ RV strain (e.g. due to pulmonary embolism)	▪ LBBB
▪ Ostium Secundum ASD	▪ Ostium Primum ASD
▪ Chronic lung disease like COPD	▪ Ventricular pacing
▪ Left sided Pneumothorax	▪ Right sided pneumothorax
▪ Dextrocardia	▪ Normal variant
▪ Left Posterior Fascicular Block	▪ **L**eft **A**nterior Fascicular Block (**LA**FB has **LA**D)

P WAVE

	II	V₁
Normal	∿	∿
RAE	∿	∿
LAE	∿	∿
RAE + LAE	∿	∿

- P wave represents **atrial depolarization**
- The initial 1/3ʳᵈ of the P wave represents RA activation, the final 1/3ʳᵈ represents LA activation.
- **P *mitrale*** (bifid P waves) – seen with left atrial enlargement.
- **P *pulmonale*** (peaked P waves) – seen with right atrial enlargement.
- P wave inversion – seen with ectopic atrial and junctional rhythms.
- Variable P wave morphology – seen in multifocal atrial rhythms (MAT).

P pulmonale

- The presence of tall, peaked P waves in lead II is a sign of **right atrial enlargement**, usually due to **pulmonary hypertension** (e.g. *cor pulmonale* from chronic respiratory disease).
- A similar picture can be seen in hypokalaemia (known as "pseudo p-pulmonale").

P mitrale

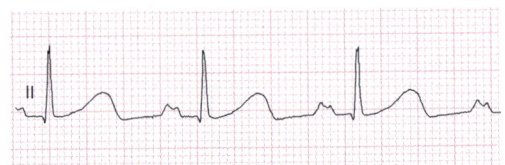

- The presence of broad, notched (bifid) P waves in lead II is a sign of **left atrial enlargement**, classically due to **mitral stenosis**.

QT INTERVAL

- It represents the time taken for ventricular depolarization and repolarization, effectively the period of ventricular systole from ventricular isovolumetric contraction to isovolumetric relaxation.
- The QT varies with heart rate. It shortens at faster heart rates and lengthens at slower heart rates.
- An abnormally prolonged QT is associated with an increased risk of **Torsades de Pointes.**
- **Bazett's formula** to estimate QTc. $QT_C = QT / \sqrt{RR}$. The RR interval is given in seconds (RR interval = 60 / heart rate).

Shortened QT interval	Prolonged QT
▪ Hypercalcemia ▪ Digitalis / Digoxin ▪ Thyrotoxicosis - ↑ sympathetic activity ▪ Hyperthermia	▪ Hypokalemia; Hypomagnesemia; Hypocalcemia ▪ Class IA antiarrhythmics – Quinidine, Procainamide, Disopyramide ▪ Class III antiarrhythmics – Amiodarone, Sotalol, Ibutilide ▪ Hypothermia ▪ Chloroquine ▪ Romano-Ward syndrome – Congenital long QT syndrome without deafness

ST SEGMENT

ST Segment Elevation		ST Segment Depression
▪ Acute ischemia ▪ Myocardial infarction ▪ Prinzmetal Angina ▪ LV aneurysm ▪ Acute pericarditis ▪ Myocarditis	▪ Pulmonary embolism ▪ Hyperkalemia ▪ Hypercalcemia ▪ Hypothermia ▪ Early repolarization ▪ Brugada syndrome	▪ Ischemia ▪ LVH with strain ▪ Digoxin ▪ Hypokalemia

AV BLOCK

Feature	1° AV Block	2° AV Block (Mobitz Type I/Wenckebach)	2° AV Block (Mobitz Type II)	3°AV Block
Pathology	▪ Delay in conduction from AV node	▪ Intermittent failure of conduction via AV Node		▪ Complete block of conduction via AV Node
PR interval	▪ Prolonged (>0.20s) and Constant	▪ Progressive prolongation of PR interval till a QRS is dropped	▪ Normal and constant PR interval with intermittent QRS dropping	▪ Dissociation between P and QRS wave
Treatment	▪ No treatment in asymptomatic	▪ Pacemaker if symptomatic	▪ Pacemaker if symptomatic	▪ Implantable cardioverter defibrillator (ICD)

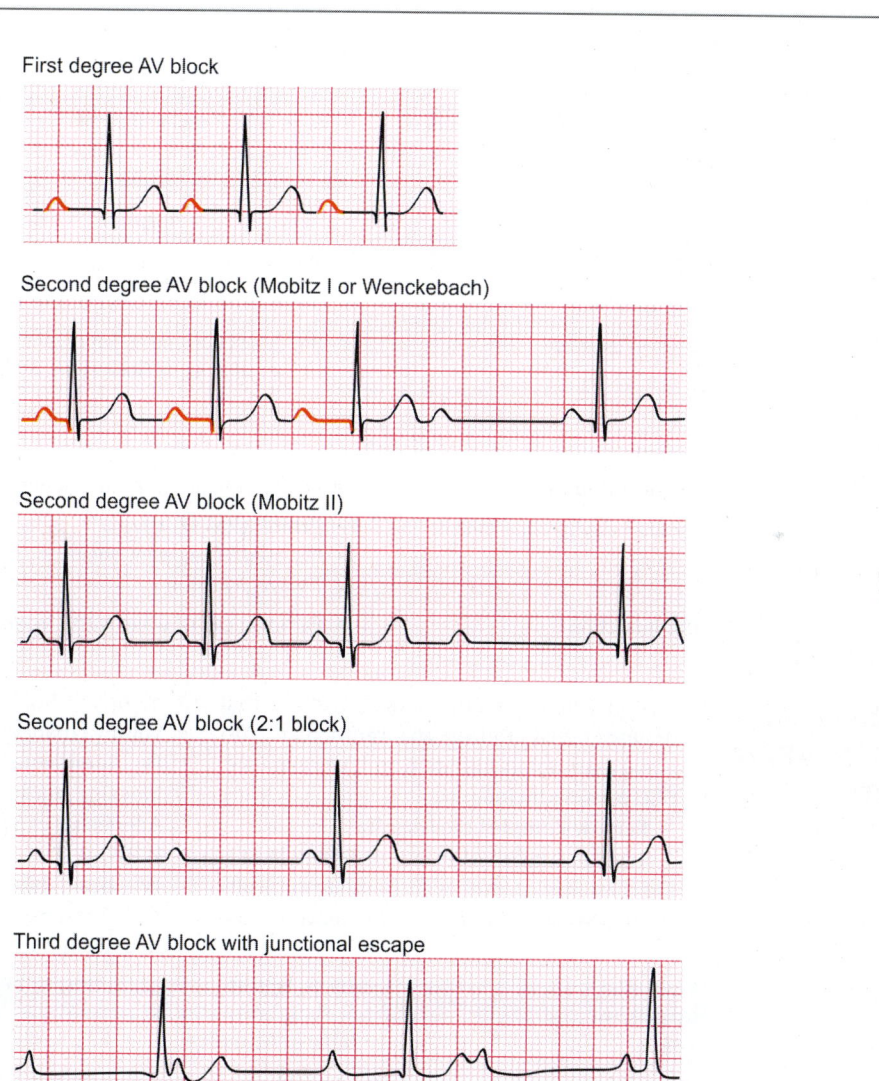

First degree AV block

Second degree AV block (Mobitz I or Wenckebach)

Second degree AV block (Mobitz II)

Second degree AV block (2:1 block)

Third degree AV block with junctional escape

FREQUENTLY ASKED ECGS

Cardiac tamponade	■ Electrical alternans, Low voltage ECG
Pericarditis (Acute)	■ Diffuse ST segment elevation with upwards concavity, usually present in all leads ■ PR segment depression or elevation is 'hallmark'
RBBB	■ **rSR'** seen in lead V_1, M pattern in V_1, Wide QRS
LBBB	■ Wide QRS complex with negative deflection
WPW syndrome	■ Short 'PR' interval (<120 ms) ■ Wide QRS with slurred slowly rising upstroke – **delta waves**
Right atrial enlargement (COPD, Acute PE, Cor pulmonale)	■ Tall, peaked P wave aka '**P-pulmonale**'
Left atrial enlargement (Mitral and Aortic valvular disease, Hypertension Cardiomyopathy)	■ Wide and notched 'P' wave aka 'P' mitrale
Atrial flutter	■ **Saw toothed** appearance
Brugada syndrome	■ RBBB like pattern with ST elevation in V_1-V_3
Wellens syndrome	■ Symmetrical deep T wave inversion in precordial leads esp. V_1-V_2
Ventricular premature complex (VPC)	■ Wide (>0.12 sec) and Bizarre premature QRS complex ■ Premature QRS is not preceded by a 'P' wave and is followed by a compensatory pause
Torsades de pointes	■ Marked **QT prolongation** → aka polymorphic VT
Hypothermia	■ **Osborne** waves/J waves
Digoxin effect	■ Reverse check or reverse tick or **Hockey stick** sign
Digoxin toxicity	■ VPC (Most Common), Supraventricular Tachycardia, Sinus bradycardia, Atrial fibrillation, AV block

ECG Evolution in Acute STEMI

Within minutes (Early acute phase)	■ Tall peaked T wave
Minutes – hours	■ Progression of ST segment elevation
Hours – days (Fully evolved)	■ Pathological 'Q' wave ■ Elevated ST segment begins to resolve ■ T wave inversion
Old infarction	■ Pathological 'Q' wave with T wave normalisation

SUPRAVENTRICULAR TACHYCARDIA [SVT/PSVT]

- SVT in general is any tachyarrhythmia that requires atrial and/or atrioventricular (AV) nodal tissue for its initiation and maintenance.
- ECG features include:
  - **Narrow-complex** tachycardia
  - Regular, rapid rhythm except AF and MAT
- The first-line treatment in hemodynamically stable patients includes vagal maneuvers, such as breath-holding, Carotid massage and the Valsalva maneuver.
- IV A**denosine** (**DOC**) acts by transiently blocking conduction in the AV node.
- Adenosine can precipitates AF in patients with WPW syndrome
- IV beta blockers and CCB (verapamil or diltiazem) can be given for long term management.

SVT vs VT

Features	Supraventricular Tachycardia	Ventricular Tachycardia
Origin	■ Atrial or AV node	■ Distal to bundle of his
Intensity of S_1	■ Constant	■ Fluctuates
QRS complex	■ <120 msec	■ >120 msec
Axis	■ Normal	■ Extreme axis deviation
Response to vagal maneuver	■ Yes	■ No
Response to Adenosine	■ Yes	■ No
Others	■ Triggered by premature P wave ■ No AV dissociation	■ Capture & fusion beat present ■ AV dissociation seen

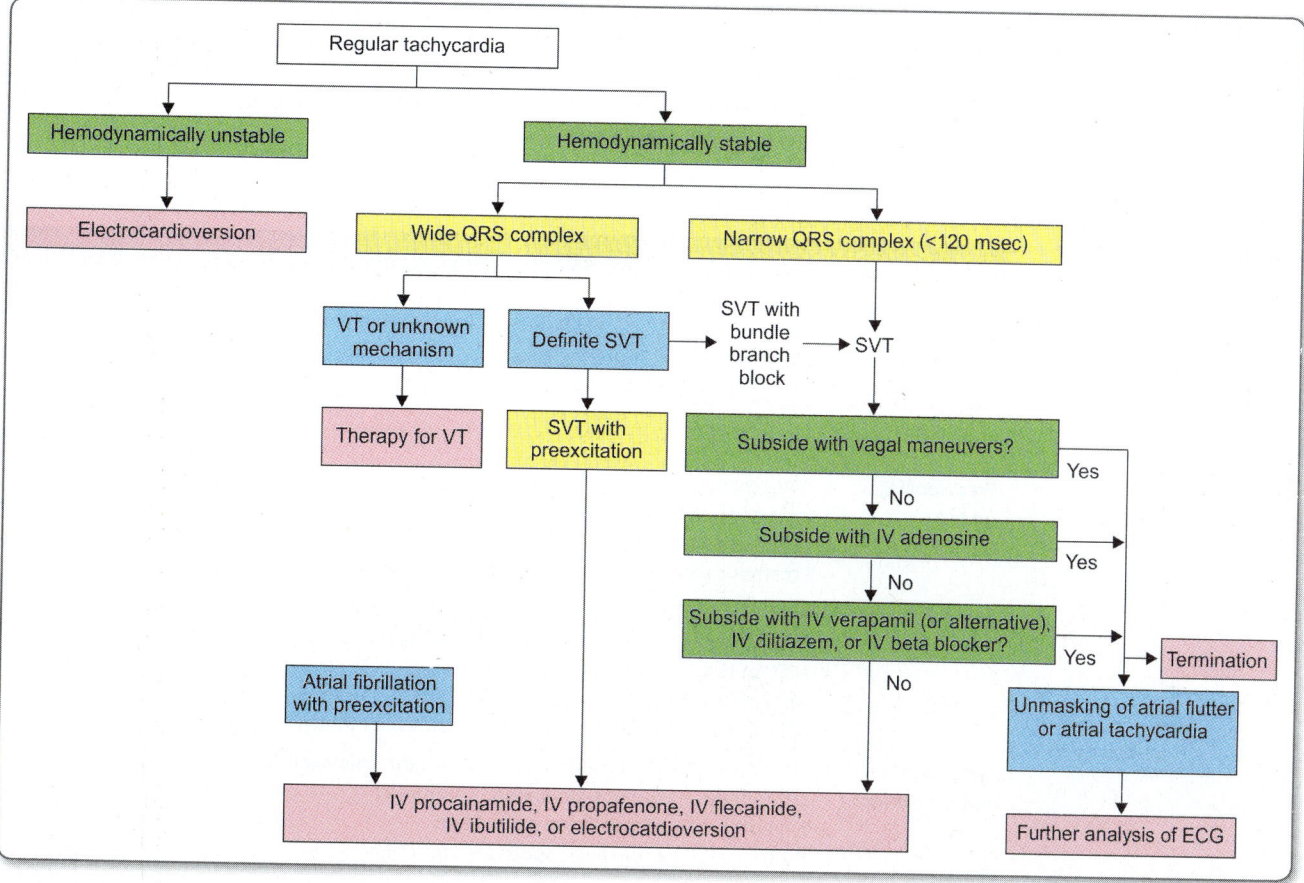

Multifocal Atrial Tachycardia (MAT)
- HR >100 bpm with irregular rhythm
- ECG – presence of ≥3 different P wave morphology

Atrial Flutter
- Atrial rate is around 250-350 bpm
- ECG – saw tooth flutter waves
- AV conduction block of 2:1 is usually seen

Atrial Fibrillation (AF)
- MC source of origin: pulmonary veins
- MC sustained arrhythmia in adults
- Etiology: CAD, Acute alcohol intoxication, cocaine, hyperthyroidism, Diabetes, Hypertension, Valvular heart diseases, Pulmonary embolism
- If duration of AF is unclear or is >48 hr, anticoagulation is done before cardioversion
- Drugs for rate control include beta blocker, CCB like Verapamil and Diltiazem and Digoxin
- Oral anticoagulants approved for stroke prevention in AF include Warfarin, Dabigatran, Rivaroxaban, Apixaban and Edoxaban.
- CHA_2DS_2-VASc scoring helps to estimate the risk of stroke in patients with non-rheumatic AF.

CARDIOMYO PATHY AND MYOCARDITIS

Features	Dilated	Restrictive	Hypertrophic
Ejection fraction	Usually <30%	25–50 %	>60%
Etiology	<ul><li>Alcohol</li><li>Chemotherapeutic agents<ul><li>Anthracyclines</li><li>Trastuzumab</li></ul></li><li>Nutritional deficiencies<ul><li>Thiamine</li><li>Selenium</li></ul></li><li>Trichinella spiralis</li><li>Peripartum cardiomyopathy</li></ul>	<ul><li>Amyloidosis</li><li>Hemochromatosis</li><li>Fabry's disease</li><li>Carcinoid syndrome</li><li>Hypereosinophilic syndrome (Loffler's endocarditis)</li><li>Sarcoidosis</li></ul>	<ul><li>Familial HCM<ul><li>AD disease</li></ul></li><li>Abnormal sympathetic stimulation</li></ul>

Takotsubo Cardiomyopathy

- Aka stress induced cardiomyopathy/apical ballooning syndrome / broken heart syndrome
- Occurs typically in older women after sudden intense emotional or physical stress
- Mechanism → stress induced catecholamines release

- Clinical presentation mimics ACS – chest pain, ST elevation & elevated cardiac biomarkers
- Angiography → LV apical ballooning without coronary artery stenosis

Alcohol Cardiotoxicity

Holiday Heart Syndrome	Dilated Cardiomyopathy
• Appears after an acute binge of alcohol • Present with arrhythmia. • MC arrhythmia: Atrial fibrillation • No previous history of heart disease	• With **C**hronic consumption of alcohol • Presents with heart failure

INFECTIVE ENDOCARDITIS

Predisposing factors	• IV drug abusers • Indwelling catheter • Bicuspid aortic valve • Prosthetic valve – risk of PVE is greatest during first 6–12 months
Etiology	• MCC of Infective Endocarditis (overall): **S. aureus** • MCC of Native Valve Endocarditis: *Streptococcus species* • MCC of IE in IV drug abusers: *S. aureus* • MCC of Prosthetic valve endocarditis: CoNS • MCC of early Prosthetic valve endocarditis (<2 months of valve surgery): *S. aureus*
Non cardiac manifestation	• Janeway lesions – Non-tender macule on the palms and soles • Osler nodes – Painful subcutaneous nodule • Splinter hemorrhage – seen on nail bed • Roth's spot – hemorrhagic spots seen in retina

Modified Duke Diagnostic Criteria

Definitive diagnosis of endocarditis:
- 2 Major criteria or
- 1 Major + 3 Minor criteria or
- 5 Minor criteria

Major criteria	• **Positive blood culture:** Typical organism from 2 separate blood cultures OR persistently positive blood culture drawn 12 hrs apart OR single positive blood culture for *C. burnetti*
	• **Evidence of endocardium involvement:**
	  ○ Echocardiogram evidence: mass, abscess or dehiscence of prosthetic valve
	  ○ Development of new valvular regurgitation

Minor criteria	• Predisposing heart conditions or IV drug use • Fever ≥38.0°C (≥100.4°F) • Vascular phenomena: Major arterial emboli, septic pulmonary infarcts, mycotic aneurysm, intracranial hemorrhage, conjunctival hemorrhages, janeway lesions • Immunologic phenomena: glomerulonephritis, Osler's nodes, Roth's spots, rheumatoid factor • Microbiologic evidence: Positive blood culture but not meeting major criterion.

IE Prophylaxis Indications

- Presence of prosthetic heart valve
- Prior h/o endocarditis

- Valvulopathy developing after cardiac transplantation
- Unrepaired cyanotic heart disease

CARDIAC FEATURES OF

Hypothyroidism	Hyperthyroidism	Pheochromocytoma	Cushing Syndrome
• **Bradycardia** • Raised DBP • Narrowed pulse pressure • Pericardial effusion • AV Block	• Tachycardia • Systolic hypertension with wide pulse pressure • **Atrial fibrillation**	• Severe hypertension • Postural hypotension	• Hypertension • LV hypertrophy

PERICARDIAL DISEASES

Features that distinguish cardiac tamponade from constrictive pericarditis and similar disorders

	Characteristic	Cardiac Tamponade	Constrictive Pericarditis	Restrictive Cardiomyopathy	RVMI
Clinical Examination	Pulsus paradoxus	Common	Usually absent	Rare	Rare
	Prominent y descent	Absent	Usually present	Rare	Rare
	Prominent x descent	Present	Usually present	Present	Rare
	Kussmaul's sign	Absent	Present	Absent	Present
	Third heart sound	Absent	Absent	Rare	May be present
	Pericardial knock	Absent	Present	Absent	Absent
ECG	Low ECG voltage	May be present	May be present	May be present	Absent
	Electrical alternans	May be present	Absent	Absent	Absent
Echocardiography	Thickened pericardium	Absent	Present	Absent	Absent
	Pericardial effusion	Present	Absent	Absent	Absent
	Pericardial calcification	Absent	Present	Absent	Absent
	RV size	Small	Normal	Normal	Enlarged
	Myocardial thickness	Normal	Normal	Usually increased	Normal
	Right atrial collapse	Present	Absent	Absent	Absent
CT	Thickened/calcific pericardium	Absent	Present	Absent	Absent

JONES CRITERIA (2015)

		Low-risk population	Moderate/High-risk population
	Definition	• ARF incidence ≤2 per 100000 school-aged children or all-age RHD prevalence of ≤1 per 10000 population year	• Children not clearly from a low-risk population
Major criteria	**Carditis**	• Clinical and/or **subclinical***	• Clinical and/or **subclinical***
	Arthritis	• Polyarthritis	• **Monoarthritis, Polyarthritis** and/or **Polyarthralgia**
		• Chorea	• Chorea
		• Erythema marginatum	• Erythema marginatum
		• Subcutaneous nodules	• Subcutaneous nodules
Minor criteria	**Carditis**	• Prolonged PR interval**	• Prolonged PR interval**
	Arthralgia	• Polyarthralgia	• **Monoarthralgia**
	Fever	• ≥38.5°C	• ≥38°C
	Markers of inflammation	• Peak ESR ≥60 mm in 1 h and/or CRP ≥3.0 mg/dL	• Peak ESR ≥30 mm in 1 h and/or CRP ≥3.0 mg/dL

Change compared with the 1992 revision are highlighted in bold
*Subclinical carditis → Seen only on echocardiography without ausculatory findings.
**Only if carditis is not counted as a major criteria

Evidence of Recent Group A Streptococcal Infection

- Positive throat culture or rapid streptococcal antigen test
- Elevated or increasing streptococcal antibody titre:
  ○ ASO titer >240 Todd U in adults and >320 Todd U in children
- Recent scarlet fever

2 Major or 1 Major + 2 Minor criteria along with evidence of recent infection makes the diagnosis of ARF.

ACUTE RHEUMATIC FEVER

Etiology	▪ Due to only pharyngeal (not skin) infection ▪ Caused by Group-A beta hemolytic streptococci (*S pyogenes*)
Sex	▪ F > M
Age group	▪ 5-15 Yrs
Pathology	▪ Immunologically mediated condition ▪ M protein is believed to be the virulence factor ▪ More common in low socioeconomic status
Clinical features	**MAJOR CRITERIA:** ▪ **Carditis:** 　○ Early clinical feature 　○ Occurs in 50-60% patient 　○ It is pancarditis i.e. involve all layers of heart 　○ Aschoff bodies are seen in atrial myocardium – Pathognomonic 　○ Most serious complication of ARF 　○ Mitral valve is almost always involved leading to MR and later MS. 　○ Associated with **C**arey **C**oomb's murmur (which is a **D**DM) **[Mn: CCD]** ▪ **Arthritis:** 　○ **Earliest** and **MC** clinical feature – present in 60-75% cases 　○ Classically described as **asymmetric** painful **Migratory** polyarthritis typically involving the large joints. 　○ Also include monoarthritis or polyarthralgia 　○ Non erosive/Non deforming 　○ Dramatic response to NSAIDS and salicylates ▪ **Erythema marginatum:** 　○ Early clinical feature 　○ Rarest manifestation 　○ Never present on face 　○ Transient & migratory in nature ▪ **Subcutaneous nodule:** 　○ Late manifestation 　○ Appears on bony prominences 　○ Non tender 　○ Almost always associated with Carditis ▪ **Chorea:** aka Sydenham chorea / St. Vitus' dance 　○ Late manifestation 　○ Aggravated by pregnancy 　○ Disappears during sleep **MINOR CRITERIA:** ▪ Fever ▪ Monoarthralgia (in the absence of arthritis)
Treatments	▪ Inj. Benzathine Penicillin single dose OR inj. Procaine penicillin BD for 10 days ▪ If Carditis present – steroids for 12 weeks ▪ In Penicillin allergic patient – Erythromycin ▪ None of the treatment is known to alter the likelihood of developing RHD ▪ DOC for secondary prophylaxis: Benzathine Penicillin every 4 or 3 weeks / Erythromycin (in allergic patient) **Duration of Secondary Prophylaxis:** ▪ *Only RF present:* 　○ 5 years or until age of 21, whichever is longer ▪ *RF + Carditis (with no residual heart disease):* 　○ 10 years ▪ *RF + Carditis + residual heart disease:* 　○ At least for 10 years after last episode 　○ At least till the age of 40 years 　○ Lifelong prophylaxis

ACUTE CORONARY SYNDROME

	Unstable Angina | NSTEMI	STEMI
Chest pain	▪ Severe & associated with sweating, dyspnea, epigastric discomfort, nausea etc ▪ Occurs at rest or with minimal exertion ▪ Lasts > 10 minutes ▪ Crescendo pattern ▪ Do not respond to rest or NTG	▪ Heaviness, squeezing or crushing type ▪ Occurs at rest ▪ Lasts > 30 min ▪ Typical radiation ▪ Levine sign +
ECG	▪ New ST segment depression ▪ New onset T wave inversion	▪ ST elevation
Biomarkers	▪ Normal | Increased in NSTEMI	▪ Increased

Treatment	▪ **M**orphine, **O**xygen, **N**itrates, **A**ntiplatelet
	▪ Beta blockers, Statins
	▪ Reperfusion therapy:
	  ○ PCI
	  ○ Thrombolysis – Contraindicated
		▪ **M**orphine, **O**xygen, **N**itrates, **A**ntiplatelet
		▪ Beta blockers, Statins
		▪ Reperfusion therapy:
		  ○ Primary PCI – preferred
		  ○ Thrombolysis within 12 hours

Cardiac Biomarkers

Cardiac Markers	Time of Elevation	Peaks	Normalize
Myoglobin	2-4 hrs	6-12 hrs	24-36 hrs
Troponin I/T	4-6 hrs	12-24 hrs	7-10 days
CK-MB	4-8 hrs	12-24 hrs	2-3 days

Thrombolysis in Acute MI

Absolute Contraindications	Relative Contraindications
▪ Prior intracranial hemorrhage ▪ Ischemic stroke within 3 months ▪ Head trauma within 3 months ▪ Severe hypertension uncontrolled with medications ▪ Suspected aortic dissection ▪ Active internal bleeding or bleeding diathesis excluding menses	▪ Prolonged CPR (>10 minutes) ▪ Major surgery within 3 weeks ▪ SBP > 180 mm Hg or DBP > 110 mm Hg ▪ Internal bleeding within 2-4 months ▪ Active peptic ulcer ▪ On anticoagulant with INR > 1.7

Prinzmetal's Variant Angina

- It is a syndrome of severe ischemic chest pain that usually occurs at rest
- Caused by focal spasm of an epicardial coronary artery resulting in transmural ischemia & abnormal LV function

- ECG – transient ST segment elevation.
- Pharmacotherapy – Nitrates and calcium channel blockers
- Aspirin can increase the severity of ischemic episodes

AORTIC DISSECTION

- Defined as separation of the layers within the aortic wall.
- Tears in the intimal layer → entry of blood between the intima and media → propagation of dissection
- **Etiology:**
  ○ Marfan syndrome
  ○ Ehlers Danlos syndrome
  ○ Bicuspid Aortic valve
  ○ Hypertension – MI factor
- **Sign and Symptoms:**
  ○ Sudden onset severe chest pain that has a tearing or ripping quality
  ○ Neck or jaw pain

  ○ Tearing or ripping intrascapular pain – may indicate dissection involving the descending aorta
  ○ Syncope
- **Physical examination:**
  ○ Asymmetrical pulses
  ○ Interarm BP difference ≥ 20 mm Hg
  ○ Signs of AR
- **Investigations:**
  ○ CXR: Widening of the mediastinum is the classic finding
  ○ Hemothorax → if dissection has ruptured
  ○ Contrast CT: definitive test
  ○ Echocardiography:
  ○ MRI: most sensitive method

HYPERTENSION GUIDELINES

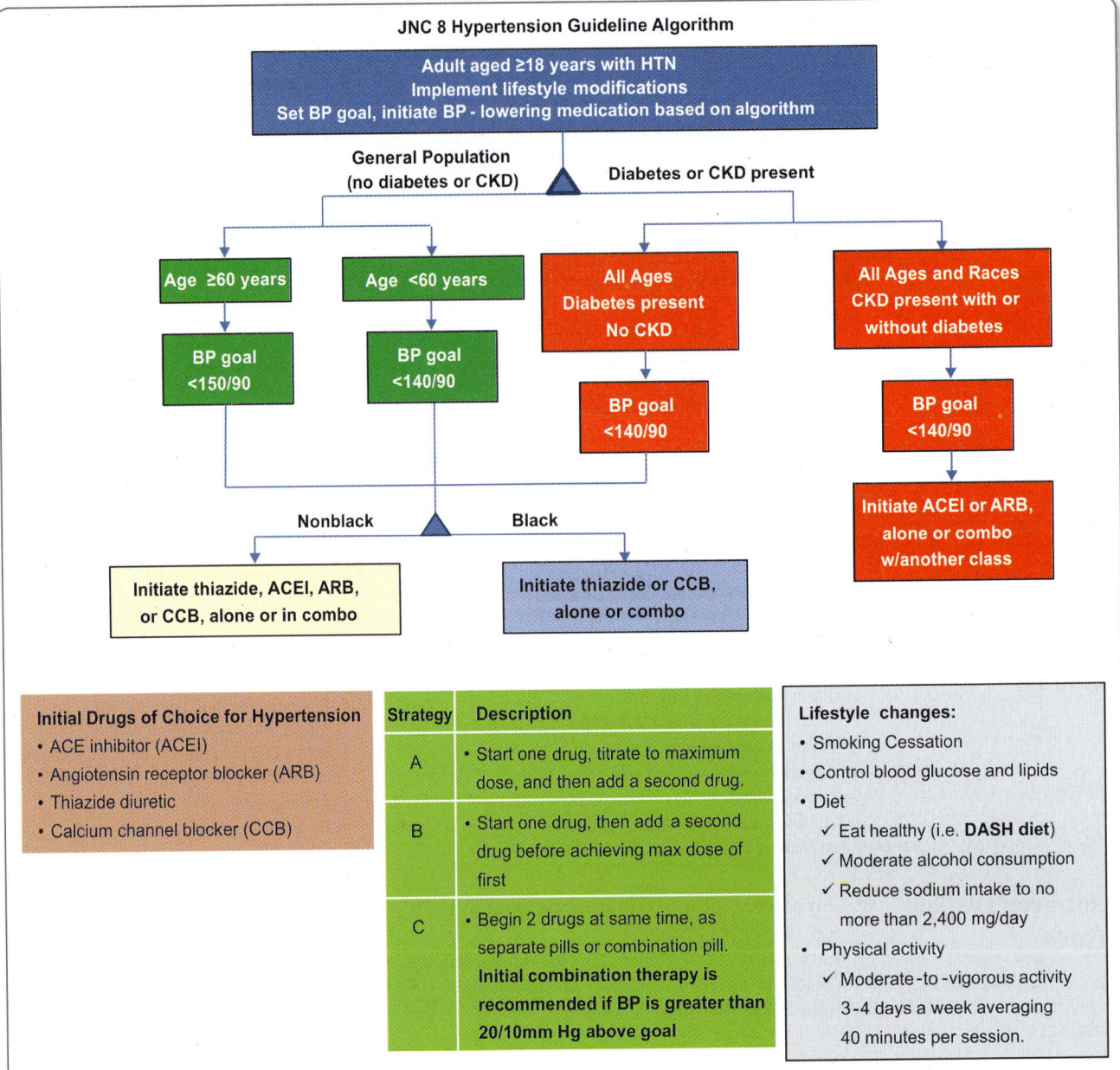

JNC 7

JNC 7		
	Systolic (mm Hg)	Diastolic (mm Hg)
Normal Blood Pressure	<120	<80
Prehypertension	120-139	80-89
Stage 1 hypertension	140-159	90-99
Stage 2 hypertension	≥160	≥100

ACC/AHA 2017

ACC/AHA 2017			
	Systolic (mm Hg)		Diastolic (mm Hg)
Normal Blood Pressure	<120	and	<80
Elevated	120-129	and	<80
Stage 1 hypertension	130-139	or	80-89
Stage 2 hypertension	≥140	or	≥90
Hypertensive Crisis	>180	and/or	>120
Target BP	<130/80 mm Hg for all patients		

PULMONARY HYPERTENSION

- Defined as mean PA pressure >25 mm Hg
- *Etiology*:
  - Idiopathic
  - BMPR2 & ALK 2 mutation
  - Scleroderma, COPD, ILD
- *Clinical features:*
  - Dyspnea – MC
  - Loud P2
  - Prominent A wave on JVP
- **MI screening test:** 2D echo with bubble study

Treatment

Class	Drugs	Mechanism of Action
Prostacyclin (PGI₂) analogues	Epoprostenol Treprostinil Iloprost	• cAMP mediated vasodilation • Antiproliferative effects on smooth muscle • Inhibits platelet aggregation.
Prostacyclin agonist	Selexipag	• Activates Prostacyclin receptor
PDE-5 inhibitors	Sildenafil Tadalafil Vardenafil	• cGMP mediated vasodilation and platelet inhibition
Endothelin (ET-1) receptor antagonist	Bosentan Macitentan	• Non-selective endothelin receptor antagonist
	Ambrisentan	• Selective ET-A receptor antagonist
	Riociguat	• Soluble guanylyl cyclase stimulator

CONGENITAL HEART DISEASE

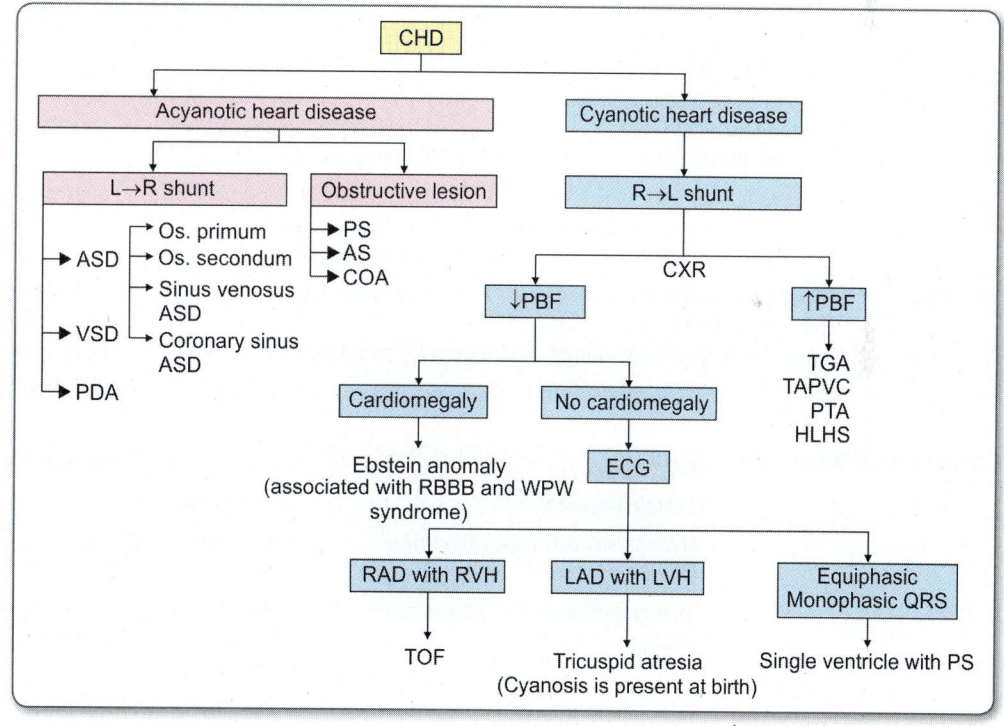

*PBF = Pulmonary blood flow

Nada's Criteria

Major	Minor
▪ Systolic murmur ≥ grade 3 (thrill)	▪ Systolic murmur <grade 3
▪ Diastolic murmur	▪ Abnormal S₂
▪ Cyanosis	▪ Abnormal BP
▪ CHF	▪ Abnormal ECG
*Presence of 1 Major or 2 minor criteria indicates high probability of CHD	▪ Abnormal CXR

ACYANOTIC HEART DISEASE

	Ostium Secundum ASD	Ostium Primum ASD	VSD
General	▪ MC type of ASD ▪ Located at fossa ovalis ▪ Usually asymptomatic in infancy and childhood	▪ Defect present in lower portion of atrial septum and in anterior leaflet of mitral valve ▪ Therefore ASD + MR are seen	▪ MC congenital heart disease ▪ Located mostly in membranous part of inter ventricular septum ▪ VSD in muscular part has good prognosis
Associated Conditions	▪ Lutembacher syndrome (ASD + MS) ▪ Holt-Oram syndrome (ASD+1° AV block+ hypoplastic /absent radius) ▪ TAR syndrome ▪ Ellis van Creveld syndrome	▪ DOWN syndrome is associated with endocardial cushion defect.	▪ Associated with risk of AR. Max. risk is seen in supra crystal type of VSD ▪ One of the components of TOF
Clinical features	▪ Mostly asymptomatic ▪ No risk of CCF during infancy	▪ Features of MR present ▪ CCF in infancy	▪ Recurrent chest infection (d/t ↑PBF) ▪ CCF around 6-10 weeks
Infective endocarditis	▪ Rare	▪ Rare	▪ MC CHD to be complicated by IE ▪ Clubbing in a patient with VSD suggests IE
S_1	▪ Loud	▪ Loud	▪ Masked by PSM
S_2	▪ Widely split and fixed ▪ Loud P_2	▪ Widely split and fixed ▪ Loud P_2	▪ Wide and variable split ▪ Loud P_2 suggest PAH
Murmur	▪ Shunt murmur-Absent/ silent ▪ ESM at pulmonary area	▪ Apical PSM of MR	▪ Shunt murmur-PSM
CXR	▪ Relatively small aortic shadow ▪ Plethoric lung field	▪ Plethoric lung field	▪ Prominent main PA segment ▪ Plethoric lung field
Heart size	▪ LA – normal (if LA is enlarge then exclude the diagnosis) ▪ RA and RV enlarged	▪ LA – increase in size d/t MR ▪ Marked cardiomegaly d/t MR ▪ RA and RV enlarged	▪ Normal ▪ LA enlarged in moderate to large VSD
ECG	▪ RVH with RAD, Tall P wave ▪ rSR pattern in the precordial leads is the hallmark feature	▪ LAD (d/t mal development of Left Bundle Branch) ▪ 1° AV block	▪ Suggestive of LVH ▪ In large VSD – biventricular hypertrophy
Treatments	▪ Surgery at 1-4 yrs of age, earlier if $Q_p : Q_s$ (Pulmonary to systemic blood flow ratio) > 1.5 ▪ Development of Eisenmenger syndrome is C/I to surgery		▪ Small holes close spontaneously ▪ Small, hemodynamically insignificant VSD is not an indication for surgery ▪ Supracrystal VSD – operate ASAP

Corrective Procedure

CHD	Corrective Procedure
Ebstein anomaly	▪ Starnes procedure
Hypoplastic Left Heart Syndrome [HLHS]	▪ Norwood/Sano procedure
Transposition of the Great Arteries [TGA]	▪ Jantene's repair → Arterial switching is done ▪ Mustard or Senning operation in dTGA → Atrial switching done
Tricuspid atresia [TA]	▪ Bidirectional Glenn shunt ▪ Modified Fontane operation
Double Outlet Right Ventricle with PS	▪ Rastelli procedure

Important Signs

Signs	Congenital Heart Disease
Reverse 3 sign on barium meal	**COA**
Box shaped cardiomegaly	**Ebstein anomaly**
Coeur-en-sabot / boot shaped heart	**TOF**
Egg on end appearance	**TGA**
Snowman/ figure of 8 appearance o CXR	**TAPVC**

	Patent Ductus Arteriosus	Coarctation of Aorta	Aortic Sclerosis

General	▪ F > M
	▪ It is a risk factor for the development of:
	  ○ Necrotizing Enterocolitis
	  ○ Pulmonary hemorrhage
		▪ MC located distal to left Subclavian artery
		▪ Common in Turner syndrome
		▪ Two types: - preductal or infantile type
		  -post ductal or adult type
			▪ Pulsus parvus et tardus and pulsus alternans seen

Associated condition	▪ Congenital Rubella Syndrome – MC cardiac lesion in CRS	▪ Bicuspid aortic valve in 70% ▪ Shone complex (COA+MS+AS)	▪ Supravalvular AS is associated with **William's syndrome**

Clinical features	▪ Symptoms similar to aorto-pulmonary window
	▪ Bounding arterial pulse due to ↑ stroke volume
	▪ Wide pulse pressure
	▪ CO_2 retention
	▪ Differentia cyanosis if PAH develops
	▪ CCF around 6 – 10 weeks
	▪ MCC of death → CCF
		▪ Disparity in pulse and BP (UL > LL)
		▪ Weak/ absent pulsation in LL
		▪ Radio-femoral delay present (good femoral pulse rules out COA)
		▪ Headache
		▪ Intermittent claudication
		▪ Hypertension d/t RAS
		▪ CCF
			▪ Exertional dyspnea–MC
			▪ Angina, Syncope, Heart failure
			▪ Features of severe AS:
			  ○ Narrow pulse pressure
			  ○ Later peak of ESM
			  ○ Paradoxical splitting of S_2

Infective endocarditis	▪ Seen	▪ Seen	▪ Seen
S_1	▪ Normal	▪ Loud	▪ Normal
S_2	▪ Normal or paradoxical split	▪ Loud	▪ Paradoxical split
Murmur	▪ **Continuous** machinery murmur → best heard at 2nd left ICS/ infraclavicular	▪ Continuous murmur in postductal type	▪ Systolic murmur that radiates to carotid
ECG	▪ LVH	▪ LVH	▪ Normal/LVH
CXR	▪ Plethoric lung fields ▪ Dilatation of ascending aorta ▪ Cardiomegaly ▪ Prominence of main PA segment	▪ **Reverse 3 sign** or double bulge sign on barium swallow ▪ **Inferior** rib notching is seen after 6-10 yrs d/t increase blood flow k/a **Roesler sign**. It gets autocorrected once COA is treated.	▪ Normal heart size
Treatments	▪ Medical management is done in preterm by Indomethacin/ Ibuprofen ▪ No role of medical management in term PDA ▪ Spontaneous closure is rare in term/post term infants ▪ To keep PDA patent- PGE_1 is used ▪ Development of Eisenmenger syndrome is C/I to surgery	▪ PGE_1 **(Alprostadil)** infusion to keep the ductus arteriosus open ▪ Urgent surgical intervention in symptomatic neonate	▪ Development of symptoms is an indication for AVR (AV valve replacement) ▪ Percutaneous aortic Balloon valvuloplasty in patient who cannot undergo AVR
Complication	▪ Pulmonary hypertension	▪ Dissection of aorta ▪ Rupture of berry intracranial aneurysm	▪ Sudden cardiac death

Extra edge	▪ Unmasking of DDM indicates impending Eisenmenger syndrome	▪ In post ductal COA blood flow to the LL is via collateral formation mainly through
		  ○ Intercostal artery
		  ○ Superior epigastric artery
			▪ S_4 can be present
			▪ Ejection click heard

Shunt Procedures In TOF

Shunt	Procedure
Blalock-Taussig shunt	Between Subclavian Artery & I/L Pulmonary artery
Waterston's shunt	Between ascending Aorta & right Pulmonary Artery
Potts shunt	Between descending aorta & left Pulmonary Artery

CYANOTIC HEART DISEASE

	Tetralogy of Fallot	Tricuspid Atresia	Ebstein Anomaly
General	■ **Components :** ○ Infundibular stenosis (most basic lesion) ○ RVH ○ VSD ○ Overriding/ dextraposed aorta	■ There is congenital absence of the TV therefore RV is hypoplastic ■ For exit of blood from RA, there is patent foramen ovale /ASD ■ PBF is dependent on size of VSD which is always muscular	■ Downward displacement of TV in RV l/t atrialization of RV ■ Leaflet anomaly leads to TR
Associated conditions	■ Pentalogy of Fallot (TOF + ASD) ■ Trilogy of Fallot: ASD + RVH + PS ■ Right sided aortic arch in 20% ■ CATCH-22 syndrome ■ Persistence of left SVC may be seen	■ ASD ■ VSD ■ PDA	■ ASD (leading to cyanosis) ■ Lithium intake in 1st trimester ■ WPW syndrome
Clinical features	■ MC cyanotic CHD ■ MC cyanotic CHD to be ass. with IE ■ No CCF ■ Pt. do not have cyanosis in Pink TOF (VSD + MILD PS) ■ Cyanosis is absent at birth	■ Prominent large a wave in JVP ■ Enlarged liver with presystolic pulsation ■ CCF at birth ■ Cyanosis present at birth	■ Cyanosis and clubbing ■ CCF seen ■ Cyanosis may be present at birth
S_1	■ N	■ Single loud S_1	■ Widely split, Loud T_1
S_2	■ Single, only loud A_2	■ Single or normal split	■ May be Wide and variable
Murmur	■ Shunt murmur of VSD is absent ■ Pulmonary ESM ■ Intensity of murmur is inversely proportional to severity	■ PSM (due to blood flow from VSD)	■ Holosystolic murmur of TR which increase in intensity during inspiration
CXR	■ Normal sized heart ■ Coeur-en-sabot (boot shaped heart) ■ Oligemic lung field ■ Absence of main PA segment	■ Oligemic lung fields	■ Cardiomegaly ■ Box shaped heart ■ Large Right atrium ■ Oligemic lung field
ECG	■ RVH + RAD ■ P-pulmonale	■ LVH + LAD	■ RBBB with rSR' pattern ■ P-pulmonale, P-mitrale ■ Prolonged PR interval
Treatments	■ Cyanotic spells/tet spells/hypoxic spells: ○ Knee chest position ○ **M**orphine, **O**$_2$, **N**aHCO$_3$ ○ **P**ropranolol, **E**smolol ○ **P**henyl ephrine (**Mn** : MONa PEP) ■ **Shunt procedures:** ○ Blalock taussig shunt ○ Waterston shunt ■ To keep ductusarteriosus patent: ○ PG (Alprostadil)	■ Blalock – Taussig procedure ■ Bidirectional Glenn shunt ■ Modified Fontane operation ■ (**Mn:** fon**TA**n) ■ Infusion of PGE$_1$ to keep ductus arteriosus patent	■ Starnes procedure
Complication	■ Cerebral thrombosis in <2 yrs ■ Brain abscess in >2 yrs ■ Delayed puberty	■ IE	■ IE ■ CCF
Extra edge	Ductal dependent lesion	■ Ductal dependent lesion	■ Ductal dependent lesion

Closure Time

	Ductus Arteriosus	Foramen Ovale
Functional	10-15 hours	Immediately
Anatomical	10-21 days	3rd month

	Transposition of Great Arteries	TAPVC	HLHS
General	**Types:** ○ Complete TGA (d-TGA) ○ Physiologically corrected TGA (l-TGA)	**Types:** ○ Supracardiac- MC type ○ Cardiac ○ Infra cardiac	• LV ill developed due to closed mitral valve • Marked hypoplasia of LV & ascending aorta
Clinical features	• d-TGA with intact ventricular septum: ○ Cyanosis is present within 24 hrs ○ CCF – 1st week of life • TGA with VSD : ○ CCF around 4-10th week • Loud single S_2	• TAPVC may be associated with pulmonary venous obstruction • Cyanosis is present within 24 hrs • CCF within 1 – 2 weeks of age • PaO_2 in PA > Aorta • Reverse differential cyanosis in supracardiac type • Wide and fixed spit S_2 (like ASD)	• Patient presents in Shock within the first few days of life d/t closure of ductus arteriosus
CXR	• Plethoric lung fields • Egg on string/egg in a cup appearance • Cardiomegaly with narrow base	• Plethoric lung fields • Snowman/Figure of 8 appearance in supra cardiac • Ground glass appearance if associated with pulmonary venous obstruction	• Cardiomegaly • Plethoric lung fields
Treatments	• Arterial switch (Jantene's repair) is the TOC • Atrial switch procedure (Mustard or Senning operation) – dTGA	• PGE_1 to keep ductus arteriosus patent in obstructive type	• PGE_1 to keep ductus patent • Norwood or Sano procedure
Extra edge	• Ductal dependent lesion • In d-TGA the aorta is anterior and to the right of the PA.	• Ductal dependent lesion • Infracardiac type of TAPVC is always obstructive in nature	• Ductal dependent lesion

SYNDROMES ASSOCIATED WITH CONGENITAL HEART DISEASES

Syndromes	Genetic Defect	Most Common CHD	Other Important Features
Patau syndrome	Trisomy 13	VSD	Mental retardation, Cleft lip and palate, Polydactyly, Microcephaly, Short neck
Edward syndrome	Trisomy 18	VSD	Cleft lip and palate, Microcephaly, Micrognathia
Down syndrome	Trisomy 21	Endocardial cushion defect/ AV canal defect	Mental retardation, Clinodactyly
Turner syndrome	45, XO	Bicuspid aortic valve > COA	Short stature, Webbed neck, Shield chest
Noonan syndrome	*PTPN11* mutation	Valvular PS	Hypertelorism, Triangular shaped face
Alagille syndrome	Mutation in ***JAG1*** or ***NOTCH2***	Peripheral PS	Prolonged neonatal jaundice, Dysmorphic face, Posterior embryotoxon
William's syndrome	Deletion of 7q	Supravalvular AS	Elfin facies
VACTERL	No specific defect	VSD	Vertebral defect, Anal atresia, Tracheo-esophageal fistula, Renal abnormalities
CHARGE	*CHD7* gene mutation	Conotruncal abnormalities like AS	Coloboma, Choanal atresia, growth retardation, Ear malformation
Congenital Rubella syndrome		PDA > PS > VSD	Sensorineural hearing loss (MC), Cataract, Salt and pepper retinopathy, Blueberry muffin spot
Holt-Oram syndrome		Ostium Secundum ASD	Limb deformity
DiGeorge Syndrome [Mn: CATCH 22]	Microdeletion in **22**q11	**C**onotruncal defects like TOF, Truncus arteriosus	**A**bnormal facies, **T**hymic hypoplasia, **C**left palate, **H**ypoparathyroidism, **H**ypocalcemia,

MULTIPLE CHOICE QUESTIONS

CHAPTER 1: CARDIOLOGY

CLINICAL EXAMINATION

PULSES

1. Dicrotic pulse is seen in? *(PGMEE 2014-15)*
- a. HOCM
- b. DCM
- c. RCM
- d. Left ventricular failure

[Ref: Harrison 20th ed. pg. 1670]

2. Pulsus alterans is seen in? *(PGMEE 2014-15)*
- a. Anterior wall MI
- b. Bronchial asthma
- c. Critical aortic stenosis
- d. Constrictive pericarditis

[Ref: Harrison 20th ed. pg. 1670]

JVP

3. In JVP 'y' descent is absent and 'x' wave is prominent? This is suggestive of: *(PGMEE 2015-16)*
- a. Restictive cardiomyopathy
- b. Cardiac tamponade
- c. Constrictive pericarditis
- d. Right Ventricular Failure

[Ref: Harrison 20th ed. pg. 1669]

4. Internal jugular vein pressure determines pressure of: *(PGMEE 2015-16)*
- a. RA
- b. RV
- c. LA
- d. LV

[Ref: Harrison 20th ed. pg. 1668]

5. 'a wave' in JVP is absent in: *(PGMEE 2015-16)*
- a. Atrial fibrillation
- b. Heart block
- c. Tricuspid regurgitation
- d. Complete heart block

[Ref: Harrison 20th ed. pg. 1668]

6. Canon 'a' waves are seen in: *(PGMEE 2015-16)*
- a. Atrial fibrillation
- b. Complete heart block
- c. Constrictive pericarditis
- d. Cardiac tamponade

[Ref: Harrison 20th ed. pg. 1668]

7. C- wave in jugular venous pressure curve is formed due to *(PGMEE 2018)*
- a. Contraction of atria against resistance
- b. Bulging of tricuspid valve into Rt atrium during isovolumetric contraction
- c. Due to venous filling
- d. Atria relaxed and tricuspid valve moves down

[Ref: Harrison 20th ed. pg. 1668]

HEART SOUNDS

8. Reverse split S2 is seen in *(PGMEE 2015-16)*
- a. Aortic stenosis
- b. Mitral stenosis
- c. Pulmonary artery hypertension
- d. Pulmonic stenosis

[Ref: Harrison 20th ed. pg. 1671]

9. All form boundaries of triangle of auscultation except? *(PGMEE 2014-15)*
- a. Trapezius
- b. Latissmus dorsi
- c. Scapula
- d. Rhomboid major

[Ref: PJ Mehta Clinical Methods]

10. Which is the location of Erb's point during auscultation?
- a. 2nd intercostal space right parasternal line
- b. 2nd intercostal space left parasternal line
- c. 3rd intercostal space left parasternal line
- d. 5th intercostal space left parasternal line

[Ref: PJ Mehta's Clinical Methods]

11. Which is not a high pitched heart sound: *(PGMEE 2014-15)*
- a. Mid systolic click
- b. Pericardial shudder
- c. Opening snap
- d. Tumor plop sound

[Ref: Harrison 20th ed. pg. 1672]

12. Loud P2 is found in? *(PGMEE 2014-15)*
- a. Pulmonary HTN
- b. MS
- c. MR
- d. Aortic incompetence

[Ref: Harrison 20th ed. pg. 1672]

MURMURS

13. Which murmur increases on standing? *(NEET 2019)*
- a. MS
- b. VSD
- c. HOCM
- d. MR

14. Which murmur decreases on standing *(PGMEE 2019)*
- a. HOCM
- b. Aortic Stenosis
- c. Both
- d. None

Explanation

Effect of Physiological Maneuvers on Murmur

Manuever	Aortic Stenosis	HOCM
Supine	↑	↓
Standing	↓	↑
Valsalva	↓	↑
Deep Inspiration	↑	↓
Deep Expiration	↓	↑

1.	b
2.	a
3.	b
4.	a
5.	a
6.	b
7.	b
8.	a
9.	d
10.	c
11.	d
12.	a
13.	c
14.	b

15. Severity of mitral stenosis is best identified by:
(PGMEE 2015-16)
a. Loud S1
b. Gap between S_2 opening snap
c. Duration of mid-diastolic murmur
d. Intensity of mid-diastolic murmur

[Ref: Harrison 20th ed. pg. 1672]

16. Murmur heard in aortic stenosis? *(PGMEE 2015-16)*
a. Right 2nd intercostal, low pitch murmur
b. Apex, low pitch murmur
c. Left Sternal area, low pitch murmur
d. Pan-systolic murmur, high pitch murmur

[Ref: Harrison 20th ed. pg. 1805]

17. Continuous murmur is seen in all except:
a. PDA *(PGMEE 2014-15)*
b. Ruptured sinus of Valsalva aneurysm
c. Aortic pulmonary window
d. None

[Ref: Harrison 20th ed. pg. 1674]

18. All are true about Physiological murmur EXCEPT:
(PGMEE 2014-15)
a. Only Diastolic murmur
b. Midsystolic murmur
c. Present in child with anemia
d. Not audible without stethoscope

[Ref: Harrison 20th ed. pg. 1673]

19. Systolic murmur is associated with? *(PGMEE 2014-15)*
a. Ejection click
b. Opening snap
c. S4
d. Pericardial knock

[Ref: Harrison 20th ed. pg. 1672]

DISORDERS OF RHYTHM

BASICS OF ELECTROPHYSIOLOGY

20. Normal axis of heart is? *(DNB June 2009)*
a. -30 to +90
b. 60 to –60
c. +90 to 120
d. +120 to –30

[Ref: Harrison 20th ed. pg. 1676]

21. In LVH, SV1 + RV6 is more than .... mm?
(PGMEE 2014-15)
a. 25
b. 30
c. 35
d. 40

[Ref: EGG problem 3rd edition John R. Hampton; Harrison's 20th/e pg. 1677]

22. Epsilon wave is seem in:
(PGMEE 2014-15, 2015-16, 2016-17)
a. WPW syndrome
b. Brugada syndrome
c. Hypothermia
d. Arrhythmogenic right ventricular dysplasia

[Ref: Harrison 20th ed. pg. 1720]

Explanation

■ Epsilon wave is a small positive deflection seen at the end of QRS complex, in ARVD - Arrhythmogenic Right Ventricular Dysplasia.

23. 30 to -60 degree axis deviation indicates:-
(PGMEE 2015-16)
a. Normal Cardiac Axis
b. Extreme Right Axis Deviation
c. Left Axis Deviation
d. Right Axis Deviation

[Ref: Harrison 20th ed. pg. 1676]

24. Low voltage in ECG indicates? *(PGMEE 2014-15)*
a. Pulmonary embolism
b. Cor pulmonale
c. Infective endocarditis
d. Pericardial effusion

[Ref: Harrison 20th ed. pg. 1682]

25. Low voltage ECG is seen in? *(PGMEE 2014-15)*
a. Hypothyroidism
b. Hyperthyroidism
c. Diabetes
d. Addison's disease

26. Electrical alterans is seen in? *(PGMEE 2014-15)*
a. Cardiac tamponade
b. Constrictive pericarditis
c. Severe LVF
d. Severe RVF

[Ref: Harrison 20th ed. pg. 1682]

Explanation

■ Classical triad for pericardial effusion with cardiac tamponade:
○ Sinus tachycardia
○ Low voltage QRS colplex
○ Electrial alternans

27. Left axis deviation is seen in all except?
(PGMEE 2014-15)
a. Left anterior hemi block
b. Inferior wall MI
c. ASD (Septum secundum)
d. Right pneumothorax

[Ref: Harrison 20th ed. pg. 1677]

ST SEGMENT CHANGES

28. Reciprocal changes in ECG in patients with inferior wall myocardial infarction are seen in which lead?
(NEET Pattern 2019)
a. I
b. II
c. III
d. IV

29. ECG shown below depicts *(PGMEE 2016-17)*

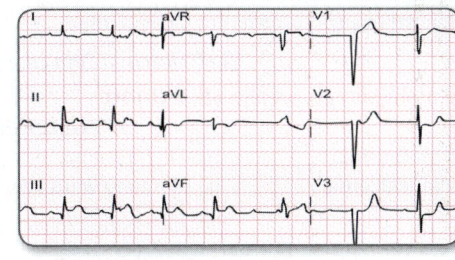

a. Lateral wall ischemia
b. Inferior wall MI with AV block
c. Anterior wall ischemia
d. Posterior wall MI

[Ref: Harrison 20th ed. pg. 1680]

30. **A 65-year old man presents with crushing chest pain for 2 hours. On examination BP = 80/60 mmHg and JVP is elevated 4 cm above the sternal angle. All are true about the condition shown EXCEPT:**
    a. ST elevation in V4R
    b. ST segment depression in lead II, III, aVF
    c. Right ventricular infarction
    d. Cardiogenic shock

    [Ref: Harrison 20th ed. pg. 1882]

Explanation

- Diagnosis → Right ventricle MI presenting with hypotention likely due to cardiogenic shock.
- ECG → ST elevation in right precordial leads (V4R)
- Note: ST depression in II, III, aVF is a reciprocal change seen in high lateral MI (a/w ST elevation in I. aVL)

31. **Persistent ST segment elevation 24 hours after treatment for MI with P.C.I is due to** *(PGMEE 2014-15)*
    a. Left ventricular aneurysm
    b. Impending cardiac rupture
    c. Dressler syndrome
    d. Coronary artery dissection

    [Ref: Harrison 20th ed. pg. 1681]

32. **ST elevation is seen in all of the following conditions EXCEPT:** *(PGMEE 2014-15)*
    a. Myocardial infarction
    b. Coronary artery spasm
    c. Constrictive pericarditis
    d. Ventricular aneurysm

    [Ref: Harrison 20th ed. pg. 1681]

33. **ST segment elevation in ECG is not seen in?**
    (DNB June 2010)
    a. Hyperkalaemia
    b. Pericarditis
    c. Hypocalcaemia
    d. Hypothermia

    [Ref: Harrison 20th ed. pg. 1681]

QT INTERVAL

34. **Congenital long QT syndrome causes death due to?**
    (PGMEE 2014-15)
    a. Complete heart block
    b. Polymorphic ventricular tachycardia
    c. Acute myocardial infarction
    d. Recurrent supraventricular tachycardia

    [Ref: Harrison 20th ed. pg. 1761]

35. **QT prolongation is seen in all, EXCEPT:**
    (PGMEE 2014-15)
    a. Hypothermia   b. Digitalis toxicity
    c. Hypocalcemia   d. Romano ward syndrome

    [Ref: Harrison 20th ed. pg. 1761]

36. **Which of the following drug causes prolongation of QT interval:-** *(PGMEE 2018)*
    a. Rifampicin   b. Quinidine
    c. Cisapride   d. Chloroquine

    [Ref: Harrison 20th ed. pg. 1761]

37. **QT interval is shortened in:** *(PGMEE 2014-15)*
    a. Hypocalcemia   b. Hypokalemia
    c. Hypercalcemia   d. Digoxin

    [Ref: Harrison 20th ed. pg. 1765]

QTC PROLONGATION (TORSADESDES POINTES)

38. **True about Torsades de pointes?** *(PGMEE 2014-15)*
    a. ST segment depression
    b. QTc prolongation
    c. Narrow qRS Complex
    d. PQ segment elevation

    [Ref: Harrison 20th ed. pg. 1760]

WPW SYNDROME

39. **Which of these statements is true for Bundle of Kent?**
    (NEET 2019)
    a. It is slower than AV nodal pathway
    b. An abnormal pathway between the two atria
    c. It is muscular or nodal pathway between atria and ventricle in WPW
    d. None

40. **Bundle of Kent is:** *(NEET 2018)*
    a. Accessory conduction pathway between the atria and ventricles
    b. Seen in WPW syndrome
    c. Responsible for formation of re-entry circuits leading to tachyarrhythmias
    d. All are true

    [Ref: Harrison's 19th/e pg. 1481]

Explanation

Bundle of Kent

- Are abnormal extra or accessory pathway between the atria and the ventricles, in addition to the AV node. This accessory pathway is k/as the bundle of Kent.
- Usually seen in WPW syndrome.
- This pathway may communicate between the left atrium and the left ventricle, in which case it is termed a "type A pre-excitation", or between the right atrium and the right ventricle, in which case it is termed a "type B pre-excitation".
- When an aberrant electrical connection is made via the bundle of Kent → tachydysrhythmias may result.
- Compared to AV node, the bundle of Kent lacks the capability of slowing the rate of conduction of electrical impulses.

41. **Which of the following statements is true about the bundle of kent?** *(PGMEE 2019)*
    a. Accessory pathway between the atria and ventricle with short refractory period
    b. Accessory pathway between the atria and ventricle with long refractory period
    c. Accessory pathway between two atria with short refractory period
    d. It is slower than the AV nodal pathway

    [Ref: Harrison's 19th/e pg. 1481]

30.	b
31.	a
32.	c
33.	c
34.	b
35.	b
36.	b,d
37.	c,d
38.	b
39.	c
40.	d
41.	a

42. ECG given below is showing:- *(PGMEE 2016-17)*

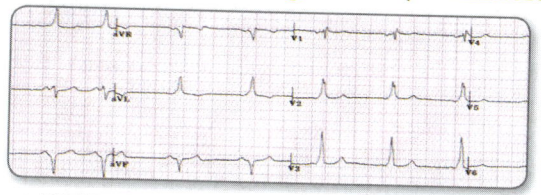

a. Wolf Parkinson White syndrome
b. PSVT
c. Long QT syndrome
d. Mobiz type 1 block

[Ref: Harrison 20th ed. pg. 1741]

Explanation

- ECG shows 'PR' interval with delta wave

43. PR interval is reduced in? *(PGMEE 2014-15)*
a. Wenckebach phenomenon
b. WPW syndrome
c. Hypothyroidism
d. Complete heart block

[Ref: Harrison 20th ed. pg. 1741]

44. All are true about WPW syndrome except?
a. More common in females *(PGMEE 2014-15)*
b. Delta wave in ECG
c. HIS bundle study is done for diagnosis
d. Can occur in a normal heart

[Ref: Harrison 20th ed. pg. 1740]

BRUGADA SYNDROME

45. What is incorrect about Brugada syndrome?
a. SCN5A defect *(PGMEE 2014-15)*
b. Asymptomatic ST segment elevation
c. Sudden death
d. Pacemaker is treatment of choice

[Ref: Harrison 20th ed. pg. 1761]

Explanation

- Brugada syndrome is SCN5A defect Sodium channelopathy that may head to sudden cardiac death. It is also known as Pokkuri Death Syndrome or SUNDS (Sudden Unexpected Nocturnal Death Syndrome). ECG shows ST elevation in leads V_{1-3}. Treatment of choice is a implantable cardiac defibrillator (ICD).

ECG CHANGES IN DYSELECTROLYTEMIA

- Discussed in General Medicine

CARDIAC ARRYTHMIAS

BASICS OF ARRYTHMIAS

46. Most common mechanism of tachyarrhythmia?
a. Late after depolarization *(PGMEE 2015)*
b. Automaticity
c. Re-entry
d. Early after depolarization

[Ref: Harrison 20th ed. pg. 1718]

47. Most common benign cardiac rhythm is?
(PGMEE 2014-15)
a. Atrial premature contraction
b. Atrial fibrillation
c. Ventricular premature contraction
d. Ventricular tachycardia

48. Which of the following is a Sino atrial disease?
(PGMEE 2014-15)
a. Atrial ectopics
b. Ventricular ectopic
c. Sinus arrest
d. A-V block

[Ref: Harrison 20th ed. pg. 1724]

49. Sinus Bradycardia is defined as heart rate of?
(PGMEE 2014-15)
a. Less than 40/min   b. Less than 50/min
c. Less than 60/min   d. Less than 70/min

[Ref: Harrison 20th ed. pg. 1735]

50. Treatment of asymptomatic bradycardia is:
(PGMEE 2014-15)
a. No treatment is required
b. Give atropine
c. Isoprenaline
d. Cardiac pacing

[Ref: Harrison 20th ed. pg. 1725]

51. While at the ward round, you see an elderly lady attendant slump to the floor. Going to her aid, you notice her to be unresponsive and apneic. Your first step in Adult Basic Life Support (CPR) should be the following? *(PGMEE 2014-15)*
a. Check for a carotid pulse
b. Assess breathing
c. Determine responsiveness
d. Institute chest compression

[Ref: Harrison's 19th/e pg. 1768]

52. The image shows presence of: *(PGMEE 2015-16)*

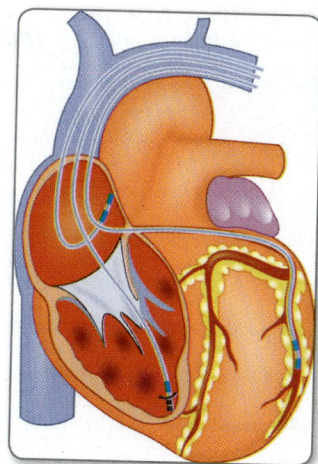

a. Implantable cardioverter defibrillator
b. Cardiac resynchronization therapy
c. Dual pacing
d. Transvenous pacemaker

[Ref: Harrison 20th ed. pg. 1777]

42.	a
43.	b
44.	a
45.	d
46.	c
47.	a
48.	c
49.	c
50.	a
51.	c
52.	b

53. Which is incorrect about a pacemaker:
(PGMEE 2014-15)

a. Deployed below skin of the chest
b. Pacing leads lie in the right atrium and right ventricle
c. Treatment of choice in Mobitz 1 heart Block
d. Biventricular pacing is useful for dilated cardiomyopathy

[Ref: Harrison 20th ed. pg. 1732]

SUPRAVENTRICULAR ARRYTHMIAS

54. A patient present in emergency with palpitation and sweating. ECG changes shown below. DOC for the reversal of this condition is:-
(PGMEE 2016-17)

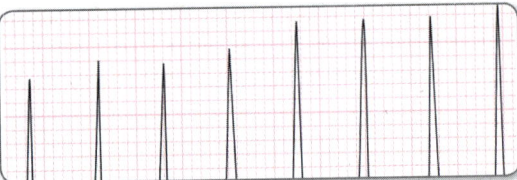

a. Metoprolol   b. Amiodarone
c. Adenosine   d. Lidocaine

[Ref: Harrison 20th ed. pg. 1742]

55. ECG given below is of :-
(PGMEE 2016-17)

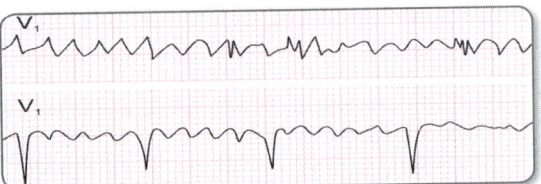

a. Atrial fibrillation   b. Atrial flutter
c. Sinus tachycardia   d. PSVT

[Ref: Harrison 20th ed. pg. 1743]

56. A 70-year old hypertensive patient with complaint of palpitations and pre-syncope. On examination, his heart rate is 72 BPM and BP was 150/100. ECG done shows
(PGMEE 2015-16)

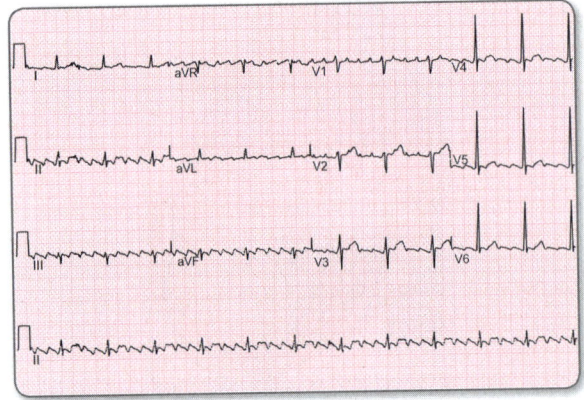

a. Atrial flutter
b. Atrial fibrillation
c. Multifocal atrial tachycardia
d. PSVT

[Ref: Harrison 20th ed. pg. 1733]

57. Identify the condition associated with the following ECG?
(PGMEE 2019)

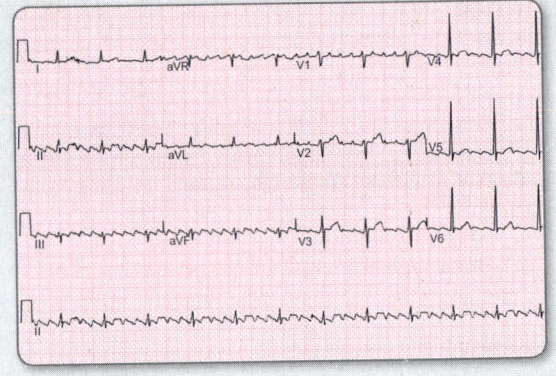

a. Atrial fibrillation
b. Arrhythmia
c. Atrial flutter
d. Cardiomyopathy

[Ref: Harrison 20th ed. pg. 1733]

58. A 62-year-old male with underlying COPD develops a viral upper respiratory infection and begins taking an over-the-counter decongestant. Shortly thereafter he experiences palpitations and presents to the emergency room, where the given rhythm strip is obtained, demonstrating:
(PGMEE 2015-16)

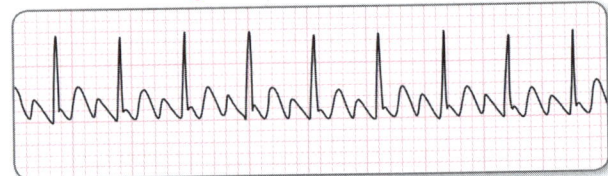

a. Junctional tachycardia
b. Atrial flutter with 2:1 atrioventricular block
c. Paroxysmal atrial tachycardia
d. Complete heart block

[Ref: Harrison 20th ed. pg. 1743]

59. All of the following are true about Atrial fibrillation, EXCEPT:
(PGMEE 2014-15)

a. Risk of thromboembolism
b. Digoxin for treatment
c. Cardioversion followed by anticoagulation
d. Ectopic originating in pulmonary vein

[Ref: Harrison 20th ed. pg. 1747]

60. A 78-year-old male with hypertension (controlled on anti-hypertensive drugs) presents with new onset of left hemiparesis and the finding of atrial fibrillation. Which of the following must be done?
(PGMEE 2014-15)

a. Close observation   b. Permanent pacemaker
c. Aspirin   d. Warfarin

[Ref: Harrison 20th ed. pg. 1749]

61. Digitalis is used in mitral stenosis when patient develops?
(PGMEE 2015-16)

a. Atrial fibrillation
b. Right ventricular failure
c. Acute pulmonary edema
d. Myocarditis

[Ref: Harrison 20th ed. pg. 1747]

53.	c
54.	c
55.	b
56.	a
57.	c
58.	b
59.	c
60.	d
61.	a

62. Most common arrhythmia in ICU patients:-
(PGMEE 2015)
a. Atrial fibrillation   b. PSVT
c. Atrial flutter   d. NPAT

[*Ref: Harrison 20th ed. pg. 1746*]

63. Atrial fibrillation may occur in all the following conditions, except: *(PGMEE 2014-15)*
a. Mitral stenosis
b. Hypothyroidism
c. Dilated cardiomyopathy
d. Mitral regurgitation

[*Ref: Harrison 20th ed. pg. 1746*]

64. Which of the following arrhythmia is most commonly associated with alcohol binge in alcoholics?
a. Ventricular fibrillation   *(PGMEE 2014-15)*
b. Ventricular premature contractions
c. Atrial flutter
d. Atrial fibrillation

[*Ref: Harrison 20th ed. pg. 1746*]

65. All of the following features can differentiate between ventricular tachycardia and supraventricular tachycardia EXCEPT: *(PGMEE 2014-15)*
a. qRS < 0.12 seconds
b. Ventricular rate >160/min
c. Variable first heart sound
d. Relieved by carotid sinus massage

[*Ref: Harrison 20th ed. pg. 1757*]

66. Patient in high dependency unit developed narrow complex tachycardia with a heart rate of 150 bpm. What is the next step in management? *(NEET Pattern 2017)*
a. Diltiazem   b. Carotid massage
c. Adenosine   d. Labetalol

[*Ref: Harrison 20th ed. pg. 1743*]

67. Drug of choice in maintenance therapy in P.S.V.T is:
(PGMEE 2014-15)
a. Amiodarone   b. Lignocaine
c. Verapamil   d. Adenosine

[*Ref: Harrison 20th ed. pg. 1743*]

68. Drug of choice for paroxysmal supraventricular tachycardia is? *(DNB June 2010)*
a. Metoprolol   b. Lidocaine
c. Adenosine   d. Amiodarone

[*Ref: Harrison 20th ed. pg. 1742*]

69. A female presents with chest pain and palpitations. Systolic BP is 80 mmHg. ECG is shown. What is the best management of this patient *(PGMEE 2019)*

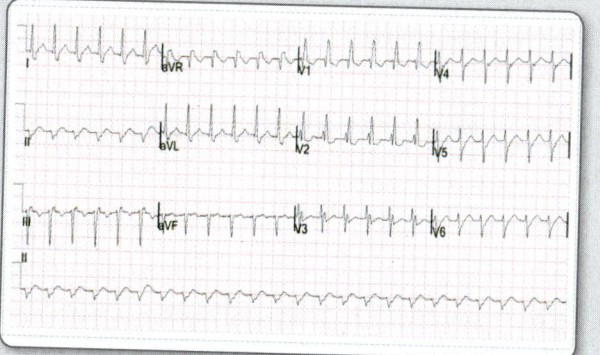

a. Metoprolol
b. Adenosine
c. Defibrillation Cardioversion
d. Amiodarone

70. The ECG image was given. What is the finding seen in this ECG. *(NEET Pattern 2017)*

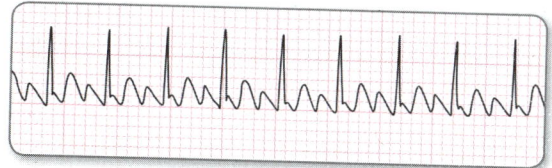

a. Ventricular bigeminy   b. PSVT
c. Electrical alternans   d. Calibration error

Explanation

- Above ECG shows consecutive, normally-conducted low voltage QRS complexes alternating in height. This is termed electrophysiologically as Electrical alternans that describes alternate-beat variation in the direction, amplitude, and duration of any component of the ECG waveform. Electrical alternans associated with cardiac motion is due to alternation in the position of the heart with relation to recording electrodes. The most common underlying disorder is an enlarged pericardial sac. In patients with large effusions.

Massive pericardial effusion produces a triad of:
  ○ Low QRS voltage
  ○ Tachycardia
  ○ Electrical alternans

71. Frog sign is seen in: *(PGMEE 2014-15)*
a. AVNRT   b. Diabetic nephropathy
c. Medullary sponge kidney d. Budd Chiari syndrome

Explanation

- In patients with AV Nodal re-entrant tachycardia (AVNRT), ventricles and atria are activated simultaneously at the rate of 160 to 180 beats/minute. This dissociation causes atria to contract against closed mitral & tricuspid valves, that produces rapid and regular pounding in the neck, known as Frog sign.

VENTRICULAR ARRHYTHMIAS

72. In the ICU, a patient suddenly becomes unresponsive, pulseless, and hypotensive, with cardiac monitor indicating ventricular tachycardia. The first therapeutic step among the following should be: *(PGMEE 2014-15)*
a. Amiodarone 300 mg IV push
b. Lidocaine 1.5 mg / kg IV push
c. Defibrillation at 200 joules biphasic
d. Defibrillation at 360 joules uniphasic

[*Ref: ACLS algorithm 2019*]

73. Broad complex tachycardia, due to ventricular tachycardia is suggested by all except?
(PGMEE 2014-15)
a. Fusion Beats
b. A V dissociation
c. Capture Beats
d. Termination of tachycardia by carotid Sinus massage

62.	a
63.	b
64.	d
65.	b
66.	b
67.	c
68.	c
69.	b
70.	c
71.	a
72.	c
73.	d

74. If a person is having ventriular tachycardia,extra systoles appears to- *(PGMEE 2015)*
   a. P wave
   b. QRS complex
   c. T wave
   d. R wave

[Ref: Harrison 20th ed. pg. 1757]

75. A 40-year-old male presents to the office with a history of palpitations that last for a few seconds and occur two or three times a week. There are no other symptoms. ECG shows a single unifocal premature ventricular contraction. The most likely cause of this finding is: *(PGMEE 2014-15)*
   a. Underlying coronary artery disease
   b. Valvular heart disease
   c. Hypertension
   d. Idiopathic

[Ref: Harrison's 19th/e pg. 1492]

76. In a patient with wide-complex tachycardia, the presence of all of the following in the ECG indicates ventricular tachycardia except? *(PGMEE 2014-15)*
   a. Atrio-ventricular dissociation
   b. Fusion beats
   c. Typical right bundle branch block
   d. Capture beats

[Ref: Harrison 20th ed. pg. 1757]

77. Which of the following statements about premature ventricular beat is false? *(PGMEE 2014-15)*
   a. Sequential depolarization of ventricles
   b. Wide, Bizarre, Notched qRS complexes
   c. Prevalence decreases with age
   d. Palpitations is a common presenting feature

[Ref: Harrison 20th ed. pg. 1755-56]

HEART BLOCKS

78. Which of the following causes AV block?
(NEET Pattern 2019)
   a. Hypothyroidism
   b. Carcinoid
   c. Pheochromocytoma
   d. Hyperthyroidism

79. Infective organism causing AV block: *(NEET 2018)*
   a. Ixodes scapularis
   b. Dermacentor variabilis
   c. Amblyomma americanum
   d. Ixodes ricinus

[Ref: Harrison's 19th/e pg. 1471]

Explanation
   - Various infections, as well as inflammatory and connective tissue disorders of the heart, can lead to AV block.
   - These include Lyme disease, Pinta, sarcoidosis, hemochromatosis, and ankylosing spondylitis.

80. Classic 'rsr' pattern in V1 as shown in ECG is seen in:- *(PGMEE 2016-17)*

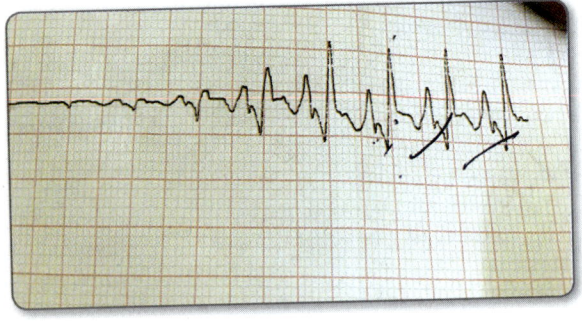

   a. Left bundle branch block
   b. Right bundle branch block
   c. Hypothermia
   d. Aortic regurgitation

[Ref: Harrison 20th ed. pg. 1679]

81. Most common cause of heart block in infants is? *(PGMEE 2015-16)*
   a. SLE
   b. Surgery for congenital heart disease
   c. Viral myocarditis
   d. Rheumatic fever

82. Patient of 1st degree heart block complains of dizziness. Best treatment for this patient is? *(All India Dec 2015 Pattern)*
   a. Isoprenaline
   b. Pacemaker
   c. Atropine
   d. Adrenaline

[Ref: Harrison 20th ed. pg. 1732]

Explanation
   - Treatment of first degree AV block
     ○ Asymptomatic → No treatment
     ○ Symptomatic → Pacemaker implantation (Class IIa recommend)

83. AV block is commonly seen in : *(PGMEE 2018)*
   a. Pheochromocytoma
   b. Hyperthyroidism
   c. Hypothyroidism
   d. Cushing syndrome

[Ref: Harrison 20th ed. pg. 1728]

Explanation
   - Endocrine causes of AV block include hypothyroidism and adrenal insufficiency

84. Which of the following is the most common heart block in neonatal lupus. *(PGMEE 2014-15)*
   a. 1st degree heart block
   b. Mobitz 2A heart block
   c. Mobitz 2B heart block
   d. 3rd degree heart block

[Ref: Internet]

74.	b
75.	d
76.	c
77.	c
78.	a
79.	a
80.	b
81.	b
82.	b
83.	c
84.	d

85. ECG tracing showing which heart block:-

(PGMEE 2016-17)

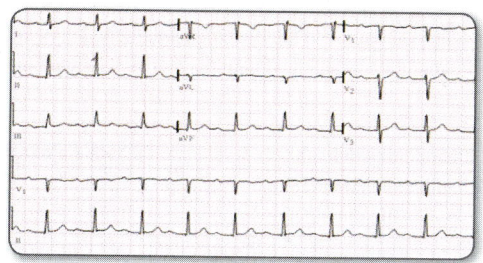

a. First degree heart block
b. Second degree heart block
c. Third degree heart block
d. Right bundle branch block

[Ref: Harrison 20th ed. pg. 1729]

86. Which of the following is cause of RBBB?

(PGMEE 2014-15)

a. It can occur in a normal person
b. Pulmonary embolism
c. Corpulmonale
d. All of the above

87. QRS duration greater than 0.16 seconds is seen in?

(PGMEE 2011)

a. Bundle branch block　　b. Sick sinus syndrome
c. Mobitz 1　　　　　　　　d. Mobitz 2

[Ref: Harrison 20th ed. pg. 1678]

88. Alternating RBBB with Left anterior hemiblock is seen in?

(PGMEE 2014-15)

a. 1st degree heart block　b. Complete heart block
c. Mobitz type II block　　d. Bifascicular block

89. What is not correct about LBBB? *(PGMEE 2014-15)*

a. Can occur after MI
b. ST segment elevation is seen
c. A-V dissociation
d. Cardiomyopathy is associated

[Ref: Harrison 20th ed. pg. 1679]

MISCELLANEOUS

90. Osborn J waves is seen in *(PGMEE 2019)*

a. Hypothermia
b. Hyperkalemia
c. Hypocalemia
d. Hypokalemia

91. Permanent cardiac pacing is helpful in: *(NEET 2018)*

a. Transient AV block
b. Brugada syndrome
c. Post-myocardial infarction AV block
d. Ventricular fibrillation

92. All of the following electrocardiographic findings may represent manifestations of digitalis intoxication, EXCEPT:

(PGMEE 2014-15)

a. Ventricular Bigeminy
b. Junctional tachycardia
c. Bidirectional tachycardia
d. Multifocal Atrial tachycardia

[Ref: Harrison's 19th/e pg. 1485]

93. A person with mitral regurgitation and atrial fibrillation presents with syncope. On examination the person has a heart rate of 46 bpm What is the most probable cause?

(PGMEE 2014-15)

a. Digitalis toxicity
b. Junctional Tachycardia
c. Stroke
d. Subarachnoid Hemorrhage

94. ECG changes in Digoxin toxicity are:- *(PGMEE 2016-17)*

a. Prolonged QT interval
b. Prolonged PR interval
c. ST segment elevation
d. Tall T-waves

[Ref: Internet]

95. In left sided massive pneumothorax, ECG shows all, EXCEPT:

(PGMEE 2014-15)

a. Left axis deviation
b. Absent R wave
c. Pathological Q waves
d. Precordial T wave inversion

[Ref: Harrison 20th ed. pg. 1761]

96. Inverted T waves are seen in? *(PGMEE 2014-15)*

a. Hyperkalemia　　　　　b. Hyperthermia
c. Wellen syndrome　　　　d. Coronary syndrome X

[Ref: Harrison 20th ed. pg. 1680]

VALVULAR HEART DISEASE

MITRAL VALVE DISEASES

97. Which of the following is not a cause if mitral stenosis?

a. Systemic lupus erythematosus *(NEET Pattern 2019)*
b. Cryoglobulinemia
c. Atrial myxoma
d. Cor triatriatum

98. In mitral stenosis "the double shadow" on X-ray chest PA view is due to enlargement of: *(NEET Pattern 2019)*

a. Left atrial enlargement
b. Left ventricular enlargement
c. Right atrial enlargement
d. Right ventricular enlargement

99. Contraindication for percutaneous balloon mitral valvotomy include the following *except*:

a. Severe mitral regurgitation *(NEET Pattern 2019)*
b. Left atrial thrombus
c. Commissural calcification
d. Presence of pulmonary hypertension

100. In pregnancy which valvular disease is most dangerous?

(PGMEE 2015-16)

a. MR　　　　　　　　　　b. MS
c. AS　　　　　　　　　　d. AR

[Ref: CMDT 2016, pg. 3441]

Explanation

- MS is most likely associated with worst outcome during pregnancy. Other valvular diseases like MR, AR & AS are associated with syndrome risk of CCF due to pregnancy induced decrease in SVR.

85.	a
86.	d
87.	a
88.	d
89.	c
90.	a
91.	c
92.	d
93.	a
94.	b
95.	a
96.	c
97.	b
98.	b
99.	d
100.	b

101. CXR showing cardiomegaly, straightening of left heart border which valve is involved, what disease:- *(PGMEE 2016-17)*

a. MS
b. MR
c. AS
d. AR

[Ref: Harrison 20th ed. pg. 1815]

102. In mitral stenosis double atrial shadow is due to enlargement of? *(PGMEE 2015)*

a. Right atrium
b. Left atrium
c. Both atria
d. Left auricle

103. In a patient of mitral stenosis, decreased 1st heart sound is seen in all except: *(NEET Pattern 2017)*

a. Aortic regurgitation
b. Mild mitral stenosis
c. Calcified mitral valve
d. 1st degree heart block

[Ref: Harrison's 20th/e pg. 1815]

Explanation

Soft S$_1$	Loud S$_1$
▪ MR	▪ MS
▪ TR	▪ TS
▪ Severe MS or TS (valve calcification)	▪ High cardiac output states
▪ Prolonged PR interval (1° heart block)	▪ Short PR interval
▪ Acute AR	

Split S$_1$	Variable
▪ Ebstein anomaly	▪ Atrial fibrillation
▪ RBBB with pulmonary hypertension	▪ Extrasystoles
▪ LV pacing	▪ Complete heart block.
▪ Ectopic beats and idioventricular rhythms from LV	

104. Criteria for mitral Valvotomy includes all except? *(PGMEE 2014-15)*

a. Significant symptoms
b. Isolated mitral stenosis
c. Mobile non calcified valve
d. Left atrial thrombus

[Ref: Harrison's 20th/e pg. 1816]

105. Histopathology of mitral valve prolapse shows which type of degeneration? *(PGMEE 2012)*

a. Fibrous degeneration
b. Granulomatous changes
c. Myxomatous degeneration
d. Fibrinoid necrosis

[Ref: Harrison 20th ed. pg. 1822]

106. Mitral valve vegetations do not embolise usually to- *(DNB Dec. 07)*

a. Spleen
b. Brain
c. Liver
d. Lungs

[Ref: Harrison 20th ed. pg. 1814]

AORTIC VALVE DISEASES

107. A patient came with early diastolic murmur in the second intercostal space and had differential BP recording in the upper limb with one arm showing measurement of 150/110 mmHg and the other showing 90/60 mmHg. All of the following can be a cause except:

a. Aortic dissection *(NEET Pattern 2017)*
b. Takayasu arteritis
c. Coarctation of aorta
d. Supravalvular aortic stenosis

[Ref: Harrison 19/e, P.1445]

Explanation

Blood Pressure Measurement

- Blood pressure should be measured in both arms, and the difference should be less than 10 mmHg. A blood pressure differential that exceeds this threshold may be associated with **atherosclerotic or inflammatory subclavian artery disease, supravalvular aortic stenosis, coarctation of aorta, or aortic dissection**. Systolic leg pressures are usually as much as 20 mmHg higher than systolic arm pressures. Greater leg–arm pressure differences are seen in patients with chronic severe AR as well as patients with extensive and calcified lower extremity peripheral arterial disease.
- All the options can have differential BP in upper limb on examination. Patient presents with murmur suggestive of AR. Among the options, SVAS is least likely to be associated with AR. Hence, it is the answer.

108. Dicrotic nature of aortic pulse is lost in? *(DNB Dec'2010)*

a. Aortic stenosis
b. Arteriosclerosis
c. PDA
d. Aortic Regurgitation

[Ref: Harrison 20th ed. pg. 1670]

109. Duroziez's sign in seen in? *(PGMEE 2015)*

a. Aortic Regurgitation
b. Mitral Regurgitation
c. Aortic Stenosis
d. Mitral Stenosis

[Ref: Harrison 20th ed. pg. 1810]

110. Which of the following is a cause of wide pulse pressure- *(PGMEE 2015)*

a. Mitral stenosis
b. Aortic regurgitation
c. Tricuspid stenosis
d. Aortic stenosis

[Ref: Harrison 20th ed. pg. 1810]

111. A patient with angina, exertional syncope and Left ventricular hypertrophy is diagnosed as aortic stenosis. What is the predicted life span of this patient? *(PGMEE 2014-15)*

a. 1 year
b. 2 years
c. 3 years
d. 4 years

[Ref: Harrison 20th ed. pg. 1806]

112. Incorrect about chronic aortic regurgitation is: *(PGMEE 2014-15)*

a. Chest pain
b. Wide pulse pressure
c. Quincke's sign
d. Late systolic murmur

[Ref: Harrison 20th ed. pg. 1810]

101.	b
102.	b
103.	b
104.	d
105.	c
106.	d
107.	d
108.	a
109.	a
110.	b
111.	c
112.	d

113. Dyspnea, syncope and angina pectoris occur most commonly in? *(PGMEE 2014-15)*
a. MS
b. AS
c. MR
d. AR

[Ref: Harrison 20th ed. pg. 1810]

PULMONARY & TRICUSPID VALVE DISEASES

114. Most common valvular lesion seen with carcinoid syndrome is? *(PGMEE 2014-15)*
a. Tricuspid stenosis and pulmonic stenosis
b. Tricuspid insufficiency and pulmonic stenosis
c. Mitral stenosis and aortic stenosis
d. Mitral insufficiency and aortic stenosis

[Ref: Harrison 20th ed. pg. 1823, 1826]

115. Pulsatile liver is seen with *(PGMEE 2014-15)*
a. Tricuspid regurgitation
b. Tricuspid stenosis
c. Dilated cardiomyopathy
d. Pulmonic stenosis

[Ref: Harrison 20th ed. pg. 1824]

116. Vitum's Sign is seen in:- *(PGMEE 2015-16)*
a. Aortic Stenosis
b. Tricuspid Regurgitation
c. Pericardial effusion
d. Mitral Stenosis

[Ref: Sapira's Art and Science of Bedside Diagnosis 4th/e pg. 360]

Explanation

- The murmur of Tricuspid regurgitation may increase with compression of Liver, known as Vitums sign.

117. Carvallo's Sign representing a Diagnostic Murmur that increases on inspiration is seen in:- *(PGMEE 2015-16)*
a. Mitral Stenosis
b. Tricuspid Stenosis
c. Aortic Regurgitation
d. Tricuspid Regurgitation

[Ref: Harrison 20th ed. pg. 1673]

HEART FAILURE

118. Heart failure is seen in which heart disease in infant:- *(PGMEE 2016-17)*
a. Endocarditis
b. Hypertrophic cardiomyopathy
c. VSD
d. Rheumatic fever

[Ref: Nelson's 20th/e pg. 2284]

119. A patient with CHF with LVEF<40% should be given? *(PGMEE 2015-16)*
a. ACEI + beta blocker
b. ACEI + furosemide
c. ACEI + CCB
d. ACEI + ARB

[Ref: Harrison 20th ed. pg. 1772, 1774]

Explanation

- Drugs associated with reduced mortality in heart failure:
  ○ ACEI & ARB
  ○ Angiotensin receptor neprilysin inhibitors (ARNIs)
  ○ β-blockers
  ○ Mineralocorticoid antagonist
  ○ Hydralazine + nitrates

120. Cheyne stokes breathing is seen in: *(PGMEE 2014-15)*
a. Intracranial hypotension
b. Congestive heart failure
c. Left atrial myoxma
d. Pickwinian syndrome

[Ref: Harrison 20th ed. pg. 1766]

121. Displacement of cardiac apex to left and downwards indicates? *(PGMEE 2014-15)*
a. Right ventricular hypertrophy
b. Left ventricular hypertrophy
c. Right atrial hypertrophy
d. Left atrial hypertrophy

[Ref: Harrison 20th ed. pg. 1670]

122. Acute pulmonary edema due to acute LVF. Drug of choice is :- *(PGMEE 2016-17)*
a. Nitrate
b. Digitalis
c. Furosemide
d. Milrinone

[Ref: Harrison 20th ed. pg. 1770]

123. Factor responsible for Cardiac Hypertrophy is? *(DNB Dec. 10)*
a. TGF beta
b. TNF alpha
c. c-myc
d. ANF

[Ref: Robbin's 8th/e pg. 532]

124. Concentric hypertrophy of left ventricle is seen in- *(PGMEE 2013-14)*
a. Aortic regurgitation
b. Hypertension
c. Mitral stenosis
d. None

[Ref: Robbins 9th/e pg. 568; 490]

125. Heart failure cells are seen in- *(PGMEE 2013; 2014, 2016-17, 2008)*
a. Heart
b. Brain
c. Kidney
d. Lungs

[Ref.: Robbins 9th/e pg. 529]

126. Heart failure cells are- *(PGMEE 2013-14)*
a. Pigment cells seen in liver
b. Pigmented alveolar macrophages
c. Lipofuscin granules in cardiac cells
d. Pigmented pancreatic acinar cells

[Robbins 9th/e pg. 529]

MYOCARDITIS AND CARDIOMYOPATHY

127. Parasitic infestation causing myocarditis- *(PGMEE 2012-13, 2014)*
a. Enterobius
b. Trichinella spiralis
c. Strongyloides
d. Trichuris

[Ref: Harrison 20th ed. pg. 1786]

128. Which one of the following is not a cause for restrictive cardiomyopathy- *(DNB Dec. 11)*
a. Alcohol
b. Amyloidosis
c. Hemochromatosis
d. Sarcoidosis

[Ref: Harrison 20th ed. pg. 1792]

113.	b
114.	b
115.	a
116.	b
117.	b
118.	c
119.	a
120.	b
121.	b
122.	c
123.	c
124.	b
125.	d
126.	b
127.	b
128.	a

129. Tigered effect in myocardium is due to-
(PGMEE 2016-17, PGMEE 2012-13)
a. Seen in rheumatic fever
b. Fatty degeneration
c. Associated with myocarditis
d. Malignant change

Explanation

- Tigered heart is a heart, on the inside of which stripes of yellowish or white myocardium caused by fatty degeneration can be seen alternate with stripes of normal myocardium. It is seen in prolonged moderate hypoxia. Dipthertic Myocarditis and Fatty degeneration

130. Most common cause of dilated cardiomyopathy:-
(PGMEE 2016-17)
a. Alcohol
b. Hypertension
c. Thiamine deficiency
d. Diabetes mellitus

[Ref: Robbin's 9th/e pg. 565]

131. The most common type of cardiomyopathy in India is-
(PGMEE 2015)
a. Dilated Cardiomyopathy
b. Toxic Cardiomyopathy
c. Hypertrophic Cardiomyopathy
d. Restrictive Cardiomyopathy

[Ref: API textbook of Medicine 9th/e p. 728]

132. Which cardiomyopathy is commonly associated with alcohol consumption
(PGMEE 2019)
a. RCM
b. DCM
c. HCM
d. None of the above

133. Hypertrophic cardiomyopathy is due to
(PGMEE 2019)
a. Asymmetrical septal hypertrophy
b. Endocardial fibrosis
c. Myofiber disarray
d. Left ventricular hypertrophic

134. Double apical impulse is seen in?
(PGMEE 2012)
a. HOCM
b. Pulmonary hypertension
c. Aortic regurgitation
d. Cardiac tamponade

[Ref: Harrison's 19th/e pg 1568]

135. A 25-year-old footballer is elbowed in the chest by the rival defender during ball possession. Following the chest trauma the player collapses and dies. The most probable cause of death is:
(PGMEE 2014-15)
a. HOCM
b. Commotio cordis
c. Hemothorax
d. Aortic transection

[Ref: Harrison 19th p 289 e-3]

136. Cardiomyopathy does not occur in
(PGMEE 2014-15)
a. Duchenne muscular dystrophy
b. Alkaptonuria
c. Pompe disease
d. Fabry's disease

[Ref: Harrison 20th ed. pg. 1781]

Explanation

- Genetic defects associated with cardiomyopathy
  ○ Friedreich's ataxia - AR
  ○ Fabry's disease - XLR
  ○ Duchenn's & Becker's dystrophy - XLR

137. RCM is caused by all EXCEPT:
(PGMEE 2014-15)
a. Fatty infiltration of myocardium
b. Amyloidosis
c. Daunorubicin
d. Carcinoid syndrome

[Ref: Harrison 20th ed. pg. 1792]

138. Banana shaped left ventricle is seen in?
(PGMEE 2014-15)
a. HOCM
b. DCM
c. RCM
d. Takotsubo cardiomyopathy

139. Incorrect about restrictive cardiomyopathy:
a. Kussmaul's sign
(PGMEE 2014-15)
b. Pulsatile liver
c. Pedal edema
d. Dip and spike configuration in ventricular systolic pressure

[Ref: Harrison 20th ed. pg. 1791]

140. In case of sudden death in a young football player, the first clinical suspicion would rest on which of the following differentials?
(PGMEE 2014-15)
a. Arrthymogenic right ventricular dysplasia
b. Takotsubo cardiomyopathy
c. Atrial septal defect
d. Eisenmenger complex

[Ref: Harrison 20th ed. pg. 2061]

Explanation

- Causes of sudden death in young people include : HCM, Coronary artery anomalies, arrhythmogenic right ventricular cardiomyopathy and Long QT syndromes.

141. Drug contraindicated in HOCM is?
(DNB Dec'2010; PGMEE 2014-15)
a. Propranolol
b. Verapamil
c. Digoxin
d. None of the above

[Ref: Harrison 20th ed. pg. 1796]

142. Stunning of myocardium without any acute coronary syndrome changes are seen in
(PGMEE 2018)
a. Dilated cardiomyopathy
b. Tako Tsubo cardiomyopathy
c. Restrictive cardiomyopathy
d. Rt heart arrythmogenic dysplasia

[Ref: Harrison 20th ed. pg. 1790-91]

Explanation

Takotsubo Cardiomyopathy aka Broken Heart Syndrome

- Takotsubo cardiomyopathy (apical ballooning syndrome or stress-induced cardiomyopathy) is a transient cardiac syndrome that involves left ventricular apical akinesis and mimics acute coronary syndrome (ACS).
- When the patient undergoes cardiac angiography, left ventricular (LV) apical ballooning is present, and there is no significant coronary artery stenosis.

129.	b
130.	a
131.	a
132.	b
133.	c
134.	a
135.	b
136.	b
137.	a,c
138.	a
139.	d
140.	a
141.	c
142.	b

143. Incorrect about Broken heart syndrome:
(PGMEE 2014-15)
a. Catecholamine toxicity
b. ST elevation
c. Apical ballooning
d. Dobutamine for cardiogenic dysfunction

[Ref: Harrison 20th ed. pg. 1790-91]

ENDOCARDITIS

144. Dukes criteria for infective endocarditis include which of the following as essential major criteria: *(NEET 2019)*
a. Single positive culture of coxiella
b. Single positive culture of Corynebacterium
c. Single culture positive for S viridians
d. Single positive culture of HACEK

145. Libman sack's endocarditis is seen in?
(PGMEE 2016-17; 2015, 2012-13)
a. SLE
b. Infective endocarditis
c. Carcinoid
d. Syphilis

[Ref: Harrison 20th ed. pg. 2520]

146. Which type of endocarditis has vegetation on both sides of the valves: *(PGMEE 2015, 2013)*
a. Infective endocarditis
b. Libman Sack'endocarditis
c. RF
d. None

[Ref: Robbins 9th/pg 560]

147. Flat vegetations in pockets of valves are due to-
(DNB Dec. 11)
a. NBTE
b. Rheumatic heart disease
c. Infective endocarditis
d. Libman sacks Endocarditis

[Ref: Robbin's 8th/e pg. 567; Harsh Mohan 4th/e pg. 307]

148. Vegetations in Libman sac endocarditis are-
(PGMEE 2012-13)
a. Small bland vegetations
b. Large and fragile
c. Small or medium sized on either or both sides of valve
d. Small warty vegetations along the line of closure of valve

[Ref: Robbin's 8th/e pg. 567]

149. Small warty vegetations seen on the under surfaces of AV valves, valvular endocardium, chords or mural endocardium of atria or ventricles is characteristic of
a. Libman sack endocarditis *(PGMEE 2015]*
b. Nonbacterial thrombotic endocarditis
c. Infective endocarditis
d. Rheumatic fever

[Ref: Robbins 9th/pg 560]

150. Large warty vegetation are characteristic of-
(DNB June 07)
a. SLE
b. SABE
c. Both
d. None

[Ref: Robbin's 8th/e pg. 598]

151. Libman-Sacks endocarditis most commonly causes
(PGMEE 2015)
a. Mitral regurgitation
b. Mitral stenosis
c. Tricuspid regurgitation
d. Aortic regurgitation

[Ref: Robbins 9th/pg 560]

152. Vegetations on the under surface of heart is seen in
a. Rheumatic heart disease *(PGMEE 2015)*
b. Infective endocarditis
c. Libman-Sacks endocarditis
d. Subacute bacterial endocarditis

[Ref: Robbins 9th/pg 560]

153. Sterile vegetations are seen in all except-
a. Libmann sack's endocarditis *(PGMEE 2015; 2012)*
b. Marantic endocarditis
c. Infective endocarditis
d. None

[Ref: Harrison 20th ed. pg. 921]

154. Vegetations of the following endocarditis has the maximum chances of embolization *(PGMEE 2015)*
a. Rheumatic heart disease
b. Infective endocarditis
c. Libman-sacks endocarditis
d. Subacute bacterial endocarditis

[Ref: 9th/pg 560; 8th/pg 567]

155. Non-bacterial thrombotic endocarditis is seen in
a. Rheumatic fever *(PGMEE 2015)*
b. Systemic lupus erythematosus
c. Rheumatoid arthritis
d. Mucinous adenocarcinoma of pancreas

[Ref: Harrison 20th ed. pg. 923]

156. Which of the following is associated with destruction of valves? *(PGMEE 2012-13)*
a. Acute infective endocarditis
b. Rheumatic Heart disease
c. Libman sack's endocarditis
d. All

[Ref: Harrison 20th ed. pg. 923]

157. All are true about non- bacterial thrombotic endocarditis, except- *(PGMEE 2013-14)*
a. No inflammatory reaction
b. Vegetation >5 mm
c. Locally nondestructive
d. Cause emboli

[Ref: Robbins 9th/e pg. 561]

158. Changing character of a murmur in a patient with joint pain and embolic phenomenon indicates the diagnosis of: *(PGMEE 2014-15)*
a. Mitral stenosis
b. SABE
c. Aortic regurgitation
d. Rheumatiod arthritis

[Ref: Harrison 20th ed. pg. 923]

159. Diagnostic criterion for infective endocarditis includes all EXCEPT: *(DNB June 2011)*
a. Rheumatoid factor
b. ESR
c. Positive ECG
d. Positive blood culture

[Ref: Harrison 20th ed. pg. 923]

143.	d
144.	d
145.	a
146.	b
147.	d
148.	c
149.	a
150.	b
151.	a
152.	c
153.	c
154.	b
155.	b
156.	a
157.	b
158.	b
159.	b,c

CHAPTER-1 ♦ CARDIOLOGY

160. Osler's nodes are seen in? *(PGMEE 2014-15)*
a. Rheumatoid arthritis
b. Rheumatic heart disease
c. Subacute bacterial endocarditis
d. Typhoid

[Ref: Harrison 20th ed. pg. 924]

161. Potentially serious complication in a pateint with prosthetic valve replacement:- *(PGMEE 2016-17)*
a. Infective endocarditis   b. Myocarditis
c. Pericarditis   d. Pancarditis

[Ref: Harrison 20th ed. pg. 921]

162. Incorrect about prosthetic valve endocarditis is:
a. Embolism   *(PGMEE 2014-15)*
b. Strept. Viridans > 1 year of operation
c. Mitral valve mostly involved
d. C.O.N.S < 1 year of operation

[Ref: Harrison's 19th/e pg. 817]

163. Roth's spot is seen in? *(PGMEE 2015, DNB June 2010)*
a. Infective endocarditis   b. Typhoid
c. CRAO   d. Rheumatic Carditis

[Ref: Harrison 20th ed. pg. 924]

164. Left sided endocarditis is associated with:
(PGMEE 2014-15)
a. Endocardial cushion defect
b. Osteum secondum ASD
c. Patent Fossa Ovalis
d. Osteum primum ASD

[Ref: CMDT-14/ch:33/pg:143]

165. Most common cause of infective endocarditis in I.V drug user is:- *(PGMEE 2016-17)*
a. Streptococcus viridians
b. Staphylococcus aureus
c. Pseudomonas aurigenosa
d. Coagulase negative staphylococci

[Ref: Harrison 20th ed. pg. 922]

166. Most common cause of infective endocarditis is?
(PGMEE 2014-15)
a. Staphylococcus aureus   b. Streptococcus viridians
c. Streptococcus pyogenes d. Streptococcus mutilan

[Ref: Harrison 20th ed. pg. 922]

167. Valve affected in infective endocarditis due to septic abortion? *(PGMEE 2014-15)*
a. Mitral   b. Aortic
c. Pulmonary   d. Tricuspid

[Ref: Harrison's 19th/e pg. 819]

168. Infective endocarditis where lifelong treatment is required:
(PGMEE 2014-15)
a. Aspergillus endocarditis b. Libman sacks endocarditis
c. Fusarium solani   d. Enterococci

[Ref: Current diagnosis and treatment in Cardiology 2nd edition, chapter 29]

169. Bacterial endocarditis is most commonly seen in:
(PGMEE 2014-15)
a. VSD   b. PDA
c. ASD   d. AS

170. In which of the following lesion infective endocarditis is least common? *(PGMEE 2012)*
a. Severe MR
b. Severe AR
c. Small ASD
d. Small VSD

[Ref: Nelson 20th/e/p 437]

PERICARDITIS

171. Aetiology of Dressler Syndrome is? *(PGMEE 2015-16)*
a. Viral
b. Autoimmune
c. Idiopathic
d. Toxin mediated

[Ref: Harrison 20th ed. pg. 1841]

172. Most common presentation of cardiac lupus?
a. Aortic regurgitation   *(PGMEE 2015)*
b. Pericarditis
c. Libman sacks endocarditis
d. Myocarditis

[Ref: Harrison 20th ed. pg. 2520]

173. Which is incorrect about Dressler syndrome?
a. Post MI pericarditis   *(PGMEE 2014-15)*
b. Post MI pleuritis
c. Autoimmune
d. Treatment with steroids is necessary

[Ref: Harrison 20th ed. pg. 1845]

174. Dressler's syndrome is characterized by?
a. Onset within 72 hours   *(PGMEE 2014-15)*
b. Treatment of choice is steroids
c. Pericardial effusion
d. Angina

[Ref: Harrison 20th ed. pg. 1841]

175. Restrictive and constrictive pericarditis occurs together in: *(PGMEE 2014-15)*
a. Radiation
b. Adriamycin
c. Amyloidosis
d. Post cardiotomy syndrome

[Ref: Harrison 20th ed. pg. 1845]

176. Fibrinous pericarditis is seen in? *(PGMEE 2012)*
a. Myxoma
b. Post cardiac surgery
c. Infectious mononucleosis
d. TB

[Ref: Harrison 20th ed. pg. 1845]

Explanation
- Causes of fibrinous pericarditis:
  ○ Acute MI
  ○ Dresser syndrome
  ○ Cardiac surgery
  ○ Radiotherapy
  ○ Acute rheumatic fever
  ○ RA, SLE

160.	c
161.	a
162.	c
163.	a
164.	c
165.	b
166.	a
167.	d
168.	a
169.	a
170.	c
171.	b
172.	b
173.	d
174.	c
175.	a
176.	b

CARDIAC TAMPONADE

177. Hypotension with muffled sounds and congested neck veins is seen in? *(PGMEE 2015-16)*
a. Cardiac tamponade
b. Pericardial effusion
c. Constrictive pericarditis
d. Acute congestive heart failure

[Ref: Harrison 20th ed. pg. 1843]

178. Becks triad is seen in- *(PGMEE 2015)*
a. Restrictive cardiomyopathy
b. Constrictive pericarditis
c. Cardiac tamponade
d. All of the above

[Ref: Harrison 20th ed. pg. 1843]

ACUTE RHEUMATIC FEVER

179. Most common symptom of acute rheumatic fever in adults? *(PGMEE 2015)*
a. Migratory polyarthritis
b. Carditis
c. Chorea
d. Rash

[Ref: Harrison 20th ed. pg. 2542]

180. Not a feature of rheumatic heart disease- *(PGMEE 2014)*
a. Carditis
b. Chorea
c. Janeways lesion
d. Arthritis

[Ref : Robbin's 8th/e pg. 566]

181. Which is not a major criteria for diagnosis of rheumatic fever? *(PGMEE 2013-14)*
a. Carditis
b. Arthritis
c. Increased ASLO
d. Subcutaneous nodules

[Ref: Harrison 20th ed. pg. 2544]

182. All are minor Jones criteria except- *(PGMEE 2012-13)*
a. Chorea
b. Fever
c. Prolonged PR interval
d. Arthralgia

[Ref: Harrison 20th ed. pg. 2544]

183. ASO Titres are used in the diagnosis of- *(DNB June 08)*
a. Ankylosing spondylitis
b. Acute rheumatic fever
c. Osteoarthritis
d. Acute rheumatoid arthritis

[Ref: Harrison 20th ed. pg. 2543]

184. In Rheumatic carditis, Mc callums patch is seen in subendothelium of? *(PGMEE 2015)*
a. Right atrium
b. Right Ventricle
c. Left atrium
d. Left ventricle

[Ref: Robbins 9th/e pg. 529]

185. Mc Callum's patch is diagnostic of- *(PGMEE 2012-13)*
a. Tetralogy of Fallot (ToF)
b. Rheumatic endocarditis
c. Infective endocarditis
d. Myocardial infarction

[Ref: Robbins 9th/e pg. 529]

Explanation
- Mc Callum's Patch is seen on posterior wall of Left atrium above the mitral valve, it often forms nidus for endocarditis. It is very specific for Rheumatic Endocarditis.

186. Anitschkow cells are seen in- *(PGMEE 2013-14)*
a. Rheumatic myocarditis
b. Infective endocarditis
c. Myocardial infraction
d. None

[Ref: Robbins 9th/e pg.558]

187. 30-year-old male presented with severe dyspnoea and fatigue. X-ray showed left atrial enlargement. Physician suspects the patient of having mitral stenosis and gets a histopath exam ination done, the image of which is shown, it shows? *(NEET Pattern 2017)*

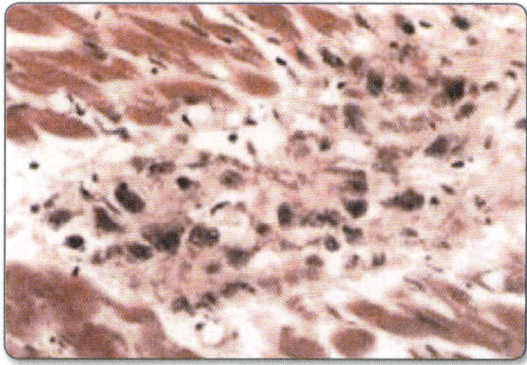

a. Sarcoidosis
b. Tuberculosis
c. Aschoff bodies
d. Fungal granuloma

Ref: Robbins 9th edition pg 558

Explanation
- Microscopic appearance of Aschoff body in a patient with acute rheumatic carditis. The myocardial interstitium has a circumscribed collection of mononuclear inflammatory cells, including some large macrophages with prominent nucleoli and a binuclear macrophage, associated with necrosis.
- In given scenario patient had left atrial enlargement and mitral stenosis, which favour diagnosis of rheumatic heart disease as other options does not present with same clinical scenarios. Also given slide shows Aschoff's bodies.
- In macrophages chromatin condensed into long wavy ribbons (caterpillar cells), which is diagnostic of Aschoff's body.

188. Aschoff's bodies are seen in- *(DNB June 07)*
a. Rheumatic myocarditis
b. Marantic endocarditis
c. Rheumatic arthritis
d. Bacterial endocarditis

[Ref: Robbins 9th/e pg.558]

189. Cells forming aschoff nodules are all the following except *(PGMEE 2015)*
a. T cells
b. B cells
c. Plasma cells
d. Activated macrophages

[Ref: Robbins 9th/e pg.558]

190. Causative organism of rheumatic fever
(PGMEE 2014-15)
a. Staphylococci
b. Group A Streptococci
c. Group B Streptococci
d. Group D Streptococci
[Ref: Robbins 9th/e pg.557]

191. The probable interval between throat infection and onset of rheumatic fever is- *(DNB June 07)*
a. 2-4 days
b. 2-4 months
c. 2-4 weeks
d. 2-4 hours
[Ref: Nelson 18th/e pg. 1141]

192. Following are major criteria of rheumatic fever, except- *(DNB Dec. 07)*
a. Carditis
b. Chorea
c. Arthritis
d. Prolonged P-R interval
[Ref: Harrison 18th/e pg. 2755; Robbin's 8th/e pg. 566]

193. MC valve involved in Rheumatic fever- *(DNB Dec. 08)*
a. Mitral
b. Pulmonary
c. Tricuspid
d. Aortic
[Ref: Robbin's 8th/e pg. 566; Textbook of Cardioogy 2nd/e pg. 877]

194. Valve usually not involved in rheumatic fever- *(DNB Dec.08)*
a. Aortic
b. Tricuspid
c. Pulmonary
d. Mitral
[Ref: Robbin's 8th/e pg. 566; Textbook of Cardiology 2nd/e pg. 877]

195. Sequele of rheumatic heart disease in a 5 year old child is? *(PGMEE 2014-15)*
a. Mitral regurgitation
b. Mitral stenosis
c. Tricuspid stenosis
d. Tricuspid regurgitation
[Ref: Harrison's 19th/e pg. 2150-51]

196. Rheumatic Heart disease diagnostic criteria includes: *(PGMEE 2015-16)*
a. Oral ulcer
b. Malar rash
c. Erythema Marginatum
d. Nail telangiectasia
[Ref: Harrison 19th ed. / 2149]

197. Which of the following regarding rheumatic nodules is false? *(PGMEE 2014-15)*
a. Found over extensor surface
b. Tender on palpation
c. Associated with carditis
d. Pea size nodules
[Ref: Harrison's 18th ed. ch.322]

198. Earliest valvular lesion in acute rheumatic fever: *(PGMEE 2014-15)*
a. Mitral stenosis
b. Mitral insufficiency
c. Aortic stenosis
d. Aortic regurgitation
[Ref: Harrison's 18th ed. pg. 2752]

199. The most characteristic murmur of rheumatic carditis is: *(PGMEE 2014-15)*
a. Apical high-pitched early diastolic murmur
b. Apical high-pitched holosystolic murmur
c. Apical low-pitched mid-diastolic murmur
d. Systolic ejection murmur along the left stenal border
[Ref: Harrison's 19th/e pg. 2150]

200. Consider the following clinicopathological changes in the Rheumatic Carditis: *(PGMEE 2014-15)*
i. Mitral regurgitation
ii. Aortic regurgitation
iii. ASLO rise
iv. Left atrial enlargement
The correct chronological sequence of these events is
a. iii, i, iv, ii
b. i, ii, iii, iv
c. iv, ii, i, iii
d. iii, iv, i, ii
[Ref: Ch 322, Harrison's 18th ed.]

201. Features of rheumatic carditis are all except?
a. Aschoff nodule *(PGMEE 2014-15)*
b. Commisural involvement
c. PR segment prolongation
d. Fourth heart sound heard
[Ref: Harrison's 19th/e pg. 2150-51]

202. Steroids are given in rheumatic fever when there is: *(PGMEE 2014-15)*
a. Carditis
b. Subcutaneous nodules
c. Chorea
d. All of the above
[Ref: Harrison's 19th/e pg. 2153]

203. A Carey-Coomb's murmur heard in a child with multiple joint pains is suggestive of: *(PGMEE 2014-15)*
a. Infective endocarditis
b. Rheumatoid arthritis
c. Rheumatic fever
d. Libman-Sacs endocarditis
[Ref: Harrison's 19th /e pg. 2153]

204. Intra-cardiac calcifications indicate: *(PGMEE 2014-15)*
a. SBE
b. Rheumatic valves
c. Old MI
d. Chronic pericarditis
[Ref: Harrison's 19th/e pg. 2138]

MISCELLANEOUS

205. Pericardical cyst is seen at: *(PGMEE 2015-16)*
a. Cardiophrenic angle
b. Middle mediastinum
c. Posterior mediastinum
d. Lingula
[Ref: Harrison 19th ed. / 1719]

206. Most common cause of unilateral pedal edema? *(PGMEE 2015-16)*
a. Pregnancy
b. Lymphedema
c. Venous insufficiency
d. Milroy disease
[Ref: Harrison 19th ed. / 253]

207. A Patient presented with deficiency of thiamine. What could be possible outcome: *(PGMEE 2015-16)*
a. Delayed wound healing
b. Cardiac abnormality
c. Memory loss
d. Gingival bleeding
[Ref: Harrison 19th ed. / 96e-1t]

208. Dresseler syndrome is associated with all EXCEPT: *(PGMEE 2014-15)*
a. Eosinophilia
b. Myocarditis
c. Endocarditis
d. Encephalitis
[Ref: Harrison's 19th/e pg. 382]

209. Who invented the stethoscope: *(PGMEE 2014-15)*
a. Rene Laennec
b. Leeuwenhoek
c. Joseph Littmann
d. William Osler
[Ref: Medical Encyclopedia]

190.	b
191.	c
192.	d
193.	a
194.	c
195.	a
196.	c
197.	b
198.	b
199.	c
200.	a
201.	d
202.	a
203.	c
204.	b
205.	b
206.	c
207.	b
208.	c
209.	a

210. A 60-year-old female patient with cardiac prosthetic valve has serum creatinine of 3 mg % with pyo-nephrosis. Investigation of choice for determining prosthetic valve damage is? *(PGMEE 2014-15)*
a. Blood culture
b. Cinefluorography
c. Over penentrated CXR
d. T.E.E.

[Ref: Harrison's 19th ed. p 820]

211. Angiography image is given below. Identify the marked vessel:- *(PGMEE 2016-17)*

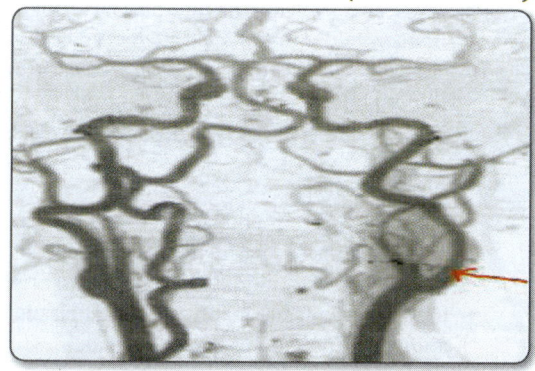

a. Vertebral artery
b. Basilar artery
c. External carotid artery
d. Internal carotid artery

[Ref: Internet]

212. Pharmacological stress testing is done by using all EXCEPT:- *(PGMEE 2016-17)*
a. IV Dopamine
b. Dipyridamole
c. IV Dobutamine
d. IV Adenosine

[Ref: Textbook of Cardiovascular Medicine edited by Eric J. Topol, Robert M. Califf pg. 887]

213. P.S.T is: *(PGMEE 2014-15)*
a. Phenol sulfotransferase deficiency
b. Post traumatic stress disorder
c. Protein S deficiency
d. Paroxysmal supraventricular tachycardia

[Ref: Net Source: Pubmed]

214. A 12 year old wheel chair bound boy with scoliosis has presented with Dyspnea. ECG shows sinus tachycardia with tall R in lead V1 and deep Q wave in V5, V6. Probable diagnosis: *(PGMEE 2014-15)*
a. Amyotrophic lateral sclerosis
b. Duchenne muscular dystrophy
c. Pott's paraplegia
d. Myotonic dystrophy

[Ref: www.ahajournals.com]

215. In a patient there is dyspnea in upright position which is relieved in supine position. Diagnosis? *(PGMEE 2015-16)*
a. Tachypnea
b. Orthopnea
c. Paroxysmal nocturnal dyspnea
d. Platypnea

[Ref: Harrison 20th ed. pg. 228]

210.	d
211.	d
212.	a
213.	a
214.	b
215.	d

ATHEROSCLEROSIS

1. Atheromatous changes of blood vessels affects earliest in the- *(PGMEE 2012-13, 2014)*
- a. Heart
- b. Liver
- c. Kidney
- d. Spleen

[Ref: Robbin's 9th/e pg. 499]

2. Infective agent causing atherosclerosis- *(PGMEE 2015)*
- a. C. Diptheriae
- b. C. Pneumoniae
- c. H. influenza
- d. M. Pneumoniae

[Ref: Robbin's 8th/e pg. 1182]

3. Atheromatous plaque don't contain- *(PGMEE 13; 16)*
- a. Monocytes
- b. Neutrophils
- c. Smooth muscle fibres
- d. Platelets

[Ref: Robbin's 9th/e pg. 496]

4. Cleft like space in atheromatous plaque mainly contains? *(PGMEE 2016)*
- a. Smooth muscle cell
- b. Fibrous tissue
- c. Cholesterol
- d. Macrophages

[Ref: Robbin's 9th/e pg. 498]

5. Needle shaped empty space on the histopathological slide of an atheromatous plaque represents? *(PGMEE 2015-16)*
- a. Foam cell
- b. Glycogen tissue
- c. Cholesterol clefts
- d. Smooth muscle cells

[Ref: Robbin's 9th/e pg. 498]

6. The following arteries are usually spared from extensive atherosclerosis *(PGMEE 2015)*
- a. Popliteal artery
- b. Internal carotid artery
- c. Arteries of circle of willis
- d. Mesenteric arteries

[Ref: Robbin's 9th/e pg. 498-499]

7. The necrotic core of an atherosclerotic plaque contains
- a. T cells
- b. Collagen
- c. Lipid
- d. None of the above

[Ref: Robbin's 9th/e pg. 498]

8. True about atherosclerosis *(PGMEE 2014-15)*
- a. Chronic inflammatory disorder of vessel wail
- b. Not lead to complications of vessel wall
- c. Thoracic aorta more than abdominal aorta
- d. Atherosclerostic plaques do not demonstrate extracellular matrix deposition

[Ref: Robbin's 9th/e pg. 494]

9. The coronary artery most commonly involved in atherosclerosis *(PGMEE 2015)*
- a. Left anterior descending artery
- b. Left main coronary artery
- c. Right coronary artery
- d. Circumflex coronary artery

[Ref: Robbin's 9th/e pg. 498-499]

10. Medial calcification is seen in- *(PGMEE 2012-13)*
- a. Dissecting aneurysm
- b. Arteriolosclerosis
- c. Monckebergs sclerosis
- d. Atherosclerosis

[Ref: Robbin's 9th/e pg. 491]

11. Not true about Monkeberg's medial sclerosis *(PGMEE 2015)*
- a. Calcification of the walls of muscular arteries
- b. Typically involving the internal elastic membrane
- c. Persons older than age 50 are most commonly affected
- d. Calcifications cause significant narrowing of vessel lumen

[Ref: Robbins 9th/pg 491-492]

Explanation

- Monckeberg's medial sclerosis is a form of arteriosclerosis, in which calcium deposits are found in the muscular middle layer of walls of arteries (tunica media). It typically involves internal elastic membrane andaffects individuals aged >50 years.

12. Foamy macrophage cells in atherosclerosis contain lipid in the form of *(PGMEE 2014-15)*
- a. Oxidized LDL
- b. Reduced LDL
- c. Oxidized VLDL
- d. Reduced VLDL

[Ref: Robbin's 9th/e pg. 496]

13. Following are the modifiable risk factor of atherosclerosis except *(PGMEE 2014-15)*
- a. Physical inactivity
- b. Family history
- c. Diabetes
- d. Hypertension

[Ref: Robbin's 9th/e pg. 496]

14. True about the basic structure of artherosclerosis plaque is- *(PGMEE 2014-15)*
- a. Concave part formed by fibrous cap
- b. Convex part formed by tunica media of the vessel
- c. Convex part formed by fibrous cap
- d. Necrotic core contains collagen, elastin and proteoglycans

*[Ref: Robbin's 9th/e pg. **496**]*

15. Atherosclerosis initiation by fibroblast plaque is mediated by injury to *(PGMEE 2014-15)*
- a. Smooth muscle
- b. Media
- c. Adventitia
- d. Endothelium

[Ref: Harrison's 20th ed. pg. 1851]

16. Changes seen in atherosclerotic plaque at the time of rupture are all except- *(PGMEE 2013-14)*
- a. Cell debris
- b. Thin fibrosis cap place in
- c. Smooth muscle cell hypertrophy atherosclerosis
- d. Multiple foam cap

[Ref: Robbin's 9th/e pg. 499 fig.11-15]

1.	a
2.	b
3.	b
4.	c
5.	c
6.	d
7.	c
8.	a
9.	a
10.	c
11.	d
12.	a
13.	b
14.	c
15.	d
16.	c

ISCHEMIC HEART DISEASES/CAD

ANGINA PECTORIS

17. **Which of the following is not true about Prinzmetal's angina?** *(NEET Pattern 2019)*
a. Aspirin treatment decreases the episodes of angina
b. Severe ischemic pain at rest with ST segment elevation
c. Focal spasms are common in eight coronary artery
d. Nitrates and calcium channel blockers are the mainstay of management

18. **Wellen's syndrome is seen with:** *(PGMEE 2014-15)*
a. Stable angina
b. Unstable angina
c. Prinzmetal angina
d. Ludwig angina

Explanation

- Wellen's Syndrome is a pattern of deeply inverted or biphasic T waves in V_{2-3}, which is seen in unstable angina. Specific for critical stenosis of Left anterior descending artery (LAD).

19. **Unstable angina is characterized by?** *(PGMEE 2014-15)*
a. Decrescendo pattern of symptoms
b. Crescendo pain with ECG findings
c. ST segment elevation
d. Normal cardiac biomarkers

[Ref: Harrison 20th ed. pg. 1868]

20. **Usual duration of chest pain in chronic stable Angina is?** *(PGMEE 2014-15)*
a. 1-3 minutes
b. 2-5 minutes
c. 15 minutes
d. 30 minutes

[Ref: Harrison 20th ed. pg. 1853]

21. **Nitrates are used in Angine pectocis:-** *(PGMEE 2016-17)*
a. Intravenous
b. Sublingually
c. Orally
d. Intradermally

[Ref: Harrison 20th ed. pg. 1861]

22. **ROSE questionnaire is used for?** *(PGMEE 2015-16)*
a. Alcohol addiction
b. Sex addiction
c. Angina assessment
d. Deep Vein thrombosis Assessment

[Ref: Braunwald 8th edn Ch 57]

Explanation

- ROSE Questionaire is used to evaluate the subjective severity of ischemic heart pain and intermittent claudication in patients with CAD.

23. **Characteristic of pain of Angina Pectoris are all EXCEPT:-** *(PGMEE 2016-17)*
a. Stabbing type
b. Sharp excruciating pain
c. Radiates to left arm, neck and jaw
d. Confined in precordial region

[Ref: Harrison 20th ed. pg. 1853]

24. **Which is the best way to differentiate between stable angins and NSTEMI?** *(PGMEE 2015)*
a. Multi uptake gated A cquisition scan
b. Trans thoracic Echocardiography
c. ECG
d. Cardiac-biomarker

[Ref: Harrison 20th ed. pg. 1866]

ACUTE CORONARY SYNDROME

25. **Infarcts involving which portion of myocardium cause aneurysm as post-MI complication?** *(NEET 2019)*
a. Inferior wall
b. Anterior transmural
c. Subendocardial
d. Posterior transmural

26. **Which is best for plaque morphology?** *(PGMEE 2015-16)*
a. CCTA
b. MRI
c. Optical Coherence Tomography
d. IVUS

[Ref: Evidence based cardiology consult, Page 217, 2014 edition; CMDT 2015, p 354; Harrison's 19th/e pg.1465]

27. **All are true about right ventricular infarct EXCEPT:** *(DNB December 2011)*
a. Nocturia
b. Normal JVP
c. Ascites
d. Hepatomegaly

[Ref: Harrison 20th ed. pg. 1882]

28. **Which of the following is not a contraindication to thrombolysis?** *(PGMEE 2014-15)*
a. BP>180/110 mm Hg
b. Diabetic retinal flame shaped hemorrhage
c. History of previous cerebral bleed
d. Aortic dissection

[Ref: Harrison 20th ed. pg. 1879]

29. **Dose of streptokinase to be used in MI is?** *(PGMEE 2014-15)*
a. 0.15 Million units
b. 1.5 Million units
c. 15 Million units
d. 150 Million units

[Ref: Harrison 20th ed. pg. 1879]

30. **Dose of reteplase for management of MI is?** *(PGMEE 2014-15)*
a. 5 IU
b. 10 IU
c. 15 IU
d. 50 IU

[Ref: Harrison 20th ed. pg. 1879]

31. **Not recommended in coronary artery disease patients:** *(PGMEE 2015)*
a. Statins
b. Vitamin-E
c. Daily exercise
d. Potassium

[Ref: Harrison 20th ed. pg. 1879, 1884]

32. **Which one of the following is not an early complication of acute myocardial infarction?** *(PGMEE 2015)*
a. Papillary muscle dysfunction
b. Pericarditis
c. Ventricular septal defect
d. Dressler's syndrome

[Ref: Harrison 20th ed. pg. 1882-84]

17.	a
18.	b
19.	b,d
20.	b
21.	b
22.	c
23.	d
24.	d
25.	b
26.	c
27.	b
28.	b
29.	b
30.	b
31.	b
32.	d

33. A patient of acute Myocardial infarction with ECG showing ST segment elevation has severe hypotension. Immediate management of the patient is: *(PGMEE 2014-15)*

a. Intra-aortic balloon pump
b. PCI with angioplasty
c. Thrombolysis
d. Intravenous fluids

[Ref: Harrison 20th ed. pg. 1881]

34. Half- life of alteplase? *(PGMEE 2014-15)*

a. 3 min b. 5 min
c. 9 min d. 12 min

35. CAD is related to decreased levels of which HDL: *(PGMEE 2014-15)*

a. HDL1 b. HDL 2
c. HDL 3 d. HDL 4

36. All are associated with increased risk of coronary events EXCEPT: *(PGMEE 2014-15)*

a. High sensitivity CRP
b. High Agatson score
c. Intravascular IVUS showing lumen reduction
d. Ability to complete stage 3 of Bruce protocol treadmill

[Ref: Harrison 20th ed. pg. 1858]

Explanation

- Development of angina and/or severe ST segment depression before completion of stage II of the Bruce protocol suggest severe IHD & high risk of future adverse events.
- Agatston score is used to quantify coronary artery calcification on cardiac CT. High Agatston score is associated with increased risk of major adverse cardiac event.

37. In myocardial infarction, the correct sequence of increase in enzyme levels is: *(PGMEE 2014-15)*

a. CPK, AST, LDH b. CPK, LDH, AST
c. AST, CPK, LDH d. LDH, CPK, AST

[Ref: Harrison 20th ed. pg. 1875]

38. Which of the following is associated with atherosclerosis? *(PGMEE 2014-15)*

a. Chlamydia trachomatis b. Chlamydia pneumoniae
c. Chlamydia psittaci d. Chlamydia gingivalis

[Ref: Harrison 20th ed. pg. 1324]

39. A 65-year-old male had MI one year ago. Now the same patient presents with hypertension. Which of the following drug is best suited for this patient? *(PGMEE 2015)*

a. Lisinopril b. Metoprolol
c. Clonidine d. Thiazide

[Ref: Harrison 20th ed. pg. 1904]

40. All are used for secondary prevention of MI EXCEPT: *(PGMEE 2015)*

a. Aspirin b. Beta blockers
c. Warfarin d. Statins

[Ref: Harrison 20th ed. pg. 1884]

41. Which of the following is given to decrease Serum Tri-glycerides? *(PGMEE 2015)*

a. Niacin b. Statins
c. Fibrates d. Ezetimibe

[Ref: Harrison 20th ed. pg. 2901]

42. A patient with anterior wall MI was thrombolysed within 6 hours with STK. On day 3 he had fever with chills and platelet count of 60,000. Which of the following is responsible for this presentation? *(PGMEE 2015-16)*

a. Aspirin b. Ranolazine
c. STK d. Clopidogrel

[Ref: Harrison's 19th/e pg. 745]

43. A 50-year old man who had recently joined a gym collapsed on the treadmill. He was rushed to the hospital where an ECG shows presence of: *(PGMEE 2015-16)*

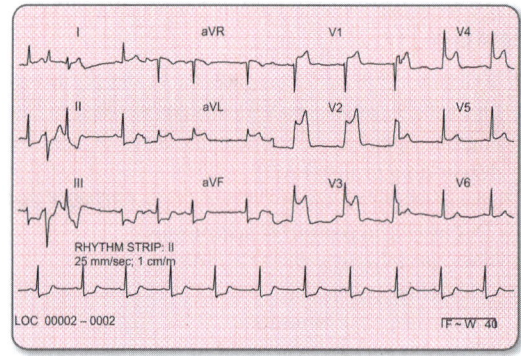

a. Acute extensive anterior wall MI
b. Brugada syndrome
c. Catecholamine sensitive ventricular tachycardia
d. Arrhythmogenic right ventricular dysplasia

44. Which scan shows Hot-spot in myocardial infarction :- *(PGMEE 2016-17)*

a. Thallium b. Tc labelled RBCs
c. Tc-99 Pyrophosphate d. Gd

Explanation

- Myocardial perfusion studies is done by
  ○ Thallium 201 → ischemic myocardium appears as cold area
  ○ 99m - Technetium sestamibi → myocardium appears as cold area
  ○ 99m - Technetium pyrophosphate → infarct appears as hot area

45. Levine's sign is seen in:- *(PGMEE 2016-17)*

a. Pericarditis
b. Dresseler syndrome
c. Acute coronary syndrome
d. Saggital sinus thrombosis

[Ref: Harrison 20th ed. pg. 1853]

46. Most common cause of sudden death (< 24 hours) in MI is? *(PGMEE 2014-15)*

a. Cardiogenic shock
b. Ventricular fibrillation
c. Mobitz 1 heart block
d. Cardiac rupture

[Ref: Harrison 20th ed. pg. 1882]

33.	d
34.	b
35.	b
36.	d
37.	a
38.	b
39.	a
40.	c
41.	b,c
42.	d
43.	a
44.	c
45.	c
46.	b

47. Persistent ST segment elevation 24 hours after treatment for MI with P.C.I is due to *(PGMEE 2014-15)*
a. Left ventricular aneurysm
b. Impending cardiac rupture
b. Dressler syndrome
c. Coronary artery dissection

[Ref: Harrison 20th ed. pg. 1681]

48. Infarcts involving which part of the myocardium cause aneurysm as a post-Myocardial infarction complication? *(PGMEE 2019)*
a. Subendocardial MI
b. Anterior transmural MI
c. Posterior transmural MI
d. Inferior wall MI

Explanation
- A left ventricular aneurysm can form after a transmural myocardial infarction and involves dilation of the left ventricular wall in an abnormal fashion. Most commonly, the apex of the heart is involved however, the inferior wall can form an aneurysm as well.

49. False positive troponin I can be seen in all except? *(PGMEE 2014-15)*
a. **Blunt trauma chest**
b. Pulmonary embolism
c. Chronic liver failure
d. Renal failure

[Ref: Cardiac intensive care 2nd edition, pg. 199]

50. Most common arrhythmia seen after reperfusion strategy in MI? *(PGMEE 2014-15)*
a. A.I.V.R
b. V.T
c. V.fibrillation
d. P.S.V.T

[Ref: Harrison 20th ed. pg. 1882]

51. Correct sequence of ECG changes in acute MI is? *(PGMEE 2014-15)*
a. T inversion, ST elevation, Q wave
b. ST elevation, T inversion, Q wave
c. ST elevation, Q wave, T inversion
d. Q wave, ST elevation, T inversion

[Ref: Harrison 20th ed. pg. 1680]

52. Coronary artery disease is associated with all EXCEPT: *(PGMEE 2015-16)*
a. Alcohol
b. Poor dental hygiene
c. Smoking
d. None

[Ref: Harrison 20th ed. pg. 1859]

53. Which one of the following sets of components of cigarette smoke is a casual agent of coronary artery disease- *(PGMEE 2012-13)*
a. Carbon monoxide and Tar
b. Nicotine and carbon monoxide and tar
c. Carbon dioxide
d. Tar and nicotine

[Ref: Park 21st/e pg. 339]

54. Most common site of artery of atherosclerosis- *(PGMEE 2012-13)*
a. LAD
b. LCX
c. Diagonal branch of LAD
d. RCA

[Ref: Robbin's 8th/e pg. 549-550]

55. Recurrent ischaemic events following thrombosis have been pathophysiologically linked to *(PGMEE 2016)*
a. Antibodies to thrombolytic agents
b. Fibrinopeptide A
c. Lipoprotein A
d. Triglycerides

[Ref: Circulation June 29, 2004 vol. 109 no. 25 suppl 1 IV-6- IV-19]

56. Which of the following is a non-modifiable risk factor for CHD- *(PGMEE 2013-14)*
a. Hypertension
b. Diabetes
c. Smoking
d. Age

[Ref: Harrison 18th/e pg. 1987; Robbins 9th/e pg. 492,494]

57. Post mortem finding in a case of death due to myocardial infarction is? *(PGMEE 2015)*
a. Fat necrosis
b. Caseous necrosis
c. Liquefactive necrosis
d. Coagulative necrosis

[Ref: 9th/pg 544; 8th/pg 550]

58. In myocardial infarction, microscopic picture of coagulation necrosis with neutrophilic infiltration is seen in- *(DNB Dec. 08)*
a. 4-12 hours
b. 3-7 days
c. 1-3 days
d. 12-24 hours

[Ref: Robbins 9th/pg 544]

59. Approximate time, at the end of which the quantity, of ATP within ischemic cardiac myocytes is reduced to 10% of original is- *(DNB Dec. 08)*
a. 10 minutes
b. 20 minutes
c. <2 minutes
d. 40 minutes

[Ref: Robbins 9th/pg 544]

60. Most common site of myocardial infarction is *(DNB Dec. 07)*
a. Ant. wall of left ventricle
b. Inferior Wall of left ventricle
c. Post. Wall of right ventricle
d. Post. Wall of left ventricle

[Ref: Robbins 9th/pg 544]

61. Myocardial infraction shows fibrosis. What is the duration? *(PGMEE 2014)*
a. 2 days
b. 5 days
c. 1 week
d. 3 weeks

[Ref: Robbins 9th/pg 544]

62. In myocardial infraction, dense neutophilic infilteration is seen in how much time- *(PGMEE 2014)*
a. 24 hours
b. 2 days
c. 5 days
d. One week

[Ref: Robbins 9th/pg 544]

63. Cells seen in MI at 48 hours are- *(DNB June 07)*
a. Polymorphs
b. Macrophages
c. Fibroblasts
d. Lymphocytes

[Ref: Robbins 9th/pg 544]

64. Diagnostic Troponin I value for Myocardial infarction is? *(PGMEE 2012)*
a. >0.2 ng/ml
b. >0.6 ng/ml
c. >0.8 ng/ml
d. >0.4 ng/ml

[Ref: Robbins 9th/pg 544]

47.	a
48.	b
49.	c
50.	a
51.	c
52.	d
53.	b
54.	a
55.	c
56.	d
57.	d
58.	c
59.	d
60.	a
61.	d
62.	b
63.	a
64.	a

65. **Autopsy diagnosis of myocardial infarction can be done by immersion of tissue slices in a solution of**
   a. Triphenyl tetrazolium chloride   *(PGMEE 2015)*
   b. 100% alcohol
   c. Orcein stain
   d. Crystal violet

   [Ref: Robbins 9th/pg 544]

66. **Due to ischemia, irreversible cell injury to cardiac myocytes occur in**   *(PGMEE 2015)*
   a. <2 minutes   b. 10-20 minutes
   c. 20-40 minutes   d. >1 hour

   [Ref: Robbins 9th/pg 544]

67. **Earliest light microscopic change seen in myocardial infarction**   *(PGMEE 2015; 2013-14)*
   a. Waviness of fibres   b. Neutrophilic infiltration
   c. Coagulation necrosis   d. Contraction band necrosis

   [Ref: Robbins 9th/e pg. 544]

68. **First enzyme to be raised in MI is-**   *(PGMEE 2013-14)*
   a. LDH   b. Troponin- I
   c. Myoglobin   d. CPK- MB

   [Ref: Textbook of comprehensive coronary case-151]

69. **Creatinine kinase is elevated in MI after-**   *(PGMEE 2013-14)*
   a. 2-4 hours   b. 12-24 hours
   c. >24 hours   d. 4-8 hours

   [Ref: Robbins 9th/pg 544]

70. **The cells seen between 24-72 hours in the infarcted area in MI are**   *(PGMEE 2015)*
   a. Neutrophils   b. Lymphocytes
   c. Macrophages   d. Monocytes

   [Ref: Robbins 9th/pg 544]

71. **Inferior wall MI-**   *(PGMEE 2012-13)*
   a. Post interventricular artery
   b. Nodal branch
   c. Ant interventricular artery
   d. Atrial branch

   [Ref: BDC Vol 1 5th/e pg. 252, 253; Robbin's 8th/e pg. 550]

72. **The cells seen after 72 hours in the infarcted area in MI are-**   *(PGMEE 2012-13)*
   a. Lymphocytes   b. Monocytes
   c. Macrophages   d. Neutrophils

   [Ref: Chandrasoma Taylor 3rd/e pg. 364]

73. **7 days old MI the most sensitive biochemical marker-**   *(PGMEE 2012-13)*
   a. Troponin I T   b. LDH
   c. Myoglobin   d. CPK MB

   [Ref: Robbins 9th/pg 544]

74. **Post MI day 10 which enzyme is raised-**   *(PGMEE 2012-13)*
   a. LDH   b. Troponin
   c. Myoglobin   d. CPK

   [Ref: Robbins 9th/pg 544]

75. **Fatal arrythmias are seen if myocardial infarction is-**   *(PGMEE 2012-13)*
   a. Anterolateral   b. Inferior
   c. Subendodardial   d. Posterior

   [Ref: Robbins 9th/pg 544]

65.	a
66.	c
67.	a
68.	c
69.	d
70.	a
71.	a
72.	c
73.	a
74.	a
75.	b
76.	c
77.	a
78.	b
79.	d
80.	b
81.	d

AORTIC DISSECTION

76. **Most common predisposing factor for aortic dissection**   *(PGMEE 2015)*
   a. Atherosclerosis   b. Syphilis
   c. Hypertension   d. Smoking

   [Ref: Harrison's 20th ed. pg. 1920]

Explanation

- Factors predisposing to aortic dissection:
  ○ Hypertension (~70%)
  ○ Marfan's syndrome
  ○ Ehlers - Danlos syndrome
  ○ Bicuspid aortic valve
  ○ Coarctation of the aorta
  ○ Takayasu arteritis
  ○ Giant cell arteritis
  ○ Pregnancy
  ○ Cocaine use

77. **Most common cause of dissecting hematoma is because of-**   *(PGMEE 2015; 2012-13)*
   a. Hypertension   b. Trauma
   c. Mafan syndrome   d. DM

   [Ref: Harrison's 20th ed. pg. 1920]

78. **Classification of aortic dissection depends upon-**   *(PGMEE 2013-14)*
   a. Percentage of aorta affected
   b. Level of aorta affected
   c. Cause of dissection
   d. None

   [Ref: Harrison's 20th ed. pg. 1920]

79. **Aortic dissection is not common in the following disease**   *(PGMEE 2015)*
   a. Marfan syndrome   b. Hypertension
   c. Cystic medial necrosis d. Secondary syphilis

   [Ref: Harrison's 20th ed. pg. 1920]

80. **Cystic medial necrosis is seen in**   *(PGMEE 2014-15, 2012-13)*
   a. Hypertension   b. Marfan's syndrome
   c. Kawasaki disease d. Friedrichs ataxia

   [Ref: Harrison's 20th ed. pg. 1918]

Explanation

- Cystic medial necrosis, now k/a Medial degeneration describes the degeneration of collagen and elastic fibers in the tunica media of aorta.
- It characteristically affects the proximal aorta & l/t aneurysm of ascending aorta.
- It occur in patients with Marfan's syndrome, ehler-Danlos syndrome.

ANEURYSM

81. **Surgery is indicated in asymptomatic abdominal aortic aneurysm if the size of aneurysm is more than**   *(PGMEE 2015)*
   a. 4 cm   b. 4.5 cm
   c. 5 cm   d. 5.5 cm

   [Ref: Harrison's 20th ed. pg. 1919]

82. Visceral aneurysm is most commonly seen in-
(PGMEE 2012-13)
a. Splenic artery   b. Hepatic
c. Coronary   d. Renal

[Ref: Textbook of interventional radiology pg. 740]

83. Risk of abdominal aortic aneurysm rupture is > 25% per year when the size is greater than *(PGMEE 2015)*
a. 4 cm   b. 6 cm
c. 7 cm   d. 8 cm

[Ref: Guidelines for the treatment of abdominal aortic aneurysms. J Vasc Surg. 2003; 37[5]:1106]

84. Most common complication following open repair of abdominal aortic aneurysm *(PGMEE 2015)*
a. Paraplegia   b. Acute renal failure
c. Myocardial infarction d. Pulmonary embolism

[Ref: Guidelines ...J Vasc Surg. 2003;37[5]:1106]

85. Most common cause of aortic aneurysm is-
(PGMEE 2015)
a. Atherosclerosis   b. Cystic medial necrosis
c. Syphilis   d. Trauma

[Ref: Harrison's 20th ed. pg. 1917]

86. Ascending aorta involvement is the commonest site of which aneurysm- *(DNB June 09)*
a. Syphilitic   b. Atherosclerotic
c. Mycotic   d. None of the above

[Ref: Harrison's 20th ed. pg. 1918]

87. Syphilitic aneurysm mostly involve- *(PGMEE 2013-14)*
a. Abdominal aorta below the renal arteries
b. Abdominal aorta above the renal arteries
c. Descending aorta
d. Ascending aorta

[Ref: Harrison's 20th ed. pg. 1918]

88. Which of the following causes pseudoaneurysm?
(PGMEE 2015)
a. Trauma   b. Atherosclerosis
c. Infection   d. Inflammation

[Ref: Robbin's 9th/e pg. 501]

89. In Marfan syndrome, rupture of aortic aneurysm usually occurs at *(PGMEE 2015)*
a. Ascending aorta   b. Descending aorta
c. Arch of aorta   d. Abdominal aorta

[Ref: Harrison's 20th ed. pg. 1918]

90. True regarding fibromuscular dysplasia are all except-
(PGMEE 2013-14)
a. Irregular hyperplasia
b. Use of OCPs predisposes this condition
c. Medium size vessels are affected
d. Aneurysm may occur   *[Ref: Robbins 9th/e pg. 485]*

91. Dissecting aneurysm is seen in? *(PGMEE 2014-15)*
a. Takayasu disease b. Atherosclerosis
c. Syphilis aortitis d. Marfan syndrome

[Ref: Harrison's 20th ed. pg. 1920]

92. Investigation of choice for aortic dissection with hypotension is ? *(PGMEE 2014-15)*
a. CT scan   b. Technetium 99 scan
c. MRI   d. T.E.E.

[Ref: Harrison's 20th ed. pg. 1921]

HYPERTENSION

93. Which of the following is not used in hypertensive emergency? *(DNB December 2011)*
a. Nitroglycerin   b. Fenoldopam
c. Nitroprusside   d. Clonidine

[Ref: Harrison 20th ed. pg. 1905]

94. Indications of giving IV antihypertensive:-
(PGMEE 2016-17)
a. Acute pulmonary edema
b. Subarachnoid hemorrhage
c. Pergnancy induced hypertension
d. Type 1 DM

[Ref: Harrison 20th ed. pg. 1905]

95. Management of essential hypertension is?
(DNB Dec 2009)
a. No need to treat
b. Invasive surgery
c. Diet modification and drugs
d. Diet modification alone

[Ref: Harrison 20th ed. pg. 1900-01]

96. Most common cause of Secondary hypertension is?
a. Renovascular disease   *(PGMEE 2014-15)*
b. Pheochromocytoma
c. Renal parenchymal disease
d. Hyperthyroidism

[Ref: Harrison 20th ed. pg. 1985]

97. A lady on anti hypertensive medication comes with hemiparesis and speech difficulty for 2.5 hours. BP is 180/100. What is the best treatment for this patient?
(NEET Pattern 2013)
a. Aggressive Reduction of BP
b. Modest Lowering of BP
c. Thrombolysis with tissue plasminogen activator
d. Aspirin and Clopidogrel loading dose

[Ref: American stroke association 2018 guidelines]

98. Pregnant lady with Hypertension with diabetes mellitus requires which drug to control her BP?
(PGMEE 2014-15)
a. ACE inhibitors
b. Beta blocker
c. ARB
d. Diuretics

[Ref: Harrison 20th ed. pg. 3441]

99. Most common cause of hypertension is?
(PGMEE 2014-15)
a. Renal artery stenosis
b. Essential hypertension
c. Pheochromocytoma
d. Chronic Glomerulonephritis

[Ref: Harrison 20th ed. pg. 1896]

100. Blood pressure is difficult to measure in a patient with:
(PGMEE 2014-15)
a. Mitral stenosis   b. Aortic stenosis
c. Complete heart block d. Atrial fibrillation

[Ref: Harrison's 19th/e pg. 1486]

82.	a
83.	c
84.	c
85.	a
86.	a
87.	d
88.	a
89.	a
90.	b
91.	b,d
92.	d
93.	d
94.	c
95.	c
96.	c
97.	b
98.	b
99.	b
100.	d

101. A female has a SBP = 130 mm Hg and DBP = 100 mm Hg on two consecutive occasions. Best treatment is?

(PGMEE 2015-16)

a. Life style modification
b. Sedative
c. Anti –hypertensive drugs
d. Error in BP Machine

[Ref: Harrison 20th ed. pg. 1904]

102. Hypertension patient has presented with BP of 220/130 mm Hg in the emergency with headache but no CNS deficit. What is the goal BP for this patient?

(PGMEE 2014-15)

a. 200/150
b. 180/110
c. 160/100
d. 140/90

[Ref: Harrison 20th ed. pg. 1905]

103. Most common cause of Resistant hypertension is?

a. Non-compliance of patient   *(PGMEE 2014-15)*
b. Obstructive sleep apnea
c. Pheochromocytoma
d. Renovascular disease

[Ref: Harrison 20th ed. pg. 1905]

104. Male patient suffering from headache, profuse sweating, palpitations and BP of 160/110. Which drug will be useful?   *(DNB June 2009)*

a. Phenxybenzamine
b. Labetalol
c. Prazosin
d. Nifedipine

[Ref: Harrison's 19th/e pg 2582,2643, 463e-1]

PULMONARY HYPERTENSION

105. A 35-year-old lady with idiopathic pulmonary artery hypertension. Which findings best describe this patient

(PGMEE 2014-15)

a. Elevated JVP, normal S1 S2, diastolic murmur
b. Elevated JVP, singular loud S2, systolic murmur
c. Elevated JVP, wide fixed split S2, systolic murmur
d. Elevated JVP, barrel chest reverse split S2

[Ref: Harrison 20th ed. pg. 1937]

106. Pulmonary hypertension is defined as pulmonary arterial pressure:-   *(PGMEE 2016-17)*

a. >15 mm Hg   b. > 25 mm Hg
c. >30 mm Hg   d. >40 mmHg

[Ref: Harrison 20th ed. pg. 1938]

107. Extremely bad prognosis is seen in which heart disease in pregnancy?   *(PGMEE 2014-15)*

a. Repaired TOF
b. Bicuspid aortic valve
c. ASD
d. Pulmonary artery hypertension

[Ref: Table 31-3, current diagnosis and treatment in cardiology 2nd edition]

108. Which of the following does not cause pulmonary hypertension?   *(DNB Dec 2009)*

a. Scleroderma
b. Fenfluramine
c. Hyperventilation
d. Sickle cell anemia

[Ref: Harrison 20th ed. pg. 1936-39]

101.	a
102.	c
103.	a
104.	b
105.	b
106.	b
107.	d
108.	c

1. **The fetal circulation changes to normal circulation at birth with-** *(PGMEE 2015)*
   a. Opening of fossa Ovalis
   b. Closure of ductus arteriosus
   c. Increased activity of right Ventricle
   d. Closure of ductus venosus

   [Ref: Ghai 9th/e/ p. 400]

2. **Not true about Fetal circulation is-** *(PGMEE 2013-14)*
   a. Maternal blood enters fetus through umbilical vein
   b. Fetal hemoglobin has higher affinity for O_2 than adult hemoglobin
   c. Pulmonary blood has low O_2
   d. All

   [Ref: Ghai 9th/e/p. 399]

3. **NADA's criteria are used for-** *(PGMEE 2015)*
   a. Assessment of child for degree of dehydration
   b. Assessment of child for degree of malnutrition
   c. Assessment of chid for presence of heart disease
   d. Assessment of child for degree of mental retardation

   [Ref: Ghai 9th/e/p. 403]

4. **Ductus arteriosus complete closure occurs at how many weeks in a term baby?** *(PGMEE 2014-15)*
   a. 1 week   b. 2 week
   c. 3 week   d. 4 week

   [Ref: O.P. Ghai 9th/e/p. 400]

5. **First line of treatment in pediatric congestive cardiac failure:** *(PGMEE 2016-17)*
   a. Loop diuretics   b. Digoxin
   c. Beta agonists   d. ACE inhibitors

   [Ref: Ghai 9th/e/p. 397]

6. **Common cause of congestive cardiac failure is seen in neonates is** *(PGMEE 2016)*
   a. Ostium Primium ASD
   b. TOF
   c. PDA
   d. VSD

   [Ref: Ghai 9th/e/p. 395]

7. **'Differential cyanosis' seen in:** *(PGMEE 2012-13)*
   a. PDA + PAH
   b. PPHN
   c. Interrupted aortic arch
   d. All

   [Ref: Nelson 20th/e/p 2164]

Explanation

- Differential cyanosis: Cyanosis present only in lower limbs
- Examples
  - PDA with pulmonary hypertension (Eisenonenger)
  - PDA with PPHTN
  - Interrupted aortic arch
  - Severe COA with VSD & PDA

ACYANOTIC CONGENITAL HEART DISEASES

ATRIAL SEPTAL DEFECT

8. **Most common cardiac lesion in Down's syndrome is?**
   a. VSD
   b. Coarctation of aorta
   c. Atrioventricular Septal Defect
   d. Transposition of great vessels

   [Ref: Ghai 9th/e/p. 398]

9. **Partial anomalous pulmonary venous connection is associated with which of the following defects?** *(PGMEE 2014-15)*
   a. Sinus venosus ASD
   b. Ostium primum ASD
   c. Endocardial cushion defect
   d. Tricuspid atresia

   [Ref: Ghai 9th/e/p. 409]

10. **Which ASD is common -** *(PGMEE 2013-14)*
    a. Sinus venosus   b. Coronary sinus ASD
    c. Ostium primum   d. Ostium secondum

    [Ref: Nelson 20th/e/p 2189]

11. **Hilar dance on fluoroscopy is seen in-** *(PGMEE 2013-14)*
    a. PS   b. ASD
    c. TR   d. VSD

    [Ref: Textbook of Paediatrics – by Desai pg. 518]

12. **Holt Oram syndrome is characterized by** *(PGMEE 2013-14)*
    a. ASD   b. TAPVC
    c. TGA   d. VSD

    [Ref: Nelson 20th/e/p 2189]

13. **Wide fixed S_2 is seen in-** *(PGMEE 2012-13)*
    a. ASD   b. PDA
    c. VSD   d. All of the above

    [Ref: Ghai 9th/e/p. 410]

14. **ASD with murmur similar to MR and left axis deviation-** *(PGMEE 2012-13)*
    a. ASD secondum with rheumatic MR
    b. ASD primum
    c. ASD Floppy mitral valve
    d. ASD secondum

    [Ref: O.P. Nelson 20th/e/p 2192]

15. **ASD is associated with all except-** *(PGMEE 2012-13)*
    a. Arrhythmia   b. Pulmonary hypertension
    c. Stroke   d. Infective endocarditis

    [Ref: Ghai 9th/e/p. 407]

16. **In atrial septal defect, the aorta is-** *(PGMEE 2012-13)*
    a. Small   b. Aneurysmal
    c. Normal   d. Enlarged

    [Ref: Nelson 20th/e/ pg. 2210; Ghai 9th/e/p 411]

1.	b
2.	c
3.	c
4.	c
5.	a
6.	d
7.	d
8.	c
9.	a
10.	d
11.	b
12.	a
13.	a
14.	b
15.	d
16.	a

17. Heart lesion not seen in Congenital Rubella Syndrome- *(PGMEE 2012-13)*

   a. ASD
   b. PS
   c. PDA
   d. VSD

   [Ref: Nelson 20th/e/ p 1549 table 247-1]

VENTRICULAR SEPTAL DEFECT

18. Most common heart abnormality in child-

   a. Tetralogy of Fallot   *(PGMEE 2015)*
   b. Atrial septal defect
   c. Total anomalous pulmonary venous connection
   d. Ventricular septal defect

   [Ref: Ghai 9th/e/p. 411]

PATENT DUCTUS ARTERIOSUS

19. Drug used to keep PDA open   *(PGMEE 2013-14)*

   a. PGE1 (Misoprost)
   b. PGI2
   c. PGE2 (Dinoprostone)
   d. PGH2

   [Ref: Nelson 20th/e/p 2207]

20. Which drug is used to treat PDA?   *(PGMEE 15)*

   a. Oxaceprol
   b. Medical treatment Is ineffective
   c. Dopamine
   d. Indomethacin

   [Ref: O.P. Ghai 9th/e/p. 416]

21. Not true regarding PDA:-   *(PGMEE 2016-17)*

   a. Asymptomatic at birth
   b. Connection Aorta & pulmonary artery
   c. Severity depends on diameter
   d. Continuous murmur

   [Ref: Ghai 9th/e/p. 416]

22. Large PDA (Patent ductus arteriosus) leads to-

   a. CHF   *(PGMEE 2012-13)*
   b. Endocardial valvulitis
   c. Eisenmenger syndrome
   d. All

   [Ref: Nelson 20th/e/p 2197]

23. In patent ductus arteriosus connection is between-   *(PGMEE 2012-13)*

   a. Aorta and subclavian artery
   b. Aorta and coronary artery
   c. Pulmonary artery and subclavian artery
   d. Aorta and pulmonary artery

   [Ref: Nelson 20th/e/ p 2197]

COARCTATION OF AORTA

24. Turner syndrome is associated with?   *(PGMEE 2015)*

   a. Aortic regurgitation
   b. Pulmonic stenosis
   c. Coarctation of aorta
   d. Aortic dissection

25. Notching of ribs occurs in all EXCEPT: *(DNB Dec 2009)*

   a. Coarctation of aorta
   b. Neurofibromatosis
   c. Hypothyroidism
   d. Osteogenesis imperfect

   [Ref: Fundamentals of Diagnostic Radiology edited by William E. Brant, Clyde A. Helms 3rd/e pg. 542]

26. Which of the following conditions causes both superior as well as inferior notching of the ribs?

   a. Coarctation of aorta   *(PGMEE 2014-15)*
   b. Hyperparathyroidism
   c. Interrupted aortic arch
   d. Blalock Taussig shunt

   [Ref: Principles of cardiovascular radiology, pg. 86, ch. 7]

27. All of the following are seen in Coarctation of Aorta, except-   *(PGMEE 2015)*

   a. Left ventricular Hypertrophy
   b. High incidence of associated Bicuspid aortic valve
   c. Boot Shaped Heart
   d. Diminution of femoral pulsations

   [Ref: Chest Radiographic Interpretation in Pediatric Cardiac Patients (Thieme) 2011 p. 81]

28. In coarctation of aorta, site of rib notching is?   *(PGMEE 2015-16)*

   a. Superior to rib
   b. Inferior to rib
   c. At sternum
   d. At Vertebra

   [Ref: Pg 218, Chetst X Ray solutions, H. Singh Ist ed.]

29. All are causes of sudden death in infant EXCEPT: *(PGMEE 2014-15)*

   a. Romano ward syndrome
   b. Aortic stenosis
   c. Hypoplastic left heart syndrome
   d. Kawasaki disease

   [Ref: Nelson, ch. 436, table 436.1; Sudden Death in Children], Harrison's 19th/e pg. 2192]

30. Coarctation of aorta in most commonly seen with-   *(PGMEE 2013-14)*

   a. ASD
   b. VSD
   c. Bicuspid aortic valve
   c. PDA

   [Ref: Nelson 20th/e/p 2205; Ghai 9th/e/p. 428]

CYANOTIC HEART DISEASES

TETRALOGY OF FALLOT

31. Components of TOF are all except-   *(PGMEE 2014)*

   a. Right ventricular hypertrophy
   b. VSD
   c. Subpulmonary stenosis
   d. PDA

   [Ref: Ghai 9th/e/p. 417]

32. Which is not a component of Tetralogy of Fallot-   *(PGMEE 2012-13)*

   a. Ventricular septal defect
   b. Pulmonary stenosis
   c. Overriding aorta
   d. Left ventricular hypertrophy

   [Ref: O.P. Ghai 9th/e pg. 417]

33. Fallot physiology includes all except- *(PGMEE 2012-13)*

   a. TA with VSD with PS
   b. TGA with VSD and PS
   c. Eisenmenger complex
   d. Single ventricle with pulmonic stenosis

   [Ref: Ghai 9th/e/p. 402]

17.	a
18.	d
19.	a
20.	d
21.	a
22.	d
23.	d
24.	c
25.	c
26.	b
27.	c
28.	b
29.	d
30.	c
31.	d
32.	d
33.	c

34. 'Pentology of Cantrell' include all except- *(PGMEE 2013)*
a. VSD
b. Ectopia cordis
c. Trisomy 21
d. TOF

[Ref: Nelson 20th/e/p 2238]

35. Which of the following is most common type of congenital cardiac cyanotic anomaly? *(PGMEE 2012-13)*
a. Transposition of great vessels
b. Tetralogy of Fallot
c. Ebstein's Anamoly
d. TAPVC

[Ref: O.P. Ghai 9th/e pg. 417; Nelson 20th/e pg 2211]

36. When does crying stop in cyanotic spells? *(PGMEE 2015)*
a. Mid inspiration
b. Crying is continuous
c. Forced inspiration
d. Forced Expiration

[Ref: Ghai 9th/e/p. 408]

37. Brain abscess in Cyanotic heart disease is commonly seen in- *(PGMEE 2016-17)*
a. Parietal lobe
b. Temporal lobe
c. Occipital hemisphere
d. Frontal lobe

[Ref: Internet]

EBSTEIN ANOMALY

38. Not present in Ebstein anomaly: *(PGMEE 2013-14, 12)*
a. Left ventricular enlargement
b. Left atrial enlargement
c. Right atrial enlargement
d. Right ventricular enlargement

[Ref: Nelson 20th/e/p 2221]

39. WPW syndrome is associated with- *(PGMEE 2012-13)*
a. VSD
b. TOF
c. TAPVC
d. Ebstein anomaly

[Ref: Nelson 20th/e/p 2254]

TOTAL ANOMALOUS PULMONARY VENOUS CONNECTION

40. Most common site for opening of TAPVC is: *(PGMEE 2015)*
a. Cardiac
b. Mixed
c. Infracardiac
d. Supracardiac

[Ref: Nelson 20th/e/p 2227]

41. Snow man appearance or figure of 8 appearance is seen in? *(PGMEE 2015-16)*
a. Total anomalous pulmonary venous connection
b. Transposition of great arteries
c. Tetralogy of fallot
d. Tricuspid atresia

[Ref: Ghai 9th/e/p. 424]

42. Alprostadil is contraindicated in: *(PGMEE 2014-15)*
a. Tricuspid atresia
b. Transposition of great arteries
c. Tetralogy of Fallot
d. Total anomalous pulmonary venous connection (TAPVC)

[Ref: Cloherty Manual of Neonatal Care: 7th ed., ch. 41]

Explanation

■ Alprostadil (PGE) is indicated as palliative measure to maintain patency of ducts arteriosus in ductal dependent lesions like Tricuspid atresia, TOF, TGA, PS etc.

TRANSPOSITION OF GREAT VESSELS

43. Pulmonary oligaemia is seen in which of the following congenital cardiac disease- *(PGMEE 2015)*
a. Persistent truncus arteriosus
b. Transposition of great vessels with pulmonary stenosis
c. Transposition of great vessels with TAPVC
d. Transposition of great vessels with VSD

[Ref: O.P. Ghai 9th/e 422]

44. Neonate with cyanosis, heart failure and systolic murmur is suffering from: *(PGMEE 2014-15)*
a. TOF
b. VSD
c. TGA
d. Rheumatic fever

[Ref: Ghai 9th/e/p. 422]

45. A 2 week baby having central cyanosis, on auscultation has grade 2 murmur, normal S1 and single S2. X-Ray shows cardiomegaly with a narrow base and plethoric lung fields. The Diagnosis is? *(PGMEE 2012-13)*
a. TAPVC
b. TOF
c. Pulmonary atresia
d. TGA

[Ref: Ghai 9th/e/p. 422]

MISCELLANEOUS

46. What is the cardiothoracic ratio in children is- *(PGMEE 2015)*
a. 30-35%
b. 40-45%
c. 50-55%
d. 60-65%

[Ref: Nelson 20th/e/p 2170]

47. Umbilical cord has- *(PGMEE 2012-13)*
a. 1 vein and 2 arteries
b. 2 vein and 2 arteries
c. 1 vein and 1 artery
d. 2 veins and 1 artery

[Ref: Nelson 20th/e pg. 797]

48. All are true regarding tricuspid atresia except- *(PGMEE 2012-13)*
a. Split S2
b. Pulmonary oligemia in chest X-ray
c. Left axis deviation in ECG
d. Patent foramen ovale

[Ref: Nelson 20th/e/p 2218, Ghai 9th/e/p 420]

49. The most common presentation of double aortic arch in infants is? *(PGMEE 2013)*
a. Dysphagia
b. Positional hyperemia with right upper arm oedema
c. Bleeding
d. Tracheal compression symptoms

[Ref: Nelson 20th/e/p 2236 table 432-1]

50. Coarctation of the aorta is common in which syndrome- *(PGMEE 2012-13)*
a. Down's
b. Noonan's
c. Klinefelter's
d. Turner's

[Ref: Nelson 20th/ e/p 2205, Ghai 9th/e/p 398]

34.	c
35.	b
36.	d
37.	d
38.	d
39.	d
40.	d
41.	a
42.	d
43.	b
44.	c
45.	d
46.	c
47.	a
48.	a
49.	d
50.	d

Gastroenterology

FACTS

- Serosa is absent in → Esophagus (except in intra abdomen portion)
- Strongest layer of gut: Submucosa
- Usual site of foreign body impaction in the esophagus → above cricopharynx
- H. pylori is a risk factor for intestinal type of CA stomach
- Most serious extra-intestinal manifestation of ulcerative colitis → Primary sclerosing cholangitis (do not resolve after colectomy).
- Extraintestinal manifestation of IBD which worsen with exacerbation of disease → Peripheral arthritis

- Massive colonic bleeding in a patient of diverticulosis is from → Superior mesenteric artery
- Pacemaker cells of GIT: Interstitial cells of Cajal
- Maximum intestinal adaptation is seen at → Ileum.
- *Cecum:*
  - Widest portion of the colon
  - Thinnest muscular wall
  - Most vulnerable to perforation
  - Least vulnerable to obstruction

MOST COMMON

- MC cause of diarrhea in children of age 6-24 months: Rotavirus
- MC cause of traveler's diarrhea: Enterotoxigenic *E. coli*
- MC pathogenic parasitic infection in the human: *Giardia*
- MC organism associated with pseudomembranous colitis: *Clostridium difficile*

- MC cause of entero-enteral fistula: Crohn's disease
- MC extraintestinal manifestation of Crohn's disease: Peripheral Arthritis
- MC extraintestinal manifestation of Ulcerative colitis: Uveitis
- MC cause of upper GI bleed → Peptic ulcer disease
- MC cause of lower GI bleed → Diverticulosis.

Esophagus

- MC risk factor for the development of Adenocarcinoma of esophagus: Barrett's esophagus
- MC site of Mallory Weiss tear → below the squamo-columnar junction at the cardia.
- MC site of spontaneous rupture → gastroesophageal junction

- MC cause of esophageal perforation → medical instrumentation
- MC site of iatrogenic esophageal perforation → hypopharynx
- MC site of perforation in Boerhaave syndrome → Left posterolateral wall of lower third of esophagus above G-E junction

Peptic Ulcer Disease

- MC site of gastric ulcer → Lesser curvature near incisura.
- MC type of gastric ulcer → Type I
- MC complication of PUD → Bleeding
- MC complication of duodenal ulcer → Bleeding (from gastroduodenal artery)

- MC complication of gastric ulceration → Perforation. (MC site → Anterior aspect of lesser curvature).
- MC cause of death → Perforation

CLASSIFICATION AND SCORE

- Rockall score & Blatchford score → prediction score for upper GI bleeding

- Forest classification → Endoscopic grading of risk of re-bleeding in peptic ulcer.

INVESTIGATIONS

- Screening test for Achalasia: CCK test
- CXR in Achalasia Cardia shows: Absent gastric bubble
- Most confirmatory investigation for Achalasia: Manometry
- Gold standard for detection of *H. pylori*: Histology/Staining
- Best test for confirmation of *H. pylori*: Urea breath test
- Test to assess success of treatment against *H. pylori*: Urea breath test & Stool Antigen test
- 24 hours pH manometry is IOC for → reflux esophagitis

REMEMBER

Dysphagia Lusoria:
- Dysphagia caused by compression of the esophagus by an aberrant right subclavian artery arising from the descending aorta & passing behind the esophagus.

Diuelafoy's Lesion:
- Presence of large aberrant tortuous arteriole most commonly in the stomach wall with potential for bleeding.

Zenker Diverticulum:
- It is a false diverticulum of hypopharynx
- Type of pulsion diverticulum
- MC location: Killian's triangle – between the inferior constrictor and cricopharyngeus muscle
- Observed in elderly population
- MC presenting symptom: dysphagia
- IOC: Barium swallow with videofluoroscopy
- Treatment: Surgical diverticulectomy and cricopharyngeal myotomy or a Marsupialization procedure

Barrett's Esophagus:
- Metaplasia of squamous epithelium into columnar epithelium
- Commonly associated with GERD
- More common in males (2:1)
- Usually affects the lower 1/3rd of esophagus
- Risk factor for esophageal adenocarcinoma
- IOC: Esophagogastroduodenoscopy and biopsy
- Rx: Endoscopic mucosal ablation

Features of Plummer Vinson Syndrome:
- Middle aged female
- Proximal esophageal webs
- Iron deficiency anemia
- Koilonychia
- Associated with development of Squamous cell carcinoma of esophagus

***H. pylori* Associated Conditions:**
- Chronic active gastritis
- Peptic ulcer disease
- Gastric cancer
- MALTomas
- GERD

Cushing's Ulcer:
- Stress ulceration after head trauma

Curling's Ulcer:
- Stress ulceration after severe burns

GI Ulcers in:
- **T**uberculosis → **T**ransverse
- Typhoid → Longitudinal [**Mn**: Long tie]
- Amebiasis → Flask shaped ulcer

Rat Tail Appearance *on Barium Swallow:*
- CA Esophagus
- Achalasia Cardia

Pulled up Caecum *on Barium Studies:*
- Intestinal tuberculosis

ESOPHAGEAL INJURY

	Mallory Weiss Tear	Boerhaave Syndrome
Pathology	▪ Longitudinal mucosal tear at the gastroesophageal junction or gastric cardia ▪ Nontransmural tear of esophageal mucosa	▪ Spontaneous rupture at the lower esophagus, proximal to GEJ ▪ Transmural perforation of esophagus
Mechanism	▪ Rapid rise in intragastric pressure	▪ Sudden rise in intraluminal esophageal pressure against a closed cricopharyngeus
Precipitant	▪ Vigorous coughing, Vomiting and retching following an alcohol binge	▪ Forceful vomiting or retching following alcohol binge
Clinical presentation	▪ Upper gastrointestinal bleeding ▪ Hematemesis	▪ Chest pain radiating to back ▪ Subcutaneous emphysema ▪ Hematemesis not seen
Diagnosis	▪ IOC – Endoscopy	▪ Esophagogram using gastrografin
Treatment	▪ Bleeding usually stops spontaneously ▪ Active bleeding tear may be treated with electrocoagulation with or without epinephrine	▪ Resuscitation ▪ Surgical intervention is the standard of care
Prognosis	▪ Good	▪ High morbidity and mortality

|GEJ - Gastroesophageal junction|

PEPTIC ULCER DISEASE

	Duodenal Ulcers	Gastric Ulcers
MC location	• 1st part of duodenum	• Gastric body along lesser curvature
Epidemiology	• More common • Peak incidence: 3rd – 4th decade	• Less common • Peak incidence – 6th decade
Pathophysiology	• *H. pylori* (90%), NSAIDs induced mucosal damage • Increased basal & nocturnal gastric acid secretion	• *H. pylori* (80%), NSAIDs induced mucosal damage • Variable basal & nocturnal gastric acid secretion
Clinical features	• Epigastric pain – 2-3 hours after meal • Night pain which can awaken the patient • Relieving factor – food, antacids	• Epigastric pain shortly after meals • Night pain is less common
Complication	• GI bleeding, Perforation – less common • Pancreatitis due to posterior perforation • Gastric outlet obstruction	• GI bleeding, Perforation – more common • Perforation into the left hepatic lobe
Investigation	• IOC: Upper GI endoscopy • Biopsy – not required	• IOC: Upper GI endoscopy • Biopsy to rule out malignancy

Dumping Syndrome

- Seen in patients who have undergone vagotomy and drainage procedures (especially Billroth)
- Most noticeable after meals rich in simple carbohydrates and high osmolarity
- **Preferred therapy:** Dietary modifications like small, frequent meals devoid of simple carbohydrates, avoiding liquids during meals.

	Early Dumping Syndrome	Late Dumping Syndrome
Onset	• 15–30 minutes after meals	• 1 – 3 hours after meals
Symptoms	• Diarrhea, abdominal cramps, belching, tachycardia, palpitations	• Light-headedness, diaphoresis, palpitations, tachycardia, and syncope
Mechanism	• Rapid emptying of hyperosmolar gastric contents into the small intestine	• Due to reactive hypoglycemia from excessive insulin release
Hormones involved	• Vasoactive intestinal polypeptide, neurotensin, motilin	• GLP-1

CHRONIC GASTRITIS

Type A	Type B
• Less common • Involves body and fundus • **A**utoimmune gastritis • Associated with pernicious **A**nemia • Vitamin B_{12} deficiency + • Achlorhydria ++ • Hypergastrinemia + • Antibodies against parietal cells and IF + • Increased risk of gastric carcinoma	• More common • Involves antrum • Chronic inflammatory gastritis • Associated with H. pylori infection • Normal Vitamin B_{12} levels • Increase acid production • Normal gastrin levels • Antibodies to *H. pylori* + • Increased risk of gastric carcinoma

DIARRHEA

- Acute diarrhea is defined as an episode that has acute onset and last <2 weeks, persistent if 2–4 weeks, and chronic if >4 weeks in duration.
- MC cause of diarrhea in adults: Norovirus/ Norwalk virus
- MC cause of diarrhea in children: Rotavirus
- MC cause of traveler's diarrhea: Enterotoxigenic *E. coli*
- MC complication of acute diarrhea is dehydration.

Etiology

Acute Diarrhea	
▪ Enterotoxigenic or Enteroaggregative *E. coli* ▪ *Salmonella* ▪ *Campylobacter* ▪ *Shigella* ▪ *Giardia* ▪ Enterohemorrhagic *E. coli* (O157:H7) ▪ *Bacillus cereus*	▪ *Staphylococcus aureus* ▪ *Vibrio* ▪ *Cryptosporidium* ▪ *Isospora belli* ▪ *Microsporidia* ▪ *C. difficile* ▪ *Norovirus*

Chronic Diarrhea	

▪ Hormone-producing tumors:
  ○ Carcinoid
  ○ VIPoma
  ○ Medullary cancer of thyroid
  ○ Gastrinoma
▪ Gluten and FODMAP intolerance
▪ Lactase deficiency
	▪ Inflammatory bowel disease
	▪ Irritable bowel syndrome
	▪ Hyperthyroidism
	▪ Drugs (Prokinetic agents)
	▪ Post vagotomy

Hydration

Assessment	0-5% dehydration (Mild)	5-10% dehydration (Moderate)	10% or more (Severe)
General	▪ Well	▪ Restless	▪ Lethargic
Eyes	▪ Normal	▪ Sunken	▪ Very sunken
Tears	▪ Present	▪ Absent	▪ Absent
Mouth	▪ Moist	▪ Dry	▪ Very dry
Thirst	▪ Drinks normally	▪ Thirsty	▪ Drinks poorly
Skin Pinch	▪ Retracts immediately	▪ Retracts slowly	▪ Pinch stays folded

Management

- Most episodes of acute diarrhea are mild and self-limited. Indications for evaluation are:
  - Profuse diarrhea with dehydration
  - Grossly bloody stools
  - Fever ≥101°F or severe abdominal pain
  - No improvement in ≥48 h
  - Recent antibiotic use
  - Elderly (≥70 years) or immunocompromised.
- In most cases, the best option for treatment of acute-onset diarrhea is the early use of oral rehydration therapy (ORT).
- In moderately severe nonfebrile and nonbloody diarrhea, antimotility and antisecretory agents such as loperamide can be useful adjuncts to control symptoms.
- Such agents should be avoided with febrile dysentery which may be exacerbated or prolonged by them.
- Prophylactic antibiotic is indicated in patients who are immunocompromised, have mechanical heart valves or recent vascular grafts, or are elderly.
- Antibiotic prophylaxis is also indicated for certain patients traveling to high-risk countries.

INFLAMMATORY BOWEL DISEASE

Features	Crohn Disease	Ulcerative Colitis
Age of onset	▪ 15-30 years & 60-70 years	▪ 15-25 years & 55-65 years
Earliest lesion	▪ Aphthoid ulcers	▪ Proctitis
MC site of lesion	▪ Ileum	▪ Rectum / rectosigmoid
Involvement	▪ Usually the entire wall thickness (transmural) ▪ Entire length of GIT	▪ Usually confined to mucosa and submucosa ▪ Only colon (Pancolitis)
Distribution	▪ Segmental with skip lesions + ▪ Rectal sparing +	▪ Continuous involvement ▪ Proctitis +
Inflammation	▪ Noncaseating granuloma (specific)	▪ Granuloma are characteristically absent
Pseudopolyp	▪ Less frequent	▪ Common
Smoking	▪ Increase recurrence [**C**igarette **C**ause **C**rohn]	▪ Protective
Oral contraceptives	▪ Increase in risk	▪ No increase in risk
Appendectomy	▪ Not protective	▪ Protective
Bleeding	▪ Uncommon	▪ Common
Fissure / Fistula / Abscess	▪ Common	▪ Rare
Obstruction & perineal disease	▪ Common	▪ Uncommon
Toxic megacolon	▪ Rare	▪ Relatively common
Stricture formation	▪ Frequently	▪ Occasionally
Antibody	▪ ASCA positive (60%) > ANCA (40%)	▪ pANCA positive (60–80%) > ASCA
Radiology	▪ Barium → String sign of Kantoor	▪ Barium → lead pipe/Hose pipe colon
Named features	▪ **C**obblestone appearance of mucosa ▪ **C**reeping fat	▪ Backwash ileitis (Involvement proximally from rectum) ▪ Collar button ulcer
Extraintestinal manifestation	▪ Ankylosing spondylitis ▪ Psoriatic arthritis ▪ Erythema nodosum ▪ Aphthous ulceration	▪ Uveitis – MC ▪ Erythema nodosum ▪ Primary sclerosing ▪ Ankylosing spondylitis cholangitis ▪ Pyoderma gangrenosum

Treatment	▪ Steroids
	▪ Methotrexate
	▪ TNF α-blockers: Infiximab, Adalimumab, Certolizumab
	▪ Natalizumab → binds α4β7 and α4b1
	▪ Vedolizumab
		▪ Mild disease: Topical measlazine
		▪ Acute, severe disease:
		  ○ Intravenous high-dose conticosteroids
		  ○ Cyclosporine, Tacrolimus
		  ○ TNF α-blockers: Infiximab, Adalimumab
		  ○ Tofacitinib (JAK inhibitor)
		▪ Maintenance therapy
		  ○ Mesalamine → Drug of choice
		  ○ Azathioprime → Steroid sparing drug

Indication of surgery	▪ Intractable or fulminant disease ▪ Perianal disease unresponsive to medical therapy ▪ Refractory fistula ▪ Massive hemorrhage ▪ Stricture and obstruction ▪ Cancer prophylaxis ▪ Colon dysplasia or cancer	▪ Intractable or fulminant disease ▪ Toxic megacolon ▪ Extracolonic disease ▪ Steroid dependent disease ▪ Perforation or massive hemorrhage ▪ Obstruction ▪ Cancer prophylaxis ▪ Colon dysplasia or cancer
Surgical procedure of choice	▪ Conservative resection	▪ Ileal pouch anal anastomosis (IPAA)
Recurrence after surgery	▪ Common	▪ Rare
Malignant transformation	▪ Colon carcinoma	▪ Colon carcinoma

MALABSORPTION SYNDROME

	Celiac Disease	Tropical Sprue	Whipple Disease
Also Known as	▪ Gluten sensitive enteropathy ▪ Celiac sprue ▪ Non tropical sprue	▪ Malabsorption syndrome with infectious cause & no systemic features	▪ Malabsorption syndrome with infectious cause & systemic features
Pathology	▪ ↑ Sensitivity to gliadin/gluten present in wheat, oat, barley & rye	▪ Microbial infection with *Klebsiella, E. coli*	▪ Etiology → *Tropheryma whipplei* (Gram +ve AFB)
Association	▪ HLA DQ2 or DQ8 ▪ Type I DM, Dermatitis Herpetiformis		▪ Culture negative endocarditis
Age group	▪ 8 – 12 months & 3rd – 4th decade	▪ Adult onset disease	▪ Middle aged and elderly
Clinical features	▪ Weight loss, chronic diarrhea ▪ Malabsorption ▪ Steatorrhea ▪ Deficiency of Iron, Folate, Niacin, Calcium, Vitamin B_2 & B_{12}, Vitamin D	▪ Weight loss, chronic diarrhea ▪ Malabsorption ▪ Steatorrhea ▪ Iron, Vitamin B12 and folate deficiencies	▪ Weight loss, diarrhea ▪ Non deforming arthralgia ▪ Steatorrhea ▪ Supranuclear ophthalmoplegia ▪ Cerebellar ataxia ▪ Dementia, Nystagmus

Workup	▪ Biopsy is **not** diagnostic
	  ○ Lymphocyte & Plasma cell proliferation in Lamina propria.
	  ○ **Hyperplastic crypts**
	  ○ Markedly atrophic or absent villi
	  ○ Decreased villous to crypt ratio (Flat appearance)
	  ○ No mucosal atrophy
		▪ Biopsy is **not** diagnostic
		  ○ Atrophy of villi
		  ○ Similar to celiac disease
		▪ Mucosal malabsorption of fat & D-Xylose
			▪ Biopsy is diagnostic
			  ○ Intestinal mucosa laden with macrophage in lamina propria
			  ○ **Presence of PAS +ve diastase resistant granules in macrophages**
			  ○ Lymphatic blockage leading to lymphatic dilatation & lipid deposition in the villi

Antibody	▪ IgA Anti**gli**adin ▪ IgA Anti**en**domysial – most useful ▪ IgA Anti **tissue** transglutaminase antibody (Anti t-TG) is the most useful screening test	▪ None	▪ IgG for *T. whipplei* (no diagnostic utility)
Complications	▪ Intestinal T Cell Lymphoma ▪ Increased risk of cancer	▪ Malnutrition ▪ No associated risk of malignancy	▪ CNS related Whipple disease
Treatments	▪ Gluten free diet ▪ Corticosteroids in refractory patient	▪ Antibiotics – Tetracyclines ▪ Nutritional supplements	▪ Antibiotics

MOST COMMON SITES IN GIT

- Polyps in Peutz Jeghers syndrome → Jejunum
- Typhoid ulcer → Terminal ileum
- TB ulcer → Terminal ileum
- Amebiasis: Caecum

- Ischemic colitis → Splenic flexure
- Colonic diverticula → Sigmoid colon
- Hirschsprung disorders → Rectum

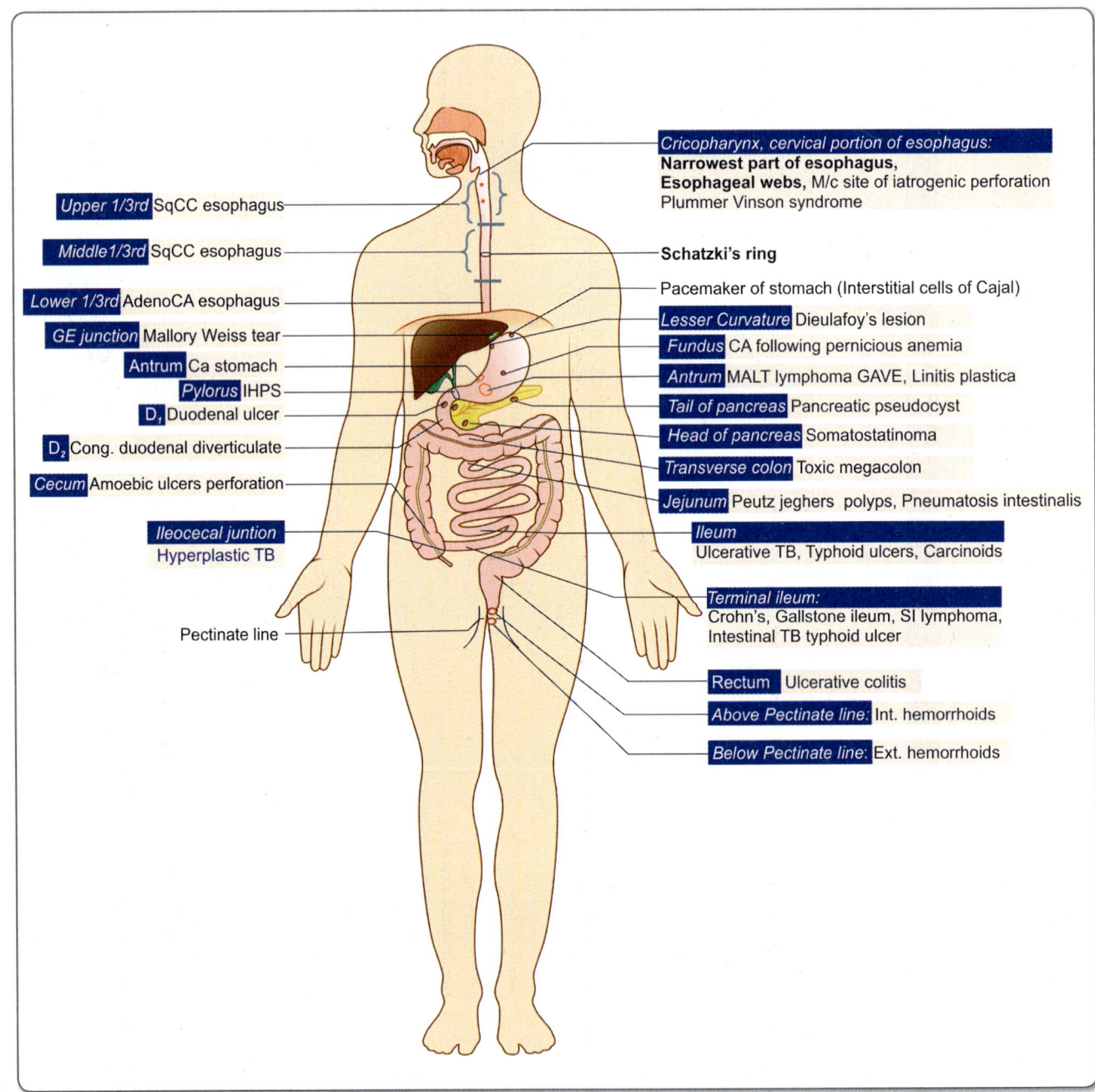

Cricopharynx, cervical portion of esophagus:
Narrowest part of esophagus,
Esophageal webs, M/c site of iatrogenic perforation
Plummer Vinson syndrome

Upper 1/3rd SqCC esophagus

Middle 1/3rd SqCC esophagus

Schatzki's ring

Lower 1/3rd AdenoCA esophagus

Pacemaker of stomach (Interstitial cells of Cajal)

Lesser Curvature Dieulafoy's lesion

GE junction Mallory Weiss tear

Fundus CA following pernicious anemia

Antrum Ca stomach

Antrum MALT lymphoma GAVE, Linitis plastica

Pylorus IHPS

Tail of pancreas Pancreatic pseudocyst

D₁ Duodenal ulcer

Head of pancreas Somatostatinoma

D₂ Cong. duodenal diverticulate

Transverse colon Toxic megacolon

Cecum Amoebic ulcers perforation

Jejunum Peutz jeghers polyps, Pneumatosis intestinalis

Ileocecal juntion
Hyperplastic TB

Ileum
Ulcerative TB, Typhoid ulcers, Carcinoids

Terminal ileum:
Crohn's, Gallstone ileum, SI lymphoma,
Intestinal TB typhoid ulcer

Pectinate line

Rectum   Ulcerative colitis

Above Pectinate line: Int. hemorrhoids

Below Pectinate line: Ext. hemorrhoids

MULTIPLE CHOICE QUESTIONS

CHAPTER 1: ESOPHAGUS

ESOPHAGUS

DYSPHAGIA

1. Patient complains of dysphagia for solids and liquids. The level of lesion is at: **(PGMEE 2014-15)**
   a. Cortical level
   b. Esophagus
   c. Brainstem damage
   d. Cranial nerve palsy
   [Ref: Harrison's 19th/e pg. 257]

2. The investigation of choice for dysphagia is- **(PGMEE 2015)**
   a. CT Scan
   b. Endoscopy
   c. Barium Swallow
   d. Manometric Study
   [Ref: Harrison's 19th/e pg. 257]

3. Investigation of choice for dysphagia for liquids:-
   a. Barium swallow **(PGMEE 2016-17)**
   b. Endoscopy
   c. Manometry
   d. 24 hr pH monitoring
   [Ref : Sabiston's 20th /e pg. 1017]

4. A patient presents with difficulty in swallowing liquids but not solids. The best investigation to make a diagnosis is- **(PGMEE 2015)**
   a. PET CT
   b. Endoscopic ultrasound
   c. Manometry
   d. Endoscopy
   [Ref: Sabiston's 20th /e pg. 1017; Schwartz 10th/e pg. 990; Maingot's 10th/e pg. 846; Bailey & Love 26th/e pg. 1014]

5. 24 hour pH manometry is gold standard investigation for **(DNB June' 2011)**
   a. Hiatal hernia
   b. Barrett's esophagus
   c. Reflux esophagitis
   d. Esophageal ulcers
   [Ref: Sabiston 18th/e p. 1112]

6. Treatment of Duodenal atresia is **(DNB June' 2011)**
   a. Duodenojejunostomy
   b. Duodenoduodenostomy
   c. Duodenal canalization
   d. Roux-en-y procedure
   [Ref: Bailey and love 24th/e p. 1198]

7. Dysphagia for fluids but not for solids is seen in: **(PGMEE 2012-13)**
   a. Carcinoma oesophagus
   b. Achalasia
   c. Reflux oesopagitis
   d. Stricture
   [Ref: Dhingra 6th/e pg. 344]

8. Dysphagia lusoria is mostly due to- **(PGMEE 2015)**
   a. Compression by retrostrenal thyroid
   b. Compression by mediastinal thymoma
   c. Compression of esophagus by the arch of aorta
   d. Compression by the aberrant right subclavian artery
   [Ref: Dhingra 6th/e pg. 347]

9. Non progressive dysphagia in a lady with a sensation of something stuck in the throat and worsened by intake of cold drinks is suggestive of? **(PGMEE 2014-15)**
   a. Diffuse esophageal spasm
   b. Upper esophageal web
   c. Achalasia
   d. Scleroderma
   [Ref: Harrison's 19th/e pg. 1905]

10. Cork-screw appearance of esophagus is seen in: **(PGMEE 2016-17; DNB 2008)**
    a. Achalasia cardia
    b. Diffuse esophageal spasm
    c. Carcinoma esophagus
    d. Reflux oesophagitis
    [Ref: Sabiston's 20th /e pg. 1015]

> **Explanation**
> - Cork-screw shaped → Diffuse/distal esophageal spasm
> - Bird's Beak appearance → Achalasia cardia

ACHALASIA CARDIA

11. Pseudoachalasia is seen with all except?
    a. Esophageal tumor **(PGMEE 2014-15)**
    b. Paraneoplastic
    c. Carcinoma fundus
    d. Rosary esophagus
    [Ref: Harrison's 19th/e pg. 1904]

12. In achalasia cardia, there is - **(PGMEE 2012-13; 2015)**
    a. Absence of nerves
    b. Hypertrophy of nerves
    c. Absence of muscles
    d. None
    [Ref: Robbin's 9th/e pg. 753]

13. Gold standard test for achalasia cardia?
    a. Esophageal Manometry **(PGMEE 2015-16)**
    b. Barium swallow
    c. Endoscopy
    d. Endoscopic ultrasound
    [Ref: Bailey and love's 26th /e pg. 1014; Harrison's 19th/e pg. 1904, 257]

14. Most common complication of achalasia is: **(PGMEE 2014-15)**
    a. Recurrent pulmonary infections
    b. Stricture of esophagus
    c. Pleurisy
    d. Peptic ulcer
    [Ref: Harrison's 19th/e pg. 1904]

1.	b
2.	b
3.	c
4.	c
5.	c
6.	b
7.	b
8.	d
9.	a
10.	b
11.	d
12.	a
13.	a
14.	a

15. **Triple A syndrome is all except?** *(PGMEE 2014-15)*
   a. Alacrimia
   b. Addison disease
   c. Achlorhydria
   d. Achalasia

   [Ref: Harrison's 19th/e pg. 2324t]

Explanation

Triple A syndrome/Allgrove syndrome

- Triple A syndrome/Allgrove syndrome (AAA syndrome), also known as achalasia-addisonianism-alacrima syndrome or Allgrove syndrome, is a rare autosomal recessive congenital disorder characterized by:
  ○ Achlalasia
  ○ Primary adrenal insufficiency (Addison disease)
  ○ Alacrima (insufficiency of tears)

16. **Achalasia cardia due to:** *(PGMEE 2016-17)*
   a. Degeneration of myentric plexus due to toxin
   b. Disintegration & absence of ganglion cells in auerbach' Plexus
   c. Selective destruction of inhibitory neurons
   d. Absence of cholinergic neurons

   [Ref: Sabiston's 20th/e pg. 1017]

Explanation

Achalasia cardia

- It is a primary esophageal motility disorder characterized by loss of peristaltic activity of esophagus.
- It is caused by loss of inhibitory ganglion cells within the myenteric plexus of esophagus

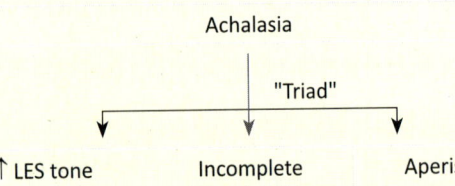

Myenteric plexus inflammation/neurodegeneration
↓
Loss of inhibitory ganglion cells i.e. NO producing cells
↓
↓ inhibitory neurotransmitter (NO)
↓
Intact cholinergic (excitatory) transmission (Ach)
↓
Imbalance of neurotransmittors (↑ Ach/↓ NO)
↓
Achalasia
"Triad"
↑LES tone | Incomplete LES relaxation | Aperistalsis

- Etiology: Infective, Autoimmune etc
- Most patient presents with dysphagia to both solid & liquid food

- Barium swallow → bird beak appearance
- Esophageal manometry → IOC
- Medical treatment
  ○ Calcium channel blockers, Nitrates
  ○ Botulinum toxin
- Surgical treatment
  ○ Heller's myotomy

17. **Oesophageal manometry is used in:** *(PGMEE 2016-17)*
   a. DES
   b. Barett Oesophagus
   c. GERD
   d. Achalasia cardia

   [Ref: Sabiston's 20th/e pg. 1017]

18. **Achalasia cardia all are true except:-** *(PGMEE 2016-17)*
   a. Selective loss of inhibitory neuron of lower oesophagus
   b. Dysphagia solid> liquid
   c. Bird beak appearance in barium study
   d. Treatment is Hellers myotomy

   [Ref: Sabiston's 20th/e pg.1017]

19. **About LES true statement is:-** *(PGMEE 2016-17)*
   a. Length 3-5 cm and pressure 30 cm H_2O
   b. Length 3-5 cm and pressure 10 cm H_2O
   c. It is a anatomical sphincter
   d. Tone is increase by tea addiction

   [Ref: Sabiston's 20th/e pg.1016]

20. **Pencil tip deformity in barium study is seen in:** *(PGMEE 2016-17)*

   a. Carcinoma esophagus
   b. Diffuse esophageal spasm
   c. Gastroesophageal reflux
   d. Achalasia cardia

   [Ref: Internet; should be achalasia. No other option fits in; ca esophagus – apple core / asymmetrical bulge DES - corkscrew.]

21. **"Bird's beak sign" as shown in the image is characteristic of:** *(PGMEE 2016-17)*

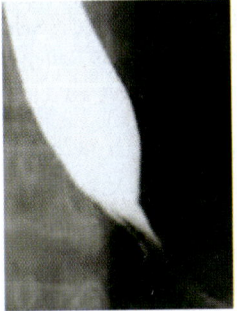

   a. Achalasia cardia
   b. Barret's esophagus
   c. Diffuse esophageal spasm
   d. Ca esophagus

   [Ref: Sabiston's 20th/e pg.1018]

22. **Per-oral endoscopic myotomy (POEM) is the treatment modality for the management of:**
   a. Achalasia cardia *(Recent Pattern June 2018)*
   b. GERD
   c. Esophageal spasm
   d. Pseudoachalasia

   [Ref: Sabiston's 20th/e pg. 1018]

15.	c
16.	c
17.	d
18.	b
19.	b
20.	d
21.	a
22.	a

Explanation

- Per-oral endoscopic myotomy (POEM) has emerged as an efficacious treatment modality for the management of achalasia cardia (AC) and non-achalasia spastic esophageal motility disorders

23. Heller's myotomy is done in   **(PGMEE 2018)**
   a. Zenker diverticulum
   b. Achalasia cardia
   c. GERD
   d. Duodenal stenosis

   [Ref: Maingots abdominal operations 12th/e, pg. 303]

24. Heller's myotomy operation is done for:
   (PGMEE 2016-17,2015; 2011, PGMEE 2012)
   a. Achalasia cardia   b. GERD
   c. Berret's oesophagus   d. Sliding hernia

   [Ref: Harrison's 19th/e pg. 1905, Schwartz 10th /e pg.990]

25. Achalasia presents with: **(PGMEE 2016-17)**
   a. Progressive dysphagia for solid
   b. Progressive dysphagia for liquid
   c. Intermittent dysphagia for liquid
   d. Intermittent dysphagia for solid

   [Ref: SABISTON 20TH /E PG. 1017]

26. Progressive dysphagia for solids and liquids is found in carcinoma of   **(DNB June' 2011)**
   a. Oropharynx
   b. Hypopharynx
   c. Nasopharynx
   d. All

   [Ref: Harrison's 19th/e pg.257, Schwartz 10th /e pg.990]

GERD

27. Which of the following staging is used for GERD?   **(PGMEE 2014-15)**
   a. Ranson   b. Gleason
   c. Savary miller   d. Hunter scale

   [Ref: Grading and staging in gastroenterology by tytgat pg. 108]

28. Ambulatory pH monitoring is indicated in-   **(PGMEE 2016-17)**
   a. GERD   b. Achalasia cardia
   c. Peptic ulcer   d. Pyrosis

   [Ref: Harrison's 19th/e pg. 1902]

29. A 70-year-old male patient presented to the emergency department with pain in epigastrium and difficulty in breathing for 6 hours. On examination, his heart rate was 56 per minute and the blood pressure was 106/60 mm Hg. Chest examination was normal. The patient has been taking omeprazole for gastroesophageal reflux disease for last 6 months. What should be the initial investigation: **(PGMEE 2014-15)**
   a. An ECG
   b. An upper GI endoscopy
   c. Urgent ultrasound of the abdomen
   d. An X-ray chest

   [Ref: Harrison's 18th ed. ch. 243]

30. Nissen fundoplication is done for: **(PGMEE 2016-17)**
   a. Achalsia cacdia
   b. Oesophagel structure
   c. GERD
   d. Diffuse esophageal spasm

   [Ref: Sabiston's 20th/e pg. 1023; Schwartz 10th /e pg.990]

31. All of the following are true about Nissen Fundoplication except-   **(PGMEE 2015)**
   a. Upper part of stomach is plicated around the lower esophagus
   b. It is done for GERD
   c. It is done for paraesophagal hiatus hernia
   d. Reinforcment is done only in the anterior half

   [Ref: Sabiston's 20th/e pg. 1023; Minjarez, Renee c.; Jobe, Blair a. (2006). "Surgical therapy for GERD". GI Motility online]

ESOPHAGITIS

32. The most common cause of drug induced esophagitis is   **(PGMEE 2014-15)**
   a. Metronidazole
   b. Indomethacin
   c. Doxycyline
   d. Steroids

   [Ref: Harrison's 19th/e pg. 1910]

33. Investigation of choice for dysphagia lusoria is?   **(PGMEE 2014-15)**
   a. Barium studies   b. X-ray
   c. CT angiography   d. Esophageal manometry

   [Ref: Harrison's 18th ed. ch. 292]

34. Volcano ulcers in esophagus are seen in: **(PGMEE 2014-15)**
   a. Herpetic esophagitis   b. HIV esophagitis
   c. Apthous ulcer in crohn d. Candida esophagitis

   [Ref: Mayo clinic gastroenterology and Hepatology Board review-5th ed. by Stephen C. Hauser]

35. Serpigenous like ulcerative lesion at distal end of esophagus is due to   **(PGMEE 2019)**
   a. Reflux esophagitis
   b. CMV esophagitis
   c. Candida
   d. Herpes

Explanation

- In patients with HIV, various infections can cause this disease, including herpes simplex virus (HSV), cytomegalovirus (CMV), varicella-zoster virus (VZV), Candida, and HIV itself. ... CMV classically causes serpiginous ulcers in the distal esophagus that may coalesce to form giant ulcers.

36. Reflux esophagitis is defined as pH of esophagus to be less than: **(PGMEE 2014-15)**
   a. 1   b. 2
   c. 3   d. 4

   [Ref: Grading and staging in gastroenterology by page 108, Harrison's 19th/e pg. 1894]

23.	b
24.	a
25.	b
26.	b
27.	c
28.	a
29.	a
30.	c
31.	d
32.	c
33.	c
34.	a
35.	b
36.	d

37. All of the following are correct statements regarding reflux esophagitis, EXCEPT: *(PGMEE 2014-15)*

a. Water brash
b. Weight gain
c. Mediastinitis
d. Infant apnea

[Ref: CMDT, ch. 15, pg. 594, Harrison's 19th/e pg. 1906]

38. All are true about Plummer-Vinson syndrome EXCEPT: *(PGMEE 2014-15)*

a. Esophageal webs
b. Premalignant
c. Common in elderly male
d. Dysphagia

[Ref: CMDT, ch. 15, pg. 600, Harrison's 19th/e pg. 237/532]

39. Feline esophagus is seen in: *(NEET 2018)*

a. Reflex esophagitis
b. Radiation-induced esophagitis
c. Herpetic esophagitis
d. Eosinophilic esophagitis

BARRET'S ESOPHAGUS

40. Which is true regarding Barrett's esophagus? *(PGMEE 2014-15)*

a. Squamous metaplasia of lower esophagus
b. Seen mainly in females
c. Premalignant
d. Responds to conservative management

[Ref: Harrison's 19th/e pg. 1907]

Explanation

- Barret's esophagus:
  ○ Metaplasia of squamous epithelium into columnar epithelium
  ○ Commonly associated with GERD
  ○ May transform into esophageal adenocarcinoma
  ○ M : F = 2 : 1
  ○ Investigation of choice: Esophagogastro duodeno scopy (EGD) & biopsy (to confirm intestinal metaplasia).

41. False regarding Barrett esophagus *(PGMEE 2019)*

a. Columnar to squamous metaplasia
b. It is a premalignant condition
c. Due to reflux
d. It is an acquired condition

[Ref: Sabiston's 20th /e pg. 1047]

42. True about Barret's esophagus:- *(PGMEE 2016-17)*

a. Squamous epithelium replaced by columnar epithelium
b. Endoscopic mucosal resection prevents occurence of Ca esophagus
c. It is a risk factor for adenocarcinoma
d. All of the above

[Ref: Harrison's 19th/e pg. 1907]

43. Features of Barrett's esophagus are: *(NEET June 2018)*

a. Metaplasia
b. Always gastric type of epithelium
c. Adenocarcinoma more common
d. A & c

[Ref: Sabiston's 20th /e pg. 1047]

37.	b
38.	c
39.	a
40.	c
41.	a
42.	d
43.	d
44.	a
45.	c
46.	a
47.	b
48.	c
49.	a
50.	b

Explanation

- In barrett's esophagus red, velvety metaplastic mucosa is seen between the smooth pale pink esophageal squamous mucosa and the lusher light brown gastric mucosa. It may present as patches or as a broad irregular circumferential band.

44. Endoscopic mucosal resection in Barrett's esophagus results in: *(PGMEE 2014-15)*

a. Stricture esophagus
b. Peptic ulceration
c. Reflux esophagitis
d. Achalasia cardia

[Ref: Harrison's 19th/e pg. 1907]

45. NOT true about Barrett's oesophagus:- *(PGMEE 2016-17)*

a. Endoscopy is gold standard in otherwise healthy individuals.
b. Most severe histological consequence of GERD
c. Laser ablation 100% protective from ca
d. The Seattle biopsy protocol is widely accepted for mapping of Barret's esophagus with high grade dysplasia.

[Ref: Harrison's 19th/e pg. 1907; Sabiston's 1st SAE pg.1035]

46. Most frequent site of ectopic gastric mucosa is: *(PGMEE 2015)*

a. Upper third of esophagus b. Middle third of esophagus
c. Duodenum
d. Lower third of esophagus

[Ref: Robbin's 9th/e pg. 752]

PLUMMER VINSON SYNDROME

47. A 40 year old female presents with koilonychias, iron defiency anemia & dysphagia, diagnosis is *(PGMEE 2013)*

a. Achalasia cardia
b. Plummer Vinson syndrome
c. Zollinger Ellison syndrome
d. Sipple syndrome

[Ref: Dhingra 6th/e pg. 346, 449; Schwartz 8th/e p. 918]

48. All statement about Plummer Vinson Syndrome are true except- *(PGMEE 2012)*

a. Common in females
b. Common with iron deficiency
c. Commonly leads to carcinoma in lower third of esophagus
d. Premalignant

[Ref: Dhingra 6th/e pg. 449]

49. Web constriction is seen in which part of esophagus, in Plummer Vinson syndrome – *(PGMEE 2014)*

a. Cervical
b. Abdominal
c. Thoracic
d. Any of the above

[Ref: Dhingra 6th/e pg. 346, Schwartz 8th/e p. 918]

50. Which of the following region is involved in Plummer-Vinson sydrome – *(PGMEE 2012)*

a. Valleculae
b. Post cricoid region
c. Pyriform sinus
d. Posterior pharyngeal wall

[Ref: Dhingra 6th/e pg. 346, Bailey & Love 25th/e p. 304]

51. Which is not true about Plummer Vinson syndrome:-
  (PGMEE 2016-17)
  a. Oesophageal web
  b. Megaloblastic anemia
  c. Dysphagia
  d. Glossitis

  [Ref: Sabiston's 20ᵗʰ/e pg. 798]

ESOPHAGEAL DIVERTICULA

52. True statement about a 6 cm Zenker's diverticulum is:
  (PGMEE 2014-15)
  a. It is a true diverticulum
  b. Occurs in the mid oesophagus
  c. Treatment is CP myotomy
  d. It occurs in children

  [Ref: CMDT, ch. 15, pg. 601, Harrison's 19th/e pg. 1903]

53. Patient complaint of bad breath with regurgitation of food three day ago :
  (PGMEE 2016-17)
  a. Zenkers diverticulum
  b. Achalsia cardia
  c. DES
  d. GERD

  [Ref: Sabiston's 20ᵗʰ /e pg. 1019]

54. Zenker's diverticulum presents with: *(PGMEE 2014-15)*
  a. Dysphonia
  b. Reflux esophagitis
  c. Dysphagia
  d. It is found in stomach

  [Ref: CMDT, ch. 15, pg. 601, Harrison's 19th/e pg. 1903]

55. Incorrect about Zenkers diverticulum?
  a. Located in killian triangle *(PGMEE 2015-16)*
  b. Regurgitation of previous day food
  c. Premalignant
  d. Dysphagia

  [Ref: Harrison's 19th/e pg. 1903]

56. Zenker's diverticulum – all are false except:
  a. True diverticulum *(PGMEE 2016-17)*
  b. Lies in mid- esophagus
  c. Treatment is by diverticulo-esophagostomy
  d. Senile change

  [Ref: Sabiston's 20ᵗʰ/e pg. 1020]

57. Which of the following is located in Laimer's triangle:
  (PGMEE 2014-15)
  a. Esophageal diverticulum
  b. Colonic diverticulosis
  c. Meckel's diverticulum
  d. Peri-ampullary diverticulum

  [Ref: www.ncbi.nlm.nih.gov ; CMDT, ch. 15, pg. 601]

58. Schatzki's Ring is present at – *(PGMEE 2013)*
  a. Upper end of trachea
  b. Lower end of trachea
  c. Upper end of esophagus
  d. Lower end of esophagus

  [Ref: Dhingra 6ᵗʰ/e pg. 345]

59. Traction diverticula is most commonly seen in:
  a. Middle 3rd esophagus *(PGMEE 2016-17)*
  b. Between upper esophagus and pharynx
  c. Supra diaphragmatic
  d. All sites are equally common

  [Ref Sabiston's 20ᵗʰ/e pg. 1020]

ESOPHAGEAL TEAR

60. Which of the narrowest portion of the esophagus?
  a. At the diagphragmatic aperture *(PGMEE 2015)*
  b. At the crossing of the left main bronchus
  c. At the level of the aortic arch
  d. Al the cricopharyngeal sphincter

  [Ref: Dhingra's 6ᵗʰ/e pg. 340]

61. Food can commonly get obstructed in the esophagus at all of the following locations except- *(PGMEE 2015)*
  a. Crossing of the hemiazygous vein
  b. Crossing of left bronchus
  c. Crossing of arch of aorta
  d. Diagphragmatic aperture

  [Ref: Butter P. Applied radiological anatomy, Cambridge University Press. (1999) ISBN: 0521481104]

62. Esophageal tear is best detected with:
  a. CT *(PGMEE 2014-15)*
  b. Angiography
  c. UGI endoscopy
  d. Barium swallow

  [Ref: CMDT, ch. 15, pg. 599]

63. Spontaneous esophageal rupture is most common in-
  a. Pharyngoesophagal junction *(PGMEE 2015)*
  b. Below the diagphragmatic aperture
  c. At the crossing of the arch of aorta
  d. Above the diagphramatic aperture

  [Ref: Curci JJ, Horman MJ. Boerhaave's syndrome: The importance of early diagnosis and treatment. Ann Surg. 1976 Apr. 183(4): 401-8]

64. Most common site for iatrogenic rupture of esophagus:
  (PGMEE 2014-15)
  a. Cervical esophagus
  b. Thoracic below aortic arch
  c. Thoracic above aortic arch
  d. Abdominal

  [Ref: Harrison's 19th/e pg. 1910]

65. Most common site of spontaneous rupture of esophagus is
  a. Cricopharyngeal junction *(DNB Dec' 2009)*
  b. After the crossing of arch of aorta
  c. Cardio esophageal junction
  d. Mid esophagus

  [Ref: Cole and Zollinger textbook of surgery 9ᵗʰ/e p. 719]

66. Most common site of tear in Boerhaave syndrome:
  a. Lower end of oesophagus *(PGMEE 2014-15)*
  b. At Gastroesophageal junction
  c. Upper esophagus
  d. Mild oesophagus

  [Ref: Harrison's 19th/e pg. 1910]

51.	b
52.	c
53.	a
54.	c
55.	c
56.	c
57.	a
58.	d
59.	a
60.	d
61.	a
62.	c
63.	d
64.	a
65.	c
66.	a

Explanation

Features	Boerhaave syndrome	Mallary - Weiss syndrome
Involvement	Transmural perforation of esophagus	Longitudinal mucosal laceration
MC site	Left posterolateral wall of the lower ⅓rd of esophagus	Gastroesophageal junction > gastric cardia
Precipitating factor	Forceful emesis	Persistent retching and vomiting
Associated factor	Food/Alcohol binge	Alcohol binge
See ratio	M > F	F > M
Mortality	High	Less

67. Boerhaave syndrome is: *(PGMEE 2016-17)*

   a. Partial tear of stomach after binge drinking
   b. Complete tear of lower esophagus in postero lateral wall
   c. Commonly occure after heavy exercise
   d. No treatment required

   [Ref: Sabiston's 20th/e pg.1025]

68. All of the following are true about Boerhave syndrome expect- *(PGMEE 2015)*

   a. Spontaneous perforation of the esophagus occurs due to violent contraction against a close glottis
   b. It has a lower mortality rate compared to a Mallory Weiss tear
   c. It may follow a bout of heavy drinking
   d. All layers of the esophageal musculature are ruptured

   [Ref: internet]

69. Which of the following is true about Mallory weiss tear *(All India Dec. 15 pattern)*

   a. It is a mucosal tear not extending through the muscle layer
   b. It is more common in women than men
   c. It is associated with achalasia cardia
   d. It is common in young individuals

   [Ref: Internet]

70. A patient after heavy drinking of alcohol presents with too much vomiting & haematemesis. Most likely diagnosis could be: *(NEET June 2018)*

   a. Mallory Weiss syndrome
   b. Oesophageal carcinoma
   c. Achalasia cardia
   d. Boerhaave syndrome

   [Ref: Sabiston's 20th/e pg.1026]

Explanation:

Esophagus Disorders & Presentation

   ■ In Mallory Weiss syndrome, vigorous vomiting produces a vertical split in gastric mucosa, immediately below

67.	b
68.	b
69.	a
70.	a
71.	d

the squamo-columnar junction at the cardia in 90% of cases. The condition presents with haematemesis

   ■ Most oesophageal neoplasms presents with mechanical symptoms, principally dysphagia, but sometimes also regurgitation, vomiting, odynophagia & weight loss
   ■ Achalsia cardia presents with dysphagia, although pain (often mistaken for reflux) is common in the early stages.
   ■ In Boerhaave's syndrome, vomiting occurs against a closed glottis, and pressure builds up in the oesophagus

ESOPHAGEAL VARICES

71. Which of the following is true for upper gastrointestinal endoscopy: *(PGMEE 2018)*

   a. MCC of upper GI bleed is Variceal bleed
   b. Used to diagnose active bleeding
   c. Upper GI bleed is defined as GI bleed proximal toampulla of vater
   d. Rock hall scoring is done to identify patients at risk of adverse outcome (risk stratification)

   [Ref: Bailey & Love 26th/e pg. 1042]

Explanation

   ■ Hemorrhage can originate from any region of the GI tract and is typically classified based on its location relative to the ligament of Treitz. Upper GI hemorrhage from proximal to the ligament of Treitz accounts for more than 80% of cases of acute bleeding. (Ref: Sabistons 19th/e, pg 1160)
   ■ A number of scoring systems have been advocated for the assessment of rebleeding and death after upper gastrointestinal haemorrhage. Perhaps the most useful of these is the Rockall score. This can be used in a pre-endoscopy format to stratify patients to safe early discharge and postendoscopy it can relatively accurately predict rebleeding and death.

Causes of Upper Gastrointestinal Bleeding

Condition	%
Ulcers	60
○ Oesophageal	6
○ Gastric	21
○ Duodenal	33
Erosions	26
○ Oesophageal	13
○ Gastric	9
○ Duodenal	4
Mallary-weiss fear	4
Oesophageal varices	4
Tumour	0.5
Vascular lesions, e.g. Dieulafay's disease	0.5
Other	5

H. PYLORI DISEASE

1. H. Pylori causes all EXCEPT: *(PGMEE 2015-16)*
a. Peptic ulcer
b. Maltoma
c. Carcinoid tumor
d. Gastric CA

[Ref: Harrison's 19th/e pg. 1039-1040]

2. Best test for determining eradication of H.Pylori infection: *(NEET 2019)*
a. Urease test
b. Serum ELISA
c. Tissue biopsy
d. Breath urea test

[Ref: CMDT-14/chap: 33/PG:1462 and Harrison's 19th/e pg. 1040]

Explanation

- IOC to diagnose H. pylori ELISA.
- IOC to diagnose H. pylori, if you do endoscopy: Rapid urease kit.
- IOC to look for eradication: C^{13} and C^{14} urea breath test.
- Gold standard to diagnose H. pylori: culture in Skirrow medium.

3. Indications to eradicate H. pylori: *(PGMEE 2014-15)*
a. Low grade B cell lymphoma
b. Family history of gastric cancer
c. Duodenal ulcer
d. Gastric outlet obstruction

[Ref: Harrison's 19th/e pg. 1041]

4. The following statements are correct for Helicobacter pylori EXCEPT: *(PGMEE 2014-15)*
a. It shows positive urease test
b. It is spiral gram negative flagellate
c. It is linked with duodenal ulcer
d. It can invade tissue to a great depth

[Ref: CMDT-14/ch. 15/pg: 609, Harrison's 19th/e pg. 1039]

Explanation

- Around 90% of patients of duodenal ulcer and 70% of gastric ulcer are infected with H. pylori.
- Organism gets localized deep beneath the mucus layer closely adherent to epithelial cells.

5. CLO test is used for: *(PGMEE 2014-15)*
a. H. pylori
b. Brucella
c. Gonorrhoea
d. EBOLA

[Ref: Harrison's 19th/e pg. 1040]

Explanation

- CLO test is better k/as Rapid urease test which is done to confirm the presence of H.pylori

6. Which drug is not effective against H. pylori?
a. Colloidal bismuth *(PGMEE 2014-15)*
b. Metronidazole
c. Amoxycilline
d. Erythromycin

[Ref: CMDT, ch. 15, pg. 613, Harrison's 19th/e pg. 1039]

7. All of the following are indications for surgery in a case of duodenal ulcer EXCEPT: *(PGMEE 2014-15)*
a. Acute perforation of ulcer
b. Pyloric stenosis
c. Massive haemorrhage
d. Multiple large ulcers

[Ref: CMDT, ch. 15, pg. 617, Harrison's 19th/e pg. 1925]

8. Which of the following statements about peptic ulcer disease is true? *(PGMEE 2014-15)*
a. Helicobacter pylori eradication increases the likelihood of occurrences of complication
b. The incidence of complication has remained unchanged
c. The incidence of Helicobacter pylori infection in India is very low
d. Helicobacter pylori eradication does not alter the recurrence ratio

[Ref: Harrison's 18th ed. ch. 293, Harrison's 19th/e pg. 1911]

9. Helicobacter pylori is associated with following EXCEPT: *(PGMEE 2014-15)*
a. Type A gastritis
b. M.A.L. Toma
c. Gastric adenocarcinoma
d. Hyperchlorhydria

[Ref: CMDT, ch. 15, pg. 609, Harrison's 19th/e pg. 1039]

Explanation

Association of H. Pylori

- Type-B gastritis
- Lymphoma: MALToma
- Cancer stomach (Intestinal variant)
- Peptic ulcer (Duodenal and gastric)

10. True about MALToma is- *(PGMEE 2015)*
a. Commonly seen in gastric cardia
b. H. Pylori infection is risk factor
c. They are secondary gastric lymphomas
d. They are a type of T cell lymphoma

[Ref: Bailey & Love 26th/e pg. 1054; Harrison 17th/e pg. 573; Schwartz 10th/e pg. 1084]

11. Eradication of infection by anti-H.Pylori antibiotics is best determined by *(PGMEE 2014-15)*
a. S. ELISA
b. Breath urea test
c. Rapid urease test
d. Biopsy

[Ref: Harrison's Internal Medicine, 18th ed. Figure 151-2, Harrison's 19th/e pg. 1039]

12. H. pylori causes: *(PGMEE 2014-15)*
a. Type A gastritis
b. Type B gastritis
c. Autoimmune
d. Allergic gastritis

[Ref: CMDT, ch. 15, pg. 609, Harrison's 19th/e pg. 1039]

1.	c
2.	d
3.	d
4.	d
5.	a
6.	d
7.	d
8.	b
9.	a
10.	b
11.	b
12.	b

GASTRITIS

13. Phlegmonous gastritis occurs due to: *(PGMEE 2014-15)*
- a. H. pylori
- b. E.coli
- c. Drugs
- d. Reflux of acid

[Ref: Harrison's 19th/e pg. 1930]

14. Most common viral cause of gastritis *(PGMEE 2014-15)*
- a. H. Pylori
- b. CMV
- c. Hepatitis A
- d. Enterovirus

[Ref: Harrison's 19th/e pg. 1930]

15. Erosive gastritis commonly occurs at: *(PGMEE 2014-15)*
- a. Cardia
- b. Fundus
- c. Greater curvature
- d. Antrum

[Ref: Harrison's 19th/e pg. 1930]

16. Not true in type A fundal gastritis is: *(PGMEE 2014-15)*
- a. Low gastric PH
- b. Hyperchlorhydria
- c. Antibody against parietal cells and presence of autoimmunity
- d. Antibody against intrinsic factor

[Ref: Harrison's 19th/e pg. 1931]

Explanation
- Atrophy of parietal cell mass leads to hypochlorhydria and decrease intrinsic factor.

17. Chronic gastiritis is caused by all except:- *(PGMEE 2015; 2012-13)*
- a. Gastrectomy with gastroenterostomy
- b. Pernicious anaemia
- c. H. Pylori
- d. Overuse of salicylates

[Ref: Robbin's 9th/e pg. 763]

18. True in Menetrier's disease are A/E: *(PGMEE 2014-15)*
- a. Rugosities fold hypertrophy
- b. Foveolar hyperplasia
- c. Protein losing gastropathy
- d. Hypergastrinaemia

[Ref: Sabiston's 20th/e pg. 1231]

PUD

19. Prepyloric or channel ulcer in the stomach is termed as: *(DNB 2008)*
- a. Type 1
- b. Type 2
- c. Type 3
- d. Type 4

[Ref: Sabiston 20th /e pg.1208]

20. Pyloric end of a stomach can be distinguished during surgery by the presence of which structure in close proximity ? *(PGMEE 2016-17)*
- a. Nerve
- b. Vein
- c. Artery
- d. Lymph node

[Ref: Prepyloric vein of Mayo is important]

21. MC age of presentation of gastric ulcer is: *(PGMEE 2014-15)*
- a. 3rd decade
- b. 4th decade
- c. 5th decade
- d. 6th decade

[Ref: Harrison's Principles of Internal Medicine ch. 239, Harrison's 19th/e pg. 1911]

22. Most common site of peptic ulcer in duodenum- *(PGMEE 2013-14)*
- a. 1st part
- b. 4th part
- c. 2nd part
- d. 3rd part

[Ref: Robbin's 9th/e pg. 766]

23. Most common site/location of peptic ulcer is- *(PGMEE 2015)*
- a. At gastro-esophagal junction
- b. Gastric antrum
- c. 1st part of duodenum
- d. Lesser curvature of stomac

[Ref: Harrison's 19th/e pg. 1911; Bailey & Love 26th/e pg. 1033]

24. Most common site of chronic peptic ulcer disease is: *(PGMEE 2018)*
- a. Lesser curvature near cardia
- b. Greater curvature
- c. Lesser curvature near incisura angularis
- d. Pyloric antrum

Ref: Sabistons 19th/e, pg 1198

25. Most common site of type 1 gastric ulcer: *(PGMEE 2014-15)*
- a. Gastric body
- b. Antrum
- c. Pylorus
- d. Cardia

[Ref: CMDT, ch. 15, pg. 611, Harrison's 19th/e pg. 1911]

Explanation
- Gastric ulcers can occur at any location in the stomach, although they usually present on the lesser curvature, near the incisura. Approximately 60% of ulcers are located in this location and are classified as type I gastric ulcers

Gastric Ulcer Types

Types	Location	Acid level
I	Leser curve at incisura	Low to normal
II	Gastric body with duodenal ulcer	Increased
III	Prepyloric	Increased
IV	High on lesser curve	Normal
V	Anywhere	Normal, NSAID-induced

26. Most common site of curling's ulcer:- *(PGMEE 2015)*
- a. Proximal Duodenum
- b. Esophagus
- c. D. jujenum
- d. Distal duodenum

[Ref: Robbin's 9th/e pg. 762]

27. Hour glass deformity is seen in- *(DNB Dec. 11)*
- a. CHPS
- b. Peptic ulcer
- c. Duodenal atresia
- d. Carcinoma stomach

[Ref: Robbin's 9th/e pg. 766]

13.	b
14.	b
15.	c
16.	b
17.	d
18.	d
19.	c
20.	b
21.	d
22.	a
23.	c
24.	c
25.	a
26.	a
27.	b

28. All of the following are true regarding a patient with acid peptic disease EXCEPT: *(PGMEE 2014-15)*
a. Misoprostol is the drug of choice given with NSAIDs
b. DU is preventable by the use of night time H2 blockers
c. Omeprazole may help ulcers refractory to H2 blockers
d. Misoprostol is DOC in a pregnant lady

[Ref: Harrison's 19th/e pg. 1911]

Explanation

■ Misoprostol can help patients with PUD who require NSAID therapy (e.g. for arthritis).

29. Which of the following is the most outermost histological layer of peptic ulcer: *(PGMEE 2015)*
a. Necrotic zone
b. Granulation tissue zone
c. Superficial exudative zone
d. Zone of cicatrisation

[Ref: Robbin's 9th/e pg. 766]

30. When an ulcer in anterior wall of stomach perforates, it goes to which space in supine position
a. Left anterior *(PGMEE 2016-17)*
b. Lesser sac
c. Right anterior
d. Freely into intraperitoneal space

[Ref: Radiology of the Stomach and Duodenum by Alan H. Freeman, E. Sala pg. 217]

31. Where does posterior perforation of peptic ulcer drain *(DNB June' 2009)*
a. Paracolic gutter
b. Greater sac
c. Formen of winslow
d. Omental bursa

[Ref: CSDT 11th/e p. 553]

32. A 45 year old lawyer presents with pain in the abdomen more so in the epigastric region that worsens with eating spicy food and is relieved by bending forward. Complications of the above mentioned condition could be all except- *(PGMEE 2015)*
a. Bleeding
b. Perforation
c. Gastric outlet obstruction
d. Splenic vein thrombosis

[Ref: Bailey & Love 26th/e pg. 1040, 1042]

33. MC site for stress induced gastric ulcer: *(PGMEE 2016-17)*
a. Greater curvature
b. Antrum
c. Lesser curvature
d. Anywhere in stomach

[Ref: Robbin's 9th/e pg. 762]

34. MC site for gastric peptic ulcerations:-
a. Along the greater curvature *(PGMEE 2016-17)*
b. Antrum
c. Along the lesser curvature
d. Anywhere in stomach

[Ref: Robbin's 9th/e pg. 766]

35. Bleeding from lesser curvature in gastric ulcer, source of bleeding is? *(PGMEE 2014)*
a. Right gastro-epiploic artery
b. Right omento duodenal
c. Pancreatoduodenal artery
d. Left gastric artery

[Ref: Harrison's 19th/e pg. 1925]

36. Prolonged intake of PPI does not cause:
a. Hypothyroidism *(NEET Pattern 14)*
b. Pelvic fracture
c. Clostridium difficile infection
d. Increased community acquired pneumonia

[Ref: Harrison's 19th/e pg. 263/568]

37. The most common complication of vagotomy is: *(PGMEE 2014-15)*
a. Diarrhoea
b. Dryness of mouth
c. Tachycardia
d. Bleaching

[Ref: CMDT, ch. 34, pg. 1615]

38. Not a hormone causing early dumping? *(PGMEE 2014-15)*
a. VIP
b. Neurotensin
c. Motilin
d. CCK

[Ref: Harrison's 19th/e pg. 1926]

39. Dumping syndrome is due to all EXCEPT: *(PGMEE 2014-15)*
a. Motilin
b. Small stomach
c. Hypertonic fluid contents in bowel
d. Neurotensin

[Ref: Harrison's 19th/e pg. 1926]

Explanation

■ Large volume of hyperosmotic fluid in the intestine plays a major role in the development of dumping syndrome.

40. True about dumping syndrome is all EXCEPT: *(PGMEE 2014-15)*
a. Caused by early emptying of stomach
b. Medically managed
c. Controlled by small diets
d. Needs re-surgery

[Ref: Harrison's 19th/e pg. 1926; Sabiston's 20th/e pg. 1212]

ZES

41. Increased gastrin is seen in: *(PGMEE 2014-15)*
a. Zollinger-Ellison syndrome
b. Iron deficiency anaemia
c. Duodenal ulcer
d. Gastric cancer

[Ref: Harrison's 19th/e pg. 568, 1928]

42. Boundaries of gastrinoma triangle are all except: *(DNB Dec' 2011)*
a. Junction of neck and body of pancreas
b. Cystic duct and bile duct junction
c. Junction of hepatic ducts
d. Junction of second and third part of duodenum

[Ref: Sabiston 20th/e pg. 954]

28.	d
29.	d
30.	d
31.	d
32.	d
33.	d
34.	c
35.	d
36.	a
37.	a
38.	d
39.	b
40.	d
41.	a
42.	c

Explanation

- Gastrinoma triangle (Passaro's triangle)
  - Confluence of cystic & common bile ducts
  - Junction of 2nd & 3rd portion of duodenum
  - Junction of neck & body of pancreas.

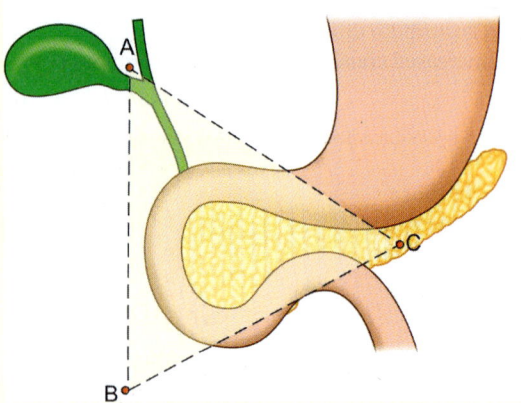

43. Not a part of gastrinoma Δ *(PGMEE 2016-17, 2015-16)*
a. Junction of cystic duct and common bile duct
b. Junction of 2nd and 3rd part of dudenum
c. Junction of head and neck of pancreas
d. Junction of neck and body of pancreas

[Ref: Sabiston's 20th/e pg.1210, 954]

44. All of the following are true about Zollinger Ellison syndrome exopect- *(PGMEE 2015)*
a. Gastrin provocation tests are a part of diagnostic work up
b. They may be associatd with insulinomas
c. It is due to the presence of a gastrinoma
d. It might be associated with ulcers in unusual locations in stomach

[Ref: Bailry & Love 26th /e pg. 790; Schwartz 10th /e pg. 392; Harrison 17th /e pg. 1868 , p.2354; CMDT 2006, P.595;]

43.	c
44.	b
45.	d
46.	d
47.	a
48.	b
49.	d

Explanation

- Zollinger-Ellison Syndrome:

Gastrin secreting tumor of pancreas

↓

Hypergastrinemia

Stimulate acid secretion   ↑ number of parietal cells

↓   ↓

↑ basal acid output   maximal acid output

Mucosal ulceration, Diarrhoea, Malabsorption

- Occurs sporadically or associated with MEN-1
- Screening test: Fasting serum gastrin level in increased
- Gastric pH < 2 is highly suggestive of ZES.
- Provocative test of choice: Secretin stimulation test

- Imaging modality of choice: Somatostatin receptor scintigraphy
- Endoscopic ultrasound (EUS) is a never modality for localizing gastrinomas.

45. Best for localization for Z-E syndrome is: *(PGMEE 2014-15)*
a. Increase in Serum gastrin with pH<2
b. Increase in serum gastrin with pH>2
c. BAO/MAO ratio
d. Octreoscan

[Ref: Sabiston 20th/e pg. 955; Harrison's 19th/e pg. 1928]

46. Which of the following have hypergastrinemia with decrease acid output? *(PGMEE 2014-15)*
a. Retained gastric antrum
b. ZES
c. G-cell hyperplasia
d. Pernicious anemia

[Ref: Sabiston 20th/e pg. 955; Harrison's 19th/e pg. 568, 1927]

47. Which one of the following is best for localization of Zollinger-Ellison syndrome? *(PGMEE 2014-15)*
a. EUS (Endoscopic ultrasound)
b. Secretin injection test
c. MRI
d. Basal gastric acid output

[Ref: CMDT, ch. 15, pg. 619,Harrison's 19th/e pg. 568, 1927]

48. Best provocative test for diagnosis of Gastrinoma is:-
a. Steroid assay *(PGMEE 2015-16)*
b. Secretion injection test
c. Ca++ infusion test
d. ACTH stimulation test

[Ref: Harrison's 19th/e pg. 1928]

49. Which of these features are present in Zollinger-Ellison Syndrome (1 = Peptic ulceration, 2 = diarrhoea 3 = reduce gastric acid secretion)
a. 1 and 3
b. 2 and 3
c. 1, 2 and 3
d. 1 and 2

[Ref: CMDT, ch. 15, pg. 619, Harrison's 19th/e pg. 1927]

Explanation

Zollinger-Ellison syndrome

- Excessive secretion of gastrin.
- Epigastric pain
- Diarrhea (caused by mucosal damage and pancreatic enzyme inactivation leading to malabsorption)

MALABSORPTION SYNDROMES

1. Malabsorption syndrome features include all, except:
(PGMEE 2014-15)
- a. Anaemia
- b. Constipation
- c. Tetany
- d. Steatorrhoea

[Ref: CMDT, ch. 15, pg. 621, Harrison's 19th/e pg. 1946]

2. Most common cause of malabsorption in our country is:
(PGMEE 2014-15)
- a. Intestinal surgery
- b. Gastric surgery
- c. Sprue
- d. Intestinal parasite

[Ref: CMDT, ch. 15, pg. 621, Harrison's 19th/e pg. 1946t]

3. Malabsorption syndrome does not result from:
- a. Parasite infestation *(PGMEE 2014-15)*
- b. Small bowel diverticulae
- c. Post-gastrectomy
- d. Anterior resection of colon

[Ref: CMDT, ch. 15, pg. 621, Harrison's 19th/e pg. 1946t]

4. A 41-year-old patient presented with chronic dirarrhea for 3 months. A D-xylose absorption test was order to look for: *(PGMEE 2014-15)*
- a. Carbohydrate malabsorption due to mucosal disease
- b. Carbohydrate malabsorption due to chronic pancreatitis
- c. Fat malabsorption due to mucosal disease
- d. Fat malabsorption due to chronic pancreatitis

[Ref: Harrison's 18th ed. ch. 46, pg. 257, Harrison's 19th/e pg. 1938]

Explanation
- D-xylose is a pentose sugar absorbed almost exclusively in the proximal small intestine and is excreted in urine. Urinary estimation of D-xylose is a surrogate indicator of carbohydrate absorption and proximal small intestine mucosal function.

5. Xylose absorption test is used to assess:
- a. Insulinoma *(PGMEE 2014-15)*
- b. Atypical carcinoid
- c. ZES
- d. Monosaccharide absorption

[Ref: Harrison's 19th/e pg. 1938]

6. Which of the following is not a malabsorption syndrome?
- a. Coeliac disease *(DNB June 2009)*
- b. Whipple's disease
- c. Tropical sprue
- d. Tangier's disease

[Ref: Harrison's 17th/e table 288-7; Harrison 19th/e pg 1946]

7. Non absorption of fat soluble vitamins is due to?
(DNB June 2009)
- a. Steatorrhea
- b. Pancreatic insufficiency
- c. Both
- d. None

[Ref: Harrison's 19th/e pg 272, 2099]

CELIAC DISEASE

8. Most sensitive and specific antibody for celiac sprue is?
(DNB December 2011)
- a. Anti endomysial
- b. Anti TTG
- c. Anti reticulin
- d. Anti Gliadin

[Ref: Harrison's 19th/e pg. 1940]

9. Most common extra-intestinal manifestation of Coeliac disease is:- *(PGMEE 2016-17)*
- a. Malabsorption
- b. Hypocalcemia
- c. Type 1 DM
- d. Anemia

[Ref: Internet link https://www.researchgate.net]

10. Which of the following vitamin deficiencies is uncommon in coeliac disease: *(PGMEE 2015-16; DNB Dec 2009)*
- a. Folic Acid
- b. Vitamin A
- c. Vitamin B12
- d. Vitamin D

[Ref: Celiac Disease for Dummies by Blumer and Crowe (John Wiaey and Sons 2010)]

11. In celiac sprue there is a deficiency of all EXCEPT:
(PGMEE 2014-15)
- a. Vitamin A
- b. Vitamin B12
- c. Folic acid
- d. Iron

[Ref: Harrison's 19th/e pg. 1897f/1940]

12. Anti endomysial antibody is seen in? *(DNB Dec' 2010)*
- a. Celiac disease
- b. Tropical sprue
- c. Collagenous colitis
- d. SLE

[Ref: Harrison's 19th/e pg 1940]

13. Celiac sprue is associated with:- *(PGMEE 2015)*
- a. HLA DQ1
- b. HLA DQ2
- c. HLA DQ3
- d. HLA DQ4

[Ref: Robbin's 9th/e pg. 795]

14. A female patient is having diarrhea and abdominal distension. Small intestinal biopsy shows villous atrophy and crypt hyperplasia. Diagnosis is- *(PGMEE 2013-14)*
- a. Celiac sprue
- b. Whipples disease
- c. Hirchsprung's disease
- d. Tropical sprue

[Ref: Robbins 9th/e pg. 782, Harrison's 19th/e pg. 1940]

15. Anti tissue transglutaminase antibody (Anti- TTG) is seen in? *(DNB Dec. 09, PGMEE 2014-15)*
- a. Celiac disease
- b. Tropical sprue
- c. Collagenous colitis
- d. SLE

[Ref: Robbin's 9th/e pg. 782]

1.	b
2.	d
3.	d
4.	a
5.	d
6.	d
7.	c
8.	a
9.	d
10.	c
11.	b
12.	a
13.	b
14.	a
15.	a

16. **Antigliadin antibodies are detectable in-** *(DNB Dec. 08)*
   a. Intestinal colitis
   b. Intestinal lymphoma
   c. Celiac disease
   d. Tropica sprue

   [Ref: Robbin's 9th/e pg. 782]

17. **Celiac disease A/E-** *(PGMEE 2014)*
   a. Increase in intraepithelial lymphocytes
   b. Increase in the thickness of the mucosa
   c. Increase in inflammatory cells in lamina propyria
   d. Crypt hyperplasia

   [Ref: Robbins 9th/e pg. 782; Harrison 18th/e pg. 2470, 2471]

18. **Which cereal is not to be given in celiac sprue?** *(PGMEE 2015-16)*
   a. Wheat
   b. Maize
   c. Corn
   d. Rice

   [Ref: Harrison's 19th/e pg.1940]

19. **In celiac disease allowed is:-** *(PGMEE 2016-17)*
   a. Rice
   b. Rye
   c. Oat
   d. Barley

   [Ref: Harrison's 19th/e pg.1940]

20. **Non-tropical sprue is characterized by:**
   a. Elongation of intestinal villi *(PGMEE 2014-15)*
   b. Currant jelly stools
   c. Hypertriglyceridemia
   d. Poor absorption of lipids

   [Ref: Harrison's 19th/e pg. 1940]

21. **Enteropathy associated T cell lymphoma is associated with:** *(PGMEE 2014-15)*
   a. M.A.L.Toma
   b. Crohn's disease
   c. Menetrier disease
   d. Celiac Sprue

   [Ref: Harrison's 19th/e pg.1942]

16.	c
17.	b
18.	a
19.	a
20.	d
21.	d
22.	a
23.	a
24.	a
25.	c
26.	b
27.	d
28.	a
29.	d
30.	d
31.	c

Explanation

- Enteropathy associated T cell lymphoma (EATL) is a rare GI non-Hodgkin's lymphoma, originating from T lymphocytes & is specifically associated with celiac disease.

WHIPPLE'S DISEASE

22. **Small intestinal biopsy of a patient reveals Periodic acid Schiff staining macrophages in lamina propria. The likely etiology is:-** *(PGMEE 2018)*
   a. Whipple disease
   b. Gluten sensitive enteropathy
   c. Abetalipoproteinemia
   d. Agammaglobulinemia

Explanation

- Whipple disease presents with arthritis, lympadenopathy, cardiac issues, PAS positive granules in lamina propria on biopsy.

23. **Characteristic histopathology finding in Whipples disease** *(PGMEE 2014-15)*
   a. PAS positive macrophages and rod shaped bacilli in lamina propria
   b. Shortened thickened villi with increased crypt depth

   c. Mononuclear infiltration at base of crypts
   d. Blunting and flattening of mucosal surface and absent villi

   [Ref: Robbin's 9th/e pg. 783]

24. **Whipple's disease is characterized by?** *(PGMEE 2013)*
   a. Foamy macrophages
   b. Villous atrophy
   c. AFB positive
   d. Papillary projections

   [Ref: Robbin's 9th/e pg. 783]

25. **Jejunal biopsy is diagnostic in:** *(PGMEE 2014-15)*
   a. Coeliac sprue
   b. Tropical sprue
   c. Whipple's disease
   d. Radiation enteritis

   [Ref: Harrison's 19th/e pg. 1091, 1944]

26. **2 yr old male presented with abdominal distension, chronic diarrhea, severe anemia and failure to thrive? Which of the following is the investigation of choice:**
   a. Anti milk protein antibody *(PGMEE 2015)*
   b. Anti endomysial antibody
   c. Intestinal biopsy
   d. Antinuclear antibody

   [Ref:http://emedicine.medscape.com/article/932104-clinical, Robbins 9th/e pg. 782]

27. **True about tropical sprue are A/E:** *(PGMEE 2014-15)*
   a. Protein losing enteropathy
   b. Steatorrhea
   c. Stomatitis
   d. Jejunal biopsy is specific

   [Ref: Harrison's 19th/e pg. 1942]

28. **Jejunal biopsy is diagnostic in:** *(PGMEE 2014-15)*
   a. Abetalipoproteinemia
   b. Giardiasis
   c. Tropical sprue
   d. Celiac sprue

   [Ref: Harrison's 19th/e pg. 2444]

MISCELLANEOUS DISEASE

29. **In giardiasis malabsorption is due to all EXCEPT:**
   a. Bacterial overgrowth *(PGMEE 2014-15)*
   b. Hypogammaglobulinaemia
   c. Lactose intolerance
   d. Mucosal injury

   [Ref: Harrison's 19th/e pg. 1406]

30. **Recurrent glardiasis is a feature of:** *(PGMEE 2015)*
   a. C3 deficiency
   b. D1 Georges syndrome
   c. C1 inhibitor deficiency
   d. Common variable immunodeficiency

   [Ref: CMDT 2013 p. 868; Harrison 19th/e p. 270]

31. **Patient with congenital lactose deficiency will experience distension, flatulence and diarrhea on ingestion of:** *(PGMEE 2014-15)*
   a. Glucose
   b. Sucrose
   c. Milk
   d. Eggs

   [Ref: CMDT, ch. 15, pg. 626, Harrison's 19th/e pg. 272]

DIARRHOEA

32. Most common cause for diarrhoea in adults associated with intake of Shell fish? *(NEET Pattern 2015)*
a. Norwolk virus
b. Calcivirus
c. Rotavirus
d. Filovirus

[Ref: Harrison's 19th/e pg.1285-86]

33. Which is not a cause of diarrhea? *(DNB December 2011)*
a. Carcinoids
b. Hypercalcemia
c. Hyperthyroidism
d. Diabetes mellitus

[Ref: Harrison's 19th/e pg. 265]

34. Which diarrhea decreases after prolonged fasting? *(PGMEE 2015-16)*
a. Osmotic diarrhea
b. Bloody
c. Infective
d. Secretory

[Ref: chapter 338, Harrison's 18th edition, Harrison's 19th/e pg. 269/303]

35. Mucosal invasion of intestine causes of which type of diarrhoea- *(PGMEE 2013-14)*
a. Rice stool
b. Watery diarrhea
c. Dysentery
d. None

[Ref: Harrison 19th/e pg. 266]

36. Diabetes induced diarrhea is best managed by which of the following? *(PGMEE 2014-15)*
a. Clonidine
b. Octreotide
c. Levosulpiride
d. Clindinium

[Ref: Current clinical practice, type 2 diabetes, 2nd ed. R.codaria pg. 200, Harrison's 19th/e pg. 270, 272]

37. All cause diarrhea except? *(PGMEE 2014-15)*
a. Diabetes
b. Hypercalcemia
c. Hyperthyroidism
d. Irritable bowel syndrome

[Ref: CMDT, ch. 15, pg. 574, Harrison's 19th/e pg. 265]

38. Which of the following does not a causes invasive diarrhea? *(DNB June 2009)*
a. Salmonella
b. Bacillus cereus
c. Shighella
d. Aeromonas

[Ref: Harrison 19th/e pg. 266]

39. Travellers diarrhea is most commonly caused by :- *(PGMEE 2016-17)*
a. ETEC
b. EHEC
c. EIEC
d. Shigella

[Ref: Harrison's 19th/e pg. 266]

Explanation

- **ETEC**: Watery diarrhea (Traveller's diarrhea)
- **EHEC**: Hemorrhagic (Bloody diarrhea)
- **EIEC**: Invasive, dysentry, clinical manifestation similar to shigella.
- **EPEC**: Diarrhea, usually in Pediatric patients

40. Causitive agent of traveler diarrhea among following? *(PGMEE 2015-16)*
a. Campylobacter
b. Aeromonas
c. Actinobacillus
d. Cryptosporidium

[Ref: Harrison's 19th/e pg. 266]

41. Large bowel colonic Diarrhea is associated with all of the following EXCEPT:- *(PGMEE 2015-16)*
a. Urgency
b. Mucus
c. Large Volume Stool
d. Tenesmus

[Ref: Mayo Clinic Medicine Review 7th/e pg. 262, 263, 264]

42. A patient with chronic diarrhoea with normal D-xylose and Schilling test. What could be the diagnosis: *(PGMEE 2014-15)*
a. Chronic pancreatitis
b. Bacterial overgrowth syndrome
c. Coeliac disease
d. Gastric disease

[Ref: CMDT, ch. 15, pg. 624, Harrison's 19th/e pg. 1944]

43. Protein losing enteropathy is characterized by all EXCEPT: *(PGMEE 2014-15)*
a. Decreased serum albumin and globulin
b. Increased lymphatic flow
c. 99mTc-dextran radionuclide study done
d. Lymphangiectasia on biopsy

[Ref: Harrison's 19th/e pg. 1945]

44. On a trip 4 hours after having lunch at a restaurant, your friend develops diarrhea, and had 5 loose stools. There are signs of minimal dehydration. What should be your management? *(NEET Pattern 2017)*
a. Buy ORS and gives after preparing according to instruction
b. ORS and antibiotics, both tinidazole and ofloxacin
c. Give only ofloxacin because tinidazole is not required as Giardia will not cause diarhea within 4 hours
d. Go to a hospital as needs to be shown immediately, as night is approaching

45. Alpha 1 anti-tryspin in stool is indicative of? *(PGMEE 2014-15)*
a. Protein losing enteropathy
b. Chronic pancreatitis
c. Acute pancreatitis
d. Whipple disease

[Ref: Harrison's 19th/e pg. 1945]

IBD

ULCERATIVE COLITIS & CROHN'S

46. Which of the following is not a feature of severe ulcerative colitis: *(NEET 2018)*
a. Spontaneous bleeding seen on endoscopy
b. 4-6 bowel movements per day
c. Pulse rate of 96 per minute
d. ESR 50 mm

47. Most characteristic difference between crohn disease and ulcerative colitis *(PGMEE 2019)*
a. Crypt abscess
b. Lymphocytic infiltration
c. Mucosal edema
d. Polyps

32.	a
33.	b
34.	a
35.	c
36.	a
37.	b
38.	b
39.	a
40.	a
41.	c
42.	b
43.	b
44.	a
45.	a
46.	b
47.	d

48. Pseudopolyps (pseudopolyposis) are seen in?
(PGMEE 2009, June 2008, 2007; 2015; PGMEE 2012-13)
a. Crohn's disease
b. Ulcerative colitis
c. Enteric fever
d. Juvenile polyposis

[Ref: Robbins 9th/e pg. 800; Harrison's 19th/e pg 1951; Bailey and Love 26th /e pg. 1145]

Explanation

- *Colonoscopy shows:*
  - UC: Diffuse and continuous rectal involvement, friability, edema and pseudopolyps.
  - CD: Aphthoid, linear, or stellate ulcers, stricture, non-caseating granulomas, "Cobblestoning" and "skip lesion".

49. Which of the finding is not a usual feature of Crohn's disease? *(PGMEE 2014-15)*
a. Granulomas   b. Pseudopolyps
c. Skip lesion   d. Right colon predominance

[Ref: CMDT, ch. 15, pg. 641, Harrison's 19th/e pg 1954]

50. Which of the following is earliest manifestation of Crohn's disease? *(PGMEE 2018)*
a. Deep ulcers involving GI mucosa
b. Aphthous ulcers
c. Cobblestone appearance
d. Discontinuous involvement of ileum

Ref: Maingots abdominal operations 12th/e, pg. 667

Explanation

- The earliest gross manifestations of Crohn's disease are the development of small mucosal ulcerations call aphthous ulcers.

51. Skip lesions of colon with epithelioid granuloma are usually seen with- *(DNB June 07)*
a. Crohn's disease   b. Sarcoidosis
c. Ulcerative colitis   d. Intestinal TB

[Ref: Robbin's 9th/e pg. 799]

52. Anti-saccharomyces cerevisiae antibodies are seen in? *(DNB June 11)*
a. Crohn's disease   b. SLE
c. Scleroderma   d. Sjogren's syndrome

[Ref: Robbin's 9th/e pg. 799]

53. Inflammatory bowel disease with transmural involvement and skip lesions is? *(DNB June 11)*
a. Crohn's disease   b. Ulcerative colitis
c. Clostridium infection d. Shigella infection

[Ref: Robbin's 9th/e pg. 799]

54. Crohn's Disease most commonly affects the- *(PGMEE 2015)*
a. Stomach   b. Rectum
c. IIeum   d. Duodenum

[Ref: Bailey & Love 26th /e pg.1013]

55. True about ulcerative colitis, all except- *(PGMEE 2012-13)*
a. Pancolitis   b. Rectum involved

c. Psedopolyps   d. Noncaseating granuloma

[Ref: Robbin's 9th/e pg. 800]

56. What is true about ulcerative colitis- *(PGMEE 2012-13)*
a. Skip lesions seen
b. Involves only colon
c. Ileum not involved
d. Involves rectum and then whole colon backwards

[Ref: Robbin's 9th/e pg. 800]

57. All are true for ulcerative colitis except: (DNB Dec' 2011)
a. Usual age of presentation is > 60 years
b. Back wash ileitis
c. Pancolitis
d. Cobble stoning

[Ref: Robbin's 9th/e pg. 800]

58. Collar button ulcer is a feature of *(PGMEE 2015)*
a. Ulcerative colitis
b. Ischamic Colitis
c. Crohn's Disease
d. Sigmoid Volvulus

[Ref: Gastrointest Radiol. The collar button ulcer. A radiologic-pathologic correlation. 1979 Jan 30; 4 (1): 79-84]

59. Toxic megacolon is most commonly associated with- *(DNB June 07)*
a. Ulcerative colitis   b. Whipple's disease
c. Reiter's disease   d. Crohn's disease

[Ref: Robbin's 9th/e pg. 800]

60. Creeping fat is a feature of: *(PGMEE 2013-14)*
a. Crohn's disease   b. Celiac disease
c. Tropical sprue   d. Ulcerative colitis

[Ref: Robbin's 9th/e pg. 799]

61. Which extraintestinal symptom of IBD worsens with exacerbation of disease activity? *(PGMEE 2014-15)*
a. Ankylosing spondylitis b. Arthritis
c. PSC   d. Uveitis

[Ref: Harrison's 17th ed. ch. 289, Harrison's 17th ed. ch. 289]

62. DOC of acute exacerbation of ulcerative colitis? *(PGMEE 2015-16)*
a. Sulfasalazine   b. Steroids
c. Infliximab   d. Cyclosporine

[Ref: Chapter 295: Harrison's 18th edition, Harrison's 19th/e pg. 1952]

63. All are complications of ulcerative colitis, EXCEPT: *(PGMEE 2014-15)*
a. Haemorrhage   b. Stricture
c. Malignant change   d. Fistula

[Ref: CMDT, ch. 15, pg. 646, Harrison's 19th/e pg. 1953]

64. Best screening test for Crohn's disease is: *(PGMEE 2014-15)*
a. A.S.C.A
b. P-ANCA
c. Fecal alpha 1 anti-trypsin
d. Fecal calprotectin

[Ref: CMDT, ch. 15, pg. 642, Harrison's 19th/e pg. 1954]

48.	b
49.	b
50.	b
51.	a
52.	a
53.	a
54.	c
55.	d
56.	d
57.	d
58.	a
59.	a
60.	a
61.	b
62.	b
63.	d
64.	a

65. A 41-year-old male patient presented with recurrent episodes of bloody diarrhea for 5 years. Despite regular treatment with adequate doses of sulfasalazine, he has had several exacerbations of his disease and required several weeks of steroids for the control of flares. What should be the next line of treatment for him?

(PGMEE 2014-15)

a. Methotrexate
b. Azathioprine
c. Cyclosporine
d. Cyclophosphamide

[Ref: CMDT, ch. 15, pg. 641]

66. Invariably involved site in ulcerative colitis:

(PGMEE 2014-15)

a. Sigmoid colon
b. Transverse colon
c. Ileum
d. Rectum

[Ref: CMDT, ch. 15, pg. 646, Harrison's 19th/e pg. 1952]

67. Treatment of choice in intractable ulcerative colitis:

(PGMEE 2014-15)

a. Mucosal proctectomy + Ileoanal pouch anastomosis
b. Proctectomy
c. Colectomy with ileostomy
d. Ileorectal anastomosis

[Ref: CMDT, ch. 15, pg. 649, Harrison's 19th/e pg. 1962]

68. Treatment of choice in ulcerative colitis is:

(PGMEE 2014-15)

a. 5 aminosalicylic acid
b. Azathioprine
c. Metronidazole
d. Salicylates

[Ref: CMDT, ch. 15, pg. 647, Harrison's 19th/e pg. 1962]

69. Best treatment of refractory peri-anal fistula in crohn's disease:

(PGMEE 2014-15)

a. Fistulectomy
b. Infliximab
c. Olasalazine
d. Mesalamine

[Ref: CMDT, ch. 15, pg. 642, Harrison's 19th/e pg. 1963]

70. Which of the following is the established biological therapy for Crohn's disease?

(PGMEE 2014-15)

a. Anti TNF alpha-antibody
b. IL-1 antagonist
c. IL-6 antagonist
d. IL-8 antagonist

[Ref: Harrison's 19th/e pg. 1961]

71. All are true about ulcerative colitis EXCEPT:

(PGMEE 2014-15)

a. Smoking may prevent the disease
b. 1:1 male female ratio
c. Presents with bloody diarrhea
d. Highly associated with infertility

[Ref: CMDT, ch. 15, pg. 646, Harrison's 19th/e pg. 1951]

72. True about ulcerative colitis:- *(PGMEE 2018)*

a. Morbidity risk after surgery is 20%
b. Extraintestinal problems of ulcerative colitis are managed medically
c. Steroid dependent cases require surgery
d. Extensive colitis and young age at diagnosis are associated with high risk of colectomy.

Ref: Maingots abdominal operations 12th/e, pg. 718; Sabistons 20th/e, pg 1339; Bailey & Love 26th/e pg. 1145

Explanation

- Morbidity rates are high following both urgent and elective procedures. Morbidity rates of 33–66% have been reported for patients having subtotal colectomy for acute colitis with the main complications being wound infection, ileus, small bowel obstruction, and a blown rectal stump
- The severity of these extraintestinal manifestations of disease may coincide with the severity of the colitis. Some of these, including arthritis and skin manifestations, tend to respond to treatment or surgical extirpation of the colon. The symptoms and progression of PSC are not aff ected by the management of the colonic disease. So all extraintestinal problems are not managed medically.

Indications for surgery in UC are:

- Severe/fulminating disease which does not respond to medical treatment
- Chronic disease with anaemia, diarrhea, urgency and tenesmus;
- Steroid-dependent disease (here, though the disease is not severe, but substantial doses of steroids are required to maintain the remission)
- Poor compliance/tolerance/complications to medical therapy (steroid psychosis or other side effects, azathioprine-induced pancreatitis), such that remission cannot be maintained;
- Patients with severe dysplasia or carcinoma on review colonoscopy (neoplastic changes)
- Extraintestinal manifestations;
- Rarely, severe haemorrhage or stenosis causing obstruction.
- One of the most serious squeal of ulcerative colitis is the development of colorectal carcinoma. The most important risk factors include prolonged duration of the disease, pancolonic disease, continuously active disease, and severity of inflammation.
- Although extensive colitis and young age at diagnosis are associated with high risk of (option D) carcinoma, which ultimately will require colectomy, but if we have to choose only one answer, then its option C.

73. A highly sensitive and specific marker for detecting intestinal inflammation in ulcerative colitis is?

(PGMEE 2014)

a. CRP
b. Fecal lactoferrin
c. Fecal calprotectin
d. Leukocytosis

[Ref: CMDT, ch. 15, pg. 642, Harrison's 19th/e pg. 1954]

Explanation

- Fecal lactoferrin & calprotectin are noninvasive markers of intestinal inflammation in IBD
  - Fecal lectoferrin is highly sensitive and specific marker for detecting inflammation.
  - Calprotectin has high sensitivity but modest specificity as gastrointestinal infiltration & colorectal malignancy can also increase fecal calprotectin

65.	b
66.	d
67.	a
68.	a
69.	b
70.	a
71.	d
72.	c
73.	b

74. Ulcerative colitis associated features include all, EXCEPT: *(PGMEE 2014-15)*
   a. Iritis
   b Arthritis
   c. Urethritis
   d. Pyoderma

   [Ref: CMDT, ch. 15, pg. 646, Harrison's 19th/e pg. 1952]

75. Chronic inflammatory bowel disease is associated with:
   a. Chronic hepatitis *(PGMEE 2014-15)*
   b. Fibrosis
   c. Cholangiosarcoma
   d. Primary sclerosing cholangitis

   [Ref: CMDT, ch. 16, Page no. 709]

MISCELLANEOUS

76. A vasopressin analogue does not produce therapeutic effect through vasopressin V2 receptor in which of the following: *(PGMEE 2014-15)*
   a. Central diabetes insipidus
   b. Bleeding oesophageal varices
   c. Type I von Willebrand's disease
   d. Primary nocturnal enuresis.

   [Ref: Harrison's 19th/e pg. 276, 2063]

77. A 25-year-old woman presents with recurrent abdominal pain and anemia. Peripheral blood smear shows basophilic stippling of the red blood cells. What is the most likely diagnosis? *(PGMEE 2014-15)*
   a. Coeliac disease
   b. Hookworm infestation
   c. Sickle cell disease
   d. Lead poisoning

   [Ref: Harrison's 19th/e pg. 2607, 472e-2t]

78. A 25-year-old woman presents with recurrent abdominal pain and anemia. Peripheral blood smear shows basophilic stippling of the red blood cells. What is the most likely diagnosis? *(PGMEE 2014-15)*
   a. Coeliac disease
   b. Hookworm infestation
   c. Sickle cell disease
   d. Lead poisoning

   [Ref: Harrison's 19th/e pg. 2607, 472e-2t]

74.	c
75.	d
76.	b
77.	d
78.	d

GI BLEED

UPPER GI BLEED

1. Forrest classification is used for evaluating:
   a. Upper GI bleeding   **(PGMEE 2014-15)**
   b. Liver transplantation
   c. Lower GI bleeding
   d. Familial adenomatous polyposis
   [Ref: CMDT 2014 2014, ch. 15, pg. 580]

Explanation

- Forrest classification used for assessing re-bleed risk of upper GI bleeding.

2. Which indicates least chances of re-bleeding after hematemesis episode: **(PGMEE 2014-15)**
   a. Adherent clot on ulcer
   b. Clean based ulcer
   c. Gastric ulcer with AV malformation
   d. Visible bleeding vessel

[Ref: Harrison's Principles of Internal Medicine ch. 41, Harrison's 19th/e pg. 276]

3. Most common site of dieulafoys lesion is:
   a. Lesser curvature of stomach   **(PGMEE 2015-16)**
   b. Greater curvature of stomach
   c. Pylorus
   d. Antrum

[Ref: CMDT, ch. 15, pg. 581, Harrison's 19th/e pg. 277, 1891]

Explanation

- Dieulafoy's lesion is characterized by dialted (1-3 mm) submucosal artery (a branch from left gastric artery) most commonly in the lesser curvature about 6cm from cardia.

4. True about upper GI bleeding is: **(NEET 2018)**
   a. Most common management is endoscopic banding
   b. Rockall scoring is used for risk stratification
   c. Most common cause is variceal bleeding
   d. It is bleeding up to ampulla of Vater

Explanation

- *Risk stratification score:-*
  ○ Rockall score: With Endoscopy
  ○ Blatchford score: Without endoscopy

LOWER GI BLEED

5. Most common cause of hematochezia in children?
   a. Rectal polyp   **(PGMEE 2014-15)**
   b. Meckels diverticulum
   c. Necrotizing enterocolitis
   d. Acute gastritis

[Ref: Table 303.12 Nelson's 18th ed., Harrison's 19th/e pg. 276, 1899]

6. Which of the following excludes a diagnosis of irritable bowel syndrome: **(PGMEE 2014-15)**
   a. Relieved by defacation
   b. Straining during stool passage
   c. Passage of blood per rectum
   d. Change of stool form
   [Ref: CMDT, ch. 15, pg. 633, Harrison's 19th/e pg. 1965]

7. Most common cause of lower GI Bleed in India is   **(PGMEE 2012)**
   a. Amoebic dysentery   b. Typhoid enteritis
   c. Tubercular enteritis   d. Bacilliary Angiomatosis

[Ref: Indian Journal of Surgery, Vol. 65, No. 2, March-April, 2003, pp. 151-155]

8. A patient presents with lower gastrointestinal bleed. Sigmoidoscopy shows ulcers in the sigmoid. Biopsy from this area shows flask-shaped ulcers. Which of the following is the most appropriate treatment:
   a. Intravenous ceftriaxone   **(PGMEE 2014-15)**
   b. Intravenous metronidazole
   c. Intravenous steroids and sulphasalazine
   d. Hydrocortisone enemas

[Ref: Harrison's 19th/e pg. 1366]

9. Most common cause of lower GI Bleed is-   **(PGMEE 2015)**
   a. Diverticulosis   b. Angiodysplasia
   c. Anal Fissure   d. CA Colon

[Ref: Sabiston 20th /e pg.1151]

Explanation

- *Etiology of Lower GI Bleeding:*
  ○ Diverticulosis (60%), angiodysplasia, IBD, hemorrhoids, fissures, neoplasms, arteriovenous malformations.

10. What is the most characteristic of congenital hypertrophic pyloric stenosis: **(DNB 2007)**
   a. Affects the first born female child
   b. The pyloric tumor is best felt during feeding
   c. The patient is commonly marasmic
   d. Loss of appetite occurs early

[Ref. Bailey and Love's 26th/e pg. 79]

11. Vertical banding gastroplasty, also known as stomach stapling is done for?   **(PGMEE 2010)**
   a. Gastric carcinoma   b. Achalsia cardia
   c. Morbid obesity   d. Perforated gastric ulcer

[Ref: Sabiston Textbook of Surgery, 18th/e chapter 17]

INTESTINE

12. Which vitamin deficiency commonly occurs in short bowel syndrome?   **(PGMEE 2015)**
   a. Vitamin B1   b. Vitamin B12
   c. Vitamin B3   d. Vitamin B6

[Ref: Harrison 17th /e pg.1882, Bailey & Love 26th /e pg.265]

1.	a
2.	b
3.	a
4.	b
5.	a
6.	c
7.	b
8.	b
9.	a
10.	b
11.	c
12.	b

Explanation

- The diagnosis of Spontaneous Bacterial Peritonitis is made when the ascitic fluid sample has an absolute neutrophil count >250/μL. MCC is E.coli. Treatment is with third generation cephalosporins like cefotaxime.

31. Which of the following is true about Ménétrier disease :-
(PGMEE 2015)
a. Atrophied mucosal folds are seen
b. It is premalignant condition
c. There is increased gastric acid secretion
d. Affects the stomach and small intestines

[Ref: Bailey & Love 26th/e pg. 1054, 1032, 1046]

Explanation

- It is a premaligant condition characterized by massive gastric folds in the fundus and body of stomach giving the gastric mucosa a cobble stone and cerebriform appearance (Brain like mucosa).

32. Rigler's sign is suggestive of-
(PGMEE 2015)
a. Pneumothorax
b. Peritonitis
c. Hemothorax
d. Pneumoperitoneum

[Ref: internet]

33. All of the following are cause of Pneumoperitoneum expect-
(PGMEE 2015)
a. Hirschsprung's Disease
b. Perforated peptic ulcer
c. Perforated Appendix
d. Laproscopic Precedure

[Ref: Usually no pneumoperitoneum in Hirschprung]

34. Immediate treatment in perforation of intestine:
(PGMEE 2016-17)
a. Conservative management
b. Immediate surgery
c. Stabilize the patient and take him for surgery as soon as possible
d. Order CT scan

[Ref: Medscape]

35. Most common cause of air under diaphragm:-
(PGMEE 2016-17)
a. Intestinal perforation
b. Gynecological investigation
c. Cholecystitis
d. Acute pancreatitis

[Ref: Internet]

36. Fistula leading to the highest electrolyte imbalance is
(DNB June' 2009)
a. Duodenal
b. Gastric
c. Sigmoid
d. Rectal

[Ref: Sabiston 17th/e p. 324, CSDT 11th/e p. 696]

37. A Newborn male child is observed to have imperforate anus. On cross table lateral film rectal gas is above the coccys. The initial treatment at choice is:
(PGMEE 2015-16)
a. Colostomy
b. PSARP without colostomy
c. Anoplasty
d. PSARP with colostomy

[Ref: Pediatric Surgery (Elsevier Health Sciences] 7th/e pg. 1291]

31.	b
32.	d
33.	a
34.	c
35.	a
36.	b
37.	a
38.	c
39.	d
40.	a
41.	a
42.	d
43.	c

38. Burst abdomen is seen on which post operative day:-
(PGMEE 2016-17)
a. 3rd day
b. 5th day
c. 7th day
d. 10th day

[Ref: Sabiston's 20th/e pg. 283]

39. All of the following statements about 'Burst Abdomen' are true, except:
(PGMEE 2015-16)
a. Suture length should be 4 times of wound length
b. High incidence if Catgut is used for closure
c. Incidence is 1-3 percent
d. Typically presents between postoperative day 3 and 5

[Ref: Bailey and Love 26th/e pg. 34, 279; Sabiston's 20th/e pg. 450]

40. Procedure shown below is:
(PGMEE 2016-17)

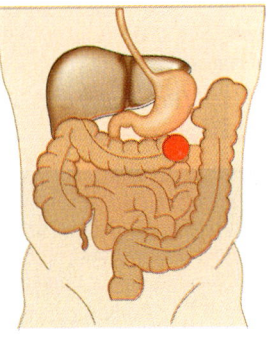

a. Transverse colostomy
b. Hartman procedure
c. Ilieostomy
d. Descending colostomy

41. 50 yr patient with Acute abdomen pain with history of not passing stool or gas since 2 days X-ray abdomen shows - dilated small bowels :-
(PGMEE 2016-17)
a. Small bowel obstruction
b. Large bowel obstruction
c. Chrons disease
d. Colon carcinoma

[Ref: Internet]

42. Paralytic ileus occurs in:
(PGMEE 2014-15)
a. Hypokalaemia
b. Hypomagnaesemia
c. Hypocalcaemia
d. All of the above

[Ref: CMDT, ch. 15, pg. 627, Harrison's 19th/e pg. 1982]

Explanation

- *Electrolyte abnormalities in paralytic ileus:-*
  - Uremia, hypokalemia, hyponatremia, hypomagnesemia and hypermagnesemia.

43. Disabling paraumbilical pain within 10 minutes of eating food with history of weight loss. Past history is positive for Myocardial infarction in last year. It is indicative of.
(New pattern 2015-16)
a. Gastric ulcer
b. Duodenal ulcer
c. Abdominal angina
d. Acute cholecytitis with stone impaction

[Ref: Harrison's, 18th ed., ch. 160, pg. 1019]

MECKEL'S DIVERTICULUM

44. Meckel's diverticulum follows 'the rule of 2s', the following are true except:- *(PGMEE 2015)*
a. Occur in approx 2% of population
b. Approx 2 inches long
c. Generally present 2 feet from ileoceacal valve
d. 2% are symptomatic

[Ref: Robbin's 9th/e pg. 751]

Explanation

- The length varies with age and not 2 inch always.
- Prevalance Rate: 2%.
- Present most commonly in <2 years age.

45. Meckels diverticulum is --- from ileocaecal junction:- *(PGMEE 2016-17)*
a. 15 cm
b. 30 cm
c. 45 cm
d. 60 cm

[Ref: Harrison's 19th/e pg. 277, 279]

46. Most common complication of Meckel's Diverticulum in children- *(PGMEE 2015)*
a. Abdominal pain
b. Peptic ulcers
c. Painless Rectal bleeding
d. Intestinal obstruction

[Ref: Nelson's 20th/e/p 1805]

47. Gastric mucosa in Meckel's diverticulum is diagnosed by: *(PGMEE 2014-15)*
a. Endoscopy
b. Occult blood in stool
c. Technetium isotope scan
d. Barium studies

[Ref: Harrison's 19th/e pg. 277, 279]

48. Meckel's diverticulum is remnant of: *(NEET June 2018)*
a. Allantois
b. Omphalomesenteric duct
c. Urachus
d. None of the above

[Ref:Sabiston's 20th/e pg. 1157]

Explanation

- Persistence of vitellointestinal (omphalomesenteric) duct can lead to Meckel's diverticulum:-
  - Proximal part → MD
  - Intermediate part → Enterocytoma.
  - Distal part → Raspberry tumour
  - Whole VID → Fecal fistula at umbilicus
- Persistent allantois/urachus leads to urinary fistula at umbilicus.

Meckel's diverticulum

- MD is a true diverticulum means it has all the 3 layers of the intestine.
- MD is situated at the anti-mesenteric border of small intestine.
- It's the MC congenital anomaly of the GIT.
- Male to female ratio is 3 : 2.
- Often,heterotopic mucosal tissue is present at the base of MD. > 60% consists of gastric mucosa followed by pancreatic tissue (acini).
- A useful but crude & traditional Mnemonic for describing MD is rule of two : i.e.
  - 2% prevalence
  - 2 inch in length
  - 2 feet proximal to ileocecal valve.
  - Half of these who are symptomatic are < 2 yrs of age

49. Acquired diverticulum most common site is:- *(PGMEE 2015)*
a. Sigmoid colon
b. Transverse colon
c. Ascending colon
d. Ileum

[Ref: Robbins 9th/e pg. 751]

50. Investigation of choice for diverticulitis:-
a. CT scan
b. USG *(PGMEE 2016-17)*
c. Barium studies
d. Angiography

[Ref: Sabiston's 20th/e pg. 1332]

VOLVULUS

51. Commonest site for volvulus is *(PGMEE 2012)*
a. Caecum
b. Proximal jejunum
c. Sigmold colon
d. Stomach

[Ref: Maingot's 10th/e p. 1404]

52. Most common site for volvulus is: *(PGMEE 2012)*
a. Centre
b. Verumontum
c. Peripheral
d. None

[Ref: Bailey & Love 24th/e p. 1380]

53. Sigmoid volvulus:- *(PGMEE 2016-17)*
a. It is almost always in clockwise direction
b. Present with constipation and fever
c. Treatment is air enema
d. The most serious complication is bowel ischemia

[Ref: Internet]Clinical feature – constipation +; but no fever

54. Most common type of intusususcption is *(DNB June' 2009)*
a. Ileo-ileal
b. Ileo colic
c. Colo-colic
d. Ileo-ileo-colic

[Ref: Bailey and love 25th/e e p. 1195]

55. Picture shown below is characteristic of what pathology:- *(PGMEE 2016-17)*

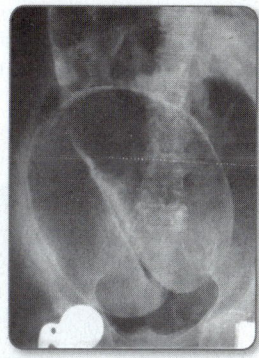

a. Sigmoid volvulus
b. Ceacal volvulus
c. Intusesseption
d. Illeal TB

[Ref: Sabiston's 20th/e pg. 1128]

56. What is the first line treatment of a 4 year old child presenting with intussusceptions? *(PGMEE 2015)*
a. Surgical correction
b. Exploratory laparotomy with resection of the affected segment
c. Conservative management with wait and watch policy
d. Immediate attempt to reduction using barium edema

[Ref: Nelson 20th/e/p 1763 table 306-9]

44.	d>b
45.	d
46.	c
47.	c
48.	b
49.	a
50.	a
51.	c
52.	c
53.	d
54.	b
55.	a
56.	d

57. Commonest cause of intestinal obstruction in children is- *(PGMEE 2012-13)*
   a. Adhesions
   b. Volvulus
   c. Hernia
   d. Intussusception

   [Ref: Nelson 20th/e/ pg. 1812]

APPENDIX

58. A 25 year old male is receiving conservative management for an appendicular mass since 3 days now presents with a rising pules rete, tachycardia and fever . The mode of management must be- *(PGMEE 2015)*
   a. Ochsner sherren regimen
   b. Continue conservative management
   c. Intravenous antibiotics
   d. Proceed to laparotomy and appendicectomy

   [Ref: Bailey & Love 26th /e pg.1211]

59. Obstruction Sign in Acute Appendicitis is most common associated with
   a. Pre-Ileal
   b. Post-Ileal
   c. Pelvic Appendix
   d. Retrocecal

   [Ref: The Washington Manual of Surgery 5th /e pg. 207]

60. In a case of retrocecal appendicitis which movement aggravates pain: *(NEET June 2018)*
   a. Flexion
   b. Extension
   c. Medial Rotation
   d. Lateral Rotation

Explanation

- In retrocecal appendicitis, inflammed appendix is in contact with psoas muscle causing flexion of the hip joint. Hyperextension of the hip joint may induce abdominal pain. This is known as `iliopsoas sign' and is typical of retrocecal appendicitis.
- Other signs seen in appendicitis:
- Obturator sign: pain on internal rotation of the hip (suggesting a pelvic appendix)
- Dunphy's sign: Any movement, including coughing (Dunphy's sign), may cause increased pain Rovsing's sign: pain in the right lower quadrant during palpation of the left lower quadrant

61. Which of the following score is used for the specimen shown below: *(NEET June 2018)*

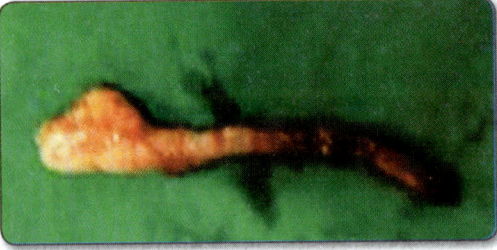

   a. Alvrado
   b. Marshal's
   c. Ranson's
   d. MPI

[Ref: Bailey & Love 26th /e pg.1211; Sabiston's 20th/e pg.1026]

Explanation

- The Alvarado scoring is used for - Appenidicitis
- Ranson's criteria are used for- Prognosis in acute pancreatitis
- Marshal's scoring is done for -Organ dysfunction

Alvarado Score:

Migratory right iliac fossa pain	1
Anorexia	1
Nausea/vomiting	1
RLQ tenderness	2
Rebound tenderness	1
Elevated temperature	1
Leukocytosis	2
Left shift	1
Total	10

62. Appendicular stump is obtained by: *(DNB 2007)*
   a. Crushing
   b. Ligation and inversion
   c. Inversion
   d. Ligation

   [Ref: Bailey & Love 26th /e pg. 1208]

63. Under what guidelines is treatment started for a patient presenting with appendicular mass on CT scan? *(PGMEE 2015)*
   a. Conservative management and discharge
   b. Immediate Laprotomy
   c. Kocher's Regimen
   d. Ochsner Sherren Regiman

   [Ref: Bailey & love 26th/e.pg. 1211]

64. Ochsner-Sherren regimen is used for *(PGMEE 2012)*
   a. Acute appendicitis
   b. Apendicular lump
   c. Apendicular perforation
   d. Apendicular abscess

   [Ref: Bailey & Love 25th/e page 1215]

65. Most common location of appendix is- *(PGMEE 2015)*
   a. Pelvic
   b. Pre IIeal
   c. Post ileal
   d. Retrocaecal

   [Ref: Bailey & Love 26th/e pg.1198]

MISCELLANEOUS

66. Which is the most frequently used gas for laproscopy? *(PGMEE 2016-17, 2015)*
   a. Oxygen
   b. Helium
   c. Carbon Dioxide
   d. Nitrogen

   [Ref: Sabiston's 20th/e pg.1498]

67. All of the following are used in cryosurgery except- *(PGMEE 2015)*
   a. Carcon dioxide
   b. Argon
   c. Helium
   d. A Liquid nitrogen

   [Ref: Internet]

57.	d
58.	d
59.	c
60.	b
61.	a
62.	d
63.	d
64.	b
65.	d
66.	c
67.	c

68. A patient undergone laproscopic surgery c/o pain in Left shoulder most common causes is *(PGMEE 2016-17)*

a. Irritation of phrenic nerve because of gas
b. Trauma from instuments
c. Injury of gall bladder
d. Because of reactionary hemorrhage

[Ref: Internet – many studies say pain is due to high pressure of CO_2 irritating diaphragm.]

69. A patient presents in coma for 20 days, what will be the best way to give him nutrition *(DNB Dec' 2009)*

a. Parenteral nutrition
b. Feeding via jejunostomy
c. Oral feeding
d. Ryle's tube feeding

[Ref: European Journal of Anaesthesiology: January 1998-Volume 15 – Isue – pp 94-96]

70. Mucoviscidosis of pancreas in newborn m/c causes:- *(PGMEE 2016-17)*

a. Meconium ileus
b. Rectal prolapse
c. Diverticulosis
d. Volvulus

[Ref: Internet]

71. Intestinal angiodyplasia involves- *(PGMEE 2013-14)*

a. AV malformation
b. Malignant tumor
c. Cavernous hemangioma
d. Capillary hemangioma

[Ref: Robbin's 9th/e pg. 780]

72. Most common site of mesenteric cyst:-

a. Mesentery of small intestine *(PGMEE 2016-17)*
b. Mesentery of large intestine
c. Mesorectum
d. Mesoappendix

[Ref: Sabiston's 1st SAE pg. 1082]

73. Commonest type of mesenteric cyst? *(PGMEE 2015)*

a. Enterogenous
b. Urogenital remnant
c. Chylolymphatic
d. Demoid

[Ref: Bailey & Love 26th /e pg.983]

74. Content of epiplocele is? *(DNB Dec' 2011)*

a. Urinary bladder
b. Intestine
c. Colon
d. Omentum

[Ref: Bailey & Love 25th/e p. 969]

75. Pain of external haemorrhoids is carried by *(DNB June' 2011)*

a. Pudendal nerve
b. Superior rectal nerve
c. Dorsal nerve of penis or clitoris
d. Perineal nerve

[Ref: Gray's anatomy 39th/e p. – 1371]

76. Most common site of internal hemorrhoids:- *(PGMEE 2016-17)*

a. 2,8,12 O'clock position
b. 3,7,11 O'clock position
c. 8,9,10 O'clock position
d. 1 and 4 O'clock position

[Ref: Bailey and Love 26th /e pg. 1250]

77. Image showsis of:- *(PGMEE 2016-17)*

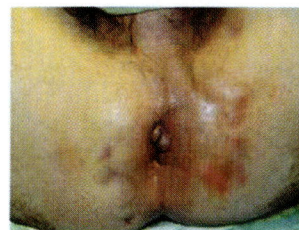
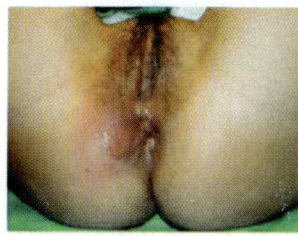

a. Peranal fistula
b. Perianal abscess
c. Hemorroids
d. Folliculitis

[Ref: Internet]

78. Image shown below is of: *(PGMEE 2016-17)*

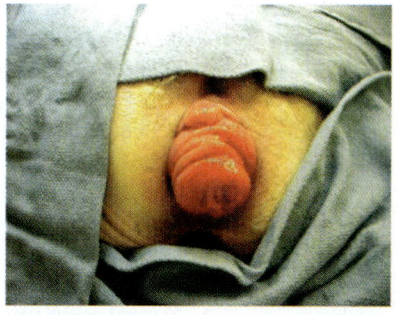

a. Rectocele
b. Rectal prolapse
c. Hemorrhoids
d. Intusussseption

[Ref: Sabiston's 20th/e pg. 1382]

79. A young male present with a midline painful fluctuant mass between the gluteal folds. On per-rectal examination there is no pain or tenderness. The most likely diagnosis is:- *(PGMEE 2015-16)*

a. Pilonidal abscess
b. Perianal abscess
c. Anal fissure
d. Perirectal abscess

[Ref: Sabiston's 20th/e pg.1408]

80. A vasopressin analogue does not produce therapeutic effect through vasopressin V2 receptor in which of the following: *(PGMEE 2014-15)*

a. Central diabetes insipidus
b. Bleeding oesophageal varices
c. Type I von Willebrand's disease
d. Primary nocturnal enuresis.

[Ref: CMDT, ch. 15, pg. 602, Harrison's 19th/e pg. 276, 2063]

81. A patient presents with lower gastrointestinal bleed. Sigmoidoscopy shows ulcers in the sigmoid. Biopsy from this area shows flask-shaped ulcers. Which of the following is the most appropriate treatment: *(PGMEE 2014-15)*

a. Intravenous ceftriaxone
b. Intravenous metronidazole
c. Intravenous steroids and sulphasalazine
d. Hydrocortisone enemas

[Ref: CMDT, ch. 35, pg. 1504, Harrison's 19th/e pg. 1366]

68.	a
69.	b
70.	a
71.	a
72.	a
73.	c
74.	d
75.	a
76.	b
77.	c
78.	b
79.	a
80.	b
81.	b

Hepatology

FACTS

- Liver contains stem cells/progenitor cells in the **canals of Hering** which give rise to precursor cells k/a **oval cells**.
- *Stellate cells or Ito cells:*
  - Located in the space of Disse
  - Required for Vitamin A metabolism
  - Inflammatory mediators stimulate these cells to produce type 1 collagen which leads to hepatic fibrosis
- Drug shown to reduce mortality from renal failure in alcoholic hepatitis: Pentoxifylline
- Normal portal vein pressure is 5–10 mm Hg/10 – 15 cm of water
- Councilman bodies are seen in acute viral hepatitis
- Councilman/apoptotic bodies represent acidophilic degeneration of hepatocytes
- Ballooning and spotty necrosis, Piecemeal necrosis of hepatocytes is seen in → Acute viral hepatitis
- Bridging necrosis/fibrosis and periportal fibrosis is seen in → Chronic hepatitis
- Ground glass hepatocytes are seen in → Chronic HBV hepatitis
- CAGE questionnaire is used in the clinical diagnosis of alcohol dependence and abuse.

- Zone of liver most sensitive to damage due to ischemia, hypoxia and drugs – Zone 3/Centrilobular
- Classification scheme used for the grading of hepatic encephalopathy – West Haven classification
- In Wilson disease, estimation of severity is done with – Nazer prognostic index
- *Conjugated hyperbilirubinemia* is seen in:
  - **D**ubin Johnson syndrome
  - **R**otor syndrome
- *Unconjugated hyperbilirubinemia* is seen in: (**Mn:** UGC)
  - **G**ilbert syndrome
  - **C**rigler-Najjar syndrome
- Alcoholic liver disease is pathologically characterized by:
  - Ballooning degeneration
  - Giant mitochondria
  - Macrovesicular steatosis
  - Mallory hyaline bodies
  - Perivenular and perisinusoidal fibrosis

Drugs	Necrosis Pattern
▪ Carbon tetrachloride	Centrilobular/Zone 3
▪ Yellow phosphorus	Periportal/Zone 1
▪ Acetaminophen	Centrilobular/Zone 3
▪ Statins	Centrilobular/Zone 3

REMEMBER

Mallory hyaline bodies are seen in:
- *Steatosis*
- *Alcoholic hepatitis – characteristic*
- *Wilson's disease*
- *Indian childhood cirrhosis*
- *NAFLD*
- *Primary Biliary cirrhosis*

Mn: Mallika Steals Alcohol to WIN Prince Bil

NAFLD/NASH is associated with:
- Obesity
- Dyslipidemia
- Hyperinsulinemia/Insulin resistance
- Diabetes

Recurrence of 1° diseases after liver transplantation occurs in:
- Autoimmune hepatitis
- Primary Biliary Cirrhosis
- Primary Sclerosing Cholangitis
- Budd Chiari syndrome
- Cholangiocarcinoma
- Hepatitis A, B and C

MOST COMMON

- MC autoimmune disease of liver: PBC
- MC cause of acute liver failure in India: Acute viral hepatitis
- MC cause of acute liver failure in west: Drug induced (Acetaminophen)
- MC cause of chronic liver disease: NAFLD
- MC cause of Cirrhosis: Alcoholic liver disease
- MC cause of Portal HTN in adults: Cirrhosis

- MC cause of congestive splenomegaly: Cirrhosis with portal hypertension
- MC cause of obstructive jaundice in children: Biliary atresia
- MC cause of Budd Chiari syndrome is Polycythemia Vera
- MC cause of acute and chronic pancreatitis: Alcohol

SYNDROMES

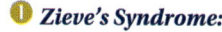

1 Zieve's Syndrome:
- Result from alcohol abuse/Alcoholic hepatitis
- Triad of:
  - Hemolytic anemia (spur cells and Acanthocytes)
  - Cholestatic jaundice
  - Hyperlipidemia

2 Mirizzi syndrome:
- Complication of gallstone.
- Due to common hepatic duct obstruction caused by an extrinsic compression from a stone impacted in cystic duct or Hartmann's pouch
- Patient presents with obstructive jaundice, fever and RUQ pain
- Diagnosis: USG, CT, MRCP, ERCP (IOC), HIDA scan.

3 Alagille syndrome:
- Inheritance: AD
- Mutation in JAG1/NOTCH 2 gene
- Features:
  - Pulmonary valvular stenosis, VSD, TOF
  - Narrow and malformed bile ducts which are either less in number or are completely absent
  - Neonatal jaundice
  - Posterior embryotoxon

4 Alpha 1- Antitrypsin Deficiency
- Inheritance: AR
- Function of α_1 AT: Inhibition of enzyme protease
- Locus of gene: chromosome 14
- Most common form of a_1 AT deficiency: PiZZ
- Clinical features:
  - Emphysema/COPD/Bronchiectasis
  - Chronic liver disease
  - Neonatal hepatitis with cholestasis
- Histology – Inclusion bodies in hepatocytes which are acidophilic PAS +ve and diastase resistant.
- Rx: Orthotropic liver transplantation.

5 Stauffer's syndrome:
- Intrahepatic Cholestasis associated with Renal cell carcinoma

SCORING

Child Pugh Scoring	Meld Scoring
▪ Useful in determining **P**rognosis of patients with chronic liver disease and **P**redict likelihood of major complications	▪ Stands for **M**odel for **E**nd stage **L**iver **D**isease ▪ To estimate prognosis in patients with liver failure and to prioritize candidates waiting for liver transplantation
Parameters	
▪ Serum bilirubin ▪ Serum albumin ▪ PT/INR ▪ Ascites ▪ Hepatic encephalopathy	▪ Serum **b**ilirubin ▪ Serum **c**reatinine ▪ **I**NR **Mn: CBI** ▪ Revised MELD also includes serum sodium ▪ PELD – **P**ediatric **E**ndstage **L**iver **D**isease Scoring

BILIRUBIN METABOLISM

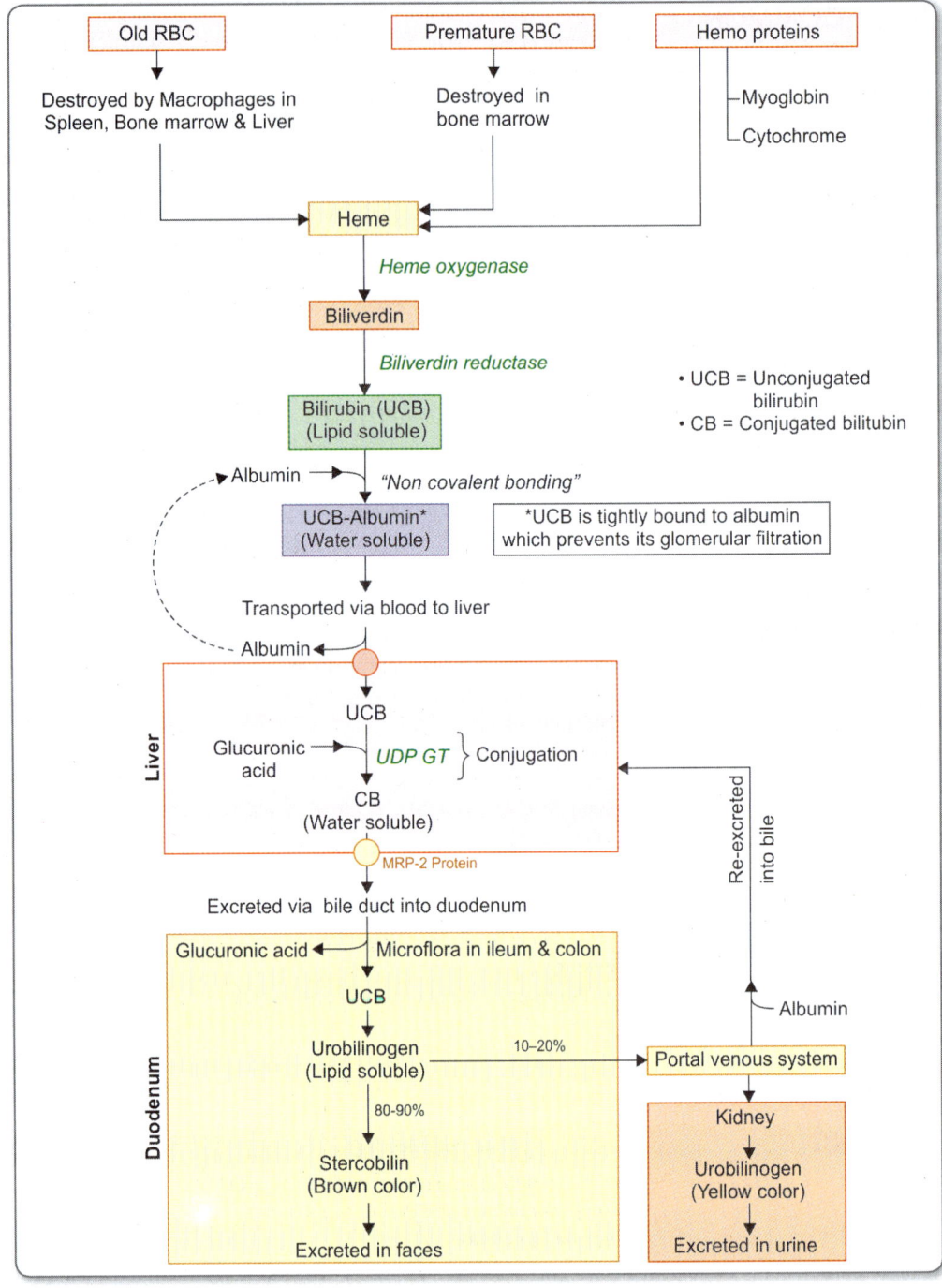

LIVER FUNCTION TESTS

- SGPT is a cytoplasmic enzyme while SGOT is found in both cytoplasm and mitochondria
- ALT is more specific indicator of liver cell injury
- In most acute liver diseases → ALT (SGPT) > AST (SGOT)
- ALT > AST is also seen in chronic viral hepatitis and NAFLD.

- AST > ALT also is seen in Cirrhosis and Alcoholic liver disease
- AST/ALT ratio > 3:1 is highly suggestive of alcoholic liver disease
- ALP, 5-nucleotidase and ϒ glutamyl transpeptidase are markers of Cholestasis.

Liver Function Test in Various Conditions

LFT	Hemolysis/Gilbert Syndrome	Acute Hepatocellular Necrosis (Viral hepatitis toxins, drug etc)	Chronic Hepatocellular disorder	Alcoholic Hepatitis / Cirrhosis	Cholestasis / Obstructive Jaundice
Bilirubinemia	↑ Indirect fraction	↑ in both fraction	↑ in both fraction	↑ in both fraction	↑ in both fraction
Bilirubinuria	No	Yes	Yes	Yes	Yes
Urobilinogen in urine	↑	↑	↑	↑	N/absent
Aminotransferases	N	↑↑(often > 500 IU)	↑↑(usually < 300)	AST: ALT > 2	N/↑
ALP	N	May be elevated (<3 times)	May be elevated (<3 times)	May be elevated (<3 times)	Elevated (>4 times)
Albumin	N	N	↓	↓	N/
PT/INR	N	N/↑	↑↑/N	↑↑/N	N/↑
Response to Vit K	No	Yes	No	No	Yes

*N = Normal

EVALUATION OF THE PATIENT WITH JAUNDICE

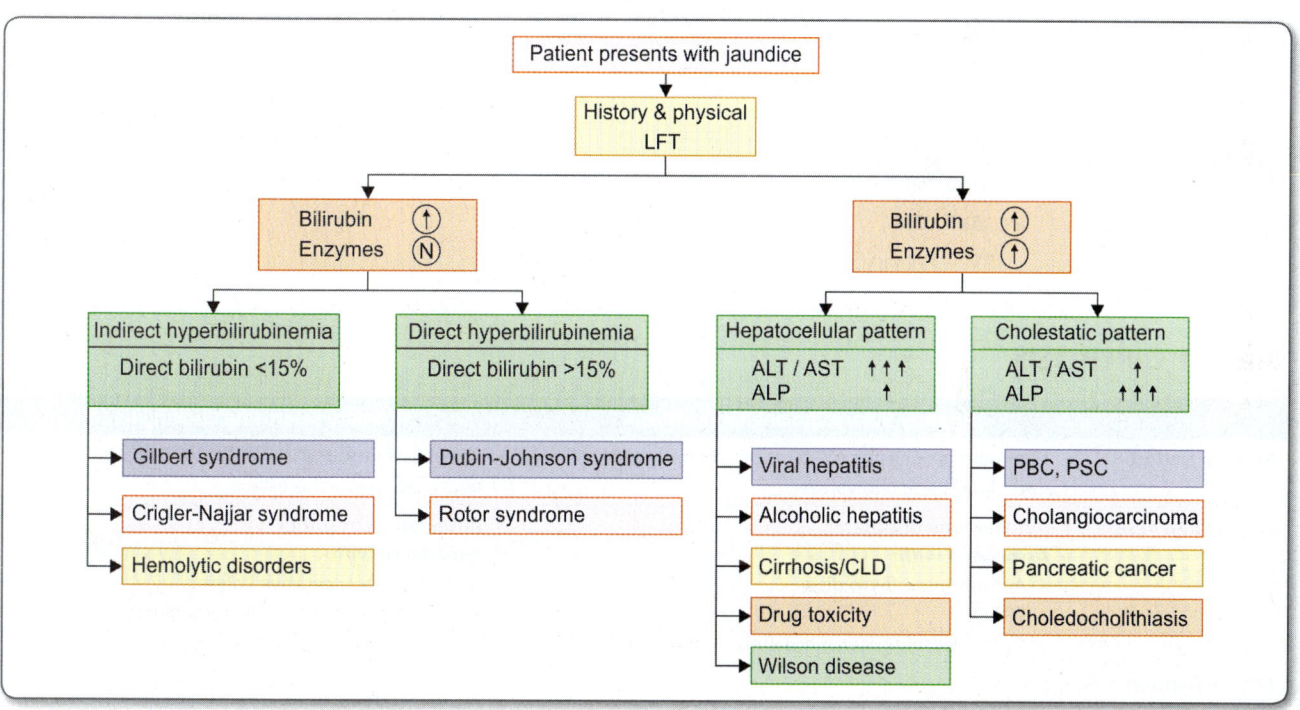

Crigler-Najjar Syndrome	Type-1	Type-2
Inheritance	▪ AR	▪ AD & AR
Hyperbilirubinemia	▪ Severe	▪ Mild – moderate
Jaundice	▪ Develops in the neonatal period	▪ Usually asymptomatic
Liver histology	▪ Normal	▪ Normal
Kernicterus	▪ Present	▪ Absent
UDP glucoronyl transferase activity	▪ Absent	▪ Depressed (<10%)
Response to Phenobarbital	▪ No	▪ Yes
Hemolysis	▪ Absent	▪ Absent
Survival	▪ Infancy/Childhood	▪ Adulthood

	Gilbert Syndrome	Dubin Johnson Syndrome	Rotor Syndrome
Inheritance	▪ AR	▪ AR	▪ AR
Hyperbilirubinemia	▪ Unconjugated (<6 mg/dL)	▪ Conjugated	▪ Conjugated
Jaundice	▪ Mild	▪ Usually symptomatic	▪ Usually asymptomatic
Pathology	▪ Reduced UDP glucoronyl transferase activity and decrease bilirubin uptake ▪ No kernicterus seen	▪ Defect in MRP-2 protein ▪ Defective bilirubin excretion into bile ▪ Reflux of BSP seen from liver to circulation	▪ Defect in drug reuptake transporter – OATP1B1 and OATP1B3 ▪ No reflux seen
Liver enzymes	▪ Normal	▪ Normal	▪ Normal
Liver histology	▪ N/increase lipofuscin	▪ Melanin deposits	▪ Normal

Mn: for **D**ubin **J**ohnson syndrome: **DJ** ya**AR** hai **ME**ra so don't ask **MRP 2** him |

AUTOIMMUNE LIVER DISEASES

Auto-antibodies	Autoimmune Hepatitis	Other Associated Conditions
Atypical pANCA	AIH Type I	Primary Sclerosing Cholangitis
Anti – Smooth muscle antibody (ASMA)	AIH Type I	Primary Biliary Cirrhosis (PBC)
Anti Mitochondrial Antibodies		Primary Biliary Cirrhosis
ANA	AIH Type I	PBC, PSC, HBV, HCV
Anti – LC1 (ALC-1)	AIH Type II	HCV
Anti - LKM 1	AIH Type II	Chronic Hepatitis C
Anti - LKM -2		Drug induced Hepatitis
Anti - LKM - 3	AIH Type II	Chronic Hepatitis D
Anti - SLA	AIH Type III	

PSC – Primary Sclerosing Cholangitis |

BILIARY CIRRHOSIS

	Primary Biliary Cholangitis /Cirrhosis	Primary Sclerosing Cholangitis
General feature	▪ Liver damage causing obliteration of intrahepatic biliary ducts leading to cholestasis	▪ Fibrosis of intrahepatic and extra hepatic bile ducts leading to cholestasis

Etiopathogenesis	▪ Autoimmune disorder
	▪ **Associated with:**
	  ○ Autoimmune thyroiditis
	  ○ CREST
	  ○ Sicca syndrome: Xerophthalmia, Xerostomia
		▪ Autoimmune disorder
		▪ **Associated with:**
		  ○ IBD mainly Ulcerative colitis
		▪ Smoking appears to have protective role

Clinical features	▪ F >> M ▪ Median age of presentation – 50 years ▪ Fatigue: MC symptom; Pruritus: 2nd MC symptom ▪ Hyperpigmentation of skin due to melanin deposition ▪ Jaundice ▪ Xanthomas and Xanthelasmas ▪ Malabsorption and deficiency of fat soluble vitamin	▪ M >> F ▪ Fatigue, Pruritus ▪ Jaundice ▪ Significant risk of development of cholangiocarcinoma
Lab features	▪ Antimitochondrial antibody (AMA) is positive in 90% ▪ Significant elevations of the ALP, GGTP, ALT, AST, 5' nucleotidase levels ▪ Lipid levels and cholesterol levels may be increased	▪ pANCA, ANA andanticardiolipin autoantibodies ▪ Serum ALP levels are usually 3-5 times of range ▪ MRCP - Imaging modality of choice
Histology	▪ Florid duct lesions	▪ Onion skin fibrosis
Treatments	▪ Ursodeoxycholic acid ▪ TOC: Liver transplantation – only lifesaving option	▪ Liver transplantation is only lifesaving option

Hepatic Failure | **Acute Liver Failure** | **Chronic Liver Disease** | **Hepatic Dysfunction without Overt Necrosis**

Chronic Liver Disease/Cirrhosis

	Chronic Liver Disease/Cirrhosis	Complications		
		Portal Hypertension	**Hepatic Encephalopathy**	**Hepatopulmonary Syndrome (HPS)**
General	▪ Fibrogenesis is stimulated by proliferation of Stellate cells and its modulation by TGF – β. ▪ Can be reversed if the underlying insult leading to fibrosis has been removed.	▪ Defined as elevation of hepatic venous pressure gradient to > 5 mm Hg	▪ Aka Portosystemic encephalopathy	▪ Characterized by shortness of breath and hypoxemia in a patient with liver disease.

Cause	▪ Alcoholism [MC Cause]
	▪ Chronic viral hepatitis
	  ○ HBV
	  ○ HCV [MCC in west]
	▪ Non Alcoholic Steatohepatitis
	▪ Autoimmune hepatitis
	▪ Primary Biliary cirrhosis
	▪ Primary Sclerosing Cholangitis
	▪ Cardiac cirrhosis
	▪ Metabolic liver disease
	  ○ Hemochromatosis
	  ○ Wilson's disease
	  ○ Cystic fibrosis
	  ○ α1 Antitrypsin deficiency
		Prehepatic:
		  ○ Portal vein thrombosis
		Hepatic:
		  ○ Presinusoidal – Schistosomiasis
		  ○ Sinusoidal – Cirrhosis (MC Cause)
		Posthepatic:
		  ○ Budd – Chiari syndrome
		  ○ CHF, Constrictive Pericarditis
			Precipitating factors:
			▪ Upper GI bleed
			▪ Increased dietary protein load
			▪ Infection
			▪ Hyponatremia/ Hypokalemia
			▪ Benzodiazepines, Anti psychotics, Diuretics
			▪ Peritoneal tap
				▪ Enhanced production of nitric oxide by the lung → Intra-pulmonary vasodilation → ventilation-perfusion mismatch.

Clinical Feature	▪ Jaundice
	▪ Parotid gland enlargement
	▪ Fetor hepaticus
	▪ Gynecomastia
	▪ Decreased body hairs
	▪ Palmer erythema, Clubbing
	▪ Duputyren contracture
	▪ Spider angiomas
	▪ Testicular atrophy
	▪ Hepatosplenomegaly
	▪ Anaemia/Leukopenia/ Thrombocytopenia
	▪ Decreased S. albumin
	▪ Hyperammonemia
	▪ Increase S. Bilirubin
	▪ Prolonged PT/INR
	▪ Elevated AST and ALT
	  ○ AST:ALT >2:1 is seen in Alcoholic Liver Disease
		▪ Hepatic encephalopathy
		▪ Gastroesophageal varices leading to UGI bleed
		▪ Hemorrhoids
		▪ Periumbilical Caput medusa
		▪ Ascites and Peripheral edema
		▪ Splenomegaly and Hypersplenism
		▪ Testicular atrophy
			▪ Asterixis/Flapping tremor/Liver Flap
			▪ Grading of symptoms is done according to the West Haven classification:
			  ○ Grade – 0 → minimal changes in memory and attention. Normal mental status but abnormal psychometric testing
				▪ **Triad of:**
				  ○ Chronic liver disease
				  ○ Oxygenation defect l/t Hypoxemia
				  ○ Intrapulmonary vasodilation
				▪ Hypoxemia and dyspnea worsen on moving from supine to upright position (k/as orthodeoxia and platypnea, respectively).

Management	▪ Treat the cause
	▪ Prolonged PT/INR do not respond to Vit K
	
	▪ **Prognostic tool and assessment of severity:**
	▪ Child-Turcotte-Pugh scoring system
	▪ MELD scoring system
		▪ **Acute Variceal hemorrhage:**
		  ○ Endoscopic Variceal band ligation
		  ○ Somatostatin or Octreotide
		▪ **Primary prophylaxis** – β-blockers or endoscopic Variceal ligation
		▪ **Refractory Ascites:**
		  ○ Repeated large volume paracentesis or TIPS
			▪ Hydration and Correction of electrolyte imbalance
			▪ Lactulose
			▪ Rifaximin > Metronidazole > Neomycin
			▪ Zinc supplementation
			▪ L- ornithine & L – aspartate (LOLA)
				▪ Liver transplantation

HEPATOLOGY ⟳ (HIGH-YIELD POINTS)

ASCITES

- Cirrhosis accounts for 84% of cases of ascites.
- The lower left quadrants are the most frequent sites for paracentesis.
- White, milky fluid indicates a triglyceride level >200 mg/dL (and often >1000 mg/dL), which is the hallmark of *chylous ascites*. Chylous ascites results from lymphatic disruption that may occur with trauma, cirrhosis, tumor, tuberculosis, or certain congenital abnormalities.
- Dark brown fluid can reflect a high bilirubin concentration and indicates biliary tract perforation.
- Black fluid may indicate the presence of pancreatic necrosis or metastatic melanoma.
- The ascitic fluid should be sent for measurement of albumin and total protein levels, cell and differential counts, and, Gram's stain and culture. A serum albumin level should be measured simultaneously to permit calculation of the *serum-ascites albumin gradient* (SAAG).
- The SAAG is calculated by subtracting the ascitic albumin concentration from the serum albumin level. It reflects the pressure within the hepatic sinusoids and correlates with the hepatic venous pressure gradient.
- The SAAG is useful for distinguishing ascites caused by portal hypertension from nonportal hypertensive ascites. A SAAG ≥1.1 g/dL reflects the presence of portal hypertension and indicates that the ascites is due to increased pressure in the hepatic sinusoids.
- A SAAG <1.1 g/dL indicates that the ascites is not related to portal hypertension.
- For high-SAAG (≥1.1) ascites, the ascitic protein level can provide further clues to the etiology. An ascitic protein level of ≥2.5 g/dL indicates that the hepatic sinusoids are normal and are allowing passage of protein into the ascites, as occurs in cardiac ascites, early Budd-Chiari syndrome, or sinusoidal obstruction syndrome.
- An ascitic protein level <2.5 g/dL indicates that the hepatic sinusoids have been damaged and scarred and no longer allow passage of protein, as occurs with cirrhosis, late Budd-Chiari syndrome, or massive liver metastases.
- Rx of refractory ascites – repeated Large Volume Paracentesis Or TIPS (Transjugular Intrahepatic Portosystemic Shunt)

Approach

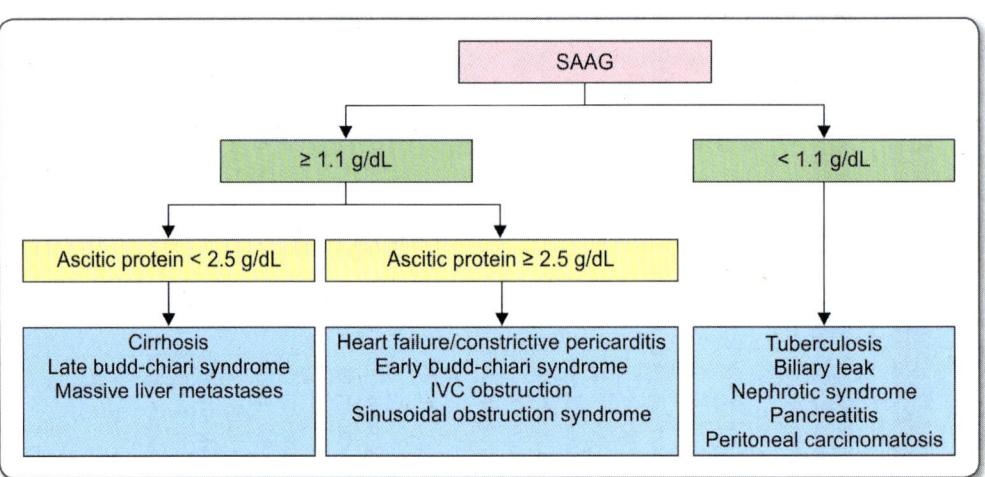

HEPATORENAL SYNDROME

- HRS is the development of renal failure in patients with advanced chronic liver disease.
- Pathophysiological hallmark → Renal vasoconstriction
- Histologically, Kidneys are normal and resume normal functioning after liver transplantation.

Diagnostic Criteria

Major Criteria (All Required)	Additional Criteria
▪ S.Cr > 1.5 mg/dL or 24 hr Cr_{CL} < 40 mL/min ▪ Absence of shock, infection of fluid loss ▪ No sustained improvement in renal function after diuretic withdrawal and expansion of plasma volume with 1.5 L of plasma expander ▪ Proteinuria < 500 mg/day ▪ No evidence of obstructive uropathy or parenchymal disease on USG	▪ Urine volume < 500 mL/d ▪ Urine sodium < 10 mEq/L ▪ Urine osmolality > Plasma osmolality ▪ Urine RBC < 50/hpf ▪ Sexrum sodium < 130 mEq/L

Types

	Type-I HRS	Type II HRS
Course	▪ Rapid deterioration of renal function and development of AKI	▪ Moderate and progressive reduction in GFR
Precipitant	▪ Volume depletion, Infection (SBP) etc	▪ Refractory, diuretic resistant ascites
Prognosis	▪ Median survival <2 weeks	▪ Median survival of 3-6 months
Treatment	▪ Liver Transplantation	▪ Liver transplantation

- Type 3 HRS: Acute renal failure occurring in cirrhotic patients with CKD
- Type 4 HRS: Acute renal failure occurring in patients with acute liver failure

CIRRHOSIS

Micronodular (<3 mm)	Macronodular	Mixed
▪ Alcoholic Liver disease ▪ Wilson's disease ▪ Primary Biliary Cirrhosis ▪ Hemochromatosis ▪ Reye's syndrome	▪ Viral hepatitis ▪ α_1 AT deficiency	▪ Alcoholic Liver disease ▪ Hepatitis C

PORPHYRIA

Porphyria	Inheritance	Deficient Enzyme	Principal Symptoms
Hepatic			
5 ALA dehydratase deficient porphyria (ADP)	AR	ALA dehydratase	Neurovisceral
Acute intermittent porphyria	AD	HMB synthase	Neurovisceral
Porphyria cutanea tarda (PCT)	AD	URO decarboxylase	Cutaneous photosensitivity
Hereditary coproporphyria	AD	COPRO oxidase	Neurovisceral + Cutaneous photosensitivity
Variegate porphyria (VP)	AD	PROTO oxidase	Neurovisceral + Cutaneous photosensitivity
Erythropoietic			
Congenital erythropoietic porphyria (CEP)	AR	URO synthase	Cutaneous photosensitivity
Erythropoietic protoporphyria	AR	Ferrochelatase	Cutaneous photosensitivity
X-linked protoporphyria	XL	ALA synthase 2	Cutaneous photosensitivity

WILSON'S DISEASE AND HEMOCHROMATOSIS

	Wilson's Disease	Hemochromatosis
General Features	- AR disorder of copper metabolism - Characterized by deposition of Copper in liver, brain and other tissues ∴ aka Hepatolenticular degeneration	- AR disorder of iron metabolism - Characterized by abnormal accumulation of iron in various organs
Genetic defect	- Mutation of a gene *ATP 7B* located on Chromosome 13q results in reduced biliary excretion of Copper	- Mutation of *HFE* gene present on chromosome 6 increase intestinal absorption of iron

Clinical Features	- ***All forms of hepatitis can occur:***
	  ○ Acute hepatitis
	  ○ Fulminant hepatic failure
	  ○ Chronic active hepatitis
	  ○ Cirrhosis – MC initial presentation
	- ***Neurological manifestations*** – Copper gets deposited in Basal ganglia leading to:
	  ○ Tremors → both resting and kinetic
	  ○ Wing beating tremor, Chorea
	  ○ Dystonia, spasticity and rigidity
	- ***Psychiatric manifestations include:***
	  ○ Emotional lability
	  ○ Impulsiveness
	- ***Musculoskeletal manifestations:***
	  ○ Degenerative arthropathy
	- ***Hematological manifestations:***
	  ○ Coombs negative intravascular hemolytic anemia
	- ***Kayser – Fleischer ring:***
	  ○ Greenish gold to brown in colour
	  ○ Formed by deposition of copper in descemet membrane
	  ○ Not a Pathognomonic features
	  ○ Almost always associated with neurological features
	- **Sunflower cataract**
	- Skin pigmentation
		- Fatigue and arthralgia are the most common symptoms
		- ***Liver***: 1st organ to be affected
		  ○ Hepatomegaly
		  ○ Splenomegaly
		  ○ Micronodular cirrhosis
		  ○ Hepatocellular carcinoma
		- ***Skin***:
		  ○ Bronze discoloration/Generalized hyperpigmentation
		- ***Diabetes mellitus – aka*** bronze diabetes
		- ***Heart:***
		  ○ Congestive heart failure
		  ○ Dilated Cardiomyopathy
		  ○ Restrictive cardiomyopathy
		- ***Musculoskeletal manifestations:***
		  ○ Arthropathy
		- Hypogonadism, Impotence and Amenorrhea:
		  ○ Due to iron deposits in pituitary

Investigations	- Serum ceruloplasmin levels < 20 mg/dl in 90% patients - Urinary copper excretion > 100 mcg/day - Hepatic copper concentration on liver biopsy > 200 mcg/g of dry weight – Gold standard test - Slit lamp to see Kayser-Fleischer ring - Brain MRI – Panda's sign - Presence of KF rings and ceruloplasmin levels <20 mg/dL in a patient with neurologic signs or symptoms suggest a diagnosis of Wilson disease.	- Serum iron increase - % Transferrin saturation is increased - Serum ferritin Increased - High Transferrin saturation is the earliest evidence of hereditary hemochromatosis - Transferrin saturation is considered best initial test for screening
Management	- Lifelong Zinc andpenicillamine/trientine - Tetrathiomolybdate Zn is a chelating drug used as an initial treatment for patients who present with neurologic or psychiatric manifestations - Trientine and Zinc is indicated in Wilson disease if the initial presentation is hepatic	- TOC → Phlebotomy (500 mL) - Chelating agents such as desferrioxamine in patients with heart disease, anemia or poor venous access - Concomitant alcohol intake increases the risk of cirrhosis

ACUTE PANCREATITS

Definitions	• **Acute pancreatitis**: inflammatory process settles down without causing any functional or morphological impairment i.e. it is a reversible process.
	• **Chronic pancreatitis**: recurrent attack occur leading to irreversible functional and morphological loss.
	• **Severe acute pancreatitis:**
	  ○ Evidence of organ failure (SBP < 90 mm Hg, $P_aO_2 \leq 60$ mm Hg, S. Creatinine ≥ 2 mg/dL, GI bleeding ≥ 500 mL in 24 hours)
	  ○ Local complications (eg, necrosis, abscess, pseudocyst)
	  ○ Ranson score ≥ 3 or APACHE score ≥ 8.

Etiology	• **Alcohol – MC Cause** • Trauma • Drugs: • Infection • **Gallstone – 2ⁿᵈ MC Cause** • CA pancreas ○ Azathioprine ○ **Mumps** (MC viral agent) • Hypertriglyceridemia • Hypercalcemia ○ 5 – amino salicylic acid ○ Coxsackie virus • ERCP • Cystic fibrosis ○ CMV, HBV • Recurrent pancreatitis is caused by Alcohol, Cholelithiasis, Hypertriglyceridemia, CA pancreas, Cystic fibrosis etc.
Clinical feature	• Pain abdomen → located in the epigastrium and radiates to back, relieves on sitting and bending forward. • **Cullen sign** → bluish discoloration around the **u**mbilicus → reflection of hemoperitoneum. • **Grey Turner sign** → reddish brown discoloration of the **F**lank [**Mn:** Girl Friend] • **Purtscher retinopathy** → due to ischemic injury of the retina.
Complications	• ARDS – leading to hypoxia and bilateral infiltrates on CXR • Pancreatic pseudocyst: If symptomatic → endoscopic or percutaneous drainage
Lab	• Serum amylase and lipase ≥ 3 times. **Lipase** is more specific and best to diagnose. • Serum amylase normalise after 3–7 days while serum lipase may remain elevated for 7–14 days (Lipase = **L**ong half life). • Degree of elevation of amylase and lipase do not correlate with severity of pancreatitis. • Leukocytosis, **Hypocalcemia**, **Hyperglycemia**.
Prognosis	• Ranson criteria, APACHE II scoring, BISAP score, Modified Marshall score • Balthazar grading system → based on CT grading • Modified Atlanta classification is currently used to define grade and severity of acute pancreatitis
Treatment	• Nil per mouth, IV fluids (Ringer lactate or Normal saline), analgesics • Prophylactic antibiotics are usually not indicated. • Targeted antibiotic therapy is indicated in infected necrotic pancreatitis.

BISAP Score	Ranson's Criteria (Obsolete now)	
Within 24 hours of hospitalization	**At admission**	**Within 48 hours**
• **B**UN > 25 mg/dL • **I**mpaired mental status (GCS < 15) • **S**IRS: ≥ 2 out of 4 criteria • **A**ge > 60 years • **P**leural effusion on CXR	• **A**ge > 55 years • **B**lood glucose ≥ 200 mg/dL • **S**GOT/AST > 250 U/L • Serum **L**DH > 350 IU/L • WBC **C**ount > 16,000 **Mn:** Admission **A**ge of **B**abies in **S**chool **L**ost its **C**ount	• Base deficit > 4 mEq/L • BUN increase > 5 mg/dL • Fluid sequestration > 6 L • Serum calcium < 8 mg/dL • Decrease in Hematocrit > 10% • Arterial pO_2 < 60 mmHg

MULTIPLE CHOICE QUESTIONS

CHAPTER 1: LIVER

PATHOPHYSIOLOGY OF LIVER INJURY

1. Liver stem cells are present in:- *(PGMEE 2016-17)*
- a. Canal of Herings
- b. Beneath liver capsule
- c. Portal triad
- d. Cords of Billroths

[Ref: Robbins 9th/e pg. 28, 102]

2. Liver damage in shock:- *(PGMEE 2015)*
- a. Centrilobular necrosis
- b. Spotty necrosis
- c. Diffuse necrosis
- d. Periportal necrosis

[Ref: Robbins 9th/e pg. 864]

3. Which of the following regions of the liver is most sensitive to ischemic injury:- *(PGMEE 2015)*
- a. Perihepatic
- b. Periportal
- c. Centrilobular
- d. Midzonal

[Ref: Robbins 9th/e pg. 863]

4. Centrilobular necrosis of liver may be seen with- *(PGMEE 2012-13)*
- a. Ethanol
- b. Phosphorus
- c. CCl_4
- d. Arsenic

[Ref: Harrison's 20th/e pg. 2367]

Explanation
- Centrilobular portion of liver is most sensitive to metabolic toxins (Ethanol, CCL_4, halothane, rifampin, acetaminophen).
  - CCL_4 (converted by cytochrome P-45 into → CCl_3 free radical) → Fatty liver → ↓ apolipoprotein synthesis → Fatty changes (centrilobular necrosis).

5. Massive hepatocellular necrosis is seen with:- *(PGMEE 2015)*
- a. Methyldopa
- b. Tetracycline
- c. Macrolides
- d. Acetaminophen

[Ref: Harrison's 20th/e pg. 2369]

6. The following is not a feature of non-cirrhotic portal Fibrosis:- *(PGMEE 2015)*
- a. Intimal fibroelastosis
- b. Portal fibrosis
- c. Lymphocytic infiltration
- d. Bridging fibrosis

[Ref: Robbins 9th/e pg. 863]

7. In cirrhosis, the proliferation and activation of the following cell results in fibrosis:- *(PGMEE 2015; 2016)*
- a. Bile duct epithelium
- b. Stellate cells
- c. Kuptter cells
- d. Hepatocytes

[Ref: Harrison's 20th/e pg. 2399]

Explanation
- Cirrhosis - Diffuse bridging fibrosis (via stellate cells) and regenerative nodules; disrupt normal architecture of liver; ↑ risk for hepatocellular carcinoma.

8. Nutmeg liver is seen in ? *(PGMEE 2016-17, 2015; 2010)*
- a. Chronic venous congestion liver
- b. Infarction of liver
- c. Amyloidosis
- d. Budd Chiari syndrome

[Ref: Robbin's 9th/e pg. 864]

Explanation
- *Nutmeg appearance of liver:-* Chronic passive congestion of liver due to:-
  - Right heart failure → ↑ central venous pressure → ↑ Resistance to portal flow → Hepatomegaly
  - Budd chiari syndrome - Mottled appearance

9. Nutmeg liver is seen in- *(PGMEE 2012-13)*
- a. Right sided heart failure
- b. Increased pulmonary resistance
- c. Decreased pulmonary resistance
- d. Left sided heart failure

[Ref: Robbin's 9th/e pg. 864]

10. Lysosome remnants after degradation of hepatocytes represent:- *(PGMEE 2016-17)*
- a. Councilman bodies
- b. Mallory bodies
- c. Cholangiocytes
- d. Kupffer cells

[Ref: Harrison's 20th/e pg. 2355]

11. Acidophil/Councilman bodies are seen in:- *(PGMEE 2016-17)*
- a. Pancreatitis
- b. Splenic necrosis
- c. Viral hepatitis
- d. Alcoholic hepatitis

[Ref: Harrison's 20th/e pg. 2355]

12. Mallory- Denk bodies are seen in all EXCEPT:-
- a. Indian childhood cirrhosis *(PGMEE 2016-17)*
- b. Wilson's disease
- c. Congenital hepatic fibrosis
- d. Alcoholic hepatitis

[Ref: Robbins 9th/e pg. 823,843, 850]

13. Mallory hyaline bodies are seen in? *(PGMEE 2012)*
- a. Hepatitis C
- b. Billiary cirrhosis
- c. Amyloidosis
- d. Hemochromatosis

[Ref: Robbin's 9th/e pg. 843]

14. Mallory hyaline changes are seen in A/E:
- a. Wilson's disease *(PGMEE 2014-15)*
- b. Indian childhood cirrhosis
- c. Primary biliary cirrhosis
- d. Hepatitis E

[Ref: CMDT 2014, 2014, ch. 16, pg. 681]

15. Histopathology of chronic hepatitis- *(PGMEE 2012-13)*
- a. Councilman bodies
- b. Balloning
- c. Bridging necrosis
- d. All

[Ref: Harrison's 20th/e pg. 2376]

1.	a
2.	a
3.	c
4.	c>a
5.	d
6.	d
7.	b
8.	a, d
9.	a
10.	a
11.	c
12.	c
13.	b
14.	d
15.	c

16. **Pathological manifestation of chronic alcoholism include all of the following except-** *(PGMEE 2012-13)*
    a. Piecemeal necrosis
    b. Central hyaline sclerosis
    c. Balloning degeneration
    d. Microvesicular fatty changes

    [Ref: Harrison's 20th/e pg. 2400]

17. **Mallory bodies contain-** *(PGMEE 2012-13)*
    a. Keratin
    b. Cytokeratins
    c. Collagen
    d. Vimentin

    [Ref: Robbin's 9th/e pg. 843]

18. **Mallory hyaline bodies are present in all of the following, except-** *(DNB Dec 09)*
    a. Alcoholic cirrhosis
    b. Primary biliary cirrhosis
    c. Indian childhood cirrhosis
    d. Secondary biliary cirrhosis

    [Ref: Robbin's 9th/e pg. 843]

19. **Mallory hyaline is characteristic features of?**
    a. Hepatocellular carcinoma *(DNB June 11)*
    b. Primary biliary cirrhosis
    c. Wilson's disease
    d. Alcoholic liver disease

    [Ref: Harrison's 20th/e pg. 2400]

20. **Which does not cause microvesicular steatosis-**
    a. Alcoholic liver disease *(PGMEE 2012-13)*
    b. Reye's syndrome
    c. Tetracycline toxicity
    d. Acute fatty liver of Pregnancy

    [Ref: Schiff's disease of liver 11th/e pg. 62, 426]

21. **Chicken wire fence pattern hepatocytes are seen in:-**
    a. Indian childhood cirrhosis *(PGMEE 2016-17)*
    b. Wilson's disease
    c. Alcoholic steatofibrosis
    d. Alcoholic hepatitis

    [Ref: Robbins 9th/e pg. 823, 843, 850]

22. **"Ground glass hepatocytes" with eosinophilic granular, glassy cytoplasm on light microscopy are seen in:-** *(PGMEE 2016-17)*
    a. Hepatitis A
    b. Chronic Hepatitis B
    c. Hepatitis C
    d. Steahepatosis

    [Ref: Harrison's 20th/e pg. 2355]

LIVER FUNCTION TESTS

23. **Bilirubin conjugation occurs in:-** *(PGMEE 2015)*
    a. Liver
    b. Duodenum
    c. Spleen
    d. Pancreas

    [Ref: Harrison's 20th/e pg. 276, 2342]

24. **Absent urobilinogen in urine with icterus indicates:-** *(NEET Pattern 2015)*
    a. Perihepatic obstruction
    b. Liver failure
    c. Hepatitis
    d. Hemolysis

    [Ref: Harrison's 20th/e pg. 2343]

25. **Regarding liver enzymes true is?** *(DNB Dec'2010)*
    a. Absolute levels of enzyme markers correlate with outcome
    b. ALT is less specific than AST
    c. Glutathione-s-transferase used as hepatic prognostic marker following surgery
    d. None

    [Ref: Harrison's 20th/e pg. 2339]

Explanation

- ALT (SGPT) is present primarily in the liver and is therefore a more specific indicator of injury to hepatocytes.
- Absolute elevation of the liver enzymes as in acute hepatocellular disorders is of no prognostic significance.
- Glutathione-S-Transferase (GSTs) is present in high concentration inside hepatocytes and it function as indicator of hepatocyte injury in viral infection, after toxin exposure and post liver transplant.

26. **Normal A:G ratio is :-** *(PGMEE 2016-17)*
    a. 1.2 – 2.2
    b. 0.8 – 2.2
    c. 0.8 – 2.0
    d. 1.2 – 2.0

    [Ref: Harrison's 19th/e pg 1997]

27. **Marker for cholestasis:** *(PGMEE 2016-17)*
    a. ALP
    b. SGOT
    c. SGPT
    d. Acid phosphatase

    [Ref: Harrison's 20th/e pg. 2340]

Explanation

- LFT pattern typically seen with cholestasis: ↑ conjugated bilirubin, ↑ cholesterol, ↑ ALP, ↑ GGT

28. **SGPT is found in_____ of hepatocytes:** *(PGMEE 2014-15)*
    a. Cytoplasm
    b. Mitochondria
    c. Nucleus
    d. All of above

    [Ref: Table 16.2 Robbins, 8th ed.]

HYPERBILIRUBINEMIA/JAUNDICE

29. **A patient presents with raised conjugated bilurubin with prolonged prothrombin time which improves with vitamin K:-** *(PGMEE 2016-17)*
    a. Hemolytic anemia
    b. Hepatocellular disease
    c. Crigler- Najjar syndrome
    d. Obstruction of bile duct

    [Ref: Harrison's 19th/e pg. 2003]

30. **Vitamin K is given to patient of jaundice but PT remains unchanged. The probable cause is?** *(PGMEE 2014-15)*
    a. Obstructive jaundice
    b. Cirrhosis
    c. Hemolytic jaundice
    d. Biliary atresia

    [Ref: Harrison's 20th/e pg. 2406]

31. **In a child surgery was done for EHBO with hepatojejunal anastomosis. Post-operatively bilirubin level after 2 weeks was 6 mg/dl from a pre-operative level 12mg/dl. The reason for this could be?** *(NEET Pattern 2015)*
    a. Normal lowering of bilirubin takes time
    b. Delta bilirubin
    c. Anastomotic stricture
    d. Mistake in lab technique

    [Ref: Harrison's 20th/e pg. 277]

16.	a
17.	b
18.	d
19.	d
20.	None
21.	c
22.	b
23.	a
24.	a
25.	c
26.	c
27.	a
28.	a
29.	b
30.	b
31.	b

32. A defect in which of the following processes give rise to bilirubinuria? *(PGMEE 2014-15)*
a. Conjugation of bilirubin to glucuronic acid
b. Conversion of biliverdin to bilirubin
c. Transport of conjugated bilirubin to bile canaliculi
d. Transport of unconjugated bilirubin into hepatocytes
[Ref: Harrison's 20th/e pg. 2342]

Explanation
- Unconjugated bilirubin is tighty bound to albumin which prevents its glomeutar filteration.
- Bilirubinuria is a feature of diseases associated with increased serum, conjugated bilirubin like viral hepatitis & intrahepatic/extrahepatic obstructive cholestatic jaundice.

33. Which of the following does not cause cholestasis in newborn:- *(PGMEE 2016)*
a. ABO incompatibility   b. Biliary atresia
c. Tyrosenemia   d. Sepsis
[Ref: Harrison's 20th/e pg. 278, Table 45-1]

Explanation
- In biliary atresia fibro - obliterative destruction of extrahepatic bile duct leads to → cholestasis

34. All of the following are autosomal recessive except:- *(PGMEE 2015)*
a. Dubin Johnson synd   b. CrigglerNajjar type I
c. Rotor Syndrome   d. CrigglerNajjar type II
[Ref: Harrison's 20th/e pg. 2344]

32.	c
33.	a
34.	d
35.	d
36.	a
37.	c
38.	a
39.	a
40.	d
41.	c,d
42.	d
43.	a

Explanation
- Autosomal recessive hyperbilirubinemia syndromes
  - Gilbert syndrome
  - Criggler - Najjar type -I
  - Dubin - Johnson syndrome
  - Rotor syndrome

35. What is true about Gilbert syndrome? *(PGMEE 2012-13)*
a. No treatment required
b. Causes indirect hyperbilirubinemia
c. Reduced activity of glucuronyl transferase enzyme
d. All of above
[Ref: Harrison's 20th/e pg. 2345]

36. Unconjugated hyperbilirubinemia is seen in all except:- *(PGMEE 2016-17)*
a. Dubin Johnson syndrome
b. Criggler Najjar syndrome type 1
c. Criggler Najjar syndrome type 2
d. Gilbert syndrome
[Ref: Harrison's 20th/e pg. 2346]

37. Conjugated hyperbilirubinemia is seen in? *(PGMEE 2013)*
a. Criggler Najjar-1   b. Criggler Najjar-2
c. Rotor syndrome   d. Gilbert's syndrome
[Ref: Harrison's 20th/e pg. 2346]

Explanation

Isolated hyperbilirubinemia

Conjugated	Unconjugated	
Defective excretion	Overproduction	Defective conjugation
↓	↓	↓
▪ Dubin - Johnson syndrome ▪ Rotor syndrome	▪ Hemolytic anemia	▪ Gilbert syndrome ▪ Criggler-Nijjar

38. Raised unconjugated hyperbilirubinemia is seen in: *(PGMEE 2014-15, 2012-13)*
a. Gilbert's Syndrome   b. Dubin Johnson syndrome
c. Drug induced cholestasis d. Hepatocellular necrosis
[Ref: Harrison's 20th/e pg. 2344]

39. Gilbert's syndrome all are true except?
a. Mild conjugated bilirubinaemia   *(PGMEE 2014-15)*
b. Normal LFT
c. Normal liver biopsy
d. Ligandin defect
[Ref: Harrison's 20th/e pg. 2344, table 331-1]

40. The following features differentiate Rotor syndrome from Dubin Johnson's syndrome EXCEPT: *(PGMEE 2015-16)*
a. Liver patients with Rotor syndrome has no increased pigmentation and appears normal
b. In Rotor syndrome Gall bladder is usually visualized on cholecystography
c. Total urinary coproporphyrin is substantially increased in Rotor syndrome
d. Fraction of corpophyrin I in urine is elevated usually more than 80% of the total in Rotor syndrome
[Ref: Harrison's 19th/e pg. 2004]

41. Normal liver microscopy is a feature of: *(PGMEE 2014-15)*
a. Wilson's disease   b. Dubin-Johnson syndrome
c. Gilbert's syndrome   d. Criggler-Najjar
[Ref: Harrison's 20th/e pg. 2344 Table 331-1]

42. Conjugated hyperbilirubinemia is seen in:- *(PGMEE 2016-17)*
a. Criggler najjer synd   b. Gilbert syndrome
c. Hypothyroidism   d. Rotor syndrome
[Ref: Harrison's 20th/e pg. 2346]

Explanation
- Hypothyroidism leads to unconjugated hyperbilirubinemia.

OBSTRUCTIVE JAUNDICE

43. Obstructive jaundice is best detected by: *(PGMEE 2014-15)*
a. Increased ALP   b. Decreased ALP
c. Increased AST   d. Decreased AST
[Ref: Harrison's 20th/e pg. 2340]

44. Marker for cholestasis are all except:- *(PGMEE 2016-17)*

   a. GGT   b. Serum bile acids

   c. ALP   d. 5'-nucleotidase

[Ref: Harrison's 20th/e pg. 2340]

Explanation

- Elevated levels & ALP, r-glutamyl transpeptidase (GGT) & 5' - nucleotidase reflect cholestatic jaundice.

45. Investigation of choice in obstructive jaundice is:

(PGMEE 2014-15)

   a. ERCP   b. Ultrasound

   c. Cholecystography   d. MRCP

[Ref: Harrison's 20th/e pg. 2341]

46. Most common cause of obstructive jaundice in children:

(PGMEE 2014-15)

   a. Biliary atresia   b. Criggler najjar syndrome

   c. Byler disease   d. Caroli cyst

[Ref: Harrison's 19th/e pg. 283]

47. Vitamin to be corrected in obstructive jaundice is

(DNB June' 2009)

   a. Vitamin K   b. Vitamin B 12

   c. Vitamin D   d. Vitamin C

[Ref: Harrison's 20th/e pg. 2340]

48. Patient with hepatic insufficiency is being planned for surgery. Which vitamin deficiency has to be treated first

(DNB June' 2009)

   a. Vitamin A   b. Vitamin D

   c. Vitamin K   d. Vitamin E

[Ref: Harrison's 20th/e pg. 2340]

VIRAL HEPATITIS

49. All of the following are true regarding chronic active hepatitis, EXCEPT: *(PGMEE 2014-15)*

   a. Common in females

   b. Progression to cirrhosis is not seen

   c. Remission with steroids

   d. May associate with autoimmune disease

[Ref: Harrison's 20th/e pg. 2375]

50. Not a complication of acute viral hepatitis?

(PGMEE 2012)

   a. Acute pancreatitis   b. Autoimmune hepatitis

   c. Aplastic anemia   d. Hepatocellular cancer

[Ref: Harrison's 20th/e pg. 2362]

51. Hallmark of chronic hepatitis:- *(PGMEE 2015)*

   a. Interface hepatitis

   b. Cholestasis

   c. Ballooning degeneration of hepatocytes

   d. Periportal fibrosis and bridging fibrosis

[Ref: Harrison's 20th/e pg. 2376]

52. Granulomatosis hepatitis is not caused by:

(PGMEE 2014-15)

   a. Blastomycosis   b. Metastatic carcinoma

   c. Tuberculosis   d. Cat scratch disease

[Ref: www.msdmanuals.com]

Explanation

- Hepatic granulomas rarely affect hepatocellular function
- These are usually asymptomatic.
- Causes of granulomatous hepatitis:
  - Mycobacterial infection
  - Cat scratch disease
  - Fungal infection
  - Sarcoidosis
  - C. burnetii (Q fever)

53. Feature of Granulomatous hepatitis: *(PGMEE 2014-15)*

   a. Jaundice is a usual feature

   b. Seen with sarcoidosis

   c. Seen with syndrome X

   d. Seen after jejuno-ileal bypass surgery in obese patients

[Ref: www.msdmanuals.com]

DRUG-INDUCED LIVER TOXICITY

54. All of the following are true of Reye's syndrome EXCEPT:

(PGMEE 2014-15)

   a. It frequently complicates viral infections

   b. Prothrombin time is prolonged

   c. Disease may by precipitated by salicylates

   d. Deep jaundice is present

[Ref: Harrison's 20th/e pg. 1355]

Explanation

Reye's syndrome:

- Typically occurs after a viral infection
- Associated with use of Aspirin/Salicylates
- Pathology: Mitochondrial dysfunction & disruption of β-oxidation of fatty acids
- Clinically Jaundice is minimally or absent
- Lab : ↑ ALT & AST, ↑ ammonia, prolonged PT/INR & aPTT

55. In Reye's syndrome hepatic change- *[PGMEE 2014]*

   a. Microvesicular steatosis   b. Macrovesicular steatosis

   c. Both   d. None

[Ref: Sheila Sherlock 11th/e pg. 62, 426; Robbins 9th/e pg. 58]

56. Microvesicular steatosis is seen in all EXCEPT:

   a. Alcoholic liver disease   *(PGMEE 2014-15)*

   b. Acute fatty liver of pregnancy

   c. Methotrexate toxicity

   d. Reye's syndrome

[Ref: CMDT 2014, ch. 16, pg. 684]

57. Microvesicular fatty liver is caused by-

(PGMEE 2013-14)

   a. Starvation   b. IBD

   c. Valproate   d. DM

[Ref: Robbin's 9th/e pg. 841]

58. Periportal fatty infiltration of liver is seen with-

(DNB Dec 07)

   a. Tetracycline   b. Malnutrition

   c. Viral hepatitis   d. Alcoholism

[Ref: Harshmohan pg. 735; Robbin's 8th/e pg. 36, 37, 864]

44.	b
45.	b
46.	a
47.	a
48.	c
49.	b
50.	d
51.	d
52.	b
53.	b
54.	d
55.	a
56.	c
57.	c
58.	b

59. Most common hepatotoxin causing acute liver injury:- *(PGMEE 2015)*

a. Acetaminophen   b. Alcohol
c. Paracetamol   d. Halothane

[Ref: Harrison's 20th/e pg. 2369]

60. Fibrin ring granuloma in liver is caused by:- *(PGMEE 2015)*

a. Sulphonamides   b. Isoniazid
c. Amlodarone   d. Allopurinol

[Ref: Robbins 9th/e pg. 863]

61. Peliosis hepatis is caused by:- *(PGMEE 2015)*

a. Contraceptives   b. Anabolic steroids
c. Ezetemibe   d. Erythromycin

[Ref: Harrison's 20th/e pg. 2369]

62. Peliosis hepatis is caused by all except- *(DNB Dec 08)*

a. Analgesics   b. Danazol
c. Anabolic steroids   d. OC pills

[Ref: Harrison's 20th/e pg. 2369]

63. Steatohepatitis with mallory-Denk bodies is caused by:- *(PGMEE 2015)*

a. Alcohol   b. Enalapril
c. Methotrexate   d. Vitamin A

[Ref: Harrison's 20th/e p 2400]

64. Periportal fibrosis is caused by:- *(PGMEE 2015)*

a. OCPs   b. Methotrexate
c. Rifampicin   d. Alcohol

65. Perivenular fibrosis is caused by:- *(PGMEE 2015)*

a. OCPs   b. Alcohol
c. Methotrexate   d. Amiodarone

[Ref: Harrison's 20th/e pg. 2400]

66. Periportal necrosis is caused by? *(PGMEE 2012)*

a. CCL₄   b. Acetaminophen
c. Phosphorous   d. Alcohol

[Ref: Harrison's 20th/e pg. 2367]

AUTOIMMUNE HEPATITIS

67. Most common antibody in autoimmune hepatitis is? *(PGMEE 2012)*

a. ul RNP   b. ANA
c. Anti-LKM   d. Anti-SMA

[Ref: Harrison's 20th/e pg. 2396-97]

Explanation

- Question should have specified specific type of AIH as different type has different autoantibody profile. In general Harrison mentions that homogenous staining pattern of ANAs are most characteristically associated with AIH.

68. Following liver transplantation, recurrence of primary disease in the liver most likely occurs in: *(PGMEE 2014-15)*

a. Wilson's disease
b. Autoimmune hepatitis
c. Alpha-1-antitrypsin deficiency
d. Primary biliary cirrhosis

[Ref: Harrison's 20th/e pg. 2420]

69. Antibody present in autoimmune hepatitis type 2:- *(PGMEE 2015)*

a. Anti-LKM1 antibody
b. Anti-mitochondrial antibody
c. Anti-endomysial antibody
d. Anti-nuclear antibody

[Ref: Harrison's 20th/e pg. 2396]

Explanation

Antibodies in Autoimmune Hepatitis

Type-I	Type-II
■ Anti-Nuclear antibody ■ Anti-Smooth muscle body	■ Anti-Liver-Kidney-Microsomal-I (Anti-LKM-I) antibodies ■ Anti-liver cytosol antibodies

70. Antibody seen in type 1 autoimmune hepatitis:- *(PGMEE 2016-17)*

a. Anti-LKM1 antibody
b. Anti-mitochondrial antibody
c. Anti-smooth muscle antibodies (ASMA)
d. Anti-liver cytosol antibody-1 (ALC-1)

[Ref: Harrison's 20th/e pg. 2396]

ALCOHOLIC LIVER DISEASES AND NAFLD

71. Following test is marker of alcohol induced liver injury: *(PGMEE 2014-15)*

a. Gamma Glutamyl Transferase
b. MCV
c. SGPT/SGOT >2
d. SGOT/SGPT >2

[Ref: Harrison's 20th/e pg. 2339]

72. Focal or confluent periportal necrosis along with ballooning degeneration of hepatocytes with or without Mallory bodies and megamitochondria is suggestive of:- *(PGMEE 2015)*

a. Chronic Hepatitis B   b. Primary HCC
c. Alcoholic liver injury   d. Acute Hepatitis B

[Ref: Harrison's 20th/e pg. 2400]

73. Friction rub may not be heard in right upper quadrant in one of the following conditions: *(PGMEE 2014-15)*

a. Fatty liver
b. Recent biopsy
c. Tumour
d. Perihepatitis

[Ref: Harrison's 19th/e pg. 2053]

74. CAGE scale is used in: *(PGMEE 2014-15)*

a. Alcohol Abuse   b. Depression
c. Suicidal intention   d. Coma

[Ref: Harrison's 20th/e pg. 2334]

75. Maddrey discriminant score is used for determining mortality due to: *(PGMEE 2014-15)*

a. Alcoholic hepatitis   b. Viral hepatitis
c. Cryptogenic hepatitis   d. Hepatic encephalopathy

[Ref: Harrison's 20th/e pg. www.mdcalc.com]

59.	a
60.	d
61.	a,b
62.	a
63.	a
64.	b
65.	b
66.	c
67.	b
68.	b
69.	a
70.	c
71.	d
72.	c
73.	a
74.	a
75.	a

76. Which is best in evaluating alcoholic hepatitis?
(PGMEE 2014-15)

a. Carbohydrate deficient transferrin
b. 5-nucleotidase
c. SGPT raised
d. MCHC

[Ref: Internet]

77. Gamma glutamyl transferase is elevated in:
(PGMEE 2014-15)

a. Liver abscess
b. Viral hepatitis
c. Alcoholic liver disease
d. Secondaries in liver

[Ref: Harrison's 20th/e pg. 2400]

78. Most common cause of non-alcoholic fatty liver disease?
(PGMEE 2014-15)

a. Reye syndrome
b. Syndrome-X
c. Cardiac syndrome-X
d. Pregnancy

[Ref: Harrison's 20th/e pg. 2401]

Explanation

- NAFLD is strongly associated with overweight/obesity, Type of II DM, Dyslipidemia & Insulin resistance (together labelled as syndrome X)

CIRRHOSIS/CLD/ LIVER FAILURE

79. Micronodular cirrhosis is seen in all, except-
(DNB June 08)

a. Indian childhood cirrhosis
b. Wilson's disease
c. Alcoholic cirrhosis
d. Budd Chiari syndrome

[Ref: Essentilas of pathology 4th/e pg. 1121]

80. Hand signs of liver cell failure are all except?
(PGMEE 2014-15)

a. Palmar erythema
b. Clubbing
c. Duputyren contracture
d. Splinter hemorrhages

[Ref: Harrison's 20th/e pg. 2400]

81. Drug requiring dose reduction in cirrhosis :-
(PGMEE 2016-17)

a. Midazolam
b. Succinylcholine
c. Atracurium
d. Isoflurane

[Ref: Internet]

82. Which of the following is not a sign of liver failure:
(DNB Dec'2010)

a. Palmar erythema
b. spider naevi
c. Testicular atrophy
d. Subcutaneous nodule

[Ref: Harrison's 20th/e pg. 2406]

83. The most frequent location for spider angiomata in cirrhosis is:
(PGMEE 2014-15)

a. Abdomen
b. Back
c. Neck and shoulders
d. Upper & lower extremities

Explanation

- A **spider angiomata (aka spider nevi)** is a type of telangiectasia caused by excess levels of estrogen in patient with liver diseases. It can be also be seen in other conditions of estrogen excess like pregnancy & in women taking OCPs. These are found only in the distribution of the SVC & are thus commonly found on face, neck and upper part of trunk.

84. All of the following are noticed in cirrhosis of liver, EXCEPT:
(PGMEE 2014-15)

a. Raised serum albumin
b. Excessive urobilinogenuria
c. Prolonged prothrombin time
d. Raised serum globulin

[Ref: Harrison's 20th/e pg. 2406]

85. First sign of hepatocellular failure is?
(PGMEE 2011)

a. Abnormal PT T
b. Increased ammonia
c. Increased PT
d. Decrease A:G ratio

[Ref: Oxfordmedicine.com]

Explanation

- Hepatocellular failure is characterized is by in bilirubin, enzyme & prolongation of PT/INR.

86. Palmar erythema is seen in:
(PGMEE 2014-15)

a. CCF
b. ARF
c. CRF
d. Hepatic failure

[Ref: Harrison's 20th/e pg. 2406]

87. Most likely cause for acute hepato-cellular failure is:
(PGMEE 2014-15)

a. Viral hepatitis
b. Large IV albumin infusion
c. Large carbohydrate meal
d. Upper GI bleeding

[Ref: Harrison's 20th/e pg. 2347]

88. On a epidemic of hepatitis; fulminant hepatic failure is seen in:
(PGMEE 2014-15)

a. Malnourished child
b. Pregnant female
c. Old age
d. Child < 15 year of age.

[Ref: Harrison's 20th/e pg. 2356, table 332-2]

89. Which of the following is False about Chronic Liver disease patient
(PGMEE 2019)

a. MELD used for Liver transplant
b. MELD has PT, INR, Albumin and Creatinine
c. CTP (Child-Turcotte-Pugh) Calculator has Grades A,B and C
d. CTP score has INR, Albumin and Bilirubin

90. MELD score includes
(PGMEE 2019)

a. Serum creatinine
b. Transaminase
c. Albumin
d. Alkaline phosphatase

91. Spider naevi can occur in:
(PGMEE 2014-15)

a. Rheumatoid arthritis
b. Cirrhosis of the liver
c. Pregnancy
d. All of the above

PRIMARY BILIARY CIRRHOSIS

92. All of the following are true about Primary Biliary Cirrhosis EXCEPT:
(PGMEE 2014-15)

a. Increase 5'- nucleotidase
b. Median age 50
c. Second most common cause of cholangitis in children
d. PBC frequently associated with CREST syndrome

[Ref: Harrison's 20th/e pg. 2408]

76.	a
77.	c
78.	b
79.	b
80.	d
81.	a
82.	d
83.	c
84.	a
85.	c
86.	d
87.	a
88.	b
89.	b
90.	a
91.	d
92.	c

Explanation
- Most commonly present in middle aged female with other auto-immune conditions.

93. M/C symptom of Primary Biliary Cirhosis? :-
(PGMEE 2016-17)

a. Itching
b. Jaundice
c. Fever
d. Weight loss

[Ref: Harrison's 20th/e pg. 2408]

Explanation
- Symptoms of primary biliary cirrhosis (PBC) :- pruritus, progressive jaundice and fat soluble vitamin deficiencies.

94. Most specific antibody in primary biliary cirrhosis:-
(PGMEE 2016-17)

a. Anti mitochondrial Ab
b. ANA
c. Anti-SLA
d. Anti-nucleolar antibody

[Ref: Harrison's 20th/e pg. 2408]

95. Antimitochondrial antibodies are seen in-
(PGMEE 2015,2014)

a. Primary biliary cirrhosis
b. Neonatal cholestasis
c. Secondary biliary cirrhosis
d. Neonatal hepatitis

[Ref: Harrison's 20th/e pg. 2408]

96. Florid duct lesions are diagnostic of:
(PGMEE 2015)

a. Primary sclerosing cholangitis
b. Secondary biliary cirrhosis
c. Primary biliary cirrhosis
d. Klatskin tumor

[Ref: Robbins 9th/e pg. 858]

97. In adults, most common autoimmune disease of liver is?
(PGMEE 2012)

a. Autoimmune hepatitis
b. α antitrypsin deficiency
c. Sclerosing cholangitis
d. Primary billiary cirrhosis

[Ref: Robbin's 8th/e pg. 867-868]

PRIMARY SCLEROSING CHOLANGITIS

98. Autoantibody +ve in primary sclerosing cholangitis :
(PGMEE 2016-17)

a. Auto antibodies against biliary ductular epithelium
b. Anti-endomyseal antibody
c. Anti-ds DNA
d. Anti cytoplasmic antibody

[Ref: Harrison's 20th/e pg. 2409]

99. Onion skin fibrosis is seen in :
(PGMEE 2015)

a. Progressive familial intrahepatic cholestasis
b. Primary biliary cirrhosis
c. Primary sclerosing cholangitis
d. Secondary biliary cirrhosis

[Ref: Robbins 9th/e pg. 859]

Explanation
- In primary sclerosing cholangitis liver biopsy reveals periductal sclerosis (onion skinning) → ductopenia.

100. Ductopenia is seen in: -
(PGMEE 2016-17)

a. Ulcerative colitis
b. Hemochromatosis
c. Primary biliary cholangitis
d. Primary sclerosing cholangitis

[Ref: Robbins 9th/e pg. 858]

101. Sclerosing cholangitis is associated with-
(PGMEE 2013-14)

a. Ulcerative colitis
b. Whipple's disease
c. Celiac sprue
d. Wilson's disease

[Ref: Harrison's 20th/e pg. 2409]

PORTAL HYPERTENSION

102. Ascitic fluid SAAG<1.1; what is the disease associated with it?
(NEET Pattern 2019)

a. Idiopathic portal fibrosis
b. Peritoneal carcinomatosis
c. Hepatic failure
c. Constrictive pericarditis

103. Cirrhosis of liver with portal hypertension occurs in all EXCEPT:
(PGMEE 2014-15)

a. Cystic fibrosis
b. Alpha 1 anti-trypsin deficiency
c. Wilson's disease
d. Schistosomiasis

[Ref: Harrison's 20th/e pg. 2405 Table 337-1]

104. Most common cause of portal hypertension in children is-
(PGMEE 2012-13)

a. Veno-occlusive d/s
b. Post necrotic
c. Extrahepatic compression
d. Budd chiari syndrome

[Ref: Ghai 8th/e/p 319]

105. Which is not characteristic of portal hypertension:
(PGMEE 2014-15)

a. Splenomegaly
b. Hypersplenism
c. Ascites
d. Gynaecomastia

[Ref: Harrison's 20th/e pg. 2410]

106. A patient presented to emergency ward with massive upper gastrointestinal bleed. On examination, he has mild splenomegaly. In the absence of any other information available. Which of the following is the most appropriate therapeutic modality?
(PGMEE 2014-15)

a. I/V propranolol
b. I/V vasopressin
c. I/V pantoprazole
d. I/V somatostatin

[Ref: Harrison's 20th/e pg. 2411]

107. Best Treatment of refractory ascites is
(PGMEE 2014-15)

a. AV shunt
b. TIPS
c. Frusemide with paracentesis
d. Distal splenorenal shunt

[Ref: Harrison's 20th/e pg. 2413]

108. Child with S.A.A.G < 1.1 gm/dl: The probable diagnosis of the child is:
(PGMEE 2014-15)

a. Cirrhosis
b. Portal hypertension
c. CHF
d. Nephrotic syndrome

[Ref: Harrison's 20th/e pg. 284, Figure 46-3]

93.	a
94.	a
95.	a
96.	c
97.	d
98.	d
99.	c
100.	d
101.	a
102.	b
103.	d
104.	c
105.	d
106.	d
107.	b
108.	d

Explanation

SAAG >1.1	SAAG <1.1
■ Related to portal hypertension ○ Pre-sinusoidal: Splenic or portal vein thrombosis, Schistosomiasis ○ Sinusoidal: Cirrhosis ○ Post-sinusoidal: Right heart failure, constrictive pericarditis, Budd-chiari syndrome	■ Not related to portal hypertension ■ Associated with ○ Nephrotic syndrome ○ TB ○ Malignancy with peritoneal carcinomatosis (ovarian cancer).

109. SAAG > 1.1% in all case of ascites except

(NEET Pattern 2017)

a. Cirrhosis
b. Peritoneal tuberculosis
c. Liver failure
d. Hepatic metastasis

Ref: Harrison 19/e, P. 287

110. Consider the following statements: *(PGMEE 2014-15)*
Ascites in cirrhosis of liver is due to
1. Portal hypertension
2. Hypoalbuminaemia
3. Inappropriate ADH secretion
4. Secondary hyper-aldosteronism

a. 1, 2 and 3 are correct
b. 1, 2 and 4 are correct
c. 2, 3, 4 are correct
d. 1, 3 and 4 are correct

[Ref: Harrison's 20th/e pg. 283]

111. Which finding suggests a SVC obstruction versus ascites?
a. Bulging flanks *(PGMEE 2014-15)*
b. Collateral flow towards umbilicus
c. Everted umbilicus
d. Pulsatile liver

[Ref: Harrison's 20th/e pg. 2413]

112. Which one of the following is NOT true about Ascites?

(PGMEE 2014-15)

a. S.A.A.G > 1.1 is seen with portal hypertension
b. S.A.A.G < 1.1 is seen with Nephrotic syndrome
c. Pseudochylous ascites is seen with hypertriglyceridemia
d. Black ascitic fluid is seen with pancreatic necrosis

[Ref: Harrison's 20th/e pg. 283]

113. In patients with cirrhosis of the liver the site of obstruction in the portal system is in the: *(DNB 2007)*
a. Hepatic vein
b. Post-sinusoidal
c. Extra hepatic portal vein
d. Sinusoids

[Ref: Robbins 9th /e pg. 828]

114. A 45-year-old cirrhotic patient presented with severe haematemesis. The management of choice is:

(PGMEE 2014-15)

a. Whole blood transfusion
b. Colloids are preferred over crystalloids
c. Normal saline infusion
d. IV fluid with diuretics

[Ref: Harrison's 20th/e pg. 2411]

HEPATIC ENCEPHALOPATHY

115. Which one of the following is least expected to precipitate hepatic encephalopathy in a liver cirrhosis patient:

(PGMEE 2014-15)

a. Peritoneal tap
b. Antibiotic treatment
c. Variceal bleed
d. Hypokalemia

[Ref: Harrison's 20th/e pg. 2413]

116. Hepatic encephalopathy is aggravated by all except?

(PGMEE 2014-15)

a. Hyperkalemia
b. Anemia
c. Hypothyroidism
d. Barbiturates

[Ref: Harrison's 20th/e pg. 2413]

117. Flapping tremors are seen in all EXCEPT:

(DNB Dec'2010)

a. Hepatic encephalopathy
b. CO_2 narcosis
c. Thyrotoxicosis
d. Uremia

[Ref: Harrison's 20th/e pg. 2413]

118. Earliest sign in hepatic encephalopathy is:

(PGMEE 2014-15)

a. Asterixis
b. Alternate constriction and dilated pupil
c. Constructional apraxia
d. Psychiatric abnormalities

119. Alzehiemer type II astrocyte are seen in:
a. Hepatic encephalopathy *(PGMEE 2014-15)*
b. Alzehiemer's
c. Parkinsonism
d. Biswanger disease

[Ref: https://radiopaedia.org]

Explanation

■ Alzheimer Type II astrocyte are glial cells seen in grey matter. They are seen most frequently in Wilson disease and other metabolic disorders such as hepatic encephalopathy.

120. Acute hepatic encephalopathy is precipitated by:
a. Lactulose *(PGMEE 2014-15)*
b. Potassium sparing diuretics
c. Excessive use of diuretics
d. High protein diet

[Ref: Harrison's 20th/e pg. 2413]

121. Acute hepatic encephalopathy is precipitated by:
a. Lactulose *(PGMEE 2014-15)*
b. Potassium sparing diuretics
c. Excessive protein intake
d. All of the above

[Ref: Harrison's 20th/e pg. 2413]

122. Which one of the following is not advocated in the management of hepatic encephalopathy? *(PGMEE 2014-15)*
a. Oral Lactulose
b. I.V. Glucose drip
c. High protein diet more than 60 grams/day
d. If tests for blood in stool are positive then give colonic washout

[Ref: Harrison's 20th/e pg. 2414]

109. b
110. b
111. b
112. c
113. d
114. a
115. b
116. a
117. c
118. d
119. a
120. c,d
121. c
122. c

123. Portacaval Encephalopathy is treated with:
a. Lactulose *(PGMEE 2014-15)*
b. Large amounts of proteins
c. Emergency portal systemic shunt surgery
d. Diuretics

[Ref: Harrison's 20th/e pg. 2413]

124. All the following drugs are used in hepatic encephalopathy EXCEPT: *(PGMEE 2014-15)*
a. LOLA   b. Rifaximin
c. Lactulose   d. Phenobarbitone

[Ref: Harrison's 20th/e pg. 2414]

125. Antibiotic of choice in cirrhotic patient to prevent encephalopathy: *(PGMEE 2014-15)*
a. Neomycin   b. Ampicillin
c. Metronidazole   d. Rifaximin

[Ref: Harrison's 20th/e pg. 2414]

126. All of the following are characterized by depletion of the intracellular water, EXCEPT: *(PGMEE 2014-15)*
a. Massive diarrhea   b. Peritonitis
c. Pancreatitis   d. Hepatic coma

[Ref: Harrison's 20th/e pg. 2413]

Explanation
- Coma is hepatic encephalopathy is associated with swelling of the neurons in grey matter.

BUDD CHIARI SYNDROME

127. A patient presents with pain abdomen, swelling, and tender hepatomegaly. What is the diagnosis *(PGMEE 2019)*
a. Portal vein thrombosis
b. Congestive hepatomegaly
c. Budd Chiari syndrome
d. Sinusiodal obstruction syndrome

[Ref: Harrison's 19th/e pg. 673]

128. The following is the least likely manifestation of acute Budd-Chiari syndrome: *(PGMEE 2014-15)*
a. Enlarged tender liver b. Ascites
c. Jaundice   d. Venous collaterals

[Ref: Harrison's 19th/e pg. 673]

129. Budd-Chiari syndrome is commonly due to: *(PGMEE 2014-15)*
a. Hepatic venous out flow obstruction
b. Portal Cavernoma
c. Left Sided portal hypertension
d. IVC thrombosis

[Ref: Harrison's 20th/e pg. 2415]

130. Most common cause of Budd-Chiari syndrome is: *(PGMEE 2014-15)*
a. Hepatic vein valves
b. Hypercoagulable state in Nephrotic syndrome
c. PNH
d. Polycythemia vera

[Ref: Harrison's 19th/e pg. 673]

123.	a
124.	d
125.	d
126.	d
127.	c
128.	d
129.	a
130.	d
131.	c
132.	a
133.	a
134.	a
135.	c

131. In Budd Chiari syndrome, the site of venous thrombosis is
a. Infrahepatic inferior vena cava *(PGMEE 2004)*
b. Infrarenal inferior vena cava
c. Hepatic veins
d. Portal veins

[Ref: Harrison's 20th/e pg. 2415]

HEPATORENAL SYNDROME

132. Not a feature of hepatorenal syndrome: *(PGMEE 2014-15)*
a. Normal GFR   b. Normal urinary sediments
c. Low Na+ in urine   d. Normal renal biopsy

[Ref: Harrison's 20th/e pg. 2413]

Explanation
- Caused by splanchnic vasodilation and decreased blood flow to the kidneys.
- Urinary sodium < 10 mEq/L

INFILTRATIVE & METABOLIC LIVER DISEASE

133. A 48 year old lady presented with hepatosplenomegaly with pancytopenia. On microscopic examination of bone marrow cells, crumpled tissue paper appearance is seen. Which is the product likely to have accumulated? *(NEET Pattern 2015)*
a. Glucocerebroside   b. Sphingomyelin
c. Sulfatide   d. Ganglioside

[Ref: Harrison's 20th/e pg. 3007]

Explanation
- Diagnosis: Gaucher's disease.
- Deficient enzyme: Glucocerebrosidase
- Accumulated product : Glucocerebroside
- Histopath: Glucocerebroside accumulates in macrophage giving it a resemblance to crumpled up paper (k/a Gaucher cell)
- Treatment: Enzyme replacement therapy.

134. A 1 month old child with conjugated bilirubinemia and intrahepatic cholestasis. On Liver biopsy and staining with PAS red coloured granules were seen inside the hepatocytes. Probable diagnosis is :-
a. Alpha1 Antitrypsin deficiency *(NEET Pattern 2015)*
b. hereditary hemochromatosis
c. Wilson disease
d. Congenital hepatic fibrosis

[Ref: Robbins 9th/e pg. 847-851]

135. PAS-positive, diastase-resistant globules in hepatocytes are seen in:- *(PGMEE 2015)*
a. Wilsons disease
b. Acute necrotic hepatitis
c. Alpha 1 antitrypsin deficiency
d. Hemochromatosis

[Ref: Harrison's 20th/e pg. 2409]

136. Which of the following leads to chronic liver disease-
(PGMEE 2015-16, 2012)
a. EBV
b. Infectious mononucleosis
c. Hepatitis A
d. α- 1- antitrypsin deficiency

[Ref: Harrison's 20th/e pg. 2405]

137. What is true about Alfa 1 antitrypsin deficiency?
(DNB June 2011)
a. Liver biopsy revealing PAS positive diastase sensitive granules
b. Manifests as neonatal cholestaisis
c. Autosomal Recessive
d. All of the above

[Ref: Nelson's 20th e/p 1941]

WILSON'S DISEASE

138. Gene of Wilson disease is- *(PGMEE 2012-13)*
a. ADP7B   b. ATP7B
c. ATP7A   d. ADP7A

[Ref: Harrison's 20th/e pg. 2982]

Explanation
- ATP7A gene mutation is seen in Menkes disease

139. Gene for Wilson's disease is located on chromosome-
(PGMEE 2013-14)
a. 17   b. 7
c. 13   d. 10

[Ref: Harrison's 20th/e pg. 2982]

140. Pencillamine is mostly used in: *(PGMEE 2014-15)*
a. Hepatolenticular degeneration
b. Penicillin anaphylaxis
c. Haemochromatosis   d. Tertiary syphilis

[Ref: Harrison's 20th/e pg. 2983]

141. Low serum copper due to ATP 7A gene is due to?
(PGMEE 2014-15)
a. Dubin-Johnson's synd   b. Wilson disease
c. Menke disease   d. Gilbert's disease

[Ref: Harrison's 20th/e pg. 2982]

142. All of the following statements about Wilson's disease are true EXCEPT:- *(PGMEE 2015-16)*
a. Liver Copper is increased
b. Total Serum Copper is increased
c. Ceruloplasmin levels are reduced
d. Urinary copper is increased

[Ref: Harrison's 20th/e pg. 2983]

143. Wilson's disease associated with :-
(PGMEE 2016-17; 2010, 2011, Aug 2013)
a. KF ring   b. Chromosome 11
c. Iron metabolism   d. ATP 7A

[Ref: Harrison's 20th/e pg. 2982]

144. Wilson's disease is diagnosed by? *(PGMEE 2010-11; 2013)*
a. ↑serum ceruloplamin   b. ↓liver copper
c. ↑urinary copper excretion   d.↓urine copper excretion

[Ref: Harrison's 20th/e pg. 2983]

145. Wilson's disease is characterized by- *(PGMEE 2013-14)*
a. Decreased copper excretion in urine
b. Increased copper in liver
c. Increased serum ceruloplasmin
d. Autosomal dominant

[Ref: Harrison's 20th/e pg. 2983]

146. A 12 years old boy suffering from hepatitis now comes with diminution of vision. Pediatrician referred to an ophthalmologist. Slit lamp examination finding of which is shown. What is the next best investigation to clinch the diagnosis? *(PGMEE 2018)*

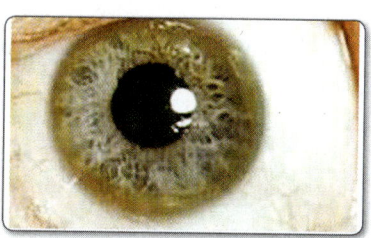

a. Chromosomal analysis   b. Rheumatoid factor
c. Serum cholesterol   d. Serum ceruloplasmin

[Ref: Harrison's 20th/e pg. 2983]

147. All the following statements about Wilson's disease are true EXCEPT: *(PGMEE 2014-15)*
a. It is an autosomal recessive disorder
b. Serum ceruloplasmin level is < 20 mcg/dl
c. Urinary copper excretion is < 100 mcg/day
d. Zinc acetate is effective as maintenance therapy

[Ref: Harrison's 19th/e pg. 2519]

HEMOCHROMATOSIS

148. Diabetic patient with liver cirrhosis and hyperpigmentation, diagnosis is- *(PGMEE 2013-14)*
a. Primary sclerosing cholangitis
b. Hemochromatosis
c. Wilson's disease
d. Hepatitis B

[Ref: Harrison's 20th/e pg. 2979]

149. In hemochromatosis pigment accumulates in all organs except- *(PGMEE 2014)*
a. Pancreas   b. Liver
c. Skin   d. Testis

[Ref: Harrison's 20th/e pg. 2980]

Explanation
- Iron accumulates in the liver, pancreas (islet cells), heart, adrenal glands, testes and pituitary glands.

150. Triad of hemochromatosis is- *(PGMEE 2014)*
a. Macronodular cirrhosis, diabetes insipidus & skin pigmentation
b. Macronodular cirrhosis, diabetes mellitus & skin pigmentation
c. Micronodular cirrhosis, diabetes mellitus & skin pigmentation
d. None

[Ref: Harrison's 20th/e pg. 2979]

| 136. d |
| 137. c |
| 138. b |
| 139. c |
| 140. a |
| 141. c |
| 142. b |
| 143. a |
| 144. c |
| 145. b |
| 146. d |
| 147. c |
| 148. b |
| 149. None |
| 150. c |

151. Not true about Hemochromatosis is? *(DNB June 2011)*
a. Hypogonadism
b. Arthropathy
c. Desferrioxamine is treatment of choice
d. Diabetes mellitus

[Ref: Harrison's 20th/e pg. 2981]

152. Term "Bronze diabetes" is used for a patient of:- *(PGMEE 2016-17)*
a. Wilson's disease   b. Hemosiderosis
c. Hemochromatosis   d. All of the above

[Ref: Internet]

153. Hemosiderosis of liver, pigment deposited is- *(PGMEE 2014)*
a. Manganese   b. Iron
c. Copper   d. Zinc

[Ref: Robbins 9th/e pg. 65 and 847]

154. All are features of primary hemochromatosis EXCEPT: *(PGMEE 2014-15)*
a. Chorea   b. Diabetes
c. Arthritis   d. Skin pigmentation

[Ref: Harrison's 19th/e pg. 2512]

155. Patient with arthritis, skin hyperpigmentation and hypogonadism is diagnosed to have: *(PGMEE 2014-15)*
a. Hemochromatosis
b. SLE
c. Ectopic ACTH secreting tumor of lung
d. Wilson's disease

[Ref: Harrison's 19th/e pg. 2516]

PORPHYRIA

156. Photosensitivity is a feature of porphyria. All the following enzyme deficiencies have photo-sensitivity except? *(PGMEE 2014-15)*
a. HMB synthase deficiency
b. Uroporphyrinogen decarboxylase deficiency
c. Protoporphyrinogen oxidase deficiency
d. Coproporphyrinogen oxidase deficiency

[Ref: Harrison 20th/e pg. 295 Table 409-I]

157. In acute intermittent porphyria, the metabolite which is elevated is: *(PGMEE 2014-15)*
a. Uroblinogen   b. Porphoblinogen
c. Coroporphyrin   d. Protoporphyrin

[Ref: Harrison 20th/e pg. 2985]

MISCELLANEOUS

158. MELD score includes: *(NEET 2019)*
a. Serum creatinine   b. Transaminase
c. Albumin   d. Alkaline phosphatase

159. Menghini's needle is used for: *(PGMEE 2014-15)*
a. Pleural aspiration   b. Lumbar puncture
c. Kidney biopsy   d. Liver biopsy

[Ref: Harrison's 19th/e pg. 336e-3f]

160. Which is the main contraindication for a liver biopsy? *(PGMEE 2015)*
a. Associated cholcysititis
b. Coagulopathy
c. Hepatitis
d. Chronic Alcoholic

[Ref: Internet]

161. Liver span is best measured by:- *(PGMEE 2016-17)*
a. Resonance and auscultation
b. Palpation
c. Percussion and palpation
d. Inspection and bimanual palpation

[Ref: Harrison's 19th/e pg. 1992]

162. Tender hepatomegaly is NOT seen in *(DNB 2007)*
a. Viral hepatitis   b. Typhoid fever
c. Right heart failure   d. Liver abscess

[Ref: Harrison's 19th/e pg. 432e]

163. Perihepatic fibrosis occurring in Fitz Hugh Curtis syndrome is due to- *(PGMEE 2015)*
a. Viral hepatitis
b. Chronic Alcoholism
c. Bile duct injury
d. Pelvic inflammatory disease

[Ref: Internet]

164. Which of the following finding is not suggestive of intrinsic hepatic fibrosis: *(PGMEE 2014-15)*
a. Bulging flanks
b. Collateral flow toward umbilicus
c. Everted umbilicus
d. Venous hum

[Ref: Harrison's 19th/e pg. 286]

165. All of the following are true about the bare area of the liver except- *(PGMEE 2015)*
a. It is not a site of portocaval anastomosis
b. Infection can spread from the abdominal to thoracic cavity at this area
c. It is triangular in shape
d. Formed by the reflections of coronary ligaments

[Ref: Gray's Anatomy 20th/e]

166. What is the Pringle Maneuver? *(PGMEE 2015)*
a. Clamping of hepatoduodenal ligament
b. Clamping of portal vein
c. Clamping of hepatic vein
d. Clamping of hepatic artery

[Ref: Schwartz 10th/e pg. 1416; Bailey 26th/e pg. 1073]

167. Which classification is used to divide the liver into segments- *(PGMEE 2015)*
a. Starzl
b. Anatomical
c. Couinaud's
d. Balthazar

[Ref: Sabiston 19th/e pg. 1414: Bailey & Love 26/e pg. 1066]

151. c
152. c
153. b
154. a
155. a
156. a
157. b
158. a
159. d
160. b
161. c
162. b
163. d
164. b
165. a
166. a
167. c

DISEASES OF GB AND BILE DUCTS

1. Acalculous cholecystitis can be seen in all the following conditions EXCEPT: *(PGMEE 2014-15)*
a. Enteric fever
b. Dengue
c. Leptospirosis
d. Malaria

[Ref: Harrison's 19th/e pg. 2081]

2. A 60 year male presented with jaundice, pale stools, dark urine and mass in the epigastric region. Which of the following diagnosis in unlikely? *(PGMEE 2015)*
a. Pancreatic cancer
b. Chronic cholecystitis
c. Biliary cancer
d. Periampullary

[Ref: Chronic cholecystitis – no mass/jaundice]

3. Which among the following is not a feature of Hemobilia? *(DNB Dec'2010)*
a. Malena
b. Jaundice
c. Fever
d. Biliary colic

[Ref: Sabiston Textbook of Surgery, 18th/e chapter 52]

Explanation

- Hemobilia:
  - Refers to the presence of blood in the biliary tree
  - Clinical feature: Triad of UGI bleed causing malena, Jaundice & Pain abdomen [Quincke's triad]
  - Mc cause: Iatrogenic > Trauma
  - IOC: CT Angiography

4. Gall stones in children is caused by all Except:
a. Prematurity *(DNB June'2010)*
b. Obesity
c. Sickle cell anemia
d. Leptospira interrogans infection

[Ref: Nelson's Pediatrics page 1566]

5. Strawberry gall bladder is also known as- *(PGMEE 2015)*
a. Gall Bladder polyp
b. Emphysematous Cholecystitis
c. Mucocoele
d. Cholesterosis

[Ref: Maingot's 11th/e pg. 684]

6. Mirizzi's syndrome is *(DNB June' 2011)*
a. Gall bladder stone compressing common hepatic duct
b. Gall bladder stone causing cholecystitis
c. Pancreatic carcinoma
d. Gall bladder carcinoma invading IVC

[Ref: Bailey and love 24th/e p. 1106]

7. A 55 old female patient with h/o recurrent episodes of RUQ abdominal pain for the last one year presented to emergency with history of jaundice and fever for 2 days. On examination ,the patient appeared toxic and had a blood pressure of 100/60 mmHg. She was started on intravenous antibiotics. Ultrasound of the abdomen showed presence of stones in the common bile duct. What would be the best treatment option for her-
a. Open surgery and bile duct stone extraction
b. ERCP and bile duct stone extractions
c. Laparoscopic cholecystectomy
d. Lithotripsy

[Ref: Schwartz 10th /e pg.1323,Maingot's 12th /e pg.1023]

8. Alagille syndrome all of the following are true expect- *(PGMEE 2015)*
a. Mutation in JAG 1 and Notch2 gene are seen
b. Can cause autoimmune hepatitis
c. Valvular anomalis of heart seen
d. Autosomal Recessive disease

[Ref: Internet]

9. Which of the following stoma is formed in Hartman's Procedure? *(PGMEE 2015)*
a. End colostomy
b. End lliostomy
c. Loop lliostomy
d. Caecostomy

[Ref: Schwartz 10th /e pg.1220]

Explanation

- Hartmann's procedure
  - Indications:- Complicated diverticulitis
  - Rectosigmoid Cancer
  - Procedure
    - Resection of retosigmoid colon
    - Formation of end colostomy

10. Treatment of retained CBD stone is *(DNB June' 2011)*
a. Endoscopic sphincterotomy
b. Laparoscopic CBD exploration
c. Percutaneous stone extraction
d. ESWL

[Ref: Maingot's 10th/e p. 1746]

11. False statement about Alagille syndrome: *(PGMEE 2015)*
a. Portal and bile ducts are absent
b. Mutation in Jag 1 gene
c. Micronodural cirrhosis of liver
d. Normal liver

[Ref: Robbins 9th/e pg. 853,859]

12. Incorrect about Mirrizi syndrome: *(PGMEE 2014-15)*
a. Jaundice
b. Cystic duct obstruction
c. MRCP for investigation
d. Hemobilia

[Ref: Harrison's 18th ed. ch. 311]

1.	d
2.	b
3.	c
4.	d
5.	d
6.	a
7.	b
8.	d
9.	a
10.	a
11.	c
12.	d

13. Most common cause of hemobilia is: *(PGMEE 2014-15)*
a. Trauma
b. Hemangioma
c. Rupture of hepatic artery aneurysm
d. Hepatitis

[Ref: Harrison's 19th/e pg. 2084]

14. A patient presented with complaints of abdominal pain, melena, jaundice, and fever of 104°F; diagnosis will be: *(PGMEE 2014-15)*
a. Carcinoma pancreas
b. CBD stones
c. Hemobilia
d. Hepatitis

[Ref: Harrison's 19th/e pg. 2089]

15. Investigation of choice in Hemobilia: *(PGMEE 2014-15)*
a. ERCP
b. Angiography
c. Upper GI endoscopy
d. Barium study

[Ref: Harrison 19th p 2089)

16. Most common site of Gallstone ileus: *(PGMEE 2014-15)*
a. Caecum
b. 2nd pt. of duodenum
c. Terminal ileum
d. Stomach

[Ref: CMDT 2014, ch. 16, pg. 703]

17. Chronic hemolytic anaemia is associated with which of the following- *(PGMEE 2015)*
a. Intestinal obstruction
b. Brown pigment stone of the gall bladder
c. Black pigment stone of the gall bladder
d. Uric acid renal calculus

[Ref: Sabiston 20th /e pg. 1491]

18. Medical treatment in gallbladder stone is amenable for: *(PGMEE 2014-15)*
a. Size of stone less than 10 mm
b. Radiopaque
c. Calcium bilirubinate oxalate
d. GB non-functioning

[Ref: Harrison's 19th/e pg. 208]

Explanation

- Medical therapy for gallstones:
  ○ Indications:
  ○ Functional gall bladder
  ○ Radiolucent stones
  ○ Size <10mm
  ○ Drug: Ursodcoxycholic acid

19. Medical treatment of gallstone indicated in A/E: *(PGMEE 2014-15)*
a. GB should be functioning
b. Gallstone should be radiolucent
c. Gallstone should be radio opaque
d. Patient is unfit for surgery

[Ref: Harrison's 19th/e pg. 2076]

20. In a patient with fever, nausea and pain in right hypochondrium for 6 hours. Liver is not palpable. Most probable diagnosis is: *(PGMEE 2014-15)*
a. Viral hepatitis
b. Acute cholecystitis
c. Gastritis
d. Pleurisy

[Ref: Harrison's 19th/e pg. 2080]

21. HIDA scan is useful in: *(PGMEE 2014-15)*
a. Acute cholecystitis
b. Meckel's diverticulum
c. Colonic angio-dysplasia
d. Diverticulitis

[Ref: Harrison's 19th/e pg. 2080]

22. Mainly cholecystokinin is secreted by: *(PGMEE 2014-15)*
a. Duodenum
b. Pancreas
c. Gallbladder
d. Ileum

[Ref: Harrison's 19th/e pg. 2053]

23. Treatment of choice for congenital biliary atresia is:- *(PGMEE 2015-16)*
a. Vitamin E
b. Roux-en-Y choledochojejunostomy
c. Kasai procedure
d. Liver transplantation

[Ref: Neonatology; A Practical Approach to Neonatal Diseases; Zakim and Boyer's Hepatology: A Textbook of Liver Disease]

24. Investigation of choice for biliary atresia in a 2 month old infant is? *(NEET Pattern 2015)*
a. Hepatic scintigraphy
b. ERCP
c. USG
d. CECT

[Ref: Page 1385-1387: Nelson 19th]

25. Contraindiction for laparoscopic Cholecystecttomy is *(DNB June' 2011)*
a. End-stage liver disease
b. Coagulopathy
c. Obstructive pulmony disease
d. All of the above

[Ref: Sabiston's 20th/e pg. 1498]

26. A female post cholecystectomy through general Anesthesia after 12 hrs she develops dyspnea and right lower lobe crackles/crepitations. Likely cause is *(PGMEE 2016-17)*
a. Drug collapse
b. Atelectasis
c. Pulmonary edema
d. Distension in abdomen

[Ref: From Sabiston 20th /e pg. 294]

13.	a
14.	c
15.	b
16.	c
17.	c
18.	a
19.	c
20.	b
21.	a
22.	a
23.	c
24.	a
25.	d
26.	c

PANCREATITIS

1. In a case of acute pancreatitis with shock, initial management is: *(NEET 2018)*
   a. Central line and isotonic crystalloid solution
   b. Urgent laparotomy
   c. Wide bore peripheral line and hypertonic colloid solution
   d. ERCP

2. MCC of Viral pancreatitis :- *(PGMEE 2016-17)*
   a. Coxsackie virus   b. Mumps
   c. CMV   d. HIV

[Ref: Harrison's 20th/e pg. 2439]

3. All of the following are causes of acute pancreatitis except- *(PGMEE 2015)*
   a. Trauma   b. Hypocalcemia
   c. Gall stones d. Mumps

[Ref: Harrison's 20th/e Table 341-1 pg. 2438]

4. In acute pancreatitis all are seen EXCEPT *(DNB Dec' 2009)*
   a. Increased serum lipase b. Hypercalcemia
   c. Hypocalcemia   d. Raised amylase

[Ref: Harrison's 20th/e pg. 2439]

5. All of the following can cause acute pancreatitis expect- *(PGMEE 2015)*
   a. Alcohol   b. Gall stones
   c. Trauma   d. Hepatitis

[Ref: Harrison's 20th/e pg. 341-1, pg. 2439]

6. An alcoholic patient present with severe epigastric pain radiating to back. Best investigation to confirm the diagnosis:- *(PGMEE 2016-17)*
   a. LDH   b. S. amylase
   c. Alkaline phosphatase d. Serum lipase

[Ref: Harrison's 20th/e pg. 2439]

Explanation

- Serum lipase is more sensitive and specific than amylase.

7. All are used in treatment of acute pancreatitis except: *(DNB Dec' 2011)*
   a. Nasojejunal feeds b. Analgesics
   c. Antibiotics   d. IV fluids

[Ref: Harrison's 20th/e pg. 2443]

Explanation

- Infected pancreatic necrosis should be treated with antibiotics, though prophylactic antibiotics are not recommended.

8. Acute and recurrent pancreatitis is reported to occur in: *(DNB 2008)*
   a. Homocystinuria
   b. Maple syrup urine disorder
   c. Isovaleremic aciduria
   d. Tyrosinemia

[Ref: Internet (Pubmed article)]

9. A 65 year old male presenting with acure pancreatitis is now having refractory hypoxia. The X-ray chest would show- *(PGMEE 2015)*
   a. Pneumatocoeles   b. Hilar lymphadenopathy
   c. Bilateral infiltrates d. Ground glass appearances

[Ref: Harrison's 20th/e Table 341-4, pg. 2444]

Explanation

- Patient has developed present with ARDS which is characterized by bilateral infiltrate.

10. A 55 years old male with a known history of gall stones presents with chief complaints of severe abdominal pain and elevated levels of serum lipase with periumbilical ecchymosis. All of the following are prognostic criteria to predict severity of the condition except- *(PGMEE 2015)*
   a. Age   b. Serum GGT
   c. Base deficit d. Serum LDH

[Ref: Harrison's 20th/e pg. 2443]

11. Difference between acute and chronic pancreatitis is? *(DNB Dec' 2011)*
   a. Acute pancreatitis has reversible changes
   b. Chronic pancreatitis shows no signs of inflammation
   c. Acute pancreatitis affects mainly younger population
   d. Alcohol causes only acute pancreatitis

[Ref: Harrison's 20th/e pg. 2444]

12. Patient of acute pancreatitis developed sudden loss of vision the most likely cause is: *(PGMEE 2014-15)*
   a. Purtscher's retinopathy b. Hyperglycemia
   c. Hypoxia   d. CRVO

[Ref: Harrison's 20th/e Table 341-4, pg. 2444]

13. The following can be associated with acute pancreatitis EXCEPT: *(PGMEE 2014-15)*
   a. Hyperparathyroidism
   b. Cystic fibrosis
   c. Hypercalcemia
   d. Hypercholestrolemia

[Ref: Harrison's 20th/e pg. 2443]

14. Which is the diagnostic test in pancreatic insufficiency: *(PGMEE 2014-15)*
   a. Schilling test   b. Serum lipase
   c. Serum amylase   d. Fecal Elastase level

[Ref: Harrison's 20th/e pg. 2433]

Explanation

- Determination of fecal elastase is highly sensitive in the diagnosis of moderate to severe exocrine pancreatic insufficiency.
- Schilling test is used to investigate Vit B_{12} deficiency.

15. Medical treatment of acute pancreatitis to reduce pancreatic damage: *(PGMEE 2014-15)*
   a. Glucagon   b. Aprotinin
   c. Calcitonin   d. Gabexate

[Ref: Harrison's 19th/e pg. 2091]

1.	a
2.	b
3.	b
4.	b
5.	None
6.	d
7.	c
8.	c
9.	c
10.	b
11.	a
12.	a
13.	d
14.	d
15.	d

Explanation

- Gabexate is a serine protease inhibitor known to decrease production of inflammatory cytokines and is found useful in acute pancreatitis.

16. A 45 year old male is brought to casualty after a night party with complaints of epigastric pain, penetrating towards back. Which is the best for diagnosis?
(PGMEE 2015-16)

a. Serum lipase
b. CPK-MB
c. ALP
d. Gamma- GGT

[Ref: Harrison's 20th/e pg. 2439]

17. Diabetic ketoacidosis mimics acute pancreatitis in all findings EXCEPT:
(PGMEE 2014-15)

a. Elevated amylase
b. Elevated lipase
c. Abdominal pain
d. Hyperglycemia

[Ref: Harrison's 20th/e pg. 2440]

18. Ranson's criteria includes all EXCEPT:
(PGMEE 2014-15)

a. Fall in hematocrit > 10%
b. Calcium < 8 mg%
c. WBC > 16,000
d. Base deficit > 2

[Ref: Harrison's 19th/e pg. 2091]

19. 35-year-old man presents with acute pancreatitis in shock. Ideal fluid of choice is:- *(PGMEE 2018)*

a. Isotonic saline
b. Hypertonic saline
c. Hypotonic solution
d. Dextrose 10%

20. Most common cause of chronic pancreatitis:-
(PGMEE 2018)

a. Alcoholism
b. Gall bladder stones
c. Trauma
d. ERCP

[Ref: Harrison's 20th/e pg. 2445]

16.	a
17.	b
18.	d
19.	a
20.	a
21.	d
22.	a
23.	c
24.	b
25.	d
26.	d
27.	b

Explanation

- Heavy alcohol consumption is the most common cause of chronic pancreatitis (90% of cases)
- Mutations in the cationic trypsinogen gene, also known as protease serine 1 (*PRSS1*) gene, are common in hereditary chronic pancreatitis. *PRSS1* is located on chromosome 7

21. All of the following are true regarding Acute pancreatitis EXCEPT: *(PGMEE 2014-15)*

a. Elevated serum amylase
b. Alcoholics are more prone
c. Ranson score is used to grade severity
d. Raised serum calcium

[Ref: Harrison's 20th/e pg. 2440]

22. Criteria for severity in acute pancreatitis includes all EXCEPT: *(PGMEE 2014-15)*

a. 3 fold increase in serum lipase
b. Serum creatinine > 2.0mg%
c. PaO2 < 60mmHg
d. SBP<90

[Ref: Harrison's 20th/e Table 341-3 pg. 2441]

Explanation

Risk Factors for Severity

- Age >60 years
- Obesity, BMI >30
- Comorbid disease (Charlson Comorbidity Index)

Markers of Severity at Admission or Within 24 h

- **SIRS**—defined by presence of 2 or more criteria:
  - Core temperature <36° or >38°C
  - Heart rate >90 beats/min
  - Respirations >20/min or Pco_2 <32 mmHg
  - White blood cell count >12,000/μL, <4000/μL, or 10% bands
- **APACHE II**
  - Hemoconcentration (hematocrit >44%)
  - Admission BUN (>22 mg/dL)
- **BISAP Score**
  - (B) BUN >25 mg/dL
  - (I) Impaired mental status
  - (S) SIRS: ≥2 of 4 present
  - (A) Age >60 years
  - (P) Pleural effusion
- **Organ failure (Modified Marshall Score)**
  - Cardiovascular: systolic BP <90 mmHg, heart rate >130 beats/min
  - Pulmonary: Pao_2 <60 mmHg
  - Renal: serum creatinine >2.0 mg%

23. Grey Turner's sign is seen in: *(PGMEE 2014-15)*

a. Myocarditis
b. Cholecystitis
c. Pancreatitis
d. Pleural effusion

[Ref: Harrison's 20th/e pg. 2439]

24. Brownish discoloration of flank seen in acute pancreatitis is referred to as? *(DNB Dec'2010)*

a. Cullen's sign
b. Grey turner sign
c. Alvaradao's sign
d. Balance's sign

[Ref: Harrison's 20th/e pg. 2439]

25. Which of the following is/are associated with pancreatic exocrine insufficiency: *(PGMEE 2014-15)*

a. Hypertriglyceridemia
b. Enterokinase deficiency
c. Malabsorption
d. All of the above

[Ref: Harrison's 19th/e pg. 2090]

26. Which of the following is associated with recurrent acute pancreatitis: *(PGMEE 2014-15)*

a. Hypertriglyceridemia
b. Cystic fibrosis
c. Pancreatic cancer
d. All of the above

[Ref: Harrison's 20th/e pg. 2444]

27. Best diagnosis of pancreatic disease: *(PGMEE 2014-15)*

a. Ultrasound
b. CT scan
c. ERCP
d. PTC

[Ref: Harrison's 20th/e pg. 2436]

Explanation

- Flank brussing: Grey Turner sign.
- Periumbilical discoloration:- Cullen sign.

28. Serum amylase is raised in: *(PGMEE 2014-15)*
   a. Rubella
   b. Measles
   c. Mumps
   d. Chickenpox

[Ref: Harrison's 20th/e pg. 2436]

29. Increased amylase seen in A/e: *(PGMEE 2014-15)*
   a. Pancreatic pseudocyst
   b. Chronic pancreatitis
   c. Perforated peptic ulcer
   d. Ruptured ectopic pregnancy

[Ref: Harrison's 20th/e pg. 2436, 2445]

30. Anti-diabetic drug causing hemorrhagic pancreatitis: *(PGMEE 2014-15)*
   a. Exenatide   b. Sitagliptin
   c. Saxagliptin   d. Canagliflozin

[Ref: Harrison's 19th/e pg. 2090]

31. Most common cause of Acute Pancreatitis is: *(PGMEE 2014-15)*
   a. Trauma   b. Hyperlipidemia
   c. Alcoholism   d. Viral infection

[Ref: Harrison's 20th/e pg. 2438]

32. Pancreatic auto-transplantation is done for: *(PGMEE 2014-15)*
   a. Chronic pancreatitis b. Carcinoma pancreas
   c. Wolfram syndrome   d. Nesidioblastosis

[Ref: Harrison's 20th/e pg. 2448]

33. Most common cause of pseudopancreatic cyst is? *(PGMEE 2015)*
   a. Pancreatitis   b. Trauma
   c. Pancreatic malignancy d. Pancreatic surgery

[Ref: Sabiston's 20th/e pg. 1530]

34. About pseudocyst pancreas false statement is *(DNB June' 2011)*
   a. Fibrous coat
   b. Has mucous lining epithelium
   c. Not a true cyst
   d. Presents as epigastric mass

35. Treatment of choice for asymptomatic pseudocyst pancreas is? *(DNB June'2010)*
   a. Drainage   b. Conservative
   c. Marsupialisation d. Cystogastrostomy

[Ref: Harrison's 20th/e pg. 2443]

36. Cut-off for Severe Acute Pancreatitis is defined by:- *(PGMEE 2015-16)*
   a. ROME Score > 3   b. Imrie Score > 6
   c. Ranson Score > 1   d. APACHE II Score > 8

[Ref: Sabiston's 20th/e pg. 1527]

37. All of the following structures are removed in Whipple's procedure except- *(PGMEE 2015)*
   a. CBD   b. Neck of Pancreas
   c. Pylorus   d. Duodenum

[Ref: Bailey & Love 26th/e pg. 1139; Schwartz 10th/e pg. 1401]

Explanation

- Ex: Head of the pancreas is removed

SPLEEN

38. Most common cause of congestive splenomegaly is: *(PGMEE 2014-15)*
   a. Chronic congestive cardiac failure
   b. Cirrhosis
   c. Hepatic vein occlusion
   d. Stenosis of splenic vein

[Ref: Harrison's 20th/e pg. 2411]

39. Splenectomy is the best treatment for:
   a. Purpura   b. Hereditary spherocytosis
   c. Leukaemia   d. Hodgkin's disease

[Ref: Harrison's 20th/e pg. 416]

40. Visceral aneurysm is most common in *(DNB 2007)*
   a. Splenic artery   b. Lt gastric artery
   c. Hepatic artery   d. Renal artery

[Ref: Sabiston's 20th /e pg. 1788]

41. Splenectomy predispose to which infection:- *(PGMEE 2016-17)*
   a. Capsulated bacterial infection
   b. Viral infection
   c. Fungal infection
   d. Parasite infection

[Ref: Sabiston's 20th /e pg. 1557]

42. Most common opportunistic infection after splenectomy is: *(DNB 2008)*
   a. E. coli   b. Pneumococci
   c. Meningococci   d. H. influenzae

[Ref: Sabiston 20th /e pg. 1567]

43. Howel-Jolly bodies may be seen after- *(PGMEE 2013-14)*
   a. Cholecystectomy   b. Splenectomy
   c. Hepatectomy   d. Pancreatectomy

[Ref: Robbins 9th/e pg. 636]

28.	c
29.	b
30.	a
31.	c
32.	a
33.	a
34.	b
35.	b
36.	d
37.	b
38.	b
39.	b
40.	a
41.	a
42.	b
43.	b

MOST COMMON

- MC hospital acquired infection → UTI
- MC agent associated with catheter associated UTI → E. coli
- MCC of complicated UTI → E. coli
- MC viral infection after renal transplant → CMV
- MC opportunistic infection in kidney transplant recipients: CMV
- MC virus associated with post-transplant lymphoproliferative disorder (PTLD) → EBV
- MC clinical presentation of Renal TB → Sterile pyuria
- MCC of Nephrotic syndrome in adults → Diabetes Mellitus
- MC Primary cause of Nephrotic syndrome in adults → FSGS
- MCC of Nephrotic syndrome in children → Minimal Change Disease
- MC cause of primary glomerulonephritis → IgA nephropathy
- MC primary glomerular disease in children → IgA nephropathy

- MC systemic vasculitis in children → HSP
- MC type of lupus nephritis → Class IV
- MCC of primary renal vein thrombosis in an adult → Nephroticsyndrome/Membranous Glomerulopathy
- MCC of primary renal vein thrombosis in a neonate → Dehydration
- MC type of ARF → Prerenal
- MCC of death in chronic dialysis patient → Cardiovascular disease
- MC hereditary nephritis → Alport's syndrome
- MC cystic disease of kidney → AD Polycystic Kidney Disease
- MC extra renal location of cyst in adult PKD → Liver
- MCC of Renal artery stenosis in young adults in India → Takayasu arteritis
- MCC of Renal artery stenosis in young female → Fibro muscular dysplasia
- MCC of Renovascular hypertension:
  ○ Elderly patient → Atherosclerosis
  ○ Young patient → Takayasu arteritis (in India)

REMEMBER

Medications associated with Renal calculi:
[Mn: SITA–G]

- **S**ulfa drugs
- **S**ilicate (present in antacids)
- **I**ndinavir
- **T**riamterene
- **A**tazanavir
- **G**uaifenesin

Glomerular lesions associated with Hepatitis B infection:

- Type I MPGN
- Membranous GN
- FSGN

Glomerular lesions associated with Hepatitis C infection:

- **C**ryoglobulinemic glomerulopathy – MC
- MPGN Type I
- Membranous nephropathy

Features of Diabetic Nephropathy:

- Microalbuminuria → Earliest clinical

manifestation of diabetic nephropathy
- Glomerular Basement membrane thickening
- Diffuse glomerulosclerosis
- Nodular Glomerulosclerosis/Kimmelstiel Wilson lesion – Eosinophilic and PAS +ve nodule
- Papillary necrosis
- Armani Ebstein cells
- Capsular drop
- Glomerular hyalinosis

Radiolucent stones [Mn: TIXU]

- **T**riamterene stones
- **I**ndinavir stones
- **X**anthine stones
- **U**ric acid stones

Triple drug immunosuppression therapy for renal allograft recipient: [Mn: PAC/PMT]

- **P**rednisolone
- **A**zathioprine/**M**ycophenolate mofetil
- **C**yclosporine/**T**acrolimus

INVESTIGATIONS

- Best test for evaluation of renal function → DTPA scan
- **S**tructure Anatomy of the kidney is assessed by → DM**S**A scan
- Water deprivation test is used to access the → function of distal tubule
- Renal artery stenosis: Screening IOC → CT / MR Angiography
- *GFR Estimation:*
  ○ Inulin clearance → Gold standard test

  ○ Creatinine clearance → Can overestimate GFR as it is also secreted into the proximal tubules
  ○ Cystatin – C estimation
- *Formulas for GFR Estimation:*
  ○ Cockcroft Gault
  ○ MDRD
  ○ CKD-EPI
- Investigation of choice for renal calculi: NCCT KUB

SUMMARY OF MAJOR GLOMERULONEPHRITIDES

Disease	Features/Etiology	EM	Staining	LM	Lab findings	Extra Edge	
Heymann Nephritis		■ Sub epithelial	■ Granular pattern			■ Ag is located on Visceral epithelium & is k/as Heymann Ag or **Megalin**	Nephritic syndrome
Post Streptococcal Glomerulonephritis or Acute proliferative Glomerulonephritis	■ Immune complex mediated condition ■ Seen1-4 wks after a skin or pharyngeal infection ■ Caused by Gp-Aβ hemolytic streptococci ■ Majority of cases recover without treatment	■ Subepithelial humps ■ Subendothelial immune deposits of IgG, IgM & C_3	■ Granular IgG& C_3 in GBM and mesangium ■ Starry sky appearance	■ Diffuse endocapillary proliferation	■ Transient hypocomplementemia – returns to normal in 6-8 weeks ■ ↓ C3 ■ ↑ ASO & Anti DNAase	**Antigen** ○ NSAP → Nephritic strain Associated Protein ■ No role of immunosuppressive therapy	
Type I RPGN (Anti GBM Anti-body)	■ Good Pasture syndrome	■ GBM disruption	■ Linear IgG& C3 deposits along GBM	■ Presence of glomerular crescents in > 50% of glomeruli ■ Crescents are composed of Parietal cells, Leukocytes Macrophages & fibrin	■ Anti GBM Antibody	■ Prognosis is related to number of crescents.	Nephritic syndrome
Type II RPGN (Immune complex disease)	■ Idiopathic ■ Post-infectious ■ SLE, HSP, IgA Nephropathy	■ Subepithelial	■ Lumpy bumpy granular pattern		■ Low C_3 in SLE / lupus nephritis		
Type III RPGN (Pauci immune)	■ ANCA associated Wegener's, MPA	■ No deposits				■ Type III RPGN has Best Prognosis	
Type I MPGN (Most Common MPGN)	■ Subacute bacterial endocarditis ■ Malignancy ■ HBV, HCV, SLE	■ Sub endothelium & Mesangium	■ Granular pattern (C_3 with IgG, C_4)	■ Tram track or double contour appearance of GBM due to mesangial interposition between GBM & endothelial cells	■ Activation of both classical & alternate complement pathway ■ Low C_3 levels		Nephritic Syndrome
Type II MPGN (Dense deposit disease)	■ C_3 nephritic factor associated ■ Partial lipodystrophy	■ Dense deposits in the GBM	■ Granular & linear pattern of C_3 with absence of IgG	■ Mesangial & endocapillary proliferation ■ GBM thickening	■ Activation of alternate pathway ■ Serum contains C_3NeF result in hypocomplementemia (↓C_3 levels)		

RPGN – Rapidly Progressive GN (Crescentic GN) | MPGN – Membranoproliferative GN (Mesangiocapillary GN) |

Disease	Features/etiology	Deposits	LM	EM	Lab	Extra edge	
Lipoid Nephrosis *(Minimal change disease)*	▪ MC cause of Nephrotic syndrome in children	▪ No immune or Complement deposits	▪ Normal ▪ Lipid in tubules	▪ Effacement of the foot process of podocyte	▪ Highly selective proteinuria ▪ **C₃** levels **Normal**	▪ Responds to steroids ▪ Selective proteinuria – urine mainly contains albumin	Nephrotic
Membranous Glomerulopathy (MGN)	▪ HBV, HCV, Syphilis, Malaria, Schistosomiasis Leprosy, NSAIDS, RA, SLE , Malignancy	Sub epithelial deposits of C_3 and IgG	▪ Thickening of GBM ▪ BM projection as **'M' spike**	▪ Effacement of the foot process of podocyte		▪ Anti PLA2R Ab have high specificity	Nephrotic
IgA Nephropathy *(Berger's disease)*	▪ Recurrent gross hematuria following an URTI OR persistent asymptomatic microscopic hematuria	▪ Mesangial deposits of IgA_1 with C_3 and properdin	▪ Mesangioproliferative glomerulonephritis		▪ ↑↑ serum IgA ▪ Normal complement levels	▪ MC GN in world ▪ Mesangial cells express CD 71 ▪ ACE inhibitors can be used	Nephritic
Focal Segmental Glomerulosclerosis	▪ Associated with ○ Renal agenesis ○ **HIV** *(Collapsing variant)* ○ Reflux nephropathy ○ Hypertensive nephropathy ○ Heroin abuse ○ Sickle cell anemia ○ Hepatitis B	▪ Focal IgM + C_3 deposits	▪ Focal and segmental sclerosis and hyalinosis	▪ Degeneration & 'focal' disruption of visceral epithelial cells – **Hallmark**	▪ Mutation in: ○ **Podocin**→ AR FSGS ○ α-4 **actinin** → AD FSGS	▪ MC primary Nephrotic syndrome in adults ▪ MC subtype: NOS variant ▪ Worst prognosis: Collapsing FSGS ▪ Responds to steroids	Nephrotic

Clinical Significance of Cast

Hyaline Cyst	▪ Normal constituent of urine ▪ Due to Tamm Horsfall protein – aka Uromodulin ▪ Produced in the TAL of loop of Henle
RBC Cast	▪ Suggestive of Glomerular injury/Glomerulonephritis
WBC cast	▪ Interstitial nephritis ▪ Pyelonephritis (If associated with bacteriuria)
Pigmented muddy brown granular cast	▪ Tubular necrosis (ATN)
Broad granular cast	▪ Chronic Renal failure
Waxy cast	
Lipid cast/Fatty cast/Fat oval bodies	▪ Nephrotic syndrome
Eosinophilic cast	▪ Allergic interstitial nephritis

	PSGN	IgA Nephropathy/Berger's Disease	Good Pasture's Syndrome	Alport Syndrome	Diabetic Nephropathy
Facts	■ It is an immune mediated disease ■ Seen 1-4 weeks after a skin or pharyngeal infection ■ Due to group A β hemolytic streptococci (M type). ■ Usually affect children	■ Respiratory/GI exposure to environmental Agents → ↑ mucosal IgA Synthesis → Formation of circulating IgA complex → gets entrapped in mesangium ■ Seen in < 1 week of URTI ■ MC cause of GN worldwide	■ Autoimmune disorder characterized by formation of Anti GBM Ab against both capillary of lungs & glomerulus (GBM) ■ Antibody formed are against noncollagenous domain of α3 chain of **Type IV collagen**	■ MC hereditary Nephritis. ■ Due to abnormality in Type IV collagen. ■ MC form of Alport syndrome is d/t mutation of the **α5 chain of Type IV collagen** ■ α5-chain gene is located on 'X' chromosome ■ MC pattern of inheritance → X linked (classical Alport syndrome) ■ Can be inherited as X-linked, AR or AD	■ MC systemic disorder associated with Nephrotic syndrome ■ Overall MCC of Nephrotic syndrome ■ MC cause of chronic renal failure
Clinical features	■ Development of Hematuria 1-4 wks after an episode of URTI or skin infection (Delayed hematuria). ■ Oliguria, Edema, HTN ■ **Complete recovery in > 95% patients** ■ One attack confers lifelong immunity	■ Synpharyngitis hematuria → Development of Hematuria within 2-4 days of pharyngitis/URTI ■ Recurrent Gross Hematuria→ MC clinical feature ■ Persistent asymptomatic microscopic hematuria may be present ■ Usual age: 2nd – 3rd decade	■ Pulmonary manifestation: ○ Hemoptysis, ○ Pulmonary hemorrhage (Diffuse alveolar hemorrhage) ■ Renal manifestation ○ Features of RPGN like hematuria, Proteinuria, Rapidly progressive renal failure etc.	■ Similar to nephrotic syndrome ■ Presents with a **triad** of → 1. **Hereditary Nephritis:** ■ Recurrent gross hematuria ■ Proteinuria ■ Progressive Renal failure by 30 years 2. **Sensorineural hearing loss:** ■ MC extrarenal manifestation 3. **Ocular abnormalities:** ■ Anterior lenticonus is characteristic ■ Cataract ■ Keratoconus	■ Passage of foamy urine ■ May present with complications like Diabetic retinopathy, CAD, neuropathy etc
Investigations	■ Transient hypocomplementemia ■ C₃ levels ↓ & then return to normal ■ ASO titer↑ ■ Subnephrotic proteinuria (1-2 g/d) ■ RBC & WBC casts in urine	■ Normal C₃ level ■ ASO titre → Normal	■ Normal complement level. ■ Circulating IgG anti GBM Antibody ■ Dysmorphic RBC & RBC cast ■ CXR → Diffuse B/L pulmonary infiltrates ■ ANCA may be +ve in up to 30% patient	■ Kidney or skin biopsy ■ High frequency audiometry for SNHL ■ Genetic analysis	■ Microalbuminuria → 1st clinically detectable sign / Earliest clinical feature ■ Spot urine sample is preferred & is Best ■ Macroalbuminuria→ Indicates established disease
Microscopy	■ Crescents ■ Hypercellularity of mesangial & endothelial cells ■ Subendothelial deposits and subepithelial humps	■ Mesangioproliferative GN ■ IF →Mesangial deposits of IgA (subclass IgA₁) often with C₃ and Properidin ■ IgG deposits may also be seen ■ EM → Electron dense deposits in mesangium	■ Diffuse crescenteric GN ■ IF → Diffuse linear IgG staining along BM	■ EM → Irregular thinning & splitting of GBM giving a basket weave appearance or split basement membrane	■ Diffuse glomerulosclerosis: ○ MC pattern ○ Thickening of GBM ○ Capsular hyaline drops or fibrin caps may be present ■ Nodular glomerulosclerosis ○ Aka Kimmelstiel Wilson lesion ○ Pathognomonic of DM.
Extra edge	■ Early systemic antibiotic therapy for throat or skin infection will not eliminate the risk of GN ■ Recurrence → rare ■ Prognosis – excellent	■ Rx: ACEI for proteinuria ■ Recurrence → Common	■ T/T → Plasmapheresis	■ Lenticonus + Hematuria is considered pathognomonic for classical Alport. ■ Recurrence of disorder in renal transplant → rare	■ Armani - Ebstein cells → Tubular cells with glycogen deposit ■ Kidney size may increase in initial stage of disease

LUPUS NEPHRITIS

Class I	Minimal mesangial	Normal histology Mesangial deposits
Class II	Mesangial proliferation	Mesangial hypercellularity Expansion of mesangial matrix
Class III	Focal nephritis	Focal proliferation Focal subendothelial immune deposit
Class IV	Diffuse nephritis	Diffuse proliferation Diffuse subendothelial immune deposits*
Class V	Membranous nephritis	Thickened basement membrane Diffuse subepithelial immune deposits
Class VI	Sclerotic nephritis	Global sclerosis of glomerulus capillaries

*Wireloop lesion→ Thickening of the capillary wall due to subendothelial deposits → Seen in class IV or III of lupus nephritis.

DISORDERS AFFECTING RENAL TUBULE

	Disease or Syndrome	Gene Defect
Disorders Involving the Proximal Tubule	▪ Proximal renal tubular acidosis (RTA Type 2) ▪ Isolated renal glycosuria ▪ Hartnup disorder ▪ Dent disease ▪ X-linked recessive hypophosphatemic rickets	Sodium bicarbonate cotransporter Sodium glucose cotransporter Neutral amino acid transporter Chloride channel Chloride channel

Disorders Involving the Loop of Henle	▪ Bartter syndrome
	  ○ Type 1
	  ○ Type 2
	  ○ Type 3
	▪ Familial hypocalciuric hypercalcemia
		
		Sodium, potassium chloride cotransporter
		Potassium channel
		Chloride channel
		Calcium-sensing receptor

Disorders Involving the Distal Tubule and Collecting Duct	▪ Gitelman syndrome	Sodium chloride cotransporter
	▪ Pseudoaldosteronism (Liddle's syndrome)	Epithelial sodium channel (ENaC) β and γ subunits
	▪ X-linked nephrogenic diabetes insipidus	Vasopressin V_2 receptor
	▪ Autosomal nephrogenic diabetes insipidus	Water channel – Aquaporin 2
	▪ Distal renal tubular acidosis (RTA Type I)	Chloride Bicarbonate exchanger

BARTTER, GITELMAN & LIDDLE'S SYNDROME

	Bartter Syndrome (Mimics loop diuretics)	Gitelman Syndrome (Mimics thiazide diuretics)	Liddle's Syndrome (Pseudoaldosteronism)
Inheritance	▪ Autosomal Recessive	▪ Autosomal Recessive	▪ Autosomal Dominant
Pathophysiology	▪ Genetic defect in the TAL of loop of Henle ▪ Defect in Na-K-2 Cl⁻ co-transporters	▪ Genetic defect in the distal tubule ▪ Defect in Na-Cl co-transporters	▪ Genetic defect in the distal tubule ▪ Constitutive activation of amiloride-sensitive epithelial sodium channels
Presentation	▪ Early in life (**Mn:** Barter Baby) ▪ No hypertension ▪ Polyuria and Polydipsia ▪ Periodic paralysis	▪ Early adulthood (**Mn:** gitel**MAN**) ▪ No hypertension ▪ Polyuria and Polydipsia	▪ Early in life [Liddle in little age] ▪ Hypertension ▪ Fluid retention
Lab	▪ Hypokalemia ▪ Metabolic Alkalosis ▪ Normal serum magnesium ▪ ↑ Urinary Ca^{+2} excretion ▪ ↑ Risk of kidney stone ▪ ↑ Renal PGE_2 production	▪ Hypokalemia ▪ Metabolic Alkalosis ▪ Hypomagnesemia ▪ ↓ urinary Ca^{+2} excretion ▪ No ↑ risk of kidney stone ▪ (N) Renal PGE_2 production	▪ Hypokalemia ▪ Metabolic Alkalosis ▪ Low plasma renin ▪ Low/Normal aldosterone ▪ Low urine sodium ▪ ↑ serum sodium

*Bartter syndrome may be associated with sensorineural hearing loss |

Hypokalemia with Metabolic alkalosis	
With hypertension	*Without hypertension*
▪ Primary Hyperaldosteronism ▪ Liddle's syndrome	▪ Bartter syndrome ▪ Gitelman syndrome

RENAL TUBULAR ACIDOSIS

Features	RTA Type I	RTA Type II	RTA Type IV
Also Known as	Classic Distal RTA	Proximal RTA	Hyperkalemic RTA
Defect	Inadequate secretion of H+ ion from the Distal tubule	Decrease re-absorption of HCO_3 from PCT	Generalised transport abnormality of DCT
Urinary anion gap	+ ve/Normal	- ve	+ve/Normal
Minimum urine pH	>5.5	<5.5	<5.5
Serum potassium	Low	Low/Normal	High
Urinary Ca^{+2} levels	High	High	
Nephrolithiasis	Yes (Mn: st**one** in 1)	No	No
Fanconi's syndrome	No	Yes	No
Urinary levels of citrate	Low (due to ↑ reabsorption from PCT)	N/High	Low
Serum HCO_3^-	<10 mEq/L	>15 mEq/L	> 15mEq/L
Other findings		Glycosuria Aminoaciduria	

RENAL PAPILLARY NECROSIS

Etiology [Mn: POST CARD]	
▪ **P**yelonephritis ▪ **O**bstruction of the urinary tract ▪ **S**ickle cell anemia ▪ **T**B / Transplant rejection	▪ **C**irrhosis / **C**LD ▪ **A**nalgesic & **A**lcohol abuse ▪ **R**enal vein thrombosis ▪ **D**iabetes Mellitus – MC Cause

ACUTE AND CHRONIC KIDNEY DISEASES

	Acute Kidney Injury	Chronic Kidney Disease
Definition	▪ Rise in S. creatinine from baseline of at least 0.3 mg/dl within 48 hrs OR at least 50% higher than baseline within 1 week OR a reduction in urine output to <0.5 ml/kg per hour for >6 hours.	▪ Abnormalities of kidney structure or function (GFR < 60 mL/min/1.73 m²), present for ≥ 3 months
Labs:	▪ Hyperkalemia ▪ Hyperphosphatemia ▪ Hypocalcemia ▪ Metabolic acidosis with ↑ anion gap ▪ Hyponatremia ▪ Low erythropoietin	▪ Hyperkalemia >>Hypokalemia ▪ Hyperphosphatemia ▪ Hypocalcemia ▪ Metabolic acidosis with ↑ anion gap ▪ High PTH & FGF-23 ▪ Low vitamin- D ▪ Hyperuricemia
Biomarkers	▪ Kidney injury molecule-1 (KIM-1): ▪ Neutrophil gelatinase associated lipocalin (NGAL, aka Lipocalin-2) ▪ IL-18 ▪ Cystatin-C ▪ Clusterin ▪ Osteopontin ▪ Alanine aminopeptidase ▪ Cysteine rich protein	**CKD stage** — **GFR (ml/min/1.73 m²)** G_1 — ≥ 90 G_2 — 60-89 G_{3a} — 45-59 G_{3b} — 30-44 G_4 — 15-29 G_5 — <15

- RIFLE, AKIN and KDIGO criteria are used to define AKI.

Renal Failure Indices

Diagnostic Index	Prerenal ARF	Intrinsic ARF	Post Renal ARF
Fractional excretion of Na$^+$ (%)	<1	>1	>1
Urine Na concentration (mEq/L)	<20	>20	>20
Urinary osmolality (mosmol/L)	> 500	< 350	< 350
Urine/Plasma Creatinine (U_{cr}/P_{cr})	> 40	< 20	< 20
Urine specific gravity	> 1.020	~ 1.010	> 1.020
Serum BUN	↑↑	↑	↑
Serum BUN / Creatinine ratio	> 20:1	< 20:1	< 20:1
Urinary sediments	Hyaline cast	Muddy brown granular cast	Cellular Cast

NEPHROSCLEROSIS

- Term used to describe the kidney changes in a patient with hypertension.
- Sclerosis of the renal arterioles leads to reduced renal blood flow and contracted kidneys

	Benign	Malignant
Features	▪ Associated with benign HTN ▪ No RAS activation ▪ Renin levels is Normal	▪ Malignant/Acceleration HTN ▪ RAS pathway is activated ▪ Renin levels ↑
Gross	▪ Grain leather appearance	▪ Flea bitten appearance
Microscopic	▪ Hyaline arteriosclerosis ▪ Fibroelastic intimal hyperplasia	▪ Fibrinoid necrosis of arterioles ▪ Intimal Hyperplasia/Onion-Skin lesion

ESWL In Renal Calculi

Most Responsive	Most Resistant
▪ Calcium oxalate Dihydrate ▪ Uric acid calculi ▪ Magnesium Ammonium Phosphate stone	▪ Calcium oxalate monohydrate ▪ Cystine calculi

Referred Pain of Ureteric/Renal Colic

Site of Stone	Pain Referred	Nerve Responsible
Renal Pelvis	Testis	
Upper ureter	Testis	
Mid ureter	Iliac fossa, Groin (mimic appendicitis on Right side or diverticulitis on left side)	Iliohypogastric nerve
Lower ureter (Pelvic brim)	Thigh, Scrotum, perineum	Ilioinguinal nerve
Intramural ureter (VU Junction)	Tip of penis	

RENAL STONES

	Calcium Oxalate Stone (75%)	Struvite/Staghorn Calculi (15%)	Uric Acid Calculi (6%)	Cystine Stone (2%)	Xanthine Stone
Facts	▪ **MC** type of renal stone	▪ Aka infectious stone, Triple PO_4 stone	▪ MC radiolucent urinary calculi	▪ Hardest calculi ∴ ESWL not useful	
Gender		▪ F > M (due to ↑ chances of UTI)		▪ F > M	
pH	▪ Acidic urine	▪ Alkaline urine	Acidic urine (pH < 5.5)	▪ Acidic urine	
Composition	▪ Ca. Oxalate dihydrate – **MC** ▪ Ca. Oxalate monohydrate,	▪ Calcium, Magnesium & Ammonium phosphate			
Etiology/Pathogenesis	▪ Hypercalciuria → MCC Ethylene glycol poisoning ▪ Hypercalcemia ▪ Hyperoxaluria ▪ High Na intake ▪ Hypocitraturia ▪ Hypomagnesuria	▪ **Organism that produces urease** – Most commonly Proteus mirabilis ▪ Neurogenic bladder ▪ Excess alkali consumption	▪ Gout ▪ Leukemia ▪ Malignancy ▪ Hyperuricemia ▪ Lesch Nyhan syndrome ▪ High purine diet	▪ Failure of renal tubular reabsorption of **C**ystine, **O**rnithine, **L**ysine and **A**rginine	▪ Xanthinuria
Clinical features	▪ **Pain** – MC symptom ▪ **Bleeding** d/t irregular shaped stone with sharp projection, ▪ Associated with hypocitraturia and **RTA-1**	▪ Usually silent ▪ May lead to destruction of renal parenchyma		▪ Change in color of urine from yellow to green on exposure to air	
Morphology	▪ Monohydrate – dumb bell/hour glass shaped ▪ Dihydrate – enveloped/bi pyramidal shaped	▪ Coffin lid, opaque and radiolucent appearance	▪ Multifaceted, irregular Plates or rosettes (Diamond/Barrel shaped)	▪ Hexagonal/ benzene ring shape	▪ Smooth, brick red color, show lamination on cross section
X-ray	▪ Radio opaque	▪ Radio **opaque**	▪ **Radiolucent** calculi (MC)	▪ Radio opaque	▪ Radiolucent stone
Treatments	▪ Ca oxalate ○ Monohydrate → PCNL ○ Dihydrate → ESWL ▪ Brushite → PCNL (needle shaped) ▪ Low Na, Low Protein but normal Ca^{+2} diet to prevent recurrence ▪ Low Ca diet ↑risk of stone formation	▪ Best: PCNL + ESWL (moderately effective) ▪ Acetohydroxamic acid (irreversible inhibitor of urease)	▪ Low purine diet ▪ Allopurinol ▪ Alkalinisation of urine ▪ Most responsive to ESWL	▪ High fluid intake ▪ D-Penicillamine ▪ α – Mercapto Propionyl Glycine (MPG) ▪ PCNL ▪ Low methionine diet ▪ Alkalinisation of urine	▪ High fluid intake ▪ Allopurinol

CYSTIC DISEASES OF KIDNEY

	Childhood PKD / ARPKD	Adult PKD / ADPKD	Nephronophthisis	Medullary Cystic Kidney Disease
General	■ Inheritance → AR ■ Defective gene → **PKHD-1** – located on chromosome 6 ■ PKHD gene encodes for protein Fibrocystin	■ Inheritance → AD ■ Mutations in gene → PKD 1 & 2 – located on chromosome 16 & 4 ■ PKD gene produces polycystin protein	■ Inheritance → AR ■ MC genetic cause of ESRD in children ■ MC form – Juvenile Nephronophthisis	■ Inheritance → AD

Clinical features	■ Majority present during infancy
	■ Hypertension present
	■ Presenting with abdominal mass
	■ Proteinuria – minor feature
	■ Renal failure
	■ **Associations:**
	  ○ Oligohydramnios
	  ○ Potter's syndrome
	  ○ Pulmonary hypoplasia due to oligohydramnios
	  ○ Hepatic cysts may be seen
		■ Usually present in 4th – 5th decade
		■ Hypertension present
		■ Hematuria
		■ Proteinuria
		■ Nephrolithiasis → 15-20%
		■ **Extra Renal manifestations:**
		  ○ Cysts →**Liver (MC)**. Pancreas, spleen (Cyst are generally asymptomatic and LFT is Normal)
		  ○ Intra cranial i.e. **Berry's** aneurysm
		  ○ Mitral valve prolapse
		  ○ Colonic diverticulosis
		  ○ MC extra renal manifestation → Hepatic cyst
			■ Usually present in childhood
			■ No hypertension
			■ **Salt wasting** → Hyponatremia
			■ Loss of concentrating ability of urine leading to Polyuria, Polydipsia & Nocturnal enuresis
			■ Extra renal abnormalities:
			  (**Mn: SCARF**)
			  ○ **S**keletal abnormality
			  ○ **C**erebellar **A**taxia
			  ○ **R**etinitis Pigmentosa
			  ○ Hepatic **F**ibrosis
			  ○ Growth retardation
				■ Present with adult onset renal failure
				■ No hypertension
				■ **Salt wasting** → Hyponatremia
				■ Loss of concentrating ability of urine leading to Polyuria, Polydipsia
				■ Extra renal manifestations:
				  ○ Hyperuricemia & gout

Pathology (Gross and Microscopic)	■ **B/L enlarged** kidney ■ Outer Surface → Smooth ■ Cyst both in cortex and medulla ■ Sponge like appearance of kidney ■ Cyst arises from the **distal tubule** and CD ■ Long axis of cyst is at right angle to capsule ■ Cyst may be present prenatally, at birth or later in life	■ **B/L enlarged** kidney ■ Outer surface → Bosselated ■ Cyst distributed uniformly throughout cortex and medulla ■ Cyst contain straw colored fluid that may become hemorrhagic	■ Kidney size → N or reduced ■ Outer Surface → Smooth ■ Multiple cysts in the medulla and corticomedullary region ■ Loss of corticomedullary differentiation	■ Kidney size → N or reduced ■ Outer Surface → Smooth ■ Multiple cysts in the medulla and corticomedullary region

Tolvaptan (selective V2 receptor antagonist) is approved to slowdown the decline in renal function in rapidly progressing ADPKD |

MULTIPLE CHOICE QUESTIONS

CHAPTER 1: NEPHROLOGY

STRUCTURE AND FUNCTIONS OF KIDNEYS

1. A urine dipstick test shows 3+ proteinuria. What's the value of protein appearing in urine is: *(NEET 2018)*
- a. 100 mg/dL
- b. >1000 mg/L
- c. 300 mg/dL
- d. 3000 g/L

[Ref: Harrison's 19th/e pg. 293; Vasudevan's biochemistry 7th/e pg. 371]

Explanation

Proteinuria

- Protein or albumin to creatinine ratio is better predictor of chronic renal disease

Dipstick results

- *Analysis of dipstick results*
  - 1+ = 30 mg/dL
  - 2+ = 100 mg/dL
  - 3+ = 300 mg/dL
  - 4+ = 1,000 mg/dL
- *Grading of severity of proteinuria*
  - < 300 mg/day → Benign proteinuria
  - 300 - 1000 mg/day → Pathological proteinuria
  - >1,000 mg/day → Glomerular proteinuria
- **Transient proteinuria:** Temporary benign, self-limited e.g. orthostatic proteinuria that results from prolonged standing, but negative U/A after recumbency.

2. Podocytes are seen in- *(PGMEE 2012-13)*
- a. Bowman's capsule
- b. Collecting tubule of the kidney
- c. Distal convoluted tubule
- d. Proximal convoluted tubule

[Ref: Harrison's 20th/e pg. 2132]

3. Uremia occurs when total GFR is reduced to- *(PGMEE 2012-13, 2014-15)*
- a. 25%
- b. 50%
- c. 60%
- d. 80%

[Ref: Robbins 8th/e pg. 907, Harrison's 19th pg. 1811]

4. Tamm Horsfall protein is produced by- *(PGMEE 2012-13)*
- a. Ureter
- b. Loop of Henle
- c. Distal tubule
- d. Collecting duct

[Ref: Harrison's 20th/e pg. 2103]

5. Normal level of serum uric acid in males is: *(PGMEE 2015)*
- a. 1.5-3.3 mmol/L
- b. 1.8-4.4 mmol/L
- c. 3.1-7 mg/dl
- d. 2.5-5.6 mg/dl

[Ref: Harrison 18th/e pg. Appendix]

6. The protein in glomerular basement membrane responsible for charge dependent filtration is- *(PGMEE 2013, 2015)*
- a. Fibronectin
- b. Collagen type IV
- c. Albumin
- d. Proteoglycan

[Ref: Robbins 9th/e pg. 900,906,910]

Explanation

- The glomerular basement membrane (GBM) consist of collagen (mostly type IV), laminin, polyanionic proteoglycans (mostly heparan sulphate), fibronectin and several other glycoproteins. The charge dependent barrier function of GBM is mainly due to the anionic moieties like proteoglycans.

7. Dysmorphic RBC with ARF is seen in? *(PGMEE 2013)*
- a. Glomerural disease
- b. Distal tubule disease
- c. Renal carcinoma
- d. Proximal tubule disease

[Ref: Harrison's 20th/e pg. 2134]

8. Glomerular hematuria does NOT clot because *(PGMEE 2014; 2013)*
- a. Plasminogen activator urokinase is synthesized in the renal tubules
- b. Heparin like substance is present in urine
- c. Glomerular filtrate is acidic in nature
- d. Rapid and down urinary flow

[Ref: Internet]

9. Polyuria with low fixed specific gravity urine is seen in? *(PGMEE 2015)*
- a. Potomania
- b. Diabetes mellitus
- c. Chronic glomerulonephritis
- d. Diabetes insipidus

10. Microalbuminuria is defined as 24 hour albumin excretion of - *(PGMEE 2012-13)*
- a. 30-150 mg/d
- b. 30-300 mg/d
- c. 201-300 mg/d
- d. 301-600 mg/d

[Ref: Harrison's 20th/e pg. 2134]

11. Cells involved in interstitial cystitis ? *(PGMEE 2012-13)*
- a. Lymphocytes
- b. Macrophagus
- c. Neutrophils
- d. Mast cells

[Ref: Harrison's 20th/e pg. 286]

12. Positive dipstick for RBC with Red color urine and clear supernatant after centrifugation is due to: *(PGMEE 2015-16)*
- a. Porphyria
- b. Hematuria
- c. Hemolysis
- d. Rhabdomyolysis

1.	c
2.	a
3.	b
4.	b
5.	c
6.	d
7.	a
8.	a
9.	c
10.	b
11.	d
12.	d

13. **RBC cast is present in:** *(PGMEE 2015-16)*
    a. Acute tubular nephritis
    b. Acute glomerulonephritis
    c. Acute Pyelonephritis
    d. Acute interstitial nephritis

    [Ref: Harrison's 20th/e pg. 2106]

14. **Which of the following best defines Microscopic Hematuria as:-** *(PGMEE 2015-16)*
    a. 3 or More RBC/HPE   b. 5 or More RBC/HPE
    c. 25 or More RBC/HPF   d. 50 or More RBC/HPE

    [Ref: Harrison's 20th/e pg. 294]

15. **Best test for determining initital stage of renal insuffi-ciency?** *(DNB June 2009)*
    a. Serum creatinine   b. Serum urea
    c. Glomerular filtration rated. Creatinine clearance

    [Ref: Internet]

16. **All of the following may be associated with massive pro-teinuria EXCEPT:** *(PGMEE 2014-15)*
    a. Amyloidosis
    b. Renal vein thrombosis
    c. Polycystic kidneys
    d. Microscopic polyangitis

    [Ref: Harrison's 20th/e pg. 2152]

17. **All are true about GFR except ?** *(PGMEE 2015)*
    a. GFR is dependent on height in children
    b. C.K.D. is defined as GFR < 30 ml/min/1.732 for 4 weeks
    c. Best estimated by creatinine clearance
    d. 30-40% decrease after 70 years of age

    [Ref: Harrison's 20th/e pg. KDIGO Guideliness 2012]

18. **The kidney in sickle cell anemia is characterized by:**
    a. Pyuria   *(PGMEE 2014-15)*
    b. Inability to concentrate urine
    c. Decrease in glomerular filtration
    d. Inability to acidify the urine

    [Ref: Harrison's 20th/e pg. 693, 2161]

19. **The cause of oedema in Nephritic syndrome is-**
    (PGMEE 2012-13)
    a. Decreased in plasma protein concentration
    b. Reduced plasma osmotic pressure
    c. Increased in plasma protein concentration
    d. Sodium and water retention

    [Ref: Harrison's 20th/e pg. 239]

13.	b
14.	a
15.	a
16.	c
17.	b
18.	b
19.	d
20.	d
21.	a
22.	c
23.	d
24.	d
25.	d
26.	c
27.	d
28.	d

Explanation

- The heavy proteinuria depletes serum albumin levels in patients with nephrotic syndrome. This results in generalized edema as a consequence of ↓ed colloid osmotic pressure. Sodium & water retention is also seen which aggravates the edema.
- However, in Nephritic syndrome damage to glomeruli causes a fall in GFR and eventually produces uremic symptoms with salt & water retention, leading to edema and hypertension.

NEPHROTIC & NEPHRITIC SYNDROME

20. **Regarding complications of nephrotic syndrome incorrect is:** *(PGMEE 2014-15)*
    a. Volume overload state   b. Hypercoagulable state
    c. Hyperlipidaemia   d. Hypocalcemia

    [Ref: Harrison's 20th/e pg. 2142]

21. **False regarding nephritic syndrome:-** *(PGMEE 2015)*
    a. Hypoalbuminemia   b. Proteinuria <3.5g/day
    c. Generalize edema   d. Hypertension

    [Ref: Harrison's 20th/e pg. 2135]

22. **Lipid casts are seen in -** *(PGMEE 2013)*
    a. Cytomegalic inclusion disease
    b. Acute tubular necrosis
    c. Nephrotic syndrome
    d. None of the above

    [Ref: Robbins 9th/e pg. 914]

23. **All are true about nephrotic syndrome in children except?** *(PGMEE 2015-16)*
    a. It is not associated with hypertension
    b. Minimal change disease in children <10 year
    c. Massive Proteinuria> 3.5gm%/24 Hours
    d. Low Complement Levels

    [Ref: Harrison's 20th/e pg. 2135]

24. **Essential feature of nephritic syndrome is** *(PGMEE 2014-15)*
    a. Proteinuria   b. Hypoalbuminaemia
    c. Hyperlipidaemia   d. Hematuria

    [Ref: Harrison's 20th/e pg. 2135]

25. **In nephrotic syndrome all of the following proteins are reduced EXCEPT:** *(DNB June 2011)*
    a. Transferrin   b. Albumin
    c. Ceruloplasmin   d. Fibrinogen

    [Ref: Harrison's 19th/e pg. 1841]

26. **All are seen in Nephrotic syndrome except-**
    a. Atherosclerosis   *(PGMEE 2015)*
    b. Thrombo-embolism
    c. Increased protein C levels
    d. Lipiduria

    [Ref: Harrison 19th/e p. 1841]

27. **Most common cause of primary nephrotic syndrome in Adult:-** *(PGMEE 2015)*
    a. Amyloidosis
    b. Minimal change disease
    c. Membranoproliferative glomerulonephritis
    d. Focal segmental glomerulosclerosis

    [Ref: Harrison's 20th/e pg. 2142]

28. **Renal vein thrombosis is associated with which underlying disease of kidney:** *(PGMEE 2014-15)*
    a. Chronic glomerulonephritis
    b. Pyelonephritis
    c. SLE
    d. Nephrotic syndrome

    [Ref: Harrison 19th/e pg. 252]

29. Muehrcke lines in nails are seen in: *(PGMEE 2014-15)*
a. Nephrotic syndrome
b. Barrter syndrome
c. Nail patella syndrome
d. Acute tubular necrosis

Explanation

- These lines are seen in conditions associated with hypoalbuminemia.

30. Nephrotic syndrome patient after a bout of diarrhea presented with acute kidney injury and serum creatinine = 4.5. All are possible reasons except? *(NEET Pattern 14)*
a. Renal vein thrombosis
b. Diarrhea water depletion
c. Frusemide water depletion
d. Steroid induced diabetes

[Ref: Nelson's19th/e pg. 1756; Harrison's 19th p 1841]

31. Edema in nephritic syndrome is due to- *(PGMEE 2015)*
a. Elavated fibrinogen
b. Proteinuria
c. Sodium and water retention
d. Cardiac decompensation

Explanation

- Morning periorbital edemia is characteristic.

32. Cyclosporine in nephrotic syndrome acts by
a. Acts as an alkylating agent *(PGMEE 2015)*
b. Inhibiting calcineurin
c. Inhibition of GMPD
d. Antibiotic

[Ref: Harrison's 20th/e pg. 2128]

33. Which is seen in nephrotic syndrome-
a. Low Serum fibrinogen *(PGMEE 2012-13)*
b. High Serum ceruloplasmin
c. Low serum calcium
d. Low lipid

[Ref: Nelson 20th/e/ch 508]

34. Nephrotic syndrome associated with malaria is due to infection of? *(PGMEE 2014-15)*
a. P. malariae
b. P. ovale
c. P. vivax
d. P. falciparum

[Ref: Harrison's 20th/e pg. 2150]

Explanation

- Malaria due to P. falciparum can present clinically as nephritic syndrome (MPGN).
- Malaria due to P. malariae can present clinically as nephrotic syndrome (MGN).

35. The most common gene defect in idiopathic steroid resistant nephrotic syndrome-
(PGMEE 08; DNB Dec 09; PGMEE 2013; 16)
a. NPHS2
b. ACE
c. PAX
d. HOX 11

[Ref: Robbins 9th/e pg. 927]

36. Protein affected in steroid resistant nephritic syndrome-
(PGMEE 08; PGMEE 2013, 16)
a. Transient receptor potential-6
b. Alpha-actinin-4
c. Nephrin
d. Podocin

[Ref: Robbins 9th/e pg. 925]

37. The finnish type of congenital nephritic syndrome occurs due to gene mutations affecting the following protein *(PGMEE 2014; PGMEE 07)*
a. Alpha-actinin
b. CD2 activated protein
c. Podocin
d. Nephrin

[Ref: Robbins 9th/e pg. 912]

38. Post streptococcal glomerulonephritis causes-
a. Chronic renal failure *(PGMEE 2015)*
b. Nephritic syndrome
c. Primary Nephrotic syndrome
d. Secondary Nephrotic syndrome

[Ref: Harrison's 20th/e pg. 2135]

39. Characteristic finding in AGN: *(PGMEE 2014-15)*
a. Red cell cast
b. Hematuria
c. Proteinuria
d. Epithelial Cells

[Ref: Harrison's 20th/e pg. 2135]

40. RBC cast in the microscopic examination of the urine is an indicator of: *(PGMEE 2014-15)*
a. Acute glomerulonephritis
b. Acute pyelonephritis
c. Chronic glomerulonephritis
d. Nephrotic syndrome

[Ref: Harrison's 20th/e pg. 2135]

41. Manifestation of acute glomerulonephritis includes each of the following EXCEPT: *(PGMEE 2014-15)*
a. Peri-orbital edema
b. Hypertensive encephalopathy
c. Acute renal failure
d. Optic atrophy

[Ref: Harrison's 20th/e pg. 2135]

42. In Wegner's glomerulonephritis, the characteristics renal changes seen in- *(DNB June 10)*
a. Nodular glomerulosclerosis
b. Granulomas in the vessels wall
c. Focal necrotizing glomerulonephritis
d. Interstital granulomas

[Ref: Harrison's 20th/e pg. 2140]

43. Pauci immune glomerulonephritis is seen in-
a. Henoch- schonlein nephritis *(DNB Dec. 09)*
b. Microscopic polyangitis
c. After transplant in Alports
d. Lupus *[Ref: Robbins 9th/e pg. 912]*

44. First pathologcal change apparent in Nephrotic syndrome is- *(PGMEE 2014)*
a. Thickening of the glomerular capillary wall and effacement of podocyte foot processes
b. Break in basement membrane
c. Mononuclear infiltration
d. Segmental sclerosis of glomerulus

[Ref: Robbins 9th/e pg. 915]

29.	a
30.	d
31.	c
32.	b
33.	c
34.	a
35.	a
36.	d
37.	d
38.	b
39.	a
40.	a
41.	d
42.	c
43.	b
44.	a

GLOMERULAR DISEASES

POST STREPTOCOCCAL GLOMERULONEPHRITIS

45. True about post streptococcal glomerulonephritis is all except *(DNB December 2011)*
- a. Subendothelial deposition of IgG and C3
- b. Immunosuppressive are not used
- c. Recurrence is very common
- d. Complement decreases

[Ref: Harrison's 20th/e pg. 2137]

46. The following type of glomerulonephritis should not be treated with prednisolone: *(PGMEE 2014-15)*
- a. Minimal change disease
- b. Lipoid nephrosis
- c. Congenital Nephrotic Syndrome
- d. Post-streptococcal GN

[Ref: Harrison's 20th/e pg. 2137]

47. Serum C_3 is persistently low in the following except- *(DNB Dec. 07)*
- a. Post- streptococcal glomerulonephritis
- b. Lupus nephritis
- c. Glomerulonephritis related to bacterial endocarditis
- d. Membranoproliferative glomerulonephritis

[Ref: Harrison's 20th/e pg. 2137]

48. Focal segmental glomerulosclerosis is characterized by? *(PGMEE 2013)*
- a. Linear IgG and C3
- b. IgM and C3
- c. IgA ± IgG
- d. Granular IgG and C3

[Ref: Robbins 9th/e pg. 910]

49. The pathogenesis of acute proliferative glomerulonephritis- *(PGMEE 2013-14)*
- a. Antibody mediated
- b. Immune complex mediated
- c. Cell – mediated (Type IV)
- d. Cytotoxic T- cell mediated

[Ref: Harrison's 20th/e pg. 2137]

50. Post streptococcal glomerulonephritis presents with:- *(PGMEE 2015)*
- a. Massive renomegaly
- b. Massive anasarca
- c. Renal failure
- d. Asymptomatic hematuria

[Ref: Harrison's 20th/e pg. 2137]

51. Not seen in Post streptococcal glomerulonephritis are all EXCEPT ?
- a. Nephrotic range proteinuria
- b. Sub epithelial deposits
- c. Linear deposits
- d. Poor prognosis

[Ref: Harrison's 20th/e pg. 2137]

52. Post-streptococcal glomerulonephritis results in:- *(PGMEE 2015)*
- a. Acute tubular necrosis
- b. Nephritic syndrome
- c. Interstitial nephritis
- d. Nephrotic syndrome

[Ref: Harrison's 20th/e pg. 2137]

53. Which is seen in Electron microscopy in PSGN?
- a. Epithelial humps *(PGMEE 2015)*
- b. Subendothelial deposits
- c. Mesangeal deposits
- d. Spike and dome appearance

[Ref: Robbins 9th/e pg. 909-912]

54. Subepithelial humps are characteristic of:- *(PGMEE 2015)*
- a. Membranoproliferative glomerulonephritis
- b. Focal segmental glomerulonephritis
- c. Acute proliferative glomerulonephritis
- d. Rapidly progressive glomerulobephritis

[Ref: Harrison's 20th/e pg. 2137]

55. Which of the following types of glomerulonephritis is most likely to cause CRF all excep- *(PGMEE 2013, 15)*
- a. Post-streptococcal glomerulonephritis
- b. Focal segmental glomerulosclerosis
- c. Membranous GN
- d. Membranoproliferative GN

[Ref: Harrison's 20th/e pg. 2137]

RAPIDLY PROGRESSIVE GLOMERULONEPHRITIS

56. Type I RPGN is seen in:- *(PGMEE 2015)*
- a. Henoch schonlein purpura
- b. IgA nephropathy
- c. SLE
- d. Good pasture syndrome

[Ref: Robbins 9th/e pg. 912]

57. The crescent forming glomerulonephritis is:-
- a. RPGN *(DNB June 2008,2007)*
- b. Membrano proliferative GN
- c. Acute GN
- d. Membranous GN

[Ref: Robbins 9th/e pg. 913]

58. Crescents are derived from- *(PGMEE 2012-13)*
- a. Epithelial cells + fibrin + macrophage
- b. Tubule + mesangiaum + fibrin
- c. Mesangiaum + fibrin
- d. Mesangium + fibrin + macrophage

[Ref: Robbins 9th/e pg. 913]

59. Which of these does not cause crescentic glomerulo nephritis- *(PGMEE 2012-13)*
- a. Goodpasture syndrome
- b. Alport syndrome
- c. Rapidly progressive glomerulonephritis
- d. Henoch schonlein purpura

[Ref: Robbins 9th/e pg. 912]

60. Triad of glomerulonephritis pulmonary hemorrhages and antibody to basement membrane is called:
- a. Goodpasture's syndrome *(PGMEE 2014-15)*
- b. Systemic Necrotising Vasculitis
- c. Mixed connective tissue disease
- d. Diabetic

[Ref: Harrison's 20th/e pg. 2135]

45.	c
46.	d
47.	a
48.	b
49.	b
50.	c
51.	b
52.	b
53.	b>c
54.	c
55.	a
56.	d
57.	a
58.	a
59.	b
60.	a

61. Rapidly progressive glomerulonephritis is histologically characterised by the presence of numerous- *(PGMEE 07)*
  a. Hyalinized small arterioles
  b. Intramembranous dense deposits
  c. Atrophic proximal convoluted tubules
  d. Epithelial cell crescent
[Ref: Robbins 9th/e pg. 913]

62. All of the following causes RPGN Except:- *(PGMEE 2015)*
  a. Microscopic polyangitis b. Polyarteritis nodosa
  c. HSP d. Wegeners
[Ref: Robbins 9th/e pg. 912]

63. Feature of RPGN are A/E: *(PGMEE 2014-15)*
  a. Rapid recovery b. Crescent formation
  c. High blood pressure d. Non-selective proteinuria
[Ref: Harrison's 20th/e pg. 2135]

64. Linear deposits along glomerular basement membrane are seen in- *(DNB June 07)*
  a. Good pasture syndrome
  b. Drug reaction
  c. HS purpura
  d. SLE
[Ref: Harrison's 20th/e pg. 2139]

65. A patient presenting with haemoptysis and renal failure with antibasement membrane antibodies has- *(PGMEE 2012-13)*
  a. Good pasture's syndrome
  b. Henoch-schlolein purpura
  c. Churg Strauss syndrome
  d. Wegener's granulomatosis
[Ref: Harrison's 20th/e pg. 2139]

66. Good pasture's syndrome is characterized by- *(PGMEE 2013-14)*
  a. Necrotisting hemorrhagic interstitial pneumonitis
  b. Patchy consolidation
  c. Pulmonary edema
  d. Alveolitis
[Ref: Robbins 9th/e pg. 700]

IGA NEPHROPATHY

67. Which of the following is not true about IgA nephropathy? *(NEET Pattern 2019)*
  a. Majority of the IgA deposited is polymeric form of IgA1 subclass
  b. Characterized by episodic hematuria and deposition of IgA in mesangium
  c. Nephrotic syndrome commonly develops
  d. Persistent proteinuria for 6 months or longer points towards bad clinical outcomes

68. A female patient presents with upper respiratory tract infection. Two days after, she develops hematuria. Probable diagnosis: *(PGMEE 2014-15)*
  a. IgA nephropathy
  b. Wegener's granulomatosis
  c. Henoch-Schnlein purpura
  d. Poststreptococcal glomerulonephritis
[Ref: Harrison's 20th/e pg. 2140]

69. Berger's nephropathy is due to mesangial deposition of- *(DNB Dec. 09)*
  a. IgA and C3 b. IgD and C3
  c. IgE and C3 d. Fibrin and C3
[Ref: Harrison's 20th/e pg. 2139]

70. All the following are true regarding IgA nephropathy except *(PGMEE 2015)*
  a. IgA 1 deposition in the mesangium
  b. Can present as persistent microscopic hematuria
  c. ACE inhibitors can be used
  d. Decreased serum IgA level
[Ref: Harrison's 20th/e pg. 2139]

71. Organised glomerular deposits in kidney seen in all except *(PGMEE 2008; PGMEE 2013)*
  a. Cryoglobulinemia b. Diabetes Mellitus
  c. IgA nephropathy d. Amyloidosis
[Ref: Harrison's 20th/e pg. 2139]

72. True regarding IgA Nephropathy: *(PGMEE 2015)*
  a. Usually in children < 10 years
  b. Decreased serum IgA
  c. Recurrent gross hematuria following respiratory infection
  d. Microscopic hematuria is the most common presentation
[Ref: Harrison's 20th/e pg. 2140]

73. In IgA nephropathy (Berger's disease) there are- *(PGMEE 2013, 16)*
  a. Subepithelial deposits
  b. Basement membrane deposits
  c. Subendothelial deposisits
  d. Mesengial deposits
[Ref: Harrison's 20th/e pg. 2140]

74. Mesangial cells of IgA Nephropathy over-express which of the following marker- *(PGMEE 2014-15)*
  a. CD51 b. CD61
  c. CD71 d. CD81
[Ref: Pubmed article]

75. True regarding IgA Nephropathy are all EXCEPT: *(PGMEE 2016-17)*
  a. Most common nephropathy in adults
  b. CD72 is an important marker
  c. Recurrent gross hematuria is characteristic
  d. C3 levels are normal
[Ref: Robbins 9th/e pg. 923]

76. Most common nephropathy in world is:- *(PGMEE 2015)*
  a. IgA nephropathy b. Adult PSGN
  c. Minimal Change ds d. FSGS
[Ref: Harrison's 20th/e pg. 2139]

77. Selective proteinuria is seen in: *(PGMEE 2014-15)*
  a. Minimal change disease
  b. Mesangio-proliferative GN
  c. Membranous glomerulonephritis
  d. Focal segmental Glomerulosclerosis
[Ref: Harrison's 20th/e pg. 2142]

61. d
62. b
63. a
64. a
65. a
66. a
67. c
68. a
69. a
70. d
71. c
72. c
73. d
74. c
75. b
76. a
77. a

111. Plasmapheresis is indicated for which of the following: *(PGMEE 2014-15)*
a. Wegener's granulomatosis
b. Henoch-Schonlein purpura
c. Goodpasture's syndrome
d. Acute transplant rejection

[Ref: Harrison's 20th/e pg. 2139]

112. Visceral Leishmaniasis cause- *(PGMEE2013)*
a. Focal segmental golomerulonephritis
b. Rapidily progressive golmerulonephritis
c. Mesangiopoliferative glomerulonephritis
d. Membranous glomerulonephritis

[Ref: Robbins 9th/e pg. 920]

113. Nephrotic syndrome is the hall mark of the following primary kidney diseases EXCEPT: *(PGMEE 2014-15)*
a. Membranous Glomerulopathy
b. IgA nephropathy
c. Minimal change disease
d. Focal segmental Glomerulosclerosis

[Ref: Harrison's 20th/e pg. 2135]

114. Membranous GN with reduced complement level is seen in? *(PGMEE 2014-15)*
a. Hepatitis B   b. SLE
c. Malaria   d. Syphilis

115. In bronchogenic carcinoma patient presenting as a case of nephrotic syndrome. If kidney biopsy is done most likely lesion will be: *(PGMEE 2014-15)*
a. Membranous GN   b. Focal proliferative GN
c. Minimal change disease
d. Focal segmental glomerulosclerosis

[Ref: Harrison's 20th/e pg. 2144]

116. Chronic reflux nephropathy causes: *(PGMEE 2014-15)*
a. Membranous nephropathy
b. Focal segmental GN
c. MPGN
d. Lipoid nephrosis

[Ref: Harrison's 20th/e pg. 2143]

117. Most common nephropathy associated with malignancy? *(NEET Pattern 2015)*
a. Membranous   b. MCD
c. IgA   d. FSGS

[Ref: Harrison's 20th/e pg. 2144]

118. In thin basement membrane disease the defect lies in:- *(PGMEE 2015)*
a. Alpha-7 chain of collagen type IV
b. Alpha-3 and alpha-4 chains of collagen type IV
c. Alpha-5 chain of collagen type IV
d. Alpha-1 and alpha-2 chains of collagen type IV

[Ref: Harrison's 20th/e pg. 2147]

NEPHROPATHY IN SYSTEMIC DISEASES

DIABETIC NEPHROPATHY

119. The intracytoplasmic vacuoles seen in the Armanni-Ebstein cell are rich in- *(PGMEE 2014)*
a. Glycogen   b. Lipids
c. Na and K⁺   d. None of the above

[Ref: Harsh Mohan 5th/e pg. 701]

120. Nodular glomerulosclerosis is seen in:- *(PGMEE 2015)*
a. Diabetes mellitus
b. Amyloidosis
c. Multiple myeloma
d. Malignant hypertension

[Ref: Harrison's 20th/e pg. 2144]

121. Most specific histological lesion in diabetic nephropathy is- *(PGMEE 2015; DNB June 2011)*
a. Occlusion of glomeruli with fibrin caps
b. Nodular glomerulosclerosis
c. Glomerular crescents
d. Immune complex deposition

[Ref: Robbins 9th/e pg. 1118]

122. Kimmelsteil- Wilson lesions in kidney consists of-
a. Hyaline sclerosis   *(PGMEE 2015; 2013)*
b. Nodular sclerosis of the glomeruli
c. Hyperplastic arteriosclerosis
d. Splitting of glomerular basement membrane

[Ref: Harrison's 20th/e pg. 2144]

123. Kimmelstiel- Wilson lesion is characteristic of? *(DNB June 2007, PGMEE Nov. 12 & Aug'13)*
a. Diabetic nephropathy
b. HIV nephropathy
c. Analgesic nephropathy
d. Hypertensive nephropathy

[Ref: Harrison's 20th/e pg. 2144]

124. All are causes of granular contracted kidneys, except-
a. Chronic PN   *(DNB June 09)*
b. Diabetes mellitus
c. Benign nephrosclerosis
d. Chronic GN

[Ref: Harrison's 20th/e pg. 2119]

LUPUS NEPHRITIS

125. Wire loop lesion seen in HPE of kidney:-
a. SLE   *(PGMEE 2016-17)*
b. Wegener's granulomatosis
c. Crescenteric glomerulonephritis
d. good pasture syndrome

[Ref: Harrison 20th/e pg. 2518]

126. Drug induced lupus antibodies are found in- *(PGMEE 2013-14)*
a. Anti- Rho   b. Ds- DNA
c. Anti- Sm   d. Anti- histon antibody

[Ref: Harrison 20th/e pg. 2517]

127. According to WHO, membranous glomerulonephritis seen in SLE, is- *(PGMEE 2013-14)*
a. Class II   b. Class III
c. Class IV   d. Class V

[Ref: Harrison 20th/e pg. 2518]

128. Most common cause of death in SLE in children
a. Lupus nephritis   *(PGMEE 2014-15)*
b. Lupus cerebrits
c. Libman sacks endocarditis
d. Anemia and infections

[Ref: OP ghai 7th ed. Pg 603]

111. c	
112. c	
113. b	
114. b	
115. a	
116. b	
117. a	
118. b	
119. a	
120. a	
121. b	
122. b	
123. a	
124. b	
125. a	
126. d	
127. d	
128. a	

129. According to WHO, membranous glomerulonephritis seen in SLE, is- *(PGMEE 2013-14)*
a. Class IV
b. Class III
c. Class II
d. Class V

[Ref: Harrison's 20th/e pg. 2138]

130. Most common type of lupus nephritis- *(PGMEE 2013-14)*
a. Focal proliferative
b. Memberanous
c. Mesangial
d. Diffuse proliferation

[Ref: Robbins 8th/e pg.218]

HIV ASSOCIATED NEPHROPATHY

131. Most common renal lesions in HIV:- *(PGMEE 2015)*
a. MPGN
b. Membranous nephropathy
c. FSGS
d. RPGN

[Ref: Harrison's 20th/e pg. 2149]

132. Renal changes seen in AIDS- *(PGMEE 2014)*
a. Berger disease
b. FSGS
c. MCD
d. MPGN

[Ref: Harrison's 20th/e pg. 2149]

DISORDERS AFFECTING RENAL TUBULE

RENAL TUBULAR ACIDOSIS (RTA)

133. Normal anion gap is seen- *(PGMEE 2015)*
a. Chronic renal failure
b. Diabetic ketoacidosis
c. Methanol toxicity
d. Renal tubular acidosis

[Ref: Harrison's 20th/e pg. 317]

134. Hyperkalemia aciduria is seen in- *(PGMEE 2015)*
a. Type 1 RTA
b. Type II RTA
c. Type IV RTA
d. Sigmoidocolostomy

[Ref: Harrison's 20th/e pg. 320]

135. Hypokalemia is seen in: *(PGMEE 2015-16)*
a. RTA- I
b. RTA- II
c. RTA- III
d. RTA- IV

[Ref: Harrison's 20th/e pg. 320]

136. Renal tubular acidosis all are true EXCEPTE:
a. Impaired acid production *(PGMEE 2014-15)*
b. Impaired bicarbonate resorbtion
c. Inability to acidify urine
d. Nephrolithiasis

[Ref: Harrison's 20th/e pg. 320]

137. R.T.A shows all EXCEPT: *(PGMEE 2014-15)*
a. Urine pH < 5.5
b. Anion gap normal
c. Bicarbonaturia
d. Vitamin D deficiency

[Ref: Harrison's 20th/e pg. 320]

138. In which renal tubular acidosis, is hyperkalemia a prominent feature: *(PGMEE 2014-15)*
a. Type I
b. Type II
c. Type III
d. Type IV

[Ref: Harrison's 20th/e pg. 320]

139. Dent disease is characterized by all EXCEPT:-
a. Affects males more than females *(PGMEE 2015-16)*
b. Distal Renal Tubule defect
c. Chloride channel defect
d. Low Molecular Weight proteinuria

Explanation

- Dent diseases
  - Disorder affecting the PCT
  - Characterized by mutation in chloride channel
  - Affects M > F
  - MC feature : LMW proteinuria
  - Inheritance: X-Linked recessive

140. Dent disease is due to defect of? *(PGMEE 2013)*
a. Calcium channel
b. Sodium channel
c. Chloride channel
d. Potassium channel

[Ref: Harrison 18th/e 284]

141. Causes of low urinary calcium include:
a. Renal tubular acidosis *(PGMEE 2014-15)*
b. Cushing's syndrome
c. Chronic glomerulonephritis/CKD
d. Paget's disease

142. True about renal tubular acidosis are A/E:
a. Increased urinary anion gap *(PGMEE 2014-15)*
b. Bicarbonaturia
c. Hyperchloremia
d. High urinary PH

[Ref: Harrison's 20th/e pg. 320]

Explanation

- Refer to General medicine section for details of anion gap.

143. Distal renal tubular acidosis is associated with:- *(PGMEE 2015-16)*
a. Calcium stones
b. Citrate stones
c. Oxalate stones
d. Uric acid stones

[Ref: Harrison's 20th/e pg. 2172]

Explanation

- Calcium phosphate stones are more common in patients with Type I RTA (Mn : Stone) & primary hyperparathyroidism

TUBULOINTERSTITIAL DISEASE

144. Interstitial nephritis is common with *(PGMEE 2015-16)*
a. NSAID
b. Black water fever
c. Rhabdomyolysis
d. Tumor lysis syndrome

[Ref: Harrison's 20th/e pg. 2157]

145. Which of the following does NOT cause Polyuria: *(PGMEE 2015-16)*
a. Interstitial nephritis
b. Hypokalemia
c. A.D.H insufficiency
d. Rhabdomyolysis

[Ref: Harrison's 20th/e pg. 294]

146. Salt losing nephritis is: *(PGMEE 2014-15)*
a. Interstitial nephritis
b. Polycystic Kidney
c. Lupus nephritis
d. R.P.G.N

[Ref: Harrison 19th p 1856]

129. d
130. d
131. c
132. b
133. d
134. c
135. a,b
136. a
137. d
138. d
139. b
140. c
141. c
142. a
143. a
144. a
145. d
146. a

147. Mercury affects which part of the kidney- *(DNB Dec. 09)*
   a. PCT
   b. Loop of Henle
   c. DCT
   d. Collecting duct

   [Ref: Robbins 9th/e pg. 927]

148. Balkan nephropathy is caused by:- *(PGMEE 2015)*
   a. Calcineurin inhibitors
   b. Lead
   c. Fungal toxins
   d. Aristocholic acid

   [Ref: Harrison's 20th/e pg. 2162]

PYELONEPHRITIS

149. Histological feature of acute pyelonephritis are all except- *(PGMEE 2014)*
   a. Tubular necrosis
   b. Hypercellular glomerulus
   c. Patchy interstitial suppurative inflammation
   d. Intratubular aggregates of neutrophils

   [Ref: Robbins 9th/e pg. 911]

150. The most common infectious agent associated with chronic pyelonephritis is- *(PGMEE 2013-14)*
   a. Staphylococcus aureus
   b. Proteus vulgaris
   c. Klebsiella pneumonia
   d. Escherichia coli

   [Ref: Harrison's 20th/e pg. 969]

151. On one side kidney is normal, while other side kidney is contracted with scar, what is the most probable diagnosis? *(DNB June 10)*
   a. Chronic pyelonephritis   b. Renal artery stenosis
   c. Tuberculosis of kidney   d. Polycystic kidney

   [Ref: Robbins 9th/e pg. 934]

BARTTER'S AND GITELMAN SYNDROME

152. Which type of Bartter's syndrome is associated with mutations in barttin? *(NEET 2016)*
   a. Type 1
   b. Type 2
   c. Type 3
   d. Type 4

153. All of following are features of Bartter's syndrome EXCEPT: *(PGMEE 2014-15)*
   a. Hypertension
   b. Periodic paralysis
   c. Alkalosis
   d. Polyuria

   [Ref: Harrison's 20th/e pg. 321]

154. True about Bartter's syndrome are all except-
   a. Hyperkalemic alkalosis   *(PGMEE 2013-14)*
   b. Presents in neonate with ototoxicity
   c. Have Bartin gene mutation
   d. Autosomal recessive

   [Ref: Harrison's 20th/e pg. 2094]

155. All of the following are true about Bartter's syndrome EXCEPT:- *(PGMEE 2016-17)*
   a. A/w hypertension
   b. Hereditary hypokalemic metabolic alkalosis
   c. Use of frusemide can cause it
   d. Calcium levels are normal

   [Ref: Harrison's 20th/e pg. 321]

156. Gitelman's Syndrome incorrect is: *(PGMEE 2014-15)*
   a. Hypokalemic metabolic alkalosis
   b. Mimics thiazide diuretics
   c. Hypercalciuria
   d. Generally milder clinical course

   [Ref: Harrison's 20th/e pg. 321]

157. All are true regarding Bartter syndrome except?
   a. Hypokalemic alkalosis   *(PGMEE 2014-15)*
   b. Hypomagnesuria
   c. Congenital SN hearing defect
   d. Associated with Barttin mutation

   [Ref: Harrison's 20th/e pg. 321]

158. Hypertension with Hypokalemia is seen in- *(PGMEE 2015)*
   a. Gitelman's syndrome   b. Liddle's syndrome
   c. Bartter syndrome   d. All of the above

   [Ref: Harrison's 20th/e pg. 2729]

159. Low Renin Hypertension is seen in all of the following, EXCEPT:- *(PGMEE 2015-16)*
   a. Liddle's syndrome
   b. Conn's syndrome
   c. Essential hypertension
   d. Renovascular hypertension

   [Ref: Harrison's 20th/e pg. 1899]

Explanation

- Vasoconstrictor form of hypertension have associated high renin levels.
- Renovascular hypertension is an example of renin mediated form of hypertension

160. ENaC mutation is seen in:- *(PGMEE 2015)*
   a. Liddle syndrome   b. Gordon syndrome
   c. Bartter syndrome   d. Gitelman syndrome

   [Ref: Harrison's 20th/e pg. 2729]

161. A 7-year-old child presents with failure to thrive, hypokalemia, hypertension and metabolic alkalosis. What is the diagnosis: *(PGMEE 2018)*
   a. Barter syndrome   b. Gitelman syndrome
   c. Liddle's syndrome   d. Fanconi syndrome

162. Defect seen in Barter syndrome *(PGMEE 2018)*
   a. Thick ascending limb of Loop of Henle
   b. Proximal convoluted tubule
   c. Thin limb of Loop of Henle
   d. Distal convoluted tubule

   [Ref: Harrison's 20th/e pg. 2094]

PAPILLARY NECROSIS

163. Renal Papillary necrosis is seen in all EXCEPT:- *(PGMEE 2016-17)*
   a. Diabetes   b. Infection
   c. Sickle cell disease   d. Rheumatoid arthritis

   [Ref: Harrison's 20th/e pg. 2162]

164. Renal papillary necrosis can be caused by: *(PGMEE 2014-15)*
   a. Phenacetin   b. Sulphonamides
   c. Gentamicin   d. Penicillin

   [Ref: Harrison's 20th/e pg. 2162]

147. a	
148. d	
149. b	
150. d	
151. a	
152. d	
153. a	
154. a	
155. a,d	
156. c	
157. b	
158. b	
159. d	
160. a	
161. c	
162. a	
163. d	
164. a	

165. Renal papillary necrosis is caused by? *(DNB June 2010)*
a. Alcohol
b. Morphine
c. Heroin
d. Cocaine

[Ref: Harrison's 20th/e pg. 2162]

166. Papillary necrosis is seen with all except?
(PGMEE 2014-15)
a. Chronic alcoholism
b. Sickle cell anemia
c. Analgesic nephropathy
d. Medullary sponge kidney

[Ref: Harrison's 20th/e pg. 2162]

167. Papillary necrosis is seen in all the following except:-
(PGMEE 2015)
a. Sickle cell anemia
b. Diabetes mellitus
c. NSAIDs
d. Shock

[Ref: Harrison's 20th/e pg. 2162]

168. Renal papillary necrosis seen in all EXCEPT:-
(PGMEE 2013)
a. Analgesic nephropathy
b. Diabetes mellitus
c. Sickle cell anemia
d. Nephrosclerosis

169. Renal papillary necrosis is almost always associated with one of the following conditions - *(PGMEE 2012-13)*
a. Diabetes-mellitus
b. Analgesic-nephropathy
c. Post streptococcal GN
d. Chronic pyelonephritis

[Ref: Dorlands Illustrated Medical Dictonary 28th/e pg. 1104; Chapman's pg. 321]

ACUTE KIDNEY INJURY

170. RIFLE criteria is used for diagnostic of:
(NEET Pattern 2019)
a. Acute liver injury
b. Acute splenic injury
c. Acute bowel injury
d. Acute kidney injury

171. Acute renal failure results in- *(PGMEE 2015)*
a. Hypokalemia acidosis
b. Hyperkalemia alkalosis
c. Hyperkalemic acidosis
d. Hypokalemic acidosis

[Ref: Harrison's 20th/e pg. 2107]

172. All of the following causes acute renal failure except-
(PGMEE 2015)
a. Snakebite
b. Pyelonephritis
c. Analgesic nephropathy
d. Rhabdomyolysis

[Ref: Harrison's 20th/e pg. 2105]

173. Marker of acute kidney injury all except- *(PGMEE 2015)*
a. Acid phosphatase
b. Osteopontin
c. Clusterin
d. Alanine aminopeptidase

[Ref: Internet]

174. Non oliguric renal failure is seen in?
(DNB December 2011, PGMEE 2014-15)
a. Aminoglycoside toxicity
b. Post streptococcal glomerulonephritis
c. NSAIDS
d. Hypovolemia

[Ref: Harrison's 20th/e pg. 2103, 2105]

175. Oliguric phase of ARF is characterized by A/E:
(PGMEE 2014-15)
a. Chest pain
b. Acidosis
c. Hypertension
d. Hypokalemia

[Ref: Harrison's 20th/e pg. 2108]

176. In renal failure, metabolic acidosis is due to?
a. Increased H+ production *(PGMEE 2014-15)*
b. Loss of HCO3–
c. Decreased excretion of ammonia
d. Use of diuretics

[Ref: Harrison 19th p 1799, 1811]

177. Biomarker not involved in acute kidney injury is?
(NEET Pattern 2013)
a. NGAL
b. KIM 1
c. Micro RNA 122
d. Cystatin C

[Ref: Harrison's 20th/e pg. 2108]

Explanation
- Micro RNA 122 (miR-122) is a associated with hepato-cellular carcinoma and HCV replication.

178. The difference between sodium and chloride is low, the metabolic disorder in the patient would be?
a. Metabolic acidosis *(PGMEE 2014-15)*
b. Metabolic alkalosis
c. Respiratory acidosis
d. Respiratory alkalosis

[Ref: Refer to general Medicine]

179. Anuria is defined as urine output less than:-
a. 0.5 ml/kg/h *(PGMEE 2016-17, 2015-16)*
b. 1.0 ml/kg/h
c. 2ml/kg/h
d. 10 ml/kg/h

[Ref: Internet]

180. Anuria in clinical practice is defined as:-
a. Urine output < 100 ml/hr *(PGMEE 2015-16)*
b. Urine output < 400 ml/hr
c. Urine output < 800 ml/hr
d. Urine output < 1200 ml/hr

[Ref: Harrison's 20th/e pg. 292]

181. Polyuria is defined as: *(PGMEE 2019)*
a. Urine output > 40ml/kg/day
b. Urine output > 50ml/kg/day
c. Urine output > 60ml/kg/day
d. Urine output > 30ml/kg/day

182. In Hepatorenal syndrome, urine shows:
a. Proteinuria *(PGMEE 2014-15)*
b. Hematuria
c. A and b
d. No abnormality

183. Low erythropoietin level is seen in? *(PGMEE 2012)*
a. Aplastic anemic
b. Renal failure
c. Obesity
d. Hematoma

[Ref: Harrison's 20th/e pg. 2108]

184. Complication of diuretic phase of acute renal failure is:
a. Convulsion *(PGMEE 2014-15)*
b. Hyperkalemia
c. Increased sodium excretion in urine
d. Metabolic acidosis

[Ref: Harrison's 20th/e pg. 2108]

165.	a
166.	d
167.	d
168.	d
169.	a
170.	d
171.	c
172.	c
173.	a
174.	a,c
175.	d
176.	c
177.	c
178.	a
179.	a
180.	a
181.	d
182.	c
183.	b
184.	c

185. **Investigations in a patient of oliguria revealed: Urine osmolality: 800 mosm/kg. Urinary sodium 10 mmol/L. BUN: creatinine = 20:1. The most likely diagnosis is?** *(PGMEE 2014-15)*
   a. Prerenal acute renal failure
   b. Acute tubular necrosis
   c. Acute cortical necrosis
   d. Urinary tract obstruction

   [Ref: Harrison's 20th/e pg. 2107]

186. **The differentiating factor between pre-renal and renal azotemia is:** *(PGMEE 2014-15)*
   a. Sodium fraction excretion
   b. Creatinine clearance
   c. Serum creatinine level
   d. Urine specific gravity

   [Ref: Harrison's 20th/e pg. 2107]

CHRONIC KIDNEY DISEASE (CKD)

187. **Patient on insulin in CKD stage 4. What is the dose adjustment of insulin required?** *(PGMEE 2015)*
   a. Add DPP-4 inhibitors
   b. Decreased insulin
   c. Normal insulin
   d. Increased insulin

   [Ref: Harrison's 20th/e pg. 2118]

Explanation
- Kidneys contribute to insulin degradation & removal from circulation Thus, patients with CKD have elevated levels of plasma insulin, both in fasting and post prandial state. Therefore, as renal function deteriorates, insulin dose must be reduced. Other agents which require cautious use in a patient with renal failure include Metformin, Sulphonylureas, SGLT-2 inhibitors and DPP-4 inhibitors (except Linagliptin)

188. **The signs and symptoms of CRF are seen when the renal function deteriorates by?** *(DNB December 2011)*
   a. > 40 %
   b. > 50 %
   c. > 60 %
   d. > 70 %

   [Ref: Harrison's 20th/e pg. 2112]

189. **Which among the following is not seen in chronic renal failure?** *(DNB Dec'2010)*
   a. Hyperkalemia
   b. Hyperphosphatemia
   c. Hypercalcemia
   d. Hyponatremia

   [Ref: Harrison's 20th/e pg. 2115]

190. **CRF is associated with?** *(PGMEE 2012)*
   a. Respiratory acidosis
   b. Metabolic alkalosis
   c. Metabolic acidosis
   d. Respiratory alkalosis

   [Ref: Harrison's 20th/e pg. 2114]

191. **The most common neurological disorder seen in CRF patients:** *(PGMEE 2014-15)*
   a. Dementia
   b. Peripheral neuropathy
   c. Restless leg syndrome
   d. Encephalopathy

   [Ref: Harrison's 20th/e pg. 2118]

192. **Patient with CRF is having a sodium level =110mEq/dl. Till what level should serum sodium be corrected in next 24 hours?** *(PGMEE 2014-15)*
   a. 120 mEq/dl
   b. 130 mEq/dl
   c. 140 mEq/dl
   d. 150 mEq/dl

Explanation
- Refer to section of hyponatremia in General Medicine"

193. **Not seen with uremic lung?** *(PGMEE 2014-15)*
   a. Alveolar injury
   b. Pulmonary edema
   c. Interstitial fibrosis
   d. Fibrinous exudate in alveoli

   [Ref: Harrison 19th p 1796]

194. **Diagnostic feature of CRF is:** *(PGMEE 2014-15)*
   a. Broad casts in urine
   b. Elevated blood urea
   c. Proteinuria
   d. Bleeding diathesis

   [Ref: Harrison 19th p 1811]

195. **Which one of the following studies is most sensitive for detecting diabetic nephropathy in early stage?** *(PGMEE 2014-15)*
   a. Microalbuminuria
   b. Creatinine clearance test
   c. Ultrasonography
   d. Serum cretinine level

   [Ref: Harrison's 20th/e pg. 2878]

196. **CRF shows all EXCEPT:** *(PGMEE 2014-15)*
   a. Hyperphosphataemia
   b. Hyperuricaemia
   c. Decreased t ½ of insulin
   d. Decreased Serum vitamin D3

   [Ref: Harrison's 20th/e pg. 2118]

197. **CRF changes are A/E:** *(PGMEE 2014-15)*
   a. Hyperkalaemia
   b. Hypophosphatemia
   c. Hypocalcaemia
   d. Hypokalemia

   [Ref: Harrison's 20th/e pg. 2116]

198. **Raised PTH is found in:** *(PGMEE 2014-15)*
   a. Pseudopseudohypoparathyroidism
   b. Renal osteodystrophy
   c. Hypercalcaemia
   d. Osteogenesis imperfecta

   [Ref: Harrison's 20th/e pg. 2114]

199. **An adult patient presents with normal or enlarged kidneys with massive proteinuria. Most likely cause is:** *(PGMEE 2014-15)*
   a. Chronic pyelonephritis
   b. Chronic glomerulonephritis
   c. Amyloidosis
   d. Renal artery stenosis *[Ref: Harrison's 20th/e pg. 2119]*

Explanation
- Enlarged kidney can be seen in
  - Diabetic nephropathy
  - Amyloidosis
  - ADPKD
  - RCC
  - Hydroureteronephrosis
  - VHL,
  - Tuberous sclerosis (Renal angiomyolipoma)

200. **Central nervous system manifestations in chronic renal failure are a result of all of the following EXCEPT:** *(PGMEE 2014-15)*
   a. Hyperosmolarity
   b. Hypocalcemia
   c. Acidosis
   d. Hyponatremia

   [Ref: Harrison 19th p 2049]

185. a
186. a,d
187. b
188. b
189. c
190. c
191. b
192. a
193. c
194. a
195. a
196. c
197. b
198. b
199. c
200. b

201. Normal sized to enlarged kidneys in a patient with chronic renal failure is indicative of: *(PGMEE 2014-15)*
  a. Benign Nephrosclerosis
  b. Chronic glomerulonephritis
  c. Chronic interstitial nephritis
  d. Primary amyloidosis

[Ref: Harrison's 20th/e pg. 2119]

202. Chronic renal failure is often complicated by all of the following EXCEPT: *(PGMEE 2014-15)*
  a. Myopathy
  b. Hemolytic uremic syndrome
  c. Peripheral neuropathy
  d. Ectopic calcification

[Ref: Harrison's 20th/e pg. 2115, 2118]

203. Dementia in patient of chronic renal failure with chronic hemodialysis is due to: *(PGMEE 2014-15)*
  a. Aluminium toxicity
  b. Uremia
  c. A Beta amyloid
  d. A Beta amyloid deposition

[Ref: Harrison's 18th ed. ch. 371, 281 Table-371.5 DDx of Dementia]

204. In chronic renal failure there is: *(PGMEE 2014-15)*
  a. Decrease anion gap
  b. Normal anion gap
  c. Increased anion gap
  d. Metabolic alkalosis

[Ref: Harrison's 20th/e pg. 2114]

205. Convulsions are commonly precipitated in terminal renal failure by: *(PGMEE 2014-15)*
  a. Hyperkalemia
  b. Hypokalemia
  c. Water intoxication
  d. Hypermagnesemia

[Ref: Harrison 19th p 332e-9]

206. Anaemia of advanced renal insufficiency is best treated by:
  a. Blood transfusions *(PGMEE 2014-15)*
  b. Recombinant human erythropoietin
  c. Parenteral iron therapy
  d. Folic acid supplementation

[Ref: Harrison's 20th/e pg. 2118]

RENAL DIALYSIS

207. In uraemia all are reversed by dialysis EXCEPT: *(PGMEE 2014-15)*
  a. Sexual dysfunction
  b. Pericarditis
  c. Uraemic lung
  d. Neuropathy

[Ref: Harrison 19th p 1823]

208. Definitive treatment of hypermagnesemia is? *(DNB June 2009)*
  a. Calcium gluconate
  b. IV fluids
  c. Exchange resins
  d. Hemodialysis

[Ref: Harrison's 20th/e pg. 2918]

209. Dialysis disequilibrium occurs due to:
  a. Cerebral edema *(PGMEE 2014-15)*
  b. Hypertension
  c. Alumunium toxicity
  d. A Beta2 amyloid deposition

[Ref: Harrison 19th p 250]

210. Dialysis disequilibrium occurs due to:- *(PGMEE 2015-16)*
  a. Aluminum toxicity
  b. Hypertension
  c. Amyloid deposition
  d. Reserve Urea effect

[Ref: Replacement of Renal Function by Dialysis (Springer) 4th/e pg. 422]

211. Most common type of renal cell cancer in dialysis patient is? *(PGMEE 2014-15)*
  a. Clear cell carcinoma
  b. Oncocytoma
  c. Bellini tumour
  d. Papillary carcinoma

[Ref: Devita, Hellman and Rosenberg's Cancer: Principles and Practice of Oncology, 8th /e ch. 40 - Cancers of the Genitourinary System, Section 3: Cancer of the Kidney]

212. Dialysis indications- *(PGMEE 2015)*
  a. Hypokalemia
  b. Hypertension
  c. Metabolic alkalosis
  d. Pericarditis

[Ref: Harrison 19th/e p. 1810, 1822]

213. Hemodialysis can be performed for long periods from the same site due to ?
  a. Arteriovenous fistula facilitates small bore needles for high flow rates
  b. Arteriovenous fistula reduces bacterial contamination of site
  c. Arteriovenous fistula reduces chances of graft failure
  d. Arteriovenous fistula results in arterialization of vein

[Ref: Harrison 19th/e 1823-23]

214. Chronic hemodialysis in ESRD patient is done- *(PGMEE 2015)*
  a. Daily
  b. Twice per week
  c. Once per week
  d. Thrice per week

[Ref: Harrison's 20th/e pg. 2124]

215. The following are the complications of haemodialysis except- *(PGMEE 2015)*
  a. Peritonitis
  b. Bleeding tendency
  c. Hypotension
  d. Hypertension

[Ref: Harrison's 20th/e pg. 2125]

216. Most common acute complication of dialysis is- *(PGMEE 2015)*
  a. Demantia
  b. Muscle carcinoma
  c. Bleeding
  d. Hypotension

[Ref: Harrison's 20th/e pg. 2124]

217. Which of the following Microorganism is incriminated in infection after Hemodialysis? *(PGMEE 2015-16)*
  a. Chlamydia
  b. Gram positive
  c. Gram negative
  d. Anaerobes

[Ref: Harrison 18th edition, chapter 281]

218. Amyloidosis protein associated with hemodialysis? *(PGMEE 2014-15)*
  a. $A\beta_2$
  b. $A\beta$
  c. A transthyretin
  d. AL

[Ref: Harrison's 20th/e pg. 804]

219. $A\beta_2$ microglobulins are deposited in: - *(PGMEE 2016-17)*
  a. Alzhiemers disease
  b. Dialysis patient
  c. Parkinsons disease
  d. Familial Mediterranean fever

[Ref: Harrison's 20th/e pg. 804]

201. d
202. b
203. a
204. c
205. c
206. b
207. a
208. d
209. a
210. d
211. d
212. d
213. d
214. d
215. a
216. d
217. b
218. a
219. b

220. A patient of ESRD is being performed hemodialysis. Central dialysis cathreter is placed at which site ?

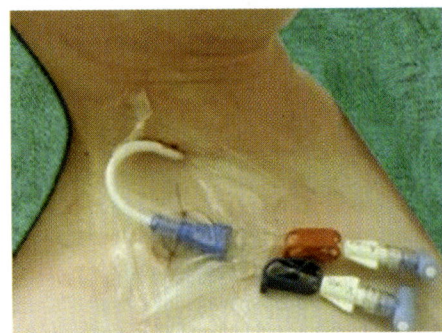

a. Right internal jugular vein
b. Left internal jugular vein
c. Right subclavian vein
d. Right subclavian artery

[Ref: KDIGO 2012 guidelines]

221. The patient is scheduled for haemodialysis. The A-V fistula is called as? *(PGMEE 2015-16)*

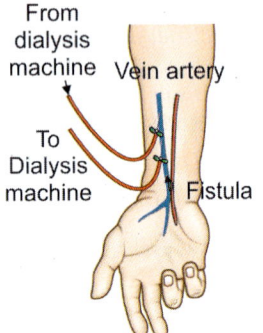

a. Cimino- Brescia fistula
b. Hughes fistula
c. SLED (sustained Low efficiency dialysis)
d. Continuous renal replacement therapy

222. The absolute indications for dialysis include the following EXCEPT: *(PGMEE 2014-15)*

a. Persistent Hyperkalaemia
b. Congestive cardiac failure
c. Pulmonary edema
d. Hyperphosphatemia

[Ref: Harrison 19th p 1810]

Explanation

Indications of dialysis:

Intractable volume overload	Uremic complications
Severe metabolic acidosis	- Asterixis
Refractory hyperkalemia	- Pericardial rub/effusion
Certain poisoning & drug overdose (Eg: Lithium)	- Encephalopathy Uremic bleeding

223. Most common complication causing death in patients on recurrent hemodialysis? *(PGMEE 2014-15)*

a. Cardiovascular
b. Adynamic osteomalacia
c. Dyselectrolytemia
d. Encephalopathy

[Ref: Harrison 19th p 1810]

224. All of the following uremic manifestations improve with dialysis EXCEPT: *(PGMEE 2014-15)*

a. Metabolic acidosis
b. Osteodystrophy
c. Asterixis
d. Nausea, vomiting and anorexia

[Ref: Harrison 19th p 291/2478]

225. Following are absolute indication for hemo-dialysis EXCEPT: *(PGMEE 2014-15)*

a. GI bleeding
b. Convulsions
c. Pericarditis
d. Hyperkalemia of 6.5 mEq/L

[Ref: Harrison 19th p 1823]

226. Dialysis patients are prone to develop: *(PGMEE 2014-15)*

a. Lead toxicity
b. Iron toxicity
c. Aluminium toxicity
d. Zinc toxicity

[Ref: Harrison's 18th ed. ch. 281]

RENAL TRANSPLANTATION

227. A patient recently underwent a renal allograft transplantation and on treatment with azathioprine and prednisolone He developed, fever and cough with thick sputum and left lower lung consolidation with a cavity. The culture specimen demonstrates gram+ve organism with beaded string appearance. Initial treatment will include: *(PGMEE 2014-15)*

a. Penicillin
b. Erythromycin
c. Ceftazidime
d. TMZ-SMX

[Ref: Harrison's 20th/e pg. 1219]

Explanation

- Diagnosis : Nocardiosis
- DOC : Trimethoprim - Sulfamethoxazole

220. A 40-year-old man underwent kidney trans-plantation for end-stage renal disease. Two months after transplantation, he developed, fever and features suggestive of bilateral diffuse interstitial pneumonia. Which one of the following is the most likely etiological agent? *(PGMEE 2014-15)*

a. Herpes simplex virus
b. Cytomegalovirus
c. Epstein-Barr virus
d. Legionella

[Ref: Harrison's 20th/e pg. 1363]

Explanation

Opportunistic infection	Pulmonary involvement
Cytomegalovirus	▪ B/L diffuse interstitial or pathy pneumonia
Pneumocystis jiroveci	▪ B/L pulmonary infiltrates s/o interstitial pneumonia on x-ray ▪ Diffuse ground glass opacification on HRCT
Legionella	▪ UL > BL involvement ▪ Nodular to multilobar involvement (interstitial involvement is rare)
Epstein-Barr virus	▪ None
Nocardia	▪ Consolidation & cavitation

220. a
221. a
222. d
223. a
224. b
225. d
226. c
227. d
228. b

229. The most common ocular infection after renal transplantation is by: *(PGMEE 2014-15)*

a. Cytomegalovirus
b. Toxoplasma
c. Herpes virus
d. EB virus

[Ref: Harrison 19th p 1190]

230. Most common cancer after kidney transplantation? *(PGMEE 2014-15)*

a. Skin cancer
b. Renal cell cancer
c. NHL
d. Hodgkins lymphoma

[Ref: Harrison's 20th/e pg. 2131]

231. After renal transplant, recurrence of the disease occurs mostly with: *(PGMEE 2014-15)*

a. Lupus nephritis
b. DM nephropathy
c. Membranous glomerulonephritis
d. Membranous proliferative glomerulonephritis

[Ref: Harrison 19th p 1841]

Explanation

Glomerulonephritis	Recurrence risk after transplant
FSGS	▪ 20-30%
IgA Nephropathy	▪ 20-60%
Membranous nephropathy	▪ 10-30%
MPGN Type I	▪ 20-30%
MPGN Type II	▪ 50-100%
Lupus nephritis	▪ 2-10%
Diabetic nephropathy	▪ 50-10%

232. All are true for transplanted kidney except- *(PGMEE 2015)*

a. Humoral antibody responsible for rejection
b. HLA identity similarity seen in 1:100 people
c. Previous blood transfusion increases chances of rejection
d. CMI is responsible for rejection

[Ref: Harrison's 20th/e pg. 2127]

233. An emerging viral pathogen causing pyelonephritis in kidney allografts:- *(PGMEE 2015; DNB Dec. 10)*

a. Polyoma virus
b. JC virus
c. Ebola virus
d. Marburg virus

[Ref: Robbins 9th/e pg. 953, Harrison's 20th/e pg. 2130]

234. First sign/symptom of renal graft rejection is ? *(PGMEE 2013)*

a. Tenderness
b. Fever
c. Increase creatinine
d. Rash

[Ref: Harrison's 20th/e pg. 2129]

Explanation

▪ In case of transplant rejection, clinical evidence in the form of fever, swelling and tenderness over the auograft in rarely appreciated. Rise in serum creatinine may be the only initial evidence which may or may not present with a reduction in urine volume.

VASCULAR INJURY

RENOVASCULAR HYPERTENSION

235. The accurate diagnostic aid in renal artery stenosis is:

a. Selective renal angiography *(PGMEE 2014-15)*
b. Ultrasound
c. CT scan
d. IVU

[Ref: Harrison's 20th/e pg. 1897]

236. Renal artery stenosis is associated with:

a. High renin Hypertension *(PGMEE 2014-15)*
b. Normal renin hypertension
c. Low renin hypertension
d. Fibrinoid necrosis of vessels

[Ref: Harrison's 20th/e pg. 1896]

237. Which is characteristic feature of malignant hypertension in kidney? *(PGMEE 2014-15)*

a. Hyaline necrosis
b. Fibrinoid necrosis
c. Medical wall hyperplasia
d. Micro-aneurysm

[Ref: Harrison's 20th/e pg. 1895]

NEPHROSCLEROSIS

238. Characteristic histological finding in benign hypertension:- *(PGMEE 2015; 2013-14, 2012-13; DNB June 07)*

a. Proliferative endarteritis
b. Cystic medial necrosis
c. Hyaline arteriosclerosis
d. Necrotizing arteriolitis

[Ref: Harrison's 20th/e pg. 1909]

239. Characteristic feature of benign nephrosclerosis:-

a. Leather grain appearance *(PGMEE 2015)*
b. Flea bitten appearance
c. Hyperplastic arteriosclerosis
d. Onion skin appearance

[Ref: Robbins 9th/e pg. 938]

240. Flea bitten appearance of the kidney is seen in- *(PGMEE 2012-13)*

a. Diabetes mellitus
b. Benign hypertension
c. Chronic pyelonephritis
d. Malignant hypertension

[Ref: Robbins 9th/e pg. 939]

241. Gross renal changes seen in malignant hypertension is

a. Flea bitten kidney *(PGMEE 2015, 2012-13)*
b. Granular contracted and irregular kidney
c. Waxy and enlarged kidney
d. No change

[Ref: Robbin's 9th/e pg. 939]

242. Onion skin thickening of arteriolar wall is seen in

a. Atherosclerosis *(DNB Dec' 2008, PGMEE 2013-14)*
b. Median calcific sclerosis
c. Hyaline arteriosclerosis
d. Hyperplastic arteriosclerosis

[Ref: Robbin's 9th/e pg. 939 , 490]

229. a
230. a
231. d
232. b
233. a
234. c
235. a
236. a
237. b
238. c
239. a
240. d
241. a
242. d

243. Onion skin lesion in vessel wall are seen in-
a. Malignant hypertension   *(PGMEE 2013-14)*
b. Peripheral vascular disease
c. Benign hypertension
d. None

[Ref: Robbin's 9th/e pg. 495-496]

244. Hyperplastic arteriolitis with necrotizing arteriolitis is seen in?   *(PGMEE 2013)*
a. Buerger's disease
b. Wegner's granulomatosis
c. Benign hypertension
d. Malignant hypertension

[Ref: Robbin's 9th/e pg. 490]

CYSTIC DISEASES OF KIDNEY

245. Least common cause of renal mass:-   *(PGMEE 2015)*
a. Wilm's tumor
b. Hydronephrosis
c. Renal cysts
d. Renal cell carcinoma

[Ref: Robbins 9th/e pg. 953]

246. Most common cystic disease of kidney is:-   *(PGMEE 2015)*
a. X linked recessive polycystic kidney disease
b. Autosomal recessive polycystic kidney disease
c. X linked dominant polycystic kidney disease
d. Autosomal dominant polycystic kidney disease

[Ref: Harrison's 20th/e pg. 2150]

247. Adult polycystic kidney disease is-   *(PGMEE 2012-13)*
a. Autosomal dominant
b. Mitochondrial
c. X-linked
d. Autosomal recessive

[Ref: Harrison's 20th/e pg. 2151]

248. PKD1 mutation associated with kidney disease shown below. Diagnosis is:-   *(PGMEE 2016-17)*

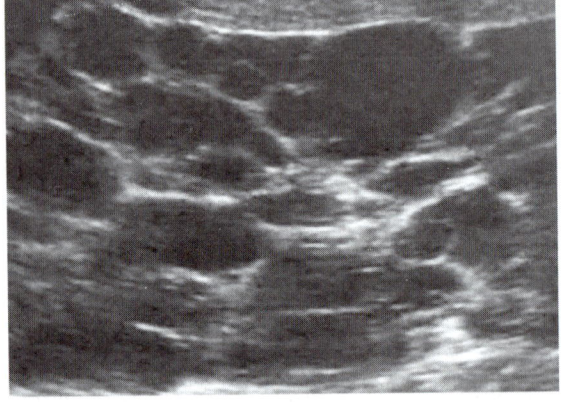

a. X linked recessive polycystic kidney disease
b. Autosomal recessive polycystic kidney disease
c. X linked dominant polycystic kidney disease
d. Autosomal dominant polycystic kidney disease

[Ref: Harrison's 20th/e pg. 2151]

249. Which of the following is most common extrarenal involvement in ADPKD-   *(PGMEE 2014, 16)*
a. Hepatic cysts
b. Splenic cysts
c. Colonic diverticulosis
d. Mitral valve prolapse

[Ref: Harrison's 20th/e pg. 2152]

250. Cyst not found in Autosomal dominant polycystic kidney (ADPKD) is-   *(PGMEE 2014; 2015)*
a. Liver
b. Kidney
c. Lung
d. Brain

[Ref: Robbins 9th/e pg. 947; Harrison 19th p 477t]

251. All can be manifestations of polycystic kidney EXCEPT: *(PGMEE 2014-15)*
a. Urine retention
b. Renal hypertension
c. Renal failure
d. Haematuria

[Ref: Harrison's 20th/e pg. 2152]

252. Commonest Symptom of medullary sponge kidney disease: *(PGMEE 2014-15)*
a. Anuria
b. Anemia
c. Azotemia
d. UTI

[Ref: Harrison's 20th/e pg. 2156]

253. Most common intra-abdominal mass in neonates is?   *(PGMEE 2014-15)*
a. Rhabdomyosarcoma
b. Wilm's tumor
c. Hydronephrosis
d. Multi-cystic dysplastic kidney

[Ref: Nelson textbook 18th /e ch. 537]

254. Chromosomal location of adult polycystic kidney disease type I and II respectively is: *(PGMEE 2014-15, 2016)*
a. Chr 16 and 5
b. Chr 16 and 4
c. Chr 11 and 5
d. Chr 21 and 18

[Ref: Robbins 9th/e pg. 945, Harrison 19th p 1851]

255. Medullary cystic kidney disease is best diagnosed by: *(PGMEE 2014-15)*
a. Radio nucleotide scanning
b. Biopsy
c. USG
d. CT Scan

[Ref: Harrison 19th p 1854]

256. Hepatic fibrosis is found in:-   *(PGMEE 2016)*
a. ADPCKD
b. Medullary cystic kidney
c. ARPCKD
d. Nephrophthosis

[Ref: Robbins 9th/e pg. 945; Refer to pretexts]

257. Gross section of kidney depicts what:-   *(PGMEE 2015)*
a. RCC
b. Hydatid cyst
c. Medullary sponge kidney
d. Polycystic kidney disease

[Ref: Robbins 9th/e pg. 945]

258. Cylindrical dilations of renal tubules is seen in-
a. Polycytic disease of kidney   *(PGMEE 2014)*
b. Medullary cystic disease
c. Lipoid nephrosis
d. Wilms' tumor

[Ref: Robbins 9th/e pg. 946]

259. Which of the following is not associated with adult polycystic kidney disease? -   *(PGMEE 2015)*
a. Autosomal dominant inheritance
b. Tricuspid valve prolapse
c. Mutations involving gene affecting cell-cell-matrix interation
d. Intracranial berry aneurysm may be present

[Ref: Robbins 9th/e pg. 946]

243. a
244. d
245. c
246. d
247. a
248. d
249. a
250. d
251. a
252. d
253. d
254. b
255. d
256. c,d
257. d
258. a
259. b

Explanation

- PKD-1 gene which is located on chromosome 16 encodes for Polycystin-1, a transmembrane protein responsible for cell to cell and cell to extracellular matrix binding.
- PKD-2 gene (located on chrosome 4) encodes for Polycystin-2 which in conjugation with polycystin-1, acts as a calcium channel.

NEPHROCALCINOSIS

260. Nephrocalcinosis is seen in all EXCEPT:
(PGMEE 2014-15)

a. Polycystic kidney   b. Hyperparathyroidism
c. Medullary sponge kidney d. Renal tubular acidosis

[Ref: Harrison 19th p 477t]

Explanation

- Nephrocalcinosis is a condition characterised by deposition of calcium salts in the renal paranchyma.
- MC form of nephrocalcinosis Renal medullary nephrocalcinosis
- Etiology:
  - Hypedrparathyroidism - Sarcoidosis
  - Medullary Sponge Kidney - Multiple myeloma
  - RTA (Type 1) - Bartter syndrome
  - Milk - alkali syndrome - Hypervitaminosis D

261. Nephrocalcinosis is common in which type of renal tubular acidosis:
(PGMEE 2014-15)

a. Type I   b. Type II
c. Type III   d. Type IV

[Ref: Harrison 19th p 332e-7t]

NEPHROLITHIASIS

262. Which of these is correct about Struvite stones?

a. Present in alkaline urine   (PGMEE 2015-16)
b. Most common kidney disease
c. Are Calcium pyrophosphate stones
d. Most common kidney stones

[Ref: Harrison 19th ed. / 1871]

263. IOC for ureteric stone?   (PGMEE 2015-16)

a. CT scan   b. USG
c. MIBG scan   d. DMSA scan

[Ref: Bailey and love 26th/e pg. 1293; Harrison 19th pg.1866]

264. Most common cause of calcium oxalate stones is?

a. Hyper-parathyrodism   (PGMEE 2014-15)
b. Idiopathic Hypercalciuria
c. Dietary intake of milk based products
d. Renal tubular acidosis type 1

[Ref: Harrison 19th p 2237]

265. Which of the following helps most in nephrolithiasis?
(PGMEE 2015-16)

a. Low sodium diet   b. Low calcium diet
c. High sodium diet   d. Low citrate diet

[Ref: Harrison 19th ed. / 1870-71]

266. Xanthogranulomatous pyelonephritis associated stones are due to infection with?

a. Proteus   b. Klebsiella
c. Pseudomonas   d. E coli

[Ref: Tarascon Pocket Urological by Pamela Ellsworth page 8]

267. Renal calculi associated with proteus infection:
(PGMEE 2016-17)

a. Struvite stone   b. Calcium oxalate
c. Calcium phosphate   d. Uric acid stone

[Ref: Sabiston's 1st SAE pg. 2083]

268. Radiolucent renal stones are composed of-

a. Calcium phosphate   b. Cysteine
c. Calcium phosphate   d. Xanthine

[Ref: Sabiston's 1st SAE pg. 2083]

269. Which of the following stones are common with infection?
(PGMEE 2015)

a. Struvite
b. Xanthine Stones
c. Calcium Oxalate stones
d. Cysteine stones

[Ref: Bailey & Love 26th /e pg.1292]

270. The following stent is placed after surgery of:-

a. Post cholecystectomy   (PGMEE 2018)
b. Post ESWL
c. Post cardiac catheterization
d. Stent for bile duct obstruction by malignancy

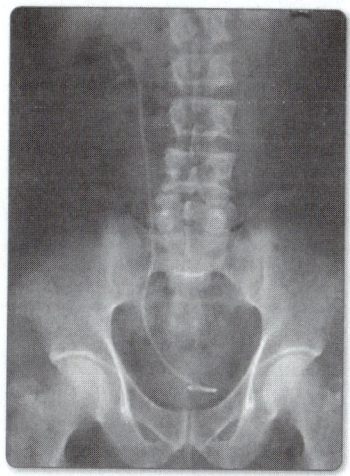

271. ESWL is contraindicated in which of the following stones-
(PGMEE 2015)

a. Cysteine stones
b. Urate Stones
c. Oxalate Stones
d. Phospate Stones

[Ref: Bailey and Love's 26th/e pg. 1294]

272. A staghorn calculus of size 4 cm was detected in a patient. What is the management?   (PGMEE 2017)

a. Retrograde intrarenal surgery
b. Ureteroscopic surgery
c. Percutaneous nephrolithotomy
d. Extracorporeal shock wave lithotripsy

[Ref: Schwartz 10th page 1666]

260. a	
261. a	
262. a	
263. a	
264. b	
265. a	
266. a	
267. a	
268. d	
269. a	
270. b	
271. a	
272. c	

Explanation

- PCNL is performed through a percutaneous tract into the kidney, where a larger scope and various energy sources (laser, ultrasound) are used to fragment and aspirate large renal calculi. This approach is well suited to staghorn calculi. ESWL is completely noninvasive and uses a device that delivers convergent shockwave energy to the calculus under fluoroscopic guidance. However, the lower efficacy rate of ESWL, when compared with ureteroscopy or PCNL, highlights the point that despite ESWL being less invasive, patients will often undergo multiple procedures to be rendered stone free.
- Smaller stones (up to 6 mm) may cause severe symptoms, such as flank pain and nausea, but typically pass without intervention beyond supportive care.
- Calculi ≥7 mm are more likely to become impacted or to have a prolonged passage through the ureter. For this reason, intervention at the time of presentation is preferred for larger stones

MISCELLANEOUS

273. **An athlete came to casualty with 4 days of passing red colored urine. Most probable cause of red coloured urine in this condition is?** *(DNB Dec'2010)*
   a. Hemosiderin
   b. Hemoglobin
   c. Hematuria
   d. Myoglobin

   [Ref: Harrison's 19th/e pg 1804]

273. d

Urology

FACTS

- Length of membranous urethra: 2-2.5 cm
- Length of male urethra: 18-20 cm
- Length of Female urethra: 4 cm
- Normal weight of prostate gland: 20 g
- Significant post void residual volume: ≥50 mL
- Fascia separating urogenital system: Denoviller's fascia
- Fascia separating rectum from coccyx: Waldeyer's fascia
- Testes reaches deep inguinal ring at the age of: 4th month of IUL
- Maximum chances of a calculi to get stuck is in: Navicular Fossa
- Widest part / most stretchable part of urethra: Prostatic Urethra
- Only fixed part/least stretchable part of urethra: Membranous Urethra
- During pelvic fracture, urethra is injured at: Superior surface of pelvis diaphragm
- Most prominent landmark of urethra during cystoscopy: Verumontanum (Ejaculatory ducts and prostatic utricle opens here)
- Corpora amylacea is seen in: Prostate
- Parasympathetic supply of bladder is from: $S_{2,3,4}$
- In horse-shoe kidney isthmus is at the level of: L3 – L4 (Below IMA)
- Renal collar is formed by: Left renal vein
- "Potter facies" and oligohydramnios are pathognomonic of: Bilateral renal agenesis
- Prostatic calculi are usually made up of: Ca phosphate
- Testis is involved but epididymis is spared in → Syphilis. [Mn: SIT → Syphilis involve Testes]
- A 13-year-old boy presents with 5 cm testicular mass, next line of management → USG scrotum → High inguinal orchidectomy
- "Bag of worms" feel in testis is characteristic of →Varicocele
- Varicocele is predominantly seen on: Left side
- Presence of barley water fluid is a feature of: Spermatocele
- Chinese lantern pattern on transillumination is seen in Epididymal cyst
- Hydrocele is a type of exudation cyst.
- Congenital hydrocele is best treated by → Herniotomy
- Cremasteric reflex is seen in acute epididymo-orchitis. Presence of reflex rules out torsion.
- Preferred kidney for renal transplant kidney: Left kidney.
- Absence of fructose in semen indicates: Obstruction to seminal vesicle
- Best laser for intracorporeal lithotripsy: Ho:YAG
- Whitaker test is done for: Hydronephrosis.
- Butterfly shape hematoma are characteristics of: Anterior urethra rupture
- Extravasation of urine in Space of Retzius (Prevesical space) occurs in: # pelvis/ extraperitoneal rupture of urinary bladder.
- Egg plant deformity and Butterfly hematoma is seen in: # Penis
- High flying (floating) prostate is a sign of → Membranous urethral injury.
- Stress urinary incontinence is more common in women.
- The Grayhack shunt connects → Corpora cavernosa and saphenous vein
- It is used for treatment of ischemic Priapism

Indications of orchidectomy:
- Prostate carcinoma
- Male breast carcinoma
- Testicular tumor
- Clotted hydrocele

Dietl's Crisis:
- Due to acute hydronephrosis
- Caused by the formation of kinks in the ureter
- Triad of:
  - Renal pain associated with chills, nausea & vomiting
  - Swelling in loin
  - Swelling disappears after passing urine

Undescended Testes

- Incidence in a newborn: 3-4%
- More common on: **R**ight side [**Mn:** RUN]
- MC location of UDT: Inguinal canal
- MC tumor in UDT: Seminoma
- MC associated congenital anomaly: Patent processus vaginalis
- IOC for UDT: Laparoscopy/inguinal exploration
- Orchidopexy in UDT do not decrease the risk of testicular tumor

Benign Prostatic Hyperplasia

- BPH mostly involves: Median lobe
- BPH develops only in: Transitional Zone.
- Earliest symptoms of prostatism: Nocturia
- IPSS / AUA scoring is used for assessment of severity of symptoms of: BPH
- In urometry, Normal max flow rate (Q_{max}) = 15 mL/s. Poor Q_{max} = <10 mL/s
- Irrigant of choice in TURP: 1.5% glycine
- Irrigant of choice in TURP with Bipolar cautery (plasmakinetics): Normal saline (NS)
- Incidence of TURP Syndrome: 2%
- In laser prostatectomy, laser of choice is: Ho: YAG laser.

Genitourinary Tuberculosis

- **T**himble bladder is characteristic of: **TB** Bladder
- Earliest radiological sign of renal TB on IVP: Moth eaten pelvis
- Auto nephrectomy is seen in: Renal TB
- Putty kidney term is used for: Renal TB
- MC/1st Site affected in TB testes: Epididymis (Globus minor)
- Earliest cystoscopic evidence of TB bladder: Mucosal pallor around ureteric orifices

Cystoscopic findings in bladder TB:
- Mucosal pallor
- Cobble stone mucosa
- Thimble bladder
- Golf hole ureter

Carcinoma Prostate

- MC type of CA prostate: Adenocarcinoma
- MC zone of origin: Peripheral zone
- MC lobe involved: Posterior lobe
- MC lymph node involved: Obturator
- MC site of metastasis: Vertebrae
- Screening is commonly done by: Digital Rectal Examination + PSA
- Normal level of PSA in male: <4 ng /mL
- Gleason scoring is done for: CA prostate
  - Score ranges from 2 – 10
  - Higher the score poorer the prognosis
- Bilateral Orchidectomy is done for: CA Prostrate

Urinary Tract Stones

- MC renal calculus: Ca Oxalate dihydrate
- Stones commonly associated with UTI/ *Proteus* infection → Struvite
- ESWL is contraindicated for → Cystine stones
- Xanthogranulomatous pyelonephritis associated stones are formed due to infection with → *Proteus*
- Jejunoileal bypass surgery leads to formation of: Ca oxalate stones
- Hardest calculi is formed by: Cystine calculi
- *Stones formed in:*
  - Acidic urine → Uric acid & cystine stones
  - Alkaline urine *Struvite & phosphate

MOST COMMON

- MC cause of acute epididymitis in sexually active young males: *Chlamydia trachomatis*
- MC cause of urethritis : *C. trachomatis*
- MC cause of bladder calcification worldwide: Schistosomiasis
- MC organism causing UTI: *E. coli*
- MC cause of emphysematous pyelonephritis: *E. coli*
- MC predisposing factor for chronic pyelonephritis: VUR
- MC congenital renal anomaly: Duplication of renal pelvis
- MCC of PUJ obstruction: Aberrant renal artery
- MC cause of palpable abdominal mass in a new born: Multicystic dysplastic kidney leading to hydronephrosis
- MCC of fetal hydronephrosis: PUJ obstruction
- MC renal fusion anomaly: Horse shoe kidney
- MC location of ectopic testes: Superficial inguinal pouch
- MC predisposing factor for torsion of testes: inversion of testes or High investment of testes
- MC cause of urethral injury : Instrumentation
- MC part of the urethra injured during instrumentation (Iatrogenic trauma): Bulbo-membranous > Bulbar
- MC cause of urethral stricture: Trauma
- MC site of stricture urethra: Bulbo-membranous > Bulbar {due to trauma}
- MC site of urethral injury due to external trauma/fall astride injury/straddle injury: Bulbar urethra

- MC type of bladder rupture → Extraperitoneal
- MC cause of extraperitoneal bladder rupture: fracture pelvis
- MC site of rupture in intraperitoneal bladder injury: Dome of bladder
- MC complication after TURP: Retrograde ejaculation OR Dry ejaculation
- MC site of stricture after TURP: Bladder neck

- MC cause of neurogenic bladder in children: Spina bifida
- MC cause of bladder outlet obstruction: Medial lobe enlargement
- MC surgically treatable cause of male infertility: Varicocele
- MC type of primary hydrocele is: Vaginal type
- MC cause of priapism in infant: Sickle cell anemia

SIGNS

- *Blue dot sign:*
  - Small bluish discoloration in the upper part of testes
  - Seen in cyst of Morgagni or torsion of the appendix of testes
- *Drooping lily sign:*
  - Seen in ectopic ureter on IVP

- *Prehn sign:*
  - Pain is relieved on lifting the affected hemiscrotum (positive sign) → in acute Epididymitis
  - If pain is increased, then test is negative → in torsion of testes

INVESTIGATION

- IOC for documentation of obstructive nature of pelvicalyceal system dilatation: DTPA scan
- Best imaging modality for zones of prostrate or capsule of prostate: T_2W MRI
- Imaging modality of choice when suspecting malignancy of prostrate: TRUS
- Most sensitive investigation for a renal calculus: NCCT Scan
- Main stay investigation for acute ureteric colic: CT Scan
- IVP/RGP finding in retroperitoneal fibrosis: Medial pulling of ureters
- IOC to see anterior urethra: Retrograde Urethrogram
- IOC to see posterior urethra: Micturating Cystourethrogram (MCU)
- Best investigation to visualize posterior urethra (membranous & prostatic urethra) is → Cystoscopy
- IOC for horse shoe kidney: IVP which reveals
  - Flowers vase pattern of ureteric curve
  - Hand joining sign
- *Pie in the sky* finding on IVP is seen in: # pelvis with posterior urethral injury (Complete disruption of posterior urethra)

- *Fetal head appearance* on radiograph is seen in: Schistosomiasis
- *Sandy patches* are cystoscopic finding in: Schistosomiasis
- *Tear drop bladder* on IVP suggest: Pelvic hematoma
- *Spider leg appearance* in IVP is suggestive of: Renal cyst
- *Adder head or cobra head* appearance on IVP: Ureterocele
- *Reverse J or fish Hook deformity* on IVP: Retrocaval ureter

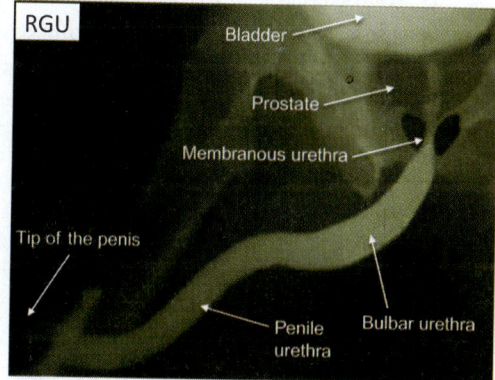

TREATMENT

- TURP Syndrome: 3% Saline
- Drug indicated for shrinking of the size of prostate: Finasteride
- Torsion of test: Bilateral orchiopexy
- In UDT, age of orchidopexy: 6 months-1year
- Difficult orchidopexy is done by: Fowler-Stephens surgery (Division of testicular artery is done)
- In case of UDT with short testicular artery (difficult orchiopexy), result are best with: Testicular auto transplantation

- **Nesbitt's operation** is done in: Peyronie's disorder (fibrous plaques or scarring in penis)
- Winter shunt: For treatment of priapism
- Anderson-Hynes operation: Dismembered pyeloplasty for PUJ operation

Treatment of hydrocele:

- Small hydrocele: Lord's operation
- Medium hydrocele: Jabulay's procedure → eversion of sac
- Large Hydrocele: Excision of sac

MULTIPLE CHOICE QUESTIONS

CHAPTER 1: UROLOGY

KIDNEY AND URETER

1. One side of kidney is normal, other side of kidney is contracted kidney with scar, what is the most probable diagnosis *(DNB June' 2011)*
- a. Chronic pyelonephritis
- b. Polycystic kidney
- c. Renal artery stenosis
- d. Tuberculosis of kidney

[Ref: Chandrasoma Taylor 3ʳᵈ/e p. 725, table 49.2]

2. In "Three Glass Test" shreds are present in 1ˢᵗ glass only. The most probablediagnosis should be *(PGMEE 2012)*
- a. Urethritis
- b. Cystitis
- c. Prostatitis
- d. Renal pathology

[Ref: Bailey & Love 25ᵗʰ/e p. 1366, Differential Diagnosis in Primary Care by R. Douglas Collins 2009e/p. 221]

3. Whitaker test is done for *(PGMEE 2012)*
- a. Renal carcinoma
- b. Hydronephrosis
- c. Renal tuberculosis
- d. Wilm's tumor

[Ref: Smith's urology 17ᵗʰ/e p. 117]

4. Image shown below is: *(PGMEE 2016-17)*

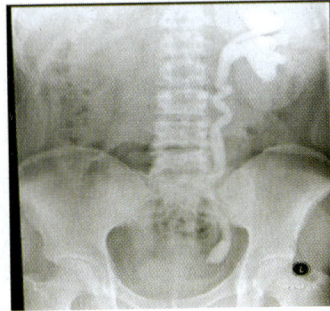

- a. Hydronephrosis of kidney
- b. Gall bladder empyma
- c. Urinary bladder stones
- d. Tuberculosis of kidney

[Ref: Robbins 9ᵗʰ/e pg. 971]

5. Best investigation to visualize posterior urethra is- *(PGMEE 2015)*
- a. IV Pyelogram
- b. Ascending urethriogram
- c. CT Scan
- d. Cystoscopy

[Ref: Internet]

6. Image shown below is of:- *(PGMEE 2016-17)*

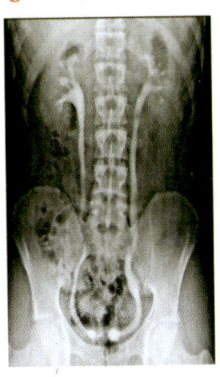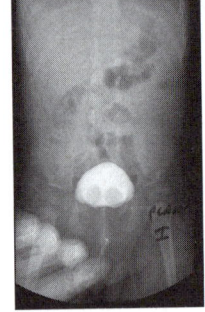

- a. Urtereocele
- b. Ectopic ureter
- c. Double ureter
- d. Vesico ureteric reflux

7. A 4-year-old girl presented with urinary infection with E. coli, pus cells in urine, dilatation of left ureter with hydro-ureter; micturating cysto-urethrogram shows filling defect in bladder, likely diagnosis is:
- a. Sacrococcygeal teratoma *(PGMEE 2014-15)*
- b. Ureterocele
- c. VUR
- d. P.U.V

[Ref: Harrison 19th]

8. About VUR all statements are true except: *(PGMEE 2016-17)*
- a. More commonly involve male children
- b. Leads to hydronephrosis of kidney
- c. Infection is primary concern
- d. Never requires surgical treatment

[Ref: Internet]

9. Image shown below is: *(PGMEE 2016-17)*

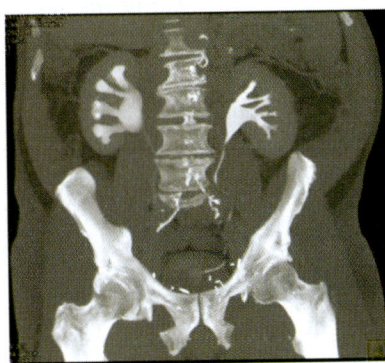

- a. PUJ obstruction
- b. Bladder stones
- c. Ureterocele
- d. Ectopic ureter

[Ref: Internet]

1.	a
2.	a
3.	b
4.	a
5.	d
6.	a
7.	b
8.	d
9.	a

10. A patient came to the trauma center, with a history of renal trauma 12 days back which had led to urine extravasation and urinoma formation and was managed conservatively. On urography, the extravastion and urinoma are still persisting. What would be the next step?
    a. Percutaneous nephrostomy   (*NEET Pattern 2017*)
    b. Surgical management
    c. Ureteric stenting
    d. Conservative management

BLADDER & URETHRA

11. **Christmas tree appearance of urinary bladder is seen in:**
    (*PGMEE 2014/15*)
    a. Enuresis   b. Stress incontinence
    c. Neurogenic bladder   d. Autonomous bladder

    [*Ref: Clinical Pediatric Nephrology, 2nd /e pg 96*]

12. **50-year-old male presents with features of bladder outflow obstruction (BOO). He has difficulty and pain during micturition. Retrograde urethrogram was performed. finding as shown in radiograph. Most likely diagnosis is:-**   (*PGMEE 2018*)
    a. Prostate calculi
    b. Benign prostatic hyperplasia
    c. Vescical calculus
    d. Urethral stone

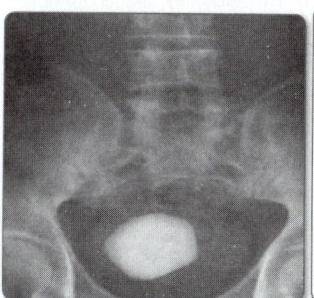 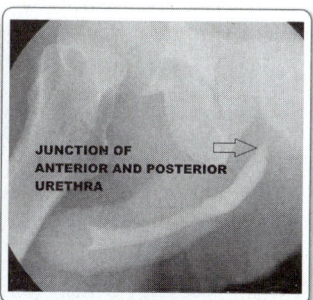

Normal RGU

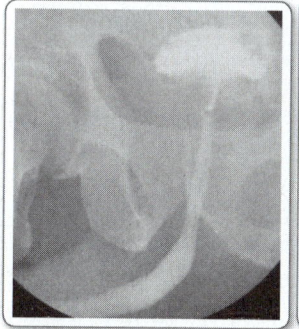 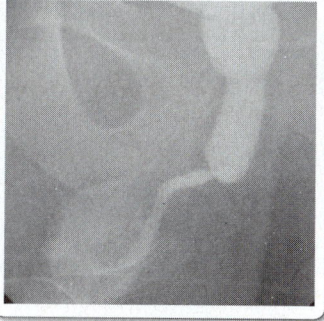

Normal RGU   **Urethral stricture**

Explanation

- Case courtesy of Dr Ian Bickle, <a href="https://radiopaedia.org/">Radiopaedia.org</a>. From the case <a href="https://radiopaedia.org/cases/30340">rID: 30340</a>

13. **Paniless haematuria is found in all except**
    (*DNB June' 2009*)
    a. Cystitis
    b. Renal carcinoma
    c. PCKD
    d. Chronic glomerulonephritis

    [*Ref: Washington Manual of Surgery 5th/e p. 597*]

14. **Most common type of bladder rupture is-**
    (*PGMEE 2015*)
    a. Equal incidence of extraperitoneal and intrtaperitoneal
    b. Extraperitoneal
    c. Intraperitoneal
    d. At the trigone

    [*Ref: internet*]

15. **False about bladder trigone is-**   (*PGMEE 2015*)
    a. Sensitive to stretch
    b. It is developed from mesonephric duct
    c. Both ureteral orifices are present ar either end
    d. Muscle fibres are loosely attached to mucosa

    [*Ref: Various websites*]

16. **Drugs used for detrusor instability are all except:**
    (*DNB 2008*)
    a. Duloxetine   b. Solifenacin
    c. Flavoxate   d. Tiaperetide

    [*Ref: Sabiston's 20th/e pg. 2076; Harrison's 19th/e pg. 81*]

17. **Which of the following are features of membranous urethral injury expect-**   (*PGMEE 2015*)
    a. Perineal butterfly hematoma
    b. Inability to pass urine
    c. High flying prostate
    d. Blood at the meatus

    [*Ref: Internet*]

PROSTATE

18. **BPH involves-**   (*PGMEE 2015*)
    a. Prostate capsule   b. Peripheral zone
    c. Central zone   d. Transitional zone

    [*Ref: Bailey and love 1341*]

19. **55-year-old man came with urinary symptoms of increased frequency and hesitation. The patient was diagnosed with benign hyperplasia of prostate. Which of the drugs will help in prevent further growth and possibly reduces the size of the prostate?**
    (*NEET Pattern 2017*)
    a. Tamsulosin   b. Finasteride
    c. Tadafil   d. Flutamide

Explanation

- α_1-antagonists (α_1-blockers) e.g. doxazosin, terazosin, tamsulosin, and alfuzosin are commonly used to treat BPH related LUTS.
- **MOA:** They treat the dynamic component of BPH by blocking α_1-mediated sympathetic stimulation to relax the smooth muscle in the prostate.
- Effects starts on voiding within hours of administration, regardless of prostate size, without altering serum PSA level or volume.

10.	a
11.	c
12.	c
13.	a
14.	b
15.	d
16.	d
17.	a
18.	d
19.	b

- Currently available α_1-blockers include
  - *Nonselective α_1-blockers* : Terazosin, doxazosin, and alfuzosin
  - *Highly selective α_{1A}-blocker*: Tamsulosin. Silodosin is a new agent.
  - α_{1D}-*blocker*: Naftopidil is α_{1D}-blocker, a/w less ejaculatory dysfunctions.

5-alpha Reductase Inhibitors

- They inhibit the conversion of testosterone to dihydrotestosterone (DHT), the primary androgen involved in both normal and abnormal prostate growth.
- Finasteride and dutasteride are used in practice.
- Dutasteride, inhibits both type 1 and type II 5 α reductase enzymes competitively, induces a more profound reduction of serum DHT in the range of 90–95% compared with 70–75% for finasteride.
- Finasteride was the first drug in this class approved by U.S. FDA. In human it decreases the prostatic DHT level by 70–90% and reduces the prostatic size.
- Epristeride, a novel 5 ARI, which belongs to class of carboxy steroid. It has been shown to be an uncompetitive inhibitor against both testosterone and NADPH.
- The long-acting PDE5 inhibitor tadalafil is approved for treatment of the signs and symptoms of BPH/LUTS.

20. High flying (floating) prostate is a sign of-
   (PGMEE 2015)
   a. Bulbar urethral injury
   b. Extraperitoneal bladder rupture
   c. Membranous urethral injury
   d. Intraperitoneal bladder rupture

   [Ref: internet]

21. A 29 year male complains of pain in the flank that radiates from the loin to the groin region. The first investigation to be done is- *(PGMEE 2015)*
   a. CECT
   b. USG abdomen
   c. Plain CT Scan
   d. X-ray Abdomen

   [Ref: Bailey & Love 26ᵗʰ /e pg. 1293]

22. Which of the following organism is NOT implicated in acute bacterial prostatitis:- *(PGMEE 2018)*
   a. Peptostreptococci
   b. Proteus
   c. Staphylococcus
   d. Serratia

Explanation

Acute bacterial prostatitis (ABP) is caused by
- **Gram-negative bacteria** - *E.coli* (the **most common** bacteria), *Klebsiella, Enterobacter*, **Proteus, Serratia** and *Pseudomonas aeruginosa*.
- **Gram positive cocci** - *Staphylococcus* aureus (due to prolonged catheterization in hospitalized patients) and Enterococci (in 5-10% cases)
- **Occasional** causative agents include *Mycobacterium tuberculosis, Salmonella* species, *Clostridium* species, those associated with sexually transmitted diseases (e.g., *Chlamydia trachomatis, Neisseria gonorrhea, Trichomonas vaginalis, and Ureaplasma urealyticum)*.
- **Obligate anaerobic bacteria** (like **Peptostreptococcus**) **rarely** cause acute bacterial prostatitis.

20.	c
21.	b
22.	a
23.	a
24.	a
25.	c
26.	a
27.	a
28.	a
29.	a
30.	b
31.	b

23. Which is false about stress urinary incontinence
   a. More common in men
   b. It is due to weakening of Pelvic floor muscles
   c. It occurs during increased abdominal pressure
   d. Prostate surgery may be a cause

   [Ref: WWW. Mayoclinic.org/urinary-incontinence /types.html]

   [Ref: S. Das short cases in Surgery]

24. Congenital hydrocele is best treated by- *(PGMEE 2015)*
   a. Herniotomy
   b. Excision of sac
   c. Eversion of sac
   d. Lords procedure

   [Ref: Bailey & Love 26ᵗʰ/e pg. 1382]

25. Congenital hydrocele is treated by *(DNB Dec' 2009)*
   a. Herniorraphy
   b. Eversion of sac
   c. Herniotomy
   d. No treatment before 5 years

   [Ref: Bailey & Love 26ᵗʰ/e pg. 1382; Fundamentals of Operative Surgery – Vipul Yagnik p. 35]

26. Testis is involved but epidydimis is spared in? *(DNB Dec' 2011)*
   a. Syphilis
   b. Gonorrhea
   c. Chancroid
   d. Chlamydia

   [Ref: Bailey and Love 24/e p. 1411]

27. What is the best time to do surgery in a case of undescended testis (cryptorchidism): - *(PGMEE 2015)*
   a. Infancy
   b. 1-2 years
   c. 5 years
   d. Puberty

   [Ref: Sabiston's 20th/e (=1ˢᵗ SAE) pg. 1885]

28. Surgery for unilateral undescended testis is recommended at what age:- *(PGMEE 2016-17)*
   a. 6 months – 1year
   b. 1-2 year
   c. 2-3 year
   d. 18 years

   [Ref: Sabiston's 20th/e (=1ˢᵗ SAE) pg. 1885]

29. "Bag of worms" feel in testis is characterstic of: *(PGMEE 2016-17)*
   a. Varicocele
   b. Hydrocele
   c. Rotation of testis
   d. Testicular malignancy

   [Ref: Sabiston's 1ˢᵗ SAE pg. 2081]

30. A 13 year old boy presents with 5 cm testicular mass, next line of management:- *(PGMEE 2016-17)*
   a. Testicular biopsy
   b. High ingunal orchidectomy
   c. Subcapsular orchidectomy
   d. Total orchidectomy followed by radiotherapy

   [Ref: Sabiston's 1ˢᵗ SAE pg. 1886]

31. Positive Prehn's sign is? *(DNB Dec'2010)*
   a. Depression of testis reduces pain of epididymitis
   b. Elevation of testis reduces pain of epididymitis
   c. Elevation of testis increase pain of epididymitis
   d. Depression of testis increases pain of epididymitis

   [Ref: Blueprints Urology by Stanley Zaslau-Page 127]

Rheumatology

FACTS

- **Target Antigen of:**
  - **C** – ANCA: **C**ytoplasmic Proteinase 3
  - **P** – ANCA: **P**erinuclear M**P**O
- Aortic arch syndrome, Nonspecific aorto-arteritis, Reversed COA and Pulseless disease are synonymous with: Takayasu arteritis
- **P**ulmonary **A**rtery is **N**ot involved in: PAN
- Most serious complication seen in Kawasaki disease → Coronary artery aneurysm
  - Usually seen in: 2nd - 3rd week of illness
  - Best test to detect: 2D ECHO
- Bony enlargement of the PIP joint in osteoarthritis is k/a: Bouchard's nodule
- Bony enlargement of the DIP joint in osteoarthritis is k/a: Heberden nodule
- Pinch purpura is seen in: Primary systemic amyloidosis
- Best marker for **D**rug **I**nduced **L**upus: Anti Histone Antibody [**Mn:** His stone DIL]
- **IgA deposition in renal mesangium is seen in:**
  - IgA nephropathy
  - Henoch Schonlein Purpura (HSP)
- IgA vasculitis (HSP) is due to immune complex deposition i.e. it is an example of type III HSR.

Causes of Hyperuricemia

Increase urate production:
- Idiopathic
- Alcohol
- Obesity
- Male gender
- Leish Nyhan syndrome
- Myeloproliferative disorders

Decrease uric acid excretion:
- Chronic kidney disease
- Alcohol
- Low dose salicylates
- Diuretics
- Pyrazinamide
- Ethambutol
- Levodopa

Mixed Connective Tissue Disease

- MCTD has overlapping features of: [**Mn:** MC Sher RAP Singer]
  - **SLE**
  - **R**heumatoid **A**rthritis
  - **P**olymyositis
  - **S**ystemic sclerosis/**S**cleroderma
- Diagnosis – Anti U1 RNP antibody

Named Lesion

Named Lesion	Seen in
▪ Strawberry **G**um	Wegener's **G**ranulomatosis
▪ Strawberry tongue	Kawasaki Disease
▪ Bouchard's Nodule and Heberden's Nodule	Osteoarthritis

HLA

HLA	Associated condition	HLA	Associated condition
HLA B 8	Myasthenia gravis (also with HLA DR3); Graves disease	HLA B 27	Spondyloarthropathies like Ankylosing spondylosis; Anterior uveitis
HLA B 5 / B 51	Behçet's disease	HLA B 57	Abacavir hypersensitivity
HLA DR 3	Myasthenia gravis Type I Diabetes Dermatitis herpetiformis SLE	HLA DR 4	Rheumatoid arthritis Type I Diabetes Pemphigus vulgaris
HLA DR 2	Narcolepsy; Multiple sclerosis	HLA B*15:02	SJS / TEN
HLA DQ 2	Celiac disease		

REMEMBER

Examples of Granulomatous Vasculitis:
- **Giant** cell/Temporal arthritis
- **W**egener's granulomatosis/GPA
- **T**akayasu arteritis
- **C**hurg Strauss syndrome/EGPA
  [**Mn: Giant World Trade Center**]

Arteries involved in Giant cell arteritis:
- **T**emporal artery (MC)
- **O**ccipital artery
- **F**acial artery
- **L**ingual artery
  [**Mn: TOeFL**]

Charcot's joint is seen in association with:
- **Di**abetes (MC)
- **L**eprosy

- **A**myloidosis
- Tabes **Dor**salis
  [**Mn: Char (4) coat DiLA Do**]

Eosinophilic Granulomatosis with Polyangiitis (Churg Strauss Syndrome) is characterized by:
- **E**osinophilia
- Extravascular **G**ranuloma
- **A**sthma
- **V**asculitis of multiple organ system

Anti Ro (SS-A) antibodies are present in:
- SLE
- Sjögren/sicca syndrome
- Neonatal lupus with congenital heart block
- Subacute Cutaneous Lupus Erythematosus

MOST COMMON

- MC site of involvement in hypersensitivity vasculitis: Post capillary venules
- MC cause of vasculitis in children: HSP
- MC class of antibody deposited in HSP: IgA
- MC artery involved in Takaya**su** arteritis: **Su**bclavian artery
- MC type of Takayasu arteritis in India: Type III
- MC site of obstruction in Takayasu arteritis: Proximal aspects of the branches of aortic arch
- MC valvular disease in RA: MR

- MC affected part of the spine in RA/only affected part of spine in RA: Cervical spine
- MC site of cardiac involvement in RA: Pericardium
- MC mechanism of hyperuricemia in gout: underexcretion of uric acid
- MC site of involvement of gout: Metatarsophalangeal joint of big toe (Podagra)
- MC chronic arthritis of childhood: Juvenile idiopathic arthritis (JIA / JRA)

OSTEOARTHRITIS (OA)

General	▪ OA is the most common type of arthritis.
	▪ **Risk factors:**
	  ○ Age – most potent risk factor for OA
	  ○ Obesity
	  ○ Female sex
	  ○ Developmental abnormalities like congenital dysplasia, acetabular dysplasia, Legg-Perthes disease, and slipped capital femoral epiphysis
	▪ The pathologic sine qua non of disease is loss of hyaline articular cartilage
	OA RA CPPD

Clinical features	▪ Joint pain from OA is activity related pain (contrasting from RA) ▪ Commonly affected joints include the cervical and lumbosacral spine, hip, knee and first Metatarsophalangeal joint (MTP). In the hands, the DIP and PIP joints and the base of the thumb are often affected. ▪ Severe osteoarthritis of the hands affects the DIP joints (**Heberden nodes**) and the PIP Joints (**Bouchard's nodes**). ▪ DIP joints are most often affected. Spares the wrist, elbow, and ankle joint
X-ray	▪ Structural changes of OA include cartilage loss (seen as joint space loss) and osteophytes
Rx	▪ Acetaminophen (paracetamol) is the initial analgesic of choice

RHEUMATOID ARTHRITIS

General	■ It is the most common form of chronic inflammatory arthritis ■ Associated with HLA DRB1 and HLA DR4 ■ F > M (3:1) ■ CD4+ T cells play a key role in pathogenesis ■ Pathological hallmark – early synovial membrane inflammation which progresses to focal bone erosions and thinning of articular cartilage. ■ TNF-α is the most important cytokine involved in synovial inflammation ■ Chronic inflammation leads to synovial lining hyperplasia and the formation of pannus
Clinical features	**Articular manifestation:** ■ Early morning joint stiffness lasting more than 1 hour that eases with physical activity ■ Earliest involved joints are the small joints of the hands and feet ■ The initial pattern of joint involvement may be monoarticular, oligoarticular (≤4 joints), or polyarticular (>5 joints), usually in a symmetric distribution. ■ Most frequently involved joints: Metacarpophalangeal (**MCP**) > Wrists > Proximal interphalangeal (PIP) > Knee > Metatarsophalangeal ■ DIP joint are typically **spared** ■ Flexor tendon tenosynovitis is a hallmark feature. Other features include periarticular and generalized osteoporosis. ■ **Swan neck deformity** – Hyperextension of the PIP joint with flexion of the DIP joint ■ **Boutonnière deformity** – Flexion of the PIP joint with hyperextension of the DIP joint ■ **Z-line deformity** – Subluxation of the first MCP joint with hyperextension of the first interphalangeal joint ■ Subluxation of the distal ulna, resulting in a "**piano-key movement**" of the ulnar styloid. ■ **Ulnar deviation** – Subluxation of the MCP joints, with subluxation of the proximal phalanx to the volar side of the hand. ■ Axial skeleton involvement is usually limited to upper cervical spine (Atlantoaxial subluxation) – can cause radicular pain and quadriparesis ■ Thoracic and lumbar spine involvement is rare **Extra-articular manifestations:** ■ Subcutaneous rheumatoid nodules → MC site: elbow ■ Secondary Sjögren syndrome – present with either dry eyes (keratoconjunctivitis sicca) or dry mouth (xerostomia). ■ Pleuritis – MC pulmonary manifestation of RA ■ Pulmonary nodules, Pleural effusions (**exudative**), ILD, Normocytic anemia ■ **Caplan's syndrome**: development of pulmonary nodules and pneumoconiosis following silica exposure ■ **Felty's syndrome**: triad of **N**eutropenia, **S**plenomegaly, and nodular **RA** (NSR) ■ Cardiac involvement – Pericarditis (MC), Mitral regurgitation ■ Nerve entrapment – median nerve (l/t carpel tunnel syndrome), Mononeuritis multiplex ■ Hypogonadism – Low serum testosterone, LH and DHEA

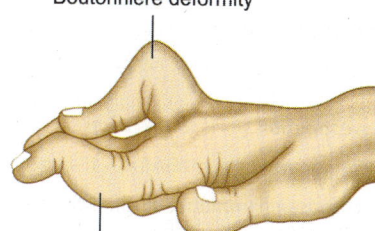

Boutonnière deformity

Swan neck deformity

Lab	■ Rheumatoid factor (RF): it is an **A**ntibody of Ig**M** class against Fc portion of Ig**G** class [**Mn: RAM G**] ○ Seen in only 75–80% of patients with RA ■ Best diagnostic test: Anti-CCP antibody (specificity – 95%) ■ Elevated titre of RF, CRP, Anti-CCP Antibody are associated with worst outcome ■ Pleural fluid contains low levels of glucose with high protein (exudative) ■ Anti MCV Antibody (modified citrullinated vimentin) → has lower diagnostic valve than anti-CCP antibody.
X-ray	■ The initial radiographic finding is periarticular osteopenia f/b narrowing of joint space ■ Abnormalities of the **temporomandibular** joint occur commonly
Management	■ Methotrexate is the DMARD of first choice for initial treatment of moderate to severe RA. ■ Failure to achieve adequate response with MTX alone → step up to combination DMARD ○ MTX + Sulfasalazine + Hydroxychloroquine OR MTX + Leflunomide OR MTX + Biological agent ■ Hydroxychloroquine and sulfasalazine are probably the safest DMARDs to use during pregnancy. ■ Methotrexate and Leflunomide therapy are contraindicated during Pregnancy ■ Switch or add DMARD therapy after **3 months** of worsening or persistent moderate/high disease activity. ■ Disease Activity Score-28 (DAS-28) is useful for classifying the states of low disease activity and remission
Newer drugs	■ Tofacitinib: Oral JAK inhibitor ■ Tocilizumab: IL-6 receptor inhibitor ■ Sarilumab: binds to IL-6 receptor ■ Abatacept: Selective costimulation modulator that binds to CD80 and CD86 → inhibit T cell activation

SPONDYLOARTHRITIDES

	Ankylosing spondylitis	Psoriatic arthritis	Reactive arthritis/Reiter syndrome	Enteropathic arthritis
General features	■ MC subtype ■ Age of onset <40 years	■ Seen in 10-30% patients with psoriasis	■ Develop 1-3 months after GI or GU infection ■ MC organism implicated – *C. trachomatis*	■ More common in CD
Skeletal involvement	■ Axial	■ Peripheral	■ Peripheral	■ Peripheral
HLA B27	■ 90%	■ 40-50%	■ 40-80%	■ 35-75%
Sacroiliitis	■ Symmetrical	■ Asymmetrical	■ Symmetrical/ Asymmetrical	■ Symmetrical
Articular features	■ Earliest joint to get involved: Sacroiliac joint ■ MC site of fracture: cervical spine	■ Distal joint involvement ■ Dactylitis with sausage digits ■ Arthritis mutilans		
Enthesitis	■ Common	■ Common	■ Common	■ Uncommon
Dactylitis	■ Uncommon	■ Most common	■ Common	■ Uncommon
Extra articular features	■ Uveitis – MC ■ Aortic insufficiency	■ Uveitis ■ Conjunctivitis	■ Triad: Arthritis, Conjunctivitis and Non Gonococcal urethritis	■ Inflammatory bowel disease ■ Uveitis
Skin manifestations	■ Uncommon	■ Psoriasis – usually precede arthritis	■ Keratoderma blennorrhagicum ■ Circinate balanitis	■ Aphthous ulcer ■ Erythema nodosum (CD) ■ Pyoderma gangrenosum (UC)
Investigation	■ X-ray: Bamboo spine	■ X-ray: Pencil in cup deformity	■ Non diagnostic	■ ASCA antibodies
Management	■ NSAIDs – 1st line	■ Diagnosis – CASPER criteria	■ NSAIDs – 1st line	■ NSAIDs, Corticosteroids

Enthesitis–inflammation at the site of insertion of ligaments and tendons on to bone | CD – Crohn disease | UC – Ulcerative colitis |

CRYSTAL INDUCED ARTHROPATHIES

	Gout	Pseudogout/Calcium Pyrophosphate Deposition Disease
General features	■ Disorder of Purine metabolism ■ Characterized by deposition of monosodium urate (MSU) crystals ■ Precipitating factors includes use of diuretics or low dose aspirin	■ Caused by Calcium pyrophosphate (CPP) crystals ■ MC cause – idiopathic
Clinical features	■ Males > Females ■ MC joint involved: Metatarsophalangeal joint of big toe (Podagra) > tarsal > ankle > knee ■ Uric acid renal stones ■ Tophaceous deposits of urate crystals along helix of ear, prepatellar bursa etc.	■ Males = Females ■ MC involved joint: Knee > wrist > shoulder > ankle ■ Associated conditions: Aging, Primary hyperparathyroidism, Hemochromatosis, Hypomagnesemia
Lab features	■ Gouty attacks are not related to serum levels of uric acid. Thus, an elevated serum uric acid level does not prove the diagnosis of acute gout ■ MSU crystals appear as **N**eedle-shaped and exhibit **N**egative birefringence. ■ X-ray → punched out erosions or lytic areas with overhanging edges – Rat bite erosions ■ **Martel sign** → overhanging margin of new bone along the edge of erosion ■ Synovial fluid → ↑ TLC in acute attack with normal glucose level	■ Normal serum uric acid levels ■ CPP crystals appear as rhomboid shaped and are positively birefringent ■ X-ray → punctate / linear radiodense deposits within hyaline cartilage = chondrocalcinosis

Management	**Acute gout/Pseudogout:** ▪ High dose <u>N</u>SAIDS are the DOC ▪ <u>C</u>orticosteroids ▪ <u>C</u>olchicines – uricosuric agent ▪ <u>C</u>osyntropin (ACTH) ▪ Allopurinol is contraindicated in acute gout	**Chronic gout:** ▪ Febuxostat and Allopurinol – Xanthine oxidase (XO) inhibitor: MC used drug ▪ Probenecid – inhibit tubular absorption of uric acid ▪ Pegloticase – recombinant uricase ▪ Benzbromarone ▪ Lesinurad – selective uric acid reabsorption inhibitor (SURI): acts by inhibiting the urate transporter, URAT1 ▪ XO inhibitors are the preferred agent in renal disease ▪ Febuxostat do not require dose adjustment in mild-moderate renal disease.

SYSTEMIC LUPUS ERYTHEMATOSUS

General feature	▪ Usually seen in female of child bearing age (90%)
Clinical features	**SLICC* Classification Criteria for Systemic Lupus Erythematosus** ▪ Requirements: ≥4 criteria (at least 1 clinical and 1 laboratory criteria) OR biopsy-proven lupus nephritis with positive ANA or Anti-DNA **Clinical Criteria / Immunologic Criteria** ▪ Acute cutaneous lupus — ▪ ANA ▪ Chronic cutaneous lupus — ▪ Anti-DNA ▪ Oral or nasal ulcers — ▪ Anti-Sm ▪ Non-scarring alopecia — ▪ Antiphospholipid Ab ▪ Arthritis — ▪ Low complement (C3, C4) ▪ Serositis — ▪ Direct Coomb's test ▪ Renal ▪ Neurological ▪ Hemolytic anemia ▪ Leukopenia ▪ Thrombocytopenia (<100,000/mm³) ▪ MC clinical feature: arthralgia/myalgia **Other features:** ▪ Shrinking lung syndrome, Pulmonary fibrosis ▪ Libman Sacks endocarditis ▪ Recurrent abortions – due to antiphospholipid antibodies ▪ Raynaud's phenomenon
Lab features	▪ Renal biopsy shows wire loop lesion in class III/ IV / V (most characteristic of IV) ▪ Spleen biopsy shows onion skin lesions ▪ Band test (IF of skin with Ab to IgG demonstrates band like deposition of immune complexes in SLE) ▪ Increase in ESR with normal CRP levels during disease flare
Treatments	▪ Hydroxychloroquine, NSAIDS, Steroids, Immunomodulators like Methotrexate, Belimumab, Rituximab etc. ▪ Hydroxychloroquine in pregnancy *Belimumab – inhibits the biological activity of B lymphocyte stimulator (BLyS)

Antibodies in SLE

ANA	▪ Most sensitive test; Best screening test
Anti dsDNA antibody	▪ High titres are specific for SLE ▪ Correlate with disease activity
Anti-Smith antibody	▪ Most specific test
Anti Ro (SS-A)	▪ Predisposes to neonatal lupus with congenital heart block and subacute cutaneous lupus
Antiphospholipid	▪ Predisposes to clotting, fetal loss and thrombocytopenia
Antiribosomal P	▪ Correlates with depression or psychosis

SLE vs Drug Induced Lupus

Features	SLE	Drug Induced Lupus
Age of onset	▪ 20-30 years	▪ 50 years
Female : Male	▪ 9:1	▪ 1:1
Kidney and CNS involvement	▪ In 1/3rd patients	▪ Less common
Cutaneous manifestations	▪ Common	▪ Uncommon
ANA	▪ >95%	▪ >95%
Anti dsDNA antibody	▪ Specific	▪ Rare
Anti histone antibody	▪ In 50%	▪ >95% [**Mn:** His Stone DIL]
Etiology/Association	▪ Autoimmune ▪ Mixed connective tissue disease	▪ **S**ulfasalazine, **S**ulfonamides, **H**ydralazine, **I**soniazid, **P**rocainamide

ANTIPHOSPHOLIIPID ANTIBODY SYNDROME/APS

General feature	▪ Disorder of blood coagulation system resulting in hypercoagulable state

Manifestations	▪ Arterial thrombosis leading to stroke, TIA, Myocardial ischemia, gangrene, renal artery thrombosis
	▪ Venous thrombosis leading to DVT, Pulmonary embolism and Budd Chiari syndrome
	▪ Arthralgia, Arthritis
		▪ Obstetric manifectations like preeclampsia and eclampsia
		▪ Recurrent spontaneous abortions:
		  ○ Early fetal loss (<10 weeks)
		  ○ Late fetal loss (≥10 weeks)

Lab features	▪ Antiphospholipid antibodies → Hallmark of APS ▪ Any one of the following should be present in serum on 2 or more occasions at least 12 weeks apart: ○ Lupus anticoagulant or Anticardiolipin antibody or Anti beta -2 glycoprotein I antibody	▪ False positive test for syphilis in presence of anticardiolipin Antibody ▪ Autoimmune Hemolytic anemia ▪ Thrombocytopenia ▪ Prolonged aPTT
Management	▪ Diagnosis is confirmed if one clinical and one lab criteria are met ▪ Treatment is anticoagulation with heparin followed by warfarin ▪ Prophylaxis during pregnancy is provided with LMWH and aspirin	

SYSTEMIC SCLEROSIS AND SJOGREN SYNDROME

	Systemic Sclerosis/Scleroderma	Sjögren syndrome
General feature	▪ More common in female ▪ Scleroderma = skin hardening + induration ▪ Renal crisis is associated with poor prognosis	▪ More common in females ▪ Immunological mediated destruction of lacrimal and salivary glands ▪ Associated with RA, SLE, Scleroderma, MCTD, Primary biliary cirrhosis, Chronic hepatitis
Manifestations	▪ Subcutaneous **C**alcinosis ▪ **R**aynaud's phenomenon ▪ **E**sophageal dysmotility/dysphagia ▪ **S**clerodactyly ▪ **T**elangiectasia	▪ Xerophthalmia (dry eyes) ▪ Xerostomia (dry mouth) ▪ Bilateral painless parotid gland enlargement ▪ Glandular MALToma – MC lymphoma
Lab features	▪ ANA +ve (Screening test) ▪ Type specific autoantibodies	▪ ANA +ve ▪ Antibodies against SSA (Ro) and SSB (La)
Rx	▪ Corticosteroids ▪ Immunosuppressants	▪ Corticosteroids ▪ Immunosuppressants

Types	Limited Cutaneous Systemic Sclerosis	Diffuse Cutaneous Systemic Sclerosis
Onset	▪ Indolent	▪ Rapid
Progression	▪ Slow	▪ Rapid
Skin involvement	▪ Limited to fingers, distal to elbow, face	▪ Diffuse: fingers, extremities, face, trunk
Raynaud's	▪ Antedate skin involvement	▪ Coincident with skin involvement
Musculoskeletal	▪ Mild arthralgia	▪ Severe arthralgia
ILD	▪ Mild and slowly progressive	▪ Severe and frequent
PAH	▪ May occur as an isolated complication ▪ Frequent and late complication	▪ Often occurs in association with ILD
Renal crisis	▪ Rare	▪ Early and fulminant
Calcinosis cutis	▪ Frequent and prominent	▪ Less common and mild
Autoantibody	▪ Anti-centromere	▪ Anti-Topoisomerase I (Scl 70) ▪ Anti RNA polymerase III

CHAPEL HILL NOMENCLATURE OF VASCULITIDES

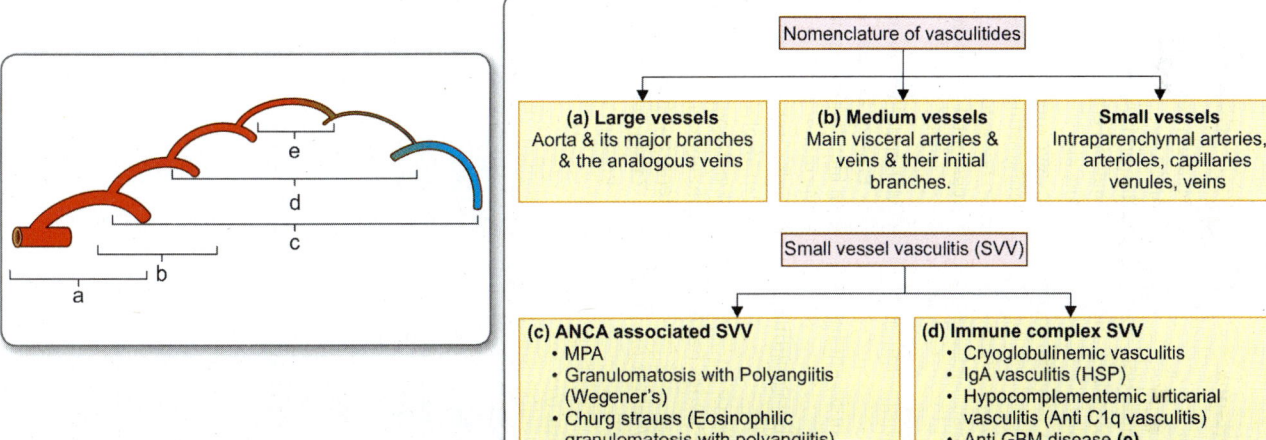

- **Large vessel vasculitis:**
  - Giant cell arteritis
  - Takayasu arteritis
- **Medium vessel vasculitis:**
  - Polyarteritis Nodosa
  - Kawasaki disorder
- **Variable vessel vasculitis:**
  - Behçet's disease
  - Cogan syndrome
- **Vasculitis associated with systemic disease:**
  - Lupus vasculitis
  - Rheumatoid vasculitis
  - Sarcoid vasculitis
- **Vasculitis associated with probable etiology:**
  - Hepatitis C associated cryoglobulinemic vasculitis
  - Hepatitis B associated vasculitis
  - Syphilis associated aortitis
  - Drug associated immune complex vasculitis

LARGE AND MEDIUM VESSEL VASCULITIS

	Giant cell arteritis/Temporal arteritis	Takayasu arteritis	Polyarteritis Nodosa / PAN	Kawasaki disease
General features	<ul><li>Large vessel vasculitis</li><li>ANCA –ve</li><li>Granulomatous inflammation</li><li>Females > Males</li><li>Exclusively in patients > 50 years</li><li>Usually involves ≥ 1 extracranial branches of Carotid artery</li><li>MC artery affected → Temporal artery</li><li>Segmental lesion of affected artery</li></ul>	<ul><li>Large vessel vasculitis</li><li>ANCA –ve</li><li>Granulomatous inflammation</li><li>Common in women of childbearing age</li><li>Age of onset < 50 years</li><li>Involves Aorta and its major branches</li><li>Association with *M. tuberculosis* +</li><li>Pulmonary artery is also involved</li></ul>	<ul><li>Medium vessel vasculitis</li><li>ANCA –ve</li><li>Non granulomatous inflammation</li><li>Male > Female</li><li>Any age</li><li>Involve medium and small muscular arteries (contrasting feature from MPA)</li><li>Do not involve Pulmonary artery</li><li>Segmental and Necrotizing vasculitis</li></ul>	<ul><li>Medium vessel vasculitis</li><li>ANCA –ve</li><li>Non granulomatous inflammation</li><li>Male > Female</li><li>Affects children < 5 years of age</li><li>Involve medium sized arteries like coronary artery</li><li>Association with TSST releasing *S. aureus* and Kawasaki has been noted</li></ul>
Clinical features	<ul><li>MC symptom → Headache</li><li>Most specific symptom → Jaw claudication</li><li>Scalp tenderness</li><li>Polymyalgia rheumatica in 40-50%</li><li>Most feared complication → sudden onset visual loss due to ischemic optic atrophy</li></ul>	<ul><li>Headache</li><li>Claudication</li><li>Decreased pulsation of one or both brachial arteries</li><li>Bruit → MC location being carotid artery</li><li>Blood pressure difference on extremities (UL < LL – hence named reversed COA)</li><li>Coronary aneurysm l/t chest pain and MI</li><li>Renal involvement:<ul><li>Renal artery stenosis l/t hypertension</li><li>Nephrotic syndrome</li></ul></li></ul>	<ul><li>Mononeuritis multiplex<ul><li>Present as weakness/numbness</li></ul></li><li>GI bleeding/Melena</li><li>Microaneurysm are typically seen</li><li>Digital ischemia and gangrene</li><li>Can involve any organ except Lung</li><li>Skin: Nodules, purpura, Raynaud phenomena</li><li>Renal involvement:<ul><li>Characterized by arteritis without GN</li><li>Present with Renovascular hypertension</li></ul></li></ul>	<ul><li>Fever is MC constitutional symptom</li><li>Associated with mucocutaneous lymph node syndrome</li><li>Mucocutaneous features:<ul><li>Erythema of palm and sole and oral mucosa</li><li>Edema of hands and feet</li><li>Strawberry tongue</li><li>Non purulent conjunctivitis</li></ul></li><li>Cervical lymphadenopathy<ul><li>Nonsuppurative</li><li>UL > BL</li></ul></li><li>Vasculitis of coronary artery l/t coronary artery aneurysm</li></ul>
Investigations	<ul><li>IOC: Temporal artery biopsy → 3-5 cm long segment of artery is excised</li><li>↑ ESR, Anemia</li><li>H/P: Panarteritis</li></ul>	<ul><li>Diagnosis established by angiography</li><li>Classified into 6 types based on angiographic involvement (MC– Type III)</li><li>↑ ESR, Anemia</li><li>H/P: Panarteritis</li></ul>	<ul><li>Hematuria, proteinuria seen but RBC cast are absent (due to absence of GN)</li><li>Presence of HbsAg</li><li>H/P: **Panarteritis**, Fibrinoid necrosis, Neutrophil infiltration in all layers</li></ul>	<ul><li>No diagnostic tests</li><li>Thrombocytosis</li><li>2D ECHO to detect aneurysm</li></ul>
Management	<ul><li>Steroids</li><li>High dose Methyl prednisolone for visual complications</li><li>Tocilizumab – Anti IL-6 receptor</li></ul>	<ul><li>Steroids remains the mainstay of treatment</li></ul>	<ul><li>Steroids + Cyclophosphamide</li></ul>	<ul><li>TOC is high dose IVIG</li><li>Excellent prognosis</li></ul>

SMALL VESSEL VASCULITIS

	Wegener's Granulomatosis/ GPA	Microscopic Polyarteritis/MPA	Churg Strauss syndrome/ EGPA	Henoch Schonlein Purpura/ IgA Vasculitis
General features	- **C** – ANCA +ve - Granulomatous inflammation - Necrotizing vasculitis - Rare in children [**Mn: C**ommon **W**ealth **G**ame]	- **P** – ANCA > C – ANCA +ve - Non granulomatous inflammation - Necrotizing vasculitis - Median age ~50 years - Involves arterioles, capillaries as well as venules (contrasting feature from PAN)	- P – ANCA +ve - Granulomatous inflammation - Necrotizing vasculitis - Mean age ~50 years	- ANCA –ve - Non granulomatous inflammation - Necrotizing vasculitis - MC vasculitis in children - IgA mediated disorder

Clinical features	Characterized by triad of –
	- Upper respiratory tract involvement:
	  ○ Septal perforation
	  ○ Otitis media
	  ○ Strawberry gum
	- Lower respiratory tract involvement:
	  ○ Hemoptysis
	  ○ Cavitary lesions in lung
	- Renal involvement:
	  ○ Type III RPGN
		- It is a dermato–pulmonary–renal syndrome
		- Skin:
		  ○ Retrospecting purpura
		- Pulmonary manifestation:
		  ○ Upper respiratory tract involvement is less frequent when compared to Wegener's
		  ○ Involves lower respiratory tract
		- Renal involvement:
		  ○ Crescentic glomerulonephritis
		  ○ Renal failure
		- Mononeuritis multiplex
			- MC presentation–Bronchial asthma
			- Allergic rhinitis
			- Sinusitis
			- Nasal polyposis
			- Peripheral neuropathy
			- Myocarditis
				- URTI may precede the clinical onset of illness by 1–3 weeks
				- Palpable purpura → MC and hallmark feature
				  ○ Symmetrical
				  ○ MC location is over buttocks and lower extremities
				- Polyarthralgia
				- Colicky abdominal pain
				- Melena and hematemesis
				- Type II RPGN and renal failure

Investigations	- Hematuria, proteinuria and RBC cast in urine (due to glomerulonephritis) - Complement levels = N/Raised - Rheumatoid factor may be positive	- Hematuria, proteinuria and RBC cast in urine (due to glomerulonephritis) - Normal complements	- Eosinophilia (>1500/μL) - Raised serum IgE - H/P: eosinophil rich granulomatous inflammation - CXR → pulmonary infiltrates	- Hematuria, proteinuria and RBC cast in urine (due to glomerulonephritis) - Normal complements - Increased serum IgA - Skin or kidney biopsy: IgA deposits - Leukocytosis with eosinophilia - Normal/increased platelet count - Benign self, limiting disorder - Excellent prognosis
Management	- Induction: Cyclophosphamide with steroids - Remission: Methotrexate, Azathioprine - Rituximab for induction	- Induction: Cyclophosphamide with steroids - Remission: Methotrexate, Azathioprine - Rituximab for induction	- Glucocorticoids - Cyclophosphamide + prednisolone if multisystem involvement	- Steroids

BEHÇET SYNDROME

- Vasculitic disorder characterized by recurrent oral ulcer, genital ulcer and uveitis
- Associated with HLA B51/B5
- Can affect small, medium and large vessels

- Oral ulcers are usually the initial clinical manifestation.
- Ulcers are painful and non scarring
- Skin → erythema nodosum

INFLAMMATORY MYOPATHIES

	Dermatomyositis	Polymyositis	Inclusion Body Myositis
Gender	▪ F > M	▪ F > M	▪ M > F
Age of onset	▪ Childhood and adults	▪ Adults	▪ Older adults
Rash	▪ Yes	▪ No	▪ No
Muscle weakness	▪ Proximal > Distal	▪ Proximal > Distal	▪ Distal > Proximal
Cellular infiltrates	▪ CD4+ T cells	▪ CD8+ T cells	▪ CD8+ T cells
Creatine kinase	▪ N/↑ 50 times	▪ ↑ 50 times	▪ Normal or mild ↑
Muscle biopsy	▪ Perivascular and perimysial inflammation ▪ Perifascicular inflammation and atrophy	▪ Minimal inflammation ▪ No vacuoles	▪ Ragged red fibers ▪ Vacuoles present

Cutaneous Manifestations of Dermatomyositis

- **Heliotrope rash** → erythematous discoloration of eyelids with periorbital edema
- **Gottron papule** → raised erythematous rash over extensor surface of joints
- **V sign** → rash on the sun exposed anterior neck and chest
- **Shawl sign** → rash over the back of neck and shoulder
- Subcutaneous calcium deposits

SARCOIDOSIS

General features	▪ Sarcoidosis is a multisystem inflammatory disease of unknown etiology ▪ Lung is involvement occur in > 90% of cases
Clinical features	▪ Lungs: Cough, chest pain, Fibrosis leading to ILD, pleural effusion ▪ Bilateral parotid enlargement ▪ Skin: Erythema nodosum, Lupus pernio ▪ Acute Sarcoidosis may present as: 　○ **Heerfordt's syndrome:** Fever, Uveitis, B/L parotid enlargement, VII CN palsy 　○ **Lofgren's syndrome:** Triad of bilateral hilar **L**ymphadenopathy, **E**rythema **N**odosum and Uveitis
Lab features	▪ ACE levels are elevated in 60% of patient at the time of diagnosis ▪ Hypercalcemia, increase 1,25 (OH) Vitamin D ▪ CXR: Bilateral hilar lymphadenopathy – hallmark ▪ Egg shell calcification of hilar lymph node ▪ **Garland sign** (1-2-3 sign) on CXR: B/L hilar and right paratracheal lymphadenopathy ▪ Gallium 67 scan: 　○ **Lambda sign** – B/L hilar and right paratracheal lymphadenopathy 　○ **Panda sign** – B/L involvement of parotid and lacrimal glands ▪ PFT: restrictive pattern with isolated decrease in DL_{CO} ▪ BAL: Increased lymphocytes with CD4: CD8 ratio >3.5 ▪ Kveim siltzbach skin test ▪ Biopsy: Noncaseating granuloma ▪ **Inclusion bodies present in granuloma:** 　○ **S**chaumann bodies 　○ **A**steroid bodies 　○ **R**esidual bodies
Staging on CXR	▪ Stage I – Bilateral hilar lymphadenopathy ▪ Stage II – Bilateral hilar lymphadenopathy + diffuse pulmonary infiltrates ▪ Stage III – Diffuse pulmonary infiltrates without hilar lymphadenopathy ▪ Stage IV – Severe fibrosis
Management	▪ Corticosteroids ▪ Methotrexate

MULTIPLE CHOICE QUESTIONS

CHAPTER 1: RHEUMATOLOGY AND VASCULITIDES

1. **Articular cause of arthritis is differentiated from non-articular cause of arthritis by all of the following signs EXCEPT:-** *(PGMEE 2018)*
   a. Presence of pain during active movement
   b. Pain during active and passive movements both
   c. Swelling near joint
   d. Presence of crepitus

   [Ref: Internal medicine essentials by American college of physicians]

Explanation

Articular and Nonarticular Disorders

- Differentiate articular from nonarticular sources of joint pain.
- Articular disorders are characterized by internal/deep joint pain that is exacerbated by active and passive motion and by reduced range of motion; joint pain may be accompanied by joint effusion, synovial thickening, joint deformity or instability, crepitations, clicking, popping, or locking.
- Periarticular (Non articular) disorders are associated with greater joint pain with active rather than passive motion; in addition, range of motion often is preserved, and tenderness and signs of inflammation are removed from the actual joint.
- Common periarticular disorders include bursitis, tendinitis, polymyalgia rheumatica, fibromyalgia, and enthesopathies (inflammation of tendinous or ligamentous attachments to bone). Enthesopathies are characteristic of spondyloarthritis; the most common are Achilles tendonitis and plantar fasciitis. Dactylitis (œsausage digits) is another classic feature of spondyloarthritis, particularly psoriatic arthritis and reactive arthritis; dactylitis is caused by synovitis and enthesitis of the fingers and toe.
- Pain also may be referred or radiate to the joints from nonarticular sources (eg, shoulder pain associated with cervical radiculopathy) or other local pathology.

2. **Glucosamine supplementation is given in:** *(NEET Pattern 2018)*
   a. Arthritis   b. Diabetes
   c. Cataract   d. Asthma

   [Ref: Glucosamines are contraindicated in Diabetes.; Maheshwari 5ed. PAGE 296]

Explanation

- Chondoprotective agents like glucosamine and chondriotin sulphate are known to result in repair of damaged cartilage. Other drugs include Sodium Hylarunon injection.

RHEUMATOID ARTHRITIS (RA)

3. **Which of the following is true regarding rheumatoid arthritis?** *(PGMEE 2014-15)*
   a. Typically involves small joints asymmetrically
   b. Causes pleural effusion with high sugar
   c. Mononeuritis multiplex is seen
   d. Enthesopathy is prominent

   [Ref: Harrison's 20th/e pg. 2529]

4. **Felty's syndrome consist of rheumatoid arthritis, splenomegaly and :-** *(PGMEE 2016-17)*
   a. Neutropenia   b. Thrombocytopenia
   c. lymphopenia   d. Neutrophilia

   [Ref: Harrison's 20th/e pg. 2530]

5. **Which of the following condition improves with pregnancy?** *(PGMEE 2014/15)*
   a. Rheumatoid arthritis   b. SLE
   c. Myasthenia gravis   d. Multiple sclerosis

   [Ref: Harrison's 20th/e pg. 2530]

6. **In rheumatoid arthritis pathology starts in:** *(PGMEE 2014-15)*
   a. Articular cartilage   b. Capsule
   c. Synovium   d. Muscle

   [Ref: Harrison's 20th/e pg. 2532]

7. **All are seen in Rheumatoid arthritis EXCEPT:**
   a. Deformities   *(PGMEE 2015-16)*
   b. Mononeuritis multiplex
   c. Peri-articular osteoporosis
   d. Sero-negative arthritis

   [Ref: Harrison's 20th/e pg.2530]

8. **In long standing rheumatoid arthritis which will be seen?** *(PGMEE 2015-16)*
   a. Milk alkali syndrome   b. Nephrolithiasis
   c. Paradoxical aciduria   d. Secondary amyloidosis

   [Ref: Harrison's 20th/e pg. 2530]

9. **Immunological factor in Rheumatoid arthritis is:-** *(PGMEE 2016-17)*
   a. HLA DR4 association   b. Anti- ds DNA antibody
   c. Anti- CCP antibodies   d. All of the above

   [Ref: Harrison's 20th/e pg.2531]

10. **Anti-CCP antibody is seen in:-** *(PGMEE 2015-16)*
    a. Crohn's disease   b. SLE
    c. Osteoarthritis   d. Rheumatoid Arthritis

    [Ref: Harrison 20th/e pg. 2535]

11. **Drug of choice for RA:-** *(PGMEE 2016-17)*
    a. Aspirin   b. Corticosteroids
    c. Nebumatone   d. Methotrexate

    [Ref: Harrison's 20th/e pg. 2536]

1. d
2. a
3. c
4. a
5. a
6. c
7. d
8. d
9. d
10. d
11. d

12. Caplan's syndrome is? *(DNB Dec 2009)*
a. Pneumoconiosis with CCF
b. Pneumoconiosis with lymphadenopathy
c. Pneumoconiosis with HIV
d. Pneumoconiosis with rheumatoid arthritis

[Ref: Harrison's 20th/e 2529]

13. Rheumatoid arthritis is seen with? *(PGMEE 2015-16)*
a. HLA DR3
b. HLA DR4
c. HLA DR 27
d. HLA B 27

[Ref: Harrison 20th/e pg. 2530]

14. Cells mainly involved in Rheumatoid arthritis:
(PGMEE 2018)
a. Macrophages
b. Dendritic cells
c. B-cells
d. T-cells

[Ref: Harrison 20th/e pg. 2532]

Explanation

- Rheumatoid arthritis is a chronic systemic inflammatory disorder that often progresses to destruction of the articular cartilage and ankylosis of the joints. Once an inflammatory synovitis has been initiated, an autoimmune reaction—in which **T cells** have the pivotal role—is responsible for the chronic destructive nature of rheumatoid arthritis. TH17 cells are important in the inflammatory reaction because they recruit neutrophils and monocytes.

15. Gold was used for management of? *(PGMEE 2015-16)*
a. Ankylosing Spondylitis
b. Rheumatoid Arthritis
c. Psoriatic arthritis
d. Rheumatic arthriitis

[Ref: Harrison 19th ed. / 2144-45]

16. Polyarticular onset JRA involves more than
(PGMEE 2014-15)
a. 3 joints
b. 4 joints
c. 5 joints
d. 6 joints

[Ref: Harrison 20th/e pg. 2528]

17. C V junction abnormalities are seen in all of the following EXCEPT: *(PGMEE 2014-15)*
a. Rheumatoid arthritis
b. Ankylosing spondylitis
c. Odontoid dysgenesis
d. Basilar invagination

[Ref: MERCK MANUAL and Williams wilkins neurosurgery pg. 2732-2735; Harrison 20th/e pg. 2528]

18. In rheumatoid arthritis the characteristic joint involvement is: *(PGMEE 2014-15)*
a. Spine
b. Knee
c. Metacarpophalangeal joint
d. Hip joint

[Ref: Harrison 20th/e pg. 2528]

19. The most common cardiac involvement in rheumatoid arthritis: *(PGMEE 2014-15)*
a. Cardiomyopathy
b. Pericarditis
c. Myocarditis
d. Endocarditis

[Ref: Harrison 20th/e pg. 2529]

20. Which of the following is the most specific test for rheumatoid arthritis? *(PGMEE 2014-15)*
a. Anti- MCV antibody
b. Anti cardiolipin antibody
c. Anti Mi-2 antibody
d. Anti Ro antibody

[Ref: Internet]

21. HLA-DR4 is a marker of: *(PGMEE 2014-15)*
a. Rheumatoid arthritis
b. Sarcoidosis
c. Sero-negative gouty arthritis
d. Psoriasis

[Ref: Harrison 20th/e pg. 2530]

22. Type of anemia seen in Rheumatoid arthritis:
a. Normocytic, normochromic *(PGMEE 2014-15)*
b. Hyperchromic, Normocytic
c. Hypochromic, normocytic
d. Hypochromic, leucopenia

[Ref: Harrison 20th/e pg. 2529]

23. Clinical manifestation of Felty's syndrome are all EXCEPT: *(PGMEE 2014-15)*
a. Rheumatoid arthritis
b. Splenomegaly
c. Neutropenia
d. Nephropathy

[Ref: Harrison 20th/e pg. 2530]

24. Rheumatoid arthritis commonly affects the:
(PGMEE 2014-15)
a. Cervical spine
b. Thoracolumbar spine
c. Lumbar spine
d. Sacral spine

[Ref: Harrison 20th/e pg. 2528]

25. Joint not involved in Rheumatoid arthritis according to 1987 modified ARA criteria? *(PGMEE 08)*
a. Knee
b. Ankle
c. Tarsometatarsal
d. Metatarsophalangeal

[Ref: Harrison 20th/e pg. 2529]

26. Caplan's syndrome is seen with ? *(PGMEE 2014-15)*
a. COPD
b. Pneumoconiosis
c. Pulmonary edema
d. Rheumatoid arthritis

[Ref: Harrison's 20th/e pg. 2528]

27. A patient of rheumatoid arthritis develops sudden onset quadriparesis increased muscle tone of limbs with exaggerated tendon jerks and worsening of gait. The investigation to be done? *(PGMEE 2014-15)*
a. Cervical spine X-ray
b. MRI brain
c. EMG and NCV
d. Carotid angiography

[Ref: Harrison 20th/e pg. 2528]

28. Which is the most common site of subcutaneous nodules in rheumatoid arthritis? *(PGMEE 2014-15)*
a. Elbow
b. Wrist
c. Achilles tendon
d. Occiput

[Ref: Harrison 20th/e pg. 2529]

29. Not seen in rheumatoid arthritis is: *(PGMEE 2014-15)*
a. Normal C.R.P
b. Juxtaarticular osteopenia
c. Cervical myelopathy
d. Hyperandrogenism

[Ref: Harrison 20th/e pg. 2530]

12.	d
13.	b
14.	d
15.	b
16.	c
17.	b
18.	c
19.	b
20.	a
21.	a
22.	a
23.	d
24.	a
25.	c
26.	d
27.	a
28.	a
29.	d

30. ANA (antinuclear antibody) is seen in all except-
(PGMEE 2013-14)
a. SLE
b. RA
c. Sjogren's syndrome
d. Systemic sclerosis

[Ref: Harrison 20th/e pg. 2535]

31. All may be true about Rheumatoid Arthritis EXCEPT:
(PGMEE 2014-15)
a. Anti- MCV antibody
b. RF positive
c. Anti- CCP antibody
d. Anti- Mi-2 antibody

[Ref: Harrison 20th/e pg. 2535]

32. Which of the following is not a seronegative spondyloarthropathy-
(PGMEE 2013-14)
a. Reiters arthritis
b. Psoriatic arthritis
c. RA
d. Ankylosing spondylitis

[Ref: Robbins 9th/e pg. 1209-1212]

33. Swan-neck deformity is-
(PGMEE 15)
a. Flexion of Metacarpophalangeal joint and extension at interphalangeal joint
b. Extension at Proximal interphalangeal joint flexion at Distal interphalangeal joint
c. Flexion at proximal interphalangeal joint and extension at distal interphalangeal joint
d. Extension at Metacarpophalangeal joint and flexion at interphalangeal joint

[Ref: Harrison 20th/e pg. 2528]

Explanation

- Swan-neck deformity: Extension of PIP + Flexion of DIP
- Boutonnier deformity: Flexion of PIP + Hyperextensoin of DIP.

34. A lady having flexion at proximal interphalyngeal joint and hyperextension at distal interphalyngeal joint of index finger is called-
(PGMEE 14)
a. Boutonniere deformity
b. Swan neck deformity
c. Wind swept deformity
d. Z deformity

[Ref: Harrison 20th/e pg. 2528]

35. Windswept deformity in foot is seen in-
(PGMEE 14)
a. Rickets
b. RA
c. Hyperparathyroidism
d. Scurvy

[Ref: Internet]

36. Periosteal reaction is NOT seen in:-
(PGMEE 13)
a. Psoriatic arthritis
b. Reactive arthritis
c. Neuropathic arthritis
d. Rheumatoid arthritis

[Ref: http://www.ajronline.org/doi/pdf/10.2214/AJR.09.3300]

37. Which joint is spared in Rheumatoid arthritis-
(DNB dec 2011; PGMEE 2012)
a. MCP joint of and
b. DIP joints of finger
c. PIP joints of finger
d. Atlanto-axial joint

[Ref: Harrison 20th/e pg. 2528]

38. Rheumatoid arthritis is associated with all except-
(PGMEE 2012)
a. Cardiac involvement
b. Bauchards nodes
c. Heberden node
d. Swan-neck deformity

[Ref: Harrison 20th/e pg. 2528]

Explanation

- Heberden node and Bauchard's node seen in osteoarthritis.
- Heberden node involves DIP, where as Bauchard's node involves PIP

39. Earliest radiological change in RA-
(PGMEE 2012)
a. Decreased joint space
b. Articular erosion
c. Periarticular osteopenia
d. Subchondral cyst

[Ref: Harrison 20th/e pg. 2535]

40. A 60 years old lady with RA complains of pain and continuous activity of the disease. She is on methotrexate, steroids and NSAIDs for last 4 months. What is the next best step
(PGMEE 2019)
a. Start monotherapy with TNF alpha inhibitors
b. Continue methotrexate and steroids
c. Change methotrexate to leflunomide
d. Add sulfasalazine

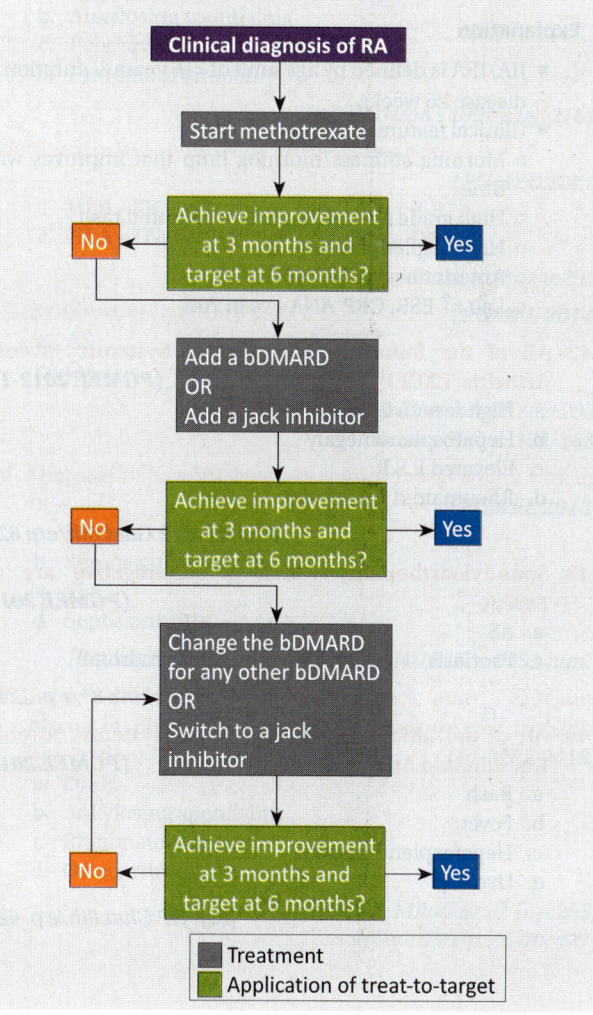

30.	b
31.	d
32.	c
33.	b
34.	a
35.	b
36.	d
37.	b
38.	b,c
39.	c
40.	c

68. A 27 year old male with back pain which is more in the morning and decreases in the evening. It is also relieved by bathing in warm water. What is the additional finding? *(NEET Pattern 2015)*
   a. Liver enlargement
   b. Decreased chest expansion
   c. Interphalangeal joint swelling
   d. Marrow fibrosis

[Ref: Harrison's 19th/e pg. 2170]

69. Joints of hand are not affected in-   *(PGMEE 2012)*
   a. AS
   b. OA
   c. RA
   d. Psoriatic arthritis

[Ref: Maheshwari & Mhaskar 5th /e p.293,4]

Explanation

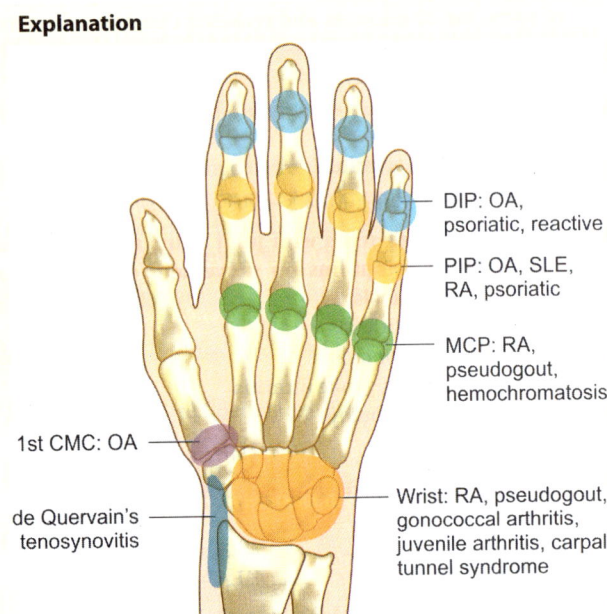

DIP: OA, psoriatic, reactive
PIP: OA, SLE, RA, psoriatic
MCP: RA, pseudogout, hemochromatosis
1st CMC: OA
de Quervain's tenosynovitis
Wrist: RA, pseudogout, gonococcal arthritis, juvenile arthritis, carpal tunnel syndrome

70. Bamboo spine with sacroilitis-   *(PGMEE 2012)*
   a. Anklosing spondylitis
   b. OA
   c. RA
   d. Psoriatic arthritis

[Ref: Maheshwari & Mhaskar 5th /e p.293-294]

71. Arthritis common with uveitis is: *(PGMEE 2014-15)*
   a. RA
   b. Ankylosing spondylitis
   c. Still's disease
   d. Reiter's disease

[Ref: Harrison's 19th/e pg. 2169]

72. In anklyosing spondylitis joint involvement is least in?   *(PGMEE 2014-15)*
   a. Wrist and hand
   b. Sacroiliac joint
   c. Acromio-clavicular joint
   d. Costochondral junction

[Ref: Harrison's 19th/e pg. 2170]

73. Schober's sign is used to evaluate: *(PGMEE 2014-15)*
   a. Flexion of lumbar spine
   b. Chest expansion
   c. Pain with motion of hip
   d. Neck pain and stiffness

[Ref: Harrison's 19th/e pg. 2170]

74. In Seronegative spondyloarthritis, what will cause maximum reduction in pain and morning stiffness?   *(PGMEE 2014-15)*
   a. Aspirin
   b. Indomethacin
   c. Corticosteroids
   d. Infliximab

[Ref: Harrison's 19th/e pg. 2172]

PSORIATIC ARTHRITIS

75. CASPAR criteria is used in diagnosis of-   *(PGMEE 2015)*
   a. Psoriatic arthritis
   b. Rheumatoid arthritis
   c. Ankyosing spondylitis
   d. Reactive synovitis

[www.rheumatologynetwork.com]

76. True about psoriatic arthritis are all except-   *(PGMEE 2012)*
   a. DOC is methotrexate
   b. Involvement of DIP joint
   c. More common in males
   d. HLA-Cw6 association

[Ref: Atlas of psoriatic arthritis p. 9]

77. Which of the following is true of psoriatic arthritis?   *(PGMEE 2014-15)*
   a. Involves distal joints of hand and foot
   b. Pencil in cup deformity
   c. Sacroilitis
   d. All of the above

[Ref: Harrison's 19th/e pg. 2175]

78. Arthritis mutilans is seen in?   *(DNB 2011 june)*
   a. Psoriatic athropathy
   b. Rheumatoid arthritis
   c. Reactive arthritis
   d. Spondyloarthroathy

[Ref: Harrison's 19th/e pg. 2175]

REACTIVE ARTHRITIS/REITER SYNDROME

79. Reactive arthritis is usually caused by: *(PGMEE 2014-15)*
   a. Shigella flexneri
   b. Shigella boydii
   c. Shigela shiga
   d. Shigela dysentriae

[Ref: Harrison 20th/e pg. 2569]

80. Keratoderma Blennorrhagica is typically seen in:-   *(PGMEE 2016-17, 2015-16; DNB June 2010)*
   a. Psoriatic Arthritis
   b. Ankylosing spondylitis
   c. Reactive arthritis (Reiter's disease)
   d. Rheumatoid Arthritis

[Ref: Harrison 20th/e pg. 2569]

81. Most common organism associated with reactive arthritis is-   *(PGMEE 2015)*
   a. Yersinia
   b. Shigella
   c. Chalmydia
   d. Staphylococcus

[Ref: Harrison 20th/e pg. 2569]

82. All are seen in Reiter's syndrome except: *(DNB pattern 2008)*
   a. Subcutaneous nodules
   b. Oral ulcers
   c. Keratoderma blenorrhagicum
   d. Circinate balanitis

(Ref. IADVL Textbook of dermatology 3rd edition pg 1861)

68.	b
69.	a
70.	a
71.	b
72.	a
73.	a
74.	d
75.	a
76.	c
77.	d
78.	a
79.	a
80.	c
81.	c
82.	a

Explanation

- Reiter's syndrome is 'oculo-urethro-synovial' syndrome-triad of conjunctivitis, urethritis and acute non-purulent seronegative arthritis. Mucocutaneous manifestations include-
  - Circinate balanitis is the most common cutaneous finding, reported in 36% pt
  - Transient painless mucosal (oral) ulcers seen in 17% of cases.
  - keratoderma blenorrhagicum are found in 15% of patients densely scattered on the soles and palms
  - psoriasiform cutaneous lesions
  - Dystrophy of nails is seen in up to 20%–30% of patients

GOUT & OTHER CRYSTAL ARTHROPATHIES

83. Saturine gout is seen with: *(NEET Pattern 2019)*
- a. Arsenic
- b. Lead
- c. Cadmium
- d. Mercury

84. Gout is a disorder of:- *(PGMEE 2018)*
- a. Pyrimidine metabolism
- b. Purine metabolism
- c. Amino acid transport defect
- d. Mismatch repair of DNA

[Ref: Harrison 20th/e pg. 2631]

85. Martel sign is seen in? *(PGMEE 2015-16)*
- a. Gout
- b. Ankylosing spondylitis
- c. Osteoarthritis
- d. Rheumatoid arthritis

[Ref: Internet]

86. True statement regarding acute attack of gouty arthritis is all EXCEPT: *(DNB June 2009)*
- a. Serum uric acid level may be absolutely normal
- b. Allopurinol should be started immediately
- c. Colchicine is known to provide relief
- d. Joint aspirate reveals negative birefringent crystlas

[Ref: Harrison 20th/e pg. 2632]

87. MC joint involved in Gout- *(PGMEE 2015)*
- a. Knee
- b. Hip
- c. MTP joint of the big toe
- d. MP joint of thumb

88. All joints are involved in acute gout EXCEPT: *(PGMEE 2014-15)*
- a. MTP
- b. Gleno-humeral joint
- c. Ankle joint
- d. Knee joint

[Ref: Harrison's 20th/e pg. 2632]

89. Tophi in gout found in all regions EXCEPT: *(PGMEE 2014-15, DNB Dec'2011)*
- a. Prepatellar bursae
- b. Muscle
- c. Helix of ear
- d. Synovial membrane

[Ref: CMDT 2014 ch.20, Pg. 812]

90. Incorrect about diagnosis of a patient of Gouty arthritis? *(PGMEE 2014-15)*
- a. High synovial fluid protein
- b. High WBC count
- c. Urate crystal in synovial fluid
- d. Normal sugar in synovial fluid

[Ref: Harrison 20th/e pg. 2632]

91. Needle shaped crystals negatively birefringent on polarized microscopy is characteristic of which crystal associated arthropathy? *(PGMEE 2015)*
- a. Gout
- b. CPPD
- c. Neuropathic arthropathy
- d. Hemophilic arthropathy

[Ref: Harrison 20th/e pg. 2632]

92. In a patient with gouty arthritis, synovial fluid aspiration will show- *(PGMEE 2009)*
- a. Monosodium Urate crystals
- b. Polymorphonuclear Leukocytosis
- c. Mononuclear Leucocytosis
- d. Calcium Pyrophosphate crystals

[Ref: Harrison 20th/e pg. 2632]

93. All drugs used in treatment of acute gout EXCEPT: *(PGMEE 2014-15)*
- a. Allopurinol
- b. Aspirin
- c. Colchicine
- d. Naproxen

[Ref: Harrison 20th/e pg. 2632-33]

94. Drug used in acute gout- *(PGMEE 2012)*
- a. Allopurinol
- b. Sulfinpyrazone
- c. Colchicine
- d. Probenacid

[Ref: Harrison 20th/e pg. 2632-33]

95. The following statements are true regarding acute gout EXCEPT: *(PGMEE 2014-15)*
- a. Acute gout is more common in males
- b. Serum uric acid is normal in acute gout
- c. First metatarsophalangeal joint is most commonly affected in acute gout
- d. Treatment with Allopurinol should be started immediately in the case of acute gout

[Ref: Harrison's 19th/e pg. 2233]

96. Prolonged allopurinol therapy in a patient with gout is NOT indicated for: *(PGMEE 2014-15)*
- a. Acute gouty arthritis
- b. Tophi
- c. Urate nephropathy
- d. Evidence of bone/joint damage

[Ref: Harrison 20th/e pg. 2632]

97. All of the following can be used to prevent gouty attack EXCEPT: *(PGMEE 2014-15)*
- a. Allopurinol
- b. Aspirin
- c. Probenecid
- d. Sulfinpyrazone

[Ref: Harrison 20th/e pg. 2633]

98. Best treatment for gout with kidney impairment? *(PGMEE 2014-15)*
- a. Allopurinol
- b. Febuxostat
- c. Uricase
- d. Benzbromarone

[Ref: Harrison 20th/e pg. 2633]

99. All are true about pseudogout except? *(PGMEE 2014-15)*
- a. Calcium pyrophosphate crystals
- b. Most commonly idiopathic
- c. Hyperparathyroidism
- d. Most common joint involved is DIP

[Ref: Harrison 20th/e pg. 2634]

83. b
84. b
85. a
86. b
87. c
88. b
89. b
90. a
91. a
92. a
93. a
94. c
95. d
96. a
97. b
98. b
99. d

100. Negatively Birefringent crystals in urine is seen with:
(PGMEE 2014-15)

a. Phosphaturia
b. Uricosuria
c. Cystinuria
d. Salicylates (low dose)

[Ref: Harrison 20th/e pg. 2632]

101. Hyperuricemia can be caused by all except-
(PGMEE 2015)

a. Salicylates (low dose)
b. Thiazide
c. Probenecid
d. Furosemide

[Ref: Harrison 20th/e pg. 2998]

102. Risk factors associated with development of Gout A/E-
(PGMEE 2015)

a. Hypertension
b. Female sex
c. Thiazide
d. Obesity

[Ref: Harrison 20th/e pg. 2998]

103. Which joint is most commonly affected in pseudogout-
(PGMEE 2015)

a. Knee
b. Hip
c. MP joint great toe
d. MP joint thumb

[Ref: Harrison 20th/e pg. 2634]

104. CPPD crystals are seen in which disease- *(PGMEE 2012)*

a. Primary hyperparathyroidism
b. Hypomagnesemia
c. Hemochromatosis
d. All of the above

[Ref: Harrison 20th/e pg. 2633]

105. A lady presents with right knee swelling. Aspiration was done in which CPPD crystals were obtained. Next best investigation is-
(PGMEE 10)

a. RF
b. ANA
c. CPK
d. TSH

[Ref: Harrison 20th/e pg. 2633]

106. Which of the following is not seen in pseudogout-
(PGMEE 09)

a. Small joints affected
b. Deposition of calcium pyrophosphate
c. Chondrocalcinosis
d. Large joints affected

[Ref: Harrison 20th/e pg. 2634]

SYSTEMIC LUPUS ERYTHEMATOSUS

107. Onion skin spleen is seen in: *(PGMEE 2014-15)*

a. ITP
b. Thalassemia
c. SLE
d. Scleroderma

[Ref: Harrison's 19th/e pg. 2127]

Explanation

- Onion skin lesions
  - Onion skin spleen - SLE
  - Onion skin fibrosis of duct - PSC
  - Onion skin periosteal reaction → Euring sarcoma
  - Onion skin lesion of artery → Scleroderma crisis & Malignant hypertension

108. Lady presents with joint pain in both knees and low grade fever off and on. On examination she has a rash on sun exposed parts. Image shown below.What is the clinical diagnosis?
(PGMEE 2016-17, 2015-16)

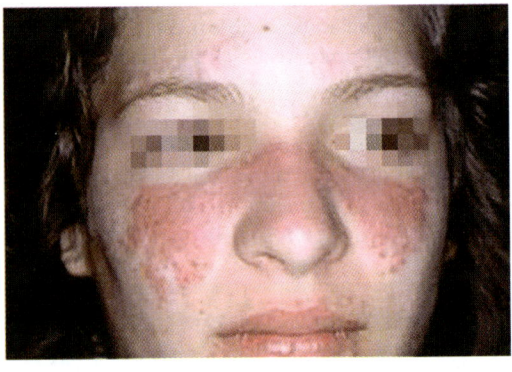

a. Lupus vulgaris
b. SLE
c. Photodermatitis
d. CREST syndrome

[Ref: Harrison 20th/e pg. 2518]

109. A 26-year old female presents with oral ulcers photosensitivity and malar rash sparing the nasolabial folds. What is the diagnosis :
(PGMEE 2019)

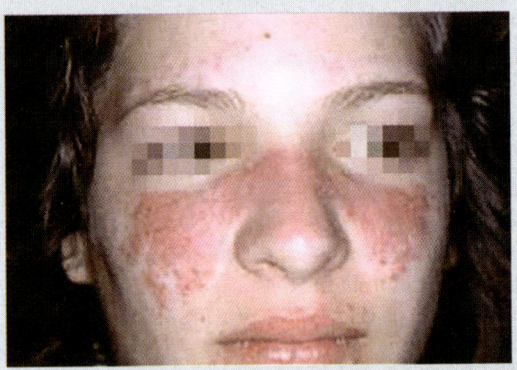

a. Stuge-Weber syndrome
b. Dermatitis
c. SLE
d. Psoriasis

[Ref: Harrison 20th/e pg. 2518]

110. Band test is done in- *(PGMEE 2013-14)*

a. RA
b. SLE
c. Scleroderma
d. PAN

[Ref: Robbins 9th/e pg. 219]

111. Best marker of SLE is ? *(DNB June 2010)*

a. Anti Sm antibodies
b. Anto Ro (ss-a) antibodies
c. Anti nucleosome antibodies
d. Anti ds DNA antibodies

[Ref: Harrison 20th/e pg. 2517]

112. Antinuclear antibody which is specific for SLE is:-
(PGMEE 2013-14)

a. Anti ds DNA
b. Anti histone Ab
c. Anti nuclear antibodies
d. Anti centromere antibody

[Ref: Robbins 9th/e pg. 219]

113. Which antibodies in mother with SLE is responsible for congenital heart disease in child - *(PGMEE 2013-14)*
   a. Anti- histone
   b. Anti- RO & Anti- LA
   c. Anti ds DNA
   d. Anti- centromere

[Ref: Harrison 20th/e pg. 2517]

114. Normal CRP with elevated ESR seen in? *(PGMEE 2015-16)*
   a. RA
   b. SLE
   c. Scleroderma
   d. Polymyalgia rheumatica

[Ref: Harrison 20th/e pg. 2522]

115. Best test for subacute cutaneous lupus Erythematosus: *(PGMEE 2014-15)*
   a. dsDNA
   b. anti-J0-1 antibody
   c. Anti-Ro/SS-A
   d. Anti-histone antibody

[Ref: Harrison 20th/e pg. 2522]

116. Characteristic cardiac lesion in SLE is: *(PGMEE 2014-15)*
   a. Verrucous endocarditis
   b. Valvular incompetence
   c. Heart block
   d. Myocardial fibrosis

[Ref: Harrison 20th/e pg. 2520]

117. Antinuclear antibodies are seen in A/E: *(PGMEE 2014-15)*
   a. Systemic sclerosis
   b. Morphea
   c. Pemphigus vulgaris
   d. SLE

118. A young girl is admitted with joint pains and butterfly rash and positive urine proteinuria. The best test for her diagnosis is? *(PGMEE 2014-15)*
   a. Anti ds-DNA antibody
   b. Anti-centromere antibody
   c. Antibodies to RNP
   d. Antibodies to tRNA synthetase

[Ref: Harrison 20th/e pg. 2517]

119. The poly-arthritic condition that is NOT common in males: *(PGMEE 2014-15)*
   a. Gout
   b. Psoriatic arthritis
   c. Ankylosing spondylitis
   d. Systemic lupus erythematosus

[Ref: Harrison 20th/e pg. 2515]

120. Coomb's positive hemolytic anemia associated with: *(PGMEE 2014-15)*
   a. TTP
   b. PAN
   c. SLE
   d. HUS

[Ref: Harrison 20th/e pg. 2518]

121. A 33-year-old woman has experienced episodes of fatigue, pleural effusion, pericardial effusion and carpal tunnel syndrome and macrocytic anemia. Best test for diagnosis shall be: *(PGMEE 2014-15)*
   a. Anti-beta 2 phospholipid antibodies
   b. Anti-smith antibody
   c. Antinuclear antibody
   d. Assay for thyroid hormones

[Ref: Harrison 20th/e pg. 2699 Table 376-3]

Explanation
   - Presenting complain suggest hypothyroidism rather than SLE.

122. Butterfly rash in SLE involves all areas except *(PGMEE 2014-15)*
   a. Cheeks
   b. Nasolabial fold
   c. Lower eylids
   d. Bridge of nose

[Ref: Harrison 20th/e pg. 2519]

123. Psychosis in SLE is caused by: *(PGMEE 2014-15)*
   a. Anti-ribosomal P antibody
   b. Anti-glutamate acid decarboxylase antibody
   c. Anti-endomysial antibody
   d. Anti-histone antibody

[Ref: Harrison 20th/e pg. 2517]

124. Lupus anticoagulant causes A/E: *(PGMEE 2014-15)*
   a. Recurrent abortion
   b. Arterial thrombosis
   c. Increase aPTT
   d. Nephritis

[Ref: Harrison 20th/e pg. 2517]

125. The following are features of SLE EXCEPT:
   a. Sterile Vegetations on valve cusps *(PGMEE 2014-15)*
   b. Raynaud's phenomenon
   c. Atherosclerosis
   d. Pulmonary fibrosis

[Ref: Harrison 20th/e pg. 2520]

126. True regarding SLE in children: *(PGMEE 2014-15)*
   a. Skin pigmentation more common
   b. No sex difference
   c. Renal involvement more common
   d. Cardiac involvement more common

[Ref: Harrison 20th/e pg. 2525]

127. Lupus anti-coagulant is associated with all EXCEPT:
   a. Recurrent abortion *(PGMEE 2014-15)*
   b. Polyhydramnios
   c. Intrauterine growth retardation
   d. Pre-eclampsia-early onset

[Ref: Harrison's 18th ed. ch.319]

128. Most common presentation of S.L.E *(PGMEE 2014-15)*
   a. Arthralgia
   b. Erosive polyarthritis
   c. Butterfly rash
   d. Autoimmune hemolytic anemia

[Ref: Harrison 20th/e pg. 2520]

129. All of the following are indicators for use of corticosteroids in SLE EXCEPT: *(PGMEE 2014-15)*
   a. Neuropsychiatric lupus
   b. Pericarditis
   c. Endocarditis
   d. Nephritic syndrome

[Ref: Harrison 20th/e pg. 2523]

130. True about drug induced SLE is except?
   a. Female: Male ratio=9:1 *(PGMEE 2014-15)*
   b. Anti-histone Antibodies
   c. CNS involvement not common
   d. Renal involvement not common

[Ref: Harrison 20th/e pg. 2525]

113.	b
114.	b
115.	c
116.	a
117.	c
118.	a
119.	d
120.	c
121.	d
122.	b
123.	a
124.	d
125.	d
126.	c
127.	b
128.	a
129.	c
130.	a

131. True about nervous system involvement in SLE are all EXCEPT: *(PGMEE 2014-15)*
a. Seizures
b. Antibodies against aquaporin-4 antibody
c. Elevated protein level in CSF
d. Pseudo-tumor cerebri

[Ref: Harrison 20th/e pg. 2520]

132. Which of the following antibodies correlates with disease activity for S.L.E *(PGMEE 2014-15)*
a. Anti Smith antibody
b. Anti dS DNA antibody
c. Anti Histone antibody
d. Anti Rho

[Ref: Harrison 20th/e pg. 2517]

133. A 23-year old woman experienced episodes of myalagias, peural effusion, pericarditis and arthralgias without joint deformity over course of several years. The best laboratory screening test to diagnosis her disease would be-
a. CD4 lymphocyte count *(PGMEE 2015)*
b. Assay for thyroid hormones
c. Erythrocyte sedimentation rate
d. Antinuclear antibody

[Ref: Harrison 18th/e p. 2730]

134. Bony erosion are seen in the following EXCEPT: *(PGMEE 2014-15)*
a. Gout
b. Psoriasis
c. SLE
d. Osteoarthritis

[Ref: Harrison 20th/e pg. 2518]

ANTIPHOSPHOLIPID ANTIBODY SYNDROME

135. A young female is suffering from, recurrent abortions and thrombosis of deep veins, thrombocytopenia, and a recent MI. The most likely diagnosis is: *(PGMEE 2014-15)*
a. Catastrophic anti-phosphilpid antibody syndrome
b. Primary anti-phospholipid antibody syndrome
c. TTP
d. Protein C deficiency

[Ref: Harrison 20th/e pg. 2526]

136. A lady with recurrent abortions and isolated prolongation of APTT. Which one of the following gives positive result? *(PGMEE 2014-15)*
a. Prothrombin time
b. Dilute Russell Viper Venom Time test
c. Bleeding time
d. Clot solubility test

[Ref: Harrison 20th/e pg. 2527]

SYSTEMIC SCLEROSIS/SCLERODERMA

137. Woman of 30-years with Raynaud's phenomenon, polyarthritis, dysphagia of 5-years and mild Sclerodactyl, blood showing Anti-centromere antibody positive, the likely cause is: *(PGMEE 2014-15)*
a. CREST
b. Mixed connective tissue disorder
c. SLE
d. Rheumatoid arthritis

[Ref: Harrison 20th/e pg. 2553]

138. All of the following are features of Scleroderma EXCEPT: *(PGMEE 2014-15)*
a. Diffuse periosteal reaction
b. Esophageal dysmotility
c. Erosion of tip of phalanges
d. Lung Nodular infiltrates

[Ref: Harrison 20th/e pg. 2554]

139. Anti-topoisomerase I is marker of: *(PGMEE 2014-15)*
a. Systemic sclerosis
b. Classic polyarteritis nodosa
c. Nephrotic syndrome
d. Rheumatoid arthritis

[Ref: Harrison 20th/e pg. 2558]

140. Screening test for scleredema: *(PGMEE 2014-15)*
a. Anti-nuclear antibody
b. U1- Ribonucleoprotein antibody
c. Anti- L.K.M antibody
d. Anti- topoisomerase antibody

[Ref: Harrison 20th/e pg. 2558]

141. X-ray finding of scleroderma are A/E: *(PGMEE 2014-15)*
a. Dilatation due to aperistalsis of oesophagus
b. Pseudo-obstruction
c. Pneumatosis intestinalis
d. Subperiosteal elevation

[Ref: Harrison 20th/e pg. 2555]

142. Recurrent aspiration pneumonia caused by:
a. Dermatomyostis/polymyositis *(PGMEE 2014-15)*
b. Rheumatoid arthritis
c. Progressive systemic sclerosis
d. Systemic lupus erythematosus

[Ref: Harrison 20th/e pg. 2554]

143. Indication of poor prognosis of systemic sclerosis is: *(PGMEE 2014-15)*
a. Calcinosis cutis
b. Renal involvement
c. Alopecia
d. Telangiectasia

[Ref: Harrison 20th/e pg. 2555]

144. In scleroderma features are all EXCEPT:
a. Decrease in tone of LES *(PGMEE 2014-15)*
b. Restrictive cardiomyopathy
c. Syndactyly
d. Halitosis

[Ref: Harrison 20th/e pg. 2556]

145. Woman presented with dysphagia and stiff fingers and leather like skin is diagnosed to have? *(PGMEE 2014-15)*
a. Buergers disease
b. Rheumatoid arthritis
c. Scleroderma
d. Osteoarthrosis

[Ref: Harrison 20th/e pg. 2547]

146. Not seen in scleroderma: *(PGMEE 2014-15)*
a. Anti-scl 70 antibody
b. Bi-basiliar fibrosis
c. Prayer sign
d. Ischemic stroke

[Ref: Harrison 20th/e pg. 2554]

131.	b
132.	b
133.	d
134.	c
135.	b
136.	b
137.	a
138.	a
139.	a
140.	a
141.	d
142.	c
143.	b
144.	c
145.	c
146.	d

SJÖGREN'S SYNDROME

147. Most common lymphoma associated with Sicca syndrome is: *(PGMEE 2014-15)*
- a. MALToma
- b. Burkitt lymphoma
- c. DLBCL
- d. Lymphoplasmacytic lymphoma

[Ref: Harrison 20th/e pg. 2561 Table 354-2]

148. Sicca syndrome is associated with all EXCEPT: *(PGMEE 2014-15)*
- a. Rheumatoid arthritis
- b. Midline granuloma
- c. Sarcoidosis
- d. Chronic active hepatitis

[Ref: Harrison 20th/e pg. 2560 Table 354-1]

149. HLA DR 52 is associated with: *(PGMEE 2014-15)*
- a. SLE
- b. Scleroderma
- c. Sjogren's Syndrome
- d. Behcet

[Ref: Internet]

150. Partoid gland enlargement is seen in all EXCEPT: *(PGMEE 2014-15)*
- a. Sjogren's syndrome
- b. Sarcoidosis
- c. Chronic pancreatitis
- d. SLE

MIXED CONNECTIVE TISSUE D/S (MCTD)

151. MCTD includes all except? *(PGMEE 2015-16)*
- a. SLE
- b. Polymyositis
- c. Rheumatoid arthritis
- d. Inclusion body myositis

[Ref: Harrison 20th/e pg. 2560]

152. About fibromyalgia all are true except? *(PGMEE 2014-15)*
- a. Associated with EEG abnormalities
- b. More common in males than females
- c. Associated with low free cortisol levels
- d. Associated with decreased blood flow to brain

[Ref: Harrison 20th/e pg. 2636]

153. MCTD incudes all excepts? *(PGMEE 2015)*
- a. Systemic sclerosis
- b. Polymyositis
- c. SLE
- d. Rheumatoid arthritis

[Ref: Harrison 20th/e pg. 2560]

154. Which of the following is diagnostic of mixed connective tissue disease (MCTD):- *(PGMEE 2013-14)*
- a. Anti- histone
- b. Anti-CCP antibody
- c. SCL-70 antibody
- d. U1-RNP antibody

[Ref: Harrison 20th/e pg. 2560]

THE VASCULITIS SYNDROMES

155. Thromboangitis obliterans is associated with- *(PGMEE 2013-14)*
- a. HLA B27
- b. HLA-DR4
- c. HLA-B5
- d. HLA-DR2

[Ref: Robbins 9th/e pg. 512; Harrison's]

156. ANCA associated vasculitis is:- *(PGMEE 2016-17)*
- a. Giant cell arteritis
- b. HSP
- c. PAN
- d. Microscopic polyangiitis [MPA]

[Ref: Harrison's 19th/e pg. 2180]

157. A 30-year-old male presented with pain in lower extremities, aggravated by walking. He gives history of cigarette smoking. In this patient prevalence of which HLA antigen is increased? *(PGMEE 2016-17)*
- a. HLA B5
- b. HLA B8
- c. HLA DR2
- d. HLA DR3

[Ref: Robbins 9th/e pg. 512; Harrison's 1645]

158. Hypersensitivity vasculitis most commonly involes *(AIIMS May 09, Nov 08; DNB June'2008)*
- a. Postcapillary venules
- b. Arterioles
- c. Veins
- d. Capillaries

[Ref: https://www.ncbi.nlm.nih.gov; Harrison 18th/e pg. 2798]

GIANT CELL ARTERITIS

159. All is true about Giant cell arteritis except- *(PGMEE 2012-13)*
- a. Segmental nature of the involvement
- b. Involves large to medium sized arteries
- c. Most commonly involved artery is abdominal aorta
- d. Granulomatous inflammation

[Ref: Harrison 20th/e pg. 2583-84]

160. True about Giant cell arteritis is all EXCEPT: *(PGMEE 2014-15)*
- a. High dose of steroid is drug of choice
- b. ESR is usually raised
- c. Intracranial ICA is particularly susceptible
- d. Mainly affects people of >50 years

[Ref: Harrison 20th/e pg. 2583-84]

161. Giant cell arteritis causes which of the following in the eye: *(PGMEE 2014-15)*
- a. Episcleritis
- b. Anterior ischemic optic neuropathy
- c. Neuroparalytic keratitis
- d. Band keratitis

[Ref: Harrison 20th/e pg. 2584]

162. What is feature of temporal arteritis? *(PGMEE 2014-15)*
- a. Giant cell arteritis
- b. Granulomatous vasculitis
- c. Necrotizing vasculitis
- d. Leucocytoclastic Vasculitis

[Ref: Harrison 20th/e pg. 2584]

TAKAYASU ARTERITIS

163. A patient having cystic medical necrosis with necrotising arteritis is suffering from? *(PGMEE 2013-14)*
- a. Malignant hypertension
- b. Kawasaki disease
- c. Temporal arteritis
- d. Aortoarteritis

[Ref: Robbin's 9th/e pg. 490]

147.	a
148.	b
149.	c
150.	d
151.	d
152.	b
153.	a
154.	d
155.	c
156.	d
157.	a
158.	a
159.	c
160.	c
161.	b
162.	a,b
163.	d

164. Absent Pulse in radial artery is seen in?
(PGMEE 2014-15)
a. Coarctation of aorta
b. Aortic regurgitation
c. Takayasu's arteritis
d. Dissection of Aorta
[Ref: Harrison 20th/e pg. 2585]

165. Aortic arch syndrome is due to-
(PGMEE 14)
a. Burger disease
b. Temporal arteritis
c. Takayasu arteritis
c. PAN
[Ref: Harrison 20th/e pg. 2585]

166. Bilateral upper limb pulse less disease is?
(PGMEE 2014)
a. Giant cell Arteritis
b. Polyarteritis Nodosa
c. Aortoarteritis
d. HSP
[Ref: Harrison 20th/e pg. 2585]

167. Incorrect about Takayasu arteritis: (PGMEE 2014-15)
a. Spares pulmonary artery
b. Renovascular hypertension
c. Blood pressure difference between left and right limbs
d. Strongly positive mantoux
[Ref: Harrison 20th/e pg. 2585]

168. In Takayasu's arteritis there is: (PGMEE 2014-15)
a. Intimal fibrosis
b. Renal hypertension
c. Coronary aneurysm
d. All of the above
[Ref: Harrison 20th/e pg. 2585]

169. Most common aortic branch involved in Takayasu Arteritis is? (PGMEE 2016-17; 2014-15)
a. Left subclavian artery
b. Common carotid artery
c. Abdominal aorta
d. Renal artery
[Ref: Harrison 20th/e pg. 2585, Table 356-7]

170. Reversed Coarctation is seen in: (PGMEE 2014-15)
a. Giant cell Arteritis
b. Polyarteritis Nodosa
c. Takayasu Arteritis
d. Kawasaki Disease
[Ref: API Textbook of Medicine 9th/ 754, Harrison's 19th/e pg. 2190]

POLYARTERITIS NODOSA

171. All of the following conditions are associated with raised ANCA except? (PGMEE 2015)
a. Churg-Strauses syndrome
b. Polyarteritis nodosa
c. Microscopic polyangitis
d. Wegener's granulomatous
[Ref: Harrison 20th/e pg. 2575]

172. Which of the following is a non granulomatous arteritis? (PGMEE 2012)
a. Wegner's granulomatosis
b. PAN
c. Takayasu arteritis
d. Chrug Strauss disease
[Ref: Harrison 20th/e pg. 2575]

173. Which is associated with vasculitis of medium size vessels- (PGMEE 2012-13)
a. Tuberous sclerosis
b. Temporal areritis
c. Classic PAN
d. Wegners granulomatosis
[Ref: Harrison 20th/e pg. 2582]

174. In PAN, cysts are seen in all except- (PGMEE 2012-13)
a. Lung
b. Liver
c. Heart
d. Pancreas
[Ref: Harrison 20th/e pg. 2582]

175. Hepatitis B virus is associated with: (PGMEE 2014-15)
a. SLE
b. Polyarteritis nodosa
c. Sjören's syndrome
d. Wegener's granulomatosis
[Ref: Harrison 20th/e pg. 2583]

176. Consider the following statements regarding classic polyarteritis nodosa: (PGMEE 2014-15)
I. It is multi-system necrotising vasculitis
II. Small and medium vessels are involved
III. Pulmonary artery involvement is a characteristic feature.
IV. Up to 30% patient may show positive test for Hepatitis B surface antigen

Which of these statements are correct?
a. I and II
b. II and III
c. I, II and IV
d. II, III and IV
[Ref: Harrison 20th/e pg. 2582-83]

177. A 30-year-old male patient presents with complaints of weakness in right upper and both lower limbs for last 4 months. He developed digital infarcts involving 2nd and 3rd fingers on right side and 5th finger on left side. On examination, BP was 160/140 mmHg, all peripheral pulses were palpable and there was asymmetrical examination showed proteinuria and RBC-10-15/hpf with no casts. What is the most likely diagnosis?
a. Polyarteritis nodosa (PGMEE 2014-15)
b. Systemic lupus erythematosus
c. Wegner's granulomatosi
d. Mixed cryoglobulemia
[Ref: Harrison 20th/e pg. 2582-83]

178. Which of the following are true about findings of Polyarteritis nodosa? (PGMEE 2014-15)
a. There is tear in the lamina Dura
b. Micro Aneurysm formation in the large blood vessel
c. Nodules are formed in skin which are clinically palpable
d. Chain of beads appearance
[Ref: Harrison 20th/e pg. 2583]

Explanation
- Neutrophil infiltration is evident in all layers of vessel wall resulting in intimal proliferation & degeneration
- Anunysmal dilation (≤1 cm) is seen in small muscular arteries
- Chain/string of beads appearance is seen d/t renal artery involvement in fibromuscular dysplasia.

164. c
165. c
166. c
167. a
168. d
169. a
170. c
171. b
172. b
173. c
174. a
175. b
176. c
177. a
178. c

179. A young female presents with rhinitis not subsiding with anti-histaminics, along with recurrent hemoptysis and glomerulonephritis. Which of the following is NOT an important differential diagnosis to be considered in the given scenario? *(NEET Pattern 2015)*
a. Goodpasture syndrome b. Wegener's granulomatosis
c. Microscopic polyangitis d. Poly-arteritis nodosa

[Ref: Harrison 20th/e pg. 2583]

180. An 18-years-old boy presents with digital gangrene in third and fourth fingers for last 2 weeks. On examination the blood pressure is 170/110 mm of Hg and all peripheral pulses were palpable. Blood and urine examinations were unremarkable. Antinuclear antibodies, antibody to double stranded DNA and anti-neutrophil cytoplasmic antibody were negative. The most likely diagnosis is:
(PGMEE 2014-15)
a. Wegner's granulomatosis
b. Polyarteritis nodosa
c. Takayasu's arteritis
d. Systemic lupus erythematosus (SLE)

[Ref: Harrison 20th/e pg. 2583]

KAWASAKI DISEASE

181. Which of the following is not true about Kawasaki disease? *(NEET Pattern 2019)*
a. 20% of the untreated patients develop cardiovascular sequel
b. 80% of the patients are 4 years old or older
c. It can result in acute myocardial infarctions
d. It is also called mucocutaneous lymph node syndrome

182. Most dreadful complication of Kawasaki disease:-
a. Lymph node *(PGMEE 2014)*
b. Thrombocytosis
c. Cardiac involvement
d. Rash

[Ref: Robbins 9th/e pg.510; Nelson's 17th/e pg. 823, 824, 825]

183. Kawasaki's disease has the following features EXCEPT:
(PGMEE 2014-15)
a. Posterior cervical lymphadenopathy
b. Conjunctival suffusion
c. Thrombocytopenia
d. Desquamation of the skin of fingers and toes

[Ref: Robbins 9th/e pg.510; Harrison's 19th/e pg 2179]

184. About Kawasaki disease all are true EXCEPT:
a. Seen in children *(DNB Dec 2009)*
b. Coronary artery is involved
c. Mucocutaneous lesions
d. Suppurative lymphadenopathy

[Ref: Harrison's 19th/e pg 2192]

185. Strawberry tongue is seen in
a. PAN
b. Kawasaki disease
c. MPA
d. Wegener's

[Ref: Harrison's 19th/e pg 2192]

186. Treatment of acute phase of Kawasaki Disease in children is- *(PGMEE 2014-15)*
a. Oral steroids b. IV Steroids
c. IV immunoglobins d. Cyclophosphamide

[Ref: Neslon's 20th/e pg. 1213, Ghai 8th/e/p 632; Harrison's 19th/e pg 2192]

GRANULOMATOSIS WITH POLYANGIITIS (WEGENER'S GRANULOMATOSIS)

187. A patient presents with recurrent episodes of sinusitis, throat pain, epistaxis and bilateral cavitatory lesions in the lungs and renal failure, what is the diagnosis and next step? *(NEET Pattern 2015)*
a. Systemic fungal infection, Biopsy
b. Miliary TB, Mantoux Test
c. Vasculitis, ANCA
d. Multiple Metastasis

[Ref: Harrison's 20th/e pg. 2579]

Explanation
■ Diagnosis → Wegener's granulomatosis

188. In Wegner's granuomatosis cytoplasmic anti neutrophilic antibodies (c-ANCA) are directed against-
(DNB June 08)
a. Proteinase 2 b. Proteinase 4
c. Proteinase 3 d. Proteinase 1

[Ref: Harrison 20th/e pg. 2575]

189. c-ANCA +ve vasculitis is :- *(PGMEE 2016-17)*
a. Takayasu arteritis
b. Microscopic polyangiitis
c. Polyarteritis nodosa
d. Granulomatosis with polyangiitis

[Ref: Harrison 20th/e pg. 2579]

190. p-ANCA is associated with *(PGMEE 2016-17)*
a. Takayasu arteritis b. Microscopic polyangiitis
c. Polyarteritis nodosa d. Giant cell arteritis

[Ref: Harrison 20th/e pg. 2575]

191. Which is not a characteristic of wegeners granulomatosis-
a. Positive for cANCA *(PGMEE 2012-13)*
b. Granuloma in vessel wall
c. Focal necrotising glomerulonephritis
d. Involves large vessels

[Ref: Harrison 20th/e pg. 2578]

192. ANCA positive vasculitis- *(PGMEE 2013-14)*
a. Behçet's syndrome
b. Henoch schonlein purpura
c. Wegner's ranulomatosis
d. None

[Ref: Harrison 20th/e pg. 2575]

193. Cavitating lesion in lung is seen in: *(PGMEE 2014-15)*
a. Wegner's granulomatosis
b. PAN
c. SLE
d. Goodpasture's syndrome

[Ref: Harrison 20th/e pg. 2579]

179. d
180. b
181. b
182. c
183. c
184. d
185. b
186. c
187. c
188. c
189. d
190. b
191. d
192. c
193. a

194. Treatment of choice in Wegner's granulomatosis is: *(PGMEE 2014-15)*

a. Cyclosporine
b. Cyclophosphamide
c. Steroids
d. Radiotherapy

[Ref: Harrison 20th/e pg. 2580]

195. Aspergilloma is commonly a complication of:

a. TB *(PGMEE 2014-15)*
b. Wegener's granulomatiosis
c. Cystic fibrosis
d. Bronchogenic carcinoma

[Ref: Harrison 20th/e pg. 2579]

196. Wegner's granulomatosis does not affect? *(DNB June 2010)*

a. Liver   b. Eye
c. Kidney   d. Lung

[Ref: Harrison 20th/e pg. 2579]

197. A person presents with involvement of kidney and respiratory tract infection with granuloma formation. Most probable diagnosis is? *(DNB June 2010)*

a. Sarcoidosis
b. Goodpasture syndrome
c. Tuberculosis
d. Wegner's granulomatosis

[Ref: Harrison 20th/e pg. 2579]

198. A 20-year-old woman presents with bilateral maxillary sinusitis, palpable purpura on the legs and hemoptysis. Radiograph of the chest shows a thin-walled cavity in left lower zone. Investigations reveal total leukocyte count 12000/mm3, red cells casts in the urine and serum creatinine 3 mg/dl. What is the most probable diagnosis?

a. Henoch.Schonlein purpura *(PGMEE 2014-15)*
b. Polyarteritis nodosa
c. Wegener's granulomatois
d. Disseminated tuberculosis

[Ref: Harrison 20th/e pg. 2578-79]

199. Intravenous immunoglobulin is given in all except? *(PGMEE 2014-15)*

a. Kawasaki disease
b. Acute ITP
c. Wegener's Granulomatosis
d. Myasthenic Crisis

[Ref: CMDT 2013 Pg. 848]

194. b
195. a,b
196. a
197. d
198. c
199. c
200. b
201. d
202. b
203. c
204. d
205. a
206. c

Explanation

- Indications of IVIG
- ITP
- GBS/AIDP
- CIDP
- Myasthenia gravis
- Kawasaki disease
- SLE

MICROSCOPIC POLYANGIITIS (MPA)

200. Which of the following is an example of small-vessel vasculitis? *(PGMEE 2014-15)*

a. Takayasu arteritis
b. Microscopic polyangitis
c. Giant cell arteritis
d. Polyarteritis nodosa

[Ref: Harrison 20th/e pg. 2581]

EOSINOPHILIC GRANULOMATOSIS WITH POLYANGIITIS (CHURG-STRAUSS SYNDROME)

201. Triad of skin lesions, mononeuritis multiplex and eosinophilia are seen in: *(NEET Pattern 2019)*

a. Alport's syndrome
b. Wegener's granulomatosis
c. Cryoglobulinemia
d. Churg-Strauss syndrome

202. Which of the following is more frequently seen in Churg Strauss Syndrome in comparison to Wegener's Granulomatosis *(PGMEE 2015)*

a. Renal involvement
b. Lower Respiratory Tract involvement
c. Eye involvement
d. Upper Respiratory Tract involvement

[Ref: Harrison 20th/e pg. 2582]

203. Not true about churg-strauss syndrome is?

a. Asthma *(DNB June 2009)*
b. Peripheral eosinophilia
c. Intravascular granulomas
d. Multisystem involvement of vessels

[Ref: Harrison 20th/e pg. 2581]

IGA VASCULITIS (HENOCH SCHÖNLEIN PURPURA)

204. Five-year-old female presents with palpable purpura over the buttocks, arthralgias, abdominal pain with diarrhea with passage of blood per rectum. Patient also has presence of proteinuria. What is the most probable diagnosis? *(NEET Pattern 2019)*

a. Nephritic syndrome
b. Thalassemia
c. Nephrotic syndrome
d. Henoch-Schonlein purpura

205. Henoch schonlein purpura is characterized by deposition of which of the following antibodies in the blood vessels? *(PGMEE 2014-15)*

a. IgA   b. IgG
c. IgD   d. IgM

[Ref: Harrison 20th/e pg. 2586]

206. Frequency of renal involvement in HSP- *(PGMEE 2012-13)*

a. 20-40%   b. >80%
c. 10-50%   d. 10%

[Ref: Harrison 20th/e pg. 2586]

207. All of the following are false about Henoch Schonlein purpura EXCEPT-   *(PGMEE 2015)*
   a. It is due to Type IV Hypersensitivity
   b. Abdominal pain is rare symptoms
   c. Deposition of IgA in vessels is seen
   d. Gross hematuria is seen in almost all cases

[Ref: Harrison 20th/e pg. 2586]

208. Investigation of choice for confirming Henoch Schonlein purpura is-   *(PGMEE 2015)*
   a. Serum IgA levels   b. CRP levels
   c. DTPA   d. Renal Biopsy

[Ref: Harrison 20th/e pg. 2586]

209. All are seen in Henoch schonlein purpura   *(PGMEE 2012-13)*
   a. Arthralagia   b. Abdominal pain
   c. Glomerulonephritis   d. Thrombocytopenia

[Ref: Harrison 20th/e pg. 2586]

210. The defective platelet function is seen in all EXCEPT:
   a. SLE   *(PGMEE 2014-15)*
   b. Acute lymphoctic leukemia
   c. Myelofibrosis
   d. Henoch-Schölein purpura

[Ref: Harrison 20th/e pg. 2586]

211. Abdominal pain in Henoch Schonelin purpura is due to-
   a. Volvulus   *(PGMEE 2015)*
   b. Gastrointestinal hemorrhage
   c. Mucosal erosions and swelling of the GI mucosa
   d. Associated pancreatic inflammation

[Ref: Harrison 20th/e pg. 2586]

212. HSP doesn't cause-   *(PGMEE 2015)*
   a. Purpura   b. Abdominal pain
   c. Arthritis   d. Hemoptysis

[Ref: Nelson 20th/e/p 1216]

213. Henoch Schonlein purpura presents with deposition of?   *(DNB Dec 2009)*
   a. Ig A   b. Ig E
   c. Ig G   d. Ig M

[Ref: Harrison's 19th/e pg 1839]

214. Important feature in Henoch Schonlein purpura?
   a. Raised IgA   *(PGMEE 2014-15)*
   b. Membranous glomerulonephritis
   c. Absent radial pulse
   d. Aneurysm of branching point

[Ref: Harrison's 19th/e pg. 2190]

215. Which antibody is incriminated in causing Henoch Schonlein Purpura?   *(PGMEE 2015-16)*
   a. IgA   b. IgG
   c. IgM   d. IgD

[Ref: Harrison 18th edition, Chapter 326]

216. All are true about Henoch Schonlein purpura EXCEPT: *(PGMEE 2014-15)*
   a. Raised IgA   b. Hematochezia
   c. Thrombocytopenia   d. Joint pain

[Ref: Harrison's 19th/e pg. 2190]

217. Regarding Henoch Schönlein purpura all are true EXCEPT: *(PGMEE 2014-15)*
   a. Associated with glomerulonephritis
   b. Non-Palpable purpura
   c. Decreased complement
   d. Normal platelet count

[Ref: Harrison's 19th/e pg. 2190]

BEHÇET'S DISEASE

218. In which of causes of oral ulcer, Auto-antibodies are not seen?   *(PGMEE 2015-16)*
   a. Behcet disease   b. SLE
   c. Pemphigus   d. Celiac disease

[Ref: Harrison 19th ed. / 2194]

219. Which of the following is the only vasculitis affecting both arteriolar and venous system?   *(PGMEE 2016-17)*
   a. Behçet's disease
   b. Polyarteritis nodosa
   c. Kawasaki disease
   d. Wegener's granulomatosis

[Ref: Harrison 18th/e pg. 2801]

220. Behcet syndrome is characterized by all of the following EXCEPT:-   *(PGMEE 2016-17)*
   a. Small to medium vessel vasculitis
   b. Recurrent oral and genital ulcers
   c. Uveitis
   d. Associated with HLA B-7

[Ref: Robbins 9th/e pg. 511]

221. Incorrect about Behçet's syndrome is: *(PGMEE 2014-15)*
   a. There is a strong association with HLA-B7
   b. The skin may be hyperactive to minor injury such as venipuncture
   c. Inflammatory reaction around large blood vessels
   d. Cortiocosteroid therapy is of definite value

[Ref: Harrison's 19th/e pg. 2194]

222. Recurrent oro-genital ulceration with arthritis is seen in: *(PGMEE 2014-15)*
   a. Behçet's syndrome   b. Gonorrhoea
   c. Reiter's syndrome   d. Syphilis

[Ref: Harrison's 19th/e pg. 2194]

223. Not Seen in Bechet's syndrome is: *(PGMEE 2014-15)*
   a. Pyoderma gangrenosum
   b. Thrombophlebitis
   c. Glans penis Apthous ulceration
   d. Panuveitis

[Ref: Harrison's 19th/e pg. 2194]

INFLAMMATORY MYOPATHIES

224. Lilac coloured (heliotrope) pigmentation over the face is characteristic of: *(PGMEE 2014-15)*
   a. Dermatomyositis   b. Polymyositis
   c. SLE   d. Systemic sclerosis

[Ref: Harrison's 19th/e pg. 2202]

207.	c
208.	d
209.	d
210.	d
211.	c
212.	d
213.	a
214.	a
215.	a
216.	c
217.	b
218.	a
219.	a
220.	d
221.	a
222.	a
223.	c
224.	a

225. **Perifascicular atrophy of muscle fibers is seen in-**
    a. Inclusion body myositis   *(PGMEE 2012-13, 2013-14)*
    b. Dermatomyositis
    c. Nemaline myopathy
    d. Steroid myopathy

    [Ref: Harrison's 20th/e pg. 2592]

226. **A 60 year old female is having proximal muscle weakness with increased serum creatinine kinase. The probable diagnosis is:**   *(PGMEE 2014/15)*
    a. Limb girdle muscle dystrophy
    b. Dermatomyositis
    c. Polymyositis
    d. Inclusion body myositis

    [Ref: Harrison's 20th/e pg. 2591]

SARCOIDOSIS

227. **Heerfordt's syndrome consists of fever, parotid enlargement, facial palsy and:**   *(PGMEE 2014-15)*
    a. Arthralgia
    b. Bilateral hilar lymphadenopathy
    c. Erythema nodosum
    d. Anterior uveitis

228. **Asteroid bodies are seen in?**   *(PGMEE 2012-13)*
    a. Sarcoidosis   b. Syphilis
    c. Chromoblastomycosis d. Sporotrichosis

    [Ref: Robbin's 9th/e pg. 693]

229. **Schaumann bodies are seen in-**   *(DNB Dec 08)*
    a. Sarcoidosis   b. Syphilis
    c. Chronic bronchitis d. Asthma

    [Ref: Robbin's 9th/e pg. 603]

230. **Bilateral hilar lymphadenopathy with non caseating granuloma is seen in-**   *(PGMEE 2013-14)*
    a. Lymphoma   b. TB
    c. Sarcoidosis   d. All of the above

    [Ref: Robbin's 9th/e pg. 693]

231. **Lupus pernio is seen in :-**   *(PGMEE 2016-17)*
    a. PAN   b. SLE
    c. Tuberculosis   d. Sarcoidosis

    [Ref: Robbin's 9th/e pg. 2207]

232. **60-year-old man presents with cough & respiratory distress. On CXR interstitial infiltrates , reticulonodular pattern was seen. What is the probable diagnosis:-**   *(PGMEE 2016-17)*
    a. Staph pneumonia   b. Atypical pneumonia
    c. Asbestosis   d. Sarcoidosis

    [Ref: Robbin's 9th/e pg. 2206]

233. **Which of the following is seen in sarcoidosis:**   *(PGMEE 2015-16)*
    a. Hypercalcemia   b. Hypocalcemia
    c. Hyperphosphatemia d. Hypophosphatemia

    [Ref: Harrison's 19th/e pg. 313, 2208]

234. **Sarcoidosis is characterized by all EXCEPT:**   *(PGMEE 2014-15)*
    a. Cavity   b. Panda sign
    c. Hilar lymphadenopathy d. Egg shell calcification

    [Ref: Harrison's 19th/e pg. 2205]

235. **Candle wax dripping sign is seen in:**   *(PGMEE 2014/15)*
    a. Rheumatoid arthritis b. SLE
    c. HIV   d. Sarcoidosis

    [Ref: Harrison's 19th/e pg. 2207]

236. **Which of the following condition does not cause multiple painful ulcers on tongue?**   *(PGMEE 2015)*
    a. Behcet disease   b. Sarcoidosis
    c. TB   d. Herpes

    [Ref: Harrison 19th/e p. 237, 417]

237. **The most common cause of sudden death in sarcoidosis is:**   *(PGMEE 2014-15)*
    a. Pneumonia   b. Cor pulmonale
    c. Arrythmias   d. Liver failure

    [Ref: Harrison's 19th/e pg. 2208]

238. **In sarcoidosis:**   *(PGMEE 2014-15)*
    a. Causes large cavitatory lesions
    b. Spontaneous remission may occur
    c. Tuberculin test is negative
    d. Caseation and necrosis may occur

    [Ref: http://www.aafp.org/afp/2004/0715/p312.html; Harrison's 19th/e pg. 2205]

239. **Most common cause of unilateral Hilar lymphadenopathy:**   *(PGMEE 2014-15)*
    a. Histoplasmosis   b. Sarcoidosis
    c. Aspergillosis   d. Tuberculosis

    [Ref: Harrison's 19th/e pg. 1102]

240. **Female patient with bilateral hilar lymphadenopathy and joint pain. ACE levels are elevated. Diagnosis is?**   *(PGMEE 2015-16)*
    a. Sarcoidosis   b. Silicosis
    c. Hodgkin's lymphoma d. Non Hodgkin's lymphoma

    [Ref: Harrison's 19th/e pg. 2206]

241. **Sarcoidosis is least likely to be associated with:**   *(PGMEE 2014-15)*
    a. Uveitis   b. Pericardial effusion
    c. Erythema nodosum d. Lymphadenopathy

    [Ref: Harrison's 19th/e pg. 2207]

242. **Following cranial nerve is involved in patients with sarcoidosis:**   *(PGMEE 2014-15)*
    a. I cranial nerve   b. II cranial nerve
    c. III cranial nerve   d. IV cranial nerve

    [Ref: Harrison's 19th/e pg. 2209]

243. **The primary involvement of which organ is so far not reported to be affected by sarcoidosis is:**   *(PGMEE 2014-15)*
    a. Heart   b. Adrenals
    c. Kidney   d. Brain

    [Ref: Harrison's 19th/e pg. 2010]

244. **All of the following are features of sarcoidosis EXCEPT:**   *(PGMEE 2014-15)*
    a. Right paratracheal lymphadenopathy
    b. Cardiomyopathy
    c. Hypercalcemia
    d. Malabsorption syndrome

    [Ref: Harrison's 19th/e pg. 2211]

225. b
226. c
227. d
228. a
229. a
230. c
231. d
232. d
233. a
234. a
235. d
236. b
237. c
238. b,c
239. d
240. a
241. b
242. b
243. b
244. d

245. True about sarcoidosis is: *(PGMEE 2014-15)*
a. Serum amyloid A is used as marker for sarcoidosis
b. Kveim test is diagnostic
c. hypocalcemia
d. Pleural effusion is common

[Ref: Harrison's 19th/e pg. 2209]

246. Lupus Pernio is a complication of: *(PGMEE 2014-15)*
a. Sarcoidosis
b. Skin TB
c. SLE complication
d. DLE and SLE

[Ref: Harrison's 19th/e pg. 2209]

247. Garland sign on CXR in sarcoidosis involves all EXCEPT:
a. Right paratracheal nodes *(PGMEE 2014-15)*
b. Right hilar nodes
c. Left hilar nodes
d. Left pretracheal lymph nodes

[Ref: Harrison's 19th/e pg. 2208]

248. A woman complaints of dyspnea at rest. Chest radiography reveals bihilar adenopathy with clear lung fields. All of the following investigations will be useful in differential diagnosis EXCEPT: *(PGMEE 2014-15)*
a. CD4/CD8 > 3.5 in B.A.L   b. Serum ACE levels
c. CECT of chest   d. Gallium scan

[Ref: Harrison 20th/e pg. 2605]

249. Which of the following condition does not cause multiple painful ulcers on tongue? *(PGMEE 2015-16)*
a. TB   b. Sarcoidosis
c. Herpes   d. Behcet disease

[Ref: Harrison 20th/e pg. 221 Table 32-1]

MISCELLANEOUS

250. Which of the following is not an autoimmune disease?
(AIIMS May 2015)
a. SLE   b. Graves disease
c. Ulcerative Colitis   d. Rheumatoid Arthritis

[Ref: Harrison 20th/e pg. 2260, 2513]

251. DOC for acute attack of Hereditary angioneurotic edema? *(PGMEE 2015-16)*
a. Danazol
b. C1 inhibitor concentrate
c. Icatibant
d. methylprednisolone

[Ref: Harrison 20th/e pg. 2502]

Explanation

- Icatibant is a selective bradykinin B2 receptor antagonist.
- DOC for acute attack of HAE is C1 INH concentrate which are commercially available

252. Type 5 Hypersensitivity mimics? *(PGMEE 2015-16)*
a. Type 1   b. Type 2
c. Type 3   d. Type 4

[Ref: Clinical microbiology and Infectious Diseases, 2nd edition, Page 30, Harrison's 19th/e pg. 232]

253. Which of the following disorders is least likely associated with progression to lymphoma? *(PGMEE 2014-15)*
a. Sjogren's syndrome
b. Ataxia telangiectasia
c. Severe combined immunodeficiency
d. Lynch II syndrome

[Ref: Harrison's 19th/e pg. 563]

254. Bilateral painless parotid enlargement is seen in all EXCEPT: *(PGMEE 2014-15)*
a. Mumps   b. Alcoholics
c. Sarcoidosis   d. Diabetes mellitus

[Ref: CMDT 2014 ch.32, Pg. 1370]

Explanation

- D/D of B/L Parotid enlargement:

Painful	Painless
- Mumps	- Alcoholism
- TB	- Cirrhosis
	- Sarcoidosis
	- Sjogren syndrome
	- Amyloidosis

255. A young man develops tiny linear wheals on exposure to sun and exercise since 6 years. Most likely diagnosis is:
a. Cholingeric urticaria *(PGMEE 2014-15)*
b. Dermatographism
c. Idiopathic chronic urticaria
d. Pressure urticaria

[Ref: Harrison 20th/e pg. 2501]

256. Best drug for bradykinin mediated Angioedema:
(PGMEE 2014-15)
a. Icatibant   b. Levocetrizine
c. Avil   d. Hydrocortisone

[Ref: Harrison 20th/e pg. 2502]

257. Which of the following can be used for confirmation of anaphyalxis: *(PGMEE 2014-15)*
a. IgE levels   b. Basophil count
c. Eosinophil count   d. Serum tryptase

[Ref: Harrison 20th/e pg. 2507]

258. Anti RO bodies are present in all EXCEPT:
a. SLE   *(PGMEE 2015-16)*
b. Sjogren syndrome
c. Neonatal lupus
d. Mixed connective tissue disorder

[Ref: Harrison 20th/e pg. 2517 Table 349-I]

259. HLA-B*1502 is a genetic marker for: *(PGMEE 2014-15)*
a. Systemic lupus erythematosus
b. Polyarteritis nodosa
c. Steven Johnson syndrome
d. Seronegative spondy-arthritis syndrome

[Ref: Harrison 20th/e pg. 365]

260. Which is not correct regarding chronic fatigue syndrome? *(PGMEE 2014/15)*
a. Fatigue>6 months   b. Myalgia/arthralgia
c. Impairment of recent memory and intelligence
d. Non tender lymph nodes

[Ref: Harrison's 20th/e pg. 3254]

245.	a
246.	a
247.	d
248.	c
249.	b
250.	c
251.	b
252.	b
253.	c
254.	a
255.	a
256.	a
257.	d
258.	d
259.	c
260.	d

MORPHOLOGICAL CLASSIFICATION OF ANEMIA

Microcytic (↓ MCV) and Hypochromic (↓ MCHC) Anemia

- **S**ideroblastic anemia
- **I**ron Deficiency Anemia (IDA)
- **T**halassemia
- **A**nemia of chronic disease (AOCD)
- **L**ead toxicity

} Low Retic Count

Condition Lab	IDA	Thalassemia	Sideroblastic anemia	AOCD
S. Iron (50-150 mg/dl)	↓↓	(N)	(N)	↓
TIBC (300-600 mg/dl)	↑	(N)	(N)	↓
Transferrin saturation (25-50%)	↓	N/↑	N/↑	↓
Ferritin (50-200 μg/L)	↓	↑	↑	N/↑
Free erythro protoporphyrin	↑	(N)	↑	↓
RDW (N ≤ 14)	↑	(N)	(N)	(N)

Sideroblastic anemia
- **Causes →** Lead poisoning, Copper deficiency, Vitamin B₆ deficiency, MDS, Chloramphenicol, Isoniazid
- Defect in incorporation of Fe into Heme molecule
- **Peripheral smear:**
  - Ring sideroblast with cytoplasmic iron → Stains +ve with Prussian blue
  - Pappenheimer bodies in siderocytes
- **Treatment:** Pyridoxine (Vitamin B₆), Folic acid
- **IDA:** Earliest/Most sensitive indicator → ↓ Ferritin
- **AOCD:** Due to inadequate iron delivery to the BM despite of normal/excess iron stores.

Normocytic Normochromic Anemia

- **↑ Reticulocyte Count**
  - Blood loss
  - Sickle cell anemia
  - Hypersplenism
  - **Hemolytic anemias:**
    - Hereditary spherocytosis
    - G6PD deficiency
    - Pyruvate kinase deficiency
    - Autoimmune hemolytic anemia
    - HUS, TTP
    - Hemoglobinopathies
    - DIC
    - PNH
- **↓ Reticulocyte Count**
  - Malignancy
  - Fanconi's anemia
  - Chronic kidney disease
  - AOCD
  - Red cell aplasia
  - Parvovirus B19 infection
  - Diamond Blackfan syndrome

WHO cut off for anemia:

Age group	Hb (g/dL)
Children aged 6-59 months	<11
Children aged 5-11 yrs	<11.5
Children aged 12-14 yrs	<12
Adule male (>15 yrs)	<13
Adult female, non pregnant (>15 yrs)	<12
Adult female, pregnant	<11

Macrocytic [MCV] Anemia

- **Vitamin B₁₂ deficiency:**
  - Pernicious anemia
  - Bacterial overgrowth
  - Fish tapeworm (*D. latum*)
  - Tropical sprue
  - Folate deficiency: Alcoholism
- **Drugs:**
  - Folate antagonists
    - Methotrexate
    - Cotrimoxazole
    - Trimethoprim
    - Pentamidine
  - 6 Mercaptopurine (6 MP)
  - Pyrimidine antagonists
  - Phenytoin
  - Zidovudine
  - Liver diseases
  - Hypothyroidism
  - Blind loop syndrome

PANCYTOPENIA

| Hypocellular Bone Marrow | Cellular Bone Marrow |

Hypocellular Bone Marrow
- **S**ome Myelodysplasia
- **A**plastic anemia: Acquired or inherited
- **Acquired:**
  - Radiation
  - Chemotherapeutics
  - Ebstein Barr Virus
  - Parvovirus B₁₉
  - HIV – 1
  - Viral hepatitis
- **Inherited:**
  - Fanconi anemia

Cellular Bone Marrow

Primary Bone Marrow diseases:
- Myelodysplasia
- PNH
- Myelofibrosis
- Hairy cell leukemia

Systemic illness:
- SLE
- Hypersplenism
- Tropical splenomegaly
- Megaloblastic anemia
  - Vit B₁₂ deficiency
  - Folate deficiency

- Malaria
- Tuberculosis
- Dengue
- Enteric fever
- Sarcoidosis
- Lymphoma

HEMOLYTIC ANEMIA

	Intravascular Hemolysis	Extravascular Hemolysis
Etiology	▪ Transfusion reactions ▪ Microangiopathic hemolytic anemia (TTP, HUS, aortic stenosis, prosthetic valve) ▪ Thermal burns ▪ Paroxysmal nocturnal hemoglobinuria ▪ Paroxysmal cold hemoglobinuria ▪ Snake bite ▪ Sepsis and DIC	▪ Malaria ▪ Hemoglobinopathy i.e. sickle cell anemia and thalassemia ▪ Autoimmune Hemolytic anemia ▪ Hereditary spherocytosis ▪ G6PD deficiency ▪ Hypersplenism
Pathogenesis	▪ Hemolysis→ Free Hemoglobin in plasma ↓ ▪ Free Hb + Haptoglobin → Plasma Haptoglobin levels ↓ ▪ Free Hb gets oxidized → Methemoglobin→ excreted as Methemoglobinuria ▪ Free Hb → renal clearance l/t Hemoglobinuria → IDA	▪ Splenomegaly is seen ▪ RBC degraded within RES ↓ ▪ Hemoglobin is released → Heme breaks down to release iron and bilirubin ▪ Iron → deposited back in bone marrow ▪ ↑ Unconjugated bilirubin
Labs	▪ Reticulocyte count ↑ ▪ Reticulocyte Index >2.5%	▪ ✓ ▪ ✓
	▪ Erythroid hyperplasia in BM	▪ ✓
	▪ Bilirubin → ↑ Unconjugated bilirubin	▪ ✓
	▪ Haptoglobin → ↓↓↓/ absent	▪ ↓
	▪ Serum LDH → ↑↑	▪ ↑
	▪ Hemoglobinuria +	▪ Negative
	▪ Hemosiderinuria +	▪ Negative
	▪ Iron deficiency → due to Hemoglobinuria	▪ No iron deficiency/Iron is preserved
	▪ PS → Schistocytes	▪ Spherocytes

AUTOIMMUNE HEMOLYTIC ANEMIA

	Warm Antibody Type	Cold Antibody Type
Pathogenesis	▪ Antibody reacts at room temperature ▪ Mainly of Ig**G** type (G = garam)	▪ Reacts at temperature <37°C ▪ Mainly Ig**M** type (CM) Except Paroxysmal Cold Hemoglobinuria → Antibodies are of IgG type known as Donath Landsteiner Antibody
Etiology	▪ Lymphoma ▪ SLE ▪ Drugs: Methyl dopa	▪ Mycoplasma infection ▪ Infectious mononucleosis ▪ Paroxysmal cold hemoglobinuria
Mechanism	▪ RBC + IgG → spleen → Extravascular hemolysis	▪ RBC + IgM → Agglutination → Fixation of C_3 to RBC surface → Intravascular hemolysis
Clinical Feature and Lab findings	Mild anemia with Jaundice Direct Coomb's test positive Spherocytosis with ↑ osmotic fragility	
	Clinical and laboratory features are same as Hereditary Spherocytosis → to differentiate → do Coombs test	

HEMOLYTIC DISORDERS

	Hereditary Spherocytosis	Paroxysmal Nocturnal Hemoglobinuria	Sickle Cell Anemia

General features	• Autosomal Dominant disorder
	• Due to mutation of gene coding for proteins on RBC membrane
	• Defect can be present in:
	  ○ Ankyrin → MC defect
	  ○ Protein 3
	  ○ Spectrin
	  ○ Paladin
		• Due to mutation in PIGA gene l/t decrease in GPI anchored proteins
		• RBC Membrane is deficient in 2 complement regulating proteins
		  ○ DAF/CD 55
		  ○ MIRL/CD 59
		• This causes uncontrolled complement activation
		• Affects all the 3 cell lines
			• Missense/Point mutation at β_6 position of HbA [Glu → Val]
			• Factors favoring sickling crisis: Hypoxia, Acidosis, Hb S concentration, Infection and Dehydration
			• Reactive BM hyperplasia lead to:
			  ○ Stunted growth
			  ○ Bossing of skull
			  ○ Fish mouth vertebrae
			• ↑ risk of infection with *H. influenza*

Clinical features	• Extravascular hemolytic anemia
	• Jaundice
	• Splenomegaly
	• Pigmented gall stone → may require cholecystectomy
		• Intravascular **H**emolytic anemia
		• Deficient Hematopoiesis leads to → Pancytopenia/**A**plastic anemia
		• Venous **T**hrombosis → due to complement mediated platelet aggregation and hypercoagulability
		  ○ Despite thrombocytopenia, thrombosis occurs
		  ○ MC site → Hepatic veins, causing Budd Chiari syndrome
			• CF are uncommon before 5-6th month
			• ↑ blood viscosity lead to:
			  ○ Bone → osteomyelitis, Bone pain
			  ○ Spleen → Hyposplenism, auto splenectomy
			  ○ Priapism, Renal papillary necrosis, Pulmonary Artery Hypertension
			• Hemolysis due to ↑ fragility:
			  ○ Anemia leading to cardiomegaly and heart failure

Lab features	• Suggestive of extravascular hemolytic anemia • MCV ↓ and MCHC ↑ • ↑ Osmotic fragility • PS → Spherocytes (also seen in AIHA ∴ to differentiate → Do Coombs test	• Suggestive of intravascular hemolytic anemia • ↓ Lap score (also a feature of CML) • Pancytopenia especially thrombocytopenia • BM → Normocellular/hypercellular • HAM test: For susceptibility of RBC to complement mediated lysis • IOC – Flow cytometry	• Reticulocytosis, ↓ ESR • ↓ Osmotic fragility • X-ray head – crew cut appearance • Gamma gandy bodies in spleen (made up of hemosiderin and calcium) • PS → Sickle cells and Target cells
Rx	• TOC → Splenectomy • Anti-Pneumococcal vaccine is given before Splenectomy	• Eculizumab (Target complement protein C5) • Steroids, Anticoagulants, Anti Thymocyte Globulin • Stem cell transplantation	• Hydroxyurea → Increases Hb F • ↑ Hb F ↓ the severity

THALASSEMIA

- An AR disorder characterized by ↓ rate of synthesis of structurally normal hemoglobin chains
- α Thalassemia can protect children against malaria
- Screening test → NESTROF (osmotic fragility test)
- Thalassemia shows ↓ osmotic fragility

α-thalassemia		β-thalassemia	
• Decrease/absent production of α chain • Formation of β and ϒ chain is normal • Most common cause → gene deletion • Gene for α-globin chain is located on chromosome 16		• Decrease (β⁺) or absent (β⁰) production of β-chain • Formation of α chain is normal • Most common cause → splicing mutation • Gene for β-globin chain is located on chromosome 11	
Excess β chain can forms tetramer in normoblast (β_4 OR HbH) ↓ • Normoblast gets trapped into spleen • Extravascular hemolysis	Excess γ-chain can form tetramer (γ_4 OR Bart Hb) ↓ • Fetus develops intrauterine hypoxia • Hydrops fetalis and fetal death	Excess α chain combines with other chains and l/t increase in the following Hb: ↓ • Hb F ($\alpha_2 \gamma_2$) • Hb A₂ ($\alpha_2 \delta_2$)	α-chain starts accumulating in normoblast which gets destroyed in BM → anemia ↓ • Repeated blood transfusion • Medullary cavity expansion • Secondary hemochromatosis • Crew cut appearance • Chipmunk facies

Types of Alpha Thalassemia

Phenotype	Genotype	Features
Normal	$\alpha\alpha/\alpha\alpha$	▪ Normal individual
Silent carrier/ α - Thalassemia-2 trait	- $\alpha/\alpha\alpha$	▪ Asymptomatic ▪ Normal or minor reductions in RBC, MCV and MCH
α - Thalassemia-1 trait/ Alpha thalassemia minor	- - / $\alpha\alpha$ or - α / - α	▪ Clinically asymptomatic ▪ Normal or mild anemia; reduced MCV and MCH ▪ Hemoglobin electrophoresis is normal
Hemoglobin H disease ▪ Accumulation of excess beta chain as tetramers (β_4)	- - /- α	▪ Often symptomatic at birth; neonatal jaundice or anemia. ▪ Hepatomegaly and splenomegaly ▪ Transfusion or Splenectomy is often necessary
Hydrops fetalis/ Bart hemoglobin (Υ_4)/ Alpha thalassemia major	- - / - -	▪ Fetuses often die either in utero or shortly after birth because of severe anemia. ▪ Infants born have massive edema with high output congestive heart failure and massive hepatomegaly

Features of β-Thalassemia

	T. major/Cooley's	T. intermediate	T. minor (T. trait)
Genotype	▪ $\beta^0\beta^0 / \beta^+\beta^+ / \beta^0\beta^+$	▪ $\beta^+\beta^+ / \beta^0\beta^0$	▪ $\beta^+\beta / \beta^0\beta$
Age of onset	▪ 6 – 9 months		▪ Usually asymptomatic
Hb levels	▪ <7 mg/dL	▪ 7-10 mg/dL	▪ >10 mg/dL
Hb F	▪ ↑↑ (becomes major Hb)	▪ ↑↑	▪ N
HbA$_2$ ($\alpha_2\delta_2$)	▪ <3.5%	▪ <3.5%	▪ 3.5 – 8 % (↑)
Peripheral smear	▪ Microcytosis, Hypochromia ▪ Anisocytosis, Poikilocytosis ▪ Target cells, Inclusion bodies		▪ Microcytosis ▪ Hypochromia ▪ Target cells
Blood transfusion	▪ Dependent	▪ Occasional	▪ Not dependent

Thalassemia Trait

	α-Thalassemia trait (T. minor)	β-Thalassemia trait (T. minor)
HBA$_2$	▪ Normal	▪ Increased (4–6%)
HbF	▪ Normal	▪ Increased
RBC count	▪ Increased	▪ Normal
Anemia	▪ Mild	▪ Mild
Blood transfusions	▪ No need	▪ No need

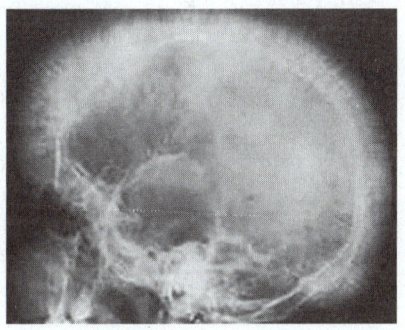

Crew cut appearance/Hair on end sign

SYNDROMES

❶ **Wiskott Aldrich syndrome:** [**Mn**: WhITE]
- ○ **X**-Linked Recessive syndrome
- ○ **I**mmunodeficiency l/t recurrent infection
- ○ **T**hrombocytopenia (the platelets are small and do not function properly)
- ○ **E**czema

❷ **Evan's Syndrome:**
- ○ Autoimmune thrombocytopenia (ITP)
- ○ Autoimmune Hemolytic anemia (Coombs positive)

❸ **Rosenthal syndrome (aka Hemophilia C):**
- ○ Inheritance → AD/AR (not 'X' linked)
- ○ Due to factor XI deficiency

(**Note:** Not to confuse with Melkersson - Rosenthal syndrome)

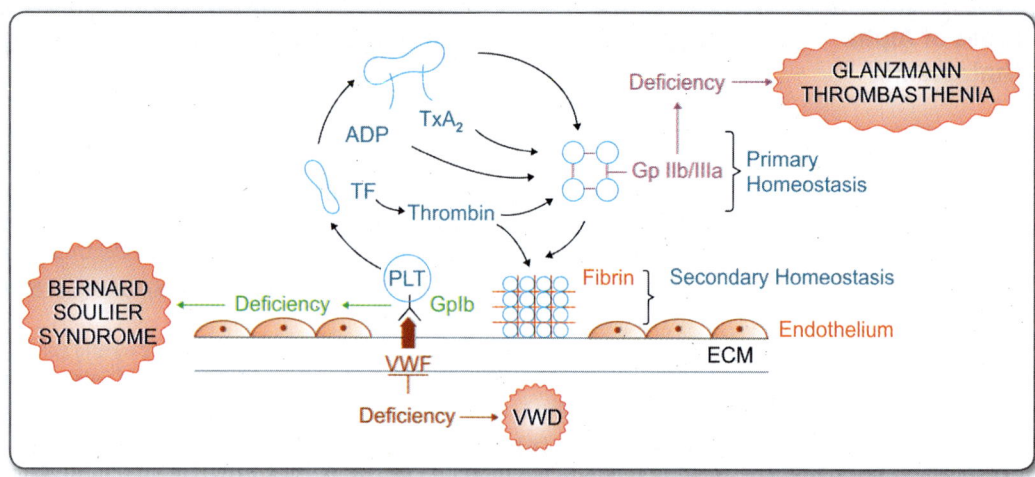

Features	Bernard Soulier Syndrome	Glanzmann Thrombasthenia
Inheritance	• AR	• AR
Defect in	• Adhesion of platelet to vessel wall	• Platelet to platelet interaction
Glycoprotein defect	• GP Ib (receptor for VMF)	• GP IIb/IIIa (receptor for fibrinogen)
Platelet count	• ↓ (Thrombocytopenia)	• Normal
Platelet morphology	• Giant platelets	• Normal
Megakaryocyte	• Increased	• Normal
Bleeding time	• Prolonged	• Prolonged
Platelet aggregation	• Ristocetin test negative	• Normal with ristocetin, but impaired with other agonists such as ADP, thrombinand collagen

VON WILLEBRAND DISEASE (VWD)

- MC inherited bleeding disorder
- MC mode of inheritance: AD
- MC type : Type I VWD
- Least common: Type III VWD
- VWF is the plasma carrier of factor VIII and is required for normal platelet adhesion and aggregation
- VWF = Factor VIII + Ristocetin cofactor (required for platelet aggregation)
- Clinical features includes Skin and mucosal bleeding; Hemarthrosis

- *Lab findings:*
  - ↓ level of factor VIII and VIIIC → Prolonged PTT, normal PT
  - Defect in platelet adhesion → prolonged BT
  - Impaired platelet aggregation in response to Ristocetin but platelet aggregation with standard agonist like ADP, collagen, thrombin are normal (differentiating feature from Glanzmann thrombasthenia
- **DOC:** Desmopressin (DDAVP) → Releases VWF and factor VIII from endothelial stores

COAGULATION DISORDER

- The prothrombin time (PT) and international normalized ratio (INR) are assays evaluating the extrinsic and common pathway of coagulation.
- PT measures factors I (Fibrinogen), II (Prothrombin), V, VII, and X (Stuart Factor). It is the earliest test to get deranged in vitamin - K deficiency (due to short t ½ of factor VII).
- The activated partial thromboplastin time (aPTT) measures the intrinsic and common pathways.
- The ristocetin-induced platelet aggregation is an ex vivo assay for live platelet function. It measures platelet aggregation with the help of von Willebrand factor (vWF) and ristocetin.

- Dilute Russell's viper venom time is a laboratory test often used for detection of lupus anticoagulant.
- The most common inherited factor deficiencies are the hemophilias, caused by deficiency of F VIII (hemophilia A) or F IX (hemophilia B). It is inherited as an X-linked condition.
- Coagulation pathway affected by heparin: Intrinsic pathway → isolated prolongation of aPTT.
- Dose of warfarin is monitored by PT/INR.
- Leiden mutation is an AD mutation in the gene coding for clotting factor V.
- Lupus anticoagulant prolongs clotting time in vitro but leads to thrombosis in vivo.

| Test result | | Conditions |
PT	aPTT	
Prolonged	*Normal*	▪ **Factor VII deficiency** ▪ **Liver disease** ▪ **Warfarin [Hence, dose is decreased in Liver disease]** ▪ Mild vitamin K deficiency [Eg: Hemorrhagic disease of Newborn]
Normal	*Prolonged*	▪ **von Willebrand disease** ▪ Heparin administration ▪ **Lupus anticoagulant** → Detected by Russell Viper venom assay ▪ Deficiency of factors VIII, IX, or XI ▪ Deficiency of factor XII, Prekallikrein, or HMW kininogen (not associated with bleeding)
Prolonged	*Prolonged*	▪ Deficiency of prothrombin (II), fibrinogen (I), or factors V or X ▪ Liver disease, Severe vitamin K deficiency, DIC ▪ Combined heparin and warfarin administration ▪ Direct factor Xa inhibitor (e.g. Rivaroxaban, Apixaban, Edoxaban) ▪ Direct thrombin inhibitor (e.g. Argatroban, Dabigatran)

Prothrombotic States

Inherited	Acquired	

▪ Factor V mutation
▪ Homocysteinemia
▪ Antithrombin III deficiency
▪ Protein C deficiency
▪ Protein S deficiency
	▪ Pregnancy
	▪ Major surgery
	▪ OCP
	▪ PNH
	▪ APLA syndrome
		▪ TTP (NOT ITP)
		  ○ Disseminated Intravascular Coagulation
		  ○ Heparin induced thrombocytopenia
		▪ Abruptio placenta
		▪ Myocardial infarction

ABNORMAL CELLS AND ASSOCIATED CONDITIONS

Image	Cell	Condition
	▪ **A**canthocytes (Spur /Spike cells)	▪ **A**betalipoproteinemia ▪ Liver disease
	▪ Bu**r**r cells (Echinocytes) *Projections are evenly spaced	▪ **R**enal failure/Uremia
	▪ Bite cells and Heinz bodies	▪ G6PD deficiency
	▪ Ringed sideroblast	▪ Sideroblastic anemia
	▪ Schistocytes (Helmet cells)	▪ Microangiopathic hemolytic anemia (HUS/TTP/DIC/APLA/ Prosthetic valve)
	▪ Spherocytes	▪ Hereditary spherocytosis ▪ Autoimmune Hemolytic anemia
	▪ **T**arget cells/Codocyte/Leptocytes	▪ **T**halassemia ▪ Post splenectomy
	▪ Tear drop cells (Dacrocytes)	▪ Condition associated with marrow fibrosis like Myelofibrosis and MDS [**Mn:** fibrosis destroys marrow, so marrow starts to cry]

THROMBOCYTOPENIA

	TTP	ITP	DIC
Introduction	■ TTP is a disorder of vessel wall ■ Characterised by lesion in arteriolar wall in various organs → leads to formation of localized platelet thrombi with fibrin deposits → Consumption of platelets causes thrombocytopenia	■ ITP is an autoimmune disease ■ Characterized by severe thrombocytopenia due to auto antibodies against platelet ■ Autoantibodies* are formed in response to previous viral infections	■ Aka consumptive coagulopathy ■ Characterized by Intravascular activation of both intrinsic and extrinsic coagulation pathways ■ Associated with M_3 type of AML, Snake bite, Sepsis, Malaria, Abruptio etc.
Clinical features	*Pentad of TTP*: [Mn: Neu MRF Tyre] ■ Disturbed **Neu**rological function ■ Intravascular hemolysis → **M**icroangiopathic hemolytic anemia ■ ↓ **R**enal function ■ **F**ever ■ **T**hrombocytopenia	■ Acute ITP is a self-limiting condition ■ Chronic ITP is more commonly seen in adult females (20-40 years) ■ Easy or excessive bruising and bleeding ■ Petechial rash ■ Spleen size → Normal ■ Hepatosplenomegaly → absent	■ MC site for thrombus formation: brain ┌─────────────────────┐ Test that correlates best and most closely with bleeding tendency is: Fibrinogen levels └─────────────────────┘ ┌─────────────────────┐ Most sensitive test for DIC is elevated FDP levels. └─────────────────────┘
Diagnostic studies	■ Coombs negative hemolytic anemia ■ ↑ LDH and Fragmentation of RBC ■ Schistocytes ■ Normal PT, aPTT, FDP and Fibrinogen ■ Deficiency of ADAMTS13 ┌─────────────────────┐ Pentad + Normal coagulation test = Pathognomic of TTP └─────────────────────┘	■ Isolated thrombocytopenia ■ Bleeding Time → prolonged ■ Coagulation profile → Normal ■ BM exam → N / ↑ in megakaryocytes ┌─────────────────────┐ *Autoantibodies are of IgG class └─────────────────────┘	■ Platelet, coagulation factors and fibrinogen gets consumed → Levels ↓ ■ BT and CT → Prolonged ■ PT, aPTT, TT → Prolonged ■ Fibrinolysis accounts for ↑ FDP ■ Thrombotic phase accounts for features of MAHA like Schistocytes
Treatment	■ Corticosteroids ■ IVIG ■ Plasmapheresis ■ Heparin and Platelet transfusion not to be done	■ Corticosteroids; IVIG ■ Rituximab – Anti CD 20 antibody ■ Eltrombopag, Romiplostim, Fostamatinib – in chronic ITP ■ Platelet transfusion is not indicated	■ Treatment of cause ■ Possibly replacement therapy (e.g. platelets, cryoprecipitate, fresh frozen plasma) ■ Low dose Heparin / EACA

BLOOD PRODUCTS

Product	Description	Indication
Whole blood	■ Deficient in factor V and VII ■ Stored at 2-4°C	■ Acute blood loss ■ Exchange transfusion
Packed RBC	■ 1 unit should raise HCT by 3%	■ In acute and chronic blood loss
Platelet concentrate	■ PCs may be stored for up to 5 days at +20°C to +24°C ■ Contraindicated in ITP and TTP	■ Thrombocytopenia (<10,000) ■ Major Surgery (<50, 000) ■ Spontaneous hemorrhage
Fresh Frozen Plasma	■ Stored at -18°C to - 20°C	■ Clotting factor replacement ■ Emergency reversal of warfarin

Cryoprecipitate	■ **Contains:**
	  ○ Fibrinogen
	  ○ vWF
	  ○ VIII and XIII
		■ Fibrinogen deficiency
		■ Von Willebrand disease
		■ Hemophilia A

FACTS

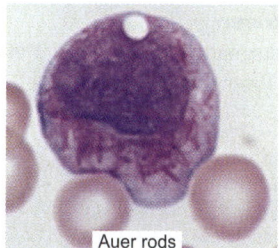
Auer rods

- Normal cellularity of BM: 50% cellular and 50% Fat
- Cells with multiple Auer rods are known as: Faggot cells
- Auer rods and Faggot cells are seen in: M-3 AML
- Subtype of AML associated with tissue infiltration and gum hypertrophy: M5 and M4
- Basophilia on PS is a typical feature of: CML
- LAP score is decreased in: CML and PNH
- Serum level of vitamin B_{12} binding protein is increased in: CML and Polycythemia Vera
- Enlarged spleen is a prognostic indicator in: CML → used in Sokel index
- **Richter's transformation:** Complication of CLL characterized by transformation of B cell CLL into an aggressive lymphoma, most commonly Diffuse Large B-Cell Lymphoma (DLBCL).
- Red pulp of spleen is characteristically involved in: Hairy cell leukemia

- Increased Expression of BCL-2 is seen in: Follicular lymphoma
- Lymphomatoid polyposis → multifocal mucosal involvement of the small bowel and colon
  - Feature of Mantle cell lymphoma
- MALToma are: Marginal zone lymphoma
- BM aspiration shows **Dry** tap in: **My**elofibrosis and **Hai**ry cell leukemia [**Mn:** Dry My Hair]

Tumors association with Polycythemia/↑ Erythropoietin Production:

- Renal Cell Carcinoma
- Hepatocellular carcinoma
- Hepatoma
- Cerebellar hemangioblastoma

Origin of lymphoid Neoplasm

Germinal center	Post germinal center
Hodgkin's lymphoma **D**LBCL **B**urkitt's lymphoma **F**ollicular lymphoma	Hairy cell leukemia

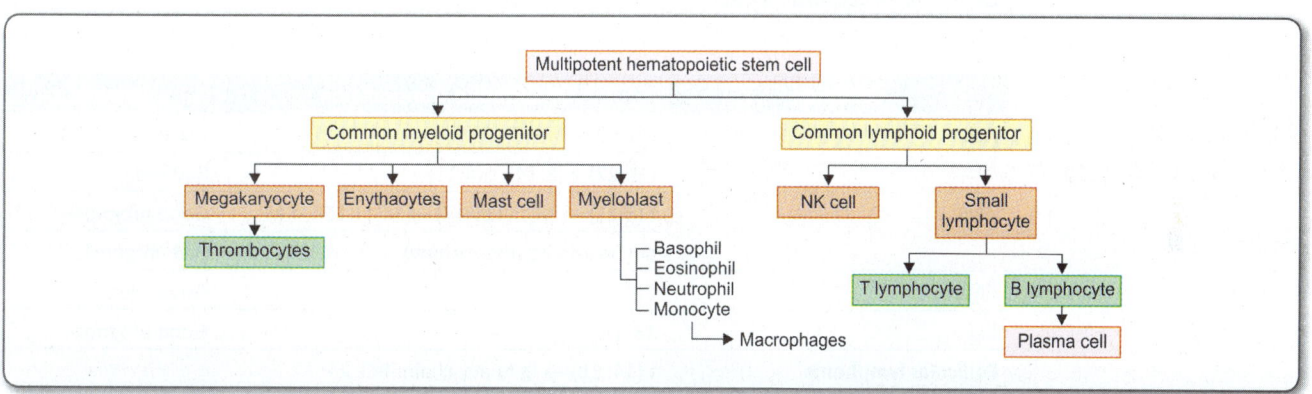

Infectious Agent	Associated Lymphoid Malignancy
Ebstein Barr virus	▪ Burkitt's lymphoma ▪ Hodgkin's lymphoma ▪ Primary CNS diffuse large B cell lymphoma ▪ Extranodal NK/T cell lymphoma ▪ Post organ transplant lymphoma
Helicobacter pylori	▪ Gastric MALToma

Infectious Agent	Associated Lymphoid Malignancy
Human Herpes virus 8	▪ Primary effusion lymphoma ▪ Multicentric Castleman's disease
HTLV-1	▪ Adult T cell leukemia/lymphoma
HIV	▪ Diffuse large B cell lymphoma ▪ Burkitt's lymphoma
Hepatitis C virus	▪ Lymphoplasmacytic lymphoma

MOST COMMON

- MC leukemia in childhood: ALL / B-ALL
- MC leukemia in >15 years: AML
- MC type of ALL: Pre B ALL
- MC subtype of AML: M_2 AML
- MC AML in Down's syndrome: M_7
- MC type of CLL : B-Cell CLL
- MC Form of cutaneous lymphoma: Mycosis fungoides
- MC Non Hodgkin Lymphoma: DLBCL
- MC type of HL: Nodular Sclerosis
- MC type of HL in India: Mixed cellularity
- MC lymph node involved in Hodgkin's lymphoma: Cervical LN
- MC lymphoma seen in HIV patient: Diffuse Large B cell Lymphoma

- MC cause of monoclonal gammopathy: MGUS → Usually asymptomatic
- MC symptomatic monoclonal gammopathy: Multiple Myeloma
- MC symptom in Multiple Myeloma: Bone Pain
- MC site of pathological fracture in Multiple Myeloma: Vertebra
- MC myeloproliferative disorder: Polycythemia Vera

Myelodysplastic Syndrome:
- MC cytogenetic abnormality: 5q-
- MC cytogenetic abnormality in children: Monosomy 7

STAINS

Stains	
Myeloid (AML)	▪ Myeloperoxidase → specific marker ▪ Sudan B Black ▪ Non Specific Enolase → M_4 and M_5
Lymphoid (ALL)	▪ PAS, TdT
Hairy cell leukemia	▪ TRAP
Epithelial cells	▪ Cytokeratin
Sarcomatous changes	▪ Vimentin
Langerhans's cell histiocytosis	▪ S-100

CONDITION/ ASSOCIATION TRANSLOCATION

Condition	Association Translocation	Remark
ALL	t (12:21)	Good prognosis
	t (9:22), t (8:14), t (4:11)	Bad prognosis
AML	t (8:21) → M_2; t (15:17) → M_3 ; i(16) → M_4	Good prognosis
	del 5q and 7q (monosomy)	Bad prognosis
CML	t (9:22)	Good prognosis
CLL	13 q del	Good prognosis
Follicular lymphoma	t (14: 18) → Ig heavy chain: BCL 2	
Burkitt's lymphoma	t (8:14) C myc : Ig heavy chain → MC t (2:8), t (8:22)	
Mantle cell lymphoma	t (11:14) → cyclin D1/bcl-1: Ig heavy chain	
Multiple myeloma	Deletion of 13 q and 17 Translocation involving Ig heavy chain locus on 14 q → MC is t (11:14)	Poor prognosis
Myelodysplastic Syndrome	Monosomy 5 and 7 (-5q, –7q, –20q); Trisomy 8	
Anaplastic large cell lymphoma	t (2:5)	Good prognosis
Marginal zone lymphoma	t (11:18)	
Diffuse Large B cell Lymphoma	t (14; 18)	

Characteristic Histological Feature	
• Pseudo gaucher cells	**pH positive CML**
• Pelger-Huet anomaly (Hyposegmented neutrophil)	**Blast phase of CML**
• Pseudo Pelger-Huet anomaly	**MDS**
• Smudge cells/Basket cells/Parachute cells • Diffuse effacement of lymph nodes by small lymphocytes • Pseudo follicular growth centers/Proliferation Centers (Pathognomic)	**CLL/SLL**
• Hairy cells (seen under phase contrast microscope) • Honey comb appearance and Fried egg appearance on BM Biopsy	**Hairy cell leukemia**
• Lymph Node Biopsy → Centrocyte and centroblast • BM Biopsy → Paratubercular lymphoid aggregate	**Follicular Lymphoma**
• Lymph Node Biopsy → Centrocyte present but Centroblast absent	**Mantle cell lymphoma**
• Lymph Node Biopsy → High mitotic index (100%) and Starry sky pattern	**Burkitt's lymphoma**
• Owl eye appearance of Reed Sternberg cells	**Hodgkin's lymphoma**
• PS → Leukoerythroblastosis; Dacrocytes/Tear drop RBC's	**Idiopathic Myelofibrosis**
• Plasma cells >30% in BM • Flame cells (Plasma cells with red cytoplasm) • Mott cells (Plasma cells with blue grape like droplets) • Russell bodies (Immunoglobulin inclusion in cytoplasm) • Dutcher bodies (Immunoglobulin inclusion in nucleus)	**Multiple Myeloma**
• Ringed sideroblasts • Pawn ball megakaryocytes • Dohle bodies in neutrophil • Pseudo Pelger-Huet cells (Neutrophil with two nuclear lobes)	**MDS**
• Sézary Lutzner cells (CD$_4$+ T$_H$ cells) • Pautrier micro abscess	**Mycosis fungoides**
• Birbeck granules	**Langerhans cell Histiocytosis**
• Hallmark cells (Horse shoe shaped nuclei and voluminous cytoplasm	**Anaplastic large cell lymphoma**
• Cells with multilobulated nuclei (cloverleaf or flower cells)	**Adult T-cell Lymphoma**

CD MARKERS

CD Markers		
• T-cell marker	CD 1,2,3,4,5,7,8	(3 → specific)
• B-cell marker	CD10, 19, 20, 21, 23	
• Monocytes/Macrophages	CD 13, CD 33	
• Stem cell	CD 34, CKIT	
• NK cell	CD 16, CD 56	(**Mn:** remember as AK 56)
• Plasma cell	CD 34 –ve, CD 38 +ve	
• Common lymphoma marker	CD 45	
• Leukocyte common Ag	CD 45 RB	
• Memory T cell	CD 45 RO	(**Mn:** memORy)
• Apoptosis	CD 95, Annexin	
• Ewing's sarcoma	CD 99	
• Histiocytosis/Langerhans cell	CD 1a, S-100 +ve	

CD Markers	
▪ Hodgkin's lymphoma/RS cells (classical)	CD 15, CD 30, PAX 5
▪ Lymphocyte predominant HL	CD 20, CD 45, Bcl-6 +ve
▪ Common AML markers	MPO (Specific), CD 13, 33, 117
▪ M_4 / M_5	CD 14, 64
▪ M_6	CD 71/ Glycophorin A
▪ $M_7 \rightarrow$ Megakaryocytic	CD 41, 61
▪ Granulocytic sarcoma/ Chloroma	CD 34, 43, 117, +ve, MPO stain +ve
▪ Paroxysmal Nocturnal Hemoglobinuria	CD55, CD59
▪ Hairy cell leukemia	CD 11c, 25, 103, 123
▪ Chronic Lymphocytic Leukemia	CD5, CD23
▪ Mantle cell lymphoma	CD5 +ve, CD23-ve
▪ Gastrointestinal Stromal Tumor	CD 117
▪ MALT Lymphoma	CD 19, 20, 79a, 43

CD 5	CD 10	CD 23	Diagnosis
+	–	–	Mantle Cell Lymphoma
–	+	–	Follicular Lymphoma
+	–	+	Chronic Lymphocytic Leukemia/SLL
–	–	–	Marginal Zone Lymphoma or MALToma

PROGNOSIS

	Good Prognosis	Bad Prognosis
AML	▪ Age <45 years ▪ No prior chemotherapy ▪ Counts <25,000 ▪ t (8:21) → M_2 ▪ t (15:17) → M_3 ▪ i (16) → M_4 ▪ NPM 1 + ▪ CEBPA + ▪ FLT-3 – ve	▪ Age >60 years ▪ Prior chemotherapy ▪ Leukocytosis > 1 lakh ▪ del 5q and 7q (monosomy) ▪ Trisomy 7 ▪ M0/M6/M7 ▪ t (12:21)
ALL	▪ Counts <1 lakh ▪ No organ involvement ▪ Hyperdiploidy ▪ t (12:21) ▪ B cell ALL	▪ Age <1 and >10 years ▪ Organ involvement (CNS, Testes) ▪ t (9:22), t (8:14), t (4:11) ▪ T cell ALL

HODGKIN'S LYMPHOMA

- HL is a malignancy of mature B lymphocytes
- Pathogenesis → activation of NF-κB by EBV infection
- Bimodal age distribution → 15-34 years and > 55 years
- Pel-Ebstein Fever is characteristic → intermittent fever having a cyclical period of 1-2 weeks
- Triad of B-symptoms : Fever, night sweats and weight loss
- MC presentation: Nontender lymphadenopathy in the neck and supraclavicular area
- Contiguous LN involvement

- Pain in the affected LN on consumption of alcohol
- Paraneoplastic cerebellar degeneration
- Prognosis is predicted by International Prognosis Score (IPS)

Newer Drugs:
- Brentuximab → Drug conjugate against CD30
  - Used in combination with AVD in classical HL
- Pembrolizumab → MAb to programmed cell death-1 protein
  - For refractory classical HL

Poor Prognostic Markers	Treatment

■ Age >45 years
■ Sex → Male
■ Presence of Group B symptoms
■ Presence of Mediastinal mass
■ Stage IV disease
■ Subtypes → Mixed Cellularity and Lymphocyte Depleted
■ Albumin <4 g/dL
■ Serum Hb <10.5 g/dL
■ WBC count ≥15,000 /mm³
■ Absolute lymphocyte count <600/mm³
	■ *Classical Hodgkin Lymphoma:*
	   ○ Stage I and II → Chemo f/b Radiotherapy
	   ○ Stage III and IV → Chemo ± Radiotherapy
	■ *Lymphocyte predominant Hodgkin Lymphoma:*
	   ○ Stage I and II → Radiotherapy
	   ○ Stage III and IV → Chemo ± Radiotherapy
	■ MC used Chemo regimen → ABVD [**A**driamycin/ Doxorubicin, **B**leomycin, **V**inblastine, **D**acarbazine]
	■ Other regimens → Stanford V, MOPP and BEACOPP

MYELOPROLIFERATIVE DISORDERS

	Polycythemia Vera	Myelofibrosis	Essential Thrombocytosis
General features	■ Over production of phenotypically normal RBC, granulocytes and platelets (Tri linear hyperplasia) ■ Predominantly RBC elevation is seen ■ ↓requirement of EPO and other growth factors ■ Arterial O_2 saturation – Normal ■ JAK-2 mutation is seen in 100% cases ■ May transform into acute leukemia	■ Neoplastic megakaryocyte → ↑ PDGF + TGF-β → leads to fibrosis ■ JAK-2 mutation is seen	■ Diagnosis of exclusion ■ Associated with Tyrosine Kinase JAK-2 mutation ■ Thrombocytosis with non functioning platelets JAK-2 mutation is seen in 50% cases

Clinical features	■ ↑ RBC and Blood viscosity leads to:
	   ○ Neurological symptoms like vertigo, dizziness, tinnitus and visual disturbances
	   ○ Thrombosis (venous or arterial) leading to DVT, Budd Chiari etc.
	   ○ Splenomegaly; Systolic Hypertension
	■ ↑ Basophil leads to ↑ secretion of histamine causing Intense pruritus and Peptic ulcer
	■ ↑ Megakaryocyte: Thrombosis
	■ May undergo Myelofibrosis in later stage
		■ Splenomegaly
		■ Extramedullary hematopoiesis
			■ Hemorrhagic tendency – Easy bruising
			■ Thrombotic tendency
			■ Mild/Moderate splenomegaly
			■ Hypercellular BM with dysmegakaryopoiesis

Lab features	■ ↑Hb% and RBC count ■ ↑ HCV/Venous HCT >55% ■ ESR ↓; EPO ↓; LAP score↑ ■ Abnormal platelet function ■ ↑ Vitamin B_{12} binding capacity ■ ↑ Uric acid ■ IOC – Red cell mass (Increased)	■ ↑ LAP score ■ PS → Tear drop cells/Dacrocytes and Pancytopenia ■ Hypercellular bone marrow ■ Dry tap on aspiration ■ BM biopsy → reticular/collagen on biopsy (IOC)	■ ↑ platelet count (>600 × 109/L) ■ Hematocrit and RBC – Normal ■ N/↑ LAP score ■ Abnormal bleeding time

Managements	■ Venesection ■ Hydroxyurea
	■ TOC for ■ Anagrelide
	  Erythromelalgia ■ Radioactive iodine P³²
	  → NSAIDS
		■ Splenectomy
		■ JAK-2 inhibitors
			■ Asymptomatic patient → No therapy
			■ Symptomatic patient → IFN and Anagrelide

CLASSIFICATION OF LYMPHOMA

Hodgkin Lymphoma

Classical HL

- **Mixed cellularity**
- **Nodular Sclerosis**
- **Lymphocyte rich**
- **Lymphocyte depleted**

○ RS cells present
○ CD 15 and 30 +ve
○ CD 20 and 45 − ve
○ PAX 5 +ve

Histological distinct HL

- **Lymphocyte predominant**
  ○ RS cells not seen
  ○ CD 15 and 30 − ve
  ○ CD 20 and 45 + ve
  ○ BCL 2 + ve

Reed Sternberg (RS) Cells:
- **Diagnostic of Classical Hodgkin Lymphoma**
- Also seen in Infectious Mononucleosis
- Derived from germinal centre B cells
- Malignant cell of HL
- Bilobed nucleus → **Owl eye appearance**
- Most sensitive marker → CD 30 (present in 100% cases)
- Most specific marker → PAX 5

Types of Hodgkin Lymphoma

Types	RS cells	Gender	EBV	Characteristics
Mixed cellularity	Classical RS cells / Mononuclear variant	M > F	+ ve	- Most Common in India - Biphasic incidence
Nodular sclerosis	Lacunar cells	M = F	- ve	- Most common type - Mediastinal involvement occurs - 2nd best prognosis
Lymphocyte depleted	Reticular variant	M > F	+ ve	- Worst prognosis - Associated with HIV
Lymphocyte Predominant	Popcorn cells / LH cells	M > F	- ve	- Best prognosis

Non Hodgkin Lymphoma

B cell Neoplasm (85%)

Neoplasm of Mature Peripheral B-Cells:
- Burkitt's lymphoma
- Follicular lymphoma
- Mantle cell lymphoma
- Hairy cell leukemia
- Diffuse Large B cell Lymphoma
- Multiple myeloma
- Waldenstrom's macroglobulinemia
- CLL/SLL
- MALToma

T cell Neoplasm

Neoplasm of Mature T cells/NK cells:
- **Mycosis fungoides**
  ○ Cutaneous T- cell lymphoma
  ○ Aka Sézary syndrome
- **Anaplastic large T cell lymphoma**
  ○ Aka Null cell lymphoma
  ○ Cells are CD 30 +ve
  ○ t (2:5) is found
  ○ ALK positivity is associated with good prognosis

Types of Non Hodgkin Lymphoma

	Burkitt's	Follicular	Mantle cell	Hairy cell
Translocation	t (8:14) → MC t (2: 8); t(8:22)	t (14:18)	t (11:14) ↑Cyclin D₁	
CD markers	CD 10, 19, 20 BCL 6 +ve BCL 2 −ve	CD 10, 19, 20 BCL 6 +ve BCL 2 +ve CD 5 and 23 −ve	CD 5 +ve CD 23 −ve FMC 7 +ve	CD 11c + ve CD 25 +ve CD 103 +ve TRAP + ve
Genes	c MYC (chromosome 8)	↑BCL 2 gene expression (chromosome 18)	↑Cyclin D₁ / BCL 1 expression (chromosome 11)	
Peripheral Smear	High mitotic index (nearly 100%) Starry sky pattern	Centrocyte + Centroblast + Paratrabecular lymphoid aggregate	Centrocyte + Centroblast −	Pancytopenia Cellular BM Honey comb and fried egg appearance
Association	EBV in endemic BL			

⬐ Ann Arbor staging system is used for staging of Hodgkin and Non Hodgkin Lymphoma

LEUKEMIA

	AML	ALL	CML	CLL / SLL
Age	▪ 15 – 40 years	▪ 1 – 5 years	▪ 25 – 50 years	▪ 60 – 80 years
Association	▪ Down's syndrome (M7) ▪ MDS ▪ DIC – Acute promyelocytic leukemia (M3)	▪ t(12:21) ▪ t (9:22) ▪ t (8: 14) ▪ t (4: 11)	▪ t (9: 22) **ABL1** gene of chromosome 9 juxtaposed onto the **BCR** gene of chromosome 22	▪ Deletion of 11, 13 or 17 chromosome ▪ Autoimmune hemolytic anemia ▪ Expression of ZAP-70 and CD 38 is associated with poorer prognosis.
Staining	▪ MPO /Sudan B black → M0-M3 ▪ NSE → M4, M5	▪ PAS → B cell ALL ▪ TdT and Acid phosphate → T cell ALL		
Markers	▪ CD 13, 33, MPO, Glycophorin-A ▪ CD 14, 64 → Monocyte series ▪ CD 41, 61 → Platelets	▪ B cell → CD 10, 19, 20, sIg ▪ T cell → CD 2, 3, 4, 5, 7, 8		▪ CD 5, 19, 20, 23 +ve ▪ CD 79B and FMC 7 – ve
Clinical features	▪ Gum hypertrophy – M4	▪ CNS features ▪ Mediastinal mass ▪ Testicular involvement	▪ Massive splenomegaly ▪ Sokel index is for prognosis	▪ More common in males ▪ MC form – B cell CLL ▪ Transformation into ALL is rare
Lab	▪ ↑ muramidase in M4/M5 ▪ ↑ FDP in M3 AML (d/t DIC)	▪ PAS and TdT positive	▪ Basophilia on PS ▪ LAP score ↓ and ↑ Vitamin B_{12} level ▪ BM is 100% cellular ▪ Pseudo gaucher cells	▪ Diagnostic criteria → ≥5000 monoclonal B lymphocytes ▪ PS – Smudge/basket/parachute cells ▪ BM – Proliferation centerand Pseudo follicular growth center

Treatments	▪ M3 AML → ATRA/ Tretinoin and As_2O_3	▪ Vincristine
		▪ Prednisolone
		▪ Cyclophosphamide
		▪ L- asparaginase
		▪ Methotrexate
		▪ Daunorubicin
		▪ Intracranial ALL → Intrathecal methotrexate/Prednisolone/ L-asparaginase/Vincristine
		▪ CNS prophylaxis → Methotrexate
			▪ Tyrosine Kinase inhibitors:
			  ○ DOC → Imatinib
			  ○ Other TKIs: Dasatinib, Nilotinib, Bosutinib, Ponatinib
			  ○ Omacetaxine – inhibits protein synthesis
				▪ Rituximab
				▪ Staging is done according to:
				  ○ Rai – Sawitsky system
				  ○ Binet staging

PLASMA CELL NEOPLASMS

Multiple Myeloma

General features
- MC symptomatic gammopathy
- Increase in plasma cell → increase production of immunoglobulins
- MC symptom → Bone pain
- MC site for lytic lesions → Vertebral column
- Most Important predictor of outcome → β_2 microglobulin

Pathology
- MI interleukin involved: IL-6 → also known as Plasma cell GF
- Metastatic calcification may be seen

Genetics
- MC translocation: t (11:14)
- Deletion of chromosome 13 and 17 and 11q abnormality is also seen

Clinical features
- Normocytic Normochromic anemia
- Lytic bone lesions (due to osteoclast) l/t bone pain, osteoporosis, fractures and cord compression,
- Hyperviscosity may lead to Neurological symptom; Headache; Visual disturbance
- Recurrent infection; Bleeding; Coagulation disorder
- Renal Failure
- Amyloidosis (AL – subtype)

Investigation
- ↑Urea/creatinine/ESR
- Hypercalcemia and metastatic calcification
- Electrophoresis → M spikes formed of IgG/IgA
- Serum Alkaline Phosphatase → Normal
- CRP → prognostic marker
- Decrease in anion gap
- Electrophoresis → Bence Jones proteinuria (made up of light chain)
- Protein cast in urine → made up of only light chains
- **Bone marrow biopsy and Histopathology shows:**
  - Flame cells
  - Mott cells
  - Russell bodies (intra/cytoplasmic inclusion)
  - Dutcher bodies (intra nuclear inclusion)
- X-ray skull → lytic lesions (Rain drop skull appearance)

Diagnosis

Major Criteria
- Plasmacytoma on biopsy
- >30% plasma cells on BM
- Monoclonal Ig spikes on electrophoresis

Minor Criteria
- Lytic bone lesions
- Monoclonal Ig spikes
- Plasma cells 10-30% in BM

Treatment

Chemotherapy regimens in use:
- Lenalidomide + Dexamethasone
- Bortezomib + Melphalan
- VAD [Vincristine, Adriamycin/ Doxorubicin, Dexamethasone]
- Melphalan + Prednisolone

Preferred regimen for Induction in transplant candidates:
- Bortezomib + Lenalidomide + Dexamethasone
- Bortezomib + Cyclophosphamide + Dexamethasone (in patients with AKI)

Preferred regimen for induction in not a transplant candidates:
- Bortezomib + Lenalidomide + Dexamethasone
- Lenalidomide + Low dose dexamethasone

Preferred regimen for maintenance chemotherapy:
- Lenalidomide ± Bortezomib

Poor prognostic factors
- Hypercalcemia (>12 mg/dL)
- Serum creatinine >2 mg/dL
- High M component
- Increase β_2 microglobulin
- ↑LDH and CRP
- t (4:14)
- Chromosome 13 and 17 deletion

Staging
- Salmon-Durie system
- International staging system

MULTIPLE CHOICE QUESTIONS

CHAPTER 1: INTRODUCTION TO HEMATOLOGY

HEMATOPOIESIS

1. Erythropoiesis in gestational age (early fetal life) takes place in *(PGMEE 2013,2015)*
   a. Yolk sac
   b. Aminotic sac
   c. Placenta
   d. Chorion

   [Ref: Ganong's 25ᵗʰ/e pg. 554;Guyton 12ᵗʰ/e p. 414]

Explanation

- Sites of Hematopoiesis:
  ○ 3ʳᵈ week to 3ʳᵈ month : Yolk sac
  ○ 3ʳᵈ month to before birth : Liver (by Hematopoietic stem cells)
  ○ Birth to puberty : Whole of skeleton (by progenitor stem cells)
  ○ Adulthood : Axial skeleton

2. Which is the earliest site of erythropoiesis in a developing foetus? *(PGMEE 2013-14)*
   a. Yolk sac
   b. Spleen
   c. Liver
   d. Bone marrow

   [Ref: Ganong's 25ᵗʰ/e pg. 554]

3. Hematopoiesis in first month of life is- *(PGMEE 2014)*
   a. Medullary
   b. Hepatic
   c. Mesoblastic
   d. Lymphatic

   [Ref: Nelson 20th/e/ch 446]

4. Common site of haematopoiesis in fetus is- *(DNB Jun. 11)*
   a. Liver
   b. Spleen
   c. Gut
   d. Bone marrow

   [Ref: Robbins 9th/e pg. 579]

5. Erythropoetin in fetus is secreted by? *(PGMEE 2016)*
   a. Spleen
   b. Kidney
   c. Liver
   d. Marrow

   [Ref: Robbins 9th/pg 618]

Explanation

- Predominant source of Erythropoietin [EPO] in:
  ○ Adults → Peritubular capillary lining cells within kidney
  ○ Fetus → Liver

6. Progenitor hematopoetic stem cells originate in- *(PGMEE 2012-13)*
   a. Bone marrow
   b. Spleen
   c. Thymus
   d. Lymph node

   [Ref: Robbins 9ᵗʰ/e pg. 580]

7. Supravital staining is used for? *(PGMEE 2015)*
   a. Nucleated RBC's
   b. Reticulocytes
   c. Myeloblasts
   d. Basophils

   [Ref: Dacie 11th/pg 34]

Explanation

Stain	Blood cell
Wright's stain	RBC, WBC (differential count)
Supravital stain	Reticulocyte [stain used New methylene blue or Brilliant cresyl blue]

8. Reticulocytes are stained with – *(PGMEE 90)*
   a. Indigo carmine
   b. Brilliant cresyl blue
   c. Sudan Black
   d. Methyl violet

   [Ref: Chaudhary 3ʳᵈ/e pg. 23]

9. Which of the following correctly describes principle of Prussian blue stain? *(PGMEE 2016)*
   a. Ferrouscyanide to ferricyanide
   b. Ferrocyanide to ferroferric cyanide
   c. Ferroferriccyanide to ferrocyanide
   d. Ferrocyanide to ferricferrocyanide

   [Ref: T. Singh 3rd ed/pg 21]

10. Periodic acid schiff stain shows block positivity in *(DNB 2008)*
   a. Myeloblasts
   b. Megakaryoblasts
   c. Monoblasts
   d. Lymphoblasts

   [Ref: Page 283 Dacie and Lewis Tenth edition]

11. Lifespan of neutrophils is? *(PGMEE 2013)*
   a. 6 hours
   b. 1 days
   c. 7 day
   d. 120 days

   [Ref: Ganongs review of medical physiology 23ʳᵈ/e p. 64]

12. Ratio of fat cells and blood cells in bone marrow is- *(PGMEE 2013)*
   a. 2:1
   b. 1:2
   c. 1:1
   d. 1:4

   [Ref: Robbins 9ᵗʰ/e pg. 582]

13. In infant, Bone Marrow biopsy is done from? *(PGMEE 2015)*
   a. Tibia
   b. Sternum
   c. Iliac crest
   d. Posterior superior Iliac Spine

   [Ref: Wintrobe's 12th/pg 10]

1.	a
2.	a
3.	a
4.	a
5.	c
6.	a
7.	b
8.	b
9.	d
10.	b
11.	a
12.	c
13.	a

48. Hemoglobin binding protein is – *(PGMEE 2014)*
- a. Haptoglobin
- b. Albumin
- c. Hemopexin
- d. All of the above

[Ref: Ganong's 25th/e pg. 563]

49. Polycythemia is seen in? *(PGMEE 2012)*
- a. Cor pulmonale
- b. Acynotic congenital heart diseases
- c. Congestive cardiac failure
- d. All of the above

50. Eosinophillia is found in? *(PGMEE 2016)*
- a. Cryptococcus
- b. Typhoid
- c. Stronglyloides
- d. HPV

[Ref: Robbins 9th/pg 583]

Explanation
- Eosinophilia is seen in conditions like Asthma, Parasitic infections, Churg strauss syndromes, Malignancy, Allergy, etc [**Mn:** Ask for PCM Allergy]

48. d
49. a
50. c

COAGULATION PATHWAY

1. True about Vitamin K is: (NEET 2018)
   a. Is a water soluble vitamin
   b. Vitamin K deficiency leads to thrombosis
   c. Prolonged antibiotic therapy for bacterial infection can cause vitamin K deficiency
   d. Helps in synthesis of factor VIII

2. All of the following are Vitamin-K deficiency features except (PGMEE 2015-16)
   a. Associated thrombocytopenia with prolonged bleeding
   b. Deficiency is rarely seen, except in infants
   c. Factor X is first to be affected
   d. Warfarin causes Vitamin K deficiency

   [Ref: Harrison 19th ed. / 96e-8]

Explanation
- Warfarin depletes functional vitamin K reserves & interfere with hepatic synthesis of vit K dependent clotting factors namely, II, VII, IX, X, Protein-C & Protein S.

3. Feature of hemorrhagic disease of new born is:
   a. Prolonged prothrombin time (PGMEE 2014-15)
   b. Defective platelet count
   c. Prolonged bleeding time
   d. Prolonged thrombin time

   [Ref: Harrison's 18th ed. pg. 980]

4. What is true about acquired disorder of coagulation?
   a. Hemarthrosis is specifically seen (PGMEE 2012)
   b. Shows defect in platelets as well
   c. Less frequent that inherited disorder
   d. Shows specific clotting deficiency

   [Ref: Wintrobe's 11th/e p. 3369]

5. Prothrombin time measures which pathway?
   (PGMEE 2015)
   a. Common pathway
   b. Extrinsic pathway
   c. Intrinsic pathway
   d. Both intrinsic and extrinsic pathway

   [Ref: Ganong's 25th /e pg. 565]

6. Common step in coagulation pathway is-
   (PGMEE 2015)
   a. Activation of factor VII
   b. Activation of factor IX
   c. Activation of factor VIII
   d. Activation of factor X

   [Ref: Ganong's 25th /e pg. 565]

7. Which clotting factor is required for stabilization of fibrin clot –
   (PGMEE 2014)
   a. XIIIa   b. IX
   c. VIII   d. V

   [Ref: Ganong's 25th /e pg. 565]

Explanation

Factor number	Common name
I	Fibrinogen
II	Prothrombin
III	Tissue factor
IV	Ca^{+2}
IX	Christmas factor
X	Stuart factor
XII	Hageman factor
XIII	Fibrin stabilizing factor

8. Clotting factors that is not affected in liver disease is?
   (DNB June 2009)
   a. Factors II   b. Factor IV
   c. Factor VIII   d. Factor IX

   [Ref: Ganong's 25th /e pg. 565]

Explanation
- All coagulation factors are produced in liver with the exception of factor VIII, VWF & Ca^{+2} (factor 4).

9. Ion which is needed for conversion of Prothrombin to thrombin is (DNB Dec 2009)
   a. Potassium   b. Sodium
   c. Magnesium   d. Calcium

   [Ref: Ganong's 25th /e pg. 565]

10. In PT test, the addition of Ca^{2+} & tissue thromboplastin activates which pathway? (NEET Pattern 2017)
   a. Extrinsic   b. Inrinsic
   c. Fibrinolytic   d. Common

   [Ref: Robbins 9th ed pg 656]

Explanation
- *Prothrombin time (PT) is used to screen the* **extrinsic and common** *pathways. In this test the clotting of plasma after addition of an exogenous source of tissue thromboplastin (e.g., brain extract) and $Ca^{[2]+}$ ions is measured in seconds.*
- A prolonged PT can result from deficiency or dysfunction of factor 5,7,10, prothrombin, or fibrinogen

Extra Points
- *Partial thromboplastin time (PTT)is used to screen the* **intrinsic and common** *pathways. The clotting of plasma after addition of kaolin, cephalin, and $Ca^{[2]+}$ ions is measured in seconds. Kaolin activates the contact dependent factor XII, and cephalin substitutes for platelet phospholipids. Prolonged PTT can be due to deficiency or dysfunction of factors V, VIII, IX, X, XI, or XII, prothrombin, or fibrinogen, or due to interfering antibodies to phospholipid.*
- *Tests of platelet function. At present, no single test provides an adequate assessment of the complex functions of platelets.*

1.	c
2.	a,c
3.	a
4.	b
5.	b
6.	d
7.	a
8.	b,c
9.	d
10.	a

- **Bleeding time**, measures the time taken for a standardized skin puncture to stop bleeding. It has some value but is time-consuming, difficult to perform well, and not a good predictor of bleeding during surgery/ hemostatic stresses.
- Other specialized tests include:-
  ○ Tests of platelet aggregation, which measure the ability of platelets to aggregate in response to agonists like thrombin;
  ○ Quantitative and qualitative tests of vWF, which play an important role in platelet adhesion to the extracellular matrix.

11. **In coagulation pathway, "Fibrin stabilizing factor" is –**
(PGMEE 2016-17)
   a. Factor IX
   b. Factor XIII
   c. High molecular Weight Kinimogen (HMWK]
   d. Factor XII

[Ref: Ganong's 23rd/e p. 542-543]

12. **Nitric oxide is produced from**　　　　**(PGMEE 2009)**
   a. Endothelium　　　b. RBC
   c. Platelets　　　　　d. Lymphocytes

[Ref: Guyton's physiology22nd edition page 199]

13. **Factor which activates factor VII in to VIIa**
(PGMEE 2015)
   a. Tissue factor　　　b. Prothrombin
   c. Fibrim　　　　　　d. Christmas factor

[Ref: Ganong 23rd/e p. 531-535]

14. **Factor which activates prekallikrein-**　**(PGMEE 2015)**
   a. Factor VIII　　　　b. Factor X
   c. Factor II　　　　　d. Factor XII

[Ref: Ganong's 25th/e pg. 565,597]

15. **All endothelial cells produce thrombomodulin except those found in-**　　　　**(PGMEE 2012-13)**
   a. Hepatic circulation
   b. Cutaneous circulation
   c. Cerebral microcirculation
   d. Renal circulation

[Ref: Ganong 21st/e p. 546]

16. **Fibrin is degraded by-**　　　　**(PGMEE 2012-13)**
   a. Plasminogen　　　b. Thromboplastin
   c. Plasmin　　　　　d. FD

[Ref: Robbin's 8th/e p. 116]

17. **Increased PT and Normal PTT are found in?**
(DNB Dec. 11)
   a. Thrombin deficiency　b. Factor 7 deficiency
   c. Factor 8 deficiency　d. Von willibrand's disease

[Ref: Robbin's 8th/e p. 973]

18. **Both APTT and PT are prolonged in which conditions?**
(PGMEE 2009)
   a. Factor II deficiency
   b. Factor XIII deficiency
   c. Thrombocytopenia
   d. Heparin administration

[Ref: Harrison's 17th/e table 59-4]

19. **Leiden mutation is associated with?**　**(PGMEE 2013)**
   a. Factor VIII　　　　b. Factor V
   c. Factor IX　　　　　d. Factor IV

[Ref: Robbin's 8th/e p. Ch. 4, Harrison 18th/e p. ch. 58, 117]

20. **Platelet Dense granules contain all except**
(DNB June 11)
   a. ADP　　　　　　　b. VwF
   c. Calcium　　　　　　d. 5-HT

[Ref: Robbin's 8th/e p. 117]

21. **Apixaban is a new drug that acts by:**　**(PGMEE 2014-15)**
   a. Inhibiting TNF alpha
   b. Inhibiting coagulation factor Xa
   c. Inhibiting platelet aggregation
   d. Activating plasminogen

[Ref: Harrison's 19th/e pg. 756]

22. **All are true about warfarin, EXCEPT:**　**(PGMEE 2014-15)**
   a. It causes inhibition of vitamin K dependent clotting factors
   b. Its half-life is 36 hours
   c. It can cross placenta
   d. Its dose is increased in liver disease

[Ref: Katzung 11th/595-596, Harrison's 19th/e pg. 7E]

HYPERCOAGULABLE STATES

23. **Thrombotic event is seen in all of following EXCEPT:**
(PGMEE 2014-15)
   a. PNH
   b. DIC
   c. ITP
   d. Heparin induced thrombocytopenia

[Ref: Harrison's 19th/e pg. 728]

24. **Thrombosis seen in which stage of lupus nephritis?**
(PGMEE 2013)
   a. Class II　　　　　　b. Class IV
   c. Class V　　　　　　d. Class I

[Ref: Robbin's 8th/e p. 218, 219]

25. **All of the following statements regarding the lupus anti- coagulant (LA) are true EXCEPT:**　**(PGMEE 2014-15)**
   a. Typically prolong the APTT
   b. A 1:1 mixing study will not correct in the presence of LA
   c. Bleeding episodes in patients with LA may be severe and life threatening
   d. Female patients may experience recurrent midtrimester abortions

[Ref: Harrison's 19th/e pg. 740]

26. **Anticoagulant of choice for coagulation testing is?**
(PGMEE 2014-15)
   a. Trisodium citrate 3.2%　b. EDTA
   c. Heparin　　　　　　d. Sodium oxalate

[Ref: Harrison's 19th/e pg. 749]

Explanation
- Discussed in biochemistry under "vacutainer tubes".

11.	b
12.	a
13.	a
14.	d
15.	c
16.	c
17.	b
18.	a
19.	b
20.	b
21.	b
22.	d
23.	c
24.	c
25.	c
26.	a

27. **Which of the following is NOT a hyper-coagulable state** *(PGMEE 2015-16)*
   a. Pregnancy
   b. MI
   c. Abruptio-placentae
   d. Cirrhosis

   [Ref: Harrison's 19th/e pg. 739]

28. **A 45 year old lady with normal PT and increased aPTT. About 2 year back, she was operated for cholecystectomy and did not have any bleeding episode. What is next investigation for clinical diagnosis?** *(PGMEE 2014-15)*
   a. Factor VIII assay
   b. Dilute russel viper venom assay
   c. Platelet aggregation test
   d. Ristocetin Cofactor assay

   [Ref: Harrison's 19th/e pg. 2131]

29. **Which one of the following platelet counts is usually associated with increased incidence of spontaneous bleeding** *(PGMEE 2014-15)*
   a. Greater than 80,000/mm³
   b. 40,000/mm3
   c. 20,000mm3
   d. Less than 20,000mm³

   [Ref: Harrison's 18th pg. 461]

30. **Purpura fulminans is associated with all except:** *(PGMEE 2014-15)*
   a. Protein C deficiency
   b. Protein S deficiency
   c. AT III deficiency
   d. Factor 5 leiden mutation

   [Ref: Harrison's 19th/e pg. 737]

Explanation

- Purpura fulminans is c/b intravascular thrombosis & hemorrhage infarction of the skin. It is associated with deficiency of the protein C, protein S & antithrombin III.

31. **A 25-year-old female presented with history of recurrent abortions. The most relevant investi-gation to identify the cause is:** *(PGMEE 2014-15)*
   a. Bleeding time
   b. Prothrombin time
   c. Dilute russel viper venom time
   d. Clot solubility test

   [Ref: Harrison's 19th/e pg. 740]

27.	d
28.	b
29.	d
30.	d
31.	c

PLATELETS

1. Which of the following is affected by platelet count-
(PGMEE 2014)
a. Bleeding time
b. Thrombin time
c. Prothrombin time
d. Partial thromboplastin time

[Ref: Robbin's 8th/e p. 670]

2. Size of platelets is (PGMEE 2015)
a. 1 A^0
b. I μm
c. 2 A^0
d. 2 μm

[Ref: Textbook of hematology 3rd/e p. 391; Ganong's 25th/e pg. 555]

3. Platelet aggregation is inhibited by: (PGMEE 2015)
a. Thromboxane A$_2$
b. PGF$_2$α
c. PGI$_2$ & PGD$_2$
d. PGE$_2$

[Ref: Goodman and Gillman's 11th/e p. 972, KDT 5th/e p. 49]

4. Platelet aggregation is caused by? (PGMEE 2013)
a. Aspirin
b. Thromboxane A2
c. PG12
d. Nitrous oxide

[Ref: Goodman and Gillman's 11th/e p. 972, KDT 5th/e p. 49]

5. Thrombocythemia is characterized by:
(PGMEE 2015-16)
a. High Platelets count
b. Low Platelets count
c. Neutrophilia
d. Monocytosis

[Ref: Harrison 18th edition, Chapter 115]

DEFECTS IN PLATELET FUNCTIONS

6. Glanzman's disease is: (PGMEE 2012-13)
a. Congenital defect of platelets
b. Clotting factor of deficiency
c. Congenital defect of RBCs
d. Defect of neutrophils

[Ref: Robbin's 8th/e p. 670]

7. All are used to screen platelet functions except
(PGMEE 10)
a. Prothrombin time
b. Bleeding time
c. Activated Clotting Time
d. PFA-100

[Ref: Clinical hematology: Theory and procedures p. 348]

8. The presence of small sized platelets on the peripheral smear is characteristic of: (PGMEE 2014-15)
a. Idiopathic thrombocytopenic purpura
b. Bernard soulier syndrome
c. Disseminated intravascular coagulation
d. Wiskott Aldrich syndrome

[Ref: Harrison's 19th/e pg. 2110]

9. A patient comes with thrombocytopenia, eczema and recurrent infections. What is the most probable diagnosis?
a. Wiskott Aldrich syndrome (DNB Dec' 2010)
b. Bruton's agammaglobulinemia
c. Job's syndrome
d. Chediak-Higashi syndrome

[Ref: Harrison's 19th/e pg 2110]

10. Platelet adhesion defect is seen in :- (PGMEE' 2010)
a. Wiskott Aldrich syndrome
b. Bernard -Soulier syndrome
c. Job's syndrome
d. Chediak-Higashi syndrome

[Ref: Robbins 9th/e pg. 661; Harrison's 19th/e pg 2110]

11. In Bernard Soulier syndrome the defect is:
(PGMEE 2018)
a. GP Ib
b. GPIIb/IIIa
c. Platelet numbers
d. None of the above

12. Bernard Soulier disease is due to (PGMEE 2019)
a. GP IIb-IIIa deficiency
b. vWF deficiency
c. Anti-hemophilic factor
d. Defect in GP1b

13. Which of the following is the finding in functional defect in platelets? (PGMEE 2014-15)
a. Normal platelet counts and prolonged bleeding time
b. Normal platelet count and bleeding time
c. Prolonged bleeding time, prothrombin time and PTT
d. Thrombocytopenia and prolonged bleeding time

[Ref: Harrison's 19th/e pg. 138e-4]

THROMBOCYTOPENIA

14. Which of the following is given to treat thrombocytopenia secondary to anti-cancer therapy and is known to stimulate progenitor megakaryocytes?
(PGMEE 2014-15)
a. Filgrastim
b. Oprelvekin
c. Erythropoietin
d. Anagrelide

[Ref: Harrison's 19th/e pg. 103e-24]

Explanation
- Oprelvekin is a recombinant IL-11 thrombopoietic growth factor.

15. Anti-coagulant of choice for heparin induced thrombocytopenia is: (PGMEE 2014-15)
a. Lepirudin
b. Aprotinin
c. Abciximab
d. Plasminogen

[Ref: Harrison's 19th/e pg. 749]

1.	a
2.	d
3.	c
4.	b
5.	a
6.	a
7.	a
8.	d
9.	a
10.	b
11.	a
12.	d
13.	a
14.	b
15.	a

16. **All the following conditions can cause thrombocytopenia except:** *(PGMEE 2012-13)*
    a. HIV infection
    b. Giant hemangioma
    c. Infectious mononucleosis
    d. Iron deficiency anemia

    [Ref: Robbin's 8th/e p. 667]

17. **Thrombocytopenia due to increased platelet destruction is seen in** *(PGMEE 2009)*
    a. Acute leukemia
    b. Aplastic anemia
    c. Systemic lupus erythematosus
    d. Cancer chemotherapy

    [Ref: Robbin's 8th/e p. 667]

18. **In a case of anemia with thrombocytopenia and PMN showing inclusions. What is the most probable diagnosis?**
    a. May Hegglin anomaly *(PGMEE 2015]*
    b. Evan syndrome
    c. Pegler Huet Anomaly
    d. Alder-Reilly anomaly

    [Ref: Wintrobe's 12th/pg 1549]

Explanation

- May Hegglin anomaly (MHA) is an AD disorder c/b thrombocytopenia & bleeding, giant platelets and inclusion bodies resembling Dohle bodies.

ITP

19. **Antibodies in ITP are:** *(PGMEE 2013-14)*
    a. IgG   b. IgE
    c. IgD   d. IgM

    [Ref: Robbin's 8th/e p. 667]

20. **Idiopathic thrombocytopenic purpura (ITP) is associated with all of the following EXCEPT:** *(PGMEE 2013-14)*
    a. Splenomegaly
    b. Mucosal bleeding
    c. Thrombocytopenia
    d. Increased megakaryocytes

    [Ref: Robbins 7th/651,652; Ghai 6th/324]

21. **Idiopathic Thrombocytopenic purpura is associated with:** *(PGMEE 2014-15)*
    a. Small megakaryoblasts   b. Non palpable purpura
    c. Massive splenomegaly   d. Evan syndrome

    [Ref: Harrison's 19th/e pg. 728]

22. **Bleeding crisis in acute Idiopathic thrombo-cytopenic Purpura is managed by all EXCEPT:** *(PGMEE 2014-15)*
    a. IVIG
    b. Prednisolone
    c. Intravenous immunoglobulin
    d. Eltrombopag

    [Ref: Harrison's 19th/e pg. 728]

Explanation

Acute ITP	Chronic ITP
▪ Corticosteroids ▪ IVIG ▪ Rituximab ▪ Splenectomy	▪ Eltrombopag > Thrombopoietin receptor agonist ▪ Romiplostin > Thrombopoietin receptor agonist
	▪ Fostamatinib > Spleen tyroxine kinase (SYK) inhibitor

23. **Which of the following intervention has maximum therapeutic benefit in ITP** *(PGMEE 2019)*
    a. Steroids
    b. IVIG
    c. Splenectomy
    d. Plasmapheresis

24. **A patient with ITP on steroids underwent splenectomy. Patient got fever on 3rd post-operative day. Next investigation is likely to reveal?** *(NEET Pattern 2015)*
    a. Left lower lobe consolidation
    b. Port site infection
    c. Focal Intra-abdominal collection
    d. UTI

    [Ref: chapter 69: Wintrobe's Hematology 12th edition and page number 1096: Bailey and love 26th edition.]

25. **A Patient has ecchymosis and petechiae all over the body with no hepato-splenomegaly. All are true except?** *(PGMEE 2014-15)*
    a. Increased megakaryocytes in bone narrow.
    b. Bleeding into the joints
    c. Decreased platelet in blood
    d. Disease resolves itself in 80% of Patients in 2-6 weeks.

    [Ref: Harrison's 18th ed. pg. 968]

DIC

26. **Cause of DIC does not include:** *(PGMEE 2014)*
    a. Carcinoma pancreas   b. Falciparum malaria
    c. Trauma   d. AML M$_1$ type

    [Ref: Robbin's 8th/e p. 673]

27. **Seen in D.I.C all EXCEPT:** *(PGMEE 2014-15)*
    a. Hyperfibrinogenimia
    b. Increase fibrin degradation products
    c. Prolonged PT
    d. Increased APTT

    [Ref: Harrison's 19th/e pg. 736]

28. **DIC is most likely characterized by:** *(PGMEE 2014-15)*
    a. Significant numbers of schistocytes
    b. A brisk reticulocytosis
    c. Decreased coagulation factor levels
    d. Significant thrombocytopenia

    [Ref: Harrison's 19th/e pg. 736]

29. **False statement regarding DIC is:** *(PGMEE 2014-15)*
    a. Thrombocytopenia   b. Decreased fibrinogen
    c. Decreased aPTT   d. Increased PT

    [Ref: Harrison's 18th ed. page- 979]

16.	d
17.	c
18.	a
19.	a
20.	a
21.	b,d
22.	d
23.	a
24.	a
25.	b
26.	d
27.	a
28.	c
29.	c

30. Disseminated intravascular coagulation can occur in all of the following EXCEPT: *(PGMEE 2014-15)*
a. Snake bite
b. Placenta praevia
c. Falciparum malaria
d. Haemophilia

[Ref: Harrison's 19th/e pg. 736]

31. Most common cause of DIC is: *(PGMEE 2014-15)*
a. Sepsis
b. Placenta previa
c. Abruption placentae
d. Snake bite

[Ref: Harrison's 19th/e pg. 736]

32. What is not associated with DIC *(PGMEE 2012-13)*
a. Increased FDP
b. Thrombocytopenia
c. Hyperfibrinogenemia
d. Increased PT

[Ref: Robbin's 8th/e p. 674]

33. Which one of the following is not used in DIC? *(PGMEE 2014-15)*

a. Heparin
b. Epsilon amino caproic acid
c. Blood transfusion
d. I.V. fluids

[Ref: Harrison's 19th/e pg. 736]

INHERITED DISORDERS OF BLEEDING

VON WILLEBRAND DISEASE (VWD)

34. The coagulation profile in a 13 year old girl with Menorrhagia having von Willebrand's disease is: *(PGMEE 2014-15)*
a. Isolated prolonged PTT with a normal PT
b. Isolated prolonged PT with a normal PTT
c. Prolongation of both PT and PTT
d. Prolongation of thrombin time

[Ref: Harrison's 19th/e pg. 732]

35. Bleeding time is increased in:- *(PGMEE 2018)*
a. Hemophilia A
b. Hemophilia B
c. Von Willebrand disease
d. Factor 13 deficiency

[Ref: Harrison 19/e, P. 862]

36. von Willebrand's disease is usually inherited as *(PGMEE 2014-15)*
a. Autosomal dominant
b. Autosomal recessive
c. X-linked recessive
d. Multicentric

[Ref: Hematology in clinical practice. 4th ed. ch. 31, Harrison's 19th/e pg. 731]

37. Most common inherited bleeding disorder: *(PGMEE 2014-15)*

a. Von willebrand's disease
b. Bernard soulier
c. Glanzmann thrombasthenia
d. ITP acute

[Ref: Harrison's 19th/e pg. 731]

38. Rarest type of Von Wille brand disease: *(PGMEE 2014-15)*

a. vWD type 1
b. vWD type 2A
c. vWD type 2N
d. vWD type 3

[Ref: Harrison's 19th p 732]

39. In Von Willebrand disease, there is: *(PGMEE 11)*
a. Factor VII deficiency
b. Factor VIII C deficiency
c. Factor X deficiency
d. vWF deficiency

[Ref: Robbin's 8th/e p. 670]

40. Bleeding time is prolonged in: *(PGMEE. 07)*
a. Von Willebrand's disease
b. Haemophilia
c. Polycythemia
d. Christmas disease

[Ref: Robbin's 8th/e p. 670-674]

41. A patient is having deficiency of Von Willebrand factor. What abnormalities he will present with? *(PGMEE. 09)*
a. Decreased PT, Increased PTT
b. Increased PTT, Increased PT
c. Normal PT, Normal PTT
d. Normal PTand Increased PTT

[Ref: Robbin's 8th/e p. 670]

HEMOPHILIAS

42. Hemophilia B is due to deficiency of: *(PGMEE 2012-13)*
a. Factor X
b. Factor VIII
c. Factor IX
d. Factor VII

[Ref: Robbin's 8th/e p. 672]

43. Not useful for treatment of hemophilia B?
a. FFP *(PGMEE 2014-15)*
b. Cryoprecipitate
c. Factor 9 concentrates
d. Prothrombin complex concentrates

[Ref: Harrison's 19th/e pg. 733, 450t]

44. Spontaneous bleeding is seen in? *(PGMEE 2009)*
a. Haemophilia
b. Scott's syndrome
c. Afibrinogeneima
d. Von willebrand's diseae

[Ref: Harrison 19th/e pg 733]

45. Feature of hemophilia *(PGMEE 2018)*
a. Epistaxis
b. Hemarthrosis
c. Hematmesis
d. Hemoptysis

46. X-linked inheritance is seen in all except: *(PGMEE 2018)*
a. Hemophilia A
b. Hemophilia B
c. Color blindness
d. Downs syndrome

47. In Hemophilia B what is most common cause of death?
a. Hemorrhage *(PGMEE 2014-15)*
b. HIV,HBV, HCV due to transfusions
c. Transfusion reactions
d. Deep vein thrombosis

[Ref: Harrison's 19th/e pg. 733]

48. Anti-factor VIII antibodies are seen in: *(PGMEE 2014-15)*

a. Postpartum
b. Hemophilia who have received infusion of plasmaconcentrates
c. Both A and B
d. None

[Ref: Hematology in clinical practice. 4th ed. ch. 32]

30.	d
31.	a
32.	c
33.	d
34.	a
35.	c
36.	a
37.	a
38.	d
39.	d
40.	a
41.	d
42.	c
43.	b
44.	a
45.	b
46.	d
47.	a
48.	c

49. Which factor deficiency is known as Hemophilia C?
(PGMEE 2013-14 & 2015-16)

a. 8
b. 10
c. 9
d. 11

[Ref: Ganong's 25th /e pg. 562]

50. The best screening test for hemophilia *(PGMEE. 11)*

a. BT
b. PT
c. PTT
d. PIT

[Ref: Robbin's 8th/e p. 672]

51. Bleeding time is increased in all EXCEPT:
(PGMEE 2014-15)

a. Thrombocytopenia
b. Thrombasthenia
c. Renal failure
d. Acquired hemophilia

[Ref: Harrison's 19th/e pg. 138e-3]

THROMBOTIC MICROANGIOPATHIES

HEMOLYTIC-UREMIC SYNDROME

52. Hemolytic uremic syndrome, false is- *(PGMEE 2014)*

a. Recurrences rare
b. Causes mild to severe coombs positive hemolytic anemia
c. Transient thrombocytopenia
d. Most commonly caused by E.Coli

[Ref: Robbin's 8th/e p. 953]

Explanation

- HUS is characterized by Microangiopathic hemolytic anemia (non immune/coombs - negative), Thrombocytopenia and Renal failure.
- HUS is the MCC of AKI in children.
- MCC of Typical HUS (Shiga like toxin-associated HUS): E coli 0157 : H7,
- MCC of typical HUS in Asia : S dysenteriae type 1.
- Lab:
  - Thrombocytopenia recovers within 2 weeks
  - PS - Schistocytes/Helmet cells
  - ADAMTS levels - Normal
- Rx
  - Typical HUS - Supportive
  - Atypical HUS - Plasma exchange

53. Most common cause of hemolytic uremic syndrome is-
(PGMEE 2012-13)

a. E. coli
b. Shigella
c. Psedononas
d. Salmonella

[Ref: Nelson 20th/e/p 2507]

54. In shigella dysentery associated hemolytic uremic syndrome, the FALSE statement is *(PGMEE 2012-13)*

a. Hepatic failure
b. Thrombotic angiopathy
c. Leucocytosis
d. Neurological abnormalities

[Ref: Nelson 20th/e/p 2508]

55. All are seen in HUS except- *(PGMEE 2015)*

a. Hemolytic anemia
b. Renal failure
c. Thrombocytopenia
d. Altered sensorium

[Ref: Harrison 18th/e p. 969, 970]

56. All of the following are associated with HUS EXCEPT:
(PGMEE 2014-15)

a. Purpura
b. Oliguria
c. Pain
d. Thrombocytopenia

[Ref: Harrison's 19th/e pg. 1863]

57. A young boy with skin rashes (Purpura), acute onset, oliguria, CNS manifestation after 5 days of diarrhea is suffering from: *(PGMEE 2014-15)*

a. D + HUS
b. D- HUS
c. Aplastic anemia
d. TTP

[Ref: Harrison's 19th/e pg. 377e-4]

Explanation

	MAHA	
	HUS	**TTP**
Age	Children	Adults
Renal failure	Common	Uncommon/mild
Neurolog symp.	Uncommon/mild	Common/severe
ADAM TS-13 activity	Normal	Deficient
Ass with Ecoli 0157:H7	Yes	Occasional
Fever	⊖	⊕
Thrombo cytopenia	+	+
Rx — Typical	Supportive	Plasma exchange
Rx — Atypical	Plasma exchange Eculizumab	

58. Which is not a feature of hemolytic-uremic syndrome:

a. Thrombocytosis *(PGMEE 2014-15)*
b. Uraemia
c. Hematuria
d. Segmented RBC's in peripheral smear

[Ref: Harrison's 19th/e pg. 1030]

59. Which of the following is not a feature of Hemolytic-Uremic syndrome? *(PGMEE 2014-15)*

a. Encephalopathy
b. Oliguria
c. Thrombocytopenia
d. Purpura

[Ref: Harrison's 19th/e pg. 1030]

60. Best treatment of atypical HUS is? *(PGMEE 2016)*

a. Plasmapheresis
b. Antibiotics
c. IvIG
d. Dialysis

[Ref: Robbins 9th/pg 941; Harrison 19th/pg 740-745]

61. Microangiopathic hemolytic anemia is seen in-
(PGMEE 2012-13)

a. TTP
b. Senile purpura
c. CML
d. ITP

[Ref: Robbin's 8th/e p. 654]

49.	d
50.	c
51.	d
52.	b
53.	a
54.	a
55.	d
56.	a
57.	d
58.	a
59.	d
60.	a
61.	a

62. All are features of haemolytic uremic syndrome, except-
   (PGMEE 2013-14)
   a. Anemia
   b. Renal microthrombi
   c. Hyperkalemia
   d. Neuro psychiatric disturbances

   [Ref: Robbins 9th/e pg. 659-661]

THROMBOTIC THROMBOCYTOPENIC PURPURA

63. All are true regarding Thrombotic Thrombocytopenia Purpura (TTP), except
   (PGMEE 2008)
   a. Complement levels are normal
   b. Microangiopathic hemolytic anemia
   c. Thrombocytopenia
   d. Thrombosis

   [Ref: Robbins 8th/e pg. 669]

64. All are true regarding Thrombotic Thrombocytopenia Purpura (TTP), except:
   (PGMEE 08)
   a. Normal levels of ADAMTS13
   b. Thrombosis
   c. Microangiopathic hemolytic anemia
   d. Thrombocytopenia

   [Ref: Robbins 9th/e pg. 660, Clinical hematology 4th/e p. 515]

65. All of the following statements about Thrombotic thrombocytopenic purpura (TTP) are true, Except:
   (PGMEE 2015)
   a. Microangiopathic Hemolytic Anemia
   b. Thrombocytopenia
   c. Normal complement levels
   d. Grossly abnormal coagulation tests

   [Ref: Harrison 18th/p 969]

62.	d
63.	a
64.	a
65.	c,d

ANEMIA

DIFFERENTIAL DIAGNOSIS OF ANEMIA

1. Plasma ferritin levels may be reduced in all of the following conditions, EXCEPT: *(PGMEE 2014-15)*
a. Iron deficiency
b. Vitamin C deficiency
c. Liver disease
d. Hypothyroidism

[Ref: Harrison's 18th /e p. 845, 846 table (103-2]

2. Anemia with reticulocytosis in serum:-
(PGMEE 2016-17)
a. Lead porsing
b. Thalassemia minor
c. Iron deficiency anemia
d. Autoimmune hemolytic anemia

[Ref: Ferri's Clinical Advisor 2015 E-Book: pg. 413]

3. 20-year-old female present with features of anemia. Blood tests: Hb-5g/dL, MCV – 52 fL, MCHC–20 g/dL, PCV – 32%. Diagnosis *(PGMEE 2015)*
a. Phenytoin toxicity
b. Fish tape worm infection
c. Hook worm infection
d. Blind loop syndrome

[Ref: Robbins 9th/pg 649]

4. Anemia with reticulocytosis is seen in *(PGMEE 2013)*
a. Hemorrhage
b. Aplastic anemia
c. Severe iron deficiency
d. Sever vitamin B12 deficiency

[Ref: Robbins 9th/e pg. 631]

5. Anemia with reticulocytosis is seen in?
(PGMEE 2013-14)
a. Hemolysis
b. Aplastic anemia
c. Iron deficiency anemia
d. Vitamin B_{12} deficiency

[Ref: Robbins 9th/e pg. 630-631]

6. What type of RBC seen in chronic renal failure?
(DNB Dec 07)
a. Macrocytic
b. Normocytic
c. Microcytic
d. None

[Ref: Harshmohan 18th/e p. 850]

7. A 20 year old female presenting with anemia, mild jaundice for 2 years, peripheral smear showing spherocytes, the best investigation to be done is:
(PGMEE 2014-15)
a. Reticulocyte count
b. Osmotic fragility test
c. Coomb's test
d. Bone marrow aspiration

[Ref: Harrison 19th p 658]

Explanation

■ Both HS & AIHA have spherocytes on PS. To differentiate both. So a coomb's test → (+ve in AIHA)

8. Reticulocytosis is seen in all EXCEPT: *(PGMEE 2014-15)*
a. P.N.H
b. Hemolysis
c. Nutritional anemia
d. Dyserythropoietic syndrome

[Ref: Harrison's 18th/pg. 449, 450, 452]

9. A patient with previously normal hemoglobin suffered a sudden massive acute hemorrhage. He is most likely to show all of the following EXCEPT *(PGMEE 2014-15)*
a. High reticulocyte count
b. High neutrophil count
c. High packed cell volume
d. Normal MCV

[Ref: Harrison's 18th/pg. 885, 886]

ANEMIA OF INFANCY

10. According to WHO cut off level for haemoglobin in child anemia is? *(PGMEE 2012)*
a. 10gm
b. 11 gm
c. 12 gm
d. 13 gm

[Ref: Wintrobe's hematology 12th/e volume 1 pg. 780]

11. Reticulocyte level in newborn is? *(PGMEE 2012)*
a. 0.2-1.5%
b. 1-1.6%
c. 2.5-6%
d. 6-10.2%

[Ref: Ghai 8th/e/ch 10]

12. Cut off value for anemia at 6 month and 6 year is-
(PGMEE 2014)
a. 10 gm/dl
b. 11 gm/dl
c. 12 gm/dl
d. 13 gm/dl of venous blood

[Ref: Ghai 8th/e/p 330]

13. True about 'Physiologic Anemia' of infant EXCEPT:
(PGMEE 2016-17)
a. Requires no treatment
b. Present for 6-8 weeks
c. Is more rapid and more severe in case of premature
d. Occurs due to less Iron content in breast milk

[Ref: Nelson 20th/e/ch 453]

14. Neonatal anemia is defined as hemoglobin-
(PGMEE 2016-17)
a. <13 g/dl
b. <12 g/dl
c. <11 g/dl
d. <10 g/dl

[Ref: Neslon 20th/e/ chapter 446]

15. Which of the following is not a cause of neonatal anemia?
(PGMEE 2015)
a. Diamond Blackfan syndeome
b. Subgaleal Hemorrhage
c. Wilson's Disease
d. Abruptio placentae

[Ref: Nelson 20th/e/ch 103]

1.	c
2.	d
3.	c
4.	a
5.	a
6.	b
7.	c
8.	c
9.	c
10.	b
11.	c
12.	b
13.	d
14.	a
15.	c

16. A 5 yr old child presents with pallor and constipation with Hb-6 gm%. Which is the most appropriate therapy? *(PGMEE 2015)*
   a. Packed cell RBC's
   b. Oral iron therapy
   c. Parenteral iron
   d. Hematologist referral

   [Ref: Robbins 9th/pg 649-652]

MICROCYTIC HYPOCHROMIC ANEMIA

17. Normal ferritin level in adult male *(PGMEE 2013)*
   a. 800 - 900 ng/ml
   b. 100 - 200 ng/ml
   c. 500 - 700 ng/ml
   d. 5 - 10 ng/ml

   [Ref: Internet]

18. Low serum iron and low serum ferritin is seen in: *(PGMEE 2015-16)*

   a. Iron deficiency anemia
   b. Chronic kidney disease
   c. Sideroblastic anemia
   d. Fanconi anemia

   [Ref: Chapter 104: Harrison 18th edition]

Explanation

Condition / Lab	IDA	Thalassemia	Sideroblastic anemia	AOCD
S. Iron (50-150 mg/dl)	↓	(N)	(N)	↓
TIBC (300-600 mg/dl)	↑	(N)	(N)	↓
% saturation (30-50%)	↓	N/↑	N/↑	↓
Ferritin (50-200 mg/L)	↓	↑	↑	N/↑
Free erythro-protoporphyrin	↑	(N)	↑	↑
RDW (N=<14)	↑	(N)	(N)	(N)

19. Hypochromic microcytic anemia is seen in all, EXCEPT: *(PGMEE 2014-15)*

   a. Thalassaemia
   b. Tropical Sprue
   c. Ancylostomiasis
   d. Chronic inflammatory disease

   [Ref: Harrison's 19th p 673]

Explanation

- Tropical sprue shows megaloblastic anemia

20. Hypochromic-microcytic anemia occurs in all EXCEPT: *(PGMEE 2014-15)*
   a. Iron deficiency
   b. Thalassaemia
   c. Lead poisoning
   d. Chronic renal failure

   [Ref: Harrison 19th p 393]

21. Which of the following is not expected in a case of micro-cytic hypochromic anemia? *(PGMEE 2015; 2009)*
   a. Reduced serum iron
   b. Reduced total RBC distribution width
   c. Normal ferritin levels
   d. Increased TIBC

   [Ref: Harrison 19th p 393]

22. Hemosiderosis is due to :- *(PGMEE 2016-17)*
   a. Abnormal copper metabolism
   b. Abnormal Iron metabolism
   c. Genetically determined disease
   d. Autoimmune disorder

   [Ref: Robbin's 9th/e pg. 65]

IRON-DEFICIENCY ANEMIA

23. First change of improvement noted after iron therapy is initiated- *(PGMEE 2012-13)*
   a. Reticulcytosis
   b. Decreased irritability
   c. Increase in serum iron levels
   d. Replenishment of iron stores

   [Ref: Ghai 8th/e/ch 10]

24. The earliest sign of iron deficiency anemia *(PGMEE 2012-13, , PGMEE 97)*
   a. Decrease in serum iron level
   b. Decrease in serum ferritin level
   c. Increase in iron binding capacity
   d. All the above

   [Ref: Chandrasoma Tayor 3rd/e p. 387; Harrison 18th/e p. 846, 847]

25. Peripheral smear is suggestive of which anemia:- *(PGMEE 2016-17)*

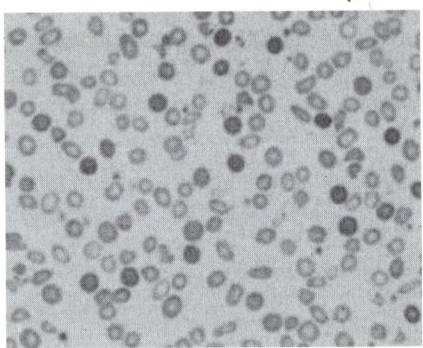

   a. Iron deficiency anemia
   b. Macrocytic anemia
   c. HUS
   d. Hereditary spherocytosis

   [Ref: Robbins 9th/e pg. 649-652]

26. Most sensitive indicator of iron deficiency anemia *(PGMEE 2015)*
   a. Packed cell volume
   b. Hemoglobin
   c. Serum ferritin
   d. Serum iron

   [Ref: Robbins 9th/e pg. 649-652]

16. b
17. b
18. a
19. b
20. d
21. b
22. b
23. b
24. b
25. a
26. c

27. Response to iron in iron deficiency anemia is assessed by- **(PGMEE 13, 14; DNB June 09)**
   a. Increase in iron binding capacity
   b. Reticulocytosis
   c. Increase in hemoglobin
   d. Restoration of enzymes

   [Ref: Robbins 9th/e pg. 649; Wintrab's clinical hematology 12th/e p. 829]

28. Iron deficiency causes: **(PGMEE 2013-14)**
   a. Microcytic hypochromic anemia
   b. Microcytic hyperchromic anemia
   c. Megaloblastic anemia
   d. Macrocytic hypochromic anemia

   [Ref: Robbins 9th/e pg. 649]

29. First sign of improvement in oral Iron therapy is? **(PGMEE 2012)**
   a. Reticulocytosis
   b. Raise in RBC count
   c. Raise of hemoglobin
   d. Increase in ESR

   [Ref: Harrison 18th/e Chapter 103]

30. Which among the following is true about Iron deficiency anemia?
   a. Increased ferritin
   b. Decreased TIBC
   c. Marrow is normoblastic
   d. Microcytic hypochromic anemia

   [Ref: Robbins 9th/e pg. 649]

31. All decrease in iron deficiency anemia except: **(NEET Pattern 2017)**
   a. Ferritin
   b. TIBC
   c. Iron
   d. Transferrin saturation

32. Which of the following is true of body iron stores? **(PGMEE 2012)**
   a. Absorption is increased in iron deficiency and reduced in iron overload
   b. Transferrin is used as a storage from in iron overload
   c. Hepcidin increases iron absorption in iron overload
   d. Normally iron iron is stored as hemosiderin

   [Ref: Robbins 9th/e pg. 649]

33. Normal transferrin is saturated with iron: **(PGMEE 2013-14)**
   a. 50 %
   b. 35 %
   c. 70 %
   d. 20 %

   [Ref: Robbins 9th/e pg. 649]

34. Iron requirement is determined from the equation: **(PGMEE 2014-15)**
   a. 2.3 x wt (kg) × Hb deficit (g/dl) + 500
   b. 3.3 x wt. (kg) × Rb deficit (g/dl) + 1000
   c. 4 x wt. (kg) × Hb deficit (g/dl) + 1000
   d. 4.3 x wt. (kg) × Hb deficit (g/dl) + 1500

   [Ref: Harrison 19th p 628]

35. Calculate iron deficit for a 50 kg person, with Hb-5g/dL. Add 1000 mg for stores. **(PGMEE 2015)**
   a. 2150 mg
   b. 1650 mg
   c. 1150 mg
   d. 1575 mg

   [Ref: Wintrobes 12ed/814]

Explanation

■ Amount of iron needed by an individual patient for parenteral therapy: 2.3 x Body weight x [15 - Patients Hb] + 500/1000 mg

36. Oral iron supplements used for iron deficiency anemia: **(PGMEE 2014-15)**
   a. Tolerable dose will deliver 40 to 60 mg of iron per day
   b. Mass of total salt is important in determining daily dose
   c. Treatment should be stopped as soon as normal hemoglobin level is reached
   d. Desired rate of hemoglobin improvement is 0.5 mg per day

   [Ref: Katzung 10th/530; KDT 6th/585-86, Harrison 19th p 398]

37. All the following are suggestive of iron-deficiency anemia EXCEPT: **(PGMEE 2014-15)**
   a. Koilonychia
   b. Pica
   c. Decreased serum ferritin
   d. Decreased total iron-binding capacity (TIBC)

   [Ref: arrison 19th p 627]

38. Earliest to improve after oral iron therapy- **(PGMEE 2015)**
   a. TIBC
   b. Reticulocyte
   c. Serum ferritin
   d. S. Transferrin

   [Ref: Harrison 19th p 627]

39. The most suitable test to assess iron stores is- **(PGMEE 2015)**
   a. Serum iron
   b. Serum ferritin
   c. Transferrin saturation
   d. TIBC

   [Ref: Harrison 18th/e p. 847]

40. Iron is mainly absorbed in the: **(PGMEE 2014-15)**
   a. Stomach
   b. Duodenum
   c. Jejunum
   d. Ileum

   [Ref: Harrison 19th p 643]

41. All of the following are characteristic features of treatment of iron deficiency anemia with oral iron supplements, EXCEPT: **(PGMEE 2014-15)**
   a. Bioavailability is enhanced with vitamin C
   b. The proportion of iron absorbed reduces as hemoglobin improves
   c. The reticulocyte count should begin to increase in two weeks and peak in 4 weeks—this suggests good response to treatment
   d. The treatment should be discontinued immediately once hemoglobin normalizes to prevent side effects of iron.

   [Ref: Harrison 19th p 628]

ANEMIA OF CHRONIC DISEASE

42. Anemia of chronic disease is due to **(PGMEE 2012-13)**
   a. Chronic blood loss
   b. Folate deficiency
   c. Decreased utilization of stored iron
   d. Vit B_{12} deficiency

   [Ref: Robbin's 8th/e p. 662, Harrison 18th/e p. 849, 850]

27.	b
28.	a
29.	a
30.	d
31.	b
32.	a
33.	b
34.	a
35.	a
36.	a
37.	d
38.	b
39.	b
40.	b
41.	d
42.	c

43. Decrease in serum iron, decrease in TIBC is seen in
(PGMEE 2012-13)

a. Sideroblastic anemia
b. Iron deficiency anemia
c. Anemia of chronic disease
d. Thallasemia

[Ref: Harrison's 18th /e pg. 849, 850 Robbins 9th/e pg 649]

44. Seen in chronic inflammatory anemia is:
(PGMEE 2014-15)

a. Serum iron↓ S. ferritin ↑ and transferrin ↓
b. Serum iron↑ S. ferritin ↑ and transferrin ↑
c. Serum iron↓ S. ferritin ↓ and transferrin ↓
d. Serum iron↑ S. ferritin ↓ and transferrin ↑

[Ref: Harrison's 18th /e pg. 849, 850 Robbins 9th/e pg 649]

45. A young female has the following lab values: Hemoglobin= 9.8 gm%, MCV = 70 serum iron = 30, serum ferritin = 100, the diagnosis is: *(PGMEE 2014-15)*

a. Thalassemia trait
b. Chronic iron deficiency anemia
c. Megaloblastic anemia
d. Anaemia of chronic infection

[Ref: Harrison's 19th/e pg. 637]

46. Epogen can be given in? *(DNB June 2010)*

a. Hemolytic anemia
b. Aplastic anemia
c. Anemia of chronic Renal disease
d. Anemia of chronic disease

[Ref: Goodman and Gilman's 11th/e pg.929]

43.	c
44.	a
45.	d
46.	c
47.	b
48.	c
49.	a>b
50.	c
51.	d
52.	b
53.	d
54.	d
55.	a
56.	c
57.	d

Explanation

▪ Epogen is recombinant human erythropoietin indicated for treatment of anemia associated with CKD and chemotherapy.

47. Anemia of chronic disease is associated with:
(PGMEE 2014-15)

a. Increased Fe, decreased Transferrin, increased Ferritin
b. Decreased Fe, decreased Transferrin, increased Ferritin
c. Decreased Fe, increased Transferrin, decreased Ferritin
d. Increased Fe, increased Transferrin, decreased Ferritin

[Ref: Harrison 19th p 393]

48. Iron deficiency anemia and anemia of chronic disease can be differentiated by the following parameter

a. Microcytic, hypochromic anemia *(PGMEE 2015)*
b. Serum iron
c. TIBC
d. Transferrin saturation

[Ref: Robbins 9th/pg 649]

49. Most important inflammatory mediator, involved in anemia of chronic disease? *(PGMEE 2015)*

a. IL-1
b. IL-6
c. TNFa
d. IFN-Y

[Ref: Wintrobes 13th ed/pg 1223]

Explanation

▪ IL-1 directly suppresses EPO production in response to anemia.

SIDEROBLASTIC ANEMIA

50. Sideroblastic anemia is seen in chronic poisoning of-
(DNB 2007, June 09)

a. Mercury
b. Copper
c. Lead
d. Arsenic

[Ref: Harshmohan 4th/e p. 345]

51. Which does not cause sideroblastic anemia-
(PGMEE 2013-14)

a. Chloramphenicol
b. Myelodysplastic anemia
c. INH
d. Mercury

[Ref: Harshmohan 4th/e p. 345]

52. Sideroblastic anemia is caused by all of the following except- *(PGMEE 2012-13)*

a. Lead poisoning
b. Iron deficit
c. Porphyria cutenea tarda
d. Collegen vascular disease

[Ref: Harsh Mohan 4th/e p. 345]

53. Lead causes following except- *(PGMEE 2012-13)*

a. Basophilic stippling
b. Uroporphyrinuria
c. Sideroblastic anemia
d. Macrocytic anemia

MACROCYTIC ANEMIA

54. Macrocytic anemia is seen in all except:
(DNB June 2010)

a. Vitamin B12 deficiency
b. Liver disease
c. Hypothyroidism
d. Anemia of chronic diseases

[Ref: Robbins 9th/e pg. 645]

55. In cobalamin deficiency which is not seen?
(PGMEE 2015-16)

a. Microcytic anemia
b. Long tract signs
c. Loss of proprioception
d. Rhomberg Sign

[Ref: Harrison 19th ed. / 640, 645]

56. Hypersegmented neutrophils are seen in
(PGMEE 2012-13)

a. Hemolytic anemia
b. Microcytic hypochronic anemia
c. Megaloblastic anemia
d. Sideroblastic anemia

[Ref: Robbins 9th/e pg. 645]

57. Macrocytosis of RBC's seen in? *(PGMEE 2012)*

a. Alcoholism
b. Phenytoin
c. Folate deficiency
d. All of the above

[Ref: Wintrobe's haematology 11th/e p. 77; Robbins 9th/e pg. 649]

58. Deficiency of the 'intrinsic factor of Castle' cause-
(PGMEE 2012-13)
a. Cooley's anemia
b. Pernicious anemia
c. Aplastic anemia
d. Megaoblastic anemia

[Ref: Robbins 9th/e pg. 647]

59. All of the following are true regarding B12 deficiency, EXCEPT: *(PGMEE 2014-15)*
a. Pernicious anemia
b. Sub-acute combined degeneration of cord
c. Carpal tunnel syndrome
d. Infertility

[Ref: Harrison 19th p 643]

60. Macrocytic anemia occurs in: *(PGMEE 2014-15)*
a. Hypothyroidism
b. CRF
c. Anemia of chronic disease
d. Vitamin-C deficiency

[Ref: Harrison's 19th p 643]

61. Which of the following types of anemia is associated with a Raised MCV and Normal MCHC?
(PGMEE 2014-15)
a. Sideroblastic anemia
b. Vitamin B12 and Folic acid deficiency
c. Beta thalassemia
d. Iron deficiency anemia

[Ref: Hematology in clinical practice. 4th ed. ch. 8, Harrison 19th p 643]

62. Megalocytic anaemia is caused by all, EXCEPT:
(PGMEE 2014-15)
a. Goat milk ingestion
b. Type A gastritis
c. Antimetabolites
d. Lead poisoning

[Ref: Harrison 19th p 643]

63. Pernicious anemia is associated with all of the following, EXCEPT: *(PGMEE 2014-15)*
a. Macrocythaemia
b. Vitamin B12 deficiency
c. Weakness, numbness and tingling of extremities
d. Increased reticulocyte count

[Ref: Harrison 19th p 2346 t]

64. In the treatment of megaloblastic anemia, vitamin B12 and folic acid should be given together because:
(PGMEE 2014-15)
a. Vitamin B12 acts as a cofactor for dihydrofolate reductase;
b. Folic acid alone causes improvement of anemic symptoms but neurological dysfunction continues.
c. Vitamin B12 deficiency may result in methylfolate trap
d. Folic acid is required for conversion of methy-malonyl-CoA to succinyl Co-A.

[Ref: Katzung 10th/532; KDT 6th /591]

65. A 40-year-old female presents with signs of heart failure. Hb-6 g/dL, MCV-112. Next step *(PGMEE 2015)*
a. Check B12 and folate levels
b. Blood transfusion
c. Start iron tablets
d. Start folate supplementation

[Ref: Robbins 9th/pg 645]

66. MCV is increased in the following anemia *(PGMEE 2015)*
a. Iron deficiency anemia
b. Sideroblastic anemia
c. Anemia of chronic disease
d. Folate deficiency anemia

[Ref: Robbins 9th/pg 645]

67. Find the false statement regarding megaloblastic anemia *(PGMEE 2015)*
a. Hypersegmented neutrophils are the earliest manifestation
b. Reticulocyte count decreased
c. Hypercellular bone marrow
d. MCHC is increased

[Ref: a 9th/pg 645; 8th/pg 654]

68. Macrocytic anemia with MCV> 110fL is seen in all except *(PGMEE 2015)*
a. Thiamine deficiency
b. B12 deficiency
c. Hypothyroidism
d. Phenytoin tocixity

[Ref: Robbins 9th/pg 645]

HEMOLYTIC ANEMIA

69. All of the following are true about Congenital Haemolytic anemia, EXCEPT: *(PGMEE 2014-15)*
a. Increased fragility
b. Splenomegaly
c. Splenectomy is useful
d. Positive direct Coomb's test

[Ref: Harrison's 18th ed. ch. 106]

Explanation

Congenital (Hereditary) Hemolytic anemia/Intrinsic cause of hemolytic anemia or Intracerpuscular cause		
Defect of RBC Membrane	**Enzyme defect**	**Hemoglobinopathies**
▪ Hereditary spherocytosis ▪ Herediatry elliptocytosis	▪ G6PD deficiency ▪ Pyncoate kinase def.	▪ Sickle cell anemia ▪ Thalassemia

70. Which of the following condition has hemolysis due to intrinsic defect *(PGMEE 2019)*
a. PNH
b. Splenomegaly
c. Transfusion related
d. G6PD deficiency

71. A patient presented with splenomegaly, anemia and shows reticulocytosis and increased bone narrow cellularity. The diagnosis is: *(PGMEE 2014-15)*
a. Pernicious anemia
b. Hemolytic anemia
c. Myelofibrosis
d. Hairy cell leukemia

[Ref: Harrison 19th p 658]

72. Hemolytic anemia are associated with all of the following, EXCEPT: *(PGMEE 2014-15)*
a. Increased indirect bilirubin in the serum
b. Decreased red cell survival
c. Increased number of reticulocytes
d. Increased fecal Urobilinogen

[Ref: Harrison 19th p 658/1649]

58.	b
59.	c
60.	a
61.	b
62.	d
63.	d
64.	b
65.	a
66.	d
67.	d
68.	a
69.	d
70.	a,d
71.	b
72.	d

73. Reticulocyte index in Hemolytic jaundice is greater than? *(PGMEE 2014-15)*

a. 0.5%
b. 1%
c. 1.5%
d. 2.5%

[Ref: Harrison's 18th ed. ch. 57]

74. When osmotic fragility is normal, RBC's begin to hemolyse when suspended in saline: *(PGMEE 2015, DNB 99)*

a. 0.33 %
b. 0.48 %
c. 0.9 %
d. 1.2 %

[Ref: Dacie 11th/pg 246]

75. Features of hemolytic anemia are all except? *(PGMEE 2015)*

a. Hemoglobinemia
b. Bilirubinemia
c. Reticulocytosis
d. Haptoglobin increased

[Ref: 9th/pg 631-632]

76. A baby born to mother who is O-ve has blood group B+ve. He developed jaundice on day 1, Peripheral blood smear is given, which cell is absent? *(PGMEE 2015)*

a. Sickle cell
b. Aniocytosis
c. Spherocytes
d. Schistocytes

[Ref: Robbins 9th/pg 635; 8th/pg 645]

77. All are features of hemolytic anemia, except: *(DNB June 08)*

a. Hemosiderinuria
b. Jaundice
c. Hemoglobinuria
d. Increased haptoglobulin

[Ref: Robbins 9th/e pg. 631]

78. Low serum haptoglobin in hemolysis is masked by: *(DNB June 10)*

a. Liver disease
b. Malnutrition
c. Pregnancy
d. Bile duct obstruction

[Ref: A manual of laboratory diagnostic test frances Fischback 7th/e p. 114, 115]

Explanation

- Haptoglobin levels are increased obstructive biliary disease

79. Intrinsic causes of hemolytic anemia are all except- *(PGMEE 2013-14)*

a. Hyperspleenism
b. Pyruvate kinase deficiency
c. G6PD deficiency
d. Hereditary spherocytosis

[Ref: Robbins 9th/e pg. 630-631]

80. Intracorpuscular hemolytic anemia is seen in: *(PGMEE 2013-14)*

a. TTP
b. Infection
c. Thalassemia
d. Autoimmune hemolytic anemia

[Ref: Robbins 9th/e pg. 630-631]

AUTOIMMUNE HEMOLYTIC ANEMIA

81. Which of the following statements about paroxysmal cold hemoglobinuria is NOT true? *(PGMEE 2014-15)*

a. Chronic autoimmune form responds well to splenectomy
b. Results from formation of Donath-Landsteiner antibody
c. Attacks are associated with hemoglobinuria
d. Can occur secondary to syphilis

[Ref: Harrison 19th p 662]

82. Direct coomb's test is positive in hemolytic anemia due to *(PGMEE 2015)*

a. Paraxysmal cold hemoglobinuria
b. Paroxysmal nocturnal hemoglobinuria
c. Idiopathic thrombocytopenic purpura
d. Hemolytic uremic syndrome

[Ref: Robbins 9th/pg 643]

83. Cold agglutinin is *(PGMEE 2012-13)*

a. IgA
b. IgM
c. IgD
d. IgG

[Ref: Robbin's 8th/e p. 654]

84. Donath landsteiner antibody is seen in- *(PGMEE 2013-14)*

a. Waldenstrom's macroglobulinemia
b. Malaria
c. Paroxysmal cold hemoglobinuria
d. PNH

[Ref: Robbin's 8th/e p. 637]

85. Test done in Autoimmune hemolytic anemia? *(PGMEE 2016)*

a. HPLC
b. Coombs test
c. Sickling test
d. Osmotic Fragility test

[Ref: 9th/pg 643-644]

86. Coombs negative hemolytic anemia is seen in: *(PGMEE 2014-15)*

a. Microangiopathic hemolytic anemia
b. SLE
c. CLL
d. Rh incompatibility

[Ref: Harrison's 19th/e pg. 658]

87. Coomb's positive hemolytic anemia associated with: *(PGMEE 2014-15)*

a. TTP
b. PAN
c. SLE
d. HUS

[Ref: API, 18th/ed. 810, Harrison's 19th/e pg. 658/138e-4]

88. Microspherocytosis in peripheral blood smear are seen in- *(DNB Dec 07)*

a. Autoimmune acquired haemolytic anaemia
b. Thalassemia
c. Sicke cell anemia
d. All of the above

[Ref: De Gruchy's 5th/e p. 184]

73.	d
74.	b
75.	d
76.	a
77.	d
78.	d
79.	a
80.	c
81.	a
82.	a
83.	b
84.	c
85.	b
86.	a
87.	c
88.	a

89. **Warm-antibody immune-hemolytic anemia is seen in all EXCEPT:** *(PGMEE 2014-15)*
   a. SLE
   b. α - Methyldopa ingestion
   c. Quinidine
   d. Infectious mononucleosis

[Ref: Harrison 19th p 658]

90. **Warm Antibodies are?** *(PGMEE 2016)*
   a. Complete Antibody
   b. Incomplete Antibody
   c. Heterophillic antibody
   d. IgM

[Ref: Wintrobes 12th/ed pg 959]

91. **A 25-year-old patient presents with the history of dyspnea on exertion for 3 weeks. Investigations revealed Hb–7g/dl, reticulocyte count 18% and positive coomb's test. Diagnosis** *(PGMEE 2015)*
   a. Autoimmune hemolytic anemia
   b. Paroxysmal nocturnal hemoglobimuria
   c. Sickle cell anemia
   d. Hereditary spherocytosis

[Ref: Robbins 9th/e pg. 643]

92. **Direct coombs test is positive in** *(PGMEE 2016)*
   a. Iron deficiency anaemia   b. PCH
   c. G6PD deficiency   d. PNH

[Ref: Robbins 9th/pg 643]

93. **Direct Coomb's test detects the presence of antibodies on the surface of erythrocytes by using:** *(PGMEE 2014-15)*
   a. Sensitization of red cells with the antibody globulin
   b. Anti-human globulin antiserum
   c. Incomplete antibody
   d. Non-agglutinating antibody

[Ref: Harrison 19th p 138e-4, 138e-4f]

PAROXYSMAL NOCTURNAL HEMOGLOBINURIA

94. **Which is not a feature of paroxysmal nocturnal hemoglobinuria-** *(PGMEE 2013-14)*
   a. Increased LAP score
   b. Hemolysis
   c. Thrombosis
   d. Thrombocytopenia

[Ref: Harrison 18th/e 883, 884; Robbin's 8th/e p. 652-653]

95. **Paroxymal noctural hemoglobinuria is due to-** *(PGMEE 2012-13)*
   a. Acquired red cell defect
   b. Lead poisoning
   c. Congential red cell defect
   d. Auto immune defect

[Ref: Robbin's 8th/e p. 652; Harrison 18th/e p. 883]

96. **Ham test is done for** *(PGMEE 2012-13)*
   a. PNH   b. Sickle cell anemia
   c. Thalassemia   d. Megaloblastic anemia

[Ref: Harrison 18th/e p. 883, 884]

97. **Not used in the treatment of PNH** *(PGMEE 2015)*
   a. Cyclosporine
   b. Eculizumab
   c. Bone marrow transplantation
   d. Leucocyte depleted blood transfusion

[Ref: Wintrobes pg 1011]

98. **All are true about paroxysmal nocturnal hemoglobinuria except** *(PGMEE 2015)*
   a. Intravascular hemolysis
   b. Deficiency of CD55 and CD59
   c. Elevated LAP score
   d. Hyperplastic bone marrow

[Ref: Robbins 9th/pg 642]

99. **P.N.H is associated with all of the following condition, EXCEPT:** *(PGMEE 2014-15)*
   a. Aplastic anemia   b. Increased LAP scores
   c. Venous thrombosis   d. Iron deficiency anemia

[Ref: Harrison 19th p 662]

100. **The gold standard test for the diagnosis of Paroxysmal Nocturnal Hemoglobinuria (PNH) is:-** *(PGMEE 2015-16)*
   a. HAM test   b. Genetic testing
   c. Flow cytometry   d. Sucrose hemolysis test

[Ref: Harrison's 18th/e pg. 884]

101. **Paroxysmal Nocturnal hemoglobinuria is due to a mutation in:** *(PGMEE 2015)*
   a. Phosphatidyl inositol group A gene
   b. CD 55 gene
   c. CD 59 gene
   d. C8 binding protein

[Ref: Robbins 9th/pg 642]

102. **CD 59 is deficient in** *(PGMEE 2018)*
   a. Paroxysmal nocturnal hemoglobinuria
   b. Chédiak-Higashi syndrome
   c. Chronic granulomatous disease
   d. Wiscott Aldrich syndrome

Explanation

- Chediak-Higashi syndrome
  ○ AR disorder due to defect in LYST gene.
  ○ Patient presents with hypopigmentation of skin, eyes and hair & are predisposed to recurrent infections.
- Chronic granulomatous disease
  ○ Inherited as an XLR
  ○ Characterized by defective NADPH oxidase activity
  ○ Patients are susceptible to severe and recurrent infections due to catalase positive organism
  ○ Catalase negative bacteria can be efficiently killed
- Wiskott Aldrich syndrome: it is an XLR disorder characterized by:
  ○ Eczema
  ○ Thrombocytopenia (the platelets are small and do not function properly)
  ○ Immunodeficiency

89.	d
90.	b
91.	a
92.	b
93.	b
94.	a
95.	a
96.	a
97.	a
98.	c
99.	b
100.	c
101.	a
102.	a

HEREDITARY SPHEROCYTOSIS

103. Most common cause of hereditary spherocytos is mutations in which gene (Most common membrane defect in hereditary spherocytosis)*(PGMEE 2016; 2011)*
  a. Spectrin
  b. Glycophorin
  c. Ankyrin
  d. Band 4

  [Ref: Robbins 9th/e pg. 633]

104. Mutation in which of the following gene correlates with the severity of anemia in hereditary spherocytosis
  (PGMEE 2016-17)
  a. Alpha spectrin
  b. Ankyrin
  c. Band 4.2
  d. Glycophorin A

  [Ref: Robbins 9th/pg 632]

105. Shape of RBC is biconcave due to?   *(DNB Dec. 09)*
  a. Band protein
  b. Spectrin
  c. Ankyrin
  d. Glycophorin- C

  [Ref: Elemental molecuar pathology 2nd/e p. 157]

106. Incorrect about osmotic fragility test is:
  (PGMEE 2014-15)
  a. Increased in hereditary spherocytosis
  b. Decreased in thalassemia
  c. Hemolysis on exposure to hypertonic saline enviornment
  d. Osmotic fragility decreased in iron deficiency

  [Ref: Harrison 19th /e pg. 651]

107. Spherocytosis is associated commonly with:
  (PGMEE 2014-15)
  a. Hypernatraemia
  b. Hyperkalaemia
  c. Hyponatraemia
  d. Hypokalaemia

  [Ref: Harrison 19th p 281, 81e-3f]

108. Not true about hereditary spherocytosis-
  (PGMEE 2013-14)
  a. Decreased MCV
  b. Reticulocytosis
  c. Decreased MCHC
  d. Defect in ankyrin

  [Ref: Robbins 9th/e pg. 632]

109. A 21-year-old male presents with complaints of fatigue and abdominal pain since birth. O/E jaundice and splenomegaly present. On USG gall stones are seen. What is your diagnosis?   *(PGMEE 2015)*
  a. Hereditary spherocytosis
  b. Cholangitis
  c. Sickle cell anemia
  d. Acute pancreatitis

  [Ref: Robbins 9th/e pg. 633]

110. Osmotic fragility is increased in-   *(PGMEE 2012-13)*
  a. Thalassemia
  b. Chronic lead poisoning
  c. Hereditary spherocytosis
  d. Sickle cell anemia

  [Ref: Robbins 9th/e pg. 633]

111. Hemolytic crisis in hereditary spherocytosis is precipitated by   *(PGMEE 2015)*
  a. Parvovirus B19 infection
  b. Infectious mononucleosis
  c. Human T-cell leukemia virus
  d. Cytomegalo virus

  [Ref: Harrison 18th/pg 1478]

G-6-PD DEFICIENCY

112. All are true about G-6-PD EXCEPT: *(PGMEE 2014-15)*
  a. Bite cells
  b. Intravascular hemolysis
  c. Favism
  d. Confers protection against plasmodium vivax

  [Ref: Harrison 19th p 656]

Explanation
- G-6-PD deficiency:
  - MC enzymatic disorder of RBC
  - Inheritance : X-linked
  - G6PD is an enzyme involved in Pentose phosphate pathway
  - Deficiency of this enzyme l/t free radical mediated oxidative damage to RBC → Produce Hemolysis
  - CF:-
    - Usually asymptomatic
    - Neonatal jaundice & Kernicterus
  - Triggers:
    - Fava beans (Broad beans)
    - Infections
    - Drugs - Primaquine, Chloroquine, Dapsone, Quinine Sulpha drugs, Acetyl salicylic acid
  - PS : Bite cells/Bliste cells, Heinz bodies.
  - G6PD confer protection aganist Plasmodium falciparum

113. Regarding G-6-PD deficiency, which of the following is FALSE:-   *(PGMEE 2015-16)*
  a. Associated with neonatal jaundice
  b. X-linked recessive disorder that does not affect heterozygous females
  c. Affects the pentose phosphate pathway
  d. Acute hemolysis can be precipitated by broad beans

114. In G6PD deficiency which cells are more prone for hemolysis   *(PGMEE 2015)*
  a. Older red cells
  b. Reticulocytes
  c. Young red cells
  d. All are susceptible

  [Ref: Robbins 9th/pg 634]

115. Drug that is safe in G6PD deficiency   *(PGMEE 2015)*
  a. Primaquine
  b. Acetanilid
  c. Quinidine
  d. Dapsone

  [Ref: 9th/pg 634-635]

116. Individuals having G6PD deficiency can be poisoned by
  (PGMEE 2015)
  a. Fava beans
  b. Soya beans
  c. Kesari dhal
  d. Maize

  [Ref: Robbins 9th/pg 634]

117. The most common trigger for hemolysis in G6PD deficiency is: *(PGMEE 2015)*
  a. Oxidant drugs
  b. Fava beans
  c. Infections
  d. Surgery

  [Ref: Robbins 9th/pg 634]

103.	c
104.	a
105.	b
106.	c
107.	b
108.	c
109.	a
110.	c
111.	a
112.	d
113.	None
114.	a
115.	c
116.	a
117.	c

118. Drug causing maximum hemolysis in G6PD deficiency is?
(PGMEE 2016)

a. Primaquine
b. Chloroquine
c. Ciprofloxacin
d. Gatifloxacin

[Ref: Robbins 9th/pg 634]

HEMOGLOBINOPATHIES

HEMOGLOBIN VARIANTS

119. Bart hemoglobin is tetramer of **(PGMEE 2015)**
a. β chain
b. α chain
c. γ chain
d. δ chain

[Ref: Robbins 9th/pg 638]

120. Hemoglobin H disease is caused by deletion
(PGMEE 2015)

a. Two α globin chains
b. Single α globin chain
c. Three α globin chains
d. All α globin chain

[Ref: 9th/pg 638; 8th/pg 648]

121. In HbM the position of point mutation **(PGMEE 2015)**
a. β chain, 87th codon, Histidine → Tyrosine
b. α chain, 87th codon, Histidine → Tyrosine
c. β chain, 6th codon, Glutamine → Valine
d. β chain, 6th codon, Glutamine → Lysine

[Ref: Wintrobes 12th ed 1060-1070]

122. HbA2 is- **(PGMEE 2012-13)**
a. Beta 2 Gamma 2
b. Alpha 2 Beta 2
c. Alpha 2 Gamma 2
d. Alpha 2 Delta 2

[Ref: Robbin's 8th/e p. 645-648]

123. Hemoglobin with zeta 2 and gamma 2 chains are seen in which of the following- **(PGMEE 15)**
a. Gower II
b. Fetal Hb
c. Portland
d. Gower I

[Ref: Harrison 19th/e p. 632]

124. Fetal hemoglobin achieves adult values by
(PGMEE 2014-15)

a. 6 months of age
b. 12 months of age
c. 24 months of age
d. 36 months of age

[Ref: Wintrobe Hematology 11th ed. pg. 442]

125. 60 year old person presents with history of angina and shortness of breath for the past week. Blood withdrawn shows thick brownish red color. Diagnosis?
(PGMEE 2015-16)

a. Sickle cell anemia
b. Hemolytic anemia
c. Meth-hemoglobinaemia
d. G-6-P-deficiency

[Ref: Harrison 19th ed. / 636]

126. All of the following are true regarding methemoglobinemia except :- **(PGMEE 2016-17)**
a. Caused by nitrites
b. Precipitated by anaesthetic agents like prilocaine and Benzocaine
c. Pulse oxymeter saturation is always >90%
d. IV Methylene blue is used in treatment

[Ref: Harrison 19th ed. / 636]

SICKLE CELL ANAEMIA

127. Gamma Gandy bodies contains hemosiderin and-
a. Na⁺
b. Cl⁻ **(DNB June 08)**
d. Mg⁺⁺
d. Ca⁺

[Ref: Robbins 9th/e pg. 639]

128. All are seen in sickle cell anemia except: **(DNB Jun. 11)**
a. Jaundice
b. Target cells
c. Reticulocytosis
d. High hematocrit

[Ref: Robbins 9th/e pg. 637]

129. In sickle cell anemia all are true except:
(PGMEE 2013-14)

a. Howell jolly bodies
b. Sickle cell
c. Target cells
d. Ringed sideroblast

[Ref: Harrison 18th/e p. 855; Robbin's 8th/e p. 6]

130. The primary defect which leads to sickle cell anemia is-
(PGMEE 2012-13, 03)

a. A nonsence mutation in the β chain of Hb A
b. Replacement of glutamate by valine in β chain of Hb A
c. Substitution of valine by glutamate in the α chain of Hb A
d. An abnormality in porphyrin part of hemoglobin

[Ref: Robbins 9th/e pg. 635]

131. Sickle cell anemia is usually associated with all, EXCEPT:
(PGMEE 2014-15)

a. Shortened RBC life span
b. Normal reticulocyte count
c. Abnormality in Hemoglobin
d. Nove of the above

[Ref: Harrison's 19th p 635]

132. Decreased ESR is seen in **(PGMEE 2016)**
a. Sickle cell Anemia
b. Hypoviscosity
c. Anemia
d. Increased fibrinogen

[Ref: Harrison's 19th p 635]

133. Mutation seen in sickle cell disease: **(PGMEE 2012-13)**
a. Point mutation
b. Frame shift mutation
c. Nonsence mutation
d. Select mutation

[Ref: Robbins 9th/e pg. 635]

134. In sickle cell anaemia defect lies in which chain:
(DNB June 09)

a. α-chain
b. β-chain
c. Both the chains
d. Gamma chain

[Ref: Robbins 9th/e pg. 635]

135. Best treatement for Sickle cell anemia is?
(PGMEE 2016)

a. Hydroxyurea
b. Blood transfusion
c. Iron Injection
d. Sulphonamide

[Ref: 9th/pg 638-642]

136. Mutation in sickle cells disease is an example of
(PGMEE 2015)

a. Frameshift mutation
b. Missense mutation
c. Nonsense mutation
d. Silence mutation

[Ref: 9th/pg 635]

118.	a
119.	c
120.	c
121.	b
122.	d
123.	c
124.	a
125.	c
126.	c
127.	c
128.	d
129.	d
130.	b
131.	b
132.	a
133.	a
134.	b
135.	a
136.	b

137. Beta globin mis-sence gene mutation seen in?
(PGMEE 2016)
- a. HbH
- b. Sickle cell anemia
- c. BART
- d. Thalassemia

[Ref: 9th/pg 635]

138. Mutation in Sickle cell anemia is? *(PGMEE 2016)*
- a. Frameshift
- b. Non sense mutation
- c. Non conservative missence
- d. Complete

[Ref: 9th/pg 635]

139. All the following features precipitate sickling of HBS except *(PGMEE 2015)*
- a. Dehydration
- b. Hypoxia
- c. Infections
- d. Alkalosis

[Ref: Robbins 9th/pg 635]

140. Sickle cell disease is less severe in *(PGMEE 2015)*
- a. Thalassemia
- b. Females
- c. HbSC
- d. All the above

[Ref: Robbins 9th/pg 635]

141. A young adult presents with history of bone pains, recurrent chest infections and dyspnea. Peripheral blood smear given. What is you diagnosis? *(PGMEE 2015)*

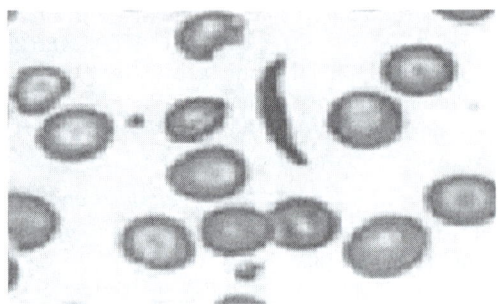

- a. Thalassemia
- b. Megaloblastic anemia
- c. Sickle cell anemia
- d. Hereditary spherocytosis

[Ref: Robbins 9th/pg 635]

137.	b
138.	c
139.	d
140.	d
141.	c
142.	c
143.	c
144.	a
145.	c
146.	a
147.	a

Explanation

- **Dactylitis**, often referred to as **hand-foot syndrome**, is often the first manifestation of pain in children with sickle cell anemia, occurring in 50% of children by their 2nd year. Need hydration and treatment with pain killers.
- Other important points about SCA:
  - Infants with sickle cell anemia have abnormal immune function and, as early as 6 mo of age, may have functional asplenia. Bacterial sepsis is one of the greatest causes for morbidity and mortality in this patient population. By 5 yr of age, most children with sickle cell anemia have functional asplenia. Regardless of age, all patients with sickle cell anemia are at increased risk of infection and death from bacterial infection, particularly encapsulated organisms such as *Streptococcus pneumoniae* and *Haemophilus influenzae* type b.

- Children with sickle cell anemia should receive prophylactic oral penicillin V until at least 5 yr of age.
- Acute infection with parvovirus B19 is associated with red cell aplasia (aplastic crisis), fever, pain, splenic sequestration, acute chest syndrome (ACS), **glomerulonephritis,** and strokes.
  - ▪ Salmonella causes osteomyelitis
  - **Acute splenic sequestration** is a life-threatening complication occurring primarily in infants and can occur as early as 5 wk of age.
  - Hydroxyurea, a myelosuppressive agent, is the only effective drug proved to reduce the frequency of painful episodes.
  - **Priapism** is defined as an involuntary penile erection lasting for longer than 30 minutes and is a common problem in sickle cell anemia.
  - ▪ Prone for stroke
  - ▪ Can develop acute chest syndrome
  - ▪ **Renal disease** among patients with sickle cell anemia is a major comorbid condition that can lead to premature death. Seven sickle cell anemia associated nephropathies have been identified: gross hematuria, papillary necrosis, nephrotic syndrome, renal infarction, hyposthenuria, pyelonephritis, and renal medullary carcinoma.

142. Autospenectomy is seen in? *(PGMEE 2012, 2010)*
- a. G6PD deficiency
- b. Thalassemia major
- c. Sickle cell anemia
- d. Hereditary spherocytosis

[Ref: Robbins 9th/e pg 637]

143. Bone infarcts are seen in *(DNB 2008)*
- a. Iron deficiency anaemia
- b. Thalassemia
- c. Sickle cell anaemia
- d. Hereditary spherocytosis

[Ref: Robbins 9th/e pg 637]

144. Painful Ischemic dactylitis is seen in:- *(PGMEE 2018)*
- a. Sickle cell anemia
- b. Thalassemia
- c. Hereditary spherocytosis
- d. G-6-PD deficiency

[Ref: Nelson 19th edition – chapter]

145. Sickle cell Red blood cells have *(DNB 2008)*
- a. Stability
- b. Altered function
- c. Decreased oxygen carrying capacity
- d. Protective against vivax malaria

[Ref: Robbins 9th/e pg 637]

146. Person having heterozygous sickle cell trait is protected from infection of *(PGMEE 2013-14)*
- a. Plasmodium falciparum
- b. Salmonella
- c. P. Vivax
- d. Pneumococcus

[Ref: Harrison 18th/e p. 855]

147. Persistent priapism is due to: *(PGMEE 2014-15)*
- a. Sickle cell anaemia
- b. Hairy cell leukaemia
- c. Paraphimosis
- d. Urethral stenosis

[Ref: Harrison 19th p 635]

148. Patient with sickle cell anemia are at increased risk of infection with all except *(PGMEE 2013-14)*
   a. Mycobacterium tuberculosis
   b. Streptococcus pneumoniae
   c. H. influenzae type b
   d. All

[Ref: Ghai 8th/e/ch 10]

149. Salmonellosis is most common in- *(PGMEE 2012-13)*
   a. Cystic fibrosis   b. Thalassemia
   c. Hemophilia   d. Sickle cell anemia

[Ref: O.P. Ghai 8th/e/ch 10]

150. Basic defect in HbS is: *(PGMEE 2014-15)*
   a. Altered function
   b. Altered solubility
   c. Altered stability
   d. Altered O2 binding capacity

[Ref: Harrison's 18th ed.pg. 854]

THALASSEMIA

151. Ischemic dactylitis is seen in: *(NEET Pattern 2019)*
   a. Hereditary spherocytes   b. Hemophilia
   c. Sickle cell anemia   d. Thalassemia

152. A 6-year-old patient with anemia, on electrophoresis shows HbF 90%, Hb A2/=3%. Which of the following will be seen on peripheral smear *(NEET Pattern 2017)*

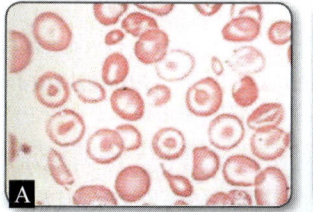 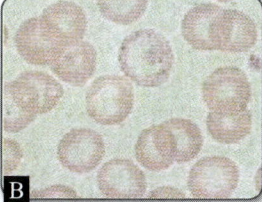

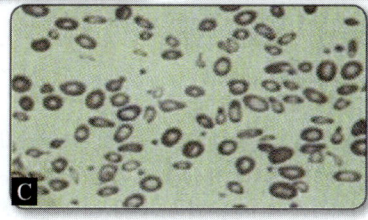

   a. A, B   b. A, C
   c. ABC   d. B, C

Explanation

- Given scenario is suggestive of beta thalassemia. Beta Thalassemia is characterized by HbF levels ranging from 10 to 100%; HbA$_2$ may be normal or increased up to 5 to 7% and the remaining percentage is constituted by HbA. HbF is heterogeneously distributed among red cells. The reticulocyte count is low, usually below 1%. MCV is typically 60 to 70 fl and MCH is 12 to 18 pg/cell. In the peripheral blood smear a great variation in size and shape of the erythrocytes is always evident. Together with large and pale target cells, microcytes, tear drop cells, and nucleated red cells are present.

- So in given scenario slide A showing Target cells, slide B showing Hypochromic cell and Slide C showing great variation in size and shape of RBCs.

153. All of the following are true about β Thalassemia trait EXCEPT *(PGMEE 2013-14)*
   a. ↑ HbF   b. ↑ HbA$_2$
   c. Microcytosis   d. Severe anemia

[Ref: Harrison 18th/e p. 859; Robbins 9th/e pg. 639]

154. Quantity of globin chain synthesis is reduced in- *(PGMEE 2014)*
   a. HbC   b. HbS
   c. Thalassemia   d. None

[Ref: Robbins 9th/e pg. 639; Harper 27th/e p. 415]

155. Thalassaemia major manifests in- *(DNB June 07)*
   a. Childhood/Infancy   b. Middle age
   c. Puberty   d. Adolescence

[Ref: Nelson 18th/e p. 2035, 2036]

156. In α- thalassemia- *(PGMEE 2012-13)*
   a. Excess β- chain   b. No α- chain
   c. No β- chain   d. Excess α- chain

[Ref: Robbins 9th/e pg. 639]

157. Screening test for thalassemia *(PGMEE 2015)*
   a. Alkali denaturation test b. Kleihauer test
   c. Hb electrophoresis   d. NESTROF

[Ref: Robbins 9th/pg 638; 8th/pg 648]

158. In α-thalassemia, Hb Barts is said when number of gene loci affected is: *(PGI May 2015)*
   a. 1   b. 2
   c. 3   d. 4

[Ref: Robbins 9th/pg 638]

159. In a patient with thalassemia major, who had received multiple blood transfusions, the serum iron overload can be detected by *(PGMEE 2015)*
   a. Serum ferritin level
   b. Blood iron level
   c. Total iron binding capacity
   d. Blood hemoglobin level

[Ref: 9th/pg 649]

160. Thalassemia shows which kind of inheritance? *(PGMEE 2012)*
   a. Autosomal recessive
   b. X-linked recessive
   c. X-linked dominant
   d. Autosomal dominant

[Ref: Robbins 9th/e pg. 639]

161. Thalassemia gives protection against: *(PGMEE 2013-14)*
   a. Kala-azar   b. Leptospirosis
   c. Malaria   d. Fiaria

[Ref: Robbins 9th/e pg. 649-652]

162. Regarding to Thalassemia minor the following is incorrect: *(PGMEE 2014-15)*
   a. Hypochromic microcytic cells
   b. Raised HbA2
   c. Severe anemia
   d. RBC count increased

[Ref: Harrison's 19th p 638]

148.	a
149.	d
150.	b
151.	c
152.	c
153.	d
154.	c
155.	a
156.	b
157.	d
158.	d
159.	a
160.	a
161.	c
162.	c

163. X-ray skull characteristically shows "Hair standing on end" appearance in one of the following disease:
(PGMEE 2014-15)
a. Still's disease
b. Scurvy
c. Thalassemia major
d. Cirrhosis of liver
[Ref: Harrison 19th p 638]

Explanation
- Hair on end sign or crewcut appearance is usually seen in sickle cell anemia & thalassemia.

164. In Beta thalassemia, the most common gene mutation is:
(PGMEE 2014-15)
a. Intron 1 inversion
b. Intron 22
c. 619 bp deletion
d. 3.7 bp deletion
[Ref: Harrison 19th p 637]

165. Which one of the following is true regarding Thalassemia Major?
(PGMEE 2014-15)
a. Normocytic normochromic anemia
b. Enlargement of medullary cavity
c. Iron deficiency anemia
d. Megaloblastic anemia
[Ref: Harrison 19th p 633, 637]

166. The most appropriate drug used for chelation therapy in beta thalassemia major is:
(PGMEE 2014-15)
a. Oral deferoxamine
b. Oral deferiprone
c. Intramuscular EDTA
d. Oral succimer
[Ref: KDT's 6th/868, Harrison 19th p 638]

PANCYTOPENIA

167. Pancytopenia is a feature of:
(PGMEE 2014-15)
a. Dengue fever
b. Enteric fever
c. SLE
d. All of the above
[Ref: Harrison 19th p 2132]

168. Pancytopenia with cellular marrow is seen in all EXCEPT:
(PGMEE 2014-15)
a. Megaloblastic anemia
b. Myelodysplasia
c. Paroxysmal Nocturnal hemoglobinuria
d. G6PD deficiency
[Ref: Harrison 19th p 656]

169. Pancytopenia may occur in the following EXCEPT:
(PGMEE 2014-15)
a. Megaloblastic anemia
b. Severe iron-deficiency anemia
c. Hypoplastic anaemia
d. Paroxysmal nocturnal haemoglobinuria
[Ref: Harrison's 19th p 662]

170. Pancytopenia with hypocellular bone marrow seen in
(PGMEE 2015)
a. Fanconi's anemia
b. Paroxysmal nocturnal hemoglobinuria
c. Hairy cell leukemia
d. Myelopthisis
[Ref: Harrison 18th/Chapter 107]

171. 2 year-old-child presents with short stature and café-au lait spots. Bone marrow aspiration yields a little material and mostly containing fat. What is your diagnosis:
(PGMEE 2015)
a. Fanconi anemia
b. Dyskeratosis congenita
c. Tuberous sclerosis
d. Osteogenesis imperfecta
[Ref: Robbins 9th/pg 653]

Explanation
- **Fanconi anemia**
- AR disorder caused by mutation in proteins required for DNA repair.
- CF:
  - Short stature
  - Cafe all lait spots.
  - Anomalies involving thumb and radius
- Bone marrow biopsy is s/o aplastic anemia ("dry tap")

172. Fanconi anemia can lead to? *(PGMEE 2015)*
a. Folate deficiency
b. Iron deficiency
c. B12 deficiency
d. Aplastic anemia
[Ref: Robbins 9th/pg 653]

173. Which of the following causes of Anemia is associated with a Hypoplastic marrow? *(PGMEE 2014-15)*
a. Fanconi's Anemia
b. Paroxysmal Nocturnal Hemoglobinuria
c. Hypersplenism
d. Myelofibrosis
[Ref: Harrison 19th p 434/664]

174. All cause aplastic anemia EXCEPT: *(PGMEE 2014-15)*
a. Hepatitis B
b. Hepatitis C
c. Hepatitis D
d. None
[Ref: Harrison 19th p 667]

175. Dry tap is a feature: *(PGMEE 2015)*
a. Anemia of chronic disease
b. Megaloblastic anemia
c. Aplastic anemia
d. Sickle cell anemia
[Ref: Robbins 9th/pg 653]

176. Which is best to prevent rejection after bone marrow transplantation in aplastic anemia? *(PGMEE 2014-15)*
a. Anti-thymocyte globulin + cyclosporine
b. Prednisolone
c. Cyclosporine
d. Tacrolimus plus prednisolone
[Ref: Harrison's 19th p 667]

177. A patient aged 65 years, is diagnosed to have severe aplastic anemia. HLA compatible sibling is available. The best option of treatment is: *(PGMEE 2014-15)*
a. Anti-thymocyte globulin followed by cyclosporine
b. A conventional bone marrow transplantation from the HLA identical sibling
c. A non-myeloablative bone marrow transplant-ation from the HLA identical sibling
d. Cyclosporine
[Ref: Harrison's 19th p 667]

163.	c
164.	a
165.	b
166.	b
167.	d
168.	d
169.	b
170.	a
171.	a
172.	d
173.	a
174.	d
175.	c
176.	a
177.	a

Explanation

- Immunosuppressive therapy (ATG + Cyclosporine) is the preferred therapy for patients with severe aplastic who are ≥ 50 years. For patients younger than 50 years, HLA matched sibling done BMT is the TOC.

MYELODYSPASTIC SYNDROME

178. False regarding myelodysplastic syndromes *(PGMEE 2015)*

a. Pawn ball megakaryocytes
b. Increased neutrophil alkaline phosphastase
c. Ringed sideroblasts
d. Hypercellular bone marrow

[Ref: Robbins 9th/pg 617]

179. Which of the following is not a characteristic feature of Myelodysplastic syndrome? *(PGMEE 2015)*

a. Leucoerythroblastic blood picture
b. Transformation to AML
c. Pseudo pelger heut cells
d. Pawn ball megakaryocytes

[Ref: Robbins 9th/pg 614- 615]

180. Leukocyte alkaline phosphatase score is decreased in *(PGMEE 2015)*

a. Polycythemia vera
b. Pregnancy
c. Infections
d. Myelodysplastic syndrome

[Ref: Robbins 9th/e pg. 614]

181. Pawn ball megakaryocytes are characteristic of: *(PGMEE 2014-15)*

a. Myelodysplastic syndrome
b. idiopathic thrombocytopenic purpura
c. Thrombotic thrombocytopenic purpura
d. Chloramphenicol toxicity

[Ref: Harrison's 19th/e pg. 669]

182. Isolated deletion of which chromosome causes myelodysplastic syndrome: *(PGMEE 2014-15)*

a. 2q
b. 5q
c. 8q
d. 11q

[Ref: Harrison's 19th/e pg. 670]

183. All of the following are WHO classified Myelodysplastic Syndromes EXCEPT: *(PGMEE 2014-15)*

a. CML
a. Refractory anemia with excess blasts
c. Refractory anemia with ringed sideroblasts
d. Refractory anemia

[Ref: Harrison's 19th/e pg. 693]

184. Pancytopenia with hypercellular marrow is due all EXCEPT: *(DNB June 2011)*

a. Myelodysplasia
b. Sarcoidosis
c. Paroxysmal nocturnal hemoglobinuria
d. Dyskeratosis congenita

[Ref: Harrison's 19th/e pg 663]

185. Dwarf megakaryocytes with unilobed nucleus is characteristic of *(PGMEE 2015)*

a. Myelodysplastic syndrome
b. Essential thrombocytosis
c. Polycythemia vera
d. Chronic myeloid leukemia

[Ref: Robbins 9th/e pg. 614- 615]

186. Pseudo pelger huet anomaly is seen in *(PGMEE 2013)*

a. Multiple myeloma
b. Hodgkin's lymphoma
c. Hairy cell leukemia
d. Myeolo dysplastic syndrome

[Ref: Wintrobe's clinical hematology 12th/e p. 1548, Harrsion 18th/e Ch. 60]

MISCELLANEOUS

187. All of the following are true regarding Hemoglobin EXCEPT:- *(PGMEE 2016-17)*

a. Hills coefficient is 2.8
b. Co-operative binding present
c. Oxygen affinity is more than myoglobin
d. Fetal hemoglobin binds O2 more avidly than does HbA

188. Which organism causes infection after splenectomy: *(PGMEE 2015-16)*

a. H. Influenzae
b. Staph aureus
c. E.coli
d. Klebsiella

[Ref: Harrison 19th ed. / 484, 652]

Explanation

- Post splenectomy infection is usually caused by the encapsulated bacteria like S. pneumoniae. Haemophilus influenza & N. meningitidis.

189. Which of the following is the most common organ of origin causing cancer related death in female <20 years? *(PGMEE 2014-15)*

a. Breast
b. Cervix
c. Bone marrow
d. Lung

[Ref: table 81.2, Harrison's 18th ed.]

190. To develop cyanosis the concentration of reduced hemogloblin should be :- *(PGMEE 2016-17)*

a. > 5 mg/dl
b. > 5gm/dl
c. > 5gm/l
d. < 5 gm/dl

[Ref: Internet]

191. The following drug is associated with pure red cell aplasia: *(PGMEE 2015)*

a. Phenytoin
b. Isoniazid
c. Erythropoietin
d. All of the above

[Ref: 9th/pg 653-655]

192. MC tumor associated with pure red cell aplasia: *(PGMEE 2015)*

a. Hepatoma
b. Hodgkins lymphoma
c. Thymoma
d. Bronchogenic carcinoma

[Ref: Robbins 9th/pg 653]

193. Bone marrow transplantation is indicated in all EXCEPT: *(PGMEE 2014-15)*

a. Osteopetrosis
b. Mucopolysaccharidosis
c. Hemochromatosis
d. Beta-Thalassemia

[Ref: Harrison's 19th p 139e-1]

178.	b
179.	a
180.	d
181.	a
182.	b
183.	a
184.	d
185.	a
186.	d
187.	c
188.	a
189.	c
190.	b
191.	d
192.	c
193.	c

LEUKEMIA

1. Marker of T -lymphocyte is? *(PGMEE 2016)*
- a. CD8
- b. CD20
- c. CD19
- d. CD45

[Ref: Robbins 9th/pg 590]

2. Marker of B-lymphocyte is? *(PGMEE 2016)*
- a. CD8
- b. CD4
- c. CD19
- d. CD21

[Ref: Robbins 9th/pg 590]

3. Pan Tell marker is *(PGMEE 2015)*
- a. CD3
- b. CD8
- c. CD19
- d. CD20

[Ref: Robbins 9th/pg 590]

4. In acute leukemia Periodic acid schiff (PAS) block positivity is shown by: *(DNB Dec 09)*
- a. Lymphoblasts
- b. Myeloblasts
- c. Monoblasts
- d. Megakaryoblasts

[Ref: www.ncbi.nlm.nih.gov/pubmed]

5. The anemia associated with leukemia is *(PGMEE 2012-13)*
- a. Megaloblastic type
- b. Iron deficiency
- c. Myelophthisic type
- d. All of above

[Ref: Robbins 9th/e pg. 655]

6. All are true about CNS leukemia EXCEPT: *(PGMEE 2015)*
- a. CNS irradiation is given
- b. Single blast in CSF is sufficient for diagnosis
- c. Seen with myeloid leukemia
- d. Intrathecal methotrexate is given

[Ref: Robbins 9th/e pg. 655]

7. Chloroma is a *(PGMEE 2015)*
- a. Carcinoma
- b. Leukemia
- c. Sarcoma
- d. Lymphoma

[Ref: Robbins 9th/pg 612]

8. Stain used for diagnosis of granulocytic sarcoma *(PGMEE 2015)*
- a. Myeloperoxidase
- b. Neuron specific enolase
- c. Nonspecific esterase
- d. Leukocyte alkaline phosphatase

[Ref: Robbins 9th/pg 612]

Explanation
- AML occasionally presents as localized soft tissue mass k/a Granulocytic sarcoma, chloroma or Myeloblastoma.
- Stains used for detection inducles Mycloperoxidase, Sudan B Black etc.
- Immunohistochemistry markers include CD 34 & CD 117.

9. Specific stain for myeloblasts *(PGMEE 2012-13)*
- a. PAS
- b. LAP
- c. Myeloperoxidase
- d. Sudan black

[Ref: healthline.com/galecontent/leukemia-stains]

10. Patient presented with h/o headaches. Hb-16g/dL, TIL-21000, Platelet—3,75000. DLC N-25, L20, Metamyelocytes myelocytes 40, E-5. What should be your next investigation? *(NEET Pattern 2017)*
- a. JAK 2 mutations
- b. EPO levels
- c. Philadelphia chromosome
- d. Bone marrow biopsy

ACUTE MYELOID LEUKEMIA (AML)

11. Most common type of acute myeloid leukemia: *(PGMEE 2014-15)*
- a. M2
- b. M3
- c. M4
- d. M5

[Ref:Harrison's 19th/e pg. 678]

12. Most common type of AML in Down's syndrome *(PGMEE 2015)*
- a. M2
- b. M3
- c. M6
- d. M7

[Ref: Robbins 9th/pg 612]

13. Auer rods are specific for *(PGMEE 2015)*
- a. Acute myeloid leukemia
- b. Acute lymphocytic leukemia
- c. Hodgkin's lymphoma
- d. Chronic lymphocytic leukemia

[Ref: Robbins 9th/e pg. 612]

14. AML is characterized by: *(PGMEE 2012-13)*
- a. Hemolytic anemia
- b. Auer rods
- c. Dohle bodies
- d. Philadelphia chromosome

[Ref: Robbin's 8th/e p. 622]

15. A 35 year old male presented with complaints of bleeding from gums. There is a history of recurrent infections in the past 1 year. On examination, pallor present. Peripheral smear of the patient is given below. Identify the arrow marked structure? *(PGMEE 2015)*

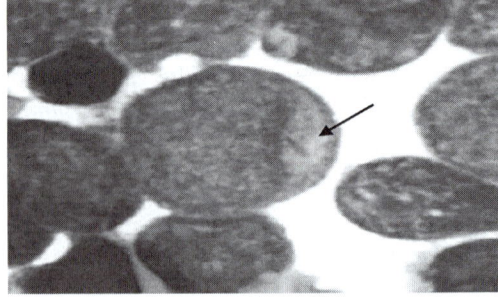

- a. Heinz bodies
- b. Normoblast
- c. Auer Rods
- d. Dohle body

[Ref: Robbins 9th/pg 590-592]

16. Good prognosis of AML is indicated by all except? *(PGMEE 2015)*
- a. t(15;17]
- b. inv 16
- c. t(8;21]
- d. t(12;21]

[Ref: Robbins 9th/pg 612]

1.	a
2.	c
3.	a
4.	a
5.	c
6.	c
7.	b
8.	a
9.	c
10.	d
11.	a
12.	d
13.	a
14.	b
15.	c
16.	d

17. Indicator of good prognosis in AML? *(PGMEE 2015)*
   a. t (15:17]
   b. Monosomy 7
   c. Deletion 5q
   d. Trisomy 7

   [Ref: Robbins 9th/pg 612]

18. D.I.C. is seen in- *(PGMEE 2012-13)*
   a. Acute promyelocytic leukemia
   b. CMC
   c. Autoimmune hemolytic anemia
   d. Acute myelomonocytic leukemia

   [Ref: Robbin's 9th/e pg. 612;Harrison's 19th/e pg. 678]

19. DIC is seen most commonly seen in which AML type? *(PGMEE 2015, 14)*
   a. M2
   b. M3
   c. M4
   d. M5

   [Ref: Robbins 9th/e pg. 612; Harrison's 19th/e pg. 678]

20. AML causing gum hypertrophy: *(PGMEE 2013-14)*
   a. M3
   b. M2
   c. M 1
   d. M4

   [Ref: Harrison 18th/e p. 908, 909]

21. Gum hypertrophy is seen in which type of AML: *(PGMEE 2014-15)*
   a. Myelogenous leukaemia
   b. Myelomonocytic leukaemia
   c. Megakaryocytic leukaemia
   d. Erthroleukemia

   [Ref: Harrison's 19th/e pg. 682]

22. According to FAB classification, promyelocytic blood picture belongs to which type of AML? *(PGMEE 2014-15)*
   a. MO
   b. Ml
   c. M2
   d. M3

   [Ref: Harrison's 19th/e pg. 683]

23. Arsenic is used in treatment of: *(PGMEE 2014-15)*
   a. Acute Promyelocytic leukemia
   b. A.L.L
   c. CML
   d. Transient myeloproliferative disorder

   [Ref: Harrison's 19th/e pg. 686]

24. Drug of choice in acute myeloid leukemia (APL):- *(PGMEE 2016-17)*
   a. ATRA
   b. Cytarabine
   c. Daunorubicin
   d. Fludarabine

ACUTE LYMPHOBLASTIC LEUKEMIA (ALL)

25. Treatment of choice of CNS leukemia is:
   a. Intra-thecal methotrexate   *(PGMEE 2014-15)*
   b. Vincristine and predinisolone
   c. Intrathecal vincristine
   d. Prednisolone

   [Ref: Ghai 7th ed. pg. 590]

26. Most common malignancy of blood is? *(PGMEE 2016)*
   a. ALL
   b. CLL
   c. CML
   d. AML

   [Ref: Robbins 9th/pg 590-592]

27. CD-10 is seen in *(DNB Dec 07)*
   a. ALL
   b. CML
   c. HCL
   d. CLL

   [Ref: Wintrobe's 11th/e p. 27]

28. Most common malignant tumor in pediatric age group is- *(PGMEE 2015)*
   a. Acute lymphoblastic leukemia
   b. Medulloblastoma
   c. Sacrococcygeal teratoma
   d. Neuroblastoma

   [Ref: O.P. Ghai 8th/e pg. 590]

29. Commonest site of extra-medullary relapse of ALL- *(PGMEE 2012-13)*
   a. CNS
   b. Testis
   c. Lung
   d. Liver

   [Ref: Ghai 8th/e/p 604]

30. True about ALL *(PGMEE 2015)*
   a. tdT positive
   b. t(8,14)
   c. Gamma globulinopathy
   d. Insidious onset

   [Ref: Robbins 9th/pg 590]

31. B -ALL is due to: *(PGMEE 2012-13)*
   a. Immature T cells
   b. Immature precursor B cells
   c. Mature peripheral B cells
   d. Both T and B cells

   [Ref: Robbins 9th/e pg. 591]

32. Good prognostic factor for ALL is presence of:- *(PGMEE 2012-13)*
   a. Hyperdiploidy
   b. T cell line
   c. Philadelphia chromosome
   d. Hypodiploidy

   [Ref: Robbins 9th/e pg. 592]

33. Bad prognostic factor of Acute Lymphoblastic Leukemia (ALL) is - *(PGMEE 2012)*
   a. WBC count < 50,000
   b. T (12:21) translocation
   c. Age > 10 years
   d. Hyperdipoidy

   [Ref: Ghai 8th/e/p 601 table 20.5]

34. Poor prognostic indicator in ALL *(DNB June 10)*
   a. Presence of testicular involvement at presentation
   b. TLC 4000-10,000
   c. Presence of blasts in peripheral smear
   d. Age <2 year

   [Ref: O.P. Ghai 6th/e p. 562, Tejinder Singh p. 170]

35. Drugs used in ALL in child are all except- *(PGMEE 2013-14)*
   a. Vincristine
   b. Methotrexate
   c. Cyclophosphamids
   d. Vinblastine

   [Ref: Ghai 8th/e/p 603]

36. Which one is best prognostic factor for ALL?
   a. Hypoploidy   *(PGMEE 2015]*
   b. TLC more than 50,000/ul
   c. Orgnomegaly
   d. Response to treatment

   [Ref: Robbin's 9th/ 590-592]

17.	a
18.	a
19.	b
20.	d
21.	b
22.	d
23.	a
24.	a
25.	a
26.	a
27.	a
28.	a
29.	a
30.	a,b
31.	b
32.	a
33.	c
34.	a>d
35.	d
36.	d

37. **The following parameter in ALL indicates poor prognosis** *(PGMEE 2015)*
   a. Age >10 years
   b. Early pre-B phenotype
   c. Hyperdiploidy
   d. WBC count <50000/mm3 at diagnosis

   [Ref: Robbins 9th/pg 590-592]

38. **Drug that is not used in the treatment of ALL** *(PGMEE 2015)*
   a. Rituximab   b. Daunorubicin
   c. Vincristine   d. Methotrexate

   [Ref: Robbins 9th/pg 590-592]

39. **Most common type of ALL in children** *(PGMEE 2015)*
   a. Pre-B cell ALL   b. Pre-T cell ALL
   c. Mature B cell ALL   d. Mature T cell ALL

   [Ref: Robbins 9th/pg 590-592]

40. **Good prognosis factors of ALL are all EXCEPT:** *(DNB June 2011)*
   a. Hyperdipoidy   b. Female sex
   c. Pre B cell ALL   d. T (12:21) Translocation

   [Ref: Devita's 6th/e pg. 2240, Nelson 17th/e pg. 1695, Wintrobe's Clinical Hematology 11th/e Table 80.2]

41. **2 year old child with ALL, which of the following has the best prognosis?** *(PGMEE 2015-16)*
   a. Age between 1-10 years
   b. TLC >1 lac
   c. Petechiae
   d. t (9:22)

   [Ref: Harrison 19th ed. / 699-700]

CHRONIC LYMPHOCYTIC LEUKEMIA (CLL)

42. **CLL/SLL arises from.** *(NEET Pattern 2017)*
   a. Mature B cell
   b. Naive B cell
   c. Centrocytes of germinal center
   d. Progenitor B-cell

   [Ref: Robbins 9th edition pg 593]

Explanation

- CLL/SLL are somatically hypermutated, whereas others are not, suggesting that the cell of origin may be either a postgerminal center memory B cell or a naive B cell. For unclear reasons, tumors with unmutated Ig segments (those putatively of naive B-cell origin) pursue a more aggressive course.

43. **Radiation exposure is not related to :** *(PGMEE 2014-15)*
   a. ALL   b. AML
   c. CML   d. CLL

   [Ref: Harrison's 19th/e pg. 701]

44. **80 year old, asymptomatic man present with a TLC of 1 lakh, with 80% lymphocytes and 20% PMCs. What is the most probable diagnosis?** *(PGMEE 2014-15)*
   a. HIV   b. CML
   c. CLL   d. TB

   [Ref: Harrison's 19th/e pg. 703]

45. **CLL is characterized by?** *(DNB June 2011)*
   a. Hepatosplenomegaly
   b. Seen commonly in age>50 years persons
   c. Small lymphocytes in peripheral smear
   d. All the above

   [Ref: Wintrobe's 9th/e 1976; Harrison's 19th/e pg 703]

46. **In Ritcher's transformation CLL transforms into:** *(PGMEE 2014-15)*
   a. Large B cell Lymphoma
   b. Anaplastic carcinoma
   c. Burkitt lymphoma
   d. Lymphoproliferative lymphoma

   [Ref: Hematology in clinical practice. 4th ed. ch. 21, Harrison's 19th/e pg. 703]

47. **CLL is characterised by following except** *(DNB Dec 07)*
   a. ZAP-70 is associated with poor prognosis
   b. Small lymphocytes in peripheral smear
   c. Hepatosplenomegaly
   d. Age > 50 years and usually females

   [Ref: Wintrobe's 2438; Robbin's 8th/e p. 631-604]

48. **A 60-year-old male presents with generalized lymphadenopathy and hepatosplenomegaly. Immunophenotype: CD5 and CD19 are positive and CD10 negative. Diagnosis** *(PGMEE 2015)*
   a. Burkitt lymphoma
   b. Follicular lymphoma
   c. Hairy cell leukemia
   d. CLL

   [Ref: Robbins 9th/pg 593]

HODGKIN'S LYMPHOMA

49. **Which of the following differentiates hodgkin's lymphoma from non hodgkin's lymphoma?** *(DNB Dec' 2011)*
   a. Elderly
   b. Fever, night sweat, weight loss
   c. Generalized lymphadenopathy
   d. Reed stern berg cells

   [Ref: Robbin's 7th/e p. 669]

50. **Most common presentation of childhood Hodgkin Lymphoma-** *(PGMEE 2016-17)*
   a. Cervical Lymphadenopathy
   b. Inguinal Lymphadenopathy
   c. Fever
   d. Weight Loss

   [Ref: Ghai 8th/e/ p 609]

51. **Bimodal age distribution in Hodgkin lymphoma:-** *(PGMEE 2016-17)*
   a. 15-30 years and > 50 years
   b. 15-34 years and > 50 years
   c. 15-30 years and > 55 years
   d. 15-34 years and > 55 years

   [Ref: Harrison's 19th p 697]

37.	a
38.	a
39.	a
40.	c
41.	a
42.	b
43.	d
44.	c
45.	d
46.	a
47.	d
48.	d
49.	d
50.	a
51.	d

52. On Bone marrow biopsy "owl's eye nucleus" was seen in cell as shown in image. The diagnosis is:-
(PGMEE 2016-17)

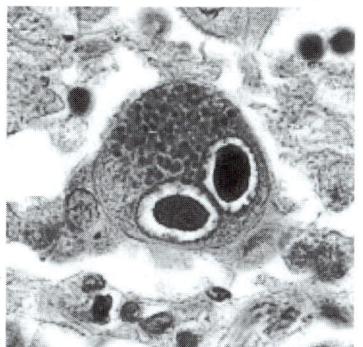

- a. Sickle cell anemia
- b. Multiple myeloma
- c. Hodgkin Lymphoma
- d. Hairy cell leukemia

[Ref: Robbin's 9th/e p. 610]

53. Ann Arbor classification is used for? *(PGMEE 2013)*
- a. Neuroblastoma
- b. Retinoblastoma
- c. Nephroblastoma
- d. Hodgkin lymphoma

[Ref: Robbin's 9th/e p. 610]

54. Which of the following malignancy is associated with underlying progression and spreads characteristically in a stepwise fashion and hence staging the disease is an important prognostic factor? *(DNB Dec 08)*
- a. Multiple myeloma
- b. Mature T cell NHL
- c. Hodgkin's lymphoma
- d. Mature B cell NHL

[Ref: Robbin's 9th/e p. 610]

55. Reed sternberg cells are: *(PGMEE 2014-15)*
- a. B cells
- b. T cells
- c. Natural killer cells
- d. All of above

[Ref: Harrison's 19th/e pg. 709f]

56. Reed strenberg cells are found in:
(PGMEE 2012-13,2013-14)
- a. Hodgkin's disease
- b. CML
- c. Sickle cell anemia
- d. Thalassemia

[Ref: Robbin's 9th/e p. 607]

57. Which Hodgkin's disease is associated with best prognosis- *(PGMEE 2012-13, 2013-14; PGMEE'2010)*
- a. Lymphocytic predominance
- b. Nodular sclerosis
- c. Lymphocyte depletion
- d. Mixed cellularity

[Ref: Robbin's 9th/e p. 607; Harrison's 19th/e pg 709]

58. Lacunar cells are seen in which type of Hodgkin's lymphoma- *(PGMEE 2012-13)*
- a. Mixed cellularity
- b. Lymphocyte depletion
- c. Nodular sclerosing
- d. Lymphocyte predominance

[Ref: Robbin's 9th/e p. 609]

59. L and H type of Reed Sternberg cells are seen in which type of Hodgkin's disease:- *(PGMEE 2018)*
- a. Nodular sclerosis type
- b. Lymphocyte predominance type
- c. Mixed cellularity type
- d. Lymphocytic depletion type

[Ref: Robbin's 9th/e p. 609]

Explanation

- "Classical" Reed-Sternberg cells are usually difficult to find in Lymphocyte Predominance Type. Instead, this tumor contains so-called L&H (lymphocytic and histiocytic) variants, which have a multilobed nucleus resembling a popcorn kernel ("popcorn cell").

60. 'ABVD' regimen is used in: *(PGMEE 2014-15)*
- a. Chronic lymphocytic leukemia
- b. Acute lymphoblastic leukemia
- c. N.H.L
- d. Hodgkin's disease

[Ref: Harrison's 19th p 697]

61. Popcorn variant of Reed-Sternberg cells are seen in: *(PGMEE 2014-15)*
- a. Follicular center lymphoma
- b. Lymphocyte depleted Hodgkin's disease
- c. Nodular sclerosis Hodgkin's disease
- d. Lymphocyte predominant Hodgkin's disease

[Ref: Robbin's 9th/e p. 609]

62. Reticular variant of Reed Sternberg found in which subtype of Hodgkin's? *(PGMEE 2015)*
- a. Nodular Sclerosis
- b. Lymphocyte depleted Hodgkins lymphoma
- c. Lymphocyte predominant Hodgkins lymphoma
- d. Lymphocyte rich Hodgkins lymphoma

[Ref: Robbins 9th/pg 606-611]

63. Which of the following statements on lymphoma is not True? *(PGMEE 2014-15)*
- a. A single classification system of Hodgkin's disease is almost universally accepted
- b. HD tends to remain localized to a single group of lymph nodes and spreads by contiguity
- c. Several types of Non-Hodgkin's lymphoma may have a leukemic phase
- d. In general follicular NHL has worse prognosis compared to diffuse NHL

[Ref: Harrison's 19th/e pg. 701]

64. All are true regarding Reed Sternburg cell immuno-phenotype in classical Hodgkin's lymphoma EXCEPT *(PGMEE 2015)*
- a. Positive for PAX 5
- b. Negative for other B-cell markers, T-cell markers, and CD45
- c. Positive for CD15 and CD30
- d. Over expression of BCL-6

[Ref: Robbins 9th/e pg. 606-611]

52.	c
53.	d
54.	c
55.	a
56.	a
57.	a
58.	c
59.	b
60.	d
61.	d
62.	b
63.	d
64.	d

65. Hodgkin's lymphoma type which presents more commonly as fever of unknown origin *(PGMEE 2015)*
- a. Lymphocyte depletion
- b. Mixed cellularity
- c. Lymphocyte predominance
- d. Nodular sclerosis

[Ref: Robbins 9th/pg 606-611]

66. Which of the following types of Hodgkin's lymphomas is not associated with Epstein Barr virus? *(PGMEE 2015)*
- a. Lymphocye rich
- b. Mixed cellularity
- c. Lymphocyte depletion
- d. Nodular sclerosis type

[Ref: Robbins 9th/e pg. 608]

67. A 35-year-old female presents with cervical and axillary lymphadenopathy. There is history of fever and drenching night sweats. She is diagnosed to have Hodgkin's lymphoma. What is the stage of the disease? *(PGMEE 2015)*
- a. II-A
- b. II-B
- c. IIE-A
- d. IIE-B

[Ref: Robbins 9th/pg 606-611]

NON- HODGKIN'S LYMPHOMA

68. CD 30 marker for
- a. Anaplastic large cell lymphoma
- b. Seminoma
- c. Embroyonal cell ca
- d. Hodgkins lymphoma

[Ref: Robbins 9th/pg 605]

69. The low grade non-Hodgkin's lymphoma is *(DNB June 08)*
- a. Diffuse large cell
- b. Lymphoblastic
- c. Follicular
- d. Large cell

[Ref: Robbin's 8th/e p. 638; Chandrasoma taylor 3rd/e p. 604]

Explanation

- **Low grade NHL:**
  - ○ Follicular lymphoma → MC type of low grade
  - ○ Mantle cell lymphoma
  - ○ Marginal zone lymphoma
- **High grade NHL:**
  - ○ Diffuse Large B Cell Lymphoma → MC NHL
  - ○ Burkitt lymphoma
  - ○ Peripheral T cell lymphoma

70. Most common extranodal site for Non-Hodgkin's lymphoma is *(DNB June 07)*
- a. Tonsils
- b. Stomach
- c. Brain
- d. Intestines

[Ref: Advance in oncology vol-3 p. 137]

71. Most Common extranodal site of Lymphoma in HIV is ? *(DNB Dec 10)*
- a. CNS
- b. Mediastinum
- c. GIT
- d. Retroperitoneum

[Ref: Advance in oncology vol-3 137; Handbook of Cancer Chemotherapy edited by Roland T. Skeel pg. 568]

65.	b
66.	d
67.	b
68.	a
69.	c
70.	b
71.	a
72.	c
73.	b
74.	d
75.	b
76.	a
77.	c
78.	c
79.	b
80.	d

72. Most common ocular lymphoma: *(PGMEE 2013-14)*
- a. Hodgkin's lymphoma
- b. Pre T-cell lymphoma
- c. B-cell NHL
- d. T-cell lymphoma

[Ref: Textbook of ophthalmological tumors p. 701]

73. CD20 is positive in all the following lymphomas except *(PGMEE 2015)*
- a. Mantle cell lymphoma
- b. Lymphocyte rich HL
- c. Follicular lymphoma
- d. Butkitt lymphoma

[Ref: Robbins 9th/e pg. 597]

74. Find the false statement about diffuse large B cell lymphoma *(PGMEE 2015)*
- a. Most common form of NHL
- b. Waldeyer ring is involved commonly
- c. Extranodal sites are also involved
- d. Bone-marrow involvement in early phase

[Ref: Robbins 9th/pg 608]

75. Neoplastic cells with multilobated nuclei (cloverleaf or flower cells) are seen in *(PGMEE 2015)*
- a. Mycosis fungoides
- b. Adult T cell leukemia
- c. Anaplstic large T cell lymphoma
- d. Diffuse large B cell lymphoma

[Ref: Robbins 9th/e pg. 605]

76. Gastric MALTomas may express all of the following except: *(PGMEE 2015)*
- a. CD5
- b. CD19
- c. CD20
- d. CD43

[Ref: Robbins 9th/pg 603]

77. CD marker of MALT lymphoma is? *(PGMEE 2015; 2013)*
- a. CD 40
- b. CD 3
- c. CD 20
- d. CD 5

[Ref: Robbins 9th/e pg .603]

78. IgA lymphoma is seen in? *(PGMEE 2016)*
- a. Spleen
- b. Large Intestine
- c. Small Intestine
- d. Lymph nodes

[Ref: WHO Hemato-lymphoid Tumors 4th/ed 2008 pg 197-199]

79. Translocation seen on follicular lymphoma is? *(PGMEE 2016)*
- a. 5;14
- b. 14;18
- c. 8;14
- d. 14;20

[Ref: Robbins 9th/pg 594]

BURKITT'S LYMPHOMA

80. A 10-yr-old boy presents with abdominal mass . On imaging the paraaortic LN is enlarged. On biopsy starry sky appearance is seen. What is the underlying abnormality? *(NEET Pattern 2015)*
- a. p53 gene mutation
- b. Translocation involving BCR-ABL genes
- c. RB gene mutation
- d. Translocation involving MYC gene

[Ref: Robbins 9th/pg 597; 8th/607]

81. **True about endemic Burkitt's lymphoma** (*PGMEE 2015*)
    a. All are associated with EBV infection
    b. Abdominal amass involving ileocaecum and peritoneum and peritoneum
    c. Bone marrow is commonly involve
    d. Most aggressive form d

    [Ref: Robbins 9th/pg 591]

82. **Translocation t(8;14) of c-MYC gene is seen in**
    a. Diffuse large B cell lymphoma   (*PGMEE 2015*)
    b. Burkitt lymphoma
    c. Mantle cell lymphoma
    d. Follicular lymphoma

    [Ref: Robbins 9th/e pg. 597]

83. **Chromosomal translocation seen in Burkitt's lymphoma is:**   (*PGMEE 2015, 2012-13, DNB June 2009*)
    a. t(9;22)   b. t(11;14)
    c. t(8;14)   d. t(14;18)

    [Ref: Robbins 9th/pg 594]

84. **Burkitt's lymphoma is positive for-**   (*PGMEE 2013*)
    a. CD 25   b. CD 5
    c. CD 20   d. CD 15

    [Ref: Robbin's 8th/e p. 606-611]

85. **Burkitt's lymphoma arises from-**   (*DNB Dec 10*)
    a. NK cell   b. T cell
    c. B cell   d. Pre B cell

    [Ref: Robbin's 8th/e p. 608]

86. **Burkitt's is associated with infection by?** (*PGMEE 2015*)
    a. HSV   b. EBV
    c. HHV-8   d. CMV

    [Ref: Robbins 9th/pg 597]

87. **Pathognomic feature of Burkitt's lymphoma**   (*PGMEE 2015*)
    a. Russel bodies   b. Howell-Jolly bodies
    c. Starry sky pattern   d. Reed Stenberg cells

    [Ref: Robbins 9th/e pg. 598-602]

MANTLE CELL LYMPHOMA

88. **Mantle cell lymphoma shows-**   (*PGMEE 2012-13*)
    a. CD5 +, CD25 –   b. CD5+, CD23 +
    c. CD 5+, CD 10 +   d. CD5+, CD23-

    [Ref: Robbin's 8th/e p. 612-613]

89. **CD5 is expressed in**   (*PGMEE 2015*)
    a. Mantle cell lymphoma
    b. Burkitt lymphoma
    c. Follicular lymphoma
    d. Chronic myeloid lymphoma

    [Ref: Robbins 9th/pg 602-603]

90. **Mantle cell lymphoma are positive for all of the following, except**   (*PGMEE 2013-14, DNB Dec'2011*)
    a. CD23   b. CD5
    c. CD 43   d. CD 20

    [Ref: Robbins 9th/pg 602-603,613]

91. **Characteristic translocation in mantle cell lymphoma**   (*PGMEE 2015*)
    a. t(11;14)   b. t(15;17)
    c. t(9;22)   d. t(8;14)

    [Ref: Robbins 9th/pg 597]

92. **Marker for Mantle cell lymphoma :-**   (*PGMEE 2016-17*)
    a. Bcl-2   b. Bcl-6
    c. GPST1   d. Cyclin D1

    [Ref: Robbin's 9th/e pg. 602]

HAIRY CELL LEUKEMIA

93. **Hairy cell leukemia is a neoplasm of?**   (*PGMEE 2015-16*)
    a. B cell   b. NK cell
    c. T cell   d. Plasma cell

    [Ref: Robbins 9th/pg 603; Harrison 19th ed. / 706]

94. **Marker for hairy cell leukaemia is?**   (*DNB June 2009*)
    a. CD 1   b. CD 4
    c. CD 30   d. CD 103

    [Ref: Robbins 9th/e pg .603]

MYCOSIS FUNGOIDES

95. **Not a B cell lymphoma:**   (*PGMEE 2014*)
    a. Mycosis fungoides   b. Hairy cell leukemia
    c. Mantle cell lymphoma   d. CLL

    [Ref: Robbin's 8th/e p. 600]

96. **Mycosis fungoides is?**   (*DNB June 2009*)
    a. T cell lymphoma   b. B cell lymphoma
    c. Plasma cell dyscrasia d. Mixed

    [Ref: Robbins 9th/e pg .605]

97. **Most common form of cutaneous lymphoma:-**   (*PGMEE 2018*)
    a. Eosinophilic granuloma
    b. Langerhans cell histiocytosis
    c. Mycosis fungoides
    d. None of the above

    [Ref: Harrison 19/e, P. 707]

Explanation

Mycosis Fungoides/Sézary Syndrome

- Mycosis fungoides and Sézary syndrome are different manifestations of a tumor of CD4 + helper T cells that home to the skin (cutaneous lymphoma).
- Mycosis fungoides is the most common type of cutaneous T-cell lymphoma (44%). Histologically, it is characterized by infiltration of the epidermis and upper dermis by neoplastic T cells, which often have a cerebriform appearance due to marked infolding of the nuclear membrane. Late disease progression is characterized by extracutaneous spread, most commonly to lymph nodes and bone marrow.

81.	a
82.	b
83.	c
84.	c
85.	c
86.	b
87.	c
88.	d
89.	a
90.	a
91.	a
92.	d
93.	a
94.	d
95.	a
96.	a
97.	c

- Sézary syndrome accounts for about 5% of all cases of mycosis fungoides. The patient with Sézary syndrome has generalized **exfoliative dermatitis or erythroderma** and lymphadenopathy, as well as associated leukemia of "Sézary" cells with characteristic cerebriform nuclei circulating in the peripheral blood. The WHO-EORTC classification for cutaneous lymphoma classifies it as one with aggressive behavior.

98. Sezary syndrome in included in category of- *(PGMEE 2013-14)*
   a. T cell leukemia skin
   b. Pigmented disorder of
   c. Lymphoma
   d. B cell leukemia

[Ref: Robbins 9th/e pg. 605]

99. Shape of berbicks granules is *(PGMEE 2012-13)*
   a. Tennis racket
   b. Bat
   c. Ball
   d. Hockey stick

[Ref: Robbins 9th/pg 622]

ANAPLASTIC LARGE T CELL LYMPHOMA

100. CD 30 positivity and t(2;5) is characteristic of *(PGMEE 2015)*
   a. Langerhans cell histiocytosis
   b. Follicular lymphoma
   c. Null cell lymphoma
   d. Lymphoplasmacytic lymphoma

[Ref: Wintrobe's 12thed/pg 2169]

101. Not true about anaplastic large T cell lymphoma *(PGMEE 2015)*
   a. CD30 (ki-1] positive
   b. t(2;5] translocation
   c. Large anaplastic cells containing horseshoe-shaped nuclei and voluminous cytoplasm
   d. ALK positive tumors carry worst prognosis

[Ref: Robbins 9th/e pg 605]

Explanation
- Anaplastic large T-cell lymphoma with ALK rearrangement carry a very good prognosis.

102. Hallmark cells are seen in: *(PGMEE 2015)*
   a. Anaplastic large cell lymphoma
   b. Mantle cell lymphoma
   c. Hairy cell leukaemia
   d. Burkitt's lymphoma

[Ref: Robbins 9th/pg 591]

103. Translocation t(2;5) is seen in *(PGMEE 2015)*
   a. Null cell lymphoma
   b. Langerhans cell histiocytosis
   c. Diffuse large B cell lymphoma
   d. Systemic mastocytosis

[Ref: Wintrobes pg 2169]

98.	a
99.	a
100.	c
101.	d
102.	a
103.	a
104.	d
105.	a
106.	d
107.	d
108.	b
109.	c
110.	a

PLASMA CELL NEOPLASMS

104. Life span of plasma cell *(PGMEE 2016)*
   a. 12 hr
   b. 24 hrs
   c. 48 hrs
   d. Days to weeks

[Ref: Robbins 9th/e pg. 598-602]

105. In POEM syndrome, E stands for: *(PGMEE 2016)*
   a. Endocrinopathy
   b. Eosinophilia
   c. Edema
   d. Erythema

[Ref: Robbins 9th/e pg. 598-602]

Explanation
- POEMS stands for Polyneuropathy, Organomegaly, Endocrinopathy, Monoclonal Gammopathy, and Skin changes.
- It is seen in the setting of a plasma cell dyscrasia.

MONOCLONAL GAMMOPATHIES

106. False statement about monoclonal gammopathy of undetermined significance (MGUS) *(PGMEE 2015)*
   a. <3g/dL of monoclonal protein
   b. Bone marrow plasma cells < 10%
   c. No bence jones proteinuria
   d. Does not progress to multiple myeloma

[Ref: Robbins 9th/pg 598-602]

107. False statement about MGUS *(PGMEE 2015)*
   a. Secrete M protein
   b. Asymptomatic
   c. Few progress to multiple myeloma
   d. Bence jones proteinuria

[Ref: Robbins 9th/e pg. 598-602]

108. Most common heavy chain disease is: *(PGMEE 2014-15)*
   a. Franklin disease
   b. Seligmann disease (Alpha heavy chain disease]
   c. Mu heavy chain disease
   d. Waldenstrom cryoglobulinemia

[Ref: Harrison's 19th/e pg. 718]

109. Which of the following is associated with Bence jones proteinuria? *(PGMEE 2014-15)*
   a. γ chain disease
   b. α chain disease
   c. λ chain disease
   d. μ chain disease

[Ref: Harrison's 19th/e pg. 721]

110. Kappa light chains in urine are seen in: *(PGMEE 2014-15)*
   a. Mu chain disease
   b. Seligman disease
   c. Franklin disease
   d. Waldenstrom macroglobulinemia

[Ref: Hematology in clinical practice. 4th ed. ch. 25 Harrison's 18th ed. ch. 111]

WALDENSTROM MACROGLOBULINEMIA (WG)

111. Which antibody is commonly elevated in Waldenstrom macroglobinemia? *(PGMEE 2012)*
- a. IgA
- b. IgD
- c. IgG
- d. IgM

[Ref: Robbins 9th/e pg. 598]

112. M splike in waldenstorm macroglobulinemia is due to *(PGMEE 2015)*
- a. IgM
- b. IgG
- c. IgA
- d. IgD

[Ref: Robbins 9th/pg 598-602]

113. In lymphoplasmacytoid lymphoma which of the following monoclonal immunoglobulin is seen: *(PGMEE 2014-15)*
- a. IgA
- b. IgD
- c. IgG
- d. IgM

[Ref: Harrison's 19th/e pg. 706]

Explanation

- Lymphoplasmacytic lymphoma is the tissue manifestation of Waldenstrom's macro globulinemia.
- It has been associated with chronic Hepatitis C infection
- Patients often have high levels of monoclonal IgM protein
- It is a B-cell neoplasm
- Cells express B-cell markers such as CD 20

MULTIPLE MYELOMA

114. A 60 years old male presented with 'punched out' lesions of the head on x ray. His routine blood and urine examination is normal. Histopathology image of lesion is shown. Diagnosis is *(PGMEE 2019)*
- a. Histiocytosis
- b. Multiple myeloma
- c. Waldenstrom's macroglobulinemia
- d. Monoclonal gammopathy

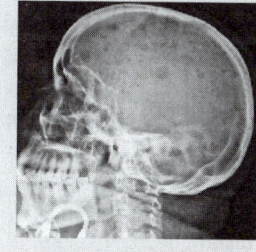 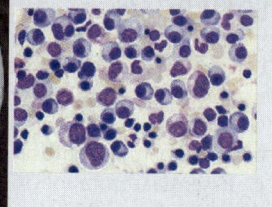

115. Drugs used in management relapsed multiple myeloma is: *(NEET Pattern 2019)*
- a. Bortezomib
- b. Lenalidomide
- c. Doxorubicin
- d. All of the above

116. Russell bodies are found in *(PGMEE 2012-13)*
- a. Intracranial neoplasm
- b. Parkinsonism
- c. Multiple Myeloma
- d. Gonadal tumor

[Ref: Robbin's 8th/e p. 610]

117. Multiple myeloma is diagnosed by *(DNB June 07)*
- a. > 10% Plasmacytosis
- b. Kidney biopsy
- c. 24 hours urine protein
- d. Rouleaux formation in blood

[Ref: Robbins 9th/e pg. 599 and Tejinder Singh p. 210, 211]

118. Which of the following metabolic abnormality is seen in multiple myeloma *(DNB Dec 08)*
- a. Hyponatremia
- b. Hyperphosphatemia
- c. Hypokalemia
- d. Hypercalcemia

[Ref: Harrison 18th/e p. 938-940; Robbins 9th/e pg. 600]

119. Large homogenous eosinophilic inclusions in plasma cells are called *(PGMEE 2015)*
- a. Mallory hyaline bodies
- b. Councilman bodies
- c. Russell bodies
- d. Dutcher bodies

[Ref: Robbins 9th/e pg. 598-602]

120. Russell bodies are seen in *(PGMEE 2015)*
- a. Histiocytes
- b. Plasma cells
- c. Mast cells
- d. Langerhan cells

[Ref: Robbins 9th/e pg. 598-602]

121. The single most important predictor of survival in multiple myeloma *(PGMEE 2015)*
- a. IL-6 levels
- b. CD 138 positivity
- c. Bence jones proteinuria
- d. Serum β2-microglobulin

[Ref: Robbins 9th/pg 598-602]

122. Russell bodies are seen in *(PGMEE 08)*
- a. Lymphocytes
- b. Neutrophils
- c. Macrophages
- d. Plasma cells

[Ref: Robbins 9th/e pg. 599]

123. All are seen in multiple myeloma EXCEPT: *(DNB June 2011)*
- a. Bleeding tendency
- b. Visual disturbance
- c. Proteinuria
- d. Dystrophic Calcification

[Ref: Harrison's 19th/e pg 713]

124. Bence Jones proteinuria is best detected by? *(PGMEE 2014-15)*
- a. Dipstick method
- b. Sulfosalicylic acid
- c. Heat test
- d. Electrophoresis

[Ref: Harrison's 19th/e pg. 721]

125. Hypercalcemia is caused by all EXCEPT *(DNB June 2010)*
- a. Multiple myeloma
- b. Lytic skeletal metastases
- c. Acute pancreatitis
- d. Total parenteral nutrition

[Ref: Harrison's 19th/e pg 313]

126. Which of the following is the least common feature of Multiple Myeloma? *(PGMEE 2014-15)*
- a. Bone pain
- b. Normocytic Normochromic Anemia
- c. Susceptibility to bacterial Infection
- d. Hyperviscosity syndrome

[Ref: Harrison's 19th/e pg. 721]

111.	d
112.	a
113.	d
114.	b
115.	d
116.	c
117.	a
118.	d
119.	d
120.	b
121.	d
122.	d
123.	d
124.	d
125.	c
126.	d

127. Classical 'Rain drop' lesions are seen in:
(PGMEE 2014-15)
a. Burkitt's lymphoma
b. Hodgkin's lymphoma
c. Multiple myeloma
d. Haemophilia

[Ref: Harrison's 19th/e pg. 72]

128. Commonest site of lytic lesion in multiple myeloma is:
(PGMEE 2014-15)
a. Vertebral column
b. Femur
c. Clavicle
d. Pelvis

[Ref: Harrison's 19th/e pg. 721]

129. Most common cause of kidney involvement in multiple myeloma:
(PGMEE 2014-15)
a. Hypercalcemia
b. Amyloid deposition
c. Tubular proteinuria
d. Hyperviscosity

[Ref: Wintrobe Hematology: pg. 5184, Harrison's 19th/e pg. 721]

130. ESR is decreased in all the following conditions except
(PGMEE 2015)
a. Sickle cell anemia
b. Polycythemia
c. Congestive cardiac failure
d. Multiple myeloma

[Ref: Dacie 11th/pg 105; Harrison's 19th/e pg. 635]

131. Most common symptom of multiple myeloma:
(PGMEE 2014-15)
a. Bone pain
b. Anemia
c. Hypercalcemia
d. Bleeding

[Ref: Harrison's 19th/e pg. 721]

132. . Immunoglobulin not affected in Multiple myeloma:
(PGMEE 2014-15)
a. IgG
b. IgA
c. IgM
d. IgD

[Ref: Harrison's 19th/e pg. 722]

133. All of the following are true about multiple myeloma EXCEPT:
(PGMEE 2014-15)
a. Lytic bone lesions
b. Back pain
c. Polycythemia
d. Viscosity of blood

[Ref: Harrison's 19th/e pg. 721]

134. Most common cause of death in multiple myeloma is:
(PGMEE 2014-15)
a. Infection
b. Bleeding
c. CHF
d. Kidney failure

[Ref: Wintrobe Hematology 11th ed. pg. 5185, Harrison's 19th/e pg. 721]

135. Maximum ESR is seen in:
(PGMEE 2014-15)
a. CHF
b. Polycythemia vera
c. Multiple myeloma
d. Sickle cell anemia

[Ref: Harrison's 19th/e pg. 721]

136. A drug not effective in multiple myeloma is?
(DNB June 2009)
a. Bortezomib
b. Hydroxyurea
c. Melphalan
d. Cyclophosphamide

[Ref: Harrison's 19th/e pg 716]

137. In multiple myeloma treatment, the following drug is avoided during induction therapy for transplant candidates
(PGMEE 2015)
a. Bortezomib
b. Thalidomide
c. Melphalan
d. Dexamethasone

[Ref: Robbins 9th/e pg. 598-602; Harrison's 19th/e pg. 721]

MYELOPROLIFERATIVE DISORDERS

138. Myeloproliferative diseases include all EXCEPT:
(PGMEE 2014-15)
a. Myelofibrosis
b. Chronic neutrophilic leukemia
c. Acute myelogenous leukemia (AML)
d. Systemic mastocytosis

[Ref: Robbin's 8th/e p. 626; Harrison's 19th/e pg. 672]

139. Mutation seen in systemic mastocytosis *(PGMEE 2015)*
a. BCR-ABL fusion gene
b. FGFR1 fusion genes
c. JAK 2 point mutation
d. c-kit point mutation

[Ref: Robbins 9th/pg 616-620]

140. Highest LAP score is seen in? *(PGMEE 2015)*
a. Acute Myeloid Leukemia
b. Polycythemia Vera
c. Paroxysmal Nocturnal Hemoglobinuria
d. Chronic myeloid Leukemia

[Ref: Wintrobe's 12th/pg 180-190]

ESSENTIAL THROMBOCYTOSIS

141. Not seen in essential thrombocytosis *(PGMEE 2015)*
a. Erythromelagia
b. Abnormally large platelets
c. Activating mutation in JAK2 gene
d. Marrow fibrosis

[Ref: Robbins 9th/pg 620/630]

142. Thrombocythemia is characterized by- *(PGMEE 2015)*
a. Monocytosis
b. Low platelets
c. Neutrophilia
d. Platelets elevation

[Ref: Harrison 18th/e ch. 115]

MYELOFIBROSIS

143. Triad of leukoerythroblastosis, tear drop erythrocytes and large platelets is seen in *(PGMEE 2015)*
a. Myelodysplastic syndrome
b. Primary myelofibrosis
c. Essential thrombocytosis
d. Langerhan cell histiocytosis

[Ref: Robbins 9th/pg 620/630]

144. Bone marrow finding in myelofibrosis is? *(PGMEE 2012)*
a. Leucoerythroblastosis
b. Tear drop cells
c. Leucocytopenia
d. All of the above

[Ref: Robbin's 8th/e Chapter 13]

145. Bone marrow finding in myelofibrosis *(PGMEE 2013-14)*
a. Dry tap (hypocellular]
b. Microcytic cells
c. Thrombocytosis
d. Megalobastic

[Ref: Robbin's 8th/e p. 630; Chandrasoma Taylor 8th/e p. 421]

127.	c
128.	a
129.	c
130.	d
131.	a
132.	c
133.	c
134.	a
135.	c
136.	b
137.	d
138.	c
139.	d
140.	b
141.	d
142.	d
143.	b
144.	d
145.	a

146. 45 year male presents with leukoerythroblastic blood picture in PBS with dry tap, What is your diagnosis? *(PGMEE 2015)*
a. AML
b. ALL
c. CML
d. Myelofibrosis

[Ref: Robbins 9th/pg]

147. All of the following are true regarding myelo-fibrosis EXCEPT: *(PGMEE 2014-15)*
a. Tear drop poikilocytes
b. Giant abnormal platelets
c. Leucoerythroblastic blood picture
d. Absent spleen

[Ref: Harrison's 19th/e pg. 675]

POLYCYTHEMIA VERA

148. Most common myeloproliferative disorder: *(PGMEE 2014-15)*
a. Polycythemia vera
b. CML
c. Chronic eosinophilic leukemia
d. Myelofibrosis

[Ref: Harrison's 19th/e pg. 673]

149. LAP score is maximum in? *(PGMEE 2013)*
a. Essential thrombocytosis
b. CML
c. AML
d. Polycythemia vera

[Ref: Wintrobe's 12th/e p. 14, 15]

150. Abnormally high LAP score is seen in *((DNB Dec 07)*
a. CLL
b. Polycythemia vera
c. PNH
d. All

[Ref: Wintrobe 16th/e 27]

151. All are true about Polycythemia vera except- *(PGMEE 2013-14)*
a. Increased platelets
b. Decreased LAP score
c. Increased vit B$_{12}$
d. Leucocytosis

[Ref: Robbin's 8th/e p. 14]

152. Which is not seen in Polycythemia vera- *(PGMEE 2012-13)*
a. Ocular congestion
b. Increased Vit B$_{12}$ binding capacity
c. Increased RBC count
d. Increased erythropoietin level

[Ref: Robbin's 8th/e p. 629; Harrison 18th/e p. 898, 899]

153. Polycythemia is not caused by *(PGMEE 2013-14)*
a. Liver carcinoma
b. Cerebellar hemangioma
c. Renal carcinoma
d. Lung carcinoma

[Ref: Harrison 18th/e p. 831, 832; Robbin's 8th/e p. 321]

154. All are true about Polycythemia vera except- *(PGMEE 2014, 2012)*
a. Increased ESR
b. Increased LAP score
c. Increased blood volume
d. Decreased erythropoietin

[Ref: Robbin's 8th/e p. 629; Harrison 18th/e p. 898, 899]

155. The following is true regarding polycythermia vera? *(PGMEE 2015)*
a. Raised ESR
b. Decrease LAP score
c. Thrombocytopenia
d. Leukocytosis

[Ref: Robbins 9th/e pg. 618- 619]

156. Not seen in polycythemia vera *(PGMEE 2015)*
a. Platelet function abnormalities
b. Low ESR
c. Abnormal oxygen saturation
d. Normal red cell morphology

[Ref: Robbins 9th/e pg. 618]

157. Erythromelalgia in polycythemia vera is a complication of *(PGMEE 2015)*
a. Lymphocytosis
b. Thrombocytosis
c. Granulocytosis
d. Erythrocytosis

[Ref: Robbins 9th/pg 618]

158. Which of the following is NOT commonly seen in polycythemia vera ? *(PGMEE 16)*
a. Hyperuricemia
b. Thrombosis
c. Prone for Acute Leukemia
d. Spontaneous severe infection

[Ref: Robbins 9th/e pg. 618]

159. Gaisbock syndrome is known as- *(PGMEE 2015)*
a. Polycythemia vera
b. Spurious Polycytemia
c. High altitude Erythrocytosis
d. Primary familial polycytemia

[Ref: Wintrobe 12th/e p. 1263]

160. Erythropoietin is increased in all of the following conditions EXCEPT: *(PGMEE 2014-15)*
a. Hepatocellular carcinoma
b. Renal cell carcinoma
c. Cerebellar Hemangioblastoma
d. Pancreatic carcinoma

[Ref: Harrison's 18th ed. pg. 899]

161. All of the following conditions may be associated with a thymoma, EXCEPT: *(PGMEE 2014-15)*
a. Erythrocytosis
b. Hypogammaglobulinemia
c. Myasthenia gravis
d. Pure red blood cell aplasia

[Ref: Harrison's 19th/e pg. 668]

162. Polycythaemia is commonly seen in: *(PGMEE 2014-15)*
a. Congestive cardiac failure
b. Hereditary spherocytosis
c. Chronic cor pulmonale
d. Uncomplicated ASD

[Ref: Harrison's 18th ed. ch. 108]

163. Which of the following statements about erythropoietin is FALSE? *(PGMEE 2014-15)*
a. It is used for the treatment of anemia due to chronic renal failure
b. It results in decrease in reticulocyte count
c. It decrease the requirement of blood transfusions
d. It can cause hypertension

[Ref: Katzung 10th/537-538;KDT's 6th/592]

146.	d
147.	d
148.	a
149.	d
150.	b
151.	b
152.	d
153.	d
154.	a
155.	d
156.	c
157.	b
158.	d
159.	b
160.	d
161.	a
162.	c
163.	b

164. Polycythemia vera is absolute venous hematocrit of >: *(PGMEE 2014-15)*

a. 45%   b. 55%
c. 65%   d. 70%

[Ref: Harrison's 19th/e pg. 674]

165. Which one of the following is not commonly seen in polycythemia vera? *(PGMEE 2014-15)*

a. Thrombosis
b. Hyperuricemia
c. Prone for acute leukemia
d. Spontaneous severe infection

[Ref: Harrison's 19th/e pg. 673]

166. True about polycythemia rubra vera is all EXCEPT: *(PGMEE 2014-15)*

a. Bleeding   b. Thrombosis
c. ↓ed ESR   d. Increased erythropoietin

[Ref: Harrison's 19th/e pg. 678]

167. Polycythaemia vera is associated with all EXCEPT: *(PGMEE 2014-15)*

a. Increased red cell mass   b. Leukocytosis
c. Splenomegaly   d. Decreased platelet count

[Ref: Harrison's 19th/e pg. 674]

168. Not related to Polycythemia Vera: *(PGMEE 2014-15)*
a. Budd chiari syndrome   b. Hypertension
c. Erythromelalgia   d. Infections

[Ref: Harrison's 19th/e pg. 672]

169. Essential WHO criteria for polycythemia vera: *(PGMEE 2014-15)*

a. Tyrosine kinase JAK2 mutation
b. Low levels of erythropoietin levels
c. Thrombocytosis
d. Increased MCV

[Ref: Harrison's 19th/e pg. 672]

170. A 59-year-old male came with Hb 18.0 gm/dl on three occasions. The resident doctor wants to exclude Polycythemia Vera. Which of the following is the most relevant investigation: *(PGMEE 04)*

a. Hematocrit   b. Total leukocyte count
c. Red cell mass   d. Reticulocyte count

[Ref: Harrison 18th/p 899;]

CHRONIC MYELOCYTIC LEUKEMIA

171. Robertsonian translocation is seen in? *(PGMEE 2016)*

a. AML   b. CML
c. CLL   d. ALL

[Ref: Robbins 9th/e pg. 616- 618]

172. True about Robertsonian translocation is? *(PGMEE 2016)*

a. Acrocentric chromosome involved
b. Poor prognosis
c. Large part is lost
d. Balanced translocation

[Ref: Robbins 9th/e pg. 160]

173. BCR ABL gene mutation is seen in? *(DNB June 09)*
a. AML   b. ALL
c. CML   d. CLL

[Ref: Robbins 9th/pg 616-618]

174. Best investigation for BCR-ABL fusion gene *(PGMEE 2015)*

a. RT-PCR (Reverse transcriptase-Polymerase chain reaction)
b. Fluorescent in situ hybridization (FISH)
c. Karyotyping
d. Flow cytometry

[Ref: Robbins 9th/e pg. 170, 616-618]

175. Increase in alkaline phosphatase is seen in *(DNB 2007, June 2009)*

a. CML   b. Leukemoid reaction
c. Eosinophilia   d. Malaria

[Ref: Page 19 Wintrobes, 11th Edition]

176. Which one of the following laboratory tests differentiates leukamoid reaction from chronic myeloid leukemia? *(PGMEE 2014-15)*

a. LAP (Leukocyte alkaline phosphatase)
b. LCA (Leukocyte common antigen)
c. MPO (Myelo-peroxidase)
d. TRAP (Tartrate resistant alkaline phosphatase]

[Ref: Harrison's 18th ed. pg. 477]

177. Chromosomal transocation seen in CML is? *(DNB June 09, Dec 2011)*

a. 2:8   b. 9:22
c. 11:14   d. 15:17

[Ref: Robbin's 8th/e p. 627]

178. Philadelphia chromosome refers: *(PGMEE 2015-16)*

a. Long arm of chromosome 9 and long arm of chromosome 22
b. Short arm of chromosome 9 and short arm of chromosome 22
c. Short arm of chromosome 9 and long chromosome 22
d. Long arm of chromosome 9 and short arm of chromosome 2

[Ref: Harrison 19th ed. / 101e-3]

179. Hyposegmented neutrophils are seen in *(PGMEE 2015)*

a. Accelerated phase of CML
b. Sideroblastic anemia
c. Megaloblastic anemia
d. Blast crisis phase of CML

[Ref: Robbins 9th/e pg. 616- 618]

180. Sea blue histiocytes are seen in *(PGMEE 2015)*

a. Chronic lymphoblastic leukemia
b. Chronic myeloid leukemia
c. Burkitt lymphoma
d. Langerhan cell histiocytosis

[Ref: Internet]

181. Priapism can be due to? *(PGMEE 2015-16)*

a. CML   b. Myelo-fibrosis
c. A.I.H.   d. Thrombocytopenia

[Ref: Harrison 19th ed. / 324, 634]

164.	b
165.	d
166.	d
167.	d
168.	d
169.	a
170.	c
171.	b
172.	a
173.	c
174.	b
175.	a
176.	a
177.	b
178.	a
179.	d
180.	b
181.	a

182. Therepeutic phlebotomy is not done in which of the following conditions? *(PGMEE 2015)*
a. CML
b. Hemochromatosis
c. Polycythemia vera
d. Porphyria cutanea tarda

[Ref: Nelson 20th/e/ch 495]

183. Not a feature of juvenile CML *(PGMEE 2012-13, 2014-15)*
a. Fetal hemoglobin is increased
b. Thrombocytopenia
c. Lymphadenopathy
d. Philadelphia chromosome is positive

[Ref: O.P. Ghai 8th/e/p 608; Harrison's 19th/e pg. 687]

184. Drug of choice for CML is? *(DNB June 2011)*
a. Imatinib
b. IFN
c. Infliximab
d. Hydroxurea

[Ref: Harrison's 19th/e pg 691]

185. Vitamin B12 level in chronic myeloid leukemia is: *(PGMEE 2014-15)*
a. Elevated
b. Decreased (slightly]
c. Normal
d. Markedly decreased

[Ref: Harrison's 19th/e pg. 687]

186. What is the most effective treatment for chronic myeloid leukaemia? *(PGMEE 2014-15)*
a. Allogeneic bone marrow transplantation
b. Heterogeneic bone marrow transplantation
c. Chemotherapy
d. Hydroxyurea and interferon

[Ref: Harrison's 19th/e pg. 694]

187. A peripheral smear with increased neutrophils, basophils, eosinophils, and platelets is highly suggestive of: *(PGMEE 2014-15)*
a. Actute myeloid leukemia
b. Acute lymphoblastic leukemia
c. Chronic myelogenous leukemia
d. Myelodysplastic syndrome

[Ref: Harrison's 19th/e pg. 687]

188. Treatment of choice for CML *(PGMEE 2015)*
a. Erlotinib
b. Imatinib mesylate
c. Sunitinib
d. Sorafenib

[Ref: Robbins 9th/pg 617]

LANGERHANS CELL HISTIOCYTOSIS (LCH)

189. In Langerhans Cell Histiocytosis (LCH), the characteristic abnormality seen in cytoplasm is:- *(PGMEE 2015; 2007)*
a. Birbecks granules
b. Macrophages
c. Giant cell
d. Plasma cell

[Ref: Wintrobe's 12th/pg 1573]

190. Localised langerhans cells histiocytosis affecting head and neck is *(PGMEE 2014)*
a. Letterer-siwe disease
b. Hand-schuller-christian disease
c. Pulmonary Langerhans cell histiocytosis
d. Eosinophilic granuloma

[Ref: Robbins 9th/e pg. 631-632]

191. Marker of Langerhan's cell histiocytosis
a. CD 100
b. CD 43
c. CD 1a
d. CD 15

[Ref: Robbins 9th/pg 621]

192. Baby has recurrent infection of ear and seborrheic dermatitis. Examination findings are hepatosplenomegaly with painless cystic skull lesions. Probable diagnosis is- *(PGMEE 2012-13)*
a. ALL
b. Multiple myeloma
c. Hemophagocytic lymphohistiocytosis
d. Langerhans cell histiocytosis

[Ref: Ghai 8th/e/p 620; Nelson 20th/e/p 507.1]

193. A 2-year old child comes with ear discharge, seborrheic dermatitis, polyuria and hepatos-plenomegaly. Which of the following is the most likely diagnosis: *(PGMEE 2014-15)*
a. Leukemia
b. Lymphoma
c. Langerhan's cell histiocytosis
d. Germ cell tumor

[Ref: O.P. Ghai 7th ed. pg. 595, Harrison's 19th/e pg. 1713]

194. CD marker of Langerhans cell histiocytosis is: *(PGMEE 2013-14)*
a. CD1a
b. CD100
c. CD1c
d. CD1b

[Ref: Robbins 9th/pg 621]

MISCELLANEOUS

195. Steroids are not indicated in the treatment of? *(NEET Pattern 2015)*
a. Kaposi Sarcoma
b. Hodgkin Lymphoma
c. CLL
d. Multiple Myeloma

[Ref: page 716: Harrison 19th edition]

196. CD marker of Angiosarcoma is? *(PGMEE 2013)*
a. CD 10
b. CD 19
c. CD 25
d. CD 31

[Ref: Textbook of dermatology surgery volume 1 by Luigi Rusciani, Rusciani-Robbins, Perry Robins p. 447]

197. All are true regarding hemophagocytic lymphohistiocytosis (HLH) except? *(PGMEE 2015)*
a. Cytopenias due to phagocytosis of progenitors in bone marrow
b. Activation of macrophages and CD 8+ T cells
c. HTLV-1 is a cause in immunodeficient patients
d. Abnormal liver function tests

[Ref: Robbins 9th/pg 239-242]

182.	a
183.	d
184.	a
185.	a
186.	a
187.	c
188.	b
189.	a
190.	d
191.	c
192.	d
193.	c
194.	a
195.	a
196.	d
197.	c

STORAGE OF BLOOD PRODUCTS

1. Fist covers surface area of ml of blood loss
(PGMEE 2014)

a. 20 ml
b. 30 ml
c. 50 ml
d. 80 ml

[Ref: Wintrobe's clinical hematology]

2. Addition of glucose to stored blood causes?
(DNB Dec. 2011)

a. Prevent Hyperkalemia
b. Increases 2,3 DPG
c. Increase acidosis of blood
d. Prevent hemolysis

[Ref: Ganong's 25th/e pg. 558]

3. Preservatives used for storing blood for transfusion is –
(PGMEE 92)

a. Heparin + dextrose
b. EDTA
c. Citrate + glucose
d. CDP-A

[Ref: Ganong's 25th/e pg. 558]

4. Blood when stored at 4⁰C can be kept for
(PGMEE 2008; DNB June 07)

a. 7 days
b. 14 days
c. 21 days
d. 35 days

[Ref: Textbook of blood bank and transfusion medicine p. 64]

Explanation

- CPDA-1 is a commonly used preservative for storage of blood required for transfusion. Shelf life of blood stored in CPDA-1 at 2-4⁰C is 35 days where as the shelf life of blood which was previously stored in CPD was only 21 days.

5. How long can blood be stored with CPD-A-
(DNB June 08)

a. 21 days
b. 28 days
c. 35 days
d. 42 days

[Ref: Textbook of blood bank and transfusion medicine p. 64]

6. Which of the following anticoagulant preservative can be used to store blood, so that it can be kept for 35 days?
(NEET Pattern 2017)

a. Acid citrate dextrose (ACD)
b. Citrate phosphate dextrose adenine (CPDA)
c. CPD Citrate phosphate dextrose
d. CP2D citrate phosphate double dextrose

[Ref: Wintrobe's clinical hematology 12th edition, chapter 23]

Explanation

- CPDA-1 is CPD supplemented with adenine. CPDA-1 is now one of the standard anticoagulant-preservative solutions in clinical use. The shelf life of RBC concentrates in CPDA-1 is 35 days

7. Citrate Phosphate Dextrose (CPD) blood is preferred to Acid Citrate Dextrose (ACD) blood in a patient with hypoxia due to
(PGMEE 2019)

a. Less fall in 2, 3 DPG
b. Less P 50
c. Less glycolysis
d. Prevention of caramelization of sugar

Explanation

- Infusion of ACD blood causes P50 and 2,3-DPG concentration to decrease significantly.
- The infusion of blood stored in CPD did not significantly increase the oxygen affinity.

Citrate Phosphate Dextrose (CPD)	Acid Citrate Dextrose (ACD)
▪ CPD is commonly used	▪ Used in apheresis procedure ▪ Citric acid, sodium citrate, and dextrose (pH 5)
▪ Alkaline pH and PO4 help in maintaining 2, 3- DPG	▪ Acid pH does not help in maintaining 2,3-DPG levels ▪ Prevents caramelization of sugar
▪ Shelf life of 28 days	▪ Shelf life of 21 days

8. Whole blood is stored at blood bank at? *(PGMEE 2015)*

a. -4°C
b. 0°C
c. 4°C
d. 8°C

[Ref: Wintrobe'ss 12thed/pg 665-666]

9. Storage temperature of platelets is: *(PGMEE 2014-15)*

a. – 4 degrees Celsius
b. + 4 degrees Celsius
c. – 20 degrees Celsius
d. + 20-24 degrees Celsius

[Ref: Wintrobe's Hematology 11th ed. 1681, Harrison's 19th/e pg. 138e-4]

10. Anticoagulant used for blood glucose estimation is?
(PGMEE 2012)

a. Sodium fluoride
b. Double oxalate
c. Oxalate
d. Citrate

[Ref: Textbook of practical physiology 2nd/e by G.K. Pal, Pravati p. 9, Manual of Basic Techniques for a health Laboratory by WHO p. 69]

11. A voluntary donor, underwent apheresis for platelet donation for the first time at a platelet count of 1.9 × 10³/ mL. He started having tingling sensation (perioral) and numbness because. *(NEET Pattern 2017)*

a. His platelet count was low for donation
b. It was his first donation
c. Due to fluid depletion
d. Due to citrate based anticoagulant

[Ref: Henry's clinical diagnosis and management by lab oratory methods 22nd edition pg 771]

1.	a
2.	b
3.	d
4.	d
5.	c
6.	b
7.	a
8.	c
9.	d
10.	a
11.	d

Explanation

- Citrate is used as the primary anticoagulant in both donor and therapeutic apheresis
- Citrate infusion can result in symptomatic hypocalcemia in a donor/patient due to decrease in ionized calcium to levels at which the nerne mebrane excitability reaches to the point where spontaneous depolarization can occur
- Sign and symptoms include perioral paresthesia, acral paresthesia, shivering, light headedness, twitching and tremors.

12. **What should be the sequence of events during collection of blood sample.** *(NEET Pattern 2017)*
a. Ask the patient his name → verify from file → collect blood → Label the sample at bedside
b. Look at the file→Collect sample → Label the sample at bedside
c. Prelabel the sample vials→Check the file patient details → Collect sample
d. Collect sample→Confirm name from file → Label the sample vial

13. **Which is best vial for sending a blood sample for serum electrolyte analysis?** *(NEET Pattern 2017)*
a. Sodium fluoride
b. Lithium heparin
c. EDTA
d. Citrate

BLOOD GROUPS

14. **There are more than 400 blood groups, we consider only ABO blood group, because:** *(PGMEE 2014-15)*
a. Presence of antibodies in the serum when the RBC lacks the corresponding antigen
b. A andB antigens are secreted by cells which are not in the circulation only.
c. Soluble blood group antigens cannot block binding of organisms to polysaccharides.
d. These antigens are lipoproteins

[Ref: Harrison's 19th/e pg. 138e-1]

15. **True about Rh factor is** *(PGMEE 2014-15)*
a. There are no natural anti-Rh antibodies in serum
b. Seen only in females
c. Approximately 15 % of Indians are Rh positive
d. D is the least powerful Rh antigen

[Ref: Harrison's 18th ed. ch. 113]

16. **Duffy antigen is associates with** *(PGMEE 2016)*
a. Plasmodium vivax
b. Falciparum
c. Ovale
d. Malaria

[Ref: Harrison 18th/pg 1014]

17. **ABO antigens are not found in-** *(DNB June 10)*
a. Plasma
b. Semen
c. CSF
d. Saiva

[Ref: Reddy 18th/e p. 369; Ganong 22nd/e p. 537]

18. **Blood group ABO antigens are located on which chromosome?** *(PGMEE 2016)*
a. Chromosome 1
b. Chromosome 3
c. Chromosome 19
d. Chromosome 9

[Ref: Dacie/pg 486, 487]

19. **Rh gene is located on which chromosome?** *(PGMEE 2016)*
a. Chromosome 1
b. Chromosome 6
c. Chromosome 9
d. Chromosome 19

[Ref: Dacie/pg 486, 487]

20. **Blood group antigen NAG transferase present but galactosyl transferase is absent is** *(PGMEE 2014)*
a. Group A
b. Group AB
c. Group B
d. Group O

[Ref: Ganong's 25th/e pg. 558]

21. **Bombay blood group contains?** *(PGMEE 2016)*
a. Anti H
b. Anti A, Anti B, Anti H
c. Anti A , Anti B
d. H antibody

[Ref: Dacie/pg 487]

22. **Patient with blood group O can receive plasma from?** *(PGMEE 2015)*
a. Group A
b. Group O
c. Group AB
d. All of the above

[Ref: Ganong's 25th/e pg. 558]

23. **Which of the following is universal donor blood group-** *(PGMEE 2014)*
a. A
b. B
c. AB
d. O

[Ref: Ganong's 25th/e pg. 558]

24. **Identify the blood group** *(PGMEE 2019)*

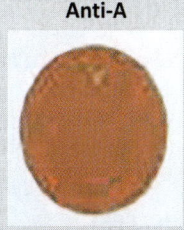 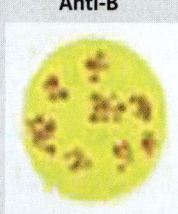

Anti-A   Anti-B

a. AB+
b. A+
c. B+
d. O+

BLOOD PRODUCTS

25. **Half life of transfused platelets is** *(PGMEE 87)*
a. 15 Days
b. 4 Days
c. 8 Days
d. 4 Hours

[Ref: Rassi's transfusion medicine]

26. **Best blood product to be given in a patient of multiple clotting factor deficiency with active bleeding is?** *(NEET Pattern 2015)*
a. Fresh Frozen Plasma
b. Whole blood
c. Packed RBCs
d. Cryoprecipitate

[Ref: Wintrobes 12thed/pg 677]

27. **Cryoprecipitate is useful in?** *(PGMEE 2013)*
a. Thrombasthenia
b. Warfarin reversal
c. Afibrinogenemia
d. Hemophilia A

[Ref: William's hematology 12th/e p. 695]

12.	a
13.	b
14.	a
15.	a
16.	a
17.	c
18.	d
19.	a
20.	a
21.	b
22.	b
23.	d
24.	c
25.	b
26.	a
27.	c,d

28. Which disease is transmitted by all the components of blood: *(PGMEE 2013-14)*
   a. Malaria
   b. H. pylori
   c. Toxoplasma
   d. Syphilis

   [Ref: Textbook of transfusion medicine 11th/e p. 743]

29. Before transplant surgery blood products are irradiated with: *(PGMEE 2016)*
   a. α Rays
   b. β Rays
   c. γ Rays
   d. X-Rays

   [Ref: Wintrobes 12thed/pg 699]

30. Rise in hemoglobin levels after one unit of whole blood transfusion is? *(DNB June 07)*
   a. 0.55%
   b. 1%
   c. 1.5%
   d. 2%

   [Ref: Textbook of Blood Banking and Transfusion Medicine 2nd/e by Sally V. Rudman p. 451]

31. Shelf life of gamma irradiated packed RBCs is? *(PGMEE 2016)*
   a. 21 d
   b. 28 d
   c. 35 d
   d. 42 d

   [Ref: Wintrobes 12thed/pg 677]

32. Blood when stored at 4°C can be kept for a duration of- *(PGMEE 2013-14)*
   a. 28 days
   b. 7 days
   c. 21 days
   d. 14 days

   [Ref: Textbook of blood bank and transfusion medicine p. 64]

33. Life span of transfused platelets is? *(PGMEE 2016)*
   a. <24 hrs
   b. 1-3 days
   c. 3-5 days
   d. 7-14 days

   [Ref: Wintrobes 12thed/pg 687]

34. Shelf life is maximum for? *(PGMEE 2015)*
   a. Whole blood
   b. FFP
   c. Platelet concenterate
   d. PRBC

   [Ref: Wintrobes 12thed/pg 677]

35. Cryoprecipitate does not contain? *(PGMEE 2014-15)*
   a. Factor 8
   b. Factor 9
   c. Von wilebrand factor
   d. Fibrinogen

   [Ref: Hematology in clinical practice. 4th ed. ch. 37]

36. Indication of Cryoprecipitate? *(PGMEE 2015)*
   a. DIC
   b. vWD
   c. Hemophilia B
   d. Severe plasma loss

   [Ref: Wintrobe's 12thed/pg695]

37. Cryoprecipitate is useful in: *(PGMEE 2013-14)*
   a. Warfarin reversal
   b. Hemophilia A
   c. Afibrinoogenemia
   d. Thrombosthenia

   [Ref: Williams hematology 12th/e p. 695; Guyton 11th/e p, 420; Choudhuri physiology 6th/e p. 32]

38. Not true regarding fresh frozen plasma: *(PGMEE 2012-13)*
   a. ABO match not required
   b. Should be used in replacement of factors in DIC/ trauma

   c. Supplies major coagulation factors
   d. To be used within 30 minutes of having trauma

   [Ref: Textbook of blood banking and transfusion medicine 8th/e p. 247-250]

39. Wrong about FFP: *(PGMEE 2014-15)*
   a. Stored at minus 18 degrees
   b. Given for reversal of warfarin toxicity
   c. ABO matching is mandatory before transfusion
   d. Deficient in factor 5 and 8

   [Ref: Hematology in clinical practice. 4th ed. ch. 37and ch. 33]

40. In massive transfusion of blood, citrate toxicity is primarily due to? *(PGMEE 2012)*
   a. Coagulopathy
   b. DIC
   c. Hemolysis
   d. Direct binding to calcium

   [Ref: Wintrobe's clinical hematology 11th/e Chapter 24]

BLOOD TRANSFUSION

41. All are true about cross-matching of blood except- *(PGMEE 2015)*
   a. Donor serum is tested against recipient packed cells
   b. Mandatory in all cases except emergency
   c. Involves visible agglutination
   d. Recipient serum is tested against donor packed cells

   [Ref: Harrison 19th/e p. 138e-2]

42. Platelets transfusion must be competed in how many hours after entering the bag- *(PGMEE 2015)*
   a. 1 hours
   b. 2 hours
   c. 3 hours
   d. 4 hours

   [Ref: Wintrobe's Clinical Hematology 13th/e p. 565]

43. The following is not true of platelet transfusion:
   a. Not Useful in ITP *(PGMEE 2014-15)*
   b. Used in D.I.C.
   c. Effective for 9-10 days
   d. Effect decrease with repeated usage

   [Ref: Harrison's 19th/e pg. 138e-1]

44. Shelf life of platelets in blood bank is: *(PGMEE 2014-15)*
   a. 5 days
   b. 7 days
   c. 10 days
   d. 21 days

   [Ref: Harrison's 19th/e pg. 138e-5]

45. Platelets transfusion must be completed in: *(PGMEE 2014-15)*
   a. 1 hour
   b. 2 hour
   c. 3 hour
   d. 4 hour

   [Ref: Wintrobe's Hematology 12th ed. 1683]

46. Platelets in stored blood do not survive after: *(PGMEE 2014-15)*
   a. 24 hours
   b. 48 hours
   c. 72 hours
   d. 96 hours

   [Ref: Wintrobe 13th ed. pg. 552 ; Harrison's 19th/e pg. 138e-4]

47. All are complications of blood transfusion except? *(PGMEE 2015-16)*
   a. Hypomagensemia
   b. Hypokalemia
   c. Hypocalcemia
   d. Metabolic alkalosis

   [Ref: Harrison's 19th/e pg. 138e-5]

28.	a
29.	c
30.	b
31.	b
32.	c
33.	c
34.	b
35.	b
36.	b
37.	c
38.	a,d
39.	d
40.	d
41.	a
42.	d
43.	c
44.	a
45.	d
46.	c
47.	b

48. Blood transfusion should be completed within _____ hours of initiation: *(PGMEE 2014-15)*

a. 1-4 hours
b. 3-6 hours
c. 4-8 hours
d. 8-12 hours

[Ref: Wintrobe's Hematology 11th ed. Pg 1679, Harrison's 19th/e pg. 138e-E]

49. Most common complication of massive transfusion: *(PGMEE 2014-15)*

a. Hypothermia
b. Acidosis
c. Hyperkalemia
d. Hypocalcemia

[Ref: Wintrobe Hematology: 11th ed. pg 1708, Harrison's 19th/e pg. 138e-5]

50. Transfusion associated lung injury (TRALI) is seen within -------- of transfusion: *(PGMEE 2018)*

a. Less than 6 hours
b. 12 hours
c. 24 hours
d. 48 hours

[Ref: Harrison 19/e, P. 728]

Explanation

Transfusion-related Acute Lung Injury

- Transfusion-related acute lung injury (TRALI) is the most common cause of transfusion related death.
- TRALI usually results from the transfusion of donor plasma that contains high-titer anti-HLA class II antibodies that bind recipient leukocytes.
- The recipient develops symptoms of hypoxia (PaO_2/FiO_2 <300 mm Hg) and signs of noncardiogenic pulmonary edema, including bilateral interstitial infiltrates on chest x-ray, either during or within 6 h of transfusion.
- Treatment is supportive.
- Testing the donor's plasma for anti-HLA antibodies can support this diagnosis

51. Which of the following is false about TRALI?

a. Develops within 24 hours *(NEET Pattern 2015)*
b. Mostly seen after sepsis and cardiac surgeries
c. It's a cause of non-cardiogenic pulmonary edema
d. Plasma is more likely to cause it than whole blood

[Ref: Wintrobes 12thed/pg 699]

52. Which one of the following is the cause of non - cardiogenic pulmonary oedema seen in immunologic blood transfusion reaction: *(PGMEE 2014-15)*

a. Antibody to IgA in donor plasma
b. Antibody to donor leukocyte antigen
c. Donor antibody to leukocyte of patient
d. RBC incomapatibility

[Ref: Harrison's 19th p 138e-5]

53. True about blood transfusion reaction: *(PGMEE 2014-15)*

a. Complement mediated severe hemolysis
b. Extravascular hemolysis
c. Transfusion should not be stopped
d. Death unlikely

[Ref: Harrison's 19th p 138e-5]

54. Complication of blood transfusion can be all EXCEPT: *(PGMEE 2014-15)*

a. Hyperkalemia
b. Citrate toxicity
c. Metabolic acidosis
d. Hypothermia

[Ref: Harrison's 19th/e pg. 138e-5]

55. Not an Indicator of mismatched Blood transfusion in patient under general anesthesia: *(PGMEE 2014-15)*

a. Fever with chills
b. Hypotension
c. Excessive oozing of blood from surgical site
d. Passage of black urine

[Ref: Wintrobe Hematology: 11th ed. pg. 1701]

56. Most common cause of febrile non haemolytic transfusion reaction? *(PGMEE 2014-15)*

a. ABO mismatch
b. Rh mismatch
c. HLA mismatch
d. All of the above

[Ref: Pg 1704: Wintrobe: Hematology: 11th ed., Harrison 19th/e pg. 138e-4/5]

57. Anti-D (Rho) Ig is used for the prevention of:

a. Sickle cell disease *(PGMEE 2014-15)*
b. Hemorrhagic disease of newborn
c. Paroxysmal haemoglobinuria
d. Hemolytic disease of newborn

[Ref: Harrison's 19th/e pg. 649]

58. Apheresis is: *(PGMEE 2014-15)*

a. Selective separation of components of blood
b. Preventing blood transfusion infections (HIV, HBV)
c. Separation of platelets from plasma
d. Isolating organisms from mixed culture

[Ref: Harrison's 19th/e pg. 138e-2]

59. Most common complication of blood transfusion: *(PGMEE 2014-15)*

a. Transfusion associated hepatitis
b. Hyperkalemia
c. Hemolysis
d. Febrile non hemolytic transfusion reaction

[Ref: Harrison's 19th/e pg. 138e]

60. Transfusing blood after prolonged storage could lead to: *(PGMEE 2014-15)*

a. Citrate intoxication
b. Potassium intoxication
c. Circulatory overload
d. Haemorrhagic diathesis

[Ref: Harrison's 19th/e pg. 138-e]

61. Acute renal failure in a patient who received incompatible blood transfusion with hemolytic reaction is best managed by: *(PGMEE 2014-15)*

a. 20% Mannitol
b. IV fluids with K+ supplementation
c. Alkalinizing the urine
d. Stopping blood transfusion

[Ref: Harrison's 19th/e pg. 138e-5]

62. Which of the following infection has highest chances of transmission by blood transfusion? *(PGMEE 2014-15)*

a. HIV
b. HBV
c. HTLV-1
d. HCV

[Ref: Wintrobe Hematology 11th ed. pg. 1712: Table 24.11, Harrison's 19th/e pg. 138e-3]

48.	a
49.	a
50.	a
51.	a
52.	c
53.	a
54.	c
55.	a
56.	c
57.	d
58.	a
59.	d
60.	b
61.	d
62.	b

CHAPTER 14

Oncology

FACTS

- *Hamartoma* → Cells with abnormal differentiation but present at normal location
- *Choristoma* → Cells with normal differentiation but present at abnormal location
- *Anaplasia* → Absence of differentiation. Hallmark of malignant transformation
- *Metastasis* → Most reliable feature of a malignant tumor
- *Examples of Oncogene:*
  - RAS, ABL, MYC, SIS, INT-2, KIT
- *Examples of Tumor suppressor gene:*
  - RB, P^{53}, NF, BRCA, APC
- MYC proto-oncogene codes for transcriptional factors that induce cell proliferation
- NF - 1 gene encodes for: Neurofibromin protein
- NF - 2 gene encodes for: Merlin protein
- The phosphorylation of this gene acts as a molecular ON - OFF switch for the cell cycle: Retinoblastoma gene
- Most carcinogenic UV rays to reach the earth: UV-B (280-320 nm)
- RET gene mutation is associated with: Medullary CA of Thyroid
- Valproate embryopathy is due to mutation in: HOX gene
- Vitamin A induced embryopathy is due to mutation in: TGF signaling pathway
- Which phase of cell cycle is considered as point of no return: S – phase
- Carcinogenic potential of a chemical is tested by: Ames test
- Almost all cancer can metastasize except:
  - Glioma
  - Rodent ulcer/Basal cell cancer of skin
- Familial Retinoblastoma is also associated with increased risk of: Osteosarcoma
- Only leukemia not associated with exposure of ionizing radiation: CLL
- Spontaneous regression of tumor is seen in: Neuroblastoma
- Glomus tumor is seen in: Fingers
- Most radiosensitive tissue of the body: Bone marrow
- Least radiosensitive cell of the body: Neurons
- Most radiosensitive blood cell: Lymphocyte
- Least radiosensitive blood cell: Platelet

- Amifostine is a: Radio protector
- In Malignant melanoma, HMB 45 is a more specific marker whereas S-100 is more sensitive marker
- Gold standard in diagnosing synovial sarcoma: t (X: 18)

Phase of cell cycle:
- Most sensitive to radiation: G2M > G2
- Most resistant to radiation: Late S phase

Adjuvant chemotherapy is of definitive value in:
- Breast CA
- Colorectal CA

Trousseau sign (Migratory thrombophlebitis) is seen in:
- Pancreatic cancer
- Bronchogenic carcinoma
- Colon cancer

Bone Metastasis:
- Purely osteolytic: Kidney (expansile mets)
- Purely osteoblastic: Prostrate
- IOC: Bone scan

Pulsatile secondaries are seen in:
- Follicular carcinoma of Thyroid
- Renal Cell Carcinoma

Sentinel LN Biopsy is usually done in:
- Breast cancer
- Penile cancer
- Malignant melanoma
- Endometrial carcinoma

Pure β - emitters:
- Strontium-90
- Yttrium-90
- Phosphorus-32
- Tritium-H_3

Isotopes used as Permanent interstitial implants:
- Palladium 103
- Gold (Au) 198
- Iodine 125

Isotopes used as temporary interstitial implant:
- Iridium 192
- Cesium 137

Intensity modulated Radiotherapy (IMRT) is most suitable for:
- Prostate cancer
- Cervical cancer

Most radiosensitive tumors:
- Lung tumor: Small cell carcinoma
- Kidney tumor: Wilms' tumor
- Bone tumor: Ewing's sarcoma and Multiple myeloma

- Brain tumor: Medulloblastoma
- Ovarian tumor: Dysgerminoma
- Testicular tumor: Seminoma

Cell Cycle Check Points

$G_1 - S$	$G_2 - M$
▪ Checks for DNA damage & inhibits its transition into the S phase ▪ Controlled by p53 & RB gene	▪ Prevent mitosis of cells with DNA damage ▪ Activation by ionizing radiation ▪ Controlled by Cyclin – B (CDK1)

Differences

Features	Metaplasia	Dysplasia	Anaplasia
Pleomorphism	▪ Absent	▪ Present	▪ Present
Reversibility	▪ Reversible	▪ Reversible in early stage	▪ Irreversible
Mitotic figure	▪ Absent	▪ Typical appearance	▪ Atypical appearance

MOST COMMON

- MC gene mutation present in human cancers: p53
- MC cancer in world: Lung cancer
- MC cancer in males: Lung cancer > Prostate cancer
- MC cancer in females: Breast cancer
- MC cancer in India: Oral cancer > Lung cancer
- MC cancer in Indian men: Oral cancer
- MC cancer among Indian women: Breast cancer > Cervical cancer
- MC malignancy of childhood: Leukemias > Brain tumor
- MC intra abdomen tumor of childhood: Neuroblastoma
- MC cancer due to excessive UV light exposure: Basal cell carcinoma
- MC site of oral cancer: Tongue
- MC tumor to produce metastasis to cervical lymphadenopathy: Nasopharyngeal Carcinoma
- MC tumor responsible for secondaries in the neck with no obvious primary malignancy: Nasopharyngeal carcinoma
- MC primary malignancy causing bone metastasis: Prostate cancer
- MC tumor metastasize to bone in females: Breast cancer

- MC cause of osteoblastic secondaries in male: Prostate cancer
- MC cause of osteoblastic secondaries in females: Breast cancer
- MC extra nodal site for lymphoma: Stomach
- MC site of gastric lymphoma: Antrum
- MC type of gastric lymphoma: Diffuse large B-cell lymphoma
- MC type of metaplasia in Barrett's esophagus: Intestinal metaplasia
- MC benign tumor of stomach: Leiomyoma
- MC retroperitoneal tumor: Liposarcoma
- MC site of Rhabdomyosarcoma: Orbit
- MC site for distant metastasis: Liver
- MC liver tumor: Metastasis / Secondaries
- MC benign tumor of liver: Hemangiomas
- MC benign tumor of urinary bladder: Leiomyoma
- MC cancer caused by ionizing radiation: Papillary CA of Thyroid and Leukemia (except CLL)
- MC cancer after kidney transplant: Squamous cell carcinoma of skin ‘
- MC Paraneoplastic syndrome: Hypercalcemia
- MC tumor associated with superior vena cava syndrome: Lung cancer

Brain Tumors

- MC tumor of the brain: Metastatic brain tumor
- MC primary malignancy associated with brain metastasis: Lung cancer > Breast cancer
- MC primary brain tumor: Meningioma
- MC malignant primary brain tumor: Glioma
- MC brain tumor in children: Pilocytic Astrocytoma → occurs typically in cerebellum
- MC intracranial tumor to calcify: Oligodendroglioma

- MC CNS neoplasm in HIV patients: Primary CNS Lymphoma
- MC cause of leptomeningeal metastasis/ Carcinomatous meningitis:
  - Hematological malignancy – Acute leukemia
  - Solid tumor – Breast cancer

CANCER PREDISPOSITION SYNDROME

	Syndromes	Gene	Chromosome	Associated Tumors
Autosomal Recessive	*Ataxia Telangiectasia*	**ATM**	11q	Breast Cancer
	Bloom Syndrome	**BLM**	15q	Multiple
	Fanconi Anemia	**FANCA**		AML, Hepatocellular Carcinoma, MDS
	Xeroderma Pigmentosum			Multiple
	Werner Syndrome	**WRN**		Hematological & Cutaneous Malignancies
Autosomal Dominant	*Cowden Syndrome*	**PTEN**	10q	Breast & Thyroid
	Gardner Syndrome	**APC**	5q	Osteomas, Thyroid Carcinoma, Pancreatic Adenocarcinoma, Desmoid Tumor
	Familial Adenomatous Polyposis	**APC**	5q	Colorectal Cancer, Stomach cancer
	HNPCC / Lynch Syndrome	**MSH2, MLH1 MSH6**		Colon, Endometrial, Ovarian, Stomach, Small Bowel Cancer
	Turcot's Syndrome			Colorectal cancer, Brain tumors
	Li-Fraumeni Syndrome	**P53**	17p13	Breast Cancer
	Neurofibromatosis type 1	**NF1**	17q	Neurofibroma, Optic Nerve Glioma
	Neurofibromatosis type 2	**NF2**	22q	Vestibular Schwannoma, Meningioma
	Tuberous Sclerosis	**TSC1**	9q	Angiofibroma, Renal Angiomyolipoma
	Peutz Jeghers Syndrome	**STK11/LKB1**	19p	Colorectal Cancer (MC), Breast Cancer, Small Bowel Cancer
	Hereditary Retinoblastoma	**RB1**	13q14	Retinoblastoma, Osteosarcoma
	VHL Syndrome	**VHL**	3p	Renal Cell Carcinoma, Pheochromocytoma Retinal & CNS Hemangioblastoma
	Wilms' Tumor	**WT1**	11p13	Renal Tumor
	Familial Melanoma	**CDKN2A**	9p	Melanoma, Pancreatic Cancer
	Multiple Endocrine Neoplasia 1	**MEN1**	11q	Parathyroid Adenoma, Pancreatic Islet Cell Tumor Pituitary Tumors
	Multiple Endocrine Neoplasia 2a	**RET**	10	Medullary Thyroid Carcinoma Pheochromocytoma

POLYPOSIS SYNDROMES

Autosomal Dominant Gastrointestinal Polyposis Syndrome					
Syndromes	**Familial Adenomatous Polyposis**	**Gardner's Syndrome**	**Turcot's Syndrome**	**Nonpolyposis Syndrome* (Lynch Syndrome)**	**Peutz Jeghers Syndrome**
Chromosome (Gene)	5q (*APC*)	5q (*APC*)			*19p (STK11/LKB1)*
Distribution of polyps	Large intestine	Large & small intestine	Large intestine	Large intestine	Small & large intestine
Histology	Adenoma	Adenoma	Adenoma	Adenoma	Hamartoma
Malignant Potential	Common	Common	Common	Common	Rare
Associated Features		Osteoma, Congenital hypertrophy of retinal pigment epithelium	Brain tumor Colorectal cancer	Endometrial & ovarian tumor	Mucocutaneous pigmentations Tumors of the ovary, breast & endometrium

*It is characterized by the presence of ≥3 relatives with documented colorectal cancer; ≥1 cases of colorectal cancer diagnosed before 50 years of age; and colorectal cancer involving at least two generations |

TUMOR MARKERS

Tumor Marker	Cancer
α - Fetoprotein	Hepatocellular carcinoma Non Seminomatous Germ cell tumor of testes
Placental Alkaline phosphatase	Seminoma
CEA	Adenocarcinoma of the Colon, Pancreas, Ovary, Lung
CA-15-3, CA 27.29	Breast cancer
CA-19-9	Pancreatic > Colorectal cancer
CA-125	Ovarian cancer
Gastrin	Gastrinoma (Pancreatic NET)
BCL-2	Follicular lymphoma
Chromogranin A	Neuroblastoma, Neuroendocrine tumors
VMA	Neuroblastoma
Neuron Specific Enolase	Neuroblastoma, Neuroendocrine tumors, Small cell lung cancer
HMB-45	Malignant melanoma
S-100	Histiocytoma, Schwannoma, Malignant Melanoma
Human Chorionic Gonadotropins	Gestational trophoblastic tumor, Choriocarcinoma, Germ cell tumor
Inhibin	Granulosa cell tumor
Calcitonin	Medullary Thyroid Cancer
Thyroglobulin	Thyroid cancer
Nuclear Matrix Protein (NMP-22)	Bladder cancer
5-HIAA	Carcinoid tumor
PSA	Prostate cancer
TMPT	ALL
Oncotype DX, Mammaprint	Breast cancer
BRCA 1 & 2	Ovarian and Breast cancer
CD 99 / MIC 2	Ewing sarcoma
CD34	GIST
CD 117 / c KIT	GIST, Mastocytosis
Cytokeratin	Carcinoma
Desmin	Sarcoma
Vimentin	Sarcoma, Renal cell carcinoma

MICRO-ORGANISMS ASSOCIATED WITH CANCERS

- HPV is associated with expression of E_6 & E_7 gene → E_6 protein causes inactivation of P_{53}
- CD-21 on B cell surface acts as a target molecule of EBV

Pathogen	Associated Malignancy	Pathogen	Associated Malignancy
H. pylori	▪ Gastric MALT Lymphoma ▪ Gastric cancer	Human Papillomavirus (HPV 16 > 18)	▪ Squamous cell carcinoma of cervix, anus, vagina ▪ Laryngeal Carcinoma
Hepatitis B Virus	▪ Hepatocellular carcinoma	Ebstein Barr Virus	▪ Post-transplant lymphoproliferative disorder ▪ Hodgkin lymphoma ▪ B-cell lymphoma ▪ Burkitt's lymphoma- African type ▪ Nasopharyngeal Carcinoma

Contd...

Pathogen	Associated Malignancy	Pathogen	Associated Malignancy
Hepatitis C Virus	• Hepatocellular carcinoma • Lymphoplasmacytic lymphoma	*HHV-8*	• Multicentric Castleman disease • Primary effusion lymphoma • Kaposi Sarcoma
HTLV-1	• Cutaneous adult T cell Lymphoma	*Merkel cell polyomavirus*	• Merkel cell carcinoma
Clonorchis sinensis	• Cholangiocarcinoma	*Opisthorchis viverrini*	• Cholangiocarcinoma
Schistosoma haematobium	• Squamous cell carcinoma of Urinary bladder	*Schistosoma japonicum*	• Colorectal carcinoma
P. falciparum	• Burkitt lymphoma		

GENES AND THEIR ASSOCIATED TUMORS

Genes		Chromosome	Associated Tumor
ABL **BCR**		9q 22q	• CML
β - *catenin*		3p	• Hepatocellular carcinoma
BRCA 1 **BRCA 2**		17q 13q	• Breast & Ovarian carcinoma
Cyclin - D		11	• Mantle cell lymphoma
E cadherin		16	• Stomach carcinoma • Colon carcinoma
Her 2 / neu or ERB B2		17	• Breast cancer • Adenocarcinoma of lung
FMS			• Leukemia
HNPCC		hMLH 1 - 3p hMSH 2 - 2p hPMSI - 2q hPSM 2 - 7q	• Colorectal carcinoma • Colon cancer • Endometrial carcinoma • Gastric Cancer
INT - 2			• Stomach CA
C – KIT / CD 117			• GIST, Seminoma
K RAS		12	• Colon carcinoma
MYC	*C – myc*	8	• Burkitt's lymphoma
	L – myc		• Small cell lung cancer
	N – myc		• Neuroblastoma
P$_{16}$INK 4a			• Malignant melanoma
PTEN		10	• Cowden syndrome • Familial endometrial carcinoma

LUNG CANCER

- MC benign tumor of lung: Hamartoma
- Hamartoma is characterized by
  - Popcorn calcification → Pathognomonic
  - Marble like feel of the tumor.
- MC cancer in the world: Lung cancer
- MC site of distant metastasis in lung CA: Liver > Bone.
- MC source of metastatic lung CA: Colon CA.
- Lung cancer MC associated with SVC syndrome: Small cell lung carcinoma.
- MC endocrine organ to be involved by metastasis from carcinoma lung: Adrenals
- Ca lung which can metastasize to opposite lung: Adenocarcinoma
- Ca lung most responsive to chemotherapy: Small cell Ca
- MC type of Ca lung associated with hypokalemia: Small cell lung carcinoma
- MC cause of hemoptysis: Bronchitis > Bronchogenic carcinoma

- MC cause of hemoptysis in India: TB
- MC cause of massive hemoptysis: Bronchiectasis (TB – in India).
- MC cause of recurrent hemoptysis: Bronchial adenoma.
- MC symptom of CA Lung: Cough.
- MC nerve involved in Pancoast tumor: C8, T1, T2
- MC site of primary in a patient presenting with secondaries to adrenals: Melanoma > Lungs

- *Risk Factors for CA lung:*
  - Tobacco smoking
  - Ionizing radiation
  - Asbestos, Arsenic
  - Nickel, Chromium, Silica
  - Primary tuberculosis
- Highest risk of lung Ca: Smoking + Arsenic exposure
- Solitary fibrous tumor → not associated with asbestosis
  - CD34 +ve & keratin -ve

Management

- IOC to look for mediastinal involvement: CT scan
- Screening test → History + Physical exam + S. alkaline phosphatase.
- MC anticancer drug for treatment of NSCLC: Etoposide + Cisplatin.
- TOC in stage I & II NSCLC → surgical resection

- Radiotherapy is indicated in:
  - Stage I & II which cannot be resected
  - Patient refuses for surgery
  - Not fit for surgical resection
  - Known mediastinal lymph node disease
- TOC of carcinoma of superior pulmonary sulcus producing Pancoast syndrome is: RT + Surgery.

Management of NSCLC (Adenocarcinoma, Squamous cell carcinoma, & Large cell carcinoma)		
N0 or N1 nodes	Stage IA	▪ Surgery – Lobectomy/Pneumonectomy/Wedge resection
	Stage IB	▪ Surgery alone if lesion is <4 cm ▪ Surgery + adjuvant chemotherapy if lesion is >4 cm
	Stage II/ III	▪ Surgery + adjuvant chemotherapy
N2 or N3 nodes		▪ Combined chemoradiation therapy

Management of Small Cell Lung Cancer	Limited stage SCLC	Stage I-III	Chemotherapy + Radiotherapy
	Extensive stage SCLC	Stage IV	Chemotherapy

Gastrointestinal Malignancies

Premalignant Conditions
- Plummer Vinson syndrome
- Chronic Atrophic gastritis
- Adenomatous polyp
- Villous adenoma

- HNPCC
- FAP

Benign Condition
- Inflammatory/Pseudo polyp
- Hamartomatous Polyps (PJ syndrome)

Hepatoblastoma

- MC liver cancer in children
- Originate from immature liver precursor cells
- Usually unifocal and affect the right lobe > > the left lobe

- Cirrhosis is not associated with this tumor.
- AFP levels are often high

Hepatocellular/ Hepatic Adenoma (HCA)

- MC in women of childbearing age
- Strongly associated with use of OCPs and anabolic steroids
- Bordeaux classification includes HNF1α HCA, β-catenin mutated HCA & inflammatory HCA (50%)
- Pregnancy should be avoided → risk of tumor growth and rupture

- Patients should stop using oral contraceptives or anabolic steroids.
- AFP levels are within the reference range
- Resection is indicated in all cases of size > 5 cm
- Caries the risk of development of HCC, especially when sized >5 cm

GISTS

- Arises from the interstitial cell of Cajal – pacemaker cells of GIT
- Characterized by mutation in c-*KIT* proto-oncogene
- MC mesenchymal tumor of the GI tract
- MC site: Stomach > Small intestine
- MC clinical manifestation: Upper GI bleed
- Diagnosis – spindle shaped cell GI tumor with positive CD117
- Other immunohistochemistry markers: Nestin & CD34

- Treatment of choice – Surgery
- Imatinib is used as an adjuvant therapy post surgical resection in patients with high-risk tumors or as neoadjuvant therapy prior to surgical resection

Carney triad: defined by coexistence of 3 tumors
- GIST
- Pulmonary chondroma
- Extra-adrenal paragangliomas

CARCINOIDS

- Carcinoid tumors arise from neuroendocrine cells, which are widespread in the human body.
- MC location: Midgut
- MC site: Small intestine (Ileum > Rectum). They are the MC neoplasm of small intestine.
- MC neoplasm of appendix → represents 90% of appendiceal tumors.
- Intestinal carcinoid originates from serotonin secreting enterochromaffin cells of intestine k/a Kulchistky cells.
- It is more frequent in whites, females & older persons (>65 years).
- Most of these tumors produce 5-hydroxytryptamine (5-HT or Serotonin).
- MC symptoms: Flushing and diarrhea.
- Flushes may be precipitated by stress; alcohol; exercise; certain foods, such as cheese; or certain agents, such as catecholamines, and serotonin reuptake inhibitors.
- Cardiac involvement is characterized by the dense fibrous deposits that can result in tricuspid insufficiency (in 90–100% cases) and tricuspid stenosis.

- Diagnosis relies on measurement of urinary or plasma serotonin or its metabolites in the urine. The biochemical diagnosis of carcinoid tumors is mainly based on the measurement of the serotonin metabolite 5-HIAA in a 24-hour urine collection.
- Platelet serotonin levels are more sensitive than urinary 5-HIAA.
- Because patients with foregut Neuroendocrine Tumors (NETs) may produce an atypical carcinoid syndrome, if this syndrome is suspected and the urinary 5-HIAA is minimally elevated or normal, other urinary metabolites of tryptophan, such as 5-HTP (5-Hydroxytryptophan) and 5-HT, should be measured.
- Most sensitive screening test: Plasma level of chromogranin A
- Plasma neuron-specific enolase levels are also used as a marker but are less sensitive than chromogranin A.
- Imaging modalities useful are Iodine-131 metaiodobenzylguanidine (MIBG) scanning and Scintigraphy with indium-111 DTPA octreotide (In-111 DTPA Octr), or OctreoScan.

NEUROBLASTOMA

- Catecholamines producing malignancy of the sympathetic nervous system
- Arises from neuroblasts (sympathetic cells).
- Typically affects infants and children <5 years of age
- MC intra-abdominal malignancy of infancy
- MC extracranial solid tumor of childhood
- **Clinical Manifestations:**
  - Constitutional features, fatigue, bone pain, nontender abdominal mass that crosses the midline (Wilms tumor does not cross the midline).
  - Hypertension is uncommon (d/t renal artery compression) & chronic diarrhea is rare (secondary to VIP secretion).

- Orbital metastasis lead to: Raccoon eye
- Cutaneous metastasis lead to: Blueberry muffin lesions
- Paraneoplastic features: Opsomyoclonus (Dancing eye, Dancing feet syndrome)
- Increase catecholamines (VMA/HVA) excretion in urine.
- Elevated Neuron-specific enolase (NSE) – nonspecific tumor markers
- H/P – Homer Wright rosette pattern
- Poor prognostic factors:
  - N-Myc gene amplification – Most important
  - Deletion of chromosome 1(-1p)
  - Loss of heterozygosity at 11q & 17q
- Stage I and II neuroblastoma – surgery
- Advanced stages: multiple agent chemotherapy

LUNG CANCERS

	Squamous Cell Carcinoma	Adenocarcinoma	Small Cell (Oat cell) Lung Cancer (SCLC)	Large Cell Carcinoma
Facts	▪ MC lung cancer in India ▪ MC lung cancer in smokers	▪ MC lung cancer worldwide; in non smokers; and in women	▪ Least common type ▪ Endobronchial growth +	▪ Aka Anaplastic carcinoma
M:F	▪ M > F	▪ F > M	▪ M > F	
Location	▪ Central	▪ Peripheral	▪ Central	▪ Peripheral
Prognosis	▪ Best prognosis		▪ Worst – most rapidly growing & most aggressive lung cancer	
Cavity	▪ Cavitations +	▪ -	▪ Cavitations +	
Genetics	▪ Over expression of EGFR & P53 mutation	▪ K-RAS mutation ▪ EGFR mutations	▪ Expression of BCl2 gene	
Associated with	▪ Smoking – strongest ▪ Pancoast Tumor (MC cause)	▪ Transbronchial spread (Bronchioalveolar type). ▪ Pleural involvement + ▪ Cells are +ve for Mucin & Thyroid transcription factor - 1 (TTF-1)	▪ Smoking ▪ Myasthenia, Lambert Eaton syndrome ▪ Least resectability rate. ▪ Most early and widely metastasizing tumor ▪ Intrathoracic spread	▪ Pleural involvement ▪ CNS involvement (MC with this variety)
Paraneoplastic syndrome	▪ MC paraneoplastic syndrome associated is hypercalcemia and hypophosphatemia due to PTHrP.	▪ MC paraneoplastic syndrome associated is Hematological syndromes like Trousseau's syndrome (Migratory venous thrombophlebitis)	▪ MC lung cancer to produce paraneoplastic syndromes and extra thoracic metastasis ▪ Hyponatremia with SIADH ▪ Ectopic secretion of ACTH leads to hypokalemia ▪ Ectopic GHRH & AVP secretion ▪ Cushing's syndrome ▪ Ectopic calcitonin, ANF	▪ Tender gynecomastia. ▪ Ectopic Gn secretion. ▪ Ectopic GH secretion.
Miscellaneous points	▪ MC lung cancer associated with clubbing. ▪ MC type of lung cancer in male ▪ MC cause of Pancoast tumor	▪ MC type of lung cancer in young patient ▪ MC cancer arising from pulmonary scar ▪ Bronchoalveolar carcinoma is a subtype of Adenocarcinoma	▪ Hilar lymphadenopathy is typical. ▪ EM shows +se of Neurosecretory granules: chromogranin, Synaptophysin, leu - 7. ▪ Azzopardi effect is frequently seen ▪ Best serum marker: NSE ▪ Most resistant to combined modality treatment ▪ Most radiosensitive lung cancer	

THYROID CANCERS

Types	Medullary Carcinoma (MCT)	Papillary Carcinoma (PCT)	Anaplastic Carcinoma	Follicular Carcinoma
Origin	▪ Neuroendocrine tumor of thyroid parafollicular 'C' cells	▪ Follicular cells	▪ Undifferentiated CA	▪ Follicular cells
General	▪ "C cells" are more on the upper pole ▪ Spindle cells +	▪ It is a well differentiated carcinoma ▪ Develop in Thyroglossal duct	▪ Very aggressive tumor of short duration ▪ Elderly females are more affected	▪ Well differentiated carcinoma ▪ Characterized by Angioinvasion & capsular invasion ▪ Most probable malignancy to develop in long standing goiter

Etiology & Types	▪ **Sporadic: (75%)**
	  ○ MC type; Usually unilateral
	  ○ Associated with RET proto-oncogene mutation on chromosome 10
	▪ **Familial: (25%)**
	  ○ Usual age group: 4th- 5th decade
	  ○ RET proto-oncogene mutation ++
	  ○ Multicentric & bilateral
	  ○ Autosomal dominant
	  ○ Least malignant potential
	▪ **MCT with MEN II syndrome:**
	  ○ More aggressive; always bilateral
	  ○ Multifocal & multicentric
	  ○ Affects younger age
	  ○ MCT associated with MEN IIb → Most aggressive type
		▪ Irradiation
		  ○ RAI (MC cancer in individuals exposed to radiation)
		  ○ RET NTRK-1 BRAF fusion gene RET/ PTC (10:17)
		  ○ Aggressive PCT is ass. with RET/ PTC3 oncogene
		  ○ Less aggressive CA is ass. with RET/ PTC1 oncogene
		  ○ Variants → Associated with worse prognosis
		    ○ Follicular
		    ○ Diffuse sclerosing
		    ○ Clear cell
			▪ Unknown
			▪ Common in iodine deficiency areas
			▪ Associated with p53 RAS P13K PTEN mutation
			▪ Associated with multinodular goiter
				▪ De novo (more common in iodine deficient area)
				▪ Associated with multinodular goiter /Endemic goiter
				▪ Types:
				  ○ Non invasive → Blood spread is not common
				  ○ Invasive → Blood spread common
				▪ Variants
				  ○ Hurthle cell carcinoma
				  ○ Insular carcinoma

Age	▪ Sporadic/Familial in 5th – 6th decade ▪ 2nd-3rd decade if associated with MEN II	▪ 20 - 40 years ▪ Common in female	▪ Elderly female >50 years	▪ 30-50 years ▪ Common in females
Hormone production	▪ Serotonin (5HT), ACTH (corticotropin) ▪ VIP, Melanin	▪ Very rare	▪ No	
Spread	▪ Lymphatic (60%) > Blood	▪ Lymphatics >>> Hematogenous	▪ Direct invasion > Lymphatics (Most malignant)	
Association	▪ MEN II A & II B syndrome, Amyloidosis ▪ Sipple's syndrome = MCT + MEN IIa + Pheochromocytoma + Mucocutaneous neuroma	▪ Lateral aberrant thyroid ▪ Dystrophic calcification		▪ H/P - follicles present but lumen devoid of colloid
TSH dependent	▪ Not dependent ▪ Does not take up radioactive iodine	▪ Yes ∴ TSH levels are high in blood	▪ No	▪ Yes
Prevalence	▪ 2-4%	▪ 80% (MC)	▪ 5%	▪ 10%

Contd...

Types	Medullary Carcinoma (MCT)	Papillary Carcinoma (PCT)	Anaplastic Carcinoma	Follicular Carcinoma
Clinical features	<ul><li>Solitary neck nodule</li><li>Thyroid swelling</li><li>Enlargement of cervical lymph node +</li><li>Diarrhea, flushing (**MC** presenting complaint)</li><li>Labile hypertension (d/t pheochromocytoma)</li><li>Mucosal neuromas & Marfanoid habitus if associated with MEN IIB</li><li>Paraneoplastic syndrome like Cushing's & carcinoid syndrome</li><li>The calcitonin excess in MTC is not associated with hypocalcemia</li></ul>	<ul><li>Slow growing painless mass</li><li>Thyroid swelling:<ul><li>Solid/Cystic</li><li>Solitary/Multinodular</li></ul></li><li>Rarely encapsulated</li></ul>	<ul><li>Hard neck swelling</li><li>Sudden ↑ in size</li><li>Stridor and Hoarseness</li><li>Dysphagia</li><li>Fixity to skin local structure</li><li>Positive Berry's sign → Absence of carotid pulse due to involvement of carotid sheath</li></ul>	<ul><li>Aggressive tumor/Rapid ↑ in size</li><li>Tracheal infiltration & stridor</li><li>Dyspnea, Hemoptysis ,Chest pain indicate lung secondaries</li><li>Hoarseness d/t RLN involvement</li><li>Berry's sign in advanced malignancy</li><li>Pulsatile secondaries in skull & long bones</li><li>LN involvement – 10% (least common)</li><li>Pathological # (d/t osteolytic bone mets)</li></ul>
Metastasis	<ul><li>Osteoblastic metastasis</li><li>MC metastasis → Liver</li></ul>	<ul><li>Enlarged LN (LN mets common)</li><li>Multifocality is a common feature</li><li>Hematogenous</li><li>Metastasis is uncommon in lungs, liver and brain</li></ul>	<ul><li>MC metastasis → Lungs</li><li>Distal metastasis → Common</li></ul>	<ul><li>MC metastasis → Bones → Pulsatile skeletal deposits</li><li>LN mets produces so called lateral aberrant thyroid</li><li>Multiple foci rarely seen</li></ul>
Marker	<ul><li>Calcitonin<ul><li>Both baseline & and following Ca++/ Pentagastrin stimulation → High</li></ul></li><li>CEA → for detecting recurrences</li></ul>	<ul><li>Thyroglobulin (T_G) level >2 ng/ml is highly suggestive of metastasis or persistence of normal thyroid tissue</li></ul>		<ul><li>Thyroglobulin immune staining is +ve</li><li>For follow up → T_G should be <2 ng/ml.</li><li>↑ in T_G signifies recurrence/ metastasis</li></ul>
Diagnosis	<ul><li>Serum calcium & PTH</li><li>CEA → ↑ in 50%</li><li>Urine → VMA, Catecholamines & metanephrines to rule out pheochromocytoma</li><li>USG neck to detect LN mets</li><li>**FNAC:**<ul><li>C cell hyperplasia</li><li>Amyloid stroma with dispersed malignant cells</li></ul></li><li>¹¹¹In octreotide scanning</li><li>I¹³¹ scan - **No use**</li></ul>	<ul><li>TSH level – high</li><li>Radio isotope → Cold nodule</li><li>Plain X-ray – fine calcification</li><li>FNAC of thyroid mass or LN</li><li>**Microscopic findings:**<ul><li>Psammoma bodies (calcified deposits)</li><li>Orphan Annie eye nuclei</li><li>Papillary projections</li><li>Diagnosis is based on nuclear characteristics (intranuclear inclusions & grooves)</li></ul></li></ul>	<ul><li>FNAC → Diagnostic<ul><li>Poorly differentiated cells</li><li>Giant & Multinucleated cells</li></ul></li><li>Incision biopsy</li></ul>	<ul><li>FNAC → Not diagnostic<ul><li>Cannot differentiate adenoma from CA</li><li>Nuclei lacks typical features of Papillary CA</li><li>RAI uptake – Cold nodule</li><li>Plain X-ray → Osteolytic lesions</li><li>⁹⁹ᵐTc sestamibi scan – very useful for Hurthle cell carcinoma</li></ul></li></ul>

Contd...

ONCOLOGY ⊙ (HIGH-YIELD POINTS)

Types	Medullary Carcinoma (MCT)	Papillary Carcinoma (PCT)	Anaplastic Carcinoma	Follicular Carcinoma

Treatment	▪ Total Thyroidectomy + central node dissection + maintenance dose of levothyroxine in symptomatic MCT
	▪ Bilateral MRND if LN palpable
	  ○ Neck LN block dissection → If LN are involved.
	  ○ Includes level → 2-6
	▪ No role of Radioactive I ^{131} or suppressive hormonal therapy
	▪ External Beam RT for residual tumor
	▪ If associated with pheochromocytoma → 1st adrenalectomy f/b total thyroidectomy
	▪ Rx of Diarrhea → Octreotide
	▪ Prophylactic thyroidectomy is indicated for carriers of RET mutation without any disease
	▪ Asymptomatic metastatic disease – watch for progression
	▪ Symptomatic metastatic disease – surgery or palliative EBRT
	▪ Chemotherapeutic agents include Vandetanib, Cabozantinib etc.
		▪ Total/Near total thyroidectomy + central node compartment dissection
		▪ Replacement dose of L-Thyroxine
		▪ MRND type III if LN are involved
		▪ RAI^{131} – for both intra & extra thyroidal carcinoma
		
		⊼ T$_G$ levels after total thyroidectomy should be <2 ng/ml, if >2 ng/mL → Highly suggestive of metastatic disease or persistence of normal thyroid tissue)
			▪ **Palliative:**
			  ○ Tracheostomy
			  ○ Isthmectomy
			  ○ Debulking surgery
			▪ Rx to prolong survival
			  ○ External Radiotherapy
			  ○ CT → Adriamycin
			▪ If mass is resectable – do thyroidectomy
			▪ No role of RAI
				▪ I: Enlarged thyroid gland & scalp swelling → Total thyroidectomy
				▪ II: MNG → Hemi/subtotal thyroidectomy→ Biopsy → FCT → Completion thyroidectomy within 7 days or > 4 weeks
				▪ III: Solitary nodule → High suspicion of malignancy on US & FNAC showing follicular cells → Total thyroidectomy
				▪ Total thyroidectomy is done with central node compartment dissection (level VI)
				▪ If nodes are present → Functional neck node dissection
				▪ Replacement dose of L-thyroxine
				▪ Secondaries→ Therapeutic RAI^{131}& Ext RT
				▪ Chemotherapy → no role
				▪ **Hurthle cell Carcinoma:**
				  ○ Does not takes up I^{131}
				  ○ Contains abundant oxyphilic cell/ Askanazy cells/ Hurthle cells
				  ○ Secretes thyroglobulinI^{131}
				  ○ Total thyroidectomy, MRND, TSH suppression is the treatment

Prognosis	▪ Sporadic /with MEN II – aggressive course
	▪ Familial → better prognosis
	▪ All familial members should be screened
	  ○ Positive RET MCT + MEN IIA & familial MET type → Prophylactic thyroidectomy within 5 years of age
	  ○ Positive RET MCT + MEN II B → prophylactic total thyroidectomy within 1 years of age
		▪ Best prognosis (Least malignant)
		▪ Encapsulated variant of PCT→ Good prognosis,
		▪ Diffuse sclerosing variant → Poor prognosis
		▪ Scoring:
		  ○ AMES
		  ○ AGES
		  ○ MACIS
			▪ Worst/most aggressive thyroid Malignancy.	▪ Good prognosis
				▪ Poor in Hurthle cell variant, Age >50 years, size >4 cm, High grade vascular & extra thyroid invasion, distant mets +
				▪ FNAC cannot distinguish it from Hurthle cell adenoma

TUMORS OF GASTROINTESTINAL TRACT

	Esophageal Carcinoma	Stomach Cancer	Colon/Colorectal Cancer

General features & Types	■ Overall MC site for CA → Middle 1/3rd
	■ **Squamous cell carcinoma:**
	  ○ MC type in India and worldwide
	  ○ MC type in upper 1/3rd
	  ○ MC type in middle 1/3rd
	■ **Adenocarcinoma:**
	  ○ MC type in western world
	  ○ MC in lower 1/3rd
	  ○ *H. pylori* CAG A strain is protective in adenocarcinoma
	  ○ *Barrett's esophagus* → replacement of the normal squamous epithelium of distal esophagus by columnar mucosa
		■ MC site in India → Distal stomach
		■ MC site of diffuse CA → Fundus
		■ MC histological type is Adenocarcinoma
		■ Overall incidence is decreasing
		■ MC Lymphatic drainage – Celiac LN
		■ **Based on Histology:**
		  ○ Intestinal type
		  ○ Diffuse type → Signet ring appearance
		■ **Based on Depth of invasion:**
		  ○ Early → Mucosa + submucosa ± LN. Better prognosis
		  ○ Late → Invasion of muscular layer. Poor prognosis
			■ MC site → Rectosigmoid (Rectum > Sigmoid colon)
			■ MC type → Adenocarcinoma
			■ Mucin producing tumor are associated with bad prognosis
			■ HIV infected persons may be at slightly ↑ risk
			■ Risk of malignancy is more in villous adenoma
			■ Cholecystectomy has been associated with a moderate ↑ risk of proximal colon cancer
			■ **Factors decreasing the risk:**
			  ○ ↑ intake of dietary fibers
			  ○ Intake of ω-3 fatty acids (fish)
			  ○ NSAIDS especially Aspirin
			  ○ Intake of folic acid and Calcium
			  ○ HRT (Estrogen)

Risk factors	■ **RF for Squamous cell carcinoma:**
	  ○ Tobacco smoking and alcohol
	  ○ Hot beverages and food
	  ○ Lye ingestion
	  ○ Prolonged esophagitis, Achalasia
	  ○ Plummer Vinson syndrome
	  ○ Nitrates, Caustics ingestion
	  ○ Deficiency of Vitamin A, C, Zn
	  ○ Tylosis et Palmaris
	  ○ Amplification of EGFR
	  ○ Radiation induced stricture
	  ○ External Beam radiation
	
	■ **RF for Adenocarcinoma:**
	  ○ Barrett's esophagus – Most important
	  ○ Tobacco/ Cigarette smoking
	  ○ Over expression of p53, amplification of C- ERB B2 & nuclear translocation of β-catenin
	  ○ Obesity, GERD, Scleroderma
	  ○ Male sex
		■ **Environmental factors:**
		  ■ **H. pylori infection** – Intestinal type
		  ○ Smoking
		  ○ Nitrites in diet, Preservatives
		  ○ Nutritional deficiency – Vit C, E
		■ **Genetic factors:**
		  ○ Blood group A
		  ○ FAP, HNPCC, Li -Fraumeni syndrome
		  ○ Familial gastric cancer syndrome due to E. cadherin mutation → Diffuse type
		  ○ Peutz Jeghers syndrome
		
		■ **Host factors:**
		  ○ Chronic gastric; Atrophic gastritis
		  ○ Intestinal metaplasia
		  ○ Ménétrier disease
		  ○ Gastric ulcer
		  ○ Barrett's esophagus
		  ○ Achlorhydria and Pernicious anemia
		  ○ Post gastrectomy
		  ○ Adenoma
			■ **Environmental factors:**
			  ○ ↑ Calorie intake and obesity
			  ○ Smoking, Alcohol & fatty diet
			  ○ Ureterosigmoidostomy, Low fiber diet
			  ○ Inflammatory bowel disease (UC > CD)
			  ○ Pelvic irradiation
			  ○ Acromegaly
			
			■ **Genetic factors:**
			  ○ Mutation in p53 & K RAS
			  ○ HNPCC (Lynch syndrome) → AD condition
			    – Mutation in DNA repair gene MSH-2 and MLH-1 leading to microsatellite instability
			    – Affects Right sided colon
			    – Better prognosis
			  ○ FAP – mutation in APC gene on long arm of chromosome 5(5q) → cancer develops in 100%
			■ **Involved Pathways:**
			  ○ APC/ β - catenin pathway
			  ○ Microsatellite instability pathway involve MSH 2 & MLH-1 gene

Contd...

Colon/Colorectal Cancer

	Right sided/Proximal	Left sided/Distal
	• Fungating/Ulcerative type	• Obstructive type
	• Bleeds readily	• Napkin ring configuration
	• Melena	• Diarrhea, constipation, tenesmus
	• Good prognosis	• Poor prognosis

- MC site → Liver >> Lung
- **Solitary liver metastasis is not a C/I to Surgery**
- Incidence of metastases is related to depth of invasion

- Tumor marker → CEA & CA-19.9
- Radiological IOC: Double contrast Ba enema → **"Apple core"** deformity
- Colonoscopy → Gold stand for diagnosis
- Colonoscopy → Napkin ring appearance in left sided CA
- Endorectal coil → MRI Radiological IOC in CA Rectum
- Immunohistochemistry → CDX 2+, CK20+, CK7 –

- Right sided colonic obstruction → Resection with ileo-transverse anastomosis
- Sigmoid colon/Descending colon →
  ○ Hartmann's operation
  ○ Sigmoidectomy with primary colorectal anastomosis
  ○ Abdominal colectomy with ileorectal anastomosis
- Chemo regimen: 5-FU, Leucovorin, Oxaliplatin (FOLFOX)
- Prophylactic colectomy is the standard therapy in patients with APC mutation but it does not ↓ risk for cancer
- MI prognostic indicator: Stage or LN status
- Screening → begins at age 50 years in asymptomatic individuals with no family history
  ○ FOBT annually & Flexible sigmoidoscopy every 5 years OR
  ○ Colonoscopy every 10 years

Stomach Cancer

- MC cause of gastric outlet obstruction (GOO)
- MC location – antrum of the stomach
- Paraneoplastic syndromes like
  ○ Trousseau's syndrome
  ○ Acanthosis nigricans
  ○ **CA stomach is the MC cause of**
  ○ Krukenberg tumor
  ○ **Sister Mary Joseph nodule**

- Liver (1st organ to be affected)
- Ovary (Krukenberg tumor)
- Periumbilical LN (Sister Mary nodule)
- Peritoneal cul-de-sac (Blumer's shelf)
- Left supraclavicular LN (Virchow's LN)

- Endoscopy with biopsy and brush cytology → IOC
- CT scan → IOC for staging
- IOC to know the depth of invasion → EUS
- Peritoneal dissemination → Best assessed by laparoscopy
- **Signet ring appearance seen in:** Diffuse type of CA Stomach

- Relatively a radio resistant tumor
- Surgery is the primary modality of treatment as it is curative
- Maintain a 5 cm surgical margin proximal & distal to primary lesion
- **Protective factors:**
  ○ Antioxidants – Vitamin A & B
  ○ Aspirin ↓ the risk
  ○ NSAIDs
- Alcohol is **not** a risk factor
- Prognosis depends on:
  ○ Lymph node status
  ○ Depth of tumor invasion

Esophageal Carcinoma

- Progressive dysphagia – more for solids
- MC symptom: Dysphagia → occurs when >60% of esophageal circumference is infiltrated
- Males > Females

- Liver

- IOC – Endoscopy and Biopsy
- Barium swallow → 'Rat-tail appearance'
- Endoscopic Ultrasound (EUS) → IOC for staging (T-stage)

- SqCC is a chemo-radio sensitive
- TOC for CA in situ: Endoscopic mucosal resection (EMR)
- Chemo → Epirubicin + **Cisplatin** + 5FU
- Best indicator of survival – TNM stage
- Prognosis depends upon:
  ○ Depth of invasion (T)
  ○ No. of LN involved (N)
  ○ Location of tumor
- Surgical options:
  ○ Ivor Lewis esophagogastrectomy
  ○ McKeown esophagogastrectomy
  ○ Transhiatal esophagectomy

Clinical features	
Metastasis	
Investigations	
Management	

TUMORS OF THE HEPATOBILIARY SYSTEM AND PANCREAS

	Hepatocellular Carcinoma	Cholangiocarcinoma	CA Gallbladder	CA Pancreas

General	■ MC primary malignant tumor of liver
	■ MC solid organ cancer
	■ MC cause of death in patient with cirrhosis
	■ Worldwide incidence of HCC parallels with the prevalence of Hepatitis B
	■ HCC derives its blood supply from Hepatic artery
	⌐ MC primary malignancy in children → Hepatoblastoma
		■ Extrahepatic – 70%
		  ○ Perihilar – 50%
		  ○ Distal – 20%
		■ Intrahepatic – 30%
			■ MC cancer of the biliary tract
			■ MC site of origin → Fundus
			■ Age: 6th – 7th decade of life
			■ Women >> Men
			■ >90% patient of CA GB have gall stone
			■ Risk of CA in patient with Gall stone → 0.3–3%
				■ MC site – Head of pancreas
				■ Male > Female

Risk factors	■ Cirrhosis: Most important
	■ Chronic Hepatitis with HBV & HCV
	■ Alcoholism
	■ Hereditary hemochromatosis
	■ Wilson's disease
	■ Smoking
	■ Non Alcoholic Fatty Liver Disease
	■ Primary Biliary Cirrhosis
	■ α_1 AT deficiency
	■ Aflatoxin → toxin B_1
	■ Thorotrast
		■ Primary Sclerosing **C**holangitis
		■ **C**holedocholithiasis
		■ **C**ontrast material - thorotrast
		■ **C**hronic alcoholic liver disease
		■ **C**holedochal cyst
		■ **C**aroli's disease
		■ Recurrent pyogenic **C**holangitis
		■ **C**igarette smoking
		■ Ulcerative **C**olitis
		■ Typhoid infection
		■ Liver flukes:
		  ○ *Clonorchis sinensis*
		  ○ *Opisthorchis viverrini*
			■ **Gall stone** → MI risk factor
			■ Choledochal cyst
			■ Porcelain Gall bladder → precancerous condition
			■ Gall bladder stone >3 cm
			■ GB polyp >10 mm
			■ Primary sclerosing cholangitis
			■ Obesity
			■ *S. typhi & paratyphi* infection
			■ *Clonorchis sinensis* infection (acquired by eating fish)
			■ *Helicobacter pylori*
				■ Smoking & Alcohol
				■ Obesity
				■ Chronic pancreatitis
				■ Diabetes mellitus
				■ **Hereditary factors:**
				  ○ PJ syndrome
				  ○ Ataxia telangiectasia
				  ○ Cystic fibrosis
				  ○ BRCA - 2
				  ○ Lynch syndrome/HNPCC
				  ○ Hereditary Pancreatitis
				■ **Genetic factors:**
				  ○ K-RAS – MC mutation
				  ○ K-RAS and Her 2 neu over-expression

Types/Variants	■ **Fibrolamellar Carcinoma:**
	  ○ Seen in young adults
	  ○ M = F
	  ○ No association with HBV or Cirrhosis
	  ○ Better prognosis
	  ○ No ↑ in AFP (differentiate from HCC)
	  ○ Affects left lobe of liver commonly
	  ○ Spread by lymphatic route
	  ○ Tumor marker → Neurotensin
	  ○ ↑ Vit B_{12} binding globulin
	  ○ Tumor is well circumscribed & easily resectable (but it is non encapsulated)
		■ MC type is Adenocarcinoma
		■ Macroscopically MC type is sclerosing
		■ **Klatskin tumor:**
		  ○ aka Hilar Cholangiocarcinoma
		  ○ MC subtype
		  ○ Located at the junction of right and left hepatic ducts
			■ Adenocarcinoma → 80-90%
			■ Histological type → Papillary has got best prognosis
				■ MC → Ductal adenocarcinoma

Contd...

ONCOLOGY ⊃ (HIGH-YIELD POINTS)

	Hepatocellular Carcinoma	Cholangiocarcinoma	CA Gallbladder	CA Pancreas

Clinical features	▪ More prevalent in Asia & Sub Sahara
	▪ MC symptom → Abdominal pain
	▪ **Paraneoplastic syndromes**
	  ○ Hypercholesterolemia – MC
	  ○ Hypoglycemia
	  ○ Hypercalcemia
	▪ Vascular bruit in 25%
		▪ Painless jaundice → MC	▪ Palpable mass in RUQ
			▪ RUQ pain mimicking cholecystitis & cholelithiasis
			▪ Jaundice
			▪ **Courvoisier sign / law** → palpable non tender gall bladder in the presence of jaundice is unlikely to be due to gall stone
				▪ MC symptom of CA head: painless jaundice
				▪ A palpable GB in 1/3rd of patient with periampullary cancer
				▪ **Troisier sign:** Left supraclavicular LN / Virchow's LN
				▪ Sister Mary Joseph node
				▪ Blummer shelf
				▪ Trousseau syndrome or Migratory thrombophlebitis

Metastasis	▪ Strong propensity for vascular invasion especially portal vein		▪ MC mode of spread → Direct invasion ▪ Direct hepatic invasion > LN mets	
Investigations	▪ ↑ αFP (Tumor marker) in ~ 70% ▪ Other marker → **PIVKA - 2** ▪ If focal lesion 1-2 cm → Both CT + MRI should be done ▪ If focal Lesion > 2 cm → Either CT or MRI done ▪ Biopsy → Usually not required	▪ Tumor marker → Cytokeratin 7, 8, 19 +ve and -ve for Cytokeratin 20 ▪ ↑CA 19-9 → Poor prognostic factor	▪ Best tumor marker → CA 19-9 ▪ Most accurate technique to define staging and invasion: MRCP	▪ Tumor marker → CA 19-9 (most sensitive) and CEA ▪ IOC → MDCT ▪ ERCP → Double duct sign ▪ Biopsy → not necessary ▪ Inverted 3 sign → Periampullary CA

Management	▪ Rx – Resection of the tumor by partial hepatectomy when size is <5 cm
	▪ **RFA** (Radio frequency ablation)
	▪ Transcatheter arterial chemoembolization (TACE)
	▪ Tyrosine kinase inhibitors like Sorafenib, Regorafenib
	▪ VEGF inhibitors like Lenvatinib
	▪ Most accepted staging system: Barcelona Clinic Liver Cancer (BCLC) classification
	▪ Okuda staging → For prognosis
	▪ **MILAN Criteria**→ For liver transplantation
	▪ CLIP system is applicable for Hep C related HCC
	▪ Barcelona staging → to guide the Rx
	▪ Recurrence → Common
		▪ Perihilar→ CBD resection + LN + Hepatic resection
		▪ Intrahepatic → Hepatic resection
		▪ Distal → Whipple's procedure
		▪ Components of Whipple's
		  ○ Pancreaticojejunostomy
		  ○ Choledochojejunostomy
		  ○ Gastrojejunostomy
			▪ Aggressive malignancy with poor prognosis
			▪ Simple or radical cholecystectomy for stage I or II
			▪ Stage III or IV → unresectable
			▪ If Δ is made after cholecystectomy:
			
			Staging / Management
			T1a: Invasion of lamina propria — Conservative & 5-FU is sufficient
			T1b: Invasion of Muscle layer — Margin –ve → FU; Margin +ve → Extended resection
			T2: Invasion of perimuscular — Extended cholecystectomy
			T3: Perforation of serosa — Radical cholecystectomy
				▪ CA Head → Pylorus preserving pancreaticoduodenectomy (Whipple procedure)
				▪ CA Body & tail → Distal pancreatectomy and en-bloc splenectomy
				▪ Best prognosis → Periampullary/ CA head of pancreas
				▪ MC complication of Whipple procedure → Delayed Gastric emptying
				▪ **Chemotherapy regimens:**
				  ○ Gemcitabine
				  ○ GTX (Gemcitabine, Docetaxel, Capecitabine)
				  ○ FOLFIRINOX (5FU + Irinotecan + Oxaliplatin)
				  ○ Erlotinib + Gemcitabine

TUMORS OF GENITOURINARY SYSTEM

	Wilms Tumor/Nephroblastoma	Renal Cell Carcinoma	Testicular Cancer

General	■ MC primary renal tumor of childhood
	 ■ MC childhood abdominal malignancy
	 ■ Median age at diagnosis: 3.5 years
	 ■ Usually unilateral (Bilateral in 5-10%)
		■ Aka Hypernephroma, Grawitz tumor & Renal adenocarcinoma
		 ■ MC malignant neoplasm of the kidney
		 ■ More commonly affects upper pole
		 ■ Arises from PCT/cortex commonly
		 ■ Males >> Females
		 ■ It is a radioresistant tumor
			■ MC testicular neoplasm: Germ cell tumor of testes
			 ■ MC in infants and children
			    <3 years: Yolk sac tumor
			 ■ MC in prepubertal children: Teratoma
			 ■ MC age of presentation: 20-40 years
			 ■ **Seminoma (MC Germ Cell Tumor):**
			   ○ MC tumor of testes
			   ○ Most radiosensitive testicular carcinoma
			 ■ **Lymphoma:**
			   ○ MC testicular cancer in patient >60 years

Etiology/Risk factors	**Syndromes associated with Wilms tumor –**
	 ❶ WAGR syndrome:
	   ○ Deletion of two genes WT-1 and PAX - 6, both located at chromosomes 11p13.
	 ❷ Denys Drash syndrome:
	   ○ Gonadal dysgenesis, male pseudohermaphroditism
	 ❸ Beckwith-Wiedemann syndrome:
	   ○ Organomegaly, Macroglossia
	   ○ Hemihypertrophy
	   ○ Genetic locus is present in band p15.5 of chromosome 11 called "WT-2"
		■ VHL syndrome – chromosome 3p
		 ■ Estrogen therapy
		 ■ Asbestos exposure
		 ■ Tuberous sclerosis
		 ■ Hypertension
		 ■ Obesity
		 ■ Tobacco smoking – MI risk factor
		 ■ Chronic Renal Failure
		 ■ Acquired **C**ystic **D**iseases
		   [**Mn:** " V EAT HOT at CCD]
		 ■ Genetics:
		   ○ t (x: 1); Trisomy 7,16, 17 in Papillary type of RCC
		   ○ VHL gene mutation in Clear cell CA
		   ○ Hypodiploidy in Chromophobe CA
			■ **For Germ Cell Tumor:**
			   ○ Cryptorchidism – strongest association
			     – Higher the testes, greater is the risk
			     – ↑ risk is seen in both the testes
			     – MC tumor seen is Seminoma
			     – Orchidopexy does not ↓ the risk
			   ○ H/o testicular intratubular germ cell neoplasia
			 ■ Testicular feminization syndrome
			 ■ Klinefelter syndrome
			 ■ Male Breast cancer

Types		■ Histologically, RCC is most often a mixed adenocarcinoma	■ MC histological type: Mixed > Seminoma

Clinical features	■ MC – Asymptomatic abdominal mass or swelling
	 ■ **Triad:**
	   ○ Abdominal mass – smooth, mobile, flank mass that does not cross the midline
	   ○ Hematuria
	   ○ Fever
		■ Classical triad includes:
		   ○ Hematuria → Earliest and MC symptom
		   ○ Palpable mass over flank or abdomen
		   ○ Flank pain
		   ○ Nonreducible varicocele (L > R)
			■ Painless swelling in one gonads
			 ■ 5% GCT may present with gynecomastia
			 ■ Secondary hydrocele

Metastasis	■ MC – Lungs	■ MC – lungs → Pulsating secondaries ■ Tendency to invade Renal vein (5-10% cases) & extend into IVC up to Right side of heart	■ GCT spread by stepwise lymphatic fashion

Contd...

	Wilms Tumor/Nephroblastoma	Renal Cell Carcinoma	Testicular Cancer
Investigations	▪ Renal USG—initial study ▪ Histopathology	▪ IOC – CECT of abdomen and pelvis ▪ Inferior venocavogram	▪ FNAC → contraindicated ▪ MC type on histopathology: classical seminoma
Management	▪ TOC: Nephrectomy f/b Chemotherapy ± post-op radiotherapy ▪ RT is given in stage III & IV, with loss of heterozygosity ▪ **SIOP approach** → Preoperative/primary chemo → Nephrectomy → Post chemo staging ▪ Presence of anaplasia leads to emergence of resistance to chemotherapy. ▪ MI prognostic factor: Histology ▪ Overall prognosis → Good	▪ TOC → Partial/Total nephrectomy ▪ Size ≤ 4 cm – Partial nephrectomy ▪ Refractory to cytotoxic agents ▪ IVC involvement does not means inoperability ▪ Metastatic RCC → **Sunitinib** ▪ Radiation therapy as palliative therapy of bone or brain mets ▪ MI prognostic factor → Pathological staging ▪ ***Paraneoplastic syndromes associated with RCC:*** ▪ Polycythemia l/t ↑ ESR (MC) ▪ **Stauffer syndrome** → non metastatic hepatic dysfunction d/t ↑ IL-6 ▪ Hypertension, Anemia, Fever ▪ Hypercalcemia – due to PTHrP ▪ Cushing's syndrome ▪ Amyloidosis, leukamoid reaction	▪ **Tumor Markers:** ○ α-FP → Yolk sac, Embryonal CA, Teratoma (YET) ○ β-hCG → Choriocarcinoma, Embryonal CA, Seminoma ○ PLAP → Seminoma (Placental ALP) ○ GGT → Seminoma ▪ Non Seminomatous GCT are more aggressive than Seminomatous GCT ▪ Schiller dual bodies → Yolk sac tumor (Endodermal sinus tumor) ▪ Chemo → BEP regimen (Bleomycin + Etoposide + Cisplatin) ▪ Teratoma are chemo resistant ▪ Spermatocytic Seminoma – indolent course; rarely metastasize ▪ Best prognosis → Yolk sac tumor ▪ Worst prognosis → Hurricane tumor (Type of choriocarcinoma testis)

Types of Renal Cell Carcinoma

Features	Clear cell Carcinoma (70-75%)	Papillary Carcinoma (10-15%)	Chromophobe Carcinoma (<5%)	Collecting duct CA (<1%)
Aka		▪ **C**hromophilic Carcinoma		▪ Bellini duct carcinoma
Origin	▪ Proximal tubule	▪ Proximal tubule	▪ Distal tubules/cortical collecting duct	▪ Medullary collecting duct (Principal cells)
Genetics	▪ Deletion of short arm of chromosome 3p i.e. VHL gene deletion	▪ ***Sporadic:*** ○ Trisomy 7, 17 ○ Loss of Y (−Y) ○ t(x:1) in children ▪ ***Familial:*** ○ Trisomy 7 → ↑ expression of MET gene	▪ Hypodiploidy ▪ Loss of multiple chromosomes 1, 2, Y ▪ Associated with Birt-Hogg-Dubé syndrome	
Histo-pathology	▪ Cells have clear cytoplasm & contain glycogen & lipid	▪ **P**apillary growth pattern is seen ▪ **P**sammoma bodies	▪ Pale eosinophilic cytoplasm with perinuclear halo	▪ Hobnail cells – cell with bulbous nucleus and nuclear projections
Features	▪ MC type ▪ Mainly sporadic ▪ Well differentiated CA	▪ 2nd MC type ▪ Sporadic and familial ▪ More likely to be bilateral and multifocal ▪ Strong tendency to invade renal vein & IVC ▪ MC RCC in patient with dialysis associated cystic disease	▪ RCC with best prognosis	▪ Rarest type ▪ Very aggressive ▪ Poorest prognosis ▪ Affects younger patients

Carcinoma of Urinary Bladder, Penis and Prostate

	Bladder Cancer	Penile Cancer	Prostrate Cancer
General	■ M >> F in 6th & 7th decade ■ MC site → Trigone and adjacent posterolateral wall ■ MC type → Urothelial carcinoma (Transitional cell cancer) – 90% ■ 2nd MC type → Squamous cell carcinoma	■ MC in 6th decade but 40% patient are <40 years. ■ MC site → Glans ■ MC type → Squamous cell carcinoma ■ Neonatal circumcision confers immunity against CA Penis, HIV & STD	■ MC cause of bone secondaries (osteoblastic) ■ MC zone of developing CA prostate: Peripheral zone ■ MC lobe involved: Posterior ■ MC type → Adenocarcinoma
Risk factors	■ *Urothelial carcinoma / Transitional cell carcinoma:* ○ Tobacco / Smoking → MI risk factor ○ Naphthylamine, Benzidine, Aniline dyes, Acrolein ○ Phenacetin, Cyclophosphamide ○ Dye leather printing industry workers ○ Analgesic Nephropathy ○ Pelvic irradiation ■ *Squamous cell carcinoma:* ○ Schistosoma haematobium ○ Urinary calculi ○ Long term indwelling catheters ○ Chronic UTI ○ Bladder diverticula ■ *Adenocarcinoma:* ○ Ectopia vesicae	■ Poor hygiene → MC risk factor ■ Phimosis ■ Smegma ■ HPV infection - 16, 18, 31, 33, ■ *Premalignant lesions:* ○ Buschke - Lowenstein tumor (verrucous CA) is a well differentiated variant of Squamous cell carcinoma. It is locally malignant; does not metastasize. ○ Leukoplakia ○ Balanitis Xerotica Obliterans ■ *Carcinoma in situ:* ○ Bowen's disease ○ Erythroplasia of Queyrat	■ Advancing age ■ Fatty diet ■ *Factors which decrease the risk:* ○ Lycopene ○ Vitamin A & E ○ Selenium ■ MC genetic alteration: hyper methylation of glutathione transferase (GSTP-1) located on chromosome 11
Clinical features	■ **MC symptom** → Painless hematuria ■ Hematuria is gross and intermittent ■ Vesical irritability leading to frequency and urgency	■ MC and earliest symptom of metastatic CA Penis: Priapism ■ MC cause of death: bleeding caused by erosion of femoral artery ■ Hypercalcemia ■ No pain	■ Being peripheral it is asymptomatic initially ■ On digital rectal examination: Median sulcus is obliterated
Metastasis	■ Lymphatic → Pelvic LN (obturator) ■ Hematogenous → Liver	■ Lymphatics → Inguinal LN (MC)	■ Local → Seminal vesicle & base of urinary bladder ■ Hematogenous → Bones (osteoblastic secondaries) ■ Lymphatics→ Obturator LN ■ Spread to vertebrae is due to Batson's internal vertebral plexus of veins

Contd...

	Bladder Cancer	Penile Cancer	Prostrate Cancer
Investigation	▪ Urine microscopy for malignant cells → for screening and to detect recurrence ▪ Best investigation → Cystoscopy & Biopsy	▪ Sentinel LN biopsy → CABANA procedure ▪ Incisional biopsy ▪ IOC for staging → MRI	▪ Best screening protocol → PSA + DRE ▪ PSA velocity >0.75 ng/mL/yr indicates carcinoma ▪ TRUS guided biopsy best investigation ▪ Increased prostatic acid phosphatase (PAP)
Staging	▪ CIS – Carcinoma in situ ▪ Ta – papillary tumor confined to epithelium ▪ T1 – invasion into the lamina propria ▪ T2 – invasion into the muscularis propria ▪ T3 – involvement of the perivesical fat ▪ T4 – involvement of the adjacent organs		▪ T1 – clinically inapparent; neither palpable nor visible ▪ T2 – confined within the prostate / prostatic capsule ▪ T3 – extents through the prostatic capsule

Management	▪ Rx of Non Muscle Invasive Bladder Cancer (NMIBC) = Ta, T1, CIS – removal of all visible tumor by TURBT + intravesical BCG
	▪ MIBC = T2-T4 – radical cystectomy or TURBT + RT + CT
	▪ Invasion of the detrusor muscle (muscularis mucosa) is associated with worst prognosis
		▪ Lesion involving glans or distal shaft → Partial penectomy with 2 cm margin
		▪ Lesion involving proximal shaft or 2 cm margins are not achieved → Total penectomy with perineal urethrostomy
		▪ B/ L illioinguinal LN dissection for metastatic LN disease
		▪ Preputial penile CA → Wide excision
			Tumor markers:
			  ○ Prostatic acid phosphatase – not specific
			  ○ Alkaline phosphatase
			  ○ PSA → prostrate specific (not cancer specific, also ↑ in BHP). Used for monitoring after radical prostatectomy
			▪ Grading is done by Gleason's scoring – Based on histological evaluation of biopsy. Helps determine the prognosis.
			▪ T1a → Incidentally found; Management – Regular follow up
			▪ For metastatic disease: GnRH analogues (Goserelin, Leuprolide, Triptorelin) are used
			▪ Antiandrogens used are Abiraterone, Bicalutamide, Degarelix, Flutamide, Nilutamide

BONE TUMORS

	Osteochondroma / Exostosis	Osteoid Osteoma	Enchondroma	Chondroblastoma
General	▪ MC benign tumor of bone ▪ Cartilaginous neoplasm ▪ Characterized by growth arising from the surface of bone ▪ Located adjacent to **growth plate** ▪ It is not at true neoplasm → growth of tumor stops with cessation of growth at epiphyseal growth plate	▪ MC true benign tumor of bone ▪ Osteoblastic tumor ▪ Can occur anywhere on bone ▪ MC occur in the cortex of the shafts of long bones	▪ Benign, cartilaginous neoplasm of hyaline cartilage ▪ Mostly solitary lesions of bone	▪ Occurs in skeletally immature persons ▪ GCT is the adult counterpart of chondroblastoma ▪ Aka Codman's tumor

Presentation	▪ Age group: Teenage or young adult (<20 years)
	▪ MC site – knee joint > Proximal humerus
	▪ Origin: Metaphysis
	▪ Presents with painless swelling
	▪ Rapid increase in size & appearance of pain is suggestive of malignant transformation into → Chondrosarcoma – MC malignancy associated with it.
	▪ *Occurrence of pain suggests:*
	  ○ Bursitis at tip of swelling
	  ○ Fracture through stalk of osteochondroma
	  ○ Tethering of neighbouring structures
	  ○ Malignant transformation
		▪ Age group: 10-30 years
		▪ MC site – Femur > Tibia
		▪ Origin: Diaphysis
		▪ Presents with nagging pain , worst at night and is relieved by salicylates or other NSAIDs
			▪ Age group: common in 20-40 years
			▪ MC site: Phalanges & Metatarsals
			▪ Origin: Growth plate
			▪ Usually asymptomatic, not painful
			▪ Other bones affected are: Femur, humerus, ribs etc.
			▪ Multiple enchondroma are seen in:
			  ○ Ollier disease
			  ○ Maffucci syndrome along with multiple hemangioma
				▪ Age group: 10-20 years
				▪ MC site: Proximal humerus
				▪ Origin: Epiphysis of long bones
				▪ Presents with the pain in the adjacent joints

Pathology	▪ Can be sessile or Pedunculated ▪ **Cartilage cap** is present surrounding the pedicle of bone ▪ Cap consist of simple hyaline cartilage	▪ Prostaglandins & other inflammatory markers have been linked ▪ Osteoid rich nidus		▪ Large collection of chondroblasts set off by the surrounding matrix of immature fibrous tissue ▪ Scattered giant cells within the stroma
X-ray	▪ Pathognomonic ▪ Well defined Exostosis emerging from metaphysis ▪ Medullary cavity of tumor is in continuation with that of bone ▪ Cartilage cap is not seen on X-ray	▪ Small radiolucent area (nidus) surround by dense sclerosis ▪ CT scan – double dot sign/ **dot within dot** sign	▪ Well defined radiolucent area at the junction of metaphysis & diaphysis ▪ In mature lesions – flecks of whips of calcification present within lucent area → Pathognomonic feature	▪ Well defined lytic lesions (radiolucent area) in epiphysis ▪ Stippled calcification which give rise to mottled appearance
Rx	▪ Asymptomatic → No treatment required ▪ Symptomatic → Excision	▪ Complete surgical excision of nidus/ En-bloc resection of the lesion	▪ Not always necessary	

	Giant Cell Tumor/Osteoclastoma	Ewing's Sarcoma	Osteogenic Sarcoma/Osteosarcoma
General	▪ It is an osteolytic tumor ▪ Origin: from epiphysis ▪ Locally very **aggressive** tumor	▪ Highly malignant sarcoma ▪ Origin: Bone marrow (medullary cavity) ▪ Derived from primitive neuroectoderm ▪ Very primitive tumor with poor differentiation	▪ Highly malignant tumor arising within bone ▪ Origin: Metaphysis ▪ Arises from primitive bone forming cells ▪ MC primary malignant tumor of bone in children & adolescent
Presentation	▪ Age group: 20-40 years ▪ MC site: lower end of femur > upper end of tibia ▪ Pain at the site of tumor ▪ Egg crackling sensation on palpation ▪ May be associated with secondary aneurysmal bone cyst (ABC)	▪ Age group: 10-15 years ▪ MC site: Diaphysis of femur, tibia & humerus ▪ Presents with fever, throbbing pain, swelling & tenderness in the mid shaft (diaphysis) → ▪ So it can mimic osteomyelitis	▪ Age group: 10-25 years ▪ MC site: lower end of femur > upper end of tibia ▪ 1st symptom – local pain with gradually ↑ in swelling ▪ 10% have pulmonary metastasis at the time of presentation ▪ Hematogenous metastasis
Pathology	▪ Presence of tumor giant cell is the hallmark ▪ Pulsatile tumor	▪ Small round blue cell tumor with scant cytoplasm ▪ Glycogen rich cytoplasm, so PAS +ve ▪ Diastase sensitive ▪ Homer Wright rosette appearance ▪ Expresses **MIC2** antigen (CD99) which differentiate it from other round cell tumors	▪ Histological hallmark – osteoid producing cells ▪ Secondary OGS is associated with Paget's disease, Bone infarction, Radiation & Chronic osteomyelitis
Radiology	▪ Solitary lytic lesions of the bone ▪ Eccentric location ▪ Expansion of overlying cortex ▪ Soap bubble appearance ▪ No calcification within tumor ▪ No/ Minimal reactive sclerosis around tumor	▪ Onion skin periosteal reaction ▪ Sunray appearance and Codman's triangle (Both are more common in Osteogenic sarcoma)	▪ Irregular periosteal reaction ▪ **Codman's triangle (due to subperiosteal new bone formation) and Sunray appearance are typical ▪ Irregular destruction in the metaphysis is overshadowed by new bone formation

Management	▪ Enbloc excision /Complete resection
	▪ Curettage & bone grafting
	▪ Excision & reconstruction by:
	  ○ Turn - O - plasty technique
	  ○ Arthrodesis using fibula
	  ○ Arthroplasty
	▪ Irradiation for spinal involvement
	▪ TOC for different sites:
	  ○ Lower end of ulna upper end of fibula → Excision of tumor
	  ○ Lower end of radius → Excision with reconstruction using I/L fibula
	  ○ Around knee → Excision with prosthesis replacement or arthrodesis
		▪ ES is highly radiosensitive – melts like snow by radiotherapy
		▪ TOC = RT+ CT+ surgery
		▪ *Poor Prognostic indicators:*
		  ○ Distant metastasis: worst prognosis
		  ○ Proximal location
		  ○ Fever, Size, Older age, Male gender
		▪ mAb to cell surface gp (p30/32) encoded by MIC2 gene is a useful screening measure
		▪ MC translocation seen in 80-95% is the t(11;22) tumor which produces the EWS-FLI1 fusion protein
			▪ Workup: X-ray, Bone scan, MRI & CT
			  ○ CT Chest: For pulmonary metastasis
			▪ Rx: It is a radio resistant tumor
			  ○ Neoadjuvant chemotherapy f/b surgery (limb salvage surgery mostly) f/b postoperative CT

OGS	Parosteal OGS	Periosteal OGS
Age	▪ In older individual (3rd – 4th decade of life)	
Origin	▪ Metaphysis	▪ Diaphysis
Location	▪ Cortical surface*	
Rx	▪ Local resection	▪ Same as OGS

*Sparing of medullary cavity for a long time – characteristic

BONE TUMOR LOCATION

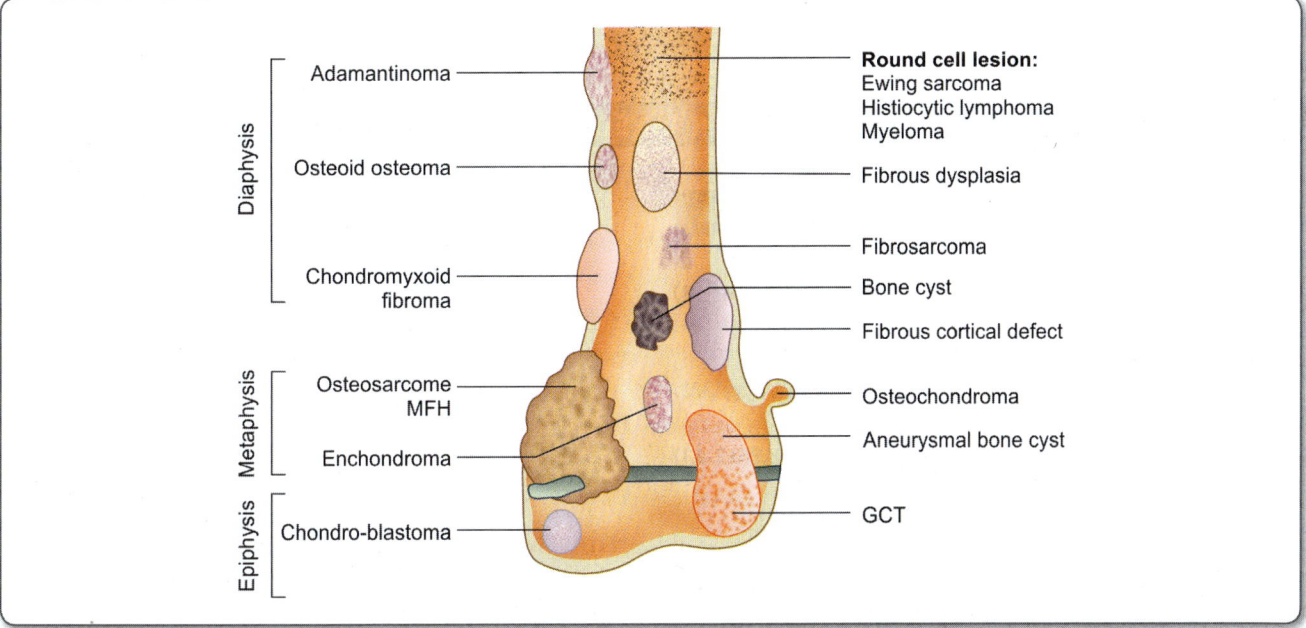

Diaphysis
- Adamantinoma
- Osteoid osteoma
- Chondromyxoid fibroma

Round cell lesion:
Ewing sarcoma
Histiocytic lymphoma
Myeloma
- Fibrous dysplasia
- Fibrosarcoma
- Bone cyst
- Fibrous cortical defect

Metaphysis
- Osteosarcome MFH
- Enchondroma
- Osteochondroma
- Aneurysmal bone cyst

Epiphysis
- Chondro-blastoma
- GCT

RADIO SENSITIVITY OF TUMORS

Highly Sensitive	Relatively Resistant	Highly Resistant
• Seminoma	• Cervical cancer	• Pancreatic carcinoma
• Ewing's sarcoma		• Osteosarcoma
• Wilms' tumor		• Melanoma
• Multiple Myeloma		
• Lymphoma & Leukemia		

MULTIPLE CHOICE QUESTIONS

CHAPTER 1: NEOPLASIA

BASIC PRINCIPLES

1. Squamous cell carcinoma spreads commonly via- *(DNB June 08)*
- a. Implantation
- b. Trancoelomic spread
- c. Lymphatic spread
- d. Hematogenous spread

[Ref: Robbin's 9th/e pg. 273]

2. The following parasitic infections predispose to malignancies- *(PGMEE 2012-13)*
- a. Guinea worm infection
- b. Pargibunuasus
- c. Clonorchiasis
- d. Schistosomiasis

[Ref: Rajesh Karyakarte pg. 239]

3. High risk of malignancy is seen in? *(DNB June 11)*
- a. Complex hyperplasia without atypia
- b. Complex hyperplasia with atypia
- c. Simple hyperplasia with atypia
- d. Simple hyperplasia without atypia

[Ref: Gynecological cancer management by Clarke Pearson pg. 463]

4. Hereditary factors are importance in- *(DNB Dec 07)*
- a. Retinoblastoma
- b. Breast carcinoma
- c. Pancreatic tumor
- d. Bronchogenic carcinoma

[Ref: Robbin's 9th/e pg. 280]

5. Centrosome duplication takes place in - *(PGMEE 2012-13)*
- a. G0 phase
- b. G2 phase
- c. S phase
- d. M phase

[Ref: Robbin's 9th/e pg.]

6. Telomerase- *(PGMEE 2012-13)*
- a. Present in somatic cell
- b. Causes carcinogenesis
- c. Absent in germ cell
- d. RNA polymerase

[Ref: Robbin's 9th/e pg. 303]

Explanation

- Telomerase is an RNA dependent DNA polymerase
- It is active in stem cells, in gametes & most cancer cells.
- Absence of telomerase activity leads to premature aging.

7. Disorganized overgrowth of a skin structure at a localized region is *(PGMEE 2012-13)*
- a. Hamartoma
- b. Polyp
- c. Malignant tumor
- d. Choriostoma

[Ref: Robbin's 9th/e pg. 267]

8. Ectopic rest of normal tissue is known as- *(DNB Dec 08)*
- a. Choristoma
- b. Lymphoma
- c. Hamartoma
- d. Pheudotumor

9. Features of dysplasia are all except- *(PGMEE 2013)*
- a. Pleomorphism
- b. Loss of architecture
- c. High nuclear- to- cytoplasmic ratio
- d. Invasion into basement membrane

[Ref: Robbin's 9th/e pg. 271]

10. Excessive fibrosis or collagenous stroma in tumor in called- *(PGMEE 2013-14)*
- a. Metaplasia
- b. Dysplasia
- c. Desmoplasia
- d. Dysplasia

[Ref: Robbin's 9th/e pg. 266]

11. Which of the following tumors show increased c-kit- *(PGMEE 2012-13)*
- a. Chriocarcinoma
- b. Yolk sac tumor
- c. Embryonal carcinoma
- d. Seminoma

[Ref: Robbin's 9th/e pg. 285; http://en.wikipedia.org/wiki/CD117]

12. Essential for tumor metastasis is- *(DNB Dec 08)*
- a. Angiogenesis
- b. Inhibition of Tyrosine kinase activity
- c. Tumorogenesis
- d. Apoptosis

[Ref: Robbins 9th/e pg. 307]

13. All the following are angiogenic factors EXCEPT-
- a. TGF- beta
- b. PDGF *(DNB Dec 10)*
- c. IFN
- d. VEGF

[Ref: Robbins 9th/e pg. 306; Wintrobe's Clinical Hematology 11th/e Table 22.1]

ONCOGENES

14. BRCA-1 gene lies on Chromosome - *(DNB Dec'2008)*
- a. 17
- b. 18
- c. 20
- d. 21

[Ref: Robbin's 9th/e pg. 108]

15. MYC gene is an example of - *(PGMEE 2012-13)*
- a. GTPase
- b. Protein kinase inhibitor
- c. Growth factor inhibitor
- d. Transcription activator

[Ref: Robbins 9th/e pg. 288]

16. BCR-ABL gene mutation is seen in? *(DNB June 2009)*
- a. CML
- b. CLL
- c. AML
- d. All

[Ref: Robbin's 9th/e pg. 317]

17. HER-2/NEU receptor gene mutation is seen in which cancer? *(PGMEE 2012)*
- a. Glioblastoma
- b. Breast cancer
- c. Squamous cell carcinoma
- d. All of the above

[Ref: Robbin's 8th/e Chapter 7]

1.	c
2.	c,d
3.	b
4.	a,b
5.	c
6.	b
7.	a
8.	a
9.	d
10.	c
11.	d
12.	a
13.	c
14.	a
15.	d
16.	a
17.	b

18. Amplification of N -MYC proto-oncogene is associated with which tumor? **(PGMEE 2012-13; DNB June 07)**
    a. Neuroblastoma
    b. Neuroma
    c. Retinoblastoma
    d. Osteosarcoma

    [Ref: Robbins 9th/e pg. 284]

19. Which among the following pairs of Oncongenes is activated by Translocation? **(DNB Dec 10)**
    a. HGF & HST-1
    b. SIS & HST-1
    c. TGF & CDK4
    d. ABL & C-MYC

    [Ref: Robbins 9th/e pg. 290]

20. Gene most commonly involved in CA endometrium:- **(PGMEE 2016-17)**
    a. p16/INK 4a   b. BRAF
    c. CD-99   d. PTEN

    [Ref: Robbin's 9th/e pg. 1015]

TUMOR SUPRESSOR GENES

21. False about p^{53} is - **(DNB June 10)**
    a. 53 KDa
    b. It causes cell cycle arrest in G1
    c. It is present on chromosomes 17
    d. Non mutated wild p^{53} is associated with neoplasm in childhood

    [Ref: Robbin's 9th/e pg. 294-296]

22. An example of a tumor suppressor gene is- **(DNB Dec 07, PGMEE 2012-13)**
    a. fos   b. ras
    c. myc   d. Rb

    [Ref: Robbin's 9th/e pg. 94, 290]

23. Tumor suppressor genes are not involved in?
    a. Neurofibromatosis **(PGMEE 2013)**
    b. Multiple endocrine neoplasia
    c. Retinoblastoma
    d. Breast carcinoma

24. Which of the following tumor suppressor gene is involved in familial endometrial carcinoma:- **(PGMEE 2012-13)**
    a. APC   b. P53
    c. PTEN   d. Rb

    [Ref: Robbins 9th/e pg. 291]

25. RET gene mutation is associated with which malignancy
    a. Renal cell carcinoma **(PGMEE 2012-13)**
    b. Medullary carcinoma thyroid
    c. Pheochromocytoma
    d. Lymphoma

    [Ref: Robbin's 9th/e pg. 283, 728-729]

TUMOR MARKERS

26. Carcinoma of lung, best marker is- **(PGMEE 2012-13)**
    a. CEA   b. hCG
    c. CA-15-3   d. AFP

    [Ref: Robbin's 9th/e pg. 337]

27. A 67-year-male smoker presents with haemoptysis and cough. Bronchoscopic biopsy revealed undifferentiated tumor. Most useful immunohistochemical marker for this malignancy is: - **(DNB June 10)**
    a. GGT   b. Calretinin
    c. Cytokeratin   d. Vimentin

    [Ref: Harrison 18th/e pg. 823]

Explanation

■ Cytokeratin can be present is variety of epithelial cancers including lung carcinoma.

28. Alpha-fetoprotein is detected in case of- **(PGMEE 2012-13)**
    a. Hepatocellular Ca   b. Renal cell Ca
    c. Tuberculoma   d. Colonic cancer

    [Ref: Robbin's 9th/e pg. 337]

29. Sqamous cell carcinoma marker is- **(PGMEE 2012-13)**
    a. Myogenin   b. Cytokeratin
    c. Vimentin   d. Desmin

    [Ref: Sternberg Diagnostic surgical pathology 4th/e Volume 1, p, 285]

30. CD 34 is a tumor marker used for- **(PGMEE 2012-13)**
    a. Inflammatory myofibroblastic tumor
    b. Ewings sarcoma
    c. GIST
    d. Myofibrosarcoma

    [Ref: Neoplastic Hematopathology 1st/e pg. 161]

31. Marker of malignant melanoma is? **(DNB June 2009)**
    a. HMB 45   b. S-100
    c. Synaptophysin   d. Both A and B

    [Ref: Anderson, 10th edition, Page 147]

32. S 100 is a marker of? **(DNB June 09)**
    a. Histiocytoma   b. Schwannoma
    c. Melanoma   d. All of the above

    [Ref: Anderson 10th e pg.147,151]

33. Tumor marker CA 15-3 is associated with? **(PGMEE 2012)**
    a. Kidney   b. Breast
    c. Ovary   d. All

    [Ref: Robbin's 9th/e pg. 337]

34. Ca 125 is used for? **(PGMEE 2012)**
    a. Follow up of ovarian cancer
    b. Diagnosis of stomach cancer
    c. Diagnosis of pancreatic cancer
    d. Diagnosis of ovarian cancer

    [Ref: Robbin's 9th/e pg. 337]

Explanation

■ CA 125 is used to monitor treatment for ovarian cancer to check recurrences & to screen women at high risk for ovarian cancer.

35. Increased LDH helps in diagnosis of? **(PGMEE 2012)**
    a. Prostate carcinoma
    b. Renal cell carcinoma
    c. Hepatocellular carcinoma
    d. Pancreatic carcinoma

    [Ref: Biochemistry M N Chatarjee, 2nd/e pg. 205, A manual of laboratory and diagnostic tests pg. 429]

18.	a
19.	d
20.	d
21.	d
22.	d
23.	b
24.	c
25.	b
26.	a
27.	c
28.	a
29.	b
30.	c
31.	d
32.	d
33.	b
34.	a
35.	a

36. MIC-2 is a marker of? *(PGMEE 2012)*
a. Chronic lymphocytic leukemia
b. Mantle cell lymphoma
c. Ewing sarcoma
d. All of these

[Ref: Diagnostic musculoskeletal surgical pathology clinico-cardiologic and cytologic correlation pg. 26]

37. CEA is a marker for all except- *(PGMEE 2014)*
a. Carcinoma lung   b. Carcinoma pancreas
c. Carcinoma colon   d. Carcinoma prostate

[Ref: Robbin's 9th/e pg. 337]

38. Elevated AFP levels are seen in all of he following except- *(DNB June 10)*
a. Hepatoblastoma   b. Seminoma
c. Teratoma   d. None of the above

[Ref: Robbin's 9th/e pg. 337]

39. Calcitonin is a marker of- *(PGMEE 2013-14)*
a. Pancreatic cancer
b. Medullary carcinoma of thyroid
c. Pheochromocytoma
d. Prostate cancer

[Ref: Robbins 9th/e pg. 337 & 1073]

40. All of the following immunohistochemical markers are positive in the neoplastic cells of granulocytic sarcoma, except- *(PGMEE 2013-14)*
a. CD45RO   b. Lysozyme
c. CD43   d. Myeloperoxidase

[Ref: Internet]

41. Alkaline phosphatase is a tumor marker of which tumor- *(PGMEE 2013-14)*
a. Seminoma   b. Yolk sec tumor
c. Embryonal carcinoma d. Embryonal sinus tumor

[Ref: Diagnosis and management of cancer pg. 554]

42. Which of the following is not a tumor marker- *(DNB Dec 10)*
a. AFP
b. Tyrosinase
c. Human leucocyte antigen A2
d. CEA

[Ref: Robbin's 9th/e pg. 337]

43. Not a marker for muscle tumor- *(PGMEE 2013-14)*
a. Actin   b. Intermediate filament
c. Neurofilament   d. Desmin

[Ref: Textbook of muscloshletal tumors pg. 786]

44. Marker of small cell cancer of lung is- *(DNB Dec' 2011)*
a. Chromogranin   b. Vimentin
c. Cytokeratin   d. Desmin

[Ref: Robbins 9th/e pg. 717; Chromogranin, synaptophysin, CD57 are neuroendocrine markers of small cell carcinoma of lung]

45. AFP and CEA both are raised in:- *(PGMEE 2016-17)*
a. Seminoma
b. Hepatocellular carcinoma
c. Colorectal carcinoma
d. Non seminoma GCT

[Ref: Robbin's 9th/e pg. 964 - 965]

36.	c
37.	d
38.	b
39.	b
40.	a
41.	a
42.	c
43.	c
44.	a
45.	b
46.	b
47.	b
48.	b
49.	b
50.	a
51.	c

CARCINOGENS

46. Most common antecedent of erythroplakia and leuko-plakia is- *(PGMEE 2013-14)*
a. Alcohol   b. Tobacco use
c. Diphtheria   c. Poor oral hygiene

[Ref: Robbins pathologic basis of disease 9th/e pg. 667]

47. Risk factors for malignant melanoma are all except- *(PGMEE 2014)*
a. Sunlight   b. Coal tar exposure
c. Dysplastic nevi   d. Xeroderma pigmentosa

[Ref: Robbin's 9th/e pg. 1147]

48. Mutation in malignant melanoma is- *(PGMEE 2012-13)*
a. RET   b. CDK2A
c. N-myc   d. None

[Ref: Robbins 9th/e pg. 1148; Textbook of carcinogenesis pg. 731]

49. Most commonly involved transcription factor in carcinogenesis? *(PGMEE 2013)*
a. GRAP   b. MYC
c. FOS   d. RAS

[Ref: Robbins 9th/e pg.18,288] Important transcription factors involved in oncogenesis are:- MYC, MYB, JUN, FOS, and REL proto-oncogenes.

50. Which chemotherapeutic agent is pro carcinogenic? *(DNB June 2009)*
a. Alkylating agents b. Monoclonal antibodies
c. Antibiotics   d. All of the above

[Ref: Robbin's 9th/e pg. 323]

PREMALIGNANT CONDITIONS

51. Which is not a premalignant condition? *(DNB Dec' 2011)*
a. Solar keratosis
b. Leukoplakia
c. Acanthosis nigracans
d. Bowen's disease

[Ref: Das text book of surgery 3rd/e p. 104, Rook's Textbook of Dermatology 4th/e volume 8th/e p. 52.29-52.37]

Explanation

- Solar keratosis/Actinic keratoses is a risk factor for skin cancer
- Bowen's ds is a risk factor for SqCa-penis
- Lesions of oral cavity a/w increased risk of malignancy (Premalignant):-

Premalignant lesions	Precancerous conditions	Doubtful association
Leukoplakia	Oral submucous fibrosis OSR	Oral lichen planus
Erythroplakia	Syphilitic glossitis	Discoid lupus erythematosus
Chronic hyperplastic candidiasis	Sideropenic dysphagia	Dyskeratosis congenita

52. All of the following are premalignant conditions except- *(PGMEE 2015)*

a. Bowen's Disease
b. Senile Keratosis
c. Pyoderma Gangrenosum
d. Xeroderma pigmentosum

[Ref: Bailey and Love's pg.]

MISCELLANEOUS

53. Acanthosis nigricans is seen in *(DNB June' 2009)*

a. GI malignancy
b. Breast cancer
c. Lung cancer
d. All above

[Ref: Internet]

54. All are seen in Carney's triad except? *(PGMEE 2014-15)*

a. GIST
b. Paraganglioma
c. Atrial myxoma
d. Pulmonary chordoma

[Ref: Harrison's 19th/e pg. 2266, 2314]

55. Tumor lysis syndrome does not have

a. Hypercalcemia *(NEET Pattern 2017)*
b. Hyperuricemia
c. Hyperphosphaturia
d. Hyperkalemia

52.	c
53.	d
54.	c
55.	a

BRAIN TUMORS

1. **"En plaque" growth pattern is seen in** *(DNB June 2010)*
   a. Astrocytoma
   b. Meningioma
   c. Glioblastoma multiforme
   d. Ependymoma
   [Ref: Robbins 9th/e pg. 1314; Sabiston's 20th/e pg. 1913]

2. **"Perivascular pseudorosettes" are classically seen in:** *(PGMEE 2015)*
   a. Ependymoma   b. Astrocytoma
   c. Oligodendroglioma   d. Medulloblastoma
   [Ref: Robbins 9th/e pg. 1310]

3. **Expression of GFAP filaments is seen in:** *(PGMEE 2016-17, 2015)*
   a. Ependymoma
   b. Astrocytoma
   c. Oligodendroglioma
   d. Medulloblastoma
   [Ref: Robbins 9th/e pg. 1310]

4. **"Fried egg cytoplasm" is characteristic of :-** *(PGMEE 2013-14)*
   a. Astrocytoma
   b. Oligodendroglioma
   c. Glioblastoma
   d. Medulloblastoma
   [Ref: Robbins 9th/e pg. 1310; Sabiston's 20th/e pg. 1913]

5. **Most common cerebellar tumor in children?** *(PGMEE 2012-13)*
   a. Astrocytoma   b. DNET
   c. Medulloblastoma   d. Ependymoma
   [Ref: Sabiston's 20th/e pg. 1911]

6. **Medulloblastoma most common metastasis is to-** *(PGMEE 2012-13)*
   a. Spleen   b. CNS
   c. Lung   d. Liver
   [Ref: Tumors of CNS pg. 72; Schwartz's 10th/e pg. 1734]

7. **Most common brain tumor are metastases. The most common primary for secondaries in brain is:- -** *(PGMEE 2016-17)*
   a. Stomach   b. Thyroid
   c. Lung   d. Liver
   [Ref: Robbins 9th/e pg. 1315]

8. **Most common site for medulloblastoma-** *(PGMEE 2012-13)*
   a. Cerebellum
   b. Pineal gland
   c. Pituitary
   d. Cerebrum
   [Ref: Robbin's 8th/e pg. 1336; Sabiston's 20th/e pg. 1913]

9. **Most common CNS neoplasm in HIV patient-** *(PGMEE 2012-13)*
   a. Astrocytoma
   b. Ependymoma
   c. Primary CNS lymphoma
   d. Medulloblastoma
   [Ref: Robbin's 8th/e pg. 1337; Sabiston's 20th/e pg. 1914]

10. **Most common site of glioblastoma multiforme is-** *(PGMEE 2012-13)*
    a. Occipital lobe
    b. Frontal lobe
    c. CP angle
    d. Brain stem
    [Ref: BRS neuroanatomy 4th/e pg. 87; Bailey & Love's 27th/e pg. 663]

11. **Commonest intracranial tumor is?** *(PGMEE 2013)*
    a. Meningioma
    b. Astrocytoma
    c. Medulloblastoma
    d. Secondaries
    [Ref: Robbin's 8th/e pg. 1330, 1333]

12. **Most common cause of leptomeningeal metastasis is adenocarcinoma arising from:** *(PGMEE 2015)*
    a. Breast   b. Thyroid
    c. Liver   d. Bone
    [Ref: Harrison 18th /ed 3390; Sabiston's 20th/e pg. 1923]

13. **Which one of the following is the most common tumor associated with type I neurofibromatosis-** *(PGMEE 2013-14)*
    a. Optic nerve glioma
    b. Low grade astrocytoma
    c. Meningioma
    d. Acoustic schwannoma
    [Ref: Nelson 17th/e pg. 2483]

14. **Most common glial tumor-** *(PGMEE 2013-14)*
    a. Neurofibroma   b. Astrocytoma
    c. Ependymomas   d. Meningioma
    [Ref: Robbins 9th/e pg. 1307]

15. **Tumour of anterior cranial fossa compresses:** *(PGMEE 2014)*
    a. Optic tract
    b. Olfactory bulb
    c. Lateral geniculate body
    d. Medial geniculate body
    [Ref: BDC 6th/e pg. 199]

16. **Most common tumor in lateral hemisphere of brain-** *(PGMEE 2013-14)*
    a. Astrocytoma   b. Medulloblastoma
    c. Meningioma   d. Ependymoma
    [Ref: Robbins 9th/e pg. 1306-1308]

1.	b
2.	a
3.	a
4.	b
5.	a
6.	b
7.	c
8.	a
9.	c
10.	b
11.	d
12.	a
13.	a
14.	b
15.	b
16.	a

17. Which chromosome mutation is associated with medulloblastoma- *(PGMEE 2014)*
- a. Chromosome 19
- b. Chromosome 17
- c. Chromosome 16
- d. Chromosome 18

[Ref: Robbins 9th/e pg. 1312]

Explanation

- Isochromosome 17 (17i) is the MC genetic abnormality present in medulloblastoma.
- Along with 17i, there is loss of genetic material from short arm of chr. 17.

18. All of the following metastatic tumors cause spinal cord compression EXCEPT: *(PGMEE 2014-15)*
- a. Lung cancer
- b. Meningioma
- c. Lymphoma
- d. Breast cancer

[Ref: Harrison's 19th/e pg. 2653]

19. Opsoclonus is seen with all except? *(PGMEE 2014-15)*
- a. Neuroblastoma
- b. Lung cancer
- c. Breast cancer
- d. Brain cancer

[Ref: Harrison's 19th/e pg. 618]

Explanation

- Paraneoplastic opsoclonus. myodonus syndrome is seen in cancer of the lung & breast, neuroblastoma & ovarian treatment

20. Brain tumor showing diffuse infiltration of brain without focal mass: *(PGMEE 2014-15)*
- a. Glioblastoma multiforme
- b. Meningioma
- c. PNET
- d. Gliomatosis cerebri

[Ref: Harrison's 19th/e pg.600]

21. Most common intracranial tumor is: *(PGMEE 2014-15)*
- a. Astrocytoma
- b. Oligodendroglioma
- c. Craniopharyngioma
- d. Meningioma

[Ref: Neurooncology by Bernstein 2nd/254; Textbook of Medical oncology 2nd/493, Harrison 19th p 598]

22. Brain tumor with worst prognosis in children: *(PGMEE 2014-15)*
- a. Cerebellar astrocytoma
- b. Pineal body tumor
- c. Craniopharyngioma
- d. Brainstem glioma

[Ref: OP. Ghai, 545, 7th ed]

23. A 5-year-old child presents with loss of vision and axial proptosis. Pupillary examination shows relative afferent pupillary defect. Probable diagnosis is? *(PGMEE 2014)*
- a. Optic nerve glioma
- b. Optic disc melanocytoma
- c. Retinoblastoma
- d. Optic nerve sheath meningioma

[Ref: Nelson Textbook of Pediatrics, ch. 620: Disorders of Vision]

24. A 14-year-old child presents with headache and visual loss. Saggital CT scan of of sella is shown below. What is the diagnosis *(PGMEE 2018)*
- a. Craniopharyngioma
- b. Pituitary microadenoma
- c. Prolactinoma
- d. Optic nerve glioma

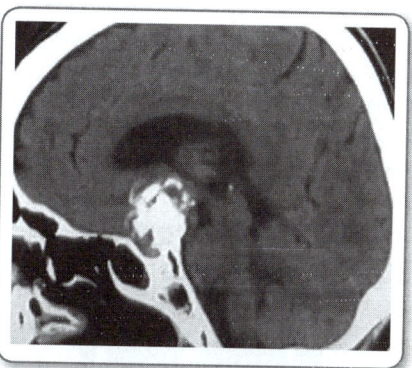

Explanation

- Suprasellar calcification in child is characteristic of craniopharyngioma.

25. The most common presentation of cranio-pharyngioma: *(PGMEE 2014-15)*
- a. Headache
- b. Visual field defects
- c. Endocrinal disturbance
- d. Cardiac disturbance

[Ref: Harrison's 19th/e pg. 2264]

26. All are true regarding cranio-pharyngioma EXCEPT: *(PGMEE 2014-15)*
- a. Derived from Rathke's pouch
- b. Contains epithelial cells
- c. Present in temporal or parietal lobes
- d. Causes visual disturbances

[Ref: Harrison's 18th ed.chpter 339, page 2883, Harrison's 19th/e pg. 2264]

27. Craniopharyngiomas are basically- *(PGMEE 2015)*
- a. Tumours resembling osteomas
- b. Tumours derived from Rathke's Pouch
- c. Adenocarcinomas
- d. Tumours similar to glottis cancer

[Ref: Garnett MR, Puget S, Grill J, Sainte-Rose C (2007). "Craniopharyngioma". Orphanet journal of arer disease]

28. Bony clival erosion with intra-cranial calcification is seen in: *(PGMEE 2014-15)*
- a. Craniopharyngioma
- b. Medulloblastoma
- c. Papilloma of the choroid plexus
- d. Sella chordoma

[Ref: Harrison's 19th/e pg. 2264]

29. True about Turcot syndrome *(PGMEE 2013-14)*
- a. Mutations in PTEN gene
- b. Associated with CNS tumors
- c. Non- neoplastic polyps
- d. Congenital hypertrophy of retinal pigment epithelium

[Ref: Robbins 9th/e pg. 1249]

17.	b
18.	b
19.	d
20.	d
21.	d
22.	d
23.	a
24.	a
25.	a
26.	c
27.	b
28.	d
29.	b

30. Most common site of brain metastasis *(DNB June' 2011)*
- a. Brainstem
- b. Thalamus
- c. Cerebellum
- d. Cerebral Cortex

[Ref: Sabiston's 20th/e pg. 1915]

31. Most common tumor which has highest propensity to develop brain metastases :- *(PGMEE 2016-17)*
- a. Lung
- b. Breast
- c. Prostate
- d. Melanoma

[Ref: Sabiston's 20th/e pg. 1915]

Explanation
- Melanoma has the highest propensity to spread to the brain

32. Image shown below is: *(PGMEE 2016-17)*

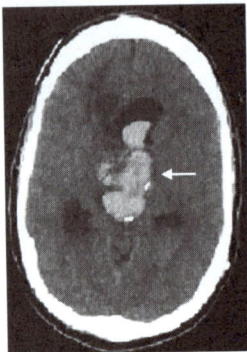

- a. Intracranial bleeding
- b. Intracranial tumor
- c. Subdural hemorrhage
- d. Cystic swelling

33. Most common brain tumor which undergoes calcification is- *(PGMEE 2014)*
- a. Medulloblastoma
- b. Glioblastoma multiformae
- c. Oligodendroglioma
- d. Ependymoma

[Ref: Robbin's 9th/e pg. 1390-1310]

RETINOBLASTOMA

34. Flexner- Wintersteiner rosette is seen in- *(PGMEE 2013-14)*
- a. Nephroblastoma
- b. Neuroblastoma
- c. Hepatoblastoma
- d. Retinoblastoma

[Ref: Robbins 9th/e pg.1339]

35. Retinoblastoma is associated with- *(PGMEE 2012-13)*
- a. Osteosarcoma
- b. SCC
- c. Osteoclastoma
- d. Hepatocellular ca

[Ref: Robbins 9th/e pg.293]

36. Retinoblastoma gene regulates- *(PGMEE 2013-14)*
- a. G_1- S phase
- b. G_0- S_1 phase
- c. S- G_2 phase
- d. G_2- M phase

[Ref: Robbin's 8th/e pg. 285, 286]

MISCELLANEOUS

37. M.C. optic nerve tumor in children causing blindness- *(PGMEE 2013-14)*
- a. Craniopharyngioma
- b. Meningioma
- c. Glioma
- d. Astrocytoma

[Ref: Nelson 20th/e/p 3022]

Explanation
- Normal adult serum PRL levels are about 10–25 mcg/L in women and 10–20 mcg/L in men. PRL secretion is pulsatile, with the highest secretory peaks occurring during rapid eye movement sleep.
- Hyperprolactinemia is the most common pituitary hormone hypersecretion syndrome in both men and women. PRL-secreting pituitary adenomas (prolactinomas) are the most common cause of PRL levels >100 mcg/L

38. Glioma of optic nerve is usually *(PGMEE 2012-13)*
- a. Gemistocytic
- b. Pilocytic
- c. Fibrillary
- d. Lamellar

[Ref: Nelson 20th/e/ pg. 3059]

39. The most common Intracranial tumor in children is- *(PGMEE 2012-13)*
- a. Lymphangioma
- b. Ependymoma
- c. Glioma
- d. Meningioma

[Ref: Nelson 18th/e pg. 2129-2133]

40. Hemangioblastoma associated with VHL are most commonly seen in: *(PGMEE 2014-15)*
- a. Pancreas
- b. Liver
- c. Kidney
- d. Cerebellum

[Ref: Harrison's 19th/e pg. 1854]

30.	d
31.	d
32.	b
33.	c
34.	d
35.	a
36.	a
37.	c
38.	b
39.	c
40.	d

1. **Preferred treatment approach for locally advanced head and neck cancers is :** *(NEET June 2018)*
   a. Radiotherapy alone
   b. Surgery alone
   c. Induction chemotherapy followed by radiotherapy / surgery
   d. Concomitant chemotherapy with radiotherapy

Explanation

- 50% patient present with locally or regionally advanced disease. In such patients combined modality therapy including surgery, radiotherapy, and chemotherapy is most successful. Concomitant (simultaneous) chemo + radiation therapy is currently MC used and supported by evidences.
- In patients with stage III and early stage IV (intermediate stages) concomitant chemoradiotherapy is given postoperatively.
- Preferred chemotherapy agents are cisplatin and cetuximab

ORAL CAVITY

2. **Which of the following is NOT a premalignant condition oral cancer-** *(PGMEE 2015)*
   a. Oral submucous fibrosis
   b. Systemic Sclerosis
   c. Leukoplakia
   d. Erythroplakia

   [Ref: Dhingra's 7th/e pg. 253; Bailey & Love 25th/e p. 735]

3. **Treatment of leukoplakia –** *(PGMEE 2012)*
   a. Excision and radiotherapy
   b. Repositioning of ill fining dentures
   c. Topical chemotherapy
   d. Local excision

   [Ref: Burket's oral medicine 11th/e p. 88; Bailey & Love's 27th/e pg. 761-762]

Explanation

- Leukoplakia regress spontaneously after removing causal agent

4. **The image of oral cavity with restricted opening of mouth is shown below from a patient who is chronic tobacco chewer. Diagnosis is?** *(PGMEE 2015)*

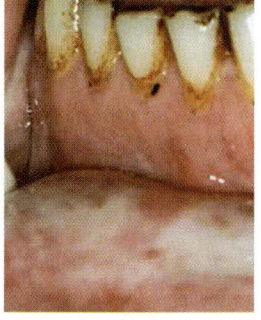

a. Squamous cell carcinoma
b. Leukoplakia
c. Erythroplakia
d. Oral submucous fibrosis

[Ref: Dhingra's 6th/e pg. 220; Bailey & Love's 27th/e pg. 763]

5. **A 50 yr old male presents with ulcerative lesion over cheek involving the mandible without any involvement of lymph nodes the most probable diagnosis is:-** *(PGMEE 2016-17)*
   a. Erythroplakia
   b. CA Buccal mucosa
   c. Carcinoma Tongue
   d. Sub mucous fibrosis

   [Ref: Dhingra's 6th/e pg. 224; Bailey & Love's 27th/e pg. 765]

6. **Which ca has best prognosis -** *(PGMEE 2014)*
   a. **Carcinoma Lip**
   b. Carcinoma Cheek
   c. Carcinoma Tongue
   d. Carcinoma palate

   [Ref: Dhingra's 6th/e pg. 224, Anderson 17th/e p. 1586; Bailey & Love's 27th/e pg. 767]

7. **Which of the following stage of lip carcinoma do not have nodal involvement?** *(PGMEE 2015)*
   a. T2N1
   b. T3N0
   c. T1N1
   d. T2N2

   [Ref: Schwartz 10th /e pg.581; Bailey & Love's 27th/e pg. 764]

8. **The commonest site of oral cancer among Indian population is -** *(PGMEE 2012)*
   a. Alveobuccal complex
   b. Floor of mouth
   c. Tongue
   d. Lip

   [Ref: ASI 1st/e p. 348; Oncology and Surgery Journal 2004, p. 161; Bailey & Love's 27th/e pg. 761]

Explanation

- Commonest site in India is→ buccal mucosa

9. **Gene mutations involved in CA buccal mucosa are all EXCEPT :-** *(PGMEE 2016-17)*
   a. p16
   b. PRAD1
   c. p18
   d. p53

   [Ref: Robbins 9th/e pg. 732]

Explanation

- Most genetic mutations in oral squamous cell carcinoma are located in chromosome 3, p16 on chromosome 9, TP53 on chromosome 17 and PRAD1 on chromosome 11.

10. **Treatment for squamous cell carcinoma stage $T_3N_0M_0$ is?** *(DNB Dec' 2011)*
    a. Maxillectomy
    b. Maxillectomy and Radiotherapy
    c. Radiotherapy
    d. Maxillectomy and chemotherapy

    [Ref: Dhingra 3rd/e p. 255; Bailey & Love's 27th/e pg. 769]

1.	d
2.	b
3.	b
4.	d
5.	b
6.	a
7.	b
8.	b
9.	c
10.	b

11. **MC pathological type of hypopaharynx cancer is:-**
    a. Squamous cell carcinma   *(PGMEE 2016-17)*
    b. Adeno carcinoma
    c. Adenosquamous carcinoma
    d. Desmid blastoma

    [Ref: Bailey & Love's 27th/e pg. 741]

12. **A 3cm tumor of the oral cavity with a single lymphnode of 2cm diameter on the same side in the neck without any metastasis is staged as-**   *(PGMEE 2015)*
    a. T2 N1 M0   b. T2 N2 M0
    c. T3 NI M0   d. TI NI M0

    [Ref: Sabiston's 1st SAE pg. 795; Bailey & Love's 27th/e pg. 764]

13. **All are true about carcinoma palate, except-**
    a. Adenocarcinoma   *(PGMEE 2015)*
    b. Presents with pain
    c. Bilateral lymphatic spread
    d. Slow growing

    [Ref: Dhingra 5th/e pg. 242; Sabiston 19th/e pg. 801]

14. **A 45 old chronic tobacco chewer presents with the chief complaints of a mass in the oral cavity of 1.5 cm with a single lymph node on ipsilateral neck. The stage of the tumor is-**   *(PGMEE 2015)*
    a. T1N1   b. T2N2
    c. T1N3   d. T3N1

    [Ref: Schwartz 10th/e pg. 581; Bailey & Love's 27th/e pg. 764]

15. **Michaelis Gutmann bodies are found in?**
    a. Malakoplakia
    b. Langerhans cell histiocytosis
    c. Xanthogranulomatous pyelonephritis
    d. Tuberculosis

    [Ref: Robbins 9th/e pg. 963]

SALIVARY GLAND TUMORS

16. **Most common parotid gland tumor:-**
       (PGMEE 2016-17; PGMEE 2012-13)
    a. Warthin tumor
    b. Mucoepedermoid carcinoma
    c. Pleomorphic adenoma
    d. Adenoid cystic carcinoma

    [Ref: Robbins 9th/e pg. 744; Schwartz's 20th /e pg. 599; Bailey & Love's 27th/e pg. 787]

17. **Most common malignant tumor of major salivary glands:-**   *(PGMEE 2016-17; 2013-14)*
    a. Adenoid cystic Carcinoma
    b. Muco epidermoid carcinoma
    c. Pleomorphic adenoma
    d. Warthin tumor

    [Ref: Robbin's 9th/e pg. 746; Bailey & Love's 27th/e pg. 787]

18. **Most common malignant tumor of parotid gland is?**
       (DNB Dec'2010)
    a. Pleomorphic adenoma (Mixed tumor)
    b. Warthin's tumor
    c. Squamous cell carcinoma
    d. Mucoepidermoid carcinoma

    [Ref: Sabiston Textbook of Surgery, 18th/e Chapter 33; Bailey & Love's 27th/e pg. 787]

19. **Variable cellularity, abundant cytoplasm, fibromyxoid form is seen in:-**   *(PGMEE 2016-17)*
    a. Adenoid cystic Carcinoma
    b. Muco epidermoid carcinoma
    c. Pleomorphic adenoma
    d. Warthin tumor

    [Ref: Robbin's 9th/e pg. 744]

20. **All the following statements are true regarding malignant salivary gland tumors except?**
    a. Cervical lymphadenopathy present   *(DNB Dec 2010)*
    b. Present with skin ulceration
    c. Simple enucleation is treatment of choice
    d. Painful

    [Ref: Sabiston 18th/e Chapter 33; Bailey & Love's 27th/e pg. 792]

Explanation

- Primary treatment of malignant salivary gland tumor: Surgery
- It is often combined with post op radiation therapy.

21. **Perineural spread is seen in**   *(DNB Dec' 2009)*
    a. Warthin's tumor
    b. Mucoepidermoid carcinoma
    c. Mixed tumors
    d. Adeoid cystic tumor

    [Ref: Sabiston Textbook of Surgery, 18th/e chapter 33; Devita 9th/e pg. 774]

22. **Lymphoid tissue is seen in which parotid tumor-**
       (PGMEE 2014)
    a. Adenoid cystic   b. Warthins tumor
    c. Pleomorphic adenoma   d. Mucoepidermoid

    [Ref: Robbins 9th/e pg. 745; Devita 9th/e pg. 774]

23. **False about pleomorphic adenoma is-**   *(PGMEE 2014)*
    a. Slow growing
    b. Large in size
    c. Commonly turns malignant
    d. Encapsulated

    [Ref: Robbins 9th/e pg. 745; Bailey & Love's 27th/e pg.788]

24. **Pleomorphic adenoma histology is characterized by-**
    a. Mesodermal component   *(PGMEE 2013-14)*
    b. Epithelial component
    c. Endothelial component
    d. Mixed epithelial and mesenchymal components

    [Ref: Robbins 9th/e pg.744; Devita 9th/e pg. 776]

25. **Pleomorphic adenoma has?**   *(PGMEE 2013)*
    a. Exclusively myoepithelial cells
    b. Nests of squamous cells & vacuolated cells containing mucin
    c. Epithelial cells in chondroid matrix
    d. Columnar cells enclosing lymphoid stroma

    [Ref: Robbins 9th/e pg. 745]

26. **Acinic cell carcinomas of the salivary gland arise most often in the-**   *(PGMEE 2013-14)*
    a. Parotid salivary gland
    b. Submandibular salivary gland
    c. Sublingual salivary gland
    d. Minor salivary glands

    [Ref: Robbins 9th/e pg. 745 ; Bailey & Love's 27th/e pg. 757]

11.	a
12.	a
13.	b
14.	a
15.	a
16.	c
17.	b
18.	d
19.	c
20.	c
21.	d
22.	b
23.	c
24.	d
25.	c
26.	a

27. Which of the following head and neck tumor has worst prognosis? *(PGMEE 2008)*
- a. Adenoid cystic carcinoma
- b. Cystadenolymphoma
- c. Mucoepidermoid carcinoma
- d. Acinic cell carcinoma

[Ref: Robbin's 9th/e pg. 746-747 ; Bailey & Love's 27th/e pg. 757-758]

MISCELLANEOUS

28. Glomus Cells are found in- *(PGMEE 2012-13)*
- a. Carotid body Tumor
- b. Liver carcinoma
- c. Thyroid carcinoma
- d. None

[Ref: Robbin's 9th/e pg. 741 ; Bailey & Love's 27th/e pg. 741]

29. Glomous tumor is seen in- *(PGMEE 2012-13)*
- a. Soft tissue
- b. Proximal portion of digits
- c. Distal portion of digits
- d. Retroperitoneum

[Ref: Robbins 9th/e pg. 517]

30. Cartoid body tumor all are true except:
- a. It is a type of paraganglioma *(PGMEE 2016-17)*
- b. Phelp sign is positive
- c. It is a rapid growing tumor
- d. Tumor of glomus cell

[Ref: Bailey and Love page 27/e, 757]

Explanation
- Cartoid body tumor is a slow growing parasympathetic paraganglioma.
- Cell of origin - Glomus cells
- Arises at the bifurcation of internal & external carotid arteries.

31. Carotid body tumor arises from? *(PGMEE 2009)*
- a. Not a tumor but called a tumor
- b. Sympathetic paraganglioma
- c. Parasympathetic paraganglioma
- d. Carotid artery

[Ref: Robbin's 9th/e pg. 741 ; Bailey & Love's 27th/e pg. 764]

Explanation
- Chemodectoma/Cartoid body tumor:
  - Arises from chemoreceptors cells
  - Non chromaffin paraganglioma
  - Long history, 5th decade

32. Zellballen pattern on histopathology is observed in? *(PGMEE 10)*
- a. Retinoblastoma
- b. GIST
- c. Carotid body tumor
- d. Astrocytoma

[Ref: Robbin's 9th/e pg. 741]

Explanation
- Zellballen pattern is diagnostic for pheochromocytoma & paragangliomas (carotid body tumour, Glomus jugulare etc)

33. Ringertz Tumor is seen commonly in- *(PGMEE 2015)*
- a. Stomach
- b. Nose and sinuses
- c. Upper part of neck
- d. Mediastinum

[Ref: "Sinonasal Inverted Papil loma; Value of Convoluted Cerebriform Pattern on MR Imaging". American Journal of Neuroradiology]

Explanation
- **Inverted papilloma** aka Ringertz carcinoma or Schneiderian carcinoma is a non keratinizing squamous cell carcinoma of sinonasal tract.
  - Age of onset: 5th-7th decade
  - More common in males
  - It grows inward into the stroma, hence called inverted tumor.
  - Wart like, arise from nasal vestibule
  - 0.5-4% of all nasal neoplasm
  - Treatment - Excision ↓ LA
- **Parotid tumors**
  - M/c salivary gland tumour s are seen in → parotid gland
  - M/c benign & overall → Pleomorphic adenoma
  - M/c malignant tumor- mucopidermoid Ca f/b adenocystic ca.

34. True about inverted papilloma is- *(PGMEE 2015)*
- a. It is commonly seen in young girls
- b. It is also known as Schnedrian papilloma
- c. It may cause basal cell carcinoma
- d. Anatomically It has an inverted appearance

[Ref: "Sinonasal Inverted Papilloma; Value of Convoluted Cerebriform Pattern on MR Imaging". American Journal of Neuroradiology]

35. Inverted papilloma of nose is called as- *(PGMEE 2015)*
- a. Klatskin's tumor
- b. Schneiderian papilloma
- c. Bowen 's Disease
- d. Pyoderma Gangrenosum

[Ref:Das text book of surgery 3rd /e pg. 104]

36. Most common malignant neoplasm of the eyelid is- *(PGMEE 2015)*
- a. Merkel Cell tumor
- b. Basal cell Carcinoma
- c. Squamous cell carcinoma
- d. Merkel Cell tumor

[Ref: Duong H-V Q, Copeland R. Basal cell carcinoma, eyelid. (2010, February 10]

27.	a
28.	a
29.	c
30.	c
31.	c
32.	c
33.	b
34.	b
35.	b
36.	b

THYROID CANCERS

1. Best test to differentiate benign from malignant thyroid disease is- *(PGMEE 2014)*

a. MRI
b. FNAC
c. Excision
d. CT scan

[Ref: Harrison's 19th/e pg.2306; Bailey & Love's 27th/e pg. 816]

2. Most common histological type of thyroid cancer :- *(PGMEE 2016-17; PGMEE 2014)*

a. Papillary CA
b. Anaplastic CA
c. Follicular CA
d. Medullary CA

[Ref: Robbins 9th/e pg. 1094; Sabiston 20th /e pg. 902; Bailey & Love's 27th/e pg. 818]

3. Most common thyroid tumor in children is? *(DNB December 2011)*

a. Papillary carcinoma
b. Thyroid lymphoma
c. Medullary carcinoma
d. Follicular carcinoma

[Ref: Nelson 20th/e/p 2685; Bailey & Love's 27th/e pg. 818]

4. Mutation seen in papillary ca thyroid: *(PGMEE 2016-17)*

a. NTRK1
b. RET
c. BRAF
d. All of the above

[Ref: Robbins 9th/e pg. 1094]

5. Thyroid cancer associated with amyloidosis:- *(PGMEE 2016-17; 2013-14)*

a. Papillary CA
b. Anaplastic CA
c. Follicular CA
d. Medullary CA

[Ref: Robbins 9th/e pg. 1094; Bailey & Love's 27th/e pg. 820]

6. A 35 years old female presents with a diffuse swelling in the neck. The swelling has increased in size gradually over the last two years and the patient feels she is has difficulty with breathing. On examination shows swelling is soft, moves with deglutition . It measures 8cm x 10 cm. is not warm to touch. Which of the following is the most appropriate management step for this mass:- *(PGMEE 2016-17)*

a. Oral thyroxine
b. Partial thyroidectomy
c. Excision biopsy
d. FNAC

[Ref: Internet]

7. Thyroid carcinoma with pulsatile vascular skeletal metastasis is seen in: *(PGMEE 2014-15)*

a. Papillary
b. Follicular
c. Medullary
d. Anaplastic

[Ref: Harrison's 19th/e pg. 2305]

8. Most common site of Primary malignancy to metastasis to thyroid :- *(PGMEE 2016-17)*

a. Breast
b. Lungs
c. Kidney
d. Prostate

9. Psammoma bodies are seen in which thyroid tumor:- *(PGMEE 2016-17)*

a. Papillary
b. Follicular
c. Anaplastic
d. Medullary

[Ref: Bailey & Love's 27th/e pg. 818]

10. Which Thyroid Carcinoma is associated with MEN? *(PGMEE 2015)*

a. Medullary Carcinoma
b. Follicular Carcinoma
c. Thyroid Lymphoma
d. Papilary carcinoma

(Ref Schwartz 10th/e pg. 1549; Bailey & Love's 27th/e pg. 820]

11. Most common malignancy in a long standing goiter is- *(PGMEE 2014-15)*

a. Colloid carcinoma
b. Medullary carcinoma
c. Pappilary carcinoma
d. Follicular carcinoma

[Ref: Schwartz 10th /e pg. 1544; Bailey & Love's 27th/e pg. 818]

12. A nodule of 2 cm in left thyroid diagnosed as papillary carcinoma. Treatment of choice is: *(DNB 2008)*

a. Hemithyroidectomy
b. Total thyroidectomy
c. Thyroidectomy with radical dissection
d. Radiotherapy

[Ref: Sabiston 20th edition; Bailey & Love's 27th/e pg. 818]

Explanation

■ Any malignant swelling → Total thyroidectomy

13. 40-year-old female presents with neck swelling. Image of histology is given below. What is the diagnosis: *(PGMEE 2018)*

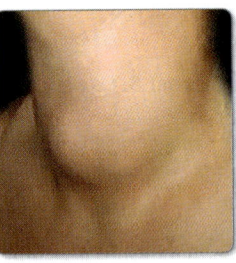 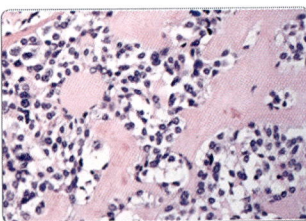

a. Non Hodgkin lymphoma
b. Hashimoto thyroiditis
c. Graves disease
d. Medullary carcinoma of thyroid

[Ref: Robbins 8th Edition Pg.No: 1099]

Explanation

■ Look for age → site → colloid
■ There is presence of amyloid like stroma and parafollicular cells, so the most likely diagnosis is medullary carcinoma of thyroid.

14. In which of the following is medullary thyroid cancer in most aggressive form: *(DNB 2007)*

a. MEN Type-l
b. MEN Type-lla
c. MEN Type-IIb
d. Sporadic cases

[Ref: Sabiston 20th edition Pg 1008]

15. FNAC is not useful in which thyroid cancer- *(PGMEE 2015)*

a. Follicular carcinoma
b. Pappilary carcinoma
c. Medullary carcinoma
d. Thyroid carcinoma

[Ref: Bailey & Love 26th /e pg.765, Schwartz 10th /e pg.1544; Sabiston 20th /e pg. 906]

1.	c
2.	a
3.	a
4.	d
5.	d
6.	d
7.	b
8.	c
9.	a
10.	a
11.	d
12.	b
13.	d
14.	c
15.	a

Explanation

- Limitations of FNAC in thyroid tumours
  - Not able to distinguish follicular adenoma from carcinoma.
  - Not for occult or malignant lesions
  - Difficult with h/o neck irradiation

16. A 65 year old female presents with swelling in the neck diagnosed as a solitary thyroid nodule. The patient is investigated and a scan shows increased uptake of iodine.Serum T3 and t4 are elevated. Most probabe dianosis- *(PGMEE 2015)*

a. Benign Colloid Nodule
b. Toxic Multinodular goitre
c. Toxic Adenoma
d. Follicular adenoma

*[Ref: **Schwartz 10th** /e pg.1533 Toxic MNG usually have enough hyperfunctioning nodules to cause hyperthyroidism]*

17. Thyroid nodule of 4 cm size, mobile but causing compressive symptoms, all are true EXCEPT *(DNB June' 2011)*

a. FNAC cannot distinguish follicular adenoma from carcinoma
b. Managed by subtotal thyroidectomy
c. FNAC is investigation of choice
d. Cold nodules are diagnostic of malignancy

[Ref: Bailey & Love's 27th/e pg. 818]

Explanation

- Hot nodules are rarely malignant
- Only 5-8% of warm or cold nodules are malignant.

18. Thyroid carcinoma with good prognosis is? *(DNB Dec'2010)*

a. Follicular
b. Papillary
c. Anaplastic
d. Medullary

[Ref: Schwartz's Principles of Surgery 9th/e chapter 38, . Thyroid cancer Springer ISBN 3 – 540-22309- 6 Page 10; ; Bailey & Love's 27th/e pg. 818]

19. Lateral Aberrant thyroid is suggestive of which thyroid carcinoma? *(PGMEE 2015)*

a. Medullary
b. Papillary
c. Thyroid Lymphoma
d. Follicular

[Ref: Schwartz 10th/e pg. 1523; Bailey & Love's 27th/e pg. 820]

20. Which of the following gene defect is associated with development of medullary carcinoma of thyroid- *(PGMEE 2012-13)*

a. RET Proto Oncogene
b. BRCA 1 gene
c. Fap gene
d. Rb gene

[Ref: Robbins 9th/e pg. 1099; Bailey & Love's 27th/e pg. 820]

21. Most common thyroid cancer which occurs after radiation exposure- *(PGMEE 2014)*

a. Medullary
b. Papillary
c. Anaplastic
d. Follicular

[Ref: Robbins 9th/e pg. 1095; Bailey & Love's 27th/e pg. 818/819]

22. Which of the following cancers tends to metastatize to the lymphnodes- *(PGMEE 2015)*

a. Thyroid Lymphoma
b. Pappilary Carcinoma
c. Medullary Carcinoma
d. Follicular Carcinoma

[Ref: Schwartz 10/e p. 1542]

23. "Orphan Annie eye nuclei" appearance is seen in?

a. Follicular carcinoma of thyroid *(PGMEE 2012)*
b. Papillary carcinoma of thyroid
c. Medullary carcinoma of thyroid
d. Paraganglioma

[Ref: Schwartz's 10th/e pg. 1542-1544]

24. Hurthle cell or oncocytic carcinoma is a variant of- *(PGMEE 2013-14)*

a. Anaplastic carcinoma
b. Medullary carcinoma
c. Follicular carcinoma
d. Papillary carcinoma

[Ref: Robbins 9th/e pg. 1098; Bailey & Love's 27th/e pg. 818]

25. Medullary ca of thyroid is associated with increase in- *(PGMEE 2013-14)*

a. Calcitonin
b. T4
c. Thyroglobulin
d. T3

[Ref: Robbins 9th/e pg. 1099; Bailey & Love's 27th/e pg. 220]

26. Which type of thyroid carcinoma is classically associated with calcitonin induced amyloid deposition? *(PGMEE 2013-14)*

a. Anaplastic
b. Papillary
c. Follicular
d. Medullary

[Ref: Robbins 9th/e pg. 1099; Bailey & Love's 27th/e pg. 220]

PARATHYROID TUMOURS

27. Most common surgically repairable cause of hyperpara-thyroidism *(DNB June' 2011)*

a. Adenoma
b. Renal disease
c. Carcinoma
d. Hyperplasia

[Ref: Blueprints Surgery by Seth J. Karp, James Morris, David I. Soybel p. 85]

28. In parathyroid carcinoma- *(PGMEE 2014)*

a. Cytology is diagnostic
b. 5-10 % incidence
c. Increased parathormone, decreased calcium
d. Metastasis is essential

[Ref: Robbins 9th/e pg. 1102; Schwartz's 10th/e pg. 1560]

Explanation

- Cytology cannot differentiate between carcinoma & adenoma
- Both S. PTH & S. Calcium levels are elevated
- In parathyroid carcinoma
  - ↑ PTH (5 times of normal)
  - ↑ Ca >14 mg/dl
  - Local invasion occurs

29. Diagnostic feature of parathyroid carcinoma is- *(PGMEE 2013-14)*

a. Clinical features
b. Metastasis
c. Cytology
d. All

[Ref: Robbins 9th/e pg. 1102]

16.	c
17.	d
18.	b
19.	b
20.	a
21.	b
22.	b
23.	b
24.	c
25.	a
26.	d
27.	a
28.	d
29.	b

1. **All are benign conditions of breast EXCEPT**
   (PGMEE 2014-15)
   a. Fibroadenoma
   b. Cystosarcoma phyllodes
   c. Pagets disease of nipple
   d. Galactocele

   [Ref: Robbins 9th/e pg. 1048; 1057; Bailey & Love's 27th/e pg. 873]

2. **CA Breast may locally spread to all of the following muscles expect-** *(PGMEE 2015)*
   a. Pectoralis Major   b. Latissimus Dorsi
   c. Pectoralis minor   d. Serratus Anterior

   [Ref:S.Das 3rd /e pg.725; Schwartz 10th /e pg. 547-549; Bailey & Love's 27th/e pg. 874]

3. **Triple assessment includes all except?** *(DNB Dec'2010)*
   a. Mammography   b. FNAC
   c. Clinical examination   d. Bone scan

   [Ref: Bailey & Love 25th/e p. 280, 290]

4. **New Mammogram Screening Guidelines Recommended Mammography should be routinely offered every two years starting at the age of:-** *(PGMEE 2015-16)*
   a. 40 years   b. 50 years
   c. 60 years   d. 70 years

   [Ref: Schwartz 10th/e pg. 513]

5. **Which of the following precancerous conditions if treated would not lead to cancer-** *(PGMEE 2015)*
   a. Vaginal intraepithelial Neoplasia
   b. Cervical intraepithelial Neoplasia
   c. Lobular Carcinoma in situ of breast
   d. Ductal carcinoma in situ of breast

   [Ref: Sabiston's 20th /e pg. 839; Bailey & Love's 27th/e pg.872]

6. **All are benign conditions except** *(PGMEE 2014-15)*
   a. Fibroadenoma   b. Cystosarcoma phyllodes
   c. Pagets disease of nipple   d. Galactocele

   [Ref: Robbins 9th/e pg. 1048; 1057; Bailey & Love's 27th/e pg. 873]

7. **Somatic mutation E17K in the PH domain of AKT-1 gene mutation is associated with ?** *(PGMEE 2016)*
   a. Ovary   b. Breast
   c. Stomach   d. Pancreas

   [Ref: atlasgeneticsoncology.org/Genes/AKT1]

8. **All are risk factor for breast ca except-** *(PGMEE 2012-13)*
   a. OCP   b. Late menopause
   c. Early mensturation   d. Family history

   [Ref: Robbins 9th/e pg. 1053; Bailey & Love's 27th/e pg. 871]

Explanation

- OCP takers have slightly increased risk of breast cancer.
  - In general population early start of OCPs increases (slightly) risk of early CA breast but protects from late onset CA breast.

1.	c
2.	b
3.	d
4.	b
5.	d
6.	c
7.	b
8.	a
9.	a
10.	a
11.	d
12.	c

- Recent studies also suggest that low dose OCPs does not increase the risk.

9. **All of the following are invasive carcinoma breast except-** *(NBE pattern 2012-13, 2015)*
   a. Comedo carcinoma
   b. Medullary carcinoma
   c. Lobular carcinoma
   d. Colloid carcinoma

   [Ref: Robbins 9th/e pg. 1065; Bailey & Love's 27th/e pg. 872]

Explanation

- Comedocarcinoma is a high grade DCIS which demonstrate central necrosis.
- It is usually non-infiltrating & intraductal tumor.

10. **ER positive status in Ca breast indicates-** *(PGMEE 2012-13)*
    a. Prognosis   b. Site
    c. Etiology   d. None

    [Ref: Robbins 9th/e pg. 1067; Bailey & Love's 27th/e pg. 872]

11. **In which patient of breast cancer, with her-2-neu positivity on IHC, is FISH recommended?** *(NEET Pattern 2017)*
    a. Her 2 neu +   b. Her 2 neu ++
    c. Her 2 neu +++   d. All of the above

    [Ref: Mahanakhan Saha]

Explanation

- An important predictive factor in breast cancer is HER-2. This protein is the product of the *erb-B2* gene and is amplified in approximately 20% of human breast cancers. HER-2 is a member of the epidermal growth factor receptor family of receptor tyrosine kinases.
- HER-2 protein overexpression is measured clinically by immunohistochemistry and scored on a scale from 0 to 3+. Alternatively, fluorescent in situ hybridization, which directly detects the number of HER-2 gene copies, can be used to detect gene amplification.
- Trastuzumab is a humanized monoclonal antibody directed against the extracellular domain of the HER-2 surface receptor and is effective treatment for HER-2-positive breast cancer
- HER-2 testing is now a standard part of pathologic reporting on the primary tumor and is a predictive marker for HER-2-directed therapies.

12. **Granulomatous mastitis is caused by all except-** *(PGMEE 2013-14)*
    a. Fungus
    b. Antibodies to milk antigens
    c. Staphylococcus
    d. TB

    [Ref: Robbins 9th/e pg. 1047; Bailey & Love's 27th/e pg. 866]

13. **BRCA-1 & BRCA-2 are associated with-**
(*NBE based DNB June 14 Pattern*)
a. Bone and testis cancers
b. Breast and ovary cancers
c. Melanoma and breast cancers
d. Testis and ovary cancers
[*Ref: Robbins 9th/e pg. 1054; Bailey & Love's 27th/e pg. 872*]

14. **Type of DCIS resulting in palpable mass in 50-60%-**
(*PGMEE 2013-14*)
a. Non comedo DCIS   b. Comedocarcinoma
c. Paget's disease   d. None of the above
[*Ref: Robbins 9th/e pg. 1057; Bailey & Love's 27th/e pg. 873*]

15. **BRCA-1 gene is located at chromosome location-**
(*PGMEE 2013-14*)
a. 13q21   b. 17q21
c. 17p21   d. 13p21
[*Ref: Harrison 17th/e pg. 494*]

16. **BRCA-1 responsible which type breast cancer-**
(*PGMEE 2014*)
a. Medullary   b. Secretory
c. Lobular   d. Colloid
[*Ref: Robbins 9th/e pg. 1065*]

17. **Which antigen is not prognostic significance in carcinoma breast-** (*NBE based DNB June 14 Pattern*)
a. PR
b. Epithelial membrane antigen
c. Her 2 neu
d. ER
[*Ref: Robbins 9th/e pg. 1067; Bailey & Love's 27th/e pg. 862*]

18. **Exemestane is used in treatment of:-** (*PGMEE 2016-17*)
a. CA testes   b. CA Breast
c. Bladder CA   d. Penile CA
[*Ref: Internet*]

19. **Which cancer detected in one breast to be screened in contralateral breast** (*PGMEE 2016*)
a. Lobular   b. Medullary
c. Ductal   d. Colloid
[*Ref: Robbins 9th/e pg. 1065; Bailey & Love's 27th/e pg. 862-863*]

20. **Male breast cancer wrong statement** (*PGMEE 2016*)
a. BRCA2 seen in 6% cases
b. Lobular carcinoma is common
c. DUCTAL carcimoma is most common subtype
d. Colloid carcinoma can be seen
[*Ref: Robbins 9th/e pg. 1054; Bailey & Love's 27th/e pg. 882*]

21. **Breast carcinoma with best prognosis is:-**(*PGMEE 2015*)
a. Mucinous   b. Medullary
c. Invasive ductal   d. Lobular Ca
[*Ref: Robbins 9th/e pg. 1064-65; Bailey & Love's 27th/e pg. 872*]

22. **Common presentation of duct papilloma of breast is**
(*DNB June' 2011*)
a. Paget's disease   b. Breast eczema
c. Mass in breast   d. Bloody nipple discharge
[*Ref: Bailey and 24th/e p. 828; Bailey & Love's 27th/e pg. 864 (table)*]

23. **Mutations in BRCA-2 gene is associated with-**
a. CA breast in Male   (*PGMEE 2016-17*)
b. CA breast in male and female both
c. CA breast in female
d. Carcinoma in situ
[*Ref: Robbins 9th/e pg. 1054; Bailey & Love's 27th/e pg. 880*]

24. **Conservative surgery in not done in breast carcinoma if there is?** (*DNB June' 2010*)
a. Lymph node metastasis
b. Sub-areolar lump
c. Lump of size 4 cms
d. Disease involving the lower quadrant only
[*Ref: Sabiston's 20th /e pg.836*]

25. **Most common site of metastasis for breast carcinoma is**
(*DNB Dec' 2010*)
a. Lung   b. Liver
c. Brain   d. Bone
[*Ref: Bailey & Love 25th/e p. 839, Schwartz's Principle of Surgery 9th/e chapter 17; Bailey & Love's 27th/e pg. 882*]

26. **All are true about Paget's disease except:**
(*DNB Dec' 2010*)
a. 97% associated with underlying invasive carcinoma of breast
b. 50% are hormone receptor positive
c. Wedge or punch is biopsy taken from nipple for diagnosis
d. Underlying tumor lying within 2cm for the nipple
[*Ref: Schwartz 9th/e chapter 17; Bailey & Love's 27th/e pg. 872*]

27. **Maximum risk of invasive breast carcinoma is seen with?** (*DNB Dec' 2010*)
a. Intraductal papilloma
b. Atypical ductal hyperplasia
c. Complex fibroadenoma
d. Sclerosing adenosis
[*Ref: Sabiston Textbook of Surgery, 18th/e Table 34-3, Schwart'z 8th/e ed. Table 17-4; Bailey & Love's 27th/e pg. 871*]

28. **Histological variety of breast carcinoma with best prognosis is?** (*DNB Dec' 2011*)
a. Lobular   b. Medullary
c. Colloid   d. Tubular
[*Ref: Sabiston 17th/e p. 891, CSDT 11th/e p. 335, Schwartz 9th/e chapter 17; Bailey & Love's 27th/e pg. 871*]

29. **The breast carcinoma with best prognosis to:**
(*DNB 2008*)
a. Schirrous carcinoma   b. Colloid carcinoma
c. Papillary carcinoma   d. Medullary carcinoma
[*Ref: Robbin's 8/e p1088, 1089; Bailey & Love's 27th/e pg. 871*]

30. **Drug of choice for estrogen receptor positive breast cancer is** (*DNB June' 2012*)
a. Transtuzumb   b. Tamopxifen
c. Cyproterone acetate d. Anastrozole
[*Ref: Sabiston 18th/e chapter 34; Bailey & Love's 27th/e pg. 878*]

13.	b
14.	c
15.	b
16.	a
17.	b
18.	b
19.	a
20.	b
21.	a
22.	d
23.	b
24.	b
25.	d
26.	d
27.	b
28.	d
29.	b
30.	b

31. Not true about medullary breast CA: *(PGMEE 2016-17)*
- a. Good prognosis
- b. Around 3rd-4th decade
- c. Associated with BRCA 1
- d. Desmoplasia less than typical breast CA

[Ref: Schwartz's 10th /e pg. 521]

32. Most common presentation of DCIS is
- a. Breast nodule
- b. Nipple discharge
- c. Peau'd orange
- d. Neck swelling

[Ref: Schwartz's 10th /e pg. 520 – table – first symptom is mass; Bailey & Love's 27th/e pg. 872]

33. Breast Ca with worst prognosis: *(PGMEE 2016-17)*
- a. Inflammatory
- b. Tubular
- c. Medullary Ca
- d. Cystosarcoma phyllodes

[Ref: Schwartz's 10th /e pg. 556; Robbins 9th/e pg. 1054] ; Bailey & Love's 27th/e pg. 872]

34. Which of the following is the treatment of choice for Cystosarcoma Phyllodes:- *(PGMEE 2015-16)*
- a. Modified radical mastectomy
- b. Lumpectomy and axillary lymphadenectomy
- c. Wide local incision
- d. Radiotherapy and/or systemic chemotherapy

(Ref. Schwartz 10th/e pg. 555; Bailey & Love's 27th/e pg. 870)

35. Most common malignant tumor of breast after radiation therapy:- *(PGMEE 2016-17)*
- a. Lobular carcinoma in situ
- b. Ductal carcinoma
- c. Comedocarcinoma
- d. Papillary cancer

[Ref: Handbook at all J. Net Cancer net 1993]

36. Most correct statement about breast cancer in male:- *(PGMEE 2016-17)*
- a. It is very common incidence
- b. More strongly associated with BRCA2 mutation
- c. ER positivity is very less
- d. 90% case associated with klinefelter syndrome

[Ref: Shwartz 10th /e pg. 515; Bailey & Love's 27th/e pg. 882]

37. Staging of breast cancer where tumor is 1.6 cm and has spread to the axillary lymph nodes: *(PGMEE 2016-17)*
- a. T0, N1, M0
- b. T1a, N1, M1
- c. T1c, N1, M0
- d. Tis, N1, M0

[Ref: Schwartz 10th /e pg. 532. T1c N1 M0]

38. In a patient undergoing breast surgery with no comorbidity has:- *(PGMEE 2016-17)*
- a. No cardiac risk
- b. Minimal cardiac risk
- c. Moderate cardiac risk
- d. High cardiac risk

[Ref: Bailey & Love 27th/e pg. 263]

39. Peau D orange and multiple ipsilateral axillary node of 3 cm without metastasis. Stage of breast cancer is :- *(PGMEE 2016-17)*
- a. T3N1MO
- b. T3N2M0
- c. T4AN1M0
- d. T4bN2m0

[Ref: Schwartz 10th /e pg. 532]

40. All are risk factors for Ca breast EXCEPT- *(PGMEE 2015)*
- a. Multiparity
- b. Family h/o breast Ca
- c. Ovarian malignancy
- d. Fibroadenosis

[Ref: Schwartz 10th/e pg. 511;Bailey & Love's 27th/e pg. 871]

41. Most common location of breast cancer is *(PGMEE 2015)*
- a. Upper outer quadrant
- b. Nipple
- c. Lower inner quadrant
- d. Upper inner quadrant

[Ref: Bailey & Love 26th/e pg. 811; Bailey & Love's 27th/e pg. 872]

42. All of the following are hormonal agents used against breast cancer, except: *(DNB 2007)*
- a. Letrazole
- b. Exemestrane
- c. Taxol
- d. Tamoxifen

[Ref: Sabiston's 20th/e pg. 857; Bailey & Love's 27th/e pg. 878]

43. Breast ca which is multicentric and bilateral- *(PGMEE 2015)*
- a. Colloid
- b. Ductal
- c. Mucoid
- d. Lobular

[Ref: Bailey and Love's 26th /e pg.810]

44. Sentinel lymph node biopsy is done if- *(PGMEE 2015)*
- a. Metastatic breast ca
- b. Breast lump with palpable axillary lymph node
- c. Breast mass but no lymph node palpable
- d. Lymph node palpable

[Ref:Schwartz 10th /e pg.305; Bailey & Love's 27th/e pg. 877]

45. A 22 year old woman comes with a non progressive mass in a left breast since 6 months. There are no associated symptoms . Examination shows a mobile mass not attached to the overlying skin or underlying tissue. The possible diagnosis- *(PGMEE 2015)*
- a. Fibroadenoma
- b. Fibroadenosis
- c. Scirrhous Carcinoma
- d. Cystasarcoma phylloides

[Ref: Sabiston 20th /e pg.836; Bailey & Love's 27th/e pg. 870]

Explanation

- Age 15-25 is fully developed breast hyperplasia of single

46. Which of the following drugs is used in management of breast cancer if it is estrogen receptor positive- *(PGMEE 2015)*
- a. Bevacizumab
- b. Adalimumab
- c. Tamoxifen
- d. Cyclophosphamide

[Ref: Sabiston 20th /e pg.841]

Breast lump with mc ALN		
US to detect axillary LN	SLNB	
	+ve	-ve
	Axillary clearance done	Axillary clearance not req.

31.	d
32.	a
33.	a
34.	c
35.	b
36.	b
37.	c
38.	b
39.	d
40.	a
41.	a
42.	c
43.	d
44.	c
45.	a
46.	c

BENIGN TUMORS OF LUNG

1. 'Popcorn' calcification in a lung nodule is pathognomic of: *(DNB 2007; PGMEE 2014-15)*
   a. Hamartomas
   b. Histoplasmosis
   c. Tuberculosis
   d. Benign nodule

   [Ref: Schwartz 10th / e pg. 622; Robbins 8th / e p 730; Harrison's 19th/e pg. 515]

2. Vanishing tumor is seen in- *(PGMEE 2015)*
   a. Lung
   b. Heart
   c. Liver
   d. Bone

   [Ref: Textbook of chest medicine Vol. 2 p. 86]

Explanation

- Phantom or vanishing tumor refers to localized transudative interlobar collection of pleural fluid in CHF.

3. Differential diagnosis of a solitary pulmonary nodule includes all of the following EXCEPT: *(PGMEE 2014-15)*
   a. Neurofibroma
   b. Hamartoma
   c. Tuberculoma
   d. Bronchial adenoma

   [Ref: Harrison's 18th ed. pg. 748]

LUNG CANCER

4. Which is not associated with Ca lung- *(DNB June 08)*
   a. Chromium
   b. Berrylium
   c. Asbestos
   d. Nickel

   [Ref: Robbin's 9th/e pg. 713; Essentials of pathology 4th/e pg. 552]

5. Most common type of carcinoma of lung is: *(PGMEE 2014-15)*
   a. Squamous cell carcinoma
   b. Small cell carcinoma
   c. Large cell carcinoma
   d. Adenocarcinoma

   [Ref: Harrison's 19th/e pg. 522]

6. The lung carcinoma most common in non-smokers is- *(DNB Dec 07)*
   a. Large cell
   b. Small cell
   c. Adenocarcinoma
   d. Sq. cell

   [Ref: Robbin's 9th/e pg. 713, 714]

7. Which is the most common tumor leading to death in aduts? *(PGMEE 2015)*
   a. Lung cancer
   b. Leukemia
   c. Prostate cancer
   d. Colorectal cancer

   [Ref: Harrison 19th/e p. 470-471; (table 99-2)]

8. Paranaeoplastic syndrome are most commonly associated with which malignancy:- *(PGMEE 2016-17)*
   a. Carcinoma lung
   b. Ca breast
   c. Ca ovaries
   d. lymphoma

9. Most common primary lung cancer in children: *(PGMEE 2014-15)*
   a. Metastasis
   b. Pulmonary blastoma
   c. Bronchial adenoma
   d. Adenocarcinoma

   [Ref: Nelson 18th /e ch. 408]

10. Which of the following statement about lung carcinoma is true? *(PGMEE 2014-15)*
   a. Squamous cell variant accounts for 70% of all lung cancers
   b. Oat cell variant typically present with cavitation
   c. Adenocarcinoma variant is typically central in location
   d. Oat cell variant presents an endobronchial growth

   [Ref: Harrison's 19th/e pg. 508]

11. Ectopic ACTH syndrome is seen most commonly with: *(PGMEE 2014-15)*
   a. Renal cell carcinoma
   b. Pituitary adenoma
   c. Bronchogenic carcinoma
   d. Lymphoma

   [Ref: Harrison's 19th/e pg. 511/609]

12. Which one of the following statements is true of systemic treatment of NSCLC? *(PGMEE 2014-15)*
   a. Chemotherapy has no effect on survival in advanced NSCLC
   b. EGFR-TKI have a higher chance of response in male smokers
   c. Adjuvant platinum-based chemotherapy confers no survival benefit
   d. Epidermal Growth Factor Receptor Tyrosine Kinase Inhibitors (EGFR-TKI) such as Erlotinib have proven active in previously treated patients with advanced NSCLC

   [Ref: Harrison's 19th/e pg. 516-17]

13. All of the following Para-neoplastic syndrome are seen in Ca lung EXCEPT: *(PGMEE 2014-15)*
   a. Hypertrophic osteodystrophy
   b. Hypoglycemia
   c. Cushing's syndrome
   d. Myasthenia gravis

   [Ref: Harrison's 19th/e pg. 511/609]

Explanation

- CA lung is associated with Lambert Eaton Myasthenia syndrome.

1.	a
2.	a
3.	a
4.	b
5.	d
6.	c
7.	a
8.	a
9.	b
10.	d
11.	c
12.	d
13.	b

14. **Which one of the following is true regarding lung cancer?** *(PGMEE 2014-15)*
    a. Adenocarcinomas tend to grow quickly
    b. 80-90% of small cell carcinomas have spread beyond the thorax at the time of diagnosis
    c. Syndrome of Inappropriate Anti Diuretic Hormone (SIADH] is associated with hypernatraemia
    d. 5% of patients with lung cancer present with, or develop complications of non-metastatic paraneoplastic syndromes

    [Ref: Harrison's 19th/e pg. 508, 11]

15. **ACTH is produced by which carcinoma?** *(PGMEE 2012)*
    a. Adenocarcinoma lung
    b. Small cell cancer Lung
    c. Bronchoaveolar carcinoma Lung
    d. Squamous cell carcinoma of lung

    [Ref: Harrison's 18th/e Table 96-1, Principles and Practice of Endocrinology and Metabolism 3rd/e pg. 957; Harrison 19th/e pg 2272]

16. **A young male presented with asymptomatic lymph node enlargement in supraclavicular region. The biopsy shows squamous cells, the likely site of carcinoma will be:** *(PGMEE 2014-15)*
    a. CA stomach   b. CA colon
    c. CA Breast   d. CA Lung

    [Ref: CMDT-2014, ch. 39, pg. 1597]

17. **Hyperglycaemia is seen in which type of bronchogenic carcinoma:** *(PGMEE 2014-15)*
    a. Squamous cell carcinoma
    b. Large cell carcinoma
    c. Oat cell carcinoma
    d. Adenocarcinoma

    [Ref: Harrison's 19th/e pg. p 511]

18. **The most radiosensitive lung cancer is:**
    a. Squamous cell carcinoma   *(PGMEE 2014-15)*
    b. Giant cell carcinoma
    c. Small cell carcinoma
    d. Adenocarcinoma

    [Ref: Harrison's 19th/e pg. 522]

19. **65 yr old man presented with hemoptysis and grade III clubbing. The probable diagnosis of the patient is?** *(PGMEE 2014-15)*
    a. Non small cell lung Ca   b. Small cell cancer of lung
    c. Tuberculosis   d. Sarcoidosis

    [Ref: Harrison's 19th/e pg. 510-511]

20. **5 year survival rate for small cell cancer lung is:** *(PGMEE 2014-15)*
    a. 1%   b. 5%
    c. 10%   d. 25%

    [Ref: Bailey and love 26th /e pg. 861]

21. **Poorest prognosis in lung cancer is associated with:**
    a. Small cell carcinoma   *(DNB 2007)*
    b. Squamous cell carcinoma
    c. Adenosquamous carcinoma
    d. None of the above

    [Ref: Sabiston 20th edition pg. 1583]

22. **Most common cancer associated with asbestosis:** *(PGMEE 2014-15)*
    a. Adenocarcinoma   b. Squamous cell carcinoma
    c. Mesothelioma   d. Bronchial adenoma

    [Ref: Harrison's 19th/e pg. 1689]

23. **Which one of the following types of bronchogenic carcinoma is most likely to cavitate:** *(PGMEE 2014-15)*
    a. Bronchoalveolar carcinoma
    b. Adenocarcinoma
    c. Oat-cell carcinoma
    d. Squamous cell carcinoma

    [Ref: Bailey & Love's 26th /e pg. 861 and DeVita 8th /e ch. 37]

24. **Most common variant of lung malignancy in woman who consume less than 10 packets cigarette per year:-** *(PGMEE 2016-17)*
    a. Squamous cell carcinoma
    b. Large cell Ca
    c. Adenocarcinoma
    d. Combined carcinoma

    [Ref: Robbin's 9th/e pg. 714]

25. **Following are increased in small cell carcinoma of lung except:** *(PGMEE 2014-15)*
    a. ACTH   b. AVP
    c. ANF   d. Growth hormone

    [Ref: Harrison's 19th/e pg. 511]

26. **A 70-year-old smoker male presents with breathlessness & facial swelling. Incorrect is?** *(PGMEE 2014-15)*
    a. Glossal edema
    b. Dilated veins have blood flow away from umbilicus
    c. Non -pulsatile elevated JVP
    d. Worse on bending forward

    [Ref: Harrison's 19th/e pg. 1787-88]

Explanation
- Given is the clinical scenario of SVC syndrome

27. **Early stage of non small cell lung cancer can be treated by-** *(PGMEE 2015)*
    a. Radiotherapy
    b. Surgical resection
    c. Surgical resection with adjuvant chemotherapy
    d. Immunotherapy

    [Ref: Schwartz 10th edition page 641]

28. **"Single coin shadow" in lung with calcification in centre is a feature of:-** *(PGMEE 2016-17)*
    a. Squamous cell carcinomab. Melanoma
    c. Oat cell tumor   d. Adenocarcinoma

    [Ref: Robbin's 9th/e pg. 717]

29. **Most common symptom of lung cancer?** *(PGMEE 2014-15)*
    a. Hemoptysis   b. Clubbing
    c. Chest pain   d. Weight loss

    [Ref: Harrison's 19th/e pg. 510; Table 107-4]

30. **Least common cause of clubbing is:** *(PGMEE 2014-15)*
    a. Adenocarcinoma   b. Squamous cell CA
    c. Small cell CA   d. Mesothelioma

    [Ref: Harrison's 19th/e pg. 506-10]

14.	b
15.	b
16.	d
17.	c
18.	c
19.	a
20.	b
21.	a
22.	a
23.	d
24.	c
25.	d
26.	b
27.	c
28.	c
29.	d
30.	c

31. Cell free DNA marker in carcinoma lung is-
(PGMEE 2016-17)
- a. TP53, APC
- b. EGFR, CA-125
- c. TP53, RAS
- d. AFP, CEA

[Ref: Robbins 9th/e pg. 337]

32. Most common type of carcinoma lung a/w TP53 mutations:- *(PGMEE 2016-17)*
- a. Small cell carcinoma
- b. Adenocarcinoma
- c. Large cell carcinoma
- d. Squamous cell carcinoma

[Ref: Robbins 9th/e pg. 714]

33. Gene responsible for development of lung cancer in non-smokers is:- *(PGMEE 2016-17)*
- a. RET
- b. c-kit
- c. EGFR
- d. c-myc

[Ref: Robbin's 9th/e pg. 714]

Explanation

- EGFR mutation is seen in ~50% of patients with adenocarcinoma.

34. A diagnosed case of lung cancer presents with sudden distress and chest pain. CXR image showing obliterated costophrenic recesses with slightly blurred lung margins of right lung. The most probable diagnosis is:--
(PGMEE 2016-17)
- a. Emphysema
- b. Pleural effusion
- c. Consolidation
- d. Lung abscess

[Ref: Robbin's 9th/e pg. 723]

PANCOAST TUMORS

35. Pancoast tumor causes: *(PGMEE 2014-15)*
- a. Wasting of muscles of hand
- b. Bony metastasis
- c. Destruction of lower ribs
- d. Increased sweating

[Ref: Harrison's 19th/e pg. 510-11]

36. True statement about pancoast tumor is:
- a. Affects left lower lobe *(PGMEE 2014-15)*
- b. Exclusively associated with adenocarcinoma
- c. Produces recurrent laryngeal nerve palsy
- d. Causes radicular pain in upper limb

[Ref: Harrison's 19th/e pg. 510-511]

MEDIASTINAL TUMORS

37. Most common mediastinal tumor is- *(PGMEE 2013-14)*
- a. Neurogenic tumors
- b. Hernia
- c. Teratoma
- d. Pericardial cyst

[Ref: Robbin's 9th/e pg. 721]

38. The commonest site for extragonadal germ cell tumor is- *(PGMEE 2013-14)*
- a. Pineal gland
- b. Retroperitoneum
- c. Sacrococcygeal region
- d. Mediastinum

[Ref: Ackerman's 9th/e pg. 485]

39. The most common posterior mediastinal mass:
(PGMEE 2014-15; 2012-13)
- a. Neurogenic tumor
- b. Lymph nodes
- c. Neurogenic parasitic cyst
- d. Teratoma

[Ref: CMDT 2014 pg. 292, Harrison's 19th/e pg. 1664-65]

40. Which of the following mass is usually not seen in anterior mediastinum *(PGMEE 2018)*
- a. Thymoma
- b. Lymphoma
- c. Retrosternal goitre
- d. Neurogenic tumour

Ref: Bailey & Love 26th/e pg. 868

Explanation

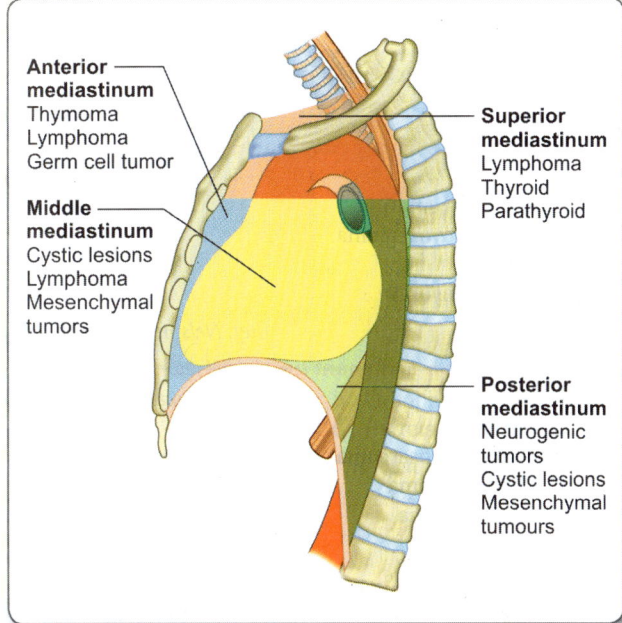

41. During exploration, a patient is found to have a tumor in the thymus that is invading the pericardium and surrounding the left and right phrenic nerves. The pathologist says that appears on frozen section to be a benign thymoma. The surgeon now should:
(NEET June 2018)
- a. Repeat frozen section
- b. Attempt as complete as resection is possible
- c. Close the chest and plan radiotherapy
- d. Close the chest and await permanent sections

Explanation

- The TOC for the patient presented in the question is as complete a resection as possible while at least one phrenic nerve is preserved.
- Thymomas are histologically benign but locally invasive tumours .The presence of a thymoma is sufficient indication for exploration by median sternotomy. The extent of resection needed can be determined on OT table.
- Postoperatively, the patient should receive x-ray therapy, and the combination of surgery + irradiation offers better control.

31.	c
32.	a
33.	c
34.	b
35.	a
36.	d
37.	a
38.	d
39.	a
40.	d
41.	b

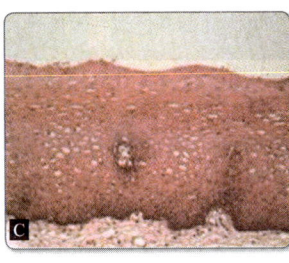
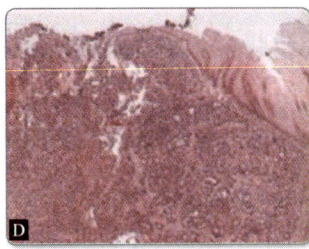

[Ref: Robbins 9th/e pg. 758; Bailey & Love's 26th/e pg. 1004]

Explanation

- In given picture there is apple core deformity seen in barium meal. Squamous cell carcinoma generally affects the upper two-thirds of the oesophagus and adenocarcinoma the lower one-third. Worldwide, squamous cell cancer is most common, but adenocarcinoma predominates in the West and is increasing in incidence.

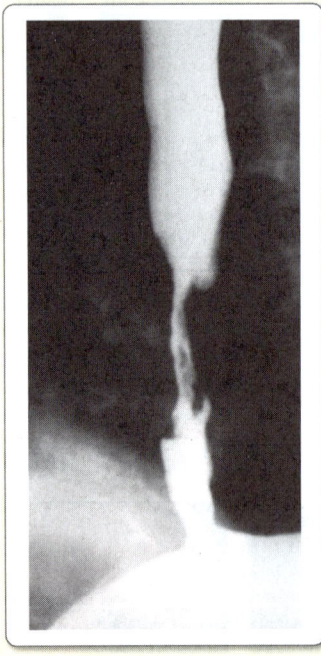

Squamous cell carcinoma of the oesophagus producing an irregular stricture with shouldered margins.

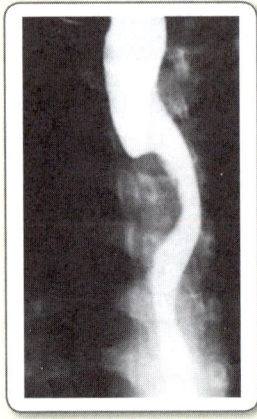

Classic appearance of a large oesophageal gastrointestinal stromal tumour on barium swallow.

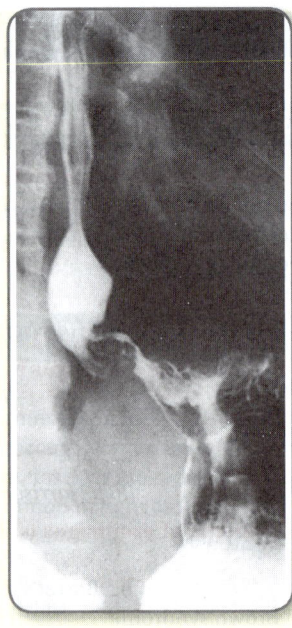

Adenocarcinoma of the lower oesophagus, spreading upwards from the cardia

- In above given situation the barium meal radiograph suggestive of both GIST and adenocarcinoma of esophagus (as per Bailey and Love 26th edition figure 62.36) but as per endoscopic finding, it seen as distorted ulcerproliferative growth. So the histopathology reports should suggest adenocarcinoma slide. That's why here answer is adenocarcinoma.

STOMACH CANCER

14. MC site for stomach Ca:- *(PGMEE 2015)*
- a. Greater curvature
- b. Antrum
- c. Lesser curvature
- d. Pylorus

[Ref: Robbin's 9th/e pg. 771]

15. Most common type of gastric polyp is: : *(PGMEE 2015)*
- a. Hyperplastic polyp
- b. Hamartomatous polyp
- c. Familial polyosis
- d. Malignant polyp

[Ref: Robbin's 9th/e pg. 769]

16. Which of the following tumour of stomach is epithelial in origin:- *(PGMEE 2018)*
- a. GIST
- b. Gastric adenoma
- c. Sarcoma
- d. Carcinoid

Ref: Maingots abdominal operations 12th/e, pg-463, 493

17. Not seen with stomach cancer? *(PGMEE 2014-15)*
- a. Microangiopathic hemolytic anemia
- b. Superficial migratory thrombophlebitis
- c. Acanthosis Nigricans
- d. Polycythemia

[Ref: Harrison's 19th/e pg. 534]

Explanation

- Unusual features associated with gastric adenocarcinoma include migratory thrombophlebitis, microangiopathic hemolytic anemia, seborrheic keratitis (Leser-Trelat sign) & Acanthosis nigricans.

14. b
15. a
16. b
17. d

18. Most common site of spread of gastric tumor?
(PGMEE 2014-15)
a. Blumer shelf
b. Ovary
c. Liver
d. Peritoneum

[Ref: Harrison's 19th/e pg. 534]

19. All the following indicates early gastric cancer, except:
a. Involvement of mucosa   (DNB 2007)
b. Involvement of mucosa and submucosa
c. Involvement of mucosa, submucosa and muscularis
d. Involvement of mucosa, submucosa and adjacent lymph nodes

[Ref: Bailey 26th/e p 1047]

20. Which vitamin deficiency is found in gastric cancer patients?   (DNB Dec' 2011)
a. Vitamin A
b. Vitamin B 12
c. Vitamin C
d. Vitamin D

[Ref: Harrison's 18th/e chapter 105]

21. Krukenberg tumor arises most commonly from which tumor-   (PGMEE 2013-14)
a. HCC
b. Carcinoma lung
c. RCC
d. Adenocarcinoma of pylorus

[Ref: Robbin's 9th/e pg. 1034]

22. True about early gastric cancer is-   (PGMEE 2014)
a. Chemotherapy
b. Lymph node metastasis present
c. Limited to serosa
d. Limited to mucosa and submucosa

[Ref: Robbins 9th/e pg. 772]

23. Linitis plastica is a type of a-   (PGMEE 2013-14)
a. GIST
b. Diffuse carcinoma of stomach
c. Plastic like lining of stomach
d. Benign ulcer

[Ref: Robbin's 9th/e pg. 772]

Explanation

- Diffuse type of Gastric adenocarcinoma develop throughout the stomach resulting in a loss of distensibility (so called linitus plastica or lether bottle appearance)
- It occur more often in younger patients & carry a poorer prognosis.

24. Most common extra-nodal site for lymphoma is?
(PGMEE 2014-15)
a. Colon
b. Waldeyer ring
c. Intestine
d. Stomach

[Ref: Harrison's 19th/e pg. 697]

25. All of the following are treatment modalities for gastric lymphoma except-   (PGMEE 2015)
a. Radical Subtotal gastrectomy for locally advanced disease
b. Chemotherapy for primary gastric lymphoma
c. Chemotherapy for secondary gastric lymphoma
d. Antibiotics treatment for H. Pylori in low grade MALToma

[Ref: Bailey & Love 26th/e pg. 1054; Harrison 17th/e pg. 573; Schwartz 10th/e pg. 1084]

TUMORS OF INTESTINE

26. Tumors of small intestinal tract in decreasing order are:-   (PGMEE 2016-17)
a. Lymphoma, adenoma, Sq cell Ca, GIST
b. AdenoCa, lymphoma, GIST, SqCC
c. Lymphoma, Sq cell Ca, adenoCa, GIST
d. Lymphoma, adenoma, Sq cell Ca, GIST

[Ref: Sabiston's 1st SAE pg.1271]

27. Aneurysmal dilation of the small bowel is seen in-
a. Duodenal Atresia   (PGMEE 2015)
b. Sjogrens Syndrome
c. Small bowel Lymphoma
d. Gall Stone Ileus

[Ref: Cancer of the upper gastrointestinal tract. PMPH-USA, 2002]

28. The highest malignant potential is seen in-
(DNB June 11, DNB 2008)
a. Ulcerative colitis
b. Infantile polyp
c. Familial polyposis
d. Crohn's disease

[Ref: Robbin's 7th/e pg. 60]

29. Most common site for gastrinoma-   (PGMEE 2013-14)
a. Duodenum
b. Antrum
c. Colon
d. Pylorus

[Ref: Robbins 9th/e pg. 1121]

NEOPLASTIC POLYPS AND COLORECTAL CANCER

30. In carcinoma of unknown primary, if the tissue marker CDX-2 is positive, it indicates: (PGMEE 2015)
a. Bladder cancer
b. Gastrointestinal cancer
c. Thyroid cancer
d. Lung cancer

[Ref: Am J Surg Pathol 2003; 27: 303]

Explanation

- CDX-2 is a fairly specific marker of adenocarcinoma of GI origin.

31. 11 year old girl presents with abdominal pain, no diarrhea, freckles on lips, nostrils, buccal mucosa & palmar surfaces of the hands. Likely diagnosis:
(PGMEE 2015)
a. Cowden syndrome
b. Cronkhite Canada sydrome
c. Peut Jeghers syndrome
d. Gardner syndrome

[Ref: Robbins 9th/e pg. 806]

32. A lady comes with polyps in intestine, melanotic pigmentation of lip and positive family history. Most probable diagnosis is?   (DNB Dec' 2011)
a. Peutz-Jeghers syndrome
b. Turcot's syndrome
c. Gartner's syndrome
d. Lynch syndrome

[Ref: Sabiston Textbook of Surgery, 18th/e p. Table 50-4]

18.	c
19.	c
20.	b
21.	d
22.	d
23.	b
24.	d
25.	b
26.	b
27.	c
28.	c
29.	a
30.	b
31.	c
32.	a

33. Among the following, the least malignant potential for colorectal cancer is seen in polyps associated with?
   a. Turcot's syndrome   *(DNB Dec' 2010)*
   b. FAP
   c. Peutz Jagher's syndrome
   d. Gardner's Syndrome

[Ref: Robbins 9th/e pg. 806]

34. All the following conditions are characterized by neoplastic polyps except: *(PGMEE 2015)*
   a. Peutz Jeghers syndrome b. Turcot syndrome
   c. Gardner syndrome   d. Lynch syndrome

[Ref: Robbins 9th/e pg. 806]

35. All are true about Peutz Jegher's syndrome except:-
   a. Autosomal dominant   *(PGMEE 2015)*
   b. Chance of fatal intussusceptions
   c. Gain of function mutation in LKB1/STK11
   d. Hamartomatous polyps do not develop into adenocarcinoma

[Ref: Robbin's 9th/e pg. 806]

36. Colon cancer is seen in people taking? *(DNB Dec' 2011)*
   a. Low fiber diet   b. High fat diet
   c. High fibre diet   d. High protein diet

[Ref: Maingot's Abdominal Operations 11th/e chapter 23]

37. Which screening test for colon cancer is proven effective in RCT?   *(DNB Dec' 2011)*
   a. Colonoscopy
   b. Upper GI endoscopy
   c. Occult blood in stool
   d. Flexible sigmiodscopy

[Ref: Sabiston 's 20th/e pg. 1364 , Maingot's Abdominal Operations 11th/e chapter 3, 23]

38. Parient having diarrhoea and colic on off with mass in right iliac fossa. Most probable diagnosis is
   a. Carcinoma rectum   *(DNB June' 2009)*
   b. Carcinoma transverse colon
   c. Carcinoma sigmoid
   d. Carcinoma caecum

[Ref: Maingot's 10th/e p. 1290]

39. A 70 year old male complaining of per rectal bleed was diagnosed of having rectal/anorectal cancer. The distal margin of the tumor was 5 cm from the anal verge. The treatment of choice would be-   *(PGMEE 2015)*
   a. Palliative Radiotherapy
   b. Abdominoperineal recection
   c. Local Excision
   d. Low anterior resection

[Ref: Sabiston page 1378]

40. Which polyp is premalignant:
   a. Familial polyposis   b. Juvenile polyp
   c. Hyperplasia   d. None

[Ref: Sabiston 26th edition Pg 1367]

41. Osteomas, adenomatous polyps of intestine & peri-ampullary carcinomas are seen in- *(PGMEE 2012-13)*
   a. Peutz Jegers syndrome b. FAP
   c. Cowden syndrome   d. Gardener syndrome

42. Inheritance of Gardner syndrome is- *(PGMEE 2012-13)*
   a. X linked
   b. Autosomal dominant
   c. Autosomal recessive
   d. None of the above

43. Not true about Cowden syndrome:-   *(PGMEE 2015)*
   a. Mutation of PTEN gene
   b. Multiple hamartomas
   c. Increased risk of Gl maliganancy
   d. Risk of follicular thyroid cancer

[Ref: Robbins 9th/e pg. 1316]

44. Which of the following is NOT associated with an increased risk of Gastrointestinal malignancy:- *(PGMEE 2015)*
   a. Cowden's syndrome   b. Lynch syndrome
   c. Gardner's syndrome   d. HNPCC

[Ref: Robbins 9th/e pg. 1316]

45. Gene mutation involved in colon cancer all except:-
   a. APC gene   b. K-RAS *(PGMEE 2016-17)*
   c. P53   d. KIT

[Ref: Sabiston's 20th/e pg. 1360]

46. Which of the following is a tumor maker for CA Colon?   *(PGMEE 2015)*
   a. Acid phosphatase   b. CEA
   c. AFP   d. Neuron specific enolase

[Ref: Sabiston's 20th/e pg. 1360]

47. Most common site of colorectal carcinoma:- *(PGMEE 2016-17)*
   a. Sigmoid colon   b. Transverse colon
   c. Ascending colon   d. Rectum

[Ref: Robbins 9th/e pg. 810]

48. Microsatellite instability is seen in:- *(PGMEE 2016-17)*
   a. Colonic CA
   b. Anal CA
   c. Small intestinal adenom
   d. Colorectal CA

[Ref: NCBI]

49. Sentinel lymph node biopsy is not done in *(PGMEE 2012)*
   a. Carcinoma breast   b. Carcinoma penis
   c. Melanoma   d. Carcinoma colon

[Ref: Mastery of surgery 5th/e pg. 1531, Schwartz 9th/e various chapters]

Explanation
- Indication of SLNB:
  - Breast cancer
  - Melanoma
  - Penile cancer
  - Endometrial cancer

50. Lynch syndrome is characterized by: *(PGMEE 2014-15)*
   a. 2 or more cases in family of polyps
   b. Defect on chromosome 10
   c. Cancer arising in recto-sigmoid junction
   d. One or more case in family of colorectal cancer < 50 years

[Ref: Harrison's 19th/e pg. 538t]

33.	c
34.	a
35.	c
36.	b
37.	a
38.	d
39.	d
40.	a
41.	d
42.	b
43.	c
44.	a
45.	d
46.	b
47.	d
48.	d
49.	d
50.	d

51. Which of the following Gastrointestinal Polyposis syndromes is associated with Congenital Hypertrophy of Retinal Pigment Epithelium (CHRPE):- *(PGMEE 2015-16)*
   a. Gardner's syndrome
   b. Cowden's syndrome
   c. Turcot's Syndrome
   d. Muir-Torre syndrome

[Ref: Quick Reference Handbook for Surgical Pathologists (Springer) 2011/111,112]

52. Most common site of spread of colorectal cancer is? *(PGMEE 2014-15)*
   a. Liver   b. Peritoneum
   c. Brain   d. Lung

[Ref: Robbins 9th/e pg. 810]

53. Peutz Jehgers syndrome is associated with: *(PGMEE 2014-15)*
   a. Lung cancer   b. Brain tumor
   c. Osteoma   d. Ovarian tumor

[Ref: Harrison's 19th/e pg. 538t]

54. All are risk factors for development of colorectal cancers except? *(PGMEE 2014-15)*
   a. Polyposis col   b. Lynch syndrome
   c. IBD   d. Intake of vegetable fat

[Ref: Harrison's 19th/e pg. 538]

55. Incorrect about colorectal cancer? *(PGMEE 2014-15)*
   a. Apple core appearance on barium study
   b. Left sided lesions associated with tenesmus
   c. Haem-occult is best screening tool
   d. Right sided lesions associated with occult bleeding

[Ref: Harrison's 19th/e pg. 541]

56. Which is rarest site of spread of colorectal cancer? *(PGMEE 2014-15)*
   a. Liver   b. Peritoneum
   c. Mesentary   d. Lung

[Ref: Harrison's 19th/e pg. 541]

57. Aspirin decreases the risk of development of which of the following: *(PGMEE 2014-15)*
   a. MALToma   b. Stomach cancer
   c. Carcinoid   d. Colorectal cancer

[Ref: Harrison's 19th/e pg.539]

58. All of the following are associated with carcinoma colon except- *(PGMEE 2013-14)*
   a. Fatty food   b. Smoking
   c. Fibre diet   d. Alcohol

[Ref: Robbin's 9th/e pg. 811-812]

CARCINOMA APPENDIX

59. Treatment of carcinoma appendix is- *(PGMEE 15)*
   a. Left hemicolectomy
   b. Right hemicolectomy with regional lymphadenectomy
   c. Appendicectomy
   d. Extended Left hemicolectomy

[Ref: Sabiston 20th /e pg. 1308]

ANAL CANCER

60. Nigro Protocol is used in:- *(PGMEE 2016-17)*
   a. Colonic CA
   b. Anal CA
   c. Small intestinal adenoma
   d. Colorectal CA

[Ref: Sabiston's 1st SAE pg. 1415]

61. Treatment of choice for squamous cell carcinoma of anal canal is *(PGMEE 2012; PGMEE 2016-17)*
   a. Chemotherapy
   b. Sphincter sparing surgery
   c. Monoclonal antibodies
   d. Chemoradiation

[Ref: Sabiston's 1st SAE pg. 1415]

GASTROINTESTINAL STROMAL TUMORS

62. Not true about GIST:- *(PGMEE 2015, 2012-13)*
   a. Stomach is the most common site
   b. High propensity of malignant change
   c. Histology shows epithelioid and spindle shaped cells
   d. Associated with c-KIT mutation

[Ref: Robbin's 9th/e pg. 775]

63. For "GIST" most common site is: *(PGMEE 2016-17)*
   a. Duodenum
   b. Pancreas
   c. Stomach
   d. Jejunum

[Ref: Sabiston's 20th/e pg. 1229]

64. Marker specific for GIST tumors? *(PGMEE 2016-17)*
   a. CD 50   b. CD117
   c. CD17   d. C-peptides

[Ref: Robbins 9th/e pg. 775; Sternberg's 4th/e pg. 1590]

Explanation

GIST

- Carcinoids are an unusual group of neoplasms that arise from cells of neuroendocrine origin. Gastric carcinoids generally arise from enterochromaffin-like (ECL) cells found in the acid-producing mucosa of the gastric body and fundus

65. Gastrointestinal stromal malignancy arises from which of the following- *(PGMEE 2013-14)*
   a. Nerve cells
   b. Vascular Endothelium
   c. Interstitial cells of Cajal
   d. Smooth muscle

[Ref: Robbin's 9th/e pg. 775]

MALTOMA

66. Tumor most commonly associated with H pylori:- *(PGMEE 2015)*
   a. MALToma   b. Squamous cell carcinoma
   c. Adenocarcinoma   d. None

[Ref: Robbin's 9th/e pg. 773]

51.	a
52.	a
53.	d
54.	d
55.	c
56.	d
57.	d
58.	c
59.	b
60.	b
61.	d
62.	b
63.	c
64.	b
65.	c
66.	a

67. Tumor exhibiting regression to anti-microbials?
a. Zollinger Ellison syndrome   *(PGMEE 2014-15)*
b. MALToma
c. Kaposi sarcoma
d. G.I.S.T

[Ref: Harrison's 19th/e pg. 573]

CARCINOIDS

68. Carcinoid tumor develops from-   *(PGMEE 2012-13)*
a. J cell   b. CAMs
c. C cells   d. Enterochromaffin cells

[Ref: Robbin's 9th/e pg. 1105]

69. Carcinoid syndrome is associated with all EXCEPT:
(PGMEE 2014-15)
a. Flushing of skin   b. Skin lesions like pellagra
c. VMA in urine   d. Bronchospasm

[Ref: Harrison's 20th/e pg. 597]

70. Carcinoid tumor:-   *(PGMEE 2016-17)*
a. Can be detect by urinary level of increased HIEE
b. Most common site is appendix
c. Flushing is never seen
d. Almost always present with carcinoid syndrome

[Ref: Harrison's 20th/e pg. 600]

71. Diagnosis of carcinoid tumor is done by?
(DNB June 2009)
a. 5-HIAA   b. Metanephrines
c. VMA   d. DHEA

[Ref: Harrison's 20th/e pg. 600]

72. Not seen with carcinoid is?   *(PGMEE 2014-15)*
a. Peyronie disease   b. Hypertension
c. Cushing disease   d. Mitral valve involvement

[Ref: Harrison's 20th/e pg. 603]

73. Flushing is most common seen with?   *(PGMEE 2014-15)*
a. Gastric carcinoid   b. Appendiceal carinoid
c. Midgut carcinoid   d. Hindgut carcinoid

[Ref: Harrison's 20th/e pg. 603]

74. Most common cardiac lesion in carcinoid syndrome is?
(PGMEE 2014-15)
a. Aortic stenosis   b. Pulmonic stenosis
c. Tricuspid regurgitation   d. Mitral regurgitation

[Ref: Harrison's 20th/e pg. 603]

75. Not used for diagnosis of carcinoid syndrome ?
(PGMEE 2014-15)
a. Neuron specific enolase
b. Chromogranin A
c. Synaptophysin
d. Somatostatin receptor scintigraphy

[Ref: Harrison's 20th/e pg. 605]

76. Most common site of carcinoid tumor leading to carcinoid syndrome?   *(PGMEE 2014-15)*
a. Appendicular carcinoid
b. Bronchial carcinoid
c. Midgut carcinoid
d. Metastatic Midgut carcinoid

[Ref: Harrison's 20th/e pg. 596]

77. Drug of choice for carcinoid crisis?   *(PGMEE 2014-15)*
a. Methysergide   b. Kentaserin
c. Cyproheptadine   d. Octreotide

[Ref: Harrison's 20th/e pg. 606]

78. Most common symptom of carcinoid syndrome is:
(PGMEE 2014-15)
a. Diarrhea   b. Flushing
c. Pellagra   d. Bronchospasm

[Ref: Harrison's 20th/e pg. 597]

79. All are correct about atypical carcinoid except?
(PGMEE 2014-15)
a. High urinary 5HTP
b. High urinary 5-HIAA
c. Seen with foregut carcinoid
d. Absent dopa decarboxylase

[Ref: Harrison's 20th/e pg. 596, 604]

80. Pellagra is seen with: *(PGMEE 2014-15)*
a. Carcinoid
b. Cronhkhite Canada syndrome
c. Phaeochromocytoma
d. Peutz Jegher syndrome

[Ref: Harrison's 19th/e pg 601]

81. In carcinoid syndrome, the part of heart mostly affected is: *(PGMEE 2014-15)*
a. Inflow tract of RV   b. Inflow tract of LV
c. Mural endocardium   d. Pericardium

[Ref: Harrison's 20th/e pg. 603]

82. Best test for diagnosis of Carcinoid tumor:
(PGMEE 2015-16)
a. 24 hour urinary 5H.I.A.A
b. 24 hour catecholamines
c. 24 hour vanilmandelic acid levels
d. 24 hour metanephrine levels

[Ref: Harrison 19th ed. / 564-65]

83. Increase excretion of 5 HIAA in urine is seen in:
(PGMEE 2018)
a. Cushing syndrome   b. Alkaptonuria
c. Carcinoid syndrome   d. Phenylketonuria

[Ref: Harrison's 20th/e pg. 604]

Explanation

Carcinoids

- Carcinoid tumors arise from neuroendocrine cells, which are widespread in the human body.
- Flushing and diarrhea are the two most common symptoms. Flushes may be precipitated by stress; alcohol; exercise; certain foods, such as cheese; or certain agents, such as catecholamines, and serotonin reuptake inhibitors.
- Cardiac involvement is characterised by the dense fibrous deposits, most commonly on the ventricular aspect of the tricuspid. This can result in tricuspid insufficiency in 90–100% cases and tricuspid stenosis in 50% cases approximately.
- The diagnosis of carcinoid syndrome relies on measurement of urinary or plasma serotonin or its metabolites in the urine. The biochemical diagnosis of

67.	b
68.	d
69.	c
70.	a
71.	a
72.	b
73.	c
74.	c
75.	c
76.	d
77.	d
78.	a
79.	b
80.	a
81.	a
82.	a
83.	c

carcinoid tumors is mainly based on the measurement of the serotonin metabolite 5-HIAA in a 24-hour urine collection.

- Platelet serotonin levels are more sensitive than urinary 5-HIAA.
- Because patients with foregut Neuroendocrine Tumors (NETs) may produce an atypical carcinoid syndrome, if this syndrome is suspected and the urinary 5-HIAA is minimally elevated or normal, other urinary metabolites of tryptophan, such as 5-HTP (5-Hydroxytryptophan) and 5-HT, should be measured.
- Serum chromogranin A levels are elevated in 56–100% of patients with GI-NETs (carcinoids), and the level correlates with tumor bulk. However, levels are not specific for GI-NETs (carcinoids) as they are also elevated in patients with other NETs.
- Plasma neuron-specific enolase levels are also used as a marker of GI-NETs (carcinoids) but are less sensitive than chromogranin A.
- Imaging modalities useful are Iodine-131 metaiodoben-zylguanidine (MIBG) scanning and Scintigraphy with indium-111 DTPA octreotide (In-111 DTPA Octr), or Oc-treoScan.

84. Which of the following is produced by Argentaffinoma of ileum? *(PGMEE 2015-16)*

a. G.A.B.A
b. Serotonin
c. Epinephrine
d. Nor-epinephrine

[Ref: Harrison's 20th/e pg. 596]

85. Most common site of carcinoid in gut is- *(PGMEE Al 2013-14, 2015)*

a. Rectum b. Esophagus
c. Ileum d. Appendix

[Ref: Robbin's 9th/e pg. 773]

86. Most common site of carcinoid tumor in hindgut:- *(PGMEE 2015)*

a. Descending colon b. Rectum
c. Transverse colon d. Caecum

[Ref: Harrison 18th ed: 350-3]

Explanation

- MC site of carcinoid tumor: Ileum > Rectum > Colon > intestinal Appendix

87. Treatment of choice for a 0.5 mm those carcinoid tumors at the tip of appendix is:- *(PGMEE 2015-16)*

a. Coecectomy b. Hepatic wedge resection
c. Right Hemicolectomy d. Appendicectomy

[Ref: Sabiston 20th /e pg. 1308]

88. All of the following about Gastrointestinal carcinoid tumors are true, Except- *(PGMEE 2015)*

a. Rectum is spared
b. Small intestine and appendix account for almost 60% of all gastrointestinal carcinoid
c. Appendicial carcinoids are more common in females than males
d. 5 year survival for carcinoid tumors is > 60%

[Ref: Sabiston 19th/e pg. 1259]

84.	b
85.	c
86.	b
87.	d
88.	a

LIVER TUMORS

1. Which of the following do not cause Hepatocellular Ca:-
(PGMEE 2016)
a. Alcoholism
b. Tyrosenemia
c. Hepatitis B
d. Non alcoholic fatty liver disease
[Ref: Robbins 9th/e pg. 870]

2. Angiosarcoma of the liver can occur due to occupational exposure to:- *(PGMEE 2015)*
a. Asbestos   b. Toluene
c. Vinyl chloride   d. Benzene
[Ref: Robbins 9th/e pg. 870]

3. Hepatic adenoma is most common in:- *(PGMEE 2015)*
a. Old females
b. Young females
c. Young males
d. Old males
[Ref: Robbins 9th/e pg. 870]

4. Which liver tumor has the best prognosis:-
(PGMEE 2015)
a. Hemangioblastoma
b. Hemangiosarcoma
c. Hepatocelluler carcinoma
d. Fibrolamellar carcinoma
[Ref: Robbins 9th/e pg. 870]

5. Not true about HNF1-α Inactivated hepatocellular adenomas:- *(PGMEE 2015)*
a. Mostly in women
b. High risk of malignant transformation
c. OCPs are implicated in pathogenesis
d. Associated with MODY-3
[Ref: Robbins 9th/e pg. 870]

6. Not true about hepatoblastoma *(PGMEE 2015)*
a. Most common in children
b. Mature hepatocytes present
c. Fatal if untreated
d. Not associated with cirrhosis
[Ref: Robbins 9th/e pg. 870]

7. Which of the following is NOT a risk factor for hepatocellular carcinoma:- *(PGMEE 2015)*
a. α1-antitrypsin deficiency
b. Chronic alcoholism
c. NASH/NAFLD
d. Hepatitis D
[Ref: Robbins 9th/e pg. 838]

8. Which malignancy is associated with liver cirrhosis:-
(PGMEE 2015)
a. Hepatocellular Ca   b. Fibrolamellar Ca
c. Cholangiocarcinoma   d. Pancreatic Ca
[Ref: Robbins 9th/e pg. 870]

9. Vinyl Chloride is associated with which Carcinoma:-
(PGMEE 2015)
a. Liver   b. Prostrate
c. Spleen   d. Lung
[Ref: Robbins 9th/e pg. 875]

10. Most common liver tumor associated with OCP:
(PGMEE 2014-15)
a. Focal nodular hyperplasia
b. Hemangioma
c. Angiomyolipoma
d. Hepatocellular adenoma
[Ref: CMDT 2014, Harrison's 18th ed. ch. 16 pg. 701, Harrison 19th p 365]

11. Best to diagnose a liver tumor? *(PGMEE 2014-15)*
a. CT
b. USG
c. MRI
d. Sulphur colloid scan
[Ref: CMDT 2014, Harrison's 18th ed. ch. 16 pg. 701, Harrison 19th p 534]

12. Which virus causes hepatocellular carcinoma-
(PGMEE 2013-14)
a. Arbo virus   b. Herpes
c. Hepatitis A   d. Hepatitis B
[Robbins 9th/e pg. 870]

13. Hepatocellular carcinoma is caused by all of the following except- *(PGMEE 2015)*
a. Primary biliary cirrhosis
b. Hepatitis B
c. Exposure to industrial dyes
d. Chronic alcohol consumption
[Ref: Harrison 17th/e pg. 580; Sabiston 19th/e pg. 1500, c.S.d.T. 13th/e pg. 520]

14. Which of the following is effective against both HCC and RCC: *(PGMEE 2014-15)*
a. Erlotinib   b. Cetuximab
c. Bortezomib   d. Sorafenib
[Ref: Harrison's 19th/e pg.550]

15. Most common benign tumor of the liver:
a. Focal nodular hyperplasia *(PGMEE 2014-15)*
b. Hemangioma
c. Angiomyolipoma
d. Hepatocellular adenoma
[Ref: Harrison's 19th/e pg.553]

16. Aflatoxin causes: *(PGMEE 2014-15)*
a. Lathyrism
b. Botulism
c. Cholangiocarcinoma
d. Hepato cellular carcinoma
[Ref: Harrison's 19th/e pg.544]

1.	b
2.	c
3.	b
4.	d
5.	b
6.	b
7.	d
8.	a
9.	a
10.	d
11.	c
12.	d
13.	c
14.	d
15.	b
16.	d

17. Most common liver tumor: *(PGMEE 2014-15)*

a. Hemangioma
b. Focal nodular hyperplasia
c. Hepatocellular carcinoma
d. Metastasis

[Ref: Robbins 8th/e pg 663-666]

18. The most common cause of hepatocellular carcinoma in India is: *(PGMEE 2014-15)*

a. Hepatitis A
b. Hepatitis B
c. Non A Non B hepatitis
d. Alcoholic cirrhosis

[Ref: Harrison's 19th/e pg. 544]

19. Hypoglycemia is seen with: *(PGMEE 2014-15)*

a. RCC
b. Breast cancer
c. Glucagonoma
d. HCC

[Ref: Harrison's 19th/e pg 545]

20. Which is a hormone dependent liver tumor:

a. Hepatocellular carcinoma *(PGMEE 2014-15)*
b. Hemangioma
c. Hepatoma
d. Hemangiopericytoma

[Ref: Harrison's 19th/e pg. 545]

21. Best for management of 10 cm hepatocellular carcinoma is: *(PGMEE 2014-15)*

a. Radiofrequency ablation
b. Transarterial catheter embolization (T.A.C.E)
c. Percutaneous ethanol
d. Orthoptic liver transplantation

[Ref: Harrison's 19th/e pg. 545]

22. In liver transplant, thromboelastography (TEG) is used for:- *(PGMEE 2016-17)*

a. Arterial embolization
b. To guide factor repletion and fibrinolytic therapy
c. To reduce anasthesia related complications
d. None of the above

[Ref: https://www.ncbi.nlm.nih]

Explanation

■ Thromboelastography (TEG) is a method of testing the efficiency of blood coagulation.

23. After hepatectomy, the level of which is elevated:- *(PGMEE 2016-17)*

a. Glucose
b. Estrogen
c. Fibrinogen
d. Lactate

[Ref: Liver Regeneration By D. Bernuau pg. 142]

GALLBLADDER CANCER

24. Focal diffuse gall bladder wal thickening with comet tail reverberation artifacts on USG is in- *(PGMEE 2012-13)*

a. Ca gall bladder
b. Xantho granuloma
c. Adenomyomatosis of gall bladder
d. Adenomatous polyps

[Ref: Biliary lithiasis: Basic Science, Current diagnosis & Management pg. 82]

25. The following condition of GB is precancerous - *(PGMEE 2012-13)*

a. Biliary atresia
b. Porcelain gall bladder
c. Choledochal cyst
d. Cholesterosis

[Ref: Robbin's 8th/e pg. 884-889]

26. Type 2 cholangiocarcinoma involves? *(PGMEE 2011)*

a. Common hepatic duct only
b. Division of both ducts and not extending outside
c. Secondary hepatic ducts
d. Extends beyond hilum

[Ref: Sabiston 18th/e p. chapter 54]

Explanation

■ Multidetector CT is the imaging study of choice for the evaluation of lesions arising in the pancreas.
■ CECT is IOC but for biopsy it is EUS
■ CT has become the imaging modality of choice for the evaluation of suspected pancreatic cancer.
■ In modern medical practice, ERCP should be reserved for cases requiring therapeutic or palliative intervention because other imaging modalities provide superior diagnostic abilities without the invasiveness of ERCP.
■ EUS is becoming widely used for the evaluation of suspected pancreatic disease. Perhaps its most important ability is to provide tissue diagnosis of suspected tumors through the use of FNA before initiation of systemic therapy.
■ Although the use of EUS is increasing for the evaluation of peritumoral vasculature and regional lymph nodes, it has not been shown to provide any significant benefit over CT alone in the absence of a need for tissue diagnosis. EUS may be beneficial for the identification of small tumors that do not appear on CT scans.
■ CT guided biopsy is not mentioned. So answer should be EUS guided biopsy (Option A).

27. Treatment of choice of mucinous carcinoma of Gall Bladder confined to the lamina propria is- *(PGMEE 2015)*

a. Simple cholecystectomy
b. Chemotherapy only
c. Cholecystectomy with wedge resection of liver
d. Extended Cholecystectomy

[Ref: Sabiston 20th /e 1514

28. All of the following are true about CA gall bladder expect- *(PGMEE 2015)*

a. Adenocarcinoma is the most common type
b. Gall stones is a common associated factor
c. Prognosis is generally poor
d. Vibrio Cholera Infection has shown an association

[Ref: Bailey & Love 26th /e pg.1116]

Explanation

■ S. typhi & S. paratyphi infection is associated with cancer of gall bladder.

17.	d
18.	b
19.	d
20.	c
21.	b
22.	b
23.	c
24.	c
25.	b
26.	b
27.	a
28.	d

29. All of the following may lead to a gall bladder carcinoma expect- *(PGMEE 2015)*
a. Gall Bladder polys
b. Exposure to carcinogens like nitrosamine
c. Thyhoid carries
d. Echinococcus Granulosus Infection

[Ref: Schwartz 10th/e pg.1334]

30. Rokitansky-Aschoff sinuses are a feature of:- *(PGMEE 2015)*
a. Adenomyomatosis of gall bladder
b. Acute Cholecystitis
c. Ca gall bladder
d. Chronic Cholecystitis

[Ref: Robbins 9th/e pg. 879]

CHOLANGIOCARCINOMA

31. Which is a risk factor for Cholangiocarcinoma:-
a. Persistent hepatitis *(PGMEE 2015)*
b. Ulcerative colitis
c. Chronic cholecystitis
d. Crohn's ds

[Ref: Robbins 9th/e pg. 874]

32. Which is risk factor for cholangiocarcinoma-
a. HBV infection *(PGMEE 2012-13)*
b. Primary sclerosing cholangitis
c. Salmonella carrier state
d. Obesity

[Ref: Robbin's 8th/e pg. 880]

33. Klatskin tumor is- *(PGMEE 2012-13)*
a. Nodular type of cholangiocarcinoma
b. Gall bladder carcinoma
c. Hepatocellular carcinoma
d. Fibrolamellar hepatocellular carcinoma

[Ref: Robbin's 8th/e pg. 880]

PANCREATIC CANCER

34. A 78 year old male presents with jaundice associated with increased itching and a palpable gall bladder, Possible diagnosis is- *(PGMEE 2015)*
a. Abdominal lymphoma
b. Hepatocellular Carcinoma
c. Gastric Carcinoma
d. Periampullary carcinoma

[Ref: Bailey & Love 26th/e pg. 1108]

35. Most common gene associated with pancreatic cancer:- *(PGMEE 2016)*
a. KRAS　　　　　b. Rb
c. P53　　　　　　d. SMAD

[Ref: Robbins 9th/e pg. 892-894]

36. Migratory superficial thrombophlebitis is seen in- *(PGMEE 07, 2008)*
a. Carcinoma pancreas　　b. Renal carcinoma
c. Astrocytoma　　　　　d. All

[Ref: Robbin's 9th/e pg. 332; Sabiston 20th/e pg. 1845]

37. Most common site of pancreatic cancer is *(PGMEE 2015)*
a. Head of pancreas　　b. Tail of pancreas
c. Neck of pancreas　　d. Body of pancreas

[Ref: Robbins 9th/e pg. 892-894 ; Harrison's 19th /e pg.554]

38. Most important presenting feature of periampullary carcinoma is- *(PGMEE 2015)*
a. Jaundice　　　　　b. Weight loss
c. Pain　　　　　　　d. Palpable mass

[Ref: Sabiston's 20th /e pg. 1544]

39. The commonest pancreatic tumor is: *(PGMEE 2007)*
a. Ductal adenocarcinoma
b. Cystabenoma
c. Insulinoma
d. Non-islet cell tumor

[Ref: Sabiston's 20th /e pg. 1541]

40. In pancratic carcinoma chemotherapy use is:- *(PGMEE 2016-17)*
a. Gemcitabine　　　　b. Cisplatin
c. Methotrexate　　　　d. Oxaliplatin

[Ref: Sabiston's 20th /e pg. 1551]

41. Pylorus preserving pancreaticodudnectomy is done in:-
a. Pancreatic head carcinoma *(PGMEE 2016-17)*
b. Gall bladder carcinmoa
c. Chronic pancreatitis
d. Duodenum adenocarcinoma

[Ref: Schwartz 10th edition page 1387]

42. Investigation of choice in carcinoma head of pancreas:- *(PGMEE 2018)*
a. Endoscopic ultrasound (EUS) guided trans-gastric biopsy
b. CECT guided biopsy
c. Percutaneous MRI guided biopsy
d. Laparoscopic biopsy

[Ref: Sabiston 20th pg 1546]

29.	d
30.	a
31.	b
32.	b
33.	a
34.	d
35.	a
36.	a
37.	a
38.	a
39.	a
40.	a,d
41.	a
42.	a

WILM'S TUMOR

1. The triad of Wilm's tumor is all EXCEPT:
a. Hamaturia   **(DNB Dec'2008)**
b. Mass abdomen
c. Pain
d. Fever

[Ref: Sabiston's 20th /e pg. 1889]

2. Most important prognostic factor of Wilms tumor-
                (PGMEE 2012-13)
a. Histopathology
b. Age<1 yr
c. Mutation of c I p gene
d. Ploidy of cells

[Ref: Sternberg Diagnostic Histopathology 4th/e vol 3 pg. 2008-2009]

3. Latest classification for Wilm's Tumor:
                (DNB 2007, 2008)
a. AJCC TNM   b. CIOS
c. CHIDC   d. NWTSG

[Ref: Sabiston's 20th /e pg. 1889]

4. The most common presentation of a child with Wilms' tumor is-   **(PGMEE 2012-13)**
a. Hypertension
b. Haematuria
c. Rhabdoid due to pulmonary secondary
d. As asymptomatic abdominal mass

[Ref: Nelson 20th/e/ ch 499; Ghai 8th/e/ p 617]

5. Not true about Wilm's tumor: **(PGMEE 2012)**
a. Mostly presents at 5 years of age
b. Spreads mainly through lymphatics
c. Presents as abdominal mass
d. Can be bilateral

[Ref: Nelson 20th/e/ ch 499; Ghai 8th/e/ p 617]

6. False about Wilm's is: **(DNB December 2011)**
a. Presents as abdominal mass
b. Hematuria is one of the presenting symptom
c. Peak age of presentation is 5 years
d. Most commonly metastasize to lung

[Ref: Nelson 20th/e/ ch 499; Ghai 8th/e/ p 617]

7. All of the following is true about Wilm's tumor except-   **(PGMEE 2015)**
a. Responds well to chemotherapy
b. It is most common renal neoplasm in children
c. It is always unilateral
d. May present with an abdominal lump

[Ref: Sabiston 20th /e pg. 1889]

8. Following are true regarding nephrogenic rests except-   **(PGMEE. 2013, 14)**
a. Increased risk for involvement of contralateral kidney with Wilm's tumor
b. Uniquely appears hyperplastic rests
c. Seen in renal parenchyma, adjacent to Wilm's tumor
d. They are putative precursor lesions of Wilm's tumor

[Ref: Robbins 9th/e pg. 1118]

Explanation

- Nephrogenic rests are fragments of residual metanephric tissues in a fully developed kidney. NR are precursor lesion of Wilm's tumor & show a strong association with bilateral Wilm's tumor.

NEUROBLASTOMA

9. N-myc gene mutation is seen in: **(DNB 2007, 2008)**
a. Neuroblastoma   b. Retinoblastoma
c. Wilm's tumor   d. Nephroblastoma

[Ref: Sabiston's 20th /e pg. 1887]

10. Most common intrabdominal solid tumor in children-
a. Rhabdomyo sarcoma   **(PGMEE 2013-14)**
b. Wilms tumor (Nephroblastoma)
c. Neuroblastoma
d. Hodgkin lymphoma

[Ref: Ghai 8th/e/p 616]

11. 4 years old child having palpable abdominal mass and hypertension with sweating and diarrhea. Most likely cause is-   **(PGMEE 2012-13)**
a. Polycystic kidney disease
b. Neuroblastoma
c. Nephroblastoma
d. None of the above

[Ref: Ghai 8th/e/p 616]

12. An USG in a 1 year old child shows a mass in abdomen which is displacing the kidney laterally. Most probable diagnosis is-   **(PGMEE 2013-14)**
a. RCC   b. Nephroblastoma
c. Neuroblastoma   d. All of the above

[Ref: Ghai 8th/e/p 616]

13. An 8-year-old child presents with a mass in the lumbar region with abdominal pain with excruciating bone pain, IVC thrombosis and fever. Possible diagnosis is-   **(PGMEE 2015)**
a. Langerhans cell Histiocytosis
b. Wilm's tumor
c. Gastric lymphoma
d. Neuroblastoma

[Ref: O.P. Ghai 8th/e pg. 616; Nelson 20th/e/ ch 493 pg. 2422]

1.	c
2.	a
3.	d
4.	d
5.	a
6.	c
7.	c
8.	b
9.	a
10.	c
11.	b
12.	c
13.	d

PROSTATE CANCER

48. The highest level of acid phosphatase in serum is found in carcinoma of which organ:- *(PGMEE 2015-16)*
- a. Thyroid
- b. Prostate
- c. Bone
- d. Liver

[Ref: A Manual of Laboratory and Diagnostic Tests 8th/e pg. 409]

49. Prostate Specifie Antigen (PSA) units are measured in- *(PGMEE 2016-17)*
- a. mg/mL
- b. microgram/mL
- c. ng/mL
- d. gm/mL

[Ref: Harrison's 19th/e pg. 581]

50. Gleason's scoring is used for- *(PGMEE 2016-17, 2012-13)*
- a. CA testes
- b. CA prostate
- c. Bladder CA
- d. Penile CA

[Ref: Sabiston's 20th/e pg.2101; Harrison's 19th/e pg. 582;Robbins 9th/e pg. 987]

51. Most commonly associated mutation in prostatic carcinoma is? *(PGMEE 2013)*
- a. p16/INK 4a
- b. APC
- c. GSTP1
- d. PTEN

[Ref: Robbins 9th/e pg. 985]

52. Most common histopathological type of CA prostate is:-
- a. Adenocarcinoma *(PGMEE 2016-17)*
- b. Squamous cell carcinoma
- c. Adenosquamous CA
- d. Transitional cell CA

[Ref: Harrison's 19th/e pg. 581]

53. Anti androgen drug used in treatment of CA prostate is:- *(PGMEE 2016-17)*
- a. Leuprolide
- b. Bicalutamide
- c. Denosumab
- d. DES

[Ref: Harrison's 19th/e pg. 585]

54. Prostate specific antigen unit ng/ml suggestive of malignancy:- *(PGMEE 2016-17)*
- a. >5
- b. >10
- c. >7
- d. >3

[Ref: Bailey & Love's 26th /e pg. 1341]

Explanation

- With a PSA level of 4-10 ng/mL, likelihood of prostate cancer is about 25%; with a level >10 ng/mL, the likelihood is much higher.

55. A 65-year-old male presents with CA prostate.The tumor is limited to the capsule and it is palpable on PR examination. The patient is diagnosed as stage T1b. The best treatment would be- *(PGMEE 2015)*
- a. Orchidectomy
- b. Radical prostatectomy
- c. Chemotherapy
- d. Palliative radiotherapy

*[**Ref:** Sabiston's 20th /e pg. 2101]*

56. Prostate cancer occurs in which part of the gland- *(PGMEE 2015)*
- a. Transitional zone
- b. Central zone
- c. Anterior portion
- d. Peripheral zone

[Ref: Campbell Urology 11th/e pg.]

57. Prostate cancer that is limited to the capsule and not involving the urethra would be satged as- *(PGMEE 2015)*
- a. Tx
- b. T1
- c. T2
- d. T3

[Ref: sabiston 20th /e pg. 2101.]

58. Prostate cancer is best diagnosed by? *(DNB Dec' 2011)*
- a. DRE
- b. Prostate specific antigen
- c. FNAC of prostate gland
- d. Trans urethral ultra sound

[Ref: Sabiston Textbook of Surgery, 18th/e p. chapter 77]

TESTICULAR CANCERS

59. Commonest germ cell tumor of testis :- *(PGMEE 2016-17)*
- a. Yolk sac tumor
- b. Lymphoma
- c. Seminoma
- d. Teratoma

[Ref: Robbins 9th/e pg. 975, Harrison's 19th/e pg. 589]

60. Commonest histological type of carcinoma testis is- *(PGMEE 2012-13)*
- a. Yolk sac tumor
- b. Chorio carcinoma
- c. Seminoma
- d. Teratoma

[Ref: Robbins 9th/e pg. 975]

61. All of the following are true about seminomas except: *(PGMEE 2015)*
- a. Most common type of germ cell tumor
- b. Anaplastic seminomas are associated with worse prognosis
- c. Spermatocytic seminoma is slow growing with good prognosis
- d. Almost never occur in infants

[Ref: Genitourinary Pathology: A Volume in the Series: pg 610]

62. A 40-year-old male was operated on scrotum for mass. Cut section and microscopic picture is shown below. Most likely cause is:- *(PGMEE 2018)*
- a. Seminoma
- b. Dysgerminoma
- c. Teratoma
- d. Yolk sac tumour

Explanation

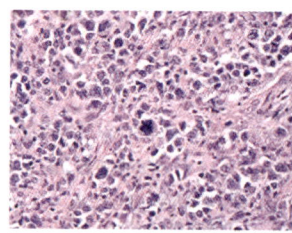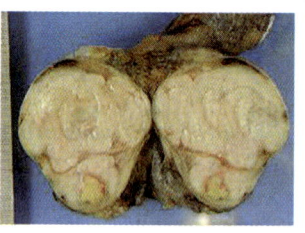

63. Intra tubular germ cell neoplasia is implicated as a cause for the following testicular tumor? *(PGMEE 2015)*
- a. Pediatric yolk sac tumors
- b. Pediatric teratomas
- c. Seminomas
- d. Adult spermatocytic seminomas

[Ref: Robbins 9th/e pg. 977]

48.	b
49.	c
50.	b
51.	c
52.	a
53.	b
54.	b
55.	b
56.	d
57.	c
58.	d
59.	c
60.	c
61.	b
62.	d
63.	c

64. Schiller- Duval bodies are seen in-
(PGMEE 2016-17; PGMEE 2012-13)
- a. Seminoma
- b. Chorio carcinoma
- c. Yolk sac tumor
- d. Teratoma

[Ref: Robbins 9th/e pg. 977]

65. All are germ cell tumors except- *(PGMEE 2012-13)*
- a. Endodermal sinus
- b. Leydig cell tumor
- c. Seminoma
- d. Embryonal carcinoma

[Ref: Robbins 9th/e pg. 978-980]

66. All are tumor markers for testicular tumors except-
(PGMEE 2014)
- a. AFP
- b. Alpha-1 antitrypsin
- c. CEA
- d. hCG

[Ref: Robbins 9th/e pg. 979]

67. Marker for seminoma testis is: *(NEET June 2018)*
- a. Alfa - fetoprotein
- b. Carcinoembryonic antigens
- c. HCG
- d. Acid phosphatase

[Ref: Sabiston's 20th /e pg. 1612]

Explanation
- "Approximately 15% of seminomas contains syncytiotrophoblasts which secret HCG"
- Seminoma is positive for placental alkaline phosphatase and keratin.
- Normally seminoma cells does not produce AFP or beta HCG.

68. The most common infantile testicular tumor is-
(PGMEE 2015)
- a. Seminoma
- b. Teratoma
- c. Embryona carcinoma
- d. Yolk sac tumor

[Ref: Robbins 9th/e pg. 978]

69. RPLND and Chemotheraphy may be used in management of- *(PGMEE 2015)*
- a. Lymphoma testis
- b. Non germ cell tumors
- c. Seminomatous germ cell tumors
- d. Non seminomatous germ cell tumors of testes

[Ref: Campbell Urology 11th/e pg. 704]

70. All of the following are NOT seen in testicular tumors expect – *(PGMEE 2015)*
- a. Oliguria
- b. Lion mass
- c. Hematuria
- d. Lion pain

*[Ref: Sabiston's 1st SAE pg. 2102; Oliguria > **hematuria**]*

71. A young male presents with a right testicular mass. The AFP is elevated while the HCG is normal. The most appropriate next step is – *(PGMEE 2015)*
- a. Wait and watch
- b. Biopsy
- c. USG
- d. Orchidectomy

[Ref: Campbell Urology 11th/e pg. 786]

72. All is true about testicular tumors expect-
(PGMEE 2015)
- a. Seminoma is the most Common testicular tumor
- b. Lymphoma may be seen in the testes
- c. Embryonal carcinoma is a non seminomatous germ cell tumor
- d. Choriocarcinoma is not a germ cell tumor

[Ref: Robbins 9th/e pg. 980]

73. A 56-year-old male is undergoing orchidectomy with inguinal lymphnode dissection for a testicular malignancy. The ideal timing of Antibiotic prophylaxis is- *(PGMEE 2015)*
- a. 1 day before surgery
- b. Onlt postoperatively
- c. 2 hours before surgery
- d. Before the time of incision

[Ref: Schwartz 10th/e pg. 141]

74. Testicular teratoma has all markers EXCEPT
(DNB June' 2011)
- a. AFP
- b. LDH
- c. CEA
- d. HCG

[Ref: Campbell Urology 11th/e pg.]

75. Testicular teratoma in adults is *(DNB June' 2011)*
- a. Broderline
- b. Benign
- c. Malignant
- d. Locally aggressive

[Ref: Robbin's 7th /e p. 1044]

76. High inguinal orchiectomy for teratoma tests with involved epididymis is what stage *(DNB June' 2011)*
- a. Stage I
- b. Stage II
- c. Stage III A
- d. Stage IV

[Ref: Campbell Urology 18th/e pg. 383]

77. Squamous cell carcinoma of scrotal skin is common among *(PGMEE 2016-17)*
- a. Wood workers
- b. Nickel industry
- c. Chimney sweepers
- d. Teratoma

[Ref: Schwartz Urology 10th/e pg.]

PENILE CANCER

78. Which of the following does not progress to carcinoma? *(PGMEE 2016)*
- a. Bowen's disease
- b. Bowenoid papulosis
- c. Erythroplasia
- d. Leukoplakia

[Robbins 9th/e pg. 970-71]

79. A 45-year-old male is diagnosed with carcinoma penis. The surgeon must look out for which lymphnodes. *(PGMEE 2015)*
- a. Internal Iliac
- b. Para aortic
- c. External iliac
- d. Inguinal

[Ref: Bailey & Love 26th /e pg.1374]

80. Most common histological type of Penis ca.
- a. Basal cell carcinoma *(PGMEE 2016-17)*
- b. Squamous cell carcinoma
- c. Bowenoid papulosis
- d. Verrucous carcinoma

[Ref: Robbins 9th/e pg. 971]

81. A 45 year old male presenting with penile cancer extending upto the glans penis is treated with –
(PGMEE 2015)
- a. Partial penectomy with 4 cm margin
- b. Partial penectomy with 2 cm margin
- c. Circumcision
- d. Partial penectomy with inguinal nodes exploration

[Ref: CSTD 13th /e pg.955; Smith's Urology 18th /e pg.390]

64.	c
65.	b
66.	b,c
67.	c
68.	d
69.	d
70.	b
71.	c
72.	d
73.	d
74.	c
75.	c
76.	a
77.	c
78.	b
79.	d
80.	b
81.	b

CLASSIFICATION & LOCATION

1. Classification system of bone tumor is- *(PGMEE 2014)*
  a. Enneking   b. Manchester
  c. Edmonton   d. TNM

[Ref: Ebnezar 4th/e p. 617]

2. Most common benign tumor of the bone is-
(PGMEE 2014)
  a. Giant cell tumor   b. Simple bone cyst
  c. Osteochondroma   d. Enchondroma

[Ref: Maheshwari & Mhaskar 5th/e p. 235]

3. Most common malignant bone tumor-
(PGMEE 2012-13)
  a. Enchondroma   b. Secondaries
  c. Osteoma   d. Osteogenic sarcoma

[Ref: Robbins 9th/e pg. 1197]

4. Tumor arising from bone marrow cells:
(PGMEE 2016-17)
  a. Ewing sarcoma   b. Osteoclastoma
  c. Multiple myeloma   d. Osteochondroma

[Ref: Robbins 9th/e pg. 1197]

5. Most common primary malignant bone tumor:
(PGMEE 2016-17)
  a. Ewing sarcoma   b. Osteoclastoma
  c. Osteosarcoma   d. Osteochondroma

[Ref: Robbins 9th/e pg. 1197]

6. Tumor with maximum bone matrix: *(PGMEE 2012)*
  a. Osteoid osteoma
  b. Enchondroma
  c. Chondrosarcoma
  d. None

[Ref: Maheshwari & Mhaskar 5th/e p. 235]

7. According to Enneking system, not true regarding an ctive benign tumors is- *(PGMEE 11)*
  a. Intracapsular
  b. Extended curettage is treatment
  c. Thick rim of reactive bone
  d. Well defined Margin of reactive bone

[Ref: Campbell's Operative Orthopaedics 11th/e

8. Epiphyseal tumor is: *(PGMEE 07)*
  a. Osteoclastoma
  b. Chondromyxoid fibroma
  c. Osteosarcoma
  d. Ewing sarcoma

[Ref: Maheshwari & Mhaskar 5th/e p. 237]

9. Commonest benign bone tumor is: *(DNB 2007)*
  a. Bony cyst   b. Chondroma
  c. Chordoma.   d. Osteoma

[Ref: Maheshwari & Mhaskar 5th/e p. 235]

1.	a
2.	c
3.	b
4.	c
5.	c
6.	a
7.	c
8.	a
9.	b
10.	b
11.	b
12.	a
13.	a
14.	b

OSTEOCHONDROMA

10. Identify the pathology depicted in the image?
(PGMEE 2015)

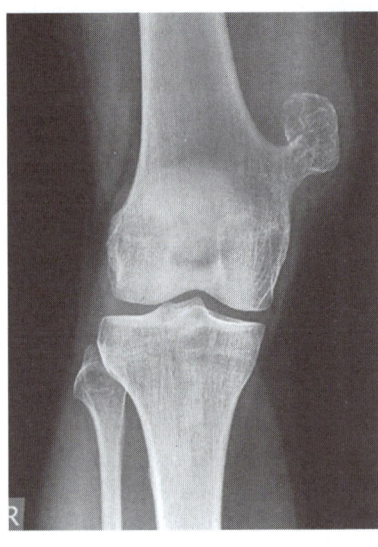

  a. Osteosarcoma   b. Osteochondroma
  c. Chondroblastoma   d. Chondrosarcoma

11. Rapid increase in the size of an osteochondroma indicates- *(PGMEE 2015)*
  a. Bursitis
  b. Malignant transformation
  c. Rupture of the stalk
  d. Dystrophy

[Ref: Internet]

12. Diaphysis achlasia is- *(PGMEE 2015)*
  a. Multiple exostosis
  b. Multiple enchondromatosis
  c. Multiple hemagioma
  d. Multiple osteoid osteoma

[Ref: Maheshwari & Mhaskar 5th/e p. 317]

OSTEOID OSTEOMA

13. Osteoid osteoma consists of- *(PGMEE 2015)*
  a. Osteoblasts   b. Osteoclasts
  c. Both of above   d. None of the above

[Ref: Robbin's pathology 6th/e p. 706]

14. A patient presents with pain in the thigh, relieved by aspirin. X-ray shows a radiolucent mass surrounded by sclerosis. Diagnosis is- *(PGMEE 2015)*
  a. Osteoma   b. Osteoid osteoma
  c. Osteoblastoma   d. Osteoclastoma

[Ref: Maheshwari & Mhaskar 5th/e p. 235]

15. **Most common site of osteoma-** *(PGMEE 2014)*
   a. Tibia
   b. Femur
   c. Humerous
   d. Skull

   [Ref: Robbin's 8th/e p. 1224]

16. **A 10 year child presented with a mid tibial swelling which on X-ray revealed a lytic lesion with sclerotic margins. What is the most likely diagnosis?** *(PGMEE 2011; 14)*
   a. Osteoid osteoma
   b. Eosinophilic granuloma
   c. Fibrocortical defect
   d. Fibrous dysplasia

   [Ref: Maheshwari & Mhaskar 5th/e p. 235]

OSTEOSARCOMA

17. **A 15 yrs old male presented with C/o sudden swelling in the Left upper arm with pain, what will be the most probable diagnosis:-** *(PGMEE 2016-17)*
   a. Osteosarcoma
   b. Ostreochondroma
   c. Osteoclastoma
   d. Enchondroma

   [Ref: Maheshwari and Mhaskar 5th e p.240]

18. **In osteogenic sarcoma predominant histological finding is-** *(PGMEE 2015)*
   a. Giant cells
   b. Osteoid forming tumor cells
   c. Fibroblastic proliferation
   d. Chondroblasts

   [Ref: Maheshwari & Mhaskar 5th/e p. 239; Apley's 9th/e pg 208]

19. **Osteogenic sarcoma arise from-** *(PGMEE 2014)*
   a. Epiphysis
   b. Metaphysis
   c. Growth plate
   d. Epiphyseal cortex

   [Ref: Maheshwari & Mhaskar 5th/e p. 239, Adam's Outline of orthopaedics 14th/e p. 113]

20. **A child is diagnosed with osteosarcoma based on Sunray appearance seen on X-ray. This is because of-** *(PGMEE 14)*
   a. Calcification along the periosteum
   b. Calcification along the blood vessels
   c. Periosteal reaction
   d. Soft tissue invasion

   [Ref: Maheshwari & Mhaskar 5th/e p. 240; Apley's system of orthopaedics and fractures 9th/e p. 207, 208]

Explanation

Sunburst/Sunray appearance

- Frequently seen in **osteosarcoma** but can also occur with other aggressive bony lesions such as an **Ewing** sarcoma or **osteoblastic** metastases (e.g. prostate, lung or breast cancer).
- When lesion grows rapidly the tiny fibers connecting the periosteum to the bone (Sharpey's fibers) become stretched out perpendicular to the bone. When these fibers ossify, they produce a pattern called "sunburst" periosteal reaction.

21. **Most common site of osteogenic sarcoma is-** *(PGMEE 2014)*
   a. Shoulder joint
   b. Wrist joint
   c. Knee joint
   d. Jaw bone

   [Ref: Robbin's 8th/e p. 1225]

22. **7 years old child presents with a lesion in upper tibia. X-ray shows radiolucent area with Codman's triangle and Sunray appearance. Diagnosis is-** *(PGMEE 2011, AI 07; 07)*
   a. Ewing sarcoma
   b. Osteosarcoma
   c. Osteoid osteoma
   d. Chondrosarcoma

   [Ref: Maheshwari & Mhaskar 5th/e p. 240]

23. **X-ray appearance of osteosarcoma are all except-** *(PGMEE 2012)*
   a. Periosteal reaction
   b. Sunray appearance
   c. Soap-bubble
   d. Codman's triangle

   [Ref: Maheshwari & Mhaskar 5th/e p. 240]

24. **Calcification in osteosarcoma is due to presence of-** *(PGMEE 2015)*
   a. Osteoid matrix
   b. Osteoblasts
   c. High Calcium levels in serum
   d. High calcitonin

   [Ref: Masculoskeletal imaging the requisites by David May p. 58]

EWING'S SARCOMA

25. **Ewing's sarcoma clinically mimics-** *(PGMEE 2015)*
   a. Osteomyelitis
   b. Osteochondroses
   c. Osteosclerosis
   d. Heterotopic ossification

   [Ref: Maheshwari & Mhaskar 5th/e p. 243; Campbell 12th/e p. 730]

Explanation

Differential diagnosis of Ewing's

- Ewing sarcoma family of tumours:-
  o PNET tumour: large soft tissue component with extension into bone.
  o Askin tumour: chest wall
- Osteomyelitis
- Osteosarcoma (ALP is not elevated in Ewing sarcoma)
- Metastases
- Eosinophilic granuloma
- Neuroblastoma (seen in age group < 5 yr)

26. **A 7 years old child comes with fever and tibial swelling exhibits on X-ray exhibits periosteal reaction. Laboratory results show raised ESR and TLC. What is the next step in diagnosis of the patient?** *(PGMEE 13)*
   a. MRI
   b. Pus culture
   c. Bone biopsy
   d. Blood culture

   [Ref: Maheshwari & Mhaskar 5th/e p. 235; Tachdjian's Pediatric Othopaedics, ch.27]

27. **Most common site of Ewing's sarcoma-** *(PGMEE 13)*
   a. Upper end of tibia
   b. Shaft of tibia
   c. Lower end of femur
   d. Shaft of femur

   [Ref: Maheshwari & Mhaskar 5th/e p. 243; Textbook of skeletal oncology p. 315]

28. **Ewings sarcoma arises from-** *(PGMEE 2012-13)*
   a. Neurons
   b. G cells
   c. Neuroectodermal cells
   d. Totipotent cells

   [Ref: Robbins 9th/e pg. 1198]

15.	b
16.	a
17.	a
18.	b
19.	b
20.	c
21.	c
22.	b
23.	c
24.	a
25.	a
26.	a
27.	d
28.	c

29. Which of the following is associated with poor prognosis in Ewings sarcoma? *(PGMEE 10)*
    a. B2 microglobulin
    b. Fever
    c. Young age
    d. Thrombocytosis

    [Ref: Campbell's Orthopaedics 11th/e p. 913]

30. The bone tumor seen in children with characteristic "onion-peel" periosteal reaction is? *(DNB DEC 2010)*
    a. Osteosarcoma
    b. Osteoid osteoma
    c. Ewing's sarcoma
    d. Giant cell tumor

    [Ref: Maheshwari & Mhaskar 5th/e p. 243]

31. A young girl presented with swelling of right thigh, with history of trauma 2 months back. Now she presented with swelling at mid-shaft of femur & low grade fever. ESR is mildly raised. X-ray shows a laminated periosteal reaction. Next line of investigation would be- *(PGMEE 09)*
    a. MRI
    b. Biopsy
    c. Bone scan
    d. Blood count & CRP

    [Ref: Maheshwari & Mhaskar 5th/e p. 243; Campbell 11th/e p. chapter 22]

32. Radiotherapy is the treatment of choice in *(DNB 2007)*
    a. Ewing's sarcoma
    b. Osteosarcoma
    c. Osteoclastoma
    d. Synovial sarcoma

    [Ref: Maheshwari & Mhaskar 5th/e p. 243]

33. Translocation seen in Ewing sarcoma :- *(PGMEE 2016-17)*
    a. t(11;22)
    b. t(q24;q11)
    c. t(11;23)
    d. t(9;22)

    [Ref: Robbin's 9th/e pg. 1203]

CHONDROBLASTOMA & CHONDROSARCOMA

34. Left hand x ray with lytic lesion of 16 yr old boy:- *(PGMEE 2016-17)*

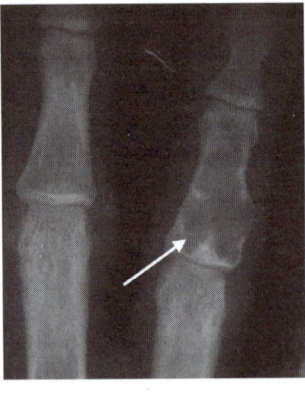

    a. Enchondroma
    b. GCT
    c. SBC
    d. Metastases

    [Ref: Internet]

35. Development of chondrosarcoma is related with- *(PGMEE 2015)*
    a. Maffucci syndrome
    b. Felty syndrome
    c. Ollier's disease
    d. None of the above

    [Ref:Maheshawari & Mhaskar 5th e pg.248; Orthopaedics pathology by Vincent PG p. 401]

Explanation

Chondrosarcam is related to

- Ollier's disease: Nonfamilial multiple enchondromas.
- Maffucci syndrome: Familial form of multiple enchondromas with cavernous hemangiomas & phlebolith.
- Multiple hereditary exostosis (diaphyseal aclasia)

36. Enchondroma commonly arises from- *(PGMEE 2014)*
    a. Ribs
    b. Vertebra
    c. Tibia
    d. Phalanges

    [Ref: Maheshawari & Mhaskar 5th e pg.248; Apley's 9th/e p. 197]

37. Variant of Giant cell tumor is- *(PGMEE 11)*
    a. Ossifying fibroma
    b. Osteosarcoma
    c. Non ossifying fibroma
    d. Chondroblastoma

    [Ref: http://emedicine.medscap.com/ article/1254949-overview]

38. Most common tumor in hand- *(PGMEE 11)*
    a. Synovial sarcoma
    b. Giant cell tumor
    c. Enchondroma
    d. Exostosis

    [Ref:Maheshawari & Mhaskar 5th e pg.248; Orthopaedics oncology 4th/e p. 69]

39. Bone tumor arising from epiphysis is? *(PGMEE 2011)*
    a. Osteoid
    b. Ewing's Sarcoma
    c. Chondrosarcoma
    d. Chondroblastoma

GIANT CELL TUMOR

40. X-ray of distal radius with characteristics appearance is given below. Most likely diagnosis is: *(PGMEE 2016-17)*

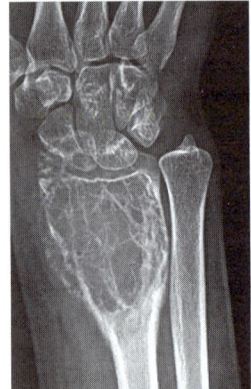

    a. Simple bone cyst
    b. Aheurysmal cyst
    c. GCT
    d. Chronic osteomylities

    [Ref: Robbins 9th/e pg. 1203]

Explanation

- Characteristic Soap-bubble appearance is seen in GCT (Giant cell tumor) or osteoclastoma.

41. Soap bubble appearance on Xray is seen in which bone tumor- *(PGMEE 2013)*
    a. Osteogenic sarcoma
    b. Giant cell tumor
    c. Multiple myeloma
    d. Chondroblastoma

    [Ref:Maheshawari & Mhaskar 5th e pg.245-6]

29.	b
30.	c
31.	a
32.	a
33.	a
34.	a
35.	a,c
36.	d
37.	d
38.	c
39.	d
40.	c
41.	b

42. Which of the following is a pulsatile tumor?
                                                    (PGMEE 2011; 10)
a. Osteosarcoma   b. Chondrosarcoma
c. Ewing's sarcoma   d. Osteoclastoma

[Ref: Clinical oncology 2nd/e p. 998]

43. 35 years male presents with lesion at proximal tibia showing egg shell crackling. Lesion is eccentric and x-ray shows osteolytic lesion just below joint line. Following is the X-ray of the patient. What is the most probable diagnosis? *(PGMEE 2015)*

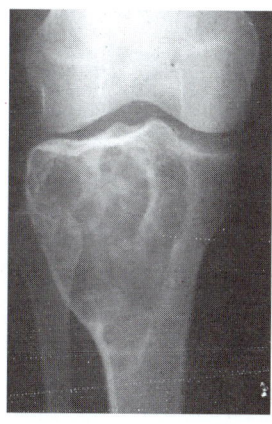

a. Giant cell tumor   b. Osteosarcoma
c. Osteoid osteoma   d. Chondromblastoma

[Ref: Maheshawari & Mhaskar 5th e pg.245-6]

44. X-ray showing: *(PGMEE 2016-17)*

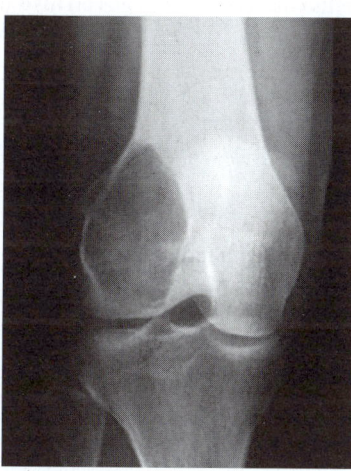

a. Osteochondroma
b. Osteosarcoma
c. Osteoclastoma
d. Osteoblastoma

[Ref: Clinical oncology 2nd/e p. 998]

45. Which of the following is true about Giant cell tumor- *(PGMEE 2012)*
a. Usually presents as a lytic lesion with sclerotic rim
b. Seen in age less than 15 years
c. Epiphyseal origin
d. Always benign

[Ref:Maheshawari & Mhaskar 5th e pg.245; GS Kulkarni 2nd/e p. 1043]

BONY METASTASIS

46. Most common tumor producing osteoblastic metastasis-
                                                    (PGMEE 2013)
a. Kidney   b. Lung
c. Prostate   d. Thyroid

[Ref: Maheshawari & Mhaskar 5th e pg.245;Orthopaedic nuclear medicine 1st/e p. 154]

47. Most common primary of metastatic bone tumor in a male among following is- *(DNB Dec' 2009)*
a. Bone   b. Brain
c. Lung   d. Liver

[Ref: Schwartz's surgery 8th/e p. 1330]

48. Metastasis not found in- *(PGMEE 2012)*
a. Femur   b. Spine
c. Fibula   d. Humerus

[Ref: Maheshawari & Mhaskar 5th e pg.247;Apley's 9th/e p. 216]

49. Predominantly osteoblastic metastasis is seen in?
a. Renal cell carcinoma   *(DNB Dec 2009)*
b. Thyroid carcinoma
c. Breast Carcinoma
d. Prostate carcinoma

[Ref: Maheshawari & Mhaskar 5th e pg.245]

BONE CYSTS

50. Aneurysmal bone cyst is most common in:-
                                                    (PGMEE 2016-17)
a. Humerus   b. Femur
c. Radius   d. Ulna

[Ref: Maheshwari and Mhaskar 5th e p.237]

51. Fallen fragment sign is a feature of- *(PGMEE 2013)*
a. Simple bone cyst   b. Aneurysmal bone cyst
c. Giant cell tumor   d. Fibrous dysplasia

[Ref:Maheshawari & Mhaskar 5th e pg.251; Textbook of musculoskeletal tumor p. 112]

52. X-ray showing

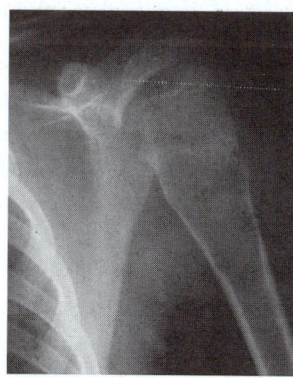

a. Simple bone cyst
b. Aneurysmal bone cyst
c. Giant cell tumor
d. Fibrous dysplasia

[Ref:Maheshawari & Mhaskar 5th e pg. 249, 251;Textbook of musculoskeletal tumor p. 112]

42.	d
43.	a
44.	c
45.	c
46.	c
47.	c
48.	c
49.	d
50.	a
51.	a
52.	a

53. All are true about aneurysmal bone cyst except-
(PGMEE 2013)

a. Eccentric
b. Expansile & lytic
c. Treated by simple curettage
d. Metaphysis of long bones

[Ref: Maheshawari & Mhaskar 5th e pg.249; Ebnezar 4th/e p. 629]

FIBROUS DYSPLASIA & ADAMANTINOMA

54. Characteristic radiological feature of fibrous dysplasia-
(PGMEE 2011; 10)

a. Thickened bone matrix
b. Cortical erosion
c. Ground glass appearance
d. Bone enlargement

[Ref: Maheshawari & Mhaskar 5th e pg.249;Orthopaedics oncology 3rd/e p. 182]

55. Shepherd crook deformity is seen in? *(DNB June 2010)*

a. Fibrous dysplasia
b. Adamantinoma
c. Non ossifying fibroma
d. Fibrous cortical defect

[www.radiologysigns.tumblr.com>post>sheperd crook]

56. All are true about fibrous dysplasia EXCEPT:-

a. Developmental disorder *(PGMEE 2016-17)*
b. Malignant tumor of bone
c. McCune-Albright syndrome is polyostotic disease
d. GNAS1 mutations

[Ref: Robbins 9th/e pg. 1206]

57. All is true about Fibrous dysplasia except-

a. Can be polyostotic *(PGMEE 2014)*
b. Benign
c. Trabeculae mimic chinese characters
d. Extramedullary

[Ref: Robbin's 8th/e p. 1231]

Explanation

- Fibrous dysplasia is a benign intramedullary fibro-osseous lesion.
- It is a bone developmental anomaly characterized by replacement of normal bone & marrow by fibrous tissue.

PAGET'S DISEASE OF BONE

58. Drug of choice of paget disease is:- *(PGMEE 2016-17)*

a. Strontium ranelate
b. Alendronate
c. Calcitonin
d. Vit d

[Ref: Maheshwari and Mhaskar 5th e p.317]

59. All of the following are true about Pagets disease except-

a. Less than 1% malignant *(PGMEE 2014)*
b. Progress to chondrosarcoma
c. Ostesclerotic phase seen
d. Virus association

[Ref: Robbins 9th/e pg. 1189]

MISCELLANEOUS

60. Moth eaten bone is seen in:- *(PGMEE 2013)*

a. Osteoid osteoma
b. Multiple myeloma
c. Eosinophilic granuloma
d. Chondromyxoid fibroma

[Ref: Maheshawari & Mhaskar 5th e pg.245]

61. Non neoplastic lesions simulating bone tumor are all except? *(PGMEE 2011)*

a. Bone island
b. Fibrous dysplasia
c. Bone infarct
d. Hurler syndrome

[Ref: Maheshwari & Mhaskar 5th ep246; Campbell's p. 885]

62. Which isotope is used for treating bone cancer?
(PGMEE 2012)

a. Sr
b. Tc
c. I 123
d. Ga

63. Striated vertebra is seen in: *(PGMEE 2012)*

a. TB spine
b. Haemangioma
c. Chordoma
d. Metastasis

[Ref: Apley's 9th/e p. 216]

SOFT TISSUE TUMORS

64. Tadpole cells comma shaped cells on histopathology are seen in: *(PGMEE 2012-13)*

a. Spideroma
b. Histiocytoma
c. Rhabdomyosarcoma
d. Trichoepithelioma

[Ref: Robbins 9th/e pg. 1222]

65. Desmoid tumor, treatment is: *(PGMEE 2015)*

a. Wide excision with radiotherapy
b. Wide excision
c. Radiotherapy
d. Local excision

[Ref: Bailey and love 26th /e pg. 969]

66. Herring bone pattern seen in: *(PGMEE 2016-17)*

a. Rhebdomyosarcoma
b. Leiomyosarcoma
c. Fibrosarcoma
d. Ependymoma

67. Multiple epidermoid cysts are seen in:

a. Peutz- Jegher syndrome *(PGMEE 2013-14)*
b. Gardner's syndrome
c. Familial polyposis coli
d. Turcot's syndrome

[Ref: Robbins 9th/e pg. 806]

68. Most common presentation of desmoid tumor:
(NEET Pattern 2017)

a. Abdominal lump
b. Abdominal pain
c. Rectal prolapse
d. Ureteric obstruction

Ref: Sabiston 20th page 1073

53.	c
54.	c
55.	a
56.	b
57.	d
58.	b
59.	a
60.	b
61.	d
62.	a
63.	b
64.	c
65.	b
66.	c
67.	b
68.	a

Explanation

Desmoid Tumor

- Most common primary malignant neoplasms of the abdominal wall are desmoid tumors and sarcomas.
- Desmoid tumor, also known as *fibromatosis, aggressive fibromatosis,* or *desmoid-type fibromatosis,*
- These tumors arise from fibroaponeurotic tissue and typically are manifested as a slowly growing mass.
- Lack metastatic potential but can be multifocal as well as locally aggressive and invasive, with a high propensity for recurrence.
- Mostly sporadic, typically in young women during pregnancy or within a year of childbirth.
- May present with an asymptomatic mass or with symptoms related to mass effect from the tumor.

- Immunohistochemistry: typically stain **+ve for** β-**catenin, actin, and vimentin** and stain negative for cytokeratin and S-100.
- Spontaneous regression occurs in up to 10% of patients.
- A conservative approach to selection of patients for surgery in desmoid type fibromatosis is becoming the new standard of care
- Radiotherapy is considered for unresectable tumors

69. Management of desmoid tumor is *(DNB June' 2009)*
   a. Growth inhibitors
   b. Wide excision
   c. Radiotherapy
   d. Local excision

[Ref: Devita 8th/e chapter 45]

69. b

FACTS

- Most abundant and the only native cell of skin → Keratinocytes (90%)
- Melanocytes are derived from → Neural crest
- *Lines of Blaschko:*
  - Represent epidermal cell migration pathway during fetal development
  - Conditions distributed along these lines:
    - Epidermal nevus
    - Nevus achromicus
    - Incontinentia pigmenti
- UV rays causing most skin diseases → UV-B
- Psoriasis associated with β-hemolytic streptococcal infection → Guttate psoriasis.
- Most characteristic finding in lichen planus → Basal cell degeneration

- Chemical present in bindi → Para tertiary butyl phenol.
- Seborrheic dermatitis is caused by → *Malassezia furfur* (Yeast form).
- Patch test is an example of → Delayed (type IV) HSR
- *Contact Dermatitis:*
  - Irritant CD is an example of → Type I HSR
  - Allergic CD is an example of → Type IV HSR

Tzanck Smear Findings	
Pemphigus	Acantholysis/Tzanck cells
Varicella Zoster virus	Multinucleated giant cells
Herpes Simplex virus	Multinucleated giant cells
Bullous pemphigoid	Predominantly eosinophils

NAMED FEATURES

Darier sign:
- Development of urticaria on light scratching with tip of pen or forceps
- Feature of Urticaria Pigmentosa

Nikolsky sign:
- Erosion or exfoliation of a normal appearing epidermis as a result of applying firm sliding pressure
- Non specific sign of Pemphigus vulgaris

Asboe-Hansen sign:
- Peripheral extension of a blister as a result of applying lateral pressure on the edge of blister
- Non specific sign of Pemphigus vulgaris

Sign of Hertoghe/Queen Anne sign:
- Thinning or loss of the outer third of the eyebrows
- Seen in:
  - Leprosy
  - Atopic dermatitis
  - Hypothyroidism

Dermatographism:
- Exaggerated whealing tendency on firmly stroking the skin

Brocq's phenomenon:
- Subepidermal hemorrhage on scraping of a lesion
- Seen in Lichen planus

Koebner/Isomorphic phenomenon:
- Development of new isomorphic lesions in the traumatized uninvolved areas of skin.
- Trauma → New lesions in otherwise normal skin
- These lesions are clinically and pathologically identical to those in the diseased skin.
- Seen in:
  - Psoriasis
  - Lichen planus
  - Vitiligo

Pseudo-Koebner/Pseudo-Isomorphic phenomenon:
- Infection arising in area of trauma.
- Seen in:
  - Molluscum contagiosum
  - Warts
  - Behçet's disease
  - Pyoderma gangrenosum

Reverse Koebner phenomenon:
- Disappearance of skin lesion after trauma.
- Seen in psoriasis

Remote reverse Koebner phenomenon:
- Spontaneous repigmentation of vitiligo patches distant from the autologous skin graft site.

Self-Limiting Papulosquamous Disorders:
- Pityriasis rosea → Heals with hypopigmentation
- Lichen planus → Heals with hyperpigmentation

MOST COMMON

- MC site of erythema nodosum→ Anterior shin of Tibia.
- MC type of psoriasis → Plaque psoriasis aka Psoriasis vulgaris.
- MC cause of drug induced **P**emphigus → **P**enicillamine.
- MC disorder associated with nail pitting → Psoriasis.
- MC endocrine abnormality associated with vitiligo → Thyroid disorder.

- MC site for Atopic dermatitis → Flexors like Antecubital fossa & popliteal fossa.
- MCC of Air borne contact dermatitis (ABCD) → Parthenium.
- MCC of metal induced allergic contact dermatitis → Nickel
- MCC of Irritant contact dermatitis in Indian women → Detergents.

MOROPHOLOGY OF SKIN

- Skin is composed of Epidermis → Dermis → Subcutaneous tissue from outer to inner.
- Epidermis serves as a barrier to water loss
- Epidermal turnover time (usually **52-75 days**) or transit time is journey of keratinocytes from basale to the surface.
- Accelerated skin turnover is seen in Psoriasis (2-4 days).
- Haascheiben cells in epidermis is responsible for touch

- **Dermis contains :**
  ○ Meissner's corpuscles – light touch & vibration receptor
  ○ Pacinian & Ruffini's corpuscles – deep pressure
  ○ Free nerve endings – nociceptors and thermoreceptor
  ○ Blood vessels & lymphatics

5-Layera of Epidermis	Features	Applied Importance
Stratum corneum (Spinous/horny/Dead layer)	■ Outermost cornified or horny cell layer. ■ **Fillagrin** protein is present. ■ Thickest on the palms and soles and thinnest on the eyelids	■ This layer is **underdeveloped in VLBW newborns.** ■ Permeable in preterm infants ■ Ringworm (Tinea) is the infection of this layer.
Stratum lucidum	■ Present as an interim layer and is responsible for transparency.	■ It is an additional layer found only in **palms and soles.**
Stratum granulosum (Granular layer)	■ It is the **thinnest** layer of skin ■ Contains filaggrin, basophilic **keratohyaline** granules.	■ Odland bodies/lamellar granules are present
Stratum spinosum (Prickle layer)	■ Thickest layer of the epidermis. ■ Contains desmosomes & **Langerhans cell (CD 1a +)**	■ Provides mechanical strength ■ Intercellular edema in stratum spinosum is k/a Spongiosis
Stratum basale/ Stratum germinativum (Basal layer)	■ Contains most important and mitotically active cells – keratinocytes, ■ Melanocytes, Merkel cells (touch corpuscles/discs) are also present	■ Acantholytic cells in **Pemphigus vulgaris** are derived from stratum basale.

Malpighian layer is composed of stratum spinosum + basale |

Stratum corneum — Lipid bilayers, cross-linked cornified envelope, FILLAGGRIN

Stratum granulosum — Tight junctions, lamellar and keratohyline granules, PROFILAGGRIN, LORICRN, LIPIDS

Stratum spinosum — K1/K10 keratin filamen bundles, intercellular junction desmosomes), Ap2, C/EBP, Hes1, Notch 1/3

Stratum basale/ germinativum — Keratin 5/K15 keratin filament bundels, intercellular junctions (Adherens rich), p63, EGFR, IGFR,TβRII, δ1(Delta1)

Hemidesmosomes, α6β4, focal adhesions α3β1
Laminin, fibronectin, collagen IV, TGFα, IGF

PAPULOSQUAMOUS DISORDERS

	Seborrheic Dermatitis	Lichen Planus	Psoriasis	Pityriasis Rosea	Pityriasis Rubra Pilaris
Etiology	• Malassezia furfur	• Autoimmune	• T – cell disorder	• ? Infection	• T-cell disorder
Onset	• Puberty – Adulthood	• Any age (usually 30-60 years)	• Any age (usually 20-30 years)	• 10-35 years	• Familial PRP – childhood
Pruritus	• ++	• ++	• +/–	• +/–	• +/–
Scales	• Greasy yellow	• No scales	• Silvery white scales	• Collarette of scales	• +
Lesion	• Follicular papule	• **P**olygonal, **P**lain, **P**urple (violaceous) **P**ruritic **P**apule	• Erythematous plaque	• Annular erythematous plaque (Herald patch)	• Reddish orange scaly plaque with papule
Distribution	• Scalp, face & trunk	• Flexor surface	• Extensor surface of knee, elbow	• Trunk & proximal extremity	• Trunk
Clinical features	• Burning, scaling and itching lesion • Severe dandruff • Cradle cap (infantile SD) • Activity increased in winters • May worsen in Parkinson disease and AIDS	• Koebner phenomenon+ • Brocq's phenomenon + • Nail – Pterygium • Healing with hyperpigmentation • Cicatricial alopecia • Wickham's striae • Lacy lesion on oral mucosa • Mucosal involvement+	• Koebner phenomenon + • Joint involvement in 10-30% • Nail changes in 10 – 50% • Ocular findings in 10% • Auspitz sign • Grattage test • Mucosal involvement uncommon	• Hanging curtain sign + • Secondary lesion – Christmas tree/Fir tree pattern • Heals with hypopigmentation	• Palmoplanter keratoderma • Cephalocaudal distribution • Keratodermic sandals • Orangish thickening of palm and sole • Keratotic follicular papules
Association		• Hep C, Alopecia areata, Vitiligo • Oral LP can transform into squamous cell carcinoma	• HLA – Cw6 • Erythroderma	• Association with HHV 6 & 7 • Drugs	• Erythroderma
Histologic findings		• Acanthosis + • Basal cell degeneration occur • Civatte/Colloid bodies • Max Joseph spaces • Band like infiltrate of lymphocytes	• Acanthosis + • Parakeratosis • Absence of granular layer • Munro microabscesses • Supra-papillary thinning • Kogoj spongiform pustules	• Acanthosis + • RPR or VDRL to rule out syphilis	• Island of normal skin in between lesions
Treatment	• 1st line – Antifungal therapy • Topical steroids	• Self limited disease • Mild cases – Topical steroids	• Psoralen with UVA (PUVA) • Retinoids, like Isotretinoin, acitretin • Apremilast	• Self-limiting disorder	• Topical steroids and retinoids

VESICO-BULLOUS DISORDERS

	Pemphigus Vulgaris	Bullous Pemphigoid	Dermatitis Herpetiformis	Erythema Multiforme
Pathology	▪ Mucocutaneous form: Autoantibodies against desmoglein 1 & 3 ▪ Mucosal form: antidesmoglein 3 antibodies	▪ IgG autoantibodies against hemidesmosomal antigen BPAg 1 & BPAg 2	▪ IgA antibodies against tissue transglutaminase (t-TG) ▪ HLA DR3, HLA DQ2	▪ Type IV HSR
Bulla characteristics	▪ Flaccid/fragile bulla ▪ Intraepidermal bulla ▪ Painful erosions	▪ Tense bulla ▪ Subepidermal bulla/DEJ ▪ Painful erosions	▪ Papulovesicular lesion ▪ Subepidermal bulla/DEJ	▪ Tense bulla ▪ Subepidermal bulla/ DEJ
Distribution	▪ Scalp, face & trunk. ▪ Asymmetric distribution	▪ Can be generalized or localized ▪ Symmetrical distribution	▪ Extensors (knee, elbow), buttocks ▪ Symmetrical distribution	▪ Face & acral extensor surfaces ▪ Symmetrical distribution
Clinical features	▪ Mean age of onset: 50 – 60 years ▪ No or minimal itching ▪ Mucous membrane involved in almost all ▪ MC presentation – painful oral erosions ▪ Asboe Hansen sign +ve ▪ Nikolsky's sign +ve	▪ Mean age of onset: 65 years ▪ Itching present ++ ▪ Mucous membrane involvement rare ▪ MC presentation – generalized bullous form ▪ Nikolsky's sign –ve	▪ Age of onset: 20-40 years ▪ Intense itching +++ ▪ Mucous membrane not involved ▪ MC presentation – pruritic eruptions on extensor surface ▪ Nikolsky's sign –ve	▪ Age of onset: 20-40 years ▪ No or minimal itching ▪ Mucous membrane involvement ± ▪ Bulla is surrounded by erythematous halo (**target** /iris/ Bull's eye lesion) ▪ Nikolsky's sign –ve
Association	▪ Myasthenia gravis ▪ Thymoma	▪ Lichen planus, Psoriasis ▪ UV rays	▪ Gluten enteropathy in > 90% ▪ Dermatomyositis, Type I DM	▪ Recurrent HSV (MCC), EBV, ▪ Drugs – Sulfa drugs
Microscopy	▪ Acantholysis + ▪ DIF: IgG deposits within epidermal intercellular substance ▪ Row of tombstones appearance	▪ Acanthosis – ▪ DIF: linear band of IgG & C3 deposits along DEJ	▪ Acanthosis – ▪ DIF: Granular IgA deposits in papillary dermis along basement membrane	▪ Acanthosis – ▪ Lymphocyte infiltrate along DEJ
Treatment	▪ Corticosteroids ▪ Immunosuppressants – Azathioprine	▪ Corticosteroids ▪ Immunosuppressants – Azathioprine	▪ Dapsone is DOC ▪ Gluten free diet	▪ Self limiting disease ▪ Topical steroids

DEJ – Dermoepidermal Junction |

DISORDERS OF PIGMENTATION

Disorders of hypopigmentation		
Localized		**Diffuse**
Decrease in pigmentation: ▪ Leprosy ▪ Pityriasis alba ▪ Atopic dermatitis ▪ Tuberous sclerosis ▪ Nevus depigmentosus	**Absence of pigmentation:** ▪ Vitiligo ▪ Piebaldism ▪ Leukoderma	▪ Albinism ▪ Chediak Higashi syndrome

Disorders of hyperpigmentation	
Localized	**Generalized**
▪ Chloasma ▪ Freckles ▪ Lentigines – Peutz Jeghers syndrome, Carney complex ▪ Café au lait macules – NF, McCune Albright syndrome ▪ Nevi	▪ Addison disease ▪ Nelson syndrome ▪ Malignancy ▪ Hyperthyroidism ▪ Primary biliary cirrhosis ▪ Chronic arsenic poisoning ▪ Hemochromatosis

	Piebaldism	Vitiligo	Albinism
Inheritance	▪ Autosomal dominant	▪ Acquired polygenic condition	▪ AR (OA 1 is XLR)
Pathology	▪ Disorder of melanocytes development	▪ Cell mediated melanocytes destruction	▪ Defective melanin production from tyrosine
Age of onset	▪ Birth	▪ Any age (usually 10-30 years)	▪ Birth
Lesion	▪ Hypopigmented macule with white forelock	▪ Well demarcated & circumscribed, depigmented macule & patches	▪ Milky white skin
Distribution	▪ Central forehead	▪ Hands, forearms, feet ▪ Face – perioral & periocular	▪ OCA: Generalized – skin, hair, eyes, optic nerve ▪ OA: only eyes are affected
Special features	▪ Islands of normal skin within white patch	▪ Trichrome pattern, segmental distribution ▪ Koebner phenomenon +	▪ Nevi, freckles, lentigenes
Associated conditions	▪ Poliosis ▪ Waardenburg syndrome	▪ Halo nevi ▪ Alopecia areata	▪ White hairs, photosensitivity ▪ Chediak Higashi syndrome
Extracutaneous associations	▪ None	▪ Hypo/Hyperthyroidism (MC) ▪ Diabetes Mellitus ▪ Addison disease,	▪ Nystagmus, Iris translucency ▪ Foveal hypoplasia l/t Reduced visual acuity ▪ Increased risk of skin cancer
Histology	▪ Melanocytes and melanin – absent in affected skin and hair follicles	▪ Melanocytes and melanin absent	▪ Melanocytes normal in number and structure
Treatment	▪ Phototherapy ± PUVA ± Grafting	▪ Phototherapy ± topical corticosteroids ▪ Laser therapy	▪ No cure

|OA – Ocular albinism| OCA – Oculocutaneous Albinism|

	Freckles	Lentigines
Etiology	▪ Genetic/Autosomal Dominant	▪ Environmental
Onset	▪ 2-3 years of age ▪ Fade with age	▪ Old age ▪ Accumulate with age
Area affected	▪ Sun exposed skin, Face, neck, chest, arms	▪ Sun exposed skin, face, hands, chest & back
Lesion	▪ Small, red or light brown macules ▪ Darker in summer, lighter in winter	▪ Large light yellow to dark brown ▪ No variation with season
At risk	▪ Individuals with fair skin with red hair	▪ Individuals with light and dark skin
Melanosome number	▪ Increased	▪ Normal
Melanosome size	▪ Large	▪ Normal

NEVUS

- Nevus cells are derived from neural crests and proliferate abnormally, resulting in blackish-brown pigmented macules.

Type	Features
Spitz nevus (Benign juvenile melanoma)	▪ Uncommon type of benign mole (benign melanocytic nevus). ▪ Affects the epidermis and dermis. ▪ Histological features may resemble melanoma
Becker's nevus (Becker melanosis or Pigmented hairy epidermal nevus)	▪ Hyperpigmented, hypertrichotic patch on the upper trunk or proximal upper extremity. The lesion is usually single and begins before puberty. ▪ Due to overgrowth of the epidermis (epidermal hyperplasia), pigment cells (melanosomes/melanocytes), keratinocytes and hair follicles ▪ Acne may develop ▪ Treated by Q switched Nd or Ir: YAG laser
Sutton nevus	▪ Nevus pigmentosus surrounded by leukodermas
Divided nevus	▪ Distribute predominantly on the upper and lower eyelids
Nevus of Ota	▪ Blue or grey coalescing macules present at birth/ adolescence. ▪ Common sites are forehead, zygomatic, **Periorbital**
Nevi of Ito	▪ Blue or grey coalescing macules present at birth/adolescence over shoulder and upper arm
Nevus achromicus (Nevus depigmentosus)	▪ Non-progressive hypopigmented macule usually seen before 3 years in segmental pattern.
Nevus anemicus	▪ Vascular malformation due to abnormal vascular tone.
Dysplastic nevus	▪ A slightly elevated, flat-topped patch >6 mm in diameter seen around puberty

HAIR GROWTH CYCLE

Phase	Anagen	Catagen	Telogen
% of hair in this phase	▪ 80-90%	▪ 1-2%	▪ 10-15%
Duration	▪ 3-4 years (approx 1000 days)	▪ 3-4 weeks	▪ 3-4 months (100 days)
Features	▪ Growth phase ▪ It decides length of the hair	▪ Transitional phase	▪ Resting phase

ALOPECIA

Non Cicatricial/Non Scarring Alopecia		Cicatricial/Scarring Alopecia	
▪ Alopecia areata ▪ Androgenic alopecia ▪ Telogen effluvium ▪ Anagen effluvium	▪ Trichotillomania ▪ Moth eaten alopecia ▪ Tinea capitis	▪ Discoid lupus ▪ Lichen planopilaris ▪ Mechanical trauma ▪ Traction alopecia	▪ Scleroderma ▪ Kerion/Flavus ▪ Tertiary syphilis

Alopecia Areata

- Characterized by localized and patchy hair loss.
- Can affect any hair-bearing area.
- Most often involved site is scalp.
- Can occur at any age. Incidence peaks between 15-29 years.
- May be associated with Atopic dermatitis, Vitiligo & Thyroid diseases
- Alopecia totalis – 100% hair loss on the scalp

- Alopecia universalis - Complete loss of hair on all hair-bearing areas
- Presence of exclamation point hairs (i.e. hairs tapered near proximal end) is pathognomonic.
- Pitting – MC nail manifestation.
- Intralesional corticosteroid if < 50% involvement.
- Minoxidil → effective in extensive disease (>50% hair loss)

Androgenetic Alopecia

- Androgenetic (or pattern) alopecia is a genetic disorder that affects both men and women.
- Pathology – shortening of Anagen phase shortens while the Telogen phase remaining constant.

- Men → gradual recession of the frontal hairline with thinning in the temporal areas
- Women → frontal hairline is often preserved but bitemporal recession is evident
- Treatment – Minoxidil, Finasteride

Effluvium

	Telogen Effluvium	Anagen effluvium
Pathology	▪ Occurs when a physiologic stress or hormonal change causes a large number of hairs to enter telogen phase	▪ Occurs after any insult to the hair follicle that impairs its mitotic or metabolic activity.
Onset of hair loss	▪ 2 – 4 months	▪ 1 – 4 weeks
Percent of hair loss	▪ 20 – 50%	▪ 80 – 90%
Characteristics	▪ Non-scarring alopecia ▪ Diffuse hair shedding, often with an acute onset ▪ Can affect hair on all parts of the body	▪ Non-scarring alopecia ▪ Tapered fracture of the hair shafts
Precipitating factors	▪ Metabolic or hormonal stress – Child birth, starvation, surgeries, emotional stress ▪ Medications, Malignancies	▪ Chemotherapeutic agents – MC Cause ▪ Pemphigus vulgaris
Stage of hair shed	▪ Normal club hairs from normal resting follicles	▪ Anagen hair
Outcome	▪ Recovery is spontaneous and occurs within 6 months	▪ Recovery is spontaneous and occurs within 6 months

EXOCRINE GLANDS

	Merocrine/Eccrine Glands	Holocrine Gland	Apocrine Gland
Secretion	▪ By exocytosis	▪ By destruction of entire cell	▪ By budding off from cell membrane
Examples	▪ Sweat glands	▪ Sebaceous gland	▪ Ceruminous gland, Moll's glands ▪ Mammary gland, Sweat glands
Diseases	▪ Hyperhydrosis ▪ Hypohydrosis ▪ Anhidrosis ▪ Miliaria ▪ Bromhidrosis	▪ Adenoma sebaceum ▪ Acne, Comedone ▪ Sebaceous cysts ▪ Milia	▪ Hidradenitis suppurativa ▪ Fox Fordyce disease ▪ Bromhidrosis – malodorous sweating ▪ Chromhidrosis - colored sweat

- **Ectopic Sebaceous Glands:**
  - Fordyce spot → Lips > Oral mucosa > Genitals
  - Montgomery tubercle → Breast
  - Tyson's glands → Glans
  - Meibomian gland → Eyes
  - Zeis gland → margin of eyelid

- Hidradenitis suppurativa is a disorder of → Apocrine Sweat glands.
- Hordeolum/stye → inflammation of zeis or Meibomian gland.
  - **F**ox-Fordyce is a disorder of **A**pocrine Sweat gland
  - **M**iliaria is a disorder of **E**ccrine Sweat gland

  [Mn: FAME]

ACNE VS ROSACEA

	Acne Vulgaris	Acne Rosacea
Pathology	▪ Blockage and/or inflammation of pilosebaceous units (hair follicles and their accompanying sebaceous gland). ▪ Follicular epidermal hyperproliferation with subsequent plugging of the follicle ▪ Excess sebum production ▪ Commensal bacteria Cutibacterium acnes (formerly P. acnes)	▪ Neurovascular disorder ▪ Flushing may be precipitated by hot drinks, heat, emotion, and other causes of rapid body temperature changes.
Age	▪ Usually adolescent but any age group	▪ Common in 30-50 years
Site	▪ Face (MC), back and chest.	▪ Central face – cheeks, nose, chin, forehead
Etiology	▪ Genetic, Steroids, CAH, PCOS	
Manifestations	▪ Open or closed comedones ▪ Inflammatory papules, pustules, and nodules.	▪ Facial flushing, erythema, telangiectasia ▪ Inflammatory papulopustular eruption resembling acne
Complications	▪ Acne conglobata	▪ Rhinophyma
Treatment	▪ 1st line therapy – topical retinoid + antimicrobial ▪ Isotretinoin – severe, recalcitrant acne vulgaris	▪ Broad spectrum sunscreen ▪ Nonablative laser

NAIL CHANGES

Condition	Description	Seen in
Pterygium	Overgrowth of proximal nail fold	Lichen Planus
20 nail dystrophy		Lichen Planus (MCC); Psoriasis
Thinning of nail plate		Lichen Planus
Pitting	Punctate depression in the nail plate	**Fine** → Alopecia areata, Atopic dermatitis **Coarse** → Psoriasis, Lichen Planus
Oil drop		Psoriasis
Onycholysis	Lifting up of nail plate	Psoriasis, Tinea
Splinter hemorrhage	Linear brown-black or red streaks	Trauma, Infective endocarditis, Psoriasis
Mee's line	Transverse white line on nail	Arsenic poisoning
Koenen periungual fibroma	Growth emerging from nail fold	Tuberous sclerosis
Terry's nail /Leukonychia	White nail	Hepatic diseases
Yellow nail syndrome		Rheumatoid arthritis Pulmonary diseases
Beau's lines	Transverse groove in the nail plate	Stressful event
Koilonychia	Spooning of nails	Iron deficiency anemia Plummer Vinson syndrome
Half and half nails/ Lindsay's nail	Leukonychia in proximal half Brownish color distal half	Renal disease
Muehrcke's lines	Double transverse white lines	Hypoalbuminemia

CHARACTERISTIC FINDINGS

- *Pityriasis rosea:*
  - Pathognomonic/Primary lesion → Herald/mother patch
  - Herald patch → Erythematous annular lesion with peripheral collarette of scales
  - Christmas tree pattern → secondary lesion
- *Lichen Planus:*
  - Wickham's striae [Mn: LPW]
  - Degeneration of stratum basale l/t formation of Civette /Colloid /Cytoid bodies.
  - Max Joseph spaces.
  - Lacy white lesion on oral mucosa
- *Psoriasis:*
  - **A**uspitz sign → pin point bleeding on scratching - d/t suprapapillary thinning
  - **B**ulkeley's membrane → Moist, red skin after removing scales
  - **C**andle grease sign → coherence of the scales can be seen as if one scratches a wax candle
  - Silvery scales
- *Pustular Psoriasis:*
  - Micro Munro's abscess in S. corneum
  - Spongiform pustule of Kogoj
  - Chain of lakes of pus → Generalized Pustular psoriasis.

- *Eczema herpeticum/Kaposi varicelliform lesion:*
  - Caused by Herpes simplex.
  - Seen in Atopic dermatitis (MC) & Darier disease
- *Pityriasis Rubra Pilaris:*
  - Palmoplanter keratoderma
  - Orange pink plaque
  - Follicular papule
- *Atopic Dermatitis:*
  - Dennie Morgan fold
  - Lichenification – thickening of skin with increased markings
- Pityriasis lichenoides → Mika like, adherent scales
- Exclamation mark hair → Alopecia areata.
- Moth eaten alopecia (Patchy hair loss) → 2° syphilis.
- Depigmented macule with white forelock → Piebaldism.
- Pinch purpura is diagnostic of → Systemic primary amyloidosis.
- Granular layer (stratum granulosum) is absent in → Ichthyosis vulgaris.
- Collodion baby & Harlequin fetus are seen in→ Lamellar Ichthyosis.
- Yellow colored honeycomb crusting is a feature of → Non bullous Impetigo/ Impetigo contagiosa.

MANAGEMENT

- DOC for Pustular psoriasis → Acitretin
- DOC for pustular psoriasis in pregnancy → Steroids.
- DOC for dermatitis herpetiformis → Dapsone.
- Spaghetti & meat ball appearance on KOH → Pityriasis versicolor.
- Apple green florescent on wood's lamp → Pityriasis versicolor.

- Patch test is done for → Allergic CD, ABCD.
- DOC for ABCD → Azathioprine.
- IgA deposits on skin biopsy → HSP
- *Excimer laser* is used in:
  - Vitiligo
  - Psoriasis

MULTIPLE CHOICE QUESTIONS

CHAPTER 1: BASICS IN DERMATOLOGY

STRUCTURE AND FUNCTIONS OF SKIN

1. All are true about skin except: *(PGMEE 2019)*
   a. Both dermis & ectoderm are derived from ectoderm
   b. Skin accounts for total of 15% of body weight
   c. Most of the cells in skin are keratinocytes derived from ectoderm
   d. Dermis is made up of type 1 and type 3 collagen in 3:2 ratio

   [Ref: IADVL Textbook of Dermatology 4th/e pg 7, 8, 26]

2. Desmosomes are helpful in connecting – *(PGMEE 2012)*
   a. Melanocytes
   b. Keratinocytes
   c. Langerhans cells
   d. Dermis and epidermis

   [Ref: IADVL Textbook of Dermatology 4th edition vol 1 pg36]

3. Haascheiben cells in epidermis are responsible: *(PGMEE 2015)*
   a. Temperature   b. Proprioception
   c. Pressure   d. Touch

   [Ref: Behl 10th/e p. 18.19; Essential of elements of embryology 16th/e p.83]

4. Extra layer of skin present in the epidermis of palms and soles is: *(PGMEE 2015-16)*
   a. Stratum Spinosum   b. Stratum Lucidum
   c. Stratum Coreum   d. Stratum Granulosum

   [Ref: Multiple References]

5. Melanocytes are present in – *(PGMEE 2014)*
   a. Stratum corneum   b. Dermis
   c. Stratum basale   d. Stratum granulosum

   [Ref: IADVL Textbook of Dermatology 4th edition vol 1 pg37]

6. Dead layer of epidermis – *(PGMEE 2013)*
   a. Stratum corneum
   b. Stratum basale
   c. Stratum granulosum
   d. Straum spinosum

   [Ref: IADVL Textbook of Dermatology 4th edition vol 1 pg33]

7. Malpighian layer is constituted by:- *(PGMEE 2018)*
   a. Corneum spinosum
   b. Stratum basale
   c. Stratum basale and spinosum
   d. Corneum lucidum

   [Ref: (IADVL's Concise Textbook of Dermatology 1s ed. pg.5)]

Explanation
- Malpighian layer of skin is constituted by stratum basale and stratum spinosum.
- Stratum Basale is the layer where the skin's most important cells, the keratinocytes, are formed

8. Odland bodies are seen in which layer of epidermis: *(PGMEE 2015)*
   a. Basal cell layer
   b. Stratum corneum
   c. Prickle cell layer
   d. Stratum granulosum

   [Ref: IADVL Textbook of Dermatology 4th edition vol 1 pg33]

9. Spongiosis involves *(PGMEE 2013)*
   a. Stratum granulosum
   b. Stratum carneum
   c. Stratum spinosum
   d. Stratum basal

   [Ref: IADVL Textbook of Dermatology 4th edition vol. 1 pg177]

10. Superficial partial thickness burn is caused due to involvement of: *(NEET Pattern 2017)*
   a. Epidermis
   b. Papillary dermis
   c. Reticular dermis
   d. Dermis

   [Ref: Rook's Textbook of Dermatology 9th edition page 126.2]

Explanation
- First-degree burns
  ○ Involves only the epidermis
  ○ Never blisters
  ○ Appears as a 'sun burn'
  ○ Is not included in the % total body surface area calculation
- Second-degree burns (dermal burns)
  ○ Superficial:
    – Involves epidermis & superficial dermis
    – Pink, homogeneous, normal capillary refill, painful, moist, intact hair follicles
  ○ Deep:
    – Epidermis & most of the dermis is destroyed, including deep follicular structures
    – Mottled or white, delayed or absent capillary refill, dry, decreased sensation or insensate, non-intact hair follicles
- Third-degree burns
  ○ Full thickness epidermal & dermal destruction
  ○ Dry, white or charred, leathery, insensate

11. Acanthosis involves- *(PGMEE 2012)*
   a. Stratum granulosum
   b. Stratum corneum
   c. Stratum Basale
   d. Stratum spinosum

   [Ref: IADVL Textbook of Dermatology 4th edition vol1 pg173]

1.	a
2.	b
3.	d
4.	b
5.	c
6.	a
7.	c
8.	d
9.	c
10.	b
11.	d

12. True about Keratinocyte is- *(PGMEE 2015)*
a. Ectoderm derived cell
b. Mature in basal layer
c. Present only in basal layer
d. Differentiate in basal layer

[Ref: IADVL Textbook of Dermatology 4th edition vol 1 pg27]

Explanation

- Keratinocytes are derived from ectoderm. They are formed in the stratum basale. As they rise up through different layers, it undergo maturation & get filled with keratin.

13. Which of these layers has abundance of desmosomes? *(NEET Pattern 2017)*

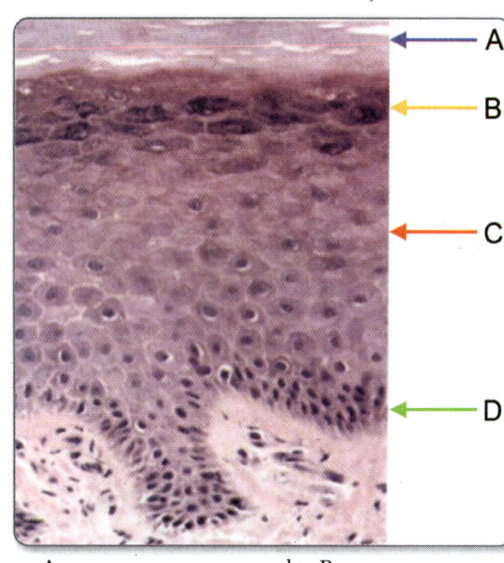

a. A
b. B
c. C
d. D

Ref: (Fitzpatrick's Dermatology in General Medicine 8th edition page 61)

Explanation

(A) *The stratum corneum:-* It the outermost skin layer. It is composed of 20 to 25 layers of cornified cells, called corneocytes, which are the largest cells in the epidermis. They are flattened and have lost their nuclei and cytoplasmic organelles.

(B) *Stratum granulosum:-* This layer, also called the granular layer due to the presence of intracellular basophilic keratohyaline granules, is 2 to 5 cells thick

(C) *The stratum spinosum,* also called the prickle cell layer, contains 8 to 10 layers of cells. The cells in the upper spinous layer are larger, more flattened and contain organelles called "lamellar granules". They are named spinous for the spine-like appearance of the cell margins in histologic sections. The "spines" of spinous cells corresponds to the abundant desmosomes, which provide a mechanical coupling between epidermal cells.

(D) *The stratum basale,* also called stratum germinativum, is a continuous layer that is generally described as only one cell thick. It is the primary site for mitotically active cells.

Answers (sidebar):
12. a
13. c
14. a
15. c
16. c
17. d
18. a
19. d

MORPHOLOGY OF SKIN LESIONS

14. Not a hemorrhagic lesion: *(PGMEE 2015)*
a. Plaque
b. Echymosis
c. Petechiae
d. None of the above

[Ref: IADVL Textbook of Dermatology 4th edition vol 1 pg. 117]

15. Which among is not a primary skin lesion–
a. Plaque *(PGMEE 2012)*
b. Abscess
c. Scales
d. Macule

[Ref: IADVL Textbook of Dermatology 4th edition vol 1 pg. 109]

16. A flat discolouration on skin as 1 cm is called– *(PGMEE 2012)*

a. Boil b. Plaque
c. Macule d. Papule

[Ref: IADVL Textbook of Dermatology 4th edition vol 1 pg. 109]

17. Linear lesion is seen in – *(PGMEE 2014)*
a. Psoriasis b. Lichen planus
c. Pemphigus d. Sporotrichosis

18. Parakeratosis is defined as: *(June 2011)*
a. Retained nuclei in stratum corneal cells
b. Elongation of rete ridge
c. Increased number of cells in Stratum spinsom
d. Increased thickness of corneal layer

(Ref: IADVL Textbook of dermatology 3rd edition pg 92)

Explanation

Parakeratosis	Retention of nuclei by the cells of the stratum corneum.
Hyperkeratosis	Thickening of the stratum corneum of epidermis
Hypergranulosis	Thickening of the granular layer of epidermis
Hypogranulosis	This is the thinning of the granular layer of epidermis
Acanthosis	Thickening of the spinous layer of epidermis
Spongiosis	Intercellular edema in the stratum spinosum seen as stretching of intercellular bridges
Acantholysis	Separation of keratinocytes due to dissolution of the intercellular bridges (desmosomes) between them.

PHENOMENA IN DERMATOLOGY

19. Koebner's phenomenon is characteristic of–
a. Pityriasis rosea *(PGMEE 2014)*
b. Pemphigus vulgaris
c. Polygonal papule
d. Psoriasis

[Ref: IADVL Textbook of Dermatology 4th edition vol 1 pg. 131]

20. In which of the following, Koebner phenomenon is NOT seen: *(PGMEE 2015)*
   a. Erythema multiforme
   b. Lichen sclerosis
   c. Lichen simplex chronicus
   d. Lichen planus
   [Ref: IADVL Textbook of Dermatology 4th edition vol 1 pg. 131]

21. Pseudoisomorphic phenomenon is seen in– *(PGMEE 2015)*
   a. Lichen planus
   b. Plane warts
   c. Vitiligo
   d. Psoriasis
   [Ref: IADVL Textbook of Dermatology 4th edition vol 1 pg131]

22. Kobner phenomenon, as a shown in the following picture, is not a feature of? *(PGMEE 2015)*
   a. Tinea corporis
   b. Viral warts
   c. Psoriasis
   d. Lichen planus
   [Ref: IADVL Textbook of Dermatology 4th edition vol 1 pg131]

23. Picture showing skin lesion, which disappears after biopsy, what is the phenomenon called as: *(PGMEE 2016-17)*

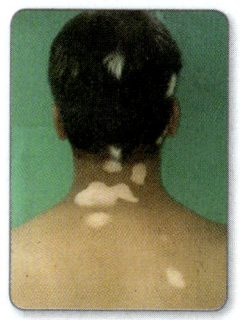

   a. Kobner phenomena
   b. Remote reverse Kobner phenomena
   c. Bulla spread phenomena
   d. Auspitz sign
   [Ref: IADVL Textbook of Dermatology 4th edition vol 1 pg128]

Explanation

Koebner's Isomorphic Phenomena

- Traumatized area often develops lesions especially over elbow, knee.
- Koebner's phenomena is characteristic of → psoriasis.
- Koebner's phenomena is NOT seen in→ Lichen simplex chronicus.

Variant	Seen in
True isomorphic phenomena	▪ **Psoriasis** ▪ **Lichen planus** ▪ **Vitiligo**
Pseudo (false) isomorphic phenomena	▪ Molluscum contagiosum, warts. ▪ Behçet syndrome ▪ Pyoderma gangrenosum
Reverse Koebner's phenomena	▪ Granuloma annulare, psoriasis

Variant	Seen in
Remote reverse Koebner's phenomena:	▪ Spontaneous repigmentation (**satellite repigmentation**) of distant patches after grafting at one site. ▪ Seen in:- ○ Vitiligo ○ Granuloma annulare
Occasional/Rare in	▪ Lichen nitidus ▪ Lichen sclerosus atrophicus ▪ Vitiligo ▪ Kaposi sarcoma ▪ Pityriasis rubra pilaris ▪ Necrobiosis lipoidica ▪ Darrier and Hailey hailey disease.

CLINICAL INVESTIGATIONS

TZANCK SMEAR

24. Tzank smear is done for all except – *(PGMEE 2014)*
   a. Herpes
   b. Psoriasis
   c. Pemphigus
   d. Varicella
   [Ref: IADVL Textbook of Dermatology 4th edition vol 1 pg 135]

25. Tzank cell is – *(PGMEE 2012)*
   a. Neutrophil
   b. Lymphocyte
   c. Fibrobalst
   d. Keratinocytes
   [Ref: IADVL Textbook of Dermatology 4th edition vol 1 pg 950]

26. In Pemphigus vulgaris, tzank smear shows – *(PGMEE 2012)*
   a. Acantholytic cells
   b. Neurtrophils
   c. Fibroblasts
   d. Macrophages
   [Ref: IADVL Textbook of Dermatology 4th edition vol 1 pg 135]

27. Tzank smear in varicella-zoster shows– *(PGMEE 2013)*
   a. Necrotic cell
   b. Multinucleated Giant cell
   c. Acantholysis
   d. Spongiosis
   [Ref: IADVL Textbook of Dermatology 4th edition vol 1 pg 135]

28. Tzank smear is positive in: *(PGMEE 2012)*
   a. Psoriasis
   b. LP
   c. Warts
   d. Herpes simplex
   [Ref: IADVL Textbook of Dermatology 4th edition vol 1 pg 135]

29. Twelve year old boy with vesicle over lip. Investigation to be done is – *(PGMEE 2014)*
   a. KOH mount
   b. Tzank smear
   c. Diascopy
   d. Woods lamp
   [Ref: IADVL Textbook of Dermatology 4th edition vol 1 pg 575]

Explanation

- Likely diagnosis is Herpes labialis

20.	**c**
21.	**b**
22.	**a**
23.	**b**
24.	**b**
25.	**d**
26.	**a**
27.	**b**
28.	**d**
29.	**b**

CHAPTER-1 ⌂ BASICS IN DERMATOLOGY

WOOD'S LAMP

30. Woods lamp is made up of – *(PGMEE 2014)*
   a. 9% nickel oxide with 6% BuSO4
   b. 9% nickel oxide with 9% BuSO4
   c. 6% nickel oxide with 6% BuSO4
   d. 9% nickel oxide with barium silicate

   [Ref: IADVL Textbook of Dermatology 4th edition vol 1 pg128]

31. Woods lamp has a wavelength of: *(PGMEE 2013)*
   a. 250 nm   b. 300 nm
   c. 320 nm   d. 360 nm

   [Ref: IADVL Textbook of Dermatology 4th edition vol 1 pg128]

32. Color of tuberous sclerosis lesions on wood lamp examination – *(PGMEE 2015)*
   a. Golden yellow   b. Milky white
   c. Blue white   d. Bright green

   [Ref: IADVL Textbook of Dermatology 4th edition vol 1 pg133]

33. Tinea versicolor shows which color under wood lamp examination? *(PGMEE 2013-14)*
   a. Yellow green   b. Red
   c. Pink   d. Blue

   [Ref: Nelson 20th/e /p 3106]

PATCH TEST

34. Patch test is done to document- *(DNB pattern 2008)*
   a. Type I hypersensitivity
   b. Delayed type hypersensitivity
   c. Autoimmune disease
   d. Immune complex deposition

   [Ref: IADVL Textbook of Dermatology 4th edition vol 1 pg.858; Rook's textbook of dermatology 8th edition pg 26.84]

Explanation

- Allergic contact dermatitis results when an allergen comes into contact with previously sensitized skin. It is due to delayed type hypersensitivity. The diagnosis of allergic contact dermatitis is made by **patch testing.**
- Indications for patch testing
  o Eczematous disorders where contact allergy is suspected or is to be excluded
  o Eczematous disorders failing to respond to treatment as expected
  o Chronic hand and foot eczema
  o Persistent or intermittent eczema of the face, eyelids, ears and perineum
  o Varicose eczema

30.	d
31.	d
32.	c
33.	a
34.	b

1. **Spongiosis is seen in-** *(PGMEE 2014)*
   a. Lichen planus
   b. Pemphigus
   c. Psoriasis
   d. Acute eczema

   [Ref: IADVL Textbook of Dermatology 4th Edition Vol 1 Pg752]

2. **Characteristic of chronic eczema-** *(PGMEE 2013)*
   a. Lichenification
   b. Induration
   c. Edema
   d. Erythema

   [Ref: IADVL Textbook of Dermatology 4th Edition Vol 1 Pg752]

3. **Lichenification occurs in which layer of skin-** *(PGMEE 2015)*
   a. Stratum lucidum
   b. Stratum corneum
   c. Stratum granulosum
   d. Stratum malpighi

   [Ref: IADVL Textbook of Dermatology 4th Edition Vol 1 Pg752]

ATOPIC DERMATITIS

4. **Identify the condition. This is child with asthmatic mother.** *(PGMEE 2019)*

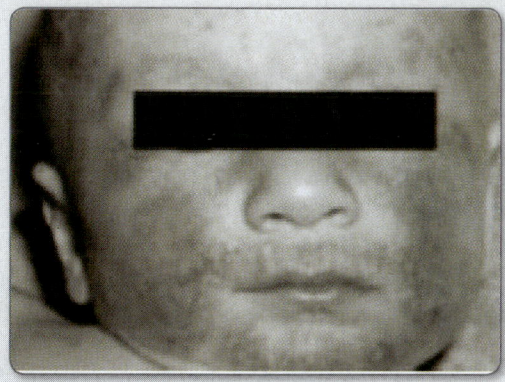

   a. Atopic dermatitis
   b. SLE
   c. Erythema infectiosum
   d. TEN

   [Ref: IADVL Textbook of Dermatology 4th/e pg 529-530]

5. **A 5 year old child presents with itchy excoriated papules and elevated Ig E levels. Most probable diagnosis is?** *(PGMEE Dec 2009)*
   a. Scabies
   b. Seborrhic dermatitis
   c. Atopic dermatitis
   d. Urticaria

   [Ref. Fitzpatrick's dermatology in general medicine 7th edition pg149-150]

Explanation

- Atopic dermatitis is a chronically relapsing skin disease that occurs most commonly during early infancy and childhood.
- Skin lesions are characterized by intensely pruritic, erythematous papules associated with excoriation.
- Serum IgE levels are elevated in 70-80 % patients

6. **A 7-year-old girl presents with lesions over flexors of arm. Similar lesions were also noted over neck and back. She has a family history of asthma. Most likely diagnosis is:** *(PGMEE 2018)*
   a. Allergic contact dermatitis
   b. Atopic dermatitis
   c. Asteototic eczema
   d. Seborrheic dermatitis

   [Ref: Rook's Textbook of Dermatology 9th edition page 41.1]

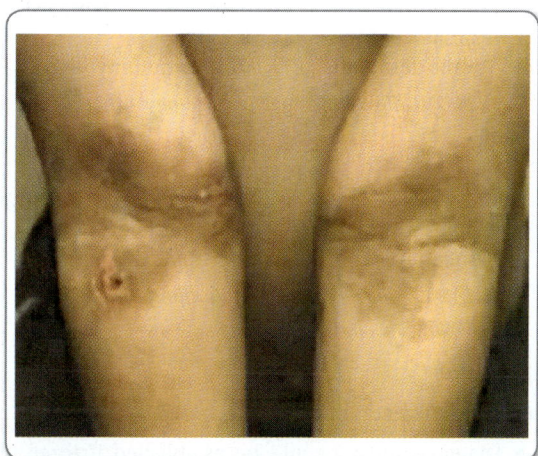

Explanation

- The rash is characterized by erythema, itchy papules/papulovesicles which may become excoriated and lichenified, and typically has a flexural distribution.
- The eruption is frequently associated with other atopic conditions in the individual or other family members.
- Classic sites of involvement in childhood AD are the flexors; antecubital and popliteal fossae, wrists, eyelids, face, and around the neck. Pruritus is a constant feature.

7. **Most common site for atopic dermatitis-** *(PGMEE 2015)*
   a. Scalp
   b. Knees
   c. Trunk
   d. Popliteal fossa

   [Ref: IADVL Textbook of Dermatology 4th Edition Vol 1 Pg 804]

1.	d
2.	a
3.	d
4.	a
5.	c
6.	b
7.	d

8. Commonest site of atopic dermatitis is:

(DNB pattern 2007)

a. Scalp
b. Elbow
c. Anti-cubital fossa
d. Trunk

[Ref. Rook's textbook of dermatology 8th edition pg 24.19; IADVL Textbook of Dermatology 4th Edition Vol 1 Pg804]

Explanation

- Atopic dermatitis- The distribution of the eruption varies with age:

Infantile phase (Birth to 2 years)	▪ Face & extensor aspects of extremities
Childhood phase (From 18 to 24 months onwards)	▪ Flexural involvement - antecubital fossae, popliteal fossae, wrists, ankles, sides of neck
Adult phase (starts from puberty)	▪ Lichenification, especially of the flexures and dorsal aspect of hands & feet.

9. Dennie-Morgan fold is seen in- *(PGMEE 2013)*

a. Psoriasis vulgaris
b. SLE
c. Atopic dermatitis
d. Dermotomyositis

[Ref: IADVL Textbook of Dermatology 4th Edition Vol 1 Pg806]

10. Hanifin & Rajke is the diagnostic criteria for-

(PGMEE 2013)

a. Contact dermatitis
b. Erythroderma
c. Urticaria
d. Atopic dermatitis

[Ref: IADVL Textbook of Dermatology 4th Edition Vol 1 Pg806]

8.	c
9.	c
10.	d
11.	a
12.	c
13.	a
14.	c
15.	c
16.	d
17.	c

Explanation

Hanifin & Rajka's diagnostic criteria of AD

- Diagnosis of AD could be established if three of the major and three of the minor criteria are present
- Major or basic features:
  ○ Pruritus - Hallmark
  ○ Typical morphology and distribution → flexural lichenification or linearity in adults and facial and extensor involvement in infants and children.
  ○ Chronic or chronically relapsing dermatitis.
  ○ Personal or family history of atopy (asthma, allergic rhinitis, or atopic dermatitis).
- Important minor or less characteristic features:
  ○ Xerosis/Dry skin
  ○ Ichthyosis, palmar hyperlinearity, keratosis pilaris.
  ○ Dennie–Morgan infraorbital folds (bilateral symmetrical folds formed by two additional creases beneath the eyelids).
  ○ Immediate (type 1) skin test reactivity.
  ○ Elevated serum IgE.
  ○ Early age of onset.
  ○ White dermographism/delayed blanch (development of a delayed white line on firm stroking of the skin, instead of the usual red line seen normally).
  ○ Pityriasis alba

11. True about atopic dermatitis are all except –

(PGMEE 2012)

a. Mica like scales
b. Scratching
c. Xerosis
d. Pruritus

[Ref: IADVL Textbook of Dermatology 4th Edition Vol 1 Pg806]

12. Identify the pathology depicted in the image?

(PGMEE 2015)

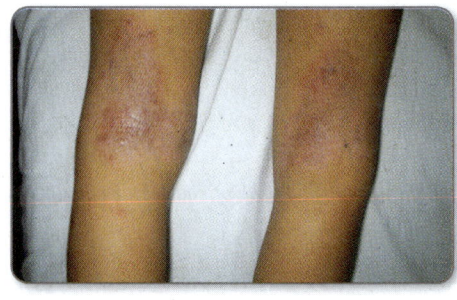

a. Contact dermatitis
b. Cutaneous
c. Atopic dermatitis
d. Hemangioma

[Ref: IADVL Textbook of Dermatology 4th Edition Vol 1 Pg.806]

13. Perioral pallor and Dennie's Morgan folds are seen in:

a. Atopic dermatitis *(DNB pattern 2008)*
b. Chronic actinic dermatitis
c. Blood dyscrasia
d. Perioral contact dermatitis

[Ref: IADVL Textbook of Dermatology 4th Edition Vol 1 Pg806; Fitzpatrick's dermatology in general medicine 7th edition pg 147)

14. A 5 year old child presents with itchy excoriated papules and elevated Ig E levels. Most probable diagnosis is?

(DNB Pattern Dec 2009)

a. Scabies
b. Urticaria
c. Atopic dermatitis
d. Seborrhic dermatitis

[Ref: IADVL Textbook of Dermatology 4th Edition Vol 1 Pg. 806]

OTHER ECZEMAS

15. Which of the following organism has a role to play in Seborrhic dermatitis- *(PGMEE 2015)*

a. Propionibacterium
b. Canida albicans
c. Malassezia
d. None

[Ref: IADVL Textbook of Dermatology 4th Edition Vol 1 Pg759]

16. Seborrhoeic dermatitis is frequently seen in-

(PGMEE 2014)

a. Lipid storage disorders
b. Psoriasis vulgaris
c. Hypertension
d. Parkinson's disease

[Ref: IADVL Textbook of Dermatology 4th Edition Vol 1 Pg760]

17. Coin shaped eczema is- *(PGMEE 2014)*

a. Endogenous eczema
b. Atopic acema
c. Nummular eczema
d. Infantile eczema

[Ref: IADVL Textbook of Dermatology 4th Edition Vol 1 Pg769]

18. Pompholyx affects – *(PGMEE 2015)*
   a. Groin
   b. Trunk
   c. Scalp
   d. Palm & soles

[Ref: IADVL Textbook of Dermatology 4th Edition Vol 1 Pg 775]

Explanation

- Pompholyx (Dyshidrotic eczema) is characterized by a pruritic vesicular eruption on the fingers, palms & soles.
- Vesicles resemble sago grain in appearance.

19. Sago grain like vesicular eruption is seen in – *(PGMEE 2015)*
   a. Atopic dermatitis   b. Seborrhoeic dermatitis
   c. Syphilis   d. Pompholyx

[Ref: IADVL Textbook of Dermatology 4th Edition Vol 1 Pg 775]

CONTACT DERMATITIS

20. Most common cause of irritant dermatitis in India: *(PGMEE 2016-17)*
   a. Detergent   b. Nickel
   c. Gold   d. Water

[Ref: IADVL Textbook of Dermatology 4th Edition Vol 1 Pg 773]

21. Most common precipitant of contact dermatitis is- *(PGMEE 2013)*
   a. Silver   b. Nickle
   c. Iron   d. Gold

[Ref: IADVL Textbook of Dermatology 4th Edition Vol 1 Pg 832]

22. Most common cause of plant induced contact dermatitis in India: *(DNB Pattern 2008; PGMEE 2015-16)*
   a. Poison ivy
   b. Parthenium
   c. Ragweed
   d. Detergents

[Ref: IADVL Textbook of Dermatology 4th Edition Vol 1 Pg 839]

23. Which of the following cause allergic contact dermatitis through air? *(DNB pattern June 2010)*
   a. House dust mite
   b. Detergents
   c. Parthenium
   d. Nickel

[Ref: IADVL Textbook of Dermatology 4th Edition Vol 1 Pg 840]

Explanation

- Most common cause of air borne contact dermatitis in India: parthenium
- Most common cause of contact dermatitis due to metal: nickel

18. d
19. d
20. a
21. b
22. b
23. c

PSORIASIS

1. First topical retinoid approved by US FDA for psoriasis: *(PGMEE 2016-17)*
   a. Isotretinoin
   b. Tazarotene
   c. Acitretin
   d. Calcipotrine

   [Ref: IADVL Textbook of Dermatology 4th edition vol 1 pg 1051]

2. Most common site affected by psoriasis is: *(Dec 2009)*
   a. Flexor surface
   b. Extensor surface
   c. Palms and soles
   d. Oral mucosa

   [Ref. IADVL Textbook of dermatology 3rd edition pg.1032]

Explanation

- In Psoriasis the extensor surfaces of the body (particularly the elbows and knees), lumbosacral area and back, scalp are commonly involved.
- Inverse psoriasis/flexural psoriasis- psoriasis affecting the flexures like axillae, groins and inframammary folds.
- The face is rarely involved in psoriasis
- Oral mucosa involvement is uncommon in psoriasis. Geographic tonque (benign migratory glossitis or glossitis areata migrans) is oral variant of psoriasis resulting in focal loss of filliform papillae.
- Nail changes seen in 20-50 % cases.
- Joint involvement (Psoriatic arthritis) is seen in 10-20% cases.

3. A lady came with red itchy and scaly plaques over bilateral submammary folds in winter season. Photograph is shown below. On treatment with steroid the lesion is now started on peripheries. What will be your diagnosis: *(Recent Pattern June 2018)*

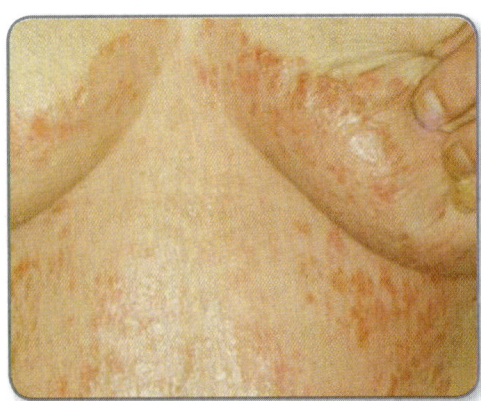

   a. Erythrodermic psoriasis
   b. Psoriasis vulgaris
   c. Inverse psoriasis
   d. Lichen planus

   [Ref:IADVL Textbook of dermatology 3rd edition pg1032]

1.	b
2.	b
3.	c
4.	c

Explanation

Psoriasis

- Inverse psoriasis is also k/as flexural psoriasis as it affects flexures → axillae, groins and inframammary folds. Flexural plaques are thin and scaling is greatly reduced or absent.
- *Chronic plaque psoriasis (psoriasis vulgaris)* is the commonest type of psoriasis, being seen in 90% of patients. It is characterized by symmetrical, erythematous, well-defined, scaly plaques. The scales are abundant, loose, dry and silvery white or micaceous.
- *Guttate Psoriasis:* Small plaque lesions with scales 2-3mm to 1 cm distributed over the trunk and proximal limbs in **children.**
- *Erythrodermic psoriasis*: Psoriasis in which most or all of the body surface is affected (>90%BSA)

4. Auspitz sign is seen in: *(PGMEE 2015)*
   a. Icthyosis
   b. Lichen planus
   c. Plaque psoriasis
   d. Pustular psoriasis

   [Ref: IADVL Textbook of Dermatology 4th edition vol 1 pg 1027]

Explanation

- Chronic plaque psoriasis (psoriasis vulgaris) is the commonest type of psoriasis, being seen in 90% of patients.
- Characterized by symmetrical, erythematous, well-defined, scaly plaques. The scales are abundant, loose, dry and silvery white or micaceous.
- Whiteness is due to the presence of air trapped in between the layers of scales.
- Scratching the psoriatic lesion with a glass slide show:
  ○ Initially accentuation of scales (grattage test)
  ○ When the scales are completely scraped off, the stratum mucosum (basement membrane) is exposed and is seen as a moist red surface (membrane of Bulkeley) through which dilated capillaries at the tip of elongated dermal papillae are seen as red spots.
  ○ On further scraping, these capillaries are torn, leading to multiple bleeding points. This is a characteristic feature of psoriasis and is known as Auspitz sign.
- Auspitz sign is attributed to parakeratosis, suprapapillary thinning of the stratum malphighii, elongation of dermal papillae and dilatation and tortuosity of the papillary capillaries.
- It is not seen in inverse psoriasis; pustular psoriasis, erythrodermic psoriasis; guttate psoriasis.
- Not specific because it is also seen in nonpsoriatic scaling disorders, including Darier's disease and actinic keratosis.

5. Tiny bleeding spots seen after removal of deep scales in plaque psoriasis are known as: *(PGMEE 2015-16)*
a. Koebner's Sign
b. Burkley's Sign
c. Candle Wax Sign
d. Auspitz Sign

[Ref: Harrison 19th/e pg. 347]

6. 45 year old male presents with scaly lesions over back. Most likely diagnosis is : *(PGMEE 2016-17)*

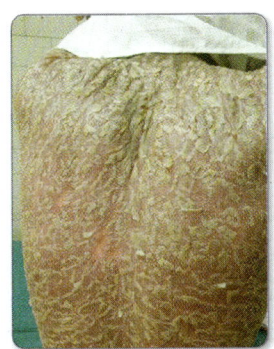

a. Lichen planus
b. Pustular psoriasis
c. Erythrodermic psoriasis
d. Psoriasis vulgaris

[Ref: IADVL Textbook of Dermatology 4th edition vol 1 pg 1027]

7. Identify the condition shown in image: *(Recent Pattern June 2018)*

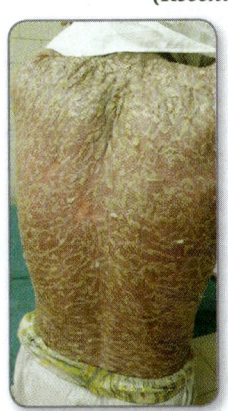

a. Nummular eczema
b. Bowen's disease
c. Lichen planus
d. Psoriasis

Explanation

- Psoriatic plaques are characterized by erythema, infiltration, and desquamation.
- Plaques are raised and easily palpable, irregular to oval in shape, well-defined, with sharply demarcated boundaries. a dry, thin, silvery-white or micaceous scaling is seen as shown in the image.

D/d of psoriatic plaques

- *Nummular eczema*: rounded, circular desquamative erythematous lesions covered with vesicles, crusts, and scales, very itchy). allergy tests are frequently positive.
- *Mycosis fungoides* is a cutaneous T-cell lymphoma erythematous patches little infiltrated and finely desquamating. Response to treatment is worst.

- *Pityriasis rubra pilaris*: follicular papules and infiltrating scales + hyperkeratosis.
- *Duhring's disease (dermatitis herpetiformis)*, its bilateral symmetric papules and vesicles on extensor surfaces. the erythematous skin. In eruptive phase with crusts full of serum and blood and lichenification due to scratching. In the chronic phase, this disease is constantly very itchy.
- *Bowen's disease* SqCC of the skin, finely desquamating mainly single patches. Showing no improvement to phototherapy and local therapy

8. True regarding munro micro abscess is all except: *(June 2009)*

a. Seen in stratum corneum
b. Debris consists of eosinophils
c. Associated pustule may be present
d. Seen in psoriasis

(Ref. IADVL Textbook of dermatology 3rd edition pg 1041)

Explanation

- Munro's microabscesses
  - A collection of neutrophils, mainly pyknotic, within the stratum corneum is classically seen in psoriasis.
- Spongiform pustule of Kogoj
  - A collection of neutrophils in stratum malpighii/ stratum spinosum.
  - Neutrophils migrate from the 'squirting papillae' to the spongiform pustules and then to the horny layer forming Munro's microabscesses.

9. In which of the following phototherapy is useful in treatment- *(PGMEE 2015)*
a. Psoriasis
b. Tinea corporis
c. PMLE
d. Pemphigus

[Ref: IADVL Textbook of Dermatology 4th edition vol 1 pg 1053]

10. This type of psoriasis is commonly seen in children and may follow a streptococcal sore throat – *(PGMEE 2014)*
a. Pustular
b. Stable plaque
c. Arthropathic
d. Guttate

[Ref: IADVL Textbook of Dermatology 4th edition vol 1 pg 1028]

11. Grattage test is used for – *(PGMEE 2014)*
a. Pemphigus vulgaris
b. Lichen planus
c. Psoriasis
d. Tinea capitis

[Ref: IADVL Textbook of Dermatology 4th edition vol 1 pg 1027]

12. Goekarman regimen used in for treatment of psoriasis is- *(PGMEE 2015)*
a. Coal tar plus anthralin
b. UVB plus coal tar
c. UVB plus anthralin
d. UVB plus methotrexate

[Ref: IADVL Textbook of Dermatology 4th edition vol 1 pg 1051]

13. Among various types of psoriatic arthritis, which variety is most common- *(PGMEE 2015)*
a. Classic
b. Spondylitis
c. Rheumatoid
d. Oligoarticular

[Ref: IADVL Textbook of Dermatology 4th edition vol 1 pg 1037]

5.	d
6.	c
7.	d
8.	b
9.	a
10.	d
11.	c
12.	b
13.	d

14. The treatment of choice for erythrodermic psoriasis is –
a. Topical corticosteroids **(PGMEE 2014)**
b. Corticosteroids
c. Coaltar topically
d. Methotrexate

[Ref: IADVL Textbook of Dermatology 4th edition vol 1 pg 1057]

15. A primigravida female presented with erythematous skin changes and lesions with multiple pus lakes. Which of the following should be the most appropriate – **(PGMEE 2010)**
a. Psorolen + PUVA b. PUVA
c. Acitretin d. Corticosteroids

[Ref: IADVL Textbook of Dermatology 4th edition vol 1 pg 1071]

Explanation
- Aciterin is contraindicated in pregnancy

16. Psoriasis is exacerbated by: **(PGMEE 2015)**
a. Antimalarials b. Lithium
c. β-blockers d. All of the above

[Ref: IADVL Textbook of Dermatology 4th edition vol 1 pg 1025]

17. The most common association with coarse pitting of nails and onycholysis is – **(PGMEE 14)**
a. Cicatricial alopecia
b. Well defined scaly plaques
c. Polygonal papule
d. Violaceous papules

[Ref: IADVL Textbook of Dermatology 4th edition vol 1 pg 1034]

18. The important feature of psoriasis is – **(PGMEE 2014)**
a. Erythema b. Crusting
c. Oozing d. Scaling

LICHEN PLANUS AND LICHENOID DERMATOSES

19. Pt developed scarring alopecia, thinning of nail, violaceous papular lesions over flexor aspect of forearms and wrist. The probable cause:- **(PGMEE 2016-17)**
a. Lichen planus b. Secondary syphillis
c. Psoriasis d. Lupus erythematosus

[Ref: IADVL Textbook of Dermatology 4th Edition Vol 1 Pg1093]

20. A male is presenting with a violaceous papule which is pruritic. There is pterygium of nail with cicatracial alopecia. Diagnosis is – **(PGMEE 2014)**
a. Lichen planus b. Pityriasis rosea
c. Seborrheic dermatitis d. Psoriasis

[Ref: IADVL Textbook of Dermatology 4th edition vol 1 pg 1093]

21. Characteristic bodies in Lichen planus:
a. Civatte bodies **(PGMEE 2016-17)**
b. HP bodies
c. Warthin Fiekendly Bodies
d. Negri bodies

[Ref: IADVL Textbook of Dermatology 4th edition vol 1 pg 1101]

22. In lichen planus all the following sites are affected except- **(PGMEE 2015)**
a. Nails
b. Extensor aspect of upper extrimities
c. Flexor aspect of upper extrimities
d. Oral mucosa

[Ref: IADVL Textbook of Dermatology 4th edition vol 1 pg 1093]

23. Which 'P' is not a feature of lichen planus- **(PGMEE 2015)**
a. Plane b. Polyhedral
c. Pruritus d. Polygonal

[Ref: IADVL Textbook of Dermatology 4th edition vol 1 pg 1090]

24. Itchy polygonal violaceous palpules seen in: **(PGMEE 2012)**
a. Lichen planus b. Pemphigus
c. Pitriasios rosea d. Psoriasis

[Ref: IADVL Textbook of Dermatology 4th edition vol 1 pg 1090]

25. Itchy purple colored papule followed by hyperpigmentation on resolution, is seen in – **(PGMEE 2014)**
a. Hypothyroidism b. DM
c. Addison's disease d. Lichen planus

[Ref: IADVL Textbook of Dermatology 4th edition vol 1 pg 1093]

26. Not a histological feature of lichen planus is – **(PGMEE 2014)**
a. Neutrophils in stratum b. Hyperkeratosis
c. Pigment incontinence d. Acanthosis

[Ref: IADVL Textbook of Dermatology 4th edition vol 1 pg 1101]

27. The most characteristic finding in lichen planus is– **(PGMEE 2013)**
a. Violaceous lesions b. Civatte bodies
c. Thinning of nail plate d. Basal cell degeneration

[Ref: Rook's Textbook of Dermatology 9th edition pg 37.14]

28. Flat topped violaceous papule, thinning of nail. Microscopic finding would be? **(PGMEE 14)**
a. Acantholysis
b. Epidermal bulla
c. Prominent necrotic cells
d. Basal cell degeneration

[Ref: IADVL Textbook of Dermatology 4th edition vol 1 pg 1101]

29. Wickham's striae seen in – **(PGMEE 2015)**
a. Lichen niditus b. Lichenoid eruption
c. Lihen striates d. Lichen planus

[Ref: IADVL Textbook of Dermatology 4th edition vol 1 pg 1093]

30. Characterstic nail finding in lichen planus –
a. Hyperpigmentation of nail **(PGMEE 2012)**
b. Pitting
c. Beau's Lines
d. Pterygium

[Ref: IADVL Textbook of Dermatology 4th edition vol 1 pg 1098]

14.	d
15.	d
16.	d
17.	b
18.	d
19.	a
20.	a
21.	a
22.	b
23.	b
24.	a
25.	d
26.	a
27.	d
28.	d
29.	d
30.	d

31. **Nail showing pterygium is seen in –**
   (PGMEE 2015)

   a. Alopecia areata   b. Lichen amyloidosis
   c. Psoriasis   d. Lichen planus

   [Ref: IADVL Textbook of Dermatology 4th edition vol 1 pg 1098]

32. **A young lady present with white lacy linear lesions in oral cavity and her proximal nail fold has extended onto the nail bed. What is the likely diagnosis –**
   (PGMEE 2012)

   a. Psoriasis   b. Lichen planus
   c. Geographic tongue   d. Candidiasis

   [Ref: IADVL Textbook of Dermatology 4th edition vol 1 pg 1098]

33. **Cicatrising alopecia with perifollicular blue-gray patches is most commonly associated with –**
   (PGMEE 2011)

   a. Pitting of nails
   b. Discoid plaques in the face
   c. Arthrtis
   d. Whitish lesions in the buccal mucosa

   [Ref: IADVL Textbook of Dermatology 4th edition vol 1 pg 1099]

34. **Treatment of choice for lichen planus–** **(PGMEE 2013)**
   a. Antihistaminics   b. Systemic corticosteroids
   c. Acitretin   d. Topical corticosteroids

   [Ref: IADVL Textbook of Dermatology 4th edition vol 1 pg 1103]

35. **A young boy presented to OPD with multiple shiny pinhead size white papules over dorsum of head, forearm and penis. What would be the diagnosis?**
   (PGMEE 14)

   a. Lichen planus   b. Lichen nitidus
   c. Scabies   d. MC

   [Ref: IADVL Textbook of Dermatology 4th edition vol 1 pg 1107]

PITYRIASIS ROSEA

36. **Hanging curtain sign and Christmas tree pattern along the ribs are seen in-** **(PGMEE 2016-17)**
   a. Pityriasis rosea
   b. Pityriasis versicular
   c. Pityriasis lichennoides chronica
   d. Pytiriasis rubra pilaris

   [Ref: Andrew's Diseases of the Skin 12th edition pg 199]

Explanation

Pityriasis rosea (PR)

- Pityriasis rosea (PR) is an acute self-limiting, papulosquamous disorder, characterized by a primary eruption (salmon or pink colored, scaly rash), the herald patch followed by a secondary eruption after 7–14 days.
- Mainly involving children and young adults (15–35 yr). Peak incidence is in spring and winter with lower incidence in the summer.
- Etiology is probably **viral**. A/w flu like prodrome (URTI).

- The disease most frequently begins with a single herald or mother patch usually larger than succeeding lesions. The characteristic rash consists of discrete, oval or round, erythematous, scaly plaques.
- The scales are fine, dry and form a collarette attached at the periphery and free edge pointing to the centre of the lesion. Lesion when stretched across the long axis, the scales tend to fold across the lines of stretch, the so-called "hanging curtain" sign.
- The histopathological features: eczematoid pattern (Unna's sign), absence or decrease of granular cell layer (Lowenbach's sign), extravasation of RBCs primarily into the papillary dermis and also partly into the epidermis (Sabouraud's sign), and homogenization of the papillary collagen.
- Eruption form a Christmas tree or fir tree pattern, the long axis of the lesions following the tension lines, running parallel to the ribs on the trunk.
- The distribution pattern is distinctive, involving the trunk and the proximal extremities. In children, the face may be involved.
- Usually itching is remarkably minimal or even absent. After 3–8 weeks they usually disappear spontaneously.

37. **Multiple erythematous annular lesions with peripheral collarette of scales arranged predominantly on trunk are seen in –** **(PGMEE 2012)**
   a. Pityriasis vesicular
   b. Pytiriasis rubra pilaris
   c. Pityriasis rosea
   d. Pityriasis lichennoides chronica

   [Ref: Andrew's Diseases of the Skin 12th edition pg 199]

38. **Christmas tree appearance in skin is seen in–**
   (PGMEE 2015)

   a. Pityriasisubrapilaris   b. Vitiligo
   c. Psoriasis   d. Pityriasis rosea

   [Ref: IADVL Textbook of Dermatology 4th edition vol 1 pg 645]

39. **Annular herald patch is seen in –** **(PGMEE 2013)**
   a. Psoriasis   b. Nocardiasis
   c. P.alba   d. P.rosea

   [Ref: Andrew's Diseases of the Skin 12th edition pg 199]

40. **Hanging curtain sign is seen in:–**
   (PGMEE 2015-16, DNB June 2010)

   a. Hordeolum externum
   b. Pityriasis rosea
   c. Measles
   d. Psoriasis

   [Ref: Andrew's Diseases of the skin 12th edition Pg 199]

MISCELLANEOUS

41. **Keratodermic sandal is a feature of–** **(PGMEE 2013)**
   a. Psoriasis
   b. Lichen planus
   c. Pityriasis rubra pilaris
   d. Pityriasis rosacea

   [Ref: IADVL Textbook of Dermatology 4th edition vol 1 pg 421]

31.	d
32.	b
33.	d
34.	d
35.	b
36.	a
37.	c
38.	d
39.	d
40.	b
41.	c

PEMPHIGUS

1. Epidermal bullae are seen in: *(PGMEE Dec 2009)*
a. Bullous pemphigoid
b. Pemphigus vulgaris
c. Pemphigoid gestationalis
d. Hailey hailey disease

[Ref: IADVL Textbook of dermatology 3rd edition pg 1088]

Explanation

Intraepidermal bullous disorders	Subepidermal (dermo-epidermal junction) bullous disorders
▪ Pemphigus vulgaris & its variant pemphigus vegetans ▪ Pemphigus foliaceus & its variants ○ Pemphigus erythematosus/Senear Usher Syndrome ○ Endemic pemphigus ▪ Paraneoplastic pemphigus ▪ IgA pemphigus ▪ Drug induced pemphigus	▪ Bullous pemphigoid ▪ Mucous membrane pemphigoid/ cicatricial pemphigoid. ▪ Linear IgA bullous dermatosis/ chronic bullous disease of childhood (CBDC) ▪ Pemphigoid gestationalis ▪ Dermatitis herpetiformis ▪ Epidermolysis bullosa acquisita

2. A middle aged female has flaccid bullae in the skin and oral erosion. Histopathology shows intraepidermal acantholytic blisters. The most likely diagnosis is–
a. Bullous pemphigoid *(PGMEE 2014)*
b. Paraneoplastic pemphigus
c. Dermatitis hepatiformis
d. Pemphigus vulgaris

[Ref: IADVL Textbook of Dermatology 4th edition vol 1 pg 941]

3. 25 year old female has palatal ulcer and skin blister most likely diagnosis is– *(PGMEE 2014)*
a. Pemphigus foliaceous
b. Pemphigoid
c. Dermatitis herpetiformis
d. Pemphigus vulgaris

[Ref: IADVL Textbook of Dermatology 4th edition vol 1 pg 941]

4. "ROW of tomb stones" appearance is a feature of-
a. Irritant dermatitis *(PGMEE 2015)*
b. Herpes
c. Pemphigoid
d. Pemphigus

[Ref: IADVL Textbook of Dermatology 4th edition vol 1 pg 951]

5. Characteristic feature of pemphigus vulgaris-
a. Sub epidermal bullae *(PGMEE 2015)*
b. Acantholysis
c. Negative Nikolsky's sign
d. Bullae on erythematous base

[Ref: IADVL Textbook of Dermatology 4th edition vol 1 pg 941]

6. Which of the following drug can lead to pemphigus-
(PGMEE 2015)
a. Isoniazid
b. Furosemide
c. Carbamazepine
d. Penicillamine

[Ref: IADVL Textbook of Dermatology 4th edition vol 1 pg 949]

7. Most common pemphigus is: *(PGMEE 2014)*
a. Pemphigus erythematosus
b. Pemphigus vegetans
c. Pemphigus vulgaris
d. Pemphigus foliaceus

[Ref: IADVL Textbook of Dermatology 4th edition vol 1 pg 936]

8. Antigen defect in pemphigus vulgaris: *(PGMEE 2015)*
a. Desmoglein – 1
b. Desmoglein – 3
c. Desmocollin – 3
d. Desmocollin – 2

[Ref: IADVL Textbook of Dermatology 4th edition vol 1 pg 937]

9. Mucocutaneous Pemphigus Vulgaris is characterized by antibodies against: *(PGMEE 2015-16)*
a. Desmoglein 1
b. Desmoglein 3
c. Desmoglein 1 and 3
d. None

[Ref: Refer Explanatory text]

10. Acantholysis is characteristic of: *(PGMEE 2014)*
a. Dermatitis herpetiformis
b. Pemphigus vulgaris
c. Erythema multoforme
d. Pemphigoid

[Ref: IADVL Textbook of Dermatology 4th edition vol 1 pg 935]

11. Loss of Intercellular cohesion between keratinocytes is called as: *(PGMEE 2012)*
a. Acanthosis
b. Acantholysis
c. Keratinolysis
d. Spongiosis

[Ref: IADVL Textbook of Dermatology 4th edition vol 1 pg 938]

1.	b
2.	d
3.	d
4.	d
5.	b
6.	d
7.	c
8.	b
9.	c
10.	b
11.	b

12. Intraepidermal blisters are seen in all of the following conditions except – *(PGMEE 2012)*
a. Pemphigoid
b. Paraneoplastic pemphigus
c. Pemphigus foliaceous
d. Pemphigus vulgaris

[Ref: IADVL Textbook of Dermatology 4th edition vol 1 pg 935]

13. Flaccid bullae with mucosal involvement and intraepidermal acantholysis are characteristic of – *(PGMEE 2015)*
a. Psoriasis b. Pemphigus foliaceous
c. Vitiligo d. Pemphygus vulgaris

[Ref: IADVL Textbook of Dermatology 4th edition vol 1 pg 941]

14. Acantholysis is seen in all except *(PGMEE 2013)*
a. Bullous pemphigoid
b. Pemphigus vulgaris
c. SSSS
d. Darrier's disease

[Ref: IADVL Textbook of Dermatology 4th edition vol 1 pg 935]

15. Nikolsky sign is seen in – *(PGMEE 2015)*
a. Staphylococci infection
b. Salmonella infection
c. Meningococci infection
d. Gram negative bacteremia

[Ref: IADVL Textbook of Dermatology 4th edition vol 1 pg 950]

16. Nikolsky's sign is positive in – *(PGMEE 2015)*
a. Pemphigus
b. Rubella
c. Pemphigoid
d. Dermatitis herpatiformis

[Ref: IADVL Textbook of Dermatology 4th edition vol 1 pg 950]

17. Intraepidermal IgG deposition is seen in: *(PGMEE 2008)*
a. Pemphigus b. Bullous pemphigoid
c. Herpes genitalis d. None of the above

[Ref. Rook's textbook of dermatology 8th edition pg 40.4]

Explanation

- *Intraepidermal IgG deposition is seen in*
  ○ Pemphigus vulgaris & its variant pemphigus vegetans Pemphigus foliaceus & its variants
    - Pemphigus erythematosus/ Senear Usher Syndrome
    - Endemic pemphigus
  ○ Paraneoplastic pemphigus
  ○ Drug induced pemphigus

18. Tzank test is positive in each of the following conditions, except: *(PGMEE 2007)*
a. Pemphigus foliacious and pemphigus vegetans
b. Pemphigus vulgaris
c. Senear Usher syndrome
d. Bullous pemphigoid

[Ref. Rook's textbook of dermatology 8th edition pg 40.3]

Explanation

- Tzanck test is positive i.e acantholytic cells are seen in pemphigus. It is negative in all subepidermal disorders.

BULLOUS PEMPHIGOID

19. Which of the following is a sub-epidermal blistering disorder? *(PGMEE June 2009)*
a. Pemphigus vulgaris
b. Bullous pemphigoid
c. Pemphigus foliaceous
d. Darier's disease

[Ref: IADVL Textbook of dermatology 3rd edition pg 1088]

Explanation

- *Subepidermal (dermo-epidermal junction) bullous disorders*
  ○ Bullous pemphigoid
  ○ Mucous membrane pemphigoid/cicatricial pemphigoid.
  ○ Linear IgA bullous dermatosis
  ○ Pemphigoid gestationis
  ○ Dermatitis herpetiformis
  ○ Epidermolysis bullosa acquisita

20. The level of blister formation in bullous pemphigoid is- *(PGMEE 2015)*
a. Subcorneal b. Sub epidermal
c. Intra epidermal d. None of the above

[Ref: IADVL Textbook of Dermatology 4th edition vol 1 pg 935]

21. Pruritus is a feature of which of the following- *(PGMEE 2015)*
a. Pemphigus foliaceous b. Bullous Pemphigoid
c. Pityrosporum ovale d. None

[Ref: IADVL Textbook of Dermatology 4th edition vol 1 pg 963]

22. Tense sub-epidermal bullae are seen in: *(PGMEE 2016-17)*
a. Burns b. Pemphigus vulgaris
c. Bullous pemphigoid d. Herpes

[Ref: IADVL Textbook of Dermatology 4th edition vol 1 pg 963]

23. Disease of dermoepidermal junction is – *(PGMEE 2014)*
a. SSSS
b. Pemphigus vulgaris
c. Bullous pemphigoid
d. Atopic dermatitis

[Ref: IADVL Textbook of Dermatology 4th edition vol 1 pg 935]

24. A person presents with hemorrhagic fluid in tense blister at dermoepidermal junction. Most probable diagnosis is? *(PGMEE Dec 2009)*
a. Pemphigoid
b. Pemhigus vulgaris
c. Pemphigus vegetans
d. Drug induced pemphigus

[Ref: IADVL Textbook of dermatology 3rd edition pg 1080]

12.	a
13.	d
14.	a
15.	a
16.	a
17.	a
18.	d
19.	b
20.	b
21.	b
22.	c
23.	c
24.	a

DERMATITIS HERPETIFORMIS

25. A 30 year old male had severely itchy papulovesicular lesions on extermities knee, elbows and butocks for one year. Direct immunofluorescence staining of the lesions showed IgA deposition at dermoepidermal junction. The most probable diagnosis is: *(PGMEE 2012)*

a. Dermatitis herpetiforms
b. Pemphigus vulgaris
c. Nummular eczema
d. Bullous pemphigoid

[Ref: IADVL Textbook of Dermatology 4th edition vol 1 pg 982]

26. All are true about dermatitis herpetiformis except: *(PGMEE Dec 2010)*

a. The lesions are intensely itchy
b. Lesions have epidermal bullae
c. IgA in papillary tips
d. Associated with gluten enteropathy

[Ref: Fitzpatrick's dermatology in general medicine 7th edition pg 504]

Explanation

- Direct immunofluorescence, demonstrates granular IgA deposition at the tips of the dermal papilla, has now become the gold standard for a diagnosis of DH.

27. One of the following is the treatment of choice for dermatitis herpetiformis – *(PGMEE 2014)*

a. Dapsone   b. Retinoids
c. Mtx   d. Corticosteroids

[Ref: IADVL Textbook of Dermatology 4th edition vol 1 pg 985]

28. Dapsone is used in the treatment and therapeutic diagnosis of: *(PGMEE Dec 2010)*

a. Leprosy
b. Dermatitis herpetiformis
c. Acne vulgaris
d. Lupus vulgaris

[Ref. Fitzpatrick's dermatology in general medicine 7th edition pg 504]

Explanation

- Dapsone is so consistently effective that the therapeutic response to it was once considered to be a major diagnostic criterion. It has an effect on neutrophil chemotaxis and attachment to IgA in vitro.

EPIDERMOLYSIS BULLOSA

29. In congenital dystrophic variety of epidermolysis bullosa, mutation is seen in the gene conding for– *(PGMEE 2015)*

a. Laminin 4
b. Collagen type 7
c. Alpha 6 integerin
d. Keratin 14

[Ref: IADVL Textbook of Dermatology 4th edition vol 1 pg 1006]

25.	a
26.	b
27.	a
28.	b
29.	b

DISORDERS OF HYPOPIGMENTATION

1. A child presents with white lesion (depigmented macule) of 2 × 2 cm with irregular margin over forehead and glabella. There is white forelock over forehead since birth. Diagnosis is: *(PGMEE 2016-17)*

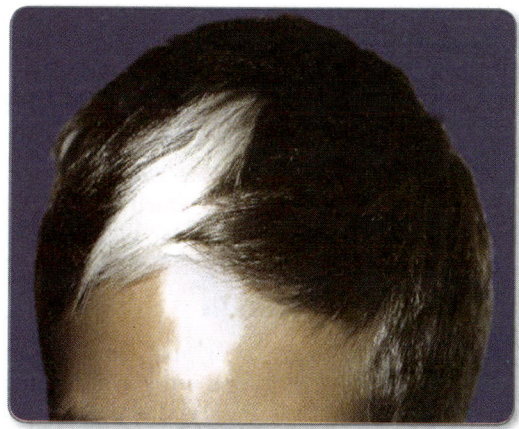

a. Piebaldism　　　　b. Dermatitis
c. Vitiligo　　　　　　d. Nevus of Ito

[Ref: Andrew's Diseases of the Skin 12th edition pg 873]

2. Piebaldism is – *(PGMEE 2014)*
a. Associated with white forelock
b. Erythema nodosum leprosum
c. Androgenetic alopecia
d. None of the above

[Ref: Andrew's Diseases of the Skin 12th edition pg 873]

3. Which of the following is untrue regarding piebaldism- *(PGMEE 2012)*
a. Amelanotic skin associated with a white forelock
b. Islands of normal or hypermelanotic skin
c. Usually improves with age
d. Autosomal dominant condition

[Ref: Andrew's Diseases of the Skin 12th edition pg 873]

4. Which of the following is/are the differential diagnosis of congenital disorders of pigmentation– *(PGMEE 2015)*
a. Piebaldism
b. Tuberous sclerosis
c. Vitiligo
d. All the above

[Ref: IADVL Textbook of Dermatology 4th edition vol2 pg 1296]

5. Causes of localized hypopigmented macule or patch are all except- *(PGMEE 2015)*
a. Pityriasis alba
b. Piebaldism
c. Freckle
d. Vitiligo

[Ref: IADVL Textbook of Dermatology 4th edition vol2 pg 1296]

Explanation

Piabaldism

- AD disorder of skin
- There is absence of melanocytes in affected areas due to dysfunction of Neural Crest --- Thus No melanocytes and No melanin
- Localised white patch and White forelock. Islands of normal skin within white patch may be seen
- **Treatment:** Phototherapy ± PUVA ± Grafting

Freckle

- AD disorder of people with fair skin and red hairs
- Melanocytes are normal but produce more melanosomes resulting in hyperpigmentation
- Rx: Photoprotection + Topical depigmenting agents like Hydroquinone or Azelaic acid

6. Identify the pathology depicted in the image? *(PGMEE 2015)*

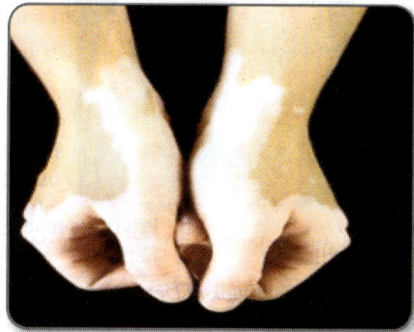

a. Vitiligo　　　　　　b. Fungal infection
c. Albinism　　　　　　d. Contact leukoderma

7. Identify the condition in the image: *(PGMEE 2019)*

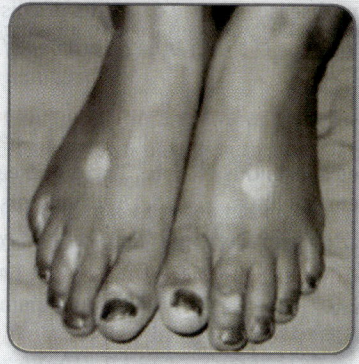

a. Leukoderma　　　　b. Piebaldism
c. Vitiligo　　　　　　d. DLE

[Ref: IADVL Textbook of Dermatology 4th/e pg 594]

VITILIGO

8. Commonest type of vitiligo– *(PGMEE 2014)*
a. Segmental　　　　　b. Facial
c. Acrofacial　　　　　d. Vulgaris

[Ref: Andrew's Diseases of the Skin 12th edition pg 865]

1.	a
2.	a
3.	c
4.	d
5.	c
6.	d
7.	a
8.	d

URTICARIA AND ANGIOEDEMA

9. A child scratches his hand with a pen. A red wheal appears which persists for 30 minutes. What would be the diagnosis? *(PGMEE 14)*

a. Contact urticaria   b. Dermographism

c. Pressure urticaria   d. Atopy

[Ref: IADVL Textbook of Dermatology 4th edition vol2 pg 1214]

10. Identify the phenomena depicted in the image in a patient with urticaria in the image? *(PGMEE 2015)*

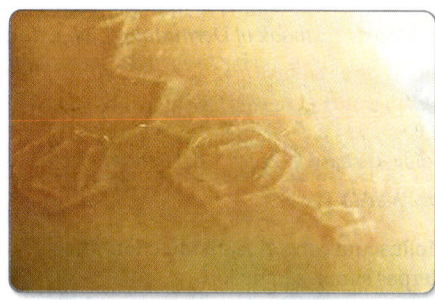

a. Koebner phenomenon

b. Christmas tree appearance

c. Heliotrope sign

d. Dermographism

[Ref: IADVL Textbook of Dermatology 4th edition vol2 pg 1214]

11. A child developed multiple lesions over face, neck and trunk as shown in picture after eating strawberry. These lesions are best described as: *(PGMEE 2016-17)*

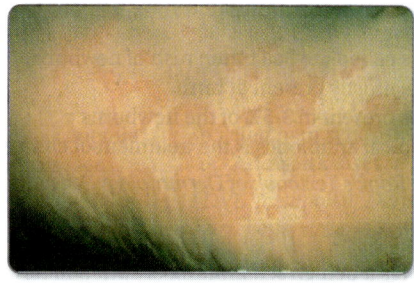

a. Papule   b. Petichae

c. Wheal   d. Purpura

[Ref: Andrew's Diseases of the Skin 12th edition pg 146]

12. Urticarial lesions are best described as- *(PGMEE 2014)*

a. Nonpruritic   b. Bullous

c. Macular   d. Evanescent

[Ref: Andrew's Diseases of the Skin 12th edition pg 146]

13. All of the following are true about solar uriticaria EXCEPT: *(DNB Pattern June 2011)*

a. Common in females between age group 20-40 yrs.

b. Some cases may develop serve urticarial/broncho-spasm

c. Lesions subsides spontaneously on avoiding exposure within 24 hours.

d. All cases are idiopathic

[Ref: IADVL Textbook of Dermatology 4th edition vol2 pg 1216; Rook's textbook of dermatology 8th edition pg 29.19]

Explanation

Solar Urticaria

- Solar urticaria (SU) may be primary (idiopathic) or secondary to porphyrias, phototoxic drugs and chemicals. Idiopathic SU is an uncommon whealing disorder induced by UVB, UVA and visible wavelengths.
- It occurs at any age, but has a peak onset between 20 and 40 years. Occurs more commonly in women. Multiple erythematous wheals appear 5–10 minutes after exposure to sunlight, though sometimes the onset of lesions is delayed by several hours.
- Individual lesions usually disappear within a day, lasting for just a few minutes, or hours, and rarely last for longer than 24 hours even if further exposure to the causative light is avoided.
- If the skin reaction is severe and extensive it may be associated with nausea, bronchospasm, light-headedness and syncope

PURPURA & CUTANEOUS VASCULITIS

14. Palpable purpura is caused by – *(DNB Pattern December 2011)*

a. Microscopic polyangitis   b. PAN

c. HSP   d. All of the above

[Ref: IADVL Textbook of Dermatology 4th edition vol2 pg 1191]

15. Schamberg's purpura are seen on *(PGMEE 2013)*

a. Chest   b. Feet

c. Arms   d. Face

[Ref: Andrew's Diseases of the Skin 12th edition pg 828]

16. Palpable purpura are seen in all except: *(DNB pattern 2011)*

a. Giant cell arteritis   b. Polyarteritis nodosa

c. Wegner granulomatosis   d. HSP

[Ref: IADVL Textbook of Dermatology 4th edition vol2 pg 1191; Rook's textbook of dermatology 8th edition pg 50.2]

Explanation

Palpable Purpura

- Palpable purpura is seen in Small vessel vasculitis and medium vessel vasculitis. It is not seen in large vessel vasculitis.

17. Periungual desquamation, which is a characteristic feature of Kawasaki syndrome, occur at- *(PGMEE 2015)*

a. 1st- 2nd week   b. 2nd – 3rd week

c. 3rd – 4th week   d. 4th – 5th week

[Ref: IADVL Textbook of Dermatology 4th edition vol2 pg 1235]

BEHCET SYNDROME

18. Pathergy test is used for – *(PGMEE 2013)*

a. Lichen planus

b. Atopic dermatitis

c. Reither's syndrome

d. Bechet's syndrome

[Ref: IADVL Textbook of Dermatology 4th edition vol2 pg 1269]

9.	b
10.	d
11.	c
12.	d
13.	d
14.	d
15.	b
16.	a
17.	b
18.	d

19. Oculoorogenital ulcers are a feature of– *(PGMEE 2012)*
- a. Psoriasis
- b. Behcet disease
- c. Lichen planus
- d. SLE

[Ref: IADVL Textbook of Dermatology 4th edition vol2 |pg 1269]

20. All are seen in Behchets syndrome except –
- a. Uveitis   *(PGMEE 2013)*
- b. Pyoderma gangrenosum
- c. Oral ulcers
- d. Genital ulcers

[Ref: IADVL Textbook of Dermatology 4th edition vol2 pg 1269]

21. Pathergy test is positive in?   *(DNB Pattern Dec 2009)*
- a. Richter's disease
- b. Behcet's disease
- c. Erythema multiforme
- d. Ritter's disease

[Ref: IADVL Textbook of Dermatology 4th edition vol2 pg 1269; Fitzpatrick's dermatology in general medicine 7th edition pg 1624]

Explanation

Pathargy test

- A positive pathergy test (hyper-reactivity reaction) manifests within 48 hours as an erythematous papule (> 2 mm) or pustule at the site of skin needle prick or after intracutaneous injection of 0.1 ml isotonic salt solution
- Positive pathergy reaction is a sign of Behcet disease. It is not pathognomic, as it can also occur in patients with pyoderma gangrenosum, rheumatoid arthritis, Crohn disease, and genital herpes infection.

DRUG REACTIONS

22. Lichenoid drug eruption is caused by   *(PGMEE 2014)*
- a. Nitrofurantoin
- b. Erythromycin
- c. Rifampicin
- d. Chloroquine

[Ref: IADVL Textbook of Dermatology 4th edition vol 1 pg 1092]

23. Drug not causing exanthematous skin eruption–   *(PGMEE 2015)*
- a. Ampicillin
- b. Hydrocortisone
- c. Phenylbutazone
- d. Phenytoin

[Ref: Andrew's Diseases of the Skin 12th edition pg 112]

24. Fixed drug eruption can be seen more frequently with –
- a. Cetrizine   *(PGMEE 2013)*
- b. Penicillin
- c. Roxithromycin
- d. Sulfonamide

[Ref: Andrew's Diseases of the Skin 12th edition pg 118]

25. Toxic epidermal necrolysis [TEN] involves body surface area: *(PGMEE 2013)*
- a. < 10%
- b. 10-20%
- c. 20-30%
- d. > 30%

[Ref: Fitzpatrick's Dermatology in General Medicine 8th edition pg 442]

Explanation

- TEN involves >30% of BSA.
- SJS involves <10% of BSA.

MISCELLANEOUS

26. A 13 year old child presents multiple lesions around lips and chest with excoriations of lips as shown in photograph. Similar lesions are also present over oral mucosa. Neck nodes are enlarged. What is the diagnosis: *(Recent Pattern June 2018)*

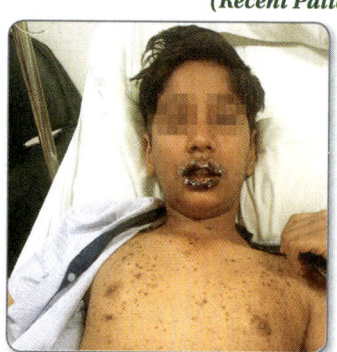

- a. Stevens-Johnson syndrome
- b. Kawasaki syndrome
- c. Impetigo contagiosa
- d. Toxic epidermal necrolysis

[Ref: IADVL Textbook of Dermatology 4th edition vol.2 pg ..1179]

Explanation

Stevens Johnson syndrome

- Also called erythema multiforme major.
- Drugs are the major precipitating factor. A/w sulfonamides, nevirapine, allopurinol, lamotrigine, aromatic anticonvulsants, oxicam NSAIDS, ATT (thioacetazones), lamotrigine etc.
- Mycoplasma pneumoniae infection associated in children and teens
- CF:
  - 1–14 day prodrome of high fever, sore throat, malaise
  - Rapid onset of cutaneous blisters with epidermal detachment beginning with target lesions.
  - Involvement of ≥2 mucosal sites
  - Fever, lymphadenopathy, toxic symptoms
  - Total body surface area of epidermal detachment ≤10% classified as SJS; 10–30% classified as SJS–TEN overlap and >30% as TEN

27. Acute febrile neutrophilic dermatosis is seen in:
- a. Haberman syndrome   *(PGMEE 2014)*
- b. Kasabach merit syndrome
- c. Sweet syndrome
- d. Bechets syndrome

[Ref: IADVL Textbook of Dermatology 4th edition vol2 pg 1253]

Explanation

- Sweet syndrome = Acute febrile neutrophilic dermatosis is characterized by fever & abrupt onset off tender or painful erythematous eruption.

28. Erythema nodosum is seen in all except:
- a. SLE   *(PGMEE 2014)*
- b. Sulfonamide use
- c. TB
- d. Pregnancy

[Ref: Andrew's Diseases of the Skin 12th edition pg 480]

19.	b
20.	b
21.	b
22.	d
23.	b
24.	d
25.	d
26.	a
27.	c
28.	a

CHAPTER-6 ⌒ CUTANEOUS VASCULAR DISORDERS AND ...

HAIR AND SCALP DISORDERS

HAIR CYCLE

1. **Hair growth seen in which phase of the hair cycle-**
   (PGMEE 2015)
   a. Catagen
   b. Anagen
   c. Telogen
   d. None

   [Ref: IADVL Textbook of Dermatology 4th ed. vol2 p1473]

2. **Telogen phase of hair growth lasts for–** *(PGMEE 2015)*
   a. 1 day
   b. 10 days
   c. 100 days
   d. 1000 days

   [Ref: IADVL Textbook of Dermatology 4th ed. vol2 pg1473]

3. **Eyebrows don't grow beyond certain length as they have a short –** *(PGMEE 2013)*
   a. Catagen phase
   b. Telogen phase
   c. Anagen phase
   d. Exogen phase

   [Ref: IADVL Textbook of Dermatology 4th ed. vol2 pg1473]

ALOPECIA

4. **Exclamation mark alopecia is seen in:**
   (PGMEE 2016-17)
   a. Infective alopecia
   b. Androgenetic alopecia
   c. Alopecia areata
   d. Trichotillomania

   [Ref: IADVL Textbook of Dermatology 4th ed. vol2 pg1511]

5. **Which of the following condition cause alopecia without scarring –** *(PGMEE 2014)*
   a. Herpes Zoster
   b. Lichen planus pilaris
   c. Alopecia areata
   d. DLE

   [Ref: IADVL Textbook of Dermatology 4th ed. vol2 pg1480]

6. **Alopecia areata is –** *(PGMEE 2012)*
   a. Fungal infection
   b. Cicatricial alopecia
   c. Non cicatricial alopecia
   d. None

   [Ref: IADVL Textbook of Dermatology 4th ed. vol2 pg1480]

7. **A child presenting with localized patches of complete hair loss with normal appearance of scalp as shown in image. Diagnosis is-** *(PGMEE 2013, 2019)*

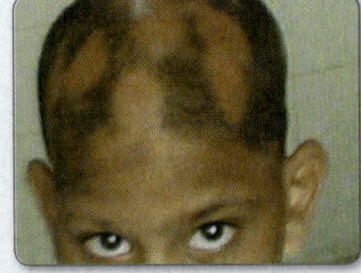

   a. Alopecia areata
   b. Cradle cap
   c. Telogen effluvium
   d. Tinea capitis

   [Ref: IADVL Textbook of Dermatology 4th ed. vol2 pg. 1511]

1.	b
2.	c
3.	c
4.	c
5.	c
6.	c
7.	a
8.	d
9.	c
10.	b
11.	d
12.	c
13.	d

8. **Scarring alopecia is seen in:** *(PGMEE 2007)*
   a. Androgenic
   b. Alopecia areata
   c. Tinea capitis
   d. Traction

   [Ref: Fitzpatrick's dermatology in general medicine 7th ed. pg 770, Rook's textbook of dermatology 8th ed. pg 66.40]

Explanation

- Traction alopecia is caused by inadvertent prolonged traction on the scalp by the physical pressure of hair styling (e.g., pony tail, tight braids, foam rollers, etc.). Although potentially reversible in its early stages, loss of hair follicles leads to permanent hair loss if the traction is unrelenting over months to years
- Causes of non cicatricial alopecia
  ○ Androgenetic alopecia alopecia areata telogen effluvium, anagen effluvium, trichotilomania, moth eaten alopecia (secondary syphilis), tinea capitis

9. **A patient presents with increased sweating, patchy hair loss with velvety skin . It points to the diagnosis of–** *(PGMEE 2015)*
   a. Alopecia aereata
   b. Trichotilomania
   c. Hyperthyroidism
   d. Adenoma sebacicum

   [Ref: IADVL Textbook of Dermatology 4th ed. vol2 pg1514]

10. **Rapid, diffuse, excessive hair loss after 3 months of pregnancy is due to?** *(PGMEE June 2011)*
    a. Androgenic alopecia
    b. Telogen effluvium
    c. Anagen effluvium
    d. Alopecia areata

    [Ref: IADVL Textbook of dermatology 3rd ed. pg 897]

Explanation

- *Postpartum Alopecia:* Hair loss occurs 1–3 months after parturition in most women. This is a loss of telogen hairs that are retained during pregnancy because of the influence of high circulating estrogens that are "withdrawn" after delivery.

DISORDERS OF SEBACEOUS GLANDS

11. **Sebaceous gland activity is mainly controlled by which hormone –** *(PGMEE 2014)*
    a. Estrogen
    b. Cortisol
    c. Progesterone
    d. Androgens

    [Ref: IADVL Textbook of Dermatology 4th ed. vol2 pg1367]

12. **A 18 year old girl presents with predominantly comedonal acne. First line of treatment will be-** *(PGMEE 2015)*
    a. Systemic antibiotics
    b. Topica steroids
    c. Topical retinoids
    d. Systemic retinoids

    [Ref: IADVL Textbook of Dermatology 4th ed. vol2 pg1390]

13. **Which hormone is responsible for acne-** *(PGMEE 2013)*
    a. Gonadotropins
    b. Thyroid
    c. Estrogen
    d. Testosterone

    [Ref: IADVL Textbook of Dermatology 4th ed. vol2 pg1367]

14. All of the following are related to sebaceous glands, except: *(PGMEE 2015-16)*
a. Zeis glands
b. Fordyce spots
c. Meibomian glands
d. Glands of Moll

[Ref: Multiple References]

Explanation

- Diseases of sebceous gland
  - Adenoma sebaceum
  - Acne, Comedone
  - Sebaceous cyst
  - Milia

15. In sebaceous glands accumulation of sebum leads to – *(PGMEE 2013)*

a. Epidermoid cyst　　b. Millia
c. Acne　　d. Milliria

[Ref: IADVL Textbook of Dermatology 4th ed. vol2 pg1369]

16. A young person is having comedones and papulopustular acne over face and trunk and back. How will you manage the patient? *(PGMEE 14 Nov 14; PGMEE 2014)*
a. Topical clindamycin
b. Oral doxycycline + topical acid
c. Oral retinoic acid
d. Topical retinoic acid

[Ref: IADVL Textbook of Dermatology 4th ed. vol2 pg1391]

17. Difference in acne rosacea & acne vulgaris– *(PGMEE 2013)*
a. Erythema
b. Absence of comedone
c. Papule
d. Pustule

[Ref: IADVL Textbook of Dermatology 4th ed. vol2 pg1377]

18. Oral retinoid is indicated in the treatment of: *(PGMEE 2007)*

a. Acne vulgaris　　b. Pemphigus vulgaris
c. Lupus vulgaris　　d. Erythema multiforme

[Ref. Comprehensive dermatologic drug therapy by Wolverton 2nd ed. pg 281]

Explanation

- Three dermatoses have FDA approval for systemic retinoid use in severe subsets:
  - Acitretin for psoriasis
  - Isotretinoin for acne vulgaris
  - Bexarotene for selected cases of mycosis fungoides
- Systemic retinoids:
  - 1st generation- isotretinoin,tretinoin
  - 2nd generation-acitretin, etretinate
  - 3rd generation-bexarotene

19. Acid that is increased in acne comedones is? *(PGMEE June 2011)*
a. Linolenic acid
b. Palmitic acid
c. Acetic acid
d. Linoleic acid

[Ref. International journal of dermatology 2001 issue10 pg 640-3]

Explanation

- In acne comedones the proportion of linoleic acid is markedly decreased, while palmitic acid is significantly increased.

20. SAPHO syndrome components are all except –
a. Osteitis　　*(PGMEE 2015)*
b. Acantholysis
c. Hyperostosis
d. Acne

[Ref: IADVL Textbook of Dermatology 4th ed. vol2 pg1376]

Explanation

- SAPHO is an acronym for **S**ynovitis, **A**cne, **P**ustulosis, **H**yperostosis and **O**steitis.

21. Identify the pathology depicted in the image? *(PGMEE 2015)*

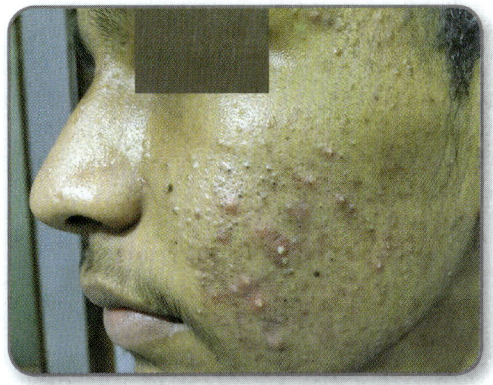

a. Acne rosacea
b. Photosensitivity
c. SLE
d. Acne vulgaris

[Ref: IADVL Textbook of Dermatology 4th ed. vol2 pg1398]

22. Rhinophyma complicates – *(PGMEE 2012)*
a. Acne rosacea
b. Phemphigus
c. Acne vulgais
d. Psoriasis

[Ref: IADVL Textbook of Dermatology 4th ed. vol2 pg1398]

23. Potato nose is seen in – *(PGMEE 2013)*
a. Acne rosacea
b. Rhinosporoidosis
c. Lupus vulgaris
d. Acne vulgaris

[Ref: IADVL Textbook of Dermatology 4th ed. vol2 pg1398]

DISORDERS OF SWEAT GLANDS

24. Disease of sweat gland- *(PGMEE 2013)*
a. Fox-Fordyce's disease
b. Acne vulgaris
c. Fordyce's spot
d. None

[Ref: IADVL Textbook of Dermatology 4th ed. vol2 pg1449]

14.	d
15.	c
16.	b
17.	b
18.	a
19.	b
20.	b
21.	d
22.	a
23.	a
24.	a

25. Fox Fordyce disease is a disorder of?

(PGMEE June 2011)

a. Sebaceous glands   b. Eccrine glands
c. Pilosebaceous units   d. apocrine glands

[Ref. Rook's textbook of dermatology 8th ed. pg 44.21]

Explanation

Fox–Fordyce disease or apocrine miliaria

- Chronic, pruritic papular eruption of the apocrine areas, principally the axillae and the pubis.
- Women > men in a ratio of 10:1.
- not generally seen before puberty onset is usually between 13 and 35 years.
- Itching is a constant feature
- Apocrine glands are seen in the axillae, areolae (Montgomery's tubercles), periumbilical, perineal and circumoral areas, prepuce, mons pubis, and labia minora.
- Fox–Fordyce spots – ectopic sebaceous glands on vermilion border of lip

26. Bromhidrosis affects which glands   *(PGMEE 2015-16)*

a. Eccrine Swept glands
b. Apocrine Sweat Glands
c. Both Apocrine and Eccrine Glands
d. Sebaceous glands

[Ref: Ref.: IADVL Textbook of Dermatology 4th ed. vol2 pg 1451]

27. Hidradenitis suppurativa is a disease of? *(PGMEE 2012)*

a. Eccrine glands   b. Apocrine glands
c. Holocrine glands   d. None of the above

[Ref: IADVL Textbook of Dermatology 4th ed. vol2 pg1451]

28. Miliaria is a disorder of –   *(PGMEE 2012)*

a. Eccrine glands   b. Apocrine glands
c. Holocrine glands   d. Sebaceous glands

[Ref: IADVL Textbook of Dermatology 4th ed. vol2 pg1436]

DISORDERS OF NAILS

29. "Oil drop sign" in nails is characteristic of:

(PGMEE 2016-17)

a. Lichen planus   b. Psoriasis
c. Tuberus sclerosis   d. Arsenic poisoning

[Ref: IADVL Textbook of Dermatology 4th ed. vol2 pg1603]

30. Characteristic nail changes from a patient of Lichen plannus are shown in the image . Most likely diagnosis is: *(PGMEE 2016-17)*

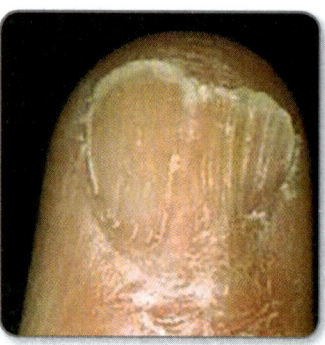

25.	d
26.	c
27.	b
28.	a
29.	b
30.	b
31.	d
32.	a
33.	c
34.	b
35.	c
36.	b
37.	d

a. Pitting of nail   b. Pterygium
c. Onchylosis   d. Mee's line

[Ref: IADVL Textbook of Dermatology 4th ed. vol2 pg1607]

31. Nails are involved in all except   *(PGMEE 2014)*

a. Taenia   b. Lichen planus
c. Psoriasis   d. DLE

[Ref: IADVL Textbook of Dermatology 4th ed. vol2 pg1612]

32. Thimble pitting of nails is seen in–   *(PGMEE 2015)*

a. Psoriasis   b. Pemphigus
c. Lichen planus   d. Alopecia areata

[Ref: IADVL Textbook of Dermatology 4th ed. vol2 pg1603]

33. Nail pitting is caused by all except   *(PGMEE 2015)*

a. Pityriasis Rosacea   b. Lichen planus
c. Fungal infection   d. Hyperthyroidism

[Ref: IADVL Textbook of Dermatology 4th ed. vol2 pg1604, Rook's Textbook of Dermatology 9th ed. pg 32.49]

34. Pitting of nails can be seen in   *(DNB pattern 2007)*

a. Tinea unguium   b. Alopecia areata
c. Androgenic alopecia   d. Peripheral vascular disease

[Ref: IADVL Textbook of dermatology 3rd ed. pg 959]

Explanation

- Pits result from a focal parakeratosis of the abnormally keratinizing cells of the proximal nail matrix.
- Causes of nail pitting:
  ○ Psoriasis (pits are coarse and irregularly placed)
  ○ Alopecia areata (pits are fine and regularly placed)
  ○ Early lichen planus
  ○ Rheumatoid arthritis
  ○ Chronic eczematous dermatitis
  ○ In some individuals with no apparent disease

35. Pterygium of nail is characteristically seen in –

(PGMEE 2012)

a. Alopecia areata   b. Psoriasis
c. Lichen planus   d. Tinea unguium

[Ref: IADVL Textbook of Dermatology 4th ed. vol2 pg1607]

36. Koenen's periungual fibroma is seen in- *(PGMEE 2015)*

a. Psoriasis
b. Tuberous sclerosis
c. Alopecia areata
d. Neurofibromatosis

[Ref: IADVL Textbook of Dermatology 4th ed. vol2 pg 1599]

37. Which of the following are known as gift spots

(DNB pattern 2007)

a. Paronychia
b. Koilonychia
c. Onycholysis
d. Leuconychia

[Ref: IADVL Textbook of dermatology 3rd ed. pg 981]

Explanation

- Punctate leukonychia: White spots of 1–3 mm size occur singly or in groups on one or several nails. They often occur without any apparent cause (fortune or gift spots) or follow minor matrix trauma, as with aggressive manicuring.

NUTRITIONAL AND METABOLIC DISEASES

1. True about Acrodermatitis enteropathica is?
(DNB Pattern June 2011)
a. Lifelong treatment required
b. Autosomal dominant disorder
c. Wound healing is not affected
d. Zinc absoption is normal

[Ref: Fitzpatrick's dermatology in general medicine 8th ed. pg 1523]

Explanation

Acrodermatitis Enteropathica

- Acrodermatitis enteropathica is an autosomal recessive disorder results from specific malabsorption of zinc
- There is defect in an intestinal zinc transporter, the human **ZIP4** protein, which prevents appropriate enteral zinc absorption.
- AE onsets soon after weaning in affected infants or during the fourth to tenth week of life in infants who are not breast-fed.
- The classic features of AE include alopecia, diarrhea, lethargy, and an acute eczematous and erosive dermatitis favoring acral areas-perioral, periocular, anogenital, hands, and feet.
- Delayed wound healing, acute paronychia, conjunctivitis, blepharitis, and photophobia may also be observe
- Patients also appear to be predisposed to systemic infections as a result of impaired cell-mediated immunity, and superinfection with Candida albicans and bacteria, usually Stayhylococcus aureus, is common
- AE require lifelong treatment. In children 0.5 to 1.0 mg/kg of elemental zinc given as one to two daily dose

2. Dose of zinc used in acrodermatitis enteropathica is?
(DNB Pattern June 2009)
a. 0.5mg/kg   b. 3mg/kg
c. 5mg/kg   d. 7mg/kg

[Ref: Andrew's diseases of skin 12th/e pg. 477; Fitzpatrick's dermatology in general medicine 8th ed. pg 1523]

Explanation

- AE require lifelong treatment. In children 0.5 to 1.0 mg/kg of elemental zinc given as one to two daily dose

3. Follicular hyperkeratosis is related to deficiency of?
(DNB Pattern Dec 2010)
a. Vitamin A   b. Vitamin C
c. Vitamin E   d. Zinc

[Ref: IADVL Textbook of Dermatology 4th ed. vol2 pg1818; Rook's textbook of dermatology 8th ed. pg 59.60]

Explanation

- Classical manifestations of vitamin A deficiency include xerophthalmia, follicular hyperkeratosis and generalized xerosis. Follicular papules are seen especially on the dorsal and lateral areas of the extremities, so-called phrynoderma.

- Histologically, there is lamellated hyperkeratosis around the hair follicles and atrophy of the sebaceous glands
- Diagnosis is confirmed by the finding of a low vitamin A level in blood and a positive response to vitamin A supplementation.

4. Vitamin D is synthesized by?
(DNB Pattern December 2011)
a. Keratinocytes   b. Granular cells
c. Melanocytes   d. Prickle cells

[Ref: Fitzpatrick's dermatology in general medicine 8th ed. pg 1507; IADVL Textbook of dermatology 3rd ed. pg 1270]

Explanation

Forms of vitamin D	Chemical name	Comment
7-dehydro cholesterol	Provitamin D3	- Precursor molecule present in epidermis
Cholecalciferol/ calciol	Vitamin D3	- Synthesized in epidermis(keratinocytes) - Obtained from diet (animal sources)
Calcidiol	25-hydroxy vitamin D	- Biologically inactive form - Circulating form of vit D - Storage form of vit D - Used to evaluated vit D status
Calcitriol	1,25-dihydroxy vitaminD	- Active form - Binds to vitD receptors in tissues

GENODERMATOSES

5. Incontinentia pigmenti involves all except:
(PGMEE 2015)
a. Skin   b. Heart
c. Bones   d. Teeth

[Ref: Andrews' Diseases of the Skin 12 th ed. pg 543]

6. Café an lait spots seen in?   *(PGMEE 2012)*
a. Cockayne syndrome
b. Down syndrome
c. Gardner syndrome
d. NF

[Ref: IADVL Textbook of Dermatology 4th ed. vol 1 pg218]

7. Earliest feature of tuberous sclerosis is?
(DNB Pattern June 2009, dec 2011)
a. Facial angiofibroma
b. Gingival fibroma
c. Ash leaf spot
d. Shagreen patch

[Ref: IADVL Textbook of Dermatology 4th ed. vol 1 pg222]

Explanation: *See the table given at the end this chapter*

1.	a
2.	b
3.	a
4.	a
5.	b
6.	d
7.	c

CONNECTIVE TISSUES DISEASES

8. Carpet tack sign seen in –   *(PGMEE 2015)*
   a. DLE
   b. Psoriasis
   c. Syphilis
   d. Lupus vulgaris

   [Ref: Andrews' Diseases of the Skin 12 th ed. pg 153]

9. All of the following are causes of "Lupus" except–
   a. Chlorpromazine   *(PGMEE 2014)*
   b. Hydralazine
   c. Penicillamne
   d. Clofibrate

   [Ref: Andrews' Diseases of the Skin 12 th ed. pg 159]

10. A girl of 19 years with arthritis and photosensitive rash on cheeks, likely diagnosis is –   *(PGMEE 2014)*
   a. Steven's Johnson syndrome
   b. Chlosma
   c. SLE
   d. Lyme's disease

   [Ref: Andrews' Diseases of the Skin 12 th ed. pg 157]

11. A child with history of fever, photosensitivity, rash sparing nasolabial fold presents to OPD. Identify the condition?   *(PGMEE 2019)*
   a. SLE
   b. Polymorphous light eruption
   c. Discoid lupus
   d. Skin tuberculosis

   [Ref: IADVL Textbook of Dermatology 4th/e pg 1225-28]

12. Which of the following not photosensitive
                                              (PGMEE 2012)
   a. Porphyria
   b. Lichen planus
   c. DLE
   d. SLE

   [Ref: IADVL Textbook of Dermatology 4th ed. vol2 pg 1705, 1902]

DERMATOMYOSITIS

13. Shawl sign is seen in–   *(PGMEE 2014)*
   a. Cutaneous scleroderma
   b. Dermatomyositis
   c. SLE
   d. Neonatal lupus

   [Ref: Andrews' Diseases of the Skin 12 th ed. pg 163]

14. All of the following are cutaneous manifestations of Dermatomyositis: *(PGMEE 2015-16)*
   a. Shawl Sign
   b. Mechanic Hands
   c. Gorlin's Sign
   d. Heliotrope Rash

15. Heliotrope rash is seen in?
                          (DNB Pattern June 2010; PGMEE 2013)
   a. Polymyositis
   b. Dermatitis herpetiformis
   c. Inclusion body myositis
   d. Dermatomyositis

   [Ref: Andrews' Diseases of the Skin 12th ed. pg 163;Fitzpatrick's dermatology in general medicine 7th ed. pg 1542]

16. Gorton's sign is seen in?   *(PGMEE June 2011)*
   a. Dermatomysitis
   b. SLE
   c. Scleroderma
   d. MCTD

   [Ref: Fitzpatrick's dermatology in general medicine 7th ed. pg 1542)

17. Localised scleroderma is –   *(PGMEE 2013)*
   a. Heliotrope erythema
   b. Shagreen patch
   c. Gottron's papule
   d. Morphea

   [Ref: Andrews' Diseases of the Skin 12 th ed. pg 166]

DIABETES

18. The following skin condition is associated with:
                                          (NEET Pattern 2017)

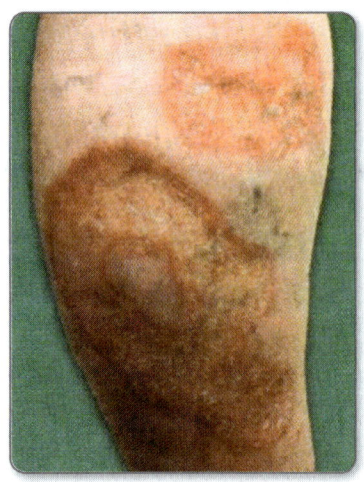

   a. Diabetes
   b. Hypothyroidism
   c. Hyperthyroidism
   d. Sarcoidosis

   [Ref: Andrew's diseases of the Skin 12th ed. pg. 533]

Explanation

- Necrobiosis lipoidica (NL) is characterized by well circumscribed, firm, depressed, waxy, yellow-brown plaques, usually of the anterior shin.
- Non-diabetics with NL should be followed up for the development of diabetes.
- It is also more frequent in type 1 DM (6.5%) than in type 2 (0.4%) or maturity-onset (2.8%) diabetes.
- Control of the diabetes does not influence the course of the NL.

19. Most common site of necrobiosis lipioidica dibeticorrum is?   *(DNB Pattern June 2011)*
   a. Face
   b. Back of leg
   c. Front of leg
   d. Neck

   [Ref: Andrews' Diseases of the Skin 12 th ed. pg 533; IADVL Textbook of dermatology 3rd ed. pg 1370]

Explanation

Necrobiosis lipoidica (NL)

- NL starts as an erythematous, slowly enlarging, irregular plaque that then turns into a yellowish-brown, telangiectatic and depressed plaque

8.	a
9.	d
10.	c
11.	a
12.	b
13.	b
14.	c
15.	d
16.	a
17.	d
18.	a
19.	c

- Classically, NL appears on the pretibial or medial malleolar skin.
- Histologically, the dermis shows degenerated collagen (necrobiosis) with a horizontal palisade of histiocytes, minimal mucin deposition, and interspersed lymphocytes, plasma cells, and giant cells.
- Topical potent corticosteroids or intralesional steroids form the mainstay of treatment.

20. Which of the following regarding the condition depicted in the image? *(PGMEE 2019)*

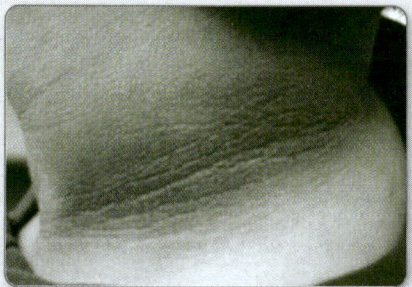

a. May be an indication of skin malignancy
b. Hypopigmentation
c. May be associated with Insulin resistant diabetes mellitus
d. Commonly occurs in lean and thin.

[Ref: IADVL Textbook of Dermatology 4th/e pg 1009-1010]

ACANTHOSIS NIGRICANS

21. A 16 year old obese female with history of PCOD and deranged lipid profile consults a dermatologist for the hyperpigmentation in the neck as shown in the photograph. Identify the condition shown in the image: *(Recent Pattern June 2018)*

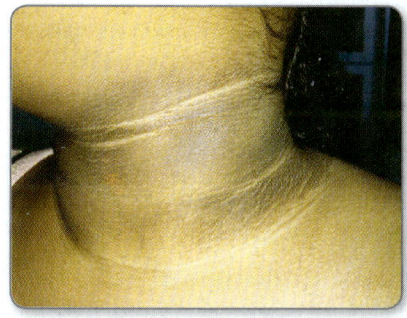

a. Epidermal nevus
b. Dowling-Degos disease
c. Acanthosis nigricans
d. Tinea corporis

[Ref: IADVL Textbook of Dermatology 4th edition vol 1 pg 396]

Explanation

Acanthosis Nigricans (AN)

- Acanthosis nigricans is common in obese people, have darker skin, and have diabetes or pre diabetic conditions.
- Associated with thick skin with hyperpigmentation seen in both men and women. there are thick black velvety areas in flexures/neck.
- It is NOT a disorder of melanin, occurs due to **insulin resistance**.

- Histology: papillomatosis & hyperkeratosis.
- Children who develop acanthosis nigricans are at a higher risk of developing type 2 diabetes later in life.
- Types:-
  - AN with insulin resistance Type A & type B (*HAIR-AN syndrome* is **H**yper**A**ndrogenism, **I**nsulin **R**esistance, and **A**canthosis **N**igricans)
  - Benign Acquired AN: Obesity associated, **most common type**
  - Drug-induced AN → Steroids, OCPs, nicotinic acid
  - Hereditary AN → Steroids, OCPs, nicotinic acid
  - Malignancy related → May be a sign of internal malignancy e.g. Adenocarcinoma stomach.
  - Pseudoacanthosis Nigricans

22. Most common association with Acanthosis nigricans-
a. Obesity *(PGMEE 2015)*
b. DM
c. Hypothyroidism
d. Hypertension

[Ref: IADVL Textbook of Dermatology 4th ed. vol 1 pg 396]

23. Acanthosis nigricans is seen in- *(PGMEE 2013)*
a. GIT cancer
b. Hypothyroidism
c. Diabetes
d. All of the above

[Ref: IADVL Textbook of Dermatology 4th ed. vol 1 pg 396]

24. Identify the pathology depicted in the image? *(PGMEE 2015)*

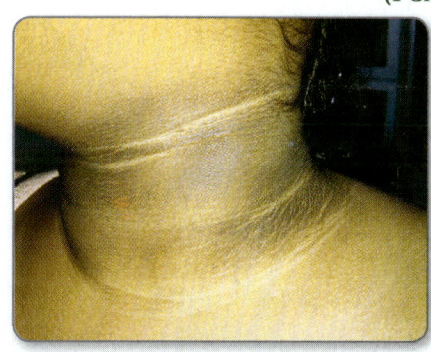

a. Dermatitis   b. Eczema
c. Urticaria   d. Acanthosis nigricans

[Ref: IADVL Textbook of Dermatology 4th ed. vol 1 pg 396]

25. Acanthosis nigricans is characterized by all of the following except: *(PGMEE 2015)*
a. Common in obese people
b. May be a sign of internal malignancy
c. Associated with thick skin with hyperpigmentation
d. Histologically there is hypermelanosis

[Ref: IADVL Textbook of Dermatology 4th ed. vol 1 pg 396]

Explanation

- Histology reveals hyperkeratosis with minimal or no hyperpigmentation.
- Blackening is secondary to hyperkeratosis & not due to increased melanocytes or melanin deposition.

20.	c
21.	c
22.	a
23.	d
24.	d
25.	d

26. Acanthosis nigrans is most common due to carcinoma of:- *(DNB pattern 2007)*
- a. Bronchus
- b. Breast
- c. Colon
- d. Testis

[Ref. Rook's textbook of dermatology 8th ed. pg 62.31]

Explanation

- Most cases of malignant acanthosis nigricans are associated with adenocarcinomas.
- The commonest site is the gastrointestinal tract (70–90%); of which gastric adenocarcinoma is most frequent (60%) > other parts of the intestine > liver or bile duct. Other tumour sites include lung, breast, endometrium, kidney, bladder, prostate, testis, cervix, thyroid and adrenal.

MISCELLANEOUS

27. Icthyosis is associated with – *(PGMEE 2012)*
- a. Hypothyroidism
- b. AIDS
- c. Hodgkins disease
- d. All

[Ref: IADVL Textbook of Dermatology 4th ed. vol 1 pg378]

28. Not true about Skin tag – *(PGMEE 2012)*
- a. Most common site is neck and axilla
- b. Associated with seborrhoeic keratosis
- c. Premalignant
- d. Pedunculated

[Ref: IADVL Textbook of Dermatology 4th ed. vol2 pg1927]

29. A patient presented with fever and joint pain for which he was put on NSAIDS. After 10 days the patient developed the following skin lesion.
(NEET Pattern 2017)

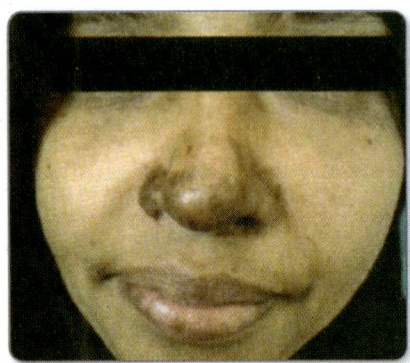

- a. Chikungunya
- b. Dengue
- c. Fixed drug eruption
- d. Melasma

[Ref: Andrew's diseases of the Skin 12th ed. pg. 398]

Explanation

Chikungunya

- It is usually a self-limiting illness, but the joint pain and some of the skin symptoms may persist after the defervescence.
- The dermatological manifestations:
  - **Morbilliform eruptions are MC** and they appears 3 to 5 days after the onset of fever and subsides within 3 to 4 days usually without any sequelae
  - In many patients, hypermelanosis of the skin may develop soon after the rash has resolved. It appears to be postinflammatory in nature and may develop rapidly. The hyperpigmentation may be of different types including centrofacial (involving nose & cheeks) and freckle-like, diffuse pigmentation of face, pinna, and extremities, flagellate pigmentation, and pigmentation of existing acne lesions.

30. Which of the following ultra-violet radiation cause most skin disorder- *(PGMEE 2013)*
- a. UV-A
- b. UV-B
- c. UV-C
- d. None

[Ref: Andrews' Diseases of the Skin 12 th ed. pg 24]

31. Erythroderma %of skin involved is – *(PGMEE 2013)*
- a. < 30%
- b. 30- 60 %
- c. 60- 70 %
- d. ≥ 90%

[Ref: IADVL Textbook of Dermatology 4th edition vol 1 pg 782]

Explanation

- Erythroderma or Exfoliative dermatitis refers to a scaling erythematous dermatitis involving ≥90% of skin.

26.	c
27.	d
28.	c
29.	a
30.	b
31.	d

NEVI

1. Epidermal nevus follows- *(PGMEE 2015)*
- a. Lymphatics
- b. Langer's lines
- c. Blaschko's lines
- d. Vasculature

[Ref: IADVL Textbook of Dermatology 4th ed. vol 1 pg287]

2. Lines of Blaschko represent- *(PGMEE 2015)*
- a. Dermatomal Patterns
- b. Epidermal cell migration pathway
- c. Vasculature pathways
- d. Lymphatic pathways

[Ref: IADVL Textbook of Dermatology 4th ed. vol 1 pg286]

3. Lines of Blaschko's are related to– *(PGMEE 2013)*
- a. Bones
- b. Keratinocytes
- c. Nerves
- d. Blood vessels

[Ref: IADVL Textbook of Dermatology 4th ed. vol 1 pg286]

4. Lines of Blaschko represent *(PGMEE 2013)*
- a. Lines of development
- b. Lines along lymphatics
- c. Lines along nerves
- d. Lines along blood vessels

[Ref: IADVL Textbook of Dermatology 4th ed. vol 1 pg286]

5. Which of the following is not a NEVUS of melanocyte- *(PGMEE 2012)*
- a. Becker nevus
- b. Nevus of ota
- c. Mongolian spot
- d. Nevus of Ito

[Ref: IADVL Textbook of Dermatology 4th ed. vol 1 pg287]

6. A 15cm hyperpigmented macule on an adolosent male undergoes changed such as coarseness, growth of hair & acne. Diagnosis is – *(PGMEE 2013)*
- a. Becker nevus
- b. Comedo nevus
- c. Sebaceous nevus
- d. Melanocytic nevus

[Ref: IADVL Textbook of Dermatology 4th ed. vol 1 pg296]

7. Maximum malignant potential is in – *(PGMEE 2014)*
- a. Intradermal naevus
- b. Superficial naevus
- c. Junctional naevus
- d. Epidermal naevus

[Ref: IADVL Textbook of Dermatology 4th ed. vol 1 pg303]

8. A 44-year-old male presents with history of hyperpigemntation and lesion over right side of chest as shown in the picture. There is growth of hairs in the lesion. Likely diagnosis is:- *(PGMEE 2018)*

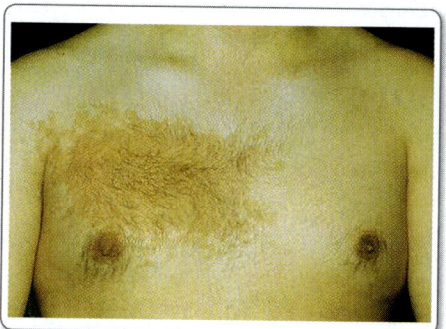

- a. Spitz nevus
- b. Café au Lait spot
- c. Bicker's nevus
- d. Congenital melanocytic nevus

[Ref: Andrew's diseases of the Skin 12th edition page 682]

Explanation

Becker Nevus

- Becker nevus presents as a hyperpigmented, hypertrichotic patch on the upper trunk or proximal upper extremity. The lesion is usually single & begins before puberty.
- Co-existence of underlying connective tissue nevi smooth muscle hamartomas and structural abnormalities of bone and soft tissue is known.
- The male predominance (M:F ratio, 5:1), onset at or after puberty and hypertrichosis suggest that local androgen hypersensitivity may be an etiological factor.

PREMALIGNANT SKIN LESIONS

9. The premalignant skin lesions are all except – *(PGMEE 2015)*
- a. Miliaria
- b. Bowen's disease
- c. DLE
- d. Actinic keratoses

[Ref: Fitzpatrick's dermatology in general medicine 8th ed. pg 1262 and IADVL Textbook of Dermatology 4th ed. vol2 pg 1710]

10. True statement about Oral leukoplakia... *(PGMEE 2016-17)*
- a. It is not a procarcinogenic condition
- b. It is more carcinogenic then erythroplakia
- c. It occures due to constant irritation of oral mucosa
- d. It will always need excision

[Ref: Fitzpatrick's dermatology in general medicine 8th ed. pg 1279]

11. Which of the following is not a premalignant condition of skin: *(PGMEE 2012)*
- a. Actinic Keratitis
- b. Xeroderma pigmentosa
- c. Bowen disease
- d. Psoriasis

[Ref: Fitzpatrick's dermatology in general medicine 8th ed. pg 1262]

Explanation

- ***Premalignant epithelial lesions***
  - Actinic keratosis
  - Bowen's disease or squamous cell carcinoma in situ
  - Arsenical keratosis
  - Chronic radiation keratosis
  - Thermal keratosis
  - PUVA keratosis
  - Hydrocarbon/tar keratosis
  - Viral keratosis
  - Bowenoid papulosis
  - Epidermodysplasia veruciformis

1.	c
2.	b
3.	b
4.	a
5.	a
6.	a
7.	c
8.	c
9.	a
10.	c
11.	d

- ○ Erythroplasia of Queyrat
- ○ Erythroplakia
- ○ Leucoplakia
- ■ Familial cancer syndromes having susceptibility to NMSC (non melanoma skin cancer) development are: naevoid basal cell carcinoma syndrome, Gorlin's syndrome, Bazex's syndrome and xeroderma pigmentosum.
- ■ *Genetic syndromes associated with skin cancers* Bloom syndrome, Rothmund–Thomson syndrome, xeroderma pigmentosum.

12. True regarding Bowen's disease is (PGMEE 2015)

- a. In situ BCC
- b. HSV infection plays a role
- c. More common in dark skinned people
- d. Chronic sun damage plays a role

[Ref: IADVL Textbook of Dermatology 4th ed. vol2 pg 2084]

Explanation

Bowen disease

- ■ Bowen disease is a squamous cell carcinoma in situ.
- ■ It is a malignant tumor of keratinocytes (intraepidermal carcinoma)
- ■ It is MC in whites over sun exposed sites
- ■ Etiological association:
  - ○ Chronic UV exposure
  - ○ Arsenic exposure
  - ○ HPV-16 (MC), 18, 31, 33
- ■ Rx: Simple excision is MC & preferred treatment for smaller lesions
- ■ Prognosis - favourable

MALIGNANT TUMORS

13. The patient came with an ulcer on the side of the nose as shown, which bleeds on itching. What is the diagnosis?
(NEET Pattern 2017)

- a. Squamous cell ca
- b. Basal cell ca
- c. Marjolin's ulcer
- d. Nevus

[Ref: Dhingra 5th ed. Pg-160]

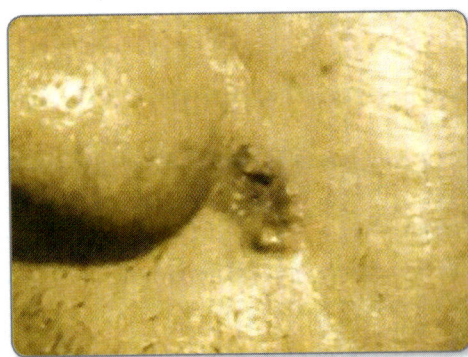

Explanation

BCC (Basal cell carcinoma)

- ■ BCC is the most common malignant tumor involving skin of nose
- ■ Male = female
- ■ Age : 40 to 60 yrs

12.	d
13.	b
14.	c
15.	a
16.	d
17.	d
18.	a

- ■ Common site on nose are tip and ala of nose
- ■ Very slow growing
- ■ Bleed on touch
- ■ Nodal metastasis is extremely rare

14. FDA approved drug for the treatment of superficial basal cell carcinoma is – (PGMEE 2015)

- a. Acyclovir
- b. Terbinafine
- c. Imiquinod
- d. Clobesterol

[Ref: IADVL Textbook of Dermatology 4th ed. vol2 pg2089]

15. Mycosis fungoides is a: (PGMEE 2014)

- a. T-cell lymphoma
- b. T-cell and B-cell lymphoma
- c. Same as Hodgkin's lymphoma but seen only in skin
- d. Derived from stem cell

[Ref: IADVL Textbook of Dermatology 4th ed. vol2 pg 2163]

Explanation

Mycosis fungoides

- ■ Mycosis fungoides is the most common type of cutaneous T-cell lymphoma and accounts for almost 50% of all primary cutaneous lymphomas. It is generally classified as a type of non-Hodgkin's lymphoma.
- ■ It primarily present in the skin and are composed of malignant clonal skin homing helper T lymphocytes.
- ■ Arising in mid to late adulthood (median age at diagnosis, 55 to 60 years) with a male predominance of 2:1.
- ■ Clinically MF is categorized as being in the patch, plaque, or tumor stage, but patients may simultaneously have more than one type of lesion.
- ■ On histopathology there is an epidermotropic bandlike infiltrate of neoplastic T lymphocytes with hyperconvoluted cerebriform nuclei involving the upper dermis with exocytosis and formation of intraepidermal Pautrier's microabscesses.

16. Patient with pruritic lesion over Left shoulder showing cigarette paper atrophy and poikiloderma with generalized lymphadenopathy. Histopathology examination of lesion shows CD4 positive sezary leutzner cells. What is the dermo-epidermal manifestation of this disease? (PGMEE 2015)

- a. Discharging sinus
- b. Pin point ulcers
- c. Miliaria
- d. Pautrier's micro abscess

[Ref: IADVL Textbook of Dermatology 4th ed. vol2 pg2168]

17. Stage 1 cutaneous T cell lymphoma treatment is:

- a. Biological response modifiers (PGMEE 2015)
- b. Extracorporial photopheresis
- c. Systemic chemotherapy
- d. PUVA

[Ref: IADVL Textbook of Dermatology 4th ed. vol2 pg2173]

18. Total Skin Electron Irradiation is used for the treatment of – (PGMEE 2012)

- a. Mycosis Fungoides
- b. Psoriasis
- c. Brain Metastasis
- d. Sezary Syndrome

[Ref: IADVL Textbook of Dermatology 4th ed. vol2 pg2173]

19. A Retro virus positive patient, developed erythematones plaque over ankle, sole of foot, The HPE shows – abnormal vascular endothelial cells with a typical spindle cells (Picture showing patient foot and microscopic slide view): *(PGMEE 2016-17)*

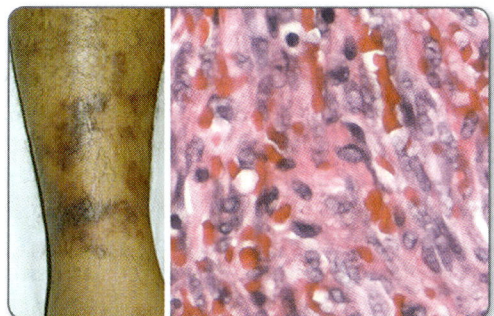

- a. Hemangioma
- b. Kaposi's sarcoma
- c. Reticulum cell carcinoma
- d. Basal cell carcinoma

[Ref: IADVL Textbook of Dermatology 4th ed. vol2 pg 2127]

MASTOCYTOSIS

20. Darier's sign is seen in – *(PGMEE 2013)*
- a. Darrier's disease
- b. Atopic dermatitis
- c. Allergic vasculitis
- d. Urticaria pigmentosa

[Ref: IADVL Textbook of Dermatology 4th ed. vol2 pg 2204]

Explanation

- Darrier's sign - changes of urtication such as edema, erythema & pruritus on stroking the skin lesion of a person with systemic mastocytosis or urticaria pigmentosa.

21. Urticaria pigmentosa is a disorder of? *(DNB June 2009)*
- a. Mast cells
- b. Lymphocytes
- c. Eosinophils
- d. Neutrophils

[Ref: IADVL Textbook of Dermatology 4th ed. vol2 pg2204; Rook's textbook of dermatology 8th ed. pg 22.31]

Explanation

Mastocytosis

- Mastocytosis is a heterogeneous group of disorders characterized by abnormal growth and accumulation of mast cells in the skin and sometimes other organs such as the bones, gastrointestinal tract, liver, and spleen.
- Cutaneous mastocytosis includes:
  - Urticaria pigmentosa.
  - Solitary mastocytoma.
  - Diffuse cutaneous mastocytosis.
  - Telangiectasia macularis eruptiva perstans

MISCELLANEOUS

22. A patient presents with lesion over chest 3 months after cyst removal. Most likely diagnosis is: *(PGMEE 2016-17)*

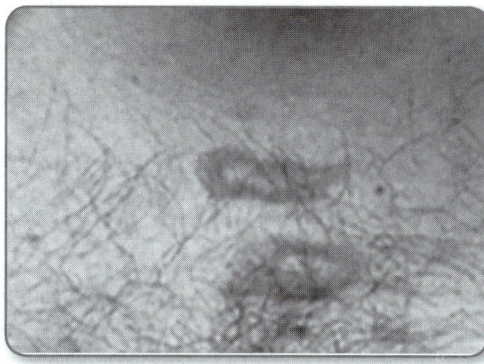

- a. Keloid
- b. Galactocel
- c. Hypertrophied scar
- d. Recurrence of cyst

[Ref: IADVL Textbook of Dermatology 4th ed. vol2 pg 2115]

MELANOMA

23. The smallest recommended margin for whole local incision of a melanoma measuring 0.5 mm in depth should be: *(PGMEE 2015-16)*
- a. 1 cm
- b. 2 cm
- c. 3 cm
- d. 5 cm

[Ref: Evidence based and Problem Oriented Surgical Treatment]

24. Melanoma staging is done according to which classification? *(DNB Dec' 2009)*
- a. Clark
- b. Breslow
- c. Both
- d. Bethseda

[Ref: Devita, Hellman, and Rosenberg's cancer: principles & practice of oncology – 8th/e p. 1908, Schwartz's Principles of Surgery 9th/e chapter 16]

19.	**b**
20.	**d**
21.	**a**
22.	**a**
23.	**a**
24.	**c**

BACTERIAL INFECTIONS

1. A 6 year old child presents with lesions on face, covered with honey coloured crusts. Pruritus is present. The possible cause can be: *(PGMEE 2016-17)*
   a. Impetigo
   b. Herpes
   c. Chickenpox
   d. Molluscum contagiosum

   [Ref: IADVL Textbook of Dermatology 4th Edition Vol 1 Pg 437]

2. Bullous impetigo is caused by – *(PGMEE 2013)*
   a. Y.Pestis
   b. Staphylococcus
   c. Streptococcus
   d. Pseudomonas

   [Ref: IADVL Textbook of Dermatology 4th Edition Vol 1 Pg 438]

3. The causative organism for the condition depicted in image is? *(PGMEE 2019)*

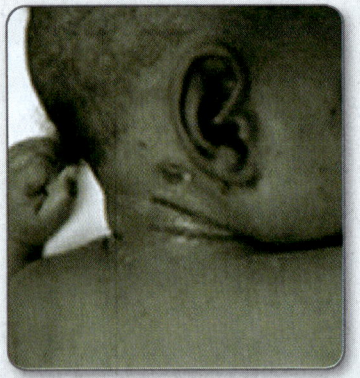

   a. Staphylococci
   b. Candida
   c. Streptococcus
   d. Actinomycetes

   [Ref: IADVL Textbook of Dermatology 4th/e pg 226]

4. Ecthyma gangrenosum is cause by? *(DNB pattern Dec' 2009)*
   a. Fungal infection
   b. Pseudomonas aeruginosa
   c. Stephylococcus
   d. Streptococcus

   [Ref: Andrews's diseases of skin- clinical dermatology 11th/e /p 273]

Explanation

- Pseudomonas infections
  - Ecthyma gangrenosum
  - Green nail syndrome
  - Pseudomonas aeruginosa folliculitis (hot tub folliculitis)
  - External otitis
  - Blastomycosis-like pyoderma
  - Gram-negative folliculitis
- **Ecthyma** is an ulcerative staphylococcal or streptococcal pyoderma, nearly always of the shins or dorsal feet.
- **Ecthyma contagiosum**/Orf is a zoonotic poxvirus infection

CUTANEOUS TUBERCULOSIS

5. Most common type of cutaneous tuberculosis is: *(PGMEE 2014)*
   a. Scrofuloderma
   b. Erythema induratum
   c. Lupus vulgaris
   d. T.B. verruca cutis

   [Ref: IADVL Textbook of Dermatology 4th Edition Vol 1 Pg 450]

6. Tuberculides are seen in? *(DNB pattern Dec' 2008)*
   a. Lupus vulgaris
   b. Scrofuloderma
   c. Lichen scrofulososum
   d. Erythema nodosum

   [Ref: Fitzpatrick's dermatology in general medicine 7th/e /p 1774]

Explanation

- Tuberculids
  - Tuberculids are skin lesion in a patient with tuberculosis, often occult, elsewhere in body.
  - Tuberculids are hypersensitivity reaction to M. tuberculosis or its products in a patient with significant immunity.
- Main features-
  - Positive tuberculin test
  - Absence of bacilli in skin biopsy specimen & culture.
  - Positive response to antitubercular therapy.
  - Evidence of manifest or past TB

Terminology/relationship to tuberculosis	Entities
Tuberculids : Condition in which M. tuberculosis/bovis appears to play significant role	Lichen scrofulosorum, Papulonecrotic tuberculid
Facultative tuberculids: conditions in which M. tuberculosis/bovis may be one of several pathogenic factors	Nodular vasculitis/erythema induratum of Bazin, Erythema nodosum
Non-tuberculids (conditions formerly designated as tuberculids ; there is no relation to tuberculosis)	Lupus miliaris disseminatus faciei (LMDF), Rosacea – like tuberculid Lichenoid tuberculid

7. Match stick test is positive in – *(PGMEE 2013)*
   a. P. versicolor
   b. Rhinophyma
   c. Lupus vulgaris
   d. Rhinosporiodosis

   [Ref: IADVL Textbook of Dermatology 4th Edition Vol 1 Pg 452]

8. Apple jelly nodules are characteristic of *(PGMEE 2015)*
   a. Neurofibroma
   b. Angiomatosis
   c. Tuberculous verrucous cutis
   d. Lupus vulgaris

   [Ref: IADVL Textbook of Dermatology 4th Edition Vol 1 Pg 452]

1.	a
2.	b
3.	a
4.	b
5.	c
6.	c
7.	c
8.	d

LEPROSY

9. Single hypopigmented hypoaesthetic patch shown below in image is suggestive of: *(PGMEE 2016-17)*

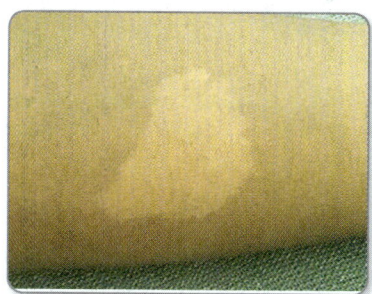

a. Post kala azar patient   b. Leprosy
c. Pityriasis alba   d. Neavus anemicus.

[Ref: IADVL Textbook of Dermatology 4th Edition Vol 3 pg 3092]

10. Image shown below is diagnostic of: *(PGMEE 2016-17)*

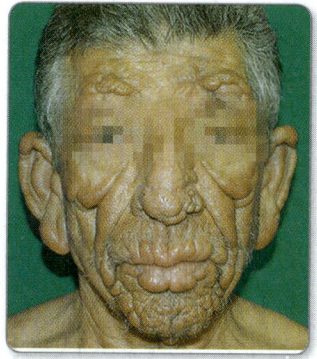

a. Leprosy
b. Kala azar
c. Multiple warts over face
d. All are true

[Ref: IADVL Textbook of Dermatology 4th Edition Vol 3 pg 3099]

11. A 7 years old child from Bihar is having hypopigmented anesthetic patch on his face. What is the most probable diagnosis? *(Dec 2009)*

a. Indeterminate leprosy   b. Pityriasis alba
c. Nevus anemicus   d. Nevus achromicus

[Ref. IADVL Textbook of dermatology 3rd edition pg 2035]

Explanation

- **Indeterminate Leprosy**
  - it is an early stage in the evolution of leprosy where histological and immunological responses have not yet evolved completely.
  - It is observed only in endemic areas, especially during surveys of the population or the school children. 1 to 3 ill-defined hypopigmented macules ranging in size from 1 to 5 cm are commonly seen on the outer side of the extremities, buttocks, face, and trunk. Their surface is smooth. The sensations may be impaired and nerve thickening may be present.
  - In Pityriasis alba, Nevus anemicus, Nevus achromicus – sensations are intact

12. Leprosy will affect all organs except? *(DNB pattern 2008)*

a. Ovary   b. Uterus
c. Nerves   d. Eye

[Ref: IADVL Textbook of dermatology 3rd edition pg 2075, IAL textbook of Leprosy 1st edition pg 299]

Explanation

- In contrast to the male organs, the ovaries are only rarely involved in leprosy.
- Uterus never involved in leprosy. In various studies the biopy findings from endometrium did not reveal any involvement. The menstrual fluid was found to be free of leprosy bacilli even in patients having bacillemia.

13. Most infective stage of leprosy is? *(June 2009)*

a. Tuberculoid   b. Lepromatous
c. Borderline tuberculoid   d. Borderline lepromatous

[Ref. IADVL Textbook of dermatology 3rd edition pg 2039]

Explanation

- Lepromatous leprosy is a multisystem disease that develops in individuals who are unable to mount a cell-mediated immune response against M. leprae. It leads to massive multiplication of M. leprae that infiltrate the skin, nerves, reticuloendothelial system, upper respiratory tract, eyes, testes, adrenals, and other viscera. It is an infectious form of leprosy and a large number of bacilli are discharged from the upper respiratory tract. The disease develops very insidiously and is virtually asymptomatic until late in the course of the disease.

14. Thickened nerve in a patient of Leprosy (?Plague) as shown in the image is:- *(PGMEE 2018)*

a. Supra-orbital nerve   b. Supratrochlear nerve
c. Facial nerve   d. Greater auricular nerve

[Ref: IAL Textbook of leprosy 1st edition page 133]

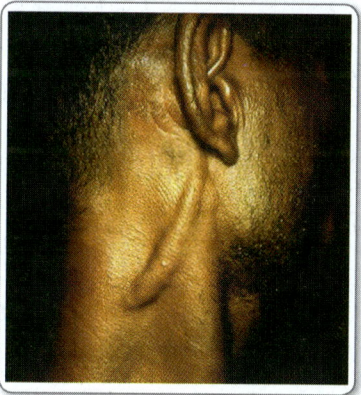

Explanation

Peripheral nerves of head & neck area which may be thickened in leprosy

Nerve	Site/bony landmark
Supraorbital	Supraorbital notch
Supratrochlear	Medial to supraorbital nerve
Infraorbital	Infraorbital formen

9.	b
10.	a
11.	a
12.	b
13.	b
14.	d

Nerve	Site/bony landmark
Branches of facial nerve- zygomatic & temporal	Zygomatic arch
Greater auricular nerve	Lateral side of neck, crosses sternomastoid muscle, from lateral side to infra-auricular area

Greater Auricular Nerve

- The greater auricular nerve is a cutaneous branch of the cervical plexus which arises from the ventral rami of C2 and C3 spinal nerves .
- It emerges along the posterior aspect of the sterno-cleidomastoid muscle at the punctum nervosum (Erb point) and ascends vertically across the oblique sternocleidomastoid muscle. When the greater auricular nerve approaches the inferior pole of the parotid gland it divides into anterior and posterior terminal branches.

15. Ulnar nerve and sural nerve are involved, what is t/t of leprosy? *(PGMEE 2016)*

- a. MBT x 9 month
- b. MBT x 12 month
- c. MBT x 24 month
- d. PBT x 6 month

[Ref: IADVL Textbook of Dermatology 4th Edition Vol 3 pg 3159]

16. Single hypoasthetic patch over trunk with bilateral ulnar nerve thickening. Patient require: *(PGMEE 2016-17)*

- a. Pancibacillary treatment for 6
- b. Multi bacillary treatment for 12 month
- c. Paucibacillary treatment for 12 wk
- d. Multi bacillary treatment for 12 wk

[Ref: IADVL Textbook of Dermatology 4th Edition Vol 3 pg 3159]

17. Most common type of leprosy in India – *(PGMEE 2014)*

- a. LL
- b. TT
- c. BL
- d. BT

[Ref: IADVL Textbook of Dermatology 4th Edition Vol 3 Pg 3097]

18. Satellite lesion are seen in – *(PGMEE 2014)*

- a. Histoid leprosy
- b. Lepromatous leprosy
- c. Tuberculoid leprosy
- d. Borderline tuberculoid leprosy

[Ref: IADVL Textbook of Dermatology 4th Edition Vol 3 Pg 3098]

19. Nerves are not involved in – *(PGMEE 2013)*

- a. Borderline tuberculoid leprosy
- b. Tuberculoid leprosy
- c. Lepromatous leprosy
- d. Indeterminate leprosy

[Ref: IADVL Textbook of Dermatology 4th Edition Vol 3 Pg 3096]

20. Symmetrical multiple lesions are seen in which type of leprosy – *(PGMEE 2014)*

- a. Lepromatous
- b. Neuritic
- c. Tubercular
- d. Borderline

[Ref: IADVL Textbook of Dermatology 4th Edition Vol 3 Pg 3099]

15.	b
16.	b
17.	d
18.	d
19.	d
20.	a
21.	b
22.	a
23.	d
24.	a
25.	b

21. Biopsy from the face lesions of this patient showed perineural invasion. What is the most probable diagnosis? *(PGMEE 2015)*

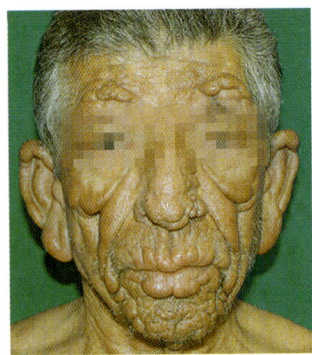

- a. Anaphylaxis
- b. Lepromatous leprosy
- c. Tuberculoid leprosy
- d. Soft tissue sarcoma

[Ref: IADVL Textbook of Dermatology 4th Edition Vol 3 Pg 3085]

22. Which of the following is not used in lepra reaction? *(DNB pattern Dec 2011)*

- a. Chloroquine
- b. Rifampicin
- c. Clofazimine
- d. Thalidomide

(Ref.IADVL Textbook of dermatology 3rd edition pg 2089)

Explanation

- Drugs Used for Treating Reactions:
  - Corticosteroids are effective against both types of reactions.
  - Clofazimine- This anti-leprosy drug has a special role in the management of patients with ENL
  - Thalidomide -This potent and fast acting anti-reaction compound is able to control practically all manifestations, including neuritis, of ENL reaction
  - Antimony Compounds- Both tri- and pentavalent compounds are useful in patients with mild to moderate ENL, particularly in relieving bone and joint symptoms. These drugs are not commonly used on account of several toxic effects and also because of their parenteral route of administration.
  - Chloroquine has been widely used in the treatment of ENL.

23. DOC for lepra II reaction is – *(PGMEE 2014)*

- a. Clofazimine
- b. Thalidomide
- c. Dapsone
- d. Steroids

[Ref: IADVL Textbook of Dermatology 4th Edition Vol 3 Pg 3172]

24. Drug of choice in type I lepra reaction with severe neuritis is: *(PGMEE 2014-15)*

- a. Systemic steroid
- b. Chloroquine
- c. Thalidomide
- d. Clofazimine

[Ref: Harrison's 19th/e pg. 1125]

25. In severe cases Lucio phenomenon is treated with: *(PGMEE 2014-15)*

- a. Steroids
- b. Exchange transfusion
- c. Clofazimine
- d. Lenalidomide

[Ref: Harrison's 19th/e pg. 1125]

26. Lucio reaction is seen in – *(PGMEE 2012)*
   a. LGV   b. Syphillis
   c. TB   d. Leprosy
    [Ref: IADVL Textbook of Dermatology 4th Edition Vol 3 Pg 3107]

27. Ulceronecrotic nodule is seen in – *(PGMEE 2013)*
   a. Indeterminate leprosy
   b. Tuberculoid leprosy
   c. Histoid leprosy
   d. Lucio leprosy
    [Ref: IADVL Textbook of Dermatology 4th Edition Vol 3 Pg 3103]

28. In multibacillary leprosy the follow up examination after adequate treatment should be done yearly for – *(PGMEE 2014)*
   a. 3 years   b. 3 years
   c. 5 years   d. 10 years
    [Ref: IAL Textbook of leprosy 2nd edition pg 562]

VIRAL INFECTION

29. Eczema herpeticum is- *(PGMEE 2015)*
   a. Viral infection   b. Bacterial infection
   c. A form of eczema   d. Fungal infection
    [Ref: IADVL Textbook of Dermatology 4th Edition Vol 1 Pg 573]

30. Eczema herpeticum is most commonly associated with-
   a. Lichen planus   *(PGMEE 2015)*
   b. Vaicella zoster
   c. Atopic dermatitis
   d. Contact dermatitis
    [Ref: IADVL Textbook of Dermatology 4th Edition Vol 1 Pg 573]

31. Herpes zoster vesicles characteristics are all EXCEPT: *(PGMEE 2016-17)*
   a. Always unilateral
   b. Pleomorphic lesions present
   c. Classical lesions are grouped vesicles on an erythematous base
   d. Recurrent lesions are uncommon
  [Ref: IADVL Textbook of Dermatology 4th Edition Vol 1 Pg 584]

32. An eight year old boy presents with multiple umbilicated papules on trunk. Diagnosis is- *(PGMEE 2015)*
   a. Dermatophytosis
   b. Molluscum contagiosum
   c. Harper zoster
   d. Chicken pox
  [Ref: IADVL Textbook of Dermatology 4th Edition Vol 1 Pg 589]

33. Infection by which of the following agents leads to wart formation- *(PGMEE 2015)*
   a. HPV
   b. Molluscum contagiosum virus
   c. Herps simplex virus
   d. Varicella zoster virus
    [Ref: IADVL Textbook of Dermatology 4th Edition Vol 1 Pg 595]

34. A patient presents with non-itchy papular lesions over dorsum of hand. One of the family member has similar history in the past. Most likely cause is:- *(PGMEE 2018)*
   a. HSV
   b. Human papilloma viruses
   c. Scabies
   d. CMV

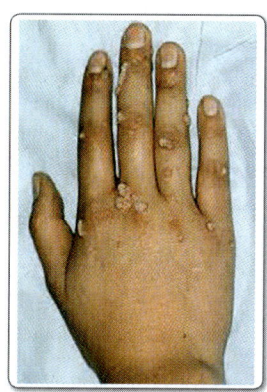

Explanation

The lesions shown in image are typically warty lesions over dorsum of hand. Cardinal features suggestive of warts are:
- Raised papular warty lesions. Lesions may be smooth and papular or keratotic/cauliflower-like.
- Lesions are usually non-itchy
- The characteristic distribution pattern of lesions : ano-genital are most common.
- History in one of the family members of the household or other contacts may be there.

The cardinal features in the clinical diagnosis of scabies are:
- The presence of the burrow, especially on the hands or penis;
- The characteristic distribution pattern of lesions (papules/ papulovesicles)---Scabies characteristically involves the webs of the fingers, flexor aspects of the wrists, elbows, anterior axillary folds, the nipple and areola, umbilicus and periumbilical region, genitalia & upper thighs, knees and ankles.
- The presence or history of similar illness in other members of the household or other contacts; and
- Intense pruritus, which tends to worsen at night.

Features	Warts	Scabies
Caused by	HPV	Sarcoptes scabiei (Itch mite)
Lesions	Anogenital area, dorsum of hand	Interdigital clefts are usually involved
Family history	Rare	Common, most of the family members have similar lesions
Pruritus	Non-itchy	Intense itchy lesions

35. Exanthems are caused by all except– *(PGMEE 2014)*
   a. Rubella   b. Malaria
   c. Measles   d. Typhoid
  [Ref: Andrew's Diseases of the skin 12th edition Pg 269, 393]

26.	d
27.	d
28.	c
29.	a
30.	c
31.	b
32.	b
33.	a
34.	b
35.	b

FUNGAL INFECTION

36. Skin scrapping & KOH mounting is done for:
(PGMEE 2013)

a. Fungus   b. Varicella
c. HSV   d. Leprosy

[Ref: IADVL Textbook of Dermatology 4th Edition Vol 1 Pg 488]

37. Best diagnosis test for fungal skin infection
(PGMEE 2012)

a. Wood's lamp   b. Patch test
c. Diascopy   d. KOH test

[Ref: Rook's Textbook of Dermatology 9th edition Pg 32.6]

38. Dermatophyes affect: *(PGMEE 2013)*

a. Dermis of skin   b. Stratum spongiosum
c. Stratum basal   d. Keratin

[Ref: Rook's Textbook of Dermatology 9th edition Pg 32.21]

39. Dermatophytes involve: *(PGMEE 2015)*

a. Stratum malpighi   b. Stratum lucidum
c. Stratum basal   d. Stratum corneum

[Ref: Rook's Textbook of Dermatology 9th edition Pg 32.20]

40. Ring worn infection affects: *(PGMEE 2014)*

a. Stratum corneum   b. Papillary layer
c. Prickle cell layer   d. Dermis

[Ref: Rook's Textbook of Dermatology 9th edition Pg 32.20]

41. Which of the following infection involves hair:
(PGMEE 2015)

a. Malasezia furfur   b. Epidermophyton
c. Trichophyton   d. All of the above

[Ref: IADVL Textbook of Dermatology 4th Edition Vol 1 Pg462]

42. Kerion is seen in – *(PGMEE 2014)*

a. Dermatophytosis
b. Candida infection
c. Pityriasis
d. Trichomoniasis

[Ref: IADVL Textbook of Dermatology 4th Edition Vol 1 Pg 462]

43. A child presents with indurated boggy swelling with crusts and hair loss over scalp as shown in the image. Most likely cause is: *(PGMEE 2016-17)*

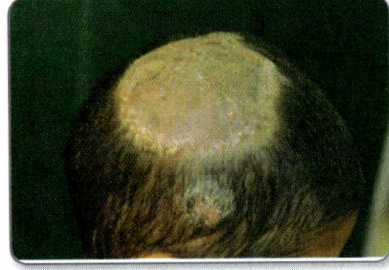

a. Trichophyton
b. Epidermophyton
c. Microsporum
d. Staph aureus

[Ref: IADVL Textbook of Dermatology 4th Edition Vol 1 Pg 462]

44. Baby brought to mother with history of hair fall with boggy scalp hair easily pluckable. There was similar history 6 months back. What is the treatment:
(PGMEE 2016-17)

a. Oral ketoconazole   b. Oral griesofulvin
c. Topical cotrimoxaxol   d. Intralesional steroid

[Ref: IADVL Textbook of Dermatology 4th Edition Vol 1 Pg 470]

45. Hair infection with scutula formation is seen in case of –
(PGMEE 2015)

a. Tenia glabrosa   b. Jock itch
c. Tenia barbae   d. Tenia capitis

[Ref: IADVL Textbook of Dermatology 4th Edition Vol 1 Pg 466]

Explanation

- Tinea favosa (favus) is a chronic fungal infection of the scalp most commonly caused by T. schoenleinii.
- The infection is characterized by the formation of large matted crusts – scutula – over the scalp.

46. Onychomycosis is most commonly caused by:

a. Epidermatophyton floccosum   *(PGMEE 2015)*
b. Trichophyton mentagrophytes
c. Trichophyton rubrum
d. Candida

[Ref: Andrew's Diseases of the skin 12th edition Pg 292]

47. Pic -boy developed itchy lesion and applied steriod ointment and developed following lesion:
(PGMEE 2016-17)

a. Tinea incognito
b. Discoid eczema
c. Erythema annulare centrifugum
d. Granuloma annulare

[Ref: IADVL Textbook of Dermatology 4th Edition Vol 1 Pg 485]

48. Picture showing skin lesion which subsides with the use of steroids for 5 days but reappears after stopping the drug. Most likely diagnosis is: *(PGMEE 2016-17)*

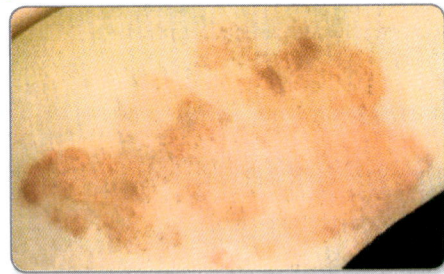

a. Tinea incognito   b. Contact dermatitis
c. Taenie corporis   d. Pityriasis rosea

[Ref: IADVL Textbook of Dermatology 4th Edition Vol 1 Pg 485]

49. Tinea incognito is seen with – *(PGMEE 2014)*

a. Antibiotics
b. 1% BHi3
c. 5% permethrin
d. Steroid treatment

[Ref: IADVL Textbook of Dermatology 4th Edition Vol 1 Pg 485]

36.	a
37.	d
38.	d
39.	d
40.	a
41.	c
42.	a
43.	a
44.	b
45.	d
46.	c
47.	a
48.	a
49.	d

50. **Drugs used topically for dermatophytes-** *(PGMEE 2014)*
   a. Terbinafine
   b. Cyclopirox oleamine
   c. Econazole
   d. All of the above

   [Ref: IADVL Textbook of Dermatology 4th Edition Vol 1 Pg 467]

51. **Black piedra is caused by –** *(PGMEE 2015)*
   a. Trichosporon ovoides
   b. Trichosporon asahii
   c. Trichosporon inkin
   d. Piedraia hortae

   [Ref: IADVL Textbook of Dermatology 4th Edition Vol 1 Pg 493]

52. **Definitive diagnosis of sporotrichosis generally depends on?** *(DNB pattern Dec' 2007)*
   a. Serology
   b. Culture
   c. Biopsy
   d. KOH preparation from the lesion

   [Ref:IADVL Textbook of dermatology 3rd/e p 305]

Explanation

- Sporotrichosis is subacute or chronic fungal infection caused by Sporothrix schenckii (dimorphic fungus).
- Direct microscopy of clinical material is of little or no value in confirming a diagnosis because very few organisms are found in the lesions.
- Diagnosis is possible only by isolation of S. schenckii. The specimens should be inoculated on Sabouraud's dextrose agar with antibiotics at 260C – moist white colonies which darkens with age because of melanin production. Conversion into the yeast form on brain heart infusion agar at 370C is important for specific identification of S. schenckii. Cigar bodies seen microscopically.
- Biopsy: mixed granulomatous reaction with neutrophil microabcesses. Demonstration of S. schenckii in tissue sections is very difficult. The organism if present, is usually in form of the asteroid body consisting of cigar shaped or oval basophilic yeast-like body (3–5 μm) surrounded by radiating elongation of a homogeneous eosinophilic material (7–20 μm). Asteroid body is considered characteristic of sporotrichosis.
- Serological tests are useful in establishing the diagnosis of extracutaneous or systemic form of sporotrichosis, when distinct clinical features are lacking.
- An intradermal sporotrichin skin test is useful for determining exposure to the fungus.

PITYRIASIS VERSICOLOR

53. **Pityriasis versicolor is caused by?** *(DNB pattern June' 2011)*
   a. Malassezia furfur
   b. T. Rubrum
   c. E. flocculosum
   d. Candidiasis

   [Ref: IADVL Textbook of dermatology 3rd/e /p 285]

Explanation

- Tinea versicolor/Pityriasis versicolor is caused by Malassezia furfur/Pityrosporum spp. Previously the term M. furfur was used to describe the mycelial phase, whereas the yeast form was called either P. ovale or P. orbiculare depending upon the shape of the budding cells. Malassezia furfur/ Pityrosporum ovle or P.orbicularis are same organism. The chief lesion is a macule that may be hypopigmented or hyperpigmented and covered with fine branny (furfuraceous) scales. Commonly present on upper trunk (chest, shoulders, upper back) upper arms and neck. Face may be sometimes involved.

Hyperpimentation attributed to	Hypopigmentation has been attributed
thicker stratum corneum	dicarboxylic acid(azelaic acid) produced by fungi, that might inhibit the dopa-tyrosine reaction
larger singly distributed hypertrophic melanocytes	Inhibition of normal tanning due to overlying scale
and inflammatory reaction against the fungus.	abnormally small melanosomes

- *Laboratory Diagnosis*
  - Direct examination of a lesion under Wood's lamp shows yellow green fluorescence.
  - Direct microscopic examination of scales in 10% KOH or Parker Quink stain shows yeast and mycelia in characteristic "bananas and grapes" or "spaghetti and meat ball" appearance.
  - Biopsy will demonstrate a thick basket-weave stratum corneum with hyphae and spores. PAS staining is confirmatory
- *Treatment*
  - Topical therapy-2.5% selenium sulfide lotion/ Sodium hyposulfite/ Zinc pyrithione 1%/ whitfield ointment. Topical antifungal like clotrimazole, miconazole, econazole, ciclopirox olamine and tolnaftate also work well. Shampoos containing Ketoconazole, selenium sulfide, Zinc pyrithione
  - Systemic therapy-One oral dose of fluconazole 400 mg/ Ketoconazole and itraconazole are very effective griesofulvin is not effective.

54. **Which of the following is not a part of P. versicolor treatment-** *(PGMEE 2015)*
   a. Griseofulvin
   b. Clotrimazole
   c. Ketocanazoe
   d. Selenium sulfide

   [Ref: IADVL Textbook of Dermatology 4th Edition Vol 1 Pg 508]

55. **Selenium sulfide is indicated for treating?** *(DNB pattern Dec' 2007)*
   a. Tinea versicolor
   b. Mixed mycotic infections
   c. Tinea corporis
   d. Candidiasis only

   [Ref: Comprehensive dermatologic drug therapy by Wolverton 2nd/e /p 557]

50.	d
51.	d
52.	b
53.	a
54.	a
55.	a

Explanation

- Selenium sulfide is a liquid antiseborrheic, antifungal preparation for topical application only. Indicated for treatment of tinea versicolor and seborrheic dermatitis. Available as 2.5% lotion and shampoos

56. Spaghetti and meat ball appearance is seen with:
a. Pityriasis versicolor   *(PGMEE 2013)*
b. Lichen planus
c. Acne rosacea
d. Pityriasis rosacea

[Ref: IADVL Textbook of Dermatology 4th Edition Vol 1 Pg 507]

57. A 11 year old boy presents with hypopigmented patches over skin of face and chest as shown in the image. Most likely diagnosis is:
(PGMEE 2016-17; Recent pattern June 2018)

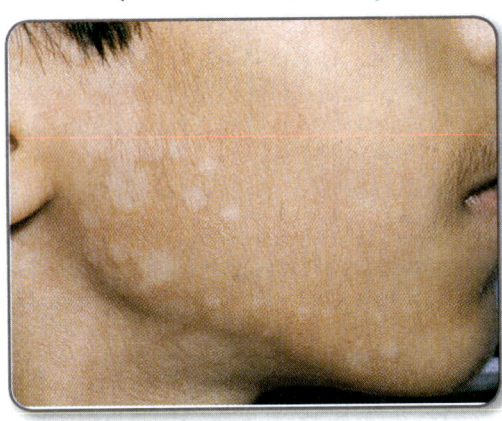

a. Photogenic dermatitis
b. Cholesma
c. Pityriasis versicolor
d. Pityriasis alba

[Ref: IADVL Textbook of Dermatology 4th Edition Vol 1 Pg 507]

Explanation

Approach to Pityriasis Related Lesions

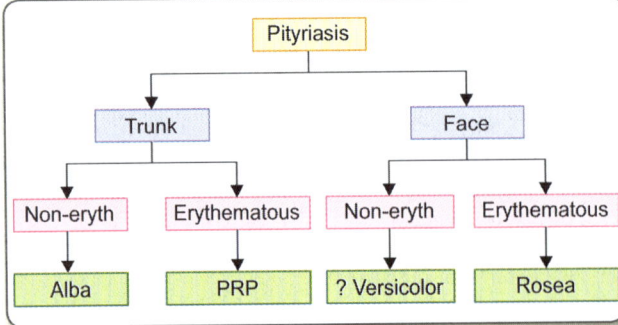

- Pityriasis alba is a benign self limiting skin disorder that mostly affects children and young adults.
- Condition may be associated with eczema, a common skin disorder that causes scaly, itchy rashes.
- It appears as light-colored patches, especially on the cheeks.

58. Adult patient with multiple scaly macules over chest and back, test which can diagnose this condition is/are –
a. Skin biopsy   *(PGMEE 2015)*
b. 10% KOH mount
c. Wood Lamp examination
d. All the above

[Ref: IADVL Textbook of Dermatology 4th Edition Vol 1 Pg 507]

59. The following drug is effective in treatment of pityriasis versicolor –   *(PGMEE 2013)*
a. Griseofulvin   b. Ketoconazole
c. Metronidazole   d. Chloroquine

[Ref: IADVL Textbook of Dermatology 4th Edition Vol 1 Pg 508]

SCABIES

60. A middle aged man come to you with an itchy rash. The clinical picture and the causative organism are shown. Identify the condition.   *(NEET Pattern 2017)*

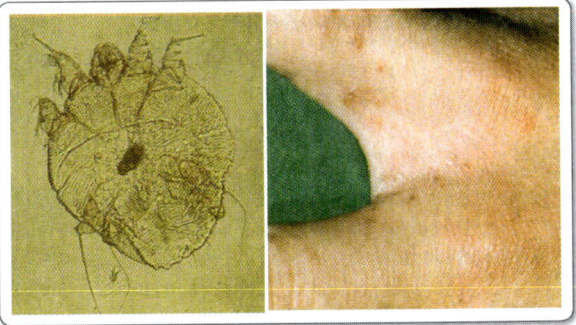

a. Scabies
b. Pediculosis
c. Insect bite hypersensitivity
d. Tinea

[Ref: Andrew's diseases of the Skin 12th edition page 445]

Explanation

- Scabies is caused by *Sarcoptes scabiei var. hominis*. They are whitish hemispherical mites. The female is about 0.4 × 0.3 mm. They have four pairs of legs. In the female the front two pairs end in 'suckers' and the hind two pairs in long trailing bristles. The body of is marked by transverse corrugations with spines and bristles on the dorsal surface.
- The cardinal features in the clinical diagnosis of scabies are:
  ○ The presence of the burrow, especially on the hands or penis;
  ○ The characteristic distribution pattern of lesions (papules/ papulovesicles)---Scabies characteristically involves the webs of the fingers, flexor aspects of the wrists, elbows, anterior axillary folds, the nipple and areola, umbilicus and periumbilical region, genitalia & upper thighs, knees and ankles.
  ○ The presence or history of similar illness in other members of the household or other contacts; and
  ○ Intense pruritus, which tends to worsen at night.

56.	**a**
57.	**c**
58.	**d**
59.	**b**
60.	**a**

61. Patient presents with pruritus of inter digital clefts of left hand as shown in the image. Identify the condition? *(PGMEE 2019)*

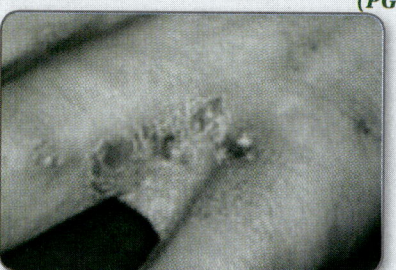

a. Sarcoptes scabiei   b. Dermatitis herpetiformis
c. Xerotic dermatitis   d. Erythema multiforme

[Ref: IADVL Textbook of Dermatology 4th/e pg 422-424]

62. Parasite shown in the photograph can cause which of the following disease: *(PGMEE 2016-17)*

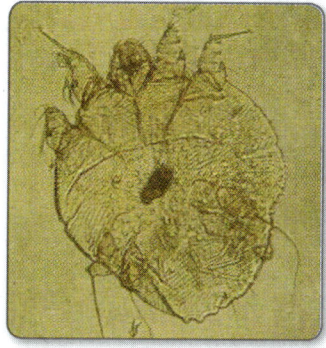

a. Babesia   b. Scabies
c. Dracunculosois   d. Filariasis

[Ref: IADVL Textbook of Dermatology 4th Edition Vol 1 Pg655]

63. The Burrows in scabies is in the: *(PGMEE 2015)*
a. Stratum corneum   b. Stratum granulosum
c. Dermis   d. Stratum basale

[Ref: IADVL Textbook of Dermatology 4th Edition Vol 1 Pg 655]

64. Treatment of choice for scabies: *(PGMEE 2015)*
a. Permethrin (5%)
b. Crotamiton (10%)
c. Malathion (0.5%)
d. Benzyl benzoate (25%)

[Ref: IADVL Textbook of Dermatology 4th Edition Vol 1 Pg 662]

65. Ivermectin in indicated in the treatment of? *(DNB pattern 2008)*
a. Syphilis   b. Scabies
c. Tuberculosis   d. Dermatophytosis

[Ref: Comprehensive dermatologic drug therapy by Wolverton 2nd/e /p 586]

Explanation

- Ivermectin, a macrolide without antibacterial activity has both ecto and endo parasiticidal activities. FDA approved indications-Strongyloidiasis, Onchocerciasis. Off label uses –Scabies, pediculosis

○ FDA approved indications-Strongyloidiasis, Onchocerciasis. Off label uses –Scabies, pediculosis
○ The dosage of ivermectin is 200 mcg/kg orally Lack of ovicidal activity.
- The dosage of ivermectin is 200 mcg/kg orally
  ○ Lack of ovicidal activity.
- Higher cure rates are obtained with two doses separated by 1-2 weeks interval
- It binds selectively and with strong affinity to glutamate-gated chloride ion channels which occur in invertebrate nerve and muscle cells. This leads to increased permeability of cell membranes to chloride ions, hyperpolarization of the nerve or muscle cell and death.
- Scabies treatment :

TOPICAL	ORAL
Precipitated sulphur	Ivermectin 200microgram/kg
Benzyl benzoate	
1% lindane (BHC)	
Crotamiton 10%	
5% permethrin	

66. All of the following are part of the treatment of scabies except- *(PGMEE 2015)*
a. Topical Permathrin
b. Long term oral steroids
c. Oral Ivermectin
d. Oral antihistamines

[Ref: IADVL Textbook of Dermatology 4th Edition Vol 1 Pg 661]

67. All of the following are part of the treatment of scabies except- *(PGMEE 2015)*
a. Topical Permathrin
b. Oral ivermactol
c. Long term oral steroids
d. Oral antihistamines

[Ref: IADVL Textbook of Dermatology 4th Edition Vol 1 Pg 507]

68. Characteristic lesion of scabies is – *(PGMEE 2012)*
a. Burrow   b. Papule
c. Vesicle   d. Fissure

[Ref: IADVL Textbook of Dermatology 4th Edition Vol 1 Pg 656]

69. Scabies in children differs from that in adults in that it affects – *(PGMEE 2014)*
a. Genitalia   b. Face
c. Webspace   d. Axilla

[Ref: IADVL Textbook of Dermatology 4th Edition Vol 1 Pg 656]

70. Scalp and face are involved in –
a. Nodular scabies   b. Infantile scabies
c. Adult scabies   d. None

[Ref: IADVL Textbook of Dermatology 4th Edition Vol 1 Pg 657]

71. Circle of hebra is associated with – *(PGMEE 2013)*
a. Lichen planus   b. Syphilis
c. Leprosy   d. Scabies

61.	a
62.	b
63.	a
64.	a
65.	b
66.	b
67.	c
68.	a
69.	b
70.	b
71.	d

72. Not a feature of scabies – *(PGMEE 2012)*
   a. Fever is a common finding
   b. Family history is found
   c. Burrows are seen in Stratum Corneum
   d. Itching is more severe at night

   [Ref: IADVL Textbook of Dermatology 4th Edition Vol 1 Pg 656]

73. A 15 years old female patient presented with history of severe itching, especially at night. There was family history of similar symptoms. One examination there were popular eruptions all over body. Close examination also showed following 'S' shaped burrows formation on wrists. Diagnosis is – *(PGMEE 2015)*
   a. Pyoderma
   b. Scabies
   c. Tinea corporis
   d. None of the above

   [Ref: IADVL Textbook of Dermatology 4th Edition Vol 1 Pg 656]

74. Treatment of choice of scabies in pregnancy– *(PGMEE 2013)*

   a. Gama-benzen hexachloride
   b. Permethrin
   c. Ivermectin
   d. None

   [Ref: IADVL Textbook of Dermatology 4th Edition Vol 1 Pg 663]

75. 8 year old boy has itchy rash all over the body, all family members are affected. What is the drug of choice– *(PGMEE 2013)*
   a. Prednisolone
   b. Topic permethrin
   c. Antibiotics
   d. Ivermectin

   [Ref: IADVL Textbook of Dermatology 4th Edition Vol 1 Pg 662]

MISCELLANEOUS

76. Maculae ceruleae is seen in- *(PGMEE 2015)*
   a. Scabies
   b. Lupus erythematosus
   c. Phthirus pubis
   d. Pediculosis capitis

   [Ref: Andrew's Diseases of the skin 12th edition Pg 441]

77. Rakesh, a 7-year old boy had itchy, excoriated papules on the arms and legs for 3 years. The disease was most severe in the rainy season and improved completely in winter. Most likely diagnosis is- *(PGMEE 2015)*
   a. Scabies
   b. Atopic dermatitis
   c. Insect bite hypersensitivity
   d. Urticaria

   [Ref: IADVL Textbook of Dermatology 4th Edition Vol 1 Pg 672]

72.	a
73.	b
74.	b
75.	b
76.	c
77.	c

GONORRHOEA

1. Patient presents with discharge perurethrum and microscopy shows presence of intracytoplasmic gram negative bacilli; what is the most probable diagnosis?
a. Donovanosis   **(PGMEE 2015)**
b. Bacterial vaginosis
c. Gonorrhea
d. Syphilis

[Ref: IADVL Textbook of Dermatology 4th ed. vol 3 pg 2900]

2. A patient presents with profuse purulent discharge from urethral meatus, 2 weeks after having sex with CSW. Most likely etiologic agent is:
a. H. ducrei   **(Recent Pattern June 2018)**
b. Neisseria gonorrhoeae
c. Chlamydia trachomitis
d. Trepanoma pallidum

[Ref: IADVL Textbook of Dermatology 4th edition vol 3 pg 2900]

Explanation

- Profuse purulent discharge per urethrum is characteristic of gonorrhoea. Causative agent is Neisseria gonorrhoeae bacterium.
- Incubation period: usually 1-14 days for symptomatic disease.
- Microscopy shows presence of intracytoplasmic gram negative bacilli

3. TOC for penicillin resistant gonorrhoea –
a. Ceftriaxone   **(PGMEE 2013)**
b. Erythromycin
c. Streptomycin
d. Ciprofloxacin

[Ref: IADVL Textbook of Dermatology 4th ed. vol 3 pg 2902]

4. In a patient of both gonococcal & non-gonococcal urethritis, what is the management? (NEET Pattern 2017)
a. Ceftriaxone 250 mg IM single dose
b. Cefixime 400 mg oral single dose
c. Azithrocycin 2 gm single dose
d. Ciprofloxacin 500 mg single dose

Explanation

- Sexually Transmitted Diseases Treatment Guidelines, 2015 by CDC
  - Monotherapy with Azithromycin 2 g as a single dose orally is effective against uncomplicated gonococcal infection, but concerns over the ease with which *N. gonorrhoeae* can develop resistance to macrolides should restrict its use to limited circumstances. Causes (35%) gastrointestinal distress
  - Since it is active against both N. gonorrhea and C. trachomatis, it is most useful in therapy of acute cervicitis and urethritis where there is no microbiological back up.

SYPHILIS

5. Rhagades are found in: **(PGMEE 2016-17)**
a. Primary syphilis
b. Secondary syphilis
c. Early stage of congenital syphilis
d. Postnatal congenital syphilis

[Ref: IADVL Textbook of Dermatology 4th ed. vol 3 pg 2799]

6. Bilateral symmetrical maculopapular rash on palms and soles is a feature of –   **(PGMEE 2015)**
a. Primary syphilis
b. Secondary syphilis
c. Tertiary syphilis
d. Congenital syphilis

[Ref: IADVL Textbook of Dermatology 4th ed. vol 3 pg 2783]

7. 19 year old male develops painless penile ulcers 9 days after sexual intercourse with a professional sex worker likely diagnosis is –   **(PGMEE 2014)**
a. Chancre   b. Herpes
c. Traumatic ulcer d. Chancroid

[Ref: IADVL Textbook of Dermatology 4th ed. vol 3 pg 2780]

8. In secondary syphilis all are seen except:
a. Proteinuria   **(PGMEE 2014)**
b. Condyloma lata
b. Arthritis
d. Interstitial keratitis

[Ref: IADVL Textbook of Dermatology 4th ed. vol 3 pg 2785, 2789]

9. Chancre redux' is a clinical feature of
a. Early relapsing syphilis   **(DNB pattern 2008)**
b. Late syphilis
c. Chancroid
d. Recurrent herpes simplex infection

(Ref. Sexually transmitted diseases and HIV/AIDS by V.K. Sharma 2nd ed. pg 276)

Explanation

- Occurrence of a relapsing lesion resembling a primary chance at the site of initial primary chancre has been reffered as 'Chancre redux'.
- It results of proliferation of residual treponemes at initial site.

10. Which of the following is characterized by a solitary painless ulcer on genitalia-   **(PGMEE 2015)**
a. Hard chancre   b. Herpes
c. Soft chancre (chancroid) d. Traumatic ulcer

[Ref: IADVL Textbook of Dermatology 4th ed. vol 3 pg 2780]

11. DOC in primary syphillis is –   **(PGMEE 2014)**
a. Benzathine penicilline
b. Oral penicilline
c. Crystalline penicilline
d. Corticosteroid

[Ref: IADVL Textbook of Dermatology 4th ed. vol 3 pg 2813]

1.	c
2.	b
3.	a
4.	c
5.	c
6.	b
7.	a
8.	d
9.	a
10.	a
11.	a

12. Jarisch-Herxheimer reaction is caused by all except – *(PGMEE 2014)*

   a. Typhoid fever   b. Brucellosis
   c. Legionellosis   d. Syphilis

[Ref: Harrison's 19th/e pg. 1140, 1147]

13. Best confirmatory serological test for syphilis is? *(PGMEE 2012)*

   a. VDRL   b. TPHA
   c. MHA-TP   d. FTA-ABS

[Ref: Harrison 19th/e pg 1132]

14. Most specific test for diagnosis of Syphilis *(DNB pattern 2008)*

   a. VDRL   b. FTA-ABS
   c. RPR   d. Kahn test

(Ref. sexually transmitted diseases and HIV/AIDS by V.K. Sharma 2nd ed. pg 304)

Explanation

- Serological tests for syphilis (STS):
- Non-treponemal tests: Antigen: Cardiolipin, cholesterol and lecithin; Antibody: Reagin (Nonspecific)
  - Complement fixation tests, e.g. Wassermann reaction, Kolmer test
  - Flocculation tests, e.g. VDRL slide test, rapid plasma reagin RPR) card test, automated reagin test (ART), reagin screen test (RST).
- Treponemal tests: Antigen: The entire organism (T. pallidum living/dead) or its components; Antibody: Specific antibodies
  - Treponema pallidum immobilization test (TPI)
  - Fluorescent treponemal antibody absorption test (FTA-Abs), and FTA-Abs double staining test (FTA-Abs DS)
  - Treponema pallidum hemagglutination assay (TPHA), microhemagglutination for T. pallidum (MHA-TP) and hemagglutination treponemal test for syphilis (HATTS)
  - Enzyme-linked immunosorbent assay (ELISA)
- Most sensitive test- VDRL
- Most specific test - Fluorescent treponemal antibody absorption test (FTA-Abs)

15. Test done to diagnosis syphilis in newborn if mother is syphilitic- *(PGMEE 2015)*

   a. ZN staining
   b. Syphilis Capita M test
   c. Fluoroescent antigen test
   d. Detection of IgG

[Ref: Harrison 16th/e pg. 982]

16. Treponema pallidum crosses placenta: *(PGMEE 2014-15)*

   a. After 36 weeks   b. After 28 weeks
   c. After 2nd trimester   d. At any stage of pregnancy

[Ref: Harrison's 19th/e pg.1133]

17. Hutchison's Triad is seen in- *(PGMEE 2015)*

   a. Congenital Syphilis   b. Primary syphilis
   c. Tertiary syphilis   d. Secondary Syphilis

[Ref: Nelson 20th/e/p 1472 table 218-1]

12.	c
13.	d
14.	b
15.	b
16.	d
17.	a
18.	a
19.	d
20.	d
21.	c

18. Doc of HIV with syphilis: *(Recent Pattern June 2018)*

   a. Benzathine penicillin G
   b. Cefazolin
   c. Indomethacin
   d. NTG

[Ref: IADVL Textbook of Dermatology 4th edition vol 3 pg 2813]

Explanation

Treatment of syphilis

Stage	Preferred T/t	Alternative T/t
primary, secondary, and early latent syphilis	Benzathine penicillin G 2.4 million units IM in a single dose	doxycycline 100 mg PO BID x 2 weeks or tetracycline 500 mg PO QID x 2 weeks.
late latent syphilis or syphilis of unknown duration & normal CSF study	benzathine penicillin G 2.4 million units weekly for 3 weeks	doxycycline 100 mg PO BID x 4 weeks or tetracycline 500 mg PO QID x 4 weeks

- HIV-infected patients who have syphilis may be at increased risk for neurologic complications and may have higher rates of treatment failure with currently recommended regimens.

CHANCROID

19. Soft sore is caused by? *(PGMEE 2012)*

   a. T. Pallidum
   b. Calymmatobacterium granulomatis
   c. Chlamydia trachomitis
   d. H ducreyi

[Ref: IADVL Textbook of Dermatology 4th ed. vol 3 pg 2835]

20. Causative agent of chancroid- *(DNB pattern June 2010, dec 2010 ; PGMEE 2015)*

   a. LGV   b. Chlamydia trachomitis
   c. T. palladium   d. Hemophillus ducrey

[Ref: IADVL Textbook of Dermatology 4th ed. vol 3 pg 2835]

Explanation

H. Ducrei	Chancroid
N. Gonnerea	Gonorrhea
T. Pallidum	Syphilis

DONOVANOSIS

21. Donovanosis is caused by: *(PGMEE 2014)*

   a. H. ducreyi
   b. T. pertenue
   c. Calymmatobacter granulomatis
   d. Chlamydia trachomatis

[Ref: IADVL Textbook of Dermatology 4th ed. vol 3 pg 2848]

22. In which of the following diseases "pseudobubo" is feature- *(PGMEE 2015)*
a. LGV
b. Donovanosis
c. Gonorrhea
d. Syphilis

[Ref: IADVL Textbook of Dermatology 4th ed. vol 3 pg 2851]

23. Pseudo bubo is seen in – *(PGMEE 2015)*
a. LGV
b. Syphilis
c. Donovanosis
d. Chancroid

[Ref: IADVL Textbook of Dermatology 4th ed. vol 3 pg 2851]

LGV

24. Lymphogranuloma venereum (LGV) is caused by: *(Recent Pattern June 2018)*
a. Chlamydia trachomatis
b. Calymmatobacterium donovani
c. H. influenzae
d. H. ducrei

[Ref: IADVL Textbook of Dermatology 4th edition vol 3 pg 2900]

Explanation
- LGV is a sexually transmitted chronic infection of the lymphatic system.
- It is caused by any of 3 different types (serovars) of *Chlamydia trachomatis*. The infection is not caused by the same bacteria that cause genital chlamydia.

25. Groove sign is seen in – *(PGMEE 2015)*
a. Genital herpes
b. Donovanosis
c. LGV
d. Chancroid

[Ref: IADVL Textbook of Dermatology 4th ed. vol 3 pg 2860]

26. LGV, treatment of choice is- *(PGMEE 2015)*
a. Azithromycin
b. Doxycycline
c. Benzathine penicillin
d. Cefalosporins

[Ref: IADVL Textbook of Dermatology 4th ed. vol 3 pg 2868]

27. Drug of choice for bubos in a pregnant female is-
a. Ceftriaxone *(PGMEE 2015)*
b. Erythromycin
c. Doxycycline
d. Tetracycline

[Ref: IADVL Textbook of Dermatology 4th ed. vol 3 pg 2868]

28. Genital elephantiasis is caused by- *(PGMEE 2015)*
a. LGV
b. Syphilis
c. Gonorrhea
d. Herpes genitalis

[Ref: IADVL Textbook of Dermatology 4th ed. vol 3 pg 2862]

HERPES GENITALIS

29. Genital Herpes simplex lesion is characterized by:
a. Single vesicle *(PGMEE 2016-17)*
b. Multiple small ulcers
c. Non-tender inguinal lymph nodes
d. Painless lesions

[Ref: IADVL Textbook of Dermatology 4th ed. vol 3 pg 2873]

30. A young sexually active old man presents with 3-4 vesiculo bullous lesion over shaft of penis. He also complaints of pain in defecation but there are no GI symptoms. On scrapping the base of vesicles smear reveals multinucleate giant cells. Biopsy is shown below. Most likely causes of this condition is:
(Recent Pattern June 2018)

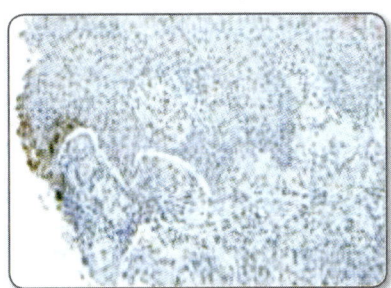

a. Hemophilus ducrei
b. HSV-2
c. Varicella zoster virus
d. Leishmania donovani

[Ref: IADVL Textbook of Dermatology 4th edition vol 3 pg 2835]

Explanation
- *HSV type 2* causes usually affects genitalia. Genital herpes causes lesions in the form of blisters or groups of small ulcers (open sores) over penis in men. Tzanck smear test is mainly used to rapidly detect a herpes infection or to distinguish SJS/TEN from SSSS. **Multinucleate giant cells** are seen from scrapped/opened up vesicle.
- *Hemophilus ducrei* causes soft sore multiple excavated ulcers over penis which bleed on touch. Prepucial margin is the MC site.
- Other important D/d of perianal ulcers:-
  ○ Gonorrhea is characterized by acute anterior arthritis associated with thick yellow urethral discharge. Perianal ulceration is not a feature of gonorrhea.
  ○ Although HIV can be considered in the differential diagnosis of Perianal ulcers, but is usually associated with GIT symptoms.

31. Blistering, painful unilateral vesicles after unprotected sexual intercourse in the genital area is suggestive of – *(PGMEE 2015)*
a. Syphilis
b. Gonorrhoea
c. Herpes genitalis
d. Donovanosis

[Ref: IADVL Textbook of Dermatology 4th ed. vol 3 pg 2873]

32. A 32 year old male presents with painful genital ulcer which started as vesicle 4 days back. Which kit should be used for treatment at peripheral heath facility: *(PGMEE 2016-17)*
a. Kit-1
b. Kit-2
c. Kit-3
d. Kit-5

33. Homosexual man with pain in defecation, no gastrointestinal symptoms, clustered ulcers extending into anal canal. Diagnosis- *(PGMEE 2013)*
a. Herpes genitalis
b. Gonorrhea
c. HIV
d. CMV

[Ref: IADVL Textbook of Dermatology 4th ed. vol 3 pg 2873]

22.	b
23.	c
24.	a
25.	c
26.	b
27.	b
28.	a
29.	b
30.	b
31.	c
32.	d
33.	a

34. Frei's test is diagnostic of *(DNB pattern 2007)*
a. Lymphogranuloma venerum
b. Lymphogranuloma inguinale
c. Donovanosis
d. Soft chancre

[Ref: sexually transmitted diseases and HIV/AIDS V.K. Sharma 2nd ed. pg 392]

Explanation

- The test consists of the intradermal injection of 0.1 ml antigen into the skin of the volar aspect of one forearm and a similar quantity of yolk sac material into the skin of the other forearm as control.
- The test is read at 48 h; a positive reaction is the development of a papule at least 6 mm in diameter, provided that the papule produced by the control is 5 mm or less in diameter.
- The test usually becomes positive after the appearance of buboes, i.e. 2–8 weeks after infection. Because the Frei antigen is common to all Chlamydia, it produces cross-reaction in infections caused by other chlamydial organisms.
- The test also tends to remain positive for several years, possibly for life, despite treatment.

GENITAL WARTS

35. A young female complains of genital wart. The agent implicated is: *(2007)*
a. Treponema pallidum
b. Adenovirus
c. Human papilloma virus
d. Pox virus

[Ref. Sexually transmitted diseases and HIV/AIDS by V.K. Sharma 2nd ed. pg 430]

Explanation

Human papilloma virus	Anogenital warts
Treponema pallidum	Syphilis
Pox virus	Molluscum contagiosum

36. Cervical warts are seen with which HPV:
a. 11, 13 *(PGMEE 2013)*
b. 6, 11
c. 17, 18
d. 5, 8

[Ref: IADVL Textbook of Dermatology 4th ed. vol 3 pg 2884]

37. Low risk type of HPV *(PGMEE 2014)*
a. Type- 6
b. Type – 16
c. Type – 18
d. Type – 31

[Ref: IADVL Textbook of Dermatology 4th ed. vol 3 pg 2884]

38. Drug of choice for genital warts is: *(PGMEE 2015)*
a. Acyclovir
b. Interferon alpha
c. Minocycline
d. Podophyllin

[Ref: IADVL Textbook of Dermatology 4th ed. vol 3 pg 2884]

39. Imiquimod is used in the treatment of: *(PGMEE 2015)*
a. Psoriasis
b. Lichen planus
c. Molluscuma contagiousum
d. Condyloma acuminata

[Ref: IADVL Textbook of Dermatology 4th ed. vol 3 pg 2885]

MISCELLANEOUS

40. Not A sexually transmitted disease – *(PGMEE 2014)*
a. Trichomonisis
b. HBV
c. Pinta
d. Candidiasis

[Ref: IADVL Textbook of Dermatology 4th ed. vol 3 pg 2831]

34.	a
35.	c
36.	b
37.	a
38.	d
39.	d
40.	c

TOPICAL THERAPY

1. Least potent topical steroid: *(PGMEE 2014)*
a. Hydrocortisone 1%
b. Clobetasol propionate 0.5%
c. Halobetasol propionate 0.05%
d. Betamethasone dipropionate 0.05%

[Ref: IADVL Textbook of Dermatology 4th ed. Vol 3 Pg 2257]

2. Depigmenting agent of choice in treatment of dermatological disorders is: *(PGMEE 2015)*
a. Kojic acid
b. Hydroquinone
c. Azelaic acid
d. Zinc

[Ref: IADVL Textbook of Dermatology 4th ed. Vol 3 Pg 2291]

3. Whitfield's ointment consists of : *(PGMEE 2015)*
a. 2% salicylic acid + 6% benzoic acid
b. 2% benzoic acid + 6% salicylic acid
c. 3% salicylic acid + 6% benzoic acid
d. 3% benzoic acid + 6% salicylic acid

[Ref: Wikipedia]

SYSTEMIC THERAPY

4. Maximum cumulative does of isotretinoin shouldn't exceed for acne treatment: *(PGMEE 2012)*
a. 30-60 mg/kg
b. 60-90 mg/kg
c. 90-120 mg/kg
d. 120-150 mg/kg

[Ref: IADVL Textbook of Dermatology 4th ed. Vol 3 Pg 2331]

PHYSICAL TREATMENTS- PHOTOTHERAPY, PHOTOCHEMOTHERAPY, LASERS

5. Machine shown below in the image is use for: *(PGMEE 2016-17)*

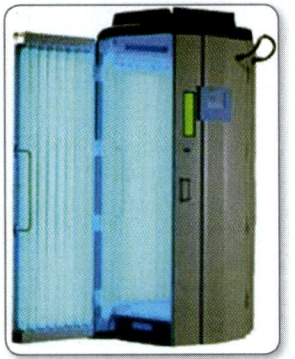

a. Psoriasis
b. Vitiligo
c. Lichen planus
d. a and b both

[Ref: IADVL Textbook of Dermatology 4th ed. vol 1 pg 1053]

Explanation

■ Image shown is of a phototherapy unit for UVA light therapy.

6. Photochemotherapy is useful in: *(DNB pattern 2007)*
a. Pityriasis rosea
b. Psoriasis
c. Lichen planus
d. Ichthyosis vulgaris

[Ref. Comprehensive dermatologic drug therapy by Wolverton 2nd ed. pg 324]

Explanation

Photochemotherapy (PUVA):

■ FDA approved indications
  ○ Psoriasis
  ○ Vitiligo
  ○ Increasing tolerance to sunlight/ enhancing pigmentation
■ Off-label dermatological uses
  ○ Mycosis fungoides/ sezary syndrome
  ○ Palmoplantar pustulosis
  ○ Atopic dermatitis
  ○ Chronic hand dermatitis
  ○ Pityriasis lichenoides
  ○ Alopecia areata
  ○ Morphea

7. Tumor not caused by PUVA is: *(DNB pattern June 2009)*
a. Melanoma
b. BCC
c. Cutaneous T cell lymphoma
d. SCC

[Ref. Comprehensive dermatologic drug therapy by Wolverton 2nd ed. pg 329]

Explanation

■ Long term adverse effects of PUVA therapy
  ○ Photoaging of skin
  ○ Nonmelanoma skin cancer: SCC > BCC, keratoacanthoma
  ○ Melanoma

1.	a
2.	b
3.	c
4.	d
5.	d
6.	b
7.	c

CHAPTER 16

Surgery

BREAST

BENIGN BREAST DISEASES

- *Acute bacterial mastitis*
  - MC cause → Staphylococcus aureus.
  - Breastfeeding should be withheld. Fréquent emptying is advised.
  - DOC is cloxacillin.
- Granulomatous mastitis is caused by → Fungus, Antibodies to milk antigens, TB [But NOT caused by Staphylococcus].
- Intramammary abscess is treated by → Radial incision & drainage.
- *Mondor's disease (String phlebitis)*
  - It is thrombophlebitis of the superficial veins of breast.
  - Lateral thoracic vein is MC involved.
  - Rx: supportive. Resolves spontaneously in 4-6 weeks.
- *Duct Ectasia (Periductal Mastitis)*
  - Dilatation of breast ducts with periductal inflammation.
  - A/w smoking.
  - Nipple discharge may be of any colour.
  - Rx: Hadfield's operation
- "Peau d'orange" appearance of breast is due to → Obstruction of dermal lymphatic.
- *Zuska's disease:*
  - Aka "lactiferous fistula"

- A rare but painful breast disorder.
- It is a form of epithelial squamous breast metaplasia.
- Treatment is antibiotics, I & D.
- *Fibroadenoma breast:*
  - Aka "Breast mouse"
  - MC benign tumour of breast.
  - A/w increased sensitivity of a focal area of breast to estrogen.
  - Usually painless
  - MC site → Lower part of breast
  - X-ray/mammography → Popcorn calcification.
  - No discharge from nipple, No axillary LN.
  - Rx: Enucleated/excised using Gaillard Thomas (submammary), periareolar or radial/curved incisions.
- *Fibroadenosis:*
  - Usually painful
  - MC site → Upper & outer quadrant of breast
- *Fibrocystic Disease of the Breast:*
  - Aka Cooper's/Reclus disease or fibroadenomatosis
  - No risk of malignancy.

INVESTIGATIONS

- Triple assessment of breast includes:-
  - Clinical examination
  - Radiological imaging (USG in young females/mammography in elderly)
  - Pathological examination (FNAC/ Core biopsy)
- *Breast Imaging:*
  - *Mammography is investigation of choice for*
    - Females >35 yrs & for screening purposes.
    - Detecting DCIS
    - Microcalcifications
  - *MRI is investigation of choice in*
    - High risk females >35
    - Implanted breasts

- Breast conservative surgery in CA breast
- Scarred breasts
- *USG (Ultrasound) is investigation of choice in*
  - Females <35 yrs of age.
  - To distinguish solid from cystic lesions.
- Features suggestive of cancer in mammography:-
  - Mass effect
  - Distortion of architecture
  - Spicules, branching calcification, microcalcification
  - Clustering
  - Loss of symmetry

MASTECTOMY

	Procedure & Structures Removed	Structures Preserved
Total/Simple Mastectomy	▪ Removal of all breast tissue, nipple areolar complex & skin without dissecting axilla (except axillary tail) ○ Prophylactic SM done in BRCA 1 & 2 mutation ○ Toilet SM: in case of ulcerated CA breast	▪ Axilla
Extended Simple Mastectomy	▪ Removal of all breast tissue, nipple areolar complex & skin & level 1 axillary nodes	▪ Level 2 axillary nodes
Modified Radical (MRM)	▪ Breast & associated structures (including nipple, areola) dissected 'en bloc' + Axillary LN. ▪ 3 types:- ○ **Patey's:** Pectoralis minor (but NOt the pectoralis major) is divided & removed to dissect level 1,2 & 3 LN. ○ **Auchincloss:** Preservation of both pectoralis major & minor. **Only level 1 & 2 LNs are dissected** after retraction of pectoralis minor. ○ **Scanlon's:** Pectoralis minor is **divided** (but not removed). Level 1,2 & 3 LN are removed.	**A**xillary vein **B**ell's long thoracic nerve **C**ephalic vein Nerve to latissimus **D**orsi & pectoralis major
Halstaed's Radical Mastectomy	▪ Same as MRM + **Pectoralis major & minor are removed** ▪ *Haagenson & Stiles RM* are traditional radical mastectomy techniques.	ABC & D
Extended RM	RM + Ribs, LN (Internal mammary lymph nodes)	
Super RM	▪ ERM + removal of supraclavicular and mediastinal LN	

BREAST RECONSTRUCTION

- The easiest type of reconstruction is done using a silicone gel implant under the pectoralis major muscle.
- Commonly used flaps in breast reconstruction include:
  ○ TRAM flap: Transverse rectus abdominis muscle
  ○ LD FLAP : Latissimus dorsi flap
  ○ DIEP : Deep inferior epigastric perforator flap
  ○ SEIA : Superficial inferior epigastric artery perforator flap
- Flap/Muscles NOT used → Pectoralis major myocutaneous flap.

- If a patient is likely to need postoperative radiotherapy then a delayed reconstruction using a flap often gives a better result. Radiotherapy onto a prosthesis often leads to a high incidence of capsular contracture and unacceptable results.
- Nipple reconstruction is a relatively simple procedure that can be performed under a local anesthesia.
- During breast reconstruction surgery the structure which is preserved → Pectoralis major.
- Patey's mastectomy involves removal of all of the following expect → Pectoralis major.

MISCELLANEOUS

- "Peau d'orange" appearance of breast is due to → Obstruction of dermal lymphatic.
- Granulomatous mastitis is caused by → Fungus, Antibodies to milk antigens, TB [But NOT caused by Staphylococcus].
- *Papilloma* is a proliferating breast mass.
- *Nerve injured in modified radical mastectomy with axillary clearance for CA breast:*

  ○ Long thoracic nerve of Bell (Winging of scapula and inability to carry weight above shoulders)
  ○ Intercostobrachial neuralgia (Pain/ tingling along medial aspect of arm). Intercostobrachial nerve is likely to be injured during **Sentinel node biopsy.**
- CA Breast local spread does not involve → Latissimus dorsi becoz it is most lateral.

- MC cause of cellulitis is → Streptococcus.
- MC nosocomial infection → Respiratory infection.
- MCC of septicemia → Gram-positive bacteria.
- Which of the following is not an immediate cause of death → Septicemia.
- *Lymphedema*
  - Lymphedema precox is MC type of primary lymphedema .
  - Primary lymphedema may be a/w many other congenital or genetic abnormalities.
  - MC bacterial infection in lymphedema → Streptococcus.
- *Milroy's disease* is primary lymphedema usually seen in females. May also be a/w arterial-venous abnormalities such as hemangioma or lymphangioma, or other genetic conditions such as
  - Klippel-Trenaunay syndrome or
  - Park-Weber Syndrome
- *Stewart – Treves syndrome* is a angiosarcoma (cutaneous) developing in long standing chronic lymphedema. Seen mostly after MRM (Modified radical mastectomy).
- The severe lymphedema seen in arms, legs, or genitalia is also called **elephantiasis**. It is seen in **Filariasis**.
- A *Felon* is an abscess between the specialized fingertip septae in the distal pulp. Most common site of felon is → Thumb. During Felon drainage incision taken as → From tip of finger to 1 cm distal to DIP.
- Pulp space infection is very painful condition.
- *Ainhum* is most commonly seen at → Base of a toe.
- *Abscesses*
  - Drained by giving **cruciate incision** at the site of maximum pointing (Hilton's method).
  - Collar stud abscess is acute suppurative infection of a LN presenting as a stud-like blister. Seen in- Tubercular cold abscess/ cervical lymphadenitis, felon, deep palmar space infection
  - Cold abscess: No sign of acute inflammation is seen (i.e. it is not red/ warm/tender). Seen mainly in TB and rarely in staphylococcal infection.
- Ganglion is → Collection of neurons outside CNS.
- *Hemorrhage after surgery:-*
  - Primary (1°) hemorrhage is hemorrhage occurring **immediately** as a result of an injury (or surgery).
  - Reactionary hemorrhage is delayed hemorrhage (**within 24 hours**) and is usually caused by **dislodgement of clot** by resuscitation, normalization of BP and vasodilatation, from technical failure such as slippage of a ligature.
  - Secondary (2°) hemorrhage is caused by sloughing of the wall of a vessel. It usually occurs **7-14 days** after injury and is precipitated by factors such as infection, pressure necrosis (such as from a drain) or malignancy.
- Best way to control external hemorrhage → Direct pressure.
- For reimplantation digits are stored in plastic bags with ice.
- A patient undergone laparoscopic surgery complaints of pain in left shoulder, most common causes is → subdiaphragmatic migration of gas and irritation of phrenic nerve.
- Carbon dioxide (CO_2) & N_2O are preferred gases for creating pneumoperitoneum during laparoscopy.
- CO_2 is the most frequently used gas for laparoscopy.
- All of the following are used in cryosurgery except → Helium.
- The bipolar cautery is NOT preferred over monopolar cautery in → Surgery of the Hip.
- All of the following drugs causes hirsutism except → Mefepristone.
- Organ most damaged in bomb explosion → Ear.
- Phantom limb is based upon → Law of projection (Feel that amputated limb is still there).
- Potato nodes are features of → Sarcoidosis.
- For parenteral nutrition, a peripheral venous catheter is preferred for short-term parenteral nutrition (less than 14 days). Tunneling subclavian line is recommended for long-term use (more than 30 days).
- *Choice of fluid/Best fluid for*
  - Resuscitation during shock state → Crystalloids (NS preferred > RL).
  - In case of burn in first 24 hours is → Ringer lactate.
  - Treatment of Dengue shock → Ringer lactate.
- Which of following is hypertonic → 3% normal saline.
- Operation theater fire is most commonly due to → Electrosurgical equipment.

- Bayonet artifacts seen during USG guided nerve block of → Axillary nerve block.
- Hypoglycemia not caused by → Pheochromocytoma.
- In TPN vein cannulated is → Internal jugular vein.
- *VAP – scoring (PIS Score) system* contains
  - Tracheal secretions
  - Chest radiography
  - Culture of tracheal aspirate
  - Body temperature
  - TLC
  - Oxygenation
- A patient on clopidogrel had severe bleeding mode of transfusion → Platelet.
- *Hormones raised in postoperative patient (Stress hormones):*
  - Cortisol
  - Epinephrine, NE
  - Glucagon
  - ACTH
  - Renin, Angiotensin-II, Aldosterone

- MCC of pulmonary emboli originate during surgery → Femoral vein.
- Antibiotics should be given within 1 hour prior to surgery or at the time of induction of anesthesia.
- MC cause of catheter induced UTI → E.coli.
- NOT a medical use of erythropoietin → Megaloblastic anemia.
- Type of shock which usually have warm peripheral extremities → Neurogenic Shock.
- *Crush syndrome:*
  - Feature of crush syndrome → Myoglobinuria.
  - NOT associated with → hypercalcemia.
- High tension injuries & electric burns damage to underlying muscle and cause rapid onset of compartmental syndrome → release of myoglobin → Renal dysfunction → Myoglobinuria.
- Compartment syndrome is confirmed when intracompartmental pressure is > 40 mm Hg.

WOUND HEALING

- *Wound Healing:*
  - More granulation tissue and fibrosis is seen in 2° healing compared to 1° healing.
  - An Incisional wound heals by → 1° Healing.
  - A full thickness wound that is not sutured heals by → 2° Healing.
- *Wound Closure:*
  - Each suture is separated by gap of **twice the thickness of skin**.
  - **Jenkin's Rule** - Suture material length must be in the ratio of 4: 1 to the wound length.
  - **Lembert Suture**: It's a **sero muscular suture** used for bowel anastomosis. It's done above the inner layer of anastomosis with the intent of holding the inner sutures.
  - **Cheatle Split**: Making a cut in the anti mesentric border for enlarging the lumen of distal collapsed bowel in case of bowel to bowel anastomosis.
  - Bowel anastomosis leaks on **7th** post operative day.
- *Wound Dehiscence (Burst Abdomen):*
  - Partial or total disruption of operative wound
  - 1st sign of burst abdomen - Serous/ Serosanguinous drainage.
  - MC observed between 6th and 8th post operative days.
  - Evisceration-extrusion of bowel after rupture.

  - Rx: Thorough Saline wash & elective closure using tension sutures at the earliest.
- *Predisposing factors for Wound Dehiscence*
  Local Risk factors:
  - Inadequate closure (Absorbable suture, Multilayer > Single layer in causing dehisence)
  - Midline Incisions > Transverse incision
  - Increased Intra-abdominal pressure.
  - Poor/no wound healing due to infections, seroma, hematoma and presence of drain.

  Systemic Risk factors:
  - Old age.
- Drainage of cervical abscess is an example of → Dirty infected wound.
- Correct management of abdominal compartment syndrome → Urgent Opening of the surgical wound and application of the Bogota bag.
- All of the following are principles of negative pressure wound therapy except → Clearance of infection.
- *Vaccum assisted wound closure is contraindicated in*
  - Chronic osteomyelitis.
  - Eschar
  - Ureterostomy
  - Malignancy

CLASSIFICATION OF SURGICAL WOUNDS

Class	Features	Example
Clean Wounds (Class I)	▪ Include those in which no infection is present; only skin microflora potentially contaminates the wound. No hollow viscus is entered. ▪ No inflammation	▪ Hernia repair, breast biopsy.
Clean/ contaminated Wounds (Class II)	▪ Those wounds in which a hollow viscus such as the respiratory, alimentary or genitourinary tracts with indigenous bacterial flora is opened but under controlled circumstances without significant spillage of contents. ▪ No inflammation.	▪ Cholecystectomy, elective GI surgery.
Contaminated Wounds (Class III)	▪ Include open accidental wounds encountered early after injury, those with extensive introduction of bacteria into a normally sterile area of the body due to major breaks in sterile technique (e.g. open cardiac massage); uncontrolled spillage of viscus contents such as from the intestine. ▪ Inflammation is apparent.	▪ Penetrating abdominal trauma, large tissue injury.
Dirty Wounds (Class IV)	▪ Traumatic wounds with significant delay in treatment ▪ Necrotic tissue /pus is present. Includes those wounds created to access a perforated viscus accompanied by a high degree of contamination. ▪ Severe inflammation is seen	▪ Perforated diverticulitis, necrotizing fascitis.

WOUND CLOSURE AND HEALING

Classification of Wound Closure and Healing			
Primary intention	▪ Wound edges opposed	▪ Normal healing	▪ Minimal scar
Secondary intention	▪ Wound left open	▪ Heals by granulation contraction and epithelialisation ▪ Increased inflammation and proliferation	▪ Poor scar
Tertiary intention (also called delayed primary intention)	▪ Wound initially left open	▪ Edges later opposed when healing conditions favourable	

BARIATRIC SURGERY

- *Bariatric surgical procedures include:*
  - Vertical banded gastroplasty.
  - Intragastric balloon (IGB) placement
  - Endoscopic sleeve gastroplasty (ESG)
  - Adjustable gastric banding
  - Roux-en Y gastric bypass
  - Biliopancreatic diversion
  - Duodenal switch
- *Indications for bariatric surgery*
  - Morbid obesity
    - BMI > 40
    - BMI > 35 with serious comorbid conditions
  - Acceptable operative candidate
  - Motivated to adhere to the postoperative lifestyle changes
  - Well informed regarding risks of surgery
  - Able to participate in long-term follow-up
  - No substance abuse issues
  - No (or under control) significant psychiatric conditions

DAMAGE CONTROL SURGERY (DCS)

- Coordinating staged operative interventions with periods of aggressive resuscitation to salvage trauma patients sustaining major injuries.
- Damage control includes an abbreviated laparotomy, temporary packing, and closure of the abdomen in an effort to blunt the physiologic response to prolonged shock & massive hemorrhage.
- In these patients limited physiological reserve & persistent operative stress results in exacerbation of their underlying **hypothermia, coagulopathy** & **acidosis** (*The trauma triad of death*) initiating a vicious cycle that culminates

in death. This combination is commonly seen in patients who have sustained severe traumatic injuries.

- In these situations, abrupt termination of the procedure after control of surgical hemorrhage & contamination, followed by ICU resuscitation & staged reconstruction, can be life saving.
- **Phase of Damage Control Surgery**
  - Phase I (initial exploration) - Consists of an initial operative exploration to attain

rapid control of active hemorrhage & contamination
  - Phase II (Secondary resuscitation) - Following completion of initial exploration, critically ill patients are transferred to ICU.
  - Phase III (definitive operation) - It consists of planned re-exploration & definitive repair of injuries
- The essential components of damage control surgery are all except → Definitive reconstruction.

ULCERS

- *Some punched out ulcers:*
  - Mortorell's ulcer found in leg in poorly controlled HTN.

  - Deep trophic ulcer
  - Peptic ulcer
  - Syphilitic/gummatous ulcer (thin base + wash leather slough)

Ulcers	Description
Martorell's ulcer	▪ Due to HTN and atherosclerosis ▪ Seen in calf region
Marjolin's ulcer	▪ Ulcer developed in chronic scars or malignant cells most commonly squamous cell CA.
Decubitus ulcer	▪ Also k/as Bed sores/Pressure sores. ▪ They develop when external pressure is **>30 mm Hg**. ▪ Sites: **Ischium** (M/c site) > greater trochanter > sacrum > heel > malleolus (lateral > medial) > occiput.
Trophic ulcers (Neuropathic ulcers)	▪ Painless, punched out ulcers d/to impaired nutrition, defective blood supply, neurological deficit ▪ (so also k/as **neurogenic ulcer).** ▪ Important causes are: Diabetes, peripheral neuritis, tabes dorsalis, spina bifida, *leprosy* (Hensen's d/s), spinal injury, paraplegia, syringomyelia.
Cortisol ulcers	▪ Formation due to long-term application of steroid creams. ▪ Callous ulcers with no healing tendency
Collar button/ Collar stud ulcer	▪ Seen in mucosa & submucosa of colon ▪ In Crohn's d/s and UC

	Ulcer		Edges
Ulcer edges	Everted (rolled out edge)/ heaped up		SqCC, epithelioma, Carcinomatous ulcer
	Undermined edge		Tuberculous ulcer Pressure injury e.g. bed score
	Sloping edge		Healing ulcer, Basal cell carcinoma
	Punched out edges		Peptic Ulcer, Trophic ulcers, Arterial ulcer
	Punched out edge with thin base + wash leather slough		Syphilis (Gummatous ulcer)
	Raised & beaded edge (pearly white)		BCC (Rodent ulcer)

SUTURES

Absorbable sutures	Non-absorbable Sutures	Monofilamentus Sutures	Polyfilamentus Sutures
▪ Catgut ▪ Chromic catgut ▪ Collagen ▪ Dexon (Polyglycolate) ▪ Vicryl (polyglactin 910) ▪ PDS (polydioxone)	▪ Silk ▪ Linen ▪ Nylon ▪ Prolene (polypropylene)	▪ Polypropylene ▪ Polyethylene, PDS, Catgut ▪ Steel	▪ Polyester ▪ Polyamide ▪ Vicryl ▪ Dexon ▪ Silk ▪ Cotton

	Types	Raw Material	Tensile Strength	Absorption Time	Remark
Silk	Braided or twisted multifilament	Natural protein raw silk form silkworm	▪ Loses 20% when wet; 80-100% lost by 6 months	Slowly over 1-2 years (Non absorbable)	Most tissue reactions are seen
Catgut	Plain	Collagen derived from submucosa of **sheep** or cattle gut (NOT from cat submucosa)	Lost within 7-10 days	7-10 days by phagocytosis & enzymatic degradation	For circumcision in children
Catgut	Chromic	Tanned with chromium salts to improve handling & resist degradation in tissue	Lost within 21-28 days	90 days	Used for suturing muscle, fascia
Polyglactin (Vicryl)	Braided multifilament	Copolymer of lactide & glycolide in a ratio of 90:10, coated with polyglactin & calcium stearate;	Remains 60% at 2 weeks & 30% at 3 weeks	60-90 days	Useful in bowel anastomosis
Polyglyconate	Monofilament	Copolymer of glycolic acid & trimethylene carbonate	Remains 70% at 2 weeks & 55% at 3 weeks	180 days	
Polyglycarpone	Monofilament	Copolymer of glycolite & caprolactone	21 days maximum	90-120 days	
Polyglycolic acid (dexon)	Braided multifilament	Polymer of polyglycolic acid	Approx., 40% remains at 1 week; 20% remains at 2 weeks	Hydrolysis minimal at 2 weeks; significant at 4 weeks; Complete absorption 60-90 days	
Polydioxane (PDS)	Monofilament dyed or undyed	Polyester polymer	Approx., 70% remains at 2 weeks; 50% remains at 4 weeks; 14% remains at 8 weeks	6 months (180 days); longest absorbable suture material	▪ Good for closing peritoneal cavity

- For vascular anastomosis - Prolene is used.
- For rectal and esophageal anastomosis - unabsorbable suture is best.
- Good for bowel anastomosis - Vicryl.
- Good for closing peritoneal cavity - PDS (Polydioxane)
- For circumcision in children - Catgut is used.
- For suturing muscle, fascia - Chronic catgut is used.
- For hernioplasty = Prolene.
- Isopropyl alcohol is used as preservative while packing sutures.
- EtO (Ethylene oxide) is used to sterilize suture material.

SURGICAL BLADES

Blade No	Image	Description
10	10	▪ Traditional blade ▪ Generally used for making small incisions in skin and muscles.
11	11	▪ Used for stab incisions. ▪ Used in procedures such as arteriotomy, creating incisions for chest drains, opening coronary arteries, opening the aorta and removing calcifications in the aortic or mitral valves.
15	15	▪ The most popular blade ▪ Ideal for making short and precise incisions. ▪ Used for minor procedures, for excision of skin lesion or recurrent sebaceous cyst and for opening coronary arteries.
22	22	▪ Used for abdominal incisions.

SURGICAL KNOTS

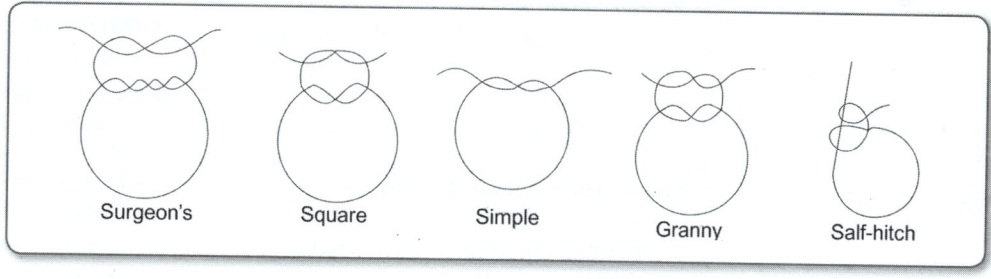

Surgeon's   Square   Simple   Granny   Salf-hitch

CLASSIFICATION OF HERNIAS

Nyhus Classification of Groin Hernia	
Type I	▪ Indirect hernia with normal deep (internal) ring (e.g. Pediatric hernia)
Type II	▪ Indirect hernia with **dilated** deep (internal) ring but posterior inguinal wall intact. Inferior deep epigastric vessels not displaced
Type III	▪ Posterior wall defect 　○ Type 3A (Direct inguinal hernia) : With posterior floor defect only 　○ Type 3B (Pantaloon hernia): Indirect inguinal hernia with posterior floor defect or a combination of direct & indirect hernia 　○ Type 3B (Femoral hernia)
Type IV	▪ All types of recurrent hernia (Direct/Indirect/Femoral/Combined)

Gilbert classification			
Type I	▪ Small, indirect	**Type V**	▪ Diverticular, direct
Type II	▪ Medium, indirect	**Type VI**	▪ Combined, pantaloon
Type III	▪ Large, indirect	**Type VII**	▪ Femoral
Type IV	▪ Entire floor, direct		

OTHER FACTS

- Hernia with highest rate of strangulation is → Femoral hernia.
- Collis gastroplasty is done for short esophagus.
- Paraesophageal hernia is also called giant hiatal hernia.
- *Hiatus hernia*
  ○ Usually presents in elderly female with recurrent pneumonia, regurgitation of food and feeling of fullness.
  ○ MC complication → Esophagitis.
- Hydrocele is a type of **exudation cyst**.
- Lumbar hernia is more common through → Grynfeltt triangle.
- *Richter's hernia:*
  ○ Seen most commonly in → Femoral hernia.
  ○ Only a portion of the bowel wall gets herniated

  ○ Strangulation is common but obstruction is not seen
  ○ Common sites are femoral ring & inguinal ring
- Spigelian hernia → abdominal hernia occurring along the semilunar line
- Most common type of hiatal hernia is Sliding hernia.
- The foramen of Morgagni. A hernia in the anterior part of the diaphragm with a defect between the sternal and costal attachments. The most commonly involved viscus is the transverse colon.
- **The foramen of Bochdalek**: Through the dome of the diaphragm posteriorly.

TREATMENT

- **Stoppa's preperitoneal repair**
  ○ Based on Pascal's law
  ○ Open preperitoneal large mesh repair for complex inguinal hernia.
  ○ It is a tension free type of hernia repair.
- *Femoral Hernias*
  ○ There is no alternative to surgery.
  ○ Surgical approaches are
    – **Lockwood** - low approach – simplest but should not be used if there is risk of bowel strangulation

    – **Lotheissen** – Inguinal approach
    – **McEvedy – High approach** – ideal in emergency situation when the risk of bowel strangulation is high
  ○ Use of a truss is not advisable as chances of complications are more with the use of truss.
- Nerves most likely to be injured during laparoscopic hernia surgery → Lateral femoral cutaneous nerve.

CYSTIC LESIONS OF HEAD & NECK

	Thyroglossal Cyst	Branchial Cyst
Etiology	▪ A fibrous cyst that formed from a persistent thyroglossal duct. ▪ Thyroglossal cyst are the m/c cause of midline neck masses.	▪ **Congenital** epithel**ial** cyst ▪ Wall consists of lymphoid tissue. ▪ Arises on the lateral part of the neck usually due to failure of obliteration of the 2nd branchial cleft (or failure of fusion of the second and third branchial arches)
Location	▪ Can occur anywhere along the path of the thyroglossal duct, from the base of the tongue to the suprasternal notch. ▪ MC site → Suprahyoid.	▪ Commonly located in the posterior triangle of neck.
Clinical Presentation	▪ M/c presentation: a palpable asymptomatic midline neck mass in suprahyoid location. Some patients may have neck or throat pain, or dysphagia.	▪ Non translucent ▪ Soft cystic swelling
	▪ Moves during swallowing or on protrusion of the tongue because of its attachment to the tongue (foramen of cecum) via the tract of thyroid descent. ▪ Only midline neck swelling mass/lump which moves with both deglutition and swallowing.	
Treatment	▪ Rx: "Sistrunk operation" which consists of en bloc cystectomy and excision of the central hyoid bone to prevent recurrence.	

Other swelling which move with swallowing - Thyroid, ectopic thyroid, subhyoid bursitis, enlarged lymph nodes fixed to trachea, dermoid cysts and laryngocele.

	Ranula	Cystic Hygroma
Etiology	▪ Mucous extravasation cyst of sublingual gland. ▪ Less commonly, a mucous retention cyst (mucocele) e.g. plunging ranula. ▪ Originates in the body of the sublingual gland, in the ducts of Rivini and, infrequently from the minor salivary glands.	▪ Develops from jugular lymphatic sequestration. ▪
Location	▪ Develops in the floor of the mouth.	▪ MC site → Lower third of neck.
Clinical Features	▪ Translucent ▪ It is called "Plunging ranula" when it extends into and past the mylohyoid muscle.	▪ Translucent, fluctuant, ill defined
Treatment	▪ Excision of the cyst & gland is TOC. ▪ Possess risk of damage to → Submandibular duct.	▪ TOC: Complete surgical excision > Injection sclerotherapy.
	▪ Most common site of dermoid cyst of → Midline.	
	▪ Hydrocele is a type of exudation cyst.	

SALIVARY GLANDS

- **Sialolithiasis:**
  - Sialolithiasis means stones in salivary glands.
  - MC site → Submandibular gland.
  - The diagnostic method of submandibular sialolithesis is → USG.
  - Dye study to find out stone is salivary gland → Sialography.
- MC site for salivary tumors – Parotid gland (m/c in parotid gland)

- MC surgery performed for parotid gland pathology – Superficial parotidectomy
- MC location of ectopic salivary gland is → Cervical lymph nodes.
- Bilaternal parotid enlargement does not occur in → SLE.
- Costen's syndrome refers to neurological pain associated with → Temporomandibular joint.
- Anterior mediastinal nodes are included in which level of lymph nodes → VII.

FREY'S SYNDROME

	Frey's Syndrome
Caused by	▪ Frey syndrome is associated with surgery of → Parotid. ▪ Nerve involved/damaged in Frey's syndrome is → Ariculo- temporal branch of mandibular nerve (postganglionic parasympathetic nerve) from otic ganglion which synapse with sympathetic nerve resulting in gustatory sweating.
Clinical features	▪ Manifests 2-3 months after surgery. ▪ Characterized by *gustatory sweating* (sweating occurs during eating)/erythema over parotid's bed as a result of autonomic stimulation of salivation by smell or taste of food.
Investigation	▪ Starch iodine test
Treatment	▪ Anti-perspirants ▪ Denervation (Jacobson's tympanic neurectomy) ▪ Botulinum toxin.

THYROID & PARATHROID

- During parathyroid surgery, whenever multiple parathyroids are resected, it is preferable to cryopreserve tissue, so that it may be autotransplanted before the patients become hypoparathyroid.
- After resection of parathyroid gland in slices 3-4 grafts are implanted into separated muscle pockets in the anterior forearm (non-dominant) muscles (in **brachioradialis** muscle), then the muscle is closed with nonabsorbable sutures.
- 1% of thyroglossal cyst harbor tumor and 85% of these tumors are papillary.

- MC thyroid Ca is Papillary CA and has best prognosis among thyroid cancers.
- Anaplastic CA of thyroid is least common (Incidence <1.1%) thyroid Ca and has worst prognosis among thyroid cancers.
- Chvostek sign could be seen after → Total thyroidectomy.
- **Signs of hypocalcemia**
  - Chovstek sign
  - Trousseau sign
  - Carpopedal spasm
- In subtotal thyroidectomy, both lobes are removed leaving behind 6-8 grams of tissue.

NECK DISSECTION

	Procedure & Structures removed	Remark/ Structures preserved
Supraomohyoid neck dissection (SOHD)	▪ Most conservative neck dissection. ▪ Selective neck dissection of level I to III.	
Classical Radical neck dissection (Classical RND) Criles	▪ Resection of the cervical lymphatics and lymph nodes (level I to level V) and closely associated structures; the IJV (internal jugular vein), the accessory nerve, the submandibular gland, sternocleidomastoid muscle, tail of the parotid and omohyoid muscle. ▪ These structures are all removed en bloc and in continuity with the primary disease, if possible.	▪ Drooping of the shoulder due to paralysis of the trapezius muscle as a consequence of excision of the accessory nerve.
Radical neck dissection (RND)	▪ Dissection of level I to V + AIS (All 3 structures) removed. A= Accessory nerve, I= IJV, S = SCM muscle	▪ Vagus nerve preserved
Modified radical neck dissection type 3 (MND-III)	▪ Dissection of all major lymph node groups and lymphatics from level I to V ▪ AIS (All 3 structures) preserved.	▪ AIS

MISCELLANEOUS FACT

- Nerves which are NOT at risk during submandibular gland excision → Auriculotemporal nerve, glossopharyngeal nerve.
- Dentigerous cysts originate from → Epithelium around the crown of unerupted teeth.
- Tooth is fixed in its socket by the → Peridontal membrane.
- What erupts from unerupted tooth → Dentigenous cyst.
- Epulis arises from → Gingiva.
- A person was brought to the emergency room after his dinner with c/o something sticking in his throat which later progressed to dyspnea . Likely diagnosis is → Foreign body.
- Management for CSF rhinorhea is → Antibiotics and observation.
- *Treatment of pituitary adenomas:*
  - Transsphenoidal surgical resection is the preferred primary treatment for both microadenomas and macroadenomas.
  - Transsphenoidal surgery + craniotomy is done for large tumors with suprasellar extension.
- T/t of Ca maxilla:-
  - Combined Surgery and radiotherapy is used for SqCC.
  - For adenocarcinoma, radiotherapy is ineffective, so only surgery is done.
- Weber-Fergusons incision is used for tumors of maxillary alveolus.
- Management plan for locally advanced (local bone invasion) tongue carcinomas includes subtotal glossectomy + selective neck dissection + mandibulectomy. Selective neck dissection is advisable for all oral tongue cancers as these patients have early lymph node involvement.
- Retro pharyngeal space lies between → Base of skull to bifurcation of trachea.

PEDIATRIC SURGERY

FACTS

- LAHSAL code is used to represent congenital malformation of Lip, Alveolus and Hard palate.
- "Double-bubble" sign is pathognomonic of → Duodenal atresia.
- Anomaly associated with duodenal atresia is → Down syndrome.
- A cystic mass at the base of umbilical cord in a neonate could be → Allantoic Cyst.
- Hormonal therapy is NOT effective in undescended testes.
- KASAI Procedure is used in the treatment of → Congenital Biliary Atesia.
- MC urethral anomaly → Hypospadias.
- Common cause of intussusception is → Hypertrophy of submucous peyer's patches.
- Fever is NOT a clinical feature suggestive of tracheo-esophageal fistula.

VENTRAL WALL DEFECTS

- Developmental defects due to failure of rostral fold closure [e.g., sternal defects [ectopia cordi)], lateral fold closure (e.g., omphalocele, gastroschisis), or caudal fold closure (e.g., bladder exstrophy)

	Gastroschisis	Omphalocele (Exomphalos)

Etiology	▪ Extrusion of abdominal contents through abdominal folds (typically right of umbilicus)	▪ Failure of lateral walls (all or part of midgut) to migrate at umbilical ring & to return into the coelom (body cavity) → persistent mid line herniation of abdominal contents into umbilical cord
		▪ Classification
		  ○ <4 cm (Exomphalos minor): Called congenital umbilical hernia of umbilical cord → A single bowel loop may be the content which if mistaken as a normal umbilical cord. Can cause an umbilical enteric fistula
		  ○ >4 cm (Exomphalos major): May contain liver, spleen, stomach, pancreas, colon and bladder, need staged approach for closure
		▪ Incidence: 1 in 5000 live births

Covering	▪ Not covered by peritoneum or amnion	▪ Surrounded by peritoneum (light gray shiny sac)

Associations	▪ Not associated with chromosome abnormalities	▪ Associated with congenital anomalies. e.g.,
		  ○ Trisomies 13 and 18
		  ○ Beckwith-Wiedemann syndrome
		  ○ Structural abnormalities of other organ systems (e.g. cardiac, genitourinary, neural tube)

CONGENITAL HYPERTROPHIC PYLORIC STENOSIS

- Also called as **IHPS (infantile hypertrophic pyloric stenosis)**
- Metabolic abnormalities a/w IHPS are:
  ○ Hypochloremia, hypokalemia,
  ○ hyponatremia,
  ○ hypocalcemia (sometimes)
  ○ Metabolic alkalosis
  ○ Paradoxical aciduria (not seen in early phase).

- **Exposure to which drugs is incriminated in IHPS → Erythromycin.**
- What is the most characteristic of congenital hypertrophic pyloric stenosis → The pyloric tumor (olive) is best felt during feeding.
- All of the following are true about congenital hypertrophic pyloric stenosis except → Metabolic acidosis occurs.

HIRSCHSPRUNG DISEASE

- All of the following are true about Hirschsprung disease expect → The nonperistaltic affected segment is dilated.
- NOT true about Hirschsprung Disease → Autosomal dominant.

- Hirschsprung's colon is due to → Loss of intrinsic enteric plexuses.
- In Hirschsprung's disease, staining used for diagnosis is → AChE.

VARIOUS GRAFTS

Terminology	Definition	Remark
Autograft	▪ Tissue transplanted from one part of the body to another in the same individual (Also called an autotransplant).	▪ Example includes:- ○ Most of the flaps used in plastic surgery
Isograft	▪ Graft of tissue between two individuals who are genetically identical (i.e. monozygotic twins)	▪ Example includes graft between monozygotic twins. ▪ Transplant rejection between two such individuals virtually never occurs (i.e Chance of recipient failure are least).
Allograft	▪ An organ or tissue transplanted from one individual to another	▪ Example includes:- ○ Renal transplantation.
Xenograft	▪ Living cells, tissues or organs transplanted from one species to another	▪ Also called heterologous transplant. ▪ Example includes:- ○ Bovine/pig heart valves transplant into humans.

LIVER TRANSPLANT

- First liver transplant was done by → Starzl.
- ***Common indications***
  ○ Cirrhosis with end stage liver disease and decompensation
  ○ Hepatocellular carcinoma
  ○ Hepatoblastoma in children
  ○ Alcoholic Liver Disease
  ○ Hepatitis - Autoimmune, chronic hepatitis B and C
  ○ Metabolic diseases - Hemochromatosis, Wilson disease
  ○ Cholestatic diseases - Primary biliary cirrhosis, Primary sclerosing cholangitis, Biliary atresia
  ○ Fulminant hepatic failure - Viral/toxin/drug induced
  ○ Others - Hepatic venous outflow tract obstruction, Polycystic liver disease.
- In modified Pugh's classification score of 8, what to do → Orthotopic liver transplant.
- Milan criteria is used for → Liver transplantation.

MISCELLANEOUS

- Transplanted kidney is relocated to which region in the recipient body → Retroperitoneal region.
- In a diabetic patient insulin deficiency was attributed to non-functional islet cells. The preferred site of pancreatic islet cell transplant in a this patient would be → Portal vein.
- Pancreatic autotransplantation is done for → Chronic pancreatitis.
- Dr. Christian Bernard is associated with → Heart transplant.

PLASTIC SURGERY

- Ideal timing of repair of isolated cleft lip is → 4-6 months.
- Cleft lip repair minimum age → 3-4 months.
- Vascularity of graft is maintained by → Through capillary plexus.
- Sun-burns are → Third degree burns.
- In a 6-year-old child with burns involving the whole of head and trunk, the estimated body surface area of burns is → 44%.
- 2nd degree burn involves → Epidermis + dermis.
- Blisters are classified as which type of burn → Superficial second degree burn.
- Skin grafts stored at 4°C can survive up to → 2 weeks.
- Silver sulfadiazine is effective against pseudomonas and is used in burns patients.
- The most commonly used myocutaneous pedicle graft for pelvis surgeries contains muscle segments from Rectus abdominis muscle.
- Full thickness skin graft (Wolfes graft) - it includes all epidermis + dermis;
- Partial thickness skin graft (Thiersch graft) - it includes all epidermis + part of dermis.

BURNS

Classification of Burns				
Degree of Burns	First Degree	**Second Degree (Partial thickness)** two types:- superficial and deep	**Third Degree** (full thickness)	Fourth Degree
Involvement of Skin	Epidermis alone	Epidermis plus some part of dermis • Superficial second degree:- Injury to the epidermis and superficial dermis. • Deep second degree: deep dermal involvement	Full thickness involving the subcutaneous fat	Underlying muscles, tendons, bone and brain are involved
Characters	Erythema	• Blister for superficial, weepy and painful • Reddish for deep, decreased sensation	• White waxy appearance • Lack of sensation • Leathery texture • Lack of capillary refill	
Resolution	Resolves in 48-72 hrs Heals uneventfully No scaring	Superficial heal with minimal scarring in 10-14 days Deep takes 25-35 days for healing, produces hypertrophic scar and skin grafting may be required	No potential for reepithelia lization Need skin grafting	

Rule of Nine Wallace	
Each upper limb	9% of TBSA (Total Body Surface Area)
Each lower limb	18% of TBSA (9% of anterior half and 9% of posterior half)
Head and Neck	9% of TBSA
Front and back of trunk	18% each
Genitalia	1%

- **Note:** The patients' whole hand (digit and palm) represents 1% of TBSA. In children the area of head and neck is amended to 18% and lower limb to 12%

BUERGER'S DISEASE

- Buerger's disease is also known as **Thrombo-angiitis obliterans.**
- Characterized by occlusion of the small and medium-size arteries, thrombophlebitis of superficial and deep veins and Raynaud's phenomenon.
- Buerger's disease involves → Artery, vein and nerve [Lymphatics are NOT affected].
- Affects male of <30 years.
- Smoking is a risk factor.
- Angiography shows 'corrugation of femoral arteries'.
- Gangrene of toes and fingers is common and is progressive
- Histology – Panangitis

MISCELLANEOUS

- Superolateral boundary of axillary dissection is → **Axillary vein.**
- *Hemangioma*
  - It is a compressible swelling.
  - Best method to treat a large port-wine hemangioma is → Pulsed dye laser.
- Blood born spread is a feature of → Sarcoma.
- NOT a features of acute ischemia of limb → Cyanosis.
- Butcher's thigh is → Accidental injury to major **vessels in thigh or groin.**
- Allens test for integrity of palmar arch tests ulnar collateral flow.
- *Varicose veins*
  - MC site of venous ulcers in varicose vein is → Gaiter area of leg.
  - Sx include → Trendelenburg's operation.
  - "Bisgaard regime" is used for the t/t of → Venous ulcer.
  - CEAP scoring system is used for clinical staging of varicose veins.

CEAP Clinical Score	Description
C0	No varicose veins
C1	Telangectasia (Thread veins/Spider veins/ Broken veins)
C2	Asymptomatic VV
C2S	Varicose veins with symptoms

CEAP Clinical Score	Description
C3	Edema
C4	Skin changes
C5	Healed ulceration
C6	Non healing ulcer

- Ankle Brachial Pressure Index (ABPI) Suggesting imminent Necrosis is → <0.3.
- Cirsoid aneurysms of the scalp are typically derived from → Superficial temporal artery.
- Commonest site of peripheral arterial aneurysm → Popliteal.
- The size beyond which the risk of rupture of an abdominal aneurysm significantly increases is greater than → 5.5 cm. Immediate surgery indicated.
- Pseudoclaudication is due to the compression of → Cauda equina.
- Pseudoclaudication occurs due to → Lumbar canal stenosis.
- Intermittent claudication means → Pain in leg only on exercise.
- Claudication due to popliteofemoral incompetence is primary seen in → Calf.
- MC Presentation of DVT is → Charley Horse Cramp.
- MC site of subclavian artery obstruction is → 1st part.
- Adson's test is positive in → Thoracic outlet syndrome.

CARDIOTHORACIC

- Flail chest with multiple injury in casualty, further management → Start positive pressure ventilatory support.
- A pleural fluid analysis confirms an exudates by → Ratio of pleural fluid to serum protein > 0.5.
- Heimlich valve is used for drainage of → Pneumothorax.
- Aberrant right subclavian artery leads to compression of esophagus known as arteria lusoria (dysphagia lusoria).
- Pain from parietal pericardium is transmitted through → Vagus nerve

MULTIPLE CHOICE QUESTIONS

CHAPTER 1: BREAST

1. A blood stained discharge from the nipple indicates:
(NEET June 2018)

a. Breast abscess
b. Fibroadenoma
c. Duct papilloma
d. Fat necrosis of breast

[Ref: Schwartz 10th /e pg. 547-549]

Explanation

- Bloody discharge is more suggestive of cancer but is usually caused by a benign papilloma in the duct." - CSDT
- "Intraductal papilloma is the most common cause of bloody nipple discharge.
- "Nipple discharge is suggestive of cancer if it is spontaneous, unilateral, localized to a single duct, occurs in women age 40 years or more, is bloody, or is associated with a mass.
- Nipple discharge is suggestive of a benign condition if it is bilateral or multiductal in origin, occurs in women age 39 years or less, or is milky or blue green in colour.

2. BI-RADS Stage 4 indicates: *(NEET June 2018)*

a. Benign Findings
b. Malignancy
c. Suspicious abnormality
d. Biopsy proven malignancy

Explanation

- BIRADS stands for Breast Imaging-Reporting and Data System. It's a quality assurance tool developed by American college of Radiology.
- The system is designed to standardize both the reporting of imaging findings and the recommendations for further management (ie, routine screening, short interval follow-up, or biopsy).
- It is important to note that the BI-RADS category only refers to the imaging findings and does not take clinical findings or presentation into account.

BENIGN DISEASES

3. All are benign conditions of breast EXCEPT

a. Fibroadenoma *(PGMEE 2014-15)*
b. Galactocele
c. Pagets disease of nipple
d. Cystosarcoma phyllodes

[Ref: Bailey & Love's 27th/e pg. 870; Robbins 9th/e pg. 1048; 1057]

Explanation

Benign breast disorder classification

Congenital disorders
- Inverted nipple

- Supernumerary breasts/nipples
- Non breast disorders including Tietze's disease (costochondritis)
- Sebaceous cysts and other skin conditions

Injury

Inflammation/infection
- ANDI (aberations of normal differentiation and involution):
  - Cyclical nodularity and mastalgia
  - Cysts
  - Fibroadenoma
  - Duct ectasia/periductal mastitis
- Pregnancy/lactation-related:
  - Galactocele
  - Lactational abscess

4. "Peau'd orange" appereance of breast is due to
(PGMEE 2012; 2009)

a. Post operative scarring
b. Obstruction of dermal lymphatic
c. Tumour necrosis involving skin
d. Infiltration of lactiferous ducts

[Ref: Bailey & Love's 27th/e pg. 879 & 873]

5. Granulomatous mastitis is caused by all except-

a. Fungus *(PGMEE 2013-14)*
b. Antibodies to milk antigens
c. Staphylococcus
d. TB

[Ref: Robbins 9th/e pg. 1047]

6. Drug of choice for severe mastitis? *(PGMEE 2019)*

a. Cefphalosporins b. Augmentin
c. Cloxacillin d. Erythromycin

7. A 14 week post natal woman presents with fluctuant breast swelling, what would be the treatment

a. Incision and Drainage *(PGMEE 2019)*
b. Continue Breast feeding with antibiotics
c. Analgesics
d. Repeated aspirations under antibiotic cover.

[Ref: Bailey and Love 27th/e pg. 866]

8. Mondor's disease is- *(PGMEE 2015)*

a. Carcinoma of the breast
b. Thrombophlebitis of the superficial veins of breast
c. Filariasis of the breast
d. Premaligment condition of the breast

[Ref: Bailey & Love's 27th/e pg. 867; Schwartz 10th /e pg.507]

Explanation

- *Mondor disease:-* Thrombophlebitis of superficial veins of breast and anterior chest wall.

1.	c
2.	c
3.	c
4.	b
5.	c
6.	c
7.	d
8.	b

9. Mainstay of treatment of for Zuska's Disease is:-
   a. Antibiotics, Incision and Drainage *(PGMEE 2015-16)*
   b. Hadfield operation
   c. Mastectomy
   d. Observation and NSAID'S

[Ref: Schwart'z 9th/e pg. 433]

Explanation

- Hadfield operation done for duct ectasia (major/central duct excision).

10. Which of the following is a proliferating breast mass-
   (PGMEE 2013-12)
   a. Adenosis   b. Duct ectasia
   c. Fibroadenoma d. Papilloma

[Ref: Bailey & Love's 27th/e pg. 871; Robbins 9th/e pg. 1049]

Explanation

Relative risk of invasive breast carcinoma based on pathological examination of benign breast tissue (American College of Pathologists Consensus Statement).[a]	
No ↑ed risk	Adenosis, sclerosing of florid
	Apocrine metaplasia
	Cysts, macro and/or micro
	Duct ectasia
	Fibroadenoma
	Fibrosis
	Hyperplasia
	Mastitis (inflammation)
	Periductal mastitis
	Squamous metaplasia
Slightly ↑ed risk (1.5-2 times)	Hyperplasia, moderate or florid, solid or papillary
	Papilloma with a fibrovascular core
Moderately ↑ed risk (5 times)	Atypical hyperplasia (ductal or lobular)
Insufficient data to assign a risk	Solitary papilloma of lactiferous sinus
	Radial scar lesion

11. 20-year-old female presents with non-painful reddish lesion over breast which bleeds on touch but there is no increase in size for past 2 years. Excision biopsy is most likely going to reveal:- *(PGMEE 2018)*
   a. Fibroadenoma
   b. Hemangioma
   c. Lipoma
   d. Phyllodes tumour

Explanation

- Fibroadenoma, lipoma and phyllodes tumor neither appear red nor will these bleed on touch.

MASTECTOMY

12. Halsteds mastectomy is:- *(PGMEE 2016-17)*
   a. Simple mastectomy
   b. Wide local excision
   c. MRM
   d. Radical mastectomy

[Ref: Bailey & Love's 27th/e pg. 876; Schwartz 10th/e pg. 547]

Explanation

Lumpectomy	Removal of only breast lump as done in case of fibroadenoma
BCS (breast conservation surgery)	Also known as wide local excision. In this condition lump excised with 1-2 cm margin eg. Carcinoma of breast but radiotherapy mandatory
Halsted mastectomy (Radical mastectomy)	Radical mastectomy (Surgery for breast cancer in which the breast, chest muscles, and all of the lymph nodes under the arm are removed) with removal of chest wall muscle which onclude pectoralis minor and major includes
Patey's mastectomy (classical MRM)	after putting a transverse elliptical incision enclosing the nipple areolar complex and the skin overlying the tumor, the entire breast is removed **with removal** of pectoralis minor and level I, II and III axillary lymph node. Pectoralis major preserved
Scanlon MRM	Same as above except pectoralis minor **divided** but not removed (level I, II and III still removed)
Auchincloss MRM	Same as above except surgeon retract pectoralis minor to facilitate level III lymph node dissection but this limits its dissection (now a days this is preferred as only 2% of the patients potentially benefit by removal of the highest level of nodes and therefore it is justified)

13. Patey's mastectomy involves removal of all of the following expect- *(PGMEE 2015)*
   a. Pectoralis major
   b. Skin of the breast
   c. Ductular system of the breast
   d. Pectoralis Minor

[Ref: Bailey & Love's 27th/e pg. 876; Schwartz 10th /e pg.549]

Explanation

- *Patey's modification:-* Divide and remove of pectoralis minor. Hence all the level I, II, III nodes can be removed.

9.	a
10.	d
11.	b
12.	d
13.	a

14. During breast reconstruction surgery which of the following structure is preserved? *(PGMEE 2016-17)*
   a. Pectoralis minor
   b. Paectoralis major
   c. Serratus anterior
   d. Nipple areola complex

[Ref: Oncoplastic and Reconstructive Surgery for Breast Cancer: By a. Fitoussi, M.G. Berry, b. Couturaud, R.J. Salmon Page 45]

15. A 45 year old female underwent modified radical mastectomy with axillary clearance for Ca breast. After surgery she could not lift her arm above head. Which nerve is likely to be injured? *(PGMEE 2015)*
   a. Nerve to latissimus Dorsi
   b. Intercostobrachial nerve
   c. Long thorasic nerve of Bell
   d. Nerve to pectoralis major

Explanation

- Thoracodorsal nerve is injured.

16. Tingling and Numbness over the posteromedial part of upper arm after Modified Radical Mastectomy is most likely to be caused as result of injury to:-
   a. Thoracodorsal Nerve   *(PGMEE 2015-16)*
   b. Long thoracic nerve of Bell
   c. Intercostobrachial nerve
   d. Medial Cutaneous nerve of arm

Explanation

Post mastectomy syndrome

- Post mastectomy syndrome is a multifaceted disorder in which the patient experiences a wide range of sensations, not only in the area of the surgical scar, but also in the axilla, chest, and upper arm. It is characterized by tightness, aching, stabbing, and burning sensations, and is most likely associated with damage to the intercostobrachial nerve.
  - In PMPS, pain is typically localized to the axilla, medial upper arm, and/or the anterior chest wall on the affected side (Stevens et al., 1995).
  - Damage to the intercostobrachial nerve, which can occur with axillary node dissection, has been considered the most common cause of PMPS.

17. Pain along medial aspect of arm in a post mastectomy patient is due to *(DNB Dec 2009)*
   a. Other nerve injury pain
   b. Phantom breast pain
   c. Neuroma pain
   d. Intercostobrachial neuralgia

[Ref: Medical care of cancer patients by Sai-ching Jim Yeung, Carmen P. Escalante, Robert F. Gagel p.415]

14.	b
15.	a
16.	c
17.	d
18.	a

Explanation

- Classification of chronic neuropathic pain syndromes following breast cancer surgery Syndrome Description

Phantom breast pain	A Sensory experience of a removed breast that is still present and is painful
Intercostobrachial neuralgia	(Includes post-mastectomy pain syndrome) Pain, typically accompanied by sensory changes, in the distribution of the intercostobrachial nerve following breast cancer surgery with or without axillary dissection
Neuroma pain (includes scar pain)	Pain in the region of a scar on the breast, chest, or arm that is provoked or exacerbated by percussion
Other nerve injury pain	Pain outside the distribution of the intercostobrachial nerve consistent with damage to other nerves during breast cancer surgery (e.g. medial and lateral pectoral, long thoracic, thoracodorsal, and other intercostal nerves)

18. Nerve not damaged in breast surgery is
   a. Median nerve   *(DNB June' 2009)*
   b. Nerve to serratus anterior
   c. Nerve to latissimus dorsi
   d. Medial pectoral nerve

[Ref: Breast surgery by William G. Cance page 95]

Explanation

Axillary dissection poses risks to the:-

- *Intercostobrachial nerve* is damaged from stretch during retraction as well as from frank transection. There is an area of numbness on the upper inner arm, usually painless.
- *Medial cutaneous nerve* of the arm, which contains fibers from C8 and T1 and arises from the medial cord of the brachial plexus. It can be harmed during section of the tributaries of the axillary vein, leaving patients with sensory loss on the lower medial skin of the upper arm.
- *Vulnerable motor nerves* in the area include the medial and lateral pectoral nerves, which innervate the pectoralis minor and major muscles and are lost during resection of these muscles.
- *The long thoracic nerve* to the serratus anterior muscle runs along the posterior part of the medial wall of the axilla behind the axillary nodes. Damage produces **'winging'** of the scapula.
- *The thoracodorsal nerve* to the latissimus dorsi muscle runs vertically through the axilla in close proximity to the subscapular artery and vein. Preservation of these neurovascular structures is required if a latissimus dorsi flap is needed for reconstructive breast surgery. Weakness of the latissimus dorsi (which adducts the upper arm) can usually be compensated for by the teres major and pectoralis major muscles.

19. Supero-lateral boundary of axillary dissection is?
a. Axillary artery   *(DNB June'2010)*
b. Clavi-pectoral fascia
c. Brachial plexus
d. Axillary vein

[Ref: Gray's anatomy, 39th/e pg. 841]

MISCELLANEOUS

20. CA Breast may locally spread to all of the following muscles expect-   *(PGMEE 2015)*
a. Pectoralis major
b. Latissimus dorsi
c. Pectoralis minor
d. Serratus anterior

[Ref: S.Das 3rd /e pg.725; Schwartz 10th/e pg. 547-549]

21. All of the following are used for reconstruction of breast except-   *(PGMEE 2015)*
a. Transversus rectus abdominis free flap
b. Transverse rectus abdominis myocutaneous flap
c. Pectoralis major myocutaneous flap
d. Latissimus dorsi myocutoneous flap

[Ref: Bailey & Love's 27th/e pg. 879]

22. Triple assessment includes all except?   *(DNB Dec'2010)*
a. Mammography   b. FNAC
c. Clinical examination   d. Bone scan

[Ref: Bailey & Love 27th/e pg. 863]

23. A female presents with discharge from nipple. A lacrimal probe wire has been passed through the discharging duct and blood stained discharge was found through the nipple. This procedure is known as:-   *(PGMEE 2018)*
a. Microdochotomy
b. Macrodochotomy
c. Conservative breast surgery
d. Ductoscopy

[Ref: Bailey & Love 26th/e pg. 802]

Explanation

Microdochectomy/ Microdochotomy

- This procedure is done for the intolerable discharge from the nipple duct.
- A lacrimal probe or length of stiff nylon suture is inserted into the duct from which the discharge is emerging. A tennis racquet incision can be made to encompass the entire duct or a periareolar incision used and the nipple flap dissected to reach the duct. The duct is then excised.

24. Van nuys staging for ductal carcinoma in situ includes all except: *(PGMEE 2018)*
a. Age
b. Size
c. Margins
d. Estrogen and progesterone receptor status

[Ref: Bailey & Love 26th/e pg. 810]

Explanation

- DCIS may be classified using the Van Nuys system, which combines the patient's age, type of DCIS and presence of microcalcification, extent of resection margin and size of disease. Patients with a high score benefit from radiotherapy after excision, whereas those of low grade, whose tumour is completely excised, need no further treatment.
- The Van Nuys Prognostic Index is based on size & grade of DCIS, margins and age of patient.

Summary of the Von nuys prognostic index scoring system

VNPI scoring system	1	2	3
Tumor size diameter (in mm)	Less of equal to 15	16-40	Greater or equal to 41
Margin width (in mm)	Less of equal to 10	1-9	<1
Pathological Classification	Non-high grade, (nuclear grades 1 and 2) no necrosis	Non-high grade, (nuclear grades 1 and 2) with necrosis	High grade, (nuclear grade 3) with or without necrosis
Overall VNPI score	3 or 4	5-7	8 or 9
8 year local recurrence-free survival rate. (statistics from the original study, not a predication)	97%	77%	20%
8 year breast-cancer specific survival rate. (statistics from the original study, not a predication)	100%	97%	100%

19.	d
20.	b
21.	c
22.	d
23.	a
24.	d

1. **Flail chest with multiple rib injury presents in casualty, further management:-** *(PGMEE 2016-17)*
   a. Insert endotracheal tube then strapping of chest
   b. Start positive pressure ventilatory support
   c. Give morphine intramuscularly
   d. Put a chest drain and start PEEP

   [Ref: Bailey & Love 27th/e pg. 368; Sabiston's 1st SEA/e/ 1603; Schwartz's 10th /e pg. 164]

2. **A pleural fluid analysis confirms an exudates by-** *(PGMEE 2015)*
   a. Pleural fluid LDH value less than 0.45 of the upper limit of normal serum values
   b. Ratio of pleural fluid to serum LDH less than 0.6
   c. Ratio of pleural fluid to serum protein greater than 0.5
   d. Pleural fluid LDH less than two thirds of the upper limits of normal serum value

   [Ref: Harrison's 19th/e pg. 1717]

3. **A 40 year old male with chest trauma presents with breathlessness, decreased respiratory sounds on the right side, hyperresonance on percussion and distended neck veins. The possible diagnosis is-** *(PGMEE 2015)*
   a. Myocardial Infarction
   b. Tension Pneumothorax
   c. Cardiac Tamonade
   d. Flail Chest

   [Ref: Bailey & Love 27th/e pg. 367; Schwartz's 10th /e pg.163]

Explanation

- The above clinical history is typical of Tension pneumothorax
  - In tension pneumothorax there will be history of trauma followed by dyspnea.
  - On clinical examination ipsilateral ↓ breath sound, heperresonance on percussion and distended/ engorged neck veins.
- Tension pneumothorax and simple pneumothorax have similar signs, symptoms, and examination findings, but **hypotension qualifies the pneumothorax as a tension pneumothorax.**
- *Myocardial infarction:* patient present with chest pain,, sweating , left shoulder pain
- *Flail chest:* Flail chest occurs when ⩾ 3 contiguous ribs are fractured in at least two locations. **Paradoxical movement** of this free-floating segment of chest wall is usually evident in patients with spontaneous ventilation. Patients mainly gives history of trauma followed by dyspnoea and bone pain due to fracture rib. Tension pneumothorax may be associate with flail chest but its not compulsory.

4. **A patient complaints of breathlessness following a trauma. On examination trachea shifted to opposite side, Resonant percussion note seen with absent breath sounds. Regarding insertion of ICD this patient, false statement is:** *(PGMEE 2019)*
   a. Done in upper part of lower rib to avoid vessel and nerve injury
   b. Direction of insertion in posterior and superior
   c. Inserted into the 4th or 5th ICS along the scapular line
   d. Insertion area must be palpated digitally to confirm the position

   [Ref: Bailey and Love 27th/e pg. 920]

5. **Lung injury with bad prognosis is** *(DNB June' 2009)*
   a. Open pneumothorax
   b. Closed pneumothorax
   c. Tension pneumothorax
   d. All have same prognosis

   [Ref: Handbook of practical medicine: Volume 1 by Hermann Eichorst p 29]

Explanation

The 'deadly dozen' threats to life from chest injury.

Immediately life threatening	• Airway obstruction • Tension pneumothorax • Pericardial tamponade • Open pneumothorax • Massive haemothorax • Fail chest
Potentially life threatening	• Aortic injuries • Tracheobronchial injuries • Myocardial contusion • Rupture of diaphragm • Oesophageal injuries • Pulmonary contusion

6. **A 40 year old male presented with a penetrating trauma to chest. He is dyspnoeic with distended neck veins with hypotension and mediastinum is shifted to opposite side. There is a sucking wound over the chest . The most appropriate management would be-** *(PGMEE 2015)*
   a. Starting Inotropic support
   b. Insertion of a large bore needle in the 2nd ICS in the mid clavicular line
   c. Fluid Resuscitation
   d. Endotracheal intubation

   [Ref: Bailey & Love 27th/e pg. 368]

1.	b
2.	b
3.	b
4.	c
5.	c
6.	b

Explanation

- Sterile occlusive & plastic dressing chest tube insertion may require.

7. What is the best sign indicating adequate functioning of the intercostal drain?   *(NEET Pattern 2017)*
   a. Bubbling in IC bottle
   b. Movement of column in IC bottle
   c. Bubbling in suction tube
   d. No bubbling

   [Ref: Source - net]

Explanation

- Intercostal neurovascular bundle i.e. intercostal vessels and nerve follow the inferior margin of each rib. Incision and tunneling should be performed over the rib.
- Chest tube should be inserted immediately above and as close to the superior rib margin as possible in order to reduce the risks of injury to the neurovascular bundle.
- A "triangle of safety" is the preferred site of insertion of chest tube. Boundries of this triangle are:- Anterior border of the latissimus dorsi, the lateral border of the pectoralis major muscle, a line passing superior to the horizontal level of the nipple, and an apex below the axilla.

8. In mid axillary pleural tapping all structures pierced EXCEPT: *(NEET June 2018)*
   a. External intercostal muscle
   b. Internal intercostal muscle
   c. Costal pleura
   d. Pulmonary pleura

Explanation

- The thoracocentesis or the pleural tap is done to remove the excess fluid from the pleural cavity. The needle passes in succession of the skin, fascia, serratus anterior, intercostal muscles, endothoracic fascia and the costal pleura before entering the pleural cavity.

- The Transversus thoracis (Sternocostalis) is situated upon the inner surface of the front wall of the chest. Thus it is not pierced by needle for pleural tapping in mid axillary line.

9. Heimlich valve is used for drainage of: *(DNB 2008)*
   a. Pneumothorax   b. Hemothorax
   c. Empyema   d. Malignant pleural effusion

10. All of the following may lead to pneumatocoele formation except-   *(PGMEE 2015)*
   a. Staphylococcal pneumonia
   b. ARDS
   c. Positive pressure ventilation
   d. Hydrocarban inhalation

   [Ref: Harrison's 19th/e pg. 1717]

11. Which of the following is an indication for thoracotomy in case of hemothorax?   *(PGMEE 2015)*
   a. >1500 ml drained on chest tube insertion
   b. Shift of mediastimum to the opposite side
   c. <500 ml total output
   d. Falling blood pressure

   [Ref: Bailey & Love 27th/e pg. 371; Sabiston's 1st SAE pg. 427]

12. Pain from parietal pericardium is transmitted through   *(DNB June' 2009)*
   a. Phrenic nerve
   b. Greater splanchnic nerve
   c. Intercostal nerve
   d. Cardiac plexus

   [Ref: Gray's anatomy 39th/e p. 996]

Explanation

- Visceral pericardium is insensitive to pain
- Pain from parieral pericardium is transmitted by the phrenic nerve.

7.	a
8.	d
9.	a
10.	b
11.	a
12.	a

1. **Most common cancer metastasis to bone:-**
   (PGMEE 2016-17)
   a. Breast
   b. Lung
   c. Renal cell carcinoma
   d. Prostate
   [Ref: Sabiston's 20th /e pg. 785]

2. **Most common cause of leptomeningeal carcinomatosis:-**
   (PGMEE 2016-17)
   a. Liver cancer
   b. Lung and breast cancer
   c. Head and neck cancer
   d. Melanoma
   [Ref: lung. Schwartz 10th /e pg. 1732]

3. **Sarcoma botryoides is also known as?** *(DNB June '2010)*
   a. Embryonal Rhabdomyosarcoma
   b. Leiomyosarcoma
   c. Lipoblastomatosis
   d. Alveolar Rhabdomyosarcoma
   [Ref: Devita's oncology 6th/e p. 1325, Gynaecologic Pathology By Marisa R. Nucci, Esther Oliva page 325]

4. **Most common soft tissue tumor of adults is?**
   a. Embryonal rhabdomyosarcoa
   (DNB Dec '2010)
   b. Liposarcoma
   c. Synovial sarcoma
   d. Malignant fibrous histiocytoma
   [Ref: Sabiston 19th/e chapter 69]

5. **The most common retroperitoneal sarcoma is?**
   (DNB Dec' 2011)
   a. Leomyo sarcoma
   b. Neural sheath sarcoma
   c. Fibrosarcoma
   d. Liposarcoma
   [Ref: Principles and Practice of Surgical Oncology: A Multidisciplinary Page 539 Howard Silberman, Allan W. Silberman]

6. **Which is the investigation of staging of a lower limb sarcoma?** *(PGMEE 2015)*
   a. MRI
   b. CT scan
   c. PET scan
   d. PET CT
   [Ref: https://www.hindawi.com/journals sarcoma/2010/506182/]

7. **True about lymphangioma is** *(DNB June' 2011)*
   a. Common in puberty
   b. Respond in low doses to radiotherapy
   c. Lymphangioma progress slowly and may invade local tissue
   d. Predispose to cancers
   [Ref: Sabiston 18th/e chapter 69]

8. **Lymphangiosarcoma occurs in?** *(DNB June'2010)*
   a. Lymphangiomas
   b. Lymphomas
   c. Lymphedema
   d. Serous cavity tumors
   [Ref: Sabiston 18th/r chapter 69]

9. **Most common type of primary lymphedema is?**
   (DNB Dec'2010)
   a. Lymphedema tarda
   b. Lymphedema precox
   c. Lymphedema congenita
   d. None
   [Ref: Sabiston 18th/e chapter 69]

10. **Most common bacterial infection in lymphedemia is?**
    (DNB Dec'2010)
    a. Pseudomonas
    b. Streptococcus
    c. Staphylococcus
    d. E. Coli
    [Ref: Differential diagnosis in internal medicine: from symptom to diagnosis by Water Siegenthaler page 388]

11. **A man presents with multiple painless swelling all over the body and coffee brown patches in trunk he condition is:-** *(PGMEE 2016-17)*
    a. Multiple Lipoma
    b. Multiple neurofibroma
    c. Melanoma
    d. Colleginoma
    [Ref: Sabiston 20th /e pg. 985 table]

12. **Which of the following is seen in tumor lysis syndrome?**
    (DNB Dec 2011)
    a. Hypokalemia
    b. Hypercalcemia
    c. Hyponatremia
    d. None
    [Ref: Harrison's 18th/e chapter 276, figure 276-4]

13. **Which of the following is most malignant tumour?**
    (PGMEE 2015)
    a. Giant cell tumour
    b. Glioblastoma Multiform
    c. Osteochondroma
    d. Meningioma
    [Ref: Osborn's Diagnostic Neuroradiology 1994/e pg.529]

14. **Chimeric chemotherapy is being investigated for the treatment of which malignancy?**
    a. Leukemia
    b. Glioblastoma multiforme
    c. CA pancreas
    d. Renal cell carcinoma
    [Ref: https://www.cancer.gov/about-cancer/treatment/ research/car-t-cells/]

15. **Hypoglycaemia not caused by:-** *(PGMEE 2016-17)*
    a. Pheochromocytoma
    b. Insulinoma
    c. Hepatocellular carcinoma
    d. Renal cell carcinoma
    [Ref: all three can cause hypoglycemia Insulinoma – sabiston 20th /e pg. 952; HCC – Sabiston's 20th /e pg. 1459; RCC – internet]

1.	d
2.	b
3.	a
4.	b
5.	d
6.	a
7.	c
8.	c
9.	b
10.	b
11.	b
12.	d
13.	b
14.	a
15.	a

SURGICAL INFECTIONS

1. Most common cause of cellulitis is *(PGMEE 2012)*
   a. Streptococcus
   b. Kleibsella
   c. Proteus
   d. Pseudomonas

   [Ref: Rook's 8th/e chapter 30.17]

2. Most common nosocomial infection:-
   a. Urinary tract infection - 14% *(PGMEE 2016-17)*
   b. Surgical site infection - 22%
   c. Respiratory infection
   d. None

Explanation

- In nosocomial infection, incidence of
  o UTI - 14%
  o Respiratory infections 22%

3. Most common cause of catheter induced UTI:-
   (PGMEE 2016-17)
   a. E Coli
   b. Klebsiella
   c. Pseudomonas
   d. Staphylococci

   [Ref: Sabiston 20th /e pg. 250]

4. In current scenario which is the most common cause of septicemia *(PGMEE 2012)*
   a. Gram negative bacteria
   b. Fungus
   c. Parasite
   d. Gram positive bacteria

   [Ref: Harrison's Schwartz 10th e pg 147; CDC guideline for prevention of SSI]

5. Which of following is not useful the preventing septicemia:- *(PGMEE 2016-17)*
   a. Washing hands
   b. Daily dressing
   c. Hypothermia
   d. Antibiotic lotions

   [Ref: Schwartz 10th /e pg. 149]

6. Degloving injury is characterised by *(Recent Pattern 2019)*
   a. Loss of Skin only
   b. Loss of Skin and Subcutaneous tissue with intact fascia
   c. Loss of Skin and Subcutaneous tissue along with Fascia
   d. Loss of Skin, Subcutaneous Tissue and Muscle

   [Ref: Bailey and Love's 27th/e pg. 27]

7. Smallest recommended margin for wide local excision in melanoma:- *(PGMEE 2016-17)*
   a. 3 mm
   b. 5 mm
   c. 1 cm
   d. 2 cm

   [Ref: Sabiston's 20th /e pg. 734]

SURGICAL SAFETY

8. Not a part of personal protective kit:
   (Recent Pattern 2019)
   a. Face mask
   b. Gloves
   c. Goggle
   d. Lab coat

9. All of the following are components of safety checklist prior to an operative procedure except:
   a. Signature of the doctor *(NEET Pattern 2017)*
   b. Verification of patient
   c. Verification of procedure
   d. Oral consent

   [Ref: Bailey and Love's 27th /e pg. 183]

Explanation

- Important question can be regarding sign in, time out and sign out
- *Check 1:* check patient's identity, check site marked, and check correct patient labels. Check 1 is then signed by a member of the ward staff, and a member of the reception staff.
- *Check 2:* check patient's identity, check documentation to ascertain site, operation surgeon/senior member of team check, and marks site if not completed on ward. Check 2 is then signed by the consultant surgeon or senior member of the team.
- *Check 3:* time out procedure is conducted to confirm the correct patient, marking of the correct site, agreement on procedure to be performed, correct patient position, and the availability of correct implants/imaging studies/histology (as appropriate). Check 3 is signed by the consultant surgeon/senior team member, senior anaesthetist, and circulating nurse

10. Antibiotics to be given before surgery:-
   a. 6 hrs *(PGMEE 2016-17)*
   b. 12 hrs
   c. Just before the incision
   d. Within 1 hr before the incision

   [Ref: Ref: Bailey and Love's 27th /e pg. 53; Sabiston 20th /e pg. 252]

11. Antibiotic Prophylaxis is best given- *(PGMEE 2015)*
   a. I day before surgery
   b. Before the time of incison
   c. 2 hour before surgery
   d. Only postoperatively

   [Ref: Sabiston 20th /e pg. 287]

1.	a
2.	c
3.	a
4.	a
5.	d
6.	b
7.	b
8.	d
9.	d
10.	d
11.	b

12. An intern while doing scalp suture injured his index finger. Which is not done? *(PGMEE 2019)*
   a. Should inform authorities
   b. HIV transmission high in surgical needle injury
   c. Injury during Suturing more common in Non Dominant Index Finger
   d. Show the finger in Running Water

13. The essential components of damage control surgery are all except- *(PGMEE 2015)*
   a. ICU resuscitation
   b. Arterial embolization/clamping
   c. Initial laparotomy
   d. Definitive reconstruction

[Ref: Sabiston's 20th /e pg. 2095]

14. The Bipolar cautery is preferred over monopolar cautery is the following surgeries except- *(PGMEE 2015)*
   a. Surgery around Penis
   b. Surgery of the Hip
   c. Surgery around the face
   d. Hand Surgery

HAND & FOOT SURGERY

15. Most common site of felon is? *(DNB Dec' 2011)*
   a. Ring finger   b. Little finger
   c. Index finger   d. Thumb

[Ref: Schwartz's Principles of Surgery 9th/e chapter 44, Bailey & Love 25th/e p. 507-508]

16. All of the following are true about pulp space infection except- *(PGMEE 2015)*
   a. It may lead to necrosis of finger pulp
   b. It is also called as felon
   c. It is a painless condition
   d. It is infection of small compartments in the pulp formed by vertical septa

[Ref: Franko OI, Abrams RA. Hand infections. Orthop Clin North Am. 2013 Oct. 44(4):625-34]

17. Tense – non tender cystic swelling (as shown below) over dorsums of wrist-

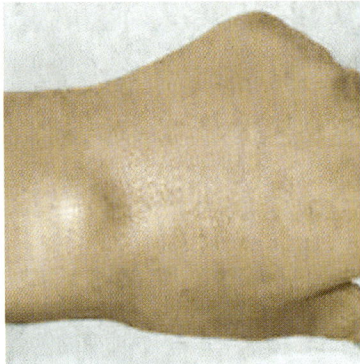

   a. Dermoid cyst   b. Lipoma
   c. Ganglion   d. Sebaceous cyst

[Ref: s das clinical surgery]

18. During Felon drainage incision taken as:- *(PGMEE 2016-17)*
   a. From tip of finger to 1 cm distal to DIP
   b. Ventral aspect of finger
   c. Cruciate incision on pulp of finger
   d. No need to excise

[Ref: A felon is an abscess between the specialised fingertip septae in the distal pulp. Internet source for answer.

19. Ainhum is most commonly seen at *(PGMEE 2015)*
   a. Base of a toe   b. Tongue
   c. At the ankle joint   d. Base of the thumb

WOUND HEALING & TISSUE REPAIR

20. Difference between primary and secondary healing is- *(PGMEE 2015)*
   a. Scar is more cosmetic in secondary healing
   b. More granulation tissue and fibrosis is seen in secondary healing
   c. Secondary healing occurs faster
   d. Surgical wound heal commonly by secondary healing

[Ref: Bailey & love 27th/e, pg 25]

21. An Incisional wound heals by- *(PGMEE 2015)*
   a. Primary Healing   b. Secondary Healing
   c. Reepithelization   d. Delayed primary Healing

[Ref: Bailey & love 27th/e, pg 25]

22. Which of the following is correct management of abdominal compartment syndrome- *(PGMEE 2015)*
   a. Urgent Fasciotomy
   b. Wait and monitor for 24 hours
   c. Antihypertensives
   d. Urgent Opening of the surgical wound and application of the Bogota bag

[Ref: Schwartz 10th/e pg. 217, 389]

23. Negative pressure wound healing technique is used in all EXCEPT: *(Recent Pattern June 2018)*
   a. Pressure sore
   b. To drain breast abscess after modified radical mastectomy
   c. Diabetic neuropathic wounds
   d. Untreated osteomyelitis

[Ref: Sabiston's 20th/e]

Explanation

Negative pressure wound healing

Indications	Contraindications
Pressure ulcers/bed sores	Eschar
Diabetic/neuropathic ulcers	Untrated osteomyclitis
Venous insufficiency ulcers	Unexplored fistulas
Traumatic wounds	Malignancy in the wound
Post operative and dehsced surgical wounds	Untreated malnutrition
Explosed fistulas	Exposed arteries, veins, or organs
Skin flaps and skin grafts	

12.	b
13.	d
14.	b
15.	d
16.	c
17.	c
18.	a
19.	a
20.	b
21.	a
22.	d
23.	d

24. A full thickness wound that is not sutured heals by-
(PGMEE 2015)
a. Delayed primary Healing
b. Primary Healing
c. Secondary Healing
d. Reepithelization

[Ref: Bailey & love 27th/e, pg 25]

25. Vaccum assisted closure is contraindicated in which of the following conditions- *(PGMEE 2015)*
a. Large amount of necrotic tissue with eschar
b. Chronic osteomyelitis
c. Surgical wound dehiscence
d. Abdominal wound

[Ref: Sabiston's 20th/e pg. 1958]

26. A 8-year-old child with obstructed inguinal hernia was taken for surgery. On exploration, Bowel was found gangrenous. Which of the following is true regarding anostomosis:- *(PGMEE 2018)*
a. Should be done by continuous layers as it takes less time
b. Done with cat gut
c. Done with single layer sero muscular lambert suturues
d. Single layer taking submucosa

Ref: Bailey & Love 26th/e pg.42

Explanation

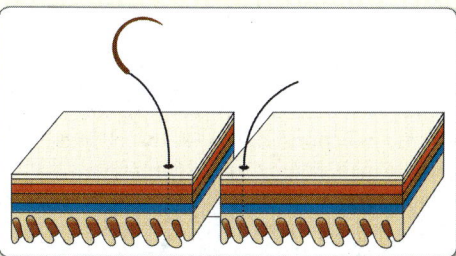

- *Halsted method:* Single layer extramucosal closure is a/w least tissue necrosis or luminal narrowing. This technique has now become widely accepted, although it is essential that this is not confused with a seromuscular suture technique.
- The extramucosal suture must include the submucosa as this has a high collagen content and is the most stable suture layer in all portions of the GI tract.
- The catgut and silk have been replaced by synthetic, usually absorbable, polymers.

27. Reactionary Hemorrhage occurs due to- *(PGMEE 2015)*
a. Damage to a blood vessel
b. Dislodgement of clot
c. Infection
d. Pressure necrosis

[Ref: Bailey and Love's 26th/e pg. 19]

28. Which hormone raised in post operative patient:-
(PGMEE 2016-17)
a. Cortisol   b. Insulin
c. Thyroxin   d. Angiotensin

[Ref: Bailey 26th/e pg. 6]

29. Drainage of cervical abscess is an example of-
a. Dirty infected wound   *(PGMEE 2015)*
b. Clean contaminated wound
c. Clean Uncontaminated wound
d. UnClean Uncontaminated wound

[Ref: Bailey and Love's 26th /e pg. 63]

30. A 10-year-old boy with difficulty and pain during walking for the past 10 days. There is no fever currently. On examination right hip is flexed and there is fullness in the right lumbar region. X-ray showed soft tissue shadow in the right side of abdomen. What is the most probable diagnosis? *(NEET Pattern 2017)*
a. Psoas abscess
b. Testicular torsion in an undescended testis
c. Pyonephrosis
d. Appendicular lump in Retrocaecal appendix

Explanation

Psoas Abscess

- Usually secondary to direct spread of infection from the inflamed and or perforated GI or urinary tract. Now a days, a primary psoas abscess due to haematogenous spread from an occult source is more common, especially in immunocompromised and older patients as well as in association with IV abuse of drugs.
- Cl/F: Back pain, lassitude and fever are cardinal symptoms. A swelling may point to the groin as it tracks along ileopsoas. Pain may be elicited by passive extension of the hip or a fixed flexion of the hip evident on inspection.
- IOC: CT scan
- T/t: Percutaneous CT-guided drainage and appropriate antibiotic therapy.

CYSTS

31. Image shown below is swelling which is sliping below fingers when surgeon tries to palpate – most likely diagnosis is:- *(PGMEE 2016-17)*

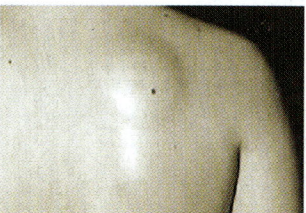

a. Lipoma
b. Sebaceous cyst
c. Dermoid cyst
d. Fibroadenoma

[Ref: s das clinical surgery]

24.	c
25.	b
26.	d
27.	b
28.	a
29.	a
30.	a
31.	a

32. What is the swelling shown here in Image?

(PGMEE 2019)

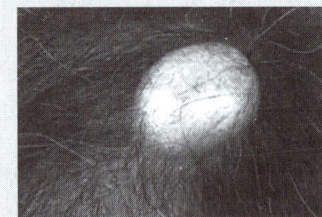

- a. Dermoid Cyst
- b. Sebaceous cyst
- c. Cysticercosis
- d. Meningioma

33. Which of the following is a compressible swelling?

(DNB June'2010)

- a. Lipoma
- b. Hemangioma
- c. Sebaceous cyst
- d. Hernia

[Ref: Bedsides Clinics in Surgery By M.I. Saha Page 314]

SUTURES

34. Catgut is made from intestine of:
- a. Cat
- b. Human
- c. Sheep
- d. All of the above

[Ref: Bailey and Love's 26ᵗʰ/e pg. 38]

Explanation

Catgut Chromic

- Catgut Chromic (TRUGUTTM) is made of collagen derived from healthy sheep or cattle (not cat or rabbit). It is tanned with chromium salts to improve handling and to resist degradation in tissue.
- It is self-degraded by phagocytosis and enzymatic degradation within 90 days.
- It causes moderate amount of tissue reaction (not very less).
- It is used to ligate superficial vessels, suture subcutaneous tissues, Stomas and other tissues that heal rapidly.

35. Which of the is an absorbable suture- *(PGMEE 2015)*
- a. Silk
- b. Polyglactin
- c. Polyester
- d. Ethilon

36. What information do you infer from surgical material shown in the image? *(PGMEE 2018)*

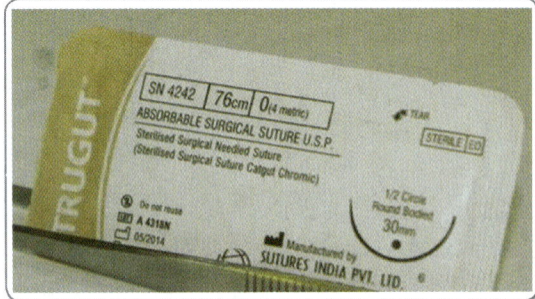

- a. Derived from mucosa of rabbit gut
- b. Very less tissue reaction
- c. Derived from mucosa of gut of Cat
- d. Self degradable over time by enzymatic action

[Ref: Bailey & Love 26th/e pg. 38]

37. Polydiaxonone suture is normally absorbed in-
- a. 2 weeks
- b. 4 weeks *(PGMEE 2015)*
- c. 6 weeks
- d. 6 months

[Ref: Examples of Surgical Suture Materials". Tom Rabinson]

38. Most commonly tissue reaction is seen with-

(PGMEE 2015)
- a. Chromic catgut
- b. Polydiaxonone
- c. Plain Catgut
- d. Silk

[Ref: Ann Surg, 1975 Feb; 181(2): 144-150, Human tissue reaction to sutures]

39. All of the following are medical uses of erythropoietin expect- *(PGMEE 2015)*
- a. Treatment of anaemia associated with renal disease
- b. Chemotherapy induced anemia
- c. Megaloblastic Anaemis
- d. Anaemis associated with Crohn's disease

[Ref:Witt S, Sinclair AM (2012)."The effect of erythropoietin on normal and neoplastic cells ."Biologics 6:163-89]

40. True statement regarding keloid are all EXCEPT?
- a. Wide local excision *(PGMEE 2018)*
- b. It will have more collagen and vascularity
- c. Will not spread beyond the wound site
- d. Can be treated with steroids

[Ref: Bailey & Love 26th/e pg. 30]

Explanation

Keloid

- Keloids tend to occur 3 months to years after the initial insult, and even minor injuries can result in large lesions. Injections, vaccines, insect bites, ear piercing may provoke or may arise spontaneously.
- Keloids vary in size from a few mm to large, pedunculated lesions with a soft to rubbery or hard consistency.
- Project as raised lesions but they rarely extend into underlying subcutaneous tissues.
- Common sites are skin of the earlobe, deltoid, presternal, and upper back regions. They rarely occur on eyelids, genitalia, palms, soles, or across joints.
- Spontaneous involution is rare. Surgical intervention can lead to recurrence, often with a worse result.
- *A keloid scar* is defined as excessive scar tissue that extends beyond the boundaries of the original incision or wound. Its aetiology is unknown, but it is a/w ↑ed levels of growth factor, deeply pigmented skin, an inherited predisposition and certain areas of the body (e.g. a triangle whose points are the xiphisternum and each shoulder tip).

Hypertrophic Scar

- A hypertrophic scar is defined as excessive scar tissue that does not extend beyond the boundary of the original incision or wound. It is a result of prolonged inflammatory phase of wound healing and from unfavorable scar siting (i.e. across the lines of skin tension). In the face, these are known as the lines of facial expression.
- The histology of both keloid & hypertrophic scars shows excess collagen with hypervascularity, but this is more marked in keloids where there is more type III collagen.

32.	b
33.	b
34.	c
35.	b
36.	d
37.	d
38.	d
39.	c
40.	c

- Treatment of hypertrophic and keloid scars
  - Pressure – local moulds/ elasticated garments
  - Silicone gel sheeting
  - Excision and steroid injections
  - Excision and postop external beam or brachytherapy
  - Intralesional excision (keloids only)
  - Intralesional steroids (triamcinolone) injection
  - Laser to ↓ redness
  - Vitamin E or palm oil massage (unproven)
- All excisions have high rates of recurrence.

Hypertrophic Scar vs Keloid

Point	Hypertrophic scar	Keloid
Association with dark skin	No	Yes, Genetic predisposition+
Spread beyond the boundary of original incision/wound.	Does not extend	Extend beyond it
Develop	Soon after Sx	Months after trauma
Improvement with time	Seen	Rare
Site	Occurs when scar crosses joints or skin creases at right angle	Occurs over ear lobe, shoulder, sternal notch but rarely across joints
Result of Sx	Improves	Often worsens after Sx

PRACTICAL ASPECT

41. An adult patient with leg pain and gangrene of toe. His ankle to brachial arterial pressure ratio would be less than *(DNB June' 2011)*

a. 1
b. 0.3
c. 0.5
d. 0.8

[Ref: Sabiston 18th/e p. chapter 66]

42. If you are asked to put a 22 gauge cannula in a patient, which of the following cannula will you pick? *(NEET Pattern 2017)*

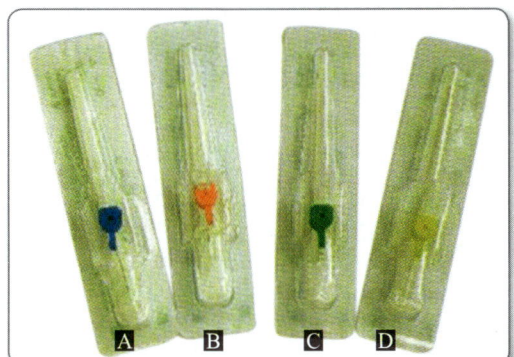

a. A
b. B
c. C
d. D

Explanation

IV Cannula Colour Coding

Size	Colour coding	Flow Rate
14G	Orange	240 ml/min
16G	Gray	180 ml/min
17 G	White	125 ml/min
18 G	Green	90 ml/min
20 G	Pink	60 ml/min
22 G	Blue	36 ml/min
24 G	Yellow	20 ml/min

Foley's Catheter Coding

Colour Code	Size
White	12Fr
Green	14Fr
Orange	16Fr
Red	18Fr
Yellow	20Fr
Purple	22Fr
Blue	24Fr

43. 'Fr' in foleys denotes: *(NEET Pattern 2017)*

a. Outer circumference
b. Inner circumference
c. Radius
d. Diameter

[Ref: Makhan lal saha 2nd edition page 926]

41. b
42. a
43. d

Explanation

- It indicate the outer diameter of tube french scale of measurement. This indicates the circumference of the catheter in millimeter. Diameter of the catheter in mm is calculated by = No. of catheter in French scale/3.

However, from Other Internet Sources

- Most common classification used for sizing of catheter in medical field is the French (Fr) scale, aka the *"Charrière's system."* It is **based on the outer diameter**. French sizing has uniform increments starting with 1Fr with no upper end point. Each increment of French sizing equals 0.33mm, for example, a 3Fr catheter equals 1mm outer diameter.
- Another method of sizing catheters is the *gauge (G) measurement* originally developed for wire sizing in the early 19th century by Peter Stubs which was later incorporated into needle sizing. Gauge is a descending scale, the higher the gauge size the smaller the tubing.
- Seems answer is outer dia only. Except M L Saha, nowhere its used for circumference. Even in an article on Dr. J. F. B. Charrier, there is no mention of circumference. Only outer diameter.

44. The length of nasogastric tube to the inserted is calculated by measuring the distance between: *(NEET Pattern 2017)*

a. Ear lobe to tip of nose to the umbilicus
b. Ear lobe to mouth of the mid point between xiphoid process and umbilicus
c. Ear lobe to tip of nose to midpoint between xiphoid process and umbilicus
d. Ear lobe to tip of nose to the xiphoid process of sternum

[Ref: BDC 4th edition pg 267]

Explanation

- The oesophagus is about 25 cm long
- Estimate the length required for insertion: run the tube from tip of nose to behind the ear and up to the midway between xiphisternum and umbilicus

45. If you need to give 180 mg drug available as 500 mg/5 ml via 2 ml syringe. Up to how many division will you fill the syringe? *(NEET Pattern 2017)*

a. 18 division
b. 1.8 division
c. 12 division
d. 8 division

Explanation

- In 2 ml syringe there are total 20 divisions. In this case 5ml = 500 mg so 2 ml = 200 mg and we have to give 180 mg so 18 small divisions will be equal to 180 mg.

46. Identify the Knot shown here: *(PGMEE 2019)*

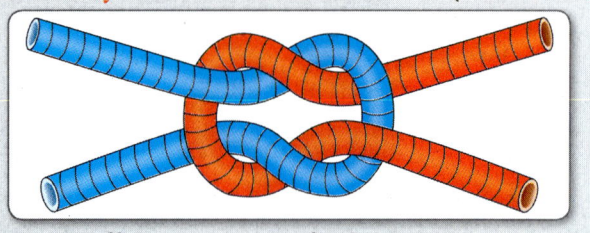

a. Reef knot
b. Granny Knot
c. Surgeon knot
d. Aberdeen knot

47. What is the Size of this blade used in incision and Drainage? *(PGMEE 2019)*

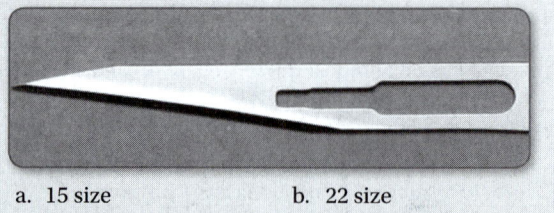

a. 15 size
b. 22 size
c. 11 size
d. 13 size

MISCELLANEOUS

48. Which of the following is a feature of crush syndrome- *(PGMEE 2015)*

a. Hypophosphatemia
b. Hypokalemia
c. Myoglobinuria
d. Hypercalcemia

[Ref: Bailey and Love's 27th/e pg. 421]

49. Crush Syndrome is associated with all of the following features expect- *(PGMEE 2015)*

a. Hypercalcemia
b. Hyperkalema
c. Myoglobinuria
d. Increased serum creatinine

[Ref: Bailey and Love's 27th/e pg. 421]

50. Phantom limb is based upon *(DNB June' 2009)*

a. Low of projection
b. Renshaw cell inhibition
c. Munro kellie doctrine
d. Weber's law

[Ref: Ganong's 22nd/e p. 125]

44.	d
45.	a
46.	b
47.	c
48.	c
49.	a
50.	a

1. Balanced resuscitation means. *(NEET Pattern 2017)*
   a. Equal use of crystalloids and colloids
   b. Permissive hypotension and limited crystalloid use
   c. Management of ariway breathing and circulation
   d. Maintaining acid base balance

Explanation

- Balanced resuscitation includes permissive hypotension, limiting crystalloid use, and the transfusion of blood products in ratios similar to whole blood. Advantages of Balanced resuscitation are:-
  - Minimizes the impact of trauma-induced coagulopathy,
  - Limits blood product waste
  - Reduces the complications that occur with aggressive crystalloid resuscitation
- Prompt initiation of transfusion with plasma; platelets and red blood cells in a 1:1:1 product ratios have improved the morbidity and mortality of patients with trauma in hemorrhagic shock.

2. Which is the best initial fluid for resuscitation during shock state *(PGMEE 2012)*
   a. Crystalloids   b. Colloids
   c. 5% dextrose   d. Plasma substitutes

   [Ref: Schwartz's Principles of Surgery 9th/e p. chapter 5; Bailey & Love 27th/e pg. 16]

3. Choice of fluid in case of burn in first 24 hour is *(PGMEE 2012)*
   a. Normal saline   b. Dextrose 5%
   c. Whole blood   d. Ringer lactate

   [Ref: Schwartz's 9th/e chapter 8 table 8-2, Bailey & Love 27th/e pg. 624]

4. 35-year-old man presents with acute pancreatitis in shock. Ideal fluid of choice is:- *(PGMEE 2018)*
   a. Isotonic saline   b. Hypertonic saline
   c. Hypotonic solution   d. Dextrose 10%

Explanation

- Intravenous fluids of lactated Ringer's or normal saline are initially bolused at 15–20 cc/kg (1050–1400 mL), followed by 3 ml/kg per hour (200–250 mL/h), to maintain urine output >0.5 cc/kg per hour. Serial bedside evaluations are required every 6–8 h to assess vital signs, oxygen saturation, and change in physical examination.
- Lactated Ringer's solution has been shown to decrease systemic inflammation and may be a better crystalloid than normal saline.
- A decrease in hematocrit and BUN during the first 12–24 h is strong evidence that sufficient fluids are being administered.
- A rise in hematocrit or BUN during serial measurement should be treated with a repeat volume challenge with a 2-L crystalloid bolus followed by increasing the fluid rate by 1.5 mg/kg per hour.

Risk Factors for Severity

- Age >60 years
- Obesity, BMI >30
- Comorbid disease (Charlson Comorbidity Index)

Markers of Severity at Admission or Within 24 h

- **SIRS**—defined by presence of 2 or more criteria:
  - Core temperature <36° or >38°C
  - Heart rate >90 beats/min
  - Respirations >20/min or Pco_2 <32 mmHg
  - White blood cell count >12,000/µL, <4000/µL, or 10% bands
- **APACHE II**
  - Hemoconcentration (hematocrit >44%)
  - Admission BUN (>22 mg/dL)
- **BISAP Score**
  - (B) BUN >25 mg/dL
  - (I) Impaired mental status
  - (S) SIRS: ≥2 of 4 present
  - (A) Age >60 years
  - (P) Pleural effusion
- Organ failure (Modified Marshall Score)
- Cardiovascular: systolic BP <90 mmHg, heart rate >130 beats/min
- Pulmonary: Pao_2 <60 mmHg
- Renal: serum creatinine >2.0 mg%

Markers of Severity During Hospitalization

- Persistent organ failure
- Pancreatic necrosis

5. Which of following is hypertonic *(DNB June' 2009)*
   a. 0.45% normal saline   b. 0.9% normal saline
   c. 3% normal saline   d. 5% dextrose

   [Ref: Fluids & electrolytes by By Lippincott Williams & Eilkins p 264]

6. Modified shock index is ratio of: *(NEET Pattern 2017)*
   a. Heart rate by systolic blood pressure
   b. Heart rate by diastolic blood pressure
   c. Heart rate by mean arterial pressure
   d. Heart rate by pulse pressure

Explanation

- SI is calculated by dividing HR by systolic blood pressure (SBP). SI can be used to predict the severity of hypovolemic shock. Previous studies have found that patients with SI more than 0.9 had a greater mortality rate.
  - SI = HR/SBP
  - MSI = HR/MAP
  - MAP = [(DBP × 2) + SBP]/3
- (Where; HR = Heart rate; SBP = Systolic Blood pressure; DBP = Diastolic blood pressure; MAP = Mean arterial pressure)
- High MSI shows a value of stroke volume and low systemic vascular resistance, a sign of hypodynamic circulation. However, low MSI indicates a hyperdynamic

1.	b
2.	a
3.	d
4.	a
5.	c
6.	c

state. Therefore, both high and low MSI indicates the serious state of the emergency patients. MSI was considered as a better marker for mortality rate prediction.

7. VAP scoring (CPIS Score) system contains all except:- *(PGMEE 2016-17)*
a. Body temprature
b. Total leucocyte count
c. Oxygenation
d. Blood pressure

[Ref: anaesthesia question Tracheal secretions; chest radiography; culture of tracheal aspirate; body temp; TLC; oxygenation]

8. What is the drug given for management of anaphylactic shock? *(NEET Pattern 2017)*
a. Epinephrine 0.5 mg, 1:1000
b. Atropine 3 mg
c. Adenosine 12 mg
d. Epinephrine 1 mg, 1:1000

[Ref: Harrison 19/e pg. 2117]

Explanation

Anaphylactic Shock

- Anaphylaxis is a medical emergency that requires immediate recognition and intervention.

Nonpharmacotherapy

- Supportive care for patients with suspected anaphylaxis includes the following:
  o Airway management (eg, ventilator support with bag and mask, endotracheal intubation)
  o High-flow oxygen
  o Cardiac monitoring
  o Intravenous access (large bore)
  o Fluid resuscitation with isotonic crystalloid solution
  o Supine position with legs elevated

Pharmacotherapy

- The primary drug treatments for acute anaphylactic reactions are epinephrine and H1 antihistamines. **Epinephrine is the drug of choice** for treating anaphylaxis. Its beta-agonistic effects include bronchodilatation, chronotropic effect on heart, and +ve inotropic effects.
- Mild symptoms such as pruritus and urticaria can be controlled by administration of 0.3–0.5 mL of 1:1000 (1 mg/mL) epinephrine SC or IM, with repeated doses as required at 5- to 20-min intervals for a severe reaction. In cases of intractable hypotension, an IV infusion should be initiated to administer epinephrine, diluted 1:10,000, along with normal saline, and vasopressor agents such as dopamine

9. Which of the following types of shock will usually have warm peripheral extremities- *(PGMEE 2015)*
a. Neurogenic Shock
b. Hypovolemic Shock
c. Cardiogenic Shock
d. Anaphylactic Shock

[Ref: Sabiston 20th /e pg. 420]

7.	d
8.	a
9.	a
10.	c
11.	d
12.	d
13.	c
14.	c
15.	b
16.	b
17.	c

10. Which of the following is not an immediate cause of death? *(DNB Dec' 2011)*
a. Thromboembolism
b. Shock
c. Septicemia
d. Ventricular fibrillation

[Ref: Harrison's 18th/e chapter 233, 270, http://en.wikipedia.org/wiki/Sepsis]

11. A patient on clopidogrel had severe bleeding mode of transfusion:- *(PGMEE 2016-17)*
a. Whole Blood
b. FFP
c. Cryoprecipitate
d. Platelet

[Ref: Clopidogrel act on platelet and inhibit its aggregation, so in its toxicity (bleeding) platelet will be transfused]

12. What is the best way to control external hemorrhage *(PGMEE 2012)*
a. Elevation
b. Artery forceps
c. Proximal tourniquet
d. Direct pressure

[Ref: Surgical Pitfalls: Prevention and Management by Stephen R. T. Evans page 762, Advanced Assessment and Treatment of Trauma by American (AAOS) 2010 ed page 71;Bailey & Love's Surgery , 25th Edn., Pg. 19]

13. Maintenance level of Mixed Venous Oxygen Saturation in shock must be: *(PGMEE 2019)*
a. < 40%
b. 40-50%
c. 50-70%
d. >70%

MISCELLANEOUS

14. All of the following are correct regarding emphysematous cholecystitis Except: *(DNB Dec' 2010)*
a. It is more common in males
b. In many cases, the gall bladder doesn't contain any stones
c. It is caused most commonly by pseudomonas
d. It is more common in diabetics

[Ref: Sabiston 18th ed Chapter 54, Schwartz 9th/e Chapter 32]

15. In Total parenteral nutrition vein cannulate is:- *(PGMEE 2016-17)*
a. Subclavian vein
b. Internal juglar vein
c. Brachial vein
d. Femoral vein

[Ref: Bailey & Love Page 268]

16. MC source of pulmonary emboli during surgery:- *(PGMEE 2016-17)*
a. Poplitial vein
b. Femoral vein
c. Abdominal aorta
d. Inferior vena cava

[Ref: sabiston 20th /e pg. 294]

17. Ideally which gas is used for laparoscopy
a. NO
b. AIR *(PGMEE 2012)*
c. CO_2
d. N_2O

[Ref: Schwartz's Principles of Surgery 9th/e chapter 14, Mastery of endoscopic and laparoscopic surgery edited by Nathaniel J. Soper, Lee L. Swanstrom, M. Stephen Eubanks 3rd/e p. 7, Palanivelu's Textbook of Surgical Laparoscopy 1st/e p. 21]

18. Which is the most frequently used gas for laproscopy?
(PGMEE 2016-17, 2015)

a. Oxygen
b. Helium
c. Carbon Dioxide
d. Nitrogen

[Ref: Sabiston's 20th/e pg.1498]

19. All of the following are used in cryosurgery except-
(PGMEE 2015)

a. Carcon dioxide
b. Argon
c. Helium
d. A Liquid nitrogen

20. A patient undergone laproscopic surgery c/o pain in Left shoulder most common causes is
(PGMEE 2016-17)

a. Irritation of phrenic nerve because of gas
b. Trauma from instuments
c. Injury of gall bladder
d. Because of reactionary hemorrhage

[Ref: Internet – many studies say pain is due to high pressure of CO_2 irritating diaphragm.]

21. Bayonet artefacts seen during USG guided nerve block of:-
(PGMEE 2016-17)

a. Femoral nerve block
b. Axillary nerve block
c. Sciatic nerve block
d. Brachial plexus block

18. c
19. c
20. a
21. b

NECK MASSES/CYST

1. Most common site of intracranial dermoid cyst:-
(PGMEE 2016-17)
- a. Midline
- b. Supra orbital
- c. Infraorbital
- d. Any of the above

[Ref: Bailey & Love 27th/e pg.667; S. Das short Cases in surgery]

Explanation
- Dermoid and epidermoid cysts are epithelial lined structures arising from displaced ectodermal remnants.
- Typically the dermoid cysts are located in the posterior fossa (midline) & epidermoid cysts in cerebellopontine angle.

2. Most common site of thyroglossal cyst is:
(DNB 2007, Dec' 2009)
- a. Suprahyoid
- b. Subhyoid
- c. Sublingual
- d. Lower neck

[Ref: Bailey & Love's 27th/e pg. 7545;Dhingra 7th/e pg. 446]

Explanation
- Thyroglossal duct cyst is a cystic midline, usually affecting young children but can occur at any age.
- It moves with protrusion of tongue.
- Can occur anywhere in the course of thyroid duct. M/c location – juxtaposition to the hyoid bone.
- T/t: complete surgical excision.

RANULA

3. Regarding Ranula all are true except -
(PGMEE 2013; DNB Dec' 2009)
- a. Plunging may be a feature
- b. Arises from submandibular gland
- c. Translucent
- d. Retention cyst of minor salivary glands

[Ref: Bailey & Love's 27th/e pg. 754;Dhingra 7th/e pg. 447]

4. Ranula is a -
(PGMEE 2014)
- a. Submandibular gland swelling
- b. Tumor
- c. Mucous retention cyst
- d. Swelling on dorsum of tongue

[Ref: Dhingra's 6th/e pg. 224,392]

5. Structure damaged most commonly during surgery on Ranula is?
(DNB Dec'2010)
- a. Lingual Artery
- b. Lingual nerve
- c. Submandibular duct
- d. Sublingual duct

[Ref: Clinical surgery: Volume 9 Head and neck edited by Charles Rob, Rodney, Smith page 56]

BRANCHIAL CYST

6. What is the swelling shown in the Image? (PGMEE 2019)

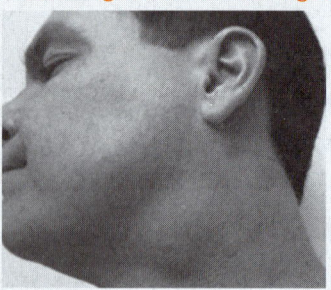

- a. Branchial cyst
- b. Pharyngeal pouch
- c. Dermoid Cyst
- d. Pretracheal Bursa

7. True about branchial cyst is-
(PGMEE 2015)
- a. Seen deep to lower 1/3 of sternocleidomastoid
- b. Wall consists of lymphoid tissue
- c. Presents at birth
- d. Filled with thick red coloured fluid

[Ref: Bailey & Love 27th /e pg.753]

8. All of the following are true about branchial cysts expect-
(PGMEE 2015)
- a. They are commonly located in the posterior triangle of neck
- b. It may contain granulation tissue
- c. They are lined by squamous epithelium
- d. They are remnants of branchial apparatus that is persistent

[Ref: Bailey & Love 27th/e pg.753; Sabiston 19th/e pg.1833; Schwartz 10th /e pg. 1414]

9. The most common site of the branchial cyst is:
(PGMEE 2019)
- a. Posterior border of sternocleidomastoid
- b. Anterior border of sternocleidomastoid
- c. Digastric muscle
- d. Omohyoid muscle

[Ref: PL Dhingra 7th/e pg. 446 , neck masses, pg. 446-447]

CYSTIC HYGROMA

10. Most common site for cystic Hygroma is-
(PGMEE 2015)
- a. Post auricular
- b. Overlying the parotid gland
- c. Lower third of neck
- d. Along the Zygomatic Prominence

[Ref: Bailey & Love's 27th/e pg. 754;Dhingra 7th/e pg. 447]

1.	a
2.	b
3.	b
4.	c
5.	c
6.	a
7.	b
8.	a
9.	b
10.	c

11. All of the following statements are false about cystic hygroma expect *(PGMEE 2015)*
   a. Seen in adults more commonly
   b. Does't transilluminate
   c. Develops from jugular lymphatic sequestration
   d. Lined by stratified squamous epithelium

[Ref: Bailey & Love's 27th/e pg. 754;Dhingra 7th/e pg. 447]

SALIVARY GLANDS

12. Most common site of sialolithiasis is *(PGMEE 2016-17)*
   a. Equally common in all salivary glands
   b. Sublingual Gland
   c. Submandibular gland
   d. Parotid Gland

[Ref: Bailey & Love 27th/e pg. 780]

13. The diagnostic method of submandibular sialolithiasis is:- *(PGMEE 2016-17)*
   a. USG   b. Sialography
   c. Plain radiograph   d. CT scan

[Ref: Bailey and Love 27th/e pg. 780]

Explanation

- The most common cause of obstruction within the submandibular gland is stone formation (sialolithiasis) within the gland and its associated duct system.
- **80%** of all salivary stones occur in the submandibular glands because their secretions are relatively viscous.
- **80%** of submandibular stones are radio-opaque and can be identified on plain radiography. Stones are mainly composed of phosphate and oxalate salts.
- **80%** cases can be diagnosed with X-ray alone hence it is investigation of choice. But for parotid gland IOC is ultrasonography.

14. Investigation using dye to find out stone is salivary gland- *(PGMEE 2015)*
   a. USG   b. Sialography
   c. MR angiography   d. Mammography

[Ref: Dhingra 6th /e pg. 233]

15. Most common site of sialolithiasis (salivary gland stones) is- *(PGMEE 2016-17, 015)*
   a. Submandibualr glands
   b. Equally common in all salivary glands
   c. Sublingual gland
   d. Parotid Gland

[Ref: Bailey & Love 27th /e pg. 787]

16. Most common location of ectopic salivary gland is-
   a. Cervical lymph nodes *(PGMEE 2015)*
   b. Posterior mandibular region & Aana parotid region
   c. Anterior mediastinum
   d. Parathyroid gland

[Ref: Witt RL (1 January 2011).Salivary Gland Disease: Surgical and Medical Management.Thieme. 50-51; Bailey & Love 27th/e pg. 780]

Explanation

- Most common site of ectopic salivary gland is hard palate (which is not in option). Amongst the options (a) is better answer as given.

17. Identify the swelling having variable consistency with no pain: *(PGMEE 2019)*

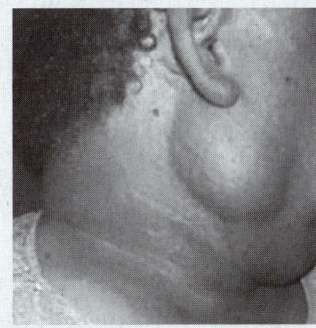

   a. Pleomorphic Adenoma
   b. Warthin tumor
   c. Abscess parotid   d. Parotid stone

18. Bitaternal parotid enlargement does not occur in- *(PGMEE 2015)*
   a. SLE   b. Chronic pancreatits
   c. Sarcoidosis   d. Sjorgen's syndrome

[Ref: Harrison 14th /e pg.1903]

FREY SYNDROME

19. Frey syndrome is associated with surgery of?
   a. Adrenal   b. Parotid
   c. Parathyroid   d. Pituitary

[Ref: Bailey and love 27th/e pg. 794]

20. Which of the following nerve is involved/damaged in Frey's syndrome: *(Recent Pattern June 2018; DNB Dec' 2011)*
   a. Facial Nerve
   b. Mandibular nerve
   c. Auriculotemporal nerve
   d. Trigeminal nerve

[Ref: Bailey & Love 27th/e pg.794; Dhingra's 7th/e pg. 265]

Explanation

- Frey's syndrome (also known as Baillarger's syndrome, Dupuy's syndrome, auriculotemporal syndrome, or Frey-Baillarger syndrome) is a rare neurological disorder resulting from damage to or near the parotid glands responsible for making saliva, and from damage to the auriculotemporal nerve often from surgery on parotid (Parotidectomy).

21. Frey's Syndrome is due to injury of which of the following nerve branch? *(PGMEE 2019)*
   a. Trigeminal nerve   b. Vagus nerve
   c. Facial Nerve   d. Glossopharyngeal nerve

[Ref: Bailey & Love 27th/e pg.794]

Explanation

- It results from damage to the autonomic innervation of the salivary gland with inappropriate regeneration of the postganglionic parasympathetic nerve fibres of the auriculotemporal nerve that aberrantly stimulate the sweat glands of the overlying skin. The clinical features include sweating and erythema (flushing) over the region of surgical excision of the parotid gland

11.	**c**
12.	**c**
13.	**a**
14.	**b**
15.	**a**
16.	**b**
17.	**a**
18.	**a**
19.	**b**
20.	**c**
21.	**a**

22. Which of the following is false regarding Frey's syndrome? **(PGMEE 2015)**
    a. It is also called gustatory sweating
    b. It is caused by injury to auriculotemporal nerve
    c. It is caused by aberrant regeneration of post ganglionic parasympathetic secretomotorfibres
    d. It occurs immediately after the parotid surgery

[Ref: Dhingra's 7th/e pg. 265 & LB 794]

Explanation

- It usually manifests several months after operation.

23. Frey's syndrome is caused by - **(PGMEE 2012)**
    a. Greater auricular with auriculotemporal nerve
    b. Facial nerve with greater auricular nerve
    c. Mixing of post trematic nerve fibres of facial nerve with parasympathetic of auriculotemporal nerve
    d. None

24. Frey's syndrome include - **(PGMEE 2014)**
    a. Gustatory sweating
    b. Merciful anosmia
    c. Crocodile tears
    d. None of the above

[Ref: Dhingra's 7th/e pg. 265]

25. Frey's Syndrome- False statement is
    (Recent Pattern 2019 Question)
    a. Auriculo temporal nerve carrying Post ganglionic Sympathetic fibres is injured
    b. Gustatory sweating
    c. Botulinum Toxin injection is the treatment.
    d. Less chances in Enucleation of lesion than in parotidectomy

[Ref: Bailey & Love 27th/e pg.794]

26. In submandibular gland excision all of the following nerves may be affected except:- **(PGMEE 2016-17)**
    a. Lingual nerve
    b. Hypoglossal nerve
    c. Glossopharyngeal nerve
    d. Marginal mandibular branch of the facial nerve

[Ref: Bailey and Love 27th/e pg. 783]

THYROID & PARATHYROID

27. Parathyroid gland accidentally removed and found after surgery is implanted in **(PGMEE 2019)**
    a. Sartorius
    b. Biceps
    c. Brachioradialis
    d. Triceps

28. Retrosternal goiter approach through: **(PGMEE 2019)**
    a. Transthoracic 2nd ICS
    b. Transthoracic 4th ICS
    c. Trans sternal via Anterior mediastinum
    d. Transcervical approach

29. Chovstek sign could be seen after- **(PGMEE 2015)**
    a. Sub total Thyroidectomy
    b. Gastrojejunostomy
    c. Total thyroidectomy
    d. Hellers Cardiomyotomy

[Ref: Schwartz 10th/e pg. 1574; Bailey & Love 27th /e pg. 831]

30. In subtotal thyroidectomy, What is true- **(PGMEE 2015)**
    a. Removal of one lobe and isthmus
    b. Removal of both lobes leaving behind 6-8 grams of tissue
    c. Removal of 1 lobe with isthmus and second lobe partially
    d. Removal of entire thyroid with cervical lymphnodes

[Ref: Bailey & Love 26th /e pg.762; Sabiston 1st SEA/e pg. 912]

Explanation

Total thyroidectomy	Involves excision of all visible thyroid tissue
Near-total thyroidectomy	Is completely resection on one side while leaving a remnant of thyroid tissue on the contralateral side, leaving less than 1 g of tissue adjacent to the RLN at the ligament of Berry
Subtotal thyroidectomy	Leaves a remnant of thyroid tissue bilaterally
Thyroid lobectomy	Typically includes removal of the thyroid isthmus and pyramidal lobe (if present)
Thyroid isthmusectomy	Removes only the isthmus and is infrequently indicated

TEETH

31. Dentigerous cyst originate from- **(PGMEE 2015)**
    a. Tooth pulp
    b. Epithelium around the crown of unerupted teeth
    c. Paranasal sinuses
    d. Retention cyst

[Ref: Scott-Brown's Otorhinolaryngology 7th/e pg. 1924, 1925]

32. Tooth is fixed in its socket by the: **(DNB 2007)**
    a. Cementocytes
    b. Peridontal membrane
    c. Cement
    d. Dentine

[Ref: BDC-III pg. 220]

33. What erupts from unerupted tooth: **(DNB 2008)**
    a. Dental cyst   b. Dentigenous cyst
    c. Both   d. None

(Ref.: Bailey and Love 26th edition pg 648)

34. Epulis arises from- **(PGMEE 2015)**
    a. Pulp   b. Root of teeth
    c. Gingiva   d. Enamel

[Ref: S.Das text of surgery 7th /e pg.422]

Explanation

- Odontogenic cysts
  ○ Dentigeroas cyst:- Treated by marsupialization
- Epulis: Rare tumour of females newborns arises from gingival mucosa

22.	d
23.	c
24.	a
25.	a
26.	c
27.	c
28.	d
29.	c
30.	b
31.	b
32.	b
33.	b
34.	c

NECK DISSECTION

35. Which of the following is the most conservative neck dissection – *(PGMEE 2015)*
   a. Supraomohyoid neck dissection
   b. Modified redical neck dissection
   c. Radical neck dissection
   d. All are conservative

[Ref: Sabiston 1st SEA/e pg. 794]

36. Structures removed in radical lymphnode dissection are all exepect *(PGMEE 2015)*
   a. Vagus nerve
   b. Sternocleidomastoid
   c. Neck lymphnodes
   d. Cranial nerve XI

[Ref: Sabiston 20th /e pg.794]

37. Superior Mediastinal nodes are included in which level of lymphnodes- *(PGMEE 2015)*
   a. I   b. V
   C. III   d. VII

[Ref: Sabiston 1st SEA/e pg.792]

38. Supraomohyoid dissection is a type of- *(PGMEE 2015)*
   a. Posterolateral dissection
   b. Selective neck dissection
   c. Modified dedical dissection
   d. Radical neck dissection

[Ref: Sabiston 19th /e pg. 797; Schwartz 10th /e pg.582]

MISCELLANEOUS

39. A person was brought to the emergency room after his dinner with c/o something sticking in his throat which later progressed to dyspnoea . Likely diagnosis is *(DNB 2008)*
   a. Myocardial Infarction   b. Foreign body aspiration
   c. Acid peptic disease   d. Ca stomach

[Ref.Scotts Brown ENT; Dhingra 7th/e pg. 366]

40. Costen's syndrome refers to neurological pain associated with? *(DNB June'2010)*
   a. Sphenopalatine ganglion
   b. Temporomandibular joint
   c. Lingual nerve
   d. Glossopharyngeal nerve

[Ref: Dhingra's 7th/e pg. 508]

Explanation

   ■ Also known as mandibular joint neuralgia

35.	a
36.	a
37.	d
38.	b
39.	b
40.	b

1. Pascal's law is used in which technique of hernia repair?　　　*(DNB June'2010)*
a. Darning repair
b. Stoppa's preperiotoneal repair
c. Lichtenstein's mesh repair
d. Bassini's repair

[Ref: Recent Advances in Surgery-10 by Jaypee Brothers, Medical Publishers, Gupta page 166]

Explanation

Mesh Repair Techniques

Techniques	Examples/Other Name
Onlay or overlay repair	Lichtenstein tension free repair
Inlay repair	Mesh at myopectineal level
Sublay or Underlay	Open Preperitoneal repair (Stoppa's technique)
Onlay-Subway sandwitch technique	Gilbert Patch & plug repair

- Application of Pascal's law will allow us to understand the biomechanics of mesh placement of abdominal wall hernias. When there is a leak in a hot air balloon or a bathtub, it is best repaired by sealing the defect from the inside.
- In Sublayhernioplasty, the prosthetic mesh is placed in the preperitoneal plane in retro-rectus space. The mesh placement is best engineered so as to be more physiological and abides by Pascal's law. It is recommended to place the mesh with at least 5-6 cm of overlap from defect margin, which allows even distribution of pressure over a wider area (Pascal's principle), and the pressure-induced apposition fixes the mesh.
- Pascal's law makes a basis for **Inlay** mesh repair Hernioplasty.

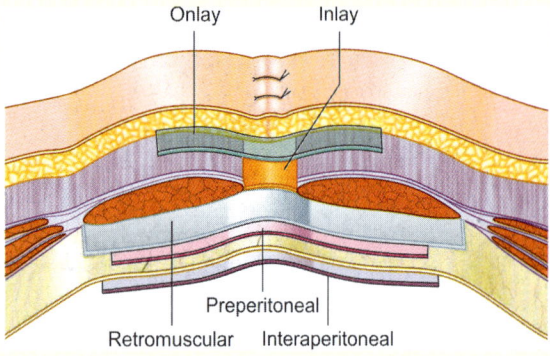

Fig. Location of mesh is in different type of hernioplasties

2. Open pre-peritoneal large mesh repair for complex inguinal hernia:-　　*(PGMEE 2015-16)*
a. Mac-Vay Operation
b. Shouldice operation
c. Lichtenstein operation
d. Stoppa operation

[Ref: Sabiston's 20th/e pg. 1101; Essentials of General Surgery 5th/e pg. 209; Bailey & Love's 27th/e pg. 1033]

3. Omphalocele is caused by?　　*(DNB Dec 2010)*
a. Failure of gut to return to the body cavity from its physiological herniation
b. Reversed rotation of the intestinal loop
c. Duplications of intestinal loops
d. Abnormal rotation of the intestinal loop

[Ref: Langman's Medical Embryology 9th/e 212, Bailey & Love 25th/e pg. 980]

4. Hernia with highest rate of strangulation is
a. Indirect inguinal hernia　　*(DNB June' 2011)*
b. Direct inguinal hernia
c. Incisional hernia
d. Femoral hernia

[Ref: Sabiston's 20th/e pg. 1104]

5. In Nyhan's classification type 3A is?　*(DNB Dec' 2011)*
a. Inguinal hernia with enlarged ring
b. Recurrent hernia
c. Direct inguinal hernia
d. Femoral and inguinal hernia both

[Ref: Sabiston's 20th/e pg. 1098]

6. What is giant hiatal hernia?　　*(DNB Dec' 2011)*
a. Bochdalek hernia
b. Sliding hernia
c. Incisional hernia
d. Paraesophageal

[Ref: Sabiston's 20th/e pg. 1059]

7. A 61 year old female presents with recurrent pneumonia, regurgitation of food and feeling of fullness. Most probable diagnosis is?　*(DNB Dec' 2011)*
a. Hiatus hernia
b. Achalasia cardia
c. Carcinoma esophagus
d. Tracheoesophageal fistula

[Ref: Sabiston's 20th/e pg. 1059]

8. Most common complication of hiatal hernia is?
　　(DNB Dec' 2011)
a. Aspiration pneumonitis
b. Volvulous
c. Esophageal stricture
d. Esophagitis

[Ref: Maingot's 11th/e p. 203; CSDT 11th/e p. 482-485]

9. Hydrocele is a type of ------- cyst　*(DNB 2007)*
a. Retention
b. Distension
c. Exudation
d. Traumatic

[Ref: Bailey & Love's 25/e p. 1502]

10. Lumbar hernia is more common through:
a. Grynfeltt triangle　　*(PGMEE 2016-17)*
b. Petit triangle
c. Gastrinoma traingle
d. Through rectus sheath

[Ref: Bailey & Love's 27th/e pg. 1042; Sabiston's 20th/e pg. 1115]

Explanation

- Most primary lumbar hernias occur through the inferior lumbar triangle of Petit bounded below by the crest of the ilium, laterally by the external oblique muscle

Answers:

1. b
2. d
3. a
4. d
5. c
6. d
7. a
8. d
9. c
10. a

and medially by latissimus dorsi. Less commonly, the sac comes through the superior lumbar triangle, which is bounded by the twelfth rib above, medially by sacrospinalis and laterally by the posterior border of the internal oblique muscle. Primary lumbar hernias are rare, but may be mimicked by incisional hernias arising through flank incisions for renal operations, or through incisions for bone grafts harvested from the iliac crest.

- Lumbar hernias can be congenital or acquired after an operation on the flank and occur in the lumbar region of the posterior abdominal wall. Hernias through the superior lumbar traingle (Grynfelt triangle) are more common. The superior lumbar triangle is counded by the 12th rib, paraspinal muscles, and internal oblique muscle. Less common are hernias through the inferior lumbar triangle (Petit triangle), which is bounded by the iliac crest latissimus dori muscle, and external oblique muscle.

- Its clear that primary tumor is common inferiorly but this is rare and overall superiorly hernias are common. Hence if question is about the commonest lumber hernias then answer would be superior and if question is about the most common primary lumber hernia then answer would be inferior triangle.

11. An asymptomatic patient presents with a reducible hernia below the inguinal ligament. Which of the following is the most appropriate management in this patient to consider:- *(PGMEE 2015-16)*
a. Emergency surgical repair of hernia
b. Emergency surgical repair with exploration of the bowel
c. Watchful waiting and follow up if symptomatic
d. Surgical repair on the next elective list

[Ref: European Hernia Society Guidelines]

12. About Spigelian hernia true statement is:-
(PGMEE 2016-17)
a. Mostly develops at 2nd and 3rd decade of life
b. Buldging is very common feature
c. After surgery recurrence in uncommon
d. Most of the hernia occure at or below the arcuate line

[Ref: Bailey & Love's 27th/e pg. 1041;
Sabiston's 20th/e pg. 1113]

13. Picture showing is characterstic of:- *(PGMEE 2016-17)*

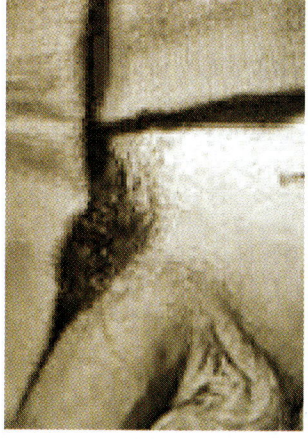

a. Varicocele
b. Hydrocele
c. Rotation of testis
d. Testicular malignancy

14. Which of the following nerves is most likely to be injured during Laparoscopic hernia surgery *(PGMEE 2015-16)*
a. Genital branch of genitofemoral nerve
b. Ilioinguinal nerve
c. Iliohypogastric nerve
d. Lateral femoral cutaneous nerve

[Ref: Sabiston's 20th/e pg. 1102]

Explanation

- Lateral femoral cutaneous nerve & femoral branch of genitofemoral nerve are likely to be injured.

15. A 50 yr old male presented with swelling of right groin. While occluding the deep inguinal ring the swelling reappears. What kind of Hernia it is:- *(PGMEE 2016-17)*

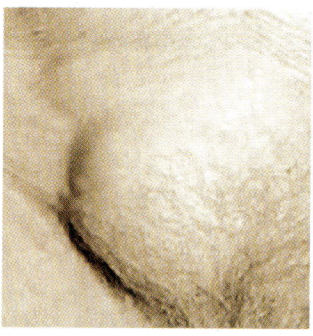

a. Direct inguinal hernia
b. Indirect inguinal hernia
c. Femoral hernia
d. Lumbar hernia

[Ref: Sabiston's 20th/e pg. 1097]

16. Richter's hernia is seen most commonly in *(DNB 2007)*
a. Direct inguinal hernia   b. Femoral hernia
c. Umbilical hernia   d. Indirect inguinal hernia

[Ref: Bailey & Love's 27th/e pg. 1024]

17. Which should not be advised as the treatment of a femoral hernia: *(DNB 2007)*
a. Lockwood's operation   b. Lotheissen's operation
c. Use of a TRUSS   d. Mc Evedy's operation

[Ref: Bailey & Love's 27th /e pg. 1036]

18. Traingle of Doom is bounded by all of the following except:- *(PGMEE 2015-16)*
a. Vas Deferens
b. Inguinal ligament
c. Gonadal vessels
d. Peritoneal reflection

[Ref: Endoscopic repair of Abdominal
wall Hernias 2nd/e pg. 41]

11.	d
12.	d
13.	a
14.	d
15.	a
16.	b
17.	c
18.	b

1. **Management of epidural abscess is** *(DNB June' 2011)*
   a. Immediate surgical evacuation
   b. Aggressive debridement
   c. Antibiotics
   d. Conservative management

   [Ref: Bailey and Love's 27th/e pg. 481]

2. **Ganglion is?** *(DNB Dec' 2011)*
   a. Collection of neurons in CNS
   b. Collection of neurons outside CNS
   c. Any collection of neurons
   d. Collection of dendrites

   [Ref: Gray's anatomy 39th/e pg. 56]

TRAUMATIC BRAIN INJURY (TBI)

3. **Common site for extradural hematoma is**
   a. Frontal *(PGMEE 2012)*
   b. Brain stem
   c. Occipital
   d. Squamous temporal bone

   [Ref: Bailey and Love's 27th/e pg. 333]

4. **In case of TBI (Traumatic brain injury) which of the following is not true:** *(NEET June 2018)*
   a. EDH & SDH with mass effects will be benefited by decompression
   b. Depressed # require early surgical intervention
   c. MRI will be able to diagnose most cases and is used as imaging modality
   d. Best motor response prognosticate the outcome

   [Ref: Bailey & Love's 26th/e pg. 315]

Explanation

Traumatic brain injury (TBI)

- Symptoms of a TBI can be mild, moderate or severe, depending on the severity and extent of brain damage to the brain.
- Mild cases may result in a brief change in sensorium and consciousness, while severe cases may result in prolonged unconsciousness, coma or even death.
- "Mass lesion" is an area of localized injury that may cause pressure within the brain. The MC mass lesions related to TBI are hematomas (epidural/subdural).
- Contusions are seen most commonly at the base of the front parts of the brain.
- The neurological examination includes an assessment using the Glasgow Coma Scale (GCS).
- The presence of a dilated pupil on only one side suggests presence of a large mass lesion on the same side of dilated pupil.
- CT scan (**not MRI**) is the gold standard for the radiological assessment of a TBI patient.

- Decompressive craniotomy is one of the available treatments for patients with TBI especially in cases of intracranial hematoma more than in cases of diffuse brain edema.
- Depressed # require early surgical intervention. Timely surgical management gives excellent results by decreasing morbidity and mortality.

5. **Image shown below is:** *(PGMEE 2016-17)*

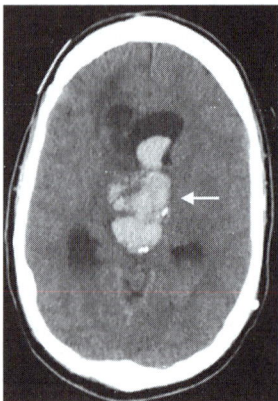

   a. Intracranial bleeding   b. Intracranial tumor
   c. Subdural hemorrhage   d. Cystic swelling

6. **A 60 year old alcoholic who sustained blunt trauma to his head due to assaults appears confused. He opens his eyes and speaks incomprehensible words on when his sternum is pressed. He withdraws his hand when approached. His Glasgow Coma Score is-** *(PGMEE 2015)*
   a. 6   b. 8
   c. 10   d. 12

   [Ref: Sabiston's 1st SAE pg.411; Bailey and Love's 27th/e pg. 331]

7. **A 50-year-old man with subdural hematoma following RTA is brought to casualty. On examination he is confused, eye opening on pain with flexion on left arm. There is localization of pain on right. His GCS is:-** *(PGMEE 2018)*
   a. 8   b. 9
   c. 10   d. 11

   [Ref: Bailey & Love's 27th/e pg. 331]

Explanation

Glasgow Coma Score

- The GCS is the sum of scores on three components as detailed in Table.
- Remember that the score represents the best performance elicited, so a patient flexing in response to a painful stimulus on the left and localising on the right scores 'M5'.
- [In this patient EVM will be 2 + 4 + 5 = 11]

1.	a
2.	b
3.	d
4.	c
5.	b
6.	b
7.	d

8. A patient opens eye to painful stimulus, saying inappropriate sentences and is able to spontaneously move all four limbs. What is the GCS score?
   a. 11
   b. 10   *(NEET Pattern 2017)*
   c. 8
   d. 15

   [Ref: Bailey and Love's 27th/e pg. 331; Sabiston (20th edition) page 411]

Explanation
- ■ **Eye Opening**
  - ○ Spontaneous 4
  - ○ To voice 3
  - ○ To pain 2
  - ○ None 1
- ■ **Verbal Response**
  - ○ Oriented 5
  - ○ Confused 4
  - ○ Inappropriate 3
  - ○ Incomprehensible 2
  - ○ None 1
- ■ **Motor Response**
  - ○ Obeys commands 6
  - ○ Localizes pain 5
  - ○ Withdraws to pain 4
  - ○ Flexion 3
  - ○ Extension 2
  - ○ None 1
- ■ **Total Glasgow Coma Scale Score** = 3-15
- ■ Injury Severity Score (ISS), calculated by summing the squares of the AIS(Abbreviated Injury Scale) severity codes for the three most severely injured body parts
- ■ The ISS ranges from 1 to 75, with severity groupings being defined as minor injury (ISS less than 9), moderate injury (ISS between 9 and 16), serious injury (ISS between 16 and 15), and severe injury (ISS more than 25).

9. All are componnets of GCS except   *(DNB June' 2009)*
   a. Eye opeining
   b. Respiration
   c. Conversation
   d. Motor response

   [Ref: Bailey and Love's 27th/e pg. 331]

10. A young male comes to emergency room following an accident in an unconscious state. A CT is done, shown below. The neurosurgeon orders immediate surgical decompression. As a surgery interne the probable diagnosis based on clinical scenario and the CT is:
    (PGMEE 2016-17)

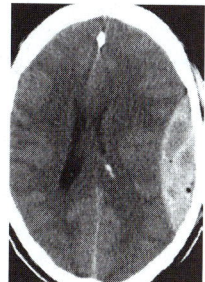

   a. Subdural hematoma
   b. Epidural hematoma
   c. Subarachnoid bleed
   d. Isolated brain contusion

   [Ref: Bailey & Love's 27th/e pg. 333]

11. Which of the following requires emergency operation in setting without tertiary care facilities:
    a. Subdural hemorrhage   *(PGMEE 2016-17)*
    b. Subarachnoid hemorrhage
    c. Extradural hemorrhage
    d. Intracerebral hemorrhage

    [Ref: Bailey & Love's 27th/e pg. 333]

12. In treatment of head-injuries one of the following is contraindicated:-   *(PGMEE 2016-17)*
    a. Mannitol
    b. Diuretics
    c. Antibiotics
    d. Narcotics

13. Lucid interval is most commonly seen in-   *(PGMEE 2015)*
    a. Acute Subdural Hemorrhage
    b. Chronic Subdural hemorrhage
    c. Acute extradural hemorrhage
    d. Subarachnoid hemorrhage

    [Ref: Bailey & Love's 27th/e pg. 333]

14. MRI of brain shown below identify the structure:-
    (PGMEE 2016-17)

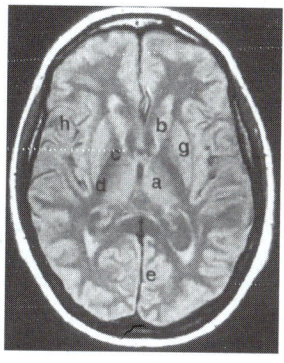

    a. a- thalamus b- caudate nucleus c – genu of internal capsule d – posterior limb
    b. a- thalamus b- caudate nucleus c– posterior limb d– genu of internal capsule
    c. a - caudate nucleus b- thalamus c – genu of internal capsule d – posterior limb
    d. a- posterior limb b- caudate nucleus c – genu of internal capsule d –thalamus

15. Subdural hematoma is due to rupture of-
    a. Retromandibular vein   *(PGMEE 2015)*
    b. Middle meningeal artery
    c. Saccular berry Anuerysm
    d. Communicating veins to superior sagittal sinus

    [Ref: Bailey & Love's 27th/e pg. 333]

16. The most common neurologic abnormality that occurs with head injury is   *(DNB 2007)*
    a. Hemiplegia
    b. Ocular nerve palsy
    c. Altered consciousness
    d. Convulsions

17. A patient has an accident with resultant transection of the pituitary what will not occur
    a. Diabetes mellitus   *(DNB 2007; PGMEE 2016-17)*
    b. Diabetes insipidus
    c. Hyperprolactinemia
    d. Hypothyroidism

    [Ref: Bailey and Love's 27th/e pg. 337]

8.	a
9.	b
10.	b
11.	c
12.	d
13.	c
14.	a
15.	d
16.	c
17.	a

1. **A newborn delivered to a mother with polyhydramnios. After birth regurgitate feeds & shows continuous drooling of saliva. Most likely diagnosis is:**
   (Recent Pattern June 2018)
   a. Oropharyngoesophageal disorders
   b. Esophageal atresia
   c. Congenital webs
   d. Meckel's diverticulum
   [Ref: O.P. Ghai 8th/e pg. 176; Nelson's 20th/e pg. 1783]

Explanation

- Neonates born to mother with polyhydramnios have higher chances of **esophageal atresia**. Neonates with esophageal atresia usually present with drooling of saliva which is noted soon after birth and is a/w frothing.
- Symptoms in **Oropharyngoesophageal disorders** in young children may thus include subtle prolongation of feeds, delay in milestones of feeding abilities, impairment of normal weight gain, excessive drooling of saliva, increases of regurgitation beyond that expected physiologically, unexplained fussiness, or chronic/recurrent respiratory symptoms.

IHPS

2. **In congenital hypertrophic pyloric stenosis (IHPS), which of the following is true regarding palpable mass:-**
   (PGMEE 2018)
   a. The mass is best felt right to left in epigastrium while crying
   b. It is best felt after feeding
   c. Olive shaped mass is felt
   d. Mass is felt in right hypochondrium
   [Ref: Nelson 19th edition – chapter 321; Bailey & Love 27th/e pg. 127-128]

Explanation

- The diagnosis is usually made with a test feed : In this the baby is breastfed or fed with the bottle by a nurse in lap of mother and surgeon palpates the abdomen with a warm hand to detect the lump observes the characteristic peristaltic waves pass across the upper abdomen. After feeding, there may be a visible gastric peristaltic wave that progresses across the abdomen.
- Pathologically musculature of pylorus adjacent to antrum is grossly hypertrophied. There is **P**alpable tumour (Olive) in mid epigastrium, The mass is firm, movable, ~2 cm in length, olive shaped, hard, best palpated from the left side. The olive is easiest palpated after an episode of vomiting.

3. **Metabolic abnormalities associated with congenital pyloric stenosis in the early phase include all except?**
   (DNB Dec'2010)
   a. Hypokalemia
   b. Alkalosis
   c. Hypochloremia
   d. None of these
   [Ref: Sabiston's 20th/e pg.1869]

4. **Which metabolic abnormality is seen in congenital hypertrophic pyloric stenosis?** *(PGMEE 2015)*
   a. Metabolic Acidosis
   b. Metabolic Alkalosis
   c. Respiratory Alkalosis
   d. Respiratory Acidosis
   [Ref: Sabiston's 20th/e pg.1869]

5. **Exposure to which of the following drugs is incriminated in IHPS (infantile hypertrophic pyloric stenosis):**
   (PGMEE 2014-15)
   a. Erythromycin
   b. Lithium
   c. Warfarin
   d. Carbimazole
   [Ref: ch. 326 Nelson's 18th ed.]

6. **Paradoxical aciduria seen in** *(DNB June' 2012)*
   a. Intestinal obstruction
   b. Vesico vaginal fistula
   c. Enterocutaneous fistula
   d. Pyloric obstruction
   [Ref: Sabiston's 20th/e pg.1869; Bailey and love 27th/e pg. 128]

7. **What is the most characteristic of congenital hypertrophic pyloric stenosis:** *(DNB 2007)*
   a. Affects the first born female child
   b. The pyloric tumor is best felt during feeding
   c. The patient is commonly marasmic
   d. Loss of appetite occurs early
   [Ref: Bailey and Love's 27th/e pg. 128]

8. **All of the following are true about congenital hypertrophic pyloric stenosis except-** *(PGMEE 2015)*
   a. Metabolic acidosis occurs
   b. Non Billous vomiting is seen
   c. RamStedt Pyloromyotomy is the treatment of choice
   d. More common in males
   [Ref: Bailey & Love 27th/e pg. 128]

DUODENAL ATRESIA

9. **Anomaly associated with duodenal atresia is?**
   (DNB June'2010)
   a. Down syndrome
   b. Autoimmune disorders
   c. Duodenal adenomas
   d. Limb defects
   [Ref: Sabiston 1st SEA/e pg. 1870]

10. **"Double-bubble" sign is pathognomonic of:**
    a. Hypertrophic pyloric stenosis
    b. Duodenal atresia
    c. Jejunal atresia
    d. Ileal stenosis
    [Ref: Sabiston's 20th/e pg. 1870]

1.	b
2.	c
3.	d
4.	b
5.	a
6.	d
7.	b
8.	a
9.	a
10.	b

HIRSCHSPRUNG DISEASE

11. All of the following are true about Hirschsprung disease expect- *(PGMEE 2015)*
a. Absence of Ganglion cells in the involved segment
b. Swenson, Duhamel and soave are surgical procedures for this condition
c. The non peristaltic affected segment is dilated
d. Mainly presents in family

[Ref: Sabiston 20th/e pg. 1876]

12. All of the following are true about Hirschsprung Disease expect- *(All india Dec. 15 pattern)*
a. Autosomal dominant
b. Absent ganglionic cell in submucus plexus
c. Rectal biopsy is diagnostic
d. Absent ganglionic cell in myentric plexus

[Ref: Sabiston 20th /e pg. 1876; In familial HD, inheritance may be XR/AD]

13. Hirschsprung's colon is due to- *(PGMEE 2013-14)*
a. Loss of extrinsic nerve supply
b. Loss of intrinsic enteric plexuses
c. Muscle atrophy in muscularis mucosa
d. None

[Ref: Robbin's 9th/e pg. 751]

14. In Hirschsprung's disease, staining used for diagnosis is? *(DNB Nov. 13 Pattern)*
a. Auramine Rhodamine stain
b. Fontana stain
c. AChE (Acetylcholine esterase) and calretinin
d. Trichome stain

[Ref: Robbin's 9th/e pg. 751; Sabiston's 20th/e pg. 1876]

MISCELLANEOUS

15. Common cause of intussusception is- *(PGMEE 2015)*
a. Polyp
b. Submucocus lipoma
c. Meckel's diverticulum
d. Hyperplasia of submucous peyer's Patches

[Ref: Bailey & Love 27th /e pg. 1283; Sabiston's 20th/e pg. 1879]

16. Omphalocele is caused by: *(Recent Pattern 2019)*
a. Duplication of Intestinal loops
b. Abnormal rotation of the intestinal loop
c. Failure of GUT to return to the body cavity from its physiological herniation
d. Reversed rotation of intestinal loop

[Ref: Sabiston 20th/e pg. 1071]

17. Turricephaly is: *(Recent Pattern June 2018)*
a. Premature fusion of frontal sutures
b. Premature fusion of coronal, sphenofrontal and frontoethmoidal sutures
c. Premature fusion of only sagittal sutures
c. Premature fusion of occipital sutures

[Ref: Nelson's 20th/e pg. 2818]

Explanation

Turricephaly

- Also known as Acrocephaly, Hypsicephaly, Oxycephaly, Steeple head, Tower head, Tower skull, High-head syndrome and Turmschädel, Oxycephaly is the most severe of the craniosynostosis.
- Early fusion of a combination of the bilateral coronal, sagittal & sometimes lambdoid sutures.
- Oxycephaly is a form of craniosynostosis that involves the fusion multiple sutures. Isolated oxycephaly is a late-appearing form of nonsyndromic craniosynostosis characterized by premature fusion of both the coronal and sagittal sutures
- The coronal, sagittal & lambdoid sutures are normally involved.
- This fusion gives a high, conical head with sharp bossing in the region of the anterior fontanelle.

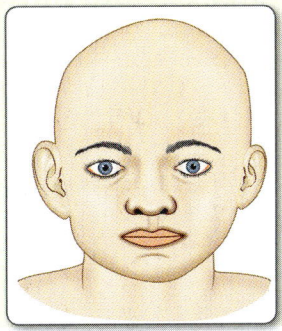

18. A cystic mass at the base of umbilical cord in a neonate could be- *(PGMEE 2015)*
a. Cystic Hygroma b. Meckel's Diverticulum
c. Allantoic Cyst   d. Ventral mesogastrium

[Ref: Amano Y, Hayashi T. Takahama K et-al. MR imaging of umbilical cord urachal (allantoic. cyst in utero. AJR Am J Roentgenol. 2003; 180 (4): 1181-2]

19. Which of the following is false about undescended testis? *(PGMEE 2015)*
a. More common on the right side
b. Secondary sexual characteristics are normal
c. Hormonal therapy is effective
d. Increased risk of malignancy

[Ref: Campbell's urology 10th /e pg.3561; Bailey & Love 27th/e pg. 125; Sabiston 20th/e pg. 1885]

20. KASAI Procedure is used in the treatment of- *(PGMEE 2015)*
a. Congenital Biliary Atesia
b. Carcinoma of gall bladder
c. Cholangiocarcinoma
d. Primary Sclerosing

[Ref: Sabiston 20th/e pg. 1880]

21. Which is the most common urethral anomaly? *(PGMEE 2015)*
a. Epispadias   b. Bladder Exstrophy
c. Urethral stenosis d. Hypospadias

[Ref: Bailey & Love 27th/e pg.1478]

11.	c
12.	a
13.	b
14.	c
15.	b
16.	c
17.	b
18.	c
19.	c
20.	a
21.	d

1. **Ideal timing of repair of isolated cleft lip is:-**
   a. 4-6 months   *(PGMEE 2016-17; 2015)*
   b. 1-2 months
   c. After 2 years
   d. Pre-school age

   [Ref: Sabiston's 20th /e pg. 1946]

2. **Cleft lip repair minimum age:-**   *(PGMEE 2016-17)*
   a. 3-4 months   b. 6 months
   c. 12 months   d. 2 years

   [Ref: Sabiston's 20th /e pg. 1946]

BURNS

3. **A patient suffered from 2nd degree burn of right upper limb, 3rd degree burns of right lower limb and 2nd degree burn of whole of the back. Total percentage of burn will be**   *(DNB June' 2011)*
   a. 27%   b. 36%
   c. 45%   d. 54%

   [Ref: Schwartz's 9th/e chapter 8 table 8-2, Bailey & Love 25th/e p. 382, Practical plastic surgery by Zol B. Kryger, Mark Sisco page 155]

4. **Myoglobinuria is seen in which type of burns**
                                      (PGMEE 2012)
   a. Contact burn   b. Scald burn
   c. Flame burn   d. Electric

   [Ref: Principles and practice of burn surgery p. 27]

5. **Operation theatre fire is most commonly due to?**
   a. Argon beam coagulators
   b. Laser
   c. Fiber optic illumination
   d. Electrosurgical equipment

   [Ref: BJA Volume 50, Issue 7 p. 659-664, Current Opinion in Anaesthesiology: December 2008 Volume 21 Issue 6 p. 790-795]

6. **Sun-burns are**   *(DNB 2007)*
   a. First Degree Burns
   b. Second Degree Burns
   c. Third Degree Burns
   d. Could be any of the above

   [Ref: Sabiston's 20th /e pg. 506; Schwartz Surgery 9/e p195, Bailey 25/2 p382]

7. **In a 6 year old child with burns involving the whole of head and trunk, the estimated body surface area of burns is:**   *(DNB 2008)*
   a. 41%   b. 52%
   c. 55%   d. 58%

   [Ref: Sabiston's 20th /e pg. 508]

8. **2nd degree burn involve:-**   *(PGMEE 2016-17)*
   a. Epidermis only
   b. Dermis only
   c. Epidermis + upper dermis
   d. Epidermis + dermis

   [Ref: Sabiston's 20th /e pg. 506]

9. **Blisters are classified as which type of burn**
   a. Deep first degree   *(DNB Dec' 2009)*
   b. Superficial second degree burn
   c. Superficial first degree burn
   d. Third degree

   [Ref: Sabiston's 20th /e pg. 506]

10. **Skin grafts stored at 4° C can survive up to**
                                      (DNB Dec 2009)
   a. 1 week   b. 2 weeks
   c. 3 weeks   d. 4 weeks

   [Ref: Facial Plastic and Reconstructive Surgery by Ira d. Papel p. 44 http://sydney.edu.au/medicine/foundation/sydneyburns/research/msg.php; Fundamental technique of plastic surgery page 47]

Explanation

- Because no preservative has mention in question reference
- By storage at a low temperature, skin cut inn excess of current requirement can be preserved viable for Later use as needed. The increase in the use of delayed exposed grafting has greatly increased the need for storage within the temperature range 0-37^{0}C the survival time of a stored graft is a function of its temperature the lower the temperature the longer the survival time.
- The graft is wrapped in gauze moistened with saline and placed in a sterile, sealed container. Unless specially long survival, e.g. up to 21 days, it's needed the storage temperature is not ol paramount important, but it seems probable that 4^{0}C is likely to give the best results.

11. **Which of the following is effective against pseudomonas and is used in burns patients**   *(DNB June' 2009)*
   a. Silver sulphadiazine
   b. Silver suplhazine
   c. Sulfamethoxozole
   d. Sulfadoxne

   [Ref: KDT 6th/e p. 643]

12. **A patient weighing 50 kg presents with 40% burn. What is the volume of fluid to be given in the first 8 hours using Parkland's formula:**   *(PGMEE 2018)*
   a. 4 litre   b. 1 litre
   c. 2 litre   d. 8 Litres

   [Ref: Sabiston's 19th/e pg. 530]

1.	a
2.	a
3.	c
4.	d
5.	d
6.	a
7.	a
8.	d
9.	b
10.	c
11.	a
12.	a

Explanation

- Parkland Formula = 4ml/kg per % TBSA burn (for 24hrs)
- Fluid requirement = 4 x 50kg x 40% = 8000 ml
- Fluid requirement for first 8 hrs = half the total requirement = 4 L

Resuscitation formulas

Volume			
Formula	Crystalioid	Colloid	Free water
Parkland	4 mL/kg per % TBSA burn	None	None
Brooke	1.5 mL/kg % TBSA burn	0.5 mL/kg per % TBSA burn	20 liters
Galveston (pediatric)	500 mL/m² burned area + 1500 mL/m² total area	None	None

1. A patient with blunt abdominal trauma presented to casualty with BP 90/60 mm Hg. His pulse rate is 124. The investigation to be done in this patient is?

(DNB Dec'2010)

a. DPL   b. FAST sonogram

c. CT abdomen   d. MRI abdomen

[Ref: Bailey and love 25th/e e p. 143-144]

2. A patient presents with internal bleeding after blunt trauma abdomen. Next management in unstable patient:- *(PGMEE 2016-17)*

a. Diagnostic peritoneal lavage

b. CECT

c. FAST

d. Immediate surgery

[Ref: Sabiston's 20th/e (=1st SAE) pg. 433]

3. Tripod fracture is seen in? *(DNB June'2010)*

a. Zygomatic bone

b. Temporo-mandibular joint

c. Frontoal bone

d. Maxilla

[Ref: Dhingra's 6th/e pg. 183]

Explanation

- Zygomaticomaxillary complex (ZMC) fractures, also known as tripod, tetrapod, quadripod, malar or trimalar fractures, are seen in the setting of traumatic injury to the face. They comprise fractures of the:
  ○ Zygomatic arch
  ○ Inferior orbital rim, and anterior and posterior maxillary sinus walls
  ○ Lateral orbital rim
- Account for ~40% of midface fractures.

4. What is the treatment for blunt trauma of kidney *(DNB June' 2011)*

a. Conservative   b. Nephrectomy

c. Nephrotomy   d. Nephroplexy

[Ref: Sabiston's 20th/e pg. 1896]

Explanation

Most genitourinary injuries involve the kidney, most are due to blunt mechanisms, and most are low grade.

- Most blunt renal injuries, including all grade 1 and 2 and most grade 3 and 4 injuries, can be safely managed conservatively. Patients should be maintained on strict bed rest until the gross hematuria has resolved.
- Obtain CECT for suspected moderate or severe injury (eg, gross hematuria, hypotension, mechanism or findings suggesting a significant renal injury).
- Consider surgical intervention or therapeutic angiography for patients with:

  ○ Persistent bleeding (ie, enough to necessitate repeated transfusions)
  ○ Expanding perinephric hematoma
  ○ Renal pedicle avulsion or other significant renovascular injuries
- Consider a ureteral stent for persistent urinary extravasation

5. After trauma, hypovolemic shock can be due to all EXCEPT *(DNB June' 2011)*

a. Blunt trauma to abdominal viscera

b. Head injury

c. Hemothorax

d. Pelvic fracture

[Ref: Fluid and Electrolyte Balance by Nomra Milligan Metheny Page 221]

Explanation

Common causes of hypovolemic shock	Nonhemorrhagic	■ Burns ■ Emesis ■ Diarrhoea
	Hemorrhagic (trauma)	■ Major vessel rupture ■ Solid abdominal organ injury ■ Pelvic and femoral fractures ■ Arterial lacerations
	Hemorrhagic (nontrauma)	■ Esophageal varices ■ Mallory-Weiss tears ■ Peptic ulcers ■ Aneurysm rupture ■ Arteriovenous malformations

6. Perineal hematoma after trauma is due to

a. Pelvic organ blunt trauma   *(DNB June' 2011)*

b. Rupture of bulbar urethra

c. Rupture of membranous urethra

d. Rupture of bladder

[Ref: Sabiston Textbook of Surgery, 18th/e p. Chapter 77]

Explanation

- On examination, patients with injuries to the urethra distal to the urogenital diaphragm and not contained by the Buck fascia typically have a butterfly hematoma, which forms as blood collects in the superficial perineum.
- Any type of trauma may affect any part of the urethra but much the commonest is iatrogenic trauma (~3%) due to catheterisation, instrumentation or surgery of the urethra.
- Non-iatrogenic trauma to the urinary tract accounts for ≈1.5% of all traumas.

1.	b
2.	c
3.	a
4.	a
5.	b
6.	b

- Pelvic fracture-related urethral injuries (PFUIs) of the posterior urethra are the commonest non-iatrogenic injuries and are usually due to motor vehicle accidents.
- Penile swelling is usually limited to the attachments of Buck's fascia and only the shaft of the penis will be ecchymotic; a localized hematoma has been termed as an "eggplant deformity." A perineal butterfly hematoma or scrotal bleeding can occur when the deep investing fascia of the penis has been ruptured by penetrating or blunt trauma.
- Posterior urethral injury is usually at the bulbo-membranous junction

7. Most common organ injury in sharp penetrating trauma:- *(PGMEE 2016-17)*

a. Liver
b. Small Bowel
c. Spleen
d. Bladder

[Ref: Sabiston's 1st SAE 20th pg.437]

Explanation

- In penetrating abdominal trauma due to gunshot wounds, the most commonly injured organs are as follows :
  - Small bowel (50%)
  - Colon (40%)
  - Liver (30%)
  - Abdominal vascular structures (25%)
- The reported incidence of internal organ injury after penetrating trauma has been reported to be as high as 70%
- Penetrating injuries are more frequent on the left side, especially in the case of stab wound .
- The most commonly injured intra-abdominal organs are the small intestine, liver and colon. Of these only one third will penetrate the peritoneum & only 50% of these will require surgical intervention. In contrast, 85% of abdominal gun-shot wounds (GSW) penetrate the peritoneum & 95% of these require a surgical intervention.

8. Best investigation to be done immediately when a patient comes with blunt abdominal trauma is- *(PGMEE 2015)*

a. USG
b. Abdominal Xray
c. CT Scan
d. Complete Hemogram

[Ref: Schwartz 10th/e pg. 181]

9. A Child presented with blunt trauma abdomen, the first investigation to be done is- *(PGMEE 2015)*

a. CT scan
b. USG
c. Abdominal Xray
d. Complete Hemogram

[Ref: Schwartz 10th /e pg.181]

10. MESS score includes all except:- *(PGMEE 2016-17)*

a. Shock
b. Age
c. Velocity of trauma
d. Blood pressure

[Ref: Sabiston's 1st SAE pg.484]

11. In Acute trauma:- *(PGMEE 2016-17)*

a. T_3 T_4 decreases, insulin decreases, cortisol & glucogon increases
b. T_3 T_4 decreases, insulin increase, cortisol & glucogon increase
c. T_3 T_4 increase, insulin increase, cortisol & glucogon increase
d. T_3 T_4 increase, insulin decreases, cortisol & glucogon increase

[Ref: Sabiston's 1st SAE pg.242]

12. TRISS incluses all of the following expect- *(PGMEE 2015)*

a. Urine output
b. Injury severity score
c. Revised Trauma score
d. Age

13. A 25 year old male presents with road traffic accidents with a BP of 100/80mm Hg and a pulse of 84/min. Best fluid for resuscitation is- *(PGMEE 2015)*

a. Packed RBCs
b. Crystalloid
c. Colloid
d. Whole Blood

[Ref: Sabiston's 1st SAE pg.416]

14. A 30 year old male is hit by an iron rod resulting in a Gr IIIA open fracture of the tibia. The Protocol for tetanus immunization in this patient who had last taken tetanus toxoid 12 years back is- *(PGMEE 2015)*

a. TT one dose + Ig
b. Full dose of Human tetanus Ig
c. Only one dose of TT
d. Complete course of TT

[Ref: Park's 23rd/e pg. 314; Sabiston 20th/e pg. 515]

Explanation

Prevention of Tetanus

- Wounds contaminated with soil can harbor tetanus spores, and active immunisation is indicated by administering 0.5 mL of tetanus toxoid intramuscularly.
- Patients with gross contamination of cavitating wounds should also receive 250–500 U of human anti-tetanus globulin (ATG) intramuscularly to provide passive immunization and to neutralise the circulating toxin. In full-administered. Wound manipulation should be avoided for 2–3 hours after ATG administration to minimise tetanospasmin release.
- *Local wound care:-* This includes a thorough wound debridement to eliminate the anaerobic environment. Intravenous administration of 10–24 × 106 U per day of penicillin G should be continued for 10–14 days. Thewound should be closed using the delayed primary or secondary closure techniques.
- Supportive care for established disease. These patients are nursed in an intensive care unit (ICU) environment, free from strong sensory stimuli. Diazepam is useful in preventing the onset of spasms but if these become sustained, the patient is paralysed, intubated and placed on a ventilator. The patient is then gradually weaned off the ventilator under cover of anticonvulsants. The overall mortality rate is around 45%, prognosis being determined by theincubation period and the time from the first symptom to the first tetanic spasm. In general, shorter intervals indicate a poorer prognosis.

7.	a
8.	a
9.	b
10.	d
11.	a
12.	a
13.	b
14.	a

- Recommendations for tetanus prophylaxis are based on th condition of the wound and the patient's immunization history. All patients with burns of more than 10% TBSA should receive 0.5 mL of tetanus toxoid. If prior immunization is absent or unclear or the last booster dose was more than 10 years ago, 250 units of tetanus immune globulin are also given.

Tetanus Wound Management

Vaccination History	Clean, minor wounds		All other wounds[*]	
	Tdap or Td[‡]	TIG	Tdap or Td[‡]	TIG
Unknown or fewer than 3 doses	Yes	No	Yes	Yes
3 or more doses	No[£]	No	No[¶]	No

- [*]Such as, but not limited to, wounds contaminated with dirt, feces, soil and saliva; puncture wounds; avulsions; and wounds resulting from missiles, crushing, burns, and frostbite.
- [‡]Tdap is preferred to Td for adults who have never received Tdap. Single antigen tetanus toxoid (TT) is no longer available in the United States.
- [£]Yes, if more than ten years since the last tetanus toxoid-containing vaccine dose.
- [¶]Yes, if more then five years since the last tetanus toxoid-containing vaccine dose.

15. In case of polytrauma with multiple injuries to the chest, neck and abdomen, highest priority is given to- *(PGMEE 2015)*
   a. Vasopressors
   b. Crystalloids
   c. Stabilizing of cervical spine
   d. Assesing disability

   [Ref: Sabiston's 1st SAE pg. 413]

16. Organ most damaged in bomb explosion: *(DNB 2008)*
   a. Heart   b. Liver
   c. Ear   d. Skeletal muscles

   [Ref: Bailey 25th/e pg. 423; Sabiston's 1st SAE pg. 594]

17. The least common organ injured by blast injury is- *(PGMEE 2015)*
   a. Tympanic membrane
   b. Stomach
   c. Spleen
   d. Alveoli of Lungs

   [Ref: Love & Bailey 26th /e pg. 430]

15. c
16. c
17. c

1. Features of acute ischemia of limb are all except ?

(DNB Dec'2010)

a. Pain b. Cyanosis

c. Paralysis d. Perishing cold

[Ref: Sabiston 1st SEA/e pg. 1777]

Explanation

- Presentation of an acutely ischemic leg is referred to as the five or six *p*'s, *poikilothermia; pain, pallor, pulselessness, paresthesias,* and *paralysis.*

2. Butcher's thigh is? **(DNB Dec'2010)**

a. Vastus lateral rupture

b. Accidental injury to major vessels in thigh or groin

c. Sabctaneous lipodermatosclerosis

d. Bursa in adductor canal

[Ref: Bailey & Love's Short practice of surgery 18th/e p. 147, 69 (in older editions]

3. Best method to treat a large port-wine hemangioma is?

a. Excision with skin grafting **(DNB Dec'2010)**

b. Radiotherapy

c. Tatooing

d. Pulsed dye laser

[Ref: Bailey and Love 27th/e pg.613]

4. Allens test for integretiy of palmar arch tests which of the following? **(DNB Dec' 2011)**

a. Radial artery b. Ulnar artery

c. Both d. None

[Ref: Bailey and Love 27th/e pg.444]

5. Trendelenburg's operation is done for **(PGMEE 2012)**

a. Deep vein thrombosis

b. Varicose veins

c. Burger's disease

d. Obturator hernia

[Ref: SRB's Manual of Surgery by Sriram Bhat 3rd e p. 199]

Explanation

- It is the surgical procedure for t/t of varicose veins.
- It is the juxtafemoral flush ligation of the great saphenous vein to the femoral vein.

BUERGER'S DISEASE

6. Buerger's disease involves **(PGMEE 2012)**

a. Arteries and veins

b. Arteries only

c. Veins only

d. Artery, vein and nerve

[Ref: Sabiston's 20th/e pg. 1780]

Explanation

- Thromboangitis obliterans, or Buerger disease, predominantly affects young male smokers in their 30s, presenting with distal limb ischemia and localized digital gangrene.
- Onset before 45 years.

7. In Buerger's disease all are affected except

(DNB June' 2009)

a. Lymphatics b. Veins

c. Nerves d. Small vessels

[Ref: SRB manual of surgery edition 4th/e pg. 185; Sabiston's 20th/e pg. 1780 ; Internet]

Explanation

Smoke contain **carbon monooxide** and **nicotinic acid**

↓ ← Carboxyhaemoglobin

Causes initially vasospasm and hyperplasia of intima

↓

Thrombosis and so obliteration of vessels occur commonly medium sized vessels are involved

↓

Panarteritis is common

Usually involvement is **segmented**

↓

Eventually artery, vein and nerve are together involved

↓

Nerve involvement causes rest pain

↓

Patient presents with features of ischaemia in the limb

↓

Once blockage occurs, plenty of collaterals open up depending on the site of blockage either around knee joint or around buttock

Once collaterals open up, through these collaterals, blood supply is maintained to the ischaemic area

↓

It is called as compensatory peripheral all vascular disease.

↓

If patient continues to smoke, disease progresses into the collaterals, blocking them eventually, leading to severe ischaemia and is called as **decompensatory** peripheral vascular disease. It is presently called as **critical limb ischaemia**. It causes rest pain, ulceration, gangrene.

- So lymphatics not involve.

1.	b
2.	b
3.	d
4.	c
5.	b
6.	a
7.	a

VARICOSE VEINS

8. Image of a surgical condition is shown below. Spot the diagnosis *(PGMEE 2016-17)*

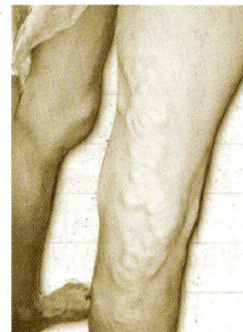

a. Arterio-venous malformation
b. Filariasis
c. Congenital vascular malformation
d. Varicosity of veins

[Ref: Sabiston's 1st SAE pg. 1831]

9. A patient presents with heaviness of leg with veins of diameter less than 1mm over the posterior part of the calf- Under CEAP , classification it comes under *(Recent Pattern 2019)*

a. C1   b. C2
c. C3   d. C0

10. Most common site of venous ulcers in varicose vein à:-
a. Gaiter area of leg   *(PGMEE 2016-17)*
b. Below toe
c. In between knee and gaiter area
d. Above thigh

[Ref: Sabiston's 1st SAE pg. 1831]

11. "Bisgaard regime" is used for the treatment of:- *(PGMEE 2016-17)*

a. Arterial ulcer   b. Venous ulcer
c. Cock's peculiar ulcer   d. Pott's puffy ulcer

[Ref. Bailey and Love]

MISCELLANEOUS

12. In aortic dissection DeBakey classification Type I involves which part of aorta: *(PGMEE 2016-17)*
a. Ascending aorta
b. Ascending aorta, aortic arch, and descending aorta
c. Descending thoracic aorta
d. Abdominal aorta

[Ref: Sabiston's 1st SAE pg. 1746]

13. Most common precipitant of Raynaud's phenomenon is- *(PGMEE 2015)*
a. Exertion   b. Exposure to Cold
c. Exposure to heat   d. Psychosocial triggers

[Ref: Bailey and Love 27th/e pg. 967]

14. Ankle Brachial Pressure Index (ABPI) Suggesting imminent necrosis is: *(PGMEE 2015-16)*
a. < 0.3   b. < 0.5
c. < 0.9   d. < 1

[Ref: Bailey and Love 26th/e pg. 880, 935]

15. Ankle brachial index (ABPI) may be falsely high in:- *(PGMEE 2018)*

a. Aorto ileitis/calcified vessels
b. Claudication/Chronic venous insufficiency
c. Acute limb ischemia
d. Deep venous thrombosis

[Ref: Bailey & Love 27th/e pg. 945]

Explanation

- Quantitative assessment can be performed at the bedside by measuring the ankle-brachial pressure index (ABPI); the ratio of systolic pressure at the ankle to that in the ipsilateral arm. The highest pressure in the dorsalis pedis, posterior tibial or peroneal artery serves as the numerator, with the highest brachial systolic pressure being the denominator. is.

ABPI	Inference
0.9-1.3	The normal resting ABPI
Below 0.9	Indicate some degree of arterial obstruction (claudication)
<0.5	Rest pain
<0.3	Indicates imminent necrosis

- Artificially high ABPI values can be caused by calcified, incompressible arteries which are often found in diabetics.

ANEURYSMS

16. Abdominal aortic aneurysm is operated when the size is more than (size beyond which risk of rupture increases) *(PGMEE 2018)*
a. 35 mm   b. 45 mm
c. 65 mm   d. 55 mm

[Ref: Bailey & Love 27th/e pg. 961]

Explanation

- An asymptomatic abdominal aortic aneurysm in an otherwise fit patient should be considered for repair if >55 mm in diameter (measured by ultrasonography).

17. Cirsoid aneurysms of the scalp are typically derived from:- *(PGMEE 2015-16)*
a. Occipital artery
b. External carotid artery
c. Superficial temporal artery
d. Internal carotid artery

Explanation

- In 90% of the patients the superficial temporal a is the main supply of fistula

18. Which of the following is the commonest site of peripheral arterial aneurysm: *(PGMEE 2015-16)*
a. Popliteal
b. Subclavian
c. Superficial femoral
d. Axillary

[Ref: Bailey & Love 27th/e pg. 966]

8.	d
9.	a
10.	a
11.	b
12.	b
13.	b
14.	a
15.	a
16.	d
17.	c
18.	a

CLAUDICATION

19. Pseudoclaudication is due to the compression of:
(PGMEE 2016-17, DNB 2007)

a. Femoral artery b. Femoral nerve
c. Cauda equina d. Popliteal artery

[Ref: Sabiston's 1st SAE pg. 1757]

20. Pseudoclaudication occurs due to- *(PGMEE 2015)*

a. Lumber canal stenosis
b. Poplitear thrombosis
c. Femoral artery thrombosis
d. Leriche syndrome

[Ref: Oxford text book of surgery vol.lll pg.2865]

21. Intermittent claudication means:
(PGMEE 2016-17; DNB 2008)

a. Pain in leg on walking
b. Pain in leg on rest
c. Pain in leg only on exercise
d. Cyanosis of leg

[Ref: Harrison 19th/e pg. 1643]

22. Claudication due to popliteo-femoral incompetence is primary seen in- *(PGMEE 2015)*

a. Thigh b. Calf
c. Feet d. Buttocks

[Ref: Rutherford's 8th /e pg. 204]

23. Material used for femoro-popliteal graft:-

a. PTFE *(PGMEE 2018)*
b. Reverse saphenous vein
c. Polypropylene
d. Dacron

[Ref: Bailey & Love 27th/e pg. 949]

Explanation

Femoro-popliteal Bypass

- Used for superficial femoral artery d/s.
- **Autogenous saphenous vein** gives the best results and can be used reversed or in situ after valve disruption. If the long saphenous vein is not available from either leg, short saphenous or arm veins may be used.
- If no vein is available, a prosthetic polytetrafluoroethylene (**PTFE**) graft may be employed, although patency rates are less.
- Long-term patency of graft is determined by following factors:-
  - The quality of inflow and outflow
  - Length of graft length (whether the distal anastomosis is above or below the knee)
  - Conduit used for the bypass.

SUBCLAVIAN ARTERY OBSTRUCTION

24. Most common site of subclavian artery obstruction is:
(DNB 2008)

a. 1st part b. 2nd part
c. 3rd part d. 4th part

[Ref: Bailey & Love 27th/e pg. 952]

25. Adson 's test is positive in- *(PGMEE 2015)*

a. Thoracic Outlet Syndrome
b. Harner's Syndrome
c. Axillary artery thrombosis
d. Carpal Tunnel thrombosis

[Ref: Sabiston's 1st SAE pg. 1604]

26. A 17-year-old boy presented with complaint of difficulty in breathing. There was venous congestion of face and neck. A clinical diagnosis of SVC syndrome was made. The X-ray showed mediastinal widening. What is next step? *(NEET Pattern 2017)*

a. CT scan of chest
b. Peripheral smear
c. IV cyclophosphamide
d. Initiate radiation therapy

THRMBOEMBOLISM & DVT

27. Factor V Leiden mutation is commonly associated with:-
(PGMEE 2018)

a. Hematmesis b. Hemarthrosis
c. Epistaxis d. Deep vein thrombosis

28. Most common Presentation of DVT is:-
(PGMEE 2015-16)

a. Edema b. Respiratory distress
c. Swelling d. Charley Horse Cramp

[Ref: Sabiston 1st SAE pg. 1841; Harrison 19th/e pg. 1632]

29. Retrograde pelvic thromboembolism lead to:
(NEET June 2018)

a. Blue leg b. Red leg
c. Purple leg d. White leg

Explanation

- Retrograde Embolism is The obstruction of a vein by a mass carried in a direction opposite to that of the normal blood current. Since the Clot moves to the legs instead of moving toward the heart , so the blood supply to the leg will be compromised leading to bluish discoloration of the leg

30. False about Deep Vein thrombosis is
(Recent Pattern 2019)

a. Leg pain is most common symptom
b. Bilateral DVT is common
c. Some People present 1st time with Pulmonary embolism
d. Clinical Evaluation is most reliable

[Ref: Bailey and Love's 27th/e pg. 987, 988 Line by line]

31. A 22 year female post LSCS has fever of 102 F for 10 days which was not responding to antibiotics. MRI pelvis was done which showed thrombophlebitis. What is the management of this patient *(PGMEE 2019)*

a. Heparin + antibiotics
b. Heparin + Stop antibiotics
c. Warfarin + Antibiotics
d. Conservative treatment only

19.	**c**
20.	**a**
21.	**a,c**
22.	**b**
23.	**b**
24.	**a**
25.	**a**
26.	**a**
27.	**d**
28.	**d**
29.	**a**
30.	**d**
31.	**a**

CHAPTER 17

Orthopedics

FACTS

- Major mineral of the bone → Calcium hydroxyapatite
- Histologically adult bone differs from fetal bone by the present of:
  ○ Lamellar structure
  ○ Haversian system
- Major blood supply of the head and neck of femur → Medial circumflex femoral artery
- Major blood supply of cruciate ligaments is by → Middle genicular artery
- *Ileofemoral ligament* (Bigelow's ligament) → Strongest ligament of the body
- *Tendoachilles* → Strongest tendon of the body
- Rotator's interval is present between → Supraspinatus and Subscapularis tendon
- Rotator's cuff is deficient → Inferiorly
- Pathognomonic clinical feature of fracture → Crepitus and abnormal mobility
- Pathognomonic sign of fracture scaphoid → tenderness and swelling in the anatomical snuff box
- Maximum shortening of lower limb is seen in → fracture shaft of femur
- Sequence of Healing in a fracture: **S**piral # > **O**blique # > **T**ransverse # [**Mn**: Surgery OT]
- Remodeling in angular # is better than rotational #
- Remodeling in metaphyseal # is better than diaphyseal #.
- Putti Platt's operation involves the tightening of: Subscapularis tendon
- Colles' fracture is associated with rupture of extensor pollicis longus tendon
- The three bony point relationship of elbow is maintained in case of supracondylar fracture of humerus
- Adduction and inversion (*varus*) deformity in CTEV is due to persistent contraction of → Tibialis posterior
- Synovial fluid is produced by → Type-B cells of synovial membrane
- Subperiosteally placed graft is called → Phemister graft
- Involucrum → reactive new bone that forms around the sequetrum
- Organism most specifically associated with osteomyelitis in sickle cell anemia patient → *Salmonella*
- Brodie's abscess → type of subacute osteomyelitis
- The earliest X-ray feature of spinal TB → reduction of intervertebral disc space
- *Dorsiflexion test* → Screening test done for CTEV
- *Stretch pain test/Stretch sign:* 1st sign of compartment syndrome → Pain on passive stretch

Synovial fluid is:
- Anti Newtonian fluid
- Thixotropic – time dependent change in viscosity
- Viscosity is variable

Age group of:
- Perthes disease → 5-10 years
- Slipped capital femoral epiphysis → 11-14 years

Malunion of fracture is commonly seen in:
- Intertrochanteric fracture of femur
- Supracondylar fracture of humerus
- Colles' fracture

Pathological hallmark of:
- Acute osteomyelitis → Abscess
- Chronic osteomyelitis → Sequestrum (dead bone)

Bone Resorption Markers: (Collagen degradation products)
- Proline, Hydroxyproline
- Deoxypyridinoline
- N - Telopeptide, C - Telopeptide
- Hydroxylysine glucoside

Healing of bone TB:
- **B**ony ankylosis → in **Sp**inal TB [**Mn**: **BSp**]
- Fibrous ankylosis → in TB of the joints elsewhere

Angle	Related to
Baumann's	Supracondylar fracture humerus
Cobb's	Scoliosis
Bohler's, Gissane's	Fracture Calcaneum (Mn: BCG)
Kite's	CTEV
Quadriceps/ Q-angle	Recurrent dislocation of patella

Conditions	Associated Nerve Injury
Supracondylar fracture humerus	Anterior interosseous nerve
Monteggia fracture	Posterior interosseous nerve
Wrist fracture	Median nerve
Fracture shaft of humerus	Radial nerve
Golfer's elbow	Ulnar nerve
Carpel tunnel syndrome	Median nerve

	Deformity	Contraction	Joints Involved
VARUS	Equinus	Tendoachilles	Tibiotalar/Ankle joint
	Inversion	Tibialis posterior	Talocalcaneal/Subtalar Joint
	Adduction	Tibialis posterior	Talonavicular/Mid tarsal joint

Dislocation of Hip	
Posterior	Anterior
▪ Position of limb → FADIR	FABER
▪ Shortening of limb (apparent + true)	Lengthening (true)

Avascular Necrosis		
Bone	Site	Cause
▪ Femur	Head	Fracture neck femur, Posterior dislocation
▪ Talus	Body	Fracture through neck of talus
▪ Scaphoid	Proximal pole	Fracture through waist of scaphoid

Scientists	Contribution
Sir Nicolas	Coined term orthopedics
Jean Andre	Father of orthopedics
Hugh Owen Thomas	Father of modern orthopedics
Methysen	POP usage for fracture
Illizarov	Principle of "Distraction Histogenesis"
Sir John Charnley	Discovered arthroplasty

Shoulder Dislocation	
Anterior (MC)	Posterior
Due to Abduction and ER	Adduction and IR
Seen after throwing ball	Epilepsy, electric shock
Very painful	Painless, Normal ROM

- Reduced by modified Kocher's technique
- Steps: **T**raction → **E**xternal rotation → **A**dduction → **M**edial rotation [**Mn:** TEAM]

Limb Attitude

Condition	Attitude
Posterior dislocation of hip	Flexion + Adduction + Internal rotation [FADIR]
Anterior dislocation of hip	Flexion + Abduction + External rotation [FABER]
Transient Synovitis of hip	Slight FABER
Fracture neck femur	External rotation < 45°
Trochanteric fracture	External rotation > 45°
Perthes disorder or Coxa Plana	Internal rotation and limitation of Abduction
Slipped Capital Femoral Epiphysis	Internal rotation and limitation of Abduction

MOST COMMON

- MC ligament injury (sprain) of body → Anterior Talofibular ligament at ankle
- MC tendon injured in the body → Tendoachilles
- MC bone to get fractured in a newborn/during childbirth → Clavicle
- MC bone to get fracture → Tibia
- MC peripheral nerve injury → Radial nerve
  - Best prognosis after peripheral nerve injury → Radial nerve
    [**Mn:** Radial Readily damages Readily heals]

- Part of the clavicle most prone to fracture: Middle 1/3rd
- MC complication of fracture clavicle → Malunion
- MC fracture due to fall on outstretched hand:
  - Elderly → Colles fracture
  - Children → Supracondylar fracture humerus
- MC bone to get fractured during childhood around elbow → Supracondylar fracture
- MC vessel injured in supracodylar fracture of humerus → Brachial artery
- MC nerve injured in supracondylar fracture of humerus→ Anterior interosseous nerve
- MC type of supracondylar fracture humerus: Extension type
- MC complication of proximal humerus fracture: Shoulder stiffness
- MC fracture during childhood → Green stick fracture
- MC bone to get fractured in a child: bones of distal forearm
- MC carpal bone to get fracture → Scaphoid.
- MC complication of fracture scaphoid → Avascular necrosis
- MC carpal bone to get dislocate → Lunate
- MC joint to undergo dislocation → Shoulder joint
- MC complication in anterior shoulder dislocation:
  - Early → Injury to axillary nerve
  - Late/overall → Recurrence
- MC complication of supracondylar fracture humerus → Malunion → leads to cubitus varus/Gunstock deformity
- MC complication of fracture Lateral condyle humerus→ Nonunion → leads to cubitus valgus
- MC complication of Colles fracture → Finger stiffness > Malunion (Dinner fork deformity)
- MC elbow injury in adolescents is → Physeal injury

- MC type of elbow dislocation: Posterior
- MC ligament injured in knee joint → Medial meniscus
- MC site of stress fracture → 2nd and 3rd metatarsal
- MC bone involved in pathological fracture → Vertebral body of thoracic spine
- MC type of spinal TB → Paradiscal type
- MC site of osteomyelitis → Tibial metaphysis
- MC cause of osteomyelitis → S. aureus
- MC complication of acute osteomyelitis → Chronic osteomyelitis
- MC cause of pathological fracture → Osteoporosis > Metastasis to bone
- MC cause of septic arthritis → S. aureus
- MC cause of septic arthritis in sexually active young adults → N. gonorrhea
- MC joint involved in septic arthritis → Hip
- MC cause of bony ankylosis → Septic arthritis
- MC cause of fibrous ankylosis → TB arthritis
- MC cause of hip pain and limp in children < 10 years age → Transient synovitis of hip.
- MC hip injury in the elderly patient → Extracapsular fracture
- MC complication of fracture neck of femur → AVN/Non union
  - MC seen in → Subcapital fracture and Garden's III and IV
- MC complication of Intertrochanteric fracture → Malunion
- MC artery to undergo injury → Popliteal artery
- MC muscle involved in VIC → FDP > FPL
- MC nerve involved in VIC → Median nerve
- MC injured ligament of knee → ACL
- MC injured in torsion of knee → ACL

Most Common site:
- Brodie abscess → Tibia (Metaphysis-diaphysis junction)
- Garre's osteomyelitis → Mandible
- Skeletal TB → Lower dorsal spine

SYNDROMES

❶ Klippel Feil Syndrome
- *Triad:*
  - Short web neck
  - Low hair line
  - Restricted mobility of the upper spine
- *Associations:*
  - Sprengel shoulder → Congenital elevation of scapula
  - Congenital fusion of ≥1 cervical vertebrae

❷ Nail Patella Syndrome
- Nail dysplasia → Most commonly thumb nail
- Small or absent patella
- Recurrent dislocation of patella
- Iliac horns
- Genu valgum (Knock knees)

EPONYMOUS FRACTURES

Named Fracture	Description
Aviator's fracture	▪ Fracture of talus
Barton fracture	▪ Intra-articular fracture of distal radius and it extends through the dorsal aspect to articular surface
Bennett fracture	▪ Intra-articular fracture of the base of the thumb as a result of forced abduction of the 1st metacarpal
Boxers fracture	▪ Fracture of neck of 5th metacarpal bone
Bumper fracture	▪ Fracture of upper end of tibia
Chauffeur's fracture	▪ Fracture of styloid process of radius
Chopart's fracture	▪ Fracture dislocation of the mid-tarsal joint i.e. talonavicular and calcaneocuboid joint
Crescent fracture	▪ Fracture of the iliac bone with disruption of the sacroiliac joint
Colles fracture/ *Pouteau fracture*	▪ Extra articular fracture of distal end of Radius with dorsal displacement ▪ Occurs at cortico-cancellous junction 2 cm above wrist as a result of fall onto an outstretched hand
Cotton fracture/Trimalleolar fracture	▪ Fracture of the ankle that involves the lateral malleolus, medial malleolus and distal tibia
Essex-Lopresti fracture	▪ Comminuted fracture of the radial head with tearing of interosseous membrane along with dislocation of the distal radioulnar joint
Galeazzi fracture	▪ Fracture *of the distal part of the radius with dislocation of distal* radioulnar *joint*
Green stick fracture	▪ Incomplete unicortical fracture seen in children ▪ Involves **R**adius and **U**lna [**Mn**: U R Green]
Holstein-Lewis fracture	▪ Fracture of upper 2/3 and lower 1/3rd of the shaft of the humerus. ▪ Radial nerve may get injured in it
Jumper's fracture	▪ Usually involving upper sacrum S1, S2
Jefferson fracture	▪ Burst fracture of C_1
Jones fracture	▪ Extra articular fracture at the base of the 5th metatarsal

Le fort fracture *Type I* *Type II* *Type III*	▪ Fracture of the midface
	  ○ Palate separated
	  ○ Maxilla separated
	  ○ Craniofacial disjunction

Lisfranc fracture	▪ Dislocation of the tarsal bone with the fracture of metatarsal base
March fracture	▪ Stress fracture of the neck of 2nd metatarsal.
Monteggia fracture dislocation	▪ Fracture shaft of ulna with dislocation of proximal radioulnar joint
Night stick fracture	▪ Isolated fracture of shaft of ulna
Potts fracture	▪ Bimalleolar ankle fracture
Rolando fracture *(Comminuted Bennett fracture)*	▪ Comminuted intra-articular fracture of the base of thumb
Smith fracture/Reverse Colles fracture	▪ Extra-articular fracture of distal end of radius with volar displacement
Tillaux fracture	▪ Salter Harries type III fracture through the anterolateral aspect of the distal tibial epiphysis

TESTS

Condition	Test	Remark
Anterior Cruciate Ligament injury	Anterior Drawer test	
	Pivot shift test	
	Lachman test	▪ Most sensitive test as it can be done in acute as well as chronic ACL injury
Injury to meniscus	Apley's grinding test	
	McMurray's test	▪ More important test
Developmental Dysplasia of Hip	Ortolani's test	▪ Reduces a dislocated hip
	Barlow's test	▪ Provocative test; used to diagnose a dislocatable hip
	Galeazzi test	▪ Allis sign – Unequal knee height
CTEV	Dorsiflexion test (screening test)	▪ Dorsum of the foot normally touches the anterior tibial surface in children
	Plumb line test	▪ Detects tibial torsion
Posterolateral instability of knee	Dial test	▪ Positive test indicates posterolateral corner injury
Carpel tunnel syndrome	Phalen's test	▪ Flexion of the wrist at 90° produces symptoms
	Tinel's sign	▪ Tapping of the nerve produces tingling
	Durkan's test	▪ Compression of the median nerve for 30 sec produces tingling and paresthesia
Median nerve palsy	Pen test	▪ Positive in palsy of Abductor Pollicis Brevis
	Oschener's test (pointing index finger)	▪ Suggest lesion in or above cubital fossa
Ulnar nerve injury	Egawa test	▪ Tests Dorsal interossei
	Card test	▪ Loss of adduction by the Palmar interossei
	Book test/ Froment sign	▪ Tests the action of Adductor Pollicis
Tennis elbow	Cozen's test	
	Wringing test	
De Quervain's tenosynovitis	Finkelstein test	▪ Ulnar deviation of wrist produces pain
Anterior shoulder dislocation	Bryant's test	▪ Anterior axillary fold is at lower level
	Dugas test	
	Callaway test	▪ Increase vertical axillary circumference
	Hamilton ruler test	
	Lift off Test aka Gerber's test	▪ Done to assess the strength of subscapularis muscle
	Jerk Test	▪ Tests the posteroinferior instability of shoulder
	Thomas test	▪ Detect flexion deformity of hip

NAMED FEATURES

- *Wandering acetabulum* → feature of TB of hip joint
- *Spina ventosa* → TB of the phalanges of the hand
- *Caries Sicca* → TB of shoulder joint that does not produce any pus
- *Clutton's joint* → Painless effusion in joints. Seen in congenital syphilis
- *Equines deformity* in CTEV is due to persistent contraction of → Tendoachilles
- *Tom Smith arthritis* → Septic arthritis of hip joint due to pyogenic infection in infancy
- *Kienbock's disease* → Avascular necrosis of the lunate bone
- *Osgood Schlatter disease* → Osteochondritis of tibial tubercle/Proximal tibia
- *Islene disease* → Osteochondritis of 5th metatarsal base
- *Perthes disease* → Osteochondritis of femoral epiphysis
- *Tennis elbow/Lateral epicondylitis:* → overuse injury involving the extensors muscles
- *Golfer's elbow/Medial epicondylitis:* → overuse injury involving the common flexor and pronator muscles

- **Pulled elbow/Nursemaid's elbow** → partial dislocation of the head of radius from the annular ligament
- **Student's elbow/Draughtsman's elbow** → chronic inflammation of the olecranon bursa
- **Thurston Holland fragment or sign** → seen in type 2 Salter-Harris fracture
- **Terry Thomas sign** → Scapho-lunate instability
- **De Quervain's tenosynovitis** affects the extensor pollicis brevis (EPB) and abductor pollicis longus (APL)
- **Lesions responsible for recurrence of anterior shoulder dislocation:**
  - Bankart's lesion → avulsion fracture of Anteroinferior glenoid rim
  - Hill-Sachs lesion → compression fracture of postero-supero-lateral aspect of head of humerus
- **Luxatio erecta** → inferior dislocation of shoulder
- **Reverse Hill Sachs lesion** → impaction fracture of head of humerus following its posterior dislocation
- **Benedict's attitude/Pointing index** → Median nerve palsy **(Oschener's test)**
- **Simian hand/Ape thumb deformity** → Median nerve palsy
- **Gamekeeper's thumb** → Ulnar collateral ligament injury of MCP (1st) joint
- **Mallet finger/Baseball finger** → avulsion of extensor tendon from distal phalanx of a finger
- **Dinner fork deformity** → occurs as a result of malunion of Colles fracture
- **Jersey finger** → avulsion injury of the FDP tendon at its point of insertion at base of distal phalanx
- **Gunstock deformity/Cubitus varus** → malunion following supracondylar fracture humerus
- **Kaplan's lesion** → dorsal dislocation of the MCP joint of fingers
- **Madelung deformity** → volar subluxation of distal radius
- **Garden spade deformity** → as a result of malunion and volar displacement of distal radius in Smith fracture
- **Dash board injury** → posterior dislocation of Hip

ORTHOPEDIC DEVICES

Splints/Casts/Traction	Use
Aeroplane splint	Brachial plexus injury
Bohler Braun splint	Universal splint used for fracture shaft of femur Skeletal traction
Colle's cast/Hand shaking cast	Colles fracture (fracture of lower end of radius)
Cylinder cast/Tube cast	Fracture Patella
Cockup splint	Radial nerve palsy (Wrist drop)
Dennis brown splint	CTEV
Dunlop's traction	Supracondylar fracture humerus
Figure of '8' bandage	Fracture Clavicle
Gallo's traction and Bryant traction	Fracture shaft femur in children < 2 years
Garden well's traction/Minerva cast /Halo device	Cervical spine injury
Glass holding cast (Scaphoid cast)	Fracture Scaphoid
Hip spica	Femur fracture
Knuckle Bender splint	Ulnar nerve palsy (Claw hand)
Milwaukee braces	Scoliosis
Patellar tendon bearing (PTB) cast	Fracture shaft of tibia
Pavlik harness/Von Rosen splint/Lorentz cast/ Frog leg cast/Bachelor's cast	Developmental Dysplasia of Hip/CDH
Perkin's traction	Fracture shaft femur in adults
Risser's cast	Scoliosis
Shoulder spica	Shoulder immobilization
Taylor's brace	Thoracic spine injury
Thomas knee splint	Immobilization for the injuries of the hip and thigh
U-Slab/Hanging cast	Fracture shaft of humerus
Velpeau bandage	Acromioclavicular joint dislocation/Shoulder dislocation

CLASSIFICATIONS

▪ **Bado classification**	Monteggia fracture	▪ **Pipkin's classification**	Femoral head fracture
▪ **Dennis classification**	Sacral fracture	▪ **Gustilo and Anderson classification**	Open fracture
▪ **Tile's classification** ▪ **Young's classification**	Pelvic fracture	▪ **Salter Thompson classification (Based on Crescent sign)**	Legg-calve-Perthes disease
▪ **Neer classification**	Proximal humerus fracture	▪ **Hawkin's classification**	Fracture neck of talus

Gartland classification	▪ Supracondylar fracture of humerus	▪ Extensor type (MC) → Dorsal displacement ▪ Flexion type → Volar displacement
Milch classification	▪ For fracture lateral condyle humerus	▪ Type I : Fracture line medial to Capitulum ▪ Type II: Lateral to capitulum
Neck of femur fracture classification	▪ Anatomic classification (Subcapital, intercervical, basicervical) ▪ Gardens classification ▪ Pauwels classification (30°, 50° 70°)	

Salter-Harris Classification for Physeal Fracture

Type	Description	Prognosis
Type I	▪ Fracture line passes through the growth plate	Good prognosis
Type II	▪ Fracture line passes through the growth plate and metaphysis ▪ Most common type	Good prognosis
Type III	▪ Fracture line passes through the growth plate and epiphysis	Poor prognosis
Type IV	▪ Fracture line passes through the metaphysis, growth plate and epiphysis	Poor prognosis
Type V	▪ Compression injury of growth plate	Poor prognosis
Type VI	▪ Injury to perichondrial structure	
Type VII	▪ Isolated injury to the epiphyseal plate	

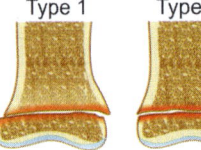 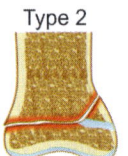 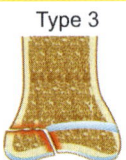 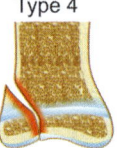 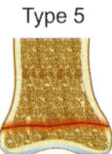

Type 1   Type 2   Type 3   Type 4   Type 5

CARPAL BONES

- Each carpel bone ossify from a single center
- Direction → counterclockwise starting with capitates

- *Carpal tunnel:*
  - Roof: Transverse carpal ligament
  - Lateral wall: Scaphoid and Trapezium
  - Medial wall: Pisiform and Hamate
  - Contents: Median nerve, flexor tendons

- *Anatomic snuffbox:* between the tendons of EPL and EPB
  - Contents: Radial artery (scaphoid directly deep to snuffbox)

- *Guyon's canal:*
  - Roof: palmer carpal ligament;
  - Floor: Transverse carpel ligaments, FDP tendons
  - Lateral wall: hook of hamate; Medial wall: pisiform
  - Contents: Ulnar nerve and artery

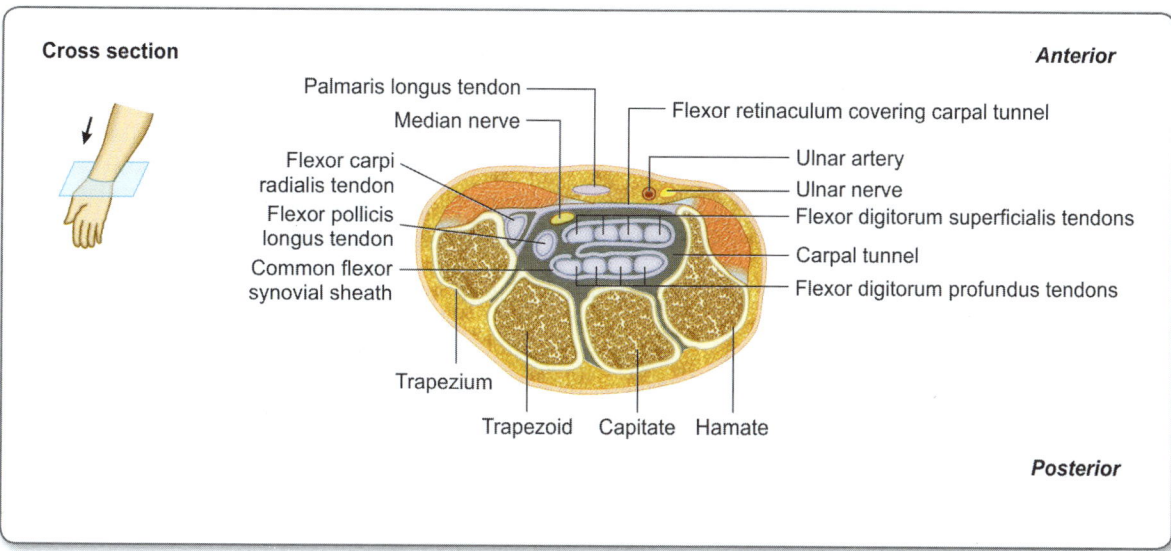

Carpal funnel, transverse section

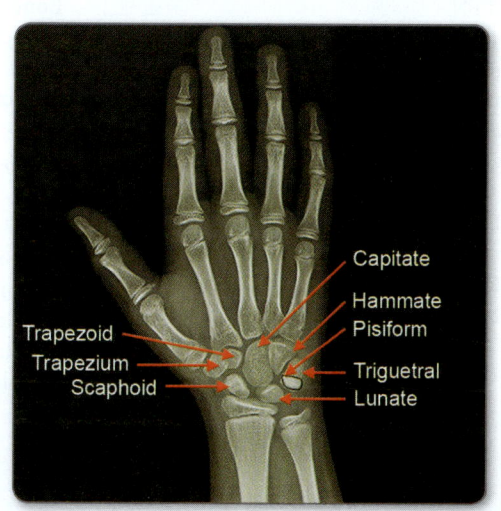

Row	Bones	Morphology	Comment
PROXIMAL ROW	Scaphoid	Boat shaped	▪ Lies beneath the anatomic snuffbox ▪ MC fractured carpel bone after fall on outstretched hand ▪ MC site of fracture – waist ▪ Major blood supply – radial artery (via retrograde blood flow ▪ Proximal pole is susceptible to avascular necrosis if injured
	Lunate	Moon/ lunar shaped (So called lunate)	▪ Dislocations often missed ▪ Fractures need ORIF to protect against avascular necrosis/osteonecrosis ▪ Dorsal fractures are treated non surgically
	Triquetrum	Pyramid shaped	▪ 2nd MC carpel bone to get fractured
	Pisiform	Pea shaped	▪ Sesamoid bone ▪ Located within the FCU tendon; TCL attaches
DISTAL ROW	Trapezium	Irregular	▪ Most radial ▪ Articulates with 1st metacarpal; TCL attaches, FCR
	Trapezoid	Wedge	▪ Articulates with 2nd metacarpal
	Capitate	Largest carpal bone	▪ First to ossify
	Hamate	Has a hook	▪ TCL, FCU attach to the hook

INVESTIGATIONS

- Rate of newly synthesized osteoid mineralization can be best estimated by → Tetracycline labeling
- 1st radiologically visible sign of fracture union → Callus formation (It is immature woven bone)
- X-ray in Pott's spine shows → Obliteration of disc space with wedge compression of adjacent vertebrae
- Occult fracture neck of femur is best diagnosed by → MRI
- IOC for Perthes disease → MRI
- Gold standard investigation for skeletal TB → CT guided biopsy
- Most reliable way of diagnosing AVN → MRI
- IOC for screening DDH → USG
- USG finding of transient synovitis of hip joint → Widening of joint space
- Electric bulb sign on X-ray → Posterior dislocation of shoulder
- **_IOC for stress fracture:_**
  - Unilateral → MRI
  - **B**ilateral → **B**one scan

Lab findings in Fat Embolism Syndrome (FES):

- ↓ Hb and Platelet count ≤ 1.5 lakh
- $PaO_2 < 60\%$
- Lipiduria
- Present of fat globules in urine.
- 1st sign of FES
- Check by Gurd test
- CXR → Snowstorm appearance

MANAGEMENT

- Implant of choice in Intertrochanteric fracture → DHS/PFN
- Transient synovitis of Hip → Conservative
- TOC in green stick fracture → Closed reduction + Cast immobilization
- Pott's paraplegia → Anterior decompression by surgical debridement f/b autogenous grafting
- CDH/DDH → Closed reduction → if fails → Salter osteotomy
- TOC of CTEV in a newborn → Serial manipulation of the deformity and above knee casting
- Fracture clavicle → "Figure of 8" bandage
- TOC in nonunion of fracture shaft femur → Bone grafting + Internal fixation
- Pulled elbow → Supination and flexion of elbow
- Watson's Jones operation is done for → Chronic ankle instability

Triple arthrodesis:

- Done in cases of neglected and persistent CTEV
- Age → After 12 years
- Fusion of →
  - Talonavicular joint
  - Talocalcenial joint
  - Calcaneocuboid joint

IMAGES

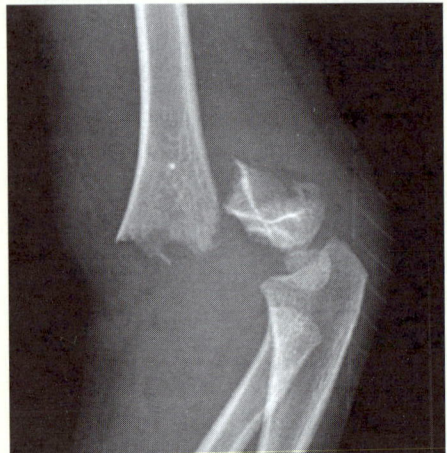

Supracondylar humerus fracture

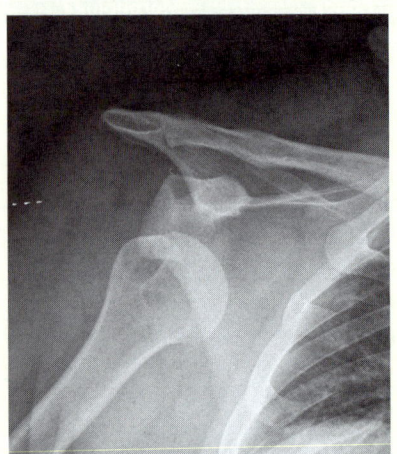

Anterior shoulder dislocation

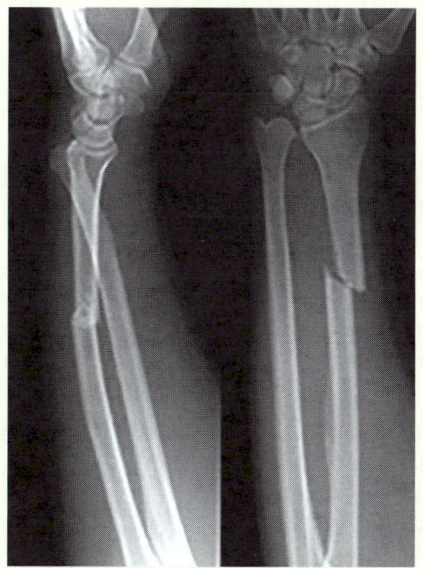

Galeazzi fracture

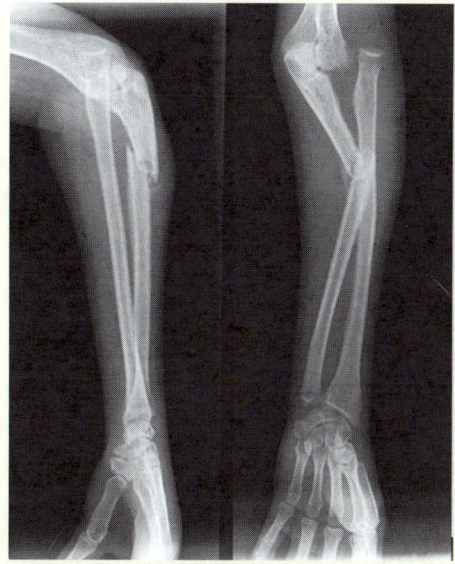

Monteggia fracture

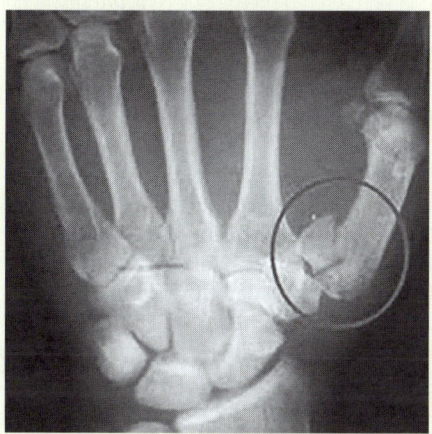

Rolando's fracture

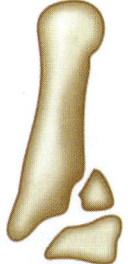
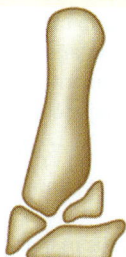

Bennett   Rolando

Bennett and Rolando fracture

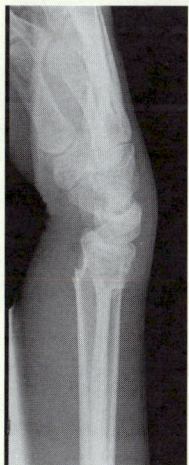

Colle's fracture

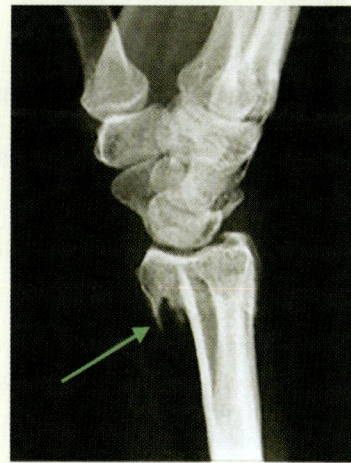

Smith fracture

MULTIPLE CHOICE QUESTIONS

CHAPTER 1: GENERAL ORTHOPEDICS

1. Most common muscle damaged in rotator cuff-
(PGMEE 2012)

   a. Supraspinatus   b. Teres minor

   c. Subscapularis   d. Infraspinatus

[Ref: Oxford handbook of orthopedics and trauma: Page 286]

Explanation

- Rotator cuff injuries most commonly effect the supraspinatus. Large tears may involve the infraspinatuus, teres minor and subscapularis in that sequence. Rotator cuff interval is found between supraspinatus and subscapularis.

2. Rotator interval is between-
(PGMEE 2002)

   a. Supraspinatus & teres monor

   b. Subscapularis & infraspinatus

   c. Supraspinatus & subcapsularis

   d. Teres major & teres minor

[Ref, Maheshwari &Mhaskar pg 88 6th edition]

3. Muscle most commonly affected by congenital absence is-
(PGMEE 09)

   a. Pectoralis major   b. Gluteus maximum

   c. Teres minor   d. Semimembranosus

[Ref: Oxford pg. 490]

Explanation

- Pectoralis major is the muscle which is MC absent congenitally.
- Upper limbs develops during intrauterine life at 4-8 weeks. Heart, eye , CNS & auditory systemic develop at this time. So associated syndromes co-exist e.g. VACTERL syndrome (vertebral + Anorectal + Cardiac + Tracheo - esophaggal + Renal + limb) & TAR (Thrombocytopenia + Absent radius) syndrome.

4. Axis of upper limb passes through-
(PGMEE 2013)

   a. Capitulum   b. Trochlea

   c. Olecranon   d. Radial styloid

[Ref: Applied biomechanics of deformity correction]

5. Spring ligament refers to-
(PGMEE 2014)

   a. Plantar calcaneo navicular ligament

   b. Short plantar ligament

   c. Long plantar ligament

   d. Deltoid ligament

[Ref: BDC Vol-II 5th/e p. 161; Maheshwari 6th/e pg. 210]

6. Osteoclasts remove bone a which of the following sites?
(PGMEE 2015)

   a. Howships lacunae   b. Resorption bays

   c. Both of above   d. None of the above

[Ref: IB singh 6th/e p. 104]

7. Marker of new bone formation is-
(PGMEE 2014)

   a. Alakaline phosphatase

   b. Hydroxyl proline

   c. Acis phosphatas

   d. None

[Ref: Robbin's 8th/e p. 1209; Harrison 18th/e p. 3126; Maheshwari 6th/e pg. 12]

Explanation

- Marker of Bone formation
  - Alkaline phosphatase
  - Osteocalcin
  - Squirm peptide collagen type 1
- Marker of Bone resorption
  - Urine & Serum cross linked 'N' telopeptide
  - Urine & Serum cross linked 'C' telopeptide
  - Urine total & free deoxypyridinoline

8. The bone matrix has the following crystals-
(PGMEE 2013)

   a. Calcium hydroxyapatite

   b. Calcium pyrophosphate

   c. Calcium phosphate

   d. Calcium sulphate

[Ref: Maheshwari 6th/e p. 9; Apley's 9th/e p. 118-119; Gray's Anatomy 40th/e p. 86-87]

9. Intramembranous ossification is seen in which bones-
(PGMEE 2013)

   a. Pelvis   b. Long bones

   c. Maxilla   d. None

[Ref: Oxford 550]

Explanation

- Intramembranous ossification:-
  - ↑ diameter of bones in - cranial & facial bones & part of clavicle
- Enchondral ossification:-
  - All other skeletal growth. Primary ossification in lay bones appear at 12 weeks of gestation & 2° centers at different times after birth. Except distal femur secondary center present at birth.

10. In Articular cartilage, most active chondrocytes are seen in-
(PGMEE 2013)

   a. Zone 1   b. Zone 2

   c. Zone 3   d. Zone 4

[Ref : Textbook of joint disorder p. 5]

1.	a
2.	c
3.	a
4.	a
5.	a
6.	c
7.	a
8.	a
9.	c
10.	c

11. Rate of newly synthesized osteoid mineralization can be best estimated by- *(PGMEE 2013)*
   a. Tetracycline labeling   b. Alizarin red stain
   c. Calcein stain   d. Van kossa stain

[Ref: Maheshwari & Mhaskar 6th e pg 12, Bone Research protocols 2003 p. 305]

12. All of the following statements about synovial fluid are true, Except- *(PGMEE 10)*
   a. Secreted primarily by type A synovial cells
   b. Follows Non- Newtonian fluid kinetics
   c. Contains hyaluronic acid
   d. Viscosity is variable

[Ref: Maheshwari & Mhaskar 6th/ed pg. 300; Gray's Anatomy 40th/e p. 100, Turek's 6th/e p. 152; Management of common Muskuloskeletal Disorders 4th/e p. 40]

Explanation
- Type A - synovial cells (phagocytes) engulf joint debris
- Type B - Secrete synovial fluid

Synovial fluid interpretation

Condition	Opacity	Leukocyte counts (per mm³)
Normal	Clear	<200
OA	Clear	1000 (<50% PMN)
RA	Cloudy	1-50,000 PMNS
Crystal disease	Cloudy	5-50,000 PMNs
Sepsis	Cloudy	10-100,000 PMNs
# (Fracture)	Cloudy + fat	-
Bleeding disorder	Bloody	-

13. Diaphysis fracture involves? *(DNB DEC 2010)*
   a. Skull bones   b. Long bone
   c. Sternum   d. Ribs

[Ref: Maheshwari 6th/e pg. 8]

14. Indicators of bone formation includes all of following except- *(PGMEE 2009)*
   a. Osteocalcin   b. Alkaline phosphatase
   c. Hydroxyproline   d. Type I procollagen

[Ref: Maheshwari & Mhaskar 6th e,pg 12
Robbin's 8th/e p. 1209]

FRACTURE HEALING

15. Callus formation is seen between what duration of fracture healing - *(PGMEE 2015)*
   a. 0-2 weeks
   b. 2-4 weeks
   c. 4-12 weeks
   d. 12-16 weeks

[Ref: Maheshwari & Mhaskar 6th/e . pg 11]

16. Initial stage of clinical union of bone is equivalent to- *(PGMEE 2014)*
   a. Callus formation   b. Woven bone
   c. Haematoma formation   d. Calcification only

[Ref: Maheshwari & Mhaskar 6th/e . 11, Apley's 9th/e p. 23, 24]{as per maheshwari callus is also called as woven bone}

17. True about fracture healing except- *(PGMEE 2012)*
   a. Nutrition affects healing
   b. Hormonal status may affect healing
   c. Compression at fracture site causes nonunion
   d. Stable fixation promotes healing

[Ref: Maheshwari & Mhaskar 6th /e pg 12]

18. Non-union is a complication of- *(PGMEE 2000)*

   a. Scaphoid #
   b. Colle's #
   c. Inter-trochanteric # of hip
   d. Supracondylor # of the humerus

[Ref: Maheshwari & Mhaskar6th/e p. 48]

MISCELLANEOUS

19. Which is a fibrous joint? *(DNB june 2011)*
   a. Inferior tibiofibular joints
   b. First costochondral joint
   c. Tooth socket
   d. Sutures of the skull

[Ref :https://en.m.wikipedia.org>wiki>fibrousjoint]

20. Ankle brachial index is pathological when:- *(PGMEE 2016-17)*
   a. Less than 0.9   b. More than 1
   c. Both a and b   d. More than 2

[Ref: Campbell 13ed: page 2310]

Explanation

Ankle brachial index

- When the patient is first seen, if the peripheral circulation in the extremity is deficient, the dislocation should be reduced as quickly as possible and the circulatory status of the limb again carefully assessed. Several authors have suggested that even if pulses are present, the ankle-brachial index (ABI) should be calculated and rechecked several times. The ABI is the systolic pressure in the ankle divided by the systolic pressure in the arm. According to proponents of this method, if the ABI is more than 0.85 to 0.90, close observation is warranted; if the ABI is less than 0.85, arteriography is indicated. In a prospective study, the sensitivity, specificity, and positive predictive value of an ABI lower than 0.90 were 100% and the negative predictive value of an ABI that reached 0.90 or higher was 100%.
- The most significant predictor of amputation in diabetics is peripheral neuropathy, as measured by insensitivity to the Semmes- Weinstein 5.07 monofilament. Other documented risk factors include prior stroke, prior major amputation, decreased transcutaneous oxygen levels, and decreased ankle-brachial blood pressure index

11.	a
12.	a
13.	b
14.	c
15.	c
16.	a
17.	c
18.	a
19.	b
20.	a

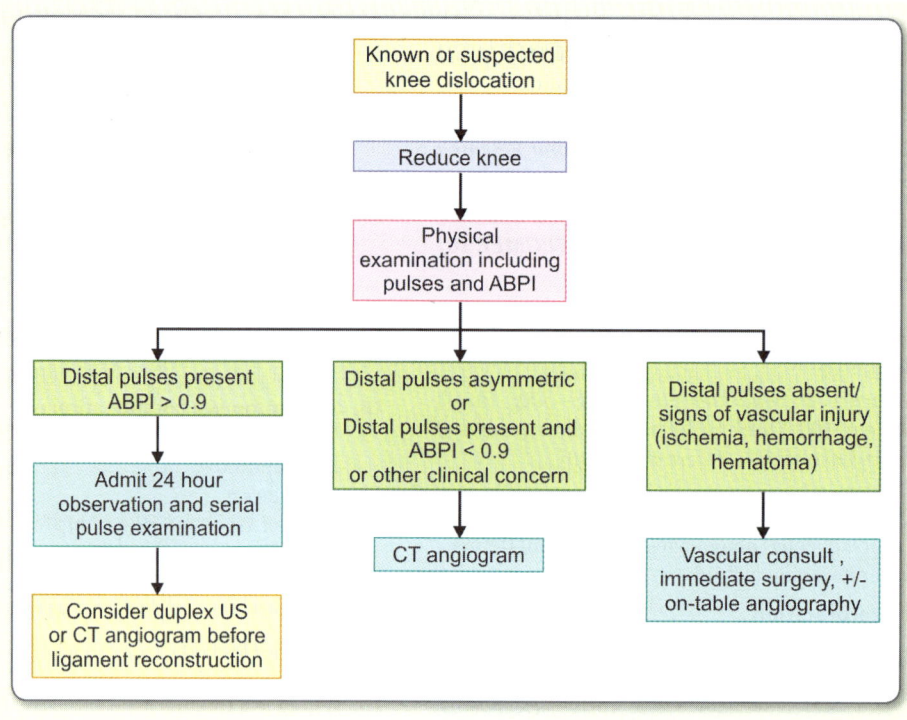

21. Which flexor comportment in hand is No man's land. :-
(PGMEE 2016-17)

a. ZONE-I
b. ZONE-II
c. ZONE-III
d. ZONE- V

[Ref: Campbell 13ed : 3750]

21. b
22. a
23. a

Explanation

- Zone I extends from just distal to the insertion of the sublimis tendon to the site of insertion of the profundus tendon.
- Zone II is in the critical area of pulleys (Bunnell's "no man's land") between the distal palmar crease and the insertion of the sublimis tendon.
- Zone III comprises the area of the lumbrical origin between the distal margin of the transverse carpal ligament and the beginning of the critical area of pulleys or first anulus.
- Zone IV is the zone covered by the transverse carpal ligament.
- Zone V is the zone proximal to the transverse carpal ligament and includes the forearm.

22. Muscle for wall climbing:-
(PGMEE 2016-17)

a. Lattisimus dorsi
b. Serratus ant
c. Deltoid
d. None of the above

Explanation

- Lattisimus dorsi causes extension, adduction and internal rotation of the shoulder joint assists in climbing.

23. Identify the X-ray:-
(PGMEE 2016-17)

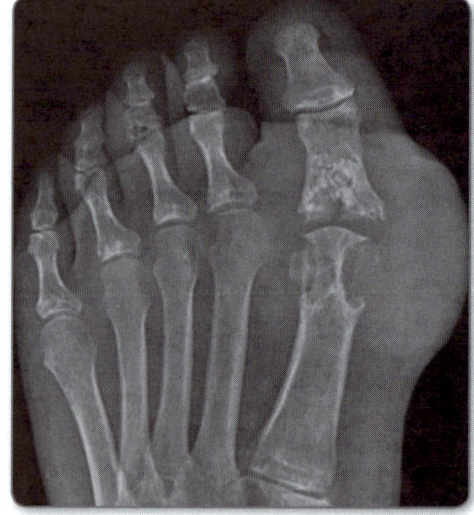

a. Gouty arthritis
b. Enchondroma
c. Metastatsis
d. None of the above

Explanation

- **Enchondromas** - Benign cartilage forming tumors. They are not associated with lysis of bone *(Maheshwari 236)*
- **Metastasis** - Most metastatic lesions are lytic. Most common involving spine, ribs, pelvic, humerus, femur. **Uncommon distal to elbow and knee.** *(Ref. Ref: Maheshwari & Mhaskar 6th/e pg. 247)*
- **Gout** - crystal arthropathy usually monoarticular. Characterized by presence of **tophi** caused by chronic

hyperuricemia. Lesion in the X ray is classical TOPHI. Aspiration shows birefringent needle shaped crystals.

- Other crystallapathies -
  - Pseudogout (calcium pyrophosphale disease): Aspiration reveals rhomboid crystals which are weakly birefringent . Most commonly involves knee. May be a/w calcification of cartilage (chondrocalcinosis)
  - Calcium hydroxy apatite deposit disease - a/w erosive arthritis usually present over tendons. *(Ref. Oxford 196)*

24. X-ray of wrist joint is given below. Identify the bone marked by the arrow :- *(PGMEE 2016-17)*

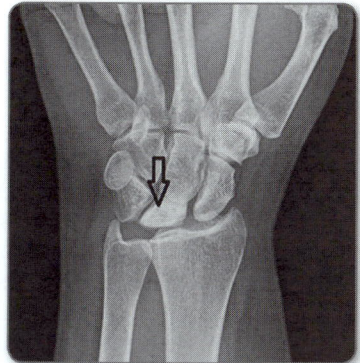

a. Capitate
b. Hamate
c. Lunate
d. Trapezoid

[Ref: Internet]

Explanation

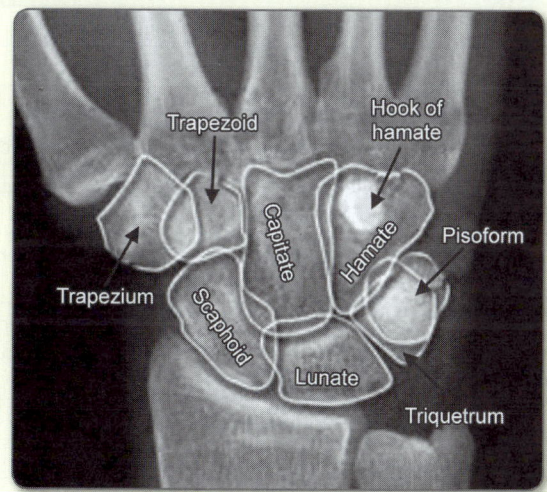

25. Most common site for fracture of mandible:- *(PGMEE 2016-17)*

a. Neck
b. Condyle
c. Angle
d. Near incisive foramen

[Ref: Internet]

26. X-ray carpal bones Indentify the marked structure:- *(PGMEE 2016-17)*

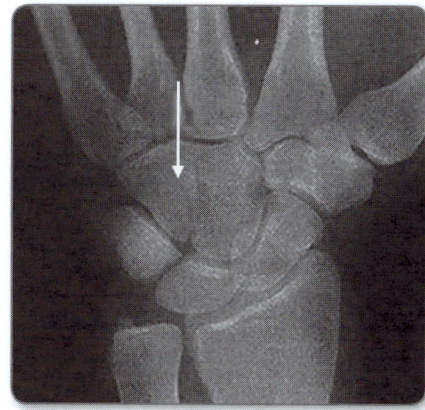

a. Scaphoid
b. Lunate
c. Hamate
d. Capitate

27. Identify arrow mark in X-ray of shoulder:- *(PGMEE 2016-17)*

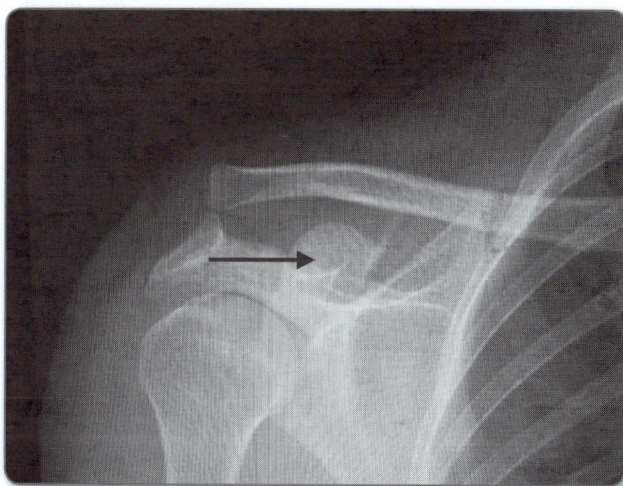

a. Acromion pr
b. Coracoid
c. Clavicle
d. Spinous process

Explanation

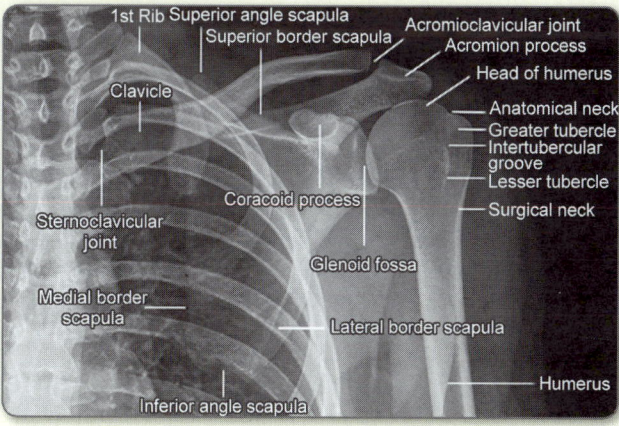

24. c
25. b
26. c
27. b

28. X ray of ankle joint with arrow at a bone. Identify the marked bone:- *(PGMEE 2016-17)*

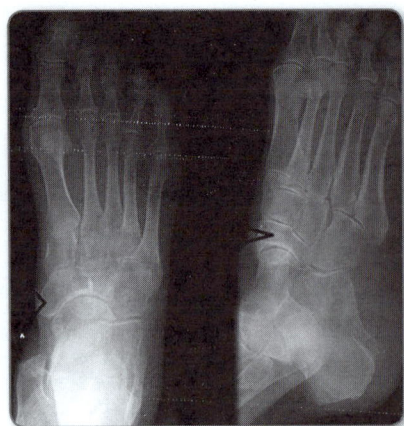

a. Calcaneus   b. Talus
c. Navicular   d. Cuboid

[Ref: Internet]

29. What is the type of fracture shown in the X-ray of left shoulder? *(NEET Pattern 2018)*

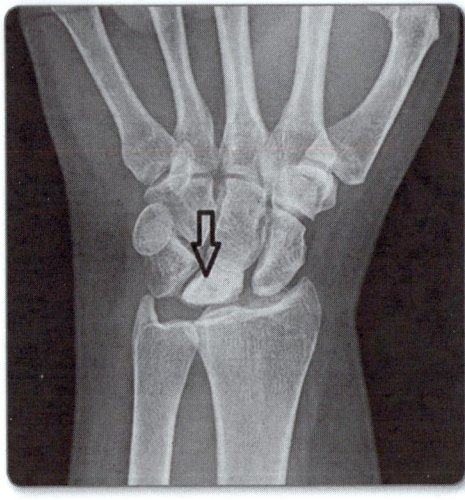

a. Neer classification grade 4
b. Ideberg classification grade 4
c. Garden classification grade 4
d. Schatzker classification grade 4

Ref: Campbell Operative Orthopedics, 13th ed. Page 2934; Campbell Operative Orthopedics, 13th ed. Page2937; Campbell Operative Orthopedics, 13th ed. Page 2817; Campbell Operative Orthopedics, 13th ed. Page 3075 tibial plateu fracture; Campbell Operative Orthopedics, 13th ed. Page3322: Schatzker classification is also for fracture of the olecronon

Explanation

Neer gave classification of fracture lateral end of clavicle and proximal humerus

28. c
29. a
30. a

Neer Classification of Lateral Clavicular Fractures

Type	Description
I	Coracoclavicular ligaments intact, attached to medial segment
II	Coracoclavicular ligaments detached from medial segment, but trapezoid intact to distal segment
IIa	Both conoid and trapezoid attached to distal segment
IIb	Conoid is torn
III	Intraarticular extension into acromioclavicular joint

- Neer's 4 -segment classification of displaced fractures and fracture-dislocations is based on pattern of displacement (two-part, three-part, or four-part) and key segment displaced. In each two-part pattern, segment named is one displaced.
- Two-part surgical neck fractures are impacted (A), unimpacted (B), and comminuted (C). All 3-part patterns have displacement of shaft segment, and displaced tuberosity identifies type of 3-part fracture. In four-part pattern, all segments are displaced. Fracture dislocations are identified by anterior or posterior position of articular segment. Large articular surface defects require separate recognition.

Ideberg Classification if for Glenoid Freactues

Femur neck fractures

Stage	Type	Description
I		Incomplete fracture line (valgus impacted)
II		Complete fracture line; nondisplaced
III		Complete fracture line; partially displaced
IV		Complete fracture line; completely displaced
	1	Pure cleavage type fracture. Occurs in young age group.
	2	Cleavage combined with depression. This tends to occur in older individuals.
	3	Pure central depression . The articular surface is driven into the plateau. These tend to occur in osteoporotic bone.
	4	Fractures of medial condyle
	5	Bicondylar fractures
	6	Plateau fracture with dissociation of metaphysis and diaphysis

30. Boston brace is used for treatment of:- *(PGMEE 2016-17)*

a. Scoliosis
b. Fracture shaft of femur
c. Trimalleolar fracture
d. Fracture shaft of tibia

[Ref: Maheshwari and Mhaskar 6ᵗʰ e p.282;From ROAMS 13ᵗʰ/e pg. 791]

31. In club foot what is the talocalcaneal angle:-

(PGMEE 2016-17)

a. Less than 15 degree
b. 15 to 35 degree
c. More than 35 degree
d. None of the above

[Ref: Maheshwari and Mhaskar 6th e p.213]

Explanation

- Normal angle is >35⁰.

32. Important support for acromioclavicular joint:-

a. Coracoclavicular ligament   *(PGMEE 2016-17)*
b. Suprascapular ligament
c. Infrascapular ligament
d. Acromioclavicular ligament

[Ref: Maheshwari and Mhaskar 6th e p.87]

Explanation

- Stability depends upon Acromio-clavicular ligament & more important is coraco-clavicular.
- So answer should be coraco-clavicular ligament if acromo-clavicular ligament is also an option.

33. Content of rotator cuff are all except:-

(PGMEE 2016-17)

a. Supraspinatus   b. Infraspinatus
c. Teres major   d. Subscapularis

[Ref: Maheshwari and Mhaskar 6th e p.88]

34. In tennis elbow,calcification starts first in:-

(PGMEE 2016-17)

a. Extensor carpi radialis bravis
b. Extensor pollices longus
c. Extensor carpi ulnaris
d. Extensor carpi radialis longus

[Ref: Campbell 13 ed page 2599]

Explanation

- Lateral epicondylitis (tennis elbow), a familiar term used to describe myriad symptoms around the lateral aspect of the elbow, occurs more frequently in nonathletes than athletes, with a peak incidence in the early fifth decade and has a nearly equal gender incidence. Lateral epicondylitis can occur during activities that require repetitive supination and pronation of the forearm with the elbow in near full extension. lateral epicondylitis is initiated as a microtear, most often within the origin of the extensor carpi radialis brevis.
- The diagnosis of tennis elbow is made by localizing discomfort to the origin of the extensor carpi radialis brevis. Tenderness typically is present over the lateral epicondyle approximately 5 mm distal and anterior to the midpoint of the condyle. Pain usually is exacerbated by resisted wrist dorsiflexion and forearm supination, and there is pain when grasping objects.

35. Muscle involved in unlocking knee joint:-

(PGMEE 2016-17)

a. Plantaris   b. Popliteus
c. Medial gastrelium   d. Lateral gatretrrium

[Ref: Maheshwari and Mhaskar 6th e p.154]

Explanation

- Unlocking involves lateral rotation of femur over tibia.
- Locking is brought about by Quadriceps.

36. Stable internal fixation with autograft required in-

a. Hypertrophic nonunion
b. Malunion
c. Psudoarthrosis
d. Compound fracture

[Ref: Maheshwari and Mhaskar 6th e p.49]

Explanation

- Both HO & pseudarthrosis need stable internal fixation. However pseudarthrosis needs extensive bone grafting.

37. In Axonotomesis all are true except:- *(PGMEE 2016-17)*

a. Tinel sign positive
b. Motor march is positive
c. Major nerve trunk intact
d. Degeneration is absent

[Ref: Maheshwari and Mhaskar 6th e p.63]

38. Nerve involved in carpal tunnel syndrome is:-

(PGMEE 2016-17)

a. Median nerve   b. Radial nerve
c. Axillary nv.   d. Ulnar nerve

[Ref: Maheshwari and Mhaskar 6th e p.302; Oxford 267-77]

Explanation

- Median n. entrapment - Anterior interosseous syndrome, Pronator syndrome, CTS.
- Unlar nerve entrapment syndrome in Guyon's canal → Cubital tunnel Syndrome.
  ○ Guttering in seen in ulnar n. entrapment
  ○ Froments test- is for ulnar nerve
- Radial nerve: Posture interosseous nerve syndrome
  ○ Saturday night palsy - seen with injury of Radial n

39. Tinel sign is elicited in:-   *(PGMEE 2016-17)*

a. Proximal to distal direction
b. Distal to proximally
c. Both directions simultaneously
d. Only distally

[Ref: Maheshwari and Mhaskar 6th e p.69]

40. Froment sign is used to detect injury of

(PGMEE 2016-17)

a. Ulnar nv.   b. Radial nv.
c. Musculocutaneous nv.   d. Median nv.

[Ref: Maheshwari and Mhaskar 6th e p.68]

31.	a
32.	a
33.	c
34.	a
35.	b
36.	c
37.	d
38.	a
39.	b
40.	a

HISTORY AND EXAMINATION

GENERAL PRINCIPLES, SPINE AND SHOULDER EXAMINATION

1. Lift off test is used to assess the function of *(PGMEE 2013)*
   a. Supraspinatus
   b. Infraspinatus
   c. Teres minor
   d. Subscapularis

   [Ref: Campbell's 11th/e p. 2607]

Explanation

- **Gerber's lift off test** - Subscapularis (dorsum of hand against buttock & lift off against nesistemice)
- **Infraspinatus & Teres minor :** arm by sided body, elbow at 90⁰, Externally rotate against resistance.
- **Supraspinatus** - Shoulder 30⁰ flexed & abducted with thumb down. Resisted abduction . Aka drop arm sign *(Oxford pg. 10)*

2. A sportsman is able to abduct his arm, internally rotate it, place the back of hand on the lumbosacral joint, but is not able to lift it from back. What is the Etiology?
   a. Subscapularis tendon tear *(PGMEE 10)*
   b. Acromioclavicular jt. dislocation
   c. Long head of biceps tendon tear
   d. Teres major tendon tear

   [Ref: Oxford pg. 10]

HIP, ELBOW, WRIST AND HAND EXAMINATION

3. Thomas test is used for testing? *(DNB Dec 2010)*
   a. Hip flexion
   b. Hip rotation
   c. Hip abduction
   d. Knee flexion

   [Ref: Maheshwari & Mhaskar 6th /e pg.349]

4. Flexion deformity is detected by- *(PGMEE 2014)*
   a. Tredenlenberg test
   b. Thomas test
   c. FABER
   d. Stinchfield

   [Ref: Maheshwari & Mhaskar 6th /e pg.349; Apley's 9th/e p. 495]

5. "Trendelenburg sign" is positive in damage og the following nerve- *(PGMEE 2013)*
   a. Inferior gluteal nerve
   b. Pudendal nerve
   c. Superior gluteal nerve
   d. Posterior tibil nerve

   [Ref: Maheshwari & Mhaskar 6th /e p. 349]

Explanation

- '**Superior gluteal nerve** supplies both gluteus medius & minimus; a.k.a **Gluteus medius gait.**

6. Trendelenberg test is positive in palsy of- *(PGMEE 2012)*
   a. Vastus medialis
   b. Gluteus medius
   c. Rectus femoris
   d. Gluteus maximus

   [Ref: Maheshwari & Mhaskar 6th /e p.349]

GAIT ABNORMALITY

7. Jaipur foot was invented by- *(PGMEE 2015)*
   a. P.K. Sethi
   b. S.K. Verma
   c. B.L. Sehgal
   d. H.R. Gupta

   [Ref: Maheshwari 6th/e pg. 28]

8. High stepping gait is seen in- *(PGMEE 2015)*
   a. TB hip
   b. Common peroneal nerve palsy
   c. Polio
   d. Cerebral palsy

   [Ref: Maheshwari & Mhaskar 6th /e p.370]

9. Scissor gait is seen in which of the following condition: *(PGMEE 2019)*
   a. Polio
   b. Cerebral palsy
   c. Hyperbilirubinemia
   d. Hyponatremia

   [Ref: Tachdjian's Pediatric Orthopaedics 3rd/e p. 83]

10. Charlie chaplin gait is seen in- *(PGMEE 2015)*
   a. Congenital coxa vara
   b. Tibial torsion
   c. DDH
   d. Genu valgus

   [Ref: Maheshwari & Mhaskar 6th /e p.370]

11. Antalgic hip gait is related to which of the following- *(PGMEE 2014)*
   a. Waddling gait
   b. Trendelenberg gait
   c. Painful hip gait
   d. Short leg gait

   [Ref: Tachdjian's Pediatric Orthopaedics 3rd/e p. 83]

12. Trendelenberg's gait is due to the weakness of- *(PGMEE 2012)*
   a. Quadriceps
   b. Sartorius
   c. Iliopsoas
   d. Gluteus medius

   [Ref: Maheshwari & Mhaskar 6th /e p.349]

MISCELLANEOUS

13. Straight leg raising test (SLRT) is done by raising leg passively in sepsis patient. All of the following are true in this patient EXCEPT:- *(PGMEE 2018)*
   a. Patient is made in passive leg position from 45 degree semirecumbent position
   b. PLR mimics a fluid challenge by autotransfusion of blood from lower extremities
   c. The test is reliable in spontaneously breathing patients. Test can be done in mechanically ventilating and on controlled ventilation patients.
   d. It is irreversible and causes significant hemodynamic changes.

   [Ref: Raising the leg usually does not cause any irreversible haemodynamic changes The Spine, Rotham. Page 182]

1.	d
2.	a
3.	a
4.	b
5.	c
6.	b
7.	a
8.	b
9.	b
10.	b
11.	c
12.	d
13.	d

Explanation

- Dural tension signs are frequently used to assess lumbar spine pathology. Many different maneuvers have been described.

Straight-leg raising test (SLRT)

- In supine SLRT is performed by elevation of the leg with knee extended and assessed for the pain into the leg:-
- SLRT is +ve if pain occurs between 30° - 70° of elevation because no true change in tension on the nerve roots is believed to occur outside of this range.
- Variations in SLRT include *Lasègue sign or Bragard sign*, which involves raising the leg to the point of symptom reproduction and then lowering the leg slightly and dorsiflexing the foot passively; a positive test results in reproduction of the patient's radiating legpain. Other tests include internally rotating the leg to increase "dural tension," raising the leg with knee flexed and then slowly extending the knee to the point of reproduction of leg pain (also sometimes referred to as Lasègue sign),
- *The bowstring sign* : pain is relieved either by flexing the already extended knee at the point of symptom reproduction or eliciting pain by pressing on the popliteal fossa of the elevated leg with the knee partially flexed.

14. **While examining a patient in supine position the examiner keeps his hand below the heel of one foot and asks the patient to flex the other hip against resistance, while keeping the week leg straight this is known as:**
    (NEET Pattern 2018)
    a. Wadell's test
    b. Donoghue's test
    c. Hoover's sign
    d. Mcmurray test

[Ref: Campbell Operative Orthopedics, 13th ed. Page 1882; Maheshwari 6th ed page 149; Maheshwari page 356]

Explanation

Wadell Test

- Waddell et al. Defined maladaptive overt illness related behavior, which is out of proportion to the underlying physical disease. It is a test of malingering. Briefly >3 nonorganic signs are diagnostic.
  - Superficial as non anatomic tenderness.
  - LBP on axial head compression.
  - Discrepancy of SLR in sitting & supine position.

  - Regional measure as non dermatomal sensory loss.
  - Patient over reaction.
- It comprises of five nonorganic signs and seven nonorganic symptom descriptions have been identified. If 3+ points are there, investigate for non-organic cause.
- *Nonorganic signs description*
  - Regional disturbances : sensory changes or weakness that is divergent from accepted neuroanatomy
  - Superficial/nonanatomic skin tenderness to light touch (pinch)
  - Depth tenderness over a widespread area not localized to one structure (nonanatomic).

- *Simulation*
  - Low back pain on axial loading of spine by pressure on the patient's head while standing.
  - Rotation Low back pain reported when shoulders and pelvis are rotated in the same plane as the patient stands.

- *Distraction*
  - Inconsistent limitation of SLR in supine and seated positions
  - Overreaction Disproportionate verbalization, facial expression, muscle tension, collapsing, sweating during examination
- *Nonorganic symptoms descriptors*
  - Do you get pain in your tailbone?
  - Do you have numbness in your entire leg (front, side, and back of leg at the same time)?
  - Do you have pain in your entire leg (front, side, and back of leg at the same time)?
  - Does your whole leg ever give way?
  - Have you had to go to the emergency department because of back pain?
  - Has all treatment for your back made your pain worse?
- ***O' Donoghue triad*** involves a triad of injury involving Anterior cruciate ligament, medial collateral ligament and medial meniscus. It is caused by twisting of the knee in semi-flexed position
- Test to detect the injury to the medial meniscus. Test is performed by passively externally rotating the knee in flexed position which reproduces the pain.
- "McMurrays test is used to detect injuries to the medial meniscus. The test is done by passive internal rotation of the leg to apply force on the injured meniscus causing pain".

14. c

1. **Which of the following is an orthopedic emergency-**
   (PGMEE 2013)
   a. Intraarticular fracture
   b. Septic arthritis
   c. Fracture lateral condyle humerus
   d. Fracture neck femur

   [Ref: GS Kulkarni 2nd/e p. 1247]

2. **A patient presents in emergency room with upper limb injury with fractured humerus. As a intern you are posted there. What will be your 1st priority:-**
   (PGMEE 2018)
   a. # with increased capillary refill time
   b. Fracture with paresthesia
   c. Displaced/communited fracure
   d. Intense pain in limb

   Ref: Campbell Operative Orthopedics 13 ed page 2662

Explanation

- ATLS developed by the American College of Surgeons is the most widely used method for evaluating trauma patients. Evaluation is based on the mnemonic ABCDE:
- Airway, which should be patent/ unobstructed
- Breathing, should be as normal as possible under the circumstances with normal oxygenation (SpO_2 should be maintained).
- Circulation both central and peripheral; the goal is good capillary filling of all limbs and maintenance of a normal BP.
- Disability, which includes neurologic, musculoskeletal, urologic, and reproductive injuries. These injuries, although rarely life threatening, can result in serious long-term disability.
- Environment. Many of these injuries do not occur in an isolated situation and may result in contamination that can expose caregivers to disease.
- Option d intense pain in the limb could indicate compartment syndrome, however this syndrome is relatively unknown in single bone limbs.

3. **Most common organism causing infection after open fracture-**
   (PGMEE 2012)
   a. Gonococcus
   b. Staphylococcus aureus
   c. Klebsiella
   d. Pseudomonas

   [Ref: Campbell 13th/e p. 2973]

Explanation

- The most common infecting organisms appear to be gram-negative and methicillin-resistant Staphylococcus aureus (MRSA), which may be hospital or community acquired

4. **There were multiple causalities in a bus accident. They are brought to your hospital. Which patient will be given the highest priority?**
   (NEET Pattern 2017)
   a. Severe head injury
   b. Airway compromise
   c. Grade 4 shock
   d. Flail chest

   [Ref: Campbell 13th/e p. 2662]

Explanation

Protocol to follow is:

- ABCDE (airway, breathing, circulation/hemorrhage, disability, and exposure/environment)
- However, at one place, catastrophic hge was given first priority, then abcde.

5. **Which of the following triage categories are correctly matched?**
   (NEET Pattern 2017)
   a. RED-Deceased/Dead
   b. BLACK-Minor injuries
   c. GREEN-Immediate intervention needed
   d. YELLOW-Stable patient, needs observation

   Ref: Bailey 26th page 422

Explanation

Triage Categories

Priority	Color	Medical need	Clinical status	Examples
First (I)	Red	Immediate	Critical, but likely to survive if treatment given early	Severe fractal trauma, tension pneumothorax, profuse external hemorrhage, haemothorax, flail chest, major intra-abdominal bleed, extradural haematomas
Second (II)	Yellow	Urgent	Critical, likely to survive if treatment given within hours	Compound fractures, degloving injuries, ruptured abdominal viscus, pelvic fractures, spinal injuries

Contd...

Answers

1. b
2. a
3. b
4. b
5. d

Priority	Color	Medical need	Clinical status	Examples
Third (III)	Green	Non-urgent	Stable, likely to survive even if treatment is delayed for hours to days	Simple fracture, sprains, minor lacerations
Last (O)	Black	Unsalvageable	Not breathing, pulseless, so severely injured that no medical care is likely to help	Severe brain damage, very extensive burns, major disruption/loss of chest or abdominal wall structures

SPLINT, CASTS, TRACTIONS

6. Cock up splint in used in-　　　　*(PGMEE 2015)*
   a. Median nerve injury
   b. Radial nerve injury
   c. Ulnar nerve injury
   d. Volkman's ischemic contracture

   [Ref: Maheshwari & Mhaskar 6th/e p. 25]

7. Functional cast bracing not used in fracture of-
　　　　　　　　　　　　(PGMEE 2015)
   a. Humerus　　　　　　b. Tibia
   c. Ulna　　　　　　　　d. Thoracolumbar spine

   [Ref: Maheshwari 6th/e p. 18]

Explanation

- Functional brace is a type of cast where the joint is not included. So that while the fracture is held in position, the joint can move.
- This is commonly used for humerus and tibia.

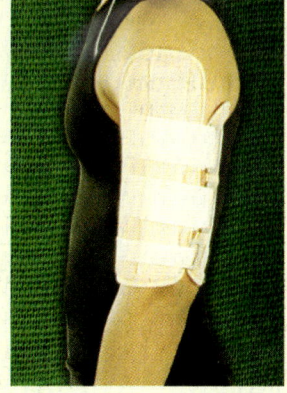

8. Milwalkee brace is used in treatment of- *(PGMEE 2015)*
   a. Scoliosis　　　　　b. Kyphosis
   c. Cubitus varus　　　d. Genu varum

   [Ref: Maheshwari & Mhaskar 6th/e p. 283;
   Apley's 9th/e p. 463]

9. What about Durham pin is true-　　　*(PGMEE 2015)*
   a. It is used to give skeletal traction
   b. It has threads in the centre of pin
   c. It is used to give skeletal traction through calcaneum
   d. All the above

   [Ref: Practical orthopaedics by Kakkad Subhosh p. 34]

10. Thomas splint is used for immobilizing fractures of-
　　　　　　　　　　　　(PGMEE 2015)
   a. Femur　　　　　　　b. Tibia
   c. Radius　　　　　　　d. Ulna

   [Ref: Maheshwari & Mhaskar 6th/e p. 25]

11. U-slab is given for fracture of-　　*(PGMEE 2014)*
   a. Femur　　　　　　　b. Radius
   c. Tibia　　　　　　　d. Humerus

   [Ref: Maheshwari & Mhaskar 6th/e p. 93; Apley's 6th/e p. 726]

12. Aeroplane splint is used in-　　　*(PGMEE 2013)*
   a. Radial nerve injury　　b. Ulnar nerve injury
   c. Brachial plexus injury　d. Scoliosis

   [Ref: Maheshwari & Mhaskar 6th/e p. 25]

13. Long compression is used for which fracture-
　　　　　　　　　　　　(PGMEE 2013)
   a. Talus　　　　　　　b. Calcaneum
   c. Fibula　　　　　　　d. Femur

14. Weight allowed in skeletal traction upto- *(PGMEE 2013)*
   a. 5 kg　　　　　　　　b. 10 kg
   c. 20 kg　　　　　　　d. 30 kg

   [Ref Maheshwari & Mhaskar 6th/e p. 27;
   Watson Jones 6th/e p. 300]

15. TT splint was not used for-　　　*(PGMEE 2013)*
   a. Injuries around knee joint
   b. Knee dislocation
   c. Infective arthritis of knee
   d. Fracture femur

   [Ref: Internet]

16. Turn-buckle cast is used for-　　*(PGMEE 2013)*
   a. Fracture shaft humerus
   b. Fracture shaft femur
   c. Scoliosis
   d. Cervical spine injury

   [Ref: Maheshwari & Mhaskar 6th/e p. 17]

17. Halopelvic traction is used for correcting which deformity-　　　　　　　*(PGMEE 2013)*
   a. Scoliosis　　　　　b. Pectus Carinatum
   c. Spondyloptosis　　　d. Coxa Vara

   [Ref: Maheshwari & Mhaskar 6th/e p. 27]

18. Maximum weight for skin traction- *(PGMEE 2012)*
   a. 1-2 kg　　　　　　　b. 4-5 kg
   c. 10-15 kg　　　　　　d. 15-20 kg

   [Ref: Maheshwari & Mhaskar 6th/e p. 27]

19. Risser Localiser cast is used in the management of-
　　　　　　　　　　　　(PGMEE 08)
   a. Kyphosis　　　　　b. Spondylolysthesis
   c. Idiopathic scoliosis　d. Lordosis

   [Ref: Maheshwari & Mhaskar 6th/e p. 17]

6.	b
7.	d
8.	a
9.	d
10.	a
11.	d
12.	c
13.	b
14.	c
15.	c
16.	c
17.	a
18.	b
19.	c

20. All of the following are used for giving skeletal traction, except- *(PGMEE 06)*

a. Steimann's pin b. Kirschner's wire
c. Bohler's stirrup d. Rush pin

[Ref: Maheshwari & Mhaskar 6th/e p. 17; Watson Jones 6th/e p. 300, 301]

NAMED FRACTURES

21. Undertaker's fracture is- *(PGMEE 2015)*

a. C23 b. C34
c. C56 d. C67

[Ref: Narayan Reddy 30th/e p. 98]

22. Which of the following fracture needs a violent force? *(PGMEE 2015)*

a. Fracture Neck of femur b. Intertrochanteric fracture
c. Clavicle fracture d. Colles fracture

[Ref: Essentials of orthopaedics 4th/e p. 719; Maheshwari 6th/e p. 4]

Explanation

- # NOF & Colle's # are examples in osteoporosis.

23. Anterolateral avulsion fracture of the distal tibial physis is known as- *(PGMEE 2015)*

a. Potts fracture b. Tillaux fracture
c. Chopart fracture d. Jones fracture

[Ref: Campbell 12th/e p.1500]

24. Posada's fracture is- *(PGMEE 2015)*

a. Transcondylar fracture of humerus
b. Fracture lateral condyle of humerus
c. Fracture medial condyle of humerus
d. Fracture anatomical neck of humerus

[Ref: www.btb.termiumplus.gc.ca]

25. Pilon fracture is- *(PGMEE 2013)*

a. Bimalleolar
b. Trimalleolar
c. Distal femur Intraarticular
d. Distal tibia Intraarticular

[Ref: Campbell 12th/e p. 2631-32; Maheshwari & Mhaskar 6th/e p. 3]

26. Lisfrans fracture dislocation- *(PGMEE 2013)*

a. Fracture dislocation through tarso-metatarsal
b. Fracture dislocation through ankle joint
c. Fracture dislocation through subtalar joints
d. Fracture dislocation through mid-tarsal joints

[Ref: Maheshwari & Mhaskar 6th/e p. 367]

27. Boxer's fracture is- *(PGMEE 2013)*

a. Radial styloid fracture b. Reverse colle's fracture
c. 5th metacarpal fracture d. 1st metacarpal fracture

[Ref.: Maheshwari & Mhaskar 6th/e p. 3]

28. Jefferson fracture is- *(PGMEE 2012)*

a. Fracture of any cervical vertebra
b. Fracture of axis - Hangman #
c. Fracture of spinous process of C_7 - Clayshover's #
d. Fracture of atlas

[Ref: Maheshwari & Mhaskar 6th/e p. 3]

CLASSIFICATION

29. Gustilo Anderson classification is used for- *(PGMEE 2015)*

a. Compound fractures
b. Closed fractures
c. Distal end radius fractures
d. Femur head fractures

[Ref: Maheshwari & Mhaskar 6th/e p. 21; Apley's 9th/e p. 706]

30. A patient with open wound with fracture of both bones of right lower limb came to the emergency. The doctor labelled the injury as 3B according to Gustillo Anderson classification. Which of the following would represent the injury? *(NEET Pattern 2018)*

a. Open wound with fracture with wound <1 cm
b. Open wound with fracture, 1 to 10 cm wound size, but mild soft tissue injury
c. Open wound >10cm, though soft tissue coverage not required
d. Open wound >10 cm, with extensive injury requiring soft tissue coverage

[Ref: Campbell Operative Orthopedics, 13th ed. Page 2659]

Explanation

Gustilo anderson classification is for open fractures:

- **Type I** open fractures have a clean wound less than 1 cm long.
- In **type II** wounds the laceration is more than 1cm long but is without extensive soft-tissue damage, skin flaps, or avulsions.
- **Type IIIA** open fractures have extensive soft-tissue lacerations or flaps but maintain adequate soft-tissue coverage of bone, or they result from high-energy trauma regardless of the size of the wound. This group includes segmental or severely comminuted fractures, even those with 1-cm lacerations.
- **Type IIIB** open fractures have extensive soft-tissue loss with periosteal stripping and bone exposure. They usually are massively contaminated.
- **Type IIIC** open fractures include open fractures with an arterial injury that requires repair regardless of the size of the soft-tissue wound.

31. Vascular repair to be done in which Gustilo Anderson type- *(PGMEE 2013)*

a. IIIc b. I
c. II d. IIIb

[Ref: Maheshwari & Mhaskar 6th/e p. 21; Apley's 19th/e p. 706]

32. The contraindication to internal fixation- *(PGMEE 2014)*

a. Physeal injury
b. Active infection
c. Intraarticular fracture
d. Fracture dislocation

[Ref: Maheshwari & Mhaskar 6th/e p. 19; Clinical orthopaedics p. 46]

20.	d
21.	d
22.	c
23.	b
24.	a
25.	d
26.	a
27.	c
28.	d
29.	a
30.	d
31.	a
32.	b

Explanation

- *CRPS I* (formally reflex sympathetic dystrophy, RSD) theoretically represents patients who have had a usculoskeletal injury without a defined neural injury.
- *CRPS II (causalgia)* includes patients who fulfill the same criteria but who have evidence of a neural injury.

33. Action of intramedullary 'K' nail is- *(PGMEE 2014)*
   a. Two-point fixation   b. Three-point fixation
   c. Compression   d. Weight concentration

[Ref: Maheshwari 6th/e p. 376]

Explanation

- K Nail has clover leaf shape & provide three point fixation.

REFLEX SYMPATHETIC DYSTROPHY

34. Sudeck's atrophy is associated with- *(PGMEE 2015)*
   a. Osteoporosis   b. Osteophyte formation
   c. Osteopenia   d. Osteochondritis

[Ref: Emergency orthopaedics 5th/e p. 61; CAMPBELL 13th/e p. 3170]

35. Sudeck's dystrophy symptoms are all except-
   (PGMEE 2012)
   a. Stiffness   b. Increased bone density
   c. Sweating   d. Pain

Explanation

- Reflex sympathetic dystrophy syndrome, also known as complex regional pain syndrome, is a distressing complication that often occurs after fractures around the wrist.
- In its early stages, this condition is characterized by extreme swelling of the soft tissues, exquisite tenderness to pressure, and pain on motion. Later, definite circulatory changes occur in the soft tissues and bone; the skin gradually becomes purplish and cold and perspires excessively. Even later, the joints of the fingers and wrist become increasingly stiff; even the shoulder and elbow can be affected secondarily from voluntary immobilization of the extremity in one position.
- Radiographs may show mottled decalcification or osteoporosis of the bones in late stages, but 30% of patients have no radiographic abnormalities.

36. A 50 year old lady sprained her ankle 2 months back from which she made a steady recovery. 2 months after the injury she gradually developed severe pain in her right ankle with significant limitation of ankle movement. Clinical examination reveals edema and shiny skin. What is the likely diagnosis? *(PGMEE 2011)*
   a. Complex regional pain syndrome TypeI {CRPS I}
   b. Complex Regional pain syndrome Type II {CRPS II}
   c. Fibromyalgia
   d. Peripheral Neuropathy

[Ref: 'Evidence Based Orthopaedics' by Wright(Saunders) 2008 p. 122; Campbell 13th/e p. 3170]

MYOSITIS OSSIFICANS

37. Treatment of myositis ossificans includes all except-
   (PGMEE 2015)
   a. Splinting elbow
   b. Gentle active movements
   c. Indometacin
   d. Vigorous passive massage

[Ref: Maheshwari & Mhaskar 6th/e p. 52-53]

38. Most common site of myositis ossificans- *(PGMEE 2013)*
   a. Knee
   b. Elbow
   c. Shoulder
   d. Wrist

[Ref: Maheshwari & Mhaskar 6th/e p. 52-53]

39. Most common site of myositis ossificans :
   a. Knee   *(Recent Pattern June 2018)*
   b. Elbow
   c. Shoulder
   d. Wrist

[Maheshwari & Mhaskar 6th/e p. 52-53]

Explanation

Myositis ossificans

- Myositis ossificans is the extraskeletal heterotropic ossification that occurs in muscles and soft tissues. It occurs in muscles which are vulnerable to tear under heavy loads, such as quadriceps, adductors, brachialis, biceps, and deltoid.
- Trauma is the most important cause of myositis ossificans. Usually there is history of severe single injury.
- More common in children.
- M/c involved joint is **elbow** > hip. There is history of trauma around the elbow, i.e.
  - Supracondylar# of humerus,
  - Dislocation of elbow or
  - Surgery with extensive periosteal stripping.
- Massage / vigorous passive stretching of elbow aggravate the condition.
- X-ray findings: shows distinct peripheral margin of mature ossification and a radiolucent center of immature osteoid & primitive mesenchymal tissue.

40. Heterotopic ossification occurs in- *(PGMEE 2012)*
   a. Bone
   b. Soft tissue
   c. Joint
   d. None

[Ref: Maheshwari & Mhaskar 6th/e p. 52-53]

41. Heterotopic ossification is a condition in which there is deposition of bone around the joints. Which of the following parameters is the most useful for this condition- *(PGMEE 11)*
   a. Serum calcium
   b. Serum PTH
   c. Serum alkaline phosphatase
   d. Serum phosphate

[Ref: Maheshwari & Mhaskar 6th/e p. 52-53; Apley's 8th/e p. 114]

33.	b
34.	a
35.	b
36.	a
37.	d
38.	b
39.	b
40.	b
41.	c

42. A 6 year old male presents with extensive heterotropic ossification over the neck, back & shoulders and decreased chest movements. He gives history of progressive immobility since the age of 3 years. Which of the following statement about his affecting condition is not true? *(PGMEE 08)*

a. They have a near normal life expectancy
b. They are predisposed to Pneumonia
c. They have short hallus
d. Increased expression of BMP4 gene is seen

[Ref: Maheshwari & Mhaskar 6th/e p. 53;Children's orthopaedics & fracture 8th/e p. 119]

Explanation

- This represents myositis ossificans progressiva (Munchmeyer's disease).
- Affects <6 years.
- Cause of death lung disease.

FAT EMBOLISM

43. Commonest site of fracture leading to fat embolism is- *(PGMEE 2014)*

a. Tibia #   b. Femur #
c. Humerus #   d. Ulna #

[Ref :Maheshwari & Mhaskar 6th/e p. 43;Caplan's stroke : a clinical approach 4th/e p. 357]

44. A person with multiple injuries develops fever, restlessness, tachycardia, tachypnea and periumbilical rash. The likely diagnosis is- *(PGMEE 08)*

a. Air embolism
b. Fat embolism
c. Pulmonary embolism
d. Bacterial pneumonitis

[Ref: Maheshwari & Mhaskar 6th/e p. 43]

CRUSH SYNDROME

45. Patient comes with crush injury to upper limb, doctor is concerned about gangrene and sepsis what can help decide between amputation and limb salvage? *(PGMEE 2015)*

a. MESS
b. Guliton score
c. Gustilo Anderson classification
d. ASIA guidelines

[Ref:https://www.ncbi.nlm.nih.gov>articles; Rockwod 7th/e p. 340; Campbell 13th/e p. 705]

Explanation

- MESS: Mangeled Extremity Severity Score: This system, which is easy to apply, grades the injury on the basis of the energy that caused the injury, limb ischemia, shock, and the patient's age.
- The system was subjected to retrospective and prospective studies, with a score of 6 or less consistent with a salvageable limb. With a score of 7 or greater, amputation was the eventual result

- ASIA: is a scale to assess spinal injuries and classify various patterns of spinal inuries
- Gustilo-Anderson classification is far open fracture classification.

COMPARTMENT SYNDROME & VIC

46. Earliest way to detect development of compartment syndrome by a nurse in a patient with cast is: *(NEET Pattern 2018)*

a. Check radial pulse by displacing the cast
b. Decreased response to analgesia
c. Change in color of fingers
d. Change in odor

[Ref: Campbell Operative Orthopedics, 13th ed. Page 2405]

Explanation

- Physical signs of acute compartment syndrome include tightness of the involved compartment, pain with passive motion of the muscles passing through the compartment, and weakness of the muscles. The most important sign is pain out of proportion to that expected with the injury. Hypesthesia or paresthesia should be evaluated by testing with pinprick, light touch, and two-point discrimination. **A variety of invasive devices are available for measurement of compartment pressures, arterial line manometer,**
- Whitesides three-way stopcock apparatus, and the wick monitor.

Treatment guideline

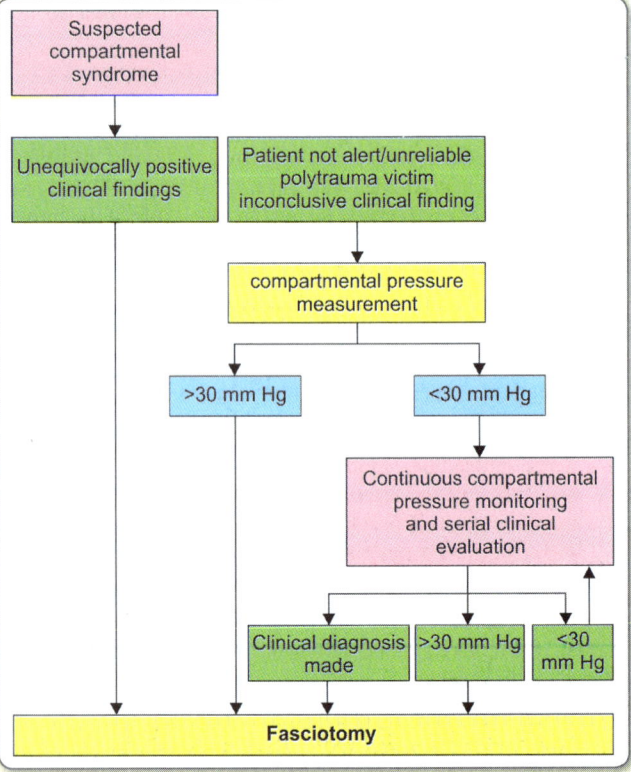

47. A person comes with fracture tibia with swelling of lower leg pulse feeble but palpable. Intracompatmental pressure is raised. What is the next step in management- *(PGMEE 2015)*

a. Fasciotomy
b. External fixation
c. Lower limb venography
d. Interlock nail

[Ref: Maheshwari & Mhaskar 6th/e p. 48]

48. The most common cause of Volkmann's ischaemic contracture [V.I.C.] in a child is- *(PGMEE 2015)*

a. Intercondylar fracture of humerus
b. Fracture both bone of forearm
c. Fracture lateral condyle of humerus
d. Supracondylar fracture of humerus

[Ref: Maheshwari & Mhaskar 6th/e p. 102]

49. Which of the following is least likely associated with vascular injury- *(PGMEE 2013)*

a. Fracture supracondylar femur
b. Fracture supracondylar humerus
c. Fracture shaft of femur
d. Fracture shaft humerus

[Ref: Maheshwari & Mhaskar 6th/e p. 94]

50. Which of the following injuries is likely to cause a severe vascular damage? *(PGMEE 2012)*

a. Closed posterior dislocation of knee
b. Elbow dislocation [posterior]
c. Tibial plateau fracture
d. Fracture middle 1/3rd of clavicle

[Ref: Maheshwari & Mhaskar 6th/e p. 48]

51. Indication for surgical compartment release in compartment syndrome in any compartment is absolute pressure greater than? *(DNB dec 2010)*

a. 15 mm Hg
b. 20 mm Hg
c. 40 mm Hg
d. Varies from compartment to compartment

[Ref: Maheshwari & Mhaskar 6th/e p. 48]

52. In posterior compartment syndrome which passive movement causes pain? *(PGMEE 08)*

a. Dorsiflexion of foot
b. Foot inversion
c. Toe dorsiflexion
d. Toe planter flexion

[Ref: Maheshwari & Mhaskar 6th/e p. 48]

53. In deep fasciotomy for compartment syndrome incision is given in:- *(PGMEE 2018)*

a. Only skin
b. Skin and subcutaneous tissue
c. Skin, subcutaneous tissue, superficial fascia
d. Skin, subcutaneous tissue, superficial and deep fascia

Ref: Capmbell Orthopedics 9th Ed page 2409

Explanation

- Techniques for release of the compartments of the lower leg:
- *Single-incision perifibular fasciotomy* useful if the soft tissue of the limb is not extensively distorted.
- *Double-incision fasciotomy* is safer and more effective and generally should be used.
- The role of selective compartment releases remains unclear.

MISCLLANEOUS

54. Which of the following is ideal site for harvesting bone graft- *(PGMEE 08)*

a. Iliac crest
b. Distal end of the humers
c. Distal end of femur
d. Fibula

[Ref: Maheshwari & Mhaskar 6th/e p. 84; Fundamentals of orthopaedics 4th/e p. 75]

47. a
48. d
49. d
50. a,b
51. c
52. a
53. d
54. a

1. Treatment of choice of anterior dislocation of shoulder:-
   (PGMEE 2016-17)
   a. Physiotherapy
   b. Reduction by Kocher's manoeuvre
   c. Manipulation under general anaesthesia
   d. Reduction followed by splinting

   [Ref: Maheshwari and Mhaskar 6th e p.91;.791]

2. Puttiplat operation is done for- *(PGMEE 2015)*
   a. Elbow instability   b. Shoulder instability
   c. Rotator cuff tear   d. Biceps Tendinitis

   [Ref: Maheswari & Mhaskar 6th e pg 91,Campbell 's pg. 2289]

3. Hill sach's lesion is most commonly seen in
   a. Recurrent shoulder dislocation *(PGMEE 2014)*
   b. Posterior shoulder dislocation
   c. Fracture neck of humrus
   d. Anterior shoulder dislocation

   [Ref: Maheshwari & Mhaskar 6th/e pg. 90]

4. Bankart's lesion involves the __ of the glenoid labrum
   (PGMEE 14)
   a. Anterior lip   b. Superior lip
   c. Antero-superior lip   d. Antero-inferior lip

   [Ref: Maheshwari & Mhaskar 6th/e pg. 90]

5. Most common dislocation is:- *(PGMEE 2016-17)*
   a. CDH   b. Subtalar
   c. Ankle   d. Shoulder dislocation

   [Ref: Maheshwari 6th/e pg 89]

6. Most common joint to undergo recurrent dislocation is-
   (PGMEE 2014)
   a. Shoulder joint   b. Patella
   c. Knee joint   d. Hip joint

   [Ref: Maheshwari & Mhaskar 6th/e pg 54, 89 Apley's Orthopaedics 9th/e p. 86, 87]

7. Luxatio erecta is-:- *(PGMEE 2016-17)*
   a. Inf dislocation of shoulder
   b. Ant dislocation of shoulder
   c. Post dislocation of shoulder
   d. None of the above

   [Ref: Maheshwari and Mhaskar 6th e p.90]

8. Anterior dislocation of shoulder is most commonly complicated by- *(PGMEE 2012, AI 97)*
   a. Axillary artery injury   b. Circumflex nerve injury
   c. Recurrent dislocation   d. Axillary nerve injury

   [Ref: Maheshwari 6th/e p. 91; Adam's 12th/e140]

9. Uncomplicated shoulder dislocation most commonly occurs in the following direction- *(PGMEE 2012)*
   a. Anterior   b. Posterior
   c. Medially   d. Superior

   [Ref: Maheshwari & Mhaskar 6th/e p. 89]

10. A 20-years old male presents with anterior shoulder dislocation. This injury is usually caused as a combination of which of the following *(PGMEE 11)*
   a. Abduction & external rotation
   b. Adduction & external rotation
   c. Abduction & internal rotation
   d. Adduction & internal rotation

   [Ref: Maheshwari & Mhaskar 6th/e p. 90]

11. Posterior glenohumeral instability can be tested by-
   (PGMEE 10, 09)
   a. Jerk test   b. Crank test
   c. Fulcrum test   d. Sulcus test

   [Ref: Orthopedic physical assessment By David J. Magee 5th/e p. 288; Oxford pg. 10, 280; Maheshwari 6th/e p. 95]

Explanation

Test	Remark
Shoulder instability test	Apprehension test
Impingement test	HAWKIN'S Test, NEER's SIGN, JOBE'S Test
Scarf Test	For pathology of AC joint.
Signs of shoulder instability	Sulcus sign, Load Shift sign.

- Jerk test is used for posterior shoulder dislocation.
   (Ref: Oxford pg. 280, 10)
- Light Bulb Sign - Radiological sign in posterior shoulder dislocation. *(Maheswari 6th/e pg. 95)*

12. Hill sach lesion is seen in? *(DNB june 2010)*
   a. Posterolateral humerus
   b. Anterior dislocation of shoulder joint
   c. Glenoid labrum tear
   d. Posterior dislocation of shoulder joint

   [Ref: Maheshwari& Mhaskar 6th/e p. 90]

13. In inferior shoulder dislocation nerve most common injured is: *(DNB dec 2010)*
   a. Axillary   b. Median
   c. Radial   d. Ulnar

   [Ref: Maheshwari& Mhaskar 6th/e p. 91]

14. Shoulder abaducts 15-90° is by which muscle:-
   (PGMEE 2016-17)
   a. Supra spinatus   b. Trapezoid
   c. Deltoid   d. Scalene anterior

   [Ref: BDC]

CLAVICLE

15. Most common bone to be fractured in children is-
   a. Distal radius   *(PGMEE 2015)*
   b. Clavicle
   c. Supracondylar humerus
   d. Radius/ulna

   [Ref: Maheshwari & Mhaskar 6th e pg 57]

16. Most common nerve involvement in fracture surgical neck humerus- *(PGMEE 2015)*
   a. Axillary nerve   b. Radial nerve
   c. Ulnar nerve   d. Median nerve

   [Ref: Maheshwari&Mhaskar 6th/e p. 92; Apley's 9th/e p. 747]

17. Proximal humerus fracture which has maximum chances of avascular necrosis- *(PGMEE 2012)*
   a. One part fracture   b. Two part fracture
   c. hree Part fracture   d. Four part fracture

   [Ref: Textbook of shoulder disorder p. 885; Oxford 414]

1.	b
2.	b
3.	a
4.	d
5.	d
6.	a
7.	a
8.	d
9.	a
10.	a
11.	a
12.	a
13.	a
14.	c
15.	c
16.	a
17.	d

Explanation

- 4 part fractures have significantly higher chance of AVN ~ 30%.

FRACTURE SHAFT HUMERUS

18. Holstein lewis fracture is related which nerve-
(PGMEE 2015)

a. Median   b. Radial
c. Ulnar   d. Axillary

[Ref: Maheshwari & Mhaskar 5th e pg 94]

19. Nerve commonly involved in fracture distal shaft of the Humerus-
(PGMEE 2012)

a. Radial nerve
b. Medial
c. Circumflex brachial nerve
d. Ulnar

[Ref: Maheshwari & Mhaskar 6th e pg. 94]

20. Fracture shaft of humerus damages which nerve?
(DNB JUNE 2009;2010)

a. Radial nerve   b. Median nerve
c. Axillary nerve   d. Ulnar nerve

[Ref: Maheshwari & Mhaskar 6th e pg. 94]

FRACTURE SUPRACONDYLAR HUMERUS

21. Most common type of supra condylar fracture in children-
(PGMEE 2015)

a. Posterio medial extension
b. Myositis ossificans
c. Anteromedial flexion
d. Anterolateral flexion

[Ref: Maheshwari & Mhaskar 6th e pg. 97]

Explanation

- A supracondyler fracture may be of extension type or flexion type depending upon the displacement of the distal fragment. The extension type is commoner (80%).
- The distal fragment may be displaced in the following directions: posterior shift, posterior tilt, proximal shift, medial shift, medial tilt, internal rotation.

22. True about deformities seen after malunited supracondylar fracture:-
(PGMEE 2016-17)

a. Gunstock deformity
b. Cubitus valgus
c. Dinner fork deformity
d. Swan neck deformity

[Ref: Maheshwari and Mhaskar 6th e p.102,104, 112, 288]

Explanation

- *Gunstock deformity* is a cubitus varus deformity with malunion of supracondyler fracture.
- *Cubitus valgus deformity* is seen with fracture of the lateral condyle humerus due to dimished growth of the lateral epiphysis]. It may be associated with ulner neuropathy called as tardy ulner nerve palsy.

- *Dinner fork defommity* it is seen with malunion of distal end radius fractures. The radial styloid lies in the same line as the ulnar styloid process.
- *Swan neck deformity* is seen in the hand affected by ra.

Other deformites in RA include

Part of body affected	Deformites
Hand	Ulnar drift of the hand Boutonniere feformity Swan neck deformity
Elbow knee	Flexion deformity Early-flexion deformity Late-triple subluxation (Flexion posterior subluxation and external rotation)
Ankle foot	Equires deformity Hallux valgus, hammer toe, etc

23. Supracondylar fracture is usually caused by-
(PGMEE 2014)

a. Hyperflexion injury   b. Axial rotation
c. Extension injury   d. Hyperextension injury

[Ref: Maheshwari & Mhaskar 6th/e p97]

24. All of the following are complications of supracondylar fracture of humerus in children, except- *(PGMEE 14)*

a. Compartment syndrome
b. Myositis ossification
c. Malunion
d. Non Union

[Ref: Maheshwari & Mhaskar 6th/e p. 100-102; Apley's 9th/e p. 760, 761]

25. All of the following are associated with supracondylar fracture of humerus, except- *(PGMEE 2012)*

a. It is uncommon after 15 yrs of age
b. Extension type fracture is more common than the flexion type
c. Cubitus varus deformity commonly results following malunion
d. Ulnar nerve is most commonly involved

[Ref: Maheshwari & Mhaskar 6th/e p.101]

26. Nerve injured in surgical neck of humerus fracture
(PGMEE 2016-17)

a. Axillary nerve   b. Ant interossei nerve
c. Radial nerve   d. Sural nerve

[Ref: Maheshwari and Mhaskar 6th e p.92]

27. Volkmanns contracture, which artery is involved-
(PGMEE 2012)

a. Radial   b. Brachial
c. Interosseus   d. Ulnar

[Ref: Maheshwari & Mhaskar 6th/e p.102]

28. Cabitus varus is most commonly seen in *(PGMEE 2012)*

a. Fracture lateral condyle humerus
b. Post inflammatory epiphyseal damage
c. Rickets
d. Malunited supracondylar fracture

[Ref: Maheshwari & Mhaskar 6th/e p.102]

18.	b
19.	a
20.	a
21.	a
22.	a
23.	d
24.	d
25.	d
26.	a
27.	b
28.	d

29. Gun stock deformity is seen in? *(DNB jun 2008)*
   a. Supracondylar fracture humerus
   b. Lateral condylar fracture of humerus
   c. Medial condylar fracture of humerus
   d. All above

   [Ref: Maheshwari & Mhaskar 6th/e p.102]

FRACTURE LATERAL CONDYLE HUMERUS

30. Most common complication of lateral condyle humerus fracture- *(PGMEE 2014)*
   a. Malunion
   b. Nonunion
   c. VIC
   d. Median nerve injury

   [Ref: Maheshwari & Mhaskar 6th/e, pg 103]

31. Cubitus valgus is due to:- *(PGMEE 2016-17)*
   a. Lateral condyle of humerus fracture
   b. Supracondylar fracture
   c. Medial condyle fracture
   d. Olecranon fracture

   [Ref: Maheshwari and Mhaskar 6th e p.104]

32. Tardy ulnar nerve palsy seen in? *(DNB December 2011)*
   a. Fracture both bones of forearm
   b. Malunited lateral condylar fracture
   c. Malunited medial condylar fracture
   d. Malunited supra condylar fracture

   [Ref: Maheshwari & Mhaskar 6th e pg104]

OTHER INJURIES

PULLED ELBOW

33. Pulled elbow means- *(PGMEE 2012)*
   a. Fracture dislocation of elbow
   b. Subluxation of head of radius
   c. Fracture of head of radius
   d. Fracture ulna

   [Ref: [Maheshwari & Mhaskar 6th/e, pg 105, Apley's 9th/e p. 765]

34. What is not true about pulled elbow? *(PGMEE 2015)*
   a. Occurs due to sudden axial pull on extended elbow
   b. Forearm is held in pronation and extention
   c. Most commonly occurs between 2-5 years of age
   d. Treatment is quick pronation and flexion of elbow

   [Ref Maheshwari & Mhaskar 6th/e, pg 105; Appley's 9th/e p. 765]

35. A child is spinned around by holding his hand by his father. While doing this the child started crying and does not allow his father to touch his elbow. The diagnosis is- *(PGMEE 14)*
   a. Pulled elbow
   b. Radial head dislocation
   c. Annular ligament tear
   d. Fracture olecranon process

   [Ref: Maheshwari & Mhaskar 6th/e, pg. 105, Apley's 9th/e p. 765]

36. A 4 year boy complaining of pain around elbow which is held in pronation with extension and normal X ray. What is the probable diagnosis? *(DNB December 2011)*
   a. Pulled elbow
   b. Cellulitis
   c. Montegia fracture
   d. None of the above

   [Ref: Maheshwari & Mhaskar 6th/e, pg 105]

DISLOCATION OF ELBOW

37. Deformity in posterior elbow dislocation- *(PGMEE 2014)*
   a. Flexion
   b. Extension
   c. Both d.   None

   [Ref: Clinical orthopaedics p. 786]

38. Commonest dislocation of elbow- *(PGMEE 2014, 2010)*
   a. Anterior
   b. Posterior
   c. Both same
   d. Medial

   [Ref: Maheshwari &Mhaskar 6th/e p 105; Ebnezar 4th/e p. 157]

39. Late complication of elbow dislocation- *(PGMEE 2013)*
   a. Median nerve injury
   b. Brachial artery injury
   c. Myositis ossificans
   d. All of the above

   [Ref: Maheshwari & Mhaskar 6th/e p 105]

40. In posterior dislocation of elbow, most prominent part- *(PGMEE 2012)*
   a. Radial head
   b. Coronoid
   c. Olecranon
   d. None

   [Ref: Maheshwari & Mhaskar 6th/e p. 105, Clinical orthopaedics p. 666; Oxford pg. 412]

Explanation

- Elbow dislocation + Coronoid # + Radial head # + medial/lateral epicondyle injury constitute *"Terrible triad"*. Prognosis is poor.

41. What is seen on x-ray with posterior elbow dislocation- *(PGMEE 2012)*
   a. Coronoid process posterior to humerus
   b. Cornoid process below humerus
   c. Coronoid process anterior to humerus
   d. None

   [Ref: Ebnezar 4th/e p. 158]

MISCELLANEOUS

42. Nerve injured in fracture of medial epicondyle of humerus- *(PGMEE 2013)*
   a. Anterior interosseous
   b. Median
   c. Ulnar
   d. Radial

   [Ref: Maheshwari & Mhaskar 6th /e p.105; Apley's 9th/e p. 760-770]

43. Tension band wiring is used for? *(DNB june 2011)*
   a. Fracture humerus
   b. Fracture spine
   c. Fracture tibia
   d. Olecranon fracture

   [Ref: Maheshwari & Mhaskar 6th e pg.106]

29.	a
30.	b
31.	a
32.	b
33.	b
34.	d
35.	a
36.	a
37.	a
38.	b
39.	c
40.	c
41.	a
42.	c
43.	d

44. Fracture of proximal forearm cast position is- *(PGMEE 2013)*
a. Pronated flexion
b. Neutral position
c. Supinated position
d. Position does not matter

[Ref: Maheshwari & Mhaskar 6th /e p.116]

45. Essex lopresti lesion in upper limb- *(PGMEE 2013)*
a. Injury to interosseous membrane
b. Radial head and DER fracture
c. Radial shaft
d. Radial shaft and radio-ulnar joint fracture

[Ref: Campbell 13 ed, page 4750, 3326]

Explanation

- Essex lopresti is a classificzation for calcaneal fractues.
- A hard fall on the outstretched hand can result in a fracture of the radial head or neck, disruption of the distal radioulnar joint, and tearing of the interosseous membrane for a considerable distance proximally called as essex lopresti injuury

COLLES FRACTURE & SMITH FRACTURE

46. Management of Smith's fracture is- *(PGMEE 2014)*
a. Open reduction and fixation
b. Plaster cast with forearm in pronation
c. Closed reduction with below – elbow cast
d. Above-elbow cast with forearm in supination

[Ref: Ebnezar 4th/e p. 180; Maheshwari 6th/e p. 114]

47. Following displacement seen in Colle's fracture EXCEPT- *(PGMEE 14)*
a. Dorsal tilt
b. Ventral tilt
c. Dorsal displacement
d. Lateral displacement

[Ref: Maheshwari & Mhaskar 6th/e p. 112]

Explanation

- The distal fragment displaces & tilts ventrally.

48. Most common complication of Colles # *(PGMEE 2014)*
a. Malunion
b. Avascular necrosis
c. Finger stiffness
d. Rupture of EPL tendon

[Ref: Maheshwari & Mhaskar 6th/e p. 114]

49. Garden spade deformity is seen in- *(PGMEE 2016-17)*
a. Barton's fracture
b. Colle's fracture
c. Smith's fracture
d. Chauffers fracture

[Ref: Maheshwari & Mhaskar 6th/e p. 112-114]

50. Most common fracture in elderly :- *(PGMEE 2012)*
a. Transcervical fracture neck of femur
b. Supracondylar fracture
c. Inter trochanteric fracture
d. Colle's fracture

[Ref: Maheshwari & Mhaskar 6th/e p. 112]

51. Dinner fork deformity is seen in- *(PGMEE 2012)*
a. Colle's fracture
b. March fracture
c. Supracondylar fracture
d. Lateral condyle fracture

[Ref: Maheshwari & Mhaskar 6th/e p. 114]

52. Smith's fracture involves which bone- *(PGMEE 2012)*
a. Distal radius
b. Proximal ulna
c. Patella
d. Metatarsal

[Ref: Maheshwari&Mhaskar 6th/e p. 114, Ebnezar 4th/e p. 180]

53. The complication of Colles fracture is:
a. Stiffness of wrist joint
b. Ulner nerve palsy
c. Radial nerve palsy
d. None of the above

[Ref: Maheshwari&Mhaskar 6th/e p. 114]

FRACTURE SCAPHOID

54. The most common nerve involvement is dislocation of Lunate is- *(PGMEE 2015)*
a. Median nerve
b. Anterior interosseu
c. Posterior interosseu
d. Ulnar nerve

[Ref: Maheshwari & Mhaskar 6th e p.122; Adam's 12th/e p. 201]

55. Fracture scaphoid is usually seen in- *(PGMEE 2013)*
a. Elderly male
b. Elderly postmenopausal female
c. Young active adult
d. Children

[Ref: Maheshwari&Mhaskar 6th/e p. 115]

56. Most common complication of scaphoid fracture- *(PGMEE 2013)*
a. Malunion
b. Avascular necrosis
c. Wrist stiffness
d. Arthritis

[Ref: Maheshwari & Mhaskar 6th/e p. 115]

57. Which part of scaphoid fracture is most susceptible to avascular necrosis? *(PGMEE 2019)*
a. Distal 1/3rd
b. Middle 1/3rd
c. Proximal 1/3rd
d. Scaphoid Tubercle

[Ref: Maheshwari & Mhaskar 6th/e p. 115]

MISCELLANEOUS

58. Barton's fracture is- *(PGMEE 2013)*
a. Fracture distal end humerus
b. Extra-articular fracture distal end radius
c. Intra-articular fracture distal end radius
d. Intra-articular fracture distal end radius with carpal bone subluxation

[Ref: Maheshwari&Mhaskar 6th/e p. 114]

59. The commonly injured carpal bone next to scaphoid is- *(PGMEE 91)*
a. Triquetrum
b. Trapezoid
c. Lunate
d. Capitate

[Ref: Maheshwari & Mhaskar 6th e p.122]

60. Muscle, pull of which can leads to failure of fixation of Benett's fracture:- *(PGMEE 2015)*
a. Extensor pollicis brevis
b. Flexor pollicis brevis
c. Adductor pollicis longus
d. Abductor pollicis longus

[Ref: Maheshwari & Mhaskar 6th e p.122]

44.	c
45.	a
46.	d
47.	b
48.	c
49.	c
50.	d
51.	a
52.	a
53.	a
54.	a
55.	c
56.	b
57.	c
58.	d
59.	c
60.	d

61. One of the common fractures that occur during boxing by hitting with a closed fist is- *(PGMEE 2015)*
   a. Monteggia fracture dislocation
   b. Galeazzi fracture dislocation
   c. Bennett's fracture dislocation
   d. Smith's fracture

   [Ref: Maheshwari & Mhaskar 6th e p.122]

62. Game Keeper's thumb is- *(PGMEE 2013)*
   a. Ulnar collateral ligament injury of MCP Joint
   b. Radial collateral ligament injury of MCP joint
   c. Radial collateral ligament injury of CMC joint
   d. Ulnar collateral ligament injury of CMC joint

   [Ref: Maheshwari & Mhaskar 6th e p.122]

63. A cricketer holds a catch and then presents with pain at the base of the right thumb. He should be examined to specifically rule out damage to which of the following structure-- *(PGMEE 11)*
   a. Extensor pollicis brevis
   b. Volar plate
   c. Abductor pollicis longus
   d. Ulnar collateral ligament

   [Ref: Maheshwari & Mhaskar 6th e p.122]

64. Carpal bone ossify first is:- *(PGMEE 2016-17)*
   a. Capitate   b. Hamate
   c. Pisiform   d. Lunate

   [Ref: Oxford pg. 550]

65. (X-ray of wrist joint with fracture scaphoid.. The most common late complication occurs due to disruption of the blood supply:- *(PGMEE 2016-17)*
   a. From proximal to distal segment
   b. From distal to proximal segment
   c. From dorsal to ventral surface
   d. From ventral to dorsal surface

   [Ref: Maheshwari and Mhaskar 6th e p.115]

66. Identify the xray:- *(PGMEE 2016-17)*

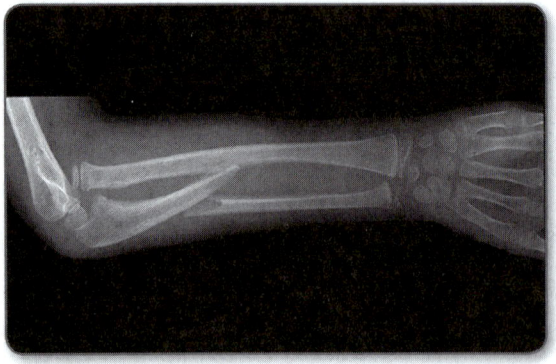

   a. Monteggia fracture
   b. Galeazzi fracture
   c. Rolando fracture
   d. Reverse smiths fracture

   [Ref: Maheshwari 6th e p.111]

Explanation

   ▪ The image shows fracture of ulna with dislocation of radial head.

67. Galeazzi fracture is
   a. Distal radio ulnar dislocation
   b. Proximal radio ulnar dislocation
   c. 1st metacarpal fracture

   [Ref: Maheshwari and Mhaskar 6th e p.111]

68. Most common cause of Compartment syndrome :-
   a. Iatrogenic   *(PGMEE 2016-17)*
   b. Closed tibial fracture
   c. Forearm bone fracture
   d. Supracondylar fracture of humerus

   [Ref: Internet]

69. Which of the following sign is present in Radial nerve injury:- *(PGMEE 2016-17)*
   a. Sign of Benediction
   b. Wrist drop
   c. Froment's sign
   d. Oschner clasp sign

   [Ref: Maheshwari and Mhaskar 6th e p.65;.17]

70. Arrow head in following X-ray shows :- *(PGMEE 2016-17)*

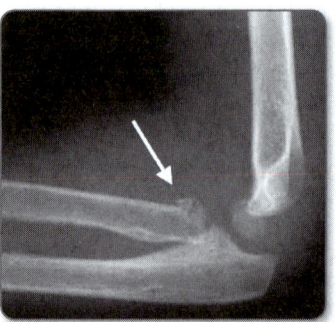

   a. Head of radius   b. Head of ulna
   c. Lateral condyle   d. Medial epicondyle

   [Ref: Internet.]

71. X-ray of wrist joint showing fracture of (image given) :- *(PGMEE 2016-17)*

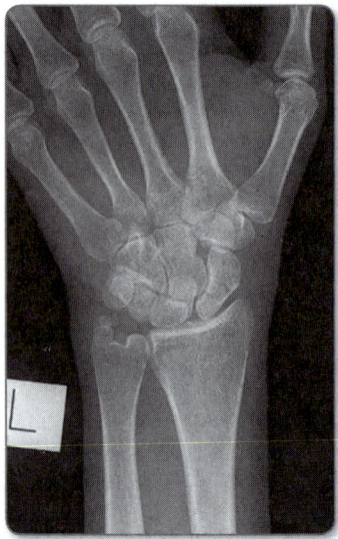

   a. Radius   b. Ulna
   c. Scaphoid   d. Capitate

   [Ref: Maheshwari and Mhaskar 5th e p.115]

61.	c
62.	a
63.	d
64.	a
65.	b
66.	a
67.	a
68.	a
69.	b
70.	a
71.	c

72. Structures of wrist and hand are numbered in the following image. The structure which is most likely to be injured due to injury by fall on outstretched hand:-

(PGMEE 2018)

a. Structure 1
b. Structure 2
c. Structure 3
d. Structure 4

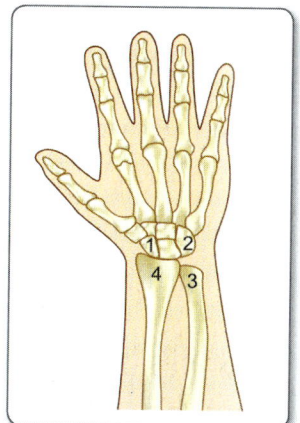

Ref: Campbell Operative Orthopedics 13 ed. Page 680

Explanation

- Most carpal bone fractures are the consequence of a fall onto an outstretched hand. The impact is transmitted on the distal carpal row when the distal radius resists tensile stresses from hyperextension. It also produces an extension moment across the proximal carpal row transmitted through the volar carpal ligaments, which may be disrupted or affected in shear stress resulting in *perilunate-pattern or "lesser arc" injuries*.
- # of the carpal bones or ligaments may occur in an arc around the lunate.
- Carpal fractures may occur on the volar aspect of the wrist from tensile stress, or dorsal cortical comminution may occur from compression shear stress.
- Fractures of the scaphoid, capitate, triquetrum, or all 3, together with perilunate instability, are known as *"greater arc" injuries*.

73. What happens in peri-lunate dislocation:-

(PGMEE 2018)

a. All the carpals and metacarpals bones displaced dorsally except Lunate
b. Only Lunate dislocates dorsally but NOT the carpal bones
c. All the carpal bones except lunate are impacted distally
d. Greater arc dislocations involves injury to scapholunate, luniocapitate and lunotriquetral ligaments.

[Ref: Maheshwari 6th Ed page 116]

Explanation

- Lunate dislocations: there are two types: Lunate discloation and perilunate discloaction. In lunate discloation which is more common the lunate dislocates anteriorly while in the latter the lunate stays in place and the rest of the carpal bones displace dorsally.

74. A young man had a fall on his outstreched hand, presented to the hospital with pain on the radial side of wrist and swelling in theanatomical snuff box. X-ray showed the following findings. What is the diagnosis?

(NEET Pattern 2018)

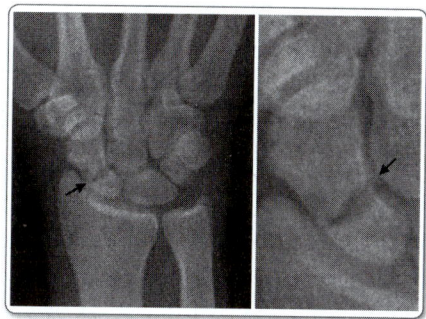

a. Scaphoid fracture
b. Trans scaphoidperilunate disruption fracture
c. Hook of hamate fracture
d. Distal radius fracture

[Ref: Campbell Operative Orthopedics, 13th ed. Page3914; Campbell Operative Orthopedics, 13th ed. Page3460]

Explanation

- Fractures of the hamate can involve the hamulus or hook, the body, and various articular surfaces. Carpal tunnel view or salute view (90-degree orthogonal from carpal tunnel view) may show the fracture.
- Transient ulnar nerve motor palsy can be caused by an undiagnosed stress fracture of the hook of the hamate. In most instances, unless the diagnosis is delayed, union is likely after immobilization, but excision of the fragment may be necessary for nonunion, persistent pain, or ulnar nerve palsy.
- *Fracture of the carpal scaphoid bone* is the **m/c** fracture of the carpus, and frequently diagnosis is delayed. Radiographs should be repeated in 2 weeks even though initial radiographs may be negative. It is caused by a fall on the outstretched palm of hand, resulting in severe hyperextension injury and slight radial deviation of the wrist. # through scaphoid waist or midportion occurs in 60% to 80% of cases. 17% of patients have other fractures of the carpus and forearm, including transscaphoid perilunar dislocations, fractures of the trapezium, Bennett fractures, fractures of the radial head, dislocations of the lunate, and fractures at the distal end of the radius.

75. 1st Carpal bone to ossify:
(NEET Pattern 2018)

a. Trapezoid
b. Capitate
c. Lunate
d. Pisiform

Ref: Netters Concise Textbook of Orthopedic Anatomy- 1st Ed

Explanation

- First carpal bone to ossify is capitate bone which tend to ossify in the 1st 1 year of life.

For details please refer discussion section in Orthopaedics

72.	d
73.	a
74.	a
75.	b

1. In Fracture acetabulum, late complication is-

(PGMEE 2014)

a. Osteoarthritis
b. Recurrent Dislocation
c. Tardy sciatic nerve palsy
d. None of the above

[Ref: Apley's 9th/e p. 840, 841]

2. Kocher Langenbeck approach for emergency acetabular fixation is done in all Except- *(PGMEE 09)*

a. Open fracture
b. Recurrent dislocation inspite of closed reduction and traction
c. Tardy sciatic nerve palsy
d. Morel-Lavallee lesion

[Ref: Essentials of orthopaedics surgery 3rd/e p. 1219]

Explanation

- *Morel-Lavallee lesions* are port traumatic degloving injuries in the subcutaneous plane. Treatment is debridement & antibiotics & plastic surgery procedures.

3. Radiological factors indicating an unstable pelvis are all except- *(PGMEE 2015)*

a. Posterior sacroiliac complex displacement by > 1cm
b. Avulsion fracture of sacral or ischial end of the sacrospinous ligament
c. Avulsion fractures of the 1.5 transverse process
d. Isolated disruption of pubic symphysis with pubic diastasis of 2 cm.

[Ref: Tile fractures of the Pelvis and acetabulum p. 139; Oxford pg. 427]

Explanation

Tiles classification for pelvic ring injuries

- 3 types
  - Type C are vertical shear & most unstable. Associated injuries include urethral (15%); Bladder (15%) vaginal & rectal injuries.

4. Jumper's fracture is seen in- *(PGMEE 2014)*

a. Calcaneum   b. Tibia
c. Pelvis   d. Neck femur

[Ref: Campbell's 11th/e p. 3348; Oxford pg. 336]

Explanation

- *Jumper's knee* is a/w
  - Traction apophysitis of patella (Larsen Jhonson disease) or
  - Injury to inferior pole of patella - Os good Schlatter disease.

5. True about Crescent fracture is- *(PGMEE 09)*

a. Anteroposterior instability with rotational stability
b. Antero-posterior compression is the mechanism of injury
c. Diastasis of pubis with pubic rami fracture
d. Fracture of the iliac bone with sacroiliac disruption

[Ref: Compbell's 11th/e p. 3339-42]

1.	a
2.	d
3.	d
4.	c
5.	d

HIP DISLOCATION

1. Posterior dislocation of hip is characterized by-
(PGMEE 2012)
  a. Marked shortening of limb
  b. Lengthening of lim
  c. Extension deformity
  d. No change in limb length

[Ref: Maheshwari & Mhaskar 6th e pg.130]

2. Sciatic nerve palsy may occur in the following injury-
(PGMEE 2012)
  a. Posterior dislocation of hip joint
  b. Anterior dislocation hip
  c. Trochanteric fracture
  d. Fracture neck of femur

[Ref: Maheshwari & Mhaskar 6th e pg.131;Adam's 12th/e p. 219]

3. Attitude of lower limb seen in posterior dislocation of hip is?
(DNB December 2011)
  a. Flexion, abduction, internal rotation
  b. Flexion, adduction, internal rotation
  c. Flexion, abduction, external rotation
  d. Flexion, adduction, external rotation

[Ref: Maheshwari & Mhaskar 6th e pg.131]

4. Pseudoflexion deformity of hip is seen in?
(DNB JUN 2009)
  a. Iliopsoas abcess
  b. Rickets
  c. Tom smith arthritis
  d. Posterior dislocation of hip

[Ref: Maheshwari & Mhaskar 6th e pg.131]

5. Vascular sign of narath is seen in? *(DNB JUN 2009)*
  a. Anterior dislocation of hip
  b. Sub trochantirc fracture of hip
  c. Posterior dislocation of hip
  d. Central dislocation of hip

FRACTURES OF FEMUR HEAD/NECK

6. Pipkin classification is for- *(PGMEE 2015)*
  a. Head of radius fracture
  b. Head of femur fracture
  c. Fracture dislocation of ankle
  d. Fracture neck of femur

[Ref: Maheshwari & Mhaskar 6th e pg.140; Apley's 9th/e p. 844]

7. Main blood supply to the head and neck of femur comes from-
(PGMEE 2011)
  a. Artery of Ligament Teres
  b. Medial circumflex femoral artery
  c. Lateral circumflex femoral Artery
  d. Popliteal Artery

[Ref: Snell's 8th/e p. 561]

8. Trabeaculae are aligned in which stage of fracture neck femur-
(PGMEE 2015)
  a. Stage 1
  b. Stage 2
  c. Stage 3
  d. Stage 4

[Ref: Maheshwari & Mhaskar 6th e pg.133;John Ebnezer's TB of orthopedics 4th/e p. 657]

9. Increase in Pauwel's angle indicate- *(PGMEE 2014)*
  a. Good prognosis
  b. Impaction
  c. More chances of displacement
  d. Trabecular alignment disrupted

[Ref: Maheshwari & Mhaskar 6th e pg.133]

10. Which of the following describes grade 2 fracture neck femur?
(PGMEE 2012)
  a. Incomplete fracture, medial trabeculae intact
  b. Complete fracture with undisplaced neck
  c. Complete fracture with ischemic head
  d. Moderate displacement of neck, vascularity damaged

[Ref: Maheshwari & Mhaskar 6th e pg.133]

CLINICAL FEATURES AND COMPLICATIONS

11. Position of leg in fracture of neck of femur is-
(PGMEE 2014)
  a. External rotation with patella facing inwards
  b. External rotation with patella facing outwards
  c. Internal rotation with patella facing outwards
  d. Internal rotation with patella facing inwards

[Ref: Maheshwari & Mhaskar 6th e pg.134]

12. Non-union in Fracture neck femur is due to:-
(PGMEE 2013)
  a. Injury to blood supply with shearing stress
  b. Poor nutrition of the patient
  c. Smoking
  d. Old age and osteoporosis

[Ref: Maheshwari & Mhaskar 6th e pg.137; Adam's 12th/e p. 228-237]

13. Complication of neck femur fracture are all except-
(PGMEE 2013)
  a. Nonunion   b. Malunion
  c. AVN   d. Osteoarthritis

[Ref: Maheshwari & Mhaskar 6th e pg.138]

14. Commonest complication of Trans-cervical fracture of femur is-
(PGMEE 2012)
  a. Non union   b. Avascular necrosis
  c. Malunion   d. All of the above

[Ref: Essentials of orthopaedic surgery 4th/e p. 311]

1.	a
2.	a
3.	b
4.	a
5.	c
6.	b
7.	b
8.	b
9.	c
10.	b
11.	b
12.	a
13.	b
14.	b

15. Most common complication of intertrochanteric fracture femur is- *(PGMEE 2014)*
a. Malunion
b. Nonunion
c. Osteoarthritis
d. Nerve injury

[Ref: Maheshwari & Mhaskar 6th e pg.1369; Adam's 12th/e p. 237]

16. AVN of femoral head is most common in- *(PGMEE 2012)*

a. Intracapsular fracture neck of femur
b. Extracapsular fracture neck of femur
c. Fracture shaft humerus
d. Subtrochanteric fracture

[Ref: Maheshwari & Mhaskar 6th e pg.138]

17. A patient who used to work out regularly at the gymgradually developed pain in the hip which is a aggravated while squatting. He gives history of regular steroid and creatine use over last six months. There is flattening of femoral head and subchondral cysts were seen on X-ray. What is the likely diagnosis? *(NEET Pattern 2018)*

a. Avascular necrosis (AVN) of hip
b. TB
c. Fracture neck of
d. Osteomalacia

Ref: Maheshwari textbook of Orthopedics, 6th ed. Page 318:

Explanation

- Causes of avascular necrosis include
  - Idiopathic (Most common),
  - Alcohol, steroid therapy
  - Sicke cell disease
  - Renal dylasis
  - Anti cancer drugs
  - Post partum necrosis
  - Gauchers disease
  - Caisson's disease.
- In later stages, an osteolytic lesion can be seen in supero-lateral part of the head. There may be diifuse osteosclerosis of the head, but the shape of the head may be maintained. In advanced stage, the head collapses.

TREATMENT

18. Treatment of choice for one week old fracture neck femur at 65 years age is- *(PGMEE 2014)*
a. Hemi-replacement arthroplasty
b. Closed reduction and internal fixation by cannulated cancellous screws
c. Closed reductions internal fixation by Austin more pins
d. Total hip replacement

[Ref: Maheshwari & Mhaskar 6th e pg.136]

15.	a
16.	a
17.	a
18.	b
19.	b
20.	c
21.	c

19. Mc Murray's osteotomy is done for- *(PGMEE 2013)*
a. Malunited intertrochantric fracture of femur
b. Nonunion transcervical neck fracture o femur
c. Nonunion lateral condyle fracture of humerus
d. Malunited supracondylar fracture of humerus

[Ref: Maheshwari & Mhaskar 6th e pg.136;Campbell's 10th/e p. 2122]

20. Best way to treat a fracture neck of femur in a child is? *(DNB june 2010)*

a. Hip Spica in abduction and internal rotation
b. Masterly inactivity
c. Open reduction
d. Traction

[Ref: Maheshwari & Mhaskar 5th e pg.135; Oxford pg. 576]

Explanation

- Treatment options
  - Closed reduction & pinning if anatomical reduction otherwise ORIF In children <2 years of age;
  - Closed reduction in hip spica is reasonable
- Since age is not mentioned ORIF is the best option.

21. Meyers muscle graft is ideal in: *(Recent Pattern June 2018)*
a. Delayed presentation of fracture neck of femur
b. Nonunion of fracture neck femur
c. Both of the Above
d. None of the Above

[Ref: Maheshwari & Mhaskar 5th /e p.141]

Explanation

- *Meyers muscle pedicle graft* has been used in delayed presentation and non-union of neck femur fracture in adults with good results.
- It is a novel procedure in t/t of neglected # NOF in pediatric age group.
- The vascularised graft like quadratus femoris muscle pedicle bone graft as used in Meyers procedure

FRACTURE SHAFT FEMUR

1. Golden hour of fracture femur is- *(PGMEE 2015)*
   a. 1 hr after injury
   b. 1 hr prior to injury
   c. 1 hr after reaching the hospital
   d. 1 hr after surgical procedure

[Ref: Emergency care and transportation of the sick and injury p. 829]

2. True about proximal fragment in supratrochanteric fracture is- *(PGMEE 2013)*
   a. Flexion   b. Abduction
   c. External rotation   d. All of the above

[Ref: J. Schatzker 3ʳᵈ/e p. 368]

3. Treatment of choice for fracture shaft femur in a 4 years old child- *(PGMEE 2014)*
   a. Gallow's traction   b. Hip spica
   c. Russel traction   d. Intramedullary nail

[Ref: Clinical orthopaedics p.786; Maheshwari & Mhaskar 6ᵗʰ/e pg. 143]

4. Treatment of choice for old non-united fracture of shaft of femur- *(PGMEE 2014)*
   a. Compression plating
   b. Bone grafting
   c. Nailing
   d. Compression plating with bone grafting

[Ref: Maheshwari & Mhaskar 6ᵗʰ/e p. 144; Adam's 12ᵗʰ/e p. 247]

5. In fracture of femur popliteal artery is common damaged by- *(PGMEE 2014)*
   a. Proximal fragment
   b. Distal fragment
   c. Muscle haematoma
   d. Tissue swelling

[Ref: Maheshwari & Mhaskar 6ᵗʰ/e p. 143; Apley's 9th/e p. 865]

6. Why fracture shaft femur is early stabilized- *(PGMEE 2012)*
   a. To prevent blood loss
   b. ARDS
   c. Compartment syndrome
   d. Non union

[Ref: Clinical orthopaedics p. 786]

7. Gallow's traction is used for fracture- *(PGMEE 10, 11)*
   a. Shaft femur
   b. Neck femur
   c. Tibial tuberosity
   d. Shaft tibia

[Ref: Maheshwari & Mhaskar 6ᵗʰ/e p. 143 ; Apley's 9ᵗʰ/e p. 86]

8. The traction that is applied for fracture shaft of the femur in children below 2 years is- *(PGMEE 2012)*
   a. Russell's traction
   b. Bryant fraction
   c. Gallow's traction
   d. Smith's traction

[Ref: Maheshwari & Mhaskar 6ᵗʰ/e p. 143]

PATELLA

9. The classical example of muscular violence is- *(PGMEE 2014)*
   a. # of fibula   b. # of patella
   c. # of clavicle   d. All of the these

[Ref: Maheshwari & Mhaskar 6ᵗʰ/e p. 147; Adam's 12ᵗʰ/e p. 253]

10. Tension band wiring is done in all except- *(PGMEE 2012)*
   a. Fracture patella   b. Fracture olecranon
   c. Colle's fracture   d. Fracture medial malleolus

[Ref: Manual of orthopaedics-pg. 786]

11. Jumpers knee is because of:- *(PGMEE 2016-17)*
   a. Patellar tendon tear
   b. Achilles tendinitis
   c. MCL tear
   d. Lateral collateral ligament tear

[Ref: Oxford pg. 336]

Explanation

- Jumper's knee is a/w inferior pole of patellar apophysis (Osgood Schatter disease)

ACL AND PCL INJURIES

12. Which of the following is incorrect about PCL? *(NEET Pattern 2018)*
   a. It is the main restraint in posterior drawer test
   b. It is an extrasynovial structure
   c. It the main restrain to internal rotation
   d. It originates from anterolateral aspect of medial femoral condyle in the area of intercondylar notch

Ref: Campbell Operative Orthopedics, 13ᵗʰ ed. Page 2491

Explanation

- The posterior cruciate ligament is composed of two major **parts, a large anterior part forms the bulk of the ligament and a smaller posterior part runs obliquely and attaches to the back of the tibia.**
- The posterior cruciate ligament attaches proximally to the posterior part of the lateral surface of the medial condyle.

1.	a
2.	d
3.	b
4.	d
5.	b
6.	a
7.	a
8.	c
9.	b
10.	c
11.	a
12.	d

- PCL guides the "screw-home" mechanism on internal rotation of the femur during terminal stage of extension of the knee. The PCL accounts for 89% of the resistance to posterior translation of the tibia on the femur and acts as a check of hyperextension only after the ACL has been ruptured.

13. Posterior gliding of tibia on femur is prevented by-
(PGMEE 2015)
- a. Anterior cruciate ligament
- b. Posterior cruciate ligament
- c. Medial collateral ligament
- d. Lateral collateral ligament

[Ref: Maheshwari & Mhaskar 6th/e p. 145]

14. Which among the following is not a femur of Unhappy triad of O' Donoghue? *(PGMEE 2015)*
- a. ACL injury
- b. Medial meniscus injury
- c. Medial collateral ligament injury
- d. Fibular collateral ligament injury

[Ref: Maheshwari & Mhaskar 6th /e pg149]

15. A 24 year old college student while playing hockey injured his right kee. This patient present after 3 months with instability of knee joint in full extension without instability at 90 degree of flexion. The structure most commonly damaged is- *(PGMEE 13)*
- a. Posterolateral bundle of anterior cruciate ligament
- b. Anteromedial bundle of anterior cruciate ligament
- c. Posterior cruciate ligament
- d. Anterior horn of medical meniscus

[Ref: Campbell's 12th/e ch.45]

16. The blood supply of anterior cruciate ligament is primarily derived from- *(PGMEE 2008)*
- a. Superior medial genicular artery
- b. Descending genicular artery
- c. Middle genicular artery
- d. Circumflex fibular artery

[Ref: Campbell's 11th/e p. 2497]

17. Which of the following is the SAFEST test to be performed in a patient with acutely injured knee joint- *(PGMEE 2008)*
- a. Lachmann test
- b. Pivot shift test
- c. McMurray's test
- d. Apley's grinding test

[Ref: Maheshwari & Mhaskar 6th/e p. 149]

MENISCUS INJURY

18. Unlocking of knee is caused by- *(PGMEE 2013)*
- a. Rectus femoris
- b. Quadriceps
- c. Hamstrings
- d. Popliteus

[Ref: Maheswari & Mhaskar 6th e pg 147]

19. Which of the following statements about 'Menisci' is not true- *(PGMEE 2010)*
- a. Medial meniscus is more mobile than lateral
- b. Menisci are predominantly made up of type I collagen
- c. Medial meniscus is more commonly injured than lateral
- d. Lateral meniscus covers move tibial articular surface than lateral

[Ref: Maheswari & Mhaskar 6th e pg152; Gray's 39th/e p. 1477]

20. When a patient gets up from sitting position which of the following events takes place in his knee joint?
(PGMEE 08)
- a. Medial rotation of femur on a fixed tibia
- b. Lateral rotationof femur on a fixed tibia
- c. Medial rotation of tibia on a fixed femur
- d. Lateral rotation of tibia on a fixed femur

[Ref: Maheswari 6th/e pg. 154]

Explanation
- Standing up involves locking of knee.

21. In which of the following meniscal tears will meniscetomy be a more suitable option for meniscal repair-
- a. Tears in the outer zone *(PGMEE 2008)*
- b. Tears in the middle zone
- c. Tears in the inner zone
- d. Tears at the junction of anterior horn of medial meniscus & tibial collateral ligament

[Ref: Campbell's 11th/e p. 2427, 2428]

MISCELLANEOUS KNEE INJURIES

22. Which of the following structure are not normally visualized during the arthroscopy of the knee?
(PGMEE 2015)
- a. Meniscus
- b. Cruciate ligament
- c. Collateral ligament
- d. Patella articular surface

[Ref: Maheshwari & Mhaskar 6th/e p. 326]

23. Commonest dangerous complication of posterior dislocation of knee is- *(PGMEE 2014)*
- a. Popliteal artery injury
- b. Sciatic nerve injury
- c. Ischaemia of lower leg compartment
- d. Femoral artery injury

[Ref: Maheshwari & Mhaskar 6th/e p. 152]

24. Insal-Salvati index is used for- *(PGMEE 2014)*
- a. Olecranon
- b. Patella
- c. Talus
- d. Scaphoid

[Ref: Campbell 13 ed, page 2625]

Explanation

Insall salavti index

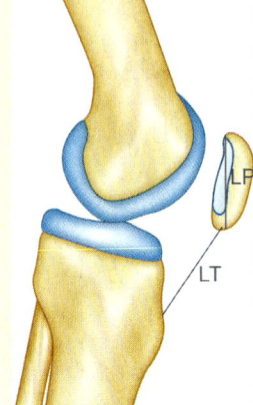

13.	b
14.	d
15.	a
16.	c
17.	a
18.	d
19.	a
20.	a
21.	c
22.	c
23.	a
24.	b

- Insall method of diagnosing patella alta. Length of patellar tendon (LT) and length of patella (LP) have normal LT-to-LP ratio of 1.0. Variation of more than 20% indicates abnormal position.

25. Mechanism of injury in lateral condylar fracture of proximal tibia- *(PGMEE 2013)*
a. Strain of valgus knee
b. Loose body varus knee joint
c. Strain of valgus knee with axial loading
d. Rotational injury

[Ref: Apley's 19th/e p. 890]

26. Bulge sign in knee joint is seen after how much fluid accumulation- *(PGMEE 2013)*
a. 100ml
b. 400ml
c. 200ml
d. <30ml

[Ref: Internet]

27. An athletic teenage girl complains of anterior knee pain on climbing stairs and on getting up after prolonged sitting. Which of the following is the most likely diagnosis?
(PGMEE 2011)
a. Chondramalacia Patellae
b. Patellofemoral osteoarthritis
c. Bipartite Patella
d. Plica Syndrome

[Ref: Apley's 9th/e p. 564-565]

28. In "bounce home" test of knee joint, end feel is described as all except? *(PGMEE 11)*
a. Firm
b. Empty
c. Springy
d. Bony

[Ref: Clinical Examination in orthopaedics 1st/e p. 71; Campbell's Orthopaedics 13th/e p. 2418]

Explanation
- Tibial External Rotation (Dial) Test. When an injured knee is tested for posterolateral instability, external rotation of the tibia on the femur is measured at both 30 and 90 degrees of knee flexion.
- The test can be done with the patient supine or prone. More than a 10-degree increase in external rotation compared with that of the contralateral side at 30 degrees of knee flexion, but not at 90 degrees, indicates an isolated injury to the posterolateral corner. An increase in external rotation of more than 10 degrees compared with that on the contralateral side at both 30 and 90 degrees of knee flexion indicates injury of both the posterior cruciate ligament and the posterolateral corner.

29. A patient met with Road Traffic Accident with injury to the left knee. Dial test was positive. What could be the cause? *(PGMEE 10)*
a. Lateral Meniscus Tear
b. Posterolateral Corner Injury
c. Medial Collateral Ligament Injury
d. Medial Meniscal Injury

[Ref: Turek's Orthopaedics 6th/e p. 599]

30. Treatment of choice for non-united fracture of lower 1/4th tibia with multiple discharging sinuses & various puckered scar with 4 cm shortening of leg-
(PGMEE 09)
a. Plating
b. Intramedullary nail
c. Ilizarov's fixator
d. External fixator

[Ref: Maheshwari & Mhaskar 6th/e p. 158; Ebnezar 4th/e p. 269]

31. The most commonly affected component of the lateral collateral ligament complex in an "ankle sprain" is the-
(PGMEE 2012)
a. Deeper component
b. Anterior component
c. Posterior component
d. Middle component

[Ref: Maheshwari &Mhaskar 6th/ep. 163]

32. Most common ligament injured in ankle sprain-
(PGMEE 2012)
a. Deltoid
b. Posterior talofibular
c. Anterior talofibular
d. Calcaneofibular

[Ref: Maheshwari& Mhaskar 6th/e p. 163]

33. Watson Jones operation is done for- *(PGMEE 08)*
a. Polio
b. Muscle paralysis
c. Neglected clubfoot
d. Chronic ankle instability

[Ref: Campbell's Orthopaedics 13th/e p. 4840]

Explanation
- Lateral repair of chronic instability of ankle: satisfactory results have been obtained from the Watson-Jones, Evans, and Elmslie operations.

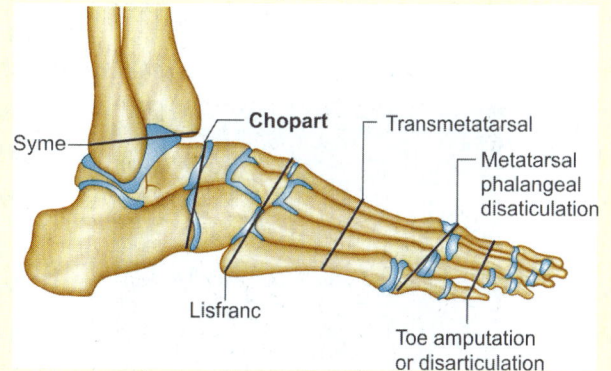

34. Recurrent dislocations are least commonly seen in-
(PGMEE 2009)
a. Ankle
b. Hip
c. Patella
d. Shoulder

[Ref: Campbell's Orthopaedics 11th/e p. 2717, 2670, 2665, 2677]

TALUS FRACTURE

35. Hawkins sign- *(PGMEE 2014)*
a. Unlikely to develop AVN
b. Non union
c. Decreased vascularity
d. Osteoarthritis

[Ref: Essential of orthopaedics 3rd/e p. 788]

25.	c
26.	d
27.	a
28.	b
29.	b
30.	c
31.	b
32.	c
33.	d
34.	a
35.	a

MISCELLANEOUS

36. Most commonly injured tarsal bone- *(PGMEE 2013)*
   a. Talus
   b. Navicular
   c. Cunieform
   d. Calcaneum

[Ref: Maheshwari & Mhaskar 6th /e p.164, Apley's 9th/e p. 924]

37. Jone's fracture is? *(DNB june 2010)*
   a. Avulsion fracture of base of fifth metatarsal
   b. Avulsion fracture of the medial femoral condyle
   c. Burst fracture of 1st cervical vertebra
   d. Bimalleolar fracture of the ankle

[Ref: Maheshwari&Mhaskar 6th/e p. 166]

38. Cotton's fracture involves: *(DNB DEC 2010)*
   a. Ankle
   b. Foot
   c. Spine
   d. Knee

[Ref: Maheshwari&Mhaskar 6th/e p. 367]

39. Most common site of march fracture is?
   (DNB june 2009)
   a. Shaft of 2nd and 3rd metatarsals
   b. Olecranon
   c. Calcaneus
   d. Avulsion fracture of fifth metatarsal

[Ref: Maheshwari&Mhaskar 6th/e p. 166]

40. Which of the following is false about Oblique Ligament:-
   (PGMEE 2016-17)
   a. It is pierced by middle genicular artery
   b. Degenerated part of semimembranous muscle
   c. Provides support to the knee posteriorly
   d. Attaches to the lateral surface of medial femoral condyle

[Ref: BDC]

41. X-ray picture of femur bone showing:- *(PGMEE 2016-17)*

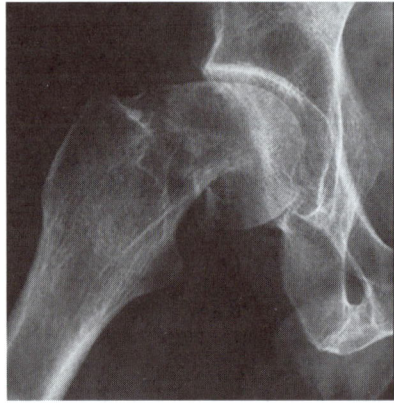

   a. # NOF
   b. # Femoral head
   c. # Shaft of femur
   d. # Acetabulum

[Ref: From internet]

42. Intercondylar # in a young adult, true is :-
   (PGMEE 2016-17)
   a. ORIF is needed
   b. Three point relationship maintained
   c. Conservation management
   d. k wire

[Ref: Maheshwari and Mhaskar 6th e p.46]

43. A patient with pain over left leg with foot drop Nerve involved is:- *(PGMEE 2016-17)*
   a. Common peroneal nerve
   b. Sural nerve
   c. Tibial nerve
   d. Radial nerve

[Ref: Maheshwari and Mhaskar 6th e p.46]

44. Cobra plating is use to stablise fracture of:-
   (PGMEE 2016-17)
   a. Hip fracture
   b. Tibia fracture
   c. Calcaneal fractute
   d. Patellar fracture

[Ref: : Maheshwari and Mhaskar 6th e p.19]

Explanation

- Amputations through the middle of the foot include:-
  ○ Lisfranc amputation at the tarsometatarsal joints and
  ○ Chopart amputation at the transverse tarsal joints,
- Both of these may lead to severe equinovarus deformity, and Pirogoff amputation, in which the calcaneus is rotated forward to be fused to the tibia after vertical section through its middle.

45. Chopart amputation is done along:- *(PGMEE 2016-17)*
   a. Tarsometatarsal joint
   b. Midtarsal joint
   c. Talo-navicular joint
   d. Tarsometaphalangeal joint

[Ref: Maheshwari and Mhaskar 6th e p.329]

36.	d
37.	a
38.	a
39.	a
40.	d
41.	a
42.	a
43.	a
44.	a
45.	b

OSTEOMYELITIS

ACUTE OSTEOMYELITIS

1. Acute Osteomyelitis is most commonly caused by-
(PGMEE 2015)

a. Staphylococcus aureus   b. Actinomyces bovis
c. Nocardia asteroids   d. Borrelia vincentii

[Ref: Maheshwari & Mhaskar 6th/e p. 168]

2. The organism causing osteomyelitis in sickle cell anemia:
(PGMEE 2014-15)

a. Salmonella   b. Staphylococcus
c. H. influenzae   d. E. coli

[Ref: CMDT 2014 ch.12, Pg. 503, Harrison's 19th/e pg. 840t]

3. Acute Osteomyelitis most commons site involved is:-
(PGMEE 2016-17)

a. Upper end femur   b. Lower femur
c. Upper tibia   d. Pelvis bone

[Ref: Maheshwari and Mhaskar 6th e pg.169]

4. 14 year old boy presents with high grade fever with pain and swelling in the thigh. X-Ray of lower limb is showing middle part of bone is swollen and periosteal reaction present. The most probable diagnosis is :-
(PGMEE 2016-17)

a. Osteosarcoma
b. Bone cyst
c. Ewing sarcoma
d. Osteomyelitis

[Ref: Maheshwari and Mhaskar 6th e pg.170]

5. The most common organism causing osteomyelitis in drug abusers is-
(PGMEE 2014)

a. E coll
b. Pseudomonas
c. Klebsiella
d. Staph Aureus

[Ref: Maheshwari & Mhaskar 6th/e p. 168]

6. Earliest site of bone involvement in hematogenous osteomyelitis-
(PGMEE 10, May 09,

a. Metaphysis
b. Diaphysis
c. Epiphysis
d. Point of entry of the nutrient artery

[Ref: Maheshwari & Mhaskar 6th/e p. 168]

CHRONIC OSTEOMYELITIS

7. Chronic discharging sinus with bone particle is seen in-
(PGMEE 2015)

a. Chronic osteomyelitis   b. Acute osteomyelitis
c. Subacute osteomyelitis   d. Garre's osteomyelitis

[Ref: Maheshwari & Mhaskar 6th/e p. 172-173]

8. Most Common cause of chronic osteomyelitis-
(PGMEE 2015)

a. Staphylococcus aureus
b. Streptococcus pyogenes
c. Mycobacterium tuberculosis
d. Staphylococcus epidermidis

[Ref: Maheshwari & Mhaskar 6th/e p. 168]

9. 25 years old male presents with pain in right leg. He had a RTA 2 years back. X ray of limb is shown. What is the diagnosis
(PGMEE 2018)

a. Chronic osteomyelitis
b. Ewings sarcoma
c. Giant cell tumor
d. Osteogenic sarcoma

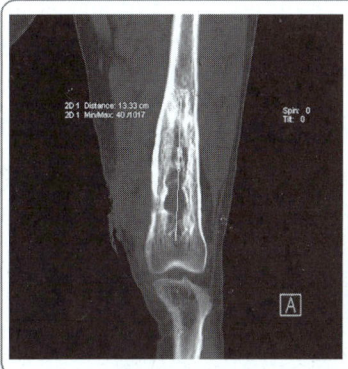 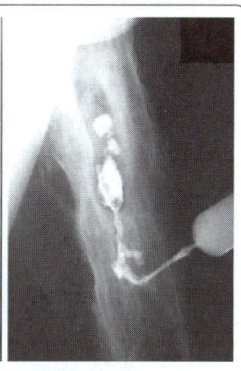

Explanation

- Injury due to right leg is associated with a compound injury. Most often Chronic osteomylitis is secondary to acute osteomyelitis.
- Delayed and inadequate treatment is the commonest cause of persistence if an osteomylitis. Delay causes spread of the pus within the medullary cavity and subperiosteally.
- Radiological examination in chronic osteomylitis involve
  ○ Thickeining and irregularity of cortices
  ○ Patchy sclerosis
  ○ Bony cavity
  ○ Sequestrum:this appears denser than the surrounding normal bone because of decalcification.
  ○ Involucrum and cloacae may be visible.

10. Cloacae are present in-
(PGMEE 2014)

a. Sequestrum
b. Involucrum
c. Normal bone
d. Myositis

[Ref: Maheshwari & Mhaskar 6th/e p. 172]

1.	a
2.	a
3.	b
4.	d
5.	d
6.	a
7.	a
8.	a
9.	a
10.	b

11. All are true about chronic osteomyelitis except- *(PGMEE 2013)*
   a. Reactive new bone formation
   b. Cloaca is an opening in involucrum
   c. Involucrum is dead bone
   d. Sequestrum is hard and porus

   [Ref: Maheshwari & Mhaskar 6th/e p. 172]

12. Sequestrum is best defined as- *(PGMEE 2012)*
   a. A piece of bone with poor vascularity
   b. A piece of dead bone surrounded by infected tissue
   c. A piece of dead bone
   d. None

   [Ref: Maheshwari & Mhaskar 6th/e p. 172]

13. Chronic persistent neutrophilic discharge is seen in- *(PGMEE 2012)*
   a. Chronic osteomyelitis   b. Septic arthritis
   c. Acute osteomyelitis   d. None

   [Ref: Maheshwari & Mhaskar 6th/e p. 173]

14. Brodie's abscess is- *(PGMEE 2012)*
   a. Acute osteomyelitis   b. Spetic arthritis
   c. Chronic osteomyelitis   d. Subacute osteomyelitis

   [Ref: Maheshwari & Mhaskar 6th/e p. 175]

15. Identify the condition as shown: *(PGMEE 2019)*

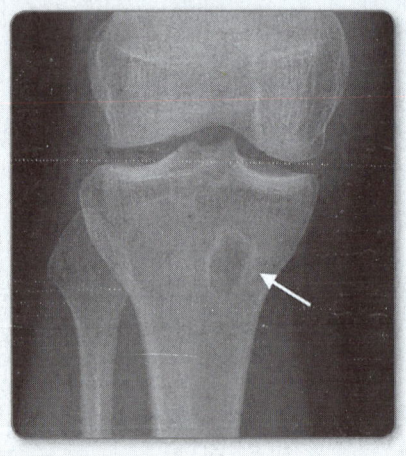

   a. Brodie abscess
   b. Osteoid osteoma
   c. Intracortical hemangioma
   d. Chondromyxoid fibroma

   [Ref: Maheshwari & Mhaskar 6th/e p. 175]

16. Sequestrum is a:- *(DNB 2007)*
   a. Infected bone   b. New bone
   c. Dead bone   d. Woven bone

   [Ref: Maheshwari & Mhaskar 6th/e p. 172]

TIS

17. Potts puffy tumor is- *(PGMEE 2014)*
   a. Osteomyelitis of frontal bone
   b. Osteomyelitis of maxilla
   c. Osteomyelitis of mandible
   d. Osteomyelitis of ethmoid

   [Ref: Dhingra's ENT 7th/e pg. 224]

18. Pott's puffy tumor: *(PGMEE 2019)*
   a. Subperiosteal abscess of frontal bone
   b. Subperiosteal abscess of ethmoid bone
   c. Mucocele of frontal bone
   d. Mucocele of ethmoid bone

   [Ref: Dhingra's ENT 7th/e pg. 224]

19. Salmonella osteomyelitis is common in: *(DNB dec 2010)*
   a. Sickle cell disease   b. HIV
   c. Pregnancy   d. IV drug abusers

   [Ref: Maheshwari & Mhaskar 6th e pg 175]

SKELETAL TUBERCULOSIS

20. Which of the following statements about tubercular osteomyelitis is not true? *(PGMEE 08)*
   a. It is type of secondary osteomyelitis
   b. Sequestrum is unknown
   c. Periosteal reaction is characteristic
   d. Inflammation is minimal

   [Ref: Maheshwari & Mhaskar 6th e pg 183]

SPINAL TUBERCULOSIS/POTT'S SPINE

21. Poor prognostic indicator of Pott's paraplegia- *(PGMEE 2013)*
   a. Early onset   b. Active disease
   c. Healed disease   d. Wet lesion

   [Ref: Maheshwari & Mhaskar 6th e pg 194;Skeletal tuberculosis by Tuli p. 222]

22. Pott's spine is commonest in spine- *(PGMEE 2012; DNB JUNE 2009)*
   a. Cervical   b. Thoracic
   c. Lumbar   d. Sacral

   [Ref: Maheshwari & Mhaskar 6th e pg 185]

23. The most common sequelae of tuberculous spondylitis in an adolescent is- *(PGMEE 2012)*
   a. Fibrous Ankylosis   b. Bony-Ankylosis
   c. Pathological dislocation d. Chronic osteomyelitis

   [Ref: Apley's 9th/e p. 472]

24. False about Pott's spine- *(PGMEE 2012)*
   a. Back pain is an early symptoms
   b. Always heals by chemotherapy
   c. Commonest at dorsolumbar junction
   d. There is disc space narrowing on x-ray

   [Ref: Maheshwari & Mhaskar 6th e pg. 194]

25. A 35 yr old lady with chronic backache. On X ray she had a D12 collapse. But Intervertebral disc space is maintained. All are possible except- *(PGMEE 10)*
   a. Multiple myeloma   b. Metastasis
   c. Osteoporosis   d. Tuberculosis

   [Ref Maheshwari & Mhaskar 6th e pg 195]

26. Pott's spine is commonest at which spine: *(DNB june'2010)*
   a. Thoracolumbar   b. Lumbosacral
   c. Cervical   d. Sacral

   [Ref: Maheshwari & Mhaskar 6th e pg 185]

11.	c
12.	b
13.	a
14.	c
15.	a
16.	c
17.	a
18.	a
19.	a
20.	c
21.	c
22.	b
23.	b
24.	b
25.	d
26.	a

OTHER SITES OF SKELETAL TUBERCULOSIS

27. Triple deformity of knee includes following except-
(PGMEE 2015)
- a. Flexion of knee
- b. External rotation of tibia
- c. Posterior subluxation of tibia
- d. Extension of knee

[Ref: Maheshwari & Mhaskar 6th /e p.201;Ebnezar 4th/e Various pages]

28. Apparent lengthening is seen in which stage of TB Hip -
(PGMEE 2012)
- a. Stage I
- b. Stage II
- c. Stage III
- d. None

[Ref: Maheshwari & Mhaskar 6th e pg 196]

29. Caries sicca is seen in-
(PGMEE 2012)
- a. Hip
- b. Shoulder
- c. Knee
- d. None of the above

[Ref: Maheshwari & Mhaskar 6th /e p.202]

30. The deformity of tibia in triple deformity of the knee is?
(DNB JUN 2009)
- a. Extension, posterior subluxation & external rotation
- b. Extension, anterior subluxation & internal rotation
- c. Flexion, posterior subluxation & external rotation
- d. Flexion, posterior subluxation & internal rotation

[Ref: Maheshwari & Mhaskar 6th e pg 201]

31. In Bony ankylosis, there is-
(PGMEE 2014)
- a. Painless, No movements
- b. Painful complete movements
- c. Painless complete movement
- d. Painful incomplete movement

[Ref: Essentials of orthopaedics 3rd/e p. 668]

32. Spina ventosa is the name given to radiographic picture of?
(DNB December 2011, PGMEE 2014)
- a. Ventral spinal cord affected in tuberculosis
- b. TB lumbosacral joint
- c. TB sacrococcygeus joint
- d. Tubercular dactylitis

[Ref: Maheshwari & Mhaskar 6th e pg 203]

33. Frozen pelvis is seen in-
(PGMEE 2013)
- a. Osteoarthritis
- b. Pott's disease
- c. Actinomycosis
- d. Reiters disease

[Ref: http://medial-dictionary.thefreedictionary.com/frozen+pelvis]

SEPTIC ARTHRITIS

34. Aspirated synovial fluid in septic arthritis will have-
(PGMEE 2013)
- a. Clear color
- b. High viscosity
- c. Markedly increased polymorphonuclear leukocytes
- d. None of the above

[Ref: Clinical Orthopaedics 2nd/e p. 712]

35. Tom smith arthritis affects: *(Recent Pattern June 2018)*
- a. Acetabulum of femur
- b. Capital epiphysis
- c. Multiple joints in children
- d. Head of femur

[Ref: Maheshwari & Mhaskar 6th /e p.178]

Explanation

Septic Arthritis in Infancy (Tom Smith Arthritis)
- It is a acute septic arthritis of the hip in infancy.
- The onset is acute with rapid pyogenic abscess formation, which may burst out or be incised and heals rapidly.
- There is rapid destruction of **head of femur** by pyogenic process. X-ray shows complete loss of head & neck of femur. **Acetabulum is well developed.**
- Telescopy of hip is positive.
- May present later as **painless limp** and unstable gait (trendelenberg gait) in adults.
- Clinically, this condition closely resembles a congenital dislocation of the hip (CDH)

36. Tom Smith arthritis involves- *(PGMEE 2014)*
- a. Knee
- b. Hip
- c. Ankle
- d. Wrist

[Ref: Maheshwari & Mhaskar 6th /e p.178]

37. Most common joint involved in septic arthritis-
(PGMEE 2013, 2019)
- a. Knee
- b. Hip
- c. Shoulder
- d. Elbow

[Ref: Maheshwari & Mhaskar 6th /e p.176]

38. Septic arthritis is diagnosed by- *(PGMEE 2012)*
- a. MRI
- b. Joint aspiration
- c. USG
- d. X-ray

[Ref: Maheshwari & Mhaskar 6th /e p.176]

MISCELLANEOUS

39. Non traumatic amputation is seen in? *(DNB dec 2009)*
- a. Sickle cell anemia
- b. Leprosy
- c. Diabetes mellitus
- d. All of the above

27.	d
28.	a
29.	b
30.	c
31.	a
32.	d
33.	b
34.	c
35.	d
36.	b
37.	a
38.	b
39.	a

METABOLIC BONE DISEASES

RICKETS AND OSTEOMALACIA

1. Identify the pathology shown in the X-ray- *(PGMEE 2015)*

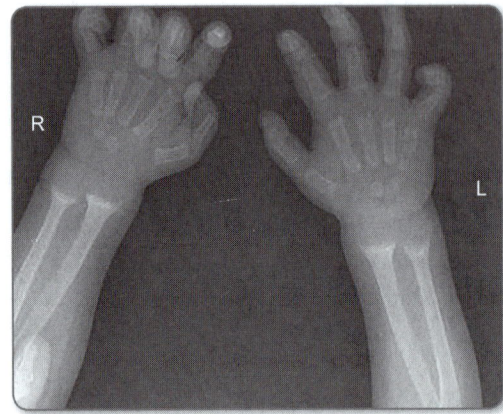

 a. Rickets
 b. Scurvy
 c. Achondroplasia
 d. Epiphyseal tumour

[Ref: Grainger and Allison Diagnostic Radiology 6th/e p. 1923]

2. Osteomalacia is associated with- *(PGMEE 2012)*
 a. Vitamin C deficiency
 b. Vitamin D deficiency
 c. Vitamin D deficiency
 d. None

[Ref: Maheshwari & Mhaskar 6th /e p312]

3. Rickets in infant present as all except-
 (PGMEE 2012, 07)
 a. Cranitabes
 b. Widened Fontanel
 c. Rachitic Rosary
 d. Bow legs

[Ref: O.P.Ghai 6th/e p. 128 & 7th/e p. 82]

4. Windswept deformity is seen in- *(PGMEE 2012)*
 a. Scurvy
 b. Ankylosing spondylitis
 c. Rickets
 d. Achondroplasia

[Ref : Nelson 18th/e p. chapter 48]

5. Alkaline phosphatase is elevated in all except-
 (PGMEE 2014)
 a. Rickets
 b. Osteomalacia
 c. Hypoparathyroidism
 d. Hypophosphatemia

[Ref: Tachdian's 3rd/e p.1687]

6. Looser's zones are seen in- *(PGMEE 2013)*
 a. Osteomalacia
 b. Paget's disease
 c. Renal osteodystrophy
 d. All of the above

[Ref : Internet]

7. Milkman's Fracture is a type of- *(PGMEE 2009)*
 a. Metacarpal fracture
 b. Clavicular fracture
 c. Humeral fracture
 d. Pseudofracture

[Ref: Maheshwari & Mhaskar 6th/e p 315; Grainger's Diagnostic Radiology 4th/e p. 1933, 1949]

SCURVY

8. Wimburger sign is seen in- *(PGMEE 2013)*
 a. Scurvy
 b. Rickets
 c. Osteoporosis
 d. Osteomalacia

[Ref: Maheshwari & Mhaskar 6th /e p 315;Radiology recall p. 912]

HYPERPARATHYROIDISM

9. Absence of lamina dura in the alveolus occurs in-
 (PGMEE 2014)
 a. Rickets
 b. Osteomalacia
 c. Deficiency of Vitamin C
 d. Hyperparathyroidism

[Ref: Maheshwari & Mhaskar 6th /e p313]

10. Hyperparathyroidism causes- *(PGMEE 2012)*
 a. Subperiosteal bone resorption
 b. Multiple bone cysts
 c. Brown's tumour
 d. All of the above

[Ref: Maheshwari & Mhaskar 6th /e p 313;Textbook of essentials In orthopaedics p. 1129]

11. (Characteristic subperiosteral bone resorption in hyperparathyroidism is best seen at? *(PGMEE 2011)*
 a. Rib margins
 b. Lamina dura
 c. Radial border of middle phalanx
 d. Medial margin of proximal humerus

[Ref: Maheshwari & Mhaskar 6th /e p 313]

12. Brown Tumor is seen in- *(PGMEE 10, 06)*
 a. Hypothyroidism
 b. Hypoparathyroidism
 c. Hyperthyroidism
 d. Hyperparathyroidism

[Ref: Maheshwari & Mhaskar 6th /e p313]

1.	a
2.	b
3.	d
4.	c
5.	c
6.	d
7.	d
8.	a
9.	d
10.	d
11.	c
12.	d

OSTEOPOROSIS

13. Most common site for the osteoporotic vertebral fracture is- *(PGMEE 2015)*
a. Dorsolumbar spine
b. Cervical spine
c. Lumbosacral spine
d. Dorsal spine

[Ref: Maheshwari & Mhaskar 6th /e p308; Apley's 9th/e p. 133

14. True about osteoporosis- *(PGMEE 2014)*
a. Low calcium
b. Low phosphate
c. Cod fish vertebrae
d. Raised alkaline phosphatase

[Ref: Maheshwari & Mhaskar 6th /e p308; Appley's 6th/e p. 133]

15. Osteoporosis is characterized by- *(PGMEE 2014)*
a. Increased serum alkaline phosphatase
b. Decreased bone density
c. Wasting of muscles
d. Looser's zone seen

[Ref: Maheshwari & Mhaskar 6th /e p308; Appley's 9th/e p. 133]

16. Z score measures the bone mineral density computed to- *(PGMEE 2015)*
a. Age, Race and sex matched individuals
b. Race and sex matched individuals
c. Sex matched individuals
d. None of the above

[Ref: Post graduate osthopaedics of paul p. 450]

Explanation

Using T-scores vs. Z-scores

T-scores	Z-scores
▪ WHO diagnostic classification in post menopaused women and men age 50 and older	▪ For use in reporting BMD in healthy premenopausal women, men under age 50, and children
▪ WHO classification with T-score cannot be applied to healthy premenopausal women, men under age 50, and children	▪ Z-core -2.0 or less is defined as below the expected rang for age
	▪ Z-score above -2.0 is within the expected range for age

▪ As per who guidelines. T score is used to define osteoporosis:
  ○ >1: Normal
  ○ 1 to -2.5: Osteopenia
  ○ < -2.5 or low: osteoporosis

17. Gold standard for diagnosis of osteoporosis- *(PGMEE 2013)*
a. DEXA
b. Single beam densitometry
c. Quatitative computed tomography
d. Bone histomorphometry

[Ref: Maheshwari & Mhaskar 6th /e pg. 309]

18. Most common site of osteoporosis- *(PGMEE 2012)*
a. Humerus
b. Vertebrae
c. Flat bones
d. Scapula

[Ref: Maheshwari & Mhaskar 6th /e p 308; Clinical orthopaedics p. 786]

19. All of the following agents decrease bone resorption in osteoporosis, Except- *(PGMEE 11)*
a. Etidronate
b. Alendronate
c. Strontium
d. Teriparatide

[Ref: Maheshwari & Mhaskar 6th /e p310]

20. Intranasal calcitonin is given for the treatment of? *(DNB Dec 2010)*
a. Paget's disease
b. Osteoporosis
c. Osteopetrosis
d. Hypercalcemia

[Ref: Internet]

PAGET'S DISEASE

21. Increased urinary hydroxyproline is seen in? *(PGMEE 2014-15)*
a. Paget's disease
b. Ehler Danlos syndrome
c. Hypo-parathyroidism
d. Osteoporosis

22. Picture frame vertebra is seen in- *(PGMEE 2013)*

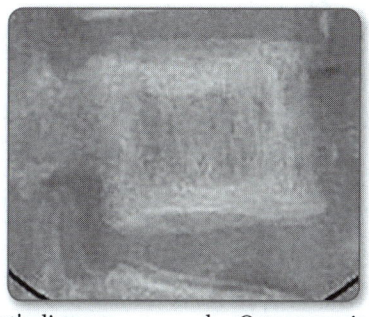

a. Paget's disease
b. Osteoperosis
c. Osteoporosis
d. Ankylosing spondylitis

[Ref: Turek 6th/ p. 274-275]

Explanation

▪ Pagete a.k a osteitis deformans.
▪ Lab - ↑ Alkaline phosphatase & ↑ urine hydroxyproline.

23. All are features of Paget's disease except- *(PGMEE 2013)*
a. Defect in osteoclasts
b. Common in female
c. Can cause deafness
d. Can cause osteosarcoma

[Ref: Maheshwari & Mhaskar 6th /e p317; Turek 6th/e p. 274-275; campbell 13th ed p 1358]

Explanation

▪ Osteogenesis imperfecta is a disease apparently of the mesodermal tissues with abnormal or deficient collagen that has been shown in bone, skin, sclerae, and dentin. The so-called diagnostic triad of blue sclerae, dentinogenesis imperfecta, and generalized osteoporosis in a patient with multiple fractures or bowing of the long bones usually is used clinically. The most used classification noted in the literature is by Sillence.

CHAPTER-9 ⬥ METABOLIC BONE DISEASES …

13.	a
14.	c
15.	b
16.	a
17.	a
18.	b
19.	d
20.	b
21.	a
22.	a
23.	b

- Besides pulmonary problems other anesthetic complications can occur such as difficulty in positioning the patient, malignant hyperthermia, basilar invagination, cardiac abnormalities, or bleeding from platelet dysfunction. The disorder is of type 1 collagen in most cases.
- **Silence classification of Osteogenesis Imperfecta (Simplified)**

Type	Inheritance	Sclerae	Features
I	AD	Blue	Mildest form, Presents at preschool age (tarda). Hearing deficit at 50%. Divided into type A & type B based on tooth involvement
II	AR	Blue	Lethal in perinatal period
III	AR	Normal	Fractures at birth. Progressively short stature. Most severe survivable form
IV	AD	Normal	Moderate severity. Bowing bones and vertebral fractures are common Hearing normal. Divided into type A and type B based on tooth involvement Hypertonic callus after fracture. Ossification of IOM between radius and ulna and tibia and fibula
V			
VI			Moderate severity similar to type IV
VII			Associated with rhizomella and coxa vara

24. Paget's disease after 10 years develops into-
(PGMEE 2012)
a. Osteosarcoma
b. Ankylosing spondylitis
c. Osteroid osteoma
d. Fibrous cortical defect

[Ref: Maheshwari & Mhaskar 6th /e p 317; Turek Orthopaedics th/e p. 274-275]

NEUROPATHIC JOINT

25. Most common cause of neuropathic joint-
(PGMEE 2013; DNB 2007)
a. Nerve injury
b. Tabes dorsalis
c. Diabetes
d. Leprosy

[Ref: Harrison 17th/e p. 2180-2181; Miller's p. 56]

26. False about Charcot's joint in diabetes mellitus is-
a. Limitation of movements with bracing   *(PGMEE 08)*
b. Arthrodesis
c. Total ankle replacement
d. Arthrocentesis

[Ref: Miller: Review of orthopaedics 4th/e p. 56; Oxford 227]

Explanation

- *Charcot Arthropathy has 4 stages:-*
  - Stage 0 & 1 - Rx is non weight bearing in mall fitted cartilage.
  - Stage 2 & 3 - gradual ↑ in weight bearing in ankle foot orthosis.
  - Surgery - for deformity correction once inflammation has settled.

27. Neuropathic joints are seen in all EXCEPT:
(PGMEE 2014-15)
a. Diabetes mellitus
b. Tabes dorsalis
c. Syringomyelia
d. Frederich's ataxia

[Ref: Harrison's 19th/e pg. 2629]

MISCELLANEOUS

28. In renal osteodystrophy skeletal abnormality is most commonly due to?   *(PGMEE 2011)*
a. Hyperphosphatemia
b. Hypocalcemia
c. Impaired synthesis of D3
d. Loss of vitamin D and calcium through dialysis

29. Boutonniere deformity is:-   *(PGMEE 2016-17)*
a. Flexion of metacarpophalyngeal joint & extension of interphalyngeal joint
b. Seen in osteo arthritis
c. Flexion of metacarpophalyngeal joint & flexion of interphalyngeal joint
d. None

[Ref: Maheshwari and Mhaskar 6th e p.288]

30. Gold salts are used in :-   *(PGMEE 2016-17)*
a. Gout
b. Rheumatoid arthritis
c. Osteoarthritis
d. Psoriatic arthritis

[Ref: Maheshwari and Mhaskar 6th e pg.288]

31. Rheumatoid arthritis with pneumoconiosis
(PGMEE 2016-17)
a. Caplan's syndrome
b. Feltys synd
c. Brodies abscess
d. Wiskott Aldrich synd

[Ref: Maheshwari and Mhaskar 6th e pg.288]

32. X-ray showing deformities of hands are typical of:-
(PGMEE 2016-17)

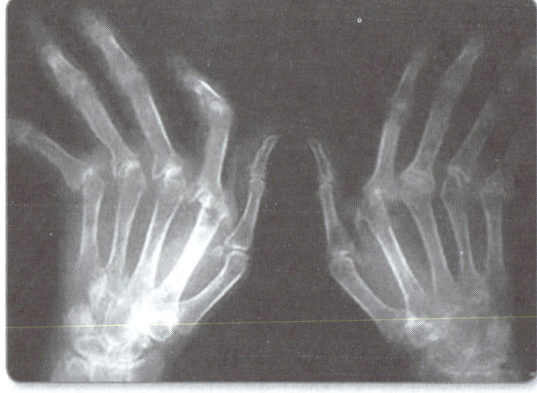

a. Gout
b. Rheumatoid arthritis
c. Osteoarthritis
d. Psoriatic arthritis

[Ref: Maheshwari and Mhaskar 6th e pg.288]

Answers

24.	a
25.	c
26.	c
27.	d
28.	c
29.	a
30.	b
31.	a
32.	b

33. Symptoms of inflammatory Arthiritis are all except:- *(PGMEE 2016-17)*

a. Pain
b. Swelling
c. Limitation of joint movement
d. With activity symp increases

[Ref: Maheshwari and Mhaskar 6th e pg.288]

34. OA spares wrist:- *(PGMEE 2016-17)*

a. Wrist
b. PIP
c. DIP
d. None of the above

[Ref: Maheshwari and Mhaskar 6th e p.300]

35. First complication arising after Menopause :- *(PGMEE 2016-17)*

a. Osteoporosis
b. Psychosis
c. Fozen arc synd
d. Supraspinatus tendinitis

[Ref: Maheshwari and Mhaskar 6th e p.308]

36. The most common presentation of osteoporosis is:- *(PGMEE 2016-17)*

a. Spine fracture
b. Weight loss
c. Back pain
d. Renal osteodystrophy

[Ref: Maheshwari and Mhaskar 6th e p.308]

AVASCULAR NECROSIS

AVN OF FEMORAL HEAD

37. Sectoral sign is positive in- *(PGMEE 2015)*

a. Avascular necrosis of femur head
b. Osteoarthritis of hip
c. Protrusio acetabuli
d. Slipped capital femoral epiphyses

[Ref: orthopedicprinciples.blogspot.com]

Explanation

- Sectoral sign also called as differential roataion is seen in avascular necrosis. There is difference in the arc of hip rotation of the hip joint when checked in hip extension and hip flexion, this is because of sectoral involvement of the femoral head from avn that results in different arc of rotation of the ball and socket joint due to difference in opposing congruity of surfaces.

38. After chronic use of steroids severe pain in right hip with immobility is due to- *(PGMEE 2012)*

a. Avascular necrosis
b. Perthes disease
c. Osteoarthritis
d. Hip dislocation

[Ref: Maheshwari & Mhaskar 6th /e p 318;Apley's 9th/e p. 105,106]

39. Avascular necrosis of hip, investigation of choice- *(PGMEE 2012)*

a. MRI
b. CT
c. USG
d. XRAY

[Ref : Maheshwari & Mhaskar 6th /e p 319;Apley's 8th/e p. 437, 683]

40. Avascular necrosis for patients can be retarded by? *(DNB june 2009)*

a. 500 mg Ca daily
b. 1000 mg Ca daily
c. 1500 mg Ca daily
d. 2000 mg Ca daily

[Ref: https://www.ncbi.nlm.nih.gov]

OSTEOCHONDRITIS DESICANS

41. Which joint is commonly involved in osteochondritis dessicans- *(PGMEE 2014)*

a. Ankle joint
b. Knee joint
c. Wrist joint
d. Elbow joint

[Ref: Oxford 533]

Explanation

- Most common site is knee - lateral aspect of medial femur condyle.

42. Most common involved in osteochondritis dessicans of elbow- *(PGMEE 2014)*

a. Radial head
b. Captitulum
c. Olecranon
d. Trochlea

[Ref: Apley's 9th/e p. 567]

OSTEOCHONDROSES

43. Osgood Shlatter's disease is osteochondritis of- *(PGMEE 2015)*

a. Tibial tuberosisty
b. Lunate
c. Calcaneum
d. Navicualr

[Ref: Maheshwari & Mhaskar 6th /e p 318;Turek's 6th/e p. 582, 583]

44. Frieberg's disease involve- *(PGMEE 2014)*

a. Tibial tuberosity
b. Calcaneal tuberosity
c. 2nd metatarsal
d. 5th metatarsal

[Ref: Maheshwari & Mhaskar 6th /e p318; Apley's 8th/e p. 723]

45. Kinebock's disease is due to avascular necrosis of- *(PGMEE 2014)*

a. Femoral neck
b. Medial cuneiform bone
c. Lunate bone
d. Scaphoid bone

[Ref : Maheshwari & Mhaskar 6th /e p318]

46. Osteonecrosis is not seen in- *(PGMEE 2012)*

a. Olliers disease
b. Kienbock
c. Kohlers disease
d. Perthes disease

[Ref: Maheshwari & Mhaskar 6th /e p318]

33.	d
34.	a
35.	a
36.	a
37.	a
38.	a
39.	a
40.	c
41.	b,d
42.	b
43.	a
44.	c
45.	c
46.	a

PRIMES ⚕ (VOLUME II)

PAINFUL CONDITIONS AROUND SHOULDER

1. Causes of painful arc syndrome is/are- *(PGMEE 2015)*
 a. Supraspinatus tendinitis
 b. Subacromial bursitis
 c. Fracture of greater tuberosity
 d. All the above

 [Ref: Maheshwari & Mhaskar 6th /e p.305]

2. Painful arc syndrome is caused by impingement of-
 (PGMEE 2013)
 a. Sub acromial bursa   b. Sub deltoid bursa
 c. Rotator cuff tendon   d. Biceps tendon

 [Ref: Maheshwari & Mhaskar 6th /e p.305]

3. Painful arc syndrome pain is felt during ? *(PGMEE 2019)*
 a. Mid abduction
 b. Initial abduction
 c. Full range of abduction
 d. Overhead abduction

 [Ref: Maheshwari & Mhaskar 6th /e p.305]

PAINFUL CONDITIONS AROUND ELBOW & WRIST

4. Cozen test is done for *(PGMEE 2015, Dnb JUNE 2011)*
 a. Little leaguer's elbow   b. Tennis elbow
 c. Golfer's elbow   d. Frozen shoulder

 [Ref : Maheshwari & Mhaskar 6th e pg.302]

5. Golfers elbow- *(PGMEE 2015)*
 a. Medial epicondylitis
 b. Lateral epicondylitis
 c. Posterior elbow dislocation
 d. Lateral collateral ligament injury

 [Ref: Maheshwari & Mhaskar 6th e pg.302, Apleys 9th/e p. 379]

6. Finkelstein's test is used for- *(PGMEE 2015)*
 a. CDH
 b. De Quervain's tenovaginitis
 c. Trigger finger
 d. Tennis elbow

 [Ref: Maheshwari & Mhaskar 6th e pg.303]

7. DeQuervain's disease classically affects the-
 a. Flexor pollicis longus and brevis *(PGMEE 2015)*
 b. Extensor carpi radialis and extensor pollicis longus
 c. Abductor pollicis longus and brevis
 d. Extensor pollicis brevis and abductor pollicis longus

 [Ref: Maheshwari & Mhaskar 6th e pg.303]

8. The following structure is involved in Dupuytren's contracture- *(PGMEE 2014)*
 a. Thickening of the palmar fascia
 b. Thickening of the dorsal fascia
 c. Contracture of the flexor tendons
 d. Post burns contracture

 [Ref: Maheshwari & Mhaskar 6th e pg.302;Adam's Outline of orthopedics 14th/e p. 321

9. Earliest finger to be involved in Duputren's contracture-
 (PGMEE 2014)
 a. Little finger   b. Ring finger
 c. Middle finger   d. Index finger

 [Ref: Maheshwari & Mhaskar 6th e pg.302;Textbook of musculoskeletal disorder p. 786]

10. Dupuytren's contracture can be caused by-
 (PGMEE 2013)
 a. Eptoin   b. Alcoholism
 c. Diabetes   d. All of the above

 [Ref: Maheshwari & Mhaskar 6th e pg.302; Textbook of musculoskeletal disorder p. 786]

11. A-65 years alcoholic suffering from diabetes has a flexion deformity at the right little finger over the metacarpophalangeal joint of around 15 degree. The ideal management for him would be- *(PGMEE 11)*
 a. Observation
 b. Total fasciectomy
 c. Subtotal fasciectomy
 d. Percutaneous fasciotomy

 [Ref: Maheshwari & Mhaskar 6th e pg.302;Apley's 8th/e p. 423; Campbells-3754]

12. Dupuytren's contracture most often involves
 (DNB 2007)
 a. Little finger   b. Thumb
 c. Ring finger   d. Any of the above

 [Ref : Maheshwari & Mhaskar 6th e pg.302]

13. Most common cause of trigger finger- *(PGMEE 2012)*
 a. Trauma   b. Smoking
 c. Alcohol   d. Drug abuse

 [Ref: Clinical orthopaedics p. 786]

14. Pulp space infection painful due to- *(PGMEE 2015)*
 a. Dense fibrous space
 b. Small phalynx
 c. Rich blood supply
 d. Rich nerve supply

 [Ref: Maheshwari & Mhaskar 6th e pg.206; Love & Bailey 25th/e p. 507]

15. Felon most common complication- *(PGMEE 2014)*
 a. Osteomyelitis   b. Subungual hematoma
 c. Infective arthritis   d. None

 [Ref: Maheshwari & Mhaskar 6th e pg.206;Ebnezar 4th/e p. 454]

16. Felon is- *(PGMEE 2012)*
 a. Infection of nail fold
 b. Infection of DIP joint
 c. Infection of pulp space
 d. Infection of ulnar bursa

 [Ref: Maheshwari & Mhaskar 6th e pg.206; Ebnezar 4th/e p. 454]

1.	d
2.	c
3.	a
4.	b
5.	a
6.	b
7.	d
8.	a
9.	b
10.	d
11.	a
12.	c
13.	a
14.	a
15.	a
16.	c

17. **Infection of ulnar bursa is diagnosed by-** *(PGMEE 2015)*
    a. Kanavel's sign
    b. Chowstek's sign
    c. Gower's sign
    d. Ludloff's sign

    [Ref: Maheshwari & Mhaskar 6ᵗʰ e pg.209]

Explanation

- *Kanavel sign* - infection of hand
  - Fusiform swelling.
  - Flexed posture.
  - Tenderness along tendon sheath.
  - Pain on passive extension.
- *Gowers sign* - Proximal muscle weakness in Duchenne muscle dystrophy
- *Ludloffi sign* - iliopsoas inflammation an tendinitis.

18. **Melon seed bodies are found in which of the following condition?** *(PGMEE 2012)*
    a. Osteoarthritis of the wrist
    b. Gout
    c. Tuberculous tenosynovitis
    d. Chondrocalcinosis

    [Ref: www.ncbi.nlm.nih.gov> pubmed;Ebnezar 4ᵗʰ/e p. 396; GS Kulkarni 2ⁿᵈ/e p. 396]

BURSITIS

19. **Housemaids knee is bursitis of-** *(PGMEE 2014)*
    a. Prepatellar bursa
    b. Infrapatellar bursa
    c. Olecranon
    d. Ischial bursa

    [Ref: Maheshwari & Mhaskar 6ᵗʰ e pg.301]

20. **Usual site of TB bursitis-** *(PGMEE 2014)*
    a. Prepatellar
    b. Subacromial
    c. Subdeltoid
    d. Trochanteric

    [Ref: Maheshwari & Mhaskar 6ᵗʰ e pg.301;Modern surgery by Da Costa p. 1269]

21. **Ischial bursitis is also known as-** *(PGMEE 2013)*
    a. Clergyman's knee
    b. Housemaid's knee
    c. Weaver's bottom
    d. Students elbow

    [Ref: Maheshwari & Mhaskar 6ᵗʰ e pg.301]

22. **Bunion is commonly seen at-** *(PGMEE 2013)*
    a. Great toe MTP joint
    b. Medial malleolus
    c. Lateral Malleolus
    d. Shin of tibia

    [Ref: Maheshwari & Mhaskar 6ᵗʰ e pg.301]

MISCELLANEOUS

23. **The primary pathology in Athletic Pubalgia is-** *(PGMEE 2013)*
    a. Abdominal muscle strain
    b. Rectus femoris strain
    c. Gluteus medius strain
    d. Hamstring strain

    [Ref: Practical Orthopaedic Sports Medicine & Arthroscopy 2006p. 532, 533; Mannual of sports Medicine 1998p. 429]

24. **24 yr old woman waking up experiences pain in heel which decreases on walking down. X-ray shows bone spur. Diagnosis-** *(PGMEE 2015)*
    a. Plantar fasciitis
    b. Calcaneal exostosis
    c. Osteomyelitis of calcaneum
    d. Achillis tendinitis

    [Ref: Essentials sports medicine 4ᵗʰ/e p. 65]

25. **Most common cause of insertional tendonitis of tendoachilles is-** *(PGMEE 08)*
    a. Overuse
    b. Improper shoe wear
    c. Runners and jumpers
    d. Steroid injections

    [Ref: Essentials sports medicine 4ᵗʰ/e p. 65]

26. **Snowstorm appearance of knee joint with multiple loose bodies is seen in?** *(DNB june 2011)*
    a. Fracture involving articular surface
    b. Ewing's sarcoma of knee joint
    c. Chondromalacia patellae
    d. Synovial chondromatosis

    [Ref: Maheshwari & Mhaskar 6ᵗʰ e pg.326]

27. **Flexor tendon graft repair graft is taken from-** *(PGMEE 2013)*
    a. Plantaris
    b. Palmaris longus
    c. Extensor digitorum
    d. Extensor indicis

    [Ref: Maheshwari & Mhaskar 6ᵗʰ e pg.94; Campbell 12th/e p.3276]

17.	a
18.	c
19.	a
20.	d
21.	c
22.	a
23.	a
24.	a
25.	a
26.	d
27.	b

1. **Which group of muscles is most commonly affected in Poliomyelitis:-** *(DNB 2007)*
   a. Dorsiflexors of the ankle
   b. Flexors of the knee
   c. Flexors of the hip
   d. Extensors of the hip

   [Ref: Maheshwari &Mhaskar 6th /e p.227]

2. **Genu valgum deformity is seen in all except-**
   a. Rickets *(PGMEE 2015)*
   b. Bone Dysplasia
   c. Rheumatoid arthritis
   d. Medial compartment osteoarthritis

   [Ref: Maheshwari &Mhaskar 6th /e p.325]

3. **Most common cause of genu valgum in children is-** *(PGMEE 2013)*
   a. Osteoarthritis   b. Rickets
   c. Page's disease   d. Rheumatoid arthritis

   [Ref: Maheshwari & Mhaskar 6th /e p.325; Ebnezar 4th/e p. 418]

4. **Blount's dsease is associated with all of the following, except-** *(PGMEE 11)*
   a. Genu varum   b. Internal Tibial Torsion
   c. Genu Recurvatum   d. External Tibial Torsion

   [Ref: Campbell's 10th/e p. 1180; Campbell 13th/e p. 1345]

Explanation

- In Blonts Disease the clinical and radiographic findings are consistent. The abnormality is characterized by varus and internal torsion of the tibia and genu recurvatum. The exact cause is unknown, but enchondral ossification seems to be altered. Suggested causative factors include infection, trauma, osteonecrosis, and a latent form of rickets, although none of these has been proved. A combination of hereditary and developmental factors is the most likely cause.

5. **Genu valgus deformity seen when?** *(DNB December 2011)*
   a. Long axis of tibia n fibula moves medial to long axis of femur
   b. Long axis of femur is anterior to tibia and fibula
   c. Long axis of femur is posterior to tibia and fibula
   d. Long axis of tibia n fibula moves lateral to the long axis of femur

   [Ref: emedicine.medscape.com]

6. **Marble bone disease is better known as? -** *(PGMEE 2012; DNB dec 2009)*
   a. Osteochondritis   b. Osteoprosis
   c. Osteopetrosis   d. Osteogenesis imperfecta

   [Ref: Maheshwari & Mhaskar 6th e p.317]

7. **Not seen in osteopetrosis-** *(PGMEE 08)*
   a. Compression of cranial nerve
   b. Osteomyelitis of mandible
   c. Pancytopenia
   d. Delayed healing of bone

   [Ref: Maheshwari & Mhaskar 6th e p.317]

8. **Caffey's disease is-** *(PGMEE 2014)*
   a. Renal osteodystrophy
   b. Infantile cortical hyperostosis
   c. Osteomyelitis of jaw in children
   d. Chronic osteomyelitis in children

   [Ref: Maheshwari & Mhaskar 6th /e p.319,Pediatric orthopaedics Vol 3 p. 477]

9. **Brittle bone disease is-** *(PGMEE 2013)*
   a. Osteogenesis imperfecta
   b. Osteopetrosis
   c. Laxity of joints
   d. Fragile fracture

   [Ref: Maheshwari &Mhaskar 6th /e p.316]

10. **Blue sclera is feature of-** *(PGMEE 2012)*
    a. Osteogenesis imperfecta
    b. Osteopetrosis
    c. Achendroplasia
    d. Cleidocarnial dysostosis

    [Ref: Maheshwari &Mhaskar 6th /e p.316]

TRANSIENT SYNOVITIS OF HIP

11. **Deformity in transient synovitis of Hip-** *(PGMEE 2013)*
    a. Abduction
    b. Flexion
    c. External rotation
    d. All of the above

    [Ref: Paediatrics Orthopaedics Vol-2 p. 1319]

12. **A 6 year old boy presents to the emergency with a painful limp. Clinical examination reveals tenderness in the femoral triangle and some limitation of hip movements. An X-ray was done which was normal. Which of the following should be the next course of action?** *(PGMEE 2011)*
    a. Aspiration
    b. Ultrasonography
    c. Wait and Watch/Observation
    d. MRI Scan

    [Ref: Maheshwari &Mhaskar 6th /e p.323]

1.	a
2.	d
3.	b
4.	d
5.	a
6.	c
7.	d
8.	b
9.	a
10.	a
11.	d
12.	c

13. A 7 yr. old boy with abrupt onset of pain in hip with hip held in abduction. Hemogram is normal. ESR is raised. What is the next line of management- *(PGMEE 09)*
- a. Ambulatory observation
- b. Hospitalize and observe
- c. Intravenous antibiotics
- d. USG guided aspiration of hip

[Ref: Maheshwari &Mhaskar 6ᵗʰ /e p.177]

14. Pseudoarthrosis is seen in all of the following except- *(PGMEE 2014)*
- a. Idiopathic
- b. Fracture
- c. Osteomyelitis
- d. Neurofibromatosis

[Ref: Maheshwari &Mhaskar 6ᵗʰ /e p.317,327Adam's Outline of orthopaedics 14ᵗʰ/e p. 55]

LIMB DEFECT

15. Madelung's deformity involves- *(PGMEE 2013)*
- a. Humerus
- b. Proximal ulna
- c. Distal radius
- d. Carpals

[Ref: Maheshwari & Mhaskar 6ᵗʰ/e p.225, Clinical Orthopaedics p.182]

KLIPPEL-FIEL SYNDROME & TORTICOLLIS

16. Sprengel's deformity is- *(PGMEE 2014)*
- a. Absence of clavicle
- b. Acomioclavicular dislocation
- c. Congenital elevation of scapula
- d. Recurrent dislocation of shoulder

[Ref: Maheshwari &Mhaskar 6ᵗʰ /e p.224, Adam's Outline of orthopaedics 14ᵗʰ/e p. 189]

17. Block vertebrae seen in- *(PGMEE 2013)*
- a. Pagets disease
- b. Leukemia
- c. TB
- d. Klippel-Feil syndrome

[Ref: Textbook of musculoskeletal radiology p. 786]

Explanation
- **Klippel-Feil syndrome** is characterized by - Block vertebrae + low lying hair line + limited range of motion.

18. The characteristic triad of Klippel-Feil syndrome includes all of the following, Except- *(PGMEE 10)*
- a. Short neck
- b. Low hair line
- c. Limited neck movements
- d. Elevated scapula

[Ref: Maheshwari &Mhaskar 6ᵗʰ /e p.224;Nelson 18ᵗʰ/e p. 2823; Harrison 15ᵗʰ/e p. 2174]

19. All are true about klippel-feil syndrome except: *(DNB December 2011)*
- a. Bilateral neck webbing
- b. BilateraL shortening of sternocleidomastoid
- c. Low hair line
- d. Restriction of neck movements

[Ref: Maheshwari &Mhaskar 6ᵗʰ /e p.224]

20. About congenital torticollis all are true except- *(PGMEE 07)*
- a. Always associated with breech extraction
- b. Spontaneous resolution in most cases
- c. 2/3ʳᵈ cases have palpable neck mass at birth
- d. Uncorrected cases develops plagiocephaly

[Ref: Maheshwari &Mhaskar 6ᵗʰ/e p. 321, Tachdjian p. 273, 274]

21. Sprengel's deformity is associated with all except: *(NEET Pattern 2018)*
- a. Congenital scoliosis
- b. Dextrocardia
- c. Diastematomyelia
- d. Klippelfeil syndrome

Ref: Campbell Operative Orthopedics, 13th ed. Page . 1292

Explanation

Sprengel Deformity
- Sprengel deformity is characterized as a congenital upward elevation of the scapula in relation to the thoracic cage.
- Other congenital anomalies may be present, such as cervical ribs, malformations of ribs, and anomalies of the cervical vertebrae (Klippel-Feil syndrome); rarely, one or more scapular muscles are partly or completely absent*sh Classifcation*
- *Brachial plexus palsy is the most severe complication of surgery for Sprengel deformity*
- Surgical correction include WOODWARD OPERATION and green procedure. Done for cosmetic reasons only.

PERTHE'S DISEASE

22. What is the diagnosis of the patient in the image? *(PGMEE 2015)*

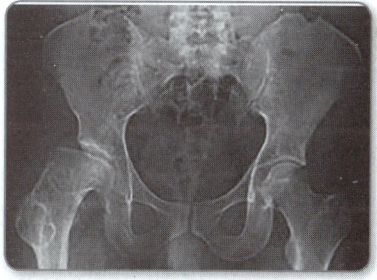

- a. Perthes disease
- b. Slipped capital femur epiphyses
- c. Developmental dysplasia of hip
- d. Fracture transcervical neck femur

23. Perthes disease etiology is- *(PGMEE 15)*
- a. Pyogenic
- b. Tubercular
- c. Traumatic
- d. Unknown

[Ref: Maheshwari & Mhaskar 6ᵗʰ /e p.318]

24. Which of the following movements is restricted Perthe's disease- *(PGMEE 2013)*
- a. Adduction & external rotation
- b. Abduction & external rotation
- c. Adduction & internal rotation
- d. Abduction & internal rotation

[Ref: Textbook of pediatric orthopaedics; Maheshwari & Mhaskar 6ᵗʰ /e p.318]

13.	d
14.	c
15.	c
16.	c
17.	d
18.	d
19.	b
20.	a
21.	b
22.	a
23.	d
24.	d

25. Radiological sign in case of Perthe's disease-
(PGMEE 2013)
a. Epiphyseal calcification
b. Organized calcification
c. Lateral subluxation femur head
d. Restriction of abduction

[Ref: Pediatric orthopaedics Vol-2 p. 1131]

Explanation
- Radiological stages of Perthe's disease
  ○ Initial or osteonecrosis
  ○ Fragmentation
  ○ Re-ossification
  ○ Residual disease
- Stage 2 & 3 show characteristic "creeping substitution"
(Ref. Oxford pg. 520)

26. Perthe's disease is- (PGMEE 2012; 94)
a. Fracture of femoral shaft
b. Osteochondritis of femoral epiphysis
c. Infraction of femoral head
d. Fracture dislocation of femoral neck

[Ref: Maheshwari &Mhaskar 6th /e p.318]

SLIPPED CAPITAL FEMORAL EPIPHYSIS

27. Slipped capital femoral epiphysis is seen most commonly in which age group- (PGMEE 12)
a. Infants   b. Adolescents
c. Old age   d. Childhood

[Ref: Ebnezar 4th/e p. 416; Maheshwari &Mhaskar 6th /e p.323,324]

28. True about Slipped femoral capital epiphysis is?
a. Seen in thin children   (DNB june 2010)
b. Trethowan sign seen
c. Major Traumatic condition
d. Seen in adults

[Ref: Maheshwari &Mhaskar 6th /e p.,324]

CONGENITAL DISLOCATION OF HIP

29. Breech presentation is a risk factor for the following condition- (PGMEE 2015)
a. CTEV   b. SCFE
c. DDH   d. Perthes disease

[Ref: Maheshwari & Mahaskar 6th /e pg219]

30. Congenital dislocation of hip in older child most common sign appreciated is- (PGMEE 2015)
a. Barlow test
b. Ortolani test
c. Painful ROM
d. Limited abduction of Lower Limb

[Ref: Maheshwari & Mahaskar 6th /e pg221]

31. Patients with bilateral CDH walk with the following gait-
a. Waddling   (PGMEE 2015)
b. Stumbling
c. Knock knee
d. Antalgic

[Ref: Maheshwari & Mahaskar 6th /e pg221]

32. Perkin's line on X-ray is used for diagnosis of-
(PGMEE 2015)
a. Perthe's disease   b. CDH
c. CTEV   d. AVN Hip

[Ref: Oxford handbook of orthopaedic surgery p. 454]

33. Ortolani test is positive when the examiner hears the-
(PGMEE 2015)
a. Clunk of entry on abduction and flexion of hip
b. Clunk of entry on extension and adduction of hip
c. Click of exit on abduction and flexion of hip
d. Click of exit on extension and adduction of hip

[Ref: Maheshwari & Mahaskar 6th /e pg221]

34. Which of the following test is useful in diagnosis of congenital dislocation of hip? (PGMEE 2014)
a. Barlow's test
b. Thomas test
c. Hibb's test
d. Laguerres test

[Ref: Maheshwari & Mahaskar 6th /e pg221]

35. 2 year old child with congenital dislocation of hip treatment of choice- (PGMEE 2014)
a. Closed reduction
b. Hip spica
c. Open reduction
d. Acetabular osteotomy

[Ref: Adam's 14th/e p. 346; Maheshwari & Mahaskar 6th /e pg221]

36. Bachelors' cast is used in- (PGMEE 2013)
a. Fracture radius   b. Club foot
c. DDH   d. Fracture calcaneum

[Ref: Maheshwari & Mahaskar 6th /e pg222]

37. Von-Rosen's sign is positive in- (PGMEE 2013)
a. Perthe's disease   b. SCFE
c. DDH   d. CTEV

[Ref: medicinembbs.blogspot.com>2013/04]

38. Salter's pelvic osteotomy is done for treatment of-
(PGMEE 2013)
a. CTEV   b. SCFE
c. DDH   d. None

[Ref: Maheshwari & Mahaskar 6th /e pg223; Pediatric orthopaedics Vol-2 p. 1823]

39. Primary pathology in CDH- (PGMEE 2012)
a. Large head of femur   b. Everted limbus
c. Excessive retroversion   d. Shallow acetabulum

[Ref: Maheshwari & Mahaskar 6th /e pg220; Adam's 14th/e p. 343]

40. Provocative Test for detecting CDH? (PGMEE 2012, 10)
a. Peterson test   b. Barlow test
c. Von Rosen tests   d. Perkin's test

[Ref: Maheshwari & Mahaskar 6th /e pg220]

41. Dysplastic hip in a child, investigation of choice-
(PGMEE 2012)
a. MRI   b. X-ray
c. USG   d. CT Scan

[Ref: Maheshwari & Mahaskar 6th/e pg222; Oxford handbook of orthopaedic surgery p. 454]

25.	c
26.	b
27.	b
28.	b
29.	c
30.	d
31.	a
32.	b
33.	a
34.	a
35.	c
36.	c
37.	c
38.	c
39.	d
40.	b
41.	c

CONGENITAL TALIPUS EQUINO VARU (CTEV)

42. Green extra articular arthrodesis done for-
(PGMEE 2015)
   a. Genu Valgum
   b. Coxa vara
   c. Congenital vertical talus
   d. Cubitus varus

[Ref: Campbells 13th/e p. 1128]

43. Treatment of partially corrected CTEV with cavus deformity is- *(PGMEE 2015)*
   a. Posteromedial release
   b. Lateral release
   c. Planter release
   d. Medial release

[Ref: Maheshwari & Mahaskar 6th /e pg215]

44. Most common cause of CTEV- *(PGMEE 2013)*
   a. Arthrogryposis multiplex congenita
   b. Spina bifida
   c. Idiopathic
   d. Neural tube defect

[Ref: Maheshwari & Mahaskar 6th /e pg211;Pediatric orthopaedics Vol-2 p. 888]

45. Early CTEV is treated by: *(DNB dec 2010)*
   a. Observation till 6 months of age
   b. Corrective splint only
   c. Manipulation only
   d. Manipulation and corrective splint both

[Ref: Maheshwari & Mahaskar 6th /e pg216]

46. Which is not true about CTEV shoe? *(DNB june 2009)*
   a. Raise outer portion
   b. Straight outer border
   c. No heel
   d. Used only from the age the child starts walking

[Ref: Maheshwari & Mahaskar 6th /e pg216]

47. Splint used in CTEV after correction- *(PGMEE 2013)*
   a. Bohler-Brown splint
   b. Thomas splint
   c. Dennis Brown splint
   d. None pf the above

[Ref:Maheshwari & Mahaskar 6th /e pg216; Adam's 14th/e p. 436]

48. Rocker bottom foot is due to- *(PGMEE 2013)*
   a. Overtreatment of CTEV
   b. Malunited fracture calcaneum
   c. Horizontal talus
   d. Neural tube defect

[Ref: Mercer 9th/e p.1217, 183]

49. Triple arthrodesis involve- *(PGMEE 2012)*
   a. Ankle joint, calcaneocuboid and talonavicular
   b. Tibiotalar, calcaneocuboid and talonavicular
   c. Calcaneocuboid, talonavicular and talocalcaneal
   d. None of the above

[Ref: Maheshwari & Mahaskar 6th /e pg216]

FRACTURE IN CHILDREN

50. Which is the commonest fracture in children?
   a. Fracture clavicle *(PGMEE 2014)*
   b. Supracondylar fracture
   c. Green stick fracture of lower end of radius
   d. All of the above

[Ref: dams notes]

51. Common fractures in children are all except-
   a. Lateral condyle humerus *(PGMEE 2013)*
   b. Supracondylar humerus
   c. Fracture of hand
   d. Radius-ulna fracture

[Ref: Pediatric orthopaedics Vol-2 p. 314]

52. Green stick fracture is- *(PGMEE 2012)*
   a. Fracture in adults   b. Fracture spine
   c. Incomplete fracture   d. Complete fracture

[Ref: Skeletal trauma in children Vol. 3 p. 161]

Explanation

- Type I fractures occur through the physis only, with or without displacement.
- Type II fractures have a metaphyseal spike attached to the separated epiphysis (Thurston-Holland sign) with or without displacement.
  - Type III fractures occur through the physis and epiphysis into the joint with joint incongruity when the fracture is displaced.
  - Type IV fractures occur in the metaphysis and pass through the physis and epiphysis into the joint. Joint incongruity occurs with displaced fractures.
  - Type V fractures, which are usually diagnosed only in retrospect, are compression or crush fractures of the physis, producing permanent damage and growth arrest. Rang added a Type VI fracture that is caused by a shearing injury to the peripheral aspect of the physis (perichondral ring)

PHYSEAL INJURIES

53. Metaphyseal fracture touching physis but not crossing it, comes under which type of Salter Harris physeal injury? *(PGMEE 2015)*
   a. I   b. II
   c. III   d. IV

[Ref: Campbell 13th/e p. 1593]

54. Type VI Rang's injury induces *(PGMEE 2015)*
   a. Transverse fracture of metaphysis with longitudinal extension into physis
   b. Open injury with loss of physis
   c. Thurston Halland's sign
   d. Perichondrial ring injury

[Ref: Essentials of orthopaedics Vol-I p. 282]

55. Thurston Halland sign is seen in- *(PGMEE 2013)*
   a. Type I   b. Type II
   c. Type III   d. Type IV

[Ref: Pediatric orthopaedics Vol-2p. 282]

42.	c
43.	c
44.	c
45.	d
46.	b
47.	c
48.	a
49.	c
50.	c
51.	c
52.	c
53.	b
54.	d
55.	b

MISCELLANEOUS

56. Tabes dorsalis +gen. paralysis:- *(PGMEE 2016-17)*
- a. Syphilis
- b. Dibatets
- c. Amyloidosis
- d. None of the above

57. All are features of osteogenesis imperfecta except:- *(PGMEE 2016-17)*
- a. Blue sclera
- b. Delayed dentition
- c. Mvp
- d. Type 4 collagen disorder

[Ref: Campbell 13th/e p. 358]

58. Rocker bottom foot is characterstic of:- *(PGMEE 2016-17)*
- a. Trisomy 18
- b. Trisomy 16
- c. Trisomy 21
- d. Monosomy 7

59. Identify the x ray:- *(PGMEE 2016-17)*

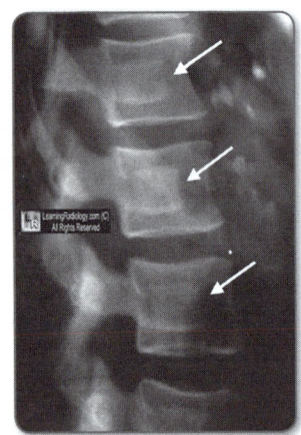

- a. Osteopetrosis
- b. Osteoporosis
- c. Osteonecrosis
- d. Pagets ds

[Ref: Maheshwari and Mhaskar 6th e p.317]

60. Components of club foot are all except:- *(PGMEE 2016-17)*
- a. Cavus
- b. Adduction
- c. Valgus
- d. Equinus

[Ref: Maheshwari 6th/e pg. 212]

61. (Image showing x-ray of hip joint with femoral necrosis). Identify the condition leading to this radiographic appearance:- *(PGMEE 2016-17)*

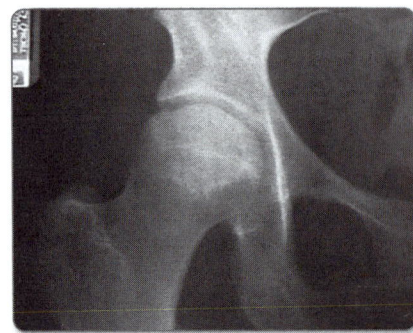

- a. Perthes disease
- b. Von-reckling hausen disease
- c. SCFE
- d. Osteoarthritis

62. All are features of achondroplasia except- *(PGMEE 2016-17)*
- a. Autosomal recessive
- b. Trident hand
- c. Rizomelic dwarfism
- d. Champagne glass pelvis

[Ref: Maheshwari and Mhaskar 6th e p.316]

63. CTEV boot is characterize by all excpet:- *(PGMEE 2016-17)*
- a. Straight inner
- b. Outer raised
- c. No heel
- d. Presence of metatarsal bar

Characterized by straight inner border,outer raised,and no heel.[Ref: Maheshwari and Mhaskar 6th e p.212]

64. Congenital dislocation of hip screening investigation of choice:- *(PGMEE 2016-17)*
- a. USG
- b. MRI
- c. CT
- d. X-ray

[Ref: Maheshwari and Mhaskar 6th e p.222]

65. A child presents with FTT and wrist widening. Xray of wrist joint showing cupping,fraying. The most likely condition causing this appearance can be:- *(PGMEE 2016-17)*

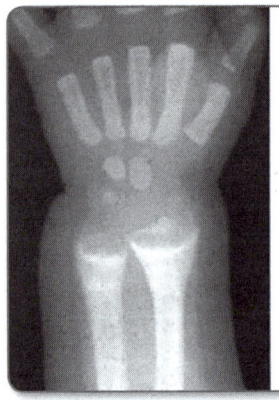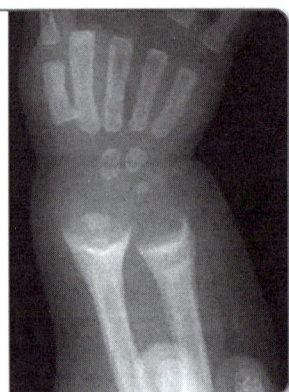

- a. Rickets,
- b. Scurvy,
- c. Osteomalacia
- d. Osteoporosis

[Ref: Maheshwari and Mhaskar 6th e p.311]

66. X-ray of both legs of a child showing windswept deformity. This appearance can be seen in:- *(PGMEE 2016-17)*
- a. Rickets
- b. Scurvy
- c. Osteogenesis Imperfecta
- d. Osteomalacia

67. Osteochondritis is diagnosed by :- *(PGMEE 2016-17)*
- a. Decrease in joint space
- b. Increase in joint space
- c. Intense inflammation
- d. Loose bodies in joint space

[Ref: Maheshwari and Mhaskar 6th e p.318]

56.	a
57.	d
58.	a
59.	a
60.	c
61.	a
62.	a
63.	d
64.	a
65.	a
66.	a
67.	b

68. Fibrous dysplasia of maxilla – true is:- *(PGMEE 2016-17)*
   a. Occurs in young females
   b. Medullary bone is replaced by cancellous bone
   c. Radiotherapy
   d. Mostly benign/malignant

   [Ref: Maheshwari and Mhaskar 6ᵗʰ e p.249]

69. The commonest cause of limp in a child of seven years is- *(PGMEE 2014)*
   a. T.B. hip
   b. C.D.H.
   c. Perthe's disease
   d. Slipped upper femoral epiphysis

   [Ref: Pediatric orthopaedics vol 2 p. 1135]

70. Painless effusion in joints in Congenital syphilis are called- *(PGMEE 2014)*
   a. Clutton's joint   b. Charcot's joint
   c. Barton's joint   d. Chronic osteomyelitis

   [Ref:Maheshwari & Mhaskar 6th e p.178]

71. Fairbank triangle is seen in- *(PGMEE 2012)*
   a. CDH
   b. SCFE
   c. Perthe's disease
   d. Congential coxa vara

   [Ref: Maheshwari & Mahaskar 6ᵗʰ /e pg323;Ebnezar 4ᵗʰ/e p. 410]

72. Which is the line of management for congenital pseudoarthrosis of Knee :- *(DNB 2008)*
   a. Amputation
   b. Chaenye's implant
   c. Immobilization
   d. Vascularised fibular graft

Explanation

- Treatment may include
  ○ Intramedullary nailing
  ○ Ilizarov frames
  ○ Resection & filling void with free vascularized fibula
  ○ Use of Bone morphagenic protein (BMP-2)

73. Siffert-katz sign is seen in: *(DNB dec 2009)*
   a. Legg-Calve-Perthes disease
   b. Blount's disease
   c. Pulled elbow
   d. Osteogenesis imperfecta

   [Ref: www.findeen.co.uk]

74. Tom-Smith's arthritis NOT true is:- *(PGMEE 2018)*
   a. Epiphysis of hip involved
   b. Epiphysis of capitulum of femur involved
   c. Greater trochanter is involved
   d. X-ray hip shows complete absence of head and Neck of femur

   Ref: Nelson Orthopedics:

Explanation

- Septic arthritis of the hip is called Tom Smith Arthrtits. Hunka's classification is used for classifiying and Choi classification for treatment planning. Greater Trochanter is not involved

Hunka Classification

- **Type I:** There is minimal collapse of the femoral head, which is later followed by reossification
- **Type II:** Deformity of the femoral head. In subtype IIa there is no evidence of physeal damage, while in Subtype IIb there is premature physeal closure, resulting in deformity of the femoral neck as well.
- **Type III:** A pseudarthrosis of the femoral neck is observed
- **Type IV:** Destruction of the femoral head, with retention of a variable portion of the femoral neck
- **Type V:** Destruction of both the femoral head and the femoral neck is seen

68.	**a**
69.	**c**
70.	**a**
71.	**d**
72.	**d**
73.	**b**
74.	**c**

1. Sunderland classification is used for- *(PGMEE 2015)*
 a. Nerve injury   b. Muscle injury
 c. Tendon injury   d. Ligament injury

[Ref: Maheshwari & Mhaskar 6th/e p. 63]

2. Physiological interruption of transmission is-
 (PGMEE 2015)
 a. Neuropraxia   b. Neurotmesis
 c. Axonotmesis   d. None of the above

[Ref: Maheshwari & Mhaskar 6th/e p. 63]

3. Saturday night palsy is which type of nerve injury-
 (PGMEE 2013)
 a. Neuropraxia   b. Axonotemesis
 c. Neurotemesis   d. Complete section

[Ref: Maheshwari & Mhaskar 6th/e p. 63; Clinical Orthopaedics p. 781]

4. Tinel sign is used for-   *(PGMEE 2012)*
 a. To locate the site of nerve injury
 b. To classify the type of nerve injury
 c. To assess the severity of damage of nerve
 d. To assess the recovery

[Ref: Maheshwari & Mhaskar 6th/e p. 69]

MEDIAN NERVE INJURY

5. Pen test is done for which nerve injury- *(PGMEE 2015)*
 a. Median   b. Ulnar
 c. Radial   d. Axillary

[Ref: Maheshwari & Mhaskar 6th/e p. 67]

6. Inability to pronate forearm is due to injury to which nerve   *(PGMEE 2015)*
 a. Ulnar   b. Radial
 c. Median nerve   d. Musculocutaneous

[Ref: Maheshwari & Mhaskar 6th/e p. 66]

7. Nerve damaged due to lunate dislocation [in carpal tunnel]-   *(PGMEE 2015)*
 a. Median & ulnar   b. Median
 c. Ulnar   d. Radial

[Ref: BDC Vol-I 5th/e p. 132]

8. Pointing index sign is seen in ----- nerve palsy-
 (PGMEE 2014)
 a. Ulnar   b. Radial
 c. Median   d. Axillary

[Ref: Maheshwari & Mhaskar 6th/e p. 64]

9. Ape thumb deformity is seen in involvement of-
 (PGMEE 2012, AI 2K)
 a. Median nerve   b. Ulnar nerve
 c. Radial nerve   d. Axillary nerve

[Ref: Maheshwari & Mhaskar 6th/e p. 64]

10. Median nerve lesion at the wrist causes all of the following except-   *(PGMEE 10)*
 a. Thenar atrophy
 b. Weakness of Adductor pollicis
 c. Weakness of 1st and 2nd lumbricals
 d. Weakness of Flexor pollicis Brevis

[Ref: Maheshwari & Mhaskar 6th/e p. 66;]

ULNAR NERVE INJURY

11. Froment's sign is positive due to loss of- *(PGMEE 2015)*
 a. Adduction of thumb due to ulnar nerve palsy
 b. Adduction of finger due to median nerve palsy
 c. Abduction of finger due to ulnar nerve palsy
 d. Extension of thumb due to radial nerve palsy

[Ref: Maheshwari & Mhaskar 6th/e p. 66; Apley's 8th/e p. 242]

12. Wasting of the intrinsic muscles of the hand can be expected to follow injury of the-   *(PGMEE 2014)*
 a. Ulnar nerve   b. Radial nerve
 c. Brachial nerve   d. Axillary nerve

[Ref: Maheshwari & Mhaskar 6th/e p. 64-70]

13. Ulnar paradox' is seen in-   *(PGMEE 2012)*
 a. Low ulnar lesion
 b. High ulnar lesion
 c. Triple nerve disease
 d. Combined ulnar and median nerve injury

[Ref: Last's anatomy 11th/e p. 101]

Explanation

 o *Ulnar paradox:* If the ulnar lesion is proximal near elbow, FDP (flexor digitorum profundus) is also denervated. It reduces the claw like appearance of head.

14. Froment's sign is characteristically seen in-
 (PGMEE 2012)
 a. Ulnar nerve injury
 b. Median nerve injury
 c. Radial nerve injury
 d. Intercostobrachial nerve injury

[Ref: Maheshwari & Mhaskar 6th/e p. 68]

15. Claw hand is caused by lesion of-   *(PGMEE 07)*
 a. Ulnar nerve   b. Median nerve
 c. Axillary nerve   d. Radial nerve

[Ref: Maheshwari & Mhaskar 6th/e p. 68 Ebnezar 4th/e p. 336]

16. The 'Card Test' detect the function of:-   *(DNB 2007)*
 a. Median nerve
 b. Ulnar nerve
 c. Axillary nerve
 d. Radial nerve

[Ref: Maheshwari & Mhaskar 6th e pg 68]

1.	a
2.	a
3.	c
4.	d
5.	a
6.	c
7.	b
8.	c
9.	a
10.	b
11.	a
12.	a
13.	b
14.	a
15.	a,b
16.	b

17. In Froment's sign ---------- muscle is tested

(DNB 2007,08)

a. Adductor pollicis
b. Opponens pollicis
c. Flexor pollicis brevis
d. Abductor pollicis

[Ref: Maheshwari & Mhaskar 6th e pg 68]

RADIAL NERVE INJURY

18. All of the following are affected in low radial nerve palsy except- *(PGMEE 11)*

a. Extensor carpi radialis longus
b. Sensation on dorsum of hand
c. Finger extensors
d. Extensor carpi radialis brevis

[Ref: Maheshwari & Mhaskar 6th/e p. 65]

19. Mr X met with road traffic accident. On examination, there is angular deformity in mid of arm. Abduction of finger possible but he is unable to dorsiflex the wrist. Possible nerve injury : *(Recent Pattern June 2018)*

a. Median nerve
b. Ulnar nerve
c. Radial nerve
d. Posterior interosseous nerve

[Ref: Maheshwari & Mhaskar 6th/e p. 65]

Explanation

- ○ Dorsiflexion of wrist not possible-extension of wrist not possible-wrist drop
- ○ Wrist drop is seen in Radial nerve injury
- ○ Finger drop is seen in Posterior interosseous nerve injury

Symptoms of an injury to the radial nerve

- Usually causes symptoms in dorsum of hand, near thumb, and in index and middle fingers.
- Sensory symptoms may include a sharp or burning pain, numbness, tingling.
- Motor: There is trouble straightening the arm. There is difficulty to extend or straighten wrist and fingers ("**wrist drop" or "finger drop**,") in severe cases.

BRACHIAL PLEXUS INJURY

20. Klumpkes paralysis- *(PGMEE 2014)*

a. Water tip deformity
b. Intrinsic hand muscle weakness
c. Elbow extended and wrist extended
d. Olny elbow is extended

[Ref: Ebnezar 4th/e p. 349; Oxford 488]

Explanation

- Brachial plexus injury include C5-T1. Three main types:-
  - ○ Upper trunk- Erb's palsy (C5-6 palsy)- Waiter's tip position
  - ○ Lower trunk- Klumpke's palsy (C8-T1 palsy)- Involves intrinsic muscles of hands.
  - ○ Whole plexus

21. Muscles paralysed in Erb's paralys are all except- *(PGMEE 2013)*

a. Biceps
b. Triceps
c. Brachioradialis
d. Brachialis

22. Investigating of choice for entrapment neuropathy is- *(PGMEE 2015)*

a. CT SCAN
b. Clinical examination
c. Ulrasonography
d. EMG NCV

[Ref: Maheshwari & Mhaskar 6th/e p.70-71]

23. Entrapment neuropathy at the arcade of frohse involves which nerve? *(PGMEE 2015)*

a. Median nerve
b. Posterior interosseous nerve
c. Ulnar nerve
d. Axillary nerve

[Ref: Maheshwari & Mhaskar 6th/e p. 65,66]

24. Most sensitive test for carpal tunnel syndrome- *(PGMEE 2014)*

a. Phalen's test
b. Tinel's sign
c. Tourniquet test
d. None

[Ref: www.physiopedia.com>phalens_test;Clinical orthopaedics p.786; Oxford 303]

Explanation

Tests for Carpal tunnel syndrome

- Weakness (typically abductor pollicis brevis)
- Tinnel test : not very reliable
- Phalen's test: Keep both wrists fully flexed for 1 minute.
- Direct compression test: Most reliable

25. Phalen's test is used in- *(PGMEE 2013)*

a. De Quervain tenosynovitis
b. Carpal tunnel syndrome
c. Trigger finger
d. Ulnar nerve injury

[Ref: Oxford's 303]

26. Meralgia paresthetica is due to involvement of-

a. Medial cutaneous nerve of thigh *(PGMEE 2013; 2007)*
b. Lateral cutaneous nerve of thigh
c. Sural nerve
d. Femoral nerve

[Ref: Maheshwari & Mhaskar 6th/e p. 305; Harrison 17th/e p. 14]

CARPAL TUNNEL SYNDROME

27. Carpal tunnel syndrome all are present except-

a. Ulnar nerve dysfunction *(PGMEE 2012)*
b. Pain & paraesthesia of wrist
c. Phalens sign
d. Tinel sign

[Ref: : Maheshwari & Mhaskar 6th/e p. 304;Harrison 17th/e p. 2153-54, Ebnezar 4th/e p. 393, 394; Oxford's 303]

17.	a
18.	a
19.	c
20.	b
21.	b
22.	d
23.	b
24.	a
25.	b
26.	b
27.	a

28. A 56-years old female presents with normal pain in the right thumb, index and middle fingers for the past 3 months. All of the provocative tests can be performed except- *(PGMEE 11)*

a. Finkelstein's test   b. Tourniquet test
c. Phalen's test   d. Tinel sign

[Ref: Adam's outline of orthopaedics 14th/e p. 320]

29. Carpal tunnel syndrome is caused by all except:
(DNB dec 2010)

a. Acromegaly   b. Tuberculosis
c. Pregnancy   d. Hypothyroidism

[Ref: Maheshwari & Mhaskar 6th/e p. 304]

30. Carpal tunnel syndrome can be caused by the following except- *(PGMEE 2009)*

a. Diabetes Mellitus   b. Hypothyroidism
c. Addison's Disease   d. Amyloidosis

[Ref: Maheshwari & Mhaskar 6th/e p. 304;Ebnezar 4th/e p. 393, 394]

MISCELLANEOUS

31. Most common cause of tarsal tunnel syndrome-
(PGMEE 09)

a. Osteoarthritis
b. Rheumatoid arthritis
c. Psoriatic arthritis
d. Ankylosing spondylitis

[Ref: McGlamry's foot & ankle surgery Vol-II p. 1267]

32. All of the following nerves are involved in entrapment neuropathy except- *(PGMEE 2009)*

a. Femoral nerve   b. Median nerve
c. ulnar nerve   d. Sural nerve

[Ref: Apley's 8th/e p. 246-252]

33. Nerve injured in fibular neck fracture- *(PGMEE 2014)*

a. Common peroneal   b. Tibial
c. Sural   d. Femoral

[Ref: Maheshwari & Mhaskar 6th e pg 46]

34. Foot drop is caused by injury to which nerve involvement: *(PGMEE 2019)*

a. Femoral nerve
b. Tibial nerve
c. Common peroneal nerve
d. Sciatic nerve

[Ref: Maheshwari & Mhaskar 6th e pg 46]

35. Extra cervical rib usually compresses which part of brachial plexus- *(PGMEE 2014)*

a. Lateral cord   b. Upper trunk
c. Middle trnlk   d. Lower trunk

[Ref: Apley's 9th/e p. 292.3]

36. Posterior dislocation of Hip can damage which nerve- *(PGMEE 2014)*

a. Superior gluteal   b. Sciatic
c. Inferior gluteal   d. Femoral

[Ref: Maheshwari & Mhaskar 6th e pg 131]

37. Limbs elevated against gravity but not against force is which power- *(PGMEE 2014)*

a. Grade I   b. Grade II
c. Grade III   d. Grade IV

[Ref: Campbell 12th/e p. 3497]

38. Most common nerve used for nerve conduction study in H reflex- *(PGMEE 2013)*

a. Median nerve   b. TB spine
c. Tibial nerve   d. Peroneal nerve

[Ref: Textbook of Neurology p. 781]

39. Trauma to neck of humerus, nerve damaged-
(PGMEE 2012)

a. Median   b. Ulnar
c. Radial   d. Axillary

[Ref: Maheshwari & Mhaskar 6th e pg 92]

40. In axillary nerve paralysis, all the following are true except- *(PGMEE 2012)*

a. Deltoid muscle is wasted
b. Small area of numbness is present over the shoulder region
c. Extension of shoulder with arm abducted to 90 degree is impossible
d. Patient cannot initiate abduction

[Ref: Maheshwari & Mhaskar 6th e pg 68;John Ebnezer's TB of orthopaedics 4th/e p. 351

28.	a
29.	b
30.	c
31.	a
32.	a
33.	a
34.	c
35.	d
36.	b
37.	c
38.	c
39.	d
40.	d

1. Column concept of spine stability was given by-
(PGMEE 2015)

a. Denis
b. Frenkel
c. Wilson
d. Todd

[Ref: Orthopaedics and Trauma for medical students and junior residents by Godwin p. 274-75]

Explanation

- Dennis: 3 column concept of spine.
- Frenkel- Grading of neurology and functional status.

2. Test used for prolapsed lumbar intervertebral disc is-
(PGMEE 2015)

a. Active straight leg raising test
b. Lasegue test
c. Thomas test
d. Apley's grinding test

[Ref: Maheshwari & Mhaskar 6th/e pg. 255]

3. After L_4-S_1 the next commonest site of intervertebral disc prolapse is-
(PGMEE 2014)

a. C_6-C_7
b. T_{12}-L_1
c. L_1-L_2
d. L_2-L_3

[Ref: Maheshwari & Mhaskar 6th/e pg.253;Apley's Outline of orthopedics 14th/e p. 236]

4. DISC prolapse is common at all site except-
(PGMEE 2013)

a. L_4-L_5
b. L_5-S_1
c. C_6-C_7
d. T_3-T_4

[Ref: Maheshwari & Mhaskar 6th/e pg.253;Apley's 9th/e p.236]

5. Investigation of choice for lumbar prolapsed disc-
(PGMEE 2012)

a. X-ray
b. Myelogram
c. MRI
d. CT Scan

[Ref: Maheshwari & Mhaskar 6th/e pg.254;Essentials of clinical orthopaedics p. 786]

6. A middle-aged lady presents with complaints of lower back pain. On examination there is weakness of extension of right great toe with no sensory impairment. An MRI of the lumbosacral spine would most probably reveal a prolapsed intervetebral disc at what level?
(PGMEE 11)

a. L3 – L4
b. L4 – L5
c. L5 –S1
d. S1 – S2

[Ref: Maheshwari & Mhaskar 6th e p.255; Essentials orthopaedics;]

7. Which of the following is not recommended in the treatment of chronic low back pain-
(PGMEE 2009)

a. Epidural steroid injection
b. Bed rest for 3 months
c. Exercises
d. NSAIDs

[Ref: Harrison 17th/e p. 115; Current Diagnosis and Treatment in Family Medicine (LANGE) 1st/e p. 257: Maheshwari & Mhaskar 5th e p.261]

8. Most common site for trauma of spine is-
(PGMEE 2012)

a. Cervical
b. Sacrum
c. Lumbar
d. Thoracic

[Ref : Clinical orthopaedics p. 786]

9. Following is true about spinal injuries except-
(PGMEE 2015)

a. Forms 65% of all trauma cases
b. Neurodeficit is present in 50% of all the cases
c. Traumatic injuries most commonly affect the cervical spine
d. Cervical spine is more prone to fracture than dislocation

[Ref: Clinical orthopaedics p. 786]

JEFFERSON'S FRACTURE AND HANGMAN'S FRACTURE

10. Hangman's fracture is-
(PGMEE 2014)

a. Subluxation of C5 over C6
b. Fracture dislocation of C2
c. Fracture dislocation of ankle joint
d. Fracture of odontoid

[Ref : Maheshwari & Mhaskar 6th e p.3; Surgical treatment of orthopaedic trauma 4th/e p. 116]

11. Jafferson's fracture is the fracture of-
(PGMEE 2012)

a. Odontoid
b. C_1
c. C_2
d. C_3

[Ref: Maheshwari & Mhaskar 6th e p.3;Apley's 9th/e p. 813, 814]

WHIPLASH INJURY

12. "Whip-lash" injury is caused due to-
(PGMEE 2014)

a. A fall from a height
b. Acute hyperextension of the spine
c. A blow on top to head
d. Acute hyperflexion of the spine

[Ref: Maheshwari & Mhaskar 6th e p. 3,269; Apley's 9th/e p. 820]

1.	a
2.	b
3.	a
4.	d
5.	c
6.	b
7.	b
8.	a
9.	d
10.	b
11.	b
12.	b

DORSAL SPINE INJURY

13. The compression fracture is commonest in-
(PGMEE 2014)
- a. Cervical spine
- b. Upper thoracic spine
- c. Lower thoracic spine
- d. Lumbosacral region

[Ref: Maheshwari & Mhaskar 6th e p.270, table 31.1; Neurotrauma & critical care of the spine 4th/e p. 81]

14. Earliest reflex to reappear after spinal shock-
(PGMEE 2013)
- a. Knee jerk
- b. Ankle jerk
- c. Bulbocavernous reflex
- d. Abdominal reflex

[Ref: Basic of Orthopaedics 2nd/e p.118

MANAGEMENT OF CERVICAL SPINE INJURY

15. On accident there is damage of cervical spine, first line of management is- *(PGMEE 2012)*
- a. X-ray
- b. Turn head to side
- c. ABCDE
- d. Stabilise the cervical spine

[Ref: Skeletal injuries 8th/e p. 71]

Explanation
- Basic principle to be followed is : ABCDE. Airway would be the first priority.

16. Patient develops myelopathy post- trauma. What does of methyl prednisolone is to be given? *(PGMEE 11)*
- a. 30 mg/kg over 15 minutes
- b. 45 mg /kg within 6 hrs.
- c. 60 mg /kg within 9 hrs.
- d. 75 mg /kg within 12 hrs.

[Ref: Campbell's operative orthopaedics vol-II 11th/e p. 1771]

MISCELLANEOUS

17. Wrist flexion and finger extension test the following nerve root- *(PGMEE 2014)*
- a. C_8
- b. C_7
- c. C_6
- d. T_1

[Ref: Rider's 1st/e p. 329]

18. What is vertebroplasty- *(PGMEE 2013)*
- a. Stabilization of vertebral compression fracture
- b. Replacement of vertebral body only
- c. Replacement of vertebral body with intervertebral disc
- d. Fusion of the adjacent vertebrae

[Ref: Maheshwari & Mhaskar 6th /epg275;Clinical orthopaedics 3rd/e p. 615]

19. Percutaneous vertebroblasty is indicated in all except- *(PGMEE 11)*
- a. Tuberculosis
- b. Metastasis
- c. Osteoporosis
- d. Hemangioma

20. A patient involved in a road traffic accident presents with quadriparesis, sphincter disturbance, sensory level up to the upper border of sternum and a respiratory rate of 35/minute. The likely level of lesion is- *(PGMEE 2010)*
- a. T_1-T_2
- b. T_3-T_4
- c. C_1-C_2
- d. C_4-C_5

[Ref: Harrison 17th/e p. 2588]

21. Material used in verterbroplasty is- *(PGMEE 08)*
- a. Isomethyl methacrylate
- b. Isoethyl methacrylate
- c. Polyethyl methacrylate
- d. Polymethyl methacrylate

[Ref: Maheshwari &Mhaskar 6th/e p.275; **The Cervical Spine' by Clarke (Lippincott-Williams)** *4th/e p. 181]*

22. Vertebral rotation in scoliosis is checked in-
(PGMEE 2015)
- a. Forward bending
- b. Backward bending
- c. Sideways
- d. Without bending

[Ref: Oski's paediatrics, Principles and pratice p. 2488]

23. Most common cause of kyphotic deformity-
(PGMEE 2013)
- a. Trauma
- b. Osteoporosis
- c. Ankylosing spondylitis
- d. Rickets

[Ref: Clinical orthopaedics 3rd/e p. 157]

24. In scoliosis degree of deformity is calculated by-
(PGMEE 2012)
- a. Cobbs method
- b. Milwaukee method
- c. Haldane method
- d. Hamburger method

[Ref: Maheshwari & Mhaskar 6th/e pg.281]

25. What should be the most likely diagnosis of this 65 year old lady presents with backache and following radiograph of the spine shown in image: *(PGMEE 2019)*

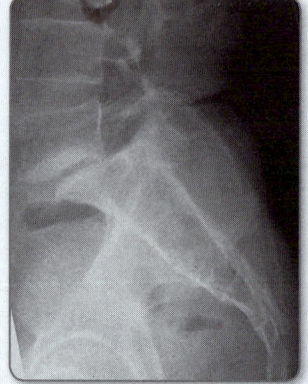

- a. Osteoporosis
- b. Spondylolisthesis
- c. Spondylolysis
- d. Discitis

[Ref: Maheshwari & Mhaskar 6th/e p.283]

26. Partial anterior dislocation of one segment of the spine over another is – *(PGMEE 2012)*
- a. Spondylosis
- b. Scoliosis
- c. Kyphosis
- d. Spondylolisthesis

[Ref: Maheshwari & Mhaskar 6th/e p.283]

27. Least helpful for the diagnosis of spondylolisthesis-
(PGMEE 11)
- a. AP x- ray of spine
- b. CT
- c. MRI
- d. Lateral x- ray of spine

[Ref: Maheshwari&Mhaskar 6th/e pg. 284; Essentials of skeletal 3rd/e p. 380]

13.	c
14.	c
15.	c
16.	a
17.	b
18.	a
19.	a
20.	d
21.	d
22.	a
23.	b
24.	a
25.	b
26.	d
27.	a

28. Progression of congenital scoliosis is least in likely in which of the following vertebral anomalies-

(PGMEE 2010)

a. Wedge vertebra
b. Fully segmented Hemivertebra
c. Block vertebra
d. Unilateral unsegmented bar with Hemivertebra

[Ref: Springer 1st/e p. 2008p. 701; Campbell 13th/e p. 2240]

Explanation

- The classification proposed by MacEwen et al. and later modified by Winter, Moe, and Eiler
- The most progressive of all anomalies is a concave, unilateral unsegmented bar with a convex hemivertebra. Next in severity of risk of progression is a double convex hemivertebra. A fully segmented hemivertebra will progress relatively slowly.

Classification of congenital Scoliosis

- Failure of formation
  - Partial failure of formation **(wedge vertebra)**
  - Complete failure of formation **(hemivertebra)**
- Failure of segmentation
  - Unilateral failure of segmentation (unilateral segmentation bar)
  - Bilateral failure of segmentation **(block vertebra)**
- Miscellaneous

29. X-ray lateral view Lumbar spine showing compression of two vertebrae. Diagnosis is:- *(PGMEE 2016-17)*

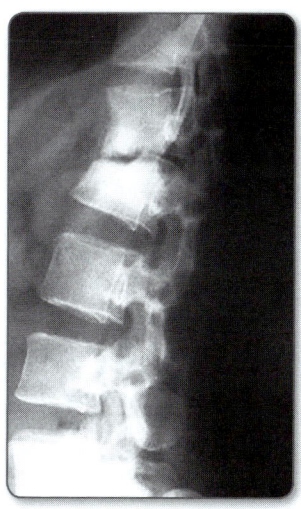

a. Spondylolisthesis
b. Spondylolysis
c. Potts spine
d. None of the above

[Ref: Maheshwari & Mhaskar 6th/e pg.284]

Explanation

- Disc is involved first in TB spine usually at slipping of vertebra.

28. c
29. c

ARTHROPLASTY

1. The father of joint replacement surgery is- *(PGMEE 13)*
   a. Manning
   b. Girdlestone
   c. Charnley
   d. Ponseti

[Ref: Internet]

2. Metal on Metal articulation should be avoided in-
(PGMEE 10)
   a. Osteonecrosis
   b. Young female
   c. Revision surgery
   d. Inflammatory arthritis

[Ref: Sauders 1st/e p.2009 p.121]

3. Most common cause of death after THR (Total Hip Replacement) is- *(PGMEE 09)*
   a. Infection
   b. Anemia
   c. Pneumonia
   d. Thromboembolism

[Ref: Campbell's 8th/e p. 548]

4. A patient developed breathlessness and chest pain, on second postoperative day after a total hip replacement. Echo-cardiography showed right ventricular dilatation and tricuspid regurgitation. What is the most likely diagnosis- *(AI 10)*
   a. Cardiac tamponate
   b. Pulmonary embolism
   c. Hypotensive shock
   d. Acute MI

[Ref: Campbell's 11th/e]

5. Watson Jones operation is done for? *(PGMEE 08)*
   a. Neglected Club foot
   b. Muscle paralysis
   c. Valgus deformity
   d. Hip replacement

[Ref: Apley's 8th/e p. 441 Turek 6th/e p. 523; http://en.wikipedia.org/wiki/Juvenile_rheumatoid_arthritis]

Explanation

- *Watson test* - scaphoid shift test.
- *Watson Jones surgery* is done far chronic lateral ankle instability.

6. Identify the pahology in the X-ray given-
(PGMEE 2015)

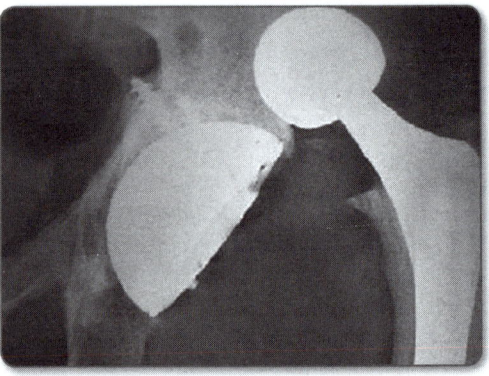

   a. Normal THR implant in situ
   b. Dislocated THR head from cup
   c. Normal bipolar hemiarthroplasty implant in situ
   d. Dislocated bipolar head

[Ref: Internet]

1. c
2. b
3. d
4. b
5. c
6. b

Anesthesia

CHAPTER 18

FACTS

- World Anesthesia Day is celebrated every year on 16th October (in memory of first successful demonstration of ether anesthesia by WTG Morton)
- Stages of Anesthesia were described by: Gudell
- Stage III of anesthesia → Surgical anesthesia
  - Plane 1 – Cessation of eye movement
- Oculocardiac reflex: bradycardia on manipulation of ocular muscles. Most common with medial rectus
- Allodynia → Perception of an ordinary non-noxious stimulus as pain.

Color Coding of IV Cannula	
Orange	14G
Grey	16G
Green	18G
Pink	20G
Blue	22G
Yellow	24G

Surface Landmark	
Nipple	T_4
Xiphisternum	T_6 (**Mn:** Si**X**)
*Inferior angle of scapula**	T_7
Umbilicus	T_{10}
Inguinal ligament	L_1
Highest point on iliac crest	L_{4-5} Interspace

*Mn: 7 letters in scapula

Airway Management

- Surest sign of tracheal intubation: End tidal CO_2 measured by Capnography
- In a capnographic waveform, the plateau phase corresponds to: Alveolar air
- In children – uncuffed ET tubes are used
- Placement of a double lumen tube for lung surgery is best confirmed by: fiber optic bronchoscopy
- Mode of mechanical ventilation cannot used for weaning off: IPPV/CMV

Airway assessment is done by:
- Mallampati scoring
- Thyromental distance
- Sternomental distance
- Neck circumference

Risk factors for difficult airway:
- Head and neck trauma
- Cervical spine disease or previous surgery
- Orofacial and neck deformity
- Obesity
- Obstructive Sleep Apnea
- Rheumatoid arthritis, Scleroderma

Laryngoscope:
- Curved blade: Macintosh → MC used
- Straight blade: Magill → used in neonates

Position for laryngoscopy/Intubation:
- Extension at Atlanto-occipital joint
- Flexion at Cervical spine

Clinical Evaluation & Monitoring

- Most accurate site for core temperature monitoring: Pulmonary artery
- Most accurate site for brain temperature monitoring: Tympanic membrane
- Bispectral index (BIS) → Measure intra-operative awareness
- Preferred artery for invasive BP monitoring: Radial artery
- Best nerve to monitor adequacy of anesthesia: Ulnar nerve
- Most sensitive indicator of myocardial ischemia in the perioperative period: Trans Esophageal Echo / TEE

- Depth of anesthesia is monitored by:
  - Bispectral Index (BIS) – MC used
  - EEG
  - Evoked potential

Perioperative ECG monitoring:
- Preferred lead for arrhythmia: Lead II
- Preferred lead for ischemia: V_5

Apnea monitoring:
- Intubated patient: Capnography
- Non intubated patient:
  - Impedance plethysmography
  - Transthoracic impedance pulmonometry

Pain assessment in children:
  - CHEOPS – Best
  - Visual Analogue Scale / Smiley scale – MC used

Inhalational Anesthesia (IA)

- *Meyer Overton rule* → Anesthetic property of inhalational anesthesia is ∞ lipid solubility (Oil gas partition coefficient).
- *Minimum Alveolar Concentration (MAC)* → estimates potency of inhalational anesthesia. Lower the MAC, higher the potency.
- *Blood gas partition coefficient* is an indicator of solubility of inhalational anesthesia in blood → determines the rapidity of induction and recovery
- Earliest induction and recovery: Xenon → lowest blood gas coefficient.
- Inhalational agent of choice (AOC) for pediatric induction: Sevoflurane
- AOC for induction among inhalational anesthetics: Sevoflurane
- Arrhythmia is side effect of: Halothane and Chloroform

Xenon:
- Inert, Non explosive, & Non Teratogenic
- Rapid induction and recovery
- No green house effect / Ozone depletion
- Does not trigger malignant hyperthermia
- Minimum cardiovascular side effects

HELIOX composition:
- 70% Helium + 30% O_2 OR
- 79% Helium + 21% O_2

Nitrous Oxide (N_2O) produces:
- Second gas effect / Concentration effect → during induction
- Diffusion hypoxia → during recovery

Epilepsy is a side effect of:
- Enflurane – Most epileptogenic
- Sevoflurane

Inhalational Agent	MAC	Blood Gas Coefficient	Comment
Halothane	0.75 %	2.4	▪ Most potent inhalational agent in use ▪ Slowest induction & recovery among IA in use
Isoflurane	1.15%	1.3	
Sevoflurane	2%	0.69	▪ Inhalational agent with smoothest induction
N_2O	104%	0.47	▪ Least potent inhalational agent
Desflurane	6%	0.42	▪ Earliest induction & recovery among IA in use
Xenon	71%	0.115	▪ IA with fastest induction and recovery
Methoxyflurane	Obsolete agent		▪ Most potent & most nephrotoxic inhalational agent

Factors Affecting MAC

Factors Decreasing MAC	Factors Increasing MAC	Neutral Factors
▪ Hypothermia ▪ Anemia ▪ Hyponatremia ▪ Hypercalcemia ▪ Hypotension ▪ Increasing age	▪ Hyperthermia (>42°C) ▪ Barometric pressure ▪ Hypernatremia	▪ Sex ▪ Obesity

Intravenous Anesthesia

- Total intravenous anesthesia (TIVA): Alfentanil + Propofol

Total Intravenous Anesthesia:
- MC used agent – Propofol
- Smooth induction & rapid recovery

- Post op nausea & vomiting – minimal
- Reduces cerebral metabolic rate & blood flow
- Safe in patients susceptible to malignant hyperthermia

Propofol Infusion Syndrome:
- Seen when Propofol infusion is > 4mg/kg/hr for > 48 hours
- Characterized by:
  - Bradycardia, Cardia failure
  - Metabolic acidosis
  - Rhabdomyolysis l/t hyperkalemia
  - Hyperlipidemia

Carbon Dioxide Absorbers

- MC used CO_2 absorbent: Soda lime
- Maximum volume of CO_2 that can be absorbed by 100g of soda lime: 23 L
- Trilene + Soda lime forms Dichloroacetylene → Neurotoxic compound
- **S**evoflurane + **S**oda lime forms compound A → Nephrotoxic compound
- Desiccated soda lime + Desflurane → Produce CO
- Desiccated soda lime + Sevoflurane → leads to heart failure
- Baralyme can absorb 9-18 L of CO_2 per 100 g

AMSORB: Aka Ca $(OH)_2$ lime
- New CO_2 absorber that does not produce compound A with Sevoflurane and CO with Desflurane
- Composition: $Ca(OH)_2 + CaCl_2 + CaSO_4$

Soda lime Composition:
- $Ca(OH)_2$ – 80%
- NaOH – 5%
- KOH – 1%
- Moisture – 15%
- Silica is added to make it hard
- Indicator – Ethyl violet

Baralyme Composition:
- $Ca(OH)_2$ = 80%
- $Ba(OH)_2$ = 20%
- It does not require silica for hardness
- Hardness is achieved by water of crystallization
- It is less efficient than soda lime

Trilene reacts with soda lime to produce:
- Dichloroacetylene – Neurotoxic compound
- Phosgene – can cause ARDS

Malignant Hyperthermia

- Observed during general anesthesia
- Due to abnormality of Ryanodine receptor (Ca^{+2} release channel)
- MC implicated drug: Succinylcholine > Halothane
- Most sensitive early sign: ↑ in Expiratory CO_2
- MCC of death → V. fib due to hyperkalemia

- Specific treatment → Dantrolene
- LA of choice in patient with history of malignant hyperthermia: Procaine
- LA not to be used: Lignocaine
- GA of choice: Thiopentone, Propofol
- Screening tool for susceptible patients: Creatinine kinase

Rapid Sequence Intubation

- Done to prevent gastric aspiration
- BMV/Mechanical ventilation is contraindicated

Steps:
- Preoxygenation for 3 minutes
- Induction with Ketamine/Thiopentone/ Propofol

- Neuromuscular blockage with Succinylcholine/ Rocuronium/Vecuronium
- ET tube intubation and cuff inflation
- Selick's manoeuvre (cricoid pressure) – controversial as it increases intubation time

Miscellaneous

- The anesthetic technique of choice to perform fast-track anesthesia: Infiltration anesthesia
- Dexmedetomidine is a centrally acting a_2 agonist that has sedative and anesthetic properties.
- MRI compatible gas cylinders are made up of: Aluminium
- Antiemetic of choice for preoperative period): Metoclopramide
- Drug useful in treatment of post-op shivering: Pethidine
- Dibucaine number is used to diagnose the presence of: Atypical pseudo cholinesterase
- Ideal gas for laparoscopy: Argon
- Most preferred gas for laparoscopy: CO_2 → easily absorbed in circulation.

- Venous air embolism is commonly seen in: Posterior Fossa surgery
- Mill wheel murmur is specific for: Air embolism
- Maximum partial pressure of O_2 in hyperbaric oxygen therapy: 2.8 atmosphere

Neurolept Anesthesia: Fentanyl + Droperidol + N_2O

Indications of premedication before anesthesia:
- Decrease anxiety – Most important
- Decrease secretions
- To provide perioperative amnesia
- Reduce post-op nausea & vomiting

Mendelson Syndrome:
- Is a chemical pneumonitis due to aspiration of gastric juices
- Critical pH to cause syndrome → < 2.5
- Critical volume to cause syndrome → > 25 mL

MEDICATIONS

Management of Drug Therapy in a Preoperative Patient			
Medications to be continued		**Medications to be stopped**	
Levodopa	▪ Discontinuation can precipitate muscle rigidity	*Diuretics*	▪ Day before surgery except thiazide diuretics
Oral Hypoglycemic Agents	▪ Minor surgery → continue omitting morning dose ▪ Major surgery → switch over to insulin therapy 48 hours prior to surgery	*Warfarin (Oral anticoagulants)*	▪ Stop 4-5 days before the procedure and switch over to LMW heparin which is to be stopped 12 – 24 hours before the surgery
Low dose Estrogen and Progesterone only pill		*Estrogen containing pills (OCP)*	▪ 4 weeks before the procedure to reduce the risk of thromboembolism
Aspirin	▪ To be continued if risk of bleeding is less	*Clopidogrel*	▪ 1 week before surgery
Anti-hypertensive/CCB / β-blockers	▪ To be continued and morning dose to be taken except ARB & ACEI where morning dose is to be omitted	*Ticlopidine*	▪ 2 weeks before surgery
		Lithium	▪ 2 – 3 days before surgery
Anti Tubercular	▪ LFT required	*Smoking*	▪ 8 weeks before surgery >> any time before surgery
Steroids	▪ Dose to be supplemented	*Herbal medication*	▪ 2 weeks before surgery
Asthma medications, Anti-depressants & Anti anxiety, Statins, Anticonvulsants & Thyroid medications		*MAO inhibitors*	▪ Stop 2 weeks before surgery

BREATHING SYSTEMS AND MEDICAL GAS CYLINDERS

- Maximum concentration of O_2 delivered by venturimask: 60 %
- Central supply of O_2 and N_2O is done at: 60 psi
- Pins are present on: Yoke of machine
- Diameter index safety system (DISS) is intended to prevent wrong fitting of central supply pipes to machine
- O_2 concentration in FGF is ensured by: Fail safe valve

- O_2 flush delivers O_2 at the rate of: 35-75 L /min

Central supply:
- Yellow pipeline → Central suction
- Black pipeline → Air
- Blue pipeline → N_2O
- White pipe/line → O_2

Composition of FGF (Free gas flow):
- Minimum O_2 – 33%
- 66% N_2O + 33% O_2 + Inhalation agent

Semi Closed/ Mapleson Circuit

Types	Comment
Type A *(Magill circuit)*	▪ Circuit of choice for spontaneous breathing patients ▪ Spontaneous ventilation: FGF = Minute Ventilation (MV) ▪ Controlled ventilation: FGF = >3 MV
Type D *(Coaxial System)*	▪ MC used semi closed circuit ▪ Bain's circuit (modification of type D) is circuit of choice for controlled ventilation
Type E *(Ayre's T – Piece)*	▪ Pediatric age group
Type F	▪ Jackson Ree's modified Type E ▪ Circuit of choice for spontaneously breathing infants & children

Cylinders	Pin Index	Filled As	Pressure	Color	Comments
O_2 Cylinders	2,5	Gas	2000 psi	Body – Black Shoulder – White	• MC used cylinders = Type E • Critical temperature of liquid O_2 = – 119°C
N_2O Cylinders	3,5	Liquid	745 psi	Blue	• Can be stored in liquid form without refrigerator • Critical temperature = 36.5°C
CO_2 Cylinders	2,6	Liquid	780 psi	Grey	
Cyclopropane	3,6	Liquid	75 psi	Orange	
Helium	2,4	Gas	2000 psi	Brown	
Air	1,5	Gas	2000 psi	Body – Grey/Black Shoulder – Black/White	
Entonox	7	Gas	2000 psi	Body – Blue Shoulder – White/Blue	• Combination gas of 50% O_2 + 50% N_2O

EFFECT OF INHALATIONAL AGENT ON SYSTEMS

System	Effect	Comment

Bronchial muscle	• All are bronchodilators	• Maximum bronchodilation in:
		  ○ Non asthmatics → Sevoflurane
		  ○ Asthmatics → Halothane

Muscular system	• Centrally acting muscle relaxant (Best – ether)	• Except N_2O (Not a relaxant)
Pulmonary vascular resistance	• All are pulmonary vasodilator	• Exception → N_2O (Pulmonary vasoconstriction)
Respiration	• All inhibit Respiration	
Cardiovascular System	• All inhibit CVS → lead to decrease CO & hypotension (Maximum - Halothane)	• Minimum ↓ in CO → Isoflurane • Deliberate hypotension → Isoflurane
Central Nervous System	• All ↓ cerebral metabolic rate & O_2 consumption • All ↑ ICT & Cerebral blood flow (CBF)	• Min. ↑ in ICT is by Isoflurane & Desflurane • Maximum ↑ in ICT is by Halothane
Liver	• All ↓ total blood flow to liver	• Maximum ↓ → Halothane (Max hepatotoxicity)
Renal	• Nephrotoxic due to fluoride production	• Desflurane does not produce fluoride → No nephrotoxicity
Uterus	• All acts as uterine relaxants	• Halothane is a potent relaxant
Analgesia	• Very poor	• Except N_2O (Good analgesic)
Metabolism	• All undergo oxidation	• Halothane → Oxidation + Reduction • N_2O → no metabolism • Xenon → not metabolized in our body • Minimum metabolism → Desflurane • Minimal Fluoride production → Desflurane

MOST COMMON

- MC complication after intubation: Sore throat
- MC cause of anesthesia related death in perioperative period: Postoperative respiratory depression
- MC respiratory complication in perioperative period: Atelectasis due to secretions
- MC drug implicated for malignant hyperthermia: Suxamethonium
- MC arrhythmia in perioperative period: Tachycardia
- MC postoperative complication: Nausea and vomiting

- MC nerve injury during anesthesia: Ulnar
- MC used approach for Brachial plexus block: Supraclavicular block
- MC complication after supraclavicular block: Phrenic nerve palsy
- MC complication of spinal anesthesia: Hypotension
- MC complication of celiac plexus block: Hypotension
- MC used drug for IV Regional Anesthesia (IVRA): Lidocaine

AGENT OF CHOICE

Agent of Choice	Inhalational	Intravenous
Electroconvulsive Therapy		▪ Methohexitone
Neurosurgery	▪ Sevoflurane > Isoflurane	▪ Propofol / Thiopentone Na
Shock / Hypotension	▪ Cyclopropane or Desflurane	▪ Ketamine ($\uparrow$BP) > Etomidate
Pediatric induction	▪ Sevoflurane f/b halothane	
Day care Surgery/Ambulatory anaesthesia	▪ Sevoflurane	▪ Propofol
$\uparrow$*risk of aspiration*		▪ Ketamine
Safest/remote location	▪ Ether	▪ Ketamine
Asthmatics	▪ Sevoflurane > Halothane	▪ Ketamine > Propofol
Cardiac patient	▪ Isoflurane (except MI $\rightarrow$ coronary steal phenomenon)	▪ Etomidate
Coronary artery disease / MI	▪ Desflurane	▪ Etomidate
Maximum analgesic	▪ Trielene/N_2O	▪ Ketamine
Obstetrics hemorrhage + flaccid uterus	▪ Isoflurane (best to maintain CO)	▪ Ketamine
Hyperthyroidism	▪ Isoflurane	▪ Thiopentone Na
Liver disorder	▪ Sevoflurane > Desflurane/Isoflurane	▪ Propofol
Renal failure, Elderly, Obese	▪ Desflurane	
Maximum nausea & vomiting	▪ Ether	
Cyanotic heart diseases		▪ Ketamine (to $\uparrow$PVR)
Malignant hyperthermia		▪ Propofol > Thiopentone

LOCAL AND REGIONAL ANESTHESIA

- 1st LA to be used clinically: Cocaine
- 1st synthetic LA: Procaine
- LA acts mainly by inhibiting: inactivated voltage gated Na+ channel
- Myelinated peripheral nerves belong to class A & B [**Mn**: MBA]
- Susceptibly of nerve fibers to local anesthesia: $B > A_\gamma > A_\delta > A_\alpha = A_\beta > C$
- Most sensitive nerve fiber to pressure: A
- Most sensitive nerve fiber to hypoxia: B
- *Sequence of blockade:* Autonomic $\rightarrow$ Sensory $\rightarrow$ Motor
- *Sequence of recovery:* Motor $\rightarrow$ Sensory $\rightarrow$ Autonomic
- Earliest sensation blocked by LA: Temperature
- Drug used to prolong action of LA in Hypertensive patient: Felypressin
- Maximum systemic absorption of LA is seen via Intercostal route
- DOC for Bier's block: Lignocaine > Prilocaine
- Needle used in Epidural anesthesia: Tuohy needle
- Gasserian ganglion blockade is done in: Trigeminal neuralgia

- Cervical plexus block is given in: Carotid endarterectomy
- The last muscle to be rendered akinetic with a retrobulbar anesthetic block: Superior oblique
- Incidence of pneumothorax is maximum with: Supraclavicular block
- In spinal anesthesia, LA is injected between the Pia & Arachnoid mater
- In epidural anesthesia, the LA is injected into the: Epidural / Extradural space
- Post neuraxial shivering: Epidural > Spinal anesthesia

Peripheral Nerve block	Nerve spared
Inter scalene approach	Ulnar nerve
Axillary approach	Musculocutaneous nerve Intercostobrachial nerve (T_2)

Use of epidural anesthesia/Extradural block:
- Postoperative analgesia
- Painless labor

Cranial nerve involvement in spinal anesthesia:
- MC : 6th CN
- Not involved: 1st , 9th, 10th

Structures pierced during spinal anesthesia:
- Skin & subcutaneous tissues
- Supraspinous ligament
- Interspinous ligament
- Ligamentum flavum
- Duramater & Arachnoid mater

LA with no topical action:
- Bupivacaine
- Procaine

Local Anesthetics (Amino esters):
- Shorter acting than amino amide
- Relatively unstable agents
- Metabolized by plasma cholinesterase except cocaine
- High incidence of allergic reaction

Signs of successful Stellate ganglion block:
- Conjunctival congestion → earliest sign
- Nasal stuffiness → Guttmann's sign
- TM Congestion → Muller sign
- Horner syndrome

Site of action of epidural analgesia
- Opioid – Substantia gelatinosa
- Local anesthetics – Nerve root

Post spinal Headache:
- Due to leakage of CSF through dural puncture site
- Seen only in sitting or standing position
- Experienced after 12-24 hours of LP
- Usually relieved in 7-10 days
- Treatment:
  - Supine position
  - Oral or IV fluids
  - Analgesics
  - Autologous blood patch

Management of spinal hypotension:
- **Prophylactic:** Preloading with 1-1.5 L of fluids
- **Curative**
  - Head low position (Trendelenburg)
  - Infusion of fluids
  - Vasopressors like Ephedrine, Mephentermine, Dopamine

Drugs	Properties	Uses	Side effects & Contraindications
Cocaine (Amino ester)	▪ Metabolized by liver ▪ Not metabolized by pseudo cholinesterase ▪ Potent vasoconstrictor		▪ Allergic reactions ▪ Abuse potential ▪ Mydriasis
Procaine (Amino ester)	▪ Metabolized by pseudo cholinesterase ▪ Least potent & short acting LA	▪ LA of choice in malignant hyperthermia	▪ Allergic reactions due to metabolite PABA
Lignocaine/ Lidocaine/ Xylocaine (Amino amide)	▪ Most commonly used LA ▪ Safe dose without Adrenaline → 4.5 mg/kg or 300 mg ▪ Safe dose with Adrenaline → 7 mg/kg or 500 mg	▪ Spinal anesthesia → 5% ▪ Topical anesthesia → 4% ▪ Nerve block → 1% ▪ Bier's block → 0.5% via IV ▪ Epidural → 2%	▪ Methemoglobinemia ▪ Neurotoxicity like Cauda Equina syndrome ▪ Contraindicated in patients with history of malignant hyperthermia
Prilocaine (Amino amide)	▪ Safest LA ▪ Metabolic by product – O toluidine	▪ Bier's block → IV regional anesthesia	▪ Methemoglobinemia – maximum
Bupivacaine (Amino amide) Long acting LA High potency LA	▪ Cannot be used topically ▪ Safe dose without adrenaline → 2.5 mg/kg or 175 mg ▪ Safe dose with adrenaline → 3 mg/kg or 200 mg	▪ Spinal anesthesia → 0.5% ▪ Painless labor → 0.1% ▪ Post operative analgesia → 0.1-0.25%	▪ Most cardiotoxic LA ▪ Can cause ventricular arrhythmia ▪ Max LA induced myotoxicity ▪ C/I in IV regional anesthesia
L – Bupivacaine (Amino amide)	▪ Less potent than Bupivacaine ▪ Potent vasoconstrictor		▪ Less cardiotoxic than bupivacaine
Ropivacaine (Amino amide) Long acting LA	▪ S enantiomer of Bupivacaine ▪ Less potent & shorter duration of action than bupivacaine	▪ LA of choice in labor analgesia	▪ Cardiotoxicity is lesser than L – Bupivacaine
Dibucaine	▪ Longest acting and most potent LA		
EMLA cream	▪ Mixture of 2.5% Lignocaine + 2.5% Prilocaine	▪ Split skin grafting ▪ Venipuncture	

INHALATIONAL ANESTHETIC AGENTS

	N_2O	Halothane	Desflurane	Isoflurane
Facts	• 1st prepared by Priestly • Stored as liquid at 745 psi • Cylinder color – Blue • $N_2O + O_2 \rightarrow$ form NO $\rightarrow$ destroy Ozone	• **Most potent IA in use**(MAC = 0.75) • Slowest indication & recovery among agents in use	• Isomer of Isoflurane • Required Tec-6 special vaporizer • Temperature of vaporizer camber is 39°C	• Inhalational AOC in Hyperthyroidism • Inhalational AOC in Cardiac patient except MI
Properties	• Least potent IA • Not metabolized in body • MAC – 104 % • Good Analgesic action • Non-irritating • Highly soluble • Given as a mixture of O_2 (33%) & N_2O (66%)	• To prevent decomposition by light, 0·01% Thymol is added as preservative • Max fat-gas coefficient $\rightarrow$ can get accumulated in obese patient • Can corrode plastic or metals in the presence of moisture • Only 20% is metabolized in body • Least fluorinated	• Lowest B:G coefficient $\rightarrow$ Fastest indication & recovery • MAC = 6% • Can produce CO with desiccated lime • Undergo minimum metabolism • Produces no/ minimum fluoride on metabolism	• Minimum ↑ in ICT
Systemic Features	• NMDA receptor antagonist • Non irritating $\rightarrow$ smooth induction • No muscle relaxant property • Pulmonary Vasoconstriction • ↑ cerebral metabolic rate	• Maximum bronchodilation in asthma • Hepatotoxicity – centrilobular necrosis • Undergo both oxidation & reduction • No analgesic action • Maximum decrease in cardiac output For known case of Halothane hepatitis, Inhalation AOC – Sevoflurane	• Inhalational AOC in ○ Renal failure ○ Old patient ○ Obese ○ Day care surgery ○ Shock/DIC ○ MI	• Max preservation of cardiac output/min ↓ in cardiac output • Inhalational AOC to produce deliberate hypotension
Side effects & contraindications	• High propensity to accumulate in cavities • Contraindicated in: ○ Pneumothorax ○ Pneumoperitoneum ○ Pneumocephalus ○ Air embolism ○ Emphysema ○ Tympanoplasty ○ Posterior Fossa surgery ○ Intestinal obstruction ○ Diaphragmatic hernia & volvulus ○ Micro Laryngeal Surgery ○ Bone marrow depression • Megaloblastic anemia, SACD	• Sensitizes the heart to Adrenaline $\rightarrow$ Can cause ventricular arrhythmias • Halothane hepatitis $\rightarrow$ Mechanism – immunogenic metabolite • Postoperative shivering $\rightarrow$ MC IA associated with postoperative shivering • C/I in pheochromocytoma • Bradycardia & ↓ cardiac output • Maximum ↑ in ICT • Avoid repeat administration at frequent interval (3 months) • Pre-existing CLD is not an absolute contraindications	• Highest vapour pressure • Not environmental safe $\rightarrow$ maximum potential for global warming	• Coronary steel phenomenon $\rightarrow$ hence not to be given in CAD • Least cardiotoxic

INTRAVENOUS ANESTHETIC AGENTS

	Thiopentone Sodium	Propofol	Ketamine

Facts	▪ First IV anesthetic agent
	▪ AOC for Neurosurgery / Head injury
	▪ Induction AOC in Hyperthyroid patient
	▪ Best site for injection – dorsum of hand
	▪ Smooth induction
		▪ IV AOC for day care surgery
		▪ Most preferred for laparoscopic surgery
		▪ Most preferred for LMA insertion
		▪ MC used agent for total IV anesthesia (TIVA)
			▪ IV AOC for shock patient
			▪ Safest agent
			▪ Agent of choice in:
			  ○ Status asthmaticus
			  ○ Cyanotic heart disease

Physical property	▪ Yellow amorphous powder
	▪ Preservative → $NAHCO_3$
	▪ pH = 10.5 i.e. highly alkaline
	▪ Used as 2.5% concentration
	▪ Injection are painful
	▪ Should not be reconstituted with RL
		▪ Contains egg lecithin & soya bean oil
		▪ Oil based ∴ Painful injection
		▪ Fospropofol → water soluble prodrug
		  ○ Injections are not painful
		  ○ Slower acting than Propofol
			▪ **Phencyclidine** derivatives
			▪ No pain on injection site
			▪ Maximum analgesic effect → decreases post op pain

MOA	▪ GABA mimetic ▪ Shows redistribution ∴ short acting with rapid recovery	▪ GABA mediated	▪ NMDA receptor antagonist ▪ Site of action: Thalamocortical projections
System effects	▪ Antithyroid agent ▪ Anticonvulsant action ▪ Cerebroprotective agent → ↓ ICT & metabolic rate of brain, ↓ Cerebral Blood Flow, O_2 consumption ▪ Anti-analgesic ∴ Painful procedure not to be done ▪ Hypotension ▪ Malignant hyperthermia ▪ ↓ Intraocular pressure ▪ Can produce rash due to hypersensitivity reaction ▪ Intra-arterial injection can cause vascular spasm leading to severe burning pain → Treatment: Lignocaine/Xylocaine	▪ Maximum inhibition of airway reflex ▪ Anticonvulsant action ▪ Cerebroprotective (↓ ICT) ▪ Antiemetic properties ▪ Anti pruritic properties ▪ Hypotension following induction ▪ Propofol as continuous infusion may lead to severe acidosis & death	▪ Pharyngeal & laryngeal reflex – Preserved ▪ ↑ ICT (cerebral vasodilatation) ▪ ↑ Cerebral O_2 consumption & metabolism ▪ ↑ Intra ocular tension ▪ ↑ Pharyngeal & respiratory secretion (salivation, lacrimation) → ↑ risk of aspiration ▪ Potent bronchodilator ▪ Dissociative anesthesia l/t vivid dreams, Hallucination and emergence delirium ▪ ↑ muscle tone ▪ ↑ **BP**, cardiac output & HR
Dose	▪ 5 mg/kg	▪ 2 mg/kg	▪ IM – 4–6 mg/kg; IV – 1–2 mg /kg
Side effects & Contraindications	**Contraindications:** ▪ Acute intermittent porphyria ▪ Status asthmaticus ▪ Shock	▪ Hyperlipidemia ▪ Pancreatitis secondary to hyperlipidemia ▪ Propofol infusion syndrome ▪ Contraindicated in Shock	▪ Head injuries as it ↑ ICT ▪ Ischemic Heart Diseases, Hypertension, Aortic aneurysm (↑Cardiac O_2 demand due to ↑ HR) ▪ Glaucoma & open eye surgery ▪ Schizophrenia
Extra edge	▪ Rapid onset of action due to high unionized fractions & lipid solubility ▪ Robin hood or Reverse steal phenomenon seen	▪ Bacterial contamination of reconstituted solution can occur can → cause life threatening infection	▪ Emergence reaction can be prevented by Benzodiazepines like Midazolam ▪ Should be avoided in hyperthyroid patients

OPIOID ANALGESICS

- Endogenous opioids acts through: Nociceptors
- Tolerance develop to all action of opioids expect: Constipation & Miosis
- Cause of death in morphine poisoning: Respiratory depression

Mechanism of action:

- μ_1 mediated – Analgesia Bradycardia, Miosis
- μ_2 mediated–Respiratory depression, Constipation

Systemic features:

- Miosis, Constipation, Truncal muscle rigidity
- Rigidity in thoracic muscle k/a wooden chest syndrome (Max – Alfentanil)
- $\uparrow$ ICT $\rightarrow$ Contraindicated in head injury
- $\uparrow$ Biliary duct pressure $\rightarrow$ C/I in biliary colic (Pethidine can be used)
- Pentazocine is C/I in MI (cause tachycardia & BP)
- Bradycardia except pethidine and pentazocine

Sufentanyl:

- Most potent opioid
- Laryngoscopy & intubation

Remifentanil:

- Shortest & rapid acting agent
- DOC in Day care surgery
- Metabolized by plasma esterase/pseudo cholinesterase
- Dose reduction is not required in hepatic or renal disease
- Opioid of choice in renal patient.

Midazolam:

- Shortest acting BZD
- Anxiolytic properties
- Causes anterograde amnesia
- Short half-life – useful in day care surgery

MUSCLE RELAXANTS

- Fading is characteristic of: Non Depolarizing Muscle relaxants (NDMR)
- Post tetanic facilitation is characteristic of: NDMR
- Train of four (T_4: T_1) in depolarizing MR – 1:1
- In train of four, time gap between two successive stimuli: **0.5 sec**
- In NDMR, T4 keeps decreasing
- Ideal muscle relaxant for intubation: Suxamethonium
- Muscle relaxant restricted to rapid sequence or difficult airways management: Suxamethonium
- Most resistant muscle to non depolarizing block is: Diaphragm
- *Clinical tests to access recovery from the effect of muscle relaxant:*
  - ○ Able to hold tongue depressor between central incisor
  - ○ Head lift for > 5 seconds
- Test for guaranteed recovery from the effect of muscle relaxant: Train of four > 0.9

Neuromuscular monitoring:

- Ideal muscle for Neuromuscular monitoring: Orbicularis oculi
- Preferred muscle: Adductor pollicis – supplied by Ulnar nerve

Phase II block (dual block):

- Seen after over dosage of Succinylcholine
- Fluorinated anesthesia agents may potentiate & even precipitate phase II block.
- Fading on train of four is diagnostic

REMEMBER

Drugs metabolized by Pseudo cholinesterase: [Mn: PSM Rat LE]	Local Anesthetics causing methemoglobinemia: [Mn: BPL]
• Succinylcholine • Mivacurium • Remifentanil • LA (Esters) except cocaine	• Benzocaine • Prilocaine – Maximum • Lignocaine
Local Anesthetics which can cause vasoconstriction: [Mn: RBC]	**EEG findings in anesthesia: [Mn: Light Bulb]**
• Ropivacaine • L-Bupivacaine • Cocaine	• β waves: Light anesthesia • θ and δ waves: Deep anesthesia

Drugs	Properties	Uses	Adverse effects & Contraindications
D – Tubocurarine	▪ Maximum tendency to release histamine		▪ Hypotension
Gallamine	▪ Only agent to cross the placenta		
Pancuronium	▪ Stimulate sympathetic system ▪ Increases BP ▪ Bronchodilator	▪ AOC in arterial surgery or hypotensive patient ▪ AOC in asthmatics	▪ Tachycardia ▪ Contraindicated in cardiac patient
Vecuronium	▪ Most cardiostable	▪ Preferred agent in shock	
Atracurium	▪ Releases histamine ▪ Metabolized by Hoffman's elimination (non-enzymatic degradation) ▪ Metabolism produces Laudanosine which can cross BBB & can produce seizure ▪ Do not require reversal	▪ Relaxant of choice in: ○ Renal failure ○ Hepatic failure ○ Neonates ○ When reversal is contraindicated	▪ To be avoided in patient with history of seizure ▪ Laudanosine decreases the MAC of Halothane
Cisatracurium	▪ More potent than atracurium ▪ No release of histamine ▪ Less production of Laudanosine		
Rocuronium	▪ Fastest onset of action ▪ AOC in day care surgery	▪ Preferred agent for rapid sequence induction	▪ Injections are painful
Mivacurium	▪ Short acting NDMR ▪ Metabolized by pseudocholinesterase	▪ Muscle relaxant of choice for day care surgery	▪ Hypotension ▪ Bronchoconstriction
Gantacurium	▪ Ultra short (Shortest) acting NDMR		

MISCELLANEOUS AGENTS

	Etomidate	Ether	Suxamethonium/Succinylcholine
General features	▪ Most cardiostable inducing agent ▪ IV AOC for cardiac & vascular surgery	▪ Stored in dark bottles ▪ Induction is very unpleasant ▪ Slow induction and recovery	▪ Ideal muscle relaxant for intubation ▪ Shortest acting skeletal muscle relaxant ▪ Rapid hydrolysis by plasma pseudo cholinesterase
Property	▪ MOA: GABA mediated	▪ Highly inflammable and explosive ▪ Pungent smelling, irritating vapour ▪ Induction is very unpleasant	▪ Depolarizing muscle relaxant ▪ Use is restricted to rapid sequence induction ▪ Fastest onset of action
Systemic effects	▪ Hemodynamic stability ▪ Adrenal suppression ▪ ↓ Intracranial pressure	▪ Do not sensitise the heart to Adrenaline → Maintenance of HR and BP ▪ Very good analgesic	▪ Bradycardia → due to muscarinic action ▪ Hyperkalemia → due to muscle fasciculation ▪ May cause ventricular arrhythmia due to hyperkalemia
Extra points	▪ Most epileptogenic IV agent ▪ Highest incidence of post op nausea & vomiting ▪ Painful injection ▪ Associated with myoclonus ▪ Can be used to treat endogenous hypercortisolemia	**Advantages** ▪ Complete anesthetic agent ▪ Safest & Best muscle relaxant ▪ Most near to ideal ▪ Cheapest ▪ Best for remote locations **Disadvantages** ▪ Irritating ▪ Inflammable and explosive ▪ Maximum incidence of N/V ▪ Laryngospasm	▪ Muscle pain in postoperative period ▪ MC implicated drug in malignant hyperthermia **Contraindications:** ▪ Hyperkalemia ▪ Head injury ▪ Glaucoma ▪ Renal failure ▪ Advance liver failure ▪ Duchenne Muscular Dystrophy ▪ 2–3 months post trauma ▪ Up to 6 months after hemiplegia/paraplegia ▪ Up to 1 years after burn

PRIMES ⓞ (VOLUME II)

MULTIPLE CHOICE QUESTIONS

CHAPTER 1: ANESTHETIC EQUIPMENT

ANESTHESIA DELIVERY SYSTEMS

1. Machine shown below is:- **(PGMEE 2016-17)**

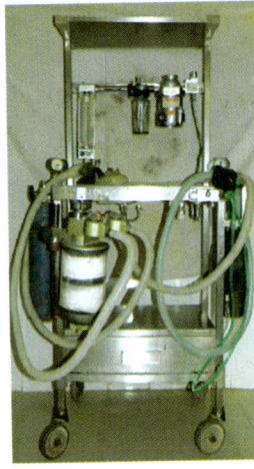

a. Ventilator
b. Boyle's anaesthesia machine
c. Simulator
d. Modern Anaesthesia work station

[Ref: Ajay Yadav's short text book of Anaesthesia 6th/e pg. 15]

2. Which of the following statements about Anesthetic Machine is true: **(PGMEE 2012)**

a. Flow-meters (Rotameters] are Interchangeable
b. Oxygen sensors are placed on the expiratory limb of the anesthesia circuit
c. Temperature of Desflurane Vaporizer Chamber is 39°C
d. All of the above

[Ref: Clinical Anesthesia by Stoelting 6th (Lippincott Williams] p. 698]

3. Which can replace N_2O as O_2 carrier – **(PGMEE 2012)**

a. Argon
b. Helium
c. Xenon
d. None

[Ref: Morgan's 5th/e p.173]

4. During anaesthesia what concentration should be of O_2 delivery- **(PGMEE 2014)**

a. 21%
b. 33%
c. 51%
d. 75%

[Ref: Ajay Yadav's 5th/e pg. 29; Morgan 6th/e]

5. Sodalime is used to absorb CO_2 in – **(PGMEE 2014)**

a. Closed circuit
b. Magilll's circuit
c. Jackson system
d. Bain's circuit

[Ref: Ajay Yadav's 6th/e pg. 27; Morgan 6th/e pg. 41]

6. For high pressure storage of compressed gases cylinders are made up of – **(PGMEE 2014)**

a. Iron + Mo
b. Cast iron
c. Steel + Cu
d. Molybdenum steel

[Ref: Ajay Yadav's 6th/e pg. 15]

7. Color of oxygen cylinder is: **(DNB Dec' 2010)**

a. Black with white color
b. Yellow with white color
c. Blue with white color
d. White

[Ref: Ajay Yadav's 6th/e pg. 15]

8. Ratio of O_2: N_2O in Entonox is – **(PGMEE 2012)**

a. 25 : 75
b. 40: 60
c. 50: 50
d. 60: 40

[Ref: Ajay Yadav's 6th/e pg. 17]

9. What is the pressure at which oxygen is stored? **(PGMEE 2015)**

a. 75 psi
b. 760 psi
c. 1600 psi
d. 2200 psi

[Ref: Ajay Yadav's 6th/e pg. 15]

10. As per ISO, color of N_2O cylinder is – **(PGMEE 2014)**

a. Red
b. Blue
c. White
d. Black

[Ref: Ajay Yadav's 6th/e pg. 17]

11. DISS is used for – **(PGMEE 2015)**

a. To monitor BP
b. To provide analgesia
c. To monitor CVP
d. Correct application of cylinder to anaesthesia machine

[Ref: Ajay Yadav's 6th/e pg. 19]

Explanation

- Like pin index system which prevent wrong fitting of cylinders to machine *Diameter index safety system (DISS)* prevent wrong fitting of central supply pipes to machine.
- As the name suggests the diameter of oxygen, nitrous oxide, air and suction pipes are different so that couplers of oxygen, nitrous oxide, air and suction can only receive their pipes.

PIN INDEX

12. Gas cylinder with single pin index – **(PGMEE 2015)**

a. Nitrogen
b. Air
c. Entonox
d. Oxygen

[Ref: Ajay Yadav's 6th/e pg. 18]

1.	b
2.	c
3.	c
4.	b
5.	a
6.	d
7.	a
8.	c
9.	d
10.	b
11.	d
12.	c

13. Pin index of N2O is – *(PGMEE 2012)*
a. 1,6
b. 2,5
c. 2,6
d. 3,5

[Ref: Ajay Yadav's 6th/e pg. 18]

14. Safety pin index for oxygen cylinder is – *(PGMEE 2013)*
a. 1,5   b. 1,4
c. 2,5   d. 3,5

[Ref: Ajay Yadav's 6th/e pg. 18]

15. Pin index for Air is – *(PGMEE 2014)*
a. 1,4
b. 1,5
c. 2,5
d. 3,5

[Ref: Ajay Yadav's 6th/e pg. 18]

BREATHING CIRCUITS

16. The most appropriate circuit for ventilating a spontaneously breathing infant – *(PGMEE 2012)*
a. Mapleson C or water's to & fro canister
b. Bain's circuit
c. Mapleson A or Magill's circuit
d. Jackson Rees modification of Ayre's T peiece

[Ref: Ajay Yadav's 6th/e pg. 26]

17. In Magill circuit airflow required for spontaneous breathing is – *(PGMEE 2014)*
a. Equal to minute ventilation (MV)
b. Half of minute ventilation (½ MV)
c. Twice the minute ventilation (2 x MV)
d. Thrice of minute ventilation (3 x MV)

[Ref: Ajay Yadav's 6th/e pg. 26; Morgan 6th/e pg. 37]

Explanation

- In Magill's circuit required fresh gas flow
  - For spontaneous breathing = Equals to minute ventilation ($\approx$80 ml/kg/min)
  - For controlled ventilation = Very high (unpredictable)
- *Fresh gas flow in various semiclosed circuits:-*

Also k/as	Fresh gas flow	
	In spontaneous breathing	**In controlled ventilation**
Type A (Magill's circuit)	= MV	3 x MV (Very high flow)
Type B	2 x MV	2.25 x MV
Type C (Water's to and Fro circuit)	2 x MV	2.25 x MV
Type D (Bain's co-axial system)	2.5 x MV	1.6 x MV (70-100 ml/kg)
Type E (Ayre's T piece)	2.5 x MV	3 x MV
Type F (Jackson Ree's)	2.5 x MV	1.5-2 x MV

18. Ayre's T-piece is which type of circuit – *(PGMEE 2012)*
a. Type A
b. Type B
c. Type D
d. Type E

[Ref: Ajay Yadav's 6th/e pg. 26; Morgan 6th/e pg. 37]

19. Mapelson circuit used in children is? *(DNB June' 2010)*
a. Mapelson A
b. Mapelson D
c. Mapelson C
d. Ayers T tube

[Ref: Ajay Yadav's 6th/e pg. 26]

13. d
14. c
15. b
16. d
17. a
18. d
19. d

Breathing Circuits

Type	Also k/as	Best suited for	Feature/Advantage
A	Magill's circuit	Spontaneous ventilation	Fresh gas flow required to prevent rebreathing is equal to alveolar minute volume (MV =70 ml/kg/min) of patient. C/b used for both spont. + controlled ventilation. **LACK's system** is modification of 'A' with co-axial circuit (tube inside tube)
B	–		Obselete
C	Water's to and Fro		Obselete
D	Bain's co-axial system	Controlled ventilation	Inspiratory limb is inside the expiratory limb, Fresh gas flow required to prevent rebreathing is 1.6 MV
E	Ayre's T piece	Controlled ventilation in Neonates	Inlet is near the face mask/ETT, used for weaning, does NOT have bag and valve.
F	Jackson Ree's	Spontaneous ventilation in Pediatric patient	Modification of Ayer's T-piece /E used in children <6 yr or <20 kg

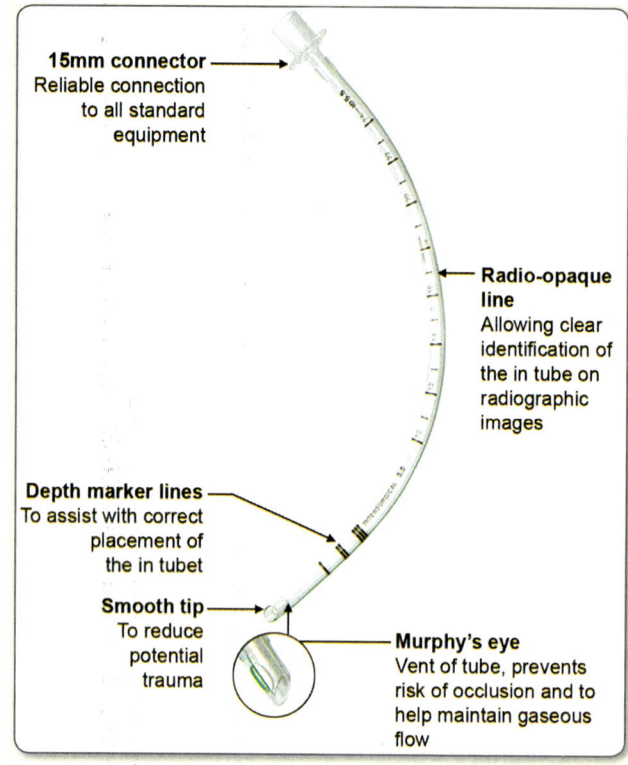

15mm connector
Reliable connection to all standard equipment

Radio-opaque line
Allowing clear identification of the in tube on radiographic images

Depth marker lines
To assist with correct placement of the in tubet

Smooth tip
To reduce potential trauma

Murphy's eye
Vent of tube, prevents risk of occlusion and to help maintain gaseous flow

O_2 DELIVERY DEVICES

37. Which of the following is low flow Oxygen delivery device– *(PGMEE 2014)*
a. Venti-mask
b. Aerosol system
c. Bag & mask ventilation
d. Nasal cannula

[Ref: Morgan 6th/e pg. 1331]

38. In hyperbaric oxygenation the maximum allowed pressure of O_2 is: *(PGMEE 2014)*
a. 1 atm
b. 3 atm
c. 5 atm
d. 9 atm

[Ref: Ganong's physiology 25th/e p. 652]

39. Maximum O_2 concentration attained in venturi mask is?
a. 60%
b. 80% *(DNB June' 2009)*
c. 90%
d. 100%

[Ref: Ajay Yadav's 5th/e pg. 50]

40. Fixed oxygen delivery device is? *(DNB June' 2010)*
a. Simple face nask
b. Nasal cannula
c. Venturi mask
d. Nasal mask

[Ref: Ajay Yadav's 6th/e pg. 42; Morgan 6th/e pg. 1333]

Explanation

- High flow system (fixed performance delivery systems) includes:-
  - Venturi mask:- Most commonly used
  - Special nebulizers
  - High airflow blenders.

41. Hyperbaric oxygen is not useful in – *(PGMEE 2015)*
a. Gas gangrene
b. Compartment Syndrome
c. Vertigo
d. CO poisoning

[Ref: Morgan 6th/e pg. 1335]

37.	d
38.	b
39.	a
40.	c
41.	c
42.	c
43.	d

Explanation

- Hyperbaric oxygen means delivering the O_2 above atmospheric pressure {>760 mm Hg or >1 atm}
- Indications of hyperbaric oxygen are:-
  - Carbon monoxide poisoning
  - Gas bubble diseases:- Decompression sickness/ Caisson's disease, Air embolism
  - Ischemia: Crush syndrome, Radiation necrosis, ischemic ulcers
  - Infections: Clostridial myonecrosis, Mucormycosis, Refractory osteomyelitis.
  - Burns, Cerebral edema.

42. Oxygen is not useful in the following condition: *(PGMEE 2018)*
a. Asthma
b. Subglottic stenosis
c. Depressed respiratory center
d. Pneumonia

[Ref: Morgan 6th/e pg. 1330]

Explanation

- COPD is the disease having respiratory depression leading to hypoventilation and CO_2 retention (hypercarbia). In these patients pulmonary vasoconstriction is the most effective way of altering V/Q ratio to improve gaseous exchange. This mechanism is counteracted by O2 therapy and accounts for largest increase in O_2 induced hypercapnea.

Role of 100% Oxygen

- **Administration of 100% O_2** ↑es the O_2 content of alveolar air and *improves the hypoxia d/ to fibrosis, hypoventilation, impaired diffusion or V/Q mismatch* by ↑ing the amount of O2 leaving the lungs.
- 100% O_2 is NOT effective in tetrology of Fallot.
- Among hypoxia O2 therapy is:-
  - Most useful in → hypoxic hypoxia
  - Limited value in → anemic hypoxia
  - Not useful in → histotoxic hypoxia as tissue enzymes can't extract O2.

43. Maximum oxygen concentration can be delivered by: *(NEET Pattern 2017)*
a. Venturi mask
b. Nasal cannula
c. Face mask
d. Face mask with reservoir

[Ref: Morgan 6th/e pg. 1332]

Explanation

- Venturi mask is variable flow fixed performance oxygen delivery system that can deliver FiO2 of 60%. It has colour codes indicating FiO2 it can deliver.

Oxygen delivery systems

- Non fixed performance device
  - *Nasal cannula-* O_2 concn up to 44%
  - *Simple face Mask-* O_2 concn up to 60%.
  - *O_2 by Mask with resrvior-* O_2 concn up to 95-100%.
- Fixed performance device
  - *O_2 by Venturi mask:* O_2 concn up to 28-60%. Based on Bernoulli's theorem. Used in patients with COPD.

PREOPERATIVE ASSESSMENT

1. For anesthesiology mild systemic disease included in ASA grade- *(PGMEE 2015)*
- a. 1
- b. 2
- c. 3
- d. 4

[Ref: Morgan 6th/e pg. 297]

2. Warfarin to be stopped _____ days before surgery- *(PGMEE 2015)*
- a. 2 to 3 days
- b. 4 to 5 days
- c. 6 to 7 days
- d. 8 to 9 days

[Ref: Morgan 6th/e pg. 299]

3. Heavy smoker for elective hernia repair, smoking should be stopped before how much period: *(PGMEE 2014)*
- a. 4 days
- b. 3-4 weeks
- c. 6-8 weeks
- d. 10 days

[Ref: Morgan's 5th/e pg. 536]

4. Preoperative fasting guidelines for solid food: *(Recent Pattern June 2018)*
- a. 10 hr
- b. 4 hr
- c. 6 hr
- d. Overnight

[Ref: Morgan's 5th/e pg.]

Explanation

Last meal time before anaesthesia (Fasting guidelines):

- Fasting guidelines recommend stoppage of
  - Clear fluid → 2 hrs before Sx.
  - Breast milk → 4 hrs before Sx.
  - Top milk/solid food → 6 hrs before Sx.
- Glucose water should be given 2 hrs prior to Sx to reduce gastric volume

5. All are features of difficult airway except:
- a. TMJ ankylosis *(PGMEE 2012; DNB Dec' 2011)*
- b. Micrognathia with macroglossia
- c. Increased thyromental distance
- d. Miller's sign

[Ref: Morgan's 5th/e p. 313]

Explanation

Difficult Airway characteristics

- Mallampati class 3&4
- Cormack and Lehane 3 &4
- Mouth opening< 3cm
- Thyromental distance <6.0 cm
- Head and neck movement restricted
- Severly receding mandible (micrognathia)
- Restricted jaw movement or restricted TMJ movement
- Miller's sign
- Oral growth

6. Mallampatti classification is used for? *(DNB Dec' 2009)*
- a. Inspection of oral cavity before intubation
- b. Size of the ET tube
- c. Size of the airway
- d. Tracheostomy tube

[Ref: Morgan 6th/e pg. 311]

Explanation

- Mallampatti classification is used for assessing the relationship of the tounge size relative to the oral cavity.
- *There are 2 important Airway Classification Systems:*

Class	Direct Visualisation (Mallampatti classification)	Laryngoscopic view (Cormack Lehane Score))
1	Soft palate, Fauces, uvula, pillars	Entire glottic opening
2	Soft palate, Fauces, uvula	Posterior commissure
3	Soft palate and base of uvula	Tip of epiglottis
4	Hard palate only	No glottic structure

- MPG zero "0" means epiglottis is seen. Ability to see any part of the epiglottis upon mouth opening and tongue protrusion.
- *Test:* The assessment is performed with the patient sitting up straight, mouth open and tongue maximally protruded, without speaking or saying "ahh."

7. Mallampatti score assist in? *(PGMEE 2018)*
- a. Assertion of induction
- b. Assessment of difficult airway during endotracheal intubation
- c. To provide assisted ventilation
- d. For socio economic status

[Ref: Morgan 6th/e pg. 311]

8. A Patient is on regular medications for co-existing medical problems. Which of the following drugs may be stopped safely with minimal risk of adverse effects before an abdominal surgery: *(PGMEE 2012)*
- a. ACE inhibitors/ACE Receptor Blockers
- b. Statins
- c. Both A and B
- d. Beta Blockers *[Ref: Morgan 6th/e pg. 389]*

9. Premedication in anaesthesia is given for:
- a. Relieving the anxiety *(PGMEE 2013)*
- b. Decreasing the dose of anaesthetic drugs
- c. Decreasing post-operative complications
- d. All of the above

[Ref: Morgan 6th/e pg. 301; KDT 7th/e p. 386]

10. Most potent antiemetic agent used in preoperative period: *(PGMEE 2014)*
- a. Hyoscine
- b. Metochlopramide
- c. Atropine
- d. Ondansetrone

[Ref: Morgan 6th/e pg. 284]

MONITORING IN ANAESTHESIA

11. Individual intraoperative awareness or depth of anaesthesia is evaluated by: *(PGMEE 2012)*
- a. Pulse oximetry
- b. End tidal CO_2
- c. Bispectral imaging
- d. Colour Doppler

[Ref: Morgan 6th/e pg. 126]

1.	b
2.	b
3.	c
4.	d
5.	c
6.	a
7.	b
8.	c
9.	d
10.	d
11.	c

12. Depth of anaesthesia is accessed by– **(NEET Jan' 2019)**
a. BIS
b. Trans thoracic echo
c. Esophageal contractility
d. Depressed responses

[Ref: Morgan 6th/e pg. 126]

13. Most sensitive non invasive monitoring of cardio-vascular ischemia in perioperative period is done by- **(PGMEE 2015)**

a. Pulse oximeter
b. EEG
c. TEE
d. NIBP

[Ref: Morgan's 5th/e p. 116]

14. Most reliable indicator to prevent oesophageal intuba-tion- **(PGMEE 2012)**
a. Direct visualization of passing tube beneath vocal cords
b. Oxygen saturation on pulse oximeter
c. Measurement of CO_2 in exhaled air ($EtCO_2$)
d. Auscultation over chest

[Ref: Morgan 6th/e pg. 122]

15. Standard method to differentiate between endotracheal and esophageal intubation is- **(PGMEE 2015)**
a. Partial pressure of O_2
b. Chest X-rays
c. End tidal CO_2
d. Auscultation

[Ref: Morgan 6th/e pg. 122]

16. Capnography basically monitors- **(PGMEE 2012)**
a. Concentration of inhaled O_2
b. Blood pressure during anesthesia
c. Concentration of exhaled CO_2
d. Central venous pressure

[Ref: Morgan 6th/e pg. 122]

17. Capnography is used for assessment of- **(PGMEE 2013)**
a. Ventilation of lung after intubation
b. Amount of CO_2 transported in blood
c. Myocardial perfusion
d. Oxygen saturation of blood

[Ref: Morgan 6th/e pg. 122]

18. In which of the following condition, flat capnogram is NOT seen: **(Recent Pattern June 2018)**
a. Apnea
b. Complete laryngospasm
c. Foreign body obstructing the upper airway
d. None of the above

[Ref: Morgan's 5th/e pg. 127]

12.	a
13.	c
14.	c
15.	c
16.	c
17.	a
18.	d
19.	d
20.	d
21.	c
22.	a

Explanation

- Capnography is a valuable monitor of the pulmonary, cardiovascular, and anesthetic breathing systems.
- Capnographs rely on the absorption of infrared light by CO_2.
- A value commonly reported on the capnography device is the end-tidal CO_2 (the maximum CO_2 concentration at the end of each tidal breath, or $ETCO_2$).
- *Flat capnograph (Flat or straight line capnogram) is seen in*
  - Apnea
  - Upper airway obstruction/ laryngeal spasm
  - Intra operative displacement of ETT
  - Disconnection of ETT /Ventilation failure,
  - Cardiac arrest
  - Esophageal intubation.

- *Progressive zeroing in $EtCO_2$ is seen in—* Esophageal intubation
- *Sudden drop (up to 0) in $EtCO_2$ is seen in—* Pulmonary venous air embolism
- *Sudden rise in $EtCO_2$ is seen in*
  - Malignant hyperthermia (up to 100 mm Hg).
  - Rise in $ETCO_2$ Pneumoperitoneum
  - Exhausted soda lime or defective valves of closed circuit.
- *Up sloping of capnograph is seen in*
  - Bronchospasm & resistance to airflow. Plateau prolonged

19. Most common cause for end tidal CO_2 falls due to – **(PGMEE 2014)**

a. Hypothermia
b. Cardiac arrest
c. Hyperthermia
d. Extubation

[Ref: Morgan 6th/e pg. 122]

20. Modern monitors to measure $ETCO_2$ make use of –
a. Ultra violet rays **(PGMEE 2015)**
b. Scatter technology
c. Laser technology
d. Infrared absorption spectroscopy

[Ref: Morgan 6th/e pg. 122]

21. Early and reliable indication of air embolism during anaesthesia can be obtained by continuous monitoring of: **(DNB 2008)**
a. Oxygen saturation
b. ECG
c. End Tidal CO_2
d. Blood pressure

[Ref: Morgan 6th/e pg. 122]

22. Neuromuscular monitoring is done by:- **(PGMEE 2018)**
a. Ulnar nerve
b. Median nerve
c. Facial nerve
d. Musculocutaneous nerve

[Ref: Morgan 6th/e pg. 134]

Explanation

Neuromuscular monitoring

- Ulnar nerve is m/c used for neuromuscular monitoring in the perioperative period.
  - **Adductor pollicis** muscle has been promoted as the most useful clinical tool and is the gold standard because of its accessibility for visual, tactile and mechanographic assessment.
  - The monitoring of **First dorsal interosseous** is preferable while using EMG.
- Other nerves which can be used for neuromuscular monitoring in the perioperative period.
  - **Facial nerve** - Orbicularis occuli
  - **Posterior tibial** - Flexor hallucis brevis.
  - **Peroneal nerve**
- The most satisfactory method for reliably monitoring neuromuscular function is the stimulation of an appropriate nerve using a peripheral nerve stimulator and observation of evoked response in the muscle supplied.
- *Train of four (TOF) ratio* has proved useful in assessing neuromuscular block in patients who exhibit prolonged response to depolarizing relaxant to diagnose and follow a dual or phase II block

1. Mechanism of action of curare is: *(PGMEE 2013)*
a. Inhibits K+ channels
b. Reducing presynaptic potential
c. Inhibits Na+ channels
d. Reducing end plate potential

[Ref: KDT's 8th/e pg. 374]

2. Mechanism of action of d- tubocurane: *(PGMEE 2018)*
a. Persistently depolarizing at Neuromuscular junction
b. Depolarizing blockade
c. Act competitively on Ach receptors blocking post-synaptically
d. Inhibit opening of chloride channels

Ref: KDT's 8th/e pg. 374]

Explanation

- D-tubocurane (d-TC) is a long acting potent non-depolarizing NMBA (neuromuscular-blocking agent).
- It competes with acetylcholine (Ach) for binding to post synaptic nicotinic receptor sites at N-M junction.
- It causes maximum release of histamine and has ganglionic blockade.
- Blockade is competitive and is reversible.

REMEMBER

- **Candocuronium** has a shorter duration and a rapid onset of action, with little or no ganglion blocking activity. It is only slightly less potent than pancuronium

3. For non depolarization block which of the following statement is correct – *(PGMEE 2014)*
a. Anticholinergic drugs potentiation of block
b. Tetanic fade is absent
c. Train of four is absent
d. Post tetanic potentiation is seen

[Ref: Morgan 5th/e p. 205]

NONDEPOLARIZING BLOCKERS

4. Site of action of vecuronium is- *(PGMEE 2014)*
a. Reticular formation   b. Myoneural junction
c. Cerebrum   d. Motor neuron

[Ref: Morgan 6th/e pg. 203]

5. Shortest acting non depolarizing muscle relaxant- *(PGMEE 2013)*
a. Vecuronium   b. Succinyl choline
c. Atracurium   d. Mivacurium

[Ref: Morgan 6th/e pg. 203]

6. Which of the following muscle relaxant has the maximum duration of action: *(PGMEE 2013)*
a. Atracurium
b. Doxacurium
c. Vecuronium
d. Rocuronium

[Ref: Morgan 6th/e pg. 212]

7. Maximum duration of action is seen with- *(PGMEE 2014)*
a. Pancuronium   b. Rocuronium
c. Rapacurium   d. Atracurium

[Ref: Goodman & Gilman 11th/e p. 222, Morgan 6th/e pg. 212]

8. Muscle relaxant contraindicated in Renal failure is- *(PGMEE 2014)*
a. Vecuronium   b. d-TC
c. Atracurium   d. Gallamine

[Ref: Lee 13th/e p. 184, Morgan 5th/e pg. 219]

Explanation

- Gallamine is excreted almost entirely by the kidneys and should be avoided in patients with renal impairment.

9. Which of the following skeletal muscle relaxants undergo Hoffman's elimination?
a. Succinylcholine   *(PGMEE 2012; 2011, 2019)*
b. Vecuronium
c. Atracurium
d. Mivacurium

[Ref: Morgan 6th/e pg. 215]

10. Which drug can be eliminated by nonenzymatic degradation – *(PGMEE 2013)*
a. Mivacurium
b. Pancuronium
c. Doxacurium
d. Atracurium

[Ref: Morgan 6th/e pg. 214]

11. Advantage of cisatracurium over atracurium is – *(NEET pattern Jan' 2019)*
a. Short duration of action
b. Rapid onset
c. Less hypersensitivity reaction
d. Release less histamine

[Ref: Morgan 6th/e pg. 214]

12. Muscle relaxant used in renal failure – *(PGMEE 2012)*
a. Ketamine   b. Fentanyl
c. Atracurium   d. Pancuronium

[Ref: Lee 13th/e p. 191; Morgan 6th/e pg. 2]

1.	d
2.	c
3.	d
4.	b
5.	d
6.	b
7.	a
8.	d
9.	c
10.	d
11.	d
12.	c

13. Which of the following can be given in hepatic as well as in renal failure – *(PGMEE 2013, DNB Dec' 2011)*

a. Pancuronium   b. Cis-atracurium
c. Vecuronium   d. Mivacurium

[Ref: Lee 13th/e p. 191, Morgan 6th/e pg. 214]

Explanation

- Enzymatic hydrolysis by plasma cholinesterase is the primary mechanism for inactivation of mivacurium
- Rocuronium is 30% protein bound in the plasma. No metabolites have been detected in plasma or urine. Excreted primarily by hepatic uptake and hepatobiliary excretion. The pharmacokinetics are not significantly altered in renal failure.
- Pancuronium has a mild vagal blocking effect on the heart and an inhibition of the re-uptake of noradrenaline by the cardiac sympathetic nerves. These result in a rise in pulse rate of about 20% and an increase in the blood pressure of 10-20%.
- Atracurium is broken down to inactive metabolites by ester hydrolysis and spontaneous Hoffman degradation. There is little change in its effects in patients with renal or liver failure.

14. Which anaesthetic agent is neither metabolished by liver nor by kidney: *(PGMEE 2012)*

a. Rocuronium   b. Atracurium
c. Pancuronium   d. Vecuronium

[Ref: Lee 13th/e p. 191; Morgan 6th/e pg. 214]

15. A patient on atracurium develops seizures due to accumulation of- *(PGMEE 2015)*

a. Vecuronium   b. Laudanosine
c. Didanosine   d. Methylated Atracurium

[Ref: Lee 13th/e p. 191, Morgan 6th/e pg. 215]

16. Laudanosine is metabolite of-

(PGMEE 2013, 11)

a. Cisatracurium   b. Atracurium
c. Gallamine   d. Pancuronium

[Ref: Morgan 6th/e pg. 215]

17. Maximum histamine is released by- *(PGMEE 2015)*

a. Pancronium
b. Succinylcholine
c. Gallamine
d. Tubocurarine

[Ref: Goodman & Gilman 11th/e p. 222, Morgan 6th/e pg. 213]

Explanation

- Atracurium & mivacurium are capable of triggering histamine release particularly at higher doses.
- Histamine release from mast cells can result in bronchospasm, skin flushing & hypotension from peripheral vasodilation.

DEPOLARIZING BLOCKERS

18. Phase II block is seen with prolonged exposure to–

(PGMEE 2013)

a. Ether   b. d-TC
c. N_2O d. Suxamethonium [Sch]

[Ref: Morgan 6th/e pg. 205]

19. Which muscle relaxant increases intracranial pressure: *(DNB 2007)*

a. Vecuronium   b. Mivacurium
c. Suxamethonium   d. Atracurium

[Ref: Morgan 6th/e pg. 210]

Explanation

- Succinylcholine may lead to an activation of the electroencephalogram and slight increases in cerebral blood flow and intracranial pressure in some patients.

20. Malignant hyperthermia is most commonly seen in:

(DNB 2008, DNB June' 2010)

a. Succinyl choline   b. Gallamine
c. Pancuronium   d. Dantrolene sodium

[Ref: Morgan 6th/e pg. 210]

21. Succinylcholine is used with caution in all except –

(PGMEE 2012)

a. Burns   b. Crush injury
c. Mysthenia gravis   d. Tachycardia

[Ref: Morgan 6th/e pg. 209]

Explanation

Conditions causing susceptibility to succinylcholine-induced hyperkalemia:

Burn injury
Massive trauma
Severe intraabdominal infection
Spinal cord injury
Encephalitis
Stroke
Guillain-Barre syndrome
Severe Parkinson's disease
Tetanus
Prolonged total body immobilization
Ruptured cerebral aneurysm
Polyneuropathy
Closed head injury
Hemorrhagic shock with metabolic acidosis
Myopatheties (e.g., Duchenne's dystrophy)

22. The use of succinylcholine is not contraindicated in:

(DNB 2007]

a. Tetanus   b. Hepatic failure
c. Cerebral stroke   d. Closed head injury

[Ref: Morgan 6th/e pg. 209]

Explanation

- The side effects of succinylcholine include:-
  - Malignant hyperthermia,
  - Muscle pains,
  - Acute rhabdomyolysis with hyperkalemia,
  - Transient ocular hypertension,
  - Constipation and

13.	b
14.	b
15.	b
16.	a,b
17.	d
18.	d
19.	c
20.	a
21.	d
22.	b

○ Changes in cardiac rhythm, including bradycardia, cardiac arrest, and ventricular dysrhythmias.
- In patients with neuromuscular disease or burns, a single injection of suxamethonium can lead to massive release of potassium from skeletal muscles, potentially resulting in cardiac arrest.
- ***Conditions having susceptibility to suxamethonium-induced hyperkalaemia are:*** burns, **closed head injury**, acidosis, Guillain–Barré syndrome, **cerebral stroke**, drowning, severe intra-abdominal sepsis, massive trauma, myopathy, and **tetanus**.

23. A 6 year old boy taken for ophthalmic examination under anaesthesia. His father told that he has lower limb weakness & his elder brother died at 14 years of age. Which anaesthetic drug has to be avoided – *(PGMEE 2013)*
- a. Pancuronium
- b. Dexacurium
- c. Atracurium
- d. Succinylcholine

[Ref: Morgan 6th/e pg. 209]

24. In pseudocholinesterase deficiency, drug to be used cautiously is – *(PGMEE 2013)*
- a. Succinylcholine
- b. Gallamine
- c. Barbiturate
- d. Halothane

[Ref: Morgan 6th/e pg. 207]

Explanation

- Prolonged paralysis from succinylcholine caused by abnormal pseudocholinesterase (atypical cholinesterase) should be treated with continued mechanical ventilation and sedation until muscle function returns to normal by clinical signs.

25. Fasciculations are seen with: *(DNB 2008)*
- a. Baclofen
- b. Succinylcholine
- c. Gallamine
- d. Mivacurium

[Ref: Morgan 6th/e pg. 205]

26. Train of fasciculations is seen in – *(DNB pattern 2008)*
- a. Mivacurium
- b. Succinylcholine
- c. Baclofen
- d. Gallamine

[Ref:, Morgan 6th/e pg. 204]

Explanation

- Sch induced depolarisation is uncoordinated skeletal muscle activity that manifest clinically as fasiculations. Presynaptic receptors are principally involved in fasiculations which can be prevented by nonparalysing dose of nondepolarising drugs.

Depolarising vs Non-depolarising Block

Depolarising (Phase I) block	Non- Depolarising (Phase II) block
Fasciculation	No fasciculation
May develop Phase 2 block	No change in character of block
No tetanic fade	Tetanic Fade
No fade on train of four stimulation	Fade on train of four stimulation

Depolarising (Phase I) block	Non- Depolarising (Phase II) block
No Post tetanic potentiation	Post tetanic fascilitation
Potentiated by anticholinesterases	Use of edrophonium antagonise block . (Antagonised by anticholinesterases)
Potentiation by other depolarisers	Antagonised by other depolarisers)

27. Dibucaine number refers to – *(PGMEE 2015)*
- a. Potency of general anesthetics
- b. Ach cholinesterase activity derangement
- c. Potency of muscle relaxants
- d. None

[Ref: Morgan 6th/e pg. 207]

NM-REVERSAL

28. Probable indicators of reversal of neuromuscular blockade are all except– *(PGMEE 2015)*
- a. Lift head for 5 seconds
- b. Ability to perform sustained tongue depressor test
- c. Sustain hand grip for 5 seconds
- d. Leg lift for 10 seconds

[Ref: Miller anaesthesia 8th/e p. 997, Morgan's 5th/e pg 232]

29. Muscle relaxing effect of Rocuronium is fastest reversed by: *(Recent Pattern June 2018)*
- a. Glycopyrrolate
- b. Sugammadex
- c. Neostigmine
- d. Cisatracurium

[Ref: Morgan's 5th/e pg. 227]

Explanation

Neuromuscular reversal

- Reversal of block is done only for NDMR (Non depolarising muscle relaxants). Reversal agents are given only when spontaneous muscular activity starts.
- Drugs used for neuromuscular reversal are:
  ○ Neostigmine/Pyridostigmine
  ○ Edrophonium + atropine/Glycopyrolate
  ○ Sugammadex
- **Edrophonium** is reversal agent of choice in mivacurium reversal as it does not inhibit pseudocholinesterase.
- **Sugammadex** is a selective relaxant binding agent for reversal of rocuronium. It is used in a dose of 2.0 mg/kg and is administered at reappearance of T2.
- Signs of adequate reversal:-
  ○ Patient is able to hold tongue depressor between central incisors . It is most reliable clinical test.
  ○ Able to hold >5 seconds

30. Which of the following muscle relaxants causes maximal pain on injection - *(PGMEE 2012)*
- a. Rocuronium
- b. Succinyl choline
- c. Cistracurium
- d. Vecuronium

[Ref: internet]

23.	d
24.	a
25.	b
26.	b
27.	b
28.	d
29.	b
30.	a

31. Drug used to reverse the effect of d- tubocuranine:

(DNB 2007)

a. Neostigmine
b. Physostigmine
c. Scoline
d. Dantrolene

[Ref: Morgan 6th/e pg. 226]

Explanation

- **Neostigmine** is anticholinesterase used for reversal of muscular relaxation produced by competitive muscle relaxant such as d-tubocurarine, pancuronium, vecuronium and gallamine
- **Dantrolene** is direct acting skeletal muscle relaxant used in the treatment of malignant hyperthermia and neuroleptic malignant syndrome.
- **Scoline** is depolarising muscle relaxant
- **Physostigmine** is anticholinesterase: nonspecific reversal of CNS side effects of BZD's, scopolamine, and ketamine.

MISCELLANEOUS

32. All statements are true about skeletal muscle relaxants EXCEPT:
(DNB June' 2011)

a. Atracurium is degraded by Hoffman's elimination
b. Mivacurium is hydrolysed by plasma cholinesterase
c. Pancuronium blocks the uptake of nor-epinephrine
d. Rocuroninum is largely eliminated by liver

[Ref: Morgan 6th/e pg. 214, 217, 218]

33. Gallamine is excreted mainly through?

(DNB June' 2011)

a. Bile
b. Liver
c. Kidney
d. Pseudocholinesterase

[Ref: Morgan's 5th/e pg 219]

34. Which muscles is most resistance to neuromuscular blockage?
(DNB June' 2011)

a. Diaphragm
b. Ocular
c. Intercostal muscles
d. Adductor pollicis

[Ref: Ajay Yadav's 6th/e pg. 123; Morgan 6th/e pg.136]

31.	a
32.	c
33.	c
34.	a
35.	d
36.	d

Explanation

- Diaphragm is considered as most resistant muscle. In clinical practice it has been seen that central muscle, i.e. muscles of face (muscle fasciculations after succinylcholine are first seen in eyelids), jaw, pharynx, larynx, muscles of respiration, abdominal and trunk muscles are blocked earlier than peripheral muscles (limb muscles)

35. Which of the following muscle relaxants is free of cardiovascular effects over the entire clinical dose range: *(PGMEE 2014)*

a. Pancuronium
b. Pipecuronium
c. Atracurium
d. Vecuronium

[Ref: Lee 13th/e p. 193, Morgan 6th/e pg. 218]

36. Muscle relaxant withdrawn due to anaphylactoid reactions: *(DNB pattern 2007]*

a. Pancuronium
b. Rocuronium
c. Atracurium
d. Alcuronium

[Ref: Lee 13th/e p. 193, Morgan's 5th/e pg 207]

Explanation

Anaphylactoid reactions with drugs

- *Neuromuscular blocking agents* are responsible for 60-75% of serious anesthetic adverse drug reactions e.g. suxamethonium, **alcuronium**, vecuronium, pancuronium and atracurium are main anaesthetic drug responsible for anaphylaxis during anesthesia.
- Reactions are mainly caused by immediate IgE mediated hypersensitivity reaction. Benzylisoquinilones (atracurium, Cis-atracurium, mivacurium) are more responsible than aminosteroids (pancuronium, vecuronium, rocuronium)
- *Anaesthetic drugs causing anaphylaxis are:*
  - Amide Local anesthetic containing preservative methylparaben
  - Ester L.A. metabolize to PABA which may produce allergic reactions
- Antibiotic used during surgery such as penicillin, cephalosporins and sulphonamides

SCIENTISTS

1. The term "balanced anaesthesia" has been given by – *(PGMEE 2013)*
a. Lundy
b. Fischer
c. Mortan
d. Simpson

2. Anaesthetic effect of ether was demonstrated by – *(PGMEE 2013)*
a. Morton
b. Priestly
c. Morgan
d. None

[Ref: Morgan 6th/e pg. 2]

3. Ether was first used as an anaesthetic by? *(DNB Dec' 2009)*
a. Wells
b. Priesly
c. Simpson
d. Morton

[Ref: Morgan 6th/e pg. 2]

Explanation

- Willam Thomas Green Morton made first public demonstration of ether use on 16th October 1846. He administered ether to Edward Gillbert Abbott for excision of vascular lesion from left side of neck.
- Father of conduction anaesthesia → Heinrich Braun
- Father of anaestheisa → John Snow
- Father of spinal anaesthesia → August Bier
- Balanced anaesthesia → John Lundy

4. Who coined term anaesthesia – *(PGMEE 2013)*
a. Morgan
b. Holmes
c. Priestly
d. Morton

[Ref: Morgan 6th/e pg. 1]

CRITICAL TEMPERATURE

5. Critical temperature of oxygen is – *(PGMEE 2013)*
a. 20°C
b. 36.5°C
c. –119°C
d. 40°C

[Ref: Morgan 6th/e pg. 11]

6. Critical temperature for liquid nitrous oxide is – *(PGMEE 2013)*
a. –20°C
b. 36.5°C
c. –147°C
d. –242°C

[Ref: Morgan 6th/e pg. 12]

7. Critical temperature for Xenon- *(PGMEE 2014)*
a. -16.6°C
b. – 36.6°C
c. -119°C
d. –147°C

STAGES OF ANESTHESIA

8. Levels of ether anesthesia were demonstrated by whom: *(PGMEE 2012)*
a. Morton
b. Thompsom
c. Guedel
d. None

[Ref: KDT 8th/e p. 400]

9. All are stages of anaesthesia except – *(PGMEE 2012)*
a. Analgesia
b. Allodynia
c. Surgical anesthesia
d. Delirium

[Ref: KDT 8th/e p. 401]

10. Stage of analgesia in anaesthesia is – *(PGMEE 2015)*
a. Stage – 1
b. Stage – 2
c. Stage – 3
d. Stage – 4

[Ref: KDT 8th/e p. 401]

11. Stage of light anesthesia is characterized by: *(Recent Pattern June 2018)*
a. ↓se in HR >20% from baseline
b. Patient have explicit memory of the period
c. ↑ in size of pin point pupil
d. ↑ Respiration is irregular and small volume

[Ref: KDT's 7th/e pg. 374]

Explanation

Light anaesthesia

- Light anaesthesia is plane 1 of stage III (surgical anaesthesia). It is characterized by:-
  - Patient has explicit memory of this period.
  - Respiration is regular, RR 12-20 bpm
  - Pulse strong , HR >90 bpm (↑ in HR >20% from baseline)
  - Normal BP
  - May respond with movement during surgery
  - Eyeball are central or rotated, nystagmus may be there.
  - Size of pupil is normal.

Guedel's stages of anaesthesia

- Described on ether by **Guedel**.

Stage	Known as	Characterized by	Respiration	Pupils
I	Stage of analgesia	Beginning of induction to loss of consciousness,	Regular, small volume	Normal
II	Excitement /delirium (pupils dilated)	loss of consciousness to onset of automatic breathing Reflexes: Eyelashes absent	Irregular	dilated

1. a
2. a
3. d
4. b
5. c
6. b
7. a
8. c
9. b
10. a
11. b

Stage	Known as	Characterized by	Respiration	Pupils
III	Stage of surgical anaesthesia (Onset of regular respiration to cessation of breathing)	**Plane I** ■ Stage of light anaesthesia ■ Moving eye become fixed ■ Reflexes: Eyelid absent, conjunctival depressed	Regular large volume	Pin point
		Plane II ■ Surgical anesthesia ■ Corneal reflex lost ■ Suitable for most surgical procedures	Regular large volume	Small
		Plane III ■ Stage of deep surgical anaesthesia. ■ Light reflex and laryngeal reflex lost so best for intubation	Changing to diaphragmatic pattern of breathing	Normal or increased
		Plane IV Fully dilated pupils	Irregular diaphragmatic	■ Dilated
IV	Medullary paralysis/ coma	Medullary paralysis/ coma	Apnea	■ fully dilated

■ Intubation can be done in Guedel's plane III of stage III.

12. Characteristic EEG pattern seen in surgical tolerance stage of anesthesia is – *(PGMEE 2015)*
   a. Alpha
   b. Beta
   c. Delta
   d. Theta

[Ref: KDT 8th/e p. 402]

MISCELLANEOUS

13. Action of which anesthetic agent is through NMDA receptors? *(PGMEE 2015)*
   a. Succinylcholine
   b. NO
   c. Etomidate
   d. Xenon

[Ref: Morgan 5th/e p. 173]

14. During rapid induction of anesthesia: *(PGMEE 2012, AI 03)*
   a. Suxamethonium is contraindicated
   b. Patient is mechanically ventilated before endotracheal intubation
   c. Pre-oxygenation is mandatory
   d. Sellick's maneuver is not required

[Ref: Morgan 5th/e p. 858]

15. Which of the following statements about Total Intra-Venous Anesthesia [TIVA] is true: *(PGMEE 12)*
   a. Reduces Cerebral Metabolic Rate
   b. Risk of Malignant Hyperthermic is high
   c. Inhibits Hypoxic Pulmonary Vasoconstriction
   d. Cause More Renal Toxicity

16. Conscious sedation is: *(PGMEE 2013)*
   a. Sedation with inability to respond to command
   b. CNS depression with uncociousness
   c. Sedation with ability to respond to command
   d. Any of the above

[Ref: KDT 8th/e p. 412]

Explanation

■ 'Conscious sedation' is a monitored state of altered consciousness that can be employed (supplemented with local/regional/dental anaesthesia), to carryout diagnostic/short therapeutic/dental procedures in apprehensive subjects or medically compromised patients, in place of general anaesthesia. It allows the operative procedure to be performed with minimal physiologic and psychologic stress.

17. Most common Gas used during laproscopic surgeries
   a. O_2
   b. CO_2
   c. NO
   d. N_2O

18. Which of the following responses is least affected by Anesthesia: *(PGMEE 12)*
   a. Visual Evoked Response [VER]
   b. Somatosensory Evoked potential [SSEP]
   c. Brainstem Auditory Evoked Response [BAER]
   d. Electroencephalogram [EEG]

19. Pre-oxygenation before Anaesthesia is best achieved by: *(PGMEE 2016-17)*
   a. 1 minute of tidal breathing with 100%
   b. 2 vital capacity breaths in 30 seconds
   c. 8 vital capacity breaths in 60 seconds
   d. 3 minutes of tidal breathing of 100% oxygen with face mask

20. The main controlling agent for respiratory drive is which of the following – *(PGMEE 2014)*
   a. Oxygen
   b. HBO_3
   c. NO
   d. CO_2

[Ref: Internet]

1. Which of the following determines the speed of recovery from IV anesthetic: *(Recent Pattern June 2018)*
a. Liver metabolism of drug
b. Protein binding of drug
c. Redistribution of the drug from sites in the CNS
d. Plasma clearance of the drug

[Ref: Morgan's 5th/e pg. 170]

Explanation

- IV anesthetics completely bypasses the absorption, because the drug is placed directly into the bloodstream. Highly perfused organs (vessel rich) including the brain take up disproportionately large amount of drug compared to less perfused areas (the muscle, fat, and vessel-poor groups).
- Drugs with high plasma protein bindings are not available for uptake by an organ. During initial distribution highly perfused organs are saturated first but the greater mass of the less perfused organs continue to take up drug from the bloodstream. As plasma concentration falls, some drug leaves the highly perfused organs to maintain equilibrium.
- This redistribution phenomena is responsible for termination of effect of anesthetic drugs.

2. Intravenous anaesthetics are all except- *(PGMEE 2014)*
a. Opioids   b. Desflurane
c. Propofol   d. Ketamine

[Ref: KDT 8th/e p. 404, Morgan 6th/e pg. 179]

Explanation

General Anaesthetics

General Anaesthetics	Inhalational	Gas	Nitrous oxide
		Volatile liquids	Ether / Halothane / Isoflurane / Desflurane / Sevoflurane
	Intravenous	Fast acting drugs	Thiopentone sod. / Methohexitone sod. / Propofol / Etomidate
		Slower acting drugs	Benzodiazepines: Diazepam / Lorazepam / Midazolam
			Dissociative anaesthetic: Ketamine
			Opioid analgesic: Fentanyl / Remifentanil

3. True about midazolam as inducing agent – *(PGMEE 2012)*
a. Does not produce pain an IV injection
b. Increase in BP
c. Increase cerebral oxygen consumption
d. Increase peripheral vascular resistance

[Ref: Morgan 6th/e pg. 179]

4. Which of the following can be used to potentiate the effect of an induction agent? *(NEET Pattern 2017)*
a. Bupivacaine   b. Neostigmine
c. Lorazepam   d. Dexmedtomidine

Explanation

Induction of anesthesia (transition from an awake to an anaesthetized state) can be done by drugs given via:
- Inhalational route
  - Gaseous - N_2O
  - Volatile liquid - Ether, Halothane, Sevoflurane.
- Intravenous route
  - Propofol/Thiopentone/Etomidate/Ketamine/Opiod agonist (Fentanyl)/alpha 2 agonist: Dexmedetomidine.

Dexmedetomidine (Dexmed)

- Dexmedtomidine is an highly selective α_2-adrenergic agonist.
- Dexmedetomidine produces sedation, sympatholysis, hypnosis, and analgesia in the locus coeruleus. It blunts the hemodynamic response such as hypertension and tachycardia induced by endotracheal intubation.
- Dexmed is notable for its ability to provide sedation without risk of respiratory depression (unlike other commonly used sedatives such as propofol, fentanyl, and midazolam) and can provide cooperative or semi-arousable sedation.
- It is a short-term sedative (<24 hours).
- Dexmed decreases sympathetic tone, with attenuation of the neuroendocrine and hemodynamic responses to anesthesia and surgery; reduce anesthetic and opioid requirements; and cause sedation and analgesia. Its role in pain management and regional anesthesia is expanding.

About Other Options

- **Bupivacaine:** A local anesthetic agent
- **Neostigmine**: A reversal agent of nondepolarizing neuromuscular blockade.
- **Lorazepan**: Is a benzodiazepines .A slow onset limits the usefulness of lorazepam for IV induction of anesthesia.

1. c
2. b
3. a
4. d

PROPOFOL

5. Regarding propofol, which one of the following is false – *(PGMEE 2013)*
- a. It is used as an intravenous induction agent
- b. It has no muscle relaxant property
- c. It causes severe vomiting
- d. It is painful on injecting intravenously

[Ref: KDT 8th/e p. 409]

6. Bradycardia during anaesthesia seen in – *(PGMEE 15)*
- a. Atracurium
- b. Vecuronium
- c. Pancuronium
- d. Propofol

[Ref: Morgan 5th/e p. 186]

7. Safe inducing agent in malignant hyperpyrexia are A/E: *(DNB 2007)*
- a. Halothane
- b. Etomidate
- c. Thiopentone
- d. Propofol

[Ref: Morgan 6th/e pg. 1220]

Explanation

Anesthesia for patients Susceptible for Malignant Hyperthermia

- Local or regional anesthesia is preferred over GA (general anesthesia).
- Safe drugs for GA are barbiturates, propofol, narcotics, BZD, nitrous oxide, non-depolarizing muscle relaxants.
- Mild hypothermia is beneficial
- Must be kept in recovery room for 4-6 hours.
- Must be instructed to avoid heat exposure as these patients are very prone for heat stroke.

8. Which of the following intravenous induction agent is most suitable for day care surgery. *(PGMEE 2013, 2016-17)*
- a. Morphine
- b. Diazepam
- c. Propofol
- d. Ketamine

[Ref: Morgan 6th/e pg. 181]

9. IV administration of which drug is most painful among the following? *(PGMEE Jan 2019)*
- a. Methohexitol
- b. Ketamine
- c. Propofol
- d. Etomidate

10. True about Propofol infusion syndrome are all except – *(PGMEE 2015)*
- a. Features are nausea and vomiting
- b. Occurs in critically ill patients
- c. Features are cardiomyopathy, hepatomegaly
- d. Occurs with infusion of propofol for 48 hours or longer

[Ref: Morgan 6th/e pg. 182]

THIOPENTONE

11. True about thiopentone – *(PGMEE 2014)*
- a. Good muscle relaxation
- b. Good analgesic action
- c. Long acting
- d. Cerebroprotective

[Ref: KDT 7the/pg.381,382]

12. Thiopentone is not used in – *(PGMEE 2015)*
- a. Medically induced coma
- b. As an antidepressant
- c. As truth serum
- d. Induction of anesthesia

[Ref: Miller 7th/e p. 756, KDT 8th/e p. 408]

13. Thiopentone is C/I in – *(PGMEE 2013)*
- a. Bronchial asthma
- b. Acute intermittent porphyria
- c. Both
- d. None

[Ref: KDT 7the/pg.382]

14. Dose of thiopentone is? *(DNB June' 2009)*
- a. 2%
- b. 2.5%
- c. 3%
- d. 5%

[Ref: KDT 8th/e p. 408; Morgan 6th/e pg. 174]

Explanation

- Thiopentone concentration used is 2.5%. Concentration >2.5% results in pain and conc <2.5% has variable response.

15. Thiopentone has cerbroprotective effect because of:
- a. Free redical removal *(PGMEE 12)*
- b. Reduction of vasospasm
- c. Decrease cerebral blood flow
- d. Calcium channel blockage

[Ref: KDT 8th/e p. 408]

ETOMIDATE

16. Induction agent that may cause adrenal cortex suppression is: *(PGMEE 2014)*
- a. Thiopentone
- b. Ketamine
- c. Propofol
- d. Etomidate

[Ref: Morgan 6th/e pg. 181]

17. Inducting agent with maximum incidence of vomiting – *(PGMEE 2014)*
- a. Thiopentone
- b. Etomidate
- c. Ketamine
- d. Propofol

[Ref: Morgan 6th/e pg. 181]

Explanation

- Postoperative nausea and vomiting are more common following etomidate than following propofol or barbiturate induction.

18. Which anaesthetic agent doesn't cause cardiac depression: *(NEET pattern Jan' 2019)*
- a. Etomidate
- b. Ketamine
- c. Thiopentone
- d. Propofol

19. Which of the following anesthetic is safe in heart failure: *(PGMEE 2012)*
- a. Ketamine
- b. Thiopentone
- c. Etomidate
- d. Propofol

[Ref: Morgan 6th/e pg. 180]

5.	c
6.	d
7.	a
8.	c
9.	c
10.	a
11.	d
12.	b
13.	b
14.	b
15.	c
16.	d
17.	b
18.	a
19.	c

20. Adverse effects of Etomidate:
(Recent Pattern June 2018)
a. Myoclonus & adrenal suppression
b. Adrenal suppression & Seizures
c. Seizures & Vomiting
d. Seizures & myoclonus

[Ref: Morgan 6th/e pg. 181]

Explanation

Adverse effects of Etomidate

- Highest incidence of nausea, vomiting (30-40% among inducing agents) and **myoclonus**.
- **Adrenal suppression**:-
  ○ ↓ed synthesis of steroids → ↑se in precursors 11-DOC and 7- OHP (hydroxyprogesterone).
  ○ The specific endocrine effect is a dose dependent **reversible inhibition of enzyme 11β - hydroxylase**.
  ○ ACTH secretion ↑ses due to loss of feedback inhibition.
- It can produce hiccups.
- Etomidate tends to reduce raised ICP, so etomidate should be considered when maintenance of cerebral perfusion is important.
- Superficial thrombophlebitis and pain on injection may occur which can be reduced by using larger vein and injecting lidocaine just before etomidate.
- Intra arterial injection is not associated with local or vascular complications.

Other peculiarities of Etomidate

- It has a briefer duration of action 4-8 minutes.
- Etomidate is the most cardiostable inducing agent. It produces little cardiovascular and respiratory depression IV agent of choice for MI patient, cardiovascular surgeries (bypass, aneurysms, valve surgery), aneurysm surgery & respiratory compromised patient.
- Coronary perfusion pressure is maintained when it is used with fentanyl.
- Vit 'C' supplementation restores cortisol levels to normal after use of etomidate.

KETAMINE

21. Ketamine acts an which receptor – *(PGMEE 2014)*
a. GABA$_A$
b. Glutamate
c. GABA$_B$
d. NMDA

[Ref: KDT 7th/e p. 384; Morgan 6th/e pg. 177]

22. Which of the following drugs produces dissociative anesthesia – *(PGMEE 2007)*
a. Thiopentone
b. Propofol
c. Enflurane
d. Ketamine

[Ref: Lee 13th/e p. 162; Morgan 6th/e pg. 177]

23. Anesthetic agent causing bradycardia are all except:
(DNB June' 2009)
a. Isoflurane
b. Thiopentone
c. Halothane
d. Ketamine

[Ref: Morgan 6th/e pg. 179]

Explanation

- **Ketamine** causes tachycardia and hypertension due to sympathetic stimulation.
- **Halothane** does not increase in heart rate. Infact, halothane cause direct myocardial suppression resulting in fall in blood pressure. It also suppress baroreceptors, thus disabling compensatory response.
- **Thiopentone**: It causes decrease in Bp and myocardial depression and compensatory increase in heart rate.
- **Propofol**: It produces more fall in Bp than thiopentone. It also decrease cardiac output, heart rate anand SVR.. It suppresses baroreceptor responses and the sympathetic stimulation.
- **Isoflurane**: Among all inhalational anesthetic, Isoflurane is most cardiostable.

24. Increased intracranial tension is seen with:
(DNB Dec 2010)
a. Ketamine
b. Thiopentone
c. Halothane
d. Propofol

[Ref: Morgan 6th/e pg. 179]

25. Contraindicated in head injury – *(PGMEE 2012)*
a. N$_2$O
b. Ketamine
c. Propofol
d. Halothane

[Ref: KDT 8th/e p. 411, Morgan 6th/e pg. 171]

26. Intraocular pressure is increased by which anesthetic –
(PGMEE 2013, May 06)
a. Propofol
b. Isoflurane
c. N$_2$O
d. Ketamine

[Ref: Miller 6th/e p. 344; Morgan 6th/e pg. 179]

27. Injection of all of the following drugs is painful except –
(NEET pattern Jan' 2019)
a. Propofol
b. Etomidate
c. Ketamine
d. ? methohexitone

28. Which of the following drugs is contraindicated in a patient with raised intracranial pressure?
(PGMEE 2012)
a. Thiopentone
b. Propofol
c. Midazolam
d. Ketamine

[Ref: Morgan 6th/e pg. 179]

29. Maximum analgesic action found in – *(PGMEE 2013)*
a. Catecholamine
b. Propofol
c. Ketamine
d. Thiopentone

[Ref: KDT 8th/e p. 411; Morgan 6th/e pg. 180]

Explanation

- Ketamine comes closet to being a "complete" anaesthetic as it induces analgesia, amnesia, and unconsciousness.

30. Benefit of ketamine – *(PGMEE 2014)*
a. Decrease IOT
b. Causes decrease in BP
c. Decrease ICT
d. Good analgesic

[Ref: KDT 8th/e p. 411; Morgan 6th/e pg. 180]

20.	a
21.	d
22.	d
23.	d
24.	a
25.	b
26.	d
27.	c
28.	d
29.	c
30.	d

31. **Emergence delirium is associated with –** *(PGMEE 2013)*
    a. Droperidol
    b. Halothane
    c. Ketamine
    d. Pentothal sodium

    [Ref: KDT 8ᵗʰ/e p. 411; Morgan 6th/e pg. 179]

Explanation

- Undesirable psychotomimetic side effects (e.g., disturbing dreams and delirium) during emergence and recovery are more common in adults then in children.

32. **Disadvantage of ketamine is:** *(PGMEE 2013)*
    a. Delirium
    b. Increased ICT
    c. Increased heart rate
    d. All of the above

    [Ref: KDT 8ᵗʰ/e p. 411; Morgan 6th/e pg. 179]

33. **Which of the following is a sympathomimetic –**
    (PGMEE 2014)
    a. Propofol
    b. Ketamine
    c. N₂O
    d. Etomidate

    [Ref: Morgan 6th/e pg. 179]

34. **Anesthetic agent of choice for status asthmaticus is?**
    (DNB June' 2011, PGMEE 2012)
    a. Ketamine
    b. Ether
    c. Thiopentone
    d. Propofol

    [Ref: Morgan 6th/e pg. 179]

Explanation

- Racemic ketamine is a potent bronchodilator, making it a good induction agent for asthmatic patients.

35. **Ketamine causes:-** *(PGMEE 2016-17)*
    a. Increase in BP
    b. Decrease in BP
    c. Increase in ICT and BP
    d. Decrease in ICT

    [Ref: Morgan 6th/e pg. 179]

36. **True about ketamine–** *(PGMEE 2012)*
    a. Causes hypotension
    b. Decreases ICT
    c. Depressed airway reflexes
    d. Bronchodilator

    [Ref: Morgan 6th/e pg. 179]

37. **Anaesthetic agent causing increase in all pressure**
    a. Propofol
    b. Ketamine
    c. Thiopentone
    d. Pancuronium

    [Ref: Morgan 6th/e pg. 179]

OPIOIDS ANAESTHESIA

38. **Muscle rigidity is caused by which anaesthetic –**
    (PGMEE 2014)
    a. Halothane
    b. Alfentanil
    c. Sevoflurane
    d. Ether

    [Ref: Miller 7ᵗʰ/e p. 788, KDT 7th/e pg.194, Morgan 6th/e pg.192]

Explanation

- Rapid administration of larger doses of opioids (particularly fentanyl, sufentanil, remifentanil, and alfentanil) can induce chest wall rigidity severe enough to prevent adequate bag-and-mask ventilation.

39. **Best drug to treat post operative shivering –**
    (PGMEE 2019)
    a. Meperidine
    b. Fentanyl
    c. Morphine
    d. Tramadol

31.	c
32.	d
33.	b
34.	a
35.	c
36.	d
37.	b
38.	b
39.	a

Uses and doses of ketamine, etomidate and propofol

Agent	Use	Route	Dose
Ketamine	Induction	IV IM	1-2 mg/kg 3-5 mg/kg
	Sedation (Almost always in combination with propofol)	IV	2.5-15 mcg/kg/min
Etomidate	Induction	IV	0.2-0.5 mg/kg
Propofol	Induction	IV	1-2.5 mg/kg
	Maintenance infusion	IV	50-200 mcg/kg/min
	Sedation infusion	IV	25-100/kg/min

Summary of nonvolatile anaesthetic effects on organ systems.

Agent	Respiratory		Cardiovascular		Cerebral		
	Vent	Bronchodilation	HR	MAP	CBF	CMRO$_2$	ICP
Barbiturates							
Thiopental	↓↓↓	↓	↑↑	↓↓	↓↓↓	↓↓↓	↓↓↓
Thiamylal	↓↓↓	↓	↑↑	↓↓	↓↓↓	↓↓↓	↓↓↓
Methohexital	↓↓↓	0	↑↑	↓↓	↓↓↓	↓↓↓	↓↓↓
Benzodiazepines							
Diazepam	↓↓	0	0/↑	↓	↓↓	↓↓	↓↓
Lorazepam	↓↓	0	0/↑	↓	↓↓	↓↓	↓↓
Midazolam	↓↓	0	↑	↓↓	↓↓	↓↓	↓↓
Etomidate	↓	0	0	↓	↓↓↓	↓↓↓	↓↓↓
Propofol	↓↓↓	0	0	↓↓	↓↓↓	↓↓↓	↓↓↓
Ketamine	↓	↑↑↑	↑↑	↑↑	↑↑^{2}	↑	↑↑^{2}

PHARMACOKINETICS

1. Index of potency of general anesthesia:
(PGMEE 2014)

a. Dead space concentration
b. Diffusion coefficient
c. Minimum alveolar concentration
d. Alveolar blood concentration

[Ref: KDT 8th/e p. 402; Morgan 6th/e pg. 158]

2. Highly lipid soluble agent would be associated with:
(PGMEE 2014)

a. Potent anaesthetic action
b. Least respiratory depression
c. Excellent muscle relaxant action
d. Potent analgesic action

[Ref: KDT 8th/e p. 403; Morgan 6th/e pg. 156]

Explanation

- All inhalation agents share a common mechanism of action at the molecular level.
- This was anesthetic potency of inhalation agents correlates directly with their lipid solubility (Meyer-Overton rule).
- Anaesthetics with higher lipid solubility (halothane) continue to enter adipose tissue for hours and laso leave it slowly.

3. Anesthetic drug with minimum blood gas partition coefficient
(PGMEE 2016-17)

a. N_2O b. Desflurane
c. Sevoflurane   d. Isoflurane

[Ref: KDT 8th/e p. 405; Morgan 6th/e pg. 151]

Explanation

Partition coefficients of volatile anesthetics at 37^0C.[1]

Agent	Blood/Gas	Brain/Blood	Muscle/Blood	Fat/Blood
Nitrous oxide	0.47	1.1	1.2	2.3
Halothane	2.4	2.9	3.5	60
Isoflurane	1.4	2.6	4.0	45
Desflurane	0.42	1.3	2.0	27
Sevoflurane	0.65	1.7	3.1	48

4. MAC stands for –   *(PGMEE 2012)*
a. Maximal alveolar concentration
b. Minimum alveolar concentration
c. Minimal anaesthetic concentration
d. Minimal analgesic concentration

[Ref: KDT 8th/e p. 402; Morgan 6th/e pg. 158]

Explanation

MAC

- Potency of inhalational agent is determined by **Minimum Alveolar Concentration (MAC)** which is the concentration of agent, at which 50% of patients will not respond to the stimulus. So agent with minimum MAC will be most potent.

$$(MAC \, \alpha \, \frac{1}{Potency})1$$

- **Methoxyflurane is most potent while N_2O is minimum in potency.**
- Factors which ↑se MAC: Children, hyperthermia, anxiety, chronic alcohol ingestion.
- MAC↓es with old age, hypothermia, anaemia, pregnancy, hypoxia, coadministration with intravenous agent, N_2O and LA, acute alcohol ingestion, hyponatremia.
- **Factors that do not affect MAC are →** Sex (male or female), thyroid disease (e.g. hypo/hyperthyroidism).
- The ↑ in alveolar anesthetic concentration (Fa) toward the inspired anesthetic concentration (Fi) is most rapid with least soluble anesthetics (nitrous oxide, desflurane and sevoflurane) and intermediate with the more soluble anesthetics (isoflurane and halothane)

5. Anaesthetic agent with minimum MAC:
(PGMEE 2016-17)

a. Desflurane   b. Isoflurane
c. N_2O d. Xenon

[Ref: Morgan 6th/e pg. 159]

6. Least MAC is of which inhalational agent –
(PGMEE 2013)

a. Xenon   b. Isoflurane
c. Sevoflurane   d. Halothane

[Ref: Morgan 6th/e pg. 156]

7. Blood: Gas partition coefficient is a measure of –
(PGMEE 2013)

a. Blood solubility of agent
b. Lipid solubility of agent
c. Potency of anaesthetic agent
d. Uptake by cerebral vasculature

[Ref: KDT 7th/e p. 375; Morgan 6th/e pg. 152]

Explanation

- Three factors affect anesthetic uptake:
  o Solubility in the blood.
  o Alveolar blood flow.
  o Difference in partial pressure between alveolar gas and venous blood.

1.	c
2.	a
3.	b
4.	b
5.	d
6.	a
7.	a

- The higher the blood/gas coefficient, the greater the anesthetic's solubility and the greater its uptake by the pulmonary circulation.

8. Fastest induction and recovery is seen with –

(PGMEE 2013)

a. Halothane
b. Isoflurance
c. Enflurane
d. Desflurane

[Ref: Morgan 6th/e pg. 166]

Explanation

- The Low solubility of desflurane in blood and body tissues causes a very rapid induction and emergence of anesthesia.
- Therefore, the alveolar concentration of desflurane approaches the inspired concentration much more rapidly than the other volatile agents.
- Wakeup times are approximately 50% less than those observed following isoflurane.
- This is principally attributable to a blood/gas partition coefficient (0.42) that is even lower than that of nitrous oxide (0.47).

9. Fast induction and recovery is seen in – *(PGMEE 2012)*

a. Halothane
b. Methoxyflurane
c. N_2O
d. Ether

[Ref: Morgan 6th/e p. 162]

Explanation

- N_2O is 35 times more soluble than nitrogen in blood. Thus, it tends to diffuse into air-containing cavities more rapidly than nitrogen is absorbed by the bloodstream.
- Because N_2O will diffuse into the cavity more rapidly than the air (principally nitrogen) diffuses out, the pneumothorax expands until it contains 100 mL of air and 100 mL of nitrous oxide.

HALOTHANE

10. Percentage of Halothane metabolized – *(PGMEE 2014)*

a. 1%
b. 5%
c. 10%
d. 20%

[Ref: KDT 8th/e p. 406]

11. True about halothane – *(PGMEE 2014)*

a. Potent bronchoconstrictor
b. Poor analgesic
c. Causes tachycardia
d. Useful in malignant hyperthermia

[Ref: Morgan 6th/e pg. 164]

Explanation

- Slowing of sinoatrial node conduction may result in a junctional rhythm or bradycardia.
- Halothane is considered a potent bronchodilator, as it often reverses asthma-induced bronchospasm.
- Like the other potent volatile anesthetics, it is a triggering agent of malignant hyperthermia.

12. Hepatotoxic agent is – *(PGMEE 2013)*

a. Ether
b. Halothane
c. N_2O
d. Ketamine

[Ref: Morgan 6th/e pg. 164]

13. Which inhalational agent is best uterine relaxant?

(DNB June' 20009)

a. Halothane
b. Isoflurane
c. Sevoflurane
d. Desflurane

[Ref: KDT 8th/e p. 407]

Explanation

- Inhalation anesthetics produce a dose-dependent uterine vasodilatation and decrease in uterine contractility.
- Uterine relaxation produced by inhalation agents may be helpful for removal of a retained placenta.

14. All are true about halothane except – *(PGMEE 2012)*

a. Bronchodilatation
b. Uterine relaxation
c. Hepatitis
d. Tachycardia

[Ref: Morgan 6th/e pg. 163; KDT 7 th e/p.379]

15. Best uterine relaxation is seen with – *(PGMEE 2015)*

a. Chloroform
b. Nitrous oxide
c. Ether
d. Halothane

[Ref: KDT 8th/e p. 407]

16. Anesthetic agent/s which have tocolytic effect are –

(PGMEE 2015)

a. Isoflurane
b. Halothane
c. Enflurane
d. All the above

[Ref: Morgan 5th/e p. 833]

17. Percentage of hepatitis after halothane use –

(PGMEE 2014)

a. 20%
b. 40%
c. 1 in 35000
d. 1 in 50000

[Ref: Morgan 5th/e p. 168]

18. A patient after giving inhalational anesthesia developed fulminant hepatitis, patient was exposed to same drug previously. Which is the drug – *(PGMEE 2013)*

a. Halothane
b. Isoflurane
c. Enflurane
d. N_2O

[Ref: Morgan 6th/e pg. 164]

Explanation

- "Halothane hepatitis" is extremely rare (1 per 35,000 cases). Patients exposed to multiple halothane anesthetics at short intervals, middle-aged obese women, and persons with a familial predisposition to halothane toxicity or a personal history of toxicity are considered to be at increased risk.

19. Which sensitizes the myocardium to catecholamines –

(PGMEE 2013)

a. Halothane
b. Ether
c. Isflurane
d. Propofol

[Ref: Morgan 6th/e pg. 163]

FLURANES

20. Which of the following inhalational anaesthetic agent causes maximum respiratory irritation–

(NEET pattern Jan' 2019)

a. Enflurane
b. Halothane
c. Sevoflurane
d. Desflurane

8.	d
9.	c
10.	d
11.	b
12.	b
13.	a
14.	d
15.	d
16.	d
17.	c
18.	a
19.	a
20.	d

ISOFLURANE

21. Inhalational agent of choice for cranial surgery– *(PGMEE 2013)*

a. Isoflurane   b. Enflurane

c. N_2O d. Halothane

[Ref: Morgan 4th/e p. 625-267]

22. All are hepatotoxic except – *(PGMEE 2014)*

a. Methoxyflurane   b. Halothane

c. Isoflurane   d. Chlorform

[Ref: Morgan 6th/e pg. 165]

SEVOFLURANE

23. Smooth induction is seen by- *(PGMEE 2013)*

a. Sevoflurane   b. Halothane

c. Ether   d. Enflurane

[Ref: Morgan 6th/e pg. 167]

Explanation

- Nonpungency and rapid increases in alveolar anesthetic concentration make sevoflurane an excellent choice for smooth and rapid inhalation inductions in pediatric and adult patients.

24. Anesthesia of choice for induction in children among the following is: *(Recent Pattern June 2018)*

a. Desflurane   b. Halothane

c. Sevoflurane   d. Isoflurane

[Ref: Morgan 6th/e pg. 167]

Explanation

- Sevoflurane is the induction agent of choice in pediatric anaesthesia.
- It is associated with less myocardial depression or arhythmias.

DESFLURANE

25. Which one of the following is the fastest acting inhalational agent: *(DNB 2007)*

a. Desflurane   b. Isoflurane

c. Halothane   d. Sevoflurane

[Ref: Morgan 6th/e pg. 166]

26. MAC of desflurane is – *(PGMEE 2014)*

a. 1.15   b. 2

c. 4   d. 6

[Ref: KDT 7th/e p. 377; Morgan 6th/e pg. 159]

27. Maximum global warming is seen with – *(PGMEE 2013)*

a. Isoflurane   b. Halothane

c. Sevoflurane   d. Desflurane

[Ref: Morgan 6th/e pg. 166]

Explanation

- For instance, because the vapor pressure of desflurane at 20^0C is 681 mm Hg, at high altitudes (eg, Denver, Colorado) it boils at room temperature.
- This problem necessiated the development of a special desflurane vaporizer.

28. Which of the following fluorinated agent does not produce fluoride to produce toxicity – *(PGMEE 2013)*

a. Methoxyflurane

b. Enflurane

c. Sevoflurane

d. Desflurane

[Ref: Morgan 5th/e p. 171]

29. Fluoride content is least in – *(PGMEE 2012)*

a. Desflurane

b. Enflurane

c. Sevoflurane

d. Isoflurane

[Ref: Ajay Yadav 6th/e p. 99; Morgan 5th/e p. 170]

Explanation

- Desflurane undergoes minimal metabolism (<0.02%) therefore does not produce any fluoride.

30. Which one of the following inhalational anesthetics is most likely to cause fluoride ion nephrotoxicity? *(PGMEE 2013)*

a. Enflurane   b. Isoflurane

c. Halothane   d. Methoxyflurane

[Ref: Ajay Yadav 4th/e p. 63]

NITROUS OXIDE

31. Diffusion hypoxia is seen during – *(PGMEE 2013)*

a. Preoperatively

b. Induction of anaesthesia

c. Postoperative

d. Recovering anaesthesia

[Ref: KDT 8th/e p. 403; Morgan 6th/e pg. 155]

32. Diffusion hypoxia is seen with – *(PGMEE 2014)*

a. Ether

b. Nitrous oxide

c. Halothane

d. Cyclopropane

[Ref: KDT 8th/e p. 403; Morgan 6th/e pg. 155]

33. N_2O – true is: *(PGMEE 2016-17)*

a. Stored as compressed gas

b. Pin index 3,5

c. Used as skeletal muscle relaxant

d. Potent agent

[Ref: KDT 8th/e p. 405; Morgan 6th/e pg. 161]

34. Second gas effect is – *(PGMEE 2015)*

a. Facilitation of inhalation of Halothane by N_2O

b. Displacement of oxygen by N_2O

c. Removal of oxygen by N_2O from alveoli during recovery from general anaesthesia

d. Displacement of N_2O by Oxygen

[Ref: KDT 8th/e p. 403; Morgan 6th/e pg. 151]

35. Poor muscle relaxant property is:- *(PGMEE 2016-17)*

a. N_2O

b. Halothane

c. Ether

d. Sevoflurane

[Ref: Morgan 6th/e pg. 161]

21.	a
22.	c
23.	a
24.	c
25.	a
26.	d
27.	d
28.	d
29.	a
30.	d
31.	d
32.	b
33.	b
34.	a
35.	a

36. Gas stored in liquid form is? *(DNB Dec' 2009)*
a. Cyclopropane   b. N_2O
c. CO_2 d. O_2

[Ref: Morgan 6th/e pg. 161]

Explanation

- Unlike the potent volatile agents, nitrous oxide is a gas at room temperature and ambient pressure. It can be kept as a liquid under pressure because its critical temperature lies above room temperature.

37. Bone marrow depression is seen with –
(PGMEE 2015, DNB June' 2011)

a. Halothene   b. Isoflurane
c. Ether   d. N_2O

[Ref: Morgan 6th/e pg. 162]

38. All are false about N_2O except – *(PGMEE 2013)*
a. Good muscle relaxant
b. No diffusion hypoxia
c. Lighter than air
d. Least potent

[Ref: Morgan 6th/e pg. 161]

39. True about N_2O – *(PGMEE 2012)*
a. High potency and poor analgesia
b. Low potency and good analgesia
c. Good muscle relaxant
d. High potency and good analgesia

[Ref: Morgan 6th/e pg. 163]

36.	b
37.	d
38.	d
39.	b

LOCAL ANESTHETICS

1. Local anaesthesia acts by – *(PGMEE 2012)*
   a. K$^+$ channel inhibition
   b. Na$^+$ channel inhibition
   c. Ca^{++} channel inhibition
   d. Mg^{++} channel inhibition

   [Ref: Morgan 6th/e pg. 263]

2. The longest acting local anesthetic is:-
   (PGMEE 2014, 2016-17)
   a. Ropivacaine
   b. Bupivacaine
   c. Procaine
   d. Dibucaine

   [Ref: KDT 7th/e pg. 366; Morgan 6th/e pg. 269]

3. Active form of local anaesthetic – *(PGMEE 2014)*
   a. Neutral
   b. Anionic
   c. Cationic
   d. Any of the above

   [Ref: Morgan 6th/e pg. 266]

4. In local anesthesia which of the following is the first sequence to go – *(PGMEE 2012)*
   a. Temperature
   b. Parasympathetic
   c. Motor
   d. Preganglionic sympathetic

   [Ref: Morgan 6th/e pg. 264]

Explanation

- Sensitivity of nerve fibers to inhibition by local anesthetics is determined by axonal diameter, myelination, and other anatomic and physiological factors.
- Small diameter increases sensitivity to local anesthetics.
  - Thus, larger, faster Aα fibers are less sensitive to local anesthetics than smaller, slower-conducting Aδ fibers, and larger unmyelinated fibers are less sensitive than smaller unmyelinated fibers.
  - Differential blockade is related to diameter of fibers (smaller fibers are inherently more susceptible to drug blockade than large fibers).
- Small unmyelinated C fibers are relatively resistant to inhibition by local anesthetics as compared with larger myelinated fibers.
- In spinal nerves
  - Local anesthetic inhibition (and conduction failure) generally follows the sequence autonomic > sensory > motor.

- Spinal anesthesia blocks small unmyelinated sympathetic fibers first, after which it blocks myelinated (sensory and motor) fibers.

5. Which of these nerve fibers is least sensitive to effect to local anaesthesia *(NEET Pattern 2017)*
   a. Aγ
   b. Aδ
   c. B
   d. C

Explanation

Susceptibility of Nerve Fibres to

1. Pressure A > B > C
2. Hypoxia B > A > C
3. Local anaesthetics C > B > A
- Sequence of blockade: Autonomic → sensory → motor.
- In sensory cold temperature sensation is lost first → Heat → pain → touch → deep pressure → Proprioception.
- Order of recovery is in the reverse order (motor → sensory → Autonomic)
- *Order of blockade of nerve fibres by LA*
- B fibers > C fibers > Aδ sensory fibers > Aα type Ia, Ib > Aβ > Aγ > Aα motor.

6. Addition of epinephrine to lignocaine – *(PGMEE 2012)*
   a. Decreases duration of LA
   b. Decreases absorption of LA
   c. Increases distribution of LA
   d. Increases metabolism of LA

   [Ref: Morgan 6th/e pg. 270]

7. Fastest route of absorption of local anaesthetic is:
   a. Intercostal *(DNB 2008)*
   b. Brachial
   c. Caudal
   d. Epidural

   [Ref: Morgan 6th/e pg. 270]

Explanation

- Systemic absorption of LA depends upon site of injection, additives to LA, doasage, volume and pharmacologic profile of the agent itself.
- When a local anesthetic solution is exposed to an area of greater vascularity, a greater rate and degree of absorption occur.
- Anesthetic drug level is **highest after intercostal nerve blockade**, followed, in order of decreasing concentration, by injection into the caudal epidural space > lumbar epidural space > brachial plexus > and subcutaneous tissue.

1.	b
2.	d
3.	c
4.	d
5.	a
6.	b
7.	a

CHAPTER-7 ◐ REGIONAL ANESTHESIA

8. **Percentage of adrenaline with lignocaine for local infiltration is –** *(PGMEE 2013)*
   a. 1:100
   b. 1:1000
   c. 1:10000
   d. 1:50000

   [Ref: KDT 8th/e p. 389]

Explanation

- Addition of a vasoconstrictor, e.g. adrenaline (1:50,000 to 1:2000,000):
  - Prolongs duration of action of LAs
  - Enhances the intensity of nerve block.
  - Reduces systemic toxicity of LAs
  - Provides a more bloodless field for surgery

11. **Which of the following is an aminoester –**

   a. Lidocaine
   b. Prilocaine
   c. Dibucaine
   d. Tetracaine

9. **Which local anesthetic does not require adrenaline –** *(PGMEE 2013)*
   a. Bupivacaine
   b. Lignocaine
   c. Cocaine
   d. Procaine

   [Ref: KDT 8th/e p. 391; Morgan 6th/e pg. 271]

10. **False about local anesthetics –** *(PGMEE 2015)*
   a. Lignocaine is used as an antiarrhythmic
   b. Lidocaine is shorter acting than bupivacaine
   c. Prilocaine is less toxic than lignocaine
   d. Mixture of ligno + prilocaine is known as eutectic

   [Ref: KDT 8th/e p. 392, 390; Morgan 6th/e pg. 267, 270]

   (PGMEE 2014)

   [Ref: Morgan 6th/e pg. 269, KDT 8th/e p. 387]

Explanation

Clinical use of local anesthetic agents

Agent	Techniques	Concentrations Available	Maximum Dose (mg/kg)	Typical Duration of Nerve Blocks
Esters				
Benzocaine	Topical	20%	NA	NA
Chloroprocaine	Epidural, infiltration, peripheral nerve block, spinal	1%, 2%, 3%	12	Short
Cocaine	Topical	4%, 10%	3	NA
Procaine	Spinal, local infiltration	1%, 2%, 10%	12	Short
Tetracaine (amethocaine)	Spinal, topical (eye)	0.2%, 0.3%, 0.5%, 1%, 2%	3	Long
Amides				
Bupivacaine	Epidural, spinal, infiltration, peripheral nerve block	0.25%, 0.5%, 0.75%	3	Long
Lidocaine (lignocaine)	Epidural, spinal, infiltration, peripheral nerve block, intravenous regional, topical	0.5%, 1%, 1.5%, 2%, 4%, 5%	4.5 7 (with epinephrine)	Medium
Mepivacaine	Epidural, infiltration, peripheral nerve block, spinal	1%, 1.5%, 2% 3%	4.5 7 (with epinephrine)	Medium
Prilocaine	EMLA (topical), epidural, intravenous regional (outside North America)	0.5%, 2%, 3%, 4%	8	Medium
Ropivacaine	Epidural, spinal, infiltration, peripheral nerve block	0.2%, 0.5%, 0.75%, 1%	3	Long

8. d
9. c
10. c
11. d

12. A patient is allergic to aminoesters. What can be used for ophthalmic purpose:- *(PGMEE 2013)*
   a. Procaine
   b. Tetracaine
   c. Cocaine
   d. Prilocaine

   [Ref: KDT 8th/e p. 387; Morgan 6th/e pg. 269 table]

13. All are amides except: ? *(DNB Dec' 2011)*
   a. Prilocaine
   b. Procaine
   c. Lignocaine
   d. Etidocaine

   [Ref: KDT 8th/e p. 387, KDT 7th e/pg.361]

14. All are used for local infiltration except – *(PGMEE 2013)*
   a. Dibucaine
   b. Ropivacaine
   c. Lidocaine
   d. Bupivacaine

   [Ref: Morgan 6th/e pg. 269]

17. Most potent local anesthetic – *(PGMEE 2014)*
   a. Procaine
   b. Prilocaine
   c. Lidocaine
   d. Bupivacaine

   [Ref: KDT 8th/e p. 386]

15. Cholinesterase metabolizes following except – *(PGMEE 2014)*
   a. Tetracaine
   b. Bupivacaine
   c. Acetylcholine
   d. Procaine

   [Ref: Morgan 6th/e pg. 268]

Explanation

- Ester local anesthetics are predominantly metabolized by pseudocholinesterase (plasma cholinesterase or butyrycholinesterase). Ester hydrolysis is very rapid, and the water-soluble metabolites are excreted in the urine.
- Procaine and benzocaine are metabolized to p-aminobenzoic acid (PABA), which has been associated with rare anaphylactic reactions.

16. Shortest acting local anaesthetics – *(PGMEE 2013)*
   a. Lignocaine
   b. Chlorprocaine
   c. Etidocaine
   d. Bupivacaine

   [Ref: KDT 8th/e p. 388]

12.	d
13.	b
14.	a
15.	b
16.	b
17.	d
18.	a
19.	a
20.	c
21.	b
22.	a

Explanation

Local Anaesthetics				
Injectable anaesthetic			**Surface anaesthetic**	
Low potency, short duration	Intermediate potency and duration	High potency, long duration	Soluble	Insoluble
Procaine Chloroprocaine	Lidocaine (Lignocaine) Prilocaine	Tetracaine Bupivacaine Ropivacaine Dibucaine	Cocaine Lidocaine Tetracaine Proparacaine	Benzocaine Butylamino-benzoate Oxethazine

18. Local anaesthetic with maximum ionized form at physiological pH – *(PGMEE 2014)*
   a. Lignocaine
   b. Chloroprocaine
   c. Bupivacaine
   d. Etidocaine

   [Ref: Morgan 5th/e p. 269, KDT 7ht e/pg.363]

COCAINE

19. Vasoconstrictor L.A. is – *(PGMEE 2014)*
   a. Cocaine
   b. Lidocaine
   c. Procaine
   d. Chlorprocaine

   [Ref: Morgan 6th/e pg. 271, KDT 7th e/pg.364]

Explanation

- Cocaine produces vasoconstriction when applied topically and is a useful agent to reduce pain and epistaxis related to nasal intubation in awake patients.

20. Local Anesthetic first used clinically – *(PGMEE 2014)*
   a. Bupivacaine
   b. Procaine
   c. Cocaine
   d. Lignocaine

   [Ref: KDT 8th/e p. 391, 392]

Explanation

- It was first used for ocular anaesthesia in 1884.
- Procaine It is the first synthetic local anaesthetic introduced in 1905.

21. Cocaine was first used as local anaesthetic by – *(PGMEE 2012)*
   a. Morton
   b. Carl kollar
   c. Holmer wells
   d. None

   [Ref: internet}

22. Effect of cocaine on blood vessels is? *(DNB June' 2011)*
   a. Vasoconstrictor
   b. First constrict then dilates
   c. Vasoineffective
   d. Vasodilator

   [Ref: Morgan 6th/e pg. 271, KDT 7 th e/pg.364]

LIGNOCAINE

23. Concentration of adrenaline used with lidocaine is?
                                                    (DNB Dec' 2011)

a. 1:200	b. 1:2000
c. 1:20000	d. 1:200000

[Ref: KDT 8th/e p. 389; Morgan 6th/e pg. 247]

24. Duration of action of Lidocaine with adrenaline –
                                                    (PGMEE 2014)

a. 15-30 minutes	b. 30-60 minutes
c. 2-3 hours	d. 3-6 hours

[Ref: Internet]

25. Maximum safe dose of lignocaine with adrenaline is:
                                            (DNB 2008, PGMEE 2013, 12)

a. 3 mg/kg wt.	b. 7 mg/kg wt.
c. 10 mg/kg wt.	d. 15 mg/kg wt.

[Ref: Morgan 6th/e pg. 269]

Explanation

- Concentration of the adrenaline is 5 microgram/ml to prepare a 1:200000
- Maximum Dose of lignocaine
  - Plain: 5mg/kg
  - With adrenaline: 7mg/kg

26. About lidocaine, all are true except –   *(PGMEE 2014)*
   a. Acts on mucous membranes
   b. Local anaesthetic effect
   c. Ester
   d. Cardiac arrhythmia

[Ref: Morgan 6th/e pg. 269]

27. Concentration of lignocaine for spinal anesthesia is?

a. 0.5%	b. 2.5% *(DNB June' 2011)*
c. 4%	d. 5%

[Ref: KDT 8th/e p. 396]

Explanation

- ***Drugs used for spinal anaesthesia and their concentrations:***
  - Procaine → 10% solution
  - Lignocaine → 5%
  - Xylocaine heavy → 5%
  - Bupivacaine → 0.75% & 0.5% hyperbaric solution (sensorcaine) in 8.25% dextrose and hypobaric solution
  - Tetracaine → 1% solution in 10% glucose or as niphanoid crystals
  - Ropivacaine → 0.5% in dextrose
  - Levobupivacaine → 0.5%

28. The best anaesthetic agent for acute paronychia is?
   a. 0.5% Xylocaine   *(DNB 2008 pattern)*
   b. 1% xylocaine
   c. Xylocaine + adrenaline
   d. 2% Xylocaine

[Ref: KDT 7th/e pg 369]

Explanation

- Paronychia infections of the nail fold can be caused by bacteria, fungi and some viruses.
- If the paronychia is more advanced, it may need to be incised and drained, a digital anesthetic block is usually necessary. If an anesthetic agent is used, it should consist of 1% lidocaine (Xylocaine) with no epinephrine for a ring block. The local injection of the anesthetic agent into the paronychia or the wound is often inadequate and more painful than the administration of drugs of a **digital ring block**.

BUPIVACAINE

29. Which one of the following local anesthetic is highly cardiotoxic-   *(PGMEE 2013)*
   a. Mepivacaine
   b. Procaine
   c. Lignocaine
   d. Bupivacaine

[Ref.: KDT 8th/e p. 393]

30. Local anesthetic that is not used topically is?
                                                    (DNB June' 2011)

a. Lignocaine	b. Dibucaine
c. Tetracaine	d. Bupivacaine

[Ref: KDT 8th/e p. 393; Morgan 6th/e pg. 269]

LOCAL ANESTHETIC TOXICITY

31. Local anaesthesia causing methemoglobinemia-
   a. Procaine   *(PGMEE 2014)*
   b. Ropivacaine
   c. Etodicaine
   d. Prilocaine

[Ref: Morgan 6th/e pg. 268]

Explanation

- Prilocaine is an oxidizing agent causing toxic methemoglobinemia.
- Methemoglobinemia **is seen with:**
  - Prilocaine
  - Lignocaine
  - Benzocaine
  - N_2O, Nitrites
  - Sulfonamides, phenacetin

32. Drug of choice for lignocaine toxicity –   *(PGMEE 2013)*
   a. Phenytoin
   b. Amiodarone
   c. Beta- blockers
   d. Phenobarbitone

[Ref: Internet]

33. Methemoglobinemia is caused by: *(DNB 2007)*
   a. Bupivacaine
   b. Lignocaine
   c. Prilocaine
   d. Procaine

[Ref: KDT 7ht e/pg.366; Morgan 6th/e pg. 268]

23.	d
24.	c
25.	b
26.	c
27.	d
28.	b
29.	d
30.	d
31.	d
32.	d
33.	c

34. Most cardio toxic local anaesthetic is? *(DNB June' 2010)*

a. Procaine
b. Bupivacaine
c. Prilocaine
d. Lignocaine

[Ref: Morgan 6th/e pg. 271]

Explanation

- All LA block the cardiac conduction system in a dose dependent block of Na⁺ channels.
- Bupivacaine has stronger binding affinity to resting and inactivated Na⁺ channels. Bupivacine dissociates slowly from Na⁺ channels during diastole. It require enough time for complete recovery of Na channels, so bupivacaine conduction block increases.
- The R(+) optical isomer of bupivacaine blocks more avidly and dissociates more slowly from cardiac Na channels than does the S(-) optical isomer. Resuscitation from bupivacaine-induced cardiac toxicity is often difficult and resistant to standard resuscitation drugs.
- Treatment of cardiotoxicity is mainly supportive. Lipid emulsion 20% should be used to remove bupivacaine from its site of action.

TOPICAL ANESTHETIC

35. The topical use of following local anesthetic is not recommended? *(PGMEE 2014)*

a. Cocaine
b. Bupivacaine
c. Ligocaine
d. Dibucaine

[Ref: KDT 7th/e p. 368; Morgan 6th/e pg. 269]

Explanation

- A topical anesthetic is a local anesthetic agent used to anesthetise the surface of a body part.
- They can be used to anesthetise any area of the skin, mucus membrane as well as the front of the eyeball, the inside of the nose, ear or throat, the ano-genital area.
- Topical anesthetics are available in creams, ointments, aerosols, sprays, lotions, and jellies.
- Examples include:- benzocaine, butamben, dibucaine, lidocaine, oxybuprocaine, pramoxine, proparacaine, proxymetacaine, and tetracaine.

36. Local Anaesthetic in wound/ulcer management- *(PGMEE 2015)*

a. Bupivacaine
b. Prilocaine
c. Benzocaine
d. Chlorprocaine

[Ref: KDT 8th/e p. 393]

Explanation

- These LAs are used as lozenges for stomatitis, sore throat; as dusting powder/ointment on wounds/ulcerated surfaces and as suppository for anorectal lesions.

37. Percentage of tetracaine used in eye surgery – *(PGMEE 2015)*

a. 0.5%
b. 1%
c. 2%
d. 4%

[Ref: Morgan 6th/e pg. 781]

Explanation

- A typical regimen for topical local anesthesia consists of application of 0.5% proparacaine local anesthetic drops, repeated at 5-min intervals for five applications.
- Ophthalmic 0.5% tetracaine may also be utilized

38. Which of the following is not primarily used to anesthetize mucosa – *(PGMEE 2015)*

a. Bupivacaine
b. Lidocaine
c. Benzocaine
d. Tetracaine

[Ref: KDT 8th/e p. 394]

39. All of the following are effective topically except – *(PGMEE 2014)*

a. Cocaine
b. Amethocaine
b. Lidocaine
d. Procaine

[Ref: KDT 8th/e p. 394]

40. True about EMLA – *(PGMEE 2015)*

a. Can be used for intubation
b. Mixture of local anesthesia
c. Faster acting
d. Used in children

[Ref: KDT 8th/e p. 392]

41. Eutectic mixture of local anaesthetic (EMLA. cream is – *(PGMEE 2013)*

a. Bupivacaine 2.0% + Prilocaine 2.5 %
b. Lidocaine 2.5% + Prilocaine 2.5%
c. Lidocaine 2.5% + Prilocaine 5%
d. Bupivacaine 0.5% + Lidocaine 2.5%

[Ref: Morgan 6th/e pg. 267]

PERIPHERAL NERVE BLOCK

42. Most commonly used approach of brachial plexus block: *(PGMEE 2013)*

a. Supraclavicular
b. Interscalene
c. Infraclavicular
d. Axillary

[Ref: Morgan 6th/e pg. 1008]

43. Supraclavicular block is used for surgery of – *(PGMEE 2015)*

a. Shoulder
b. Neck
c. Arm
d. Forearm

[Ref: Morgan 6th/e pg. 1008]

44. Not a sign of stellate ganglion block – *(PGMEE 2013)*

a. Exopthalomos
b. Conjunctival redness
c. Nasal congestion
d. Miosis

[Ref: Morgan 6th/e pg. 1097]

Explanation

- Correct placement of the needle is usually followed promptly by an increase in the skin temperature of the ipsilateral arm and the onset of Horner's syndrome
- Consists of ipsilateral ptosis, meiosis, enophthalmos, nasal congestion, and anhydrosis of the neck and face. This may be considered a side effect of the block rather than a complication.

45. Most common complication of celiac plexus block – *(PGMEE 2015)*

a. Pneumothorax
b. Intra- arterial injection
c. Retroperitoneal hemorrhage
d. Postural hypotension

[Ref: Morgan 6th/e pg. 1098]

34.	b
35.	b
36.	c
37.	a
38.	a
39.	d
40.	b,d
41.	b
42.	a
43.	c
44.	a
45.	d

46. Regarding Celiac plexus block all the following are true except- *(PGMEE 2015)*
a. Can be used to provide anesthesia for intra abdominal surgery
b. Cause hypotension
c. Can be given only by retrocrural {classic} approach
d. Relieves pain from gastric malignancy

[Ref: Morgan 6th/e pg. 1098]

BIER'S BLOCK

47. In Bier's block anaesthetic agent given by which route?
a. Retrobulbar area   *(PGMEE 2015)*
b. Peribulbar region
c. Intravenous
d. Dermal

[Ref: Morgan 6th/e pg. 1022]

48. For Bier's block drug of choice is   *(PGMEE 2013)*
a. Prilocaine   b. Bupivacaine
c. Lignocaine   d. None

[Ref: Morgan 6th/e pg. 1022]

49. Local anaesthetic contraindicated in Bier's Block is:- *(PGMEE 2016-17)*
a. Bupivacaine   b. Lignocaine
c. Prilocaine   d. Procaine

SPINAL ANESTHESIA

50. In spinal anesthesia, the needle is pierced upto- *(PGMEE 2014)*
a. Subdural space   b. Subarachnoid space
c. Extradural space   d. Epidural space

[Ref: Morgan 6th/e pg. 975]

51. Not a contraindication for spinal Anaesthesia is :- *(PGMEE 2016-17)*
a. Patient is hypovoluemic
b. Patient's refusal
c. Patient on low dose Ecopsrin
d. Infection at the back

[Ref: Morgan 6th/e pg. 969]

52. First fibres to be blocked in spinal anaesthesia is: *(DNB 2007: DNB Dec' 2011)*
a. Sympathetic preganglionic
b. Different motor nerves
c. Sensory fibres
d. Afferent motor nerves

[Ref: Morgan 6th/e pg. 967]

53. What is the indicator for reaching correct space in spinal anesthesia:- *(PGMEE 2016-17)*
a. Needle placed between duramater and arachanoid
b. Needle placed between piamater and arachanoid
c. Needle placed in epidural space
d. Needle placed in central canal

[Ref: Morgan 6th/e pg. 975]

Explanation

- During spinal anaesthesia needle is placed in subarachnoid space.

- The subarachnoid space lies between the arachanoid mater and pia mater and contains spinal cord, nerve roots and CSF. Piamater is closely adherent to spinal cord.
- Sudural space is potential space between duramater and arachnoid mater.
- Epidural space lies between the spinal meninges and sides of the vertebral canal. It contains fat and veins.

54. Spinal anesthesia should be injected into the space between- *(PGMEE 2014)*
a. $T_{12} - L_1$ b. $L_1 - L_2$
c. $L_3 - L_4$ d. $L_5 - S_1$

[Ref: Morgan 6th/e pg. 966]

55. Spinal anesthesia in children is given at which level- *(PGMEE 2013)*
a. $L_1 - L_2$ b. $L_2 - L_3$
c. $L_3 - L_4$ d. $L_4 - L_5$

[Ref: Morgan 6th/e pg. 966]

56. In high spinal anaesthesia what is seen – *(PGMEE 2013)*
a. Hypotension & Bradycardia
b. Hypertension & Tachycardia
c. Hypertension & Bradycardia
d. Hypotension & Tachycardia

[Ref: Morgan 6th/e pg. 990]

Explanation

- Spinal anesthesia ascending into the cervical levels causes severe hypotension, bradycardia, and respiratory insufficiency.
- Unconsciousness, apnea, and hypotension resulting from high levels of spinal anesthesia are referred to as a "high spinal". or when the block extends to cranial nerves, as a "total spinal".

POST DURAL PUNCTURE HEADACHE (PDPH)

57. Post spinal headache lasts for –   *(PGMEE 2015)*
a. 10 min   b. 1 hrs
c. 10 days   d. 1 week

[Ref: Morgan 6th/e pg. 992]

58. Onset of post spinal headache is usually at _ hours after spinal anesthesia – *(PGMEE 2015)*
a. 0 – 6   b. 6 – 12
c. 12 – 72   d. 72 – 96

[Ref: Morgan 6th/e pg. 992]

Explanation

- The hallmark of PDPH is its association with body position. The pain is aggravated by sitting or standing and relieved or decreased by lying down flat. The onset of headache is usually 12-72 hr following the procedure; however, it may be seen almost immediately.

59. Treatment of choice for post spinal headache – *(PGMEE 2015)*
a. Epidural blood patch
b. IV antibiotics
c. IV fluid and analgesics
d. Epidural fat patch

[Ref: Morgan 6th/e pg. 992]

46.	c
47.	c
48.	a,c
49.	a
50.	b
51.	c
52.	a
53.	b
54.	c
55.	d
56.	a
57.	c
58.	c
59.	c

60. True about post dural puncture headache is all except – *(PGMEE 2015)*

a. Timing of ambulation has no effect over its incidence
b. Orienting beveled edge needle parallel to long axis prevents it
c. It is more common in males
d. Thin bore needle prevents it

[Ref: Morgan 6th/e pg. 992]

61. For prevention of headache during spinal anesthesia- *(PGMEE 2012)*

a. Diluted solution of local anesthetic should be used
b. Preloading with crystalloids
c. Finer L.P. needle should be used
d. Head end should be elevated

[Ref: Morgan 6th/e pg. 992]

62. True about post- spinal headache are all except- *(PGMEE 2013)*

a. Can be prevented by using small bore needle
b. Frontal or occipital
c. Relieved by lying down position
d. Old age is a risk factor

[Ref: Morgan 6th/e pg. 992]

Explanation

- Factors that increase the risk of PDPH include young age, female sex, and pregnancy. The lowest incidence would be expected in an elderly male.

EPIDURAL ANAESTHESIA

63. Macintosh indicator is used for – *(PGMEE 2015)*

a. To assess degree of NM blockade
b. To monitor respiratory depression
c. To assess level of GA
d. Localization of extradural space

[Ref: Internet]

64. Patient using anticoagulants, which anesthesia not used:- *(PGMEE 2016-17)*

a. N_2O
b. Sevoflurane
c. Epidural anesthesia
d. Thiopentone sodium

[Ref: Morgan 6th/e pg. 970]

65. Anaesthesia of choice for vaginal delivery in pre-eclampsisa:- *(PGMEE 2018)*

a. Spinal anaesthesia
b. Epidural anaesthesia
c. Combined spinal and epidural anaesthesia
d. General anaesthesia

[Ref: Morgan 6th/e pg. 884]

Explanation

- Both epidural & Spinal anaesthetics are reasonable choice for cesarean section in a preeclamptic patient.
- **Continuous Epidural Anesthesia is the first choice** for patients with preeclampsia during labour, Vaginal delivery and cesarean section.

- Preeclampsia patient have a risk of severe airway edema, which makes intubation difficult
- Continuous Epidural Anesthesia can improve uteroplacental perfusion and also ↓ catecholamine secretions.
- Hypertension should be controlled and hypovolemia corrected before administration of anesthesia. In the absence of coagulopathy, continuous epidural anesthesia is the first choice for most patients with preeclampsia during labor, vaginal delivery

66. Complications of epidural anesthesia are all except:? *(DNB Dec' 2011)*

a. Hypotension
b. Headache
c. DIC
d. Epidural hematoma

[Ref: Morgan 6th/e pg. 991-993]

Explanation

- Complications of epidural anaesthesia are
  - Hypotension
  - Subdural block
  - Total spinal
  - Accidental intravascular injection
  - Dural puncture
  - Epidural Hematoma
  - Headache

67. Anesthetic agent of choice as epidural anesthesia in labour is? *(DNB June' 2009)*

a. Prilocaine
b. Bupivacaine
c. Procaine
d. Lignocaine

[Ref: Morgan 6th/e pg. 875]

Explanation

- Bupivacaine placental transfer is low. Fetomaternal ratio is 0.32 which is very less
- Placental transfer of lignocaine is very high. FM ratio of lignocaine is 0.73
- Ropivacaine readily crosses placenta.

68. Which drug can't be given in Epidural anaesthesia – *(PGMEE 2012)*

a. Fentanyl
b. Alfentanil
c. Morphine
d. Remifentanil

[Ref: Morgan 6th/e pg. 875]

69. In pediatric epidural anesthesia, volume of local anesthetic given to cause sacral dermatome block is – *(PGMEE 2013)*

a. 0.5 – 1 ml/kg
b. 2 – 4 ml/kg
c. 5 – 10 ml/kg
d. None

[Ref: Morgan's 5th/e pg. 965]

60.	c
61.	c
62.	d
63.	d
64.	c
65.	b
66.	c
67.	b
68.	d
69.	a

MISCELLANEOUS

70. Neuraxial anaesthesia is all expect:
   a. Subarachanoid block
   b. Epidural anaesthesia
   c. Caudal anaesthesia
   d. Lumbar plexus block

[Ref: Morgan 6th/e pg. 989]

71. Sphenopalatine block is given in posterior part of: *(PGMEE 2014)*
   a. Middle turbinate   b. Septum
   c. Inferior turbinate   d. Superior turbinate

[Ref: Morgan 6th/e pg. 1085]

72. Elderly patient with fracture right hip anesthetic of choice: *(PGMEE 2015)*
   a. Local infiltration   b. General anaesthesia
   c. Spinal/epidural   d. None of the above

[Ref: Morgan 6th/e pg. 941]

73. Pudendal nerve block involves – *(DNB Dec' 2009)*
   a. L1 L2 L3
   b. S1 S2 S3
   c. S2 S3 S4
   d. L3 L4 L5

[Ref: Morgan 6th/e pg. 1094]

Explanation

- Pundenal nerve block is to provide perineal anesthesia during second stage of labor. Pudendal nerves are blocked bilaterally while passing over ischial spine.
- The sensory and motor innervation of the perineum is derived from the pudendal nerve, which is composed of the anterior primary divisions of the second, third, and fourth sacral nerves.

CHAPTER-7 ⊕ REGIONAL ANESTHESIA

70.	d
71.	a
72.	c
73.	c

PRIMES ○ (VOLUME II)

1. Which does not cause malignant hyperthermia –
(PGMEE 2012)

a. Desflurane
b. Enflurane
c. N_2O
d. Isoflurane

[Ref: Morgan 6th/e pg. 1216]

2. Agent causing malignant hyperthermia –
(PGMEE 2012, DNB pattern 2007)

a. Ketamine
b. Dantrolence
c. Succinyl choline
d. Gallamine

[Ref: Morgan 6th/e pg. 1216]

Explanation

- Malignant hyperthermia (MH) or malignant hyper-pyrexia is a rare life-threatening condition that is triggered by exposure to certain drugs used for general anesthesia, specifically the volatile anesthetic agents and the neuromuscular blocking agent, succinylcholine.

3. Drug used in treatment of malignant hyperthermia-
(PGMEE 2013)

a. Paracetamol
b. Diazepam
c. Dantroline
d. Phenobarbitone

[Ref: Morgan 6th/e pg. 1218]

4. Receptor responsible for malignant hyperthermia is?
(DNB Dec' 2011)

a. Nicotinic receptor
b. Ryanodine receptor
c. Muscarinic receptor
d. None

[Ref: Morgan 6th/e pg. 1216]

POSTOPERATIVE NAUSEA & VOMITING

5. Risk factors associated with post-operative nausea and vomiting following strabismus surgery are all except –
(PGMEE 2015)

a. Personal or family history of post – op nausea and vomiting
b. Duration of anesthesia > 30 mins
c. Age < 3 year
d. Personal or family history of motion sickness

[Ref: Morgan 6th/e pg. 1292]

MALIGNANT HYPERTHERMIA

6. Which of the following drugs are believed to be effective in the treatment of post-operative shivering?
(PGMEE 2013,14)

a. Pethidine
b. Diclofenac Sodium
c. Ondansetron
d. Paracetamol

[Ref: Morgan 6th/e pg. 1123]

1.	c
2.	c
3.	c
4.	b
5.	c
6.	a
7.	d
8.	d
9.	c
10.	d

MISCELLANEOUS

7. Following are the features of persistent post operative pain except –
(PGMEE 2015)

a. Pain that develops after surgical procedure
b. Pain from pre surgical problem is excluded
c. Pain where other causes are excluded
d. Pain present for atleast 3 months

[Ref: Morgan 5th/e p. 1089]

8. A 33 year old male in post anesthesia care unit has hypertension following uncomplicated hernia repair. There is a past medical history is significant for mild anxiety & childhood asthma. Vital signs include heart rate of 95 beats /min. BP 180/90 respiratory rate 25, SpO_2 100%. Patient rates his pain as 9/10. What is most appropriate initial intervention:
(Recent Pattern June 2018)

a. Labetalol IV
b. Hydralazine IV
c. Lorazepam IV
d. Hydromorphone IV

Explanation

- As there is no significant history or other complication leading to hypertension, the most likely cause of hypertension is because of post operative pain.
- Hence I/V Hydromorphone is the correct answer

9. Ultra short acting beta blocker most commonly used in anaesthesia is –
(PGMEE 2014)

a. Propanalol
b. Nadalol
c. Esmolol
d. Atenolol

[Ref: KDT 8th/e p. 163; Morgan 6th/e pg. 250]

Explanation

- It has been used to terminate supraventricular tachycardia, episodic atrial fibrillation or flutter and arrhythmia during anaesthesia. Esmolol is also very useful for reducing HR and BP during and after cardiac surgery, in aortic dissection and in early treatment of myocardial infarction.

10. Mismatched blood transfusion mainfests intraopera-tively as –
(PGMEE 2014)

a. Hematuria
b. Rise in B.P.
c. Dyspnoea
d. Excessive bleeding

[Ref: Morgan 6th/e pg. 1201]

Explanation

- In anesthetized patients, an acute hemolytic reaction may be manifested by a rise in temperature, unexplained tachycardia, hypotension, hemoglobinuria, and diffuse oozing in the surgical field.

CARDIOVASCULAR DISEASES

1. **A 5 year old child is suffering from cyanotic heart disease. He is planed for corrective surgery. The induction agent of the choice would by –** *(PGMEE 2015)*
   - a. Thiopentone
   - b. Midazolam
   - c. Halothane
   - d. Ketamine

   [Ref: Morgan 6th/e pg. 431]

Explanation

- Ketamine (intramuscular or intravenous) is a commonly used induction agent because it maintains or increases SVR and therefore does not aggravate the right-to-left shunting.

2. **Anesthesia of choice in child with cyanotic heart disease?** *(DNB Dec' 2009)*
   - a. Thiopentone
   - b. Propofol
   - c. Sevoflurane
   - d. Ketamine

   [Ref: Morgan 6th/e pg. 431]

3. **In a patient with severe aortic stenosis which of the following anesthetic techniques is least preferred:** *(Recent Pattern June 2018)*
   - a. Propofol induction
   - b. Etomidate induction
   - c. Spinal anesthetic with 15 mg bupivacaine
   - d. Epidural anesthesia with 2%lidocaine

   [Ref: Morgan 6th/e pg. 422]

Explanation

- *In cases of severe aortic stenosis*, systemic hypotension may leads to myocardial ischaemia and a downward spiral of reduced contractility causing further falls in BP and coronary perfusion. Systemic hypotension must be avoided.
- Anaesthetic techniques that reduce systemic vascular resistance (e.g. regional neuraxial techniques-spinal anesthesia) must be avoided. Hence spinal anaesthesia is the least preferred choice in such cases.

LIVER & KIDNEY DISEASES

4. **A patient of alcoholic liver failure requires general anesthesia agent of choice is–** *(PGMEE 2014)*
   - a. Isoflurane
   - b. Halothane
   - c. Methoxyflurane
   - d. Ether

   [Ref: Morgan 6th/e pg. 743]

Explanation

- A propofol induction followed by isoflurane or sevoflurane in oxygen or an oxygen-air mixture is commonly employed for general anesthesia.

5. **Anesthesia of choice in renal failure-** *(PGMEE 2014)*
   - a. Isoflurane
   - b. Enflurane
   - c. Methoxyflurane
   - d. None

   [Ref: Morgan 6th/e pg. 683]

6. **Skeletal muscle relaxant of choice in liver and renal disease is?** *(DNB Dec' 2010)*
   - a. Mivacurium
   - b. Atracurium
   - c. Gallium
   - d. Vecuronium

   [Ref: Morgan 6th/e pg. 683]

RESPIRATORY DISEASES

7. **Best anaesthesia for status asthmaticus –** *(PGMEE 2014)*
   - a. Thiopentone
   - b. N_2O
   - c. Ether
   - d. Ketamine

   [Ref: Morgan 6th/e pg. 179]

Explanation

- Anesthetic drug of choice for status asthmaticus is ketamine because it causes bronchodialation.
- Inhalational agent of choice is halothane

OBSTETRICS ANESTHESIA

8. **Current mode of analgesia best for intrapartum pain relief–** *(PGMEE 2014)*
   - a. Inhalational
   - b. Spinal anesthesia
   - c. Local analgesia
   - d. Epidural analgesia

   [Ref: Morgan 6th/e pg. 865]

OCULAR ANESTHESIA

9. **Best local anaesthesia for ophthalmic surgery is –** *(PGMEE 2013)*
   - a. Procaine
   - b. Prilocaine
   - c. Bupivacaine
   - d. Tetracaine

   [Ref: Morgan 6th/e pg. 781]

10. **A five year old child is scheduled for strabismus {squint} correction. Induction of aneasthesia is uneventful. After conjunctival incision as the surgeon grasps the medical rectus, the anaesthesiologist looks at the cardiac monitor. Why do you think he did that?** *(PGMEE 2014)*
    - a. He wanted to see if there was an oculocardiac reflex
    - b. He wanted to be sure that the blood pressure did not fall
    - c. He wanted to check depth of anaesthesia
    - d. He wanted to make sure there were no ventricular dysarhythmias which normally accompany incision

    [Ref: Morgan 6th/e pg. 775]

1.	d
2.	d
3.	c
4.	a
5.	a
6.	b
7.	d
8.	d
9.	d
10.	a

11. **During a surgery on eyeball in a child heart rate falls to 40 from 140 baseline value when traction applied to ocular muscles. What will be your immediate action?** *(PGMEE 2018)*

   a. Give atropine
   b. Give glycopyrolate
   c. Ask the surgeon to stop surgery
   d. Lighter plane of anaesthesia

   [Ref: Morgan 6th/e pg. 776]

Explanation

- Sudden drop in heart rate during eye surgery is due to oculocardiac reflex.

Oculocardiac Reflex

- "The oculocardiac reflex" is defined clinically as a decrease in heart rate by 10% following pressure to the globe or traction of the ocular muscles.
- *Triggering Stimuli*
   ○ Traction on the extraocular muscles (especially medial rectus),
   ○ Direct pressure on the globe,
   ○ Ocular manipulation, ocular pain.
   ○ Retrobulbar block (pressure associated with local infiltration), ocular trauma, or manipulation of tissue in orbital apex after enulcleation.
- Hypoxia, hypercarbia, acidosis, and **light anesthesia can worsen the severity of the OCR**. (Option "D" ruled out).
- May occur during both local and general anesthesia.
- The retrobulbar block may prevent arrythmias by blocking the afferent limb, but may also stimulate the OCR with pressure of local injection.
- Intraoperative Management
   ○ Notify the surgeon to stop orbital stimulation. Removal of the stimulus is immediately indicated
   ○ Optimize oxygenation and ventilation.
   ○ Prevent light anesthesia.
   ○ If arrythmia/bradycardia does not resolve consider atropine 20 mcg/kg IV (or glycopyrrolate).
   ○ In extreme cases, such as asystole, CPR may be required

11.	c
12.	c
13.	d
14.	d
15.	a
16.	b
17.	c

NEURO SURGERY

12. **Inhalational agent of choice for neurosurgery –** *(PGMEE 2013)*

   a. N$_2$O
   b. Halothane
   c. Isoflurane
   d. Enflurane

   [Ref: KDT 5th/e p. 380]

13. **Which anaesthetic is cerebroprotective –** *(PGMEE 2014)*

   a. Enflurane
   b. Sevoflurane
   c. Halothane
   d. Isoflurane

   [Ref: KDT 8th/e p. 407; Morgan 6th/e pg. 165]

14. **Inhalation agent of choice in head injury with raised ICT is :** *(PGMEE 2015)*

   a. Sevoflurane
   b. Enflurane
   c. Halothane
   d. Isoflurane

   [Ref: KDT 8th/e p. 407; Morgan 6th/e pg. 165]

PEDIATRIC ANESTHESIA

15. **All of the following anesthetics are used in children except:** *(PGMEE 2015)*

   a. Desflurane
   b. Halothane
   c. Propofol
   d. Sevoflurane

   [Ref: Morgan 6th/e pg. 906]

16. **In a child with intestinal obstruction with deranged liver function test, the anesthetic of choice is –** *(PGMEE 2014)*

   a. Enflurane
   b. Sevoflurane
   c. Halothane
   d. Isoflurane

   [Ref: Morgan 6th/e pg. 906]

17. **Anesthesia of choice for induction of anesthesia in children is?** *(DNB June' 2010)*

   a. Isoflurane
   b. Halothane
   c. Sevoflurane
   d. Desflurane

   [Ref: Morgan 6th/e pg. 906]

PAIN MANAGEMENT

1. **Following group of drugs are not the first line in the management of chronic pain–** *(PGMEE 2015)*
   a. Antiepileptics
   b. Dopamine antagonist
   c. Serotonergic
   d. Opioids

   [Ref: Morgan 6th/e pg. 1078-79]

2. **↑ response to noxious stimulation is known as:** *(PGMEE 2016-17)*
   a. Allodynia
   b. Hyperalgesia
   c. Paraesthesia
   d. Hypesthesia

   [Ref: Morgan 6th/e pg. 1050]

Explanation

Terms used in pain management

Term	Description
Allodynia	Perception of an ordinarily nonnoxious stimulus as pain
Analgesia	Absence of pain perception
Anesthesia	Absence of all sensation
Anesthesia dolorosa	Pain in an area that lacks sensation
Dysesthesia	Unpleasant or abnormal sensation with or without a stimulus
Hypalgesia (hypoalgesia)	Diminished response to noxious stimulation (e.g., pinprick)
Hyperalgesia	Increased response to noxious stimulation
Hyperesthesia	Increased response to mild stimulation
Hyperpathia	Presence of hyperesthesia, allodynia, and hyperalgesia usually associated with overreaction, and persistence of the sensation after the stimulus
Hyperthesia (hypoesthesia)	Reduced cutaneous sensation (e.g., light touch, pressure, or temperature)
Neuralgia	Pain in the distribution of a nerve or a group of nerves
Paresthesia	Abnormal sensation perceived without an apparent stimulus
Radiculopathy	Functional abnormality of one or more nerve roots

3. **Visual analogue scale [VAS] most widely used to measure –** *(PGMEE 2014)*
   a. Pain intensity
   b. Sedation
   c. Depth of anaesthesia
   d. Sleep

   [Ref: Morgan 6th/e pg. 1063]

4. **Best scale to measure pain in children of 5 years age would be–** *(PGMEE 2014)*
   a. Mc Gill scale
   b. Faces scale
   c. CHEOPS
   d. VAS

   [Ref: Ajay Yadav 4th/e p. 200]

HYPOTENSIVE ANESTHESIA

5. **Hypotensive anesthesia in nasopharyngeal angiofibroma is/are given by –** *(PGMEE 2015)*
   a. Ketamine
   b. Na+ Nitroprusside
   c. Phentolamine
   d. Halothane

   [Ref: Morgan 6th/e pg. 255]

MISCELLANEOUS

6. **Intra ocular pressure rises in –** *(PGMEE 2013)*
   a. LMA
   b. Bag and mask ventilation
   c. Infusion of IV propofol
   d. Intubation & laryngoscopy

   [Ref: Morgan 6th/e pg. 335 & 775]

7. **For foreign body causing sudden choking, most appropriate first line management is?** *(PGMEE 2011)*
   a. Airway insertion
   b. Tracheostomy
   c. Laryngoscopy
   d. Heimlich maneuver

   [Ref: Harrison's 19th/e p.1768]

8. **Foley's Catheter of size 16 F means?** *(PGMEE 2010)*
   a. 16 mm inner diameter
   b. 16 mm outer diameter
   c. 16 mm diameter at the tip
   d. 16 mm circumference

9. **What is the time for which a nurse should do suction in a tracheostomised patient?** *(NEET Pattern 2017)*
   a. 10–15 sec
   b. 30 sec
   c. 45 sec
   d. 60 sec

Explanation

- There are 2 types of suctioning used in ICU:-
  1. **Open suction:** Disconnect the ventilator from ETT and do endotracheal suctioning for 10-15 sec.
  2. **Closed suction:** Suction system remains in line for 24 hours and can be used for multiple endotracheal suctioning procedures.

1.	b
2.	b
3.	a
4.	c
5.	b
6.	d
7.	d
8.	b
9.	a

Radiology

FACTS

- *Electromagnetic radiation:*
  - Include waves like light, UV, X-rays and γ rays.
  - Velocity of EM waves – 3×10^8 m/s
- *Corpuscular radiation* includes:
  - Particles like electrons, protons, neutrons, mesons, alpha α and δ beta particles.
- Maximum penetrating power → γ rays.
- Maximum biological damage is caused by (Maximum ionizing power and maximum DNA damage) → α waves.
- Maximum Linear Energy Transfer (LET) value → X-ray.
- Maximum Oxygen enhancement ratio is with → Neutrons.
- Bragg peak effect is pronounced in Proton therapy
- *PACS* → Picture Archiving and Communication System
- *DICOM* → Digital Imaging and Communication in Medicine
- *BIRADS* → Breast Imaging-Reporting and Data System
  - It applies to mammography, ultrasound, and MRI imaging of breast.
- *LIRADS* → Liver Reporting and Data System
  - For standardizing data collection and reporting of CT and MR in patients with hepatocellular carcinoma

Scientist	Contribution
W.C. Roentgen	Father of X-ray
Henri Becquerel	Father of radioactivity
Robert Egan	Father of Mammography
Sir Godfrey Hounsfield	Father of CT scan
Paul Lautenbur Peter Mansfield	Principle of MRI
John Wild	Father of medical USG
Sir Ian Donald	Father of obstetric USG

	X-rays	γ-rays
Type of	▪ EM waves	▪ EM waves
Origin	▪ Extra-nuclear	▪ Intra-nuclear
Produced by	▪ Collision of electrons with anode	▪ Isotopes by radioactive decay

REMEMBER

Contrast agents:	Risk factors for Contrast-Induced Nephropathy:
• CT – Iodinated contrast	• Dehydration
• MRI – Gadolinium	• Diabetic nephropathy
• USG – Optison, Levovist	• High osmolar agents
• Esophageal atresia – Dianosil	• Concurrent administration of nephrotoxic drugs
• Esophageal perforation – Iohexol	

X-RAYS

- X-ray was discovered on November 8, 1895
- 8th November is celebrated as International day of Radiology
- Wave length of X-ray = 0.1–1 Å.
- In an X-ray tube → Cathode is heated up → Electron particles are removed from tungsten filament → this process is known as → *Thermionic emission*.
- X-rays are produced when the electronic beam decelerates and collide with the target anode
- *In Modern X-ray tubes:*
  - Cathode is made up of Tungsten + Thorium
  - Anode is made up of Tungsten + 10% Rhenium
  - Target anode is rotating and heat loss takes place via radiation

- Anode has 2 parts:
  - Front (Target part) is made up of tungsten
  - Back part is made up of Copper as it is a good conductor of heat.
- *Photoelectric effect:* emission of inner shell electron when a light strikes a metal surface
- *Compton effect:* Scattering of the incoming X-ray by an outer atomic electron
- Photoelectric effect is due to emission of electrons from innermost shell (usually K-shell).
- *X-ray film:*
  - Double coated film made up of photosensitive emulsion (Silver bromide + Silver iodide).
  - Single coated films are used in → Mammography.
  - Most sensitive to Blue light
  - Least sensitive to red light which is considered safe light and is used in dark rooms.

- *Kilo volt peak (KV_P):*
  - Determine penetrating power of X-rays.
  - Obese/heavily built patient require ↑ in KVp.
  - Contrast inversely depends on KV_{P}.
- *MAS (Mili Ampere Second):*
  - Determines electron flows to X-ray tube
  - se MAS is directly related to no. of electron
  - Exposure depends on MAS.
- Contrast is influenced by both kVP and mAS
- kVP is inversely proportional whereas mAS is directly proportional to the contrast produced
- Penetrating power of the X-rays can be increased by increasing energy/increasing frequency or decreasing wavelength
- Protective LED apron is 0.25–0.5 mm thick.
- Radiation dose monitoring is done by using "TLD Batch" (Thermoluminescent dosimetry).

Chest X-ray

- Normal hilar shadow on CXR is produced by:
  - Pulmonary artery
  - Bronchus
  - Upper lobe veins
- Best view in CXR → PA view
- CXR (PA view) is done in erect position and in end inspiration
- Best view for pneumothorax on CXR: PA view in full expiration
- Middle lobe pathologies are best seen on: Lordotic view
- Obliteration of right cardiac border on CXR indicates pathology of: Right middle lobe
- *Lateral decubitus X-ray:*
  - Is the best view to detect minimum pleural effusion
  - Minimum amount of fluid that can be detected is 25–30 mL

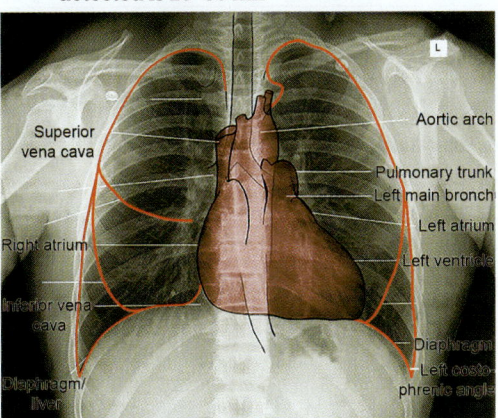

Borders of the heart

Air bronchogram:

- It is considered as a sign of alveolar pathology.
- Common cause of air bronchogram-
  - Pneumonia/Consolidation
  - Hyaline membrane disease
  - Pulmonary edema
  - Bronchoalveolar carcinoma

Signs of LA enlargement:

- Straightening of left heart border – earliest
- Double atrial shadow
- Elevation of left main bronchus and widening of carina
- Posterior displacement of esophagus

Eggshell calcification of lymph node on CXR:

- Silicosis
- Sarcoidosis
- Post radiation lymphoma
- Tuberculosis
- Histoplasmosis

D/D of Miliary shadow on CXR:

- Tuberculosis
- Histoplasmosis
- Sarcoidosis
- Coal worker pneumoconiosis
- Silicosis

Mammography

- Single-coated film is used.
- Target is made up of **M**olybdenum.
- In routine mammography, views included are → CC (crania caudal) and MLO (Medio-lateral oblique).

- All breast imaging including mammography should be reported according to BIRADS

CT SCAN

- Walls of the CT scan room is coated with lead
- *CT scan is IOC in:*
  - Pulmonary embolism → MDCT or CT angiography (in pregnancy, V/Q scan in preferred)
  - Aortic dissection → CT angiography (Gold standard is MRI)
  - Cerebral aneurysm → CT angiography
  - SAH → CT angiography
  - Stroke, Head injury, Acute brain hemorrhage, and Intracranial calcification → NCCT
  - Solitary Pulmonary Nodule → CT > PET
  - Lung malignancy
  - Urinary calculi → NCCT
- Cardiac CT is done at → Mid-diastole as heart movement is less.
- Beta blockers are used as premedication for cardiac CT to get better image.
- *Coronary calcium scoring:*
  - Estimation of calcium in coronaries (presuming atherosclerosis)

- Done with MDCT using AGATSON'S score.
- Respiratory gating in CT is used for tumor near diaphragm.
- **Swallow tail** is normal CT scan finding of Substantia nigra, it is absent in parkinsonism.
- ***Kernohan notch phenomenon*** → False localizing sign seen in ipsilateral weakness due to mid brain compression by uncal herniation.
- Hounsfield unit depends on: Attenuation coefficient

Hounsfield unit (HU) scale:

Contrast	Tissue	HU
White	Cortical Bone	+ 1000
	Hemorrhage	+ 60-70
	Brain tissue	+ 20-40
Dark	Water	0
	Fat	− 100
Black	Air	− 1000

High Resolution CT Scan (HRCT)

- Use to evaluate lung parenchyma diseases.
- HRCT takes 1–2 mm thickness of lung section
- *Investigation of Choice* for:

  - Bronchiectasis
  - Interstitial Lung Diseases
  - Miliary Tuberculosis

Spiral CT vs MDCT

	Spiral CT	**MDCT**
Aka	Single slice CT	Multi detector/Multi slice CT
Based on	*Slip ring* technology	Multiple rows of detector
Technique	• Simultaneous patient movement and X-ray tube rotation. • It can scan entire trunk in single breath hold. • No respiratory muscle registration. • Volume image acquisition.	• Cone shaped X-ray beam is used
Advantage	3D Multiplanner reconstruction is possible	Cardiovascular imaging is possible

MRI

- *Faraday cage:* Shielding of MRI room by copper to minimize electromagnetic interference
- Magnetic field strength of MRI machines is measured in Tesla.
- Human body has H^+ ions (protons) which are responsible for MR Imaging.
- Time of flight technique is employed in MR imaging
- Functional MRI is based on BOLD technique
- *FLAIR image* (Fluid Attenuated Inversion Recovery image) suppresses the bright CSF on T_2W images. Used in cerebral edema.
- Earliest diagnosis of cerebral infarct is made via Diffusion weighted MRI/DwMRI
- IOC in optic neuritis is → Gadolinium enhanced MRI brain and orbit

CT v/s MRI in Bone diseases

CT scan is IOC in	MR is IOC in
▪ Lesions of cortex of bone ▪ Ankle fracture ▪ Osteoid Osteoma	▪ Avascular necrosis ▪ Stress #, Occult # ▪ Acute osteomyelitis ▪ Marrow pathology ▪ Muscle, cartilage, and tendon pathology

Characteristics of MR Signals

Appearance of	T_1 Weighted Image (T_1W)	T_2 Weighted Image (T_2W)
Aka	▪ Spin lattice	▪ Spin-Spin
Water, CSF, Vitreous	▪ Dark (hypo intense)	▪ White (hyper intense)
Fat	▪ White	▪ Less white
White matter	▪ White	▪ Dark
Early subacute hemorrhage	▪ White	▪ Dark
Late subacute hemorrhage	▪ White	▪ White
Chronic hemorrhage	▪ Dark	▪ Dark
Ligaments/tendons, Cortical bone, Calcium	▪ Dark/Black	▪ Black
Best for	▪ Subacute hemorrhage	▪ Chronic hemorrhage

ULTRASOUND (USG)

- In medical ultrasound, very high frequencies are used [>2 MHz (>20,000 KHz) up to 30 MHz]
- Principal of USG is based on **Piezoelectric** effect.
- USG probe is made up of: "PZT crystal (Lead, Zirconium, Titanium).
- No radiation exposure.
- Contrast for USG → Sonovist.
- USG is safest investigation in obstetric patient.
- Tissue harmonic imaging is related to USG
- US elastography can tell about hardness of tissue
- Fibroscan is a type of USG elastography and helps to access early changes of cirrhosis
- *Modes in USG:*
  - A mode – used in ophthalmology
  - B mode – for all routine scans
  - M mode – echocardiography

Frequencies used in various USG probes

Type of Ultrasound	Probe Frequency
Transthoracic ECHO (TTE)	2–3 MHz
Transabdominal USG	3–5 MHz
Transesophageal ECHO (TEE), Transvaginal USG (TVS)	5–7.5 MHz
USG for breast	15 MHz
Endoscopic USG for gut wall	7.5–20 MHz
To image vessel wall via catheter	20 MHz
A-mode in eye	50–100 MHz

Important Signs on USG

Lesion/Pathology	Appearance
▪ Cyst or fluid on USG	Anechoic (Black)
▪ Stones, Bones, calcification, air	Hyper echoic (White)
▪ Water, Bile, Blood	Black
▪ Optic chiasm glioma, Hurler syndrome, Achondroplasia	Double barrel sign on USG
▪ Acute hepatitis	**Starry sky appearance**
▪ Adenomyomatosis of Gallbladder	**"Comet tail sign"**
▪ Chronic cholecystitis	**Wall Echo Shadow (WES) sign**
▪ Biliary atresia	Triangular card sign Ghost Gall bladder
▪ CBD obstruction	Double barrel sign

Doppler Ultrasound

- Principle → change in frequency of sound
- Color in doppler is based on → Direction of flow.
  - Red → Towards the USG probe
  - Blue → Away from the USG probe
- *Doppler is IOC for:*
  - DVT
  - Screening of carotid stenosis
  - Testicular torsion
  - In pregnancy to evaluate IUGR
- Reversal of diastolic flow on Doppler → Indicates impending IUGR
- Uterine artery Doppler is useful in → Pre-eclampsia.
- Increase fetal middle cerebral arterial Peak systolic velocity indicate moderate-to-severe anemia in non-hydrops fetuses
- Monophasic waveform of the venous blood flow in lower limbs is suggestive of DVT

MISCELLANEOUS

Nuclear scan
- **Tc 99m:**
  - "m" stands for meta stable isomer.
  - Half-life is 6 hours.
  - Produces gamma rays.

SPECT
- Single photon emission computed tomography.
- 3 dimensional nuclear scan using Tc 99m
- Done to assess cerebral perfusion.
- Use of Tc-HMPAD SPECT gives idea about origin of dementia.

PET
- **Positron** emission tomography.

- Cyclotron, a special machine is used to produce high speed particle accelerator proton.
- Most commonly used isotope in PET is F-18 Deoxyglucose (FDG).
  - Nonmetabolizable glucose analogue
  - $T_{1/2}$ is 110 min.
  - Brown fat (supraclavicular) and brain show high uptake of FDG.
- *PET scan is IOC for:*
  - Solitary pulmonary nodule
  - Staging for cancer patients
  - Brain tumors (C^{11} methionine PET).
- For localizing extra adrenal/abdominal pheochromocytoma F-DOPA PET is used.

Cardiac Imaging

Myocardial perfusion scintigraphy	Myocardial infarct scintigraphy
▪ Thallium scan ▪ Tc – Tetrofosmon ▪ Tc- sestamibi	Tc- pyrophosphate Infarct area is Hot spot

- Reversible myocardial ischemia is detected by: Thallium scan
- Ventricular function can also be assessed by *MUGA scan* (multi uptake gated acquisition) using Tc labeled RBCs.

- *Cardiac MRI -*
  - Most accurate assessment for ventricular function.
  - IOC for pericardial thickness assessment using Tc labeled RBCs.
  - IOC for cardiac, pericardial tumors.
- IOC for Pericardial effusion→ ECHO.
- IOC for Pericardial calcification→ CT.
- IOC for myocardial scar assessment → PET CT.
- Myocardial viability and metabolism are assessed by FDG.

Bone Scan

- Radionuclide used is → Tc 99m MDP (Methyl Di Phosphate) → has polyphosphate chain, so it selectively goes to bone.
- Bone scan is highly sensitive investigation for **metastases**. Metastases produce hot spots.

- Bone scan NOT useful for multiple myeloma because it does NOT accumulate MDP. X-ray is because sensitive in MM.
- *NaF PET (fluorinated PET)* is used now a days for metastases (it is more sensitive than Tc 99m).

DEXA Scan

- Dual Energy X ray Absorptiometry aka Bone density scanning or bone densitometry.
- Used to assess
  - Osteoporosis
  - BMD (bone mineral density)
- **T score** is used to compare BMD of young

adult of same sex. According to WHO, T score < - 2.5 is indicative of osteoporosis.
- **Z score:** Number of standard deviation above and below what's normally expected for one's age sex and weight

Miscellaneous Radionuclide Scan

- *Tc RBC scan* is used to localize site of lower GI bleeding. Can detect blood loss as low as 0.1ml/min.

- *Tc Pertechnetate scan* is used for Meckel's diverticulum. Used to localize gastric mucosa.
- *Tc sulfur colloid scan* is based on macrophage uptake in Kupffer cells of liver.

SYSTEMIC RADIOLOGY

IMPORTANT RADIOLOGICAL FINDINGS IN LUNG DISEASES

Asbestosis:
- Pleural plaques due to partial pleural calcification
- Holly leaf sign on CXR
- Comet tail/Crow feet sign on CT chest
- Round atelectasis (Asbestos Pseudotumor)

Pneumocystis Carinii Pneumonia (PCP):
- Perihilar infiltrates (Bat wing like distribution)
- Pneumatocele on CXR
- On Gallium scan – Hot nodules

Hydatid disease:
- Cart wheel appearance (USG)
- Air between pericyst and ectocyst → Air crescent sign.

- If ectocyst rupture in hydatid cyst → Onion peel sign.
- If only endocyst rupture → Water lily sign/ Camalote sign in CXR.

Pulmonary embolism:
- Focal oligemia on CXR → Westermark's sign.
- Peripheral wedge shaped infarct with convexity towards hilum produce → Hampton's hump.
- Dilated right descending pulmonary artery → Palla's sign.
- Best screening test → D-dimer assay.
- IOC → CT angiography

Important Radiological Signs in Respiratory Diseases

	Finding	Seen in
CXR	▪ Ellis curve	▪ Pleural effusion
	▪ 'D' shaped opacity along chest wall	▪ Loculated effusion
	▪ **Deep sulcus sign** (Deep costophrenic angle)	▪ Pneumothorax
	▪ **Golden 'S' sign** (Central part of tissue pushed down)	▪ Right upper lobe collapse as in Bronchogenic carcinoma
	▪ Popcorn calcification	▪ Pulmonary hamartoma
	▪ Batwing appearance	▪ Pulmonary edema
CT Scan	▪ **Tree in bud sign**	▪ Endobronchial Tuberculosis ▪ Bronchiolitis ▪ Bronchiectasis ▪ Atypical pneumonia
	▪ **Air crescent sign**	▪ Aspergillosis
	▪ **Monod sign** – Air surrounding a mass	▪ Pulmonary tuberculosis ▪ Aspergilloma
	▪ **Halo sign**	▪ Invasive aspergillosis
	▪ **Reverse Halo sign/Atoll sign**	▪ Cryptogenic organizing pneumonia
	▪ **Split Pleura sign**	▪ Empyema
USG	▪ **Barcode sign**	▪ Pneumothorax

Intracerebral Hemorrhage

	Epidural/Extradural Hemorrhage (EDH)	Subdural Hemorrhage (SDH)	Subarachnoid Hemorrhage (SAH)
Etiology	▪ Injury to Middle meningeal artery	▪ Injury to cortical bridging veins	▪ Trauma – MC cause ▪ Rupture of Berry aneurysm
CT Scan	▪ Biconvex shaped hemorrhage	▪ Crescentic (Concavo-convex)	▪ Sulcus hyperdensity
Features	▪ Hematoma limited by sutures	▪ Hematoma is limited by dural attachments	▪ Hallmark of SAH is blood in CSF detected by LP.
Other	▪ Lucid interval + ▪ It is a surgical emergency	▪ Hyperdense (<2 weeks) ▪ Isodense (2-4weeks) ▪ Hypodense (>4 weeks)	▪ NCCT is the investigation of choice ▪ Four vessels DSA (Both carotid and both vertebral artery) is the IOC

● *Hemorrhages in brain:*
  ○ Acute hemorrhages → Hyperdense (white)
  ○ CSF → Hypodense (Black)
  ○ Subacute hemorrhages → Isodense to brain (So most likely to be missed on CT scan)

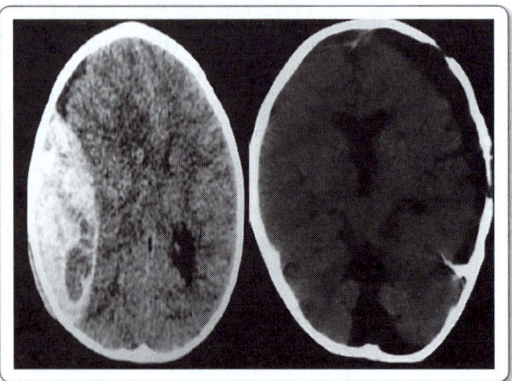

CT scan EDH (Extradural hematoma) and Chronic SDH

Aneurysmal Bleed

Source	Radiological	Clinical
SAH	▪ Blood in sylvian fissure	▪ Thunderclap headache
Basilar artery aneurysm	▪ Intraventricular bleed in 3rd ventricle	▪ Oculomotor palsy
PICA aneurysm	▪ Intraventricular bleed in 4th ventricle	▪ Lateral Medullary Syndrome

Important Radiological Signs in Brain

Sign	Modality	Diagnosis
Empty delta sign	CECT	Sagittal sinus thrombosis
Empty sella sign	Skull X-ray	Pseudotumor cerebri
Erosion of dorsum sella	Skull X-ray	Raised ICT
"J"-shaped sella	Lateral view of the skull on X-ray	Optic chiasm glioma, Hurler syndrome, achondroplasia
"Humming Bird" sign	MRI	Progressive Supranuclear palsy (PSP)
"Tiger eye" sign	MRI	Hallervorden –Spatz syndrome (Neurodegeneration with iron accumulation)
Bull's eye sign	MRI	Peripheral plexiform-neurofibromas
Racing car sign	MRI	Corpus callosum Agenesis
Banana sign *Lemon Sign*		Spina bifida associated with Arnold Chiari II malformation
Panda sign	MRI	Wilson's disease

MRI BRAIN

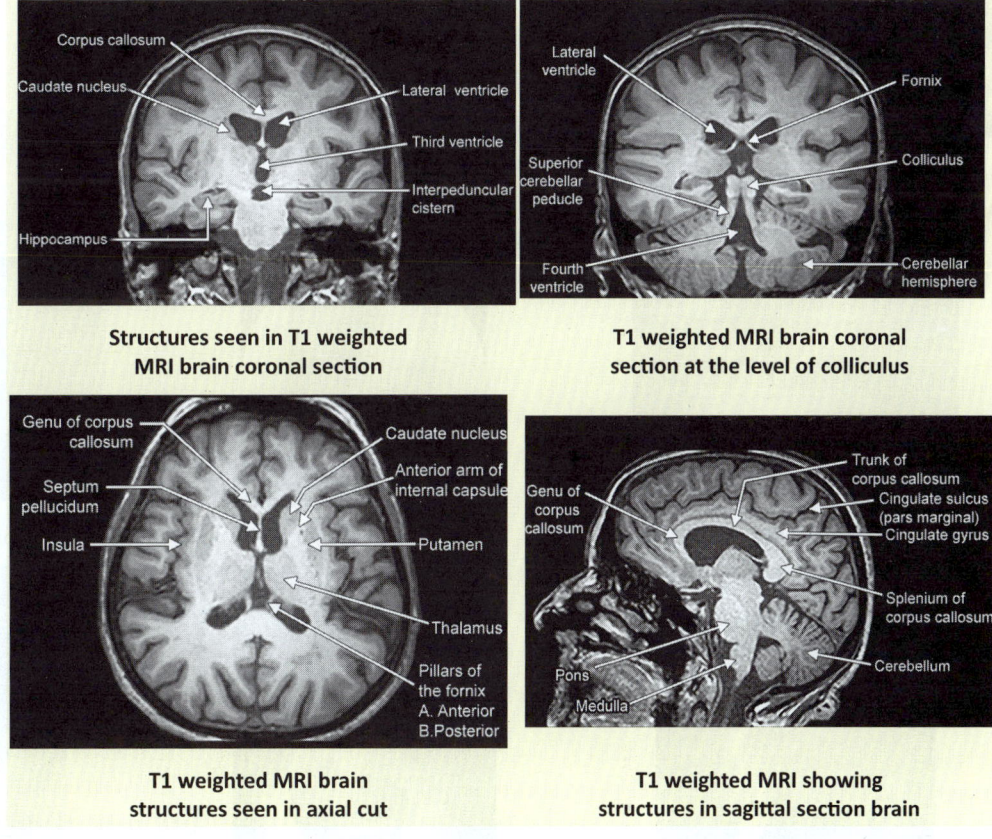

Structures seen in T1 weighted MRI brain coronal section

T1 weighted MRI brain coronal section at the level of colliculus

T1 weighted MRI brain structures seen in axial cut

T1 weighted MRI showing structures in sagittal section brain

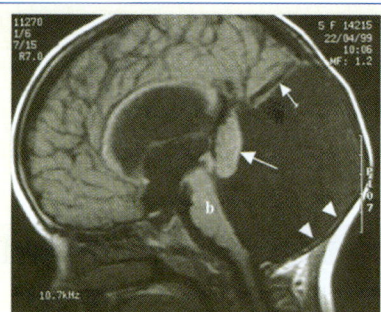

- Dandy-Walker malformation is a rare congenital malformation of cerebellum and fourth ventricle.
- The characteristic triad of Dandy-Walker malformation is:
  - Complete or partial agenesis of the vermis
  - Cystic dilatation of the fourth ventricle
  - An enlarged posterior fossa with upward displacement of lateral sinuses and tentorium.
  - It may be associated with atresia of the foramen of Luschka and Magendie and Obstructive hydrocephalus secondary to cystic dilatation of the fourth ventricle.

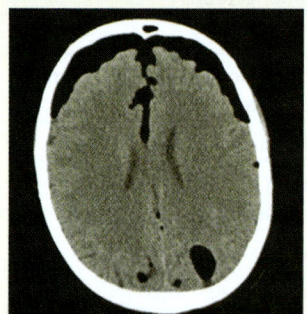

- **Pneumocephalus** refers to the presence of intracranial gas.
- Rarely a gas forming infection can result in pneumocephalus.
- CT scans of patients with a tension pneumocephalus typically show air that compresses the frontal lobes of the brain, which results in a tented appearance of the brain in the skull known as the **Mount Fuji sign.**

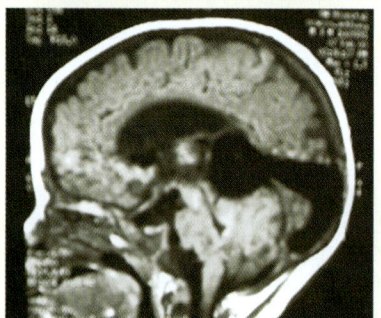

- Vein of Galen Malformation (VGAM) usually causes high-output heart failure in the newborn or may present with developmental delay, hydrocephalus, and seizures.
- It is the most common antenatal diagnosed intracranial vascular malformation.

IMPORTANT SIGNS

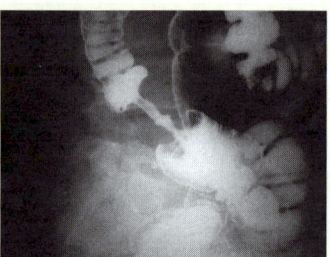

Apple core sign

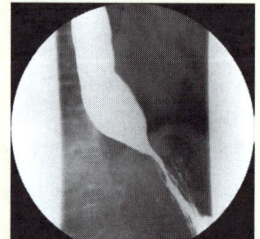

Bird beak sign

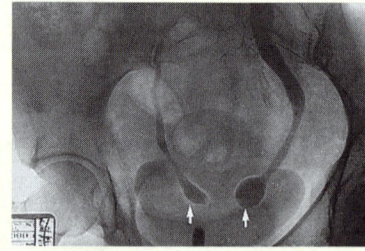

Cobra head appearance

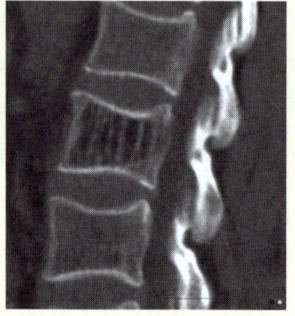

Corduroy sign

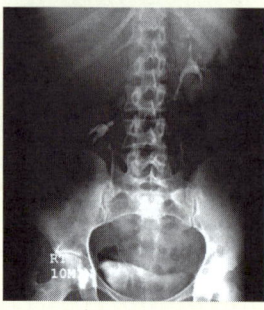

Drooping lily sign

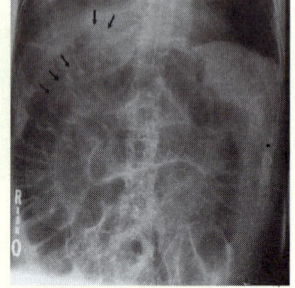

Double wall sign

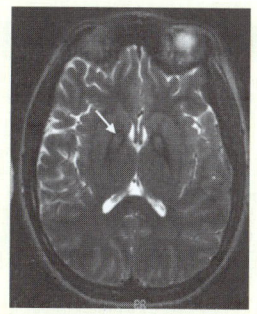

Eye of Tiger sign

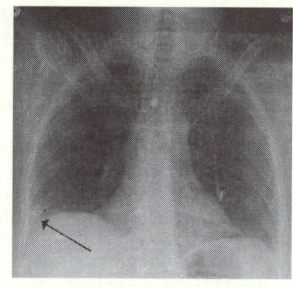

Hampton hump

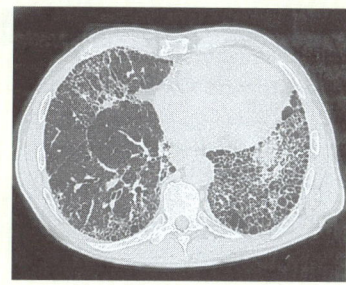

Honeycombing

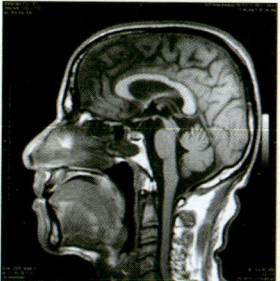

Hummingbird sign

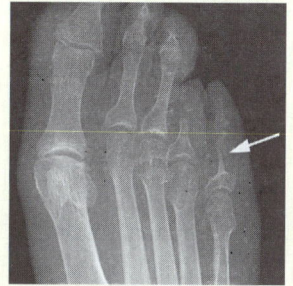

Licked candy stick appearance

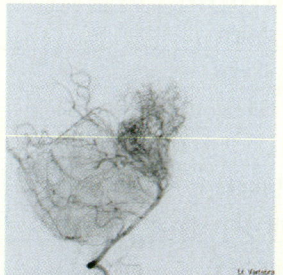

Puff of smoke sign

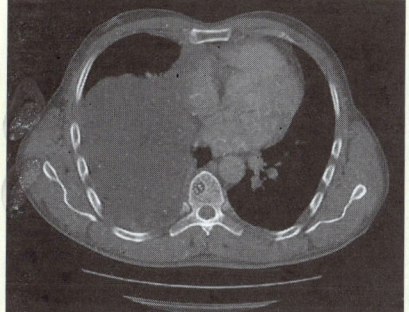

Polka dot sign

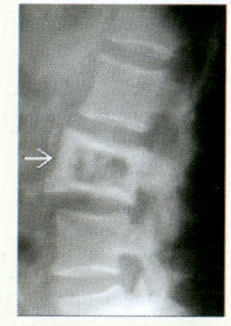

Picture frame vertebra

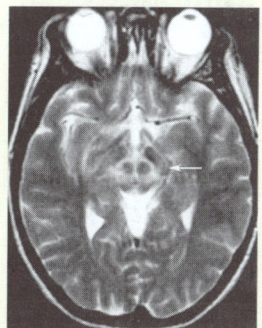

Panda sign

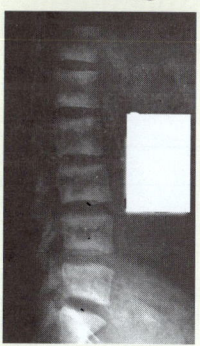

Rugger jersey spine

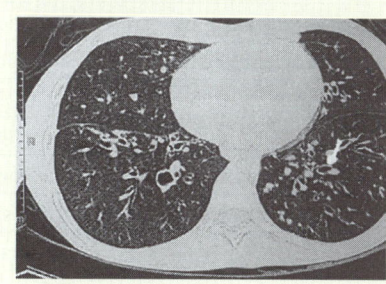

Signet ring

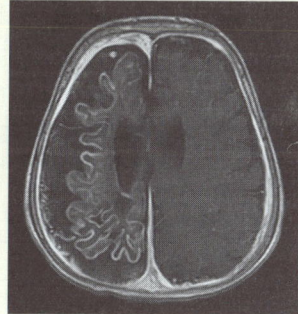

Tram track sign (Sturge-Weber syndrome)

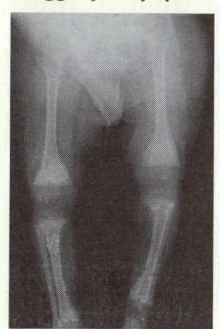

Wimberger's ring sign

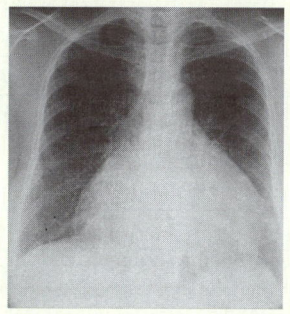

Water bottle/Money bag sign

IMPORTANT RADIOLOGICAL SIGNS

Sign	Modality	Seen in
Swirl sign	NCCT	Acute intracranial hemorrhage
Bare orbit sign	X-ray	Neurofibromatosis 1
Empty delta sign	CECT	Dural venous sinus thrombosis of superior sagittal sinus
Empty sella sign	MRI	Pseudotumor cerebri
MCA dot sign/Sylvian fissure sign	MCCT Head	Thromboembolism of distal MCA
Cingulate sulcus sign	MRI	Normal pressure hydrocephalus
Mother in law sign	Cerebral angiography	Meningioma
Spoke wheel sign	MRI	
Sunburst sign	MRI	
Dural tail sign	MRI	
Comet tail sign	CT	Lung atelectasis
Ivy sign	MRI	Moyamoya disease
Puff of smoke	Angiography	
Leopard skin sign	MRI	Metachromatic leukodystrophy
Tiger eye sign	MRI	Hallervorden Spatz syndrome
Bull's eye sign	MRI	Peripheral plexiform neurofibromas
Hummingbird sign/Penguin sign	MRI	Progressive Supranuclear Palsy
Panda sign	MRI brain	Wilson's disease
	Gallium 67	Sarcoidosis
Ice cream cone appearance	MRI	Acoustic schwannoma
Banana sign	USG	Spina bifida
Lemon sign		Chiari malformation
Racing car sign	MRI	Corpus callosum agenesis
Water bottle sign/Oreo cookie sign	CXR	Pericardial effusion
Multibarrel/Double barrel sign	USG/CT Angiography	Aortic dissection
Robert sign	USG	Gas shadow within heart or great vessel
T sign	USG	Monochorionic twin pregnancy
Lambda sign/Twin peak sign	USG	Dichorionic twin pregnancy
Lambda sign	Gallium 67 scan	Sarcoidosis
String of pearl	USG	PCOD
Snowstorm sign	USG	Complete H mole
String of pearl	Angiogram	Fibromuscular dysplasia
Bird beak sign/Rat tail sign	Barium swallow	Achalasia
Whirlpool sign/Whirl sign	USG/CT	Malrotation/Midgut volvulus Ovarian torsion
Mercedes Benz sign	CT	Gall stone
Colon cut off sign	X-ray/CT	Acute pancreatitis CA colon
Apple core sign/Napkin ring sign	Barium enema	CA colon
Inverted 3 sign	Barium meal	CA head of pancreas
Inverted V sign	X-ray (Supine)	Pneumoperitoneum
Cupola sign		
Rigler sign/Double wall sign		
Rigler notch sign		Bronchial carcinoma
Wimberger's sign	X-ray	Congenital syphilis
Wimberger's ring sign	X-ray	Scurvy

Contd...

Sign	Modality	Seen in
Target sign	USG	Pyloric stenosis
Tram track sign	MRI Brain	Sturge Weber syndrome
	Orbit	Optic nerve meningioma
	CXR	Bronchiectasis
Signet ring	HRCT	Bronchiectasis
Deep sulcus sign	CXR	Pneumothorax
Stag antler sign	CXR	Pulmonary venous hypertension
Westermark sign	CXR	Pulmonary embolism
Hampton hump	CXR	Pulmonary embolism/Lung infarction
Bulging fissure sign	CXR	Klebsiella pneumoniae – MC cause Streptococcus pneumoniae Pseudomonas Staph aureus
Honeycombing	CT	Diffuse pulmonary fibrosis
Fish hook ureter/J shaped ureter/hockey stick ureter	IVP/CT urography	Retrocaval ureter/Benign Prost Hypertrophy (BPH)
Cobra head appearance	Urography	Ureterocele
Drooping lily sign	Urography	Duplicate pelvis
Pear shaped bladder/Tear drop bladder	Urography	Pelvic hematoma
Christmas tree bladder	Cystogram	Neurogenic bladder
Molar tooth sign	CT pelvis	Extraperitoneal bladder rupture
	MRI Brain	Joubert syndrome
Champagne glass/bottle pelvis	X-ray	Achondroplasia
Bullet shaped vertebra	X-ray	Achondroplasia
Corduroy sign	X-ray	Intraosseous hemangioma
Polka dot	CT	Intraosseous hemangioma
Rugger jersey spine	X-ray	Hyperparathyroidism
Salt and pepper appearance	X ray skull	Hyperparathyroidism
Picture frame vertebra	X-ray	Paget's disease
Cotton wool skull	X ray	Paget's disease
Dinner fork deformity	X-ray	Colle's fracture
Shepherd crook deformity of femur	X-ray	Fibrous dysplasia
Gull wing appearance/seagull erosion	X-ray	Erosive osteoarthritis
Codfish vertebra	X-ray	Sickle cell anemia Osteoporosis
Sausage digit	X-ray	Psoriatic arthritis/Sickle cell anemia
Licked candy stick appearance	X-ray	Psoriatic arthritis Rheumatoid arthritis
Trethowan's sign	X-ray	Slipped capital femoral epiphysis (SCFE)
Dagger sign	X-ray	Ankylosing spondylosis
Light bulb sign	X-ray AP view	Posterior dislocation of shoulder
	MRI	Hepatic hemangioma Adrenal Pheochromocytoma
Bracket calcification	Skull X-ray	Lipoma of corpus callosum
Hockey stick sign	MRI Brain	Variant CJD
Hand shake sign	IVP	Horseshoe kidney
Moth eaten calyces	IVP	Genitourinary Tuberculosis
Cobra head/Adder head deformity	IVP	Ureterocele
Fish hook ureter	IVP	Retrocaval ureter

MULTIPLE CHOICE QUESTIONS

CHAPTER 1: GENERAL RADIOLOGY

CONTRAST AGENTS

1. Which of the following is water soluble contrast?
(PGMEE Jan 2019)

a. Barium
b. Iodine
c. Bromium
d. Calcium

Explanation

- *Contrast agents in radiology:-*
  - Iohexol, iopentol, ioxillan are → non-ionic monomer.
  - Iodixanol, Visipaque are → non-ionic dimer. (Iso-osmolar compounds)
  - Iothalamate, Gastrograffin and Urograffin are → Ionic monomer. They are high osmolar compounds.
  - Ioxoglate is → Ionic dimer.

2. All are ionic dyes EXCEPT: *(PGMEE 2015)*

a. Iohexol
b. Ioxaglate
c. Iothalamate
d. None

[Ref: Clinical radiology p. 583; Comprehensive Textbook of Diagnostic Radiology Volume 1. 2016 edition, pg. 973]

3. An MRI contrast used for imaging liver is?
(JIPMER 2018

a. Gadoteridol
b. Gadoxetate
c. Gadoterate
d. Gadopenate

X-RAYS

4. Linear accelerator is used to produce? *(DNB 2011)*

a. Gamma Rays
b. Beta rays
c. Neutrons
d. X rays

[Ref: RSNA Radiology72-242 txt]

5. X-ray Artifact is:- *(PGMEE 2013-14)*

a. A radiolucent area
b. Any abnormal opacity in the radiograph
c. Produced when patient moves while taking the shoot
d. All of the above

[Ref: Internet]

6. Kilovolt Peak (KvP) controls all of the following except:-
(PGMEE 2015-16)

a. Density (mAs)
b. Quality (KvP)
c. Penetrating Power (KvP)
d. Contrast (KvP)

[Ref: Internet]

Explanation

- *Factors controlling X-rays:-*
  - Penetrating power, Quality and contrast of X-rays are controlled by → Kilovolt peak (**KvP**).
  - Density of X-rays is controlled by → Milli amperes (**mAs**) (KvP).
- Contrast is inversely related to Kilovolt peak (**KvP**).

7. Which of the following is the most commonly used X-Ray film for Mammography:- *(PGMEE 2015-16)*

a. Dual Screen Dual emulsion
b. Single Screen-Single emulsion
c. Dual Screen Single emulsion
d. Single Screen Dual Emulsion

[Ref: Breast Imaging By Daniel B. Kopans 3rd/e pg. 259]

8. Skyline view X-ray is useful in diagnosing:
(PGMEE 2015)

a. Tibiofibular problem
b. Skull fracture
c. Radioulnars problem
d. Patellofemoral problem

[Ref: Maheshwari 4th/e/p 142]

9. X-ray view for supra orbital fissure:- *(PGMEE 2013-14)*

a. Towne's
b. AP
c. Caldwell's
d. Basal

[Ref: Dhingra 6th/e pg. 434]

10. Chest X-ray, most common view is:- *(PGMEE 2013-14)*

a. AP
b. PA
c. RAO
d. LAO

[Ref: Toriano 2nd/e p 194]

11. Rhese view is used for:- *(PGMEE 2013-14)*

a. Superior orbital foramen
b. Inferior orbital foramen
c. Optic foramen
d. Sella turcica

[Ref: Clinical Radiology 1st/e/p. 232]

12. What is the difference between x-ray and light waves:-
(PGMEE 2016-17)

a. Speed
b. Energy
c. Wavelength
d. Velocity

[Ref: Various books]

13. X-ray shield made up of:- *(PGMEE 2016-17)*

a. Lead
b. Copper
c. Iron
d. Molybdenum

[Ref: Love & Bailey 26th/e/ch 13]

MRI

14. The magnetic field in an MRI machine is measured in:-
(PGMEE 2013-14)

a. Housefield units
b. Tesla
c. MHz
d. None

[Ref: Bailey & Love's Short Practice Of Surgery 26th/e/ch 13]

15. Gyromagnetic property of proton is seen in:-
(PGMEE 2013-14)

a. MRI
b. CT
c. PET scan
d. USG

[Ref: Bailey & Love's Short Practice Of Surgery 26th/e/ch 13]

1.	b
2.	a
3.	b
4.	d
5.	c
6.	a
7.	b
8.	d
9.	c
10.	b
11.	c
12.	c
13.	a
14.	b
15.	a

16. **All are true about MRI except-** *(PGMEE 2015)*
    a. Multiple plane images
    b. Contraindicated in cardiac pacemaker
    c. Not good for bone lesion
    d. Maximum radiation exposure

[Ref: Bailey & Love's Short Practice Of Surgery 26th/e/ch 13]

17. **Which of the following is not a contraindication of MRI-**
    a. Ryle's tube *(PGMEE 2015)*
    b. Cardiac pacemaker
    c. Metallic splinter in eye
    d. Cochlear implant

[Ref: Bailey & Love's Short Practice Of Surgery 26th/e/ch 13]

18. **Following have same intensity on both T1 and T2 MRI images-** *(PGMEE 2015)*
    a. Kidney   b. Fat
    c. Gall bladder   d. CSF

[Ref: Internet]

19. **All of the following are true about T1 Weighted image, except:-** *(PGMEE 2015-16)*
    a. Short TE   b. Short TR
    c. Fluid appears bright   d. Fat appears bright

[Ref: MRI Made Easy 2nd/e pg.11]

20. **Investigation of choice for whole body imaging in metastasis is:-** *(PGMEE 2013-14)*
    a. Magnetic Resonance Imaging
    b. Angiography
    c. Venography
    d. CT scan

[Ref: Bailey & Love's Short Practice Of Surgery 26th/e/ch 13]

CT

21. **Enhancement in CT contrast is due to:-** *(PGMEE 2013-14)*
    a. Iodine   b. Gadolinium
    c. Silver   d. Mercury

[Ref: Bailey & Love's Short Practice Of Surgery 26th/e/ch 13]

22. **Amount of radiation exposure in 1 CT-scan of chest is-** *(PGMEE 2015)*
    a. 1 Msv   b. 3 Msv
    c. 5 Msv   d. 7 Msv

[Ref: Love & Bailey 26th/e/p 174]

23. **Hounsfield unit is zero for which of the following?:-** *(PGMEE 2013-14)*
    a. Fat   b. Water
    c. Air   d. Dense bone

24. **Hounsfield units used in?** *(DNB JUNE 2011)*
    a. CT Scan   b. MRI
    c. X Ray   d. USG

[Ref: Essential Radiology p.86]

25. **Use of water – soluble contrast medium in CT is indicated than Barium to prevent peritonitis in case of:**
    a. Constipation *(PGMEE 2013-14)*
    b. Perforation
    c. Ileocecal tuberculosis
    d. Gastroesophageal reflux

[Ref: Love & Bailey 26th/e/p 993]

26. **What is the Investigation of choice for focal neurologic deficit in emergency room?** *(PGMEE 2013-14)*
    a. CT   b. MRI
    c. Lumbar puncture d. CECT

[Ref: Love & Bailey 26th/e/ch 23 & 24]

27. **22-year-old female presents to the emergency with a chief complaint of severe left upper quadrant (LUQ) pain after being punched by her husband. Her blood pressure is 110/76, her pulse is 80 bpm, and her respiration rate is 24 breaths per minute. The best means to establish a diagnosis is which of the following?** *(PGMEE 2015)*
    a. Peritoneal lavage
    b. Upper gastrointestinal (GI) series
    c. Four-quadrant tap of the abdomen
    d. CT of the abdomen

[Ref: Love & Bailey 26th/e/ch 24]

28. **Identify the structure marked with arrow in the CT scan below:** *(Recent Pattern June 2018)*

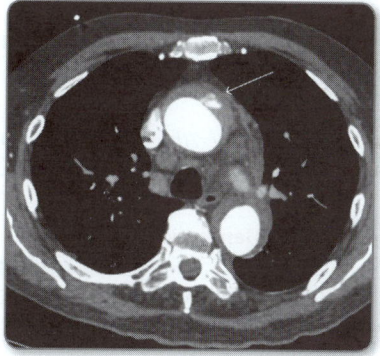

    a. Arch of aorta
    b. Inferior vena cava
    c. Superior vena cava
    d. Azygos vein

[Ref: Harrison's 19th/e pg. 1658]

Explanation

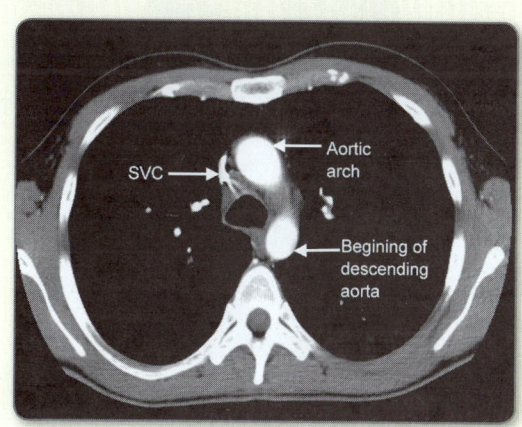

USG

29. **Posterior acoustic shadow is seen in?** *(DNB Dec 2011)*
    a. Air   b. Calculi
    c. Blood   d. All of the above

[Ref: Bailey & Love's Short Practice Of Surgery 26th/e/p 193]

16.	d
17.	a
18.	b
19.	c
20.	a
21.	a
22.	d
23.	b
24.	a
25.	b
26.	a
27.	d
28.	a
29.	b

30. Frequency of waves used in ultrasonography is-
(PGMEE 2013-14)

a. 2000 Hz
b. 5000 Hz
c. < 2 MHz
d. >2 MHz

[Ref: Bailey & Love's Short Practice of Surgery 26th/e/ch 13]

31. Doppler-effect is due to change in which parameter?
(PGMEE 2013-14)

a. Direction of sound
b. Frequency of sound
c. Amplitude of sound
d. None of the above

32. Blue colour on Colour Doppler represents?:-
(PGMEE 2015-16)

a. Venous flow pattern
b. Flow away from the transducer
c. Flow towards the transducer
d. Deoxygenated blood flow

MAMMOGRAPHY

33. Target element used in mammography is?
(DNB JUNE 2010)

a. Tungsten
b. Aluminum
c. Molybdenum
d. Copper

[Ref: Sutton's radiology 7th/ ed/p 1451; Comprehensive Textbook of Diagnostic Radiology Volume 3. 2016 edition, pg. 3323]

34. All are true about Mammography EXCEPT?
(PGMEE 2011)

a. High positive predictive value
b. Screening and diagnostic tool
c. Uses low energy X-rays
d. Specificity of mammography is 90%

[Ref: Internet]

35. Identify the condition shown on Mammography in Photograph:
(Recent Pattern June 2018)

a. Carcinoma
b. Abscess
c. Cyst
d. Fibroadenoma

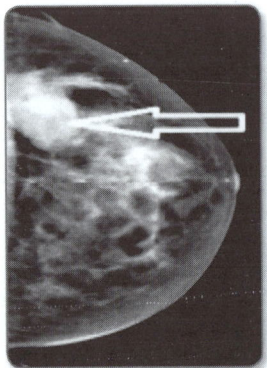

[Ref: Sabiston's 20th/e pg.836]

Explanation

- Fibroadenoma is a benign tumor of breast containing admixture of stromal and epithelial tissue.
- Diagnosis is usually made by clinical examination, ultrasound or mammography. When diagnosed confidently follow up for 6 months to assess internal growth.

- Criteria for biopsy include:-
  - Enlarging lesion
  - Atypical finding on imaging
  - Lesion above 2-5cm & no previous imaging
  - Patient's peace of mind.
- Final diagnosis rests on biopsy
- Since both fibroadenomas and CA breast can present as lumps, it is currently recommended to perform ultrasound analyses and possibly tissue sampling with subsequent histopathologic analysis in order to perform diagnosis.

PET SCAN

36. Substance used for PET scan is-
(DNB 2010; PGMEE 2015)

a. Gastrogarfin
b. Gadolinium
c. Iodine
d. 18-FDG

[Ref: Love & Bailey 26th/e/ch13]

37. PET stands for:-
(PGMEE 2013-14)

a. Positive electron tomography
b. Proton-electron therapy
c. Positron emission tomography
d. Photon emmiting tomography

[Ref: Love & Bailey 26th/e/ch 13 p 174]

38. Dye used in SPECT–
(PGMEE 2015)

a. O-14
b. Tc-99
c. Nitrogen-16
d. Iodine 124

[Ref: Love & Bailey 26th/e/ch 13]

39. PET scan uses –
(PGMEE 2012)

a. 2-Fluorodeoxyglucose
b. Technetium
c. Chromium
d. Cobalt

[Ref: Love & Bailey 26th/e/p 862]

40. Which gives a negative test on FDG PET?
(NEET Pattern 2017)

a. Small cell carcinoma
b. Large cell neuroendocrine tumor
c. Typical carcinoid
d. Atypical carcinoid

Explanation

- Bronchial carcinoids are neuroendocrine tumors of varying malignant potential.
  - low-grade typical carcinoids are well differentiated tumours. Typical carcinoids have low glucose turnover, and therefore 18F-FDG PET is not useful in evaluation intermediate-grade atypical carcinoids
  - Highly malignant large and small cell neuroendocrine tumors
- Typical carcinoids like well-differentiated NET tumors elsewere in the body (e.g. Pancreatic NETs) express of surface somatostatin receptors (STRS), allowing imaging with somatostatin receptor scintigraphy, typically with 111 indium-labeled octreotide scan and 68Ga-DOTA-labeled somatostatin analogs, called DOTANOC scan.

30.	d
31.	b
32.	b
33.	c
34.	d
35.	d
36.	d
37.	c
38.	b
39.	a
40.	c

41. Hot spots in bone scan are seen in the following conditions conditions except – *(PGMEE 2014)*
a. Osteomyelitis
b. Multiple myeloma
c. Hyperparathyroidism
d. Metastases

[Ref: Love & Bailey 26th/e/p 812]

HYSTEROSALPINGOGRAPHY

42. Identify the investigation shown in image: *(PGMEE 2018)*

a. Hysterosalpingography
b. Ultrasound guided Hysteroscopy
c. MRI hysterosalpingography
d. CT hysterosalpingography

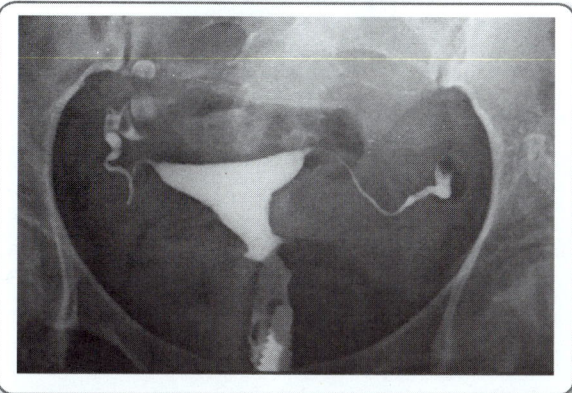

Explanation

- *Hysterosalpingography* (aka uterosalpingography) is an radiological imaging of female uterus and fallopian tubes using fluoroscopy and a contrast material.
- *Sonohysterosalpingography* (aka sono-uterosalpingography) : Endometrial cavity is visualised by TVS probeafter instillation of normal saline. Used to rule out ndometrial pathology/adhesion.
- *MRI hysterosalpingography* is an MR imaging of uterus and fallope tubes. Second line in work up for infertility. Useful in evaluating Mullerian anomalies.
- *CT hysterosalpingography* is an CT imaging of uterus and fallope tubes. Risk of radiation exposure is high.

Also Know

- *USG guided hysteroscopy* is an direct visualisation of inside of uterine cavity using ultrasound and endoscope. Useful in evaluating the endometrium in postmenopausal women or women at high risk for the development of endometrial adenocarcinoma.

43. 35 years old female presented with 2 years history of primary infertility. Identify the condition shown in hysterosalpingography: *(PGMEE 2018; NEET Pattern 2017)*
a. Septate uterus
b. Arcuate uterus
c. Bicornuate uterus
d. Unicornuate uterus

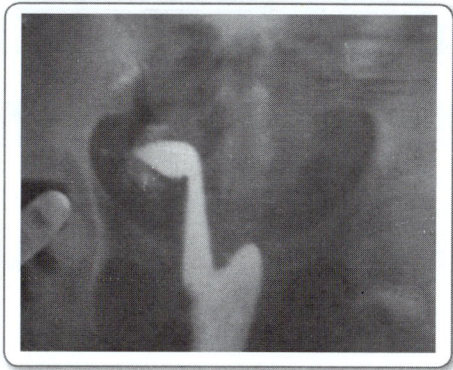

Explanation

- As the contrast is being visualised only on right side of fallopian tube this is a case of unicornuate uterus.
- *Characteristic appearances in HSG*

	Appearance
■ Hydrosalpinx	Tobacco pouch appearance
■ Endometriosis	Powder burn appearance
■ Primary infertility d/to TB	Rigid pipe stem appearance
■ TB	SIN like appearance of FT, Club like appearance of ampulla

44. Identify the investigation shown in image:
a. Hysterosalpingography *(NEET Pattern 2017)*
b. Ultrasound guided Hysteroscopy
c. MRI hysterosalpingography
d. CT hysterosalpingography

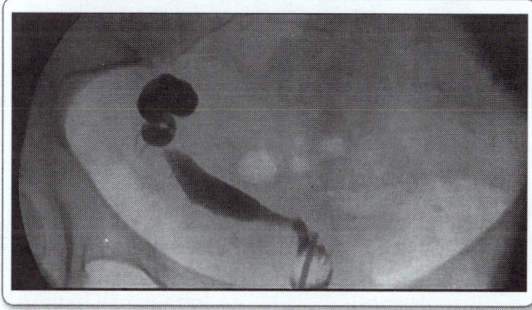

MISCELLANEOUS

45. A 40 year old male patient on long term steroid therapy for systemic disease, presents with recent onset of severe pain in the right hip. Imaging modality of choice for this problem is- *(PGMEE 2015)*
a. Bone scan
b. CT scan
c. Plain X-ray
d. MRI

[Ref: Love & Bailey 26th/e/ch 23 and 24]

46. Fluorescein angiography is used to examine- *(PGMEE 2013-14)*
a. Ciliary vasculature
b. Retinal vasculature
c. Corneal vasculature
d. Conjuctival vasculature

[Ref: Parson's]

41.	b
42.	a
43.	d
44.	a
45.	d
46.	b

NEURORADIOLOGY

1. Investigation of choice in optic neuritis is:
a. CT brain **(PGMEE 2015)**
b. MRI brain and orbit
c. MRI brain and orbit with gadolinium contrast enhancement
d. MRI brain

[Ref: Internet]

2. Tigriod pattern on MRI is seen in **(PGMEE 2015)**
a. Parkinsonism
b. Metachromatic leukodystrophy
c. Wilson's disease
d. GB syndrome

[Ref: Nelson's 20th/e/ ch 86]

3. A newborn with high output failure and left to right cardiac shunt underwent MRI of brain . Sagital section is shown below. Most likely diagnosis is:- (PGMEE 2018)
a. Pseudotumour cerebri
b. Dandy walker malformation
c. Vein of Galen malformation
d. Corpus callosum agenesis

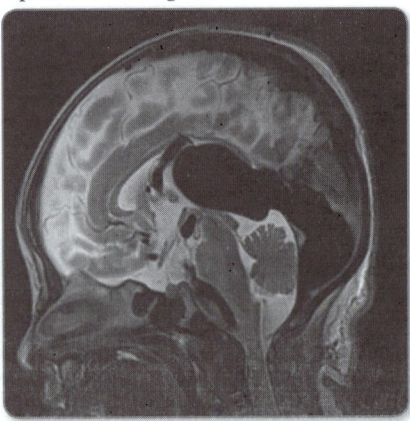

4. Ring enhancing lesion on CT is a feature of-
(PGMEE 2015)

a. Hamartoma b. Cysts
c. Toxoplasmosis d. Intracranial hemorrhage

[Ref: Nelson 20th/e/ch 290]

Explanation

- *Other cerebral ring enhancing lesions are:-*
  o Abscess
  o Metastases
  o Neurocysticercosis and tuberculoma
  o Subacute infarct
  o Tumefactive demyelinating lesions
  o Radiation Necrosis.

5. CT scan of a patient , who died of HIV, shown below. Most likely diagnosis is: **(Recent Pattern June 2018)**

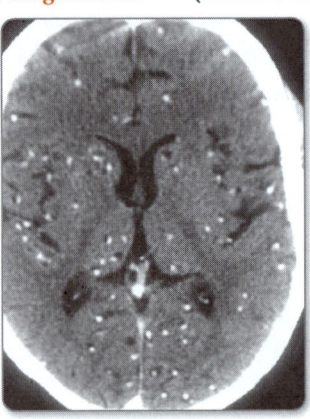

a. Toxoplasmosis b. Cryptococcosis
c. Candidiasis d. Neurocysticercosis

[Ref: Harrison's 19th/e pg.]

6. CT Scan finding in carotid cavernous sinus fistula is:-
(PGMEE 2013-14)
a. Enlarged superior ophthalmic vein
b. Enlarged inferior ophthalmic vein
c. Enlarged superior ophthalmic artery
d. Enlarged inferior ophthalmic artery

[Ref: Radiology Review Mannual 8th/e pg. 332]

7. Tram-line calcification is seen in:- **(DNB 2007)**
a. Ependymoma b. Tuberous sclerosis
c. Meningioma d. Sturge-Weber syndrome

[Ref: Nelson 20th/e/ch 596.3]

INFARCTS AND HEMORRHAGES

8. Identify the condition in the below image?
(PGMEE Jan 2019)

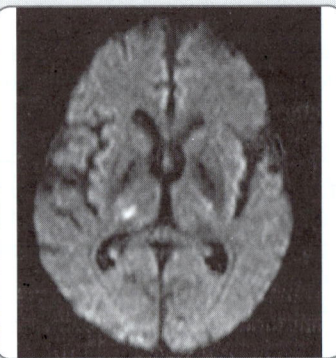

a. Lacunar infarct b. Embolic infarct
c. Thrombotic infarct d. Intracerebral hemorrhage

1.	c
2.	b
3.	c
4.	c
5.	d
6.	a
7.	d
8.	a

9. **Investigation of choice for acute intracerebral bleeding is-** *(PGMEE 2015; DNB Dec 2011)*
   a. MRI
   b. PET scan
   c. NCCT
   d. DSA

   [Ref: Love & Bailey 26th/e/ch 23]

10. **Epidural hematoma on CT scan shows-** *(PGMEE 2015)*
    a. Crescent shaped hypodense lesion
    b. Biconcave hyperdense lesion
    c. Crescent shaped hyperdense lesion
    d. Biconvex hyperdense lesion

    [Ref: Bailey & Love's 27th/e pg. 334]

Explanation

- On CT, extradural hematomas appear as a **lentiform** (lens shaped or biconvex) hyperdense lesion between skull and brain.
- Biconvex because it is limited by dural attachment at its ends.

11. **Investigation of choice for acute subarachnoid hemorrhage is-** *(PGMEE 2015)*
    a. Angiography
    b. CT scan
    c. Enhance MRI
    d. MRI

    [Ref: Bailey & Love's 27th/e pg. 335]

12. **Investigation of choice to evaluate intracranial hemorrhage of less than 48 hours is-** *(PGMEE 2015)*
    a. MRI
    b. PET
    c. CT scan
    d. SPECT

    [Ref: Love & Bailey 27th/e/ch 23]

13. **On imaging diffuse axonal injury is characterized by:-** *(PGMEE 2013-14)*
    a. Multiple small petechial hemorrhage
    b. White matter lucencies
    c. Biconcave lesion
    d. Patchy ill defined low density lesion mixed with small hyperdensity of petechial hemorrhage

    [Ref: Love & Bailey 27th/e pg. 336]

14. **DSA angiography image is shown. What is the diagnosis image** *(NEET Pattern 2017)*

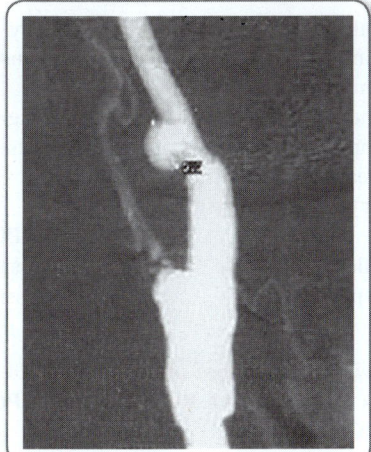

   a. Pseudoaneurysm of ICA
   b. Multiple hemangiomas
   c. Angiofibroma tumor blush
   d. Carotid cavernous fistula

Explanation

- The above image is showing a well-defined outpouching from the C1 portion of ICA, which is typical of a pseudoaneurysm.

Pseudoaneurysm of ICA

- Pseudoneurysms may arise when there is breach in the vessel wall such that blood leaks through the wall but is contained by the adventitia or surrounding perivascular soft tissue.
- Penetrating trauma is the **m/c** cause. Other causes can be infection, as an iatrogenic complication following procedures, CTDs such as Ehlers Danlos disease etc.
- Since it lacks the three layers of the arterial wall (intima, media and adventitia) it is considered as false/pseudo aneurysm. Part of the aneurysm wall is composed only of the adventitial layer, or even just by the hematoma. Therefore there is a higher risk of rupture compared to true aneurysm, leading to the need for urgent intervention.
- Pseudoaneurysms of the extracranial internal carotid artery (ICA) are rare.

15. **Earliest radiological sign of increased ICT is?**
    a. Erosion of dorsum sella *(DNB Dec 2011)*
    b. Copper beaten appearance
    c. Pineal displacement
    d. Widening of sella

16. **Fried egg appearance in brain tumour:-** *(PGMEE 2016-17)*
    a. Oligodendroglioma
    b. Astrocytoma
    c. Meningioma
    d. Ependymoma

    [Ref: Radiology Review Mannual 8th/e pg. 391]

RESPIRATORY SYSTEM

17. **On chest CT "Tree in bud appearance" is seen in which condition-** *(PGMEE 2015)*
    a. Small cell carcinoma
    b. Pulmonary hydatid cyst
    c. Silicosis
    d. Pulmonary tuberculosis

    [Ref: Nelson 20th/e/p 2066]

18. **A 45 years old bed ridden female develops sudden onset breathlessness, tachypnea and tachycardia. Her CT is given below. Most likely diagnosis is:** *(PGMEE 2018)*

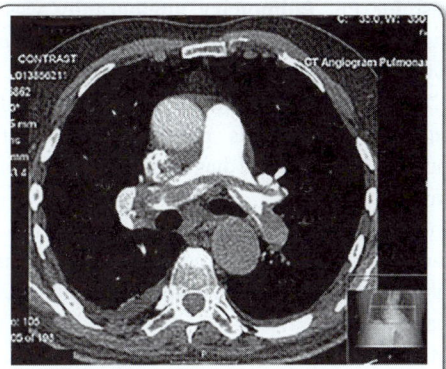

   a. Pulmonary embolism
   b. Cor pulmonale
   c. Dissection of aorta
   d. Acute myocardial infarction

9.	c
10.	d
11.	b
12.	c
13.	a
14.	a
15.	a
16.	a
17.	d
18.	a

Explanation

Pulmonary Embolism

- Patient presents with dyspnea, tachypnea, hypotension, cyanosis, cough, hemoptysis, pleuritic chest pain, syncope etc.
  - **Dyspnea** is most frequent symptom and **tachypnea** is most frequent sign.
  - Right heart failure (Cor pulmonale) is the usual cause of death from PE.
- Imaging studies:-
  - **MDCT (Multidetector CT)** is the principal imaging test now a days for the d/g of PE.
  - CXR may be normal or near normal. Some interesting signs on CXR are:-

Focal oligemia (Westermark's sign)

Wedge shaped density above diaphragm (Hampton's hump)

Enlarged right descending pulmonary artery (Palla's sign) may be seen.

- On transthoracic echo 'McConnell' s sign is seen
- **Most common** ECG finding (most cited abnormality) in pulmonary embolism is sinus tachycardia.
- The *"S1Q3T3" pattern* of acute cor pulmonale is classic/most specific (most characteristic) sign. It is termed as **McGinn-White Sign**.

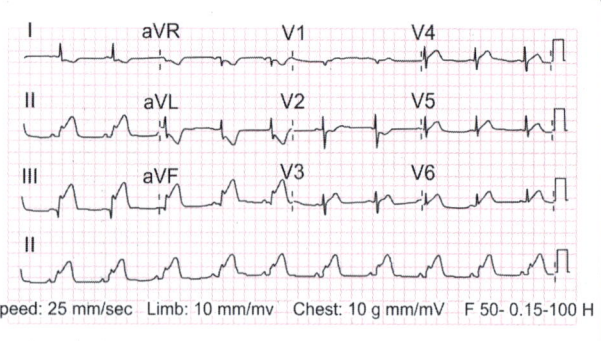

Speed: 25 mm/sec Limb: 10 mm/mv Chest: 10 g mm/mV F 50- 0.15-100 H

ECG Strip.: McGinn-White sign

- Lung scans (V/Q scan) is now the second line diagnostic test for PE. **Pulmonary angiography** was the gold standard and most specific test but now a days replaced with CTPA.
- *CT pulmonary angiogram (CTPA)* using multidetector scanners (MDCT) is preferred choice of imaging pulmonary artery and diagnosing PE due to its minimally invasive nature.
- Individuals with hypercoagulable states (esp. inherited factor V leiden) are predisoposed. The quantitative plasma D-dimer ELISA level is elevated in > 90% of patients.
- M/c source of emboli: Proximal vein of LL (femoro-popliteal/iliac).
- T/t: Anti-coagulation and thrombolysis.

Radiological signs in Pulmonary thrombo-embolism

Sign	Seen due to
Hampton hump	Shallow wedge-shaped opacity in the periphery of the lung with its base against the pleural surface and base directed towards the supplying thrombosed pulmonary artery.
Palla sign	Enlarged right descending pulmonary artery
Fleischner sign	Enlarged pulmonary artery
Chang sign	Dilated right descending pulmonary artery with sudden cut off

19. Gold standard to diagnose pulmonary thromboem-bolism:- *(PGMEE 2013-14)*
- a. CT angiography
- b. Plethysmography
- c. USG
- d. Ventilation perfusion scan

[Ref: Nelson 20th/e/p 2125]

20. Investigation of choice for lung abscess is- *(PGMEE 2015)*
- a. Chest X-ray
- b. Ultrasound
- c. MRI
- d. CECT scan

[Ref: Harrison Manual of medicine 19th/ch 132]

21. Milliary shadow in chest X ray is seen in all except- *(PGMEE 2015)*
- a. Sarcoidosis
- b. Klebsiella
- c. Tuberculosis
- d. Metastasis

[Ref: P.J Mehta 14th/e/p 309]

22. On CT chest 'halo sign' is seen in *(PGMEE 2015)*
- a. Round pneumonia
- b. Pulmonary hydatid cyst
- c. Invasion pulmonary aspergillosis
- d. Bronchiectasis

[Ref: Harrison Manual of Medicine 19th/e/p 573]

Explanation

- "Halo sign" is ground glass density surrounding a pulmonary nodule or mass and usually indicates hemorrhage.
- Other conditions which depict this sign → Pulmonary lymphoma, osteosarcoma (mets), eosinophilic lung disease, hypersensitivity pneumonitis.

23. Miliary nodules are seen in all except:- *(PGMEE 2013-14)*
- a. Silicosis
- b. Sarcoidosis
- c. Aspergillosis
- d. Anthracosis

[Ref: P.J Mehta 14th/e/p 309]

24. Best view for collapse of middle lobe of lung is seen in which view of chest X-Ray:- *(PGMEE 2013-14)*
- a. Oblique
- b. AP
- c. Lateral
- d. Lordotic

[Ref: Sutton Radiology 7th/e/177]

19.	a
20.	d
21.	b
22.	c
23.	c
24.	d

25. Differential diagnosis of solitary pulmonary nodule are all except: *(PGMEE 2013-14)*
a. Bronchogenic carcinoma
b. Mycetoma
c. Tuberculoma
d. Hamartoma

[Ref: Nelson 20th/e/p 1355]

GRANULOMATOUS DISEASES & MISCELLANEOUS

26. A 52 year old male came with a history of fever and malaise for 3-4 months & pain in the knees and ankles. On blood investigation ESR was raised. CXR showed bilateral hilar adenopathy and pulmonary infiltrates most severe in the upper and mid zones. Mantoux test was negative. What is the most probable diagnosis? *(PGMEE 2015)*
a. Berylliosis   b. Sarcoidosis
c. Asbestosis   d. Tuberculosis

[Ref: Harrison Manual of Medicine 19th/e/ch 166]

27. Identify the infection from the chest X-ray of patient with low grade fever? *(PGMEE Jan 2019)*

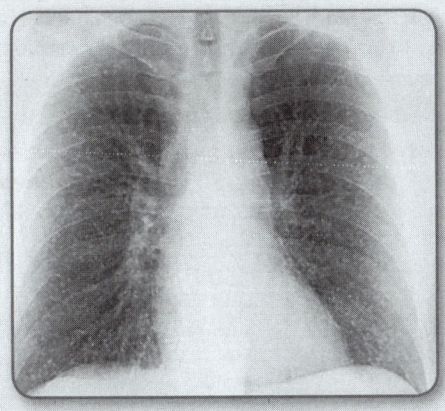

a. ILD   b. Bronchopneumonia
c. Miliary TB   d. Consolidation

28. Air bronchogram on chest Xray is suggestive of - *(PGMEE 2013-14)*
a. Intrapulmonary lesion   b. Intrathoracic lesion
c. Extrapulmonary lesion   d. Extrathoracic lesion

[Ref: Harrison Manual of Medicine19th/e/p 23]

29. Which primary carcinoma shows calcified lung metastases? *(PGMEE 2013-14)*
a. Endometrial carcinoma   b. Thyroid carcinoma
c. Pancreatic carcinoma   d. None

[Ref: Love & Bailey 26t/e/ch 51]

30. Water-lily sign on chest X-ray is seen in:- *(DNB 2007, PGMEE 2013-14)*
a. Cryptococcosis   b. Aspergillosis
c. Hydatid cyst   d. Tuberculosis

[Ref: Love & Bailey 26th/e/p 77]

31. Thick cavity in lung NOT seen in- *(PGMEE 2013-14)*
a. Lung abscess   b. TB
c. Emphysematous bulla d. Hamartoma

[Ref: Fundamentals of Radiology 2nd/e/p 314]

32. Characteristic radiological finding in sarcoidosis :- *(PGMEE 2013-14)*
a. Parenchymal disease
b. Unilateral hilar lymphadenopathy
c. Bilateral hilar lymphadenopathy
d. Miliary shadow

[Ref: Harrison Manual of Medicine 19th/e/ch 166, Nelosn 20th/e/p 1207]

33. Necrotic nodules in lung are seen in:- *(PGMEE 10' 2013-14)*
a. TB
b. Sarcoidosis
c. RA
d. All of the above

[Ref: Internet]

34. "Egg shell" calcification in hilar nodes suggest: *(DNB 2007)*
a. Asbestosis
b. Silicosis
c. Berylliosis
d. Byssinosis

[Ref: Harrison Manual Medicine 19th/e/p 716-717]

35. All of the following statements about silicosis are true, Except: *(Recent Pattern June 2018)*
a. Pleural plaques
b. Predilection for upper lobes
c. Calcific Hilar Lymphadenopathy
d. Associated with tuberculosis

[Ref: Radiology Review Mannual; 8th/e pg.670]

Explanation

- Submucosal → Subepithelial Silicosis
  - Acute Silicosis (Alveolar Silico proteinosis) → Affects periphery of lung; predominantely lower zones and is bilateral.
  - Classic Silicosis (Chronic interstitial reticulonodular disease) → Upper zones, bilateral posterior portion and produce a charachteristic "egg shell" pattern.
- Silicosis is associated with Tuberculosis. Because silica is cytotoxic to alveolar macrophages, patients with silicosis are at greater risk of acquiring lung infections particularly mycobacterium tuberculosis, atypical mycobacteria and fungi'.

36. In which variety of lung cancer cranial irradiation is also given in treatment? *(DNB Dec 2011)*
a. Adenocarcinoma
b. Small cell cancer
c. Squamous cell carcinoma
d. Non small cell cancer

[Ref: Harrison 19th/ed chapter 69]

37. Air bronchogram sign is seen? *(DNB June 2011)*
a. Cavity
b. Pneumothorax
c. Lung abscess
d. Consolidation

[Ref: Grainger 4th/e p.311]

25.	b
26.	b
27.	c
28.	a
29.	b
30.	c
31.	d
32.	c
33.	d
34.	b
35.	a
36.	b
37.	d

38. A 55-year-old non-smoker lady presented with on and off haemoptysis and productive cough for 1 year. There was no fever or constitutional symptoms. Physical examination showed clubbing of fingers and coarse crepitations over the lung base. Blood tests were essentially normal and an initial CXR was performed. CT scan was also performed. which is shown below. What is the radiological diagnosis:

(Recent Pattern June 2018)

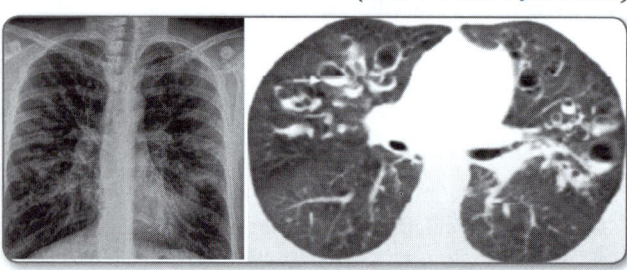

a. Pneumoconiosis
b. Bronchiectasis
c. Emphysema
d. Lung Abscess

[Ref: Harrison's 19th/e pg. 1695]

Explanation

- Frontal chest X-ray is showing clusters of cystic spaces containing air-fluid levels in the left mid and lower zones due to retained secretions in dilated bronchioles in bronchiectasis.
- A CT scan was performed to know the extent and severity of the disease. It is showing:
  ○ Cystic dilatation of bronchioles
  ○ Thickened bronchioles (inflammatory changes)
  ○ Air-fluid levels d/to retained bronchial secretions within the dilated bronchioles
- So the most likely diagnosis is cystic bronchiectasis.

Discussion on Bronchiectasis

- MC presentation is a persitsant productive cough with thick tenacious sputum. P/E includes cracles & wheezing on auscultation of lung.
- Majority of bronchiectasis occurs peripherally in lower lobes.
- Unusual sites of involvement raise the suspicion of certain aetiologies of bronchiectasis, e.g. upper zone predominance in cystic fibrosis, proximal central zone involvement in allergic bronchopulmonary aspergillosis.
- Bronchogram which was once a gold standard for diagnosis, is now replaced by HRCT.
- Radiological signs on CT due to dilated bronchioles are:-
  ○ 'Tram-track' sign
  ○ 'Signet-ring' sign

39. Best investigation for bronchiectasis is? *(DNB Dec 2010)*
a. Pulmonary function tests
b. MRI
c. Chest X ray
d. HRCT

[Ref: Harrison 19th/e/p 2082]

38. b
39. d
40. a
41. a

40. A patient who was admitted with severe dyspnoea .Chest X ray shows the following features.What can be the most possible diagnosis: *(Recent Pattern June 2018)*

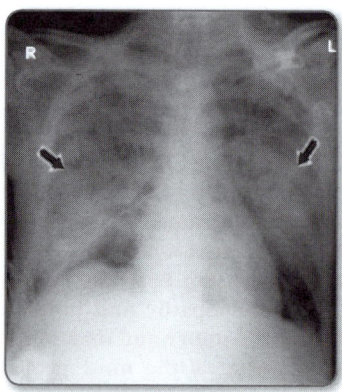

a. Pulmonary edema
b. Pulmonary atelectasis
c. Pulmonary hypertension
d. Pneumonia

Explanation

- Chest radiograph of a case of noncardiogenic pulmonary edema showing bats wing appearance (arrowheads) with air bronchogram in absence of cardiomegaly.

CVS

41. The red arrow in the chest X ray given below indicates: *(Recent Pattern June 2018)*

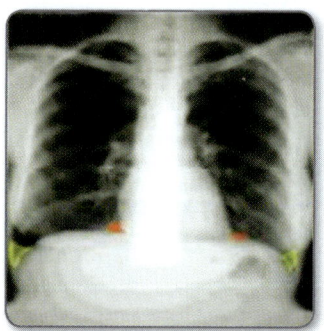

a. Cardiophrenic angle
b. Costophrenic angle
c. Cardiophrenic lymph node
d. Epicardial fat pad

Explanation

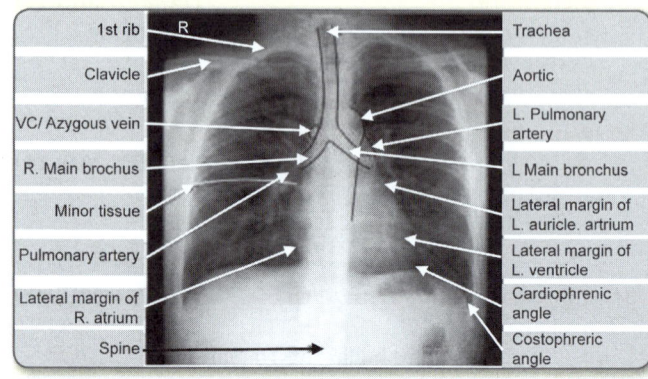

HEART BORDER

42. **Left cardiac border bulge can be seen in all, except–**
    a. Enlarged azygous vein   (PGMEE 2014)
    b. Left appendicular overgrowth
    c. Coronary artery aneurysm
    d. Pericardial defect

    [Ref: Cardiac X-ray by Chockolingam 1st/e p. 30-40]

43. **Aortic knuckle is formed from-**   (PGMEE 2016-17)
    a. Lingula
    b. Pulmonary artery
    c. Aorta
    d. Left atrium

CONGENITAL/VALVULAR HEART DISEASES

44. **Snowman's heart sign appearance on chest X-ray is seen in-**   (PGMEE2013-14, PGMEE 2016-17)
    a. Total anomalous pulmonary venous connection (TAPVC)
    b. Ebstein anomaly
    c. Tetrology of Fallot
    d. Transposition of great vessels

    [Ref: Ghai 8th/e p. 427; Radiology Review Mannual 8th/e pg. 782]

45. **Which of the following causes inferior rib notching on X-ray chest:-**   (PGMEE 2013-14)
    a. Coarctation of aorta
    b. SVC occlusion
    c. Modified Blalock Taussing shunt
    d. All of the above

    [Ref: Harrison Manual Of Medicine 19th/e/p 649]

> **Explanation**
> ■ Rib notching is deformation of superior or inferior surface of rib.

46. **Hilar dance on fluoroscopy is seen in:**   (DNB 2007)
    a. ASD   b. TOF
    c. VSD   d. TGV

    [Ref: Principles of Radiodiagnosis p. 786; Radiology Review Mannual 8th/e pg. 796]

47. **Double shadow behind right atrium and straightening of left main bronchus is seen in-**
    (DNB DEC 2010, PGMEE2013-14)
    a. Right atrium enlargement
    b. Right ventricle enlargement
    c. Left atrium enlargement
    d. Left ventricle enlargement

    [Ref: Sutton's Radioloy7th/e p.294]

48. **Left atrial enlargement is seen in:-**   (PGMEE2013-14)
    a. Mitral stenosis
    b. Tricuspid regurgitation
    c. AR
    d. None

    [Ref: O.P Ghai 8th/e/p 440-441; Radiology Review Mannual 8th/e pg. 742]

PERICARDIAL DISEASES

49. **The sign with patch of dullness beneath the angle of left scapula in a patient with pericardial effusion is named as:-**   (PGMEE2013-14)
    a. Carvallo's sign   b. Ewart's sign
    c. Hoffmann's sign   d. Homan's sign

    [Ref: Harrison 18th/e p.1971]

50. **Best investigation for pericardial effusion is:-**   (PGMEE2013-14)
    a. MRI   b. CT
    c. X-ray   d. Echocardiography

    [Ref: Sutton 7th /e p.332]

51. **Water bottle heart is seen in:-**   (PGMEE2013-14)
    a. PDA   b. Chronic emphysema
    c. Pericardial effusion   d. Constrictive pericarditis

    [Ref: Harrison 18th/e/p 1971; Radiology Review Mannual 8th/e pg. 747]

52. **"Money bag Appearance" of Heart on Chest X-ray is seen in:-**   (PGMEE 2015-16)
    a. Pericardial Effusion   b. TAPVC
    c. Tetralogy of Fallot   d. Emphysema

    [Ref: API Textbook of Medicine 9th/e pg. 740]

53. **Flask shaped heart is seen in –**   (PGMEE 2012)
    a. Ebstein anomaly   b. TAPVC
    c. TOF   d. Pericardial effusion

    [Ref: Harrison 18th/e/p 1971]

54. **For pericardial calcifications, which is the best investigation:-**   (PGMEE2013-14)
    a. MRI
    b. Transesophageal echocardiography
    c. USG
    d. CT scan

    [Ref: Textbook of Thoracic Imaging p. 803]

55. **Ground glass ventricular septum is seen in:-**   (PGMEE2013-14)
    a. TOF   b. HOCM
    c. TGA   d. CHF

    [Ref: Principle of Radiodiagnosis]

56. **Egg in cup appearance is seen in**   (PGMEE 2013)
    a. MR
    b. TOF
    c. Constrictive pericarditis
    d. Transposition of great vessels

PERIPHERAL VASCULAR DISEASES

57. **Investigation of choice for DVT is:-**   (PGMEE2013-14)
    a. Doppler USG   b. Angiography
    c. CT scan   d. MRI

    [Ref: Love & Bailey 26th/e/ch 57]

58. **Investigation of choice for DVT-**   (PGMEE 2015)
    a. Ultrasonography   b. Venography
    c. Nuclear imaging   d. MRI

    [Ref: Love & Bailey 26th/e/ch 57]

42.	a
43.	c
44.	a
45.	d
46.	a
47.	c
48.	a
49.	b
50.	d
51.	c
52.	a
53.	d
54.	d
55.	b
56.	c
57.	a
58.	a

PRIMES ∩ (VOLUME II)

PULMONARY HYPERTENSION

59. What is the earliest feature of pulmonary venous hypertension on X-Ray? *(PGMEE 2014)*
a. Upper lobar vessel dilation
b. Kerley B lines
c. Left atrial enlargement
d. Pleural effusion

[Ref: Sutton Textbook of Radiological Imaging 7th/e. pg. 288]

60. Prunning of pulmonary arteries is seen in *(PGMEE 2013)*

a. Pulmonary hypertension
b. Chronic bronchitis
c. Pulmonary infections
d. Pulmonary transplant

[Ref: Sutton Textbook of Radiological Imaging 7th/e. pg. 288]

61. Which is the objective sign of identifying pulmonary plethora in a chest radiograph? *(PGMEE 11)*
a. Diameter of the main pulmonary artery > 16 mm
b. Diameter of the left pulmonary artery > 16 mm
c. Diameter of descending right pulmonary artery > 16 mm
d. Diameter of the descending left pulmonary artery > 16 mm

[Ref: Sutton 7th/e p. 8]

62. Egg in cup appearance is seen in *(PGMEE 2013)*
a. MR
b. TOF
c. Constrictive pericarditis
d. Transposition of great vessels

[Ref: Internet]

63. Most sensitive investigation for air embolism is- *(PGMEE 2014)*
a. Decreased tidal volume of CO_2
b. Central venous pressure
c. Doppler ultrasound
d. Decreased tidal volume NO_2

[Ref: Love & Bailey 26th/e/p 890; Journal of American Society of Anesthesiologists, Inc.]

GASTROINTESTINAL TRACT (GIT)

OESOPHAGUS

64. Barium swallow is used for:- *(PGMEE 2013-14)*
a. Colon
b. Esophagus
c. Duodenum
d. Jejumum

[Ref: Bailey & Love's Short Practice of Surgery 26th/e/p.998]

65. Double bubble on abdominal X-ray sign is seen in:- *(PGMEE 2015-16)*
a. Duodenal atresia
b. Colon carcinoma
c. Perforation
d. Intussusception

[Ref: Refer explanatory text; Radiology Review Mannual 8th/e pg. 1308]

59.	a
60.	a
61.	c
62.	c
63.	c
64.	b
65.	a
66.	c
67.	a
68.	a

66. Sign seen in Hepatobiliary ascariasis on transverse scan:- *(PGMEE 2015-16)*
a. 4 Line Sign
b. Strip Sign
c. Bull's eye sign
d. Inner Tube sign

[Ref: IJRI, radiology Quiz-Hepatobiliary Imaging year 2003, volume 13, issue 2, pg. 223-224]

67. In stricture esophagus caused by corrosive poisoning investigation of choice is? *(DNB Dec 2011)*
a. Endoscopy
b. Pharyngoscopy
c. X rays
d. Barium meal

[Ref: Harrison's 18th edition chapter 292]

68. In case of suspected esophageal perforation, dye used is: *(PGMEE 2018)*
a. Iohexol
b. Methylene blue
c. Gadolinium
d. Barium sulfate

Explanation

- *Iohexol* is a water soluble iodinated contrast media. It is nonionic monomer. It is safe to used in a case of suspected esophageal perforation.
- *Barium* should not be used as it may cause mediastinitis.
- *Gastrograffin* is associated with risk of aspiration and aspiration pneumonitis. So it is contraindicated in case of esophageal peforation.

Type	Subtype of contrast media	Example	Osmolarity
Ionic	Monomer High osmolar contrast media (HOCM)	Diatrizoate, conray (Iothalamate), Ioxaglate, metrizoate	1500
Non-ionic	Monomer (LOCM)	Iohexal 300, 240, Iopamidol (Omnipaque), Metrizamide	470
	Dimer (IOCM)	Iodixanol 320 (Visipaque)	300

Contrast Agents in Radiological Procedures

Procedure	Contrast agent
- Cerebral angiography, Aortography	Conray 280
- Coronary angiography, CECT	Conray 420
- Hysterosalpingography	Conray 280/420
- DSA, Myelography Ventriculography	Iopamidol (Neopam), Iohexol(omnipaque), Myodil → Can cause arachnoiditis Metrizamide → Can cause flapping tremors
- Bronchography, esophagoscopy (Esophageal atresia)	Dionosil (Tantalum)

Procedure	Contrast agent
▪ Oral cholecystography (OCG)	Ipanoic acid (Telepaque)
▪ IV cholecystography	Biligraffin
▪ Patency of recruited Sx anastomosis (Idiopathic megacolon/ hirschprung's)	Gastrograffin enema
▪ MRI	Gadolinium
▪ IVP	Na-diatrizoate, hypaque
▪ Lymphangiography	Methylene blue, lipoidal ultrafluid

69. **Rat tail appearance in contrast radiography is seen in?**
    a. Reflux oesophagitis   *(DNB June 2011)*
    b. Carcinoma esophagus
    c. Diffuse esophageal spasms
    d. Cork screw esophagus

    [Ref: Comprehensive Textbook of Diagnostic Radiology 1st/e pg. 1146]

70. **Corkscrew appearance of esophagus is seen in:-**
    a. Carcinoma   *(PGMEE2013-14)*
    b. Achalasia
    c. Diffuse esophageal spasm
    d. Stricture

    [Ref: Bailey & Love's Short Practice Of Surgery 26th/e/p 1017]

71. **Double bubble sign is seen in?**   *(DNB June 2011)*
    a. Duodenal atresia
    b. Ileal obstruction
    c. Jejunal obstruction
    d. pyloric stenosis

    [Ref: Love and Bailey 26th /e p. 119]

STOMACH

72. **Retro cardiac shadow showing air fluid level is seen in:**
    a. Pleural effusion   *(DNB DEC 2010)*
    b. Carcinoma colon
    c. Hiatus hernia
    d. Pericardial effusion

    [Ref: Sutton Textbook of Radiology 7th/e. pg. 58]

73. **Hour glass appearance of stomach is seen in:-**
    a. Linitis plastica   *(PGMEE2013-14)*
    b. Gastric ulcer
    c. Duodenal ulcer
    d. Gastric carcinoma

    [Ref: Bailey & Love Short Practice of Surgery 26th/e/p.1034]

74. **CT of gastric Volvulus shows-**   *(PGMEE 2015)*
    a. Normal twisted stomach
    b. Shortened twisted stomach
    c. Enlarged twisted stomach
    d. None of the above

    [Ref: Love & Bailey 26th/e/ch 329]

INTESTINE

75. **The study using barium for small intestine is known as:-**
    a. Barium meal follow through   *(PGMEE2013-14)*
    b. Barium swallow
    c. Barium enema
    d. None of the above

    [Ref: Bailey & Love's Short Practice of Surgery 26th/e/p 89]

76. **String of bead sign is seen in:-**   *(PGMEE 2013-14)*
    a. Crohn's disease
    b. Ulcerative colitis
    c. Small intestine obstruction
    d. Ileocaecal TB

    [Radiology Review Mannual 8th/e pg. 1015]

77. **A 35 year-old female presented to the emergency department with the sudden onset of severe epigastric pain. She has a history of heart burn and dyspeptic symptoms for past 10 years. On physical exam, she had a temperature of 101.40F, a pulse of 118 and a blood pressure of 128/72. Abdomen was tender and rigid. Expected finding on X-ray will be-**   *(PGMEE 2015)*
    a. Air under diaphragm
    b. Prominent markings
    c. Blood under diaphragm
    d. Pseudopneumoperitoneum

    [Ref: Radiological recall 3rd/e p. 99]

Explanation

- Clinical findings are suggestive of perforated peptic ulcer which is characterized by air under diaphragm.
- Pseudopneumoperitoneum is seen in Chilaiditi syndrome.

78. **Following X-ray finding is associated with Chilaiditi syndrome-**   *(PGMEE 2015)*
    a. Pneumothorax
    b. Pseudopneumoperitoneum
    c. Hydropneumothorax
    d. Pseudopneumothorax

    [Ref: Love & Bailey 26th/e/p 190]

Explanation

- ***Chilaiditi syndrome*** is a rare condition when pain occurs due to transposition of a loop of large intestine (usually transverse colon) in between the diaphragm and the liver, visible on plain abdominal X-ray or chest X-ray.
- Normally this causes no symptoms, and this is called Chilaiditi's sign.

79. **Earliest sign on Barium Enema in patients with Ulcerative colitis is:-**   *(PGMEE 2015-16)*
    a. Collar Button Ulcers
    b. Mucosal Granularity
    c. Pseudo-Polyps
    d. Haustral Loss

    [Ref: Diagnostic radiology 5th/e volume 2, pg.1213; Radiology Review Mannual 8th/e pg. 1144]

69.	b
70.	c
71.	a
72.	c
73.	b
74.	c
75.	a
76.	c
77.	a
78.	b
79.	b

80. Barium enema finding shown below is characteristic of: *(Recent Pattern June 2018)*

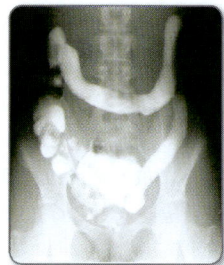

a. Polyposis coli
b. Sigmoid diverticulitis
c. Ulcerative colitis
d. Celiac disease

[Ref: Sabiston's 20th/e pg. 1341]

81. The sign as represented by an arrow in the CT abdomen picture shown below, is seen in: *(Recent Pattern June 2018)*

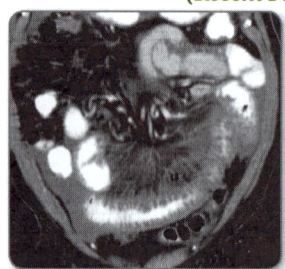

a. Crohn's disease
b. Ulcerative colitis.
c. Tuberculosis
d. Intestinal lymphoma

[Ref: Radiopedia]

80.	c
81.	a
82.	b
83.	a
84.	b
85.	b
86.	c
87.	a
88.	d
89.	d
90.	b

Explanation

- The sign shown in the CT abdomen picture above represents Comb sign i.e. dilated veins on mesenteric side of ileum.

CT finding in Crohns disease:

- Mural thickening with stratification is seen with active inflammation
- Vascular engorgement of the mesentery (comb sign)
- Hypodense lymph nodes.

CT findings in intestinal tuberculosis:

- Mural thickening with contiguous ileo-cecal involvement
- Hypodense lymph nodes with peripheral enhancement

82. A 55 years old chronic alcoholic male after having a large binge of alcohol, presented to the emergency department in subconscious state. He vomited several times, few of them mixed with blood. He had a history of heart burn and dyspeptic symptoms for past few years. On general examination, he had 102⁰F fever, a pulse of 110, respiratory rate of 20 per minute and a blood pressure of 90/60. On physical examination there was abdominal guarding and tenderness. A plane erect chest X-ray reveals air under diaphragm. Probable diagnosis is- *(PGMEE 2015)*

a. Dissected abdominal aorta
b. Perforated peptic ulcer
c. Acute MI
d. None

[Ref: Love & Bailey 26th/e/p 1032]

83. All are true about diagnostic barium follow through features of ileo cecal tuberculosis EXCEPT: *(DNB June 2011, PGMEE 2014-15)*

a. Apple core appearance
b. Pulled up or contracted cecum
c. Widening of ileocecal angle
d. Stricture involving terminal ileum

[Ref: Love & Bailey 26th/e/p. 1158]

84. Investigation done for intestinal obstruction is?

a. Barium meal *(DNB Dec 2011)*
b. X ray abdomen supine
c. X ray abdomen lateral
d. Chest X Ray

[Ref: Bailey & Love's Short Practice of Surgery 26th/e/p.1189]

85. Coffee bean sign is seen in? *(DNB JUNE 2011)*

a. Hypertrophic pyloric stenosis
b. Sigmoid volvulus
c. Gastric volvulus
d. Midgut volvulus

[Ref: SRB 4th/e/p 998; Radiology Review Mannual 8th/e pg. 1066]

86. Apple core sign in barium enema is seen with?

a. Carcinoma esophagus *(DNB JUNE 2010)*
b. Achalasia cardia
c. Colon carcinoma
d. Ileocecal tuberculosis

[Ref: Love & Bailey 26th/e/p.1165]

PANCREAS

87. On CT, Balthazar grading is for:- *(PGMEE2013-14)*

a. Acute pancreatitis
b. Choleystitis
c. Chronic pancreatitis
d. Pancreatic carcinoma

[Ref: Bailey & Love's Short Practice Of Surgery 26th/e/ p. 1129]

88. Endoscopic USG criteria for chronic pancreatitis, when echogenic lesion is:- *(PGMEE 2013-14)*

a. > 1 mm
b. 1.5 mm
c. > 2 mm
d. > 3 mm

[Ref: Textbook Of GI Endoscopy p.883]

89. Double bubble sign is seen in:- *(PGMEE 2013-14)*

a. Ladd's band
b. Annular pancreas
c. Duodenal atresia
d. All of the above

[Ref: Nelson 20th/e/p 1801]

90. To detect a 4mm nodule in pancreas what is the best investigation? *(DNB JUNE 2010)*

a. CECT
b. Endoscopic USG
c. PET scan
d. MRI

[Ref: Encyclopedia of Diagnostic Imaging Volume 1 by Albert L. Baert Page 267]

91. The typical appearance on ERCP is given below. it is seen in cases of: *(Recent Pattern June 2018)*

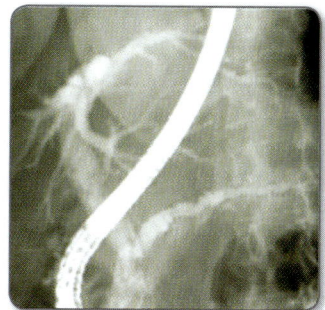

a. Chronic pancreatitis
b. Acute Pancreatitis
c. Cholelithiasis
d. Pancreatic Carcinoma

[Ref: Harrison's 19th/e pg. 2100]

Explanation

- ERCP image is showing characteristic **"chain of lake appearance"**. Main pancreatic duct is enlarged >1.5 times & is tortuous. There is severe clubbing and dilation of the side branches.
- *3 Cardinal signs of chronic Pancreatitis*
  ○ Atrophic pancreas
  ○ Main pancreatic duct (MPD) and side branches dilatation (Beaded appearance)
  ○ Intraductal calculi/Parenchynal calcification
- Surgical specimen may reveal hard, grainy, and yellowish-gray gland.

LIVER

92. Cart-wheel appearance of USG is seen in:
(DNB DEC. 2010)

a. Hydatid cyst
b. Hydatidiform mole
c. Intussusception
d. All

[Ref: Sutton's Radiology 7th/e/p771]

93. A 45 year old lady died of thromboembolism. CT scan of Her liver is shown below. Most likely cause is:-
(PGMEE 2018)

a. Cholangiocarcinoma of Liver
b. Hepatic adenoma
c. Metastases
d. Fibronodular dysplasia

Explanation

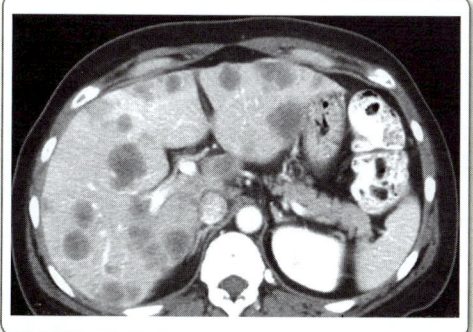

- CT scan through liver is showing multiple mets.

94. Identify the liver condition as represented in the CT scan picture below: *(Recent Pattern June 2018)*

a. Amoebic liver abscess
b. Pyogenic liver abscess
c. Hydatid disease
d. Ascending cholangitis.

[Ref: Harrison's 19th/e pg. 1433]

Explanation

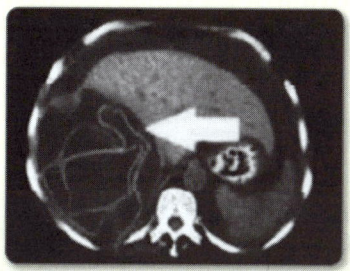

- CT scan of liver in the above radiograph is showing water lily sign , which is seen in Hydatid disease.
- Many hydatid cysts remain asymptomatic, even into advanced age. Symptoms depends upon the parasite load, the site, and the size of the cysts
- A history of living in or visiting an endemic area must be established. Also, exposure to the parasite through the ingestion of foods or water contaminated by the feces of a definitive host must be determined.
- Theoretically, echinococcosis can involve any organ. The liver is the MC organ involved, followed by the lungs. These 2 organs account for 90% of cases of hydatid cysts/echinococcosis.

GALLBLADDER

95. Investigation of choice in choledocholithiasis:-
(PGMEE 2013-14)

a. CT
b. HIDA scan
c. USG
d. PETscan

[Ref: Love & Bailey 26th/e/p 1100]

96. Mercedes Benz sign is seen in: *(DNB DEC 2010)*

a. Gall stone
b. Foreign body bronchus
c. Bladder stones
d. Renal stone

[Ref: Love & Bailey 26th/ep.1099]

97. Investigation of choice to see gall bladder

a. CT
b. USG *(PGMEE 2' 2013-14)*
c. Plain Xray
d. Oral cholecytogram

[Ref: Love & Bailey 26th/e/p 1100]

98. Radiological procedure shown below is:
(Recent Pattern June 2018)

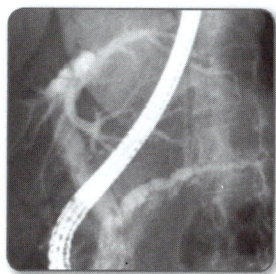

a. ERCP
b. T-tube drainage
c. PTC
d. Oral cholecystography

[Ref: Harrison's 19th/e pg. 2079]

91.	a
92.	a
93.	c
94.	c
95.	c
96.	a
97.	b
98.	a

OTHERS

99. Best investigation to detect pneumoperitoneum is?
                                                  (DNB Dec 2011)
- a. Left lateral decubitus
- b. Right lateral decubitus
- c. Plain X ray chest, erect
- d. Plain X ray abdomen, erect

[Ref: Sutton 7th/e p.663-664]

100. Identify the structure shown with arrow mark in the CT
                                                  (PGMEE 2018)

- a. Aorta
- b. Thoracic duct
- c. Inferior vena cava
- d. Superior vena cava

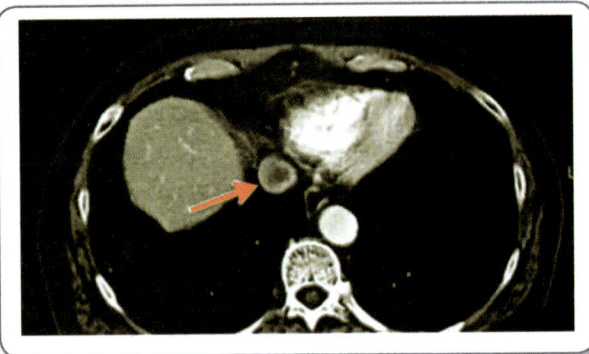

101. Identify the vascular structure shown in the CTangiogram
                                               (PGMEE 2018)
- a. Coeliac trunk
- b. Splenic artery
- c. Superior mesenteric artery
- d. Inferior mesenteric artery

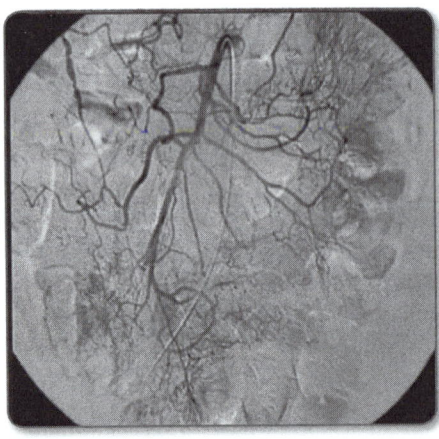

UROGENITAL SYSTEM

102. Renal GFR is estimated by-   *(PGMEE 2015)*
- a. Tc99m-DMSA
- b. Tc99m-DTPA
- c. Iodohippurate
- d. Tc99m-MAG3

[Ref: Love & Bailey 26th/e p.1276]

103. Cobra head appearance on radiograph is seen in which condition?   *(PGMEE 2015)*
- a. Bladder tumour
- b. Rectocele
- c. Ureterocele
- d. Posterior urethral valve

[Ref: Love & Bailey 26th/e/ p 1286; Sutton Textbook of Radiology 7th/e. volume2, pg. 935]

104. What is the investigation of choice for pyonephrosis:
- a. Contrast enhanced CT scan   *(PGMEE 2015)*
- b. USG
- c. Noncontrast CT scan
- d. X-ray KUB

105. 'Fir tree' appearance of bladder is seen in which condition?   *(PGMEE 2013-14)*
- a. Ureterocoele
- b. Tuberculosis
- c. Neurogenic bladder
- d. Schistosomiasis

[Ref: Love & Bailey 26th/e p.1314]

106. Most sensitive test to detect early renal TB is:-
- a. Intravenous urography   *(PGMEE 2013-14)*
- b. USG
- c. MRI
- d. CT

[Ref: Love & Bailey 26th/e/p.1302]

107. In which condition, radiographic examination reveals 'thimble bladder'?   *(DNB 2007)*
- a. Cystitis cystica
- b. Chronic tubercular cystitis
- c. Neurogenic bladder
- d. Acute tubercular cystitis

[Ref: Love & Bailey 26th/e/p.1328]

108. Which is the investigation of choice for advanced renal tuberculosis?   *(DNB June 2011)*
- a. CECT
- b. MRI
- c. USG
- d. IVP

109. In which condition the radiograph appearance is that of 'drooping water lilly':   *(DNB Dec 2010)*
- a. Splenic tumor
- b. Suprerenal mass
- c. Liver tumor
- d. Ureteral Duplication

[Ref: Nelson 20th/e/p 2572; Sutton's Radiology 7th/e. volume 2, pg. 934]

110. Most sensitive test for ureteric stones is?
                                                  (DNB June 2010)
- a. USG
- b. Non contrast CT scan
- c. X-ray
- d. Intravenous pyelogram

[Ref: Love & Bailey 26 th/e/p.1296; Sutton's Radiology 7th/e. volume 2, pg. 967]

111. Investigation of choice for posterior urethral valve is-
- a. Micturition cystouretrogram   *(DNB June 2010)*
- b. Retreograde urethrography
- c. IVP
- d. Ultrasound

[Ref: Bailey & Love's Short Practice Of Surgery 26th /e/ p1359]

112. A patient had accident 10 days before. He now presented with pain abdomen & hematuria. What investigation would you like to order: *(Recent Pattern June 2018)*
- a. Contrast CT
- b. IV Pyelography
- c. Ultrasound
- d. MRI

Explanation
- Hematuria after abdominal trauma can be due to bladder, renal or ureteric injury and resentation is acute.
- Contrast CT would be best to delineate the cause.

99.	c
100.	c
101.	d
102.	b
103.	c
104.	a
105.	c
106.	a
107.	d
108.	a
109.	d
110.	b
111.	a
112.	a

113. **The radiological procedure for studying vesico-ureteric reflux is?** *(PGMEE 2012)*
   a. Intravenous urogram
   b. Cystogram
   c. Ascending pyelogram
   d. Micturiting cystourethrogram

   [Ref: Bailey & Love's Short Practice of Surgery 26th/e/p 117]

114. **How is ureterocoele visualized on intravenous urography?** *(PGMEE 2016-17)*
   a. Adder head appearance
   b. Flower wase appearance
   c. Golf hole appearance
   d. Drooping water lilly

   [Ref: Love & Bailey 26th/e pg. 1286]

115. **A female patient presented with recurrent Urinary tract infections. Imaging shows the following picture.What can be the most probable diagnosis:** *(Recent Pattern June 2018)*

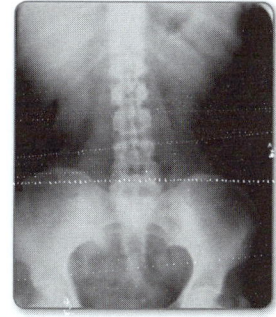

   a. Congenital Megaureter b. Duplication of Ureter
   c. Ureterocele d. Urinary Stones

Explanation

Ureterocele

- It is a submucosal cystic dilation of the terminal segment of the ureter.
- A ureterocele may be classified as:-
  ○ Intravesical (present entirely within the bladder), or
  ○ Extravesical, defined by the permanent presence of some portion of the ureterocele at the bladder neck or urethra.
- Other classification systems for ureteroceles are based on the location of insertion of the ureter into the bladder (simple orthotopic and ectopic) or based on their association with a single or duplicated system.
- Symptoms can include:
  ○ Frequent UTIs
  ○ Pyelonephritis
  ○ Obstructive/ voiding dysfunction
  ○ Retention of urine
  ○ Failure to thrive
  ○ Hematuria
  ○ Cyclic abdominal pain
  ○ Urolithiasis/urinary calculi
- **Cobra head sign** is seen in radiography
- In females: salpingitis, hydrosalpinx with sepsis or torsion may occur.
- Redundant collection systems are usually smaller in diameter than single, and predispose the patient to impassable renal stones.

OBSTETRIC & GYNEC RADIOLOGY

116. **T sign is seen in:** *(PGMEE2013-14)*
   a. Genital TB
   b. Membrane in twin pregnancy
   c. Molar pregnancy
   d. Choriocarcinoma

   [Ref: Placenta multimodality imaging RSNA]

117. **Investigation of choice in congenital uterine anomaly is:-** *(PGMEE2013-14)*
   a. MRI
   b. HSG
   c. CT
   d. Hysteroscopy

   [Ref: Placenta multimodality imaging RSNA; Imaging of Miilerion Duct Anomalies RSNA]

118. **USG is definitive investigation of:-** *(PGMEE2013-14)*
   a. Vasa previa
   b. Abruption placenta
   c. Placenta previa
   d. Imperforate hymen

   [Ref: Dutta Obs 7th/e/p.244]

119. **Fetal cardiac activity can be detected earliest by USG at which age of intrauterine life:-** *(PGMEE2013-14)*
   a. 1-2 week
   b. 2-4 week
   c. 5-6 week
   d. 6-8 week

   [Ref: Internet]

120. **Spalding sign is seen in:-** *(PGMEE2013-14)*
   a. Abortion
   b. Still birth
   c. IUD
   d. Infanticide

   [Ref: Radiology Review Mannual 8th/e pg. 1357]

Explanation

- The Spalding sign is a sign of intra-uterine fetal death (IUD).
- There is overlapping of the fetal skull bones caused by collapse of the fetal brain. It appears usually a week or more after fetal death in utero.

121. **Gas shadow in heart and great vessels appears in:**
   a. IUD *(PGMEE2013-14)*
   b. Abortion
   c. Still birth
   d. None

   [Ref: Radiology Review Mannual 8th/e pg. 1357]

122. **Snow storm appearance is seen in?** *(DNB Dec 2011)*
   a. Tubal pregnancy
   b. Abdominal pregnancy
   c. Hydatidiform mole
   d. Fibroid

   [Ref: Dutta Obs 8th ed pg]

113.	d
114.	a
115.	c
116.	b
117.	a
118.	c
119.	c
120.	c
121.	a
122.	c

123. A female patient presenting with dyspareunia with MRI lateral view is shown below. Most likely diagnosis is:
(*Recent Pattern June 2018*)

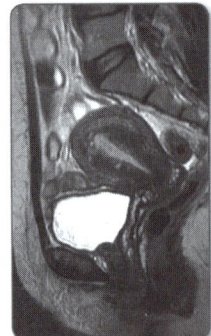

   a. Tuboovarian mass   b. Rectal carcinoma
   c. Urethral caruncle   d. Adenomyosis

[*Ref: Shaw's Gynae 15th/e pg.475*]

MUSCULOSKELETAL SYSTEM

SKULL

124. Punched out lesions in skull are seen in-
(*PGMEE 2013-14, PGMEE 2015*)
   a. Metastasis
   b. Osteomalacia
   c. Multiple myeloma
   d. Hyperparathyroidism

[*Ref: Harrison Manual of Medicine 19th/e /ch 66*]

125. Geographic skull is seen in which condition?
   a. Multiple myeloma   (*PGMEE 2015*)
   b. Pagets disease
   c. Fibrous dysplasia
   d. Eosinophilic granuloma

[*Ref: Nelson 20th/e/p 2487*]

126. 'Pepper pot' appearance of skull is seen in?
   a. Hyperparathyroidism   (*DNB JUNE 2011*)
   b. Pseudo hyperparathyroidism
   c. Hyperthyroidism
   d. Multiple myeloma

[*Ref: Yochum & Rowe's Essential of Skeletal radiology, volume 2, 3rd/ed pg. 1518*]

127. Luckenschadel skull is typically seen in:-
   a. Crouzon Syndrome   (*PGMEE 2015-16*)
   b. Sturge Weber Syndrome
   c. Arnold Chiari Malformation
   d. Paget's disease

[*Ref: Radiology Review Mannual 8th/e pg. 265*]

128. Block vertebrae are seen in:-   (*PGMEE2013-14*)
   a. Pagets disease   b. Leukemia
   c. TB   d. Klippel – Feil syndrome

[*Ref: Nelson 20th/e/ch 680*]

129. Osteolytic metastasis is seen with:-   (*PGMEE2013-14*)
   a. Lung   b. Kidney
   c. Thyroid   d. All of the above

[*Ref: Nelson 20th/e/p 3326*]

130. In fracture of nose, which view X-ray taken:-
(*PGMEE2013-14*)
   a. Waters view   b. Caldwells view
   c. Lateral view   d. Occlusive anterior view

131. Punctated lesions and floating teeth are seen in all EXCEPT:-
(*PGMEE2013-14*)
   a. Metastasis   b. Osteitis fibrosa
   c. Histiocytosis   d. Asbestosis

132. ''Bone within a Bone'' appearance is seen in:
(*DNB 2007*)
   a. Osteoporosis   b. Osteopetrosis
   c. Rickets   d. Scurvy

[*Ref: Nelson 20th/e/Ch 699 p 3375*]

133. A 50 year old male with history of bone pain presents to Hospital. X-ray lateral view Skull is shown below. Most likely cause is:-
(*PGMEE 2018*)

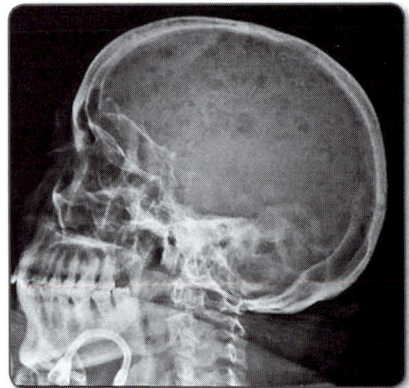

   a. Eosinophilic granuloma
   b. Paget's disease
   c. Multiple myeloma
   d. Hyperparathyroidism

Explanation

- Skull radiograph is showing characteristic multiple "punched out" lesions.
- Punched out lesions with history of bone pain in elderly points towards diagnosis of Multiple myeloma.

Radiological signs in

Sign	Seen due to
Hyperparathyroidism	Salt & pepper skull/ Pepper pot skull. Rain drop skull
Paget's disease	Tom-O Shanter sign, Widening of inner & outer tables (Increased diploic space), Cotton wool appearance, Osteoporosis-circumscripta d/to large well defined lytic lesions
Eosinophilic granuloma	Single or multiple , well defined destructive (lytic) bony lesions in boys usually <10 yr.
Multiple myeloma	Multiple lytic and punched out lesions in elderly

134. **'Sausage digits' appearance is seen in:** *(PGMEE 2015)*
 a. Rickets
 b. Rheumatoid Arthritis
 c. Psoriatic arthritis
 d. Hyperthyroidism

[Ref: Harrison 19 Manual of Medicine 19th/e/ch 161 pg 857]

135. **Acro-osteolysis is seen in:** *(PGMEE 2015)*
 a. Gout
 b. Hyperparathyroidism
 c. Amyloidosis
 d. Multiple Myeloma

[Ref: Harrison Manual Of Medicine 19th/e/p 176]

136. **All of the following are seen in Hypothyroidism except:-**
 a. Stipulated ribs *(PGMEE 2015-16)*
 b. Wormian bones
 c. Epiphyseal Dysgenesis
 d. Beaking of vertebra

[Ref: https://www.ncbi.nlm.nih.gov/pmc/articles/ PMC3830298/#!PO=42.3077]

137. **Fallen fragment sign:** *(PGMEE 2018)*
 a. Simple bone cyst
 b. Osteosarcoma
 c. Adamantinoma
 d. Aneurysmal bone cyst

[Ref: Radiology Review Mannual 8th/e pg. 200]

Explanation

- The fallen fragment sign refers to the presence of a bone fracture fragment resting dependently in a cystic bone lesion.
- Pathognomonic for a unicameral/simple bone cyst following a pathological fracture.
- Occasionally reported with other cystic lesions, e.g. eosinophilic granuloma

SOFT TISSUES

138. **Epidermoid cyst can be differentiated from arachnoid cyst by:-** *(PGMEE2013-14)*
 a. MRI
 b. USG
 c. Myelography
 d. CT scan

[Re: Love & Bailey 26th/e/p 616]

Explanation

- Epidermoid cyst shows diffusion restriction and arachnoid cyst does not show.

139. **Investigation of choice for entrapment neuropathy is?** *(DNB DEC 2010)*
 a. CT b. MRI
 c. SPECT d. Clinical exam

[Ref: Internet]

140. **Radiologically true about Lipoma is-** *(PGMEE 2015)*
 a. Hypo-intense on T1-MRI
 b. Hypo-intense on T2-MRI
 c. Anechoic on US
 d. Low attenuation on CT

141. **Prevertebral space thickness in adult at C3-C4 level is:-** *(PGMEE 2013-14)*
 a. 7 mm b. 14 mm
 c. 22 mm d. 30 mm

Explanation

Level	Flexion (mm)	Neutral (mm)	Extension (mm)
C1	11	10	8
C2	6	5	6
C3	7	7	6
C4	7	7	8
C5	22	20	20
C6	20	20	19
C7	20	20	21

CONNECTIVE TISSUE DISORDERS

142. **Radiological feature of sarcoidosis:-** *(PGMEE 2013-14)*
 a. Hilar lymphadenopathy
 b. Hilar lymphadenopathy with parenchymal lung changes
 c. No Hilar lymphadenopathy with parenchymal lung changes
 d. All of the above

[Ref: Harrison Manual Of Medicine 19th/e/ch 166]

Explanation

Stages of sarcoidosis on chest Radiograph

Stage 0	Normal chest Radiograph
Stage 1	Hilar or Mediastinal lymphadenopathy only
Stage 2	Lymphadenopathy + Parenchymal changes
Stage 3	Parenchymal Disease only
Stage 4	End stage lung disease (Pulmonary fibrosis)

143. **Most common radiological feature of sarcoidosis in Indian patients is:-** *(PGMEE2013-14)*
 a. Normal chert x-ray
 b. Bilateral hilar lymphadenopathy
 c. Bilateral hilar lymphadenopathy with parenchymal infilterate
 d. Only parenchymal infilterate

[Ref: Nelson 20th/e/ch 165]

144. **Potato nodes are feature of?** *(DNB June'2010)*
 a. Sarcoidosis b. Lymphoma
 c. Carcinoid d. Tuberculosis

[Ref: Chest radiology: the essentials By Jannette Collins, Eric J. Stern, page 165]

Explanation

- Potato nodes are a classical presentation for the large nodes seen in the lung hila and mediastinum on the chest radiograph in pulmonary sarcoidosis.

134.	c
135.	b
136.	a
137.	a
138.	a
139.	b
140.	d
141.	a
142.	d
143.	c
144.	a

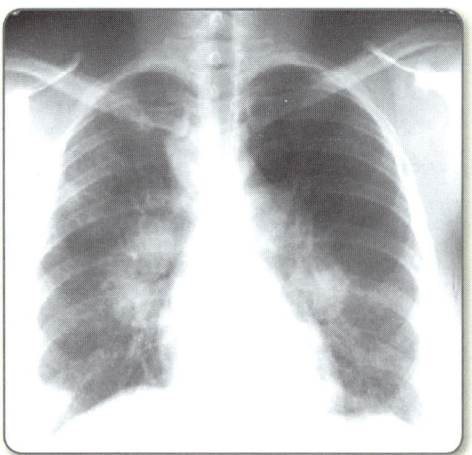

- Garland triad, also known as the 1-2-3 sign or pawnbroker's sign, is a LN enlargement pattern on CXR in sarcoidosis:
  - Right paratracheal nodes
  - Right hilar nodes
  - Left hilar nodes
- Hilar lymphadenopathy is symmetrical and usually massive. These so-called potato nodes typically do not abut the cardiac border which distinguishes the nodal enlargement from lymphoma .
- Involvement of right paratracheal nodes reflects the ease with which these nodes are identified on plain radiography.
- Left paratracheal and aortopulmonary nodes are frequently enlarged but harder to identify

145. b

RA

145. A patient suffering from morning stiffness >1 hour, presents with the following abnormality in the X-ray. What can be the most possible diagnosis:

a. Psoriatic Arthritis *(Recent Pattern June 2018)*

b. Rheumatoid Arthritis

c. Osteoarthritis

d. Relapsing polychondritis

[Ref: Harrison 19th/e, pg.2144]

Explanation

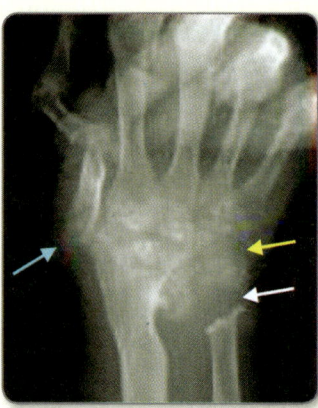

- Radiograph is characteristic of severe rheumatoid arthritis of the wrist and hand.
  - The ulnar styloid is destroyed with the rest of the distal ulna (white arrow)
  - There is destruction of the carpal bones (yellow arrow) and there is dislocation of the 1st metacarpal on the destroyed trapezium (blue arrow).
  - All of the bones are osteopenic.
- The initial radiographic finding is periarticular osteopenia
- Other findings on plain radiographs include
  - Symmetric joint space loss
  - Marginal erosions (initially bare areas) most frequently in the wrists and hands (MCPs and PIPs)

UNITS IN RADIOLOGY

1. S.I. Unit of radiation absorption is-
   (PGMEE 2015, 2016-17)
   a. Curie
   b. REM
   c. Rad
   d. Gray

[Ref: Grainger 4th/e p. 232]

Explanation

Radiation...	SI Unit	Original unit	Conversion
Exposure		Röntgen	
Activity	becquerel (Bq)	Curie (Ci)	1 Bq= 2.703 x 10^{-11} Ci
Absorbed <u>d</u>ose (Physical dose)	gray (Gy)	<u>R</u>ad	1 Gy = 100 rad
Biological dose or dose equivalent	sievert (Sv)	rem	1 Sv = 100 rem
Effective dose or Effective dose equivalent	sievert (Sv)	rem	1 Sv = 100 rem

[**Mn:** Rem with sivert Ram sita together; Red and Gray colors are together]

2. Gray equals – *(PGMEE 2012)*
   a. 100 rad
   b. 1000 rad
   c. 10000 rad
   d. 100000

[Ref: Radiation physics p. 27]

3. What is the unit of Radioactivity? *(PGMEE 2016-17)*
   a. Rad
   b. Rem
   c. Gray
   d. Curie

[Ref: Radiation Physics p. 27]

BASICS OF IONIZATION

4. Action of ionization radiation on tissues is by mechanism of- *(PGMEE 2014)*
   a. Thermal injury
   b. Excitation of electron from orbit
   c. Formation of pyramidine dimer
   d. Linear acceleration injury

[Ref: Radiation physics p. 73]

5. Which of the following statements best describes 'Background Radiation': *(PGMEE 10)*
   a. Radiation in the background of nuclear reactors
   b. Radiation from nuclear fall out
   c. Radiation present constantly from natural sources
   d. Radiation in the background during radiological investigations

[Ref: Love & Bailey 26th/e/ch 13 p 172]

6. Bragg effect is produced by:- *(PGMEE 2018)*
   a. Protons
   b. Neutrons
   c. Electrons
   d. Photons

Explanation

Special Effects in Radiology

- *Bragg effect* is seen with → Charged heavy particles like alpha particle, protons.
- *Bremsstrahlung effect* is seen with → Beta particles and X-rays.
- *Bremsstrahlung (breaking) radiation:* EM radiation produced by the deceleration of a charged particle, when deflected by another charged particle. This is the process by which X-rays are produced.
- *Photographic effect*
- X-ray film is made up of *cellulose acetate*, coated on its both sides with silver bromide emulsion. This emulsion is photosensitive and is responsible for P~ effect.
- *Fluorescent effect*
- When X-ray strikes mettalic salts like Zn, Cd, sulphides, the rays cause them to fluoresce.
- **Photoelectric effect**
  Absorption of **low energy** from radiation in tissue leads to ionization. Used in *diagnostic* radiology.
- **Compton effect** → d/to absorption of **high energy**, used in *therapeutic* radiology.

7. Which one of the following has the maximum ionization potential? *(PGMEE 13)*
   a. Electron
   b. Proton
   c. Helium ion
   d. Gamma-Photon

[Ref: Grainger Allison's diagnostic Radiology 4th/e/p39]

Explanation

- *Ionizing potential* is energy required to remove an electron from the neutral atom. It is a minimum for the alkali metals which have a single electron outside a closed shell.
- Ionizing potential is maximum with → Helium ion
- Ionizing potential is lowest with → Cesium

1.	d
2.	a
3.	d
4.	b
5.	c
6.	d
7.	c

8. **Most ionizing radiation potential is by-** *(PGMEE 10)*
   a. Alpha
   b. Beta
   c. Gamma
   d. X-rays

   [Ref: Grainger Allison's diagnostic Radiology 4th/e p. 39]

9. **Most harmful to individual cell –** *(PGMEE 2014)*
   a. X-rays
   b. α –particles
   c. β – particles
   d. X-rays

   [Ref: Grainger & Allison's diagnostic Radiology 4th/e p. 139)

10. **Radioactive energy is released from?** *(PGMEE 2011)*
    a. Electron
    b. Proton
    c. Neutrons
    d. All

    [Ref: Vasudevan Sree Kumari 3/e p.402, CSDT 10th /e p. 1256]

11. **What is NOT correct about Neutron contrast study?** *(PGMEE 2015)*
    a. Allows visualization of light elements inside heavy metallic objects
    b. Hydrogen and born have high neutron cross section
    c. Is an example of destructive testing
    d. Provides spatial resolution

    [Ref: http://www.ndt.net/article/nde-india2011/pdf/3-30C-4.pdf]

12. **Radioiodine generates which type of radiation-** *(PGMEE 2015)*
    a. Alpha and beta rays
    b. Alpha and beta rays
    c. X-rays
    d. Beta and gamma rays

    [Ref: Emergency Public Health : Preparedness and Response p. 359]

TYPES OF RADIOTHERAPY

13. **Intraoperative radiotherapy is used in-** *(PGMEE 2015)*
    a. Colon carcinoma
    b. Gastric cancer
    c. Pancreatic carcinoma
    d. All of the above

    [Ref: Internet]

Explanation

- *Intraoperative radiation therapy (IORT)* delivers a concentrated dose of radiotherapy to a tumor bed during surgery. It is a modification of external beam therapy, in which radiation is delivered by a linear accelerator.
- IORT help in killing microscopic disease, reduce radiation treatment times or provide an added radiation "boost."
- Historically, the most treated tumour locations are repre-sented by colorectal carcinoma, pancreatic carcinoma, gastric carcinoma, biliary carcinoma, soft tissue sarcoma, gyne-cologic malignancies, and bladder cancer but in the last ye-ars new indications emerged like breast cancer, head and neck tumours, prostate carcinoma, intra-thoracic malignan- cies, and brain tumours.
- IORT is beneficial in:
  o Breast conserving cancer surgery in CA breast is the main indication
  o Advanced primary or recurrent colorectal cancer
  o CA pancreas

8.	a
9.	b
10.	d
11.	c
12.	d
13.	d
14.	d
15.	b
16.	a
17.	a
18.	c
19.	b
20.	a

14. **Craniospinal irradiation is used in the Treatment of:** *(PGMEE 2014)*
    a. Oligodendroglioma
    b. Pilocytic astrocytoma
    c. Mixed oligoastrocytoma
    d. Medulloblastoma

    [Ref: Intracranial metastasis: current management strategies p.135]

Explanation

- Craniospinal Irradiation is used for t/t of medulloblas-toma and other brain tumors, which tend to spread via CSF.

15. **High dose radiation which is precisely directed is used in-** *(PGMEE 2015)*
    a. EBRT
    b. IMRT
    c. Stereotectic radiosurgery
    d. None of the above

    [Ref: Love & Bailey 26th/e/ p 141]

16. **In which of the following tumour use Stereotactic radio-surgery is made?** *(PGMEE 2015)*
    a. Brain tumor
    b. Ewing's sarcoma
    c. Osteosarcoma
    d. All of the above

    [Ref: Love & Bailey 26th/e/p 614]

17. **A female with chordoma is likely to be benefitted from:**
    a. Proton
    b. Neutron *(PGMEE 2018)*
    c. X-rays
    d. Beta radiation

18. **In brachytherapy for cervical cancer, point "A" corresponds to-** *(PGMEE 2015)*
    a. 2 cm superior to the cervical os and 2 cm medial to the uterine canal
    b. 2 cm inferior to the cervical os and 2 cm lateral to the uterine canal
    c. 2 cm superior to the cervical os and 2 cm lateral to the uterine canal
    d. None of the above

    [Ref: Shaw's Gynaecoloy 15th/e/p 436)

ADVERSE EFFECTS OF RADIATION

19. **Which of the following statements about 'Stochastic effects' of radiation is true?** *(PGMEE 10)*
    a. Severity of effect is a function of dose
    b. Probability of effect is a function of dose
    c. It has a threshold
    d. Erythema and cataract are common examples

    [Ref: Love & Bailey 26th/e/p 172]

20. **Which delivers highest dose of radiation:-**
    a. Cardiac perfusion scan (≈10msu) *(PGMEE 2013-14)*
    b. CT chest (7 msu)
    c. CT brain (2 msu)
    d. Mammogram (0.4 msu)

    [Ref: Love & Bailey 26th/e/p 172]

Explanation

Dose of Radiation in

Procedure	Dose
▪ Cardiac perfusion scan	~ 10 mSv
▪ CT chest	7 mSv
▪ CT brain	2 mSv
▪ Mammography	0.4 mSv

21. Which is a late and severe adverse effect of radiation therapy: *(PGMEE 2015)*
a. Nausea
b. Osteoradionecrosis
c. Anemia
d. Erythema

[Ref: Love & Bailey 26th/e/p721]

RADIOISOTOPES

22. Which of the following is a pure beta particle emitter? *(DNB Dec 2011, PGMEE 2013-14)*
a. Co60
b. I131
c. P32
d. Gold

[Ref: Meredith radiation physics and nuclear medicine p.28]

23. An ideal therapeutic radioisotope is:- *(PGMEE 2015-16)*
a. Low Beta; Low Gamma emitter
b. Strong Beta; Low Gamma emitter
c. Strong Beta; Strong Gamma emitter
d. Low Beta; Strong Gamma emitter

24. Route of administration of radioactive iodine- *(PGMEE 2015)*
a. Oral
b. Subcutaneous
c. Intravenous
d. All of the above

[Ref: Various books ncbi.gov.in]

25. What is the half-life of strontium in radiotherapy – *(PGMEE 2014)*
a. 8 years
b. 20 years
c. 28 years
d. 100 years

[Ref: Radiation oncology p. 239]

26. The half-life of Cobalt-60 is *(PGMEE 2014)*
a. 4.2 years
b. 5.2 years
c. 6.2 years
d. 7.2 years

[Ref: Shaw's Gynaecology 15th/e/p 436]

27. Which of the following is not used for internal radiotherapy? *(PGMEE 2015; 14)*
a. Iodine – 131
b. Cobalt-60
c. Iridium-192
d. Iodine-125

[Ref: Radiotherapy & brachytherapy by Alessandra cancer p. 191]

28. Isotope used in RAIU- *(PGMEE 2014, AI 07)*
a. I131
b. I123
c. I125
d. Either I-131 or I-123

[Ref: Love & Bailey 26th/e/ch 51]

RADIOSENSITIVITY

29. Most radiosensitive tumor among following is:- *(PGMEE 2011, 2013-14)*
a. Bronchogenic
b. Parotid carcinoma
c. Dysgerminoma
d. Osteogenic sarcoma

[Ref: Textbook of Radiotherapy 7th/e p.964, Rozer's Radiotherapy 3rd/e table 11.3]

30. Radioresistant tumor is:- *(PGMEE 2013-14)*
a. Ewings sarcoma
b. Retinoblastoma
c. Osteosarcoma
d. Neuroblastoma

[Ref: Textbook of Radiotherapy 7the p. 964]

31. Maximum radiation dose is tolerable by which tissue? *(PGMEE 2013-14)*
a. Hemopoietic tissue
b. Testis
c. Ovary
d. Bone

[Ref: Textbook of Radiotherapy]

32. Most radiosensitive organ in humans: *(Recent Pattern June 2018)*
a. Adrenal
b. Pancreas
c. Gonads
d. Uterus

[Ref: Harrison's 19th/e pg. 263e; Textbook of Radiotherapy 7th/e pg. 964]

Explanation

Most radiosensitive organs:
- Bone marrow
- Gonads
- Growing cartilage
- Prepubescent breast

Organs with lowest radiosensitivity:
- Adrenal
- Vagina
- Uterus
- Pancreas

Radiosensitivity categories

Cat		Radiosensitivity
A	Ewing's, Wilm's, Seminoma, Lymphoma	Most radiosensitive, So radiotherapy is TOC
B	Medulloblastoma, SCLC (Small cell CA of lung)	
C	CA Breast, CA bladder, CA cervix	
D	Pancreas, SqCC lung, Colorectal	
E	Melanoma, Renal cell CA, Glioblastoma, osteosarcoma	Least radiosensitive (Relatively radioresistant)

MISCELLANEOUS

33. When is oxygen administration effective in radiotherapy? *(DNB Dec 2011)*
a. Just after starting
b. Just before starting
c. After 10 min
d. After 15 min

[Ref: Medical Radiology & Radiation Oncology page 223]

34. M in $^{99}Tc^m$ stands for? *(DNB Dec 2010)*
a. Mega
b. Metastatic
c. Metastable
d. Micro

[Ref: Nuclear Physics: Principles & Aplication By Lilley Page 20]

35. Gamma knife is used in? *(DNB June 2010)*
a. Radiotherapy
b. Radioisotope scan
c. Nuclear medicine
d. Chemotherapy

[Ref: Stereotactic Radiosurgery: Technique & Evaluation p.354]

21.	b
22.	c
23.	b
24.	d
25.	c
26.	b
27.	a
28.	b
29.	c
30.	c
31.	d
32.	c
33.	b
34.	c
35.	a

36. Which element of the following on disintegration leads to daughter element in gaseous from? *(DNB June 2010)*
a. Radium
b. Iridium
c. Uranium
d. Radon

[Ref: Internet]

37. Most common cancer due to Radiation: *(PGMEE 2014)*
a. Leukaemia
b. Breast Ca
c. Thyroid Ca
d. Bronchogenic cancer

[Ref: Harrison Manual of Medicine 19th/e/ch 65]

CELL CYCLE

38. In cell cycle the most radio sensitive stage is
(PGMEE 09)
a. S phase
b. G1phase
c. G2 phase
d. G2M phase

[Ref: Bhaduri 4th/e p. 495]

39. Most radio resistant phase in cell cycle *(PGMEE 2014)*
a. G1
b. Early S
c. Late S
d. G2

[Ref: Bhaduri 4th/e p. 495]

RADIOSENSITIZERS AND RADIOPROTECTORS

40. Radioprotective drug is: *(PGMEE 01, 12)*
a. Paclitaxem
b. Etoposide
c. Amifostine
d. Vincristine

[Ref: KDT]

41. Amifostine, protects all of the following except
(PGMEE 09)
a. CNS
b. Salivary glands
c. GIT
d. Kidneys

[Ref: Radiation oncology 8th/e p. 41]

36.	a
37.	a
38.	d
39.	c
40.	c
41.	a

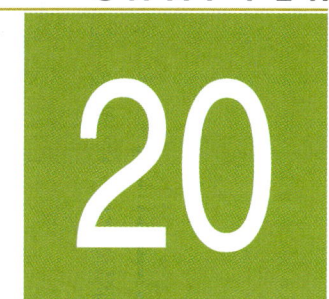
Obstetrics and Gynecology

FACTS

- Weight of nulliparous uterus is 50 – 70 g.
- Capacitation takes place in fallopian tube.
- Fertilized ovum gets implanted in the uterine cavity by 6-10 days after fertilization
- During the 5th week of gestation, gonads begin to develop as *genital ridge* from the urogenital ridges.
- By the 7th week → gonads become structurally male or female.
- By the 12th week → external genitalia become differentiated.
- At approximately 15 weeks of gestation → transabdominal ultrasonography can often distinguish between the two sexes.
- Uterus becomes abdominal organ after 12 weeks of pregnancy.
- Uterus again becomes pelvic organ post-delivery within: 2 weeks
- Incidence of breech presentation at term pregnancy is 3%.
- To say twin discordance, difference in weight should be ≥ 25%.
- Single MI determinant of survival, healthy growth and development of an infant: Birth weight
- In epidural analgesia during labor, block is from T10 to S5 dermatome.
- In epidural anesthesia for C section, block is from T4 to S1 dermatome.
- Twin gestational sacs can be detected by USG earliest at: 6–7 wks of gestation.

- Best time to detect the chorionicity of placenta by USG: 10-13 wks of gestation.
- The optimal timing for single ultrasound examination in the absence of specific indications: 18 to 20 weeks
- Modified BPP combines the use of an NST and assessment of an AFI (amniotic fluid index).
- Total iron requirement in pregnancy is 1000 mg.
- Minimum antenatal visits prescribed by WHO are four.
- Dose of levonorgestrel in emergency contraceptive pills is 1.5 mg.
- Most effective contraceptive in lactating mother: Progestin only pill.
- Most reliable marker for neural tube defect: Acetylcholinesterase.
- Adequate intake of folic acid reduces the risk of NTD
- ***Preterm labor*** → onset of labor before 37 completed weeks
- ***Post-term pregnancy*** → pregnancy continuing beyond 2 weeks of EDD
- ***Anterior/Naegele's asynclitism*** is mostly seen in multipara. Anterior parietal bone is the presenting part.
- ***Posterior/Litzman's asynclitism*** is mostly seen in nullipara. Posterior parietal bone is the presenting part.

Anatomy of Maternal Pelvis and Fetal Skull

- Shortest diameter of the true pelvis: Interspinous diameter (10 cm)
- Shortest diameter of fetal skull: Bimastoid (7.5 cm) > Bitemporal diameter (8 cm)
- Longest diameter of fetal skull: Mento-vertical
- Engagement of fetal head is related to: Biparietal diameter
- Obstetric conjugate → shortest distance between the sacral promontory and the pubis symphysis = 10 cm

- The obstetric conjugate cannot be measured directly due to the presence of the bladder.
- One Ala is absent is → Naegele's pelvis.
- Both Ala are absent in → Robert's pelvis

Triradiate pelvis is seen in:

- Osteomalacia
- Rickets in adults

Diameters of fetal skull	Measurement	Attitude of the Head	Presentation
Suboccipito-bregmatic	9.5 cm	Complete flexion	Vertex
Suboccipito-frontal	10 cm	Partial flexion	Vertex
Occipito-frontal	11.5 cm	Marked deflexion	Vertex
Mento-vertical	14 cm	Partial extension	Brow
Submento-vertical	11.5 cm	Partial extension	Face
Submento-bregmatic	9.5 cm	Complete extension	Face

Caldwell Moloy Anatomical Classification of Female Pelvis

Type	Inlet	Side Walls	Comment
Gynecoid (50%)	Rounded	Straight	▪ Normal female pelvis, MC type
Anthropoid (25%)	Oval shaped	Straight	▪ Only pelvis with AP diameter > Transverse ▪ Face to pubis delivery is MC associated
AnDroid Pelvis (20%)	Triangular/ Heart shaped	Convergent	▪ Male type of pelvis ▪ **D**eep transverse arrest/Non rotation/**D**ystocia is MC
Platypelloid (5%)	Transversally oval	Straight	▪ Transverse diameter > AP diameter

Placenta

- Umbilical cord has 2 arteries and 1 vein
- Single umbilical artery is an indicator of increased incidence of malformation
- The human placenta is discoid in shape, deciduate & hemochorial
- Placenta weight is around 1/5th of fetal weight which is roughly around 600 g.
- The uteroplacental blood flow at term is: 750 ml

- Placenta **a**ccreta → villi **a**ttached to the myometrium
- Placenta **in**creta → villi **in**vade the myometrium
- Placenta **pe**rcreta → villi **pe**netrate through the entire myometrium
- Placenta succenturiata → presence of an accessory lobe which is separated from the main placenta
- Battledore placenta → cord insertion at or near the placental margin

Etiology of IUGR

- Single most sensitive parameter to detect IUGR → Abdominal circumference.

Maternal causes:
- Constitutional
- Poor maternal nutrition during pregnancy
- Alcohol, smoking
- Heart disease; Renal disease
- Chronic hypertension, PIH
- Diabetes with vascular lesion
- Thrombophilia
- Sickle cell anemia; Hemoglobinopathy

Fetal causes:
- Trisomy 13, 18, 21
- Multiple pregnancy
- HIV, Malaria, Varicella Zoster
- Turner syndrome
- TORCH

Placental causes:
- Placental Insufficiency
- Placenta previa
- Abruption Placenta

REMEMBER

Vaginal Changes in a Normal Pregnancy:
- Increase in vascularity
- Decrease in pH – becomes acidic
- Increase in number of Lactobacilli
- Thickening of vaginal epithelial lining

Arias Stella Reaction
- Adenomatous changes in the endometrial glands.
- Due to Progesterone influence.
- Seen in:
  - Ectopic pregnancy
  - Molar pregnancy

PREGNANCY SCALE

Embryonic Age

Implantation 6th day -------
(It correspionds to the 20th day
of regular menstrual cycle)

0 FERTILIZATION (=DAY 14 AFTER OVULATION)

5th day- blastocyst formation

8 days - *Pregnancy diagnosed* earliest by presence of β-hCG
(on 22nd day from LMP or day 8 post ovulation)
using Radioreceptor assay or serum β-hCG, amnion formation

9-10 days - Pregnancy diagnosis on 25th day from LMP using
radioimmune assay (urine pregnancy test/ UPT),
implantation completed, *chorion formation*

3 wk (21 days) Fetoplacental **circulation established**

(LMP is used below)

FETAL DEVELOPMENT
↓

Glucagon	8 wk
Swallowing, fetal inulin	10 wks
Breathing movement	11 wks
Urine, Thyroid, FSH/LH	12 wks
Meconium production	16 wks
Surfactant synthesis begins, Fetal weight 300 gm	20 wks
Sucking, Hearing	24 wks
Light perception	28 wks
Surfactant appears in AF	37 wks

Genotypes, Ovary/testes distinguishable.....   4 wk ...   Gestational sac by TVS

5 wk ...   Gestatioal ring bty TVS

6 wk ...   Cardiac activity by TVS,
Gestational sac, yolk sac, fetal poles

Transabdominal USG can detect all these events 1-2 wk later

7 wk ...   Cardiac activity by TAS

8 wk ...   Embryonic movements

9 wk ...   CRL for gestational age gives best predictive value

10 wk ...

11 wk →   Chorionic villous sampling (CVS)/ biopsy

Intestines in abdomen, finger, toes, skin, nails+   12 wk ...   Uterus at L/o pubic symphysis

Sex distinguishable, externally, penis/ vagina   14 wk   1st trimester screening for NTDs, Down's (11-14 wk)

15 wk

Radiological e/o fetal skeletal shadow.........   16 wk ...   Quickening starts in multipara
-         height of uterus midway b/n P.S. & umbilicus

2nd trimester screening for NTDs →   18 wk →   Quckening starts in primi
Ideal time for USG screening of gross congenital anomaly

Anomaly scan (18-20 wk) →   20 wk ...   Iron prophylaxis in pregnancy started

Surfactant synthesis starts, lanugo hairs+   22 wk ...

Spinal cord extends to S1.................   24 wk ...   Fundal height of uterus at L/o umbilicus

Eye Opening ....   26 wk   Universal screening for GDM by GTI

Fetal weight ~ 1000 gm ....   28 wk ...

→ Prophylactic anti-D to all unsensitized Rh-ve women

30 wk

32 wk

34 wk

36 wk ...   Uterus fundal height at L/o xiphsternum
Maximum volume fo amniotic fluid

Term, maturity attained .... 37 wk   38 wk ...   **Engagement** in primi

40 wk ...   EDD

(age from LMP = gestational age)   42+ wk ...   Post term pregnancy

©VDA

PHYSIOLOGY

- IgG is the only Ig that can cross the placenta.
- Water retention at term in pregnancy → 6.5 L
- Estrogen and progesterone in the initial 2 months of pregnancy are produced by: Corpus luteum
- Physiological suppression of ovulation occurs in the lactating women due to ↑ prolactin levels.
- In lactating women, prolactin remains elevated for 6 weeks.
- In non-lactating women, prolactin levels return to normal by 3 weeks after delivery.

- Early-morning urine sample is best to perform urine pregnancy tests, as it contains highest concentration of hCG.
- The mean doubling time for hCG in pregnancy is: ~ 1.5 to 2.0 days.

Lowest value of β hCG for which G-sac is visible:
- TAS → 6000 IU/mL
- TVS → 1500 IU/mL

hCG returns back to normal:
- After delivery → 2-4 weeks
- After abortion → 4-6 weeks
- Complete mole → 9 weeks
- Partial mole → 7 weeks

CHANGES IN PREGNANCY

- ABG in pregnancy normally shows a compensated respiratory alkalosis (because of hyperventilation).
- Pregnancy is a hypercoagulable state → risk of thromboembolism ↑ during pregnancy & puerperium.
- Pregnancy produces an overall euthyroid state, despite several changes in thyroid hormones.
- Pregnancy has a diabetogenic effect on metabolism → ↑ responsiveness to insulin, hyperinsulinemia, and hyperglycemia.
- Respiratory rate, Vital capacity remains unchanged

- TSH & free T_3, T_4 levels remains unchanged
- BT & CT remains unchanged

Findings on cardiovascular examination:
- Loud S1 with splitting, Loud S2
- S3 may be heard
- Ejection systolic murmur
- Mammary soufflé → continuous murmur at 2nd – 4th ICS
- ECG – left axis deviation
- CXR – enlarged cardiac shadow

Changes in Pregnancy		
Changes	**Increased**	**Decreased**
Hematological	▪ Hb mass, WBC, Neutrophilic leukocytosis ▪ Total protein, Globulin, Fibrinogen, Plasminogen ▪ ESR, C reactive proteins ▪ Coagulation factors 2, 7, 9, 10, 8 ▪ Serum transferrin, TIBC & O_2 carrying capacity ▪ Total alkaline phosphatase	▪ Hb concentration, Hematocrit, Platelet count ▪ Plasma protein, Albumin, A : G ratio (1:1) ▪ Protein S level ▪ Coagulation factors 11 & 13 ▪ Serum iron & ferritin
Respiratory	▪ Tidal volume, Inspiratory capacity, Minute ventilation, Pulmonary blood flow	▪ Residual volume, Expiratory reserve volume, Functional residual capacity, Total lung capacity,
Renal	▪ Renal blood flow, GFR, Creatinine clearance, Renal glycosuria	▪ Urea & Creatinine, BUN, Uric acid ▪ Plasma osmolality
Cardiovascular	▪ Pulse rate by 10 bpm, Stroke volume, Cardiac output Plasma/Blood volume, ▪ Uterine blood flow (~750 mL near term)	▪ Peripheral vascular resistance ▪ Diastolic, Systolic and Mean BP
Endocrine	▪ Insulin, Prolactin, Total T3 & T4	▪ LH, FSH
Others	▪ BMR, Calorie requirement by 300 kcal/day	▪ Serum sodium and potassium

AMNIOTIC FLUID

- pH of amniotic fluid: 7.1-7.3
- *Formation of amniotic fluid (AF):*
  - ○ Early pregnancy – ultrafiltrate of maternal plasma
  - ○ 2nd trimester – fetal plasma
  - ○ >20 weeks – fetal urine
- Surfactant synthesis begins at 20 weeks of gestation. It appears in amniotic fluid at 24–28 weeks.
- Early onset oligohydramnios leads to → Potter syndrome

Grades of Polyhydramnios:
- Mild → Pocket measure. 8-11 cm
- Moderate 12-15 cm
- Severe ≥ 16 cm

Gestational Age	Amount of AF
12 weeks	50 mL
16 weeks	200 mL
20 weeks	400 mL
36-38 weeks	1 L (Maximum)
≥ 38 weeks	900 mL

Color of AF	Associated Conditions
Golden color	Rh incompatibility
Amber/saffron	Postdated pregnancy
Tobacco juice	IUFD
Green	Meconium stained
Pale straw	Near term
Dark	Hemorrhage

	Oligohydramnios	Polyhydramnios
Criteria	■ Amniotic fluid volume <200 mL ■ Amniotic fluid pocket <2 cm ■ Amniotic fluid index (AFI) <5	■ Amniotic fluid volume >2000 mL ■ Maximum vertical pocket >8 cm ■ AFI >25
Etiology	■ Renal agenesis ■ Post dated pregnancy ■ Pre eclampsia	■ Anencephaly, Neural tube defects ■ Cleft palate ■ Esophageal atresia ■ Multiple pregnancy

EVENTS IN LABOR & DELIVERY

- *Braxton Hicks contractions* (false labor) are painless, irregular, infrequent, spasmodic contraction present throughout pregnancy.
  - ○ They are not associated with dilation of the cervix.
  - ○ Also seen in submucous fibroid, hematometra
  - ○ Absent in abdominal Pregnancy.
- *Leopold maneuver* is used for initial examination of the patient's abdomen during labor. It includes a series of four palpations of the uterus and fetus therein through the abdominal wall to determine fetal lie, fetal presentation, and fetal position.
- *Zero station:* During labor, if the presenting part has reached the level of the ischial spines, it is termed as zero station. Reaching zero station means Biparietal diameter (BPD) of the fetus, which is the greatest transverse diameter of the fetal skull, has negotiated the pelvic inlet.
- *Engagement* is descent of the BPD of the fetal head below the plane of the pelvic inlet. It is clinically suggested by palpation of the presenting part below the level of 0 station (ischial spines).
- The greatest rate of descent occurs during the latter portions of the 1st stage of labor and during the 2nd stage of labor.
- *Modified Ritgen maneuver* is used as an alternate to episiotomy to support the perineal tissues and facilitate extension of the head.
- *The Friedman curve* is commonly used for assessing a patient's progress in labor and identifying abnormal labor patterns.
- Assessment of progress of labor is best done using: Partograph
- *Bishop's score* → assess the viability and success of induction of labor
- *Augmentation* of labor should be considered if:-
  - ○ The intensity of contractions is <25 mm Hg above the baseline, and/or
  - ○ The frequency of contractions is <3/10 min
- Agent C/I for induction of labor in a women with previous LSCS: Misoprostol (PGE_1)
- Gold standard agent for cervical ripening as well as for inducing labor → PGE_2 i.e. Dinoprostone.
- *Artificial Rupture of Membranes (ARM):*
  - ○ Done by using → Kocher's forceps
  - ○ Contraindications:
    - – IUD → Medical induction preferred.
    - – Chronic Polyhydramnios→ Controlled ARM done.
    - – Early deceleration of fetal HR is relative contraindication.

- Amniotomy when combined with oxytocin administration early in the active stage of labor reduces duration of labor by up to 2 hours.
- *Bandl's ring* is pathological ring felt on per abdominal examination. It is due to obstruction.
- *Schroeder's ring* is physiological, felt on P/V examination, seen due to incoordinate uterine contraction.
- If a fetus has an estimated weight >4 to 4.5 kg (LGA), the risk ↑ of:
  - Dystocia, including shoulder dystocia
  - Cephalopelvic disproportion
- Selection criteria for External cephalic version in a breech include:
  - A normal fetus with reassuring FHR tracing,
  - Adequate amniotic fluid
  - Presenting part not in the pelvis.
- Cesarean section is the preferred mode of delivery for most physicians in case of breech.
- Late decelerations are considered significantly non reassuring especially when repetitive and associated with ↓ variability.
- Variable decelerations are the most common periodic FHR pattern.
- Amnioinfusion should not be used as a preventive measure for meconium aspiration syndrome because meconium passage may predate labor.

- *Post-dated pregnancy:*
  - Induction at 41 weeks is preferred.
  - The incidence of passage of meconium increases as pregnancy becomes prolonged as does the incidence of MAS.
- *Active phase arrest* is when there is no change in cervical dilation even after 4 hours of adequate uterine contraction and 6 hours of inadequate uterine contraction.
- *A prolonged latent phase*
  - Is one that exceeds 20 hours in nullipara or 14 hours in a multipara
  - It does not necessarily predict an abnormal active phase of labor.
  - Management – observation and sedation.
- *Prolonged 1ˢᵗ stage of labor:*
  - When the cervix dilates @ <1 cm/hour in nullipara, and < 1.5 cm/hour in multiparous women.
  - Management → observation, augmentation by amniotomy or oxytocin
- *A 2ⁿᵈ stage protraction disorder* should be considered when:
  - The 2ⁿᵈ stage exceeds 3 hours if regional anesthesia has been administered
  - The 2ⁿᵈ stage exceeds 2 hours if no regional anesthesia is used, or if the rate of descent of fetus is <1 cm/hour if no regional anesthesia is used.
- *Second stage arrest* is diagnosed when there is no descent after 1 hour of pushing.

Stages of Labor

Features	First Stage	Second Stage	Third Stage	Fourth Stage
Main event	▪ Cervical dilatation	▪ Delivery of fetus	▪ Delivery of placenta and membranes	▪ Observation
Starting point	▪ Onset of true labour pain	▪ Full dilatation of cervix	▪ Expulsion of the fetus	▪ Expulsion of the afterbirth
End point	▪ Full dilatation of cervix	▪ Expulsion of the fetus	▪ Expulsion of the afterbirths (placenta and membranes)	▪ Follow up for at least 1 hour after delivery
Average duration	▪ Primigravida – 12 hours ▪ Multipara – 6 hours	▪ Primigravida – 2 hours ▪ Multipara – 30 minutes	▪ 5- 15 minutes in both primigravida and multipara	▪ At least 1 hour in all patients
Phases	▪ *Latent phase* – effacement of cervix ▪ *Active phase* – Cervical dilatation ≥5 cm ▪ Rate of dilatation – ○ Primigravida –1.2 cm/hr ○ Multipara – 1.5 cm/hr	▪ *Propulsive* – descent of the presenting part to the pelvic floor ▪ *Expulsive* – Delivery of the baby due to maternal bearing down efforts		

ANTENATAL STEROID THERAPY

- Dexamethasone and betamethasone are corticosteroids recommended for antenatal patients with preterm labor pains before 34 weeks of pregnancy

Benefits:
- Starts 24-48 hours after administration of last dose
- Lung maturation in preterm fetuses
- Reduced incidence of respiratory distress syndrome, intraventricular hemorrhage and necrotizing enterocolitis (if delivery is delayed for at least 24 hours after *initiation* of steroid therapy)

Dosage:
- Betamethasone – 12 mg I/M for 2 doses, 24 hours apart
- Dexamethasone - 6 mg I/M for 4 doses, 12 hours apart

Risks:
- Flaring up of infections (chorioamnionitis in patients with preterm PROM)
- Hyperglycemia → requires insulin dose adjustment for GDM patients
- Transient ↓ in fetal movements

MULTIFETAL GESTATION

- MC type of multifetal gestation: Dizygotic twins
- MC type of conjoined twins: Thoracophagus
- MC presentation in multifetal pregnancy: Cephalo-cephalic
- *Risk factors:*
  - ↑ maternal age
  - Assisted reproductive technologies (ARTs)
  - Ovulation induction agents e.g. Clomiphene
- *Associated morbidities include:*
  - Preterm labor (most significant)
  - Congenital anomalies, IUGR
  - Hydramnios
  - Preeclampsia
  - Placental abruption & PPH

- The most important cause of neonatal mortality in twin pregnancy is preterm labor.
- Average duration of pregnancy is inversely related to the number of fetuses
- Embryo reduction in multiple pregnancy is done at around 11-13 weeks
- In monochorionic twins, vascular anastomosis can develop between fetuses which, in turn, can lead to twin-twin transfusion syndrome.
- *Superfecundation* → fertilization of ≥2 ova in the **same cycle** by separate act of coitus
- *Superfetation* → successive fertilization of ≥2 ova released in **different cycles** by sperms from separate act of coitus

HEMORRAGE IN PREGNANCY

- MC cause of APH: Abruptio placenta
- *MC cause of:*
  - Primary PPH - Atonic uterus
  - Secondary PPH - Retained Placenta
- PPH → loss of >500 mL of blood after completion of 3rd stage of labor
- **DOC** to treat PPH: Oxytoxin
- Best drug to control PPH: Carboprost $(PGF_{2\alpha})$ → Max dose = 2 mg
- *Predisposing factors for PPH:*
  - Distended uterus – Macrosomia, Hydramnios, Multiple pregnancy
  - Uterine malformation
  - Placental abnormalities

  - Previous h/o PPH
  - HELLP syndrome
- Apt test distinguishes fetal blood from maternal blood. It can be useful if the test is rapidly available and bleeding is worrisome but not significant enough to warrant emergency delivery.

Vasa previa:
- Passage of umbilical blood vessels over the internal os below the presenting part of the fetus.
- Seen in velamentous placenta
- Diagnosis by color doppler & Apt test / Singer's alkali denaturation test

Placenta Previa

- Placenta is located close to or over the internal cervical os.
- *Classification:*
  - Minor degree – Type I, Type II anterior
  - Major degree – Type II posterior, Type III & IV
- Complete placenta previa rarely resolves spontaneously, but partial and low-lying

placenta previa often resolves by 32 to 35 weeks of gestation.
- IOC to detect abnormally located placenta: TVS

Expectant management – by Macafee & Johnson
- Mother in good health
- No active vaginal bleeding
- Assured fetal well being
- Duration of pregnancy <37 weeks

Abruptio Placenta

- The classic presentation of abruption is vaginal bleeding with abdominal pain.
- Abruption in a prior pregnancy ↑ the risk of abruption in subsequent pregnancies

- MC cause of consumptive coagulopathy in pregnancy
- Couvelaire uterus is seen in: Abruptio placentae

	Placenta Previa	Abruptio Placenta
Classification	▪ Browne's classification	▪ Page classification
Aka	▪ Warning hemorrhage ▪ Fresh revealed bleed	▪ Accidental hemorrhage ▪ Types – concealed/revealed /mixed bleed
Risk factors	▪ Previous surgery (C-section, curettage), ▪ Multiparity	▪ Smoking, Hypertensive disorders, Folate deficiency, Cocaine abuse,
Associated with	▪ Malpresentations like breech ▪ Floating head	▪ Increase age and parity ▪ Prior abruption
Placenta	▪ Lower segment (low lying)	▪ Upper segment
Uterus	▪ Soft, relaxed, non-tender ▪ Size corresponds to gestational age	▪ Tense, contracted, tender ▪ Size may be disproportionate in concealed type
Bleeding	▪ Recurrent painless, causeless	▪ Continuous and painful bleeding PV
Effect on fetus	▪ Hemorrhage is rarely fatal ▪ Normal fetal heart sounds	▪ May be fatal → Hypotension/shock → Fetal distress → Fetal demise
Diagnosis	▪ Ultrasound (IOC – TVS)	▪ Clinical
Management	▪ Conservative, PV only in OT	▪ Stabilize → Rx of shock → Deliver the baby
Complications	▪ Premature labor, Retained placenta ▪ LBW – MC	▪ Prematurity – MC

PRETERM DELIVERY

- *Premature rupture of membranes (PROM)* is the rupture of the chorioamniotic membrane before the onset of labor.
- Preterm PROM (*PPROM*) is defined as PROM that occurs before 37 weeks of gestation.
- Latency period is the time from PROM to labor. It is inversely related to gestational age.
- *Risk factors for PROM:*
  ○ Smoking
  ○ Prior PROM
  ○ Prior preterm delivery

  ○ Short cervical length
  ○ Polyhydramnios
  ○ Multiple gestations
  ○ Bleeding in early pregnancy (threatened abortion)
- The major complication of PROM is intrauterine infection.
- As cervical length ↓ in mid pregnancy, the risk of preterm birth ↑
- Tocolytic of choice to prevent preterm labor: Nifedipine

ECTOPIC PREGNANCY

- Order of ectopic pregnancy → Ampullary > Isthmic > Fimbrial > Interstitial/Cornual > Abdominal > Ovarian > Cervical
- MI and MC risk factor for ectopic pregnancy → PID (MC agent – *Chlamydia*)
- Highest risk of ectopic pregnancy is after → tubal surgery
- *The classical clinical triad:*
  ○ History of Amenorrhea
  ○ Vaginal bleeding
  ○ Abdominal pain on affected side
- Most constant sign → Tenderness.

- Pathognomonic feature of ectopic pregnancy → Decidual cast
- History of D & C is a risk factor unique to cervical pregnancy
- MC type of ectopic pregnancy associated with rupture: Isthmic.

Criteria
Abdominal pregnancy → Studiford's criteria
Ovarian pregnancy → Spiegelberg's criteria
Cervical pregnancy → Rubin's criteria

Sites of Fallopian Tube Involved In Ectopic

	Ampulla	Isthmus	Fimbriae	Interstitium
Mode of termination	▪ Abortion (between 8-12 weeks)	▪ Rupture (between 6-8 weeks – **earliest**)	▪ Abortion	▪ Rupture (between 12-16 weeks)
Comments	▪ **MC** site for fertilization ▪ **MC** site of Ectopic pregnancy ▪ **MC** site for Tubal abortion	▪ Narrowest part of fallopian tube ▪ **MC** site for tubal rupture ▪ **MC** site for Tubectomy		▪ Late clinical presentation

Diagnosis

- Inappropriately rising serum β-hCG levels i.e. low levels with prolonged doubling time
- TVS and serial measurement of serum β-hCG → most valuable tools to confirm a suspicion of ectopic pregnancy
- Best modality (Gold standard) to diagnose unruptured tubal pregnancy → direct visualization by laparoscopy

USG features of Ectopic Pregnancy:
- Pseudosac
- Fluid in POD that fails to clot
- Blob sign → Adrenal mass
- Bagel sign → Cardiac motion in unruptured ectopic
- Ring of fire appearance on color doppler
- Interstitial line sign in interstitial pregnancy

Management

- Hemodynamically unstable patients → Laparotomy
- Dose of Anti D in surgically treated case of ectopic pregnancy: 50 µg

Drugs used for Medical management:
- Methotrexate → MC used drug
- Prostaglandins (PGF$_{2\alpha}$)
- Hyperosmolar glucose
- Actinomycin
- Potassium chloride

Indications for Expectant Management:
- Asymptomatic & hemodynamically stable
- Declining β hCG levels

Indications for Medical Management:
- Hemodynamically stable
- Gestational sac <4 cm
- Absence of fetal cardiac activity
- β hCG levels <5000 mIU/mL

ABORTIONS

- MC congenital anomaly of uterus associated with abortion: Septate uterus.
- MC cause of abortion is chromosomal abnormalities (aneuploidy), most of which are trisomies.
- 2nd trimester abortions are more likely to be caused by maternal systemic diseases, abnormal placentation, or other uterine abnormalities.
- Thrombophilia are MC associated with recurrent miscarriage.

Causes of Recurrent pregnancy loss:
- Chromosomal abnormalities (aneuploidy)
- Immunological – APLA syndrome
- Anatomic uterine defect
- Endocrine – Diabetes, Thyroid, PCOS
- Infection – rare

Regimen for Medical abortion:
- Mifepristone (200 mg orally) → 48 hours later → Misoprostol (PGE$_1$) 800 mg vaginally
- Highest efficacy within 63 days of amenorrhea

Contraindications of Medical abortion:
- Active liver / kidney disease
- Uncontrolled seizure disorder
- IUCD in place
- Concurrent long term steroid therapy
- Ectopic pregnancy
- > 35 years of age
- Suction & Evacuation is the most suitable method for 1st trimester abortion (up to 12 weeks).
  ○ Hegar's dilator is used for dilating cervical os.
  ○ Instrument for evacuation → Karman suction cannula.
- Method of choice for MTP in 2nd trimester (13-20 weeks) → Prostaglandins

Cervical incompetence/Cervical insufficiency:
- Painless cervical dilatation in 2nd trimester
- Diagnosis: Cervical length <25 mm & funnelling of internal os >1 cm
- Rx: McDonald cerclage, Shirodkar cerclage

Classification of Spontaneous Abortion

Type	Clinical History	Cervical Os	USG findings
Threatened	Vaginal bleeding ± cramps	Closed	Viable fetus
Inevitable	Bleeding + cramps ± rupture of membrane	Open	Nonviable fetus
Incomplete	Bleeding + cramps ± passage of tissue	Open	Retained products of conception
Complete	Bleeding + complete passage of POC	Closed	No product of conception
Missed	Fetal death in utero	Closed	Nonviable fetus
Recurrent	≥3 consecutive spontaneous abortions		

POSTPARTUM PERIOD

- Maximum chances of cardiac decompensation: Immediate postpartum > Intrapartum > Antepartum.
- Puerperal pyrexia is fever (≥100.4°F) for 24 hours or more after child birth
- *Involution of uterus:*
  - Regeneration of endometrium → 3 weeks.
  - Placental site regeneration → 6 weeks.
- In postpartum period, vaginal muscle tone may be strengthened by the use of Kegel exercises, pelvic muscle training exercises. These exercises are also effective in treating stress incontinence.
- Episodes of ↑ vaginal bleeding b/w days 8 and 14 postpartum is most likely due to the separation and passage of the placental eschar.
- Colostrum is steadily replaced by normal milk around the 5th postpartum day.

GESTATIONAL DIABETES MELLITUS (GDM)

- *Overt Diabetes* → Preexisting diabetes in a pregnant lady
- *Babies born to mother with GDM are at ↑ risk of:*
  - Macrosomia (birth weight >4000 g), LGA ↑risk of C-section
  - Early (preterm) birth and RDS
  - Recurrent hypoglycemia because their own insulin production is high owing to islet cell hyperplasia.
  - Higher risk of developing obesity and T_2 DM later in life.
- *Gestational diabetes may also ↑ the mother's risk of:*
  - High blood pressure and preeclampsia.
  - Future type 2 diabetes

- *Complications of GDM:*
  - Spontaneous abortion
  - Polyhydramnios
  - Malformations
  - Hypocalcemia
- Malformation most specific for GDM → Caudal regression syndrome.

Anomalies seen in IDM:
- MC are cardiac anomalies like TGA, VSD, Contraction of aortic, ASD
- CNS → Anencephaly, encephalocoele
- Skeletal & Spinal → Caudal regression syndrome
- Genitourinary → Renal agenesis
- GIT → Anal atresia

Screening & Diagnosis

One Step Strategy with 75 g OGTT:
- Done at 24–28 weeks of gestation in women not previously diagnosed with diabetes.
- The diagnosis is made when any of the following plasma glucose values are met:
  - Fasting ≥92 mg/dL
  - 1 hr ≥180 mg/dL
  - 2 hr ≥153 mg/dL

Two Step Strategy:
- Done at 24–28 weeks of gestation in women not previously diagnosed with diabetes.
- **Step 1:** Perform a 50 g **non fasting** test. If the plasma glucose measured at 1 h 130, 135, or 140 mg/dL, proceed to Step 2.

- **Step 2:** Perform a 100 g **fasting** OGTT. The diagnosis is made when ≥2 of the following are met (Carpenter Coustan criteria)
  - Fasting ≥95 mg/dL
  - 1hr ≥180 mg/dL
  - 2 hr ≥155 mg/dL
  - 3 hr ≥140 mg/dL
- Target glucose levels → Fasting plasma glucose ≤95 mg/dL; 1hr postprandial glucose ≤140 mg/dL; 2 hr postprandial glucose ≤120 mg/dL; $HbA_1c < 6.5\%$

Management of GDM

- Mainstay of management of GDM is diet.
- Insulin is the preferred medication for treating hyperglycemia in GDM.
- OHA safe in pregnancy are metformin and glyburide. Both cross the placenta but are not teratogenic.
- Insulin requirements ↑ throughout the pregnancy, most markedly between 28 - 32 weeks.

HEMOLYSIS IN FETUS (FETAL HYDROPS)

- Isoimmunization can occur when an Rh D -ve woman is pregnant with a fetus that has inherited the Rh D antigen from its father and is, thus, Rh D +ve.
- Fetal-maternal hemorrhage in pregnancy can potentially lead to sensitization of maternal RBCs, which can trigger a maternal immune response.
- Anti-Lewis and anti-I antibodies are NOT associated with fetal hydrops/hemolytic disease.
- Standard practice is to administer a 300-μg dose of anti-D immunoglobulin to all Rh D-ve women at about 28 weeks of gestation.
- Minimum amount of feto-maternal hemorrhage required for sensitization of maternal RBCs → 0.1 mL.
- 300 μg of anti-D immunoglobulin will protect 30 mL of fetal whole blood.
- The extent of the fetal-maternal hemorrhage can be assessed using the Kleihauer-Betke test.
- α Thalassemia is most common cause of non-immune hydrops fetalis.

THYROID DYSFUNCTION DURING PREGNANCY

- DOC for hyperthyroidism in 1st trimester of pregnancy: Propylthiouracil
- Methimazole has been associated with fetal scalp defects k/as **aplasia cutis** and choanal atresia. So methimazole should be avoided in the 1st trimester of pregnancy.
- Hypothyroidism in pregnancy is treated by administration of levothyroxine at sufficient dosage to normalize TSH levels.

HYPERTENSION IN PREGNANCY

- Maternal vasospasm is the predominant pathophysiology in preeclampsia and gestational hypertension.
- ***Risk factors for Preeclampsia:***
  - Primigravida
  - Age >40 years
  - Twin gestation
  - Previous or family history of preeclampsia
  - APLA syndrome
- ***Preeclampsia with severe features:***
  - SBP ≥160 mm Hg or DBP ≥110 mm Hg
  - New onset cerebral or visual disturbances
  - Pulmonary edema
  - Severe persistent upper quadrant or epigastric pain; Elevated liver enzymes
  - Progressive renal insufficiency
  - Thrombocytopenia (<1 lakh)
- Biochemical marker of Preeclampsia → elevated serum uric acid level.
- In most cases, severe preeclampsia is an indication for delivery, regardless of maturity or gestational age.
- ***Eclampsia*** is the additional presence of convulsions (generalized or tonic-clonic seizures) in woman with preeclampsia.
- Most cases of eclampsia occur within 24 hours of the delivery, but up to 10% of cases are diagnosed between day 2 and day 10 after delivery.
- ***Antepartum Eclampsia:***
  - Most common type
  - Associated with worst prognosis
- ACEI/ARB are contraindicated in pregnancy
- Antihypertensive of choice for hypertension in pregnancy: Labetalol
- MC cause of death in severe preeclampsia and eclampsia: Intracranial bleeding

Classification	Maternal BP	Onset	Proteinuria	Progression/End result
Chronic hypertension	>140/90 mmHg	Before pregnancy or <20 weeks	Nil	Remains hypertensive after delivery
Preeclampsia		>20 weeks of pregnancy	Present	BP normalizes within 12 weeks of delivery
Gestational hypertension			Nil	

MgSO₄

- *Mechanism of Action:*
  - ↓ Ach release from nerve endings
  - ↓ the sensitivity of motor end plate to Ach → Neuroprotection
  - Blocks the neuronal Ca influx channel
  - Blocks NMDA receptors
  - Membrane stabilizer
- Also acts as a tocolytic → decreases uterine contractility
- Therapeutic range → 4-7 mEq/L
- *Clinical monitoring for Mg toxicity:*
  - Urine output should be at least 30 mL/hr
  - Deep tendon reflex (Patellar reflex) present
  - Respiratory rate >14/min.

- 1ˢᵗ sign of impending toxicity → disappearance of patellar reflex.
- Concentration of Mg at which patellar reflex is lost → 10-12 mEq/L.
- Best marker for Mg toxicity → Pulse oximetry.
- *Contraindications:*
  - Myasthenia Gravis.
  - Impaired renal function
- Acts synergistically with muscles relaxant → use cautiously.
- Antidote for toxicity → IV Ca Gluconate or CaCl₂
- Magpie trial → prophylactic use of MgSO₄ lowers the risk of eclampsia

CVS DISORDERS IN PREGNANCY

- MC encountered maternal arrhythmia → PSVT
- MC valvular heart disease in pregnancy → MS
- MC congenital valvular lesion in pregnancy → MVP
- Risk of cardiac failure in pregnancy: Immediate postpartum >> Labor (2ⁿᵈ stage)
- *Points for management of labor:*
  - Fluid restriction
  - Ergometrine is contraindicated to control bleeding
  - Cut short 2ⁿᵈ stage of labor by forceps or ventouse

Anticoagulation in pregnancy:
- ≤12 weeks → UFH / LMWH
- 13-36 weeks → Warfarin

- ≥36 weeks → UFH / LMWH
- Warfarin is not contraindicated during lactation

Peripartum cardiomyopathy:
- MC cardiomyopathy in pregnancy
- Development of LV systolic dysfunction towards the end of pregnancy or within 5 months after delivery

Conditions associated with worse prognosis/ Indication of termination of pregnancy:
- Pulmonary artery hypertension
- Severe ventricular dysfunction → NYHA III, IV
- Eisenmenger syndrome – worst prognosis
- Marfan syndrome with significant aortic root dilatation

GESTATIONAL TROPHOBLASTIC DISEASES

- *GTD include:*
  - Hydatidiform mole – Complete & partial mole, Invasive mole
  - Choriocarcinoma
  - Placental site trophoblastic tumors
- Incidence of Molar pregnancy → 1:400
- Irregular 1ˢᵗ trimester vaginal bleeding presenting as white currant in red currant juice is a classical feature of → H. mole.
- Most characteristic presenting symptom of molar pregnancy → Abnormal bleeding, which prompts evaluation for threatened abortion.
- Spontaneous expulsion of H. mole occurs at around → 16 weeks and rarely delayed beyond → 28 weeks.
- *Complications in molar pregnancy:*
  - Early onset preeclampsia
  - Thyrotoxicosis
  - Development of trophoblastic malignancy
- Management → evacuation of uterus by dilation & curettage

- β- hCG should be monitored for 6 months after it has reached the baseline
- The theca lutein cysts spontaneously regress within a few months of evacuation and, therefore, do not require surgical removal.
- *Gestational Trophoblastic Neoplasia (GTN) include:*
  - Hydatidiform mole – MC
  - Invasive mole
  - Choriocarcinoma
  - Placental site trophoblastic tumors (PSTT)
- Most malignant tumor of uterus: Choriocarcinoma.
- MC site of metastasis of choriocarcinoma: Lungs > Vagina
- Tumor marker of Placental site trophoblastic tumor: Placental Alkaline phosphatase
- Low risk GTN → Single agent chemotherapy with Methotrexate or Actinomycin D
- High risk GTN → EMA-CO regimen

Features	Partial Mole	Complete Mole
Karyotype	▪ Triploid (69 XXX or 69 XXY)	▪ Diploid (46 XX or 46 XY)
Presentation	▪ Missed abortion	▪ Molar gestation
Size of uterus	▪ Small for date	▪ Large for date
Fetal / Embryonic tissue	▪ Usually present	▪ Absent
Villous edema	▪ Focal	▪ Diffuse
Trophoblastic hyperplasia	▪ Focal	▪ Diffuse
Trophoblast atypia	▪ Mild	▪ Marked
Initial hCG levels	▪ <1 lakh	▪ > 1 lakh
Risk of subsequent GTN	▪ 1-5 %	▪ 15-20 %
USG		▪ Snowstorm appearance ▪ Theca lutein cyst in 25-30 %

MOST COMMON

- MC cause of thrombocytopenia in pregnancy: Benign gestational thrombocytopenia.
- MC mood disorder met during pregnancy: Depression
- MC cause of maternal mortality in India: hemorrhage.
- *Abortion:*
  - MC in 1st trimester
  - MC cause: Chromosomal abnormality, of which autosomal trisomy of chromosome 16 is MC.
  - MC single chromosomal abnormality in miscarriage: Monosomy X (45X)
- MC cause of recurrent abortions:
  - In 1st trimester – Genetic factor
  - In 2nd trimester – Cervical incompetence
- MC cause for septic abortion → Illegal induced abortion.
- MC karyotype in complete H. mole: 46,XX

- MC lie of both the fetus in twin pregnancy at term: Longitudinal (Rarest lie → both transverse).
- MC presentation of twin pregnancy: Both vertex (60%).
- MC cause of perinatal mortality in twins: Prematurity.
- MC complication of oligohydramnios: Pulmonary hypoplasia.
- MC cause of maternal death in eclampsia: Intracranial bleed
- MC cause of fetal death in eclampsia: Prematurity & fetal asphyxia.
- MC manifestation of puerperal infection: Endometriosis.
- MC cause of anemia during pregnancy and puerperium: IDA
- MC site of uterine rupture: scar of prior cesarean delivery.

IMPORTANT SYNDROMES

❶ *HELLP Syndrome:*
  - Variant of severe Preeclampsia.
  - Comprises of:
    - **He**molysis – Microangiopathic hemolytic anemia
    - Elevated **L**iver enzymes
    - Low **P**latelets
  - Microangiopathic hemolysis →↑ serum LDH & fragments of RBC on P.S.
  - PT/aPTT/ Fibrinogen – normal
  - Definitive Rx: termination of pregnancy
  - Corticosteroids – not useful

❷ *Antiphospholipid Antibody Syndrome*:
  - Autoimmune disorder associated with pregnancy related complications like:
    - Fetal loss (i.e. Recurrent abortion)
    - Preeclampsia, thrombosis
    - Autoimmune thrombocytopenia
    - Fetal growth restriction

❸ *Potter syndrome:*
  - **P**ulmonary hypoplasia
  - **O**ligohydramnios
  - **T**ampered growth (i.e. IUGR)
  - Hyper**T**elorism (low set ears) & Potter facies
  - **E**xtremity/limb deformities
  - Bilateral **R**enal agenesis

❹ *Twin to Twin Transfusion Syndrome:*
  - Complication of monozygotic twins with a monochorionic placenta
  - Donor twin develop hypovolemia, oliguria, oligohydramnios & stuck twin phenomenon
  - Recipient twin manifest features of hypervolemia, polyuria, polyhydramnios & CCF

❺ *Mirror syndrome* is polyhydramnios associated with fetal hydrops.

REMEMBER

Congenital hypothalamic syndromes which leads to Amenorrhea:
- Septo-optic dysplasia
- Laurence Moon Biedl syndrome
- Prader-Willi syndrome
- Frohlich syndrome

[**Mn:** Single Live Preterm Fetus]

Triad of symptoms in tubal/ectopic pregnancy:
- **B**leeding per vagina
- **A**menorrhea
- **P**ain abdomen → most consistent symptom

[**Mn:** BAP]

Amnioinfusion is done in:
- **P**remature rupture of membrane.
- **R**enal agenesis
- **O**ligohydramnios.
- Wash out thick **M**econium.

[**Mn:** PROM]

Absolute contraindications of induction of labor: [**Mn:** CATCH Sahi Pakdo]
- **C**ontracted Pelvis
- **A**ctive HIV and genital Herpes
- **T**ransverse lie
- **C**ord prolapse
- **H**ysterotomy
- Uterine **S**car due to previous C.S.
- **P**lacenta previa

Causes of Oligohydramnios:
[**Mn:** MILD TRAPP]
- **M**aternal conditions like Hypertension, Preeclampsia etc
- **I**UGR
- **L**eaking of fluid after amniocentesis
- **D**rugs (PG synthesis inhibitors & ACE inhibitors)
- **T**riploidy
- **R**enal abnormalities like:
  - Renal agenesis
  - Posterior urethral value
  - Multicystic dysplastic kidney
- **A**bruption of placenta
- **P**ost term pregnancy, **P**ROM

IMPORTANT SIGNS

- **Bagel sign/Tubal ring sign** → Gestational sac in the adnexa surrounded by a hyperechoic ring.
  - Diagnostic feature of ectopic pregnancy.
- **Cullen's sign** is bluish discoloration around umbilicus. Seen in **ectopic pregnancy**.
- **Lemon & Banana sign** on USG → Spina Bifida.
- **Snow storm appearance** on USG → H. mole
- **Snow storm appearance** in CXR → Lung metastasis in choriocarcinoma.
- **Cannon ball appearance on CXR** → Lung metastasis in choriocarcinoma.
- **Twin Peak sign/Lambda sign** → Seen in diamniotic dichorionic pregnancy.
- **T sign:** Seen in a monochorionic diamniotic pregnancy

- **Stallworthy sign** → Slowing of the fetal heart rate on pressing the head down into the pelvis and prompt recovery on release of the pressure.
  - It is suggestive of posterior placenta previa.
- **Weinberg Sherman's sign:**
  - Pathognomonic sign of abdominal pregnancy.
  - Superimposition of fetal skeletal shadow with maternal spinal shadow on X-ray.
- **Robert's sign** → presence of gas in areas of great vessels & Heart. Earliest conclusive evidence of IUD on X-ray
- **Placental sign:** Spotting on the expected date of period in early months of pregnancy

MISCELLANEOUS

- Risk of hyperemesis gravidarum is ↑ with:
  - Multiple gestation
  - Molar pregnancy
  - Family history or personal history of hyperemesis gravidarum in a prior pregnancy.

Genetics

- Most trisomies result from maternal meiotic non disjunction, a phenomenon that occurs more frequently with ↑ age of women.
- Detection rate for Down syndrome with:
  - Triple screen = 70%
  - Quadruple screen (Triple markers + Inhibin A) = 80%
- Cardiac malformations are the MC major congenital abnormality worldwide followed by NTDs (Neural tube defects).

Teratogens

- Exposure to <5 rad has not been associated with ↑ in fetal anomalies or pregnancy loss; therefore, it is recommended to limit accumulated exposure to <5 rad during pregnancy.
- Alcohol is the MC teratogen to which a fetus is exposed, and alcohol consumption during pregnancy is a leading preventable cause of mental retardation, developmental delay, and birth defects in the fetus.
- Tetracyclines and Fluoroquinolones are contraindicated during pregnancy.

Infections

- Cesarean delivery is recommended for active herpetic lesions identified on the cervix, vagina, or on the vulva at the time of labor or if spontaneous rupture of membranes occurs.

- Prenatal screening for IgG rubella antibody is recommended as routine test because of because of the serious fetal implications. All pregnant women should be screened, unless they are known to be immune based on previous serologic testing.
- Infants of mothers who are HBsAg positive should receive the HBV vaccine and HB Ig within 12 hours of birth.

Forceps
- **Kielland's forceps** are used in deep transverse arrest
- **Simpson's forceps** is used for primigravida and moulded head.

- **Mclane Tucker forceps** is used for multigravida and rounded head.
- **Piper forceps** use in after coming head of breech.
- **Wrigley's forceps** are outlet forceps.

Important Prostaglandin Analogues:

Prostaglandins	Use
PGE$_1$ (Misoprostol)	Induction of labor, Cervical ripening, Abortion, PPH
PGE$_2$ (Dinoprostone)	Naturally occurring PG Used for induction of labor, cervical ripening
PGF$_{2\alpha}$ (Carboprost)	PPH as it mainly acts on fundus

GYNECOLOGY

FACTS

- Angle of anteflexion (b/w cervix & uterus) is 120°-130°
- Angle of anteversion (b/w cervix & vagina) is 90°
- Peg cells are present in: Fallopian tube
- Collapsed vagina appears H-shaped in cross section.
- Normal pH of Cervix → 7.8
- Life span of corpus luteum → 12-14 days
- Size of Graafian follicle just before ovulation → 20 mm.
- **Bartholin Glands:**
  - Homologues to Cowper's gland / bulbourethral gland in males.
  - Duct is 2 cm long and opens in vestibule outside hymen at the junction of anterior 2/3rd and posterior 1/3rd in the groove b/w hymen and labia minora.
- Chocolate cyst is found in endometriosis.
- In Menorrhagia, blood loss is > 80 ml per cycle or lasting for > 7 days.
- The term *menopause* refers to the cessation of menses for >1 year.
- **Perimenopause** is the period of transition from menstrual to non menstrual life when ovarian function begins to wane, often lasting 1 to 2 years.
- **Vaginismus** is the term used to describe recurrent or persistent involuntary tightening of muscles around the vagina whenever penetration is attempted.
- Anovulation maybe a consequence of static high estrogen level.
- Maximum function of corpus luteum occurs 8-9 days after ovulation.

- Luteal phase is supported by progesterone.
- Breast tenderness and fullness in the luteal phase is due to → progesterone-mediated changes.
- Luteal phase defect is when progesterone level on day 21 is < 5 mg/mL.
- At midcycle, there is a marked ↑ in LH secretion (k/as the LH surge), which triggers ovulation.
- **Mittelschmerz** is pain at the time of ovulation.
- Secretion and ferning of cervical mucus depends on: Estrogen
- Best test for ovarian reserve: AMH
- Earliest morphological evidence of ovulation on endometrial biopsy: Subnuclear Basal vacoulization
- **Ovarian insufficiency can be primary or secondary –**
  - **Primary** if the ovary fails to function normally in response to appropriate Gonadotropin stimulation.
  - **Secondary** if the hypothalamus and pituitary fail to provide appropriate gonadotropin stimulation.
  - Primary ovarian insufficiency or premature ovarian failure is characterized by amenorrhea, hypoestrogenism, and elevated serum gonadotropin levels in women < 40 years; premature menopause, or early menopause
- **Ferriman-Gallwey score** is a method of evaluating and quantifying hirsutism in females.
- **Asherman's syndrome** is intrauterine adhesions of uterus, most commonly seen after curettage. Most commonly presents as hypomenorrhea.

- **Benson &Sneeden's criteria** are used for adenomyosis.
- **Use of Laser in gynecology:**
  - Condylomata
  - Vaginal intraepithelial neoplasia
  - Vulvar intraepithelial neoplasia.
- **Neurohormonal substances affecting sexual cycle:**
  - Positive sexual impact: Norepinephrine, dopamine, oxytocin, and serotonin
  - Negative sexual impact: Serotonin via most other receptors, prolactin, and GABA.
- Premenstrual dysphoric disorder (PMDD) is d/to serotonergic dysregulation.
- Ratio of LH/FSH in PCOS is > 2:1
- **PCOS is associated with ↑ risk of:**
  - Endometrial Hyperplasia
  - Endometrial cancer

- The most commonly used medication for ovulation induction is Clomiphene citrate.
- The use of Clomiphene is associated with ↑ risk of:
  - Multiple gestations, the majority of which are twin gestations
  - Ovarian hyper stimulation syndrome and cyst formation.
  - Ectopic pregnancy.

Structures	Measurement
Female urethra	35-40 mm
Uterus (Nulliparous)	4 x 6 x 8 cm
Cervix	2.5 - 3.5 cm
Ovary	3.5 cm
FT	10 - 12 cm
Post Vaginal Wall	11.5 cm
Ant Vaginal Wall	9 cm

Age	Vaginal pH
Newborn infant	4.5 - 7
Puberty	Change from alkaline to acid
Reproductive age	4.5 - 5.5
Pregnancy	3.5 - 4.5
Late postmenopausal	6-8

Organ	Epithelial lining
Bartholin's gland	Single layer of columnar cell
Bartholin's duct	Multilayered columnar cells
Newborn vagina	Transitional Epithelium
Cervix/Cervical Canal	High columnar epithelium
Ectocervix	Squamous epithelium
Fallopian tube	Ciliated columnar epithelium

DISORDERS OF PUBERTY

- **Delayed puberty** is when secondary sexual characteristic have not appeared by the age of 14 years, there is no evidence of menarche by age 16 years, or when menses have not begun 5 years after the onset of thelarche.
- **Normal puberty** sequence in female growth spurt is Thelarche > Pubarche > peak growth velocity > Menarche
- In male earliest sign of puberty is testicular enlargement.

- The MC cause of delayed puberty with an↑ FSH is → Gonadal dysgenesis (Turner's syndrome).
- The MC cause of familial type of delayed puberty is constitutional (physiologic) delay.
- In **Kallman syndrome**, the olfactory tracts are hypoplastic, and the arcuate nucleus does not secrete GnRH. So there is anosmia & amenorrhea.
- Craniopharyngioma is the MC tumor associated with delayed puberty.

MENOPAUSE

- Obese menopausal women have a higher risk of endometrial hyperplasia and carcinoma because of estrogenic stimulation which promotes endometrial proliferation.
- Conversely, slender menopausal women are at a higher risk for menopausal symptoms.
- Hot flush is usually the first clinical manifestation of decreasing ovarian function and is a symptom of vasomotor instability.
- The hot flushes are the MC symptom of ↓ estrogen production and are considered one of the hallmark signs of perimenopause.
- Low dose OCPs may also be used to relieve the vasomotor symptoms of menopause.

- The luteal phase of the menstrual cycle remains constant at 13 to 14 days; whereas the variation of cycle length is related to a change in the follicular phase i.e. 1st half of the menstrual cycle is variable.
- Continuous unopposed administration of estrogens can result in:
  - Endometrial hyperplasia
  - ↑ risk of endometrial adenocarcinoma.
- Therefore it is essential to advise a progestin in conjunction with estrogens in women who have not undergone hysterectomy.

ENDOMETRIOSIS

- MC site of endometriosis → ovaries and involvement is typically bilateral
- The classic symptoms of endometriosis include → progressive dysmenorrhea and deep dyspareunia.
- Uterosacral nodularity is the classic sign noted during pelvic examination.
- Because endometriosis has variable gross appearance, tissue biopsy and laparoscopic confirmation of endometrial glands and stroma are required for diagnosis.

MISCELLANEOUS

- Mullerian agenesis, or Mayer Rokitansky Kuster Hauser syndrome, is the most common cause of primary amenorrhea in women with normal breast development.
- Image shown is normal hysterosalpingography.

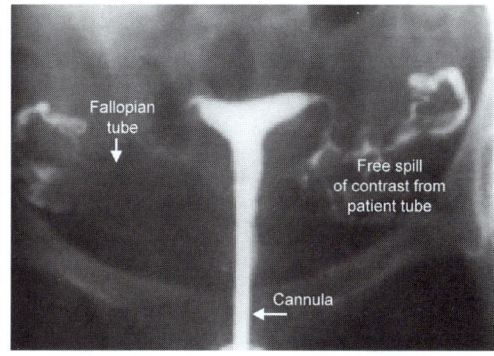

Fallopian tube

Free spill of contrast from patient tube

Cannula

IMPORTANT SYNDROMES

❶ **Asherman's Syndrome:**
- Caused by Endometrial synechiae.
- MC cause is overzealous curettage in post partum period.
- Defect is produced in the endometrium.

❷ **Stein Levinthal syndrome:**
- Also called as PCOD.
- Due to ↑ androgen levels.

❸ **Sheehan's Syndrome:**
- Ischemic necrosis of anterior pituitary.

❹ **Kallman Syndrome:**
- Defective GnRH synthesis from the hypothalamus
- Associated with:
  - Anosmia/Hyposmia due to olfactory bulb agenesis.
  - Optic atrophy
  - Color blindness
  - Cryptorchidism

❺ **Laurence Moon Biedl syndrome**
- GnRH deficiency (Hypogonadism)

❻ **MRKH Syndrome:**
- Defect lies in the development of Mullerian duct.
- FT, uterus, upper part of vagina are absent
- Secondary sexual characteristics → N
- Patient presents with primary amenorrhea

❼ **Mittelschmerz Syndrome/Ovular Pain:**
- Appears in the mid menstrual period.
- Situated in hypogastrium / iliac fossa.
- Pain is localized, does not change side.
- Lasts less than 12 hours.

MOST COMMON

- MC cause of LH surge is sustained rise of estrogen level.
- MC congenital anomaly of uterus: septate uterus > bicornuate
- MC uterine anomaly associated with abortion: septate uterus.
- MC symptom of genital TB is infertility.
- MC pathological cause of hirsutism → PCOD.
- MC cause of rapid onset hirsutism in a young female → Testosterone producing tumor.
- MC cause of CAH → 21 hydroxylase deficiency > 11β hydroxylase > 3β OH steroid dehydrogenase.
  - Diagnosis → morning sample of 17(OH)P > 800 mg/dL.
- MC cause of primary amenorrhea → Gonadal dysgenesis (MC → Turner syndrome) > Mullerian agenesis (MRKH Syndrome).
- MC cause of secondary amenorrhea in India → Endometrial TB.
- MC type of pituitary adenoma → Prolactinoma

AZOOSPERMIA

Cause	Obstructive	Hypogonadotropic	Hypergonadotropic
	Due to obstruction	Due to hypothalamic or pituitary failure	Due to testicular failure
FSH & LH level	Normal	Low	↑FSH
Testosterone	Normal	Low	Low
Volume	Normal	Reduced	Reduced

PCOS, ADRENOGENITAL SYNDROME, ANDROGEN INSENSITIVITY SYNDROME

	Polycystic Ovarian Syndrome	Adrenogenital syndrome	Androgen Insensitivity Syndrome
Aka	▪ PCOD, Stein Levinthal syndrome	▪ Congenital adrenal hyperplasia	▪ Testicular feminization syndrome
General	▪ MC cause of hirsutism in women	▪ AR trait	▪ Receptor gene is present on long arm of chromosome X (i.e. Xq)

Presentation	▪ 50% patients are obese and up to 75% have Insulin resistance → Hyperinsulinemia → Causes stromal hyperplasia →↑↑ androgens
	▪ *Diagnosis of PCOS (Rotterdam's criteria)* : *Diagnosis is made if any 2 of 3 are present:*
	1. Amenorrhea/Oligomenorrhea due to anovulation.
	2. Hyperandrogenemia (70-150 ng/mL) causing hirsutism, virilization etc
	3. USG findings of PCOS:
	a. > 12 follicles or cysts in ovary
	b. Each follicle < 10 mm (2-9 mm)
	c. Volume of ovary > 10 C.C.
		▪ *Deficiency of 21-hydroxylase (MC form)* → Clitoromegaly, which may be mistaken for a penis; an enlarged vulva, which resembles a bilobed scrotum.
		▪ *Deficiency of 11-hydroxylase* → leads to virilization and hypertension.
		▪ *Deficiency of 17-hydroxylase* → leads to deficiency of estrogens and androgens and to excess deoxycorticosterone, causing sexual infantilism and hypertension
			▪ MIS inhibits uterine development → Small atrophied vagina but clitoris and breasts are normal.
			▪ Testosterone receptors in cytoplasm of target cells are defective →
			  ○ **So axillary & pubic hairs are absent**
			  ○ Pubescence occurs normally
			  ○ Breasts are Tanner stage 4
			  ○ Internal gonads are testes which are intra-abdominal/inguinal & mimics inguinal hernia.

Pathology	▪ Theca cell hyperplasia → Excess androgens → E1 → Persistently raised LH → altered LH/FSH → Multiple Small follicles → arrest of growth of follicle → No dominant follicle → **Anovulation**	▪ Enlargement of the adrenal glands resulting primarily from excessive secretion of androgenic hormones by the adrenal cortex	
Investigations	▪ ↓ FSH, ↑ LH, LH: FSH ratio > 2:1 ▪ ↓ or absent progesterone ; ↑ Estrogen ▪ Urinary 17-Ketosteroid excretion is normal in PCOD (As adrenal is not implicated)	▪ Screening test → 17-OH progesterone ▪ Diagnostic test → ACTH stimulation test	▪ ↑ level of Gonadotropins (LH and FSH)
Treatment	▪ DOC → OCP's (low dose 3rd/4th gen progesterone) ▪ For Hirsutism & anovulation: Spironolactone – antiandrogenic action	▪ Cortisol or a synthetic glucocorticoid, such as **prednisone or dexamethasone**, and a mineralocorticoid if necessary	▪ Bilateral laparoscopic gonadectomy is preferred for removal of testes, after achieving puberty

UTERINE FIBROIDS

- MC uterine polyp is → Mucous/Endometrial/Adenomatous polyp.
- MC benign solid tumor in female → Fibroids.
- MC pelvic tumor → Fibroids
- MC type of fibroid is intramural type.
- MC presenting symptom → Menorrhagia.
- Fibroids are common in the age group of 35-45 yrs.
- Fibroids are more common in nulliparous women.
- Intramural or interstitial (75%) > Submucous (15%) > Subserous (10%).
- *Submucous fibroids:*
  - **MC** fibroid to undergo malignant change.
  - Maximum risk of abortion.
  - Maximum symptoms (Menorrhagia is common)
  - Red degeneration is most common (In 2nd trimester).
- *Subserous fibroids:*
  - Calcareous degeneration is seen most commonly.
  - Subserous pedunculated fibroid can cause → *Pseudo Meig's syndrome.*
- *Cervical fibroids:*
  - **MC** extra uterine fibroid.
  - **MC** cause of retention of urine is → Posterior cervical fibroids.
- Fibroid associated with polycythemia → Broad ligament fibroid.
- **MC** degenerative change → Hyaline degeneration.
- *Womb stone:* Calcific changes in fibroids, which starts from periphery.
- Most of the myomas remain asymptomatic for years. Most patients with myomas do not require treatment.
- Fibroids are the MC indication of hysterectomy.
- Prevalence of malignancy in fibroid is very low → 0.5% (rarest complication to occur).
- First investigation for fibroid is → USG
- Best investigation for fibroid is → MRI > USG
- *Causes of pain in fibroids:* [**Mn**: Torsion Pain Makes Me Red]
  - T → Torsion of pedunculated fibroma
  - P → Polyp formation
  - Make me → Malignancy
  - Red → Red degeneration
- *Indications for a myomectomy include:*
  - A rapidly growing pelvic mass
  - Symptoms not relieved with medical Rx, and
  - Enlargement of an asymptomatic myoma to the point of causing hydronephrosis.
- *Drugs used to ↓ the size of fibroids:* [**Mn**: GDM]
  - GnRH agonist & antagonist
  - Danazol
  - Mifepristone

OVARIAN TUMORS

- MC ovarian mass in the reproductive age group → Functional cysts
- MC ovarian tumors → Malignant epithelial cell tumors.
- MC ovarian tumors that presents with menorrhagia → Sex cord tumors.
- MC ovarian cancers in women < 20 years → Germ cell tumors.
- Ovarian cancer presents most commonly in the 5th and 6th decades of life.
- ~ 90% of all ovarian malignancies are of the epithelial cell type, derived from mesothelial cells.
- *Dysgerminomas* are usually unilateral and are the MC type of germ cell tumor seen in patients with gonadal dysgenesis. LDH is a marker of dysgerminoma.
- *Granulosa cell tumors* secrete large amounts of estrogen, which in some older women, may cause endometrial hyperplasia and endometrial carcinoma.
- *Sertoli Leydig cell tumors* (Androblastoma or Arrhenoblastoma) are the rare tumors. These are testosterone secreting counterparts to granulosa cell tumors. Testosterone results in rapid onset of acne, hirsutism (75% of patients), amenorrhea and virilization. The tumor is usually unilateral (95% of cases) and may reach a size of 7 to 10 cm in diameter.
- Krukenberg tumor is an ovarian tumor that is metastatic from sites such as the GIT (stomach being the MC site) and breast.

Important Characteristic Findings:

- Psammoma bodies → serous carcinoma of ovary
- Walthard cell nest → Brenner's tumor
- Call Exner bodies → Granulosa cell tumor
- Reinke's crystal → Leydig cell tumor
- Schiller duval bodies → Endodermal sinus tumor
- Rokitansky protuberance → Mature cystic teratoma
- Signet ring appearance → Krukenberg tumor

ENDOMETRIAL HYPERPLASIA

- Complex hyperplasia with atypia carries maximum risk of developing Ca endometrium. It represents an abnormal proliferation of primarily glandular elements without concomitant proliferation of stromal elements.
- Abnormal uterine bleeding (AUB) is the hallmark symptom of both endometrial hyperplasia and Ca endometrium.
- Tamoxifen acts as a weak estrogen and is associated ↑ risk of:
  - Endometrial hyperplasia
  - Endometrial carcinoma.
- Abnormal bleeding is the most common indication for endometrial sampling.
- Medical Rx of endometrial hyperplasia → Synthetic progesterone or other progestin.
- After initial diagnosis, D&C is indicated for sampling and to rule out coexistent endometrial Ca.
- Most endometrial polyps represent focal, accentuated, benign hyperplastic lesions.
  - MC symptom is AUB. < 5% of polyps shows malignant change.

ENDOMETRIAL CANCER

- The most common genital tract malignancy in developing countries.
- Histopathological variant of endometrial malignancy which has the poorest prognosis is → clear cell carcinoma.
- MC symptom of endometrial carcinoma is irregular bleeding and most specific symptom is post menopausal bleeding.
- Endometrial sampling, prompted by vaginal bleeding, most frequently establishes the diagnosis of endometrial cancer.
- Prognosis varies widely, depending on the **grade** of tumor and **depth** of penetration into the myometrium.
- Hysterectomy is the primary treatment of endometrial cancer.
- For women with positive lymph nodes (stage IIIc), radiation therapy provides survival benefit.
- Recurrent estrogen dependent or progestin dependent cancer may respond to high-dose progestin therapy.
- Uterine sarcomas accounts for 3% of cancers involving the body of the uterus, and only about 0.1% of all myomas.
- OC Pills are protective against endometrial cancer.

CERVICAL CANCER

- HPV is implicated in more than 90% of the cases.
- *HPV "Low-risk" subtypes* are 6 and 11 → associated with genital condyloma.
- *High risk subtypes* are 16, 18, 31, and 33 → associated with cervical dysplasia and cervical cancer.
- Gardasil (quadrivalent) & Cervarix (bivalent) vaccines are used to prevent human papilloma virus induced cervical carcinoma.
- The Squamo-columnar junction is the site where over 90% of cervical neoplasia arises.
- Colposcopy with directed biopsy has been the standard of care for detection of Ca cervix and remains the technique of choice for treatment plan.
- Radiotherapy in carcinoma cervix required at point A – 2cm lateral to uterocervical canal & 2 cm above the internal os is 8000cGY & at point B 3 cm lateral to point A is 6000c GY.

FEATURES OF CA ENDOMETRIUM, CA CERVIX & CA OVARY

	CA Endometrium	CA Cervix	CA Ovary
Risk Factors			
Age group	▪ 55-65 years	▪ 45-55 years	▪ >60 years
Mechanism	▪ Unopposed estrogen stimulation	▪ Early onset of sexual activity ▪ Frequent miscarriages	▪ Disordered ovarian function
Menstrual relation	▪ Early menarche/late menopause		▪ Early menarche/late menopause ($\uparrow$ number of ovulation years)
Parity	▪ Nulliparity	▪ Multiparity	▪ Nulliparity
Fertility Index Sexual pattern	▪ Low/Infertility	▪ Multiple sexual partners ▪ High risk male partner	▪ Low/Infertility
Socio economic status	▪ High	▪ Low	▪ –
Associations	▪ Obesity, HTN, DM	▪ Smoking, organ transplant	▪ Turner's syndrome
Personal History Associations	▪ History of breast Cancer	▪ HPV 16, 18, 31, 33; HSV2 ▪ HPV type 16 → Squamous cell carcinoma ▪ HPV type 18 → Adenocarcinoma	▪ History of breast & endometrial cancer
Family History	▪ Endometrial Ca, Breast Ca in 1st degree relatives		▪ 1st degree relatives with history of ovarian cancer
Drugs	▪ Tamoxifen ▪ HRT with estrogen	▪ OCPs, POPs, alcoholism, drug abuse, immunosuppression	▪ Clomiphene (ovulation induction)
Factors decreasing the risk	▪ Progestins added to HRT $\downarrow$ risk ▪ Use of OCPs have protective effect		▪ Risk $\downarrow$ with each pregnancy, breast feeding, & tubal ligation
Treatment			
	▪ **Stage 0** → TAH/BSO ▪ **Stage I** → Pan hysterectomy (Uterus + FT + ovaries) ▪ **Stage II** → TAH/BSO + Postoperative radiotherapy ▪ **Stage III** → TAH/BSO → LN sampling + Post op radiotherapy ⅄ Whole body radiation is required in stage IIIc & IV	▪ **Stage Ia 1** → If pregnancy required → Conization, else extrafascial hysterectomy ▪ **Stage Ia2, Ib, IIa** → Radical Hysterectomy + bilateral LN dissection OR external Radiotherapy + ICRT (Brachytherapy) ▪ **Stage IIb & III** → Primary chemoradiation ▪ **Stage IV** → Primary chemoradiation	▪ **Stage Ia & Ib, grade 1** ○ Premenopausal → staging laparotomy then U/L oophorectomy ○ Post menopausal → TAH + BSO ▪ **Stage Ia/b (grade 2/3), 1c** → TAH/BSO → Staging → **Adjuvant therapy** ▪ **Stage II,III & IV** → Cytoreductive surgery → **Adjuvant Chemotherapy for 6 cycles**

STAGING OF CA ENDOMETRIUM, CA CERVIX & CA OVARY

Stage	CA Endometrium	CA Cervix (FIGO staging revised 2009)	Ovary (FIGO 2014 & traditional TNM staging in bracket)
0	▪ In situ	▪ In situ (CIN III)	
I	▪ Limited to endometrium	▪ Limited to Cervix	▪ Limited to ovary or Fallopian tube [T1]
IA	▪ No or < ½ of myometrial invasion	▪ Invasive carcinoma diagnosed only by microscopy with Horizontal spread ≤ 7 mm ▪ Stromal invasion with depth £3 mm (IA1) or > 3mm but ≤5 mm (IA2)	▪ Limited to *one ovary or FT* (capsule intact), no tumor on external surface, PC –ve, i.e. No malignant cells in the ascites or peritoneal washings [T1a]
IB	▪ Invasion of ≥ ½ of myometrium	▪ Macroscopically visible lesion / preclinical cancer with horizontal spread >7 mm ▪ Clinically visible lesion ≤ 4 cm in greatest dimension (IB1) or >4 cm (IB2)	▪ Similar to 1A but *both ovaries involved* [T1b]
IC			▪ IA or IB + surface tumor + **PC +ve** (Tumor limited to one or both ovaries or FT)
II	▪ Tumor invades cervical stroma but does not extend beyond uterus. **	▪ Invading beyond cervix but not to the pelvic wall or lower 1/3rd of vagina	▪ Involving one or both ovaries with pelvic extension (below pelvic brim) or peritoneal cancer [T2]
IIA		▪ Tumor without parametrial invasion	▪ Extension and/or implants on the uterus and/or fallopian tubes/and/or ovaries) [T2a]
IIB		▪ Tumor with parametrial invasion	▪ Extension to other pelvic intraperitoneal tissues [T2b]
III	▪ Local &/or regional spread of tumor	▪ Extending to pelvic wall and/or lower 1/3rd vagina	▪ Tumor involves one or both ovaries, or FT, or primary peritoneal cancer, with cytologically or histologically confirmed spread to the peritoneum outside the pelvis and/or metastasis to the retroperitoneal lymph nodes) [T3]
IIIA	▪ Invasion of serosa / adnexa /peritoneal metastasis (positive cytology)	▪ Involves lower 1/3rd of vagina; no extension to pelvic sidewall	▪ Tumor extent to the pelvis /SI/ omentum / **liver surface.** Microscopic disease of A/P surface, LN –ve (Metastasis to the retroperitoneal lymph nodes with or without microscopic peritoneal involvement beyond the pelvis) (Positive retroperitoneal lymph nodes only (cytologically or histologically proven) ▪ IIIA1 (i) Metastasis ≤ 10 mm in greatest dimension (note this is tumor dimension and not lymph node dimension) T3a/T3aN1 ▪ IIIA1 (ii) Metastasis N 10 mm in greatest dimension ▪ IIIA 2 Microscopic extrapelvic (above the pelvic brim) peritoneal involvement with or without positive retroperitoneal lymph nodes) [T3a/T3aN1] [T3a/T3aN1]
IIIB	▪ Vaginal metastases &/or Parametrial invasion	▪ Tumor extends to pelvic wall &/or causes obstructive uropathy/**hydronephrosis**/non-functioning kidney	▪ A/P surface implant <2 cm, LN -ve (Macroscopic peritoneal metastases beyond the pelvic brim ≤ 2 cm in greatest dimension, with or without metastasis to the retroperitoneal lymph nodes) [T3b/T3bN1]

Contd...

Stage	CA Endometrium	CA Cervix (FIGO staging revised 2009)	Ovary (FIGO 2014 & traditional TNM staging in bracket)
IIIC	▪ Metastasis to pelvic nodes (IIIC1) ▪ Metastasis to Para-aortic nodes (IIIC2)	▪ —	▪ A/P surface but >2 cm / LN +ve (Macroscopic peritoneal metastases beyond the pelvic brim, N 2 cm in greatest dimension, with or without metastases to the retroperitoneal nodes [Note 1]) [T3c/T3cN1]
IV	▪ Tumor invasion	▪ Extending beyond the pelvis or biopsy proven involvement of the mucosa of the bladder or the rectum	▪ Distant metastasis excluding peritoneal metastases ▪ Stage IV A: Pleural effusion with positive cytology ▪ Stage IV B: Metastases to extra-abdominal organs (including inguinal lymph nodes and lymph nodes outside of abdominal cavity) [Note 2] ▪ [Any T, Any N, M1] [T3c/T3cN1]]
IVA	▪ Invasion of bladder/bowel mucosa	▪ Invasion of bladder/bowel/mucosa	▪ Distant metastasis to **liver parenchyma/**pleural effusion (stage 4)
IVB	▪ Distant metastases (lung/brain/bone)	▪ Distant organ metastasis	

A – Abdominal; P – Peritoneal; PC – Peritoneal cytology |** Endocervical glandular involvement is taken as stage I |
Note 1: Includes extension of tumor to capsule of liver and spleen without parenchymal involvement of either organ|
Note 2: Parenchymal metastases are Stage IV B |

INVESTIGATION OF CHOICE

- IOC for uterine anomaly is MRI and gold standard is laparoscopy.
- Endometrial biopsy is usually performed between 5-7th day of menstrual cycle.
- Best test for documenting ovulation: Endometrial biopsy > Follicular study (TVS) > Hormonal study.
- Investigation to identify proliferative endometrium → endometrial biopsy.

Disease/Condition	IOC
Fibroid	USG
PID	USG
Adnexal mass	USG
Molar pregnancy	USG
DUB	USG
Tubal patency	HSG
Ectopic	TVS
Mullerian anomalies	MRI
Endometriosis	Laparoscopy
Post coital bleeding	PAPS

Disease/Condition	IOC
Post menopausal bleeding	Endometrial biopsy
Primary amenorrhea	Karyotyping
Secondary amenorrhea	Hormonal assessment
Ovulation	Follicular monitoring
Hirsutism with menstrual irregularity	Serum testosterone
Adenomyosis	MRI
Ovarian reserve	AMH
VVF	Cystoscopy
Vesico-vaginal fistula	Three swab test ▪ VVF – 1 swab discoloured and wet ▪ Uretero VF – 1 swab only wet ▪ Urethro VF – Three swab wet and discolored

MULTIPLE CHOICE QUESTIONS (OBSTETRICS)

CHAPTER 1: ANATOMY OF FEMALE REPRODUCTIVE ORGANS

EXTERNAL GENITAL ORGANS

VULVA

1. Triangular area between labia minora and clitoris is?
(PGMEE 2014)

  a. Sulcus interlabiales   b. Vestibule
  c. Fourchette   d. Urogenital triangle

[Ref: Dutta's Obs. 9th/e, pg. 2]

2. Fourchette is formed by?   **(PGMEE 2014)**
  a. Joining of labia majora
  b. Joining of labia minora
  c. Joining of labia majora with minora
  d. Junction of cervix and vagina

[Ref: Dutta's Obs. 9th/e, pg. 2; Holland Brew's Obs.4th/e, pg.1; Shaw's Gynae. 16th/e, pg. 2; Jeffcoate's Gynae. 9th/e, pg. 24]

3. Gland homologous to prostate in male is?
(PGMEE 2014)

  a. Gartner's gland   b. Skene's gland
  c. Bartholin's gland   d. Cowper's gland

[Ref: Dutta's Obs. 9th/e, pg. 2; Holland Brew's Obs.4th/e, pg.1]

4. Bartholin's glands lie in relation to vaginal orifice-
(PGMEE 2012-13)

  a. Posterior   b. Anterior
  c. Anterolateral   d. Posterolateral

[Ref: Holland Brew's Obs.4th/e, pg.1; Shaw's Gynae. 16th/e, pg. 1; Jeffcoate's Gynae. 9th/e, pg. 25]

INTERNAL GENITAL ORGANS

VAGINA

5. Vestibule of the vagina develops from? *(DNB June' 2009)*
  a. Genital ridge
  b. Müllerian duct
  c. Urogenital sinus
  d. Wolffian duct

[Ref: Dutta's Obs. 9th/e, pg. 3]

6. Lower 1/5th of vagina is formed by?
(PGMEE June' 2012)

  a. Urogenital sinus
  b. Paramesonephric duct
  c. Müllerian duct
  d. Mesonephric duct

[Ref: Dutta's Obs. 9th/e, pg.4; Shaw's Textbook of Gynaecology, 16th/e, pg. 125; Jeffcoate's Principles of Gynaecology, 9th/e, pg. 233; Berek & Novak's Gynecology, 15th/e, pg. 85]

Explanation

Embryology of vagina:

- ▪ Vagina develops from the following sources-
  - ○ Upper 4/5th, above the hymen
    - - Mucous membrane is derived from the endoderm of the canalized sino-vaginal bulbs
    - - Musculature is developed from the mesoderm of the two fused Müllerian ducts
  - ○ Lower 1/5th, below the hymen is developed from the endoderm of the urogenital sinus
  - ○ External vaginal orifice is formed from the genital fold ectoderm after rupture of the urogenital membrane

7. Prepubertal vaginal pH is-   **(PGMEE 2015)**
  a. 3.5   b. 4.5
  c. 7   d. 8

[Ref: Shaw's Gynaecology 16th/e 4; Jeffcoate's Principles of Gynaecology, 9th/e, pg. 29, 31t]

8. Vaginal pH in reproductive age group is?
(DNB June' 2010)

  a. 1–3   b. 4 – 4.5
  c. 4–7   d. 7–8

[Ref: Dutta's Obs. 9th/e, pg.4; Shaw's Gynae. 16th/e, pg.4; Jeffcoate's Gynae. 9th/e, pg. 31; Novak's Gynae. 15th/e, pg. 90]

9. Vaginal pH is most acidic during?   **(DNB June' 2011)**
  a. Puerperium   b. Pregnancy
  c. Menstruation   d. Newborn

[Ref: Jeffcoate's Gynae. 9th/e, pg. 29, 31t]

10. Anaerobic bacteria commonly found in cervix or vagina?   **(DNB June' 2011)**
  a. Lactobacilli   b. Clostridium
  c. Mobilincus   d. Gardnerella

[Ref: Shaw's Gynae. 16th/e, pg.4; Jeffcoate's Gynae. 9th/e, pg. 28, 365]

11. Role of lactobacilli in vaginal secretions-
(PGMEE 2012-13)

  a. To maintain alkaline pH b. To maintain acidic pH
  c. Nutrition   d. None

[Ref: D.C.Dutta text book of gynecology 7th e.p 4-5; Shaw's Gynae 16th/e p. 4; Jeffcoate's Gynae. 9th/e, pg. 28, 365]

12. pH of vagina is lowest during: **(PGMEE 2015-16)**
  a. Puberty   b. Pre-puberty
  c. Pregnancy   d. Menopause

[Ref:Dutta's Obs. 9th/e, pg.4; Shaw's Gynae. 16th/e, pg.4; Jeffcoate's Gynae. 9th/e, pg. 29, 31t]

13. Acidic pH of vagina is due to?   **(PGMEE 2012)**
  a. Doderlein's Bacilli   b. Gardnerella
  c. Glycogen   d. Mobilincus

[Ref: Dutta's Obs. 9th/e, pg.4; Jeffcoate's Gynae. 9th/e, pg. 28]

1.	b
2.	b
3.	b
4.	d
5.	c
6.	a
7.	c
8.	b
9.	b
10.	a
11.	b
12.	c
13.	a

14. Clue cells are: *(PGMEE 2012-13)*

a. Epithelial cells
b. Lymphocytes
c. Neutrophils
d. Macrophages

[Ref: Shaw's Gynae. 16th/e, pg.384; Novak's Gynae. 15th/e, pg. 558]

CERVIX

15. The shape of external os of a nulliparous cervix is-
(DNB 91)

a. Circular
b. Transverse
c. Longitudinal
d. Fimbriated

[Ref: Dutta's Obs. 9th/e, pg.67]

16. Squamo-columnar junction is situated – mm above from cervical lip: *(Recent Pattern June 2018)*

a. 1-10 mm
b. 25 mm
c. 0.5 mm
d. 10-20 mm

[Ref: Shaw's Textbook of Gynaecology,16th/e, pg. 5-6; Jeffcoate's Principles of Gynaecology, 9th/e, pg. 34; Berek & Novak's Gynecology, 15th/e, pg.]

Explanation

Squamo-columnar junction (SCJ):

- The junction of squamous epithelium covering the portio vaginalis of cervix and the columnar epithelium lining the endocervix is called SCJ.
- Usually this change in types of epithelia is abrupt, but at times there is a gradual transition, hence the name transitional zone (the area between original SCJ & physiologically active SCJ), which is 1 – 10 mm wide
- Site of SCJ varies with varies stages of life –
  ○ Neonates – on exocervix
  ○ Puberty – squamous metaplasia advances inwards from original SCJ
  ○ Reproductive period, use of OCPs, pregnancy – exposed at the external os
  ○ Postmenopausal – moves inside the cervical canal d/t shrinkage of cervix
- Site of original SCJ can be determined by the presence of nabothian cysts
- Cytological screening for carcinoma cervix is done by Pap smear obtained from SCJ
- Colposcopy of SCJ is done in case of abnormal Pap smear & cervical biopsy obtained from abnormal areas

17. Palm leaf appearance of cervical mucus is caused by-
(PGMEE 2012-13)

a. Oestrogen
b. Progesterone
c. FSH
d. Testosterone

[Ref: Shaw's Gynae. 16th/e, pg.35]

18. Elasticity of cervical mucus max in: *(PGMEE 2015)*

a. Pre follicular phase
b. Post ovulatory phase
c. Ovulatory phase
d. Menstrual phase

[Ref: Shaw's Gynae 16th/e p. 256]

UTERUS

19. Structure preventing retroversion of uterus is?
(DNB June' 2011)

a. Uterosacral
b. Mackenrodt's ligament
c. Round ligament
d. Broad ligament

[Ref: Shaw's Gynae. 16th/e, pg. 365-367; Jeffcoate's Gynae. 9th/e, pg. 349-353]

Explanation

Supports of uterus:

- Usual position of the uterus is of anteversion & anteflexion
  ○ Version- refers to the direction of the cervical canal
  ○ Flexion- refers to the inclination of the body of the uterus on the cervix
- Retroversion: the axis of the cervix is directed upwards & backwards in relation to a line drawn through the long axis of the trunk.
- Retroflexion: the long axis of the corpus is bent backwards on the axis of the cervix.
- In clinical practice, both retroversion & retroflexion usually occur together & are collectively referred to as retrodisplacement of the uterus.
- Retrodisplacement of the uterus is found in ≈ 15% of women.
- It is most often a developmental anomaly & not congenital because uterus is without version & flexion at birth.
- The round ligaments although do not maintain the position of anteversion & anteflexion, they are used in the surgical correction of retroversion by-
  ○ Ventrosuspension
  ○ Plication of round ligaments
  ○ Baldy-Webster operation

20. Angle of anteversion of uterus is maintained by:

a. Uterosacral ligament and Broad ligament
(PGMEE 2018)
b. Pubocervical ligament and transverse cervical ligament
c. Uterosacral and Transverse cervical ligament
d. Round ligament and broad ligament

[Ref: D.C. dutta text book of gynecology p.165-166 7th e]

Explanation

- Uterus is normally placed in anteverted and anteflexed position. Uterus is held in this position by the upper tier system.
- Upper most supports of the uterus primarily maintain the uterus in anteverted position. Responsible factor are:
  ○ Endopelvic fascia covering the uterus
  ○ Round ligaments
  ○ Broad ligament with intervening pelvic cellular tissue.

21. What is cochleate uterus- *(PGMEE 2013-14)*

a. Anteflex uterus
b. Retroverted uterus
c. Uterine inversion
d. Mullerian agenesis

[Ref: Jeffcoate's Gynae. 9th/e, pg. 254, 255f, 349 f]

14.	a
15.	a
16.	a
17.	a
18.	c
19.	c
20.	d
21.	a

22. **Size of uterus in inches is** *(PGMEE 2012-13)*
    a. 5 x 4 x 2
    b. 4 x 3 x 1
    c. 3 x 2 x 1
    d. 4 x 2 x 1

[Ref: Jeffcoate's Gynae. 9th/e, pg. 32]

FALLOPIAN TUBE

23. **Thinnest part of fallopian tube is?**
    (PGMEE Nov.12 Pattern)

    a. Infundibulum
    b. Ampulla
    c. Cornual
    d. Interstitium

[Ref: Shaw's Gynae. 16th/e, pg. 10; Jeffcoate's Gynae. 9th/e, pg. 36]

24. **'Peg Cells' are seen in:**
    a. Vagina
    b. Vulva
    c. Ovary
    d. Tubes

[Ref: Dutta's Obs. 9th/e, pg. 7; Jeffcoate's Gynae. 9th/e, pg. 37; Shaw's Gynae. 16th/e, pg. 11]

OVARY

25. **Provided that one secondary oocyte is produced in each menstrual cycle. How many secondary oocytes are on an average produced during the reproductive life of a human female?** *(PGMEE June' 2012)*
    a. 4,20,000
    b. 42,000
    c. 4200
    d. 420

[Ref: Dutta's Obs. 9th/e, pg. 16; Jeffcoate's Gynae. 9th/e, pg. 59; Shaw's Gynae. 16th/e, pg.26]

26. **Number of follicles in female newborn is?**
    (PGMEE 2012)
    a. 1 million   b. 2 million
    c. 3 million   d. 4 million

[Ref: Dutta's Obs. 9th/e, pg. 16; Shaw's Gynae. 16th/e, pg.25; Jeffcoate's Gynae. 9th/e, pg. 59]

27. **Volume of ovary after menopause is:-** *(PGMEE 2015)*
    a. 3.0 cm^2 b. 5.4 cm^2
    c. 6.5 cm^2 d. 7.8 cm^2

[Ref: Ultrasound in obstetrics and gynaecology Vol. 2 by MERZ p. 105]

22. c
23. d
24. d
25. d
26. b
27. a

PHYSIOLOGY OF OVULATION

1. Ovulation can be evaluated by? *(DNB Dec' 2009)*
- a. Cervical mucous
- b. Cervical effacement
- c. Cervical dilatation
- d. Cervical colour

[Ref: Shaw's Gynae. 16th/e, pg.255-257; Jeffcoate's Gynae. 9th/e, pg.111]

2. Which is not a test for ovulation? *(DNB June' 2010)*
- a. Fern test
- b. LH surge
- c. Hysteroscopy
- d. Basal body temperature

[Ref: Shaw's Gynae. 16th/e, pg.255-257; Jeffcoate's Gynae. 9th/e, pg. 109 - 111]

3. Ovulation is associated most commonly with?
- a. LH surge   *(DNB Dec' 2010)*
- b. Increase in progesterone
- c. Increase in basal body temperature
- d. Increase in FSH

[Ref: Dutta's Obs. 9th/e, pg. 18; Shaw's Gynae. 16th/e, pg.255-257; Jeffcoate's Gynae. 9th/e, pg. 65-68, 110]

Explanation

- Definition of ovulation – a process in which an ovum, in the form of a secondary oocyte, escapes from the ovary following rupture of a mature Graafian follicle & becomes available for conception.

- 4 Ps responsible for ovulation are:
  - Proteolytic enzymes – activity increased by progesterone (produced in granulosa layer under the effect of LH)
  - Progesterone induced midcycle rise in FSH → oocyte gets free from its follicular attachments
  - Plasminogen activators → activation of plasmin → generation of active colllagenase → degeneration of collagen in cell wall especially at the follicular apex or stigma
  - Prostaglandins (ovarian content ↑ed by LH) → contraction of micromuscle cells in theca externa & stroma → follicular rupture

- **LH surge** – Most important physiological marker of imminent ovulation
  - Midcycle preovulatory LH surge precedes ovulation by 34- 36 hours
  - LH peak precedes ovulation by 10-12 hours (peak S. LH level of 75 ng / ml required for ovulation)
  - Effects of LH surge- completion of meiosis of ovum, ovulation & development of corpus luteum
  - Urinary LH detection kits available for prediction of ovulation

- ↑ in progesterone & ↑ in FSH do contribute to the process of ovulation, but it is the LH surge which is central to this process.

- BBT: ↑ in basal body temperature occurs because of thermogenic effect of progesterone
  - Measured in morning after waking up but before rising from bed
  - An ↑ of 0.5 - 1.0° F occurs in immediate postovulatory period → indicative of ovulation
  - Used for detection of ovulation in treatment of infertility patients
  - As a natural family planning (NFP) method
  - Limitation of BBT: febrile illness

4. LH Surge occurs how many hours before ovulation?
(PGMEE June' 2012)
- a. 6-8 hours
- b. 10-16 hours
- c. 18-24 hours
- d. More than 24 hours

[Ref: Shaw's Gynae.16th/e, pg. 39, 255-257; Jeffcoate's Gynae. 9th/e, pg. 67, 111]

5. Spinbarkeit is maximum at which phase-
(PGMEE 2012-13; Jeffcoate's Gynae. 9th/e, pg. 94)
- a. Menstrual phase
- b. Ovulatory
- c. Post ovulatory
- d. Pre follicular

[Ref: Shaw's Gynae. 16th/e, pg.256; Jeffcoate's Gynae. 9th/e, pg. 94]

6. For hormonal assessment, vaginal smear is taken from-
(PGMEE 2012-13)
- a. Anterior wall
- b. Lateral wall
- c. Posterior wall
- d. Fornix

[Ref: Jeffcoate's Gynae. 9th/e, pg.111]

7. Size of ovarian follicle at ovulation is?
(PGMEE Aug 13 Pattern)
- a. 0.5 to 1 cm
- b. 1 to 1.5 cm
- c. 1.5 to 2 cm
- d. 2 to 2.5 cm

[Ref: Dutta's Obs. 9th/e, pg. 17; Shaw's Gynae.16th/e, pg. 28; Jeffcoate's Gynae. 9th/e, pg. 67]

8. Mittelschemerz is- *(PGMEE 2013-14)*
- a. Pain just before menstruation
- b. Pain at the time of ovulation
- c. Pain 5 days after ovulation
- d. Pain during menstruation

[Ref: Jeffcoate's Gynae. 9th/e, pg.109]

9. In a 40 day cycle, when does ovulation takes place-
(PGMEE 2013-14)
- a. 26 day
- b. 14 day
- c. 20 day
- d. 28 day

[Ref: Shaw's Gynae. 16th/e, pg.28; Jeffcoate's Gynae. 9th/e, pg. 58, 61]

1.	a
2.	c
3.	a
4.	d
5.	b
6.	b
7.	d
8.	b
9.	a

10. Ovulation after LH surge is seen within-
                                                   (PGMEE 2013-14)
   a. 01-2 hrs   b. 12-24 hrs
   c. 24-28 hrs   d. 24-36 hrs

   [Ref: Shaw's Gynae.16th/e, pg. 39; Jeffcoate's Gynae. 9th/e, pg. 67, 111]

11. Most common cause of LH surge:-   *(PGMEE 2016-17)*
   a. ↓ FSH   b. Estradiol peak
   c. Increase FSH   d. Increase progesterone

   [Ref: Shaw's Gynae.16th/e, pg. 39; Jeffcoate's Gynae. 9th/e, pg. 67]

12. High estrogen leads to :-   *(PGMEE 2016-17)*
   a. Inhibition of LH
   b. Inhibition of FSH
   c. Secretion of prolactin
   d. Increased TSH

   [Ref: Shaw's Gynae.16th/e, pg. 39; Jeffcoate's Gynae. 9th/e, pg. 67]

13. Final maturation of follicle, ovulation is done by:-
                                                   (PGMEE 2016-17)
   a. FSH   b. LH
   c. Oestrogen   d. Oestrogen & Progesterone

   [Ref: Shaw's Gynae.16th/e, pg. 39; Jeffcoate's Gynae. 9th/e, pg. 67]

14. Menstrual cycle is 29 day regular, day of ovulation in cycle would be:-   *(PGMEE 2015)*
   a. 11th   b. 13th
   c. 15th   d. 17th

   [Ref: Shaw's Gynae.16th/e, pg. 28; Jeffcoate's Gynae. 9th/e, pg. 58, 61]

10.	d
11.	b
12.	b
13.	b
14.	c
15.	d
16.	b
17.	b
18.	a
19.	d
20.	b
21.	c
22.	c
23.	b
24.	b

PHYSIOLOGY OF FERTILIZATION AND IMPLANTATION

15. Most common site of fertilization is:
                                 (DNB Dec' 2010, PGMEE 2016-17)
   a. Cervix   b. Uterus
   c. Fimbriae   d. Ampulla

   [Ref: Dutta's Obs. 9th/e, pg. 18; Holland Brew's Obs.4th/e, pg.16; Shaw's Gynae. 16th/e, pg.10]

16. Capacitation of sperm proceeds in-   *(PGMEE 2015)*
   a. Testis   b. Female genital tract
   c. Fallopian tubes   d. Epididymis

   [Ref: Dutta's Obs. 9th/e, pg. 17; Shaw's Textbook of Gynaecology, 16th/e, pg. 240]

17. Velocity of sperms in female genital tract is?
                                                   (PGMEE 2012)
   a. 0-1 mm/min   b. 1-2 mm/min
   c. 4-5 mm/min   d. 5-6 mm/min

   [Ref: Ganong 22nd/e p. 427; Guyton 11th/e p. 999]

18. Decidual reaction is due to which hormone-
                                                   (PGMEE 2012-13)
   a. Progesterone   b. Estrogen
   c. LH   d. FSH

   [Ref: Dutta's Obs. 9th/e, pg. 21; Holland Brew's Obs.4th/e, pg.19]

19. Implantation occurs on which day of menstrual cycle-
                                                   (PGMEE 2012-13)
   a. 6th day   b. 10th day
   c. 15th day   d. 20th day

   [Ref: Dutta's Obs. 9th/e, pg. 20; Holland Brew's Obs. 4th/e, pg.17]

20. Implantation normally occurs in-   *(PGMEE 2012-13)*
   a. Ampulla   b. Body of uterus
   c. Cervix   d. Ovaries

   [Ref: Dutta's Obs. 9th/e, pg. 20]

21. At what time after fertilization the product of conception is called as "Embryo"?   *(PGMEE Aug. 12 Pattern)*
   a. 72 hours   b. 1 week
   c. 3 weeks   d. 8 weeks

   [Ref: Dutta's Obs. 9th/e, pg. 37]

22. What forms the embryo -   *(PGMEE 2016-17)*
   a. Syncytiotrophoblast b. Cytotrophoblast
   c. Inner cell mass   d. Zona pellucida

   [Ref: Dutta's Obs. 9th/e, pg. 20]

23. Post fertilization, implantation occurs on:-
                                                   (PGMEE 2016-17)
   a. D5   b. D6
   c. D8   d. D3

   [Ref: Dutta's Obs. 9th/e, pg. 20; Holland Brew's Obs.4th/e, pg.17]

24. In pregnancy heart starts contracting earliest at:-
                                                   (PGMEE 2018)
   a. 7 weeks   b. 20-22 days
   c. 20-22 weeks   d. 10-12 weeks

   Ref: Dutta's Obs. 8th / e, pg. 30, 46 734; Williams Obs. 24th / e, pg. 128, 170

Explanation

- Embryonic cardiac activity appears at MSD of 15-18 mm & embryonic CRL ≥ 4 mm.

Gestational age & fetal structures identified by TVS

Gestational age (wks)	Fetal structures
4	Choriodecidual thickness, chorionic sac
5	Gestation sac, yolk sac
6	Fetal pole, cardiac activity
7	Lower limb buds, midgut herniation (physiological)
8	Upper limb buds, stomach
9	Spine, choroid plexus

- Embryonic movements are identified as early as by 7 weeks
- The formation of 4 chambered primitive heart & the appearance of first heart beat occurs by 21-28 days post conception i.e. by 35-42 days (or 5-6 wks) of menstrual age.
- Hence, the fetal cardiac activity can be detected by TVS as early as 6 weeks.

PHYSIOLOGY OF REPRODUCTION

CHANGES IN REPRODUCTIVE TRACT DURING PREGNANCY

25. The weight of nulliparous uterus is? *(DNB Dec' 2011)*
- a. 30 to 40 gm
- b. 40 to 60 gm
- c. 60 to 80 gm
- d. 80 to 100 gm

[Ref: Dutta's Obs. 9th/e, pg. 42; William's Obs. 24th/e pg. 46]

WEIGHT GAIN DURING NORMAL PREGNANCY

26. Weight gain in normal pregnancy is?
- a. 1 to 3 kg *(PGMEE Dec' 2011)*
- b. 5 to 7 kg
- c. 10 to 12 kg
- d. 12 to 15 kg

[Ref: Dutta's Obs. 9th/e, pg. 46; William's Obs. 24th/e pg. 51, 177; Holland Brew's Obs.4th/e, pg.41]

HAEMATOLOGICAL CHANGES DURING PREGNANCY

27. Plasma volume is maximum in which week of pregnancy? *(DNB June' 2009)*
- a. 24-28 weeks
- b. 28-32 weeks
- c. 30-32 weeks
- d. 34-36 weeks

[Ref: Dutta's Obs. 9th/e, pg. 47; Holland Brew's Obs.4th/e, pg.40; William's Obs. 24th/e pg. 55]

Explanation

- Pregnancy is a state of hyperdynamic circulation with an increase in blood volume, plasma volume, RBC mass & Hb.
- Blood volume, plasma vol. & cardiac output start to increase by 5th – 6th weeks of pregnancy. Max. level by 30 – 34 weeks.
- Increase in blood volume, plasma volume & RBC mass is by 30-40%, 40-50% & 20-30% respectively above the non-pregnant level.
- Disproportionate increase in plasma volume & RBC mass → relative haemodilution → apparent fall in Hb concentration (should not be below 11.0 gm/dl) & haematocrit → physiological anaemia
- Importat functions of pregnancy-induced hypervolemia:
  - Diminished blood viscosity → optimum gaseous exchange between maternal & fetal circulation
  - To meet the ↑ed metabolic demands of the enlarged uterus with its greatly hypertrophied vascular system
  - To provide abundant nutrients & elements to support the rapidly growing placenta & fetus
  - To protect the mother & in turn the fetus against the deleterious effects of impaired venous return in the supine & erect positions
  - To safeguard the mother against the adverse effects of blood loss during delivery

28. Clotting factor that decreases during pregnancy is?
- a. Fibrinogen *(DNB Dec' 2009)*
- b. Factor XIII
- c. Factor VIII
- d. Factor X

[Ref: Dutta's Obs. 9th/e, pg. 48; Holland Brew's Obs.4th/e, pg.41; William's Obs. 24th/e pg. 57]

29. Changes in clotting factors in pregnancy:
- a. Fibrinogen level is increased *(PGMEE 2012-13)*
- b. Platelet level is increased
- c. Factor XII level is decreased
- d. Factor XI level is increased

[Ref: Dutta's Obs. 9th/e, pg. 47; Holland Brew's Obs.4th/e, pg.40-41; William's Obs. 24th/e pg. 57]

PHYSIOLOGICAL CHANGES IN CVS DURING PREGNANCY

30. By what time post delivery does the cardiac output return to pre pregnancy state? *(PGMEE June' 2012)*
- a. 4 hours
- b. 4 weeks
- c. 6 weeks
- d. 8 weeks

[Ref: Dutta's Obs. 9th/e, pg. 48]

31. Maximum cardiac output during pregnancy is seen at ? *(PGMEE 2014)*
- a. 20 weeks
- b. 30 weeks
- c. 34 weeks
- d. 36 weeks

[Ref: Dutta's Obs. 9th/e, pg. 48; Holland Brew's Obs.4th/e, pg.39; William's Obs. 24th/e pg. 59, 60]

Explanation

Cardiac output (CO)-

- Blood volume, plasma vol. & cardiac output start to increase by 5th – 6th weeks of pregnancy. Max. level by 30 – 34 weeks remains static till term
- Increase in CO is due to increase in blood volume & basal metabolic rate
- Lowest in sitting or supine position, highest in right or left lateral or knee chest position
- Increases further during labour (+ 50%) & immediately following delivery (+70%) due to auto transfusion of blood from the uterus into the maternal circulation
- Rises soon after delivery to about 60% above the pre-labour values
- Returns to - the pre-labour values by 1 hour following delivery
- The pre-pregnant level by another 4 weeks time.
- The pregnancy-induced increase is lost after delivery
- In multiple pregnancies, as compared to singletons, CO is increased further by another ≈ 20% due to greater stroke volume (15%) & heart rate (3.5%). Left atrial diameter & left ventricular end-diastolic diameter are also increased due to augmented preload. This implies that cardiovascular reserve is reduced in multiple pregnancies.

25.	b
26.	c
27.	c
28.	b
29.	a
30.	b
31.	c

32. Cardiovascular change in pregnancy is:
a. Slight right axis deviation in ECG *(PGMEE 2012-13)*
b. Slight left axis deviation in ECG
c. Diastolic murmur
d. Pulse rate is decreased

[Ref: Dutta's Obs. 9th/e, pg. 48; Holland Brew's Obs.4th/e, pg.40; William's Obs. 24th/e pg. 58]

33. Which of the following is false as physiological change in pregnancy? *(PGMEE 2019)*
a. Increase cardiac output
b. Increase total protein
c. Increase residual volume
d. Increase GFR

[Ref: William's Obs. 25th/e pg. 22, 44]

PHYSIOLOGICAL CHANGES IN RESPIRATORY SYSTEM DURING PREGNANCY

34. Which of the following is seen during pregnancy?
a. Respiratory alkalosis *(DNB June' 2009)*
b. Metabolic acidosis
c. Metabolic alkalosis
d. Respiratory acidosis

[Ref: Dutta's Obs. 9th/e, pg. 50; William's Obs. 24th/e pg. 63]

IRON AND FOLIC ACID METABOLISM DURING PREGNANCY

35. Total iron requirement during pregnancy is? *(DNB Dec' 2011)*
a. 500 mg   b. 750 mg
c. 1000 mg   d. 1500 mg

[Ref: Dutta's Obs. 9th/e, pg. 50; Holland Brew's Obs.4th/e, pg.41; William's Obs. 24th/e pg. 55, 179; Progress in Obstetrics & Gynaecology, John Studd, Vol.15, Ch.7, pg.108]

36. Daily dose of folic acid for women with history of NTDs in previous pregnancy is? *(DNB Dec' 2010)*
a. 0.4 mg   b. 40 micro gm
c. 400 micro gm   d. 4 mg

[Ref: Dutta's Obs. 9th/e, pg. 90, 252, 383, 589; Holland Brew's Obs. 4th/e pg. 71, 435, 553; William's Obs. 24th/e pg. 284]

Explanation

Folic acid supplementation in pregnancy -

- A minimum of 400 micro gm (= 0.4 mg) of folic acid supplementation with or without a multivitamin decreases the risk of fetal malformations such as neural tube defects or NTDs (anencephaly, spina bifida, meningocele or meningomyelocele), miscarriages & cardiac malformations
- To be taken at least 1-2 months prior to conception & continued through the 1st trimester of pregnancy (periconceptional supplementation)
- Higher doses recommended for special risk groups
  ○ 1 mg/ day for women with DM & epilepsy
  ○ 4 mg/ day for women with history of NTDs in previous pregnancy

○ Women with multiple fetuses also require daily supplementation of folic acid throughout pregnancy.
○ Because of its requirement in DNA synthesis, folic acid plays an important role in erythropoiesis; deficiency results in development of megaloblastic anaemia.
○ Deficiency of folic acid has also been found to be associated with abruptio placentae.

37. Folic acid supplementation leads to decreased incidence of which defect- *(PGMEE 2013-14)*
a. Neural tube defect   b. Anemia
c. Megaloblastic anemia   d. Septate uterus

[Ref: Dutta's Obs. 9th/e, pg. 252, 383; Holland Brew's Obs. 4th/e pg. 553; William's Obs. 24th/e pg. 284]

ENDOCRINE CHANGES DURING PREGNANCY

38. True about thyroid function test in pregnancy *(PGMEE 2018)*
a. Increase in Free T3   b. Increase in free T4
c. Increase in total T3   d. Increase in TSH

Ref: Dutta's Obs. 8th /e, pg.70-71; Holland Brew's Obs.4th/e, pg.138-139; Williams Obs. 24th / e, pg. 68-69

Explanation

Physiological Changes in Thyroid Gland During Pregnancy:

- Total volume of thyroid gland increases (12 ml in 1st trimester → 15 ml at the time of delivery)
- There is ↑ in –
  ○ S. protein bound iodine (from 4-8 μg% to 6.2-11.2 μg%, due to estrogenic stimulation of its synthesis and decreased hepatic clearance)
  ○ Thyroxine binding globulin (reaching a plateau at 20 weeks)
  ○ Total T3 and T4 (beginning at 6-9 weeks, reaching a plateau at 18 weeks)
  ○ Levels of free T3 and free T4 remain unchanged
- There is ↓ in TRH (due to negative feedback effect of TSH simulating α subunit of hCG)
- Transient ↓ in TSH (or may remain normal)
- TRH and T4 cross the placenta freely but TSH crosses very minimally

39. Level of prolactin in pregnancy are usually more than?
a. 50 ng/mL   b. 100 ng/mL
c. 150 ng/mL   d. 200 ng/mL

Ref: Williams obstretrics 24th/e page 1291

Explanation

- Hyperprolactinaemia is the presence of abnormally high levels of prolactin in the blood.

States	Level of prolactin
Nonpregnant	0–20 ng/mL
1st trimester	36–213 ng/mL
2nd trimester	110–330 ng/mL
3rd trimester	137–372 ng/mL

Answers:

32.	b
33.	c
34.	a
35.	c
36.	d
37.	a
38.	c
39.	d

PLACENTA AND ITS ABNORMALITIES

1. The ratio of fetal weight and placental weight at term is?
(PGMEE 2011)
a. 4 : 1
b. 5 : 1
c. 6 : 1
d. 7 : 1

[Ref: Dutta's Obs. 9th/e, pg. 26; Holland Brew's Obs.4th/e, pg.20; William's Obs. 24th/e pg. 95]

2. Placenta develops from? (PGMEE 2011)
a. Chorion frondosum
b. Decidua basalis
c. Chorion leave
d. Both A and B

[Ref: Dutta's Obs. 9th/e, pg. 25; Holland Brew's Obs.4th/e, pg.19; William's Obs. 24th/e pg. 87, 93]

3. Uteroplacental circulation is established by ____ weeks post fertilization - (PGMEE Aug 12 Pattern)
a. 1
b. 2
c. 3
d. 4

[Ref: Dutta's Obs. 9th/e, pg. 24; Holland Brew's Obs.4th/e, pg.20; William's Obs. 24th/e pg. 92]

4. Normal weight of term placenta in gms is-
(PGMEE 2012-13, 2016-17)
a. 300
b. 500
c. 700
d. 1000

[Ref: Dutta's Obs. 9th/e, pg. 26; Holland Brew's Obs.4th/e, pg.20; William's Obs. 24th/e pg. 116]

5. Which of the following is not true of placenta?
(PGMEE 2014)
a. Number of cotyledons increases with gestational age
b. Weight of fetus and placenta equal at 4 months
c. After delivery weight of placenta is 500 gm
d. At term about one fifth of placenta is of maternal origin

[Ref: Dutta's Obs. 9th/e, pg. 26; Holland Brew's Obs.4th/e, pg.200; William's Obs. 24th/e pg. 95, 116]

6. Cells seen at the junction between two layers of placenta are? (PGMEE 2014)
a. Hofbauer cells
b. Hofmann cells
c. Amniogenic cells
d. Uterine natural killer cells (UNK)

[Ref: Dutta's Obs. 9th/e, pg. 28; William's Obs. 24th/e pg. 95]

7. True about circumvallate placenta is?
(PGMEE Nov.12 Pattern)
a. Fetal plate smaller than basal plate
b. Basal plate smaller than fetal plate
c. Has accessory lobes
d. Is membraneous

[Ref: Dutta's Obs. 9th/e, pg. 205; Holland Brew's Obs.4th/e, pg.22; William's Obs. 24th/e pg. 118]

UMBILICAL CORD AND ITS ABNORMALITIES

8. Umbilical cord contains- (PGMEE 2013-14)
a. 2 artery 1 vein
b. 1 artery 2 vein
c. 1 artery 1 vein
d. 2 artery 2 vein

[Ref: Dutta's Obs. 9th/e, pg. 35; William's Obs. 24th/e pg. 100,122; Holland Brew's Obs.4th/e, pg.20]

9. Length of umbilical cord is? (PGMEE June' 2009)
a. 25-40 cm
b. 30-100 cm
c. 40-50 cm
d. 60-120 cm

[Ref: Dutta's Obs. 9th/e, pg. 36; Holland Brew's Obs.4th/e, pg.20; William's Obs. 24th/e pg. 121]

Explanation

Umbilical cord:

- Normal length of umbilical cord 40-50 cms (usual variation 30-100 cms)
- Average diameter of umbilical cord 1.5 cms (usual variation 1-2.5 cms)
- There is a spiral twist from the left to right starting as early as 12th week due to spiral turn of the vessels – vein around the arteries
- Initially, the cord has 4 vessels – 2 arteries & 2 veins, but by the end of the 4th month the right vein disappears & only left vein is left
- Normally, the insertion of the cord on the fetal surface of the placenta is eccentric (somewhere between the centre & the margin of the placenta). The insertion may be central, marginal or velamentous.
- The fetal attachment of the cord initially is to the ventral surface of the embryo close to the caudal extremity but later on it moves permanently to the centre of the abdomen at 4th month.

10. Battledore insertion of cord to placenta-
(PGMEE 2013-14)
a. Cord attached to the margin of placenta
b. Placenta attached to the margin
c. Cord attached to the membranes
d. Placenta attached to the centre

[Ref: Dutta's Obs. 9th/e, pg. 206; Holland Brew's Obs.4th/e, pg.22; William's Obs. 24th/e pg. 122]

1.	c
2.	d
3.	b
4.	b
5.	a
6.	a
7.	a
8.	a
9.	c
10.	a

11. Placenta in which vessels separate before reaching margin is? *(DNB June' 2009, PGMEE 2013)*
a. Battledore placenta
b. Velamentous placenta
c. Circumvallate placenta
d. Placenta marginata

[Ref: Dutta's Obs. 9th/e, pg. 206; Holland Brew's Obs.4th/e, pg. 22; William's Obs. 24th/e pg. 122]

12. Vasa previa may lead to- *(PGMEE 2012-13)*
a. Antepartum haemorrhage
b. Fetal exsanguination
c. Fetal death
d. All of the above

[Ref: Dutta's Obs. 9th/e, pg. 206; Holland Brew's Obs.4th/e, pg.22-23; William's Obs. 24th/e pg. 123]

Explanation

A. Abnormalities of cord insertion:

- Battledore placenta:
  - Marginal insertion of the cord on the placenta
  - If such type of placenta is low lying → chance of cord compression in vaginal delivery → fetal anoxia, IUFD
- Velamentous placenta:
  - Cord inserted on the membranes instead of the placenta
  - Branching vessels traverse between the membranes before they reach & supply the placenta
  - Vasa previa – branching vessels traverse through the membranes overlying the internal os, in front of the presenting part → vaginal bleeding → fetal exsanguination → IUFD
  - Urgent delivery (by emergency caesarean section) indicated in case of fetal bleeding
  - In IUFD, vaginal delivery is awaited.

B. Abnormalities of cord length:

- Short cord:
  - Shortening may be true (10 cm or < 8") or relative (due to entanglement of cord around any fetal part)
  - Acordia – absent cord, placenta may be attached to the liver as in exomphalos
  - Complications: failure of external version, malpresentations, separation of a normally situated placenta, prevention of descent of the presenting part & fetal distress in labour
- Long cord:
  - The cord may be unduly long (300 cm)
  - Complications: ↑ed chance of cord prolapse, cord entanglement around the neck (20-30%) or the body, true knot (rare, 1%), false knot (due to accumulation of Wharton's jelly)

C. Abnormalities of cord vessels:

- Single umbilical artery
  - Incidence 1-2%
  - Due to failure of development of one artery or due to its atrophy in later months
  - More common in twins & in babies born to women with diabetes, epilepsy, oligohydramnios, polyhydramnios, pre-eclampsia, APH.

11.	b
12.	d
13.	b
14.	b
15.	a
16.	b
17.	a
18.	b

- 20-25% cases associated with congenital malformation of the fetus (renal & genital anomalies)
- Complications: ↑ed chance of abortion, fetal aneuploidy (trisomy 18), prematurity, IUGR, ↑ed perinatal mortality

AMNIOTIC FLUID AND ITS ABNORMALITIES

AMNIOTIC FLUID

13. Amniotic fluid at 36-38 weeks- *(PGMEE 2012-13)*
a. 500 ml
b. 1000 ml
c. 1500 ml
d. 2000 ml

[Ref: Dutta's Obs. 9th/e, pg. 34; Holland Brew's Obs.4th/e, pg.26; William's Obs. 24th/e pg. 100]

14. Amniotic fluid quantity at birth (ml) - *(PGMEE 2012-13)*
a. 500   b. 1000
c. 1500   d. 2000

[Ref: Dutta's Obs. 9th/e, pg. 34; Holland Brew's Obs.4th/e, pg.26; William's Obs. 24th/e pg. 100]

15. Rate of turnover of amniotic fluid is- *(PGMEE 2013-14)*
a. 500 cc/h   b. 1L/hr
c. 1500 cc/h   d. 2L/h

[Ref: Dutta's Obs. 8th/e, pg. 43; Holland Brew's Obs. 4th/e pg. 26; Williams Obs., 23rd/e, pg. 94]

16. The major contribution of the amniotic fluid after 20 weeks of gestation : *(PGMEE 2019)*
a. Ultrafiltrate and maternal plasma
b. Fetal urine
c. Fetal lung fluid
d. Fetal skin

[Ref: Mudaliar and Menon's 12th/e pg. 28]

POLYHYDRAMNIOS

17. At 34 weeks pregnancy, polyhydramnios is present when volume is greater when- *(PGMEE 2012-13)*
a. 2000cc   b. 150cc
c. 1000cc   d. 500cc

[Ref: Dutta's Obs. 9th/e, pg. 200; Holland Brew's Obs.4th/e, pg.241]

18. Polyhydramnios is defined as a state when amniotic fluid quantity exceeds: *(Recent Pattern June 2018)*
a. 1 liter   b. 2 liter
c. 2.5 liter   d. 3 liter

[Ref: Dutta's Obs. 8th/e, pg. 246; Holland Brew's Obs.4th/e, pg.241]

Explanation

- Anatomically, polyhydramnios is defined as a state where liquor amnii exceeds 2,000 mL.

Sonographic diagnosis:

- Amniotic fluid index (AFI) is more than 24 cm (more than 95th centile for gestational age)
- Deepest vertical pocket (DVP) is more than 8 cm

19. Volume of amniotic fluid to define polyhydramnios in a normal term pregnancy: *(Recent Pattern June 2018)*
   a. 1000 ml
   b. 1500 ml
   c. 2500 ml
   d. 2000 ml

   [Ref: Dutta's Obs. 9th/e, pg. 200; Holland Brew's Obs. 4th/e pg. 241]

OLIGOHYDRAMNIOS

20. Causes of olighydramnios include - *(PGMEE 2012-13)*
   a. DM
   b. Esophagal atresia
   c. Rh isoimmunisation
   d. Renal agenesis

   [Ref: Dutta's Obs. 9th/e, pg. 203; Holland Brew's Obs.4th/e, pg.243; William's Obs. 24th/e pg. 237]

21. Oligohydraminos is associated with all except- *(PGMEE 2012-13)*
   a. Sacral agenesis
   b. Polycystic kidney
   c. Renal agenesis
   d. PROM

   [Ref: Dutta's Obs. 9th/e, pg. 203; Holland Brew's Obs.4th/e, pg.243; William's Obs. 24th/e pg. 237]

22. A 38 week mother with oligohydramnios delivers a baby with absent limb on left side. This could be because of: *(Recent Pattern June 2018)*
   a. IUGR
   b. PPROM and Chorioamnionitis
   c. Phocomelia
   d. Amniotic bands

   [Ref:Dutta's Obs. 9th/e, pg. 203; Holland Brew's Obs. 4th/e pg. 243; William's Obs. 24th/e pg. 237]

Explanation

- Congenital amputation is birth without a limb or limbs, or without a part of a limb or limbs.
- It is known to be caused by vascular insults and from amniotic band syndrome, in which there are fibrous bands of the amnion constrict foetal limbs to such an extent that they fail to form or actually fall off due to compromised blood supply.
- Congenital amputation can also occur due to maternal exposure to teratogens.

PLACENTAL ENDOCRINOLOGY

PROGESTERONE

23. At what gestational age does placenta takes over progesterone production? *(PGMEE 2014)*
   a. 4 weeks
   b. 6-8 weeks
   c. 10-12 weeks
   d. 15-18 weeks

   [Ref: Dutta's Obs. 9th/e, pg. 56; Holland Brew's Obs.4th/e, pg.47; William's Obs. 24th/e pg. 106]

24. Hormone secreted by placenta: *(PGMEE 2016-17)*
   a. Progesterone
   b. Estradiol
   c. Estrone
   d. All of the above

   [Ref: Dutta's Obs. 9th/e, pg. 55-56; Holland Brew's Obs. 4th/e pg. 46-47; William's Obs. 24th/e pg. 106, 107]

25. Precursor of progesterone from placenta is:- *(PGMEE 2016-17)*
   a. LDL cholesterol
   b. VLDL cholesterol
   c. HDL cholesterol
   d. Pregnanediol

   [Ref: Dutta's Obs. 9th/e, pg. 55, 56 b; Williams Obs., 23rd/e, P. 67-68]

HUMAN CHORIONIC GONADOTROPIN (hCG)

26. Peak hCG levels are seen by what intrauterine age? *(DNB Dec' 2011, PGMEE June' 2012)*
   a. 7–9 weeks
   b. 11–13 weeks
   c. 20 weeks
   d. 25 weeks

   [Ref: Dutta's Obs. 9th/e, pg. 54; Holland Brew's Obs.4th/e, pg. 45; Williams Obs., 23rd/e, P. 64]

19.	d
20.	d
21.	a
22.	d
23.	b
24.	a
25.	a
26.	a

CLINICAL ASSESSMENT OF A PREGNANT WOMAN

1. **Fetal heart sound can be auscultated at-**
   (PGMEE 2013-14)
   a. 10 weeks
   b. 24 weeks
   c. 18-20 weeks
   d. 6 weeks

   [Ref: Dutta's Obs. 9th/e, pg. 64; Holland Brew's Obs. 4th/e pg. 50; William's Obs. 24th/e pg. 176]

2. **Fetal trunk movements in third trimester:**
   a. Less perceived by nullipara *(PGMEE 2012-13)*
   b. Increased in IUGR
   c. Are more pronounced
   d. None of the above

   [Ref: Dutta's Obs. 9th/e, pg. 65; Holland Brew's Obs.4th/e, pg. 51; Williams Obs., 24th/e, P. 335]

3. **Most common position of fetus near term is:-**
   (PGMEE 2016-17)
   a. LOA
   b. ROA
   c. LOP
   d. ROP

   [Ref: Dutta's Obs. 9th/e, pg. 70]

4. **A patient presented at 20 weeks of gestation. The patient's LMP was 9th January. What will be the estimated date of delivery.** *(NEET Pattern 2017)*
   a. 9th January
   b. 16th September
   c. 16th October
   d. 9th October

   Ref: Dutta's Obs. 8th / e, pg. 83; Holland Brew's Obs.4th / e, pg. 52; Williams Obs. 24th / e, pg. 127

Explanation

Calculation of expected date of delivery

- *Naegele's formula*
  ○ Calculated from 1st day of last menstrual period (LMP) in a woman with regular cycles
  ○ By adding 280 days or 9 calender months and 7 days to the 1st day of LMP
  ○ A quick estimate can be made by adding 7 days to the 1st day of LMP and subtracting 3 months
  ○ Accuracy of prediction 50% within 7 days on either side
  ○ Limitations – irregular cycles, conception during lactational amenorrhoea, conception immediately following stoppage of oral contraceptives
- Pregnancy following single act of fruitful coitus – by adding 266 days to the date of coitus

- Pregnancy following ovulation induction and infertility treatment – add 266 days to date of intrauterine insemination (IUI) or in vitro fertilization- embryo transfer (IVF-ET)
- Date of quickening – by adding 22 weeks in a primigravida and 24 weeks in a multipara to the date 1st appreciating fetal movements. Limitation – all women not equally sensitive to quickening

DIAGNOSTIC SIGNS IN RELATION TO PREGNANCY

5. **Palmer's sign seen in pregnancy is?**
   (PGMEE June' 2012, PGMEE 2012-13)
   a. Pulsation in lateral fornix
   b. Rhythmic contraction of uterus
   c. Softening of uterus
   d. Bluish discolouration of vagina

   [Ref: Dutta's Obs. 9th/e, pg. 61; Holland Brew's Obs.4th/e, pg. 50]

6. **Jacquemier's sign is-** *(PGMEE 2012-13)*
   a. Softening of cervix
   b. Bluish discoloration of anterior vaginal wall
   c. Mucous discharge
   d. Increased pulsations in lateral fornix

   [Ref: Dutta's Obs. 9th/e, pg. 60; Holland Brew's Obs. 4th/e, pg. 50]

7. **Regarding Hegar's sign all are true except-**
   a. Bimanual palpation method *(PGMEE 2012-13)*
   b. Difficult in obese
   c. Can be done at 14 weeks
   d. Present in 2/3rd of cases

   [Ref: Dutta's Obs. 9th/e, pg. 61; Holland Brew's Obs. 4th/e, pg. 50]

8. **Softening of lower uterine segment on bimanual examination is known as:-** *(PGMEE 2015-16)*
   a. Goodell's sign
   b. Hegar's sign
   c. Osiander's sign
   d. Chadwick's sign

   [Ref: Dutta's Obs. 9th/e, pg. 61; Holland Brew's Obs.4th/e, pg. 50]

9. **Softening of the vaginal portion of the cervix with increased vascularity is known as:**
   (Recent Pattern June 2018)
   a. Goodell's sign
   b. Jacqemier's sign
   c. Hegar's sign
   d. Osiander's sign

   [Ref: Dutta's Obs. 9th/e, pg. 61; Holland Brew's Obs. 4th/e pg. 50]

1.	c
2.	c
3.	a
4.	c
5.	b
6.	b
7.	c
8.	b
9.	a

Explanation

The Signs in Pregnancy

Sign	Definition
Goodell's sign	Softening of the vaginal portion of the cervix due to increased vascularity which is the result of hypertrophy and engorgement of the vessels below the growing uterus.
Chadwick's sign	is a bluish discoloration of the cervix, vagina, and labia resulting from increased blood flow. It can be observed as early as 6 to 8 weeks after conception, and its presence is an early sign of pregnancy.
Hegar's sign	is a non-sensitive indication of pregnancy in women — its absence does not exclude pregnancy. Softening in the consistency of the uterus, and the uterus and cervix seem to be two separate regions.
Piskacek's sign	consists noting a palpable lateral bulge or soft prominence one of the locations where the uterine tube meets the uterus.

VARIOUS IMMUNOLOGICAL TESTS FOR DIAGNOSIS OF PREGNANCY

10. Minimum hCG level that a urine pregnancy test can detect is? *(DNB June' 2010, PGMEE 2016-17)*
   a. 5 m IU/ml
   b. 10 – 20 m IU/ml
   c. 20 – 30 m IU/ml
   d. 35 m IU/ml

   [Ref: Dutta's Obs. 9th/e, pg. 62; William's Obs. 24th/e pg. 170]

11. Most sensitive test to diagnose hCG is? *(PGMEE 2014)*
   a. Direct agglutination test
   b. Radio immunoassay
   c. Immune radiometric assay
   d. ELISA

   [Ref: Dutta's Obs. 9th/e, pg. 62, 63; William's Obs. 24th/e pg. 169]

12. Basis of urine pregnancy test: *(Recent Pattern June 2018)*
   a. β - subunit of hCG
   b. α - subunit of hCG
   c. Estrogen
   d. Progesterone

   [Ref:Dutta's Obs. 9th/e, pg. 61; Holland Brew's Obs. 4th/e pg. 50; William's Obs. 24th/e pg.]

Explanation

Immunological tests for the diagnosis of pregnancy:

- Detection of hCG (the antigen) in the maternal urine or serum with the help of the antibody (monoclonal or polyclonal, commercially available) forms the basis for immunological endocrine test for the diagnosis of pregnancy.
- With a sensitive test, the hormone (hCG) can be detected in maternal urine or serum as early as 8-9 days post conception.

- The commonly used urine pregnancy test is based on the detection of β - subunit of hCG in urine of pregnant women (card test by ELISA, sensitivity 30-50 mIU/mL of urine)
- ELISA can also detect β - subunit of hCG in serum & is more sensitive than urine ELISA (sensitivity 1-2 mIU/mL)

Various Immunological Tests for Diagnosis of Pregnancy

Test	Test sensitivity	Time taken	Inference	Positive on
Immunological tests (urine)				
Agglutination inhibition test (Latex test)	500-1000 mIU/ml	2 min.	Absence of agglutination	2 days after missed period
Direct latex agglutination test	200 mIU/ml	2 min.	Presence of agglutination	2-3 days after missed period
Two-site sandwich immunoassay (card test)	30-50 mIU/ml	4-5 min.	Colour bands in the control as well as test window	On the 1st day of the missed period (28th day of the cycle)
Immunological tests (serum)				
Enzyme-linked Immunosorbent Assay (ELISA)	1-2 mIU/ml	2-4 hrs.	-	5 days before the 1st missed period
Radioimmunoassay	2 mIU/ml	3-4 hrs.	-	25th day of the cycle
Immuno Radiometric Assay (IRMA)	0.05 mIU/ml	30 min.	-	8 days after conception

13. Urine pregnancy test detects- *(PGMEE 2013-14)*
   a. hCG
   b. Estrogen
   c. Progesterone
   d. HPL

   [Ref: Dutta's Obs. 9th/e, pg. 61; Holland Brew's Obs.4th/e, pg. 50; William's Obs. 24th/e pg. 169]

14. Basic principle of urine pregnancy test is: *(Recent Pattern June 2018)*
   a. Immunochromatography
   b. Electrophoresis
   c. Paper chromatography
   d. None

   [Ref: Dutta's Obs. 8th/e, pg. 75; Holland Brew's Obs.4th/e, pg. 50; Williams Obstetrics, 23rd/e, pg. 192]

Explanation

- HCG test utilizes the principle of Immunochromatography, a unique two-site immunoassay on a membrane.

10.	**d**
11.	**c**
12.	**a,b**
13.	**a**
14.	**a**

15. Minimum level of β–hCG for the earliest detection of intrauterine gestation sac by TVS should be:-

(PGMEE 2016-17)

a. 1500 mIU/mL
b. 5000 mIU/mL
c. 2500 mIU/mL
d. 4500 mIU/mL

[Ref: Dutta's Obs. 9th/e, pg. 601]

Explanation

- For definite sonographic diagnosis of pregnancy (at the earliest) -

	TVS	Vs	TAS
Diameter of intrauterine GS	2-3 mm		5 mm
Menstrual age at detection	4.5 wks		5 wks
S. β hCG level (mIU/ml)	1000-1200		6000

- Advantages of TVS over TAS-
  - Enhanced resolution & ↑ed proximity to pelvic organs
  - Earlier visualization of the gestational sac (GS) & its contents
  - Earlier identification of embryonic cardiac activity
  - Improved visualization of embryonic & fetal structures

15. a

ANTEPARTUM AND INTRAPARTUM ASSESSMENT OF FETAL WELL-BEING

OBSTETRIC ULTRASOUND

1. Father of obstetric ultrasound is?
(PGMEE Nov.12 Pattern)

a. Jhon Wild
b. Mc Roberts
c. Mc Donald
d. Ian Donald

[Ref: Dutta's Obs. 9th/e, pg. 599]

2. Fetal cardiac activity is detected with Transvaginal USG as early as?
(DNB June' 2010)

a. 6 weeks
b. 8 weeks
c. 10 weeks
d. 12 weeks

[Ref: Dutta's Obs. 9th/e, pg. 63, 601; William's Obs. 24th/e pg. 196]

3. Best parameter to estimate age in 1st trimester is?
(DNB June' 2011)

a. Crown rump length
b. Head circumference
c. Corrected BPD
d. BPD

[Ref: Dutta's Obs. 9th/e, pg. 63, 601; Holland Brew's Obs.4th/e, pg. 50; Arias 3rd/e, pg.9; William's Obs. 24th/e pg. 195]

4. Gestational sac on USG in first seen at _____ weeks from LMP-
(PGMEE 2012-13)

a. 2
b. 4
c. 5
d. 6

[Ref: Dutta's Obs. 9th/e, pg. 63, 601; Holland Brew's Obs. 4th/e, pg. 50; William's Obs. 24th/e pg. 196]

5. Most accurate and safest method to diagnose viable pregnancy at 6 weeks-
(PGMEE 13)

a. Doppler assessment of fetal cardiac activity
b. USG for fetal cardiac activity
c. Urinary β hCG determination
d. Per vaginal examination of uterine size corresponding to 6 weeks gestation

[Ref: Dutta's Obs. 9th/e, pg. 600, 601; Holland Brew's Obs.4th/e, pg. 50; William's Obs. 24th/e pg. 195, 196]

6. At 9 weeks best measure to calculate the gestational age-
(PGMEE 2012-13)

a. BPD
b. CRL
c. Fetal femer length
d. Embryonic movements

[Ref: Dutta's Obs. 9th/e, pg. 63, 601; Holland Brew's Obs. 4th/e, pg. 50; William's Obs. 24th/e pg. 195]

7. Gestational sac is seen on TVS at the earliest?
(PGMEE 2014)

a. 18 days
b. 21 days
c. 35 days
d. 42 days

[Ref: Dutta's Obs. 9th/e, pg. 63, 601; Holland Brew's Obs. 4th/e, pg. 50; William's Obs. 24th/e pg. 196]

8. Which of the following is not a prerequisite for transvaginal sonography (TVS) ?
(PGMEE 2014)

a. Consent
b. Full bladder
c. Empty bladder
d. Lithotomy position

[Ref: Holland Brew's Obs. 4th/e, pg. 452]

9. Nuchal translucency in USG can be detected at_____wks of gestation.
(PGMEE 2019)

a. 11-13 wks
b. 18-20 wks
c. 8-10 wks
d. 20-22 wks

[Ref: Williams Obs. 25th/e pg. 4, 73]

10. Increased nuchal translucency at 14 weeks gestation is seen in-
(PGMEE 2010)

a. Anencephaly
b. Down's syndrome
c. Hydrocephalus
d. Spina bifida

[Ref: Dutta's Obs. 9th/e, pg. 601, 604; Holland Brew's Obs.4th/e, pg. 464; William's Obs. 24th/e pg. 196]

11. Biophysical profile includes all except *(PGMEE 2012-13)*

a. NST
b. Muscle tone
c. Amniotic fluid
d. Acetyl choline level

[Ref: Dutta's Obs. 9th/e, pg. 98; Holland Brew's Obs. 4th/e pg. 84t, 460t; William's Obs. 24th/e pg. 342t]

12. Modified biophysical profile includes- *(PGMEE 2012-14)*

a. Non stress test (NST)
b. Amniotic fluid index (AFI)
c. Both
d. None

[Ref: Dutta's Obs. 9th/e, pg. 98, 601; William's Obs. 24th/e pg. 343]

13. Fetal weight at 20 weeks -
(PGMEE 2012-13)

a. 150 g
b. 200 g
c. 300 g
d. 400 g

[Ref: William's Obs. 24th/e pg. 129]

14. Best parameter for estimation of fetal age by ultrasound in 3rd trimester is-
(PGMEE 2013-14)

a. Femur length
b. BPD
c. Abdominal circumference
d. Interocular distance

[Ref: Arias' Obs. 3rd /e, pg. 10]

Explanation

Femur length:

- Not significantly affected by fetal growth alterations, hence best parameter for gestational age estimation in 3rd trimester.
- Measured from the upper to the lower end of the bone's shaft, in the bone closer to the transducer
- Head of the femur and distal epiphysis not included in the measurement

1.	d
2.	a
3.	a
4.	c
5.	b
6.	b
7.	c
8.	b
9.	a
10.	b
11.	d
12.	c
13.	c
14.	a

15. **Anencephaly is earliest diagnosed sonographically by?**
    (PGMEE 2014)
    a. 10-12 weeks
    b. 14-16 weeks
    c. 16-18 weeks
    d. 18-20 weeks

    [Ref: Dutta's Obs. 9th/e, pg. 383, 602; Holland Brew's Obs. 4th/e pg. 50, 335; William's Obs. 24th/e pg.195t, 196]

16. **Which one of the following congenital malformation of the fetus can be diagnosed in first trimester by ultrasound?**
    (PGMEE 2006)
    a. Anencephaly
    b. Inencephaly
    c. Microcephaly
    d. Holoprosencephaly

    [Ref: Dutta's Obs. 9th/e, pg. 383, 602; Holland Brew's Obs. 4th/e pg. 50, 335; William's Obs. 24th/e pg.195t, 196, 201, 203; Internet]

Explanation

Anencephaly:

- Deficient development of vault of skull & brain tissue with normal development of facial portion.
- Skull base & orbits covered by angiomatous stroma.
- Can be detected sonographically as early as 10 weeks of pregnancy.
- Incidence – 1 in 1000 births.

Microcephaly:

- Head size is smaller than normal head, d/t under development of brain.
- May be present at birth or may develop later, in first few years of life.
- May occur as part of syndromes d/t aneuploidy.
- Affected babies have poor intellectual & motor functions, poor speech, abnormal facial development, seizure disorders and dwarfism.

Holoprosencephaly:

- Failure of prosencephalon or forebrain to divide completely into 2 separate cerebral hemispheres & diencephalon.
- May be associated with abnormal development of facial structures (hypotelorism, cyclopia, micro - ophthalmia, ethmocephaly, arhinia with proboscis, median cleft lip).
- 30 – 40 % cases found to have aneuploidy (trisomy 13).
- Birth prevalence – 1 in 10000 to 15000.
- Extremely lethal, found in 1 in 250 of early abortuses.

17. **Fetal marker of growth in USG is?**
    a. Abdominal girth   *(PGMEE Aug. 12 Pattern)*
    b. Amniotic fluid index
    c. Femur length
    d. Regular serial USG bony measurements

    [Ref: Dutta's Obs. 9th/e, pg. 99, 605; William's Obs. 24th/e pg. 199; Arias' Obs. 3rd /e, pg. 10]

18. **Single best parameter to assess fetal wellbeing is?**
    a. Femur length   *(PGMEE Aug 13 Pattern)*
    b. Head circumference
    c. Abdominal circumference
    d. Amniotic fluid volume

    [Ref: Dutta's Obs. 9th/e, pg. 35; Holland Brew's Obs. 4th/e pg. 26; William's Obs. 24th/e pg. 199, 233]

15.	a
16.	a
17.	a
18.	d
19.	b
20.	c
21.	a
22.	a
23.	b
24.	a

DOPPLER

19. **As the pregnancy progresses near term, what happens to the S/D ratio of umbilical artery:**
    a. Increases   *(Recent Pattern June 2018)*
    b. Decreases
    c. Plateaues off
    d. Diastolic notch appears at term

    [Ref: Dutta's Obs. 9th/e, pg. 99; Holland Brew's Obs. 4th/e pg. 458; William's Obs. 24th/e pg. 220]

Explanation

- The umbilical artery (UA) was the first vessel to be studied by doppler ultrasound.
- At about 15 weeks of gestation, diastolic flow can be identified in the UA.
- With advancing gestation, the end-diastolic velocity increases secondary to the decrease in placental resistance.
- This is reflected in decreases in the S/D or PI (pulsatility index).

20. **Most oxygenated fetal vessel is:**   *(JIPMER 2018)*
    a. Ductus Ateriosus
    b. Umbilical Vein
    c. Umbilical artery
    d. Ductus Venosus

    [Ref: DC Dutta Obs. 7th/e, pg. 43]

ELECTRONIC FETAL MONITORING

21. **Antepartum assessment of fetal distress is indicated by all except-**   *(PGMEE 2009)*
    a. Acceleration of 15 beats/min
    b. Deceleration of 30 beats//min
    c. Variable deceleration 5-25 beats/min
    d. Fetal HR < 80 beats/min

    [Ref: Dutta's Obs. 9th/e, pg. 98, 566]

22. **Conditions associated with decreased variability of fetal heart rate are all except:**   *(DNB Dec' 2010)*
    a. Fetal movement
    b. Acidemia
    c. Sleep
    d. Chronic hypoxia

    [Ref: Dutta's Obs. 9th/e, pg. 569; Holland Brew's Obs.4th/e, pg. 473; Arias 3rd/e, pg. 53-55; William's Obs. 24th/e pg. 479]

23. **Late deceleration is due to?**   *(PGMEE 2011)*
    a. Cord compression
    b. Uteroplacental insufficiency
    c. Head compression
    d. All

    [Ref: Dutta's Obs. 9th/e, pg. 569; Holland Brew's Obs.4th/e, pg. 470; Arias 3rd/e, pg. 179; William's Obs. 24th/e pg. 483, 484]

24. **Regarding contraction stress test false is-**
    a. Oxytocin not used   *(PGMEE 2012-13)*
    b. Invasive method
    c. Detects fetal well being
    d. Negative test is associated with good fetal outcome

    [Ref: Dutta's Obs. 9th/e, pg. 466; Arias' Obs. 3rd /e, pg. 19; William's Obs. 24th/e pg. 338]

25. All are related to NST except- *(PGMEE 2012-13)*
a. Variability
b. Acceleration
c. Time period
d. Oxytocin

[Ref: Dutta's Obs. 9th/e, pg. 98, Holland Brew's Obs.4th/e, pg. 469; Arias' Obs. 3rd /e, pg. 10; William's Obs. 24th/e pg. 338]

26. NST is said to be reactive when:- *(PGMEE 2016-17)*
a. Acceleration > 10 bpm for > 10 s
b. Acceleration > 15 bpm for > 15 s
c. Acceleration > 10 bpm for > 15 s
d. Acceleration > 15 bpm for > 10 s

[Ref: Dutta's Obs. 9th/e, pg. 98; Holland Brew's Obs.4th/e, pg. 469; Arias' Obs. 3rd /e, pg. 10; William's Obs. 24th/e pg. 339]

PRENATAL GENETIC DIAGNOSIS

SCREENING OF DOWN'S SYNDROME

27. Quadruple test does not include *(PGMEE 2012-13)*
a. MSAFP
b. Total hCG
c. PAPP-A
d. Inhibin A

[Ref: Dutta's Obs. 9th/e, pg. 103; Holland Brew's Obs.4th/e, pg. 464; Arias 3rd/e, pg. 38-41; William's Obs. 24th/e pg. 289t, 291]

28. Quadruple test in pregnancy is performed at:- *(PGMEE 2018)*
a. Between 8-12 weeks
b. Between 15-18 weeks
c. Between 20-22 week
d. Between 12-14 weeks

Ref: Dutta's Obs. 8th / e, pg.129; Holland Brew's Obs.4th /e, pg.73; Arias 3rd / e, pg. 41; Williams Obs. 24th / e, pg.293

Explanation

Quadruple test

- Also known as Quad test
- Serological screening test for Down's syndrome or trisomy 21
- Performed between 15 – 22 weeks of pregnancy
- Involves detection of levels of following 4 biochemical analytes in Down's syndrome-
  o Maternal serum alpha feto protein (MSAFP) - ↓
  o Human chorionic gonadotrophin (hCG-free β subunit) - ↑
  o Unconjugated estriol (uE3) - ↓
  o Inhibin A (InhA) - ↑
- Detection rate – 85%, false-positive rate 0.9%

29. In Down's syndrome, 2nd trimester quadruple test includes all EXCEPT: *(DNB June' 2011)*
a. Inhibin A
b. hCG
c. Alpha fetoprotein
d. PAPP-A

[Ref: Dutta's Obs. 9th/e, pg. 103; Holland Brew's Obs.4th/e, pg. 464; Arias 3rd/e, pg. 38-41; William's Obs. 24th/e pg. 289t, 291]

30. Soft markers for screening of Down's syndrome are all except :- *(PGMEE 2016-17)*
a. Increased nuchal translucency
b. Absence of nasal bone
c. Cardiac defects
d. Rockerbottom foot

[Ref: Dutta's Obs. 9th/e, pg. 104t, 106t; Holland Brew's Obs.4th/e, pg. 465; Arias 4th /e, pg. 5-8; William's Obs. 24th/e pg. 292-294, 293t]

AMNIOCENTESIS

31. Amniocentesis is done at what intrauterine age? *(DNB Dec' 2011, PGMEE Aug. 12 Pattern)*
a. 10–12 weeks
b. 12–20 weeks
c. 20–25 weeks
d. 25–30 weeks

[Ref: Dutta's Obs. 9th/e, pg. 105, 607; Holland Brew's Obs.4th/e, pg. 466; Arias 3rd/e, pg. 46-47; William's Obs. 24th/e pg. 297]

32. Early amniocentesis done at- *(PGMEE 2012-13)*
a. 5-10 weeks
b. 10-15 weeks
c. 15-20 weeks
d. 20-24 weeks

[Ref: Dutta's Obs. 9th/e, pg. 105, 607; William's Obs. 24th/e pg. 299; Arias 3rd/e, pg. 46-47]

33. Amniocentesis is used to diagnose:- *(PGMEE 2016-17)*
a. Chromosomal disorders
b. Non-immune hydrops fetalis
c. Neural tube defects
d. All of the above

[Ref: Dutta's Obs. 9th/e, pg. 462, 607; Holland Brew's Obs.4th/e, pg. 466; William's Obs. 24th/e pg. 286, 287, 297, 850]

ALPHA FETO PROTEIN

34. Alpha feto protein levels are increased in all except: *(DNB June' 2009, DNB Dec' 2011)*
a. Open neural tube defects
b. Intrauterine death
c. Down's syndrome
d. Twin pregnancy

[Ref: Dutta's Obs. 9th/e, pg. 103; Holland Brew's Obs. 4th/e, pg. 464; Arias 3rd/e, pg. 53-55; William's Obs. 24th/e pg. 285]

35. Most effective in detecting neural tube defect- *(PGMEE 2012-13)*
a. AFP
b. MRI
c. CT
d. Ultrasound

[Ref: Dutta's Obs. 9th/e, pg. 103, 602; Holland Brew's Obs. 4th/e pg. 457, 463, 464; William's Obs. 24th/e pg. 285, 286; Arias 3rd/e, pg. 53-55]

Explanation

- Measurement of Alpha fetoprotein (AFP) in maternal serum or amniotic fluid is a screening test for fetal neural tube defects, elevated in ~ 85 % of fetuses with NTDs.
- USG (targeted anomaly scan) in 2nd trimester can detect ~ 99% of fetuses with open NTDs having elevated MSAFP.

36. True about Alfa feto protein (AFP) are all except:- *(PGMEE 2016-17)*
a. It is a glycoprotein
b. Produced by placenta
c. Produced by fetal liver
d. Concentration of AFP in maternal serum reaches its peak at 32 weeks of gestation

[Ref: Dutta's Obs. 9th/e, pg. 103; William's Obs. 24th/e pg. 284, 285]

25.	d
26.	b
27.	c
28.	b
29.	d
30.	d
31.	b
32.	b
33.	d
34.	c
35.	d
36.	b

FETAL PULMONARY MATURITY

37. Best method for the diagnosis of lung maturity is?
a. L/S ratio in amniotic fluid **(DNB June' 2011)**
b. Phosphtidyl glycerorl estimation in amniotic fluid
c. Amniotic fluid creatinine level
d. Bilirubin estimation in amniotic fluid

[Ref: Dutta's Obs. 9th/e, pg. 100; Holland Brew's Obs. 4th/e, pg. 466; William's Obs. 24th/e pg. 655; Internet]

Explanation

Various tests for assessment of fetal pulmonary maturity:

- Estimation of pulmonary surfactant by amniotic fluid Lecithin / Sphingomyelin (L /S) ratio-
  - Amniotic fluid L/S ratio at 31-32 wks is 1, at 35 wks is 2.
  - L/S ratio ≥ 2 indicates pulmonary maturity.
- Shake test or bubble test (Clement's)-
  - Increasing dilutions of AF mixed with 96% ethanol, shaken for 15 seconds & inspected after 15 minutes → if a complete ring of bubbles present at the meniscus → test is positive & indicates pulmonary maturity.
- Foam Stability Index (FSI)-
  - > 47 virtually excludes the risk of RDS.
- Presence of phosphatidyl glycerorl (PG) in amniotic fluid-
  - Reliably indicates pulmonary maturity.
- Saturated phosphatidyl choline-
  - > 500 ng / ml indicates pulmonary maturity.
- Fluorescence polarization-
  - Polarized light used to quantitate surfactant in the AF & the ratio of surfactant to albumin is measured by an automatic analyser.
  - Presence of 55 mg of surfactant per gram of albumin indicates pulmonary maturity.
- Amniotic fluid optical density-
  - At 650 mμ > 0.15 indicates pulmonary maturity.
- Lamellar body count in amniotic fluid –
  - > 30,000 / μl indicates pulmonary maturity.
- Orange coloured cells in amniotic fluid-
  - Presence of orange coloured desquamated fetal cells (stained with 0.1% Nileblue sulphate) > 50% s/o pulmonary maturity.
- Amniotic fluid tubidity-
  - During 1st & 2nd trimesters, AF is yellow & clear.
  - At term it is turbid d/t vernix.
- Amniotic fluid L/S (Lecithin /Sphingomyelin)ratio was considered to be "Gold standard test " in past for fetal lung maturity.
- Concentration of both in the amniotic fluid is same before 34 weeks, but at 32 – 34 weeks the concentration of lecithin begins to rise as compared to sphingomyelin.
- Although L/S ratio > 2 is indicative of fetal lung maturity, in pregnant patients with diabetes concentration of phosphatidyl glycerol in amniotic fluid is a better predictor.

38. Fetal lung maturity is signified by- **(PGMEE 2012-13)**
a. L:S > 2
b. > 37 weeks gestation
c. Level of phosphatidyl choline
d. Non reactive NST

[Ref: Dutta's Obs. 9th/e, pg. 100]

39. Which does not indicate fetal lung maturity-
a. Reactive NST **(PGMEE 2012-13)**
b. Gestation 37 weeks
c. Presence of phosphatidyl choline
d. L/S ratio

[Ref: Dutta's Obs. 9th/e, pg. 100]

40. Surfactant appears in amniotic fluid at? **(PGMEE 2013)**
a. 20 weeks
b. 32 weeks
c. 28 weeks
d. 30 weeks

[Ref: Dutta's Obs. 9th/e, pg. 443]

MISCELLANEOUS

41. Pre-implantation genetic testing (PIGT) is done:-
a. At the time of ovulation **(PGMEE 2018)**
b. After ovulation but before fertilization
c. After fertilization but before implantation of ovum
d. 1 week after implantation of ovum

[Ref: Speroff 8th e p.1362; speroff 8th e p.1199]

Explanation

Pre-Implantation Genetic Testing

- The technique requires one or more cells that may be obtained at different stages of development. The chromosomal composition of the oocyte may be inferred from that of the extruded polar bodies. One or two blastomeres may be removed from cleavage stage embryos. Biopsy of the trophoectoderm can also be performed at the blastocyst stage. In the most common scenario (cleavage stage embryo biopsy), a laser or a dilute solution of acid Tyrode's solution is used to create a small hole in the zona pellucida and one or two cells are aspirated, typically on the third day after oocyte retrieval and fertilization when embryos are at the 6–8 cell stage.
- PGD can be performed on polar bodies removed from oocytes before fertilization (preconception diagnosis) or on blastomeres or trophoectoderm removed from embryos before transfer.
- To detect abnormalities in embryos, one or two nucleated cells are removed, typically on the third day after fertilization (the 6–8 cell stage), before compaction when the blastomeres become more tightly adherent

37.	b
38.	a
39.	a
40.	c
41.	c

HEMORRHAGE IN PREGNANCY

ABORTIONS

1. Most common cause of spontaneous abortion is?
a. Chromosomal abnormality   *(DNB June' 2009)*
b. Infection
c. Immunological
d. Uterine malformations

[Ref: Dutta's Obs. 9th/e, pg. 151; Holland Brew's Obs.4th/e, pg. 197; William's Obs. 24th/e pg. 351]

2. In case of 2nd trimester recurrent abortions, most common uterine malformation seen is?
a. Mullerian fusion defects   *(DNB June' 2011)*
b. Uterine agenesis
c. Unicornuate uterus
d. Uterine synecchiae

[Ref: Dutta's Obs. 9th/e, pg. 160; William's Obs. 24th/e pg. 358, 359t]

3. In 1st trimester recurrent abortions all tests are to be done except: *(DNB Dec' 2011)*
a. Parental cytogenetics
b. TORCH infection screening
c. Antiphospholipid antibodies
d. Thyroid profile

[Ref: Dutta's Obs. 9th/e, pg. 159, 160; Holland Brew's Obs.4th/e, pg. 202; William's Obs. 24th/e pg. 358, 359]

4. Decidual cast or carneous mole expelled per vaginum is suggestive of-   *(PGMEE 2004)*
a. Inevitable abortion   b. Threatened abortion
c. Tubal abortion   d. Missed abortion

[Ref: Dutta's Obs. 9th/e, pg. 156]

5. Recurrent abortion not due to-   *(PGMEE 2012-13)*
a. Chromosomal defects
b. TORCH infection
c. Luteal phase defects
d. Poorly controlled diabetes

[Ref: Dutta's Obs. 9th/e, pg. 159, 160; Holland Brew's Obs.4th/e, pg. 202; William's Obs. 24th/e pg. 358, 359]

6. Investigation not validated for recurrent pregnancy loss is?   *(PGMEE Nov 13 Pattern)*
a. TSH
b. Hysteroscopy
c. Hysterosalphingography
d. TORCH test

[Ref: Dutta's Obs. 9th/e, pg. 159, 160; Holland Brew's Obs. 4th/e, pg. 202; William's Obs. 24th/e pg. 353, 358, 359]

Explanation
- Endocrinopathies such as uncontrolled diabetes, overt hypothyroidism & severe iodine deficiency have been found to be associated with RPL (12% of cases). Hence, screening for diabetes & hypothyroidism is required.
- Structural abnormalities of uterus, congenital (septate uterus) or acquired (Asherman's syndrome), have been implicated in 15% of cases of RPL. These can be diagnosed by HSG or hysteroscopy. Operative hysteroscopy plays a role in the management also (e.g. septal resection, adhesiolysis).
- Routine TORCH infection screening should be abandoned.
- Infections particularly speculated to play a role in RPL include Ureaplasma, Chlamydia trachomatis, L. monocytogenes, & Herpes simplex virus.
- Usually investigations for chronic infections is warranted only in immunocompromised patient with RPL & with a h/o sexually transmitted infections.

7. Most common cause of abortion in first trimester is-
a. Uterine anomaly   *(PGMEE 2013-14)*
b. Infection
c. Chromosomal abnormality
d. Hormonal disturbance

[Ref: Dutta's Obs. 9th/e, pg. 151; Holland Brew's Obs.4th/e, pg. 197; William's Obs. 24th/e pg. 351]

8. Most common cause of abortion is-   *(PGMEE 2014)*
a. Infection
b. Luteal phase defect
c. Immunological cause
d. Defective embryo

[Ref: Dutta's Obs. 9th/e, pg. 151; Holland Brew's Obs.4th/e, pg. 197; William's Obs. 24th/e pg. 351]

9. Patient with recurrent abortion diagnosed to have anti-phospholipid syndrome. What will be the treatment: *(PGMEE 2019)*
a. Aspirin only
b. Aspirin + Low molecular weight Heparin
c. Aspirin + Low molecular weight Heparin + Prednisolone
d. No Treatment

[Ref: Williams Obs. 25th/e pg. 18, 53]

10. The method of choice for termination of pregnancy between 7 and 12 weeks is: *(PGMEE 2014)*
a. Mifepristone and misoprostol
b. Dilatation and curettage
c. Suction evacuation
d. Menstrual regulation

[Ref: Dutta's Obs. 9th/e, pg. 165; Holland Brew's Obs. 4th/e pg. 580]

1.	a
2.	a
3.	b
4.	d
5.	b
6.	d
7.	c
8.	d
9.	b
10.	c

11. **A woman with 20 weeks pregnancy presents with bleeding per vaginum. On speculum examination, the os is open but no products have come out. The most likely diagnosis is-** *(PGMEE 2013)*
    a. Incomplete abortion
    b. Complete abortion
    c. Inevitable abortion
    d. Missed abortion

    [Ref: Dutta's Obs. 9th/e, pg. 154; Holland Brew's Obs.4th/e, pg. 200-201]

MTP

12. **MTP allowed till how many days as per MTP act:-** *(PGMEE 2015-16)*
    a. 70 days
    b. 120 days
    c. 140 days
    d. 160 days

    [Ref: Dutta's Obs. 9th/e, pg. 165; Holland Brew's Obs.4th/e, pg. 580]

13. **Indication of MTP:** *(Recent Pattern June 2018)*
    a. Pregnancy due to rape
    b. Contraceptive failure
    c. Pregnancy endangering mother's life
    d. All of the above

    [Ref: Dutta's Obs. 9th/e pg. 165]

Explanation

- The conditions under which pregnancy can be terminated under the MTP Act. There are 4 conditions that have been identified in the Act :
  - Medical - Where continuation of the pregnancy might endanger the mother's life or cause grave injury to her physical or mental health.
  - Eugenic - Where there is substantial risk of the child being born with serious handicaps due to physical or mental abnormalities.
  - Humanitarian - Where pregnancy is the result of rape.
  - Failure of contraceptive devices - Unwanted pregnancy resulting from a failure of any contraceptive device or method can be presumed to give a grave mental trauma/stress to the health of the mother. In these circumstances Indian law virtually allows abortion on request, in view of the difficulty of proving that a pregnancy was not caused by failure of contraception

ECTOPIC PREGNANCY

14. **The following drug is not helpful in the treatment of ectopic pregnancy-** *(PGMEE 2005)*
    a. Methotrexate
    b. Misoprostol
    c. Actinomycin-D
    d. RU 486

    [Ref: Dutta's Obs. 9th/e, pg. 174; Holland Brew's Obs.4th/e, pg. 209]

15. **Most common symptom in ectopic pregnancy-**
    a. Abdominal pain *(PGMEE 2012-13)*
    b. Bleeding per vagina
    c. Amenorrhoea
    d. Fainting attacks

    [Ref: Dutta's Obs. 9th/e, pg. 171; Holland Brew's Obs.4th/e, pg. 207; William's Obs. 24th/e pg. 379]

16. **Which is associated with least chances of ectopic pregnancy:** *(PGMEE 2012-13)*
    a. Tubectomy
    b. IUCD
    c. Oral contraceptive
    d. Tubal ligation

    [Ref: Dutta's Obs. 9th/e, pg. 169; William's Obs. 24th/e pg. 377, 378; Berek & Novak's Gynecology, 15th/e, pg. 623 - 625; Holland Brew's Obs.4th/e, pg. 206]

17. **Methotrexate is used in ectopic pregnancy when-**
    a. Patient is hemodynamically stable
    b. Serum β hCG level > 3000 IU/L *(PGMEE 2012-13)*
    c. Tubal diameter > 4cm without fetal cardiac activity
    d. When there is intraabdominal haemorrhage

    [Ref: Dutta's Obs. 9th/e, pg. 174; Holland Brew's Obs.4th/e, pg. 209; William's Obs. 24th/e pg. 384]

18. **Medical management for ectopic pregnancy is indicated in?**
    a. Detectable fetal cardiac activity
    b. Tubal diameter > 4cm
    c. Serum β hCG level < 3000 IU/L
    d. Hemodynamically unstable patient

    [Ref: Dutta's Obs. 9th/e, pg. 174; Holland Brew's Obs.4th/e, pg. 209; William's Obs. 24th/e pg. 385]

19. **Highest likely cause of ectopic pregnancy-**
    a. IUCD *(PGMEE 2012-13)*
    b. PID
    c. Artificial fertility technique
    d. Tubal damage

    [Ref: Dutta's Obs. 9th/e, pg. 169; William's Obs. 24th/e pg. 377, 378; Berek & Novak's Gynecology, 15th/e, pg. 623 - 625]

20. **Most common cause of ectopic pregnancy-** *(PGMEE 2012-13)*
    a. IUCD
    b. PID
    c. POP
    d. Peritubal adhesions

    [Ref: Dutta's Obs. 9th/e, pg. 169; William's Obs. 24th/e pg. 377, 378; Berek & Novak's Gynecology, 15th/e, pg. 623 - 625; Holland Brew's Obs.4th/e, pg. 206]

Explanation

Etiological factors for ectopic pregnancy:

- Any tubal surgery (for prev. tubal preg./tubal ligation - 15 to 50% chance of ectopic preg. in case of sterilization failure / reversal of sterilization) will cause tubal damage, conferring highest risk of ectopic pregnancy
- PID / salpingitis - 6 to 10 times increased risk of ectopic due to peritubal & intraluminal adhesions
- Contraceptives - IUCD (7 times increased risk, no protection against tubal implantation) > tubal ligation (failures) > progesterone only pills (diminished tubal motility). Least chance of ectopic with combined OCPs
- ART - 5 to 7 % increased risk (with ovulation induction, IVF-ET, GIFT)

21. **Most of ectopic pregnancies are at ampulla as-**
    a. It is narrowest part *(PGMEE 2012-13)*
    b. Tubal movements are least here
    c. Salpingitis produces least crypts here
    d. Plicae are most numerous here

    [Ref: Shaw's Gynae. 16th/e pg.295]

11.	c
12.	c
13.	d
14.	b
15.	a
16.	c
17.	a
18.	c
19.	b,d
20.	b
21.	d

22. Best modality to diagnose unruptured ectopic pregnancy- *(PGMEE 2012-13)*
   a. Laparoscopy
   b. UPT
   c. USG
   d. Culdocentesis

[Ref: Dutta's Obs. 9th/e, pg. 173; Holland Brew's Obs.4th/e, pg. 208; William's Obs. 24th/e pg. 382, 383]

23. A patient comes with 6 weeks' amenorrhoea and features of shock, most likely diagnosis is- *(PGMEE 2012-13)*
   a. Ectopic pregnancy
   b. H. Mole
   c. Twin pregnancy
   d. None of the above

[Ref:Dutta's Obs. 9th/e, pg. 171; Holland Brew's Obs.4th/e, pg. 207-208; William's Obs. 24th/e pg. 379]

24. Earliest rupture in tubal pregnancy is seen in which part of tube? *(PGMEE 2013-14)*
   a. Ampulla   b. Isthmus
   c. Interstitial   d. Fimbrial

[Ref: Dutta's Obs. 9th/e, pg. 170; Holland Brew's Obs.4th/e, pg. 207]

25. Drugs used in ectopic pregnancy- *(PGMEE 2013-14)*
   a. PGE2   b. PGI
   c. PGF2α   d. PGE1

[Ref: Dutta's Obs. 9th/e, pg. 174; Holland Brew's Obs.4th/e, pg. 209]

26. M/c site of ectopic pregnancy is *(PGMEE 2016-17)*
   a. Ampulla   b. Isthmus
   c. Interstitium   d. Cornu

[Ref: Dutta's Obs. 9th/e, pg. 168f; Holland Brew's Obs. 4th/e, 207f]

27. Least common site for extra uterine pregnancy:- *(PGMEE 2016-17)*
   a. Tubal   b. Fimbrial
   c. Ovarian   d. Interstitial

[Ref: Dutta's Obs. 9th/e, pg. 168f; Holland Brew's Obs. 4th/e, 207f]

MOLAR PREGNANCY/HYDATIFORM MOLE

28. Treatment for a 16 weeks hydatidiform mole is? *(DNB June' 2009)*
   a. Hysterectomy   b. Suction evacuation
   c. LSCS   d. Hysterotomy

[Ref: Dutta's Obs. 9th/e, pg. 184; William's Obs. 24th/e pg. 400; Holland Brew's Obs.4th/e, pg. 254]

29. Most common presenting feature of complete mole is:
   a. Vomiting   *(PGMEE 2013-14)*
   b. Amenorrhoea
   c. Headache
   d. Bleeding per vaginum

[Ref: Dutta's Obs. 9th/e, pg. 182; Holland Brew's Obs.4th/e, pg. 251; William's Obs. 24th/e pg. 398]

30. A 28 year old female presents with a pregnancy of 12 weeks (corrected LMP). However on examination, the fundal height corresponds to 14 weeks. A brownish discharge is seen on vaginal examination. Likely diagnosis is:-
   a. Missed abortion   *(PGMEE 2016-17)*
   b. Pelvic infection
   c. Molar pregnancy
   d. Meconium stained liquor

[Ref: Dutta's Obs. 9th/e, pg. 182; Holland Brew's Obs.4th/e, pg. 251; William's Obs. 24th/e pg. 398]

31. Which contraceptive should not be used after molar pregnancy? *(PGMEE 2013)*
   a. Barrier   b. Hormonal contraceptives
   c. IUCD   d. Natural method

[Ref: Dutta's Obs. 9th/e, pg. 186; William's Obs. 24th/e pg. 401]

[GTDs DISCUSSED IN DETAILS IN GYNAE SECTION]

ANTEPARTUM HEMORRHAGE: PLACENTA PRAEVIA

32. All are true about placenta previa except: *(DNB Dec' 2010)*
   a. Bright red blood loss
   b. Malpresentations usually found
   c. Increased uterine tone
   d. Painless vaginal bleeding

[Ref: Dutta's Obs. 9th/e, pg. 230; Holland Brew's Obs.4th/e, pg. 230-231]

33. Identify the type of placenta praevia as shown in the picture below? *(PGMEE 2019)*

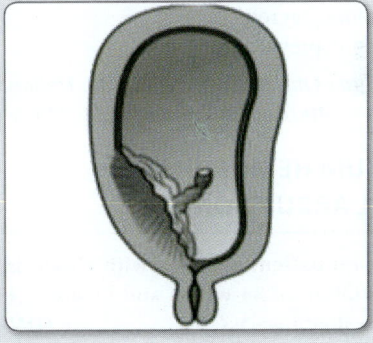

   a. I   b. II
   c. III   d. IV

[Ref: DC Dutta Obs. 7th/e pg. 242]

Explanation

Placenta previa:
- When the placenta is implanted partially or completely over the lower uterine segment
- Degree:
  ○ Type I - low lying
  ○ Type II - marginal
  ○ Type III - partial/incomplete
  ○ Type IV - complete placenta previa/central/total

22.	a
23.	a
24.	b
25.	c
26.	a
27.	c
28.	b
29.	d
30.	c
31.	c
32.	c
33.	b

34. Woman with 37 week of pregnancy comes with grade 3 placenta previa, bleeding per vaginum with uterine contractions. Treatment of choice is-
   a. Wait and watch   **(PGMEE June' 2012)**
   b. Bed rest & sedation
   c. Dexamethasome and nifedipine
   d. Emergency LSCS

[Ref: Dutta's Obs. 9th/e, pg. 235; Holland Brew's Obs.4th/e, pg. 235; William's Obs. 24th/e pg. 803]

35. 35 weeks pregnancy, painless blood discharge, most likely diagnosis is-   **(PGMEE 2012-13)**
   a. Placenta previa   b. Abruptio placenta
   c. Ectopic pregnancy d. None

[Ref: Dutta's Obs. 9th/e, pg. 230; Holland Brew's Obs.4th/e, pg. 230-231; William's Obs. 24th/e pg. 801]

36. Placenta praevia, false is-   **(PGMEE 2012-13)**
   a. Most common cause of APH
   b. Painful vaginal bleeding
   c. USG is the investigation of choice
   d. Increased maternal age is a risk factor

[Ref: Dutta's Obs. 9th/e, pg. 228, 229b, 230, 231, 232t, 238; Holland Brew's Obs.4th/e, pg. 230-232]

37. Which of the following predisposes to placenta previa?
   a. Primigravida   **(PGMEE Aug 13 Pattern)**
   b. Singleton pregnancy
   c. Diabetes mellitus
   d. Previous cesarean section

[Ref: Dutta's Obs. 9th/e, pg. 229b; Holland Brew's Obs.4th/e, pg. 230; William's Obs. 24th/e pg. 801]

38. Maximum chance of placental remnant is in:-
   a. Placenta accreta   **(PGMEE 2016-17)**
   b. Placenta increta
   c. Placenta percreta
   d. Placenta previa

[Ref: Dutta's Obs. 9th/e, pg. 235, 395; Holland Brew's Obs. 4th/e, 233t; William's Obs. 24th/e pg. 804 - 807]

ANTEPARTUM HEMORRHAGE: PLACENTAL ABRUPTION

39. A pregnant patient presents with abdominal pain with twin gestation of 34 weeks and bleeding PV. The most probable diagnosis is?   **(DNB June' 2009)**
   a. Abruptio placentae   b. Abortion
   c. Ectopic pregnancy   d. Placenta previa

[Ref: Dutta's Obs. 9th/e, pg. 232t]

40. Drug causing abruptio placentae -   **(PGMEE 2012-13)**
   a. Methadone   b. Cocaine
   c. Amphetamine   d. Fluoxetine

[Ref: Dutta's Obs. 9th/e, pg. 238; Holland Brew's Obs.4th/e, pg. 236; William's Obs. 24th/e pg. 796]

41. Couvelaire uterus is seen in   **(PGMEE 2013-14)**
   a. Vasa previa   b. Placenta previa
   c. Abruptio placentae d. Placenta accreta

[Ref: Dutta's Obs. 9th/e, pg. 238, 239; Holland Brew's Obs. 4th/e, 237t; William's Obs. 24th/e pg. 797]

42. The term Couvelaire uterus is used in relation to:-
   a. Pregnancy induced Hypertension   **(PGMEE 2015-16)**
   b. Uteroplacental Apoplexy
   c. Postpartum Haemorrhage
   d. Placenta Previa

[Ref: Dutta's Obs. 9th/e, pg. 238; Holland Brew's Obs. 4th/e, 237t; William's Obs. 24th/e pg. 797]

PRETERM LABOR

43. Risk of preterm delivery is increased if cervical length is-   **(PGMEE 2005, Nov 13 Pattern)**
   a. 2.5 cm   b. 3.0 cm
   c. 3.5 cm   d. 4.0 cm

[Ref: Dutta's Obs. 9th/e, pg. 294; Holland Brew's Obs.4th/e, pg. 357; William's Obs. 24th/e pg. 843]

44. A 34 weeks pregnant female presented with uterine contractions, with no other risk factors. Steps in management are all except -   **(DNB Dec' 2010)**
   a. Dexamethasone should be given
   b. Tocolytic for 3 more weeks
   c. Vacuum assisted delivery
   d. Expectant management

[Ref: Dutta's Obs. 9th/e, pg. 296, 539; Holland Brew's Obs. 4th/e, 358t]

45. Drug that does not prevent preterm labor is: **(DNB Dec' 2010)**
   a. Ritodrine
   b. Nitroglycerine patch
   c. Dexamethasone
   d. Atosiban

[Ref: Dutta's Obs. 9th/e, pg. 296, 472; Holland Brew's Obs. 4th/e, 359, 360t; William's Obs. 24th/e pg. 852, 853]

46. Preterm baby is born before?   **(PGMEE Nov 13 Pattern)**
   a. 28weeks
   b. 32 weeks
   c. 34 weeks
   d. 37 weeks

[Ref: Dutta's Obs. 9th/e, pg. 294, 427]

POSTDATED PREGNANCY

47. Investigation of choice for confirming postdatism?   **(PGMEE Aug. 12 Pattern)**
   a. USG
   b. Spectrophotometry
   c. Amniocentesis
   d. X-ray

[Ref: Dutta's Obs. 9th/e, pg. 300; Holland Brew's Obs.4th/e, pg. 245; William's Obs. 24th/e pg. 862]

48. Female with 41 wk gestation confirmed by radiological investigation, very sure of her LMP, no uterine contractions, no effacement and no dilatation. What should not be done?   **(PGMEE 2019)**
   a. Intracervical Foley's   b. PGE1 tab
   c. PGE2 gel   d. PGF2alpha

[Ref: DC Dutta Obs. 7th/e, pg. 523]

34.	d
35.	a
36.	b
37.	d
38.	c
39.	a
40.	b
41.	c
42.	b
43.	a
44.	c
45.	c
46.	d
47.	a
48.	d

INTRAUTERINE FETAL DEATH

49. IUFD causes all except- *(PGMEE 2008)*
- a. PIH
- b. DIC
- c. Psychological upset
- d. Infection

[Ref: Dutta's Obs. 9th/e, pg. 304; Holland Brew's Obs. 4th/e, pg. 247]

50. 1st sign of IUD - *(PGMEE 2012-13)*
- a. Spalding sign
- b. Air in heart
- c. Hyper flexion of spine
- d. Egg shell cracking feel of the fetal head

[Ref: Dutta's Obs. 9th/e, pg. 303; Holland Brew's Obs.4th/e, pg. 247]

51. Earliest sign in IUD is:- *(PGMEE 2016-17)*
- a. Robert's sign
- b. Spalding sign
- c. Hyperflexion of spine
- d. Ball sign

[Ref: Dutta's Obs. 9th/e, pg. 303; Holland Brew's Obs.4th/e, pg. 247]

52. Radiological sign in intrauterine fetal death:- *(PGMEE 2016-17)*
- a. Spalding sign
- b. Robert's sign
- c. A and B both
- d. Palmer's sign

[Ref: Dutta's Obs. 9th/e, pg. 303]

MULTIPLE PREGNANCY

53. Exclusive complication of monochorionic twins- *(PGMEE 2012-13)*
- a. Cord entanglement
- b. Twin to twin transfusion
- c. Discordant growth
- d. Abortion

[Ref: Dutta's Obs. 9th/e, pg. 194; Holland Brew's Obs. 4th/e, pg. 223; William's Obs. 24th/e pg. 904]

54. Monochorionic monoamniotic placenta develops if division takes place- *(PGMEE 2012-13)*
- a. Before 72 hrs
- b. Between 4th & 8th day
- c. After 8th day
- d. After 2 weeks

[Ref: Dutta's Obs. 9th/e, pg. 189t, 190f; Holland Brew's Obs. 4th/e, pg. 220; William's Obs. 24th/e pg. 892]

55. Least common presentation of twins:
- a. Both vertex *(PGMEE 2012-13)*
- b. Both breech
- c. Both transverse
- d. First vertex and 2nd transverse

[Ref: Holland Brew's Obs. 4th/e, pg. 223f]

56. In which condition internal podalic version is done-
- a. Transverse lie in 2nd twin *(PGMEE 2012-13)*
- b. Breech presentation
- c. Both
- d. None

[Ref: Dutta's Obs. 9th/e, pg. 197, 542; Holland Brew's Obs.4th/e, pg. 225; William's Obs. 24th/e pg. 918]

57. Least common type of twins- *(PGMEE 2012-13)*
- a. Diamniotic-dichorionic twins
- b. Diamniotic-monochorionic twins
- c. Monoamniotic-monochorionic twins
- d. Conjoined twins

[Ref: Dutta's Obs. 9th/e, pg. 189t; William's Obs. 24th/e pg. 902]

58. Sign seen in USG in monochorionic diamniotic twins is? *(PGMEE Aug. 12 Pattern)*
- a. Twin peak sign
- b. Lambda sign
- c. T sign
- d. Membrane thickness > 2 mm

[Ref: Dutta's Obs. 9th/e, pg. 192f; William's Obs. 24th/e pg. 897f]

59. Division of eggs taking place on 7th day leads to which type of twins? *(PGMEE 2012, 2015-16)*
- a. Dichorionic diamnionic
- b. Monochorionic diamnionic
- c. Monochorionic monoamnionic
- d. Conjoined twins

[Ref: Dutta's Obs. 9th/e, pg. 189t; Holland Brew's Obs.4th/e, pg. 220; William's Obs. 24th/e pg. 892]

60. In dizygotic twin there is? *(PGMEE Aug. 12 Pattern)*
- a. Always same sex
- b. Always different sex
- c. Separate chorion and amnion
- d. None

[Ref: Dutta's Obs. 9th/e, pg. 189; Holland Brew's Obs.4th/e, pg. 220; William's Obs. 24th/e pg. 892]

61. Twin peak appearance seen in:- *(PGMEE 2016-17)*
- a. Monochorionic monoamniotic
- b. Dichorionic diamniotic
- c. Monochorionic diamniotic
- d. Conjoined twins

[Ref: Dutta's Obs. 9th/e, pg. 192f; William's Obs. 24th/e pg. 897f]

62. Commonest complication of assisted reproductive technique:- *(PGMEE 2018)*
- a. Monozygotic twins
- b. Heterozygotic twins
- c. Dizygotic twins
- d. None of the above

Ref: Speroff 8th e p.1371

Explanation
- When two blastocysts are transferred, the incidence of high-order multiple gestation is markedly reduced but not altogether eliminated, because the incidence of monozygotic twinning may be increased after blastocyst transfer, and the incidence of twins is no lower than that associated with transfer of greater numbers of cleavage-stage embryos.

49.	a
50.	b
51.	a
52.	c
53.	b
54.	c
55.	c
56.	a
57.	d
58.	c
59.	b
60.	c
61.	b
62.	a

63. **Best timing to determine types of twins in case of twin pregnancy is:-** *(PGMEE 2018)*

a. 6-8 weeks
b. 12-14 weeks
c. 28-32weeks
d. 18-21 weeks

[Ref: Dutta's Obs. 8th / e, pg. 237; Holland Brew's Obs.4th/ e, pg. 224-225; Williams Obs. 24th / e, pg. 896-897]

Explanation

Determination of Type of Twin Pregnancy

- Twin gestational sacs may be seen sonographically by as early as **6-7 weeks**
- Two separate fetuses can be identified 12th week onwards
- Best time to determine chorionicity of placenta is 10-13 weeks

Features	Dichorionic placenta	Monochorionic placenta
Thickness of inter-twin membrane	≥ 2 mm	≤ 2 mm
No. of layers	Two layers of amnion with intervening chorion	Two layers of amnion only
Specific USG sign	"Lambda or twin peak" sign - due to triangular projection of chorionic tissue between 2 layers of amnion, at the base of membrane	" T " sign – due to 2 layers of amnion being at right angle with the placenta, without any placental projection or intervening chorion

MISCELLANEOUS COMPLICATIONS

HYPEREMESIS GRAVIDARUM

64. **Metabolic changes in hyperemesis gravidarum:-** *(PGMEE 2015-16)*

a. Hyperchloremia
b. Hypernatremia
c. Ketoacidosis
d. Hyperkalemia

[Ref: Dutta's Obs. 9th/e, pg. 148; Holland Brew's Obs. 4th/e, pg. 38]

63. b
64. c

HYPERTENSIVE DISORDERS IN PREGNANCY

1. **Which of the following is not a predisposing factor for preeclampsia?** *(DNB Dec' 2010)*
   a. Molar pregnancy
   b. Smoking
   c. Gestational diabetes
   d. Anti-phospholipid antibody

   [Ref: Dutta's Obs. 9th/e, pg. 208b; William's Obs. 24th/e pg. 731; Arias 3rd/e, pg. 44]

2. **Definitive treatment of severe pre eclampsia is?** *(DNB Dec' 2010, PGMEE 2012-13)*
   a. Anticonvulsants
   b. Termination of pregnancy
   c. Magnesium sulfate
   d. Antihypertensives

   [Ref: Dutta's Obs. 9th/e, pg. 216; William's Obs. 24th/e pg. 750 Holland Brew's Obs.4th/e, pg. 93; Arias 3rd/e, pg. 420-423]

3. **Not a feature of HELLP syndrome-** *(PGMEE 2012, PGMEE 14)*
   a. Hemolysis
   b. Elevated liver enzymes
   c. Low platelet count
   d. Renal failure

   [Ref: Dutta's Obs. 9th/e, pg. 209; William's Obs. 24th/e pg. 739; Holland Brew's Obs.4th/e, pg. 97]

4. **Therapeutic level of serum magnesium needed to treat pre-eclempsia-** *(PGMEE 2012-13)*
   a. 1-2 mEq / L
   b. 3-4 mEq / L
   c. 4-7 mEq / L
   d. 7-9 mEq / L

   [Ref: Dutta's Obs. 9th/e, pg. 221; William's Obs. 24th/e pg. 759; Holland Brew's Obs. 4th/e, pg. 94]

5. **Antihypertensive of choice in pregnancy is-** *(PGMEE 2012-13)*
   a. Methyldopa   b. Labetolol
   c. Hydralazine   d. CCB

   [Ref: Dutta's Obs. 9th/e, pg. 471; William's Obs. 24th/e pg. 762; Holland Brew's Obs.4th/e, pg. 93]

6. **Antihypertensive contraindicated is pregnancy-** *(PGMEE 2012-13)*
   a. Labetalol
   b. Hydralazine
   c. Methyl dopa
   d. ACE inhibitors

   [Ref: Dutta's Obs. 9th/e, pg. 471; Holland Brew's Obs.4th/e, pg. 94]

7. **DOC for eclampsia is-** *(PGMEE 2012-13)*
   a. Methyl dopa
   b. Labetalol
   c. Magnesium Sulphate
   d. Hydralazine

   [Ref: Dutta's Obs. 9th/e, pg. 221; William's Obs. 24th/e pg. 758; Holland Brew's Obs.4th/e, pg. 96]

8. **In a case of pre eclampsia Doppler USG will show?** *(PGMEE Nov 13 Pattern)*
   a. Reversed blood flow in ductus venosus at 22 weeks
   b. Absent blood flow in umbilical artery at 22 weeks
   c. Diastolic notch in uterine artery at 22 weeks
   d. Increased peak systolic flow velocity in middle cerebral artery

   [Ref: Dutta's Obs. 9th/e, pg. 214, 604; William's Obs. 24th/e pg. 746; Holland Brew's Obs.4th/e, pg. 86]

9. **First sign of magnesium sulphate toxicity is?**
   a. Loss of deep tendon reflexes *(PGMEE Nov 13)*
   b. Respiratory depression
   c. Cardiac arrest
   d. Decrease urinary output

   [Ref: Dutta's Obs. 9th/e, pg. 222b; William's Obs. 24th/e pg. 759; Holland Brew's Obs.4th/e, pg. 94]

10. **MgSO$_4$ have no role in prevention of-** *(PGMEE 2019)*
    a. Seizures in severe pre-eclampsia
    b. Recurrent seizures in eclampsia
    c. RDS in premature baby
    d. Neuroprotection

    [Ref: William's Obs. 25th/e pg. 38, 68]

11. **Management of eclampsia at 34 weeks of pregnancy is-**
    a. Continuation of convulsions and wait for 37 weeks to complete *(PGMEE 2013-14)*
    b. Wait for spontaneous labour
    c. BP monitoring
    d. Anti hypertensive, anticonvulsant and termination of pregnancy

    [Ref: Dutta's Obs. 9th/e, pg. 222, 224; William's Obs. 24th/e pg. 758; Holland Brew's Obs. 4th/e, pg. 93, 96]

12. **Not a criteria for diagnosis of superimposed pre eclempsia in a pregnant lady with pre existing chronic HTN-**
    a. Increase in systolic BP by 30 mm Hg and diastolic by 15 mm Hg *(PGMEE 14)*
    b. Platelets less than 70000
    c. New onset proteinuria
    d. New vascular changes in retinal vessels

    [Ref: Dutta's Obs. 9th/e, pg. 207t; Holland Brew's Obs.4th/e, pg. 85]

1.	b
2.	b
3.	d
4.	c
5.	b
6.	d
7.	c
8.	c
9.	a
10.	c
11.	d
12.	a

13. What feature would be helpful in differentiating chronic HTN from PIH. *(NEET Pattern 2017)*
    a. Episode of seizure
    b. Hypertension nephropathy
    c. Hypertensive retinopathy
    d. HTN at 10 weeks of gestation

    [Ref: Dutta's Obs. 8th / e, pg. 255; Holland Brew's Obs.4th / e, pg. 85, 97; Williams Obs. 24th /e, pg. 730, 1002]

Explanation

Hypertensive disorders in pregnancy

- Hypertension – BP ≥ 140/90 mm Hg (Korotkoff phase V taken as diastolic BP) measured on two occasions at least 6 hours apart)
- Delta hypertension – a sudden rise in mean arterial BP (≥ 105 mm Hg) in later pregnancy
- Gestational hypertension–BP ≥ 140/90 mm Hg for the first time after midpregnancy (20 weeks), without proteinuria
- Preeclampsia - gestational hypertension with protein-uria
- Eclampsia – preeclampsia complicated with convulsions that cannot be attributed to any other cause
- Chronic hypertension – known hypertension before pregnancy or diagnosed for the first time before 20 weeks of pregnancy
- Chronic hypertension with superimposed preeclampsia – new onset proteinuria in pregnant woman with chronic hypertension

GESTATIONAL DIABETES MELLITUS

14. Morbidities expected in baby of diabetic mother are all except: *(DNB June' 2009)*
    a. Macrosomia
    b. Hyperglycemia
    c. Caudal regression
    d. Cardiac anomalies

    [Ref: Dutta's Obs. 9th/e, pg. 265, 266t; William's Obs. 24th/e pg. 1128, 1140; Holland Brew's Obs.4th/e, pg. 130]

15. One step screening test for gestational diabetes (DIPSI criteria) is? *(DNB Dec' 2009)*
    a. Glycosylated haemoglobin measurement
    b. Fasting blood sugar
    c. Oral glucose tolerance test
    d. Random glucose (75 gms) challenge

    [Ref: Dutta's Obs. 9th/e, pg.; 263; William's Obs. 24th/e pg.; Holland Brew's Obs.4th/e, pg. 131]

16. Overt gestational diabetes is defined as random blood glucose more than_? *(PGMEE 2019)*
    a. >200 mg/dl
    b. >126 mg/dl
    c. >100 mg/dl
    d. >180 mg/dl

    [Ref: William's Obs. 25th/e pg. 4, 35]

17. All are the effects of gestational diabetes on fetus except: *(DNB Dec' 2010)*
    a. Increased perinatal mortality
    b. Hypoglycemia
    c. Congenital malformations
    d. Macrosomia

    [Ref: Dutta's Obs. 9th/e, pg. 265, 266; William's Obs. 24th/e pg. 1141, 1142; Holland Brew's Obs. 4th/e, pg. 130]

18. Glucose challenge test done with ___ grams of glucose and is seen at ___ hours according to DIPSI criteria? *(PGMEE Nov 12 Pattern)*
    a. 50 gm and 1 hour
    b. 75 gm and 1 hour
    c. 75 gm and 2 hours
    d. 100 gm and 2 hours

    [Ref: Dutta's Obs. 9th/e, pg. 263; Holland Brew's Obs.4th/e, pg.131]

19. A pregnant woman presents with normal blood sugar but urine analysis reveals glucose present in traces. What will you advise: *(Recent Pattern June 2018)*
    a. Reassurance
    b. Medical nutrition therapy
    c. Insulin
    d. Oral hypoglycemic agents

    [Ref: Dutta's Obs. 9th/e, pg. 262; Holland Brew's Obs. 4th/e pg. 129]

Explanation

- The condition mentioned in this question is called renal glycosuria.
  - Incidence 5–50 % of normal pregnancies
  - Cause – diminished renal threshold for filtration of glucose in urine (180mg/dl in non-pregnant state, whereas 155 mg/dl in pregnancy, esp. midpregnancy)
  - Increased glomerular filtration & impaired tubular reabsorption of glucose are the factors responsible for diminished renal threshold
  - The patient is reassured as the condition doesn't require treatment and disappears after delivery
  - If renal glycosuria persists → screening test for diabetes
  - Frequent urine cultures should be done in such patients as glycosuria may be a cause for asymptomatic bacteriuria

20. Oral hypoglycemic agent safely given in pregnancy is? *(PGMEE Aug 13 Pattern)*
    a. Metformin
    b. Glimepride
    c. Sitagliptin
    d. Pioglitazone

    [Ref: Holland Brew's Obs.4th/e, pg. 135; Dutta's Obs. 9th/e, pg. 267; William's Obs. 24th/e pg. 1142]

21. True about gestational diabetes is: *(PGMEE 2013-14)*
    a. These are increased chances of congenital malforma-tions
    b. Only 2% of women present with overt diabetes
    c. There is chance of macrosomia
    d. Usually diagnosed in early pregnancy

    [Ref: Dutta's Obs. 9th/e, pg. 262 - 265; Holland Brew's Obs. 4th/e, p.g. 126 - 129; William's Obs. 24th/e pg. 1136]

Explanation

- If gestational diabetes is 'first detected' during pregnancy, then fetal congenital malformations may be present if blood sugar levels are elevated during first trimester. Hence option 'a' in this ques. may also be correct in addition to option 'c'.

22. Gestational diabetes mellitus- *(PGMEE 2013-14)*
    a. Is first recognized during pregnancy
    b. Previous history of IUGR
    c. There is no recurrence of GDM in future pregnancy
    d. No risk of overt diabetes

    [Ref: Dutta's Obs. 9th/e, pg. 262 ; William's Obs. 24th/e pg. 1136; Holland Brew's Obs. 4th/e, pg. 130-131]

13.	d
14.	b
15.	d
16.	a
17.	c
18.	c
19.	a
20.	a
21.	c
22.	a

23. In 34 weeks gestation the weight of baby was 3kg. The child shows following features may indicate associated condition *(PGMEE 2019)*

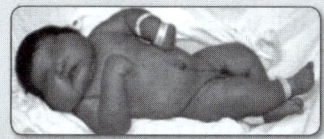

   a. Anemia   b. Diabetes
   c. APH   d. None

[Ref: William's Obs. 25th/e pg. 19, 30]

24. Cause of big baby in GDM patients- *(PGMEE 2013-14)*
   a. Hyperglycemia   b. Hyperinsulinemia
   c. Multiparity   d. Post maturity

[Ref: Dutta's Obs. 9th/e, pg. 265; William's Obs. 24th/e pg. 1129; Holland Brew's Obs. 4th/e, pg. 129-130]

Explanation

According to Pederson's hypothesis -

- Maternal hyperglycemia → fetal hyperglycemia → hypertrophy & hyperplasia of islets of Langerhan's of fetal pancreas → fetal hyperinsulinemia → increased carbohydrate utilization & fat accumulation → excessive fetal growth & adiposity (esp. on trunk & shoulders leading to shoulder dystocia)
- Hence, hyperinsulinemia is the direct cause of macrosomia or big baby in GDM patients, but hyperglycemia (maternal as well as fetal) is the indirect one.

ANEMIA IN PREGNANCY

25. Minimum hemoglobin level in pregnancy below which anaemia occurs is? *(DNB June' 2009, DNB Dec' 2009)*
   a. 9 gm %   b. 10 gm %
   c. 11 gm %   d. 12 gm %

[Ref: Dutta's Obs. 9th/e, pg. 245 ; William's Obs. 24th/e pg. 1101; Holland Brew's Obs.4th/e, pg. 104]

26. A women comes to hospital with 32 weeks of pregnancy and hemoglobin level 6.2 gm%. Most appropriate management is? *(PGMEE Aug. 12 Pattern)*
   a. Intramuscular iron   b. Iron and folic acid tablets
   c. Intravenous iron   d. Blood transfusion

[Ref: Dutta's Obs. 9th/e, pg.250-251; William's Obs. 24th/e pg. 1103; Holland Brew's Obs.4th/e, pg. 111]

Explanation

- Anaemia in pregnancy – Hb < 11 gm /dl and Hct < 33 %
- ICMR grading of anaemia-

Severtiy of anaemia	Hb level (gm/dl)
Mild	10 – 10.9
Moderate	7 – 9.9
Severe	4 – 6.9
Very severe	< 4

- Blood transfusion is recommended for women with severe or very severe anaemia at any period of gestation. Benefits are as follows:
  - Rapid correction of anaemia
  - Improvement of oxygen carrying capacity of blood
  - Patient can bear the strain of labour & blood loss following delivery

27. First sign of recovery after iron therapy- *(PGMEE 2013-14)*
   a. Reticulocytosis   b. ↑MCV
   c. ↑MCH   d. ↑Ferritin

[Ref: Dutta's Obs. 9th/e, pg. 28; Holland Brew's Obs.4th/e, pg. 109]

HEART DISEASE IN PREGNANCY

28. About NYHA grade III, IV heart disease in pregnancy which is not true regarding management? *(PGMEE 2016)*
   a. Delivery should be done in specialised hospitals
   b. Poorly tolerate major surgery
   c. Vaginal delivery is C/I
   d. Surgery (Cesarean section) done only for obstetrical indications

[Ref: Dutta's Obs. 9th/e, pg. 259, 260; Holland Brew's Obs. 4th/e, pg. 120, 121; William's Obs. 24th/e pg. 978]

29. Highest maternal mortality is seen in following congenital heart disease- *(PGMEE 2012-13)*
   a. Eisenmenger's complex
   b. Pulmonary stenosis
   c. Coarctation of aorta
   d. VSD

[Ref: Dutta's Obs. 9th/e, pg. 261; William's Obs. 24th/e pg. 985; Holland Brew's Obs.4th/e, pg. 124]

30. Which of the following drugs should not be used in the conduct of labour in a woman with rheumatic heart disease- *(PGMEE 2011)*
   a. Methylergometrine
   b. Misoprostol
   c. Synctocin   d. Carboprost

[Ref: Dutta's Obs. 9th/e, pg. 134, 260; Holland Brew's Obs.4th/e, pg. 122]

31. Heart disease with worst prognosis in pregnancy is?
   a. Aortic Stenosis   *(PGMEE 2013)*
   b. Pulmonary Hypertension
   c. Uncorrected tetralogy of Fallot
   d. Marfan's syndrome with normal aorta

[Ref: Dutta's Obs. 9th/e, pg. 261; William's Obs. 24th/e pg. 986, 987]

32. Which of the following is seen in pregnancy with heart disease, which is not seen in normal pregnancy? *(PGMEE 2013)*
   a. Distended neck veins   b. Exertional dyspnoea
   c. Pedal edema   d. Supine hypotension

[Ref: Holland Brew's Obs.4th/e, pg. 117; William's Obs. 24th/e pg. 975t]

23.	b
24.	a,b
25.	c
26.	d
27.	a
28.	c
29.	a
30.	a
31.	b
32.	a

Explanation

- Symptoms & signs in pregnancy d/t normal physiological (esp. cardiovascular) changes are:
  ○ Exercise intolerance
  ○ Easy fatiguability
  ○ Pedal edema
  ○ Exertional dyspnoea
  ○ Functional systolic murmurs
- Symptoms & signs suggestive of heart disease in pregnancy–
  ○ Chest pain
  ○ Progressive dyspnoea
  ○ Orthopnoea
  ○ Cough with / without haemoptysis
  ○ Syncopal attacks
  ○ Cyanosis
  ○ Clubbing
  ○ Distended neck veins
  ○ Persistent arrhythmia
  ○ Persistently split S2
  ○ Systolic murmur grade 3/6 or more
  ○ Diastolic murmur
  ○ Cardiomegaly
  ○ Pulmonary artery hypertension (gp II disorders secondary to pulmonary venous hypertension d/t left-sided atrial, ventricular or venous disorders are most common in pregnancy)

33. Peripartum cardiomyopathy can present at:
a. Within 3 months of pregnancy   *(PGMEE 2018)*
b. Within 5 months of pregnancy
c. Within 5 months of delivery
d. After 5 months of delivery

[Ref: Dutta's Obs. 8th / e, pg. 325; Holland Brew's Obs. 4th/e, pg. 425; Williams Obs. 24th / e, pg. 988-990]

Explanation

Peripartum Cardiomyopathy

- Diagnostic criteria –
  ○ Cardiac failure in the last month of pregnancy or within 5 months of delivery
  ○ No identifiable cause for cardiac failure
  ○ No recognizable heart disease prior to last month of pregnancy
  ○ Left ventricular systolic dysfunction as evidenced by echocardiography-
    – Ejection fraction < 45%
    – Left ventricular dilatation (end diastolic dimension > 2.7 cm/m2)
- Incidence – 1:3500 to 1:5000 deliveries
- Etiology –
  ○ Unknown
  ○ Potential causes – viral myocarditis, abnormal immune response to pregnancy, abnormal response to increased haemodynamic burden of pregnancy, oxidative stress during pregnancy, hormonal interactions, antiangiogenic factors, malnutrition, inflammation, and apoptosis
- Clinical features-
  ○ Young (20-35 years) multiparous patients

○ Symptoms – weakness, breathlessness (at night also), palpitation, cough
○ Signs – tachycardia, arrhythmia, signs of CHF
- Treatment – bed rest, digoxin, diuretics, salt restriction, oxygen, ACE inhibitors and β blockers (postpartum), anticoagulants
- Pregnancy poorly tolerated, vaginal delivery preferred

RH ISOIMMUNIZATION

34. Which is not affected in Rh isoimmunisation?
(DNB June' 2011)
a. Anti C   b. Anti D
c. Anti E   d. Anti-Lewis

[Ref: Dutta's Obs. 9th/e, pg. 311; William's Obs. 24th/e pg. 307, 308; Holland Brew's Obs. 4th/e, pg. 166]

35. Fetal cells can be detected in maternal blood using-
(PGMEE 09)
a. DCT   b. Bubble test
c. Kleihauer - Betke test   d. ICT

[Ref: Dutta's Obs. 9th/e, pg. 314; William's Obs. 24th/e pg. 313f; Holland Brew's Obs.4th/e, pg. 168]

36. Test to detect maternal sensitization- *(PGMEE 2012-13)*
a. Direct Coomb's test
b. Indirect Coomb's test
c. Both
d. None

[Ref: Dutta's Obs. 9th/e, pg. 315; William's Obs. 24th/e pg. 312; Holland Brew's Obs.4th/e, pg. 168]

37. Hydops fetalis due to-   *(PGMEE 2012-13)*
a. Rh mismatch   b. Hyperproteinemia
c. Placental hypoplesia   d. All of the above

[Ref: Dutta's Obs. 9th/e, pg. 313; William's Obs. 24th/e pg. 315; Holland Brew's Obs. 4th/e, pg. 168]

38. Non-immune hydrops fetalis is caused by:
(Recent Pattern June 2018)
a. ABO incompatibility   b. Rh incompatibility
c. Malaria   d. Parvovirus B$_{19}$

[Ref: Dutta's Obs. 9th/e, pg. 462; William's Obs. 24th/e pg.]

39. Non immune hydrops fetalis is seen In all except:
(Recent Pattern June 2018)
a. β - Thalassemia   b. Parvovirus-19
c. Rh-incompatibility   d. Chromosomal anomaly

[Ref: Dutta's Obs. 8th/e, pg, 571; Arias, 3rd/e, pg. 95-96; Williams Obstetrics, 23rd/e, pg. 626-627, 1216]

Explanation

- It is accumulation of extracellular fluid in tissues and serous cavities without evidence of circulating antibodies against RBC antigens.
  ○ It is due to conditions other than Rh isoimmunisation
  ○ It accounts for 2/3 cases of hydrops fetalis
- Non immune hydrops:
  ○ It can be caused by a number of conditions (there is an exhaustive list given on p 627 Williams 23/e, Just go through it).

33.	c
34.	d
35.	c
36.	b
37.	a
38.	d
39.	c

- Main causes
  - Cystic hygroma (associated with NIHF in 1st or early 2nd trimester)
  - Chromosomal abnormalities like Trisomies (21 1M/C), 13, 16, 15) Turner's syndrome, Triploidy etc.
  - Cardiac defects and arrhythmias.
  - Twin to Twin transfusion syndrome.
  - Hematological problems like alpha-thalassemia, 13 thalassemia G6PD deficiency etc.
  - Infections: Most common virus associated with NIHF is parvovirus B.

40. If 300 microgram anti D is given to mother, amount of fetal blood it will neutralise- *(PGMEE 2012-13)*
- a. 30 ml
- b. 40 ml
- c. 50 ml
- d. 60 ml

[Ref: Dutta's Obs. 9th/e, pg. 314;William's Obs. 24th/e pg. 311; Holland Brew's Obs. 4th/e, pg. 168]

41. Dose of Anti-D gamma globulin following first trimester abortion is- *(DNB pattern 2008)*
- a. 50 μg
- b. 100 μg
- c. 200 μg
- d. 300 μg

[Ref: Dutta's Obs. 9th/e, pg. 314; Holland Brew's Obs. 4th/e, pg.169]

Explanation

- To prevent active immunization of Rh-negative yet unimmunized mother, Rh anti-D immunoglobin (IgG) is administered intramuscularly to the mother following child birth or abortion. It should be administered within 72 hours or preferably earlier following delivery or abortion. It should be given provided the baby born is Rh-positive and the direct Coomb's test is negative.
- **DOSE:**
  - Anti D-gamma globulin is administered intramuscularly to the mother 300 microgram following delivery.
  - All Rh-negative unsensitised women should receive 50 microgram of Rh-immune globulin I.M. within 72 hours of induced abortion, spontaneous abortion, ectopic pregnancy or chorion villus biopsy in the first trimester.
  - Women with pregnancy beyond 12 weeks should have full dose of 300 microgram.

42. Regarding erythroblastosis fetalis all are true except- *(PGMEE 2012-13)*
- a. Rh haemolytic disease
- b. Severe anemia
- c. Hypoplasia of placental tissue
- d. Hypoproteinaemia

[Ref: Dutta's Obs. 9th/e, pg. 313; William's Obs. 24th/e pg. 315; Holland Brew's Obs.4th/e, pg. 168]

43. At 28 weeks gestation amniocentesis reveals ΔOD 450 in Liley's zone 3. Which of the following is the best line of management:- *(PGMEE 2015-16)*
- a. Plasmapheresis
- b. Immediate delivery
- c. Repeat amniocentesis after 1 weeks
- d. Intrauterine transfusion

[Ref: Dutta's Obs. 9th/e, pg. 316, 317; William's Obs. 24th/e pg. 310]

44. What should be done during delivery of Rh negative- *(PGMEE 2013-14)*
- a. IV Fluids
- b. IV Oxytocin
- c. Manual removal of placenta should be done gently
- d. Ergometrine to be withheld at delivery of anterior shoulder

[Ref: Dutta's Obs. 9th/e, pg. 317; Holland Brew's Obs.4th/e, pg. 173]

THYROID DISORDERS IN PREGNANCY

45. Thyroid gland is functional in the embryo by ____ weeks of pregnancy:- *(PGMEE 2016-17)*
- a. 8
- b. 9
- c. 10
- d. 11

[Ref: Dutta's Obs. 9th/e, pg. 39]

46. DOC for Hyperthyroidism in first trimester of pregnancy is :- *(PGMEE 2016-17)*
- a. Carbimazole
- b. Methimazole
- c. Lugol's iodine
- d. Propylthiouracil

[Ref: Dutta's Obs. 9th/e, pg. 269; William's Obs. 24th/e pg. 1149; Holland Brew's Obs.4th/e, pg. 139]

LIVER DISEASES IN PREGNANCY

47. LCHAD deficiency is associated with? *(DNB Dec' 2011)*
- a. Fatty liver of pregnancy
- b. HELLP syndrome
- c. Liver failure
- d. All

[Ref: William's Obs. 24th/e pg. 1086]

48. Most fatal hepatitis in pregnancy:- *(PGMEE 2016-17)*
- a. A
- b. C
- c. B
- d. E

[Ref: Dutta's Obs. 9th/e, pg. 272; William's Obs. 24th/e pg. 1092; Holland Brew's Obs.4th/e, pg. 156]

49. Fatty liver of pregnancy usually presents at:-
- a. In first trimester of pregnancy *(PGMEE 2018)*
- b. In 2nd trimester of pregnancy
- c. In 3rd trimester of pregnancy
- d. In peurperium

Ref: Holland Brew's Obs.4th/e, pg. 154; Williams Obs. 24th /e, pg. 1086-108

Explanation

Acute Fatty Liver of Pregnancy

- Rare condition (1 in 10,000) occurring in late 3rd trimester of pregnancy
- Also called acute fatty metamorphosis or acute yellow atrophy
- Commonest cause of acute hepatic failure during pregnancy with a high maternal and perinatal mortality
- Liver is small, soft, yellow and greasy with deposition of microvesicular fat droplets that 'crowds out' normal hepatocyte function
- May be due to deficiency of long chain 3-hydroxyacyl-Co A dehydrogenase (LCHAD) due to genetic mutations on chromosome 2 → accumulation of medium and long chain fatty acids
- Autosomal recessive inheritance, heterozygous mothers with homozygous fetuses

40.	a
41.	a
42.	c
43.	d
44.	d
45.	d
46.	d
47.	a
48.	d
49.	c

- **Clinical features:**
  - Non-specific: Upper abdominal pain, persistent nausea and vomiting, anorexia, progressive jaundice
  - Specific: Rapid deterioration, profound hypoglycemia, hepatic encephalopathy, hepatic failure, renal failure, severe coagulopathy and haemorrhages, coma and death
- **Differential diagnosis:**

Param-eters	Acute viral hepatitis	Acute fatty liver of pregnancy	Intra hepatic cholestasis of pregnancy	HELLP syndrome
S. transaminases	400-4000 IU/L	200-800 IU/L	< 200 IU/L	< 300 IU/L
S. bilirubin	5-20 mg/dl	4-10 mg/dl	1-5 mg/dl	2-4 mg/dl
Coagulopathy	–	+	–	+
Other specific features	Viral markers positive	Hypoglycemia, renal failure, coma	Pruritus, elevated bile acids	Hypertension, proteinuria, edema, thrombocytopenia, hyperuricemia

- Treatment – early diagnosis and aggressive supportive care
- Definitive treatment – delivery → arrests hepatic function deterioration

50. b
51. a
52. a
53. d
54. d
55. a
56. a
57. a
58. c

50. Which of the following statement is correct about acute fatty liver of pregnancy? *(PGMEE 2019)*

a. Occurs in 1 in 1000 pregnancy
b. Mostly seen in last trimester
c. Common if female fetus is present
d. May be associated with decreased uric acid

[Ref: William's Obs. 25th/e pg. 4, 28]

RENAL DISEASE IN PREGNANCY

51. Most common causative organism of acute pyelonephritis in pregnancy is? *(PGMEE 2014)*

a. E. coli
b. Klebsiella pneumonia
c. Enterobacter
d. Staphylococcus group

[Ref: Dutta's Obs. 9th/e, pg. 279]

EPILEPSY IN PREGNANCY

52. Which anti-epileptic is relatively safer during pregnancy? *(DNB Dec' 2009)*

a. Levetiracetam
b. Valproate
c. Phenytoin
d. Carbamazepine

[Ref: Dutta's Obs. 9th/e, pg. 273; William's Obs. 24th/e pg. 1190, 1191; Holland Brew's Obs.4th/e, pg. 101]

53. Which vitamin deficiency is most commonly seen in a pregnant woman who is on phenytoin therapy for epilepsy? *(PGMEE 2006)*

a. Vitamin B6
b. Vitamin B12
c. Vitamin A
d. Folic acid

[Ref: Dutta's Obs. 9th/e, pg. 273; William's Obs. 24th/e pg. 158; Holland Brew's Obs.4th/e, pg. 101]

THROMBOPHILIA IN PREGNANCY

54. Anti-phospholipid antibodies are not tested in? *(DNB Dec' 2010)*

a. Recurrent abortion
b. Mild Pre eclampsia
c. IUGR
d. Polyhydramnios

[Ref: Dutta's Obs. 9th/e, pg. 160, 322; William's Obs. 24th/e pg. 1175; Holland Brew's Obs.4th/e, pg. 584, 585]

COAGULOPATHY IN PREGNANCY

55. Consumptive coagulopathy is most commonly found in? *(DNB Dec' 2010)*

a. Abruption
b. IUCD
c. Retained products of conception
d. Dead fetus

[Ref: Dutta's Obs. 9th/e, pg. 584; Holland Brew's Obs. 4th/e, pg. 391; William's Obs. 24th/e pg. 797, 811]

56. Consumption coagulopathy is seen with- *(PGMEE 2012-13)*

a. Abruptio placentae
b. Placenta previa
c. Placenta accreta
d. Retained placenta

[Ref: Dutta's Obs. 9th/e, pg. 584; Holland Brew's Obs. 4th/e, pg. 391; William's Obs. 24th/e pg. 797, 811]

57. Pregnant women going for long journey & prolonged sitting is associated with danger of- *(PGMEE 2013-14)*

a. Thromboembolism
b. Seat belt compression
c. Preterm labor
d. Bleeding

[Ref: Dutta's Obs. 9th/e, pg. 412; Williams Obs. 23rd/e, pg. 1024, 1027]

MISCELLANEOUS

58. Antibodies in mother causing congenital heart block in fetus- *(PGMEE 2013-14)*

a. Anti-DNA
b. Anti-RNA
c. Anti-RO (SS-a)
d. Anti phospholipid

Ref: Internet

1. **Indicative of intra uterine infection is presence of:-**
   a. Ig M   b. Ig G   *(PGMEE 2016-17)*
   c. Ig A   d. Ig E

   [Ref: Dutta's Obs. 9th/e, pg. 38; Williams Obs. 24th/e,
   |pg. 1239]

TUBERCULOSIS

2. **Antitubercular drug contraindicated in pregnancy-**
   (PGMEE 2001, 2005)
   a. Streptomycin   b. Rifampicin
   c. INH   d. Ethambutol
   e. Pyrazinamide

   [Ref: Williams Obs. 24th/e, pg. 1021; Dutta's 9th/e, pg.275]

SYPHILIS

3. **Placental weight increases in which infection:**
   (Recent Pattern June 2018)
   a. Cytomegalovirus   b. Syphilis
   c. Rubella   d. Toxoplasmosis

   [Ref: Dutta Obs 7th/e p. 295]

   Explanation
   - Placentomegaly (thickness > 4cm) is an important ultrasound finding in pregnancy. It has been a/w chronic intrauterine infections, polyhydramnios, fetal hydrops, diabetes, partial mole and even fetal growth restriction as in placental mesenchymal dysplasia (PMD).
   - Hepatomegaly and placentomegaly are two MC manifestations of syphilis.

HEPATITIS

4. **Fulminant infection in pregnancy is due to:**
   (Recent Pattern June 2018)
   a. HEV   b. HDV
   c. HAV   d. HBV

   [Ref: Harrison's 19th/e pg. 2015]

   Explanation
   - In general, hepatitis E is a self-limiting viral infection followed by recovery. Prolonged viraemia or faecal shedding are unusual.
   - Fulminant hepatitis occurs more frequently in pregnancy and regularly induces a mortality rate of 20% among pregnant women in the 3rd trimester. Perinatal transmission is uncommon.
   - Fulminant hepatitis is uncommon with hepatitis-C and rare with hepatitis-A

5. **Vaccines contraindicated in pregnancy are all EXCEPT:**
   (DNB June' 2010)
   a. BCG   b. Yellow fever
   c. OPV   d. Hepatitis B

   [Ref: Dutta's Obs. 9th/e, pg, 272; Arias, 3rd/e, pg. 158, 543;
   Williams Obstetrics, 24th/e, pg. 208 & 1091]

PARVOVIRUS B 19

6. **Non immune hydrops fetalis is associated with?**
   (DNB June' 2010)
   a. Hepatitis B
   b. Parvovirus B19
   c. Tuberculosis
   d. Malaria

   [Ref: Dutta's Obs. 9th/e, pg, 462; Arias, 3rd/e, pg. 95-96;
   Williams Obstetrics, 24th/e, pg. 315, 317, 1245]

7. **Non immune hydrops fetalis is caused by all except-**
   a. Parvo virus B19   *(PGMEE 2007)*
   b. Chromosomal abnormalities
   c. Alpha thalassaemia
   d. ABO incompatibility

   [Ref: Dutta's Obs. 9th/e, pg, 462 Arias, 3rd/e, pg. 95-96;
   Williams Obstetrics, 24th/e, pg. 315, 316, 317, 1245]

HIV

8. **Least rates of HIV transmission is seen in?**
   (DNB Dec' 2010)
   a. Forceps delivery   b. Breast feeding
   c. Normal delivery   d. Cesarean section

   [Ref: Dutta's Obs. 9th/e, pg, 282; Williams Obstetrics, 24th/e,
   pg. 1282]

9. **Least teratogenic potential is of?**   *(PGMEE June' 2012)*
   a. CMV
   b. HIV
   c. Varicella
   d. Rubella

   [Ref: Dutta's Obs. 9th/e, pg, 282; Williams Obstetrics, 24th/e,
   pg. 1242, 1243]

10. **Maximum transmission of HIV occurs during-**
    (PGMEE 2012-13)
    a. Near term   b. Antepartum
    c. Labour   d. Breast feeding

    [Ref: Dutta's Obs. 9th/e, pg, 242; Williams Obstetrics, 24th/e,
    pg. 1278, 1279]

    Explanation
    - Transmission of HIV
      - Near term → 50%
      - Antepartum → 20–36%
      - Labour → 30%
      - Breast feeding → 30–40%

11. **If untreated, percentage of mother to child transmission of HIV during delivery without intervention in a non-breast fed child is-**   *(PGMEE 2013)*
    a. 40-50%   b. 10-15%
    c. 15-30%   d. 5%

    [Ref: Arias, 3rd/e, pg. 142-150, 155-156; Williams Obstetrics,
    24th/e, pg. 1278]

1.	a
2.	a
3.	b
4.	a
5.	d
6.	b
7.	d
8.	d
9.	b
10.	a
11.	c

12. **A pregnant woman has been detected with HIV in 1st trimester of pregnancy. Which of the following statements is correct according to NACO guidelines for ART for this women:- with HIV in early pregnancy, NACO guidelines suggest the use of:-** *(PGMEE 2018)*
   a. Started immediately and continued in whole pregnancy, puerperium and taken life long
   b. ART started after first trimester and continued lifetime
   c. ART started after 1st trimester, continued throughout pregnancy and stopped 6 weeks after delivery
   d. ART started immediately, continued throughout pregnancy and stopped 6 weeks after delivery

   Ref: Holland Brew's Obs.4th / e, pg.177

Explanation

NACO Guidelines

- For Prevention of Parent to Child Transmission (PPTCT) of HIV using Multidrug Anti-retroviral Regimen
- Updated in December 2013, effective from 1st January 2014
- Time for starting –
  ○ ART should be started immediately after detection
  ○ ART should be started irrespective of the following-
    – Gestational age
    – CD4 count
    – WHO clinical stage
- Eligible candidates for ART- all HIV positive pregnant and lactating women requiring ART for:
  ○ Their own sake
  ○ Prevention of mother to child transmission
- Duration of ART – should be continued lifelong

13. **Elective LSCS in a Patient with HIV is suggested in:**
   a. All patients *(Recent Pattern June 2018)*
   b. First pregnancy
   c. HIV viral copies load is >1000 copies/ml
   d. HIV viral copies load >100 copies/ml

Explanation

- Scheduled cesarean delivery at 38 weeks gestation to minimize perinatal transmission of HIV is recommended for women with HIV RNA levels >1,000 copies/mL or unknown HIV levels near the time of delivery, irrespective of administration of antepartum antiretroviral therapy (ART).

CMV

14. **Least commonly vertically transmitted organism of the following is?** *(DNB June' 2011)*
   a. Herpes simplex
   b. CMV
   c. Human papilloma virus
   d. Rubella

   [Ref: Dutta's Obs. 9th/e, pg, 280, 282; Arias 3rd/e, pg. 142-150; Williams Obstetrics, 24th/e, P. 1243, 1247, 1271, 1275]

12.	a
13.	c
14.	b
15.	a
16.	b
17.	c
18.	c

RUBELLA

15. **Maximum transmission of rubella occurs in?** *(PGMEE Nov.12 Pattern)*
   a. 1st trimester   b. 2nd trimester
   c. 3rd trimester   d. Labour

   [Ref: Dutta's Obs. 9th/e, pg, 280; Arias 3rd/e, pg. 142-150; Williams Obstetrics, 24th/e, P. 1243]

16. **An obstetrician sees a pregnant patient who was exposed to rubella virus in the eighteenth week of pregnancy. She does not remember getting a rubella vaccination. The best immediate course of action is to:** *(Recent Pattern June 2018)*
   a. Terminate the pregnancy
   b. Order a rubella antibody titer to determine immune status
   c. Reassure the patient because rubella is not a problem until after the thirtieth week
   d. Administer rubella immune globulin

Explanation

- The highest risk of fetal infection with rubella occurs during the first trimester, in the first month and in the first week of it.
- In seronegative patients, the risk of infection > 90%. However, before other measures (such as MTP/ termination of pregnancy) are considered, a rubella immune status must be performed.
- A rubella titer of 1:10 is protective.

VARICELLA

17. **6 year old son of a pregnant woman is suffering from chicken pox. Which of the following should be given to the pregnant woman-** *(PGMEE 2012-13)*
   a. Acyclovir
   b. Vaccination
   c. Only immunoglobulin
   d. Acyclovir + immunoglobulin

   [Ref: Dutta's Obs. 9th/e, pg, 281; Arias 3rd/e, pg. 142-150; Williams Obstetrics, 24th/e, P. 1241]

TOXOPLASMOSIS

18. **Vertical transmission of toxoplasmosis most commonly occurs in?** *(DNB June' 2011)*
   a. 1st trimester   b. 2nd trimester
   c. 3rd trimester   d. During delivery

   [Ref: Dutta's Obs. 9th/e, pg, 278; Arias 3rd/e, pg. 160-163; Williams Obstetrics, 24th/e, P. 1255]

Explanation

- Vertical transmission of toxoplasmosis
  ○ 1st trimester → 15%
  ○ 2nd trimester → 30%
  ○ 3rd trimester → 60%
  ○ During delivery → 0%

MALARIA

19. Malaria in pregnancy doesn't cause? *(PGMEE 2014)*
   a. HELLP syndrome   b. IUGR
   c. IUD   d. Preterm

   [Ref: Dutta's Obs. 9th/e, pg, 278b]

GYNECOLOGICAL COMPLICATIONS IN PREGNANCY

VAGINITIS

20. Most common vaginal infection in pregnancy is?
   (DNB June' 2011, PGMEE Aug. 12 Pattern)
   a. Gonorrhea
   b. Trichomoniasis
   c. Candidiasis
   d. Bacterial vaginosis

   [Ref: Dutta's Obs. 9th/e, pg, 287; Williams Obs., 24th/e, pg.1276]

FIBROID

21. Red degeneration of fibroid is seen in:
   (PGMEE 2013-14)
   a. Early pregnancy
   b. Mid pregnancy
   c. Multiparous women
   d. Nulliparous women

   [Ref: Dutta's Obs. 9th/e, pg, 289]

19. a
20. c
21. b

PHARMACOTHERAPEUTICS (DRUGS) IN OBSTETRICS

1. **All of the following are known side effects with the use of tocolytic therapy EXCEPT-** *(PGMEE 03)*
   a. Tachycardia
   b. Hypotension
   c. Hyperglycemia
   d. Fever

   [Ref: Dutta's Obs. 9th/e, pg. 472t]

2. **All of the following occur because of prostaglandin use except-** *(PGMEE 2012-13)*
   a. Excess water retention
   b. Flushes
   c. Increased motility of bowel
   d. Nausea

   [Ref: Dutta's Obs. 9th/e, pg. 465, 496t]

3. **DOC for cholera in pregnancy is-** *(PGMEE 2012-13)*
   a. Furazolidone
   b. Tetracycline
   c. Doxycycline
   d. Azithromycin

   [Ref: Internet]

4. **Tocolytics can be given in-** *(PGMEE 2012-13)*
   a. Placenta Praevia
   b. Placenta accreta
   c. Preterm labour
   d. Eclampsia

   [Ref: Dutta's Obs. 9th/e, pg. 471]

5. **Misoprostol is which prostaglandin analogue ?** *(PGMEE Aug 12 Pattern)*
   a. PGF2α
   b. PGE1
   c. PGE2
   d. PGI2

   [Ref: Dutta's Obs. 9th/e, pg. 469]

6. **Carboprost is:** *(Recent Pattern June 2018)*
   a. PGF2α
   b. PGE2
   c. PGI2
   d. None

Explanation

- Carboprost is a synthetic prostaglandin analogue of PGF2α with oxytocic properties. Carboprost induces contractions and can trigger abortion in early pregnancy. It also reduces postpartum bleeding.

7. **What is the dose of ulipristal acetate:** *(PGMEE 2019)*
   a. 300mg
   b. 30mg
   c. 300µg
   d. 30µg

   [Ref: Williams gynecology 3rd/e pg. 131]

8. **Mifepristone and misoprostol are effective upto?** *(PGMEE Nov 13 Pattern)*
   a. 49 days
   b. 70 days
   c. 90 days
   d. 120 days

   [Ref: Dutta's Obs. 9th/e, pg. 165]

9. **Decreased fetal heart sound is due to which drug-** *(PGMEE 2013-14)*
   a. Oxytocin
   b. Sodium bicarbonate
   c. IV fluids
   d. Iron

   [Ref: Dutta's Obs. 9th/e, pg. 465]

10. **Not a tocolytic-** *(PGMEE 2012-13)*
    a. Diazepam
    b. Magnesium sulphate
    c. Indomethacin
    d. Terbutaline

    [Ref: Dutta's Obs. 9th/e, pg. 472t]

11. **Regarding Atosiban all are true except:-**
    a. Inhibitor of the hormone oxytocin *(PGMEE 2016-17)*
    b. Used as tocolytic agent
    c. Given by intravenous route
    d. Given after delivery of shoulder of baby

    [Ref:Dutta's Obs. 9th/e, pg. 472t]

VACCINES IN PREGNANCY

12. **TDAP vaccine is given in between which weeks of pregnancy-** *(PGMEE 2012-13)*
    a. 10-16 weeks
    b. 17-22 weeks
    c. 22-26 weeks
    d. 27-30 weeks

13. **Which vaccine is contraindicated in pregnancy :** *(PGMEE Jan 2019)*
    a. Chicken pox
    b. Rabies
    c. Tetanus toxoid
    d. Hepatitis B

    [Ref: Williams obstetrics 25th/e pg. 10, 34]

TERATOGENS

14. **Which antibiotic can be safely used in pregnant women-** *(PGMEE 2012-13)*
    a. Tetracycline
    b. Erythromycin
    c. Isoniazid
    d. Chloremphenicol

    [Ref: Internet]

Explanation

- Tetracycline causes permanent staining & discolouration of baby's teeth.
- Chloramphenicol - category C drug, causes Gray syndrome in neonates.

15. **Which drug is not prescribed in pregnancy-** *(PGMEE 2013-14)*
    a. ACE inhibitors
    b. Hydralazine
    c. Acetaminophen
    d. Metronidazole

    [Ref: Dutta's Obs. 9th/e, pg. 471t]

16. **Not given in pregnancy-** *(PGMEE 2012-13)*
    a. Enalapril
    b. Labetalol
    c. Hydralazine
    d. Nifedipine

    [Ref: Dutta's Obs. 9th/e, pg. 471t]

17. **Fetus most radiosensitive at?** *(PGMEE Aug. 12 Pattern)*
    a. 8-15 weeks
    b. 10-15 weeks
    c. 15-20 weeks
    d. > 20 weeks

    [Ref: William's Obs. 24th/e pg. 932]

#	Ans
1.	d
2.	a
3.	d
4.	c
5.	b
6.	a
7.	b
8.	a
9.	a
10.	a
11.	d
12.	d
13.	a
14.	b,c
15.	a
16.	a
17.	a

FETAL SKULL

1. Longest diameter of fetal skull is?
(DNB June' 2009, 2011, PGMEE 2013)
a. Submentobregmatic   b. Mentovertical
c. Suboccipitofrontal   d. Occipitofrontal

[Ref: Dutta's Obs. 9th/e, pg. 78t; Holland Brew's Obs. 4th/e, pg. 56t]

2. Largest presenting diameter of brow presentation is?
(DNB June' 2010)
a. Submentobregmatic   b. Mentovertical
c. Submentovertical   d. Suboccipitofrontal

[Ref: Dutta's Obs. 9th/e, pg. 78t; Holland Brew's Obs. 4th/e, pg. 56t]

3. The smallest diameter of foetal head is:
(Recent Pattern June 2018)
a. Bitemporal   b. Biparietal
c. Occipitofrontal   d. Submentovertical

[Ref: Dutta's Obs. 8th/e, pg. 246; Holland Brew's Obs.4th/e, pg.241]

Explanation

The anteroposterior diameters of the head

Diameters	Measurement in cm (inches)	Attitude of the Head	Presentation
Suboccipito-bregmatic	9.5 cm (3 ¾")	Complete flexion	Vertex
Suboccipito-frontal	10 cm (4")	Incomplete flexion	Vertex
Occipitofrontal	11.5 cm (4 ½")	Marked deflexion	Vertex
Mento-vertical	14 cm (5 ½")	Partial extension	Brow
Submentovertical	11.5 cm (4 ½")	Incomplete extension	Face
Submentobregmatic	9.5 cm (3 ¾")	Complete extension	Face

The transverse diameters

Diameters of fetal skull	Measurement in cm (inches)
Biparietal	9.5 cm(3 ¾")
Super-subparietal	8.5 cm (3 ½")
Bitemporal	8 cm (3 ¼")
Bimastoid	7.5 cm (3")

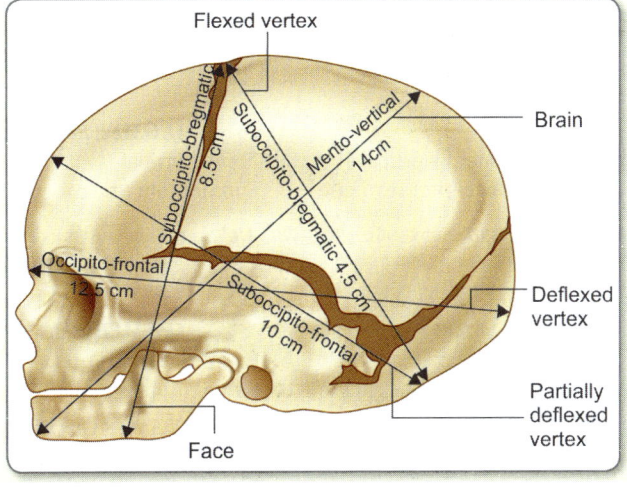

4. Markedly deflexed head of baby causes which diameter to engage-
(PGMEE 2012-13)
a. Occipitofrontal   b. Suboccipitofrontal
c. Mentovertical   d. Submentovertical

[Ref: Dutta's Obs. 9th/e, pg. 78t; Holland Brew's Obs. 4th/e, pg. 56t]

5. Mentovertical diameter of fetal skull is-
(PGMEE 2012-13)
a. 9.5 cm   b. 10 cm
c. 11.5 cm   d. 14 cm

[Ref:Dutta's Obs. 9th/e, pg. 78t; Holland Brew's Obs. 4th/e, pg. 56t]

6. Maximum diameter of fetal skull that passes through maternal pelvis-
(PGMEE 2013-14)
a. Suboccipitobregmatic
b. Biparietal
c. Suboccipitofrontal
d. Occipitofrontal

[Ref: Dutta's Obs. 9th/e, pg. 77, 78t; Holland Brew's Obs. 4th/e, pg. 56t]

7. The widest transverse diameter of the fetal skull is-
a. Biparietal diameter   *(PGMEE 2014)*
b. Bitemporal diameter
c. Suboccipitobregmatic diameter
d. Occipitofrontal diameter

[Ref: Dutta's Obs. 9th/e, pg. 77; Holland Brew's Obs. 4th/e, pg. 56t]

8. Which of the following is transverse diameter of fetal skull?
(PGMEE 2016-17)
a. Occipitofrontal   b. Suboccipitofrontal
c. Biparietal   d. Mentovertical

[Ref: Dutta's Obs. 9th/e, pg. 77; Holland Brew's Obs. 4th/e, pg. 56]

1.	**b**
2.	**b**
3.	**a**
4.	**a**
5.	**d**
6.	**d**
7.	**a**
8.	**c**

9. **Presenting diameter of full flexed head:** *(PGMEE 2019)*
   a. Suboccipito-bregmatic diameter
   b. Suboccipito-frontal diameter
   c. Occipito-frontal diameter
   d. Occipito-posterior position

   [Ref: DC Dutta Obs. 7th/e, pg. 85]

10. **In extended head, engaging diameter is:-**
    (PGMEE 2016-17)
    a. Submentovertical   b. Mentovertical
    c. Suboccipitobregmatic d. Submentobregmatic

    [Ref: Dutta's Obs. 9th/e, pg. 78t; Holland Brew's Obs. 4th/e, pg. 56t]

11. **The dimension of fetal skull which is not 9.5 cm:-**
    (PGMEE 2016-17)
    a. Biparietal   b. Occipitofrontal
    c. Suboccipitobregmatic d. Submentobregmatic

    [Ref: Dutta's Obs. 9th/e, pg. 77, 78t; Holland Brew's Obs. 4th/e, pg. 56t]

MATERNAL PELVIS

12. **Least diameter of gynecoid pelvis is-** *(PGMEE 2012-13)*
    a. Transverse   b. Oblique
    c. Diagonal conjugate   d. Obstetric conjugate

    [Ref: Dutta's Obs. 9th/e, pg. 80, 81; Holland Brew's Obs. 4th/e, pg. 10, 11t]

13. **Which of the following is most commonly clinically used-** *(PGMEE 2012-13)*
    a. Diagonal conjugate
    b. Ant post diameter of inlet
    c. Transverse diameter of outlet
    d. Oblique diameter of pelvis

    [Ref: Dutta's Obs. 9th/e, pg. 81; Holland Brew's Obs.4th/e, pg. 10]

14. **Smallest diameter of pelvis is?** *(DNB Dec' 2009)*
    a. Interspinous diameter
    b. Intertuberous diameter
    c. Diagonal conjugate
    d. True conjugate

    [Ref: Dutta's Obs. 9th/e, pg. 80-83; Holland Brew's Obs.4th/e, pg. 10-11]

15. **Interspinous diameter-** *(PGMEE 2012-13)*
    a. 10.5 cm   b. 11 cm
    c. 11.5 cm   d. 12 cm

    [Ref: Dutta's Obs. 9th/e, pg. 82; Holland Brew's Obs.4th/e, pg. 10-11]

CONTRACTED PELVIS

16. **Triradiate pelvis is seen in-** *(PGMEE 2097)*
    a. Rickets   b. Chondrodystrophy
    c. Osteomalacia   d. Hyperparathyroidism

    [Ref: Dutta's Obs. 9th/e, pg. 326]

17. **Dystocia dystrophia syndrome is seen in-**
    (PGMEE 2006)
    a. Android pelvis   b. Platypelloid pelvis
    c. Anthropoid   d. Gynaecoid pelvis

    [Ref: Dutta's Obs. 9th/e, pg. 327]

18. **Deep transverse arrest is most commonly seen in?**
    (DNB June' 2011, PGMEE 2014)
    a. Anthropoid pelvis   b. Android pelvis
    c. Gynaecoid pelvis   d. Platypelloid pelvis

    [Ref: Dutta's Obs. 9th/e, pg. 325t, 327; Holland Brew's Obs. 4th/e, pg. 12, 13t]

Explanation

- Deep Transverse Arrest (DTA) – head is arrested deep into the pelvis with sagittal suture in transverse bispinous diameter of the pelvis for > 2 hrs inspite of good uterine contractions, fully dilated cervix and ruptured membranes.
- In android pelvis –
  - The cavity is deep & narrow with convergent side walls.
  - Oblique occipito-posterior or occipito-lateral positions are common.
  - Anterior rotation is difficult → chances of deep transverse arrest.
  - Nowadays intervention is done earlier, rather than waiting for full 2 hrs, to avoid feto-maternal complications and to lessen morbidity and mortality.
  - Caesarean section is the preferred mode of intervention in current obs. Practice rather than difficult instrumental vaginal delivery.

19. **Antero-posteriorly oval pelvic inlet is seen in-**
    (PGMEE 2012-13)
    a. Android pelvis   b. Platypelloid pelvis
    c. Anthropoid pelvis   d. Gynaecoid pelvis

    [Ref: Dutta's Obs. 9th/e, pg. 325t; Holland Brew's Obs. 4th/e, pg. 12, 13t]

20. **Most suitable type of pelvis in female-** *(PGMEE 2012-13)*
    a. Gynaecoid   b. Android
    c. Anthropoid   d. Platypelloid

    [Ref: Dutta's Obs. 9th/e, pg. 325t; Holland Brew's Obs. 4th/e, pg. 12, 13t]

9.	a
10.	d
11.	b
12.	d
13.	a
14.	a
15.	a
16.	c
17.	a
18.	b
19.	c
20.	a

NORMAL LABOR

PARTOGRAPH

1. Which is true about normal partography?
(PGMEE June 2012)
a. Latent phase is till 5 cm cervical dilation
b. First stage is till the full cervical dilatation
c. Used mainly for maternal BP monitoring
d. Rate of dilatation in latent phase is 1 cm/hr

[Ref: Dutta's Obs. 9th/e, pg. 491-493]

2. What is the purpose of partogram? (PGMEE June' 2012)
a. To monitor progress of labor
b. To monitor induction of labor
c. To assess the female pelvis
d. To find CPD

[Ref: Dutta's Obs. 9th/e, pg. 493]

3. Partogram is not used to monitor- **(PGMEE 2012-13)**
a. Cervical dilatation
b. Uterine contractions
c. Descent of head
d. Fetal lung maturity

[Ref: Dutta's Obs. 9th/e, pg. 493]

4. W.H.O. modified partogram charting starts at cervical dilatation of? **(PGMEE Aug. 12 Pattern)**
a. 2 cm
b. 3 cm
c. 4 cm
d. 5 cm

[Ref: Dutta's Obs. 9th/e, pg. 491; Holland Brew's Obs.4th/e, pg. 278]

5. Mrs. S (G2 L1) presented to the hospital in labor pains. On examination she had 3 uterine contractions of 20 seconds in 10 minutes, Cervical dilation 6 cm and HR 145 bpm. What is the stage of labor? **(Neet 2017)**
a. Stage I
b. Stage II
c. Stage III
d. Stage IV

[Ref: Dutta's Obs. 8th / e, pg. 138; Holland Brew's Obs.4th / e, pg. 270-271; Williams Obs. 24th / e, pg. 412-417]

Explanation

- Uterine contractions which bring about cervical effacement and dilatation. .

Stages of Labour: Diagnostic criteria

Stage	Characteristics
1	■ From 0 cm to 10 cm dilatation. ■ Divided into latent phase and active phase. *(A) Latent phase:* The point at which mother perceives regular contractions. Prolonged latent phase is >20 hours in primi and > 14 hours in multigravida

Stage	Characteristics
	(B) Active phase: Cervical dilatation of 3 to 5 cm or more in the presence of uterine contractions. Defined as slow if <1.2 cm per hour dilatation or <1 cm descent of head in primigravida and <1.5 cm dilatation per hour or <2 cm descent per hour in multigravida.
2	Complete cervical dilatation with active expulsive efforts by the mother
3	Delivery of placenta and membranes
4	"The Golden hour" One hour after delivery of baby. The mother should be monitored for signs of post partum hemorrhage.

MECHANISM OF LABOR AND LABOR EVENTS

6. The cardinal movements during normal labor occur in following order? **(PGMEE June' 2012)**
a. Engagement, internal rotation, delivery of head, restitution, external rotation
b. Engagement, internal rotation, restitution, delivery of head, external rotation
c. Engagement, external rotation, delivery of head, internal rotation, restitution
d. Engagement, delivery of head, internal rotation, restitution, external rotation

[Ref: Dutta's Obs. 9th/e, pg. 121;Holland Brew's Obs. 4th/e, pg. 273, 276f]

7. Which of the following is a sure sign of labor?
a. Bag of waters **(PGMEE June' 2012)**
b. Cervical effacement
c. Show
d. Progressive dilatation of cervix

[Ref: Dutta's Obs. 9th/e, pg. 113]

1.	b
2.	a
3.	d
4.	c
5.	a
6.	a
7.	d

Explanation

Bag of waters:
- Bag of waters: Bag of unsupported fetal membranes (detached from lower segment due to its stretching) containing amniotic fluid. Uterine contraction → rise of intra-amniotic pressure → bag becomes tense & convex, uterine contraction passes off → bulging disappears completely, almost a certain sign of onset of labour

Cervical effacement
- Cervical effacement: taking up of cervix, muscle fibers of cervix pulled upward & merge with the fibers of lower uterine segment

Show

- Show: expulsion of cervical mucus plug mixed with blood

Progressive dilatation of cervix:

- Progressive dilatation of cervix: Actual factors responsible are- uterine contraction & retraction, bag of membranes, fetal axis pressure, vis-a-tergo.

8. Cervical effacement suggestive of onset of labor is?
(PGMEE June' 2012, PGMEE Aug. 12 Pattern)

a. 15 mm
b. 25 mm
c. 30 mm
d. 20 mm

[Ref: Dutta's Obs. 9th/e, pg. 114; William's Obs. 24th/e pg. 414, 415]

9. Percentage of women delivering on their EDD is -

a. 25% *(PGMEE 2012-13)*
b. 50%
c. 4%
d. 15%

[Ref: Dutta's Obs. 9th/e, pg. 108]

10. Pain in early labor is limited to dermatomes-
(PGMEE 2013-14)

a. T10-L1   b. S1-S3
c. L4-L5   d. L2-L3

[Ref: Dutta's Obs. 9th/e, pg. 479]

11. Active management of 3rd stage of labor includes all except:- *(PGMEE 2016-17)*

a. Early cord clamping
b. Uterine massage
c. Utererotonic drugs after delivery of anterior shoulder
d. Assisted removal of placenta

[Ref: Dutta's Obs. 9th/e, pg. 134; Holland Brew's Obs.4th/e, pg. 2711]

INDUCTION OF LABOR

12. All of the following drugs are effective for cervical ripening during pregnancy except - *(PGMEE 2004)*

a. Prostaglandins E2
b. Oxytocin
c. Progesterone
d. Misoprostol

[Ref: Dutta's Obs. 9th/e, pg. 56, 485; Holland Brew's Obs.4th/e, pg. 367-369]

Explanation

- Although oxytocin is less effective in causing cervical ripening, it is effective for inducing / augmenting labour in already ripened cervix.

13. All are true about oxytocin except - *(PGMEE 2013)*

a. Originates in the supraoptic nucleus of the hypothalamus
b. Is essential for the onset of labor
c. Stimulates the growth of uterine musculature
d. Not a good cervical ripening agent

[Ref: Dutta's Obs. 9th/e, pg. 464; Holland Brew's Obs.4th/e, pg. 369]

ASSISTED LABOR

VENTOUSE

14. In Vacuum assisted delivery cup is attached?

a. 2 cm anterior to anterior fontanelle *(PGMEE 2014)*
b. 2 cm anterior to posterior fontanelle
c. 3 cm anterior to anterior fontanelle
d. 3 cm anterior to posterior fontanelle

[Ref: Dutta's Obs. 9th/e, pg. 540; Holland Brew's Obs. 4th/e, pg. 496]

15. Vacuum delivery produces- *(PGMEE 2012-13)*

a. Chingon
b. Cephalhaematoma
c. Both
d. None

[Ref: Dutta's Obs. 9th/e, pg. 540 541]

16. Vacuum cup is placed? *(PGMEE Nov. 12 Pattern)*

a. Posterior to posterior fontanelle
b. Posterior to anterior fontanelle
c. Anterior to posterior fontanelle
d. Anterior to anterior fontanelle

[Ref: Dutta's Obs. 9th/e, pg. 540; Holland Brew's Obs. 4th/e, pg. 496]

17. All of the following complications are more common in ventouse assisted delivery than forceps except-

a. Subgaleal hemorrhage *(NEET Pattern 2013)*
b. Cephalhaematoma
c. Intracranial hemorrhage
d. Transient lateral rectus palsy

[Ref: Dutta's Obs. 9th/e, pg. 538, 541; Holland Brew's Obs. 4th/e, pg. 495]

18. Use of ventouse is preferred over forceps in the delivery of-

a. Occipito-posterior position *(PGMEE 2013)*
b. After coming head in breech
c. Face presentation
d. Fetal distress

[Ref: Dutta's Obs. 9th/e, pg. 348; Holland Brew's Obs.4th/e, pg. 296]

19. Contraindication for vacuum delivery:-

a. Fetal distress *(PGMEE 2016-17)*
b. Prolonged labor
c. Premature baby
d. Eclampsia

[Ref: Dutta's Obs. 9th/e, pg. 539; Holland Brew's Obs. 4th/e, pg. 361, 494]

FORCEPS

20. Nerve block given in forceps delivery- *(PGMEE 2013-14)*

a. Pudendal
b. Ilio inguinal
c. Genitofemoral
d. Posterior femoral

[Ref: Dutta's Obs. 9th/e, pg. 533]

8.	b
9.	c
10.	a
11.	a
12.	c
13.	c
14.	d
15.	c
16.	c
17.	d
18.	a
19.	c
20.	a

FETAL MALPOSITIONS AND MALPRESENTATIONS

OCCIPITOPOSTERIOR POSITION

21. Assisted head delivery is done in- *(PGMEE 2013-14)*
a. Brow presentation
b. Face presentation
c. Persistent occipito posterior position
d. Twin presentation

[Ref: Dutta's Obs. 9th/e, pg. 349; Holland Brew's Obs. 4th/e, pg. 295, 296]

Explanation

Mode of delivery depends on station of head:
- If at or above ischial spines - caesaren section
- If below ischial spines - face to pubis delivery (forceps application may be required, liberal mediolateral episiotomy given)

22. Which of the following is the most common occipito posterior position:- *(PGMEE 2015-16)*
a. Left occipitoposterior
b. Direct occipitoposterior
c. Indirect occipitoposterior
d. Right occipitoposterior

[Ref: Dutta's Obs. 9th/e, pg. 343; Holland Brew's Obs. 4th/e, pg. 291]

BREECH

23. Most common breech presentation is? *(DNB June' 2011)*
a. Right Sacroanterior
b. Left sacroanterior
c. Left sacroposterior
d. Right sacroposterior

[Ref: Dutta's Obs. 9th/e, pg. 352; Holland Brew's Obs. 4th/e, pg. 304]

24. Least chances of cord prolapse are seen in? *(DNB June' 2011, PGMEE 2013)*
a. Frank breech   b. Knee presentation
c. Footling   d. Complete breech

[Ref: Dutta's Obs. 9th/e, pg. 355; Holland Brew's Obs. 4th/e, pg. 303]

25. Percentage of breech presentation at term is? *(PGMEE Aug 13 Pattern, PGMEE 2011, 2016-17)*
a. 1   b. 3
c. 7   d. 10

[Ref: Dutta's Obs. 9th/e, pg. 351; Holland Brew's Obs.4th/e, pg. 303]

26. Not a method for delivery of after-coming head of breech-
a. Forceps method *(PGMEE 2012-13)*
b. Burns and Marshall method
c. Malar flexion and shoulder traction
d. Half hand method

[Ref: Dutta's Obs. 9th/e, pg. 360, 361; Holland Brew's Obs.4th/e, pg. 307-308]

27. Most common cause of breech presentation is? *(PGMEE Aug 13 Pattern, PGMEE 2015-16)*
a. Prematurity
b. Contracted pelvis
c. Oligohydramnios
d. Placenta praevia

[Ref: Dutta's Obs. 9th/e, pg. 352; Holland Brew's Obs.4th/e, pg. 304]

28. Head of baby is delivered in breech presentation by which maneuver: *(PGMEE 2013-14)*
a. Lovset's maneuver
b. Pinard's maneuver
c. Mc Robert's maneuver
d. Burns Marshall method

[Ref: Dutta's Obs. 9th/e, pg. 360; Holland Brew's Obs.4th/e, pg. 307]

29. Image showing Mauriceau procedure. The procedure shown is being done for: *(PGMEE 2016-17)*

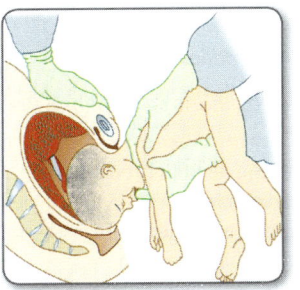

a. Face to pubes delivery
b. Second baby in twins
c. Aftercoming head of breech
d. Impacted shoulder

[Ref: Dutta's Obs. 9th/e, pg. 361; Holland Brew's Obs. 4th/e, pg. 308f]

30. A 30 year old female G2P1, presenting with a 28 weeks pregnancy. USG scan shows placenta lying partially over the os. The most common complication associated with this pregnancy can be:- *(PGMEE 2016-17)*
a. Vasa praevia   b. Placenta accreta
c. Hydramnios   d. Breech presentation

[Ref: Dutta's Obs. 9th/e, pg. 230, 352; Holland Brew's Obs. 4th/e, pg. 304]

31. External cephalic version is done after- *(PGMEE 2012-13)*
a. 34 weeks   b. 36 weeks
c. 38 weeks   d. 40 weeks

[Ref: Dutta's Obs. 9th/e, pg. 356]

32. While carrying out external cephalic version, persistent foetal bradycardia occurs, how will you proceed:-
a. Emergency LSCS *(PGMEE 2016-17)*
b. Convert to IPV
c. Revert to original position
d. Abandon the procedure

[Ref: Dutta's Obs. 9th/e, pg. 542; Holland Brew's Obs. 4th/e, pg. 482; William's Obs. 24th/e pg. 570]

21.	c
22.	d
23.	b
24.	a
25.	b
26.	d
27.	a
28.	d
29.	c
30.	d
31.	b
32.	c

33. Primigravida presents at 36 weeks of gestation with complaint of preterm premature rupture of membranes or leaking per vaginum and the following presentation. Management to be followed is? *(PGMEE Nov 13 Pattern)*

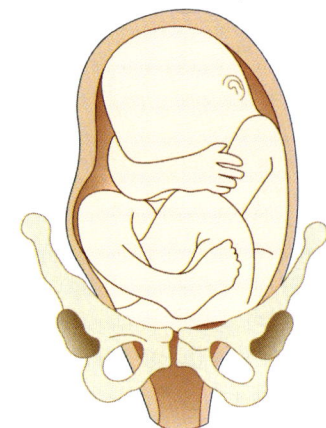

a. ECV
b. LSCS
c. Induction of labor
d. IPV (Internal podalic version)

[Ref: Dutta's Obs. 9th/e, pg. ; Holland Brew's Obs. 4th/e, pg.]

34. Prague manuever is used for- *(PGMEE 2012-13)*
a. After coming head in breech
b. Deep transverse assest
c. Extraction of extended arms
d. External cephalic version

[Ref: Dutta's Obs. 9th/e, pg. 363; William's Obs. 24th/e pg. 564, 566f]

35. Burns Marshall method is- *(PGMEE 2013-14)*
a. Method of delivering after coming head in breech
b. Head rotation is deflexed head
c. Breech extraction
d. Rotating head in D.T.A.

[Ref: Dutta's Obs. 9th/e, pg. 360; Holland Brew's Obs.4th/e, pg. 307]

TRANSVERSE LIE

36. A gravida 2 with 1 normal live birth has presented with transverse lie at 37 weeks. What should be the next step of the management? *(PGMEE June' 2012)*
a. External cephalic version
b. Wait and Watch
c. Cesarean section
d. Internal cephalic version

[Ref: Dutta's Obs. 9th/e, pg. 542; Holland Brew's Obs.4th/e, pg. 482]

37. Cord prolapse is most commonly associated with-
a. Transverse lie *(PGMEE 2096)*
b. Breech
c. Contracted pelvis
d. Prematunity

[Ref: Dutta's Obs. 9th/e, pg. 373; Holland Brew's Obs.4th/e, pg. 313]

38. Management of neglected shoulder presentation is: *(PGMEE 2012-13)*
a. Vaginal delivery   b. Caesarean section
c. External version   d. Internal version

[Ref: Dutta's Obs. 9th/e, pg. 372; Holland Brew's Obs.4th/e, pg. 313]

39. Rarest presentation is- *(PGMEE 2012-13)*
a. Cephalic   b. Breech
c. Shoulder   d. Vertex

[Ref: Dutta's Obs. 9th/e, pg. 69]

40. Presenting part in transverse lie- *(PGMEE 2012-13)*
a. Shoulder   b. Face
c. Vertex   d. Brow

[Ref: Dutta's Obs. 9th/e, pg. 69, 368; Holland Brew's Obs. 4th/e, pg. 312f]

41. During management of shoulder dystocia baby is delivered by:-
a. External cephalic version   *(PGMEE 2018)*
b. Reflexly flex hip and bend thighs over mother's abdomen
c. Traction over baby's head
d. Supra pubic pressure

Ref: Dutta's Obs. 8th / e, pg.469-470; Williams Obs. 24th/e, pg.481-485

Explanation

Shoulder dystocia

- Difficulty in delivery of fetal shoulder by gentle traction after delivery of fetal head.
- Due to impaction of anterior shoulder against pubic symphysis or posterior shoulder (rarely) against sacral promontory respectively
- Incidence – 0.2% to 1%
- Risk of recurrence – 13-25%
- Management – shoulder dystocia drill-
  - Call for help – assistant, anaesthesiologist, paediatrician
  - Drainage of bladder (if distended)
  - Generous episiotomy
  - Traction posteriorly by grasping fetal head and neck
  - Supra pubic pressure (requires only 1 assistant)
  - McRoberts maneuver (requires 2 assistants, **hyperflexion of maternal thighs over her abdomen,** increases AP diameter of the pelvis, successful in ≈ 90% of cases)
- When above techniques fail, following may be attempted:
  - Wood's corkscrew maneuver (requires general anaesthesia)
  - Extraction of the posterior arm (requires general anaesthesia)
  - Gaskin's maneuver – "All Fours" position (may be attempted in a mobile thin patient in low resource setting)
- Rarely performed techniques are:
  - Cleidotomy (deliberate fracture of clavicle – unilateral or bilateral)
  - Zavanelli's maneuver (reposition of fetal head into pelvis → cesarean section)
  - Symphysiotomy

33.	b
34.	a
35.	a
36.	a
37.	a
38.	b
39.	c
40.	a
41.	b

42. First maneuver to be done in case of shoulder dystocia is? *(PGMEE Aug 13 Pattern)*
- a. Mc Roberts
- b. Wood's corkscrew
- c. Lovset
- d. Zavanelli

[Ref: Dutta's Obs. 9th/e, pg. 381; William's Obs. 24th/e pg. 542f]

FACE PRESENTATION

43. Most unfavourable presentation for vaginal delivery is- *(PGMEE 1995)*
- a. Mento posterior
- b. Mento anterior
- c. Occipito posterior
- d. Deep transverse arrest

[Ref: Dutta's Obs. 9th/e, pg. 365; Holland Brew's Obs. 4th/e, pg. 301f]

BROW PRESENTATION

44. Presentation when the engaging diameter is Mentovertical is? *(PGMEE Aug. 12 Pattern)*
- a. Brow
- b. Breech
- c. Vertex
- d. Face

[Ref: Dutta's Obs. 9th/e, pg. 78t, 367; Holland Brew's Obs. 4th/e, pg. 302f]

COMPOUND PRESENTATION

45. The commonest cause for cephalic presentation with hand alongside the head is-
- a. Multiple Pregnancy
- b. Prematurity
- c. Contracted pelvis
- d. Polyhydramnios

[Ref:Dutta's Obs. 9th/e, pg. 372; Holland Brew's Obs. 4th/e, pg. 314]

LSCS OR C - SECTION

46. Advantage of LSCS as compared to classical C- section are all except: *(DNB June' 2009)*
- a. Lateral extension
- b. Less blood loss
- c. Less chance of gutter formation
- d. Minimal wound hematoma

[Ref: Dutta's Obs. 9th/e, pg. 552t]

47. Incidence of rupture in classical c-section is? *(DNB June' 2009)*
- a. 0.5-1.5%
- b. 2-5%
- c. 4-9%
- d. >10%

[Ref: Dutta's Obs. 9th/e, pg. 552t]

48. Classical caesarean section is done in? *(DNB Dec' 2010, PGMEE 2012-13)*
- a. Carcinoma cervix
- b. Placenta previa
- c. Previous cesarean
- d. Failed trial of labor

[Ref: Dutta's Obs. 9th/e, pg. 547]

49. Which is the commonest indication of classical cesarean section? *(PGMEE June' 2012)*
- a. Transverse lie
- b. Cord prolapse
- c. Placenta praevia
- d. Dense adhesion in lower uterine segment

[Ref:Dutta's Obs. 9th/e, pg. 547]

50. Absolute indication of Cesarean Section is? *(PGMEE Aug. 12 Pattern)*
- a. Placenta Previa
- b. Breech presentation
- c. Gross CPD
- d. Previous Cesarean section

[Ref: Dutta's Obs. 9th/e, pg. 546t]

51. Indication of caesarean section after previous caesarean section is? *(PGMEE Aug. 12 Pattern)*
- a. Hypertension
- b. Multigravida
- c. CPD
- d. Type 1 placenta previa

[Ref: Dutta's Obs. 9th/e, pg. 546t]

52. Caesarean section is recommended for- *(PGMEE 2012-13)*
- a. Rubella infected mother
- b. HSV infected mother
- c. CMV infected mother
- d. Measles infected mother

[Ref: William's Obs. 24th/e pg. 1274]

53. Definitive indication of LSCS- *(PGMEE 2012-13)*
- a. Mento anterior
- b. Persistent mento posterior
- c. Occipito posterior
- d. Vertex

[Ref: Dutta's Obs. 9th/e, pg. 365]

54. Indication of classical caesarean section- *(PGMEE 2012-13)*
- a. Cervical cancer
- b. Contracted pelvis
- c. Non re-assuring FHR
- d. None

[Ref: Dutta's Obs. 9th/e, pg. 547]

55. Chances of uterine rupture are least in- *(PGMEE 2013-14)*
- a. LSCS
- b. Classical
- c. Inverted
- d. Low vertical

[Ref: Dutta's Obs. 9th/e, pg. 308t]

56. In classical section more chances of rupture of uterus is in- *(PGMEE 2013-14)*
- a. Upper uterine segment
- b. Lower uterine segment
- c. Utero cervical junction
- d. Posterior uterine segment

[Ref: Dutta's Obs. 9th/e, pg. 308t]

57. Incomplete uterine rupture is defined as? *(PGMEE 2014)*
- a. Disruption of part of scar
- b. Disruption of entire length of scar
- c. Disruption of scar including peritoneum
- d. Disruption of scar with peritoneum intact

[Ref: Dutta's Obs. 9th/e, pg. 402]

58. What is the risk of scar rupture in LSCS? *(PGMEE Aug 13 Pattern, PGMEE 2015-16)*
- a. 1-2%
- b. 2-5%
- c. 4-9%
- d. >10%

[Ref: Dutta's Obs. 9th/e, pg. 308t]

PRECIPITATE LABOR

59. Precipitate labor is said to be when first and second stage together last for less than? *(PGMEE Nov. 13 Pattern)*
- a. 2 hours
- b. 3 hours
- c. 4 hours
- d. 6 hours

[Ref: Dutta's Obs. 9th/e, pg. 339]

42.	a
43.	a
44.	a
45.	b
46.	a
47.	c
48.	a
49.	d
50.	c
51.	c
52.	b
53.	b
54.	a
55.	a
56.	a
57.	d
58.	a
59.	b

ABNORMAL UTERINE ACTION

60. Bandl's ring is caused by- *(PGMEE 94)*
a. Uterine inertia
b. Cephalopelvic disproportion
c. Malepresentation
d. None

[Ref: Dutta's Obs. 9th/e, pg. 339, 379]

61. A lady presents at 37 weeks of gestation with uterine contraction and pain suggestive of labor for 20 hours. On examination cervix is persistently 1 cm dilated and uneffaced. What should be the next line of treatment?
a. Sedation and wait *(PGMEE 2011)*
b. Caesarean section
c. Augmentation with Oxytocin & Amniotomy
d. Induction with rupture of membranes

[Ref:Dutta's Obs. 9th/e, pg. 378]

Explanation

- This case scenario is suggestive of "Prolongation disorder", a type of dystocia or difficult labour.
- This type of abnormal labour pattern is d/t prolonged latent phase

	Primigravida	Multipara
Mean duration of latent phase	8 hrs	4 hrs
Prolonged latent phase	> 20 hrs	> 14 hrs

- Causes –
  ○ Cephalopelpic disproportion
  ○ Malpositions & malpresentations
  ○ Unfavourable Bishop's score
  ○ Premature rupture of membranes
  ○ Early onset of regional analgesia
- Management-
  ○ Expectant (rest & analgesia) – preferred treatment if fetal & maternal conditions reassuring
  ○ Augmentation with oxytocin to expedite delivery SOS
  ○ Caesarean section for urgent problems (prolonged latent phase per se is not an indication for caesarean section)

OBSTRUCTED LABOR

62. Most common cause of obstructed labor in India *(PGMEE Aug. 12 Pattern)*
a. Android pelvis
b. Anthropoid pelvis
c. Platypelloid pelvis
d. Gynecoid pelvis

[Ref: Dutta's Obs. 9th/e, pg. 325t. 327; Holland Brew's Obs. 4th/e, pg. 12]

63. Uterine rupture is most common in- *(PGMEE 2013-14)*
a. Ant lower segment scar
b. Classical C.S.
c. Placenta previa
d. Normal labor

[Ref: Dutta's Obs. 9th/e, pg. 308t]

64. In obstructed labor most important parameter is-
a. Diameter of pelvic inlet *(PGMEE 2013-14)*
b. Diameter of pelvic outlet
c. Biparietal diameter
d. Bitemporal diameter

[Ref: Dutta's Obs. 9th/e, pg. 327; Holland Brew's Obs. 4th/e, pg. 12, 13t]

COMPLICATION OF 3rd STAGE OF LABOR

65. Amount of blood passing through placenta on delayed cord clamping- *(PGMEE 2012-13)*
a. 50-100 ml   b. 100-200 ml
c. 120-150 ml   d. 150-180 ml

[Ref: Dutta's Obs. 9th/e, pg. 131]

66. Prophylactic methergine given for- *(PGMEE 2012-13)*
a. Induction of labor
b. Induction of abortion
c. To stop excess bleeding from uterus
d. All of the above

[Ref: Dutta's Obs. 9th/e, pg. 134, 467]

PPH (POSTPARTUM HEMORRHAGE)

67. Commonest cause of postpartum hemorrhage in multipara is- *(PGMEE 2012-13)*
a. Fibroid
b. Retained placenta
c. Uterine atony
d. Uterine perforation

[Ref: Dutta's Obs. 9th/e, pg. 385]

68. Active management of 3rd stage of labor is helpful in prevention of- *(PGMEE 2012-13)*
a. Atonic PPH
b. Secondary PPH
c. Uterine inertia
d. APH

[Ref: Dutta's Obs. 9th/e, pg. 134, 387]

69. Ergometrine is contraindicated in- *(PGMEE 2012-13)*
a. Third stage of labor with heart disease
b. Third stage uterine bleeding
c. Both
d. None

[Ref: Dutta's Obs. 9th/e, pg. 134, 468b]

70. Role of ergometrine to stop post partum hemorrhage is due to- *(PGMEE 2012-13)*
a. Increased uterine muscle tone
b. Vasoconstriction
c. Increased platelet aggregation
d. Increased coagulation

[Ref: Dutta's Obs. 9th/e, pg. 467]

71. Commonest cause of PPH is- *(PGMEE 2012-13)*
a. Uterine atony
b. Traumatic
c. Retained tissues
d. Blood coagulopathy

[Ref: Dutta's Obs. 9th/e, pg. 385]

60.	b
61.	a
62.	a
63.	b
64.	b
65.	a
66.	c
67.	c
68.	a
69.	a
70.	a
71.	a

72. **Which one of the following is a cause of secondary post-partum hemorrhage:-** *(PGMEE 2018)*
    a. Placenta previa
    b. Retained bits of placenta
    c. Placental abruption
    d. All of the above

    [Ref: Dutta's Obs. 8th / e, pg. 474-476; Holland Brew's Obs. 4th / e, pg. 347, 403; Williams Obs. 24th / e, pg. 670-671]

Explanation

Secondary Post-partum Hemorrhage

- Also known as delayed or late PPH
- Uterine bleeding 24 hours to 12 weeks after delivery (ACOG - 2013b)
- Common causes –
  ○ Retained products of conception (bits of placenta and membranes)
  ○ Infection of genital tract
  ○ Trauma to genital tract (lacerations and haematomas)
  ○ Uterine artery pseudoaneurysm
  ○ Placental polyp
  ○ Submucous myomas
  ○ Chronic inversion of uterus
  ○ Trophoblastic disease
  ○ Coagulopathies (including von Willebrand's disease)
- Management – clinical assessment and investigations to establish the cause of secondary PPH
  ○ Clinical assessment (vital parameters, pallor, uterine tenderness and subinvolution, offensive lochia, lower genital tract examination for signs of trauma, retained POCs, haematomas, foreign bodies viz. forgotten sponges)
  ○ Investigations (CBC, coagulation profile, vaginal swab c/s, pelvic USG to detect retained POCs)
  ○ Medical management (with oxytocin, methyl-ergonovine, prostaglandin analogue along with broad spectrum antibiotic) preferred in a stable patient with USG showing empty uterine cavity).
  ○ Surgical management (gentle suction curettage) indicated in patients with heavy bleeding, recurrent bleeding, sepsis, subinvolution.

73. **All are used in the treatment of atonic PPH except -** *(PGMEE 2012-13)*

    a. PGE2   b. PGE1
    c. PGF2 alpha   d. Oxytocin

    [Ref: Dutta's Obs. 9th/e, pg. 389]

74. **PGF2 alpha maximum dose in PPH is-** *(PGMEE 2019)*
    a. 2000 µg   b. 200 µg
    c. 2 mg   d. 20 mg

    [Ref: Williams Obs. 25th/e pg. 4, 86]

INJURIES TO THE BIRTH CANAL

75. **First sign of wound dehiscence in uterine rupture during pregnancy-** *(PGMEE 2012-13)*
    a. Tachycardia
    b. PV discharge
    c. Bloody micturition
    d. Bradycardia

    [Ref: ; Dutta's Obs. 9th/e, pg. 402, 403; Holland Brew's Obs. 4th/e, pg. 341; Internet]

76. **Most common cause of rupture uterus in India is?** *(PGMEE Nov 13 Pattern)*
    a. Multiparity
    b. Obstructed labor
    c. Precipitate labor
    d. VBAC

    [Ref: ; Dutta's Obs. 9th/e, pg. 400; Holland Brew's Obs. 4th/e, pg. 340]

77. **Complete perineal tear occurs in?**
    a. Assisted breech   *(PGMEE Nov 13 Pattern)*
    b. External breech
    c. Face to pubes delivery
    d. Occipito posterior position of head

    [Ref: Dutta's Obs. 9th/e, pg. 397]

78. **Type of suture used in complete perineal tear repair is-** *(PGMEE 2013-14)*
    a. Catgut
    b. Silk
    c. Vicryl
    d. Vicryl and catgut

    [Ref: Dutta's Obs. 9th/e, pg. 398]

79. **Hematoma during labor is not due to-** *(PGMEE 2013-14)*
    a. Improper haemostasis
    b. Extension of cervical laceration
    c. Rupture of paravaginal venous plexus
    d. Obliteration of dead space while suturing vaginal wall

    [Ref: Dutta's Obs. 9th/e, pg. 399]

72.	b
73.	a
74.	c
75.	a
76.	a
77.	c
78.	c
79.	d

NORMAL PUERPERIUM

1. After delivery upto which week is known as puerperium:
                                                  (PGMEE 2012-13)
- a. 2 weeks
- b. 4 weeks
- c. 6 weeks
- d. 8 weeks

[Ref: Dutta's Obs. 9th/e, pg. 137]

2. Uterus post pregnancy becomes a pelvic organ in-
- a. 4 weeks   *(PGMEE 2013-14)*
- b. 6 weeks
- c. 12 weeks
- d. 2 weeks

[Ref: Dutta's Obs. 9th/e, pg. 138]

3. Weight of uterus at term and just after delivery is-
- a. 1000, 500   *(PGMEE 2013-14)*
- b. 1000, 1000
- c. 1500, 1000
- d. 500, 500

[Ref: Dutta's Obs. 9th/e, pg. 42, 137; Holland Brew's Obs. 4th/e, pg.37, 395]

4. Lochia is seen for-   *(PGMEE 1998)*
- a. 1-4 days
- b. 5-10 days
- c. 10-14 days
- d. 14-21 days

[Ref: Dutta's Obs. 9th/e, pg. 139; William's Obs. 24th/e pg. 670; Holland Brew's Obs.4th/e, pg. 396]

Explanation
- Average duration of lochia is 24 - 36 days.

5. Which one of the following sets of conditions is attributed to normal physiology of puerperium-   *(PGMEE 2016)*
- a. Tachycardia and weight gain
- b. Retention of urine, constipation and weight gain
- c. Constipation, tachycardia and retention of urine
- d. Retention of urine and constipation

[Ref: Dutta's Obs. 9th/e, pg. 139; Holland Brew's Obs.4th/e, pg. 396]

6. Which of the following is correct order of lochia?
- a. Serosa, alba, rubra   *(NEET Pattern 2013)*
- b. Alba, rubra, serosa
- c. Rubra, serosa, alba
- d. Rubra, alba, serosa

[Ref: Dutta's Obs. 9th/e, pg. 139; Holland Brew's Obs.4th/e, pg. 396]

7. Immunological defense to a breastfed infant is provided by all these factors in breast milk except:
- a. Interferons   *(PGMEE 2016-17)*
- b. Lactoferrin
- c. Immunoglobulins
- d. Fat globules

[Ref: Dutta's Obs. 9th/e, pg. 140, 421]

ABNORMALITIES OF PUERPERIUM

8. In puerperal period sepsis is most commonly due to-
- a. Uterine infection   *(PGMEE 2012-13)*
- b. Ovarian infection
- c. Vaginal infection
- d. All of the above

[Ref: Dutta's Obs. 9th/e, pg. 406]

9. Commonly involved in puerperal infection are all except: *(PGMEE 2012-13)*
- a. Anerobic streptococcus
- b. Staphylococcus
- c. E. Coli
- d. None of the above

[Ref: Dutta's Obs. 9th/e, pg. 407; William's Obs. 24th/e pg. 683; Holland Brew's Obs. 4th/e, pg. 415]

Explanation
- All these organisms are involved.

10. Puerperal sepsis/infection occurs upto?
                                               (PGMEE Nov 13 Pattern)
- a. 1 week   b. 2 week
- c. 3 week   d. 4 week

[Ref: Dutta's Obs. 9th/e, pg. 406]

11. After delivery, mother has fever on the next day with temp. > 100.4 F, HR increased. What is the most probable diagnosis:-   *(PGMEE 2016-17)*
- a. Chorioamnionitis   b. Puerperal pyrexia
- c. PID   d. Retained placenta

[Ref: Dutta's Obs. 9th/e, pg. 406]

12. Organisms involved in breast abscess are all except:-
- a. Staphylococcus aureus   *(PGMEE 2016-17)*
- b. Staphylococcus epidermidis
- c. Streptococcus viridians
- d. β hemolytic Streptococcus

[Ref: Dutta's Obs. 9th/e, pg. 411]

13. First line of treatment of mastitis in a lactating mother is: *(PGMEE 2019)*
- a. Cloxacillin   b. Cefazolin
- c. Ceftriaxone   d. Ampicillin

[Ref: Williams Obs 25th/e pg. 4, 22]

14. Cause of post partum depression:-   *(PGMEE 2016-17)*
- a. Changes in the hypothalamo-pituitary-adrenal axis
- b. Decreased tryptophan level
- c. Puerperal pyrexia
- d. Positive family history

[Ref:Dutta's Obs. 9th/e, pg. 415]

15. Which of the following is not true about puerperal fever
- a. Temp > 38 (100.4°F)   *(PGMEE 2016)*
- b. S. aureus is a most common cause
- c. Anaerobic Streptococcus predominant pathogen
- d. Instrumental delivery increases risk

[Ref: Dutta's Obs. 9th/e, pg. 406, 407]

1.	c
2.	d
3.	b
4.	c
5.	d
6.	c
7.	d
8.	a
9.	d
10.	b
11.	b
12.	d
13.	a
14.	a
15.	b

NEONATOLOGY

NORMAL TERM NEWBORN

1. **New born can be given breast milk after how much time following normal delivery:** *(PGMEE 2012-13)*
   a. Half hour
   b. 1 hours
   c. 2 hours
   d. 3 hours

   [Ref: Dutta's Obs. 9th/e, pg. 421]

2. **Ballard's score is used to assess-** *(PGMEE 2012-13)*
   a. Brain development of child
   b. Gestational age of child
   c. Lung maturation of the child
   d. Viability of the child

   [Ref: Dutta's Obs. 9th/e, pg. 417; Williams Obs., 23rd/e, pg. 600]

3. **Caput succedaneum indicates that fetus was alive till-**
   a. Immediately after birth *(PGMEE 2012-13)*
   b. Till 2-3 days after birth
   c. 2-3 weeks after birth
   d. 2-3 months after birth

   [Ref: Dutta's Obs. 9th/e, pg. 78]

IUGR

4. **IUGR babies on delivery are called?** *(DNB Dec' 2010)*
   a. Growth retarded
   b. Preterm
   c. Low birth weight
   d. Small for date

   [Ref: Dutta's Obs. 9th/e, pg. 431]

5. **On Doppler studies, which is an ominous sign of IUGR?**
   a. Increase S/D ratio *(PGMEE Aug 13 Pattern)*
   b. Reverse diastolic flow
   c. Diastolic notch
   d. All of the above

   [Ref: Dutta's Obs. 9th/e, pg. 433]

6. **⬜ placental height is seen in:** *(Recent Pattern June 2018)*
   a. Malaria
   b. Syphilis
   c. Rh isoimmunization
   d. IUGR

   [Ref: Dutta's Obs. 9th/e, pg.276, 277, 313, 432; Holland Brew's Obs. 4th/e pg.147, 168, 184, 213-215]

BLEEDING PV IN NEONATE

7. **Most common cause of vaginal bleeding in neonate is?**
   a. Sarcoma botryoides *(DNB Dec' 2009)*
   b. Bleeding disorder
   c. Birth trauma
   d. Hormone withdrawal

   [Ref: Dutta's Obs. 9th/e, pg. 419]

8. **Treatment of a neonate with vaginal bleeding is?**
   a. Wait and watch *(DNB Dec' 2009)*
   b. Cryoprecipitate
   c. Progesterone
   d. Estrogen

   [Ref: Dutta's Obs. 9th/e, pg. 419]

HESS'S RULE

9. **Hess's formula used in pregnancy to?** *(DNB June' 2011)*
   a. Estimate fetal age
   b. Identify fetal blood group
   c. Identify fetal congenital malformations
   d. Identify fetal sex

   [Ref: Dutta's Obs. 9th/e, pg. 37; Forensic Medicine & Toxicology, K.S.N. Reddy 33rd/e pg. 84]

Explanation

Hess's rule:

- Used in pregnancy to estimate fetal age from the fetal length.
- States that the square of the number of calendar months of gestation gives the length of the fetus in centimeters upto 5th month.
- The length of the fetus is determined by:
  ○ Crown-rump length (from the vertex to the coccyx) in earlier weeks
  ○ Crown-heel length (from the vertex to the heel) from the end of 20th week onwards
- After 5th month, however, the number of months should be multiplied by 5, which gives the length in centimeters.
- Thus, the fetal age can be estimated from the fetal length as follows:
  ○ Upto 5th month or 20th week— by square root of the crown-rump length
  ○ After 5th month— by dividing the crown-heel length by 5

EPIDEMIOLOGY IN OBSTETRICS

10. **True about ANC visit in India is?** *(PGMEE 2014)*
    a. 1st visit at 16 weeks and 3rd in between 20th week and term
    b. 1st visit at 16 weeks and 4th in between 36th week and term
    c. 2nd visit at 16 weeks and 3rd in between 20th week and term
    d. 2nd visit at 16 weeks and 4th in between 36th week and term

    [Ref: Dutta's Obs. 9th/e, pg. 557b]

1.	a
2.	b
3.	a
4.	a
5.	b
6.	d
7.	d
8.	a
9.	a
10.	a,b

11. Minimum antenatal visits prescribed by WHO are :-
(PGMEE 2016-17)

a. 2
b. 3
c. 4
d. 5

[Ref: Dutta's Obs. 9th/e, pg. 557b]

12. Which is not true about high risk pregnancy-
(PGMEE June 14 Pattern)

a. Breech
b. Previous LSCS
c. Previous scar dehiscence
d. Height of female 150 cm

[Ref: Dutta's Obs. 9th/e, pg. 588]

MATERNAL MORTALITY

13. Most common cause of maternal mortality in India is?
(DNB Dec' 2010, PGMEE 2014, 2016-17)

a. Sepsis
b. Abortion
c. Hemorrhage
d. Anemia

[Ref: Dutta's Obs. 9th/e, pg. 560]

PERINATAL MORTALITY

14. Most common cause of perinatal mortality in twins is?
(DNB Dec' 2011, PGMEE 2016-17)

a. Intra uterine growth restriction
b. Twin to twin transfusion syndrome
c. Prematurity
d. Single fetal demise

[Ref: Dutta's Obs. 9th/e, pg. 194, 562]

INFANT MORTALITY

15. According to registrar society of India commonest cause of IMR in India is-
(PGMEE 1997)

a. Prematurity
b. Diarrhoea
c. Malnutrition
d. Acute Respiratory Infection

[Ref: Park's Textbook of Preventive & Social Medicine 23rd/e pg.569]

INSTRUMENTS

16. Obstetric instrument shown in the photograph:-

a. Jolls retractor
b. Czerny retractor
c. Morris retractor
d. Deaver's retractor

Ref: Internet

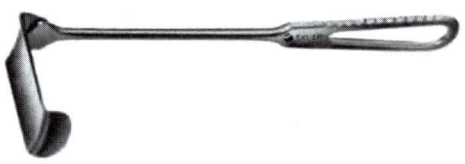

11.	c
12.	d
13.	c
14.	c
15.	a
16.	c
17.	a

Explanation

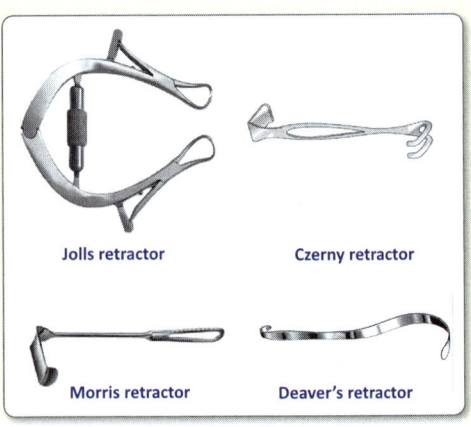

Jolls retractor   Czerny retractor

Morris retractor   Deaver's retractor

17. In the gynae labor room, the scissors shown in the diagram was used: Identify *(NEET Pattern 2017)*

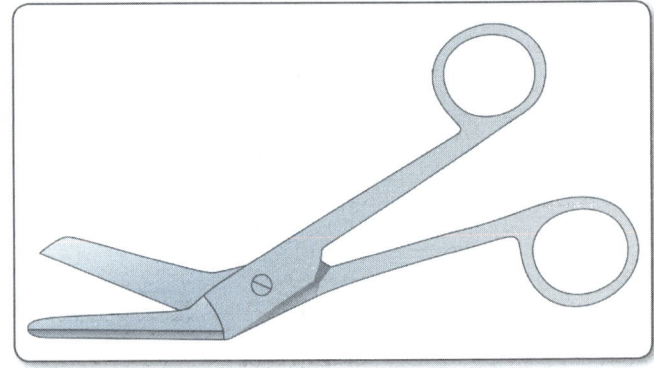

a. Episiotomy scissors
b. Dissection scissors
c. Stitch scissors
d. Mayo scissors

[Ref: Dutta's Obs. 8th / e, pg. 755; Holland Brew's Obs.4th / e, pg. 646; Internet]

Explanation

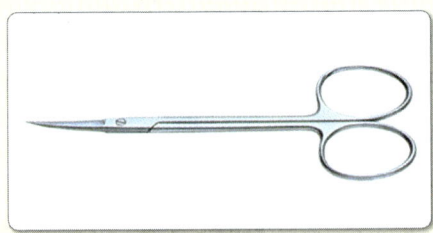

Dissection scissors

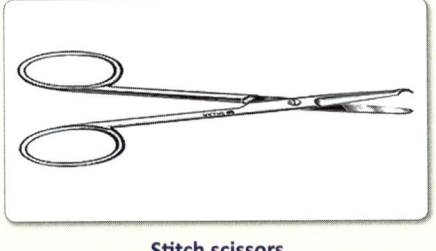

Stitch scissors

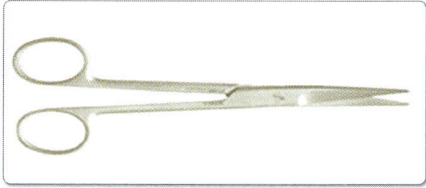

Mayo scissors

18. Which of the following leopold's grip is shown in the image: *(NEET Pattern 2017)*

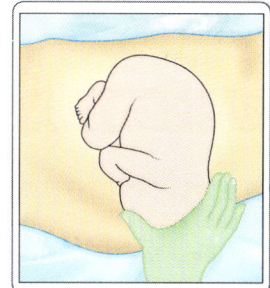

a. Pawlik's grip   b. Pelvic
c. Fundal   d. Abdominal

[Ref: Dutta's Obs. 8th/e, pg. 88-89; Holland Brew's Obs.4th /e, pg. 67]

18. a

Explanation

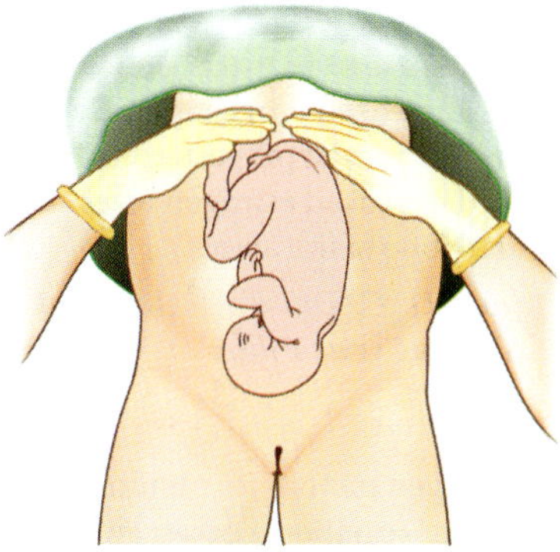

First maneuver

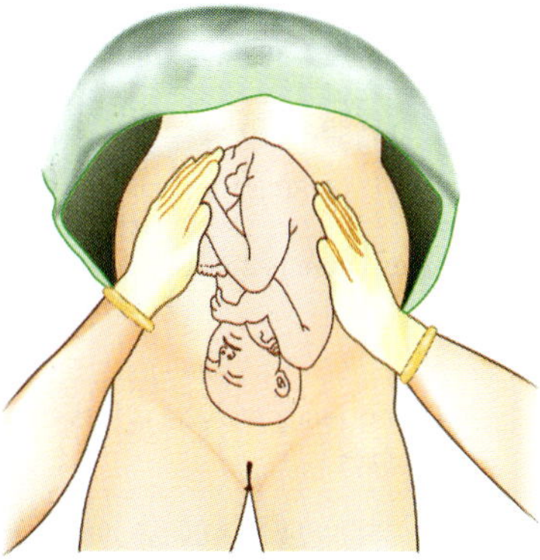

Second maneuver

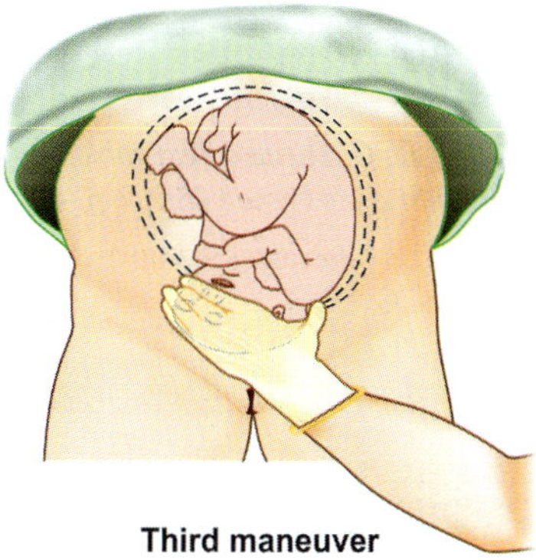

Third maneuver

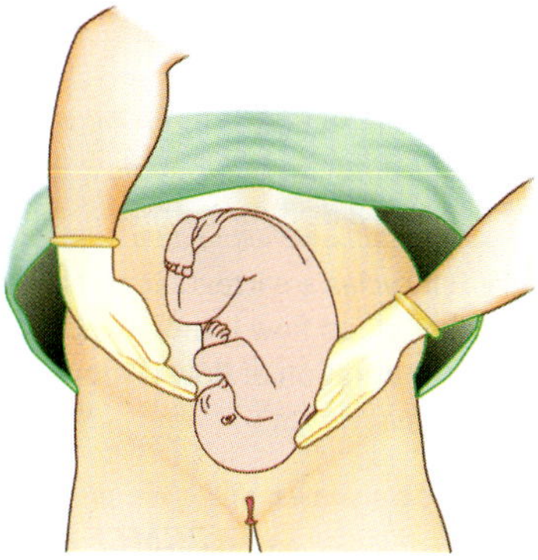

Fourth maneuver

Leopold's Maneuvers *(Obstetric Grips)*

- A systematic and codified manner of obstetric examination
- Described by Leopold and Sporlin in 1894
- Help to identify fetal landmarks and fetomaternal relationships
- Various maneuvers are as follows
  ○ First maneuver Fundal grip
  ○ Second maneuver — Abdominal grip
  ○ Third maneuver — Pawlik's grip
  ○ Fourth maneuver — Pelvic grip

MULTIPLE CHOICE QUESTIONS (GYNECOLOGY)

CHAPTER 1: DISORDERS OF MENSTRUATION AND AUB

PHYSIOLOGY OF MENSTRUATION

1. The amount of blood loss in each menstrual cycle is about- *(PGMEE 2012-13)*
a. 10cc
b. 35cc
c. 50cc
d. 100cc

[Ref: D. C. Dutta's Textbook of gynaecology, 7th/e, P. 66;Guyton 12th/e p. 996; Ganong 24th/e p. 404; Berek & Novak's Gynecology 15th/e page 404, table 14.9 and 14.10]

Explanation

In normal menstrual cycle

Menstrual cycle frequency	24-38 days
Duration of flow	4-8 days
Volume of flow	4-80 ml

■ The average blood flow per cycle is 35 ml.

Disorders of mensuration

Polymenorrhoea	If frequency of cycle is less than 21 days.
Oligomenorrhoea	If frequency of cycle is less than 35 days.
Amenorrhoea	If no menstruation has occurred in 90 days.
Menorrhagia	If cycles are regular and amount of blood flow is more than 80 ml, or duration of blood flow is more than 8 days, or both.
Menometrorrhagia	If cycles are irregular and amount of blood flow is more than 80 ml, or duration of flow is more than 8 days, or both.

2. Maximum estrogen level in menstrual Cycle is- *(PGMEE 2012-13)*
a. 100-200 pg/ml
b. 200-300 pg/ml
c. 300-400 pg/ml
d. 400-500 pg/ml

[Ref: Shaw's Gynae 15th/e p. 47]

3. Normal blood loss in menstruation is? *(PGMEE Aug 13 Pattern)*
a. 20 to 40 ml
b. 40 to 80 ml
c. 80 to 120 ml
d. 120 to 150 ml

[Ref: Guyton 12th/e p. 996; Ganong 24th/e p. 404; Dutta's Obs. 8th/e, pg. 23-27,30,46; Holland Brew's Obs.4th/e, pg.16-19,28; Shaw's Gynae. 16th/e, pg.10]

Explanation
■ See question 1

4. Regeneration of Endothelium after menstruation takes about- *(PGMEE 2012-13)*
a. 2 days
b. 5 days
c. 10 days
d. 15 days

[Ref: D. C. Dutta's Textbook of gynaecology, 7th/e, P. 71; Shaw's Gynae 15th/e p. 35]

5. Day 20 of menstrual cycle falls under which phase? *(PGMEE 2019)*
a. Menstrual phase
b. Follicular phase
c. Ovulation phase
d. Luteal phase

[Ref: Shaw's text book of Gynae 16th/e pg. 43]

6. What is seen in luteal phase- *(PGMEE 2012-13)*
a. Increased progesterone levels
b. Decreased progesterone levels
c. Decreased estrogen level
d. None of the above

[Ref: D. C. Dutta's Textbook of gynaecology, 7th/e, P. 74 Shaw's Gynae 15th/e p. 46]

Explanation
■ Regeneration of endometrium starts even before menstruation ceases and is completed 2-3 days after end of menstruation. Thickness of endometrium at this time is 2 mm.

7. Estrogen Level in follicular phase of menstrual Cycle- *(PGMEE 2012-13)*
a. 100-200 pg/ml
b. 200-300 pg/ml
c. 300-400 pg/ml
d. 400-500 pg/ml

[Ref: D. C. Dutta's Textbook of gynaecology, 7th/e, P 74 fig 8.10;Shaw's Gynae 15th/e p. 48]

8. Rescue hormone for corpus leutum is?
a. hCG
b. Progesterone
c. hPL
d. Estrogen

[Ref: D. C. Dutta's Textbook of gynaecology, 7th/e, P. 70]

DYSMENORRHOEA

9. Which of the following is a cause of dysmenorrhea: *(PGMEE 2015)*
a. Adenomyosis
b. Fibroid
c. Endometriosis
d. All of the above

[Ref: Shaw's Gyanecology 16th/e p. 471]

10. Dysmenorrhoea is due to? *(PGMEE 2014)*
a. Ovulation
b. Decreased progesterone
c. Increased progesterone
d. Secretory epithelium

1. b
2. d
3. a
4. a
5. d
6. a
7. a
8. a
9. d
10. c

[Ref: D. C. Dutta's Textbook of gynaecology, 7th/e, P. 147; Berek & Novak's Gynecology 15th/e p. 481]

Explanation

- Etiology of dysmenorrhea includes excessive or imbalanced amount of prostanoids secreted from the endometrium during menstruations.
- Decline in progesterone levels in late luteal phase triggers released of lytic enzymes, resulting in release of phospholipids with generation of arachidonic acid and COX pathway resulting in synthesis of prostanoids. This increased synthesis of prostanoids lead to higher uterine tone with high amplitude uterine contractions – thus causing dysmenorrhea.

11. Mittelschemerz is: *(PGMEE 2013-14)*
   a. Pain just before menstruation
   b. Pain at the time of ovulation
   c. Pain 5 days after ovulation
   d. Pain during menstruation

[Ref: Jeffcoate's Gynae. 8th/e, pg. 90]

12. Mainstay of treatment for primary dysmenorrhea is: *(PGMEE 2014)*
   a. Non-steroidal anti-inflammatory drugs
   b. Dicyclomine
   c. Hyoscine
   d. Paracetamol

[Ref: D. C. Dutta's Textbook of gynaecology, 7th/e, P. 148]

13. Drug of choice in premenstrual syndrome: *(PGMEE 2012-13)*
   a. Antipsychotics   b. SSRI
   c. OCP   d. Depo progesterone

[Ref: D. C. Dutta's Textbook of gynaecology, 7th/e, P. 150; Shaw's Gynae 15th/e p. 297]

ABNORMAL UTERINE BLEEDING

14. Endometrial biopsy is usually performed between: *(PGMEE 2016-17)*
   a. 1-5 days of menstrual cycle
   b. 7-14 days of menstrual cycle
   c. 5-7 days of menstrual cycle
   d. 21-28 days of menstrual cycle

[Ref: D.C Dutta text book of gynaecology 7th e p 156-158

15. Metrorrhagia is produced by the following except: *(PGMEE 2013-14)*
   a. Polyp
   b. CA endometrium
   c. IUD
   d. Intramural fibroid

[Ref: D. C. Dutta's Textbook of gynaecology, 7th/e, P153]

16. Anovulatory DUB is due to? *(PGMEE 2013-2014; PGMEE Aug 13 Pattern)*
   a. Absence of progesterone
   b. Excess of estrogen
   c. Hypothalamic pituitary defect
   d. High progesterone

[Ref: D. C. Dutta's Textbook of gynaecology, 7th/e, P. 155]

17. Most common cause of AUB is? *(PGMEE 2014)*
   a. Anovulatory   b. Ovulatory
   c. Coagulopathy   d. Pregnancy related

[Ref: D. C. Dutta's Textbook of gynaecology, 7th/e, P. 154]

18. Oligomenorrhoea means: *(PGMEE 2013- 14)*
   a. Cycle <20 days   b. Cycle more than 45 days
   c. Cycle more than 28 days
   d. Cycle more than 35 days

[Ref: D. C. Dutta's Textbook of gynaecology, 7th/e, P. 153; Shaw's Gynae 15th/e p. 283]

19. Age of metropathia hemorrhagica is- *(PGMEE 2013-14)*
   a. 20-25 years   b. 50-55 years
   c. 60-65 years   d. 40-45 years

[Ref: D. C. Dutta's Textbook of gynaecology, 7th/e, P. 155; Shaw's Gynae 15th/e p. 302]

20. Swiss cheese pattern endometrium is seen in
   a. Carcinoma endometrium   *(PGMEE 2015)*
   b. Metropathia hemorrhagica
   c. Hydatidiform mole
   d. Halban's disease

[Ref: Textbook of gynecology by Rao:65]

21. Drug not used commonly for menorrhagia: *(PGMEE 2012-13)*
   a. Methergin   b. Ormiloxifene
   c. Danazol   d. NSAIDS

[Ref: D. C. Dutta's Textbook of gynaecology, 7th/e, P. 157; Shaw's Gynae 15th/e p. 304]

Explanation

- A only, ormeloxifen or centchroman or Saheli is non hormonal drug used for contraception and also for menorrhagia.

POST MENOPAUSAL BLEEDING

22. Post menopausal endometrial thickness is: *(PGMEE 2012-13)*
   a. 1-3 mm   b. 8-9 mm
   c. 5-7 mm   d. 6-8 mm

[Ref: D. C. Dutta's Textbook of gynaecology, 7th/e, P463; Shaw's Gynae 15th/e p. 36]

23. Most common cause of post-menopausal vaginal bleeding is? *(PGMEE 2010)*
   a. Endometrial carcinoma
   b. Ovarian tumor
   c. Carcinoma vulva
   d. Carcinoma cervix

[Ref: Shaw's Textbook of Gynaecology, 15th/e, Page no. 71, Jeffcoate's Principles of Gynaecology, 8th/e, Page no. 576-578]

24. Investigation of choice in post-menopausal bleeding is? *(PGMEE 2010)*
   a. Fractional curettage   b. Coagulation profile
   c. Endometrial biopsy   d. D and C

[Ref: D. C. Dutta's Textbook of gynaecology, 7th/e, P463; Shaw's Textbook of Gynaecology, 15th/e, Page no. 71-72; Jeffcoate's Principles of Gynaecology, 7th/e, P. 13, 613-614; Berek & Novak's Gynecology, 15th/e, P. 1251]

11.	b
12.	a
13.	b
14.	d
15.	d
16.	a
17.	a
18.	d
19.	d
20.	b
21.	a
22.	a
23.	a
24.	c

CAUSES

MALE INFERTILITY

1. Which of the following is true about obstructive azo-ospermia- *(PGMEE 2009)*
   a. FSH and LH
   b. Normal FSH and Normal LH
   c. FSH, Normal LH
   d. LH, Normal FSH

[Ref: D. C. Dutta's Textbook of gynaecology, 7th/e, P191;Shaw 15th/e p. 210 & 13th/e p. 203; Oxford textbook of Medicine 4th/e p. 283; Dewhurst Obs & Gynaec 10th/e p. 449; Obstetrics & Gynaecology by James Draycott 1999 p. 137; Berek & Novak's Gynecology 15th edition page 1146.]

2. Pt. with low testosterone & low count can show all except- *(PGMEE 2012-13)*
   a. Decreased FSH
   b. Decreased LH
   c. Increased FSH
   d. Obstruction of spermatic duct

[Ref: D. C. Dutta's Textbook of gynaecology, 7th/e, P190-191 Shaw's Gynae 15th/e p. 204]

FEMALE INFERTILITY

3. What is the % of tubal causes of female infertility? *(PGMEE 2014)*
   a. 7%   b. 19%
   c. 26%   d. 52%

[Ref: D. C. Dutta's Textbook of gynaecology, 7th/e, P188; Berek & Novak's Gynecology 15th edition page 1134.]

Explanation

- Tubal factors account for 30-40% causes for female infertility.

4. Basic test for Infertility is: *(Recent Pattern June 2018)*
   a. FSH test   b. Anatomical diagnostic test
   c. HSG   d. All

[Ref: Speroff 8th e p.1162; D.C Dutta text book of gynaecology 7th/ e pg.. 193]

Explanation

- FSH test is a basic test to evaluate female ovum supply. It is performed on the 3rd day of the menstrual cycle. For men, FSH is present and regulates the production and transportation of sperm. Therefore, an FSH test would determine male sperm count.
- LH test measures a woman's ovum supply or **ovarian reserve**. The test occurs during a woman's menstrual cycle to see if she is ovulating. LH testing can also measure a male's sperm count, as LH is a testosterone stimulator, which in turn affects sperm production.
- Progesterone is helpful to **determine whether or not ovulation is occurring.** Progesterone causes thickening of uterine lining, preparing it to receive a fertilized egg.
- Testosterone is a hormone produced by both men and women. In women, a testosterone test could be useful in determining the cause of irregular periods and to evaluate decreased sex drive.
- Estradiol test is used to evaluate the quality of the eggs and a woman's ovarian function.
- Prolactin is a pituitary hormone. Measuring prolactin may give insight into why women aren't menstruating. Prolactin can be measured in men as well.

5. In hypergonadotropic hypogonadism FSH level is? *(PGMEE 2014)*
   a. <20 m IU/ml   b. >20 m IU/ml
   c. <40 m IU/ml   d. >40 m IU/ml

[Ref: Speroff's Clinical Gyaecologic Endocrinology and Infertility 8th/e p. 443; D. C. Dutta's Textbook of gynaecology, 7th/e, P374

6. A patient with infertility was prescribed bromocriptine by the gynecologist? What would be the cause?
   a. Hypogonadotropic hypogonadism *(NEET Pattern 2017)*
   b. Premature ovarian failure
   c. Hyperprolactinemia
   d. PCOS

[Ref: Speroff 8th e.p.1328}

Explanation

- Dopamine agonists are the treatment of choice for hyperprolactinemic infertile women with ovulatory dysfunction who wish to conceive.

7. In hypogonadotropic hypogonadism, what all can be seen except. *(NEET Pattern 2017)*
   a. Low GNRH   b. Low LH & FSH
   c. Low estradiol   d. Hyperprolactinemia

Ref: Speroff 8th e p.1295

Explanation

- **WHO Group I: Hypogonadotropic Hypogonadal Anovulation.** The group accounts for approximately 5–10% of anovulatory women and includes those with low or low-normal serum follicle-stimulating hormone (FSH) concentrations, and low serum estradiol levels, due to absent or abnormal hypothalamic gonadotropin-releasing hormone (GnRH) secretion or pituitary insensitivity to GnRH. Examples include women with hypothalamic amenorrhea relating to physical, nutritional, or emotional stress, weight loss, excessive

1.	b
2.	d
3.	c
4.	a
5.	b
6.	c
7.	d

exercise, anorexia nervosa and its variants, Kallmann syndrome, and isolated gonadotropin defi ciency. Women in the group may require hypothalamic-pituitary imaging to exclude a mass lesion.

- **WHO Group II: Eugonadotropic Euestrogenic Anovulation.** This group is the largest, including 75–85% of anovulatory women, and is characterized by normal serum FSH and estradiol levels and normal or elevated LH concentrations.7 The most common examples are women with polycystic ovary syndrome (PCOS), some of whom ovulate at least occasionally. Women with PCOS should be screened for type 2 diabetes mellitus before treatment, due to the fetal risks associated with untreated diabetes.8 Weight loss generally is the best initial treatment for those who are obese because it can, by itself, restore ovulatory function

- **WHO Group III: Hypergonadotropic Anovulation.** The group accounts for approximately 10–20% of anovulatory women and includes those with elevated serum FSH concentrations; most, but not all, have amenorrhea. The classic example is premature ovarian failure, due to follicular depletion, and few respond to treatment aimed at ovulation induction.

- **Hyperprolactinemic Anovulation.** Approximately 5–10% of anovulatory women have hyperprolactinemia, which inhibits gonadotropin secretion. Consequently, serum FSH concentrations generally are low or low-normal and serum estradiol levels also tend to be relatively low. Most hyperprolactinemic women have oligomenorrhea or amenorrhea. When hyperprolactinemia cannot be attributed confi dently to coexisting hypothyroidism or to medications, hypothalamic-pituitary imaging is indicated to exclude a mass lesion.

8. Cause of infertility in hypothyroidism-
(PGMEE 2012-13)
a. Decrease prolactin
b. Increased prolactin
c. Both
d. None

[Ref: D. C. Dutta's Textbook of gynaecology, 7th/e, P385]

Explanation
- Reasons for infertility in females with hypothyroidism –
  - Anovultion
  - hyperprolactinemia
  - Luteal phase defect
  - Sex hormone imbalance
  - Autoimmune factors.

9. A 35 year old nulliparous women with primary infertility presents with adenexal mass and CA -125 level of >60 U/mL. What is the most likely diagnosis?
(PGMEE 2010)
a. Ovarian cancer
b. Endometrioma
c. Borderline ovarian tumour
d. Tuberculosis

Explanation

D/d of infertility in adenexal masses

Clinical condition	Age & parity	Cl/f	CA 125
Ovarian Ca	Elderly	Abdominal distension, mass abdomen	↑ in 50% of epithelial tumours
Borderline ovarian tumours	Middle age		Normal
Endometrioma	Middle age	Painful adenexal mass, 1° infertility	↑ in > 80%
TB	Any age	↑ Painless adenexal mass 1° infertility	May be ↑

INVESTIGATIONS

10. Aspermia: **(PGMEE 2016-17)**
a. No semen
b. No sperm in semen
c. Dead sperm in semen
d. Low semen volume

[Ref: D.C Dutta text book of gynaecology 7th e p190]

11. Anovulation may be diagnosed with: **(PGMEE 2016-17)**
a. Low LH
b. High FSH
c. Static elevated estrogen
d. Low progesterone

[Ref: speroff 8th e p.1162; D.C Dutta text book of gynaecology 7th e p 193]

12. All of the following are markers of ovarian reserve except: **(PGMEE 2015)**
a. Inhibin A
b. Estradiol concentration
c. Inhibin B
d. Ovarian volume

[Ref: C. Dutta's Textbook of gynaecology, 7th/e, P 437;Speroff's Clinical Gyaecologic Endocrinology and Infertility 8th/e p. 1147]

13. Ovarian reserve is measured by- **(PGMEE 2013-14)**
a. FSH
b. LH
c. FSH & LH
d. ESTRADIOL

[Ref: D. C. Dutta's Textbook of gynaecology, 7th/e, P437; Shaw's Gynae 15th/e p. 47, 216; Speroff 7th/e p. 444-448]

14. In low ovarian reserve,anti mullerian hormone level will be **(PGMEE 2019)**
a. <1
b. 1-4
c. >7
d. >10

[Ref: Williams gynecology 3rd/e pg. 436]

15. Semen examination can be done: **(PGMEE 2013-14)**
a. Immediately in semi solid form
b. After liquefaction
c. Within 15-30 minutes of liquefaction
d. 1½-2 hr irrespective of liquefaction

[Ref: D. C. Dutta's Textbook of gynaecology, 7th/e, P190, Shaw's Gynae 15th/e p. 203]

8.	b
9.	b
10.	a
11.	d
12.	a
13.	a
14.	a
15.	d

16. On which day LH & FSH should be measured-
(PGMEE 2013-14)
a. 1-3rd day
b. 7th day
c. 1-4th day
d. 10th day

[Ref: D. C. Dutta's Textbook of gynaecology, 7th/e, P]

17. Normal sperm motility normal according to WHO is-
(PGMEE 2012-13)
a. > 20%
b. > 30%
c. > 40%
d. > 50%

[Ref: C. Dutta's Textbook of gynaecology, 7th/e, P 190; Shaw's Gynae 15th/e p. 204; Berek & Novak's Gynecology 15th edition page 1141, table 32.2.]

Explanation

WHO Guidelines for semen analysis-

	1992 guidelines	2010 guidelines
▪ Volume	2 ml	≥ 1.5 ml
▪ Sperm concentration	20 million/ml	≥ 15 million/ml
▪ Sperm motility	50% progressive, or >25% rapidly progressive	≥ 32% progressive
▪ Morphology (strict criteria)	>15% normal forms	≥ 4% normal forms
▪ White blood cells	< 1 million/ml	< 1 million/ml
▪ Immunobead or mixed antiglobulin reaction test	< 10% coated with antibodies	< 50%

18. The confirmatory test for presence of semen is?
(PGMEE Nov. 13 Pattern)
a. P 30
b. Casein
c. Amylase
d. Alpha feto protein

19. Fertile period of female is measured by-
(PGMEE 2012-13)
a. LH
b. FSH
c. Estrogen
d. Oxytocin

[Ref: Shaw's Gynae 15th/e p. 297]

20. Inhibin B levels as test of ovarian reserve is measured on?
(PGMEE 2011)
a. Day 2 of menstruation
b. Day 3 of menstruation
c. Day 4 of menstruation
d. Day 5 of Menstruation

[Ref: Shaw's Textbook of Gynaecology, 15th/e, P. 45; Berek & Novak's Gynecology 15th edition page 1149.]

Explanation

▪ Inhibin B levels are measured on 5th day of ovarian stimulation.

21. Best diagnosis of ovulation is by? *(PGMEE 2012)*
a. Ultrasound
b. Chromotubation
c. Endometrial biopsy
d. Laparscopy

[Ref: D. C. Dutta's Textbook of gynaecology, 7th/e, P194 Novak's Gynae 14th/e p. 1207; Shaw's 13th/e p. 33]

22. Best test for ovulation-
(PGMEE 2012-13; PGMEE Nov 12 Pattern)
a. Serum estrogen
b. Serum progesterone
c. Both
d. None

[Ref: D. C. Dutta's Textbook of gynaecology, 7th/e, P196; Shaw's Gynae 15th/e p. 216]

23. Dye used in Hysterosapingography- *(PGMEE 2012-13)*
a. Conray 420
b. Renografin-60
c. Toluidine blue
d. None of the above

[Ref: D. C. Dutta's Textbook of gynaecology, 7th/e486]

TREATMENT

24. Vasectomy reversal in primary infertility is done within how many years of vasectomy- *(PGMEE2012-13)*
a. 5 yrs
b. 6 yrs
c. 7 yrs
d. 8 yrs

[Ref: speroff 8th p.936; Shaw's Gynae 15th/e p. 205]

25. Drug of choice for ovulation induction-
(PGMEE 2012-13)
a. Clomiphene
b. FSH
c. LH
d. hCG

[Ref: D. C. Dutta's Textbook of gynaecology, 7th/e, P199; Shaw's Gynae 15th/e p. 217]

26. Treatment of immunological infertility is?
(PGMEE Nov 13 Pattern)
a. ICSI
b. GIFT
c. IVF
d. IUI

[Ref: D. C. Dutta's Textbook of gynaecology, 7th/e, P203; Novak 15th/e ch. 32p. 1134; Harrison 17th/e ch. 341; Danforth's Obs & Gynae 10th/e p. 706; Berek & Novak's Gynecology 15th edition page 1163.]

Explanation

▪ Immunological factors for infertility have not been found to affect IVF outcomes.

27. All are indications of intra uterine insemination except:
a. Vicid cervical mucus *(PGMEE 2010)*
b. Immune factor of sperms
c. Tubal blockade
d. Oligozoospermia

[Ref: D. C. Dutta's Textbook of gynaecology, 7th/e, P203; Shaw's Textbook of Gynaecology, 15th/e, Page no. 207 Jeffcoate's Principles of Gynaecology, 7th/e, P. 724-6 Berek & Novak's Gynecology, 15th/e, P. 1145, 1153]

28. AID the term used to describe the artificial insemination achieved by using sperms of- *(PGMEE 2012-13)*
a. Husband
b. Donor
c. Both
d. None

[Ref: D. C. Dutta's Textbook of gynaecology, 7th/e, P204]

ASSISTED REPRODUCTIVE TECHNIQUES

29. Which of the following is not an assisted reproductive technique (ART)? *(PGMEE Aug 12 Pattern)*
a. ZIFT
b. GIST
c. IVF
d. Artificial insemination

[Ref: D. C. Dutta's Textbook of gynaecology, 7th/e, P204; COGT 2009/e Chapter 58; Danforth's 10/e p. 710]

16.	a
17.	d
18.	a
19.	a
20.	d
21.	a
22.	b
23.	b
24.	a
25.	a
26.	c
27.	c
28.	b
29.	d

METHODS

1. **Which of following is/are not sexual awareness method of contraception?** *(PGMEE 2016)*
   a. Withdrawal method   b. Barrier methods
   c. Cervical mucus   d. MTP kit
   e. Symptothermal method

[Ref: D.C Dutta text book of gynaecology 7th e p 414]

2. **Knaus-Ogino method is what type of contraceptive method?** *(PGMEE Aug 13 Pattern)*
   a. Calender method
   b. Withdrawal method
   c. Barrier method
   d. Cervical mucous rhythm method

3. **Billing's method of contraception is a:** *(PGMEE 2010; PGMEE Aug 12 Pattern)*
   a. Barrier method
   b. Hormonal method
   c. Behavioral method
   d. None

[Ref: Shaw's Textbook of Gynaecology, 15th/e, P. 223 Jeffcoate's Principles of Gynaecology, 7th/e, P. 787-788 Berek & Novak's Gynecology, 15th/e, P. 218]

4. **Contraception failure defined in terms of?** *(PGMEE 2009)*
   a. Per woman years   b. Per 10 woman years
   c. Per 100 woman years   d. Per 1000 woman years

[Ref: Shaw's Textbook of Gynaecology, 15th/e, P. 223; Jeffcoate's Principles of Gynaecology, 7th/e, P. 787-788; Berek & Novak's Gynecology, 15th/e, P. 218]

TEMPORARY METHODS

BARRIER METHODS

5. **Identify the contraceptive device shown in the picture.** *(PGMEE 2016-17)*

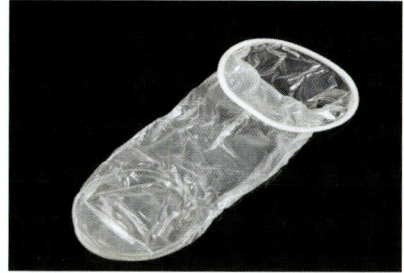

   a. Diaphragm   b. Male condom
   c. Female condom   d. Diva cup

[Ref: D.C Dutta text book of gynaecology 7th e p 412]

6. **HIV positive couple with pregnant female, contraceptive of choice is-** *(PGMEE 2012-13)*
   a. Abstinence   b. Condoms
   c. No restrictions   d. OCPs

[Ref: D. C. Dutta's Textbook of gynaecology, 7th/e, P412; Dutta Obs 7th/e p. 303]

7. **Ideal contraceptive in RHD-** *(PGMEE 2012-13)*
   a. Barrier   b. IUCD
   c. OCPs   d. DMPA

[Ref: Park 20th/e p. 425; Shaw's Gynae 15th/e p. 244; Dutta Obs 7th/e p. 545]

8. **Today vaginal sponge failure rate is?** *(PGMEE Nov 12 Pattern)*
   a. 5%   b. 9%
   c. 16%   d. 20%

[Ref: D. C. Dutta's Textbook of gynaecology, 7th/e, P413; speroff clinicalgynaecologic endocrinology& infertility 8th ep.1123]

Explanation

Lowest expected in nulliparous is 9%, lowest expected in multiparous is 20%

IUCD

9. **Pregnancy occurred with IUCD in situ, the strings are however not visible, all of the following can be done except-** *(PGMEE 2015)*
   a. Leave in situ
   b. Remove under USG guidance
   c. Remove using hysteroscope
   d. Remove using IUCD hook

[Ref: D. C. Dutta's Textbook of gynaecology, 7th/e, P396; Speroff's Clinical Gynaecologic Endocrinology and Infertility 8th/e p. 1109]

10. **IUD in situ does not cause-** *(PGMEE 2015)*
   a. Pregnancy
   b. Ectopic pregnancy
   c. Pain in abdomen
   d. Intrauterine malformation

[Ref: D. C. Dutta's Textbook of gynaecology, 7th/e, P395-6]

11. **Which IUCD has the maximum chances of development of ectopic pregnancy:-** *(PGMEE 2015)*
   a. Levenogestrol
   b. Cu T 380 A
   c. Progestasert
   d. Cu T 200

[Ref: Speroff's Clinical Gynaecologic Endocrinology and Infertility 8th/e p. 1105]

1.	d
2.	a
3.	c
4.	c
5.	c
6.	b
7.	a
8.	b
9.	d
10.	d
11.	c

12. When is copper T inserted- *(PGMEE 2013-14)*
a. 3 days after periods are over
b. Within 10 days of menstrual cycle
c. PID just before menstruation
d. Just after menstruation

[Ref: D. C. Dutta's Textbook of gynaecology, 7th/e, P393]

Explanation

- Best time for Cu-T insertion is during menses, reason – pain due to Cu-T insertion is masked by dysmenorrhea and confirmation of non pregnant state occurs.
- Else it can be inserted any time after exclusion of PID or Pregnancy.

13. Absolute contraindication for IUCD is-
(PGMEE 2013-14)
a. Menorrhagia   b. Vaginal bleeding
c. Fibroid   d. Purulent discharge

[Ref: D. C. Dutta's Textbook of gynaecology, 7th/e, P393; Shaw's 15th/e p. 227]

14. About IUCD all are true except:
(PGMEE Nov 13 Pattern)
a. Multiload 375 is a third generation IUCD
b. Lippes loop and Cu T 200 have same pregnancy rate
c. IUCD can be used as emergency contraception
d. LNG IUD has half life of 10 years

[Ref: D. C. Dutta's Textbook of gynaecology, 7th/e, P392-393; Novak's 14th/e ch. 10t. 102; William's 22nd/e ch. 32]

15. Levonorgestrel (52mg) containing IUCD releases it @:
(Recent Pattern June 2018)
a. 10 µg/day   b. 20 µg/day
c. 30 µg/day   d. 40 µg/day

[Ref: Dutta's Obs. 9th/e, pg. 497; Holland Brew's Obs. 4th/e pg. 569]

Explanation

- Mirena contains 52 mg of LNG (Levonorgestrel) and releases @ 20 microgram/d and is effective upto 5 years.
- Fibroplant contains 52 mg of LNG (Levonorgestrel) and releases @ 14 microgram/d.
- Skyla is another IUCD which contains 13.5 mg of LNG.

16. Women with menorrhagia IUCD of choice:
(PGMEE 2012-13)
a. NOVA T   b. LNG IUD
c. Mirena   d. Gyne fix

[Ref: D. C. Dutta's Textbook of gynaecology, 7th/e, P397; Shaw's Gynae 15th/e p. 303]

17. Intrauterine contraceptive device with effective life of 10 years is? *(PGMEE Nov. 12 Pattern)*
a. Cu T 380A   b. Progestasert
c. Cu T 200   d. Mirena

[Ref: D. C. Dutta's Textbook of gynaecology, 7th/e, P393; Novak's 14th/e Chapter 10]

18. Cu T 380A IUCD should be replaced once in-
(PGMEE pattern 2008)
a. 4 yrs   b. 6 yrs
c. 8 yrs   d. 10 yrs

[Ref: Park's textbook of PSM 22nd/e p. 458]

12.	a
13.	d
14.	a
15.	b
16.	c
17.	a
18.	d
19.	a
20.	a

Explanation

- Cu-T-380A is approved for use for 10 years. However, the Cu-T-380A has been demonstrated to maintain its efficacy over at least 12 years of use. The CuT-200 is approved for 4 years and the Nova T for 5 years. The progesterone-releasing IUD must be replaced every year because the reservoir of progesterone is depleted in 12-18 months. The levonorgestrel IUD can be used for at least 7 years, and probably 10 years.

Device	Pregnancy rate(%)	Expulsion rate (%)	Life span (years)
First generation: Lippe's loop	3.0	19.1	-
Second generation:			
Cu T-200	3.0	7.8	3
CuT-380A	0.5-0.8	5	10
NovaT	0.7	5.8	5
Multiload 250	0.5	2.2	3
Third generation :			
Progestasert	1.8	3.1	1

19. The most common side effect of IUD insertion is-
(DNB 2007)
a. Bleeding   b. Pain
c. Pelvic infection   d. Ectopic pregnancy

[Ref: Park's textbook of PSM 22nd/e p. 459]

Explanation

- Side effects and complications of IUDs
  ○ Bledding –most common
  ○ Pain – second major side effect
  ○ Pelvic infection- PID
  ○ Uterine perforation
  ○ Pregnancy
  ○ Ectopic pregnancy
  ○ Expulsion
  ○ Mortality – extremely rare
- Most common side effect requiring removal of the device - pain
- The commonest complaint of women fitted an IUCD (inert or medicated) is increased vaginal bleeding. It accounts for 10-20 percent of all IUCD removals. The bleeding may take one or more of all the following forms: greater volume of blood loss during menstruation, longer menstrual periods or mid-cycle bleeding. Copper devices seem to cause less average blood loss. Menstrual blood loss is consistently lower when hormone-releasing devices are used. If the bleeding is heavy or persistent or if the patient develop anemia despite the iron supplement the IUCD should be removed.

20. Mirena releases _____ microgram of LNG/day?
(PGMEE Nov. 12 Pattern)
a. 20   b. 55
c. 65   d. 380

[Ref: D. C. Dutta's Textbook of gynaecology, 7th/e, P393; Novak's 14th/e Chapter 10]

21. Which of the following has the least risk of ectopic pregnancy? *(PGMEE 2011)*
- a. Condoms
- b. OC pills
- c. Copper T
- d. Tubectomy

[Ref: Shaw's Textbook of Gynaecology, 15th/e, P. 230, 267; Jeffcoate's Principles of Gynaecology, 7th/e, P. 789, 799; Berek & Novak's Gynecology, 15th/e, P. 224]

STEROIDAL CONTRACEPTIVES

ORAL CONTRACEPTIVE PILLS

22. OCP are protective against:- *(PGMEE 2016-17)*
- a. Ovarian carcinoma
- b. Breast cancer
- c. Cervical cancer
- d. Liver cancer

[Ref: D.C Dutta text book of gynaecology 7th e p 402]

23. Regarding OCPs all are true EXCEPT? *(PGMEE 2016)*
- a. Can increase thromboembolic events
- b. Protects from benign conditions of breast
- c. Protects against endometrial cancer
- d. Decreases bone mineral density

[Ref: D.C Dutta text book of gynaecology 7th e p 401-2]

24. Absolute contraindications of OCP are all except- *(PGMEE 2015)*
- a. Sickle cell disease
- b. Breast cancer
- c. Ischemic heart disease
- d. Hepatoma

[Ref: Dutta's Obstetrics 8th/e p. 623]

25. Which of the following is not a mechanism of action of OCPs- *(PGMEE 2015)*
- a. Inhibition of ovulation
- b. Alteration of cervical mucus
- c. Out of phase endometrium
- d. None of the above

[Ref: Dutta's Obstetrics 8th/e p. 622]

26. Lowest amount of estrogen in OCP is- *(PGMEE 2015)*
- a. 15 microgram
- b. 20 microgram
- c. 30 microgram
- d. 35 microgram

[Ref: Speroff 8the p.966; Practical Obstetrics and Gynaecology, Virkhud p. 188]

27. What is to be done if 2 OCP is missed on day 17-18 of the cycle- *(PGMEE 2015)*
- a. Use back up contraceptive
- b. Take 2 pills on the next 2 days
- c. Continue taking single pill per day
- d. Both a and b

[Ref: Dutta's Obstetrics 8th/e p. 624; Speroff's gynecology – Section III- contraception-]

Explanation

If 2 pills are missed

- In first 2 weeks – take 2 pills daily for 2 days and then finish the pack + use of back up method advised for 7 days.

- During 3rd week – 2 options –
  - Start new pack and use back up method immediately and for 7 days, or
  - Take daily pill upto next Sunday and then start new pack and use back up method immediately and for 7 days.

28. OCP causes? *(PGMEE 2015; Nov 13 Pattern)*
- a. Simple hyperplasia
- b. Atypical hyperplasia
- c. Endometrial proliferation
- d. Endometrial atrophy

[Ref: speroff 8the p.974; Endometrial cytology with tissue correlations-John A. Maksem, Stanley J. Robby, John W. Bishop p. 94]

29. OCP does not prevent? *(PGMEE 2015; Nov 13 Pattern)*
- a. Breast cancer
- b. Endometrial cancer
- c. Ovarian cancer
- d. Ovarian cysts

[Ref: D. C. Dutta's Textbook of gynaecology, 7th/e, P401; Novak's gynae 14th/e p. 275]

30. OC pills decrease the risk of- *(PGMEE 2012-13)*
- a. Stroke
- b. CVD
- c. Endometrial ca
- d. Hepatic adenoma

[Ref: D. C. Dutta's Textbook of gynaecology, 7th/e, P401]

31. Side effects of oral contraceptive pills are all except: *(Recent Pattern June 2018)*
- a. Weight gain
- b. Breast discomfort
- c. Ovarian malignancy
- d. DVT

[Ref: D. C. Dutta's Textbook of gynaecology, 7th/e, P401; Novak's gynae 14th/e p. 275]

Explanation

Adverse effects of OCPs

- Nausea, vomiting, headache (migraine may be worsened).
- Breakthrough bleeding or spotting, Amenorrhoea o Breast discomfort (mastalgia)
- Weight gain, acne and increased body hair.
- Chloasma, pruritus vulvae
- Carbohydrate intolerance
- Mood swing, abdominal distention (especially with mini pill)
- Leg vein and pulmonary thrombosis.
- Coronary & cerebral thrombosis → MI, stroke , Estrogen component is responsible for venous thromboembolism.
- Both estrogen and progesterone are responsible for the arterial phenomena.

32. OC pills must be started on- *(PGMEE 2012-13)*
- a. 5th day
- b. 3rd day
- c. 1st day
- d. When menses cease

[Ref: D. C. Dutta's Textbook of gynaecology, 7th/e, P399]

33. Non-contraceptive metabolic effect of estrogen are all except- *(PGMEE 2012-13)*
- a. Increased fatty acids
- b. Increased plasma lipid and lipoproteins
- c. Increased total cholesterol
- d. Decreased HDL

[Ref: D. C. Dutta's Textbook of gynaecology, 7th/e, P402]

21.	a
22.	a
23.	d
24.	a
25.	d
26.	b
27.	a
28.	d
29.	a
30.	c
31.	c
32.	c
33.	d

34. OCPs are contraindicated in? *(PGMEE 2011)*
a. Heart disease b. Breast cancer
c. Thromboembolism d. All of the above

[Ref: Shaw's Textbook of Gynaecology, 15th/e, P. 232;[Ref: D. C. Dutta's Textbook of gynaecology, 7th/e, P401;Jeffcoate's Principles of Gynaecology, 7th/e, P. 801-804;Berek & Novak's Gynecology, 15th/e, P. 215]

35. Which of the following is an absolute contraindication to OCP use: *(PGMEE 2019)*
a. Chronic renal disease
b. DVT
c. Diabetes mellitus
d. History of amenorrhea

[Ref: Shaw's Textbook of Gynaecology, 15th/e, P. 232;[Ref: D. C. Dutta's Textbook of gynaecology, 7th/e, P401;Jeffcoate's Principles of Gynaecology, 7th/e, P. 801-804;Berek & Novak's Gynecology, 15th/e, P. 215]

36. Least failure rate is of- *(PGMEE 2012-13)*
a. OC pills b. IUDs
c. Condom d. DMPA

[Ref: D. C. Dutta's Textbook of gynaecology, 7th/e, P397,401; Speroff's gynecology – Section III- contraception and Berek & Novak's Gynecology 15th edition page 215.]

37. OCP decrease risk of - *(PGMEE 2012-13)*
a. Cervical ca b. Endometrial ca
c. Vaginal ca d. Liver carcinoma

[Ref: D. C. Dutta's Textbook of gynaecology, 7th/e, P401]

38. OC pills decrease risk of- *(PGMEE 2012-13)*
a. Stroke b. CVD
c. Endometrial ca d. Hepatic adenoma

[Ref: D. C. Dutta's Textbook of gynaecology, 7th/e, P401]

39. Which of the following causes OCP failure? *(PGMEE Nov. 12 Pattern)*
a. Carbamazepine b. Rifampicin
c. NSAIDS d. Ethambutol

[Ref: D. C. Dutta's Textbook of gynaecology, 7th/e, P400;KDT 7th/e p. 317]

40. Which of the following progesterones is preferred in combination with estrogen in Low dose Oral contraceptive pills- *(PGMEE 2011)*
a. Desogestrel b. Norethisterone
c. Norgestrel d. Levonorgestrel

[Ref: D. C. Dutta's Textbook of gynaecology, 7th/e, P398;Harrison's Endocrinology 2nd/e p. 199; CMDT 2011/e p. 743; Drug Benefits and Risk: International Textbook of clinical Pharmacology 2nd/e p. 462]

41. Which of the following methods of contraception should be avaoided in women with epilepsy- *(PGMEE 2011)*
a. Oral contraceptive pills
b. IUCD
c. Condoms
d. Diaphragm

[Ref: D. C. Dutta's Textbook of gynaecology, 7th/e, P400;Shaw's 13th/e p. 228; Berek & Novak's Gynaecology 14th/e p. 286; Wyllie's Treatment of Epilepsy: Principles & Practice (Lippincott Williams & Wilkins) 2010/e p. 657]

34.	d
35.	b
36.	a
37.	b
38.	c
39.	b
40.	a
41.	a
42.	a,c
43.	a
44.	a
45.	a
46.	d

42. Role of OCP in cervical cancer is-
a. Predisposes to squamous cell carcinoma of the cervix
b. Increases chances of Human Papilloma virus infection
c. Predisposes to adenocarcinoma of the endocervix
d. Has a preventive effect towards the carcinoma of cervix

[Ref: Speroff clinical endocrinology 8th e pg 996;CGDT 10th/e p. 834; Shaw Gynae 14th/e p.

CENTCHROMAN

43. Dose of centchroman is- *(PGMEE June 14 Pattern)*
a. 30 mg b. 60 mg
c. 90 mg d. 20 mg

[Ref: D. C. Dutta's Textbook of gynaecology, 7th/e, P415]

44. Centchroman is a? *(PGMEE 2009)*
a. Female oral contraceptive
b. Oxytocic
c. Tocolytic
d. Male contraceptive

[Ref: D. C. Dutta's Textbook of gynaecology, 7th/e, P415]

PROGESTERONE ONLY PILL (POP)

45. Progesterone only pills act by:- *(PGMEE 2018)*
a. Cervical mucous thickening
b. Prevention of implantation
c. Inhibition of ovulation
d. Interfering sperm motility

[Ref speroff 8th p.1037; d.c. dutta text book of gynecology p.403 7th]

Explanation

POP

- POP works mainly by making cervical mucous thick and viscous . thereby prevents sperm penentration. Endometrium becomes atrophic, so blastocyst implantation is also hindered. In about 2 % cases ovulation is inhibhited and 50% ovulate normally.
- After taking a progestin-only minipill, the small amount of progestin in the circulation (about 25% of that in combined oral contraceptives) will have a significant impact only on those tissues very sensitive to the female sex steroids, estrogen and progesterone. The contraceptive effect is more dependent on endometrial and cervical mucus effects, because gonadotropins are not consistently suppressed. The endometrium involutes and becomes hostile to implantation, and the cervical mucus becomes thick and impermeable. Approximately 40% of patients will ovulate normally. Tubal physiology may also be affected

46. Pelvic inflammatory Disease prevented by:- *(PGMEE 2016-17)*
a. Tubal block
b. IUC
c. Progesterone only pill
d. Condom

[Ref: D.C Dutta text book of gynaecology 7th e p403; Berek & Novak's Gynecology 15th edition page 219]

47. Which is not a side effect of POP (Progestin only pill)-
   (PGMEE 2015)
   a. Ectopic pregnancy
   b. Increased risk of diabetes mellitus
   c. Ovarian cysts
   d. Venous thromboembolism

[Ref: Dutta's Obstetrics 8th/e p. 627; Speroff's Clinical Gyanecologic Endocrinology and Infertility, 8th/e p. 1037]

48. Contraceptive of choice during lactation is-
   (PGMEE 2013-14)
   a. POP   b. PC pills
   c. IUD   d. Minena

[Ref: D. C. Dutta's Textbook of gynaecology, 7th/e, P403]

49. Minipill, side effect is-   **(PGMEE 2012-13)**
   a. Break through Bleeding
   b. PID
   c. Endometrial CA
   d. Thromboembolism

[Ref: D. C. Dutta's Textbook of gynaecology, 7th/e, P403]

50. Lactating mother OCP of choice-   **(PGMEE 2012-13)**
   a. Progestin only pil   b. Combined OCP
   c. Estrogen only pill   d. None

[Ref: D. C. Dutta's Textbook of gynaecology, 7th/e, P403]

51. Side effect of progesterone only pill are all except-
   (PGMEE 2012-13)
   a. Irregular bleeding   b. Amenorrhea
   c. Decreased lactation   d. Weight gain

[Ref: D. C. Dutta's Textbook of gynaecology, 7th/e, P403Shaw's Gynae 15th/e p. 233]

52. Progesterone only pill not given after- **(PGMEE 2012-13)**
   a. 24 hrs   b. 48 hrs
   c. 72 hrs   d. 96 hrs

[Ref: D.C. Dutta's Textbook of gynaecology, 7th/e, P403]

53. The most common side effect of POP (progesterone only pills) is?
   (PGMEE 2012)
   a. Hypertension   b. Irregular bleeding
   c. Acne   d. DVT

[Ref: Shaw's Textbook of Gynaecology, 15th/e, P. 233, Jeffcoate's Principles of Gynaecology, 7th/e, P. 811, [Ref: D. C. Dutta's Textbook of gynaecology, 7th/e, P403

INJECTABLE CONTRACEPTIVES AND IMPLANTS

54. DMPA 150 mg subcutaneous is to be repeated every:-
   (PGMEE 2016)
   a. 1 month   b. 2 months
   c. 3 months   d. 1 year

[Ref: D.C Dutta text book of gynaecology 7th e p403; From ROAMS 13th/e pg. 652]

55. Contraceptive failure is minimum with?
   (PGMEE Nov. 12 Pattern)
   a. Combined oral contraceptive
   b. Injectable hormonal contraceptive
   c. Hormonal IUCD
   d. Subdermal implant (Norplant]

[Ref: D. C. Dutta's Textbook of gynaecology, 7th/e, P404]

56. Which of the following is not an adverse effect of DMPA?
   (PGMEE Nov. 12 Pattern)
   a. Slight blood glucose elevation
   b. Disturbance of lactation
   c. PID
   d. Bone loss

[Ref: Speroff 8th e. p.1085]

57. Depot MPA (DMPA), all are true except
   (PGMEE 2012-13)
   a. Dysmenorrhea
   b. Dyslipidemia
   c. Do not prevent STDs
   d. Can be given in breast cancer

[Ref: D. C. Dutta's Textbook of gynaecology, 7th/e, P404; Shaw's Gynae 15th/e p. 234]

58. Duration of contraception after DMPA is-
   (PGMEE 2012-13)
   a. 21 months   b. 1-3 months
   c. 3-6 months   d. >6 months

[Ref: D. C. Dutta's Textbook of gynaecology, 7th/e, P404]

59. Long acting revesible contraceptives (LARC) are all except-   **(PGMEE 2015; Nov 13 Pattern)**
   a. Implanon   b. DMPA
   c. IUCD   d. OCPs

[Ref: D. C. Dutta's Textbook of gynaecology, 7th/e, P398, speroff 8th e p1059.

EMERGENCY CONTRACEPTION

60. Single dose of drug used in emergency contraception -
   a. Levonorgestrol 0.75 mg   **(PGMEE 2015)**
   b. Levonorgestral 1.5 mg
   c. Desogestrel 1.5 mg
   d. Ethinyl estradiol + levonorgestrel

[Ref: Shaw's Gyanecology 16th/e p. 279; Speroff's Clinical Endocrinology and Infertility 8th/e p. 1040]

61. Not an emergency contraception?   **(PGMEE 2013-14)**
   a. IUCD
   b. LNG
   c. Mifepristone
   d. Combined estrogen and progesterone

[Ref: D. C. Dutta's Textbook of gynaecology, 7th/e, P404 Shaw's Gynae 15th/e p. 551]

62. I pill is used when-   **(PGMEE 2012-13)**
   a. Accidental sexual exposure
   b. OCP forgotten
   c. Of choice in young
   d. All of the above

[Ref: D. C. Dutta's Textbook of gynaecology, 7th/e, P405]

63. Emergency contraceptive should must be started with in how much time after unprotected intercourse-
   (PGMEE 2012-13)
   a. 24 hrs   b. 48 hrs
   c. 72 hrs   d. 96 hrs

[Ref: D. C. Dutta's Textbook of gynaecology, 7th/e, P404]

47.	d
48.	a
49.	a
50.	a
51.	c
52.	a
53.	b
54.	c
55.	d
56.	b
57.	d
58.	c
59.	d
60.	b
61.	a
62.	a
63.	c

64. Emergency contraceptive contains? *(PGMEE 2009)*
  a. Estradiol
  b. Levonorgestrel
  c. PGE$_2$
  d. Estrone

  [Ref: D. C. Dutta's Textbook of gynaecology, 7th/e, P404

65. Following unprotected intercourse, Emergency Contraceptive levonorgestrel 0.75 mg is taken by the patient. What are the doses that she should take subsequently?
  a. 1 dose of 0.75 mg after 12 hours *(NEET Pattern 2017)*
  b. 2 dose of 0.75 mg after 12 hours
  c. 3 dose of 0.75 mg after 12 hours
  d. 4 dose of 0.75 mg after 12 hours

  [Ref: Dutta 7th e p. 405]

Explanation

■ **Levonorgestrel (e.**pills) 0.75 mg two doses given at 12 hrs interval. The two tablets 1.5 mg can be taken as a single dose also. The first dose should be taken within 72 hours may be taken up to 120 hrs.

STERILIZATION

66. Most common site of tubectomy is:- *(PGMEE 2016-17)*
  a. Isthumus
  b. Ampulla
  c. Interstitial
  d. Infudibular

  [Ref: D.C Dutta text book of gynaecology 7th ep.408]

67. Contraceptive failure rate of Pomeroy's method is? *(PGMEE Nov. 12 Pattern)*
  a. 1/1000 cases
  b. 2/1000 cases
  c. 3/1000 cases
  d. 4/1000 cases

  [Ref: speroff 8th p.912; Berek & Novak's Gynae 14th/e p. 287; Shaw's 13th/e p. 236]

68. Which of the following is not a ligation technique? *(PGMEE 14)*
  a. Irving
  b. Parkland
  c. Pomeroy
  d. Essure

  [Ref: D. C. Dutta's Textbook of gynaecology, 7th/e,p.416

69. Pomeroy technique is for- *(PGMEE 2012-13)*
  a. Tubal ligation
  b. Laprscopy
  c. Hysteroscopy
  d. Minilaparotomy

  [Ref: D. C. Dutta's Textbook of gynaecology, 7th/e,409

70. Maximum success of reversal after tubal ligation with- *(PGMEE 2012-13)*
  a. Cauterization
  b. Pomeroy's technique
  c. Clip method
  d. Fimbriectomy

  [Ref: speroff 8th e p.935]

71. Laparoscopic tubal ligation contraindication-
  a. Post partum state *(PGMEE 2012-13)*
  b. Post MTP
  c. Gynaecologic malignancies
  d. 3 pervious child birth

  [Ref: D. C. Dutta's Textbook of gynaecology, 7th/e,p.409]

72. Which one of the following techniques of tubectomy is depicted in the diagram below? *(PGMEE 2015)*

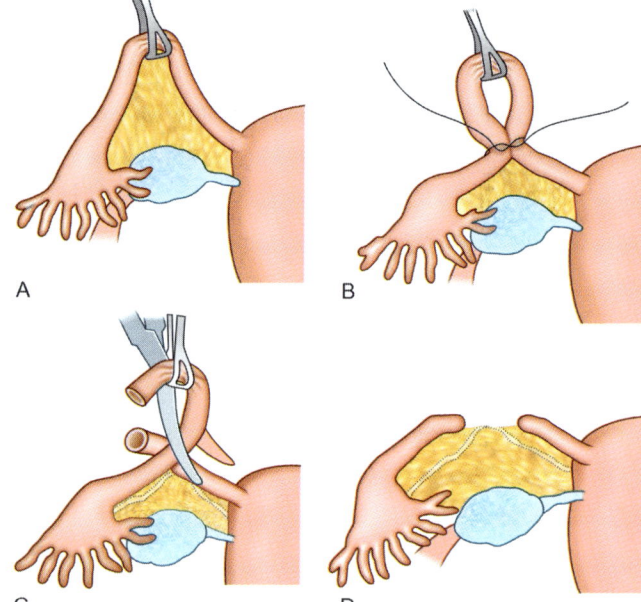

A   B

C   D

  a. Kroener technique
  b. Irving technique
  c. Pomeroy technique
  d. Uchida technique

  [Ref: D. C. Dutta's Textbook of gynaecology, 7th/e, 409, speroff 8th ep921

73. Technique in which fimbriectomy is done:- *(PGMEE 2018)*
  a. Uchida technique
  b. Irving's method
  c. Modified Pomeroy method
  d. Kroener

  [Ref: D.C. dutta text book of gynecology p.408-409 7th e; Speroff 8th e p.921-931]

Explanation

■ Fimbriectomy is done in *Kroener procedure* : ampullary end of tube is ligated and dissected .

■ *Pomeroy* : a loop is made by holding the tube by an allis forceps such a way that the major part of loop consist mainly of isthumuns and ampullary part . about 1-1.5 cm of loop is excised (Loop-ligate-cut)

■ *Modified Pomeroy* : Loop-ligate-cut and crush the end.

■ *Uchida* : a saline solution is injected subserosaly in the mid portion of tube to create bleb. The serous coat is incised along the antimesentric border to expose the muscular tube about 3-5 cm of tube is excised. The ligated proximal stump is buried beneath the serous coat. Distal stump is open in peritoneal cavity.

■ *Irving* : the tube is ligated on ethier side and mid ortion of tube is excised. The free medial end is turned back and buried in posterior uterine wall creating a myometrial tunnel.

■ *ESSURE*: Hysteroscopic tubal ligation with nickel titanium alloy.

64.	b
65.	a
66.	a
67.	d
68.	d
69.	d
70.	c
71.	a
72.	c
73.	d

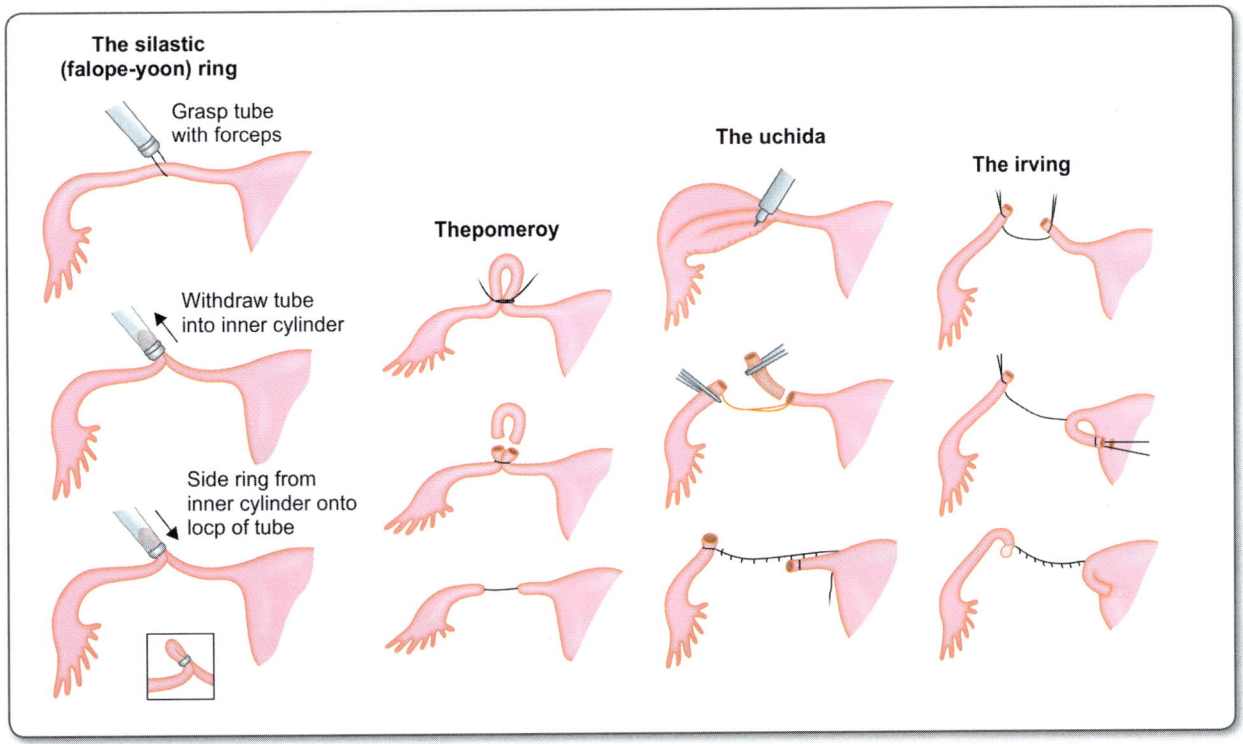

The silastic (falope-yoon) ring

Grasp tube with forceps

Withdraw tube into inner cylinder

Side ring from inner cylinder onto locp of tube

Thepomeroy

The uchida

The irving

BENIGN LESIONS OF VULVA AND VAGINA

1. In what condition does vulvectomy has to be performed sometimes- *(PGMEE 2012-13)*
   a. Granuloma inguinale
   b. Chlamydia trachomitis
   c. Herpes simplex
   d. Candidial infection

   [Ref: D.C Dutta text book of gynaecology 7th e p.124]

2. Lichen sclerosis of vulva false is *(PGMEE 2012-13)*
   a. It is infective
   b. Usually occurs in old age
   c. May b associated with autoimmune disease
   d. Due to decreased estrogen

   [Ref: D.C Dutta text book of gynaecologyp7th e.211 Shaw's Gynae 15th/e p. 124-125]

BENIGN LESIONS OF CERVIX

3. True about nabothian cyst all except- *(PGMEE 2015)*
   a. It is pre-malignant
   b. It is a pathology of the cervix
   c. It is seen in chronic irritation and inflammation
   d. Squamous epithelium occludes the mouth of the glands

   [Ref: Shaw's Textbook of Gyanecology 16th/e p. 172]

BENIGN LESIONS OF UTERUS

FIBROID

4. Red degeneration of fibroid is seen in:- *(PGMEE 2015)*
   a. First trimester   b. Second trimester
   c. Third trimester   d. Any of the above

   [Ref: D.C Dutta text book of gynaecology 7th ep.224]

5. Red degeneration of fibroid is seen in- *(PGMEE 2013-14)*
   a. Early pregnancy   b. Mid pregnancy
   c. Pueperium   d. Nulliparous women

   [Ref: D.C Dutta text book of gynaecology 7th ep.224]

6. Torsion of fibroid depends upon- *(PGMEE 2012-13)*
   a. Infection   b. Site of origin
   c. Both   d. None

   [Ref: D.C Dutta text book of gynaecology 7th e p.225; Shaw's Gynae 15th/e p. 355-356]

7. Most common degeneration of fibroids- *(PGMEE 2012-13)*
   a. Calcareous   b. Hyaline
   c. Red   d. Cystic

   [Ref: D.C Dutta text book of gynaecology 7th e p.224; Jeffcoate 7th/e p. 501]

8. Pain in fibroid is due to all except: *(PGMEE 2011)*
   a. Red degeneration
   b. Sarcomatous degeneration
   c. Hyaline degeneration
   d. Torsion

   [Ref: D. C. Dutta's Textbook of gynaecology, 7th/e, P224; Shaw's Textbook of Gynaecology, 15th/e, P. 353-355; Jeffcoate's Principles of Gynaecology, 7th/e, P. 500-502]

9. Fibroid uterus may present with all of the following except- *(PGMEE 2007)*
   a. Amenorrhoea   b. Pelvic mass
   c. Infertility   d. Polymenorrhea

   [Ref: D.C Dutta text book of gynaecology 7th ep.225; Shaws 15th/e p. 356]

10. A 40 year old female presents with history of abnormal uterine bleeding underwent hysterectomy. Post hysterectomy specimen is shown below. Most likely diagnosis is:- *(PGMEE 2018)*
   a. Lipoma   b. Endometrial carcinoma
   c. Adenomyosis   d. Leiomyoma

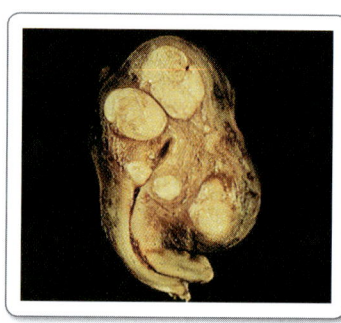

11. Treatment of choice of a 28 weeks pregnant female with pain due to fibroid of fundus of size 10 × 10 cm is? *(PGMEE Pattern 2015)*
   a. Myomectomy   b. Hysterectomy
   c. Conservative   d. Arterial embolization

   [Ref: D.C Dutta text book of gynaecology 7th ep.224]

12. 45 years female with 3 months menorrhagia. USG showing 2 cm submucosal fibroid. First line of management is: *(PGMEE Jan 2019)*
   a. Ocp for 3 months
   b. Progesterone for 3 months
   c. Endometrial sampling
   d. Hysterectomy

   [Ref: Williams gynecology 3rd/e pg. 184]

13. Treatment of choice of a 28 weeks pregnant female with pain due to fibroid of fundus of size 10 × 10cm is? *(PGMEE Pattern 2015)*
   a. Myomectomy   b. Hysterectomy
   c. Conservative   d. Arterial embolization

   [Ref: D.C Dutta text book of gynaecology 7th ep.224]

1.	a
2.	a
3.	a
4.	b
5.	b
6.	b
7.	b
8.	c
9.	a
10.	d
11.	c
12.	c
13.	c

14. **Drugs given for fibroid-** *(PGMEE 2013-14)*
    a. GnRH agonist
    b. Multivitamins
    c. Mesoprost
    d. Isoxsuprine hydrochloride

    [Ref: D.C Dutta text book of gynaecology 7th ep. 229; Shaw's Gynae 15th/e p. 359]

BENIGN LESIONS OF OVARY

15. **Ovarian fibroma develops from?** *(PGMEE Pattern 2015)*
    a. Germ cells
    b. Sex cord
    c. Epithelium
    d. Stroma

    [Ref: D.C Dutta text book of gynaecology 7th ep.237]

16. **Most common complication of dermoid cyst is-** *(PGMEE 2015)*
    a. Malignant degeneration
    b. Torsion
    c. Cyst Rupture
    d. None of the above

    [Ref: Shaw's Gynaecology 16th/e p. 439, William's Gynaecology 2nd/e p. 267]

17. **Meig syndrome is associated with-** *(PGMEE 2013-14)*
    a. Brenner tumor
    b. Fibroma
    c. Choriocarcinoma
    d. Teratoma

    [Ref: D.C Dutta text book of gynaecology 7th ep.241;Shaw's Gynae 15th/e p. 381]

CHAPTER-4 ● BENIGN DISORDER OF REPRODUCTIVE TRACT

14.	a
15.	d
16.	b
17.	b

CERVIX

1. **Most common cause of Cervical neoplasia is?**
   a. HPV-6   b. HPV-11   *(PGMEE 2015)*
   c. HPV-16   d. HHV

   [Ref: https://aidsinfo.nih.gov/guidelines/html/]

2. **100/0/0 maturation index denotes**   *(PGMEE 2015)*
   a. Atrophic smear
   b. Pregnancy
   c. Reproductive age female
   d. None

   [Ref: Dutta Gyne 4th ed:105]

3. **Most common chemotherapeutic agent used in cervical cancer:-**   *(PGMEE 2016-17)*
   a. Etoposide   b. Cisplatin
   c. Ironotecan   d. Methotrexate

   [Ref: Harrison's 19th/e pg. 596]

4. **How many years once pap smear done in female accoprding to ACOG 2013 guidelines:** *(PGMEE 2016-17)*
   a. Cervical cancer screening should start at age 21 yrs
   b. Women 21-29 yrs pap test every 3 yrs
   c. Women 30-65 paptest and HPV test (cotesting]every 5yrs or pap alone every 3yrs
   d. None

   [Ref: Internet]

5. **Gardasil vaccine used to prevent:-**   *(PGMEE 2016-17)*
   a. Ca of cervix   b. Breast ca
   c. Colon ca   d. Ovary ca

   [Ref: D.C Dutta text book of gynaecology 7th e p268]

6. **Gardasil vaccine for HPV contains which strains of virus?**   *(PGMEE 2015)*
   a. HPV 6, 11   b. HPV 6, 11, 16, 18
   c. HPV 16, 18   d. HPV 16, 18, 31, 33

   [Ref: Shaw's Gynaecology 16th/e p. 495]

7. **Treatment options for CIN III include all of the following except-**   *(PGMEE 2015)*
   a. Hysterectomy
   b. Wertheim's hysterectomy
   c. LLETZ
   d. Conization

   [Ref: Shaw's Gynaecology 16th/e p. 494]

8. **40 yr female with abnormal cervical cytology, pap smear suggestive of CIN III, next step in management is-**
   a. Surgery with adjuvant chemoradiation *(PGMEE 2015)*
   b. Colposcopy and biopsy
   c. Test for HPV and follow up after 3 months
   d. Hysterectomy

   [Ref: Shaw's Gyanecology 16th/e p. 485]

9. **Green filter is used to visualize the following in colposcopy:-**   *(PGMEE 2015)*
   a. Necrotic areas
   b. Measure actual size of lesion
   c. Vascular pattern of cervix
   d. None of the above

   [Ref: Advanced health assessment of women By Helen 2nd/e p. 531]

10. **Magnification obtained by colposcopy is-**   *(PGMEE 2013-14)*
    a. 1-2 times   b. 2-5 times
    c. 15-25 times   d. 10-20 times

    [Ref: D.C Dutta text book of gynaecology 7th e p.93]

11. **A 35-year-old multiparous woman came with post coital bleeding. What is the next step.?**   *(NEET Pattern 2017)*
    a. Pap smear   b. Cryotherapy
    c. Cone biopsy   d. 4 quadrant biopsy

    [Ref: Berek and Hacker's G. Oncology 15th e p.]

Explanation

- Pap smear is the initial screening method for pre invasive cervical lesions.
- After getting pap smear report, the patient can undergo HPV DNA testing, colposcopy, or may require to repeat the Pap smear.
- If on initial examination the patient has a grossly visible lesion, cervical biopsy may be taken at the junction of the lesion and normal cervical tissue.
- *Cryotherapy:* Women with persistent cervical discharge in whom pre invasive lesions have been ruled out, who have received antibiotic therapy.
- *Cone Boiopsy (Conization):* Performed in women with cervical intra epithelial neoplasia as a diagnostic procedure to rule out invasive cancer which cannot be seen with a simple biopsy.
- *4 quadrant biopsy:* Done in colposcopy with abnormal findings (diffuse aceto-white or reduced iodine uptake areas) but no definite lesion. Colposcopy should be done in women with unexplained post coital bleeding or discharge not responding to antibiotic therapy.

12. **A 38 year old female's pap smear shows HSIL. What will be the next step?**   *(PGMEE 2013)*
    a. Repeat pap   b. Colposcopy
    c. Currentage   d. Hysterectomy

    [Ref: Shaw's Gyanecology 16th/e p. 485]

13. **PAP smear from cervix shows HSIL grade CIN, next step is-**   *(PGMEE 2012-13)*
    a. Coagulation   b. Conization
    c. Colposcopy & biopsy   d. Cryosurgery

    [Ref: D.C Dutta text book of gynaecology 7th e p.267; Shaw's Gynae 15th/e p. 470]

1.	c
2.	a
3.	b
4.	b
5.	a
6.	b
7.	b
8.	b
9.	c
10.	c
11.	a
12.	b
13.	c

14. Cervical cytology smear reveal CIN2- next step-
(PGMEE 2012-13)

a. Colposcopy
b. Cryocautery
c. Hysterectomy
d. Laser ablation

[Ref: D.C Dutta text book of gynaecology 7th e p.267; Shaw's Gynae 15th/e p. 404]

15. HPV infects first which cells in cervix- *(PGMEE 2012-13)*

a. Basal and parabasal cells
b. Corneal cells
c. Granulosa cell
d. Spinus cells

[Ref: D.C Dutta text book of gynaecology 7th e p.265;Shaw's Gynae 15th/e p. 84; Internet]

16. Unsatisfactory colposcopy refes to failure to visualize:
(PGMEE 2010)

a. Fallopian tubes
b. Transformation zone
c. Fornices
d. Ectocervix

[Ref: D. C. Dutta's Textbook of gynaecology, 7th/e, P94;Shaw's Textbook of Gynaecology, 15th/e, P. 85, 403, 497-499; Berek & Novak's Gynecology, 15th/e, P. 575-579

UTERUS

17. Treatment of simple hyperplasia of endometrium is-
(PGMEE 2013-14)

a. Progesterone
b. Estrogen
c. Hysterectomy
d. Cryosurgery

[Ref: D. C. Dutta's Textbook of gynaecology, 7th/e, P271]

CARCINOMA VULVA

18. Most common malignancy of vulva is- *(PGMEE 2015)*

a. Squamous cell carcinoma
b. Melanoma
c. Bartolin's gland tumor
d. Adenocarcinoma

[Ref: D. C. Dutta's Textbook of gynaecology, 7th/e, P275; Shaw's Gyane 16th/e p. 478; Berek & Novak's Gyane 15th/e p. 1432]

19. Predisposing factor for Carcinoma vulva are all except:

a. Smoking
(PGMEE 2015)
b. Human papilloma virus (HPV) infection
c. Fibroepithelial polyps
d. Leukoplakia

[Ref: Robbins 9th/e pg. 997]

20. Most common extra-mammary site of Paget's disease:-
(PGMEE 2018)

a. Vagina
b. Vulva
c. Uterus
d. Fallopian tubes

Ref : D.C. Dutta text book of gynecology p.212 7th e

Explanation

- Extramammary pagets disease of vulva is a rare condition seen in postmenopausal female. It present with pruritus. On examination, the lesion appears florid ,eczematous with erythem and excoriation. It can be associated with underlying adenocarcinoma of GI tract, urinary tract and the breast. Treatment is surgical excision.

21. True regarding vulval cancer is all except-*(PGMEE 2015)*

a. HPV virus is causative factor
b. Iliac group of nodes are primary site of metastasis
c. Smoking is a risk factor
d. Vulectomy is the treatment for Bowen's disease

[Ref: D. C. Dutta's Textbook of gynaecology, 7th/e, P275-6; Shaw's Gyanecology 16th/e p. 478]

22. First symptom of vulval cancer is-
(PGMEE Pattern 2015)

a. Ulcerated lesion
b. White discharge
c. Mass in the groin
d. Pruritis

[Ref: D. C. Dutta's Textbook of gynaecology, 7th/e, P275; Shaw's Gyane 16th/e p. 475; berek & Novak's Gyanecology 15th/e p. 1432]

23. Vulval carcinoma accounts for what percentage of genital tract malignancies? *(PGMEE 2015)*

a. 0.5-1%
b. 3-5%
c. 7-11%
d. 13-15%

[Ref: D. C. Dutta's Textbook of gynaecology, 7th/e, P274]

24. Uethral involvement of Vulval carcinoma without inguino femoral nodes is seen in?
(PGMEE Pattern 2015)

a. Stage I
b. Stage II
c. Stage III
d. Stage IV

[Ref: D. C. Dutta's Textbook of gynaecology, 7th/e, P276]

25. Uethral involvement of Vulval carcinoma with inguino femoral nodes is seen in? *(PGMEE Pattern 2015)*

a. Stage I
b. Stage II
c. Stage III
d. Stage IV

[Ref: D. C. Dutta's Textbook of gynaecology, 7th/e, P276]

26. Treatement of choice of early vulvar carcinoma is?
(PGMEE Pattern 2015)

a. Radiotherapy
b. Hormone therapy
c. Radical vulvectomy
d. Chemotherapy

[Ref: D. C. Dutta's Textbook of gynaecology, 7th/e, P277]

27. Vulval carcinoma treatment during early stage:
(Recent Pattern June 2018)

a. Radiotherapy
b. Chemotherapy
c. Surgery
d. None of the above

[Ref: D. C. Dutta's Textbook of gynaecology, 7th/e, P277]

Explanation

- Treatment of choice of early vulvar radical vuivectomy.
- Radiation therapy and chemotherapy may be used if the cancer cannot be entirely removed with surgery, if the cancer has a high risk for recurrence, and/or if the lymph nodes are involved with cancer.

CARCINOMA VAGINA

28. Sarcoma botryoides in vagina is seen in which age-
(PGMEE 2012-13)

a. Less than 8 yrs
b. 8-16 yrs
c. 16-24 yrs
d. > 24 yrs

[Ref: D.C Dutta text book of gynaecology 7th e p.323]

14.	a
15.	a
16.	b
17.	a
18.	a
19.	c
20.	b
21.	b
22.	d
23.	b
24.	b
25.	c
26.	c
27.	c
28.	a

58. Cervical cancer 4mm deep invasion and 7 mm spread, stage is- *(PGMEE 2012-13)*
- a. IA
- b. IA 1
- c. IA 2
- d. IB

[Ref: D.C Dutta text book of gynaecology 7th e p.282;Shaw's Gynae 15th/e p. 412]

59. Ca cervix staging done by- *(PGMEE 2012-13)*
- a. CT
- b. MRI
- c. Clinical findings
- d. Histopathology

[Ref: D.C Dutta text book of gynaecology 7th e p.281; Shaw's Gynae 15th/e p. 409]

60. Treatment of stage IIB of cervix is- *(PGMEE 2012-13)*
- a. Chemoradiation
- b. Hysterectomy
- c. Radiation
- d. Chemotherapy

[Ref: D.C Dutta text book of gynaecology 7th e p.290;Shaw's Gynae 15th/e p. 415]

61. Radiation to point A in cervix is- *(PGMEE 2012-13)*
- a. 8000 rad
- b. 6000 rad
- c. 10000 rad
- d. 4000 rad

[Ref: D.C Dutta text book of gynaecology 7th e p.289;Shaw's Gynae 15th/e p. 436]

62. A women is diagnosed with cervical carcinoma stage 2b, treatment of choice is- *(PGMEE 2012-13)*
- a. Hysterectomy
- b. Chemoradiation
- c. Primary radiation
- d. None of the above

[Ref: D.C Dutta text book of gynaecology 7th e p.290;Shaw's Gynae 15th/e p. 414]

63. In Brachytherapy for Carcinoma cervix, dose of radiation at point A is? *(PGMEE 2013)*
- a. 1000 rad
- b. 4000 rad
- c. 8000 rad
- d. 10000 rad

[Ref: D. C. Dutta's Textbook of gynaecology, 7th/e, P289; Novak's gynaw 13th/e ch. 31]

64. Rate limiting dose of radiotherapy to rectum and bladder in gynaecologic malignacies- *(PGMEE 2012-13)*
- a. 4000cGy
- b. 5000cGy
- c. 6000cGy
- d. 7000cGy

[Ref: Shaw's Gynae 15th/e p. 438]

65. Ca cervix IIIB is treatment of choice is: *(PGMEE 2012-13)*
- a. Radiotherapy
- b. Chemotherapy
- c. Chemoradiation
- d. Surgery

[Ref: D.C Dutta text book of gynaecology 7th e p.290; Shaw's Gynae 15th/e p. 414]

66. Vaccine preventable cancer is? *(PGMEE 2012)*
- a. Ovarian cancer
- b. Breast cancer
- c. Cancer cervix
- d. Endometrial cancer

[Ref: D.C Dutta text book of gynaecology 7th e p.268; Novak's gynae 15th/e Chapter 19 p. 581]

67. A case of carcinoma cervix who earlier received radiotherapy, relapses with new lesion, what should be the next line of management? *(PGMEE 2010)*
- a. Repeat radiotherapy
- b. Complete hysterectomy
- c. Pelvic exenteration
- d. Chemotherapy

[Ref: Shaw's Textbook of Gynaecology, 15th/e, P. 415, 438-439 Jeffcoate's Principles of Gynaecology, 8th/e, P. 443-444, 449-450]

68. About vaccination for carcinoma cervix, all are true EXCEPT: *(PGMEE 2010)*
- a. Does not require further examinations
- b. Administered intramuscularly at 0, 2 and 6 months
- c. Bivalent vaccine is more efficient than Quadrivalent
- d. Can be taken with other live vaccines at different site

[Ref: D. C. Dutta's Textbook of gynaecology, 7th/e, P268; Shaw's Textbook of Gynaecology, 15th/e, P. 406-407 Berek & Novak's Gynecology, 15th/e, P. 581-582; Progress in Obstetrics & Gynaecology, John Studd, Vol. 18, Ch. 19, P. 293-295]

69. Most commonly associated human papilloma virus with cancer cervix is? *(PGMEE 2011)*
- a. HPV 16
- b. HPV 24
- c. HPV 32
- d. HPV 36

[Ref: D. C. Dutta's Textbook of gynaecology, 7th/e, P265]

70. Koilocytes with perinuclear halo on pap smear is pathognomonic of? *(PGMEE 2010)*
- a. HPV infection
- b. Bacterial vaginosis
- c. Dysplasia
- d. Metaplasia

[Ref: D. C. Dutta's Textbook of gynaecology, 7th/e, P265]

71. Management of stage II$_B$ cancer cervix is? *(PGMEE 2009)*
- a. Hysterectomy
- b. Radiotherapy in combination with chemotherapy
- c. Chemotherapy
- d. Radiotherapy

[Ref: D. C. Dutta's Textbook of gynaecology, 7th/e, P290]

CARCINOMA ENDOMETRIUM

72. Which histopathological variant of endometrial malignancy has the poorest prognosis:- *(PGMEE 2016-17)*
- a. Clear cell carcinoma
- b. Adenocarcinoma
- c. Adenosquamous CA
- d. Mucinous adenocarcinoma

[Ref: D.C Dutta text book of gynaecology 7th e p293]

73. Most common histological subtype of cancer endometrium is? *(PGMEE Pattern 2015)*
- a. Endometrioid adenocarcinoma
- b. Mucinous carcinoma
- c. Clear cell carcinoma
- d. Squamous cell carcinoma

[Ref: D. C. Dutta's Textbook of gynaecology, 7th/e, P293]

74. Treatment of stage –I endometrial carcinoma is? *(PGMEE Pattern 2015)*
- a. Radiotherapy
- b. Chemotherapy
- c. Hormone therapy
- d. Surgery

[Ref: D. C. Dutta's Textbook of gynaecology, 7th/e, P296]

75. Most common histological variety of uterine carcinoma is? *(PGMEE 2014)*
- a. Squamous cell carcinoma
- b. Columnar cell carcinoma
- c. Adeno carcinoma
- d. Mixed carcinoma

[Ref: D. C. Dutta's Textbook of gynaecology, 7th/e, P293]

58.	c
59.	c
60.	a
61.	a
62.	b
63.	c
64.	b
65.	c
66.	c
67.	c
68.	a
69.	a
70.	a
71.	b
72.	a
73.	a
74.	d
75.	c

76. Serous carcinoma of endometrium is associated with which mutation? *(PGMEE Aug 13 Pattern)*

a. p53   b. PTEN
c. K ras   d. p 16k

[Ref: D.C Dutta text book of gynaecology 7th e p.294; Robbin's 8th/e p. 1034]

77. Carcinoma endometrium is not associated with- *(PGMEE 2011-2013)*

a. Fibromyoma   b. Dysgerminoma
c. Granulosa cell tumor   d. Endometrial hyperplasia

[Ref: D.C Dutta text book of gynaecology 7th e p.294; Shaw's Textbook of Gynaecology, 15th/e, P. 378, 380, 416-418; Jeffcoate's Principles of Gynaecology, 8th/e, P. 473, 500, 501, 507]

78. Staging of endometrial ca with involvement of paraaortic lymph node involvement- *(PGMEE 2012-13)*

a. IIIC   b. IIB
c. IIIA   d. IIIB

[Ref: D.C Dutta text book of gynaecology 7th e p.295 Shaw's Gynae 15th/e p. 420]

79. Endometrial carcinoma involving cervix, stage is- *(PGMEE 2012-13)*

a. 1   b. 2
c. 3   d. 4

[Ref: D.C Dutta text book of gynaecology 7th e p.295 Shaw's Gynae 15th/e p. 420]

80. The following are risk factors for carcinoma endometrium EXCEPT- *(PGMEE 2012)*

a. Early menopause
b. Endometrial cell carcinoma
c. Nulliparity   d. Obesity

[Ref: D.C Dutta text book of gynaecology 7th e p.294; Shaw's Gynecology 15th/e p. 420]

81. A 53-year post-menopausal female, with endometrial hyperplasia with atypia what is the management.

a. Hysterectomy (Type I)   *(NEET Pattern 2017)*
b. Progesterone
c. MIRENA
d. Endometrial

[Ref: Dutta 7th e p.271-272]

Explanation

- In young premenopausal patients with endometrial hyperplasia
  - Without atypia : cyclic progestogen therapy for 6 to 9 months
  - With atypia : therapy with progestin for 6 to 9 months. Periodic endometrial sampling every 3 months is essential. Hysterectomy is best treatment at any age with atypical endometrial hyperplasia because of risk of invasive cancer.(ACOG)
- In perimenopausal and postmenopausal women
  - Hyperplasia with atypia : hysterectomy with bilateral salpingo-oophorectomy.
  - Hyperplasia without atypia : continuous progestin therapy may be considered. However , hysterectomy with bilateral salpingo-oophorectomy is done as an alternative as isk of carcinoma increases with age.

OVARIAN TUMOURS

CA OVARY

82. M/C ovarian cancer with menorrhagia: *(PGMEE 2016-17)*

a. Sex cord tumors   b. Germ cell tumors
c. Epithelial cell tumors   d. None

[Ref: D.C Dutta text book of gynaecology 7th e p316-317]

83. AFP is a marker of:- *(PGMEE 2016-17)*

a. Liver cancer   b. Yolk sac cancer
c. Pancreas cancer   d. Dysgerminoma

[Ref: D.C Dutta text book of gynaecology 7th e p 316]

84. All are Sex cord stromal tumor except:- *(PGMEE 2016)*

a. Granulosa cell tumor   b. Leydig cell tumor
c. Yolk sac tumor   d. Thecoma

[Ref: D.C Dutta text book of gynaecology 7th e p 316]

85. Call exner body seen in:- *(PGMEE 2012-17)*

a. Granulosa cell tumor   b. dysgerminoma
c. Volk sac tumor   d. Sertoli-leydig cell tumor

[Ref: D.C Dutta text book of gynaecology 7th e p 316]

86. Call Exner bodies are seen in: *(PGMEE 2012-17)*

a. Dysgerminoma
b. Mucinous cystadenoma
c. Sex cord stromal tumour
d. Yolk sac tumour

[Ref: D.C Dutta text book of gynaecology 7th e p 316; Robbins 9th/e pg. 1029]

87. A lady with abdominal mass was investigated. On surgery, she was found to have b/l ovarian masses with smooth surface. On microscopy they revealed mucin secreting cells with signet ring shapes. What is your diagnosis? *(PGMEE 2015)*

a. Dysgerminoma
b. Krukenberg tumour
c. Primary Adenocarcinoma of the ovaries
d. Dermoid cyst

[Ref: Robbins Pathology 9th Ed/Pg 1032; Robbins Pathology 8th ED/PG 1050; Shaw's Textbook of Gynaecology 15/e pg 425]

88. One of the following is a germ cell tumor of ovary: *(PGMEE 2015-2016)*

a. Granulosa cell tumor   b. Mucinous cystadenoma
c. Brenner tumor   d. Benign cystic teratoma

[Ref: Robbins 9th/e pg. 1023]

89. Rokitansky protuberance is associated with which of the following tumor of ovary: *(PGMEE 2016-17)*

a. Dysgerminoma   b. Mucinous cystadenoma
c. Sex cord stromal tumour d. Mature teratoma

[Ref: Robbins 9th/e pg. 1029]

90. Which of these tumors is unique to pregnancy? *(PGMEE 2015)*

a. Luteoma   b. Serous cystadenoma
c. mucinous cystadenoma d. Teratoma

[Ref: Robbins 9th/e pg. 1044-1070]

76.	a
77.	b
78.	a
79.	b
80.	a
81.	a
82.	a
83.	b
84.	c
85.	a
86.	c
87.	b
88.	d
89.	d
90.	a

91. Most common ovarian tumor in pregnancy is?
(PGMEE 2015)
a. Dermoid cyst
b. Serous cysyadenoma
c. Gonadoblastoma
d. Theca cell tumor

[Ref: Shaw's 16th/e p. 439]

92. Not an epithelial cancer of ovary- *(PGMEE 2015)*
a. Granulosa cell tumor
b. Choriocarnioma
c. Teratoma
d. Endodermal sinus tumor

[Ref: D. C. Dutta's Textbook of gynaecology, 7th/e, P237]

93. AFP is raised in- *(PGMEE 2015)*
a. Choriocarcinoma
b. Endodermal sinus tumor
c. Teratoma
d. Dysgerminoma

[Ref: D.C.Dutta's Textbook of gynaecology, 7th/e, P315;Shaw's Textbook of Gynaecology 16th/e p. 522]

94. Sex cord ovarian tumors are all except- *(PGMEE 2015)*
a. Thecoma
b. Sertoli – Leydig cell tumors
c. Teratoma
d. Granulosa cell tumors

[Ref: D. C. Dutta's Textbook of gynaecology, 7th/e, P237]

95. Torsion as a complication is seen with which tumor-
(PGMEE 2015)
a. Dysgerminoma
b. Teratoma
c. Serous cystadenoma
d. Granulosa cell tumor

[Ref: D. C. Dutta's Textbook of gynaecology, 7th/e, P240; Shaw's Gynaecology 16th/e p. 445; Break and Novak's Gynaecology 15th/e p. 1457]

96. Cut-off value for Ca-125 is? *(PGMEE Pattern 2015)*
a. 15 units/ml
b. 25 units/ml
c. 35 units/ml
d. 45 units/ml

[Ref: D. C. Dutta's Textbook of gynaecology, 7th/e, P311]

97. Which of the following ovarian tumors is most radiosensitive- *(PGMEE 2015)*
a. Brenner tumor
b. Carcinoid
c. Serous CystadenoCA
d. Dysgerminoma

[Ref: D. C. Dutta's Textbook of gynaecology, 7th/e, P315; Shaw's Gynaecology 16th/e p. 441]

98. Bilateral ovarian carcinoma + capsule involvement + ascites + paraaortic LN. Identify the stage:- *(PGMEE 2013-14)*
a. 1C
b. 2C
c. 3C
d. 4C

[Ref: D.C Dutta text book of gynaecology 7th e p307; Shaw's Gynae 15th/e p. 427]

99. Best to defect early ovarian Ca- *(PGMEE 2013-14)*
a. CT
b. TCS
c. USG
d. X-ray pelvis

[Ref: D.C Dutta text book of gynaecology 7th e p 310; Shaw's Gynae 15th/e p. 427]

100. 51 yr f with abdominal mass & ascites. On H/P ovarian Ca is +ve for- *(PGMEE 2012-13)*
a. Ca 125
b. Ca 19-9
c. AFP
d. hCG

[Ref: D.C Dutta text book of gynaecology 7th e p311; Harrison 16th/e p. 554; Novak's 15th/e p. 1371]

91.	a
92.	a
93.	b
94.	c
95.	b
96.	c
97.	d
98.	c
99.	c
100.	a
101.	d
102.	d
103.	a
104.	c
105.	c

Explanation
- Women with BRCAI gene mutation have 45% lifetime risk of ovarian cancer and those with BRCAII mutation have 25% risk.
- These women should be screening annually with TVS and CA 125 testing, and prophylactic oophorectomy is recommended by age 35year whenever child bearing is completed b/c of the high risk of disease.
- Confusion clears after reading these lines: "For patients with genetic mutations predisposing them to increase risk, prophylactic oophorectomy is performed with or without mastectomy "as well".

101. Ovarian cancer drugs used are- *(PGMEE 2012-13)*
a. Paclitaxel + doxorubicin
b. Cisplatin + doxorubicin
c. Docetaxel + doxorubicin
d. Paclitaxel + cisplatin

[Ref: D. C. Dutta's Textbook of gynaecology, 7th/e, P312; Shaw's Gynae 15th/e p. 442]

102. Chemotherapy for epithelial ovarian carcinoma -
(PGMEE 2012-13)
a. BEC
b. CHOP
c. MOPP
d. None of the above

[Ref: Shaw's Gynae 15th/e p. 442]

[Ref: D.C Dutta text book of gynaecology 7th e p312]

103. Ca ovary with left supraclavicular LN, stageis-
a. IV
b. III *(PGMEE 2012-13)*
c. II
d. I

[Ref: D.C Dutta text book of gynaecology 7th e p307;Shaw's Gynae 15th/e p. 427]

104. Most common malignant ovarian tumor-
a. Dysgerminoma *(PGMEE 2012-13)*
b. Germ cell tumour
c. Serous cystadenocarcinoma
d. Yolk sac tuomour

[Ref: D.C Dutta text book of gynaecology 7th e p305;Shaw's Gynae 15th/e p. 374]

105. Pseudomyxoma peritonei is seen in which ovarian tumor- *(PGMEE 2012-13)*
a. Dysgerminoma
b. Germ cell tumour
c. Mucinous cystadenoma
d. Serous cystadenoma

[Ref: D.C Dutta text book of gynaecology 7th e p305;Shaw's Gynae 15th/e p. 374]

Explanation
- *Pseudomyxoma peritonei*
  Seen in mucinous cystadenoma. If tumour ruptures, it may lead to formation of pseudomyxoma peritonei & the viscera show extensive adhesions.
- Other causes are:
  - Rupture of mucocele of appendix
  - Mucinous ovarian cysts
  - Mucin secreting intestinal adeno carcinoma
  - Mucin secreting ovarian adenocarcinoma (Mucinous cystadenoma)
  - Colloid carcinoma of stomach/colon

106. Initial drug for ovarian cancer- *(PGMEE 2012-13)*
   a. Carboplatin
   b. Doxorubicin
   c. Ifosfamide
   d. Methotrexate

[Ref: D.C Dutta text book of gynaecology 7th e p312;Shaw's Gynae 15th/e p. 442]

107. True about dysgerminoma- *(PGMEE 2012-13)*
   a. Highly aggressive
   b. Managed conservatively in young girls
   c. Usually seen in old patients
   d. Secrets male sex hormones

[Ref: D.C Dutta text book of gynaecology 7th e p314-15; Shaw's Gynae 15th/e p. 378-379]

108. AFP is increased in which ovarian tumor-
   a. Choriocarcinoma *(PGMEE 2012-13)*
   b. Granulose cell tumour
   c. Sarcoma
   d. Endodermal sinus tumour

[Ref: D.C Dutta text book of gynaecology 7th e p315;Shaw's Gynae 15th/e p. 424]

109. Age group for dysgerminoma is- *(PGMEE 2012-13)*
   a. 10-20 yrs
   b. 30-40 yrs
   c. 50-60 yrs
   d. > 60 yrs

[Ref: D.C Dutta text book of gynaecology 7th e p314: Shaw's Gynae 15th/e p. 378]

110. MC ovarian tumors originate from- *(PGMEE 2012-13)*
   a. Mullerian epithelium
   b. Stroma
   c. Germ cells
   d. Connective tissue

[Ref: D.C Dutta text book of gynaecology 7th e p305;Shaw's text book of gynaecology 15th/e p. 373]

111. Recent biomarker for early detection of surface epithelial tumours of ovary- *(PGMEE 2012-13)*
   a. Ca 125,
   b. Ca 19-9
   c. Ca 15-5
   d. Osteopontin

[Ref: D.C Dutta text book of gynaecology 7th e p311; Harrison 16th/e p. 554; Novak's 15th/e p. 1371]

112. A unilateral ovarian tumor spreads to peritoneum but not to uterus. Its stage would be? *(PGMEE Aug 12 Pattern)*
   a. Stage IB
   b. Stage IC
   c. Stage IIA
   d. Stage IIB

[Ref: D.C Dutta text book of gynaecology 7th e p307]

113. What is the FIGO staging of carcinoma ovary with negative nodes, limited to true pelvic microscopic implants on peritoneal surface? *(PGMEE 2011)*
   a. III A
   b. III B
   c. III C
   d. None

[Ref: D. C. Dutta's Textbook of gynaecology, 7th/e, P307]

114. Bilateral ovarian carcinoma with breech in capsular wall with ascites peritoneal washings and positive cytology. What is the stage of the carcinoma?
   a. Ic *(PGMEE 2010)*
   b. IIc
   c. IIIc
   d. IVc

[Ref: D. C. Dutta's Textbook of gynaecology, 7th/e, P307]

115. Most common germ cell tumor ovary is? *(PGMEE 2009)*
   a. Dysgerminoma
   b. Dermoid
   c. Carcinoids
   d. Struma ovary

[Ref: D. C. Dutta's Textbook of gynaecology, 7th/e, P239

116. Drug used in ovarian carcinoma? *(PGMEE 2009)*
   a. Cisplatin
   b. Dacarbazine
   c. Cycloposphamide
   d. Methotrexate

[Ref: D. C. Dutta's Textbook of gynaecology, 7th/e, P312]

GESTATIONAL TROPHOBLASTIC DISEASE

117. A 30 yr old primigravida patient presents with PV bleeding at 14 wks of amenorrhoea. Fundal height was 24 cm. USG exam reveals snow storm appearance & both ovaries are cystic most likely cause: *(Recent Pattern June 2018)*
   a. Ovarian malignancy
   b. Molar pregnancy
   c. Fibroid
   d. Multiple pregnancy

[Ref: Dutta's Obs. 9th/e, pg. 182, 183; Holland Brew's Obs. 4th/e pg. 252]

Explanation

- The most benign form gestational trophoblastic neoplasia (GTN) is the hydatidiform mole.The diagnosis of GTN is greatly facilitated by ultrasonography.
- In the 1st trimester the entire uterine cavity is filled with more or less refringent masses and, almost always, a total absence of fetal signs.
- There is a USG appearance of "snowflakes", "television interference", "honeycombing" or "spicule-like radiation".

118. Partial mole is :- *(PGMEE 2016-17)*
   a. Diploid
   b. Triploid
   c. Gynogenesis
   d. Organs are not form at all

[Ref: Williams Obstetrics 24th e p.397From ROAMS 13th/e pg. 682]

119. Gestational Trophoblastic neoplasm does not include: *(PGMEE Jan 2019)*
   a. Choriocarcinoma
   b. Placental site trophoblastic tumour
   c. Invasive mole
   d. Partial mole

[Ref: Williams gynecology 3rd/e pg. 785]

120. Risk factors for molar gestation are all of the following except- *(PGMEE 2015)*
   a. Oriental countries
   b. Disturbed maternal immune mechanism
   c. Faculty nutrition
   d. Higher ratio of maternal/paternal chromosomes

[Ref: William's Obs 24th/e p. 397]

121. Common misdiagnosis of partial mole is- *(PGMEE 2015)*
   a. Ectopic pregnancy
   b. Choriocarcinoma
   c. Complete mole
   d. Threatened abortion

[Ref: Dutta's Obstetrics 8th/e p. 230]

106.	a
107.	b
108.	d
109.	a
110.	a
111.	a
112.	b
113.	a
114.	a
115.	b
116.	a
117.	b
118.	b
119.	d
120.	d
121.	d

122. True about placental site trophoblastic disease is-
a. Secretes human placental lactogen   *(PGMEE 2015)*
b. Highly Malignant behavior
c. Contains syncytiotroblasts mainly
d. Hysterectomy followed by chemoradiation is the treatment of choice.

[Ref: Shaw's Gyane 16th/e p. 313; Dutta's Obstetrics 8th/e p. 231]

123. A left side ovarian tumor with HCG 4 IU/L, Normal AFP, LDH raised. Which of the following is the most likely diagnosis?   *(NEET Pattern 2017)*
a. Dysgerminoma
b. Endodermal germ cell tumor
c. Mixed germ cell tumor
d. Teratoma   *[Ref: Dutta 7th e p.314-316]*

Explanation

- Dysgerminoma : tumor markers alpha feto orotein, HCG, lactate dehydrogenase may be positive .
- Endodermal sinus tumor: tumor marker alpha feto protein
- Mixed germ cell tumor : tumor markers HCG and AFP
- Teratoma : tumor marker AFP others are CA125, CA 19-9, CEA.

124. True about hydatidiform mole is:-   *(PGMEE 2015)*
a. Highest incidence in India
b. It is principally a disease of amnion
c. Embryo is present
d. Vesicle fluid is rich in hCG

[Ref: Dutta's Obs 7th/e p. 190]

125. Hydatidiform mole follow up reliable test: *(PGMEE 2015)*
a. Clinical examination   b. USG
c. Serum estradiol levesl   d. Beta HCG

[Ref: Williams obstetrics 24the p.400]

126. Poor prognostic factor for hydratidiform mole is-
a. WHO score > 8   *(PGMEE 2015)*
b. Prior molar pregnancy
c. No prior chemotherapy
d. Metastasis to lung

[Ref: Williams obstetrics 24th e p402; Dutta's Obstetrics 8th/e p. 221, Shaw's Gyanecology 16th/e p. 517]

127. In complete mole karyotype not seen-   *(PGMEE 2013-14)*
a. XXX chromosome   b. YYY
c. 46XX   d. 46XY

[Ref: Williams Obstetrics 24th e pg 397-398]

128. Chromosome number of partial hydatidiform mole is-   *(PGMEE 2019)*
a. 46 XX   b. 45 XO
c. 46 XXY   d. 69 XXX

[Ref: Williams Obs 25th/e pg. 5, 15]

129. Most common presenting feature of complete mole is-   *(PGMEE 2013-14)*
a. Vomiting   b. Amenorrhoea
c. Headache   d. Bleeding per vaginum

[Ref: Williams Obstetrics 24th e pg 398; Shaw's Gynae 15th/e p. 254, 255]

130. Androgenic XX chromosome is-   *(PGMEE 2013-14)*
a. Partial mole   b. Complete mole
c. Turner's syndrome   d. Stein leventhal syndrome

[Ref: Williams Obs 24th e pg 397-8 Dutta Obs 7th/e p. 191]

131. Partial mole is?   *(PGMEE Aug 13 Pattern)*
a. Haploid   b. Diploid
c. Triplod   d. Polyploid

[Ref: Williams Obstetrics 24th e pg 397;Danforth's obstetrics and hynecology 10th/e p. 1074; Dutta Obs 6th/e p. 200]

132. Most common site of metastasis in choriocarcinoma is?   *(PGMEE Aug 13 Pattern; june 2011)*
a. Liver   b. Lungs
c. Ovaries   d. Brain

[Ref: D.C Dutta text book of gynaecology 7th e p300; Shaw's 14th/e p. 233

133. Which is distinguishing feature of complete mole from partial mole-   *(PGMEE 2012-13)*
a. Hydropic changes in proliferating villi
b. Proliferation of blood vessels into villi
c. Mutation of p-57 gene in chorionic cells
d. Presence of fetus

[Ref: Dutta's Obs. 8th/e, pg. 230; Holland Brew's Obs.4th/e, pg. 250; Williams Obs., 23rd/e, pg. 258]

134. What distinguishes placental site trophoblastic tumor from choriocarcinoma-   *(PGMEE 2012-13)*
a. Low β hCG
b. Low β hCG and low HPL
c. High β hCG and low HPL
d. High β hCG and high HPL

[Ref: Dutta's Obs. 8th/e, pg. 231; Holland Brew's Obs.4th/e, pg. 254-255; Williams Obs., 23rd/e, pg. 262]

135. Partial mole, not true is:-   *(PGMEE 2012-13)*
a. Fetus is present
b. Diffuse trophoblastic hyperplesia
c. Theca lutein cysts uncommon
d. Uterine size is more than the period of amenorrhoea

[Ref: Dutta's Obs. 8th/e, pg. 224,230; Holland Brew's Obs.4th/e, pg. 250-251; Williams Obs., 23rd/e, pg. 258]

136. Karyotype of complete mole is?   *(PGMEE 2009, 2011,2012-13)*
a. 46XX   b. 46YY
c. 69 XXX   d. 69 XXY

[Ref: Dutta's Obs. 8th/e, pg. 222; Holland Brew's Obs.4th/e, pg. 250; Williams Obs., 23rd/e, pg. 258]

137. Choriocarcinoma diagnosis is by-   *(PGMEE 2012-13)*
a. USG   b. CT
c. MRI   d. X-RAY

[Ref: D.C Dutta text book of gynaecology 7th e p301;Dutta Obs 7th/e p. 193]

138. Chemotherapy for choriocarcinoma, DOC is-   *(PGMEE 2012-13)*
a. Methotrexate   b. Cyclophosphamide
c. Cisplatin   d. Doxorubicin

[Ref: D.C Dutta text book of gynaecology 7th e p302;Dutta Obs 7th/e p. 196]

122.	a
123.	a
124.	d
125.	d
126.	a
127.	a
128.	d
129.	d
130.	b
131.	c
132.	b
133.	a
134.	a
135.	b
136.	a
137.	a
138.	a

139. High risk gestational trophoblastic disease according to WHO is a pre treatment hCG level higher than? *(PGMEE 2012)*

a. 100 IU/L
b. 1000 IU/L
c. 10,000 IU/L
d. 1,00,000 IU/L

[Ref: Holland Brew's Obs.4th/e, pg. 254; Novak's Gynae. 15th/e, pg. 1464, 1469]

140. Best prognostic indicator of gestational trophoblastic disease is: *(PGMEE Nov. 12 Pattern)*

a. Uterine size
b. Theca lutein cysts
c. β-hCG
d. Stage of disease

[Ref: Holland Brew's Obs.4th/e, pg. 254; Novak's Gynae. 15th/e, pg. 1469]

141. Which of the following is bad prognostic factor for choriocarcinoma? *(PGMEE 2011)*

a. Full term pregnancy
b. Short duration
c. Abortion
d. Low beta hCG

[Ref: D . C. Dutta's Textbook of gynaecology, 7th/e, P301]

142. Which of the following is a risk factor for choriocarcinoma? *(PGMEE 2011)*

a. β hCG < 40,000 mlU/mL
b. After full term pregnancy
c. Lung metastasis
d. None

[Ref: D. C. Dutta's Textbook of gynaecology, 7th/e, P301]

143. Most common gestational trophoblastic disease following hydatidiform mole is? *(PGMEE 2011)*

a. Invasive mole
b. Placental nodule
c. Placental site trophoblastic tumor
d. Choriocarcinoma

[Ref: Williams Obs., 23rd/e, pg. 262]

144. In case of hydatidiform mole, investigation used for diagnosis is? *(PGMEE 2011)*

a. Chest X- ray
b. USG
c. hCG titer
d. All of the above

[Ref: Dutta's Obs. 8th/e, pg. 225; Holland Brew's Obs.4th/e, pg. 252; Williams Obs., 23rd/e, pg. 260]

139.	d
140.	c
141.	a
142.	b
143.	a
144.	b

ACUTE AND CHRONIC PELVIC INFECTION

1. **Most common cause of pelvic inflammatory disease is-**
   a. Sexually transmitted disease   **(PGMEE 2015)**
   b. Puerperal sepsis
   c. Pelvic peritonitis
   d. IUCD   *[Ref: Shaw's 16th/e p. 177]*

2. **Pelvic inflammatory disease commonly complicates as:-**   **(PGMEE 2018)**
   a. Pyometra
   b. Senile endometritis
   c. Uterine adhesions/synachiae
   d. Hematocolpos

   [Ref: D.C. Dutta text book of Gynecology pg.108 7th e; Speroff 8th e p.921-931]

Explanation

Pelvic Inflammatory Disease (PID): Diagnostic criteria

Criteria	Parameters
Minimal criteria	1. Tenderness in lower abdomen & adenexa 2. Cervical motion tenderness
Additional criteria	1. Oral temp > 38.3°C 2. Mucopurulent Cx/vaginal discharge 3. Leukocytes abundance in cervical smear 4. Raised CRP and or ESR 5. Laboratory evidence of +ve cervical infection with gonorrhea or chlamydia trachomatis
Definitive criteria	1. Histopathologically evidence of endometritis on biopsy. 2. Radiological evidence (TVS/MRI) of thickened fluid filled tubes 3. Laparoscopic evidence of PID
Complications of PID	1. Early: Ectopic pregnancy, abortions, endometritis, infertility 2. Late: Secondary amenorrhea, **pyometra**

3. **PID after insertion of IUD is seen in how many weeks-**   **(PGMEE 2013-14)**
   a. 3   b. 5
   c. 7   d. 14
   [Ref: D. C. Dutta's Textbook of gynaecology, 7th/e, P395]

4. **Criteria for PID is?**   **(PGMEE Nov 13 Pattern)**
   a. Tubo ovarian abscess on USG
   b. Cervical erosion
   c. Temperature more than 37.5 C
   d. Infertility

   [Ref: D. C. Dutta's Textbook of gynaecology, 7th/e, P108;Danforth's obstetrics and gynecology 10th/e ch. 34]

5. **Most common cause of pyometra-**   **(PGMEE 2012-13)**
   a. Endometritis   b. CA endometrium
   c. Ca cervix   d. Radiation

   [Ref: D. C. Dutta's Textbook of gynaecology, 7th/e, P138 Shaw Gynae 15th/e p. 324]

6. **PID is most commonly caused by-**   **(PGMEE 2013; Nov.12 Pattern)**
   a. Chlamydia   b. Mycoplasma
   c. Tubercular bacillus   d. E. Coli

   [Ref: D. C. Dutta's Textbook of gynaecology, 7th/e, P107; Shaw's Gynae 15th/e p. 445-446]

7. **PID is not aggravated by?**   **(PGMEE 2012)**
   a. Cervical cap   b. Diaphragm
   c. IUCD   d. OCP

   [Ref: D. C. Dutta's Textbook of gynaecology, 7th/e, P401

8. **Gold standard for diagnosis for PID is:**   **(PGMEE 2010)**
   a. Clinical triad of pain, fever and cervical tenderness
   b. USG
   c. Diagnostic laparoscopy
   d. Histologic confirmation of endometritis

   [Ref: Shaw's Textbook of Gynaecology, 15th/e, Page no. 449, 450;Jeffcoate's Principles of Gynaecology, 7th/e, P. 359, 360; Berek & Novak's Gynecology, 15th/e, P. 565]

9. **Posterior colpotomy is done for?**   **(PGMEE 2010)**
   a. Pelvic abscess   b. Ovarian abscess
   c. Pelvic haematocele   d. All

   [Ref: Shaw's Textbook of Gynaecology, 15th/e, P. 453;Te Linde's Operative Gynecology, 9th/e, P. 1084 683-684

10. **Contraindication to dilatation and curettage (D & C):**
    a. Abnormal uterine bleeding (AUB)   **(PGMEE 2018)**
    b. Post menopausal bleeding
    c. Tuberculosis
    d. Pelvic inflammatory disease

    [Ref: Dutta 7th e p.484]

Explanation

Indications of Dialatation and Curettage:

- Diagnostic
  - Infertility
  - AUB
  - Pathologic amenorrhea
  - Endometrial tuberculosis
  - Postmenopausal bleeding
  - Chorionepithelioma
- Therapeutic
  - AUB   - Removal of IUD
  - Endometrial polyp   - Incomplete abortion
- Combined
  - AUB   - Endometrial polyp

1.	a
2.	a
3.	a
4.	a
5.	a
6.	a
7.	d
8.	a
9.	a
10.	d

GENITAL TUBERCULOSIS

11. Most common site involved in genital TB-

(PGMEE 2015)

a. Vulvo-vaginal part   b. Endometrium
c. Ovaries   d. Fallopian tubes

[Ref: D. C. Dutta's Textbook of gynaecology, 7th/e,114; Shaw's Textbook of Gyanecology 16th/e p. 188]

12. Vulvo vaginal tuberculosis is seen in how much percentage genital tuberculosis-

(PGMEE June 14 Pattern)

a. 10-15%   b. 20-30%
c. 50-60%   d. 1-2%

[Ref: D. C. Dutta's Textbook of gynaecology, 7th/e,114; Shaw's Gynae 15th/e p. 154]

13. Most common presentation of genital TB-

(PGMEE 2013-14)

a. Infertility   b. Polymenorrhoea
c. Vaginal discharge   d. Pelvic pain

[Ref: D. C. Dutta's Textbook of gynaecology, 7th/e,115; Shaw's Gynae 15th/e p. 154-156; William's Gynae 1st/e p. 423]

14. Most common symptom of uterine tuberculosis is?

a. Asymptomatic   *(PGMEE Nov 13 Pattern)*
b. Abnormal uterine bleeding
c. Infertility
d. Foul smelling discharge

[Ref: D. C. Dutta's Textbook of gynaecology, 7th/e,115; Current progress in obstetrics and gynaecology vol-1 ch. 18, p. 306-309; Danforth's obstetrics]

Explanation

Tuberculosis

- Tuberculosis is the **m/c** cause of primary infertility with adenexal mass in India. CA 125 c/b raised. Ovarian cancer or borderline tumours of ovary are rare cause of primary infertility. Distension of abdomen, ascites, and pain abdomen are common presenting features in these situations.
  - Endometrioma is a/w cyclical pain.
- *D/d of infertility in adenexal masses:*

Clinical condition	Age & parity	Cl/f	CA 125
Ovarian Ca	Elderly	Abdominal distension, mass abdomen	↑ in 50% of epithelial tumours
Borderline ovarian tumours	Middle age		Normal
Endometrioma	Middle age	Painful adenexal mass, 1⁰ infertility	↑ in > 80%
TB	Any age	↑ Painless adenexal mass 1⁰ infertility	May be ↑

15. Genital tuberculosis most commonly disseminates by?

(PGMEE Aug 13 Pattern)

a. Lymphatic route   b. Hematogenous route
c. Local spread   d. None

[Ref: D. C. Dutta's Textbook of gynaecology, 7th/e,113; A comprehensive textbook of obs & gynae by Sadhna Gupta 1st/e p. 215]

16. TB uterus all is true except-   *(PGMEE 2012-13)*

a. Mostly secondary
b. Increase incidence of ectopic pregnancy
c. Involvement of endosalpinx
d. Most common is ascending infection

[Ref: D. C. Dutta's Textbook of gynaecology, 7th/e,113-115; Shaw's Gynae 15th/e p. 154-155]

17. Fallopian tube tuberculosis-   *(PGMEE 2012-13)*

a. Most common type of genital TB
b. Size of the tubes is unchanged
c. Is asymptomatic
d. Primary focus of infection is always in fallopian tubes

[Ref: D. C. Dutta's Textbook of gynaecology, 7th/e,113-114; Shaw's Gynae 15th/e p. 154]

18. Beaded feel of fallopian tube on HSG is seen in-

(PGMEE 2012-13)

a. TB   b. Chlamydia
c. Gonococcal infection   d. Syphillis

[Ref: D. C. Dutta's Textbook of gynaecology, 7th/e, P116; Shaw's Gynae 15th/e p. 157]

19. Beading is seen in case of genital TB in women in-

(PGMEE 2012-13)

a. Tubes   b. Ovary
c. Cervix   d. Vagina

[Ref: D. C. Dutta's Textbook of gynaecology, 7th/e,116; Shaw's Gynae 15th/e p. 157]

20. Genital tuberculosis spreads through: *(PGMEE 2010)*

a. Hematogenous route   b. Ascending infection
c. Direct contact   d. Lymphatic route

[Ref: D. C. Dutta's Textbook of gynaecology, 7th/e, 113; Shaw's Textbook of Gynaecology, 15th/e, P. 154; Jeffcoate's Principles of Gynaecology, 7th/e, P. 323; Progress in Obstetrics & Gynaecology, John Studd, Vol. 18, Ch. 27, P. 397

21. Most common site of genital tuberculosis is?

a. Fallopian tubes   b. Ovary   *(PGMEE 2010)*
c. Uterus   d. Fimbriae

[Ref: D. C. Dutta's Textbook of gynaecology, 7th/e,114; Shaw's Textbook of Gynaecology, 15th/e, P. 154-5; Jeffcoate's Principles of Gynaecology, 7th/e, P. 324; Progress in Obstetrics & Gynaecology, John Studd, Vol. 18, Ch. 27, P. 400

SEXUALLY TRANSMITTED INFECTION

TRICHOMONAS

22. Strawberry cervix is seen in-   *(PGMEE 2015; 2012-13)*

a. Ureaplasma urealyticum
b. Trichomoniasis
c. Bacterail vaginosis
d. Chalmydia

11.	d
12.	d
13.	a
14.	c
15.	b
16.	d
17.	a
18.	a
19.	a
20.	a
21.	a
22.	b

[Ref: Shaw's Gyanecology 16th/e p. 163; William's Gyanecology 2nd/e p. 84]

23. A 28 year old primigravida with 32 weeks of gestation comes with complain of thin, frothy, profuse discharge through the vagina since yesterday. She was advised USG which showed Single live intrauterine gestational sac with FL and AC as adequate. What is the diagnosis?
(PGMEE 2015)

a. PPROM
b. Candidiasis
c. Normal finding
d. Trichomoniasis

[Ref: Shaw's Textbook of Gynaecology 16th/e p. 163, William's Gyanecology 2nd/e p. 84]

24. Which of the following leads to greenish discharge per vaginum-
(PGMEE 2015)

a. Chlamydia
b. Bacterial vaginosis
c. Ureaplasma urealyticum
d. Trichomoniasis

[Ref: Shaw's Textbook of Gynaecology 16th/e p. 163, William's Gynaecology 2nd/e p. 84]

25. Green frothy vaginal discharge is produced by –
(PGMEE 2019)

a. Herpes simplex
b. Candida albicans
c. Trichomonas vaginalis
d. Normal vaginal flora

[Ref: William's gynecology 3rd/e pg. 61]

26. All of the following cause endometritis except-
(PGMEE 2015)

a. IUCD
b. Septic abortion
c. Trichomoniasis
d. Gonorrhea

[Ref: Shaw's Gynaecology 16th/e p. 175]

27. Strawberry vagina causative organism is?

a. Trichomonas vaginalis *(PGMEE June14 Pattern)*
b. Candida albicans
c. H. vaginalis
d. Syphilis

[Ref: D. C. Dutta's Textbook of gynaecology, 7th/e,134 ; Shaw 15th/e p. 146; William Gynae 1st/e p. 64]

28. A lady presents with greenish discharge and strawberry cervix is due to infection of?
(PGMEE 2014)

a. Trichomonas vaginalis
b. Hemophilus vaginalis
c. Candida
d. Herpes simplex

[Ref: D. C. Dutta's Textbook of gynaecology, 7th/e,134

29. A young sexually active female has intensive pruritus and watery discharge, smear shows- *(PGMEE 2013-14)*

a. Trichomonas vaginalis
b. Candidia vaginitis
c. Gardenlla vaginalis
d. HIV

[Ref: D. C. Dutta's Textbook of gynaecology, 7th/e, 134]

30. Treatment for trichomonas vaginalis is-
(PGMEE 2013-14)

a. Metronidazole
b. Azithromycin
a. Ciprofloxacin
d. Abortions

[Ref: D. C. Dutta's Textbook of gynaecology, 7th/e, 134; Shaw's Gynae 15th/e p. 121]

31. History of yellow green watery discharge and pruritus-
(PGMEE 2013-14)

a. Trichomonas vaginalis
b. Candida
c. Bacterial vaginosis
d. Clamydia trachomatis

[Ref: D. C. Dutta's Textbook of gynaecology, 7th/e,134; Shaw's Gynae 15th/e p. 145, 131]

32. Surest sign of salpingitis is-
(PGMEE 2012-13)

a. Discharge of seropurulent pus from fimbrial end of tubes
b. Low back pain
c. Pyuria
d. Flank tenderness

[Ref: D. C. Dutta's Textbook of gynaecology, 7th/e,134; Shaw's Gynae 15th/e p. 145]

Explanation

- These lines from Shaw's give us an idea about the answer.
- 'The sure sign of salpingitis is the discharge of seropurulent fluid from the fimbrial end of the tube, without which the diagnosis cannot be justified at laparotomy as the peritoneal surface may be inflamed in pelvic peritonitis due to any other cause.'
- As Fallopian tube is the first site to be involved and simultaneously there is also involvement of ovary as it lies in close proximity to the fimbrial end of fallopian tube.
- Laparoscopic Examination are not use in routine, the pus extruded from the fimbrial end and adhesions are sure sign of PID.

33. Hanging drop preparation used for? *(PGMEE 2009)*

a. Trichomonas vaginalis
b. Gardenella vaginalis
c. Mobilincus
d. Candida albicans

[Ref: D. C. Dutta's Textbook of gynaecology, 7th/e,134]

CHLAMYDIA

34. Drug of choice for chlamydia in pregnancy is-
(PGMEE 2015)

a. Metronidazole
b. Azithromycin
c. Doxycycline
d. Erythromycin

[Ref: De Swiet's Textbook of Medical Disorders in Obstetric Practice 5th/e p. 407; Berek & Novak's Gynecology 15th edition page 564, table 18.3]

Explanation

- Both Azithromycin and Doxycycline are 1st line drugs for Chlamydia.

35. Bacteria responsible for ectopic pregnancy is-
(PGMEE 2015)

a. Staphylococcus
b. Peptostreptococcus
c. Trichomonas vaginalis
d. Chlamydia

[Ref: Dutta's Obstetrics 8th/e p. 207]

36. Usual causative organism of endocervicitis is?
(PGMEE Aug. 13 Pattern)

a. Herpes simplex virus
b. Chlamydia
c. Trichomoniasis
d. Candida

[Ref: D. C. Dutta's Textbook of gynaecology, 7th/e,123; Harrison 17th/e p. 124]

23.	d
24.	d
25.	c
26.	c
27.	a
28.	a
29.	a
30.	a
31.	a
32.	a
33.	a
34.	c
35.	d
36.	b

37. Most common cause of salpingitis- (PGMEE 2012-13)
a. Chlamydia   b. Mycoplasma
c. Tubercular bacillus   d. E. Coli

[Ref: D. C. Dutta's Textbook of gynaecology, 7th/e, P139, Shaw's Gynae 15th/e p. 445-446]

38. Woman presenting with chlamydial vaginal discharge. DOC is- (PGMEE 2012-13)
a. Ciprofloxacin   b. Doxycyclin
c. Metronidazole   d. Azithromycin

[Ref: D. C. Dutta's Textbook of gynaecology, 7th/e,123Shaw's Gynae 15th/e p. 145]

39. Which of the following is not caused by Chlamydia? (PGMEE Nov. 12 Pattern)
a. Vulvitis   b. Salpingitis
c. Urethritis   d. Cervicitis

[Ref: D. C. Dutta's Textbook of gynaecology, 7th/e, pg.123; Harrison 18th/e Chapter 176]

40. Fitz-Hugh-Curits syndrome is associated with- (PGMEE Aug. 12 Pattern)
a. Chlamydial infection   b. Genital tuberculosis
c. Syphilis   d. Candida infection

[Ref: D. C. Dutta's Textbook of gynaecology, 7th/e, 107; Harrison 17th/e p. 1073, 830]

Explanation

- Fitz hugh Curtis syndrome is caused by both Chlamydia and Gonorrhoea, but 90% is caused by chlamydia

41. Chlamydia can cause infertility due to? (PGMEE 2009)
a. Salpingitis   b. Endometritis
c. Oophritis   d. Cervicitis

[Ref: D. C. Dutta's Textbook of gynaecology, 7th/e,123

CANDIDIASIS

42. Curdy vaginal discharge is seen in which infection- (PGMEE 2012-13)
a. Bacterial vaginosis   b. Candidiasis
c. Trichomoniasis   d. Chlamydia

[Ref: D. C. Dutta's Textbook of gynaecology, 7th/e,134 Shaw's Gynae 15th/e p. 146]

43. Smear of vaginal discharge shows budding yeast cells. Causative agent is? (PGMEE 2011)
a. Candida   b. Mobilincus
c. Trichomonas   d. Chlamydia

[Ref: D. C. Dutta's Textbook of gynaecology, 7th/e,135]

GONORRHOEA

44. Most common organism causing salpingitis? (PGMEE June 14 Pattern)
a. N. gonorrhoeae   b. C. trachomatis
c. HSV   d. Mycoplasma

[Ref: William's Gynaecology 2nd/e p. 594]

45. Fitz Hugh Curtis syndrome is seen in- (PGMEE 2013-14)
a. Gonorrhoea   b. Trichomonas
c. T.B.   d. Herpes

[Ref: D. C. Dutta's Textbook of gynaecology, 7th/e,107;Shaw's Gynae 15th/e p. 486]

46. Uretheral discharge is seen in- (PGMEE 2012-13)
a. Gonorrhoea   b. Chlamydia
c. Herpes   d. Candida

[Ref: D. C. Dutta's Textbook of gynaecology, 7th/e,121; IADVL Textbook of Dermatology 3rd/e p. 1849]

47. Gonorrhoea first involves? (PGMEE Nov.12 Pattern)
a. Uterus   b. Cervix
c. Vulva   d. Vagina

[Ref: D. C. Dutta's Textbook of gynaecology, 7th/e,120;Novak's 14th/e p. 549; Danforth's 10th/e p. 614]

SYPHILIS

48. Syphilis causes- (PGMEE 2013-14)
a. Still births   b. Macrosomia
c. IUGR   d. Abortions

[Ref: Dutta Obs 7th/e p. 295]

49. Drug of choice in pregnant women with Secondary Syphilis is? (PGMEE Nov.12 Pattern)
a. Doxycycline   b. Benzathine penicillin
c. Ceftriaxone   d. Cotrimoxazole

[Ref: D. C. Dutta's Textbook of gynaecology, 7th/e,123; Danforth's Obstetrics & Gynecology 10th/e p. 613]

50. Hutchinson's traid in congenital syphilis include: (NEET Pattern 2017)
a. Interstitial keratitis, eighth nerve involvement, Hutchinson's teeth
b. Interstitial keratitis, mulberry teeth, periostitis
c. Periostitis, mulberry teeth, eighth nerve involvement
d. Hutchinson's teeth eighth nerve involvement, peritonitis

[Ref: Nelson 19th edition – chapter 210; Avery diseases of newborn – page 517]

Explanation

- Syphilis is caused by infection with the spirochete *Treponema pallidum*. In adults, this spirochete is transmitted through sexual contact, but infants acquire the infection from their mothers, either in utero or during delivery.
- Syphilis in infants is acquired primarily by transplacental transmission, which can occur at any time during pregnancy but ordinarily **occurs during 16 to 28 weeks' gestation.**
- **Classical triad in syphilis include** Deafness (SNHL) + interstitial keratitis + Hutchinson's teeth (notched upper central incisors) & mulberry molars (lower molars). *Also k/as Hutchinson's triad*
- *Details given in discussion section***90**

INFECTION OF INDIVIDUAL ORGANS

51. Bartholin cyst treatment of choice- (PGMEE 2012-13)
a. Excision   b. Antibiotics
c. Marsupialization   d. Drainage

[Ref: D. C. Dutta's Textbook of gynaecology, 7th/e,133;Shaw's Gynae 15th/e p. 125]

37.	a
38.	d
39.	a
40.	a
41.	a
42.	b
43.	a
44.	a
45.	a
46.	a
47.	b
48.	a
49.	b
50.	a
51.	c

52. Treatment of choice for Bartholin's abscess is?

(PGMEE 2012)

a. Incision drainage
b. Marsupialisation
c. Vulvectomy
d. Cystectomy

[Ref: D. C. Dutta's Textbook of gynaecology, 7th/e, 132; Jeffcoate's Principles of Gynaecology, 8th/e, P. 307-308, 418-419; Te Linde's Operative Gynecology, 9th/e, P. 872-874]

BACTERIAL VAGINOSIS

53. Amsel criteria is for-   (PGMEE 2015)

a. HELLP Syndrome
b. Bacterial vaginosis
c. Ovarian ectopic pregnancy
d. Antiphospholipid antibody syndrome

[Ref: D. C. Dutta's Textbook of gynaecology, 7th/e, 125 DeSwiet's Medical Disorders in Pregnancy 5th/e p. 405]

54. Malodorous vaginal discharge is due to- (PGMEE 2015)

a. Neisseria gonorrhea
b. Bacterial vaginosis
c. Trichomonas vaginalis
d. Chlamydia trachomatis

[Ref: D. C. Dutta's Textbook of gynaecology, 7th/e,125; DeSwiet's Medical Disorders in Pregnancy 5th/e p. 405; Berek & Novak's Gynecology 15th edition page page 560]

Explanation

■ Trichomonas vaginalis causes malodourous discharge, Bacterial vaginosis causes fishy odour discharge.

55. Fishy odor is seen in vaginitis by?

(PGMEE June 14 Pattern)

a. Trichomonas
b. Candidia
c. Chylamdia
d. Gardnerella

[Ref: D. C. Dutta's Textbook of gynaecology, 7th/e,125;Shaw 15th/e p. 131, 132; Williams Gynae 1st/e p. 51]

56. Amsel criteria for the diagnosis of bacterial vaginosis does not include? (PGMEE AUG. 13 Pattern)

a. Plenty of lactobacilli
b. pH > 4.5
c. Whiff's test positive
d. Clue cells

[Ref: D. C. Dutta's Textbook of gynaecology, 7th/e,125;Shaw's 13th/e p. 129; Novak's Gynae 12th/e p. 192; CGDT 9th/e p. 654]

57. True about genital infection is?

(PGMEE Aug 12 Pattern)

a. Thin frothy secretions associated with monilial infection
b. Tetracycline is drug of choice for trichomonas vaginalis
c. Patients and partners are given metronidazole for monilial infection
d. Clue cells are associated with gardenella vaginalis

[Ref: D. C. Dutta's Textbook of gynaecology, 7th/e, 134, 125, 135-136 Shaw's 14th/e p. 132]

58. Investigation for bacterial vaginosis is?

(PGMEE Nov. 12 Pattern)

a. KOH test
b. Culture
c. Gram stain
d. Microscopy

[Ref: D. C. Dutta's Textbook of gynaecology, 7th/e,125;Novak's 14th/e p. 544]

59. Not required for the diagnosis of vaginosis is?

(PGMEE 2012)

a. Whiff's test positive
b. pH > 4.5
c. Plenty of lactobacilli
d. Clue cells

[Ref: D. C. Dutta's Textbook of gynaecology, 7th/e,125; Shaw's Textbook of Gynaecology, 15th/e, P. 131-132; Jeffcoate's Principles of Gynaecology, 7th/e, P. 345-346; Berek & Novak's Gynecology, 15th/e, P. 558-559; Progress in Obstetrics & Gynaecology, John Studd, Vol. 15, Ch. 12, P. 186]

60. Clue cells are seen in?   (PGMEE 2011)

a. Bacterial vaginosis
b. Toxoplasmosis
c. Syphilis
d. Herpes virus

[Ref: D. C. Dutta's Textbook of gynaecology, 7th/e,125]

61. Whiff test is done for?   (PGMEE 2011)

a. Bacterial vaginosis
b. Genital tuberculosis
c. Syphilis
d. Candida

[Ref: D. C. Dutta's Textbook of gynaecology, 7th/e,125]

62. Bacterial vaginosis does not include?   (PGMEE 2010)

a. Profuse creamy discharge
b. Absent leucocytes
c. Positive whiff test
d. Clue cells present

MISCELLANEOUS

63. Vaginal emphysematous bulla, which is false-

a. Presents with vaginal discharge   (PGMEE 2012-13)
b. Leads to ulceration
c. Usually occur in pregnant patients
d. May occur secondary to genital tract infection

[Ref: Shaw's Gynae 15th/e p. 135]

64. Most common cause of pyometra is-   (PGMEE 2015)

a. PID
b. Tubercular endometritis
c. Carcinoma cervix
d. Senile endometritis

[Ref: Dutta's Obstetrics 6th/e p. 168]

52.	a
53.	b
54.	b
55.	d
56.	a
57.	d
58.	d
59.	c
60.	a
61.	a
62.	a
63.	b
64.	d

PROLAPSE ANATOMY

1. Strongest support of uterus is *(PGMEE 2012-13)*
a. Mackenrodt's ligament
b. Broad ligaments
c. Round ligaments
d. Uterosacral ligaments

[Ref: D.C. Dutta's Textbook of gynaecology, 7th/e, P 166; Shaw's Gynae 15th/e p. 181]

Explanation

- Uterosacral/cardinal ligament is the strongest support of uterus.

2. Not a support of uterus – *(PGMEE 2012-13)*
a. Urogenital diaphragm
b. Pubocervical ligament
c. Perineal body
d. Levator ani muscle fibers

[Ref: Internet]

3. The deepest, part of the perineal body if cut/damaged can lead to rectocele, cystocele and uterine prolapse. It is due to damage of: *(NEET Pattern 2017)*
a. Ischiocavernosus
b. Bulbocavernosus
c. Pubococcygeus
d. External and sphincter

[Ref: Internet - https://www.ncbi.nlm.nih.gov/pmc/articles/PMC3353407/)

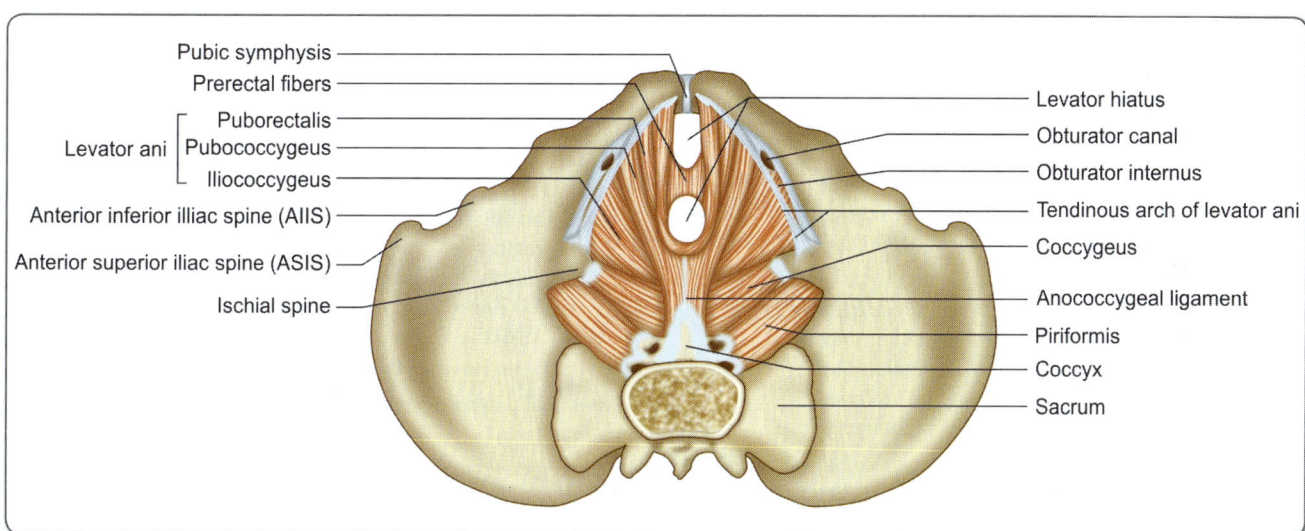

Explanation

Perineal body

- Perineal body structures are best visualized in the axial plane, revealing three distinct regions: superficial, mid and deep.
- In the superficial portion at the level of the vestibular bulb, the bulbospongiosus (BS) inserts into the lateral margins of the perineal body, while the superficial transverse perinei and external anal sphincter traverse the region.
- In the mid-region at the proximal end of the superficial transverse perinei, the puboperinealis muscle (one component of the pubovisceral muscle) inserts into the lateral margins of the perineal body and in some individuals can be seen to cross the midline.

The pubo-analis and internal anal sphincter extend into the perineal body's most deep region at the level of the midurethra.

- Weakness/injury to pubococcygeus & iliococcygeus muscles causes the elevator plate to sag down resulting in prolapse.

CLINICAL FEATURES AND DIAGNOSIS

4. Cystocele is formed by laxity and descent of:-
a. Ant upper 1/3 vagina *(PGMEE 2016-17)*
b. Post upper 1/3 vagina
c. Anterior upper 2/3rd of vaginal wall
d. Posterior upper 2/3rd of vaginal wall

[Ref: D.C Dutta text book of gynaecology 7th e p168]

1. d
2. d
3. c
4. c

CHAPTER-7 ⊙ DISPLACEMENT AND PROLAPSE...

5. Decubitus ulcers are due to -   (PGMEE 2013-14)
   a. Due to trauma
   b. Due to venous congestion
   c. Due to friction created by thighs
   d. Due to

   [Ref: D. C. Dutta's Textbook of gynaecology, 7th/e, P 170]

6. Patient with history of vaginal prolapse with ulcer on it. Diagnosis-   (PGMEE 2013-14)
   a. Carcinoma   b. Pressure erosion
   c. Syphilis   d. Decubitus ulcer

   [Ref: D. C. Dutta's Textbook of gynaecology, 7th/e, P 170; Shaw's Gynae 15th/e p. 335]

SURGICAL MANAGEMENT

7. What is the preferred treatment of complete prolapse in a female with completed family?   (PGMEE 2015)
   a. Pessary   b. Vaginal hysterectomy
   c. Sling surgery   d. Le Forte's repair

   [Ref: Shaw's Gynaecology 16th/e p. 357]

8. Le Fort repair is done for-
                (PGMEE Nov 13 Pattern; PGMEE 2015)
   a. VVF   b. RVF
   c. Vault prolapse d. Uterovaginal descent

   [Ref: Shaw's Gynaecology 16th/e p. 360][Ref: D. C. Dutta's Textbook of gynaecology, 7th/e, P180; Danforth 10th/e p. 867; Shaw's 14th/e p. 308

9. Le Fort's operation is done in?   (PGMEE Nov 13 Pattern)
   a. Young patient with utero-vaginal prolapse
   b. Elderly patient with utero-vaginal prolapse
   c. Multiparous with utero-vaginal prolapse
   d. Pregnant patient with utero-vaginal prolapse

   [Ref: D. C. Dutta's Textbook of gynaecology, 7th/e, P180; Danforth 10th/e p. 867; Shaw's 14th/e p. 308]

10. Treatment for young woman with prolapsed uterus is-
    a. Sling operation   (PGMEE 2012-13)
    b. Anterior colporrhaphy
    c. Posterior colporrhaphy
    d. Manchester operation

    [Ref: D. C. Dutta's Textbook of gynaecology, 7th/e, P182; Shaw's Gynae 15th/e p. 339]

11. Prolapse of uterus in nulliparous women, treatment is-
    a. Sling used involving rectus sheath   (PGMEE 2012-13)
    b. Anterior colporrhaphy
    c. posterior colporrhaphy
    d. Manchester operation

    [Ref: D. C. Dutta's Textbook of gynaecology, 7th/e,p.182 Shaw's Gynae 15th/e p. 339]

12. Which surgery uses rectus sheath to prevent prolapse -
                           (PGMEE 2012-13)
    a. Khanna operation   b. Purandare operation
    c. Shirodkar operation d. Le Forte repair

    [Ref: D. C. Dutta's Textbook of gynaecology, 7th/e, P182 ; Shaw's Gynae 15th/e p. 342]

13. Management of third degree utero-vaginal prolapse in woman who wants to have a child in future is?
    a. Fothergill's repair   (PGMEE 2009)
    b. Shirodkar's modified sling operation
    c. Manchester operation
    d. Le Fort's repair

    [Ref: Shaw's Textbook of Gynaecology, 15th/e, P. 339-344; Jeffcoate's Principles of Gynaecology, 8th/e, P. 266]

14. A 60 year woman comes with 3rd degree uterine prolapse. What will be the management?
                                    (PGMEE 2019)
    a. Vaginal hysterectomy with pelvic floor repair
    b. Pelvic floor repair
    c. Sacrospinous fixation
    d. Pessary

    [Ref: D. C. Dutta's Obs 7th/e pg. 211]

15. Purandare operation is indicated for?
                           (PGMEE Aug. 12 Pattern)
    a. Elongated cervix   b. Missed IUD
    c. Incompetent cervix d. Nulliparous prolapse

    [Ref: D. C. Dutta's Textbook of gynaecology, 7th/e, P182

16. A female underwent cervical encirclage. Which of the following is done to check that ring pessary is placed correctly:-   (PGMEE 2018)
    a. Insufflations of rectum between ring pessary and vagina
    b. Valsalva maneuver
    c. Ask her to urinate and look if ring is coming out
    d. All of the above

PROLAPSE IN PREGNANCY

17. 3rd degree genital prolapse is early (first trimester) of pregnancy is managed by ?   (PGMEE Aug 13 Pattern)
    a. Ring pessary
    b. Fothergill's repair
    c. Le fort's repair
    d. Right transvaginal sacrospinous colpopexy

    [Ref: D. C. Dutta's Textbook of gynaecology, 7th/e, P 173; Shaw's 14th/e p. 308; Danforth's 10th/e p. 867]

18. When ring pessary is removed during pregnancy?
                           (PGMEE Nov. 12 Pattern)
    a. Before labour
    b. 1st trimester
    c. 2nd trimester
    d. 3rd trimester

    [Ref: D. C. Dutta's Textbook of gynaecology, 7th/e, P173]

19. For uterine prolapse in pregnancy, Ring pessary can be inserted upto-   (PGMEE 2012-13)
    a. 12 weeks
    b. 14 weeks
    c. 16 weeks
    d. 18 weeks

    [Ref: D. C. Dutta's Textbook of gynaecology, 7th/e, P173]

5.	b
6.	d
7.	b
8.	d
9.	b
10.	a
11.	a
12.	b
13.	b
14.	a
15.	d
16.	b
17.	a
18.	c
19.	d

URINARY INCONTINENCE

1. Surgery for genuine stress urinary incontinence is?   *(PGMEE June14 Pattern)*
   a. Kelly's plication
   b. Retropubic urethropexy
   c. Haltain's operation
   d. Spinelli's operation

   [Ref: D. C. Dutta's Textbook of gynaecology, 7th/e, P331; Shaw's Gynae 15th/e p. 174]

2. Bonney's test is used to determine-   *(PGMEE 2013-14)*
   a. Uterine prolapsed
   b. Stress urinary incontinence
   c. Vesicovaginal fistula
   d. Uteric fistula

   [Ref: Shaw's Gynae 15th/e p. 191]

3. Continuous incontinence of urine is seen in-
   a. VVF   *(PGMEE 2013-14)*
   b. Vesicoperitoneal
   c. Ureterovaginal fistulae
   d. Uretrovaginal

   [Ref: D. C. Dutta's Textbook of gynaecology, 7th/e, P349; Shaw's Gynae 15th/e p. 185]

URINARY FISTULAS

4. VVF in obstructed labour is repaired after a gap of   *(PGMEE 2012-13)*
   a. Immediately   b. 3 weeks
   c. 3 months   d. 6 months

   [Ref: D. C. Dutta's Textbook of gynaecology, 7th/e, P346; Shaw's Gynae 15th/e p. 192]

5. 48 yr, 7 day post hysterectomy fever, burning micturition with dribbling of urine but able to pass urine voluntarily. Diagnosis is-   *(PGMEE 2012-13)*
   a. VVF   b. UVF
   c. Urge incontinence   d. Stress incontinence

   [Ref: D. C. Dutta's Textbook of gynaecology, 7th/e, P349; Jeffcoate 17th/e p. 263-265; Shaw's Gynae 15th/e p. 183]

6. A 52 years old lady presents with constant leakage of urine and dysuria two weeks after a complicated total abdominal hysterectomy. A diagnosis of Vesicovaginal fistula is suspected. The most important test for the diagnosis is: *(PGMEE 2010)*
   a. Triple swab test   b. IVP
   c. Cystoscopy   d. Urine culture

   [Ref: D. C. Dutta's Textbook of gynaecology, 7th/e, P345; William's Gynaecology 1st/e p. 574]

URINARY INFECTION

7. Genito urinary TB is characterized by:-
   a. Asymptomatic bactriuria   *(PGMEE 2016-17)*
   b. Symptomatic bactriuria
   c. Hematuria
   d. Sterile pyuria

   [Ref: D.C Dutta text book of gynaecology 7th e p 339;From ROAMS 13th/e pg. 690]

8. In a 25 year old female, cystitis is best treated by: *(PGMEE 2012)*
   a. Cephelexin   b. Amoxicillin
   c. Norfloxacin   d. Nitrofurantoin

   [Ref: Shaw's Textbook of Gynaecology, 15th/e, P. 178-179; Berek & Novak's Gynecology, 15th/e, P. 570-571]

1.	b
2.	b
3.	c
4.	c
5.	b
6.	a
7.	d
8.	d

ENDOMETRIOSIS

1. Which is the following yields definite diagnosis of endometriosis *(PGMEE 2016-17)*
   a. MRI
   b. Ca-125
   c. USG abdomen and Pelvis
   d. Laparoscopic evaluation

   [Ref.: D.C Dutta text book of gynaecology 7th e p251]

2. If endometriosis occurs in lung then what will be term use for that......:- *(PGMEE 2016-17)*
   a. Vascular theory
   b. Implantation
   c. Coelomic metaplasia
   d. Retrograde menstruation

   [Ref: D.C Dutta text book of gynaecology 7th e p249]

3. Sampson's theory is pathogenesis for *(PGMEE 2016-17)*
   a. Endometriosis
   b. Fibriod
   c. Ca endometrium
   d. Cervical intraepithelial noeplasia

   [Ref: D.C Dutta text book of gynaecology 7th e p249]

Explanation

Theory of Endometriosis

- SAMPSON'S theory (most accepted theory) is theory of retrograde menstruation
- Theory of coelomic metaplasia
- Immune mediate theory: Causes is deficiency of both cell mediated & humoral Immunity
- Genetic predisposition: Gene is **K-ras**. If 1st degree relative affected → Risk is 7 times higher
- Theory of lymphatic & vascular spread.

4. Chocolate cyst is found in *(PGMEE 2016-17)*
   a. Endometriosis   b. Ovarian mucinous cyst
   c. Fallopian cyst   d. Cornual cyst

   [Ref: D.C Dutta text book of gynaecology 7th e p252]

5. Drugs used in endometriosis - *(PGMEE 2015)*
   a. Letrozole
   b. Mifepristone
   c. Combined oral contraceptives
   d. All of the above

[Ref: D.C.Dutta text book of gynaecology 7the p.254;Shaw's Gyanecology 16th/e p. 417]

6. Not seen in endometriosis is? *(PGMEE 2012)*
   a. Vaginal discharge   b. Dysmennorrea
   c. Pelvic pain   d. Dyspareunia

   [Ref: D.C.Dutta text book of gynaecology 7the p.250]

Explanation

- Presentation → **M/c** presentation: pain
- **M/c** dysmenorrhea (secondary) > Chronic pelvic pain > dyspareunia > Lower backache.
- **M/c cause** of 2^0 dysmenorrhea: Endometriosis > PID

7. Pain in endometriosis due to- *(PGMEE 2013)*
   a. PGI   b. PG E1
   c. PG E2   d. PG F2α

   [Ref: D.C.Dutta text book of gynaecology 7the p.250-1]

8. Gold standard diagnostic technique for diagnosis of endometriosis - *(PGMEE 2013; Nov 12 Pattern; June 2009)*
   a. Laparoscopy   b. MRI
   c. Ultrasound   d. Ca 125 level

[Ref: D.C.Dutta text book of gynaecology 7the p.251; Shaw's Gynae 15th/e p. 470]

9. Most common site of endometriosis: *(PGMEE 2011-2013)*
   a. Ovary   b. FT
   c. LSCS Scar   d. Colon

[Ref: D.C.Dutta text book of gynaecology 7the p.252;Shaw's Textbook of Gynaecology, 15th / e, P. 466;Jeffcoate's Principles of Gynaecology, 7th / e, P. 370-372]

10. Drug commonly used in t/t of endometriosis- *(PGMEE 2012-13)*
   a. LH   b. GnRH
   c. MPA   d. FSH

[Ref:D.C.Dutta text book of gynaecology 7the p.254; Shaw's Gynae 15th/e p. 473]

11. 1996 ASRM classification of endometritis includes- *(PGMEE 2012-13)*
   a. Intensity of pain   b. Location
   c. Size and location both   d. Number

[Ref: Leon and speroff clinical endocrinology pg1237, 8th edition]

Explanation

ASRM classification of Endometriosis

State	Progression	Tissue description
I	Minimal (1-5)	2-3 superficial implants
II	Mild (6-15)	Appearance of more implants within deeper layers of tissue
III	Moderate (16-40)	Many deep implants in combination with minor/small endometriomas on one or both ovaries. May also present filmy adhesions.
IV	Severe (>40)	Persistence of deep implants, enlargement of endometriomas on one or both ovaries, development of dense adhesions.

1.	d
2.	a
3.	a
4.	a
5.	d
6.	a
7.	d
8.	a
9.	a
10.	b,c
11.	c

ADENOMYOSIS

12. A 30 year old woman with complaint of dysmenorrhoea, dyspareunia with chronic pelvic pain undergoes hysterectomy. From the cut section of hysterectomy specimen below identify the condition. *(PGMEE 2019)*

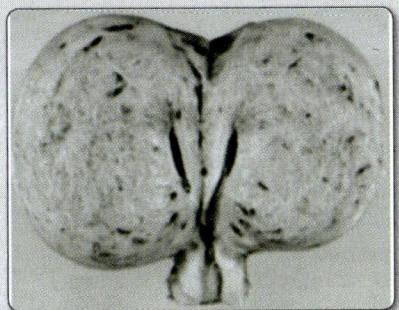

  a. Adenomyosis   b. Fibroids
  c. Leiomyoma   d. Endometriosis

[Ref: Shaw's text book of Gynaecology, 16th/e pg. 420]

13. Treatment of choice for perimenopausal adenomyosis is? *(PGMEE 2013)*
  a. OCPs
  b. GnRH agonists
  c. LNG IUS
  d. Hysterectomy

[Ref: D.C.Dutta text book of gynaecology 7the p.258; Novak's gynae 14th/e p. 521]

14. Definitive management of adenomyosis is *(PGMEE 2012-13)*
  a. GNRH analogue
  b. Danazole
  c. LH
  d. Hysterectomy

[Ref: D.C.Dutta text book of gynaecology 7the p.258; Shaw's Gynae 15th/e p. 475]

12.   a
13.   d
14.   d

ENDOSCOPY IN GYNECOLOGY

1. What is the contraindication of laparoscopic sterilization-
a. Post partum state   *(PGMEE 2012-13)*
b. Post MTP
c. Gynaecologic malignancies
d. 3 previous child birth

[Ref: D. C. Dutta's Textbook of gynaecology, 7th / e, P409]

2. Intrauterine adhesions best seen by- *(PGMEE 2013-14)*
a. USG   b. CT
c. Hysteroscopy   d. MRI

[Ref: D. C. Dutta's Textbook of gynaecology, 7th / e, P 378]

3. Which of the following cannot be treated by laparoscopy-
                          (PGMEE 2012-13)
a. Ectopic pregnancy   b. Sterilization
c. Non descent of uterus   d. Genital prolapse

[Ref: D. C. Dutta's Textbook of gynaecology, 7th / e, P506]

Explanation

- Genital prolapse. Prolapse surgeries cant be done laparoscopically.

4. Not a laparoscopy instrument-   *(PGMEE 2012-13)*
a. Trocar
b. Pneumoperitoneum needle
c. Doyen's retractor   d. Fiberoptic camera

[Ref: D. C. Dutta's Textbook of gynaecology, 7th / e, P504]

5. All of the following are used in hysteroscopy except-
                          (PGMEE 2012-13)
a. CO_2 b. O_2
c. Normal saline   d. Dextrose

[Ref: D. C. Dutta's Textbook of gynaecology, 7th / e, P511; Shaw's Gynae 15th/e p. 493]

OPERATIVE GYNECOLOGY

6. In total abdominal hysterectomy following are removed-
a. Uterus   *(PGMEE 2012-13)*
b. Uterus & cervix
c. Uterus, cervix & fallopian tube
d. Uterus, cervix, fallopian tube & ovary

[Ref: D. C. Dutta's Textbook of gynaecology, 7th / e, P 490]

7. 35 year old with history of repeated D&C. She now has secondary ammenorhea. What is your diagnosis-
                          (PGMEE 2012-13)
a. Hypothyroidism
b. Kallman syndrome
c. Sheehan's syndrome
d. Ashermann's syndrome

[Ref: D. C. Dutta's Textbook of gynaecology, 7th/e, P 378,486]

8. Which is least injured in gynaecological procedures-
a. Ureter at pelvic brim   *(PGMEE 2012-13)*
b. Renal pelvis
c. Urinary bladder
d. Ureter at infundibulopelvic ligament

[Ref: D. C. Dutta's Textbook of gynaecology, 7th/e, P493; Shaw's Gynae 15th/e p. 184]

9. Radical hysterectomy is named after- *(PGMEE 2012-13)*
a. Wertheim's   b. John clark
c. Meigs   d. Mitra

[Ref: D. C. Dutta's Textbook of gynaecology, 7th / e, P499]

10. Hysterectomy when done through broad ligament causes injury to?   *(PGMEE Aug 12 Pattern)*
a. Bladder
b. Ureter
c. Urethra
d. Transverse colon

[Ref: D. C. Dutta's Textbook of gynaecology, 7th / e, P349,496; Shaw's 13th/e p. 14; Danforth 10th/e p. 456]

11. During hysterectomy, ureter is liable for injury at?
a. Where it enters bladder wall   *(PGMEE 2010)*
b. Where it crosses pelvic brim
c. Where it crosses uterine artery
d. None

[Ref: D. C. Dutta's Textbook of gynaecology, 7th / e, P349;Te Linde's Operative Gynecology, 9th / e, P. 1084]

12. Hysterosalphingography is done during? *(PGMEE 2010)*
a. Secretory phase   b. Luteal phase
c. Follicular phase   d. During menstruation

[Ref: Shaw's Textbook of Gynaecology, 15th / e, P. 211-3, 501-4 Jeffcoate's Principles of Gynaecology, 7th / e, P. 709-14 Berek & Novak's Gynecology, 15th / e, P. 1157]

1.	a
2.	c
3.	d
4.	c
5.	b
6.	b
7.	d
8.	b
9.	a
10.	b
11.	c
12.	c

MIFEPRISTONE

1. Mifepristone can be given upto how many days-
a. 49 days   b. 63 days   *(PGMEE 2015)*
c. 78 days   d. 93 days

[Ref: Dutta's Obstetrics 8th/e p. 203]

2. Dose of mifepristone in MTP?   *(PGMEE 2013-14)*
a. 600 mg   b. 400 mg
c. 200 mg   d. 100 mg

[Ref: D. C. Dutta's Textbook of gynaecology, 7th/e, P444]

3. Mifepristone may be used for all of the following Except-
                                 (PGMEE 2011)
a. Threatened Abortion   b. Molar pregnancy
c. Fibroids   d. Ectopic pregnancy

[Ref: D. C. Dutta's Textbook of gynaecology, 7th/e, P 444]

SERM

4. Adverse effect of tamoxifen therapy is: *(PGMEE 2016-17)*
a. Ovarian cancer   b. Breast cancer
c. Endometrial cancer   d. Cervical cancer

[Ref: D.C Dutta text book of gynaecology 7th e p 441]

5. SERMs are-   *(PGMEE 2013-14)*
a. Agonist on estrogen receptor
b. Antagonist on estrogen receptor
c. Some are agonist some antagonist on estrogen receptor
d. Used due to reduced chances of hot flushes, thromboembolism

[Ref: D. C. Dutta's Textbook of gynaecology, 7th/e, P441]

6. GnRH analogue are all except-   *(PGMEE 2012-13)*
a. Soserelin   b. Gonadorlein
c. Goserelin   d. Buserelin

[Ref: D. C. Dutta's Textbook of gynaecology, 7th/e, P434]

MENOPAUSE AND HRT

7. Hot flushes in menopause is due to changes in:-
                                 (PGMEE 2016-17)
a. Prolactin   b. GnRH
c. Estrogen   d. Progesterone

[Ref: D.C Dutta text book of gynaecology 7th e p 48]

8. Hot flushes are experienced as a result of-
a. Decreased estrogen   *(PGMEE 2015)*
b. Increased noradrenaline
c. Increased noradrenaline and estrogen
d. Increased noradrenaline and decreased estrogen

[Ref: SPEROFF 8th e p.696; D. C. Dutta's Textbook of gynaecology, 7th/e, P48; Shaw 16th/e p. 68]

9. Drug of choice for vasometer symptoms in post menopausal women is?   *(PGMEE 2014)*
a. Tamoxifen   b. Medroxyprogesterone
c. Clonidine   d. Conjugates estrogen

[Ref: D. C. Dutta's Textbook of gynaecology, 7th/e, P50; Shaw's Textbook of Gynaecology, 15th/e, Page no. 63, 69; Jeffcoate's Principles of Gynaecology, 7th/e, P. 868-869; Berek & Novak's Gynecology, 15th/e, P. 1235, 1238

10. In a postmenopausal female, which hormone increases-
                                 (PGMEE 2012-13)
a. FSH   b. Estrogen
c. GH   d. None of the above

[Ref: D. C. Dutta's Textbook of gynaecology, 7th/e, P49; Shaw's Gynae 15th/e p. 62]

11. HRT is given in-   *(PGMEE 2012-13)*
a. Symptomatic postmenopausal women
b. Following hysterectomy
c. Because a women has asked for it
d. All of the above

[Ref: D. C. Dutta's Textbook of gynaecology, 7th/e, P50; Shaw's Gynae 15th/e p. 66]

Explanation

HRT (Hormone Replacement Therapy)

- HRT is required in menopausal women who are symptomatic, high risk of cardio vascular diseases, osteoporosis.
  - Estrogen component of HRT have cardioprotective effect. It increases HDL and ¯ses cholesterol and TG. So it decreases risk of CAD.
  - It is used for osteoporosis in menopausal women. Oestrogen, progesterone, tibolone and raloxifene are beneficial in osteoporosis. HRT prevents bone resorption and bone mineral density.
  - Estrogen component can cause increase risk of breast cancer in multiparous females.
  - Carcinoma of endocervix can occur. Carcinoma of endometrium occurs with increase estrogen supplementation without progesterone.
- Indications of HRT are
  - Postmenopausal women with osteoporosis
  - Adult hypopituitarism
- Remember :
  - OCPs are protective against benign diseases of breast (e.g. fibroadenoma) and malignancy of endometrium and uterus.

12. HRT improves-   *(PGMEE 2012-13)*
a. Bone density   b. Coronary artery disease
c. Dementia   d. Endometrial cancer

[Ref: D. C. Dutta's Textbook of gynaecology, 7th/e, P50]

1.	b
2.	c
3.	a
4.	c
5.	c
6.	a
7.	c
8.	d
9.	c
10.	a
11.	d
12.	a

13. Post menopausal HRT decreases incidences of which malignancy- *(PGMEE 2012-13)*

a. Breast
b. Colorectal
c. Ovarian
d. Endometrium

[Ref: speroff 8th e p.842; Shaw's Gynae 15th/e p. 66]

14. What is false about post menopausal state- *(PGMEE 2012-13)*

a. Low LH
b. Low estrogen
c. High FSH
d. High androgen

[Ref: D. C. Dutta's Textbook of gynaecology, 7th/e, P. 46; Shaw's Gynae 15th/e p. 62]

15. Which of the following is true about menopause? *(PGMEE Nov 12 Pattern)*

a. Increase progesterone
b. Increase androgens
c. Incraese FSH
d. Increase estrogen

[Ref: D. C. Dutta's Textbook of gynaecology, 7th/e, P. 47; Novak's gynae 12th/e p. 450-452]

16. Absolute contraindication of HRT is? *(PGMEE 2011)*

a. Osteoarthritis
b. Endometriosis
c. Heart disease
d. Breast carcinoma

[Ref: D. C. Dutta's Textbook of gynaecology, 7th/e, P.50; Shaw's Textbook of Gynaecology, 15th/e, P. 66-67 Jeffcoate's Principles of Gynaecology, 7th/e, P. 881-882 Berek & Novak's Gynecology, 15th/e, P. 1245]

MISCELLANEOUS

17. Vulvar atrophy and itching are treated by: *(PGMEE 2019)*

a. Estrogen ointment
b. Antihistamines
c. Tamoxifen
d. None

[Ref: Williams gynecology 3rd/e pg. 849]

13.	b
14.	a
15.	c
16.	d
17.	a

PCOS (POLYCYSTIC OVARIAN SYNDROME)

1. **Treatment of PCOD for infertility** *(PGMEE 2016-17)*
   a. Ovulation induction   b. OC pills
   c. Metformin   d. Laproscopic drilling

   [Ref: D.C Dutta text book of gynaecology 7th e p.382; From ROAMS 13th/e pg. 695]

2. **A girl presents with primary amenorrhoea with normal breast, hirsutism and acne. She MOST probably has:**
   (Recent Pattern June 2018)
   a. Klinefelter syndrome   b. PCOD
   c. Turner's syndrome   d. Gonadal dysgenesis

   [Ref: D.C Dutta 7th/e pg. 379]

Explanation

- Polycystic ovary syndrome (PCOS) is a common endocrine disorder of unknown etiology affecting 5–10% of women of reproductive age. It is characterized by chronic anovulation, polycystic ovaries, and hyperandrogenism.
- PCOS is manifested by hirsutism (50% of cases), obesity (80%), and virilization (20%). Fifty percent of patients have amenorrhea, 30% have abnormal uterine bleeding, and 20% have normal menstruation.
- In addition, they have an increased long-term risk of cancer of the endometrium because of unopposed estrogen secretion.

3. **USG ovary showing multiple small cystic structures. Ovary is increased in size and there is string of pearls appearance). The patient complains of irregular menstruation. The MOST likely diagnosis on the basis of the investigation can be:-** *(PGMEE 2016-17)*

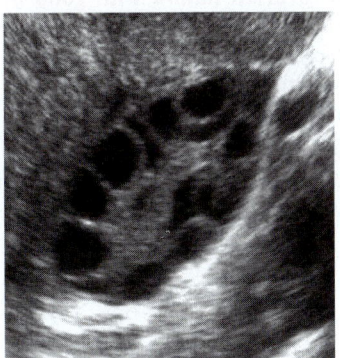

   a. Cystic adenocarcinoma ovary
   b. Chocolate cyst
   c. PCOS
   d. Ovarian cyst

   [Ref: D.C Dutta text book of gynaecology 7th e p.379]

4. **Hirsutism is graded on the basis of:-** *(PGMEE 2016-17)*
   a. Turner score
   b. Keilland score
   c. Ferriman-Galleway score
   d. Testosterone score

   [Ref: speroff 8th e p.543]

5. **Which is not increased in PCOS** *(PGMEE 2015)*
   a. Sex hormone binding globulin
   b. Estrogen
   c. Insulin
   d. Luetinizing hormone

   [Ref: D.C Dutta text book of gynaecology 7th ep.380; Shaw's Gynaecology 16th/e p. 431]

6. **Regarding PCOD all are true except-** *(PGMEE 2013-14)*
   a. High FSH/LH   b. High DHEA
   c. Raised LH   d. Estrogen

   [Ref: D. C. Dutta's Textbook of gynaecology, 7th/e, P379; Novak's Gynae 15th/e p. 1076; Shaw's Gynae 15th/e p. 217]

7. **Stein Leventhal syndrome is-** *(PGMEE 2013-14)*
   a. PCOD
   b. Turner's syndrome
   c. Swyer's syndrome
   d. Klinefelter's syndrome

   [Ref: D. C. Dutta's Textbook of gynaecology, 7th/e, P378]

8. **Stein Levinthal syndrome what hormone is raised-**
   (PGMEE 2013-14)
   a. LH   b. FSH
   c. GnRH   d. Progesterone

   [Ref: D.C. Dutta's Textbook of gynaecology, 7th/e, P378-379]

Explanation

Persistently elevated LH

- PCOD / Polycystic ovarian syndrome or disease was earlier known as Stein leventhal syndrome. 15 % of female population suffers from PCOS and the patients are mostly 15 to 25 yrs of age.
- PCOS includes chronic non ovulation and hyperandrogenemia a/w normal or raised oestrogen, **raised LH**, and low FSH/LH ratio
- In a typical case USG alone is adequate to confirm the diagnosis. In other cases, low FSH/LH ratio, raised testosterone, androstenedione, DHEA will be observed.
- DHES (Sulfated forms of DHEA) is secreted exclusively by adrenals and its secretion is increased in 50% case of PCOS and in adrenogenital syndrome esp. 3 β - HSD deficiency.
- About 25% of patients with PCOS exhibit elevated Prolactin levels. (*Ref. Novak's Gynaecology 13th/e p. 878*)

1.	a
2.	b
3.	c
4.	c
5.	a
6.	a
7.	a
8.	a

- There is an increase in LH pulse frequency as a result of GnRH pulse frequency. In some patients with PCOS, bromocriptine has reduced LH levels and restored ovulatory functions. (*Ref. Novak's Gynaecology 13th/e p. 878*)

9. A 16 years old girl came for evaluation of hirsutism, irregular bleeding and infertility, diagnosed as PCOS. Which of the following drugs should not be given? *(PGMEE 2013)*

a. Spironolactone
b. Tamoxifen
c. OCPs
d. Clomiphence citrate

[Ref: D. C. Dutta's Textbook of gynaecology, 7th/e, P382; Berek & Novak's Gynecology 15th edition – page- 1152.]

Explanation

- Clomiphene citrate is drug of choice for ovulation induction in patients with infertility secondary to PCOS, not for treatment of PCOS.

10. Commonest cause of anovulatory infertility-

a. PCOS   *(PGMEE 2012-13)*
b. TB
c. Endometriosis
d. Thyroid dysfunction

[Ref: D. C. Dutta's Textbook of gynaecology, 7th/e, P378; Shaw's Gynae 15th/e p. 209]

11. True for PCOD is-   *(PGMEE 2012-13)*

a. Increased FSH
b. Increased LH
c. Increased SHBG
d. Increased FSH/LH ratio

[Ref: D. C. Dutta's Textbook of gynaecology, 7th/e, P379; Shaw's Gynae 15th/e p. 370]

12. Enzymes responsible for conversion of androgen into estrogen are all except-   *(PGMEE 2012-13)*

a. Aromatase
b. Sulphatase
c. Fumarase
d. 3 beta hydroxy steroid dehydrogenase

[Ref: Speroff 8th e p.775]

13. Hyperstimulation syndrome, true is-   *(PGMEE 2012-13)*

a. Usually seen in late pregnancy
b. hCG is the treatment of choice
c. Raised LH is responsible in PCOD
d. Vascular permeability is decreased

[Ref: Dutta gynae 7th e p.437]

14. Which hormone is increased in PCOS?   *(PGMEE 2015)*

a. LH   b. FSH
c. Inhibin   d. Estrogen

[Ref: Robbins 9th/e pg. 1022]

PREMATURE OVARIAN FAILURE (POF)

15. Which is increased in premature ovarian failure: *(PGMEE 2015)*

a. Sr. FSH   b. Sr. Estradiol
c. Sr. Inhibin B d. Both B and C

[Ref: Shaw's Gyanecology 16th/e p. 74; Speroff's clinical Gynaecologic Endocrinology and Infertility 8th/e p. 449]

16. 35 yr old with 4 months amenorrhea with increased FSH, decreased estrogen. What is the diagnosis-

a. Premature ovarian failure   *(PGMEE 2012-13)*
b. PCOD
c. Pituitary failure
d. Hypothalamic failure

[Ref: D. C. Dutta's Textbook of gynaecology, 7th/e, P383; Shaw's Gynae 15th/e p. 70, 290]

17. Oestrogen levels in premature ovarian failure are below?   *(PGMEE Aug 12 Pattern)*

a. 10 pg/ml   b. 20 pg/ml
c. 40 pg/ml   d. 80 pg/ml

[Ref: D. C. Dutta's Textbook of gynaecology, 7th/e, P383; Principles and Practice of Endocrinology and metabolism p. 957]

18. Premature ovarian failure with good ovarian reserve next step in management-

a. Ovulation induction
b. In vitro fertilization
c. Intrauterine sperm insemination
d. Genetic counseling

[Ref: D. C. Dutta's Textbook of gynaecology, 7th/e, P200; Shaw's Gynae 15th/e p. 215]

9.	d
10.	a
11.	b
12.	c
13.	c
14.	a
15.	a
16.	a
17.	b
18.	a

PRIMARY AMENNORRHEA

1. Primary amenorrhea is called if menstruation not occurred by the age of? *(PGMEE 2014)*
a. 13 years
b. 15 years
c. 16 years
d. 18 years

[Ref: D. C. Dutta's Textbook of gynaecology, 7th/e, P. 371; Berek & Novak's Gynecology 15th edition page 1036.]

Explanation

- According to latest guidelines- primary amenorrhoea is
  - Absence of initiation of menses in female of 15 years of age with development of secondary sexual characters, or,
  - Absence of initiation of menses in females of 13 years of age without development of secondary sexual characters.

GONADAL DYSGENESIS

2. XO is seen in: *(PGMEE 2016-17)*
a. Turner's
b. Edward's
c. SuperFemale
d. Klinefelter's syndrome

[Ref : D.C Dutta text book of gynaecology 7th e p363]

3. Patient with XO syndrome attains puberty which hormone given after puberty:- *(PGMEE 2016-17)*
a. Oestrogen
b. Progesterone
c. E+P
d. Thyroid hormone

[Ref: speroff 8th e p.380]

4. Chromosomal abnormality in klinefelter's syndrome:- *(PGMEE 2016-17)*
a. 47XXY
b. 45XO
c. 46XX
d. 47XYY

[Ref: D.C Dutta text book of gynaecology 7th e p365]

5. A 16-years old female presents with primary amenorrhea and raised FSH level. On examination, her height was 58 inches. What would be the histopathological finding in the ovary? *(PGMEE 2013)*
a. Absence of oocytes in the ovaries (streak ovaries)
b. Mucinous cystadenoma
c. Psammoma bodies
d. Hemorrhagic corpus luteum

[Ref: Ref: D. C. Dutta's Textbook of gynaecology, 7th/e, P. 363; Berek's and Novak's 15th/e, Clinical gynecology Endocrionology and infertility, 8th/e]

6. A patient with amenorrhea, infantile uterus on karyotyping showed 450X0/46XY? How would you manage.
a. Bilateral orchidectomy *(NEET Pattern 2017)*
b. Vaginopathy
c. Resection of clitoris
d. Hormone replacement therapy

Ref: Speroff 8th e p 449,461-2

Explanation

- Turner syndrome is a well known and thoroughly studied disorder, classically associated with a 45,X karyotype, but also with an assortment of other structural X chromosome abnormalities (deletions, ring and iso-chromosomes), any of which may be present in all or only in some of the cells of the body (mosaicism), depending on the stage of embryonic development at the time they arise.
- The diagnosis of Turner syndrome generally can be made easily, based on the phenotype and findings of hypergonadotropic hypogonadism. A karyotype is definitive, and specifically indicated, in part because it may reveal a cell line containing a Y chromosome otherwise not suspected or identified (e.g., 45,X/46,XY); approximately 5% of women with Turner syndrome have a karyotype containing all or part of a Y chromosome.
- Whereas it is important to identify a Y chromosome because affected individuals are at significant increased risk for developing gonadoblastoma (20–30%), that risk appears lower (5–10%) in women with Turner syndrome, and limited to those having detectable Y chromosome on their karyotype.
- In all patients under age 30 with a diagnosis of ovarian failure, a karyotype should be obtained to exclude chromosomal translocations, deletions, and mosaicism that might offer an obvious explanation. A karyotype also identifies those having a Y chromosome in whom gonadectomy is indicated due to the significant risk for malignant transformation in occult testicular elements (20–30%).

ABNORMAL GENITAL ANATOMY

CYRPTOMENORRHEA

7. Cryptomenorrhoea and amenorrhoea, other symptom is:- *(PGMEE 2016-17)*
a. Abdominal lump
b. Cyclical abdominal pain
c. Short stature
d. Poor secondary sexual characters

[Ref: D.C Dutta text book of gynaecology 7th e p371]

1.	b
2.	a
3.	c
4.	a
5.	a
6.	a
7.	b

27. Investigation of choice for endometrial synechiae is-
(PGMEE Aug 13 Pattern)
a. Endometrial sampling b. Hysteroscopy
c. Colposcopy d. Ultrasound

[Ref: D. C. Dutta's Textbook of gynaecology, 7th/e, P. 378 Novak's 15th/e p. 786-2 & 14th/e p. 787; Shaw's Gynae 15th/e p. 494, Williams Gynae 1st/e p. 950-1]

28. False about Ashermann's syndrome:- *(PGMEE 2012-13)*
a. Associated with menstrual irregularities
b. Progesterone challenge test is positive
c. Synechiae formation in uterus
d. May be secondary to TB

[Ref: D. C. Dutta's Textbook of gynaecology, 7th/e, P. 378]

29. Not a cause for secondary amenorrhoea
(PGMEE 2012-13)
a. Pregnancy b. PCOD
c. Cushing syndrome d. Turner syndrome

[Ref: D. C. Dutta's Textbook of gynaecology, 7th/e, P. 371-377; Shaw's Gynae 15th/e p. 287—288]

30. Sheehan's syndrome is due to- *(PGMEE 2012-13)*
a. Ovarian necrosis b. Hypothalamus necrosis
c. Pituitary necrosis d. Thyroid necrosis

[Ref: D. C. Dutta's Textbook of gynaecology, 7th/e, P. 384]

31. Most common cause of Sheehan's syndrome:-
(PGMEE 2012-13)
a. PPH
b. Tubercular endometritis
c. Amenorrhea
d. Oligomenorrhea

[Ref D. C. Dutta's Textbook of gynaecology, 7th/e, P. 378]

32. All are causes of anovulatory amenorrhoea except-
(PGMEE 2012-13)
a. PCOD b. Hyperprolactemia
c. Gondal dysgenesis d. Drugs

[Ref: Leon & speroff 8th e pg 454]

MALFORMATIONS

33. Most common congenital uterine anomaly is-
(PGMEE 2013-14)
a. Bicronuate uterus b. Septate uterus
c. Unicornuate uterus d. Arcuate uterus

[Ref: D. C. Dutta's Textbook of gynaecology, 7th/e, P 35, Leon Speroff 7th/e p. 132]

34. Investigation of choice for septate uterus is?
(PGMEE Nov 13 Pattern)
a. HSG b. USG
c. MRI d. Laproscopy

[Ref: Internet, Danforth's obstetrics and gynecology 10th/e p. 550; William's 22nd/e ch. 40]

35. Unilateral dysmenorrhoea occurs in?
(PGMEE Aug 13 Pattern)
a. Uterus didelphys b. Bicornuate uterus
c. Septate uterus
d. Uterus with rudimentary horn

[Ref: Jeffcoates principles of gynaecology 7th/e p. 202]

36. The diagnosis of uterine anomalies is-
a. Hysterosalpingography b. MRI
c. CT Scan d. Plain radiography

*[Ref: **Shaw's Gynae** 15th/e p. 501]*

27.	b
28.	b
29.	d
30.	c
31.	a
32.	c
33.	b
34.	c
35.	d
36.	a

PUBERTY AND ITS DISORDERS

1. 1st sign of puberty:- *(PGMEE 2008, 2016-17)*
- a. Growth spurt
- b. Pubic hair growth
- c. Breast budding
- d. Menstruation

[Ref: D.C Dutta text book of gynaecology 7th e p 39]

2. All are true about precocious puberty except- *(PGMEE 2015)*
- a. Most common cause is constitutional
- b. Secondary sexual characters before the age of 6 years
- c. Menstruation before the age of 10 years
- d. Secondary sexual characters before the age of 8 years

[Ref: Shaw's Gyanecology 16th/e p. 59; Speroff Clinical Endocrinology 8th/e p. 408]

3. First sign of puberty in females is? *(PGMEE 2009)*
- a. Pubrache
- b. Thelarche
- c. Increase in height
- d. Menarche

[Ref: D. C. Dutta's Textbook of gynaecology, 7th/e, P. 39]

4. First to come in female puberty: *(Recent Pattern June 2018)*
- a. Thelarche
- b. Menses
- c. Pubarche
- d. Growth spurt

[Ref: Nelson's 20th/e pg. 2615]

Explanation
- In girls, the first visible sign of puberty is the appearance of breast buds (Thelarche), between 8-12years of age.
- In boys the first visible sign of puberty is testicular enlargement, beginning as early as 91/2 yr

5. All are true about puberty menorrhagia except: *(PGMEE 2010)*
- a. Hematinics and hormone therapy is the treatment of choice
- b. Endometrial biopsy confirms diagnosis
- c. Routine screening for bleeding disorder is done
- d. Associated with anovulatory bleeding

[Ref: D. C. Dutta's Textbook of gynaecology, 7th/e, P. 43, 156 Shaw's Textbook of Gynaecology, 15th/e, Page no. 301-2 Berek & Novak's Gynecology, 15th/e, P. 393-4; Progress in Obstetrics & Gynaecology, John Studd, Vol. 18, Ch. 20, P. 305-6]

MISCELLANEOUS

6. Most appropriate time for breast self-examination is?
- a. A week after menstruation starts *(PGMEE 2010)*
- b. A day after menstruation ends
- c. During menstruation
- d. Before ovulation

[Ref: Jeffcoate's Principles of Gynaecology, 8th/e, P. 169; Berek & Novak's Gynecology, 15th/e, P. 482 & 656]

7. Perineal tear involving all layer except anal mucosa belongs to *(PGMEE 2016-17)*
- a. 1°
- b. 2°
- c. 3°
- d. 4°

[Ref: D.C Dutta text book of gynaecology 7th e p353]

8. Following delivery, tear involves perineum, external and sphinctor with intact mucosa, grade of tear is- *(PGMEE 2015)*
- a. First degree
- b. Second degree
- c. Third degree
- d. Fourth degree

[Ref: Dutta's Obstetrics 8th/e p. 489]

9. PAP smear invented by? *(PGMEE 2013)*
- a. John papanicolaou
- b. George Papanicolaou
- c. Vladimir papanicolaou
- d. Ben papnicolau

[Ref: Cervical cancer: Current and emerging trends in detection and treatment by Heather Hasan p. 28]

10. Lithotomy position increase vaginal opening by how many cm- *(PGMEE 2013-14)*
- a. 1 cm
- b. 2 cm
- c. 3 cm
- d. 4cm

[Ref: Dutta Obs 7th/e p. 93]

11. Endometrial biopsy is usually done at *(PGMEE 2013-14)*
- a. Just before menstruation
- b. 10-12 days after menstruation
- c. Just after menstruation
- d. At the time of ovulation

[Ref: Shaw's Gynae 15th/e p. 86]

12. Best way to look at endometrial activity is by- *(PGMEE 2013-14)*
- a. HSG
- b. Biopsy
- c. USG
- d. Colposcopy

13. Pseudocyesis is common in:- *(PGMEE 2016-17)*
- a. Woman nearing menopause
- b. Young women with multiple contacts
- c. Contraceptive failure

[Ref: D.C Dutta text book of gynaecology 7th e p 471]

14. Most radiosensitive phase of cell cycle is: *(PGMEE 2016-17)*
- a. Early s phase
- b. Late s phase
- c. G2M
- d. G1S

[Ref: D.C Dutta text book of gynaecology 7th e p 412]

15. Vaginimus is:- *(PGMEE 2016)*
- a. Painful sexual intercourse
- b. Premature orgasm
- c. Inability to initiate sexual intercourse
- d. Excesscive desire

[Ref: D.C Dutta text book of gynaecology 7th e p.469]

16. Which of the following is true about vulvodynia?
- a. Surgery for localized provoked pain *(PGMEE 2016)*
- b. Pain without lesion
- c. Strong association with irritable bowel syndrome
- d. Hyperalgesia to touch

[Ref: D.C Dutta text book of gynaecology 7th e p.215] 1. (C) Imperforate hymen

1.	c
2.	b
3.	b
4.	a
5.	b
6.	a
7.	c
8.	c
9.	b
10.	b
11.	a
12.	b
13.	a
14.	c
15.	a
16.	b

21

Pediatrics

NEONATOLOGY

- Neonatal period: first 28 days after birth
- Post term infants: baby born after 42 weeks of gestation
- Perinatal period according to WHO: 22nd week of gestation to 1st 7 days after life
- Low birth weight baby: birth weight <2.5 kg
- Very low birth weight: birth weight <1.5 kg
- Extremely low birth weight baby: birth weight <1 kg
- Blood in neonate: 80-100 mL/kg
- Normal temperature of a neonate: 36.5–37.5°C
- Mild hypothermia/cold stress: 36–36.4°C
- Severe hypothermia is <32°C
- Heat production in neonates is regulated by non-shivering thermogenesis via β-oxidation of brown fat
- Appropriate for Gestational Age: between 10th and 90th percentile of weight for gestational age
- % of birth weight lost after birth in the first 7 days of life: 5-10%
- Type of breathing in a newborn: Diaphragmatic
- Neonatal reflexes are mediated through: Brain stem
- Mastitis Neonatorum is due to: maternally derived Estrogens [Mn: MEN]
- Anterior fontanelle ossifies by: 17–21 months of age
- Posterior fontanelle closes by: 6-8 weeks
- Posterior fontanel may remain open in: congenital hypothyroidism
- Hallmark feature of congenital **C**MV infection: Periventricular **c**alcification
- Most specific syndrome associated with IDM: Caudal regression syndrome
- Best stage to examine a neonate: stage 4- stage 3/ alert inactive- drowsiness

- Hyperoxia in infants can lead to: Retinopathy of prematurity/Retrolental fibroplasia
- Seizures are common in stage 2 of HIE
- Neonatal seizure with best prognosis: Focal clonic seizure
- Neonatal seizure with **wor**st prognosis: **M**yoclonic seizure [Mn: WorM]
- DOC for neonatal seizure: Phenobarbitone
- QT_c interval can be used for spot diagnosis of: hypocalcemia ($QT_c > 0.42s$)
- Hypoglycemia in a neonate is defined as:
  - Plasma glucose levels <45 mg/dL
  - Blood glucose levels <mg/dL
- Principal mode of heat exchange in an infant incubator: convection
- Dose of Vitamin K administered to a newborn: 0.5-1 mg IM

Physical signs of prematurity:
- No creases on sole
- Insignificant breast nodule
- Empty scrotum

Indicators of fetal lung maturity:
- Amniotic fluid Lecithin to Sphingomyelin (L/S) ratio <2
- Negative Shake test
- Saturated Phosphatidyl Choline levels <500 mg/dL

Features of an Infant of Diabetic Mother::
- Macrosomia
- Neural tube defects
- Hypoglycemia & hypocalcemia

Scarf sign:
- Used for the assessment of tone
- One of the neuromuscular criteria in the new Ballard score to assess maturity

Neonatal Reflex

Neonatal Reflex	Age of Appearance	Disappears by
Rooting reflex	▪ 32 weeks of GA	▪ 1 month **
Asymmetrical Tonic Neck Reflex	▪ 35 weeks of GA	▪ 6-7 months
Moro's reflex (Startle):		▪ 5-6 months
▪ Hand opening	▪ 28 weeks of GA	
▪ Extension and abduction	▪ 32 weeks of GA	
▪ Flexion	▪ 37 weeks of GA	
Symmetrical Tonic Neck Reflex	▪ 4-6 months of age*	
Landau reflex	▪ 3 months of age*	
Parachute reflex	▪ 7-9 months of age*	▪ Persist throughout life

* Appears after birth | **Earliest neonatal reflex to disappear |

Neonatal Sepsis

	Early Onset	Late Onset
Onset	▪ Before 72 hours of life	▪ After 72 hours of life
Source	▪ Maternal urogenital tract	▪ Environment, community, nursery, physician
Etiology	▪ Klebsiella, S. aureus, E. coli	▪ Klebsiella, S. aureus, E. coli
Clinical feature	▪ Pneumonia, Respiratory distress	▪ Pneumonia, Septicemia, Meningitis (MC) [Mn: PSM]
Mortality	▪ High	▪ Low

Sepsis Screen	
Total Leukocyte Count	<5000
Absolute Neutrophil Count (ANC)	<1800 (Neutropenia)
Immature: Total Neutrophil ratio	>0.2
Micro ESR	>15 mm at the end of 1 hour
CRP	Positive
*≥2 positive findings → may have sepsis	

Necrotizing Enterocolitis (NEC)

- NEC is characterized by damage to intestine, ranging from mucosa to transmural necrosis and perforation
- Most important risk factor: prematurity
- Symptoms and signs:
  ○ Vomiting, abdominal distension and tenderness, abdominal mass, abdominal wall erythema, metabolic acidosis, shock etc.
- Radiological sign: Pneumatosis intestinalis (stage IIA) → Pathognomic of NEC
- Rx: NPO & broad spectrum antibiotics

Caput & Cephalohematoma

Caput Succedaneum	Cephalohematoma
▪ Boggy diffuse edematous swelling	▪ Swelling limited to one cranial bone
▪ Soft tissue involvement	▪ Subperiosteal hemorrhage
▪ Can cross suture lines	▪ Do not cross suture lines
▪ Present at birth or immediately after	▪ Present 2-3 days after birth
▪ Disappear within few days of birth	▪ Disappear within 2 weeks to 3 months

SGA/IUGR

	Asymmetrical IUGR	Symmetrical IUGR
General	▪ MC variety of SGA	
Etiology	▪ Due to decrease in cell size but not in number	▪ Due to decrease in cell number
Ponderal index = $\dfrac{Wt\ (g)}{Ht\ (cm)^3} \times 100$	▪ <2	▪ ≥2 (Normal PI = 2-5)
Head circumference	▪ Spared	▪ Affected
Prognosis	▪ Better	▪ Poor

Scoring & Staging

Ballard's scoring	▪ Objective method of assessing gestational age
Bell's staging	▪ Neonatal Enterocolitis (NEC) [Mn: Bell around the NECk]
Modified Sarnat staging	▪ Hypoxic Ischemic Encephalopathy
Downes scoring	▪ Severity of respiratory **d**istress in neonates
Silverman Anderson Retraction Score	▪ Severity of respiratory distress in preterm infants
Brazelton scale	▪ Neonatal **b**ehavior assessment scale

REMEMBER

Ballard Scoring:
- Objective method of assessing gestational age
- **Criteria:**
  - Neuromuscular maturity
  - Physical maturity

Steroids can decrease the risk of the followings in a newborn:
- Hyaline membrane disease
- Intraventricular hemorrhage
- Mortality

Third fontanelle is seen in:
- Trisomy 21
- Preterm baby

ABO incompatibility:
- Blood group of mother: **O**
- Blood group of **BAB**y: **A/B/AB**
- Blood smear shows: Microspherocytes and Reticulocytosis

Baby born though MSL is termed vigorous if:
[Mn: HRM]
- **H**eart rate >100/min
- Strong **R**espiratory efforts*
- Good **M**uscle tone
  - ↖ Not respiratory rate

NEONATAL JAUNDICE

- First sign of congenital hypothyroidism: Persistent elevation of unconjugated bilirubin
- In kernicterus, free bilirubin gets deposit in: Basal ganglia and subthalamic nucleus
- Exclusive breast feeding can increase the chances of: Neonatal jaundice
- Most effective light for phototherapy: Blue green light (wavelength – 460-490 nm)
- MI mechanism by which phototherapy helps to reduce the bilirubin: Structural isomerism
- Infants with direct hyperbilirubinemia if given phototherapy develops: Bronze baby syndrome
- In single volume exchange transfusion,% of blood exchanged is: 69%
- In double volume exchange transfusion,% of blood exchanged is: 89-91%

Kernicterus:
- Early features → Hypotonia, stupor, seizures
- Late features → defective upward gaze, Sensorineural hearing loss & movement disorders

Important drugs involved in causation of kernicterus/hyperbilirubinemia:
- Sulfonamide
- Salicylates

Breast Feeding Jaundice	Breast Milk Jaundice
▪ Seen in 1st week of life (usually Day 1-3)	▪ Seen after 1st week of life
▪ Disappears by 3rd week	▪ Peaks during 2nd – 3rd week
▪ Due to decrease intake of milk leading to increase in enterohepatic circulation	▪ Due to Pregnanediol present in milk that inhibit UDP Glucoronyl transferase ▪ Present with unconjugated hyperbilirubinemia
▪ Treatment is increase breastfeeding	▪ Treatment is continue breast feeding

REMEMBER

Conjugated hyperbilirubinemia is seen in:
- **D**ubin Johnson syndrome
- **R**otor syndrome
[Mn: DR are conjugated]

Unconjugated hyperbilirubinemia is seen in:
- **G**ilbert syndrome
- **C**rigler-Nagger syndrome

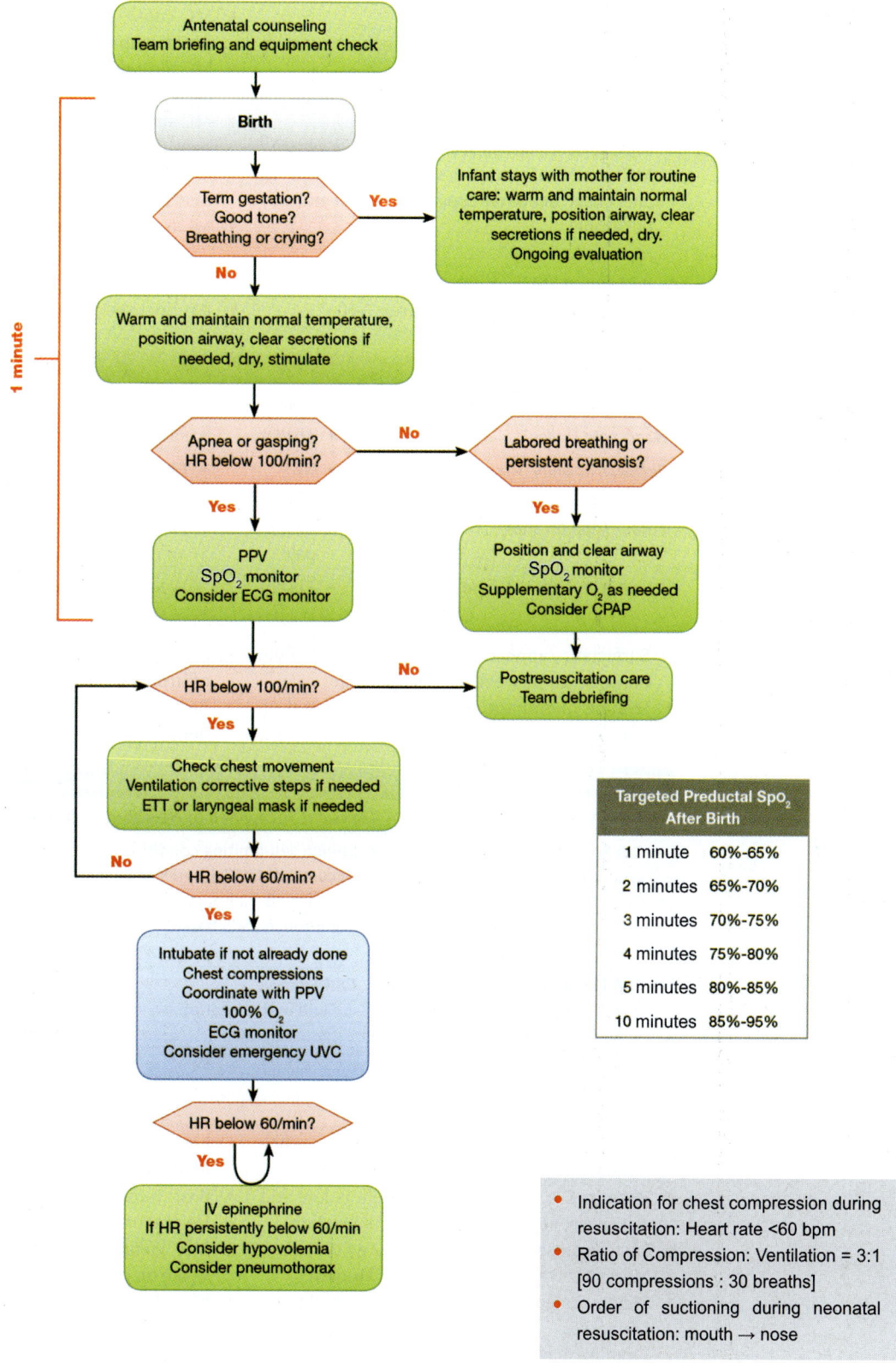

Targeted Preductal SpO$_2$ After Birth	
1 minute	60%-65%
2 minutes	65%-70%
3 minutes	70%-75%
4 minutes	75%-80%
5 minutes	80%-85%
10 minutes	85%-95%

- Indication for chest compression during resuscitation: Heart rate <60 bpm
- Ratio of Compression: Ventilation = 3:1 [90 compressions : 30 breaths]
- Order of suctioning during neonatal resuscitation: mouth → nose

MOST COMMON

- MC cause of neonatal mortality in India: LBW/prematurity
- MC cause of under 5 mortality: Pneumonia > prematurity
- MC cause of neonatal mortality in the world: Septicemia
- MC cause of neonatal sepsis: Group B *Streptococci*
- MCC of neonatal septicemia in India: *Klebsiella*
- MC mode of transmission of infection in late onset neonatal sepsis: hands of nursery personnel
- MC manifestation of late onset neonatal sepsis: Meningitis
- MC type of neonatal seizure: subtle type
- MC cause of pathological neonatal jaundice: Rh incompatibility
- MC birth defect: Neural tube defect
- MC cause of chorioretinitis: Toxoplasmosis
- MC site of diaphragmatic hernia: left posterior hemithorax via foramen of bochdalek
- MC cause of death in congenital diaphragmatic hernia: pulmonary complication
- MC bone to fracture in a neonate: Clavicle

APGAR SCORE

- Performed at 1 minutes and again at 5 minutes
- Normal Apgar score ranges from 7-10
- Score 0-3 → immediate resuscitation
- It is not used to guide resuscitation

Components	0	1	2
Muscle tone (Activity)	Floppy	Some flexion	Active movements
Heart rate (Pulse)	Absent	<100 bpm	>100 bpm
Reflex irritability (Grimace)	No response	Grimace	Cough or sneeze when stimulated
Colour (Appearance)	Blue or pale	Pink body, Blue extremities	Pink
Respiratory efforts* (and not rate)	Absent	Weak & irregular	Good strong cry

RESPIRATORY DISTRESS IN A NEWBORN

- Surfactant appears in the amniotic fluid between: 28-32 weeks of gestation age
- Hyaline membrane in HMD is composed of: Fibrin
- Neonatal alveolar proteinosis is d/t clumping of surfactant due to deficiency of: SB-B protein
- Best way to monitor breathing of a baby and to detect apnea: Impedance technique

Preterm	Term	
Hyaline Membrane Disease	**Transient Tachypnea of Newborn**	**Meconium Aspiration Syndrome**
• Aka Respiratory distress syndrome • Occurs within 1st 6 hours of life • HMD may occur in term if mother is diabetic	• Benign self-limiting condition • Occurs within 1st 6 hours of life • Lasts for 48-72 hours • Common in LSCS babies	• Seen in post term and small for date babies • May present with atelectasis and emphysema

• **CXR Findings:**
  ○ Reticulogranular opacity
  ○ Air bronchogram
  ○ Ground glass appearance
  ○ White out lung
	• **CXR Finding**
	  ○ Fluid in the interlobar fissure
		• **CXR Findings:**
		  ○ Hyperinflation
		  ○ Patchy infiltrates and coarse streaking

NUTRITION

- Main constituent of human milk: whey proteins
- Vitamin K content of human milk is low and can cause: hemorrhagic disease of newborn
- Lactose present in human milk: 7 g /100 mL
- Most sweetest mammalian milk: Human
- Major protective factor in breast milk: IgA antibodies
- Vitamins having antioxidant property: A, C & E (MI)
- Most accurate age independent criteria: Weight for Height
- Low Weight for Height (wasting) indicates: Acute malnutrition
- Best indices for chronic malnutrition: low Height for Age (stunting)
- Low Weight for Age (underweight) indicates: Acute on chronic malnutrition
- Waterlow classification of malnutrition takes into account: W/H & H/A
- X-linked dominant hypophosphatemic rickets is due to: PHEX gene mutation
- Most dangerous type of dehydration: Hypernatremic dehydration

Criteria for the diagnosis of Severe Acute Malnutrition:
- Pedal edema
- Visible severe wasting
- Weight for height less than –3 SD
- Mid upper arm circumference <11.5 cm

Mother's milk supply all the necessary nutrients except:
- Fluoride
- Vitamin K
- Vitamin D

Features of Zinc deficiency:
- Dwarfism, Diarrhea, Dermatitis
- Hypogonadism
- Impaired cell mediated immunity

Gestational Age	Initial Feeding Method
<28 Weeks **28-31 Weeks** **32-34 Weeks** **>34 Weeks**	▪ IV fluids ▪ Orogastric/Nasogastric tube feeding ▪ Feeding by spoon/paladai/cup ▪ Breast feeding

Storage of Expressed Breast Milk:
- Room temperature → 6-8 hrs
- Refrigerated → 24 hrs (4°C)
- Freezer → 3 months (-20°C)

Components of breast milk:
- Para-amino benzoic acid → protect against Plasmodium
- Bifidus factor → protects against *E. coli, Salmonella & Shigella*
- Epidermal growth factor → repair and maturation of intestinal cells
- Docosahexaenoic acid (DHA) → growth and development of CNS

Composition	Low osmolar ORS	ReSoMal*
Glucose	75	125
Sodium	75	45
Potassium	20	40
Chloride	65	70
Citrate	10	7
Osmolarity	245	300
Magnesium	—	3

* Rehydration Solution for Malnutrition

Age Independent Indices

- *Rao and Singh Index* = Weight (kg)/Height^2 (cm) × 100
- *Dugdale Index* = Weight (kg)/ Height 1.6 (cm) × 100
- *BMI/Quetlet Index* = Weight (kg)/ Height^2 (m)

- *Kanawati Index* = MAC/ Head circumference
- Ponderlal index
- *Mid upper arm circumference*
- Weight for height

SEVERE ACUTE MALNUTRITION

	Kwashiorkor	Marasmus
General	▪ Uncompensated phase of PEM ▪ Less common ▪ Body weight 60-80%	▪ Compensated phase of PEM ▪ More common ▪ Body weight <60% of expected
Clinical features	▪ Moon shaped facies ▪ Sugar baby appearance ▪ Child is lethargic, listless and apathic ▪ Psychomotor/mental changes ▪ Markedly retarded growth ▪ Hair is thin dry brittle and easily pluckable ▪ Flag sign – alternate hypopigmented and normally pigmented bands on hair ▪ Flaky paint dermatosis ▪ Appetite – impaired (child refuses to eat) ▪ Pitting edema due to hypoalbuminemia ▪ Hepatomegaly due to fatty liver ▪ Decrease IgM causing recurrent infection	▪ Monkey/Simian facies ▪ Wrinkled old man appearance ▪ Child is alert, active and irritable ▪ Gross wasting of muscle and subcutaneous tissue resulting in emaciation and marked stunting ▪ Buccal pad of fat is preserved till malnutrition becomes extreme ▪ Baggy pant appearance due to loosely wrinkled skin ▪ Voracious appetite ▪ No edema ▪ No hepatomegaly ▪ Less prone for infection

Management of SAM

- *Stabilization phase:* Day 1 to 7
  - Treat or prevent hypoglycemia and hypothermia
  - Prevent or treat dehydration with ReSoMal
  - Treat infection
  - Correct electrolyte imbalance
  - Begin feeding with F75
  - Correct micronutrient deficiencies without iron
- *Rehabilitation phase:* Weeks 2-6
  - Increase feeding
  - Correct micronutrient deficiencies with iron

- *Criteria for treatment failure:*
  - *Primary treatment failure:*
    - Failure to regain appetite by day 4
    - Failure to start losing edema by day 4
    - Presence of edema on day 10
    - Failure to gain at least 5 g/kg/day by day 10
  - *Secondary treatment failure:*
    - Failure to gain at least 5 g/kg/day for 3 consecutive days during rehabilitation phase
    - Reappearance of edema after 4 weeks

RICKETS AND SCURVY

	Rickets	Scurvy (Barlow's Disease)
Pathology	▪ Defective mineralization of normally formed osteoid, i.e. protein matrix	▪ Deficient collagen synthesis leading to defective osteoid formation
Etiology	▪ MC cause is nutritional deficiency of either calcium or phosphorus since both are requires for mineralization	▪ Vitamin C is required for hydroxylation of proline and lysine residues of collagen
Clinical features	▪ Craniotabes (soft skull) – earliest sign; Frontal bossing ▪ Rachitic rosary – Non tender swelling of costochondral junction ▪ Bow leg (genu varum) in toddlers ▪ Knock knees (genu valgum) in older children ▪ Harrison groove ▪ Pigeon chest deformity ▪ Marfan sign ▪ Hot cross bun skull ▪ String of pearls deformity ▪ Wind swept deformity ▪ Rachitic pot belly ▪ Increase tendency of fracture especially Green stick fracture	▪ Subperiosteal hemorrhage ▪ Scorbutic rosary – tender swelling ▪ Gingival bleed ▪ Petechiae, purpura, ecchymoses ▪ Epistaxis ▪ Epiphyseal separation ▪ Anemia ▪ Poor wound healing ▪ Defective dentition ▪ Generalized tenderness and pseudoparalysis ▪ Bones are brittle therefore easily fractured
X-ray	▪ Widening of the growth plate ▪ Cupping, fraying & splaying of metaphyseal end ▪ Cortical thinning ▪ White line of calcification known as Frenkel's line ▪ Double malleoli sign due to metaphyseal hyperplasia	▪ Zone of rarefaction ▪ Wimberger sign: White line surrounding the epiphysis (ringed epiphysis) ▪ White line of calcification – Frenkel's line ▪ Pelkan spurs
Lab	▪ Calcium and phosphate levels – Normal/Low ▪ Alkaline phosphate and iPTH – elevated ▪ Low levels of 25 (OH) D_3	▪ Usually not helpful ▪ Plasma or leukacyte vitamin level can confirm the diagnosis
Rx	▪ Vitamin D administered orally either in a single dose of 600,000 IU or over 10 days (60,000 IU/ day)	▪ Therapy with 100–200 mg of vitamin C orally or parentally

Types

Types of Rickets	Ca	P	ALP	iPTH	Vit D	1,25 Vit D
Hypophosphatemic /Vit D Resistant Rickets	N	↓	↑	N	N	
Nutritional/Vit D Deficiency Rickets	↓	↓	↑	↑	↓	
Type I Vitamin D Dependent Rickets	↓	↓	↑	↑		↓↓
Type II Vitamin D Dependent Rickets	↓	↓	↑			↑↑

DEHYDRATION

Symptom	Minimal or no Dehydration	Mild to Moderate Dehydration	Severe Dehydration
Loss of Body weight	▪ <3%	▪ 3-9%	▪ >9%
Mental status	▪ Well; alert	▪ Fatigued or restless, irritable	▪ Apathetic, lethargic, unconscious
Thirst	▪ Drinks normally	▪ Thirsty; eager to drink	▪ Drinks poorly; unable to drink
Heart rate	▪ Normal	▪ Normal to increased	▪ Tachycardia
Quality of pulses	▪ Normal	▪ Normal to decreased	▪ Weak, thread, or impalpable
Eyes	▪ Normal	▪ Slightly sunken	▪ Deeply sunken
Skin fold	▪ Instant recoil	▪ Recoil in <2 sec	▪ Recoil in >2 sec
Capillary refill	▪ Normal	▪ Prolonged	▪ Prolonged
Extremities	▪ Warm	▪ Cool	▪ Cold; mottled; cyanotic
Urine output	▪ Normal to decreased	▪ Decreased	▪ Minimal

Degree of dehydration	Rehydration therapy	Replacement of losses	Nutrition
Minimal or no dehydration	▪ Not applicable	▪ <10 kg body weight: 60-120 mL ORS for each diarrheal stool or vomiting episode ▪ >10 kg body weight: 120-240 mL ORS for each diarrheal stool or vomiting episode	▪ Continue breast-feeding or resume age-appropriate normal diet after initial hydration, including adequate caloric intake for maintenance
Mild to moderate dehydration	▪ ORS, 50-100 mL/kg body weight over 3-4 hr		
Severe dehydration	▪ Lactated ringer solution of normal saline in 20 mL/kg body weight IV until perfusion and mental status improve; then administer 100 mL/kg body weight ORS over 4 hr or 5% dextrose ½ normal saline IV at twice maintenance fluid rates	▪ Same; if unable to drink, administer through nasogastric tube or administer 5% dextrose in ¼ normal saline with 20 mEq/L potassium chloride IV	

GROWTH AND DEVELOPMENT

- MI hormone required for intrauterine growth: IGF-1
- % increase in the length of infant in 1st year: 50% (or 25 cm as length at birth is 50 cm)
- Term neonate looses 10% of birth weight in the 1st 7 days of life
  - Due to physiological diuresis
  - Resulting water loss is from extracellular compartment
- Microcephaly – occipitofrontal circumference >3 SD below the mean for age and sex
- Macrocephaly – occipitofrontal circumference >2 SD above the mean for age and sex
- Hydrocephalus is suspected if head circumference grows by more than 1 cm/ 2 weeks OR 2 cm/month during 1st 3 months
- Most accurate test for short stature: Bone age/ skeletal maturation
- Bone age = Chronological age in familial short stature
- Bone age >Chronological age in precocious puberty
- Bone age <Chronological age in constitutional delay, genetic and endocrine causes
- Number of ossification center present at birth: 6
- 1st carpel bone to appear: Capitate f/b Hammate

- Last carpel bone to appear: Pisciform
- Physiological hyperplasia of lymphoid tissue: 4-8 years of age
- Rett syndrome is seen due to deficiency of: Biotin
- Deficiency of cause corneal vascularization, poor growth and photophobia: Riboflavin
- In females, growth spurt is maximum in: Tanner stage III
- MC cause of short stature: Constitutional

Head Circumference

- At birth: 70% of adult head size
- At 2 yrs of age: 90% of adult head size
- Head circumference > chest circumference at birth by: 3 cm
- Head circumference = chest circumference by: 1 year

Upper segment: Lower segment ratio

- At birth: 1.7: 1
- 7-10 yrs: 1:1
- Arm span is equal to height at 10 years of age, if Arm span > Height at 10 years indicate:
  - Marfan syndrome
  - Homocysteinemia

Appearance of Ossification Center on X-ray of Elbow: [Mn: CRITOE]

- **C**apitulum – 1 year
- **R**adial head – 3 years
- **I**nternal/medial epicondyle – 5 years
- **T**rochlea – 7 years
- **O**lecranon – 9 years
- **E**xternal/lateral epicondyle – 11 years

Sequence of Puberty

Boys

- Increase in testicular size
- Appearance of pubic hair
- Growth of penis
- Spermarche – first ejaculation

Girls

- Thelarche – onset of secondary breast development
- Pubarche – appearance of pubic hairs
- Menarche – menstruation begins

Sequence of Dentition

- 1st primary teeth appears at: 6 months of age
- 1st permanent teeth appears at: 6 yrs of age
- Earliest primary teeth: lower central incisor
- Delayed dentition is said if no teeth erupts by: 13 months of age

- Teeth in the upper jaw erupts earlier than those in the lower jaw except:
  - Lower central incisor
  - 2nd molar

Primary Dentition [Mn: I M C M]	Secondary/Permanent Dentition [Mn: M I P C M]
Central Incisor (lower > upper)	1st **M**olar
Lateral Incisor (upper > lower)	Central Incisor (lower > upper)
1st **M**olar	Lateral Incisor
Canine	1st **P**remolar
2nd **M**olar	2nd **P**remolar
	Canine
	2nd **M**olar
	3rd **M**olar

IMPORTANT MILESTONES

1 month	Alert to sound	**8 months**	Sits without support
2 months	Coos Social smile	**9 months**	Stand with support Immature pincer grasps Waves bye bye Bisyllables sounds
3 months	Neck holding Recognizes mother		
4 months	Bidextrous reach Laughs aloud Can steadily hold the head	**12 months**	Stands without support Pincer grasp mature 1-2 words with meaning
5 months	Roll over	**15 months**	Walks without support Creeps upstairs Tower of 2 blocks
6 months	Sits with support/sits in tripod fashion Unidextrous reach Transfer objects Stranger anxiety Monosyllables sounds	**18 months**	Runs Scribbles Tower of 3 blocks 8-10 words vocabulary

Contd...

2 years	• Walks up and downstairs (2 feet/step) • 2-3/few word sentence • Tower of 6 blocks
3 years	• Walks upstairs with alternate foot • Rides tricycle • Tower of 9 blocks • Copies circle • Knows full name and gender • Ask questions

4 years	• Hops on one foot • Walks downstairs with alternate foot • Copies cross and square • Tells stories
4.5 years	• Copies Rectangle
5 years	• Can skip without falling • Dressing and undressing • Copies triangle
9 years	• Copies Cylinder
11 years	• Copies Cube

IMMUNIZATION

- Most thermolabile vaccine: reconstituted BCG
- Most thermostable vaccine: TT
- Most freeze sensitive vaccine is: Hepatitis–B
- Conjugation of vaccine is done to shift the non-T cell response to T cell dependent immunological response
- Temperature of an ILR is measured using: Dial thermometer
- Most important component of cold chain in India: ILR
- Cholera vaccine & yellow fever vaccine cannot be given together
- All live attenuated vaccines are contraindicated in pregnancy except: Yellow fever
- Measles and BCG are contraindicated together as measles depress cell mediated immunity

- Live influenza vaccine is given by: Intranasal route
- H_1N_1 is administered as: nasal spray
- Vaccine C/I in fever: Typhoid vaccine
- Vaccine C/I during lactation: Yellow fever
- Vaccine C/I in > 2 years age: Pertussis
- Vaccine C/I in > 1 years of age: Measles
- Adverse effect of Rotavirus vaccine: Intussusception

Vaccine	Specific Side Effects
Killed Influenza	GBS
Sabin	VAPP
MMR	Toxic shock syndrome
DPT	Shock

Live Attenuated Vaccines:
- BCG
- OPV
- MMR
- Yellow fever
- Typhoral (Ty-21a)
- Influenza vaccine
- Varicella

Cellular Fractions:
- Meningococcal
- Pneumococcal
- Hepatitis – B
- S. typhi (Vi)
- HiB – conjugate

Active + passive immunization is given in:
- Tetanus
- Hepatitis B

Vaccines not to be frozen:
- DPT, DT, TT
- Typhoid
- HBV
- HPV

Vaccines contraindicated in infants:
- Yellow fever
- Meningococcal
- Pneumococcal

Vaccines contraindicated in HIV:
- Asymptomatic: None
- Symptomatic: All live vaccines except OPV

Vaccine indicated for pneumonia patient:
- Pneumococcal vaccine
- H. influenza b
- Measles

Vaccine & Strains

Vaccine	Strain/Serotype
Varicella	▪ OKA strain
Measles	▪ Edmonston Zagreb strain
Rubella	▪ RA 27/3
Mumps	▪ Jeryl – Lynn ▪ L – Zagreb in India
BCG	▪ Danish - 1331
Yellow fever	▪ 17 D
Japanese encephalitis	▪ Nakayama stain – MC ▪ Beijing strain
Meningococcal polysaccharides	▪ Bivalent – A & C ▪ Quadrivalent – A,C,Y, W-135
Malaria	▪ SPf 66 strain ▪ Pf 25 strain

Meningococcal Vaccine

Capsular Polysaccharide Vaccine	Protein–polysaccharide Conjugate Vaccine
▪ Less immunogenic ▪ Quadrivalent – Against A, C, W-135, Y ▪ Bivalent – against A & C ▪ Administered to children ≥2 years ▪ Safe in pregnancy ▪ Useful in epidemics	▪ More immunogenic ▪ Quadrivalent – Against A, C, W-135, Y ▪ Can be given to children <2 years ▪ Safe in pregnancy ▪ Not useful

VACCINES

	Rubella/German Measles	Mumps
Type	▪ Live attenuated	▪ Live attenuated
Strain	▪ RA 27/3	▪ Jeryl-Lynn ▪ L – Zagreb (in India)
Dose	▪ 0.5 mL	▪ 0.5 mL
Schedule		▪ >1 year
Route	▪ Subcutaneous	▪ Intramuscular
Efficacy	▪ >95%	▪ 95%
Contraindication	▪ Pregnancy ▪ Recipient should not become pregnant over 3 months post vaccination	▪ Pregnancy ▪ Immunosuppression
Special points	▪ Vaccination strategy to prevent Congenital Rubella Syndrome: ○ 1st to vaccinate women of child bearing age ○ Then vaccinate children aged 1–14 years to interrupt transmission ○ Subsequently to all children 1 year of age	

REMEMBER

Vaccines that can be frozen: [Mn: OMG]
- OPV
- Measles
- BCG

Vaccines contraindicated in children with history of egg allergy:
- Yellow fever
- Influenza
  [Mn: yellow in the egg]

Post exposure active immunization done in:
- Measles
- Tetanus
- Varicella
- Hepatitis – B
- Rabies
[Mn: MTV Brings Rodies]

	BCG	OPV/SABIN	IPV/SALK
Type	▪ Live attenuated	▪ Live attenuated	▪ Killed vaccine

Strain	▪ Danish - 1331	▪ Trivalent containing virus type I, II & III	▪ Trivalent vaccine containing:-
			  ○ Salk – type-1 (40 units of D Ag)
			  ○ Salk – type-2 (8 units of D Ag)
			  ○ Salk – type-3 (32 units of D Ag)

Dose	▪ 0.1 mL	▪ 2 drops = 0.1 mL	
Schedule	▪ At birth	▪ Birth, 6 weeks, 10 weeks, 14 weeks, 12-18 months	▪ 1st three doses at the interval of 1 – 2 months, 4th dose 6 – 12 months later
Route	▪ Intradermal using 26 gauge syringe ▪ Do not use antiseptic	▪ Oral	▪ Intramuscular (preferred)/subcutaneous
Site	▪ Just above the insertion of left deltoid muscle		
Storage & usage	▪ As freeze dried form ▪ Protect from light ▪ Temperature – 2-8°C ▪ Reconstitute with NS ▪ Reconstituted vaccine to be used within 3 hours (**Mn**: BCG has 3 letters)	▪ Avoid freezing ▪ Temperature: -20°C (non stabilized) ▪ MgCl$_2$ – heat stabilizing agent ▪ Stringent storage conditions required	▪ Avoid freezing ▪ Stable at room temperature ▪ Longer shelf life ▪ Easy to store & transport
Efficacy	▪ 0 – 80%	▪ Life-long	▪ 1st dose – 90%
Complication	▪ Ulceration at the site of vaccinations ▪ Suppurative Lymphadenitis	▪ VAPP – caused by type II	▪ No risk of VAPP
Contraindication	▪ Immunodeficiency/ Immunosuppressed ▪ Pregnancy	▪ Immunocompromised ▪ Pregnancy	
Special points	▪ Offers partial protection against TB ▪ Vaccine induce cell mediated immunity ▪ Reconstituted BCG is most thermo labile vaccine	▪ Both humoral and local immunity present ▪ Useful in epidemics ▪ Widespread herd immunity results even if coverage is 66% ▪ Prevents intestinal reinfection	▪ Safe in immunocompromised ▪ Safe in pregnancy ▪ Not useful in controlling epidemics ▪ Only humoral immunity present ▪ No local immunity present ▪ Do not prevent reinfection of gut

	DPT	MEASLES/RUBEOLA	MMR
Type	▪ Diphtheria & tetanus – Toxoid ▪ Pertussis – killed acellular bacilli	▪ Live attenuated	▪ Live attenuated
Strain		▪ Edmonston – Zagreb strain	
Dose	▪ 0.5 mL	▪ 0.5 mL	▪ 0.5 mL
Schedule	▪ 6 weeks, 10 weeks, 14 weeks, 16 – 24 months f/b DT at 5-6 years of age	▪ At 9th months with Vitamin A ▪ If measles outbreak then at 6th months	▪ 15 – 18 months
Route	▪ Intramuscular, site cleaned with spirit	▪ Subcutaneous /intramuscular	▪ Subcutaneous
Site	▪ Antero-lateral aspect of thigh	▪ Antero-lateral aspect of thigh	▪ Antero-lateral aspect of thigh
Storage & usage	▪ Temperature – 2 to 8°C ▪ Should not be frozen	▪ Temperature – 2 to 8°C ▪ As freeze dried form ▪ Reconstitute with Distilled water (MD) ▪ Use within 1 hour of reconstitution	▪ Temperature – 2-8°C
Efficacy	▪ 70%	▪ 90 – 99%	▪ 90 – 95%
Complication	▪ Fever and mild local reaction ▪ Neurological like encephalopathy, convulsions & Reye's syndrome	▪ Toxic shock syndrome	
Contraindication	▪ Progressive neurological disease ▪ Reactions reported in previous dose ▪ Uncontrolled convulsion ▪ Active epilepsy	▪ Severely immunocompromised patient ▪ Pregnancy ▪ High fever ▪ H/o anaphylaxis with neomycin/gelatin	▪ Severely immunocompromised patient ▪ Pregnancy

Special points	▪ Preservative – Thiomersal
	▪ Components:
	  ○ DT – 25 lf
	  ○ TT – 5 lf
	  ○ Pertussis – 20,000 million
	▪ Adjuvant: AlPO$_4$/Al(OH)$_3$ → increases immunogenicity
	▪ Pertussis enhances the potency of DT
	▪ Unimmunised child > 5 years should be vaccinated with 2 doses of DT
		▪ Preservative – neomycin, gelatin
		▪ Sensitive to sunlight
		▪ I.P. of vaccine induced measles is 7 days
		▪ Should be routinely administered to potentially susceptible, asymptomatic HIV positive children & adults
		▪ 2nd dose of measles vaccine may be added to routine immunization if coverage of 1st dose is >80%	

	Strain	Dose (TCID)
Measles	Edmonston Zagreb	1000
Mumps	Jeryl Lynn	5000
Rubella	RA 27/3	1000

MISCELLANEOUS

- Kasai procedure is done for: Extra hepatic biliary atresia
- MC GIT malignancy of childhood is: Lymphoma
- Gas reaches colonic end in a newborn by: 8-10 hours
- MC cause of acute infantile gastroenteritis is: Rota virus
- Vitamin associated with hemolytic anemia in preterm babies: Vitamin K
- MC nephrotic syndrome in children: Minimal change disease
  - Excellent response to steroids
- MC cause of hypertension in a child: Chronic glomerulonephritis

Teratogenicity	Drugs
▪ **Neural tube defects**	Valproate, Carbamazepine
▪ **Ebstein anomaly**	Lithium
▪ **Hypoplasia of nasal bone**	Warfarin
▪ **Grey Baby syndrome**	Chloramphenicol
▪ **Pyloric stenosis**	Erythromycin
▪ **Enamel hypoplasia, teeth discoloration**	Tetracyclines

Teratogenicity	Drugs
▪ **Adenocarcinoma of vagina**	Diethylstilbestrol (DES)
▪ **Moebius syndrome**	Misoprostol
▪ **Phocomelia**	Thalidomide
▪ **Accutane embryopathy**	Isotretinoin
▪ **Fractured chromosome**	LSD

MULTIPLE CHOICE QUESTIONS

CHAPTER 1: NORMAL GROWTH AND ITS DISORDERS

ANTHROPOMETRY

1. New born doubles his weight at- *(PGMEE 2014)*
- a. 3 months
- b. 6 months
- c. 9 months
- d. 12 months

[Ref: O.P. Ghai 8th/e pg. 13 table 2.3, Nelson 21st/e/p 135]

2. Weight of a newborn quadruples at- *(PGMEE 2015)*
- a. 6 months
- b. 1 year
- c. 2 years
- d. 4 years

[Ref: O.P. Ghai 8th/e/p 13 Table 2.3]

3. Average head circumference at birth is- *(PGMEE 2015)*
- a. 35cm
- b. 30cm
- c. 45cm
- d. 40cm

[Ref: O.P. Ghai 8th/e pg. 13 Table 2.3, Nelson 21st/e/p 129]

4. Average gain of height in first year is? *(PGMEE 2013)*
- a. 25 cm
- b. 50 cm
- c. 75 cm
- d. 100 cm

[Ref: Ghai 8the/p 13, Nelson 21st/e/p 154]

5. At what age a child's height is expected to be 100 cm? *(PGMEE 2012)*
- a. 2 years
- b. 3 years
- c. 4 years
- d. 5 years

[Ref: Ghai 8th/e/p 13, Nelson 21st/e/p 154]

6. Upper segment to lower segment ratio in 3 year age child is- *(PGMEE 2012-13)*
- a. 1.2
- b. 1.3
- c. 1.4
- d. 1.5

[Ref: Ghai 8th/e/p 36]

7. What percentage of weight is lost by newborn in first week? *(PGMEE 2015)*
- a. 1-2%
- b. 5-10%
- c. 10-20%
- d. None

[Ref: Nelson 21st/e/p 154, Ghai 8th/e/p 13]

8. What is the average weight gain of the neonate per day-
- a. 5-10g *(PGMEE 2015, 2013, 2014)*
- b. 25-30g
- c. 50-60g
- d. 100-150g

[Ref: Nelson 21st/e/p 154, Ghai 8th/e/p 13]

9. The height of a child is double of the birth height at the age of- *(PGMEE 2012-13)*
- a. 1 year
- b. 2 years
- c. 4 years
- d. 6 years
- e. 8 years

[Ref: O.P. Ghai 8th/e/p 13, Nelson 21st/e/p 154]

Explanation

Age	Growth in length
0-3 mth	3.5 cm/month
3-6 mth	2 cm/month
6-9 mth	1.5 cm/month
9-12 mth	1.2 cm/month
1-3 year	1 cm/year
4-6 year	3 cm/year

10. Arm span and height becomes same at what age- *(PGMEE 2013-14)*
- a. 9 year
- b. 11 year
- c. 12 year
- d. 13 year

[Ref: Ghai 8th/e/p 36]

11. Microcephaly is defined as head circumference? *(PGMEE 2012)*
- a. <1SD for age and sex
- b. <2SD for age and sex
- c. <3SD for age and sex
- d. <4SD for age and sex

[Ref: Ghai 8th/e/p 40]

12. Which of the following parameter is best for fetal growth assessment? *(PGMEE 2016-17)*
- a. Abdominal circumference
- b. Head circumference
- c. Femur length
- d. Height

[Ref: Nelson 201st/e/ chapter 115]

Explanation

- Parameters for fetal growth assessment by USG
  - 1st Trimester → **C**rown - rump length (CRL)
  - 2nd Trimester → **B**iparietal diameter (BPD)
  - 3rd Trimester → **A**bdominal Circumference & Femoral length (AC & FL)

  [Mnemonic to remember:- CBA]

DENTITION

13. Primary dentition begins to show teeth eruption by: *(PGMEE 2013-14)*
- a. 12months
- b. 12 weeks
- c. 6 months
- d. 6 weeks

[Ref: Nelson 21st/e/p 156, Ghai 8th/e/p 11]

14. At what age do first permanent teeth appear? *(DNB Nov 13 Pattern)*
- a. 5 years
- b. 6 years
- c. 7 years
- d. 8 years

[Ref: Nelson 21st/e/p 156, Ghai 8th/e/p 11]

1.	b
2.	c
3.	a
4.	a
5.	c
6.	b
7.	b
8.	b
9.	c
10.	b
11.	c
12.	a
13.	c
14.	b

15. **Delayed dentition is seen in all except-**
    a. Down syndrome *(PGMEE 2012-13)*
    b. Rickets
    c. Congenital hypothyroidism
    d. All

    [Ref: Nelson 21st/e/p 156, internet]

Explanation

Wilm's tumour

- "Most Babies have their first primary (Milk) teeth erupt at 6 months of age and first secondary teeth erupt at age of 6 years."
- Some Important Points in dentition-
    1. Delayed eruption is usually considered when ther are no teeth by approximately 13 months of Age.
    2. Common causes of delayed Dentition are Idiopathic, hypothyroidism, Hypoparathyroidism, Trisomy 21, Familial, hypopituitarism.
    3. Central Incisors are first to develop in primary while first Molars are first to develop in secondary dentition.
    4. Second molar develops last in primary while third Molar develops last in secondary dentition.
    5. The teeth that are most commonly absent include the 3rd molars, the maxillary lateral incisors, and the mandibular 2nd premolars.

16. **Milk teeth-Total no. in human being-** *(PGMEE 2012-13)*
    a. 20   b. 28
    c. 32   d. 24

    [Ref: Nelson 21st/e/p 156, Ghai 8th/e/p 11]

17. **1st permanent teeth to appear-** *(PGMEE 2012-13)*
    a. Molar   b. Canine
    c. Premolar   d. Incisor

    [Ref: Nelson 21st/e/p 156, Ghai 8th/e/p 11]

18. **Mixed dentition present in which age group:** *(PGMEE 2016-17)*
    a. 2-6 years   b. 6-12 years
    c. 12-18 years   c. 9-12 years

    [Ref: Ghai 8th/e/p 11]

DISORDERS OF GROWTH

19. **A child has history of delayed growth and delayed growth spurt. The bone development is not according to the chronological age but corresponds to the height age. What is diagnosis?** *(PGMEE 2013)*
    a. Familial short stature
    b. Genetic
    c. Constitutional delay
    d. Psychosocial Dwarfism

    [Ref: Ghai 8th/e/p 37, Nelson 21st/e/p 155-156]

Explanation

- Constitutional growth delay is one of the **variants of normal growth** commonly encountered by the pediatrician.

- Length and weight measurements of affected children are normal at birth, and growth is normal for the 1st 4-12 mo of life.
- Height is sustained at a lower percentile during childhood.
- The pubertal growth spurt is delayed, so their growth rates continue to decline after their classmates have begun to accelerate.
- Detailed questioning often reveals other family members (often 1 or both parents) with histories of short stature in childhood, delayed puberty, and eventual normal stature.
- IGF-1 levels tend to be low for chronological age but within the normal range for bone age.
- GH responses to provocative testing tend to be lower than in children with a more typical timing of puberty.
- The prognosis for these children to achieve normal adult height is guarded.
- Predictions based on height and bone age tend to overestimate eventual height to a greater extent in boys than in girls.
- Boys with >2 yr of pubertal delay can benefit from a short course of testosterone therapy to hasten puberty after 14 yr of age.
- The cause of this variant of normal growth is thought to be persistence of the relatively hypogonadotropic state of childhood

20. **A child's growth is slower than his peers but normal when compared to his father's childhood records. If the child ultimately achieves normal height, what can be the possible diagnosis?** *(PGMEE 2016-17)*
    a. Delayed puberty   b. Hormonal imbalance
    c. GH deficiency   d. Constitutional delay

    [Ref: Ghai 8th/e/p 37]

Explanation

- See above Explanation

21. **Which of the following is TRUE about constitutional delay in growth?** *(PGMEE 2013)*
    a. Neonates with constitutional delay show anomalies at birth
    b. IGF-1 levels are low for bone age
    c. IGF-1 levels are low for chronological age
    d. Bone age is normal

    [Ref: Nelson 21st/e/p 155-156, Ghai 8th/e/p 37]

Explanation

- Constitutional delay in growth & puberty is a transient state of Hypogonadotrophic hypogonadism associated with prolongation of childhood phase of growth, delayed skeletal maturation, delayed & attenuated pubertal growth spurt & relatively low IGF-1 secretion.

22. **All are true in Constitutional Delay EXCEPT:** *(PGMEE 2016-2017)*
    a. Baseline growth hormone decreased
    b. IGF-1 levels are lower for the chronological age
    c. Growth delay occurs after 2–3 years age.
    d. Puberty is also delayed.

    [Ref: Nelson 21st/e/ chapter 573 p 2886]

15.	d
16.	a
17.	a
18.	b
19.	c
20.	d
21.	c
22.	a

23. A short stature patient with narrowed foramen magnum and rhizomelic limbs is seen in? *(PGMEE 2014-15)*

- a. Achondroplasia
- b. Laron dwarfism
- c. Hypothyroidism
- d. Morquio disease

[Ref: Harrison's 19th/e pg. 426e-7, Nelson 21st/e/p 3726]

Explanation

Achondroplasia

- Short limbs, long narrow trunk, large head with midfacial hypoplasia & prominent forehead.
- Proximal segment shortening.
- Trident configuration of fingers.
- Most joints are hyperextensible.
- X ray → Short vertebral pedicles
- Spinal canal is stenotic & spinal cord compression can occur at foramen magnum & in lumbar spine.

CRANIOSYNOSTOSIS

24. Premature closure of Lambdoid suture leads to which type of craniosynostosis? *(PGMEE 2016-17)*

- a. Occipital plagiocephaly
- b. Dolichocephaly
- c. Parietal plagiocephaly
- d. Trigonocephaly

[Ref: Nelson 21st/e/p 3081]

23. a
24. a

DEVELOPMENTAL MILESTONES

1. When does Pincer grasp develop? (PGMEE 2015, 14, 13)
  a. 2-6 months   b. 6-9 months
  c. 9-12 months   d. 12-18 months

  [Ref: Nelson 21st/e pg. 135, Ghai 8th/e/p 50 table 3.2]

2. Mature pincer grasp develops at-   (PGMEE 2016-17)
  a. 9 months   b. 10 months
  c. 11 months   d. 12 months

  [Ref: Nelson 21st/e pg. 135, Ghai 8th/e/p 50 table 3.2]

3. Which is false about developmental milestones at 6 months of age?   (PGMEE 2015)
  a. Pincer grasp   b. Monosyllable sounds
  c. Watching self in mirror   d. Sitting in tripod position

  [Ref: Nelson 21st/e pg. 135, Ghai 8th/e/p 49-53]

4. At what age child begins to use past and present tense-   (PGMEE 2015)

  a. 1 Years   b. 2 Years
  c. 18 Months   d. 36 Months

  [Ref: Nelson 21st/e pg. 273]

5. Milestones 1 year of age are all except-   (PGMEE 2015)
  a. Turn pages of book
  b. Playing a simple ball game
  c. Spontaneous scribbling
  d. Walking upstairs 1 step at a time

  [Ref: Nelson 21st/e pg. 132-133, O.P. Ghai 8th/e pg. 49 table 3.1]

Explanation

Developmental Milestones in the 1st 2 Yr of life		
Milestone	Average Age of Attainment (MO)	Developmental Implications
GROSS MOTOR		
Holds head steady while sitting	2	Allows more visual interaction
Pulls to sit, with no head lag	3	Muscle tone
Brings hands together in midline	3	Self-discovery of hands
Asymmetric tonic neck reflex gone	4	Can inspect hands in midline
Sits without support	6	Increasing exploration
Rolls back to stomach	6.5	Truncal flexion, risk of falls
Walks alone	12	Exploration control of proximity to parents
Runs	16	Supervision more difficult
FINE MOTOR		
Grasps rattle	3.5	Object use
Reaches for objects	4	Visuomotor coordination
Palmer grasp gone	4	Voluntary releases
Transfers object hand to hand	5.5	Comparison of objects
Thumb-finger grasp	8	Able to explore small objects
Turn pages of book	12	Increasing autonomy during book time
Scribbles	13	Visual-motor coordination
Builds tower of 2 cubes	15	Uses objects in combination
Builds tower of 6 cubes	22	Requires visual, gross and fine motor coordination
COMMUNICATION AND LANGUAGE		
Smiles in response to face, voice	1.5	More active social participant
Monosyllabic babble	6	Experimentation with sound, tactile sense
Inhibits to "no"	7	Response to tone (nonverbal)
Follows one-step command with gesture	7	Nonverbal communication
Follows one-step command without gesture	10	Verbal receptive language (e.g, "Give it to be")
Says "marra" or "data"	10	Expressive language
Points to objects	10	Interactive communication
Speaks firs: real word	12	Beginning of labelling

1.	c
2.	d
3.	a
4.	d
5.	d

Speaks 4-6 words	15	Acquisition of object and personal names
Speaks 10-15 words	18	Acquisition of object and personal names
Speaks 2-word sentences (e.g., "Mommy shoe")	19	Beginning grammatization corresponds with 50 word vocabulary
COGNITIVE		
Stares momentarily	2	Loss of object permanence (out of sight, out of mind [e.g., yam ball dropped])
Stares at own hand	4	Self-discovery, cause and effect
Bangs 2 cubes	8	Active comparison of objects
Uncovers toy (after seeing it hidden)	8	Object permanence
Egocentric symbolic play (e.g., pretends to drink from cup)	12	Beginning symbolic thought
Uses stick to reach toy	17	Able to link actions to solve problems
Pretend play with doll (e.g., gives doll bottle)	17	Symbolic thought

6. Stranger anxiety develops at- *(PGMEE 2015)*
- a. 3 months
- b. 4 months
- c. 7 months
- d. 11 months

[Ref: O.P. Ghai 8th/e pg. 52]

7. Milestone of 18month old child includes- *(PGMEE 2014)*
- a. Rides tricycle
- b. Ten words
- c. Knows gender
- d. Climbs steps

[Ref: Ghai 8th/e/p 49-53]

8. Two year old has vocabulary of how many words-
- a. 20
- b. 50 *(PGMEE 2014)*
- c. 100
- d. 200

[Ref: Nelson 21st/e pg. 142]

9. What is the age of the child in whom pincer grasp is present, speaks bisyllables and does 'bye-bye'?
(PGMEE 2014)
- a. 96 months
- b. 9 months
- c. 18 months
- d. 24 months

[Ref: Ghai 8th/e/p 52-53, Nelson 21st/e/chapter 22]

10. 'Red flag' sign in child development- *(PGMEE 2014)*
- a. No visual fixation at 2 months
- b. No speech at 18 months
- c. Does not walk alone at 18 months
- d. All

[Ref: Nelson 21st/e pg. 158 Table 28.2]

11. Neck holding comes at what age- *(PGMEE 2013-14)*
- a. 2 months
- b. 3 months
- c. 4 months
- d. 5 months

[Ref: Ghai 8th/e pg. 49, Nelson 21st/e pg. 133 table 22.2]

12. Bidextrous grasp is seen at *(PGMEE 2019)*
- a. 4 months
- b. 5 months
- c. 6 months
- d. 7 months

[Ref: O.P. Ghai 9th/e pg. 46, 48, 49]

13. A child identifies parts of body & builds tower of 4 cubes. Age is- *(PGMEE 2013-14)*
- a. 1 year
- b. 2 years
- c. 3 years
- d. 4 year

[Ref: Nelson 21st/e pg. 142 table 23.1, Ghai 8th/e/p 49-53]

14. An baby can make a tower of 5-6 cubes at:
(Recent Pattern June 2018)
- a. 12 month
- b. 18 month
- c. 2½ yr
- d. 3 yr

[Ref: O.P. Ghai 8th/e pg. 52; Nelson's 20th/e pg. 75]

Explanation

Stacks of Blocks

Age	Number of blocks	Findings
▪ 12-16 months	2	At this stage child can stack .... blocks without them toppling over.
▪ 16-18 months	3	
▪ 18 -22 months	4	
▪ 22-24 months	6	
▪ 23-26 months	3	Line 3 blocks end to end on the ground, and **push** them horizontally along as if they were a train
▪ 28 - 31 months	8	child can stack .... blocks without them toppling over.
▪ 31-36 months	3	child can make 3 blocks house.
▪ 32-36 months	9	child can stack 9 blocks without them toppling over.

15. Purposeful movements start at- *(PGMEE 2013-14)*
- a. 6 month
- b. 7 months
- c. 8 month
- d. 9 month

[Ref: Nelson 21st/e pg. 133 table 22.2]

16. Bidextrous grip is achieved at the age of:
(Recent Pattern June 2018)
- a. 4 months
- b. 6 months
- c. 9 months
- d. 12 months

[Ref: O.P. Ghai 8th/e pg. 52; Nelson's 20th/e pg. 75]

6.	c
7.	b
8.	c
9.	b
10.	d
11.	b
12.	a
13.	b
14.	c
15.	a
16.	a

Explanation

- 4 months- Bidextrous reach
- 6 months -Unidextrous reach
- 9 months -Immature pincer grasp
- 12 months- Mature pincer grasp
- 15 months -Imitates scribbling, tower of 2 blocks
- 18 months -Scribbles, tower of 3 blocks
- 2 years -Tower of 6 blocks, vertical & circular stroke
- 3 years - Tower of 9 blocks, draw a circle
- 4 years - Copies cross, Bridge with blocks

17. Child draws triangle at what age? *(PGMEE 2013)*
a. 3 years   b. 5 years
c. 6 years   d. 7 years

[Ref: Nelson 21st/e pg. 142 table 23.1, Ghai 8th/e/p 50 table 3.2]

18. A child speaks sentences at the age of? *(PGMEE 2012)*
a. 6 months   b. 18 months
c. 1 year   d. 2 years

[Ref: Nelson 21st/e pg. 142 table 23.1, Ghai 8th/e/p 53]

19. A child is able to say short sentences of 6 words at the age of- *(PGMEE 2012-13)*
a. 2 years   b. 3 years
c. 4 years   d. 5 years

[Ref: Nelson 21st/e pg. 142 table 23.1]

20. A child is able to build blocks of 5 Cubes Developmental age is- *(PGMEE 2012-13)*
a. 12 months   b. 15 months
c. 18 months   d. 24 months

[Ref: Nelson 21st/e pg. 142 table 23.1]

21. Which of the following cannot be done by 3 years old child- *(PGMEE 2012-13)*
a. Draw a circle
b. Can go up and down
c. Draw a triangle
d. Can arrange 9 cubes

[Ref: Nelson 21st/e pg. 142 table 23.1, Ghai 8the/p 50]

22. Child understands his sex and can build tower of 9 cubes at age- *(PGMEE 2016-17)*
a. 12 months   b. 24 months
c. 36 months   d. 48 months

[Ref: Nelson 21st/e pg. 142 table 23.1]

23. In a child milestone of scribbling and turning pages is achieved at age of- *(PGMEE 2016-17)*
a. 12-13 months   b. 18 months
c. 24 months   d. 36 months

[Ref: Nelson 21st/e pg. 142 table 23.1]

Explanation

- Scribbling and turning pages is achieved at the age of 12-13 months.

24. A child is able to draw a triangle, skip, and identify 4 different colors. Age of the child is: *(PGMEE 2016-17)*
a. 36 months   b. 48 months
c. 54 months   d. 60 months

[Ref: Nelson 21st/e pg. 142 table 23.1]

25. A child can copy a "cross" at the age of:
(Recent Pattern June 2018)
a. 24 month   b. 26 month
c. 60 month   d. 48 month

[Ref: O.P. Ghai 8th/e pg. 52; Nelson's 20th/e pg. 75]

Explanation

- A baby can draw or copy a:-
  - Horizontal/ vertical line at 2 year (scribbles)
  - Circle by 2.5 to 3 years, imitates cross
  - A plus sign at 4 years
  - Copy a cross and square by 4 years
  - A rectangle 4.5 years
  - A diamond by 6 years

26. A child can draw circle at what age- *(PGMEE 2016-17)*
a. 18 months   b. 30 months
c. 36 months   d. 48 months

[Ref: Nelson 21st/e pg. 142 table 23.1]

27. At what age can a child make a tower of 7 cubes, walk up and down the stairs, and use pronoun: *(PGMEE 2016-17)*
a. 1 year   b. 2 years
c. 3 years   d. 4 years

[Ref: Nelson 21st/e pg. 142 table 23.1]

BEHAVIORAL & PERVASIVE DEVELOPMENTAL DISORDER

28. Pica refers to- *(PGMEE 2012-13)*
a. IU sucking
b. Foreign object being put in the mouth
c. Thumb sucking
d. None

[Ref: Nelson 21st/e/p ch. 36.2, Ghai 8th/e/p 58]

29. Treatment of breath holding spells is- *(PGMEE 2013)*
a. Iron
b. Pyridoxine
c. Molybdenum
d. Zinc

[Ref: Ghai 8th/e/p 58, Nelson 21st/e pg. 3122]

30. All are characteristics of autism except- *(PGMEE 2013-14)*
a. Delayed Language development
b. Repetitive behavior
c. Severe deficit social interaction
d. Onset often at age of 6 years

[Ref: Nelson 21st/e ch. 54, Ghai 8th/e/p 61]

31. Adolescent starts at the age of- *(PGMEE 2013)*
a. 7 years
b. 10 years
c. 14 years
d. 17 years

[Ref: Nelson 21st/e ch. 132, Ghai 8th/e/p 63]

17.	b
18.	d
19.	c
20.	c
21.	c
22.	c
23.	a
24.	d
25.	d
26.	c
27.	b
28.	b
29.	a
30.	d
31.	b

PUBERTAL DEVELOPMENT

32. In females, growth spurt is maximum in?
(DNB December 2011)
a. Tanner breast stage I, axillary stage I
b. Tanner breast stage II, Axillary stage II
c. Tanner breast stage IV, Axillary stage IV
d. Tanner breast stage III, Axillary stage III

[Ref: Nelson 21st/e pg. 1014-1017, Ghai 8th/e/p 63; PHV at SMR -2, 3 NELSON pg 297]

Explanation

Pubertal development in Girls

- In girls normal age of puberty is 8-12 years.
  - Onset of puberty before 8 years → Precocious Puberty
  - After12 yrs is → delayed.
- The order of appearance is Thelarche → Pubarche (pubic hair) → Peak Growth Velocity → Menarche(*TPGM).
  - Thelarche (breast development) is first sign and occurs between 8-12 yrs.(Tanner/SMR 2).
  - Menses begin 2-21/2 yrs later (SMR3-4).
- Peak Growth Velocity occurs in SMR2-3;Just before menarche(which occurs in SMR3-4).

Pubertal development in Boys

- In boys normal age of puberty is 9-13 years.
- 1st visible sign is testicular enlargement (SMR2), beginning as early as 9yr. This is followed by penile growth during SMR3. Sperm formtion also occurs in SMR III.
- Peak growth occurs during SMR4 when testis volumes reach approximately 9-10ml.
- Sequence in boys is Testis enlargement → Penis enlargement → Pubic hair → Peak Ht. Velocity → Axillary hair → Facial Hair.

33. First Sign of Pubertal development in girls is-
(PGMEE 2013-14)
a. Pubarche   b. Adrenarche
c. Thelarche   d. Menarche

[Ref: Nelson 21st/e ch. 132 pg. 1014, Ghai 8th/e/p 63]

34. First Sign of pubertal development in boys is-
a. Enlargement of penis   (PGMEE 2013-14)
b. Enlargement of testes
c. Appearance of axillary hair
d. Appearance of pubic hair

[Ref: Nelson 21st/e/ch. 132 pg 1014, Ghai 8th/e/p 63]

35. What is thelarche?   (PGMEE 2012-13)
a. Post hormonal therapy breast enlargement in post-menopausal females
b. Breast enlargement in pregnancy
c. Hormone related breast enlargement during puberty in girls
d. Breast enlargement by implants

[Ref: Nelson 21st/e ch. 132, Ghai 8th/e/p 63]

36. Maximum growth spurt is seen in girls at time of-
(PGMEE 2012-13)
a. Menarche   b. Adrenarche
c. Pubarche   d. Thelarche

[Ref: Nelson 21st/e ch. 132, Ghai 8th/e/p 63]

37. Precocious puberty is appearance of first sign of puberty before the age of-   (PGMEE 2016-17)
a. 8 years in girls and 9.5 years in boys
b. 9.5 years in girls and 8 years in boys
c. 8 years in girls and 8 years in boys
d. 9.5 years in girls and 9.5 years in boys

[Ref: Ghai 8th/e/p 531]

Explanation

- Precocious Puberty is appearance of first sign of puberty before 8 years in girls and 9.5 years in boys (according to Nelson's pg. 2656 .

DEVELOPMENTAL DELAY

38. Patient with growth retardation, delayed milestones with kinky hair. What is the diagnosis?
(NEET Pattern 2017)
a. Menke' disease   b. Trisomy 21
c. Lesch nyhan syndrome   d. Wilson disease

[Ref: Nelson 21st/e pg. 3192]

Explanation

Menke's disease

- **Also k/as kinky hair disease**
- Progressive neurodegenerative disorder with XR inheritance.
- The Menkes gene codes for a copper-transporting, P-type ATPase, and mutations in the protein are associated with **low serum copper and ceruloplasmin levels as well as a defect in intestinal copper absorption and transport.**
- Symptoms begin in the 1st few months of life and include **hypotonia, hypothermia, and generalized myoclonic seizures.** The facies are distinctive, with chubby, rosy cheeks and kinky, colorless, friable hair. Feeding difficulties lead to failure to thrive. Severe mental retardation and optic atrophy are constant features of the disease.
- There is tortuous **degeneration of the gray matter** and **marked changes in the cerebellum** with loss of the internal granule cell layer and necrosis of the Purkinje cells. Death occurs by 3 yr of age in untreated patients.
- Microscopic examination of the hair shows (**fractures along the hair shaft (trichorrhexis nodosa)** and twisted hair (pili torti).
- **Copper-histidine therapy** if started in neonatal period may prevent neurologic deterioration. Dose is copper histidine, 250 μg by s/c injection BD to 1 yr of age and 250 μg OD thereafter.
- The **occipital horn syndrome,** a skeletal dysplasia d/ to a different mutations in the **same gene** is a relatively mild disease. Biochemical findings are same.

39. The milestones of a three year old child are considered delayed if he is unable to: (NEET Pattern 2017)
a. Hop on 1 foot   b. Use spoon effectively
c. Copy a square   d. Reliably catch a ball

Explanation

- Spoon holding develops at 15 months of age.

32.	d
33.	c
34.	b
35.	c
36.	a
37.	a
38.	a
39.	b

BASIC CONCEPTS

1. **When ICF and ECF of child becomes equal to adult person-** *(PGMEE 2012-13)*
   - a. 1 year
   - b. year
   - c. 3 year
   - d. 4 year

   [Ref: Nelson 21st/e/pg. 389]

2. **Blood volume in preterm neonate is gestation?** *(PGMEE 2013)*
   - a. 60 ml/kg
   - b. 70 ml/kg
   - c. 80 ml/kg
   - d. 60-80 ml/kg

   [Ref: Maternal, fetal and neonatal physiology by Susan Tucker Blackburn 4th/e p. 235; Advances in pediatrics by Dutta p. 154]

3. **Dose of Maintenance fluid required in a 10kg boy is-** *(PGMEE 2015)*
   - a. 1200 ml/day
   - b. 300 ml/day
   - c. 1000 ml/day
   - d. 2000 ml/day

   [Ref: Ghai 8th/e/p 72 table 5.1]

4. **What is the maintainance fluid requirement in a 6 kg child?** *(PGMEE 2015)*
   - a. 240 ml/day
   - b. 600 ml/day
   - c. 300 ml/day
   - d. 1200 ml/day

   [Ref: Ghai 8th/e/p 72 table 5.1]

5. **Child with 10 episodes of diarrhea in last 24 hours with sunken dry eyes, very slow skin pinch, and absent tear. Fluid used for management is-** *(PGMEE 2015)*
   - a. Starts Ringer's lactate
   - b. Breast feeding
   - c. ORS solution
   - d. Starts 10% dextrose

   [Ref: O.P. Ghai 8th/e pg. 294; Nelson 21st/e ch. 70 pg. 430]

Explanation

Fluid Management of Dehydration
Restore intravascular volume:
Normal saline: 20 mL/kg over 20 min
Repeat as needed
Calculate 24-hr fluid needs: maintenance + deficit volume
Subtract isotomic fluid already administered from 24 hr fluid needs Administer remaining volume over 24 hr using 5% dextrose NS + 20 mEq/L KCl
Replaced ongoing losses as they occur

- The child with dehydration needs acute intervention to ensure that there is adequate tissue perfusion.
- This resuscitation phase requires rapid restoration of the circulating intravascular volume and treatment of shock with an isotonic solution, such as normal saline (NS) or Ringer lactate (LR)
- If normal saline given in option then it would be 1st choice.

6. **Amount of fluid given in a 10 month old child is?** *(DNB December 2011)*
   - a. 2 ml/kg/hr
   - b. 4 ml/kg/hr
   - c. 8 ml/kg/hr
   - d. 10 ml/kg/hr

   [Ref: Ghai 8th/e/p 72 table 5.1]

7. **Capilary refill time in child with shock is?** *(PGMEE 2012)*
   - a. > 1 second
   - b. > 2 second
   - c. > 3 second
   - d. > 4 second

   [Ref: Internet]

8. **Maximum concentration of dextrose that can be given through peripheral vascular line in neonate-** *(PGMEE 2012-13)*
   - a. 5
   - b. 10
   - c. 12.5
   - d. 25

   [Ref: AIIMS Neonatalogy protocol-Hypoglycemia in Newborn]

Explanation

- States that we should avoid using dextrose conc. > 12.5% while infusing dextrose through peripheral cannula, as risk of thrombophlebitis increases.

9. **Requirement of potassium in child is-** *(PGMEE 2013-14)*
   - a. 1-2 mEq/kg
   - b. 4-7 mEq/kg
   - c. 10-12 mEq/kg
   - d. 13-14 mEq/lit

   [Ref: Nelson 21st/e/pg. 398]

DEHYDRATION AND ITS TREATMENT

10. **A 6 year old drowsy child came in emergency. HE was suffering from vomiting and loose motion for 3 days. On examination he had sunken eye, hypothermia, skin on pinching goes back very slowly. Diagnosis is-** *(PGMEE 2013-14)*
    - a. No dehydration
    - b. Severe dehydration
    - c. Mild dehydration
    - d. Some dehydration

    [Ref: Ghai 8th/e/p 293]

11. **A 1 year old child presents in a emergency with watery loose stools. On examination her eyes are sunken, she is thirsty and eager to drink, her skin goes back within 2 seconds. Her weight is 6 Kg. What will you instruct to Nurse:-** *(PGMEE 2018)*
    - a. Start IV Ringer Lactate solution 180 mL over 30 min.
    - b. Giver her 50 mL ORS over 30 min
    - c. 250 mL ORS over next 1-2 hour
    - d. 120 ml over 4 hours

    [Ref: Nelson 21st/e/ch. 366 acute gastroenteritis]

1.	a
2.	d
3.	c
4.	b
5.	a
6.	b
7.	c
8.	c
9.	a
10.	b
11.	c

Explanation

- Patient is mild to moderately dehydrated
- Ideal ans should be 300-600 ml ORS over 4 hrs
- Among options 250 ml ORS over 2 hrs is closest

Symptom	Minimal or no dehydration (<3% LOSS of body weight)	Mild to moderate dehydration (3-9% loss of body weight)	Severe dehydration (<9% LOSS of body weight)
Mental status	Well; alert	Normal fatigued or restless, irritable	Apathetic, lethargic, unconscious
Thirst	Drinks normally; might refuse liquids	Thirsty; eager to drink	Drinks poorly; unable to drink
Heart rate	Normal	Normal to increased	Tachycardia, with bradycardia in most severe cases
Quality of pulses	Normal	Normal to decreased	Weak, thread, or impalpable
Breathing	Normal	Normal; fast	Deep
Eyes	Normal	Slightly sunken	Deeply sunken
Tears	Present	Decreased	Absent
Mouth and tongue	Moist	Dry	Parched
Skinfold	Instant recoil	Recoil in <2 sec	Recoil in >2 sec
Capillary refill	Normal	Prolonged	Prolonged; minimal
Extremities	Warm	Cool	Cold; mottled; cyanotic
Urine outpur	Normal to decreased	Decreased	Minimal

- Summary of Treatment Based on Degree of Dehydration
- From Centers for Disease Control and Prevention: Diagnosis and management of foodborne illnesses, MMWR 53:1–33, 2004

12. a
13. a

Degree of dehydration	Rehydration therapy	Replacement of losses	Nutrition
Minimal or no dehydration	Not applicable	<10 kg body weight:60-120 mL ORS for each diarrheal stool or vomiting episode >10 kg body weight: 120-240 mL ORS for each diarrheal stool or vomiting episode	Continue breast-feeding, or resume age- appropriate normal diet after initial hydration, including adequate caloric intake for maintenance
Mild to moderate dehydration	ORS, 50-100 mL/kg body weight over 3-4 hr	Same	Same
Severe dehydration	Lactated ringer solution of normal saline in 20 mL/kg body weight IV until perfusion and mental status improve; then administer 100 mL/kg body weight ORS over 4 hr or 5% dextrose ½ normal saline IV at twice maintenance fluid rates	Same; if unable to drink, administer through nasogastric tube or administer 5% dextrose in ¼ normal saline with 20 mEq/L potassium chloride IV	Same
ORS, oral rehydration solution			

12. 1 year old child with multiple episodes of diarrhea presents with sunken eyes, depressed fontanels and very slow skin pinch. The amount of fluid to be given intravenously in the first 6 hours is- *(PGMEE 2015)*
- a. 600 ml
- b. 900 ml
- c. 1200 ml
- d. 1500 ml

[Ref: O.P. Ghai 8th/e pg. 295]

13. A child 4 month old has 10 episodes of vomiting and 2-3 episodes of loose stools and crying since the last 24 hours. There is increase thirst. Best line of management will be? *(PGMEE 2013)*
- a. ORS
- b. Intravenous fluids
- c. Intravenous fluids then ORS
- d. Hospitalise and treat

[Ref: O.P. Ghai 8th/e p. 73]

Explanation

- See IMNCI diarrhea management guidelines (in theory section)

ORS

14. Osmolarity of standard ORS solution is? *(PGMEE 2012)*
   a. 210   b. 245
   c. 311   d. 330

[Ref: O.P. Ghai 8th/e p. 293]

15. Low osmolar ORS has low content of? *(PGMEE 2012)*
   a. Glucose and sodium bicarbonate
   b. Glucose and Citrate
   c. Glucose and potassium
   d. Glucose and sodium chloride

[Ref: O.P. Ghai 8th/e/p 293]

Explanation

Low osmolarity ORS				Standard ORS
	g		**Osm**	
NaCl	2.6	Na⁺	75	90
Glucose (anhydrous)	13.5	Cl⁻	65	80
KCl	1.5	Gluc(an)	75	111
		K⁺	20	20
Trisodium Citrate dehydrate	2.9	Citrate	10	10
				10
		Total osmalarity	245	311

16. Sodium content of ReSoMal is- *(PGMEE 2013-14)*
   a. 90 mmol/lit   b. 60 mmol/lit
   c. 45 mmol/lit   d. 30 mmol/lit

[Ref: Nelson 21st/e/pg. 341 table 57.11]

17. Reduced osmolarity ORS contains all EXCEPT-
   (PGMEE 2015)
   a. Citrate   b. Potassium
   c. Lactate   d. Sodium

[Ref: O.P. Ghai 8th/e pg. 294]

18. Prepared ORS solution is stable for a period of:
   (PGMEE 2016-17)
   a. 24 hrs   b. 48 hours
   c. 72 hours   d. 7 days

[Ref: Ghai 8th/e/p 293]

14.	**c**
15.	**d**
16.	**c**
17.	**c**
18.	**a**

1. One egg (50g) contains how much proteins- *(PGMEE 2015)*

a. 6 g   b. 16 g

c. 20 g   d. 26 g

[Ref: Ghai 8th e/p 94]

2. Kwashiorkor-Triad includes all except- *(PGMEE 2015)*

a. Psychomotor changes   b. Edema

c. Growth retardation   d. Hypoglycemia

[Ref: O.P. Ghai 8th/e pg. 99-100]

3. What to give first in a severely malnourished child? *(DNB December 2011)*

a. Vitamin A   b. Dextrose

c. 10% albumin   d. RESOMAL

[Ref: Ghai 8th/e/p 102]

Explanation

- General treatment in severe acute malnutrition involves 10 steps in 2 phases.

Stabilisation Phase	Rehabilitation Phase
Initial Phase	**Subsequent Phase**
Aim is Restoration of Homeostasis and treating medical complications.	Aim is Rebuilding wasted tissues.
Takes first 2-7 days of T/T	May take several Weeks.

- *The ten steps are-Management of*
  - **Hypoglycemia**.
  - Hypothermia.
  - Dehydration.
  - Electrolytes.
  - Infection.
  - Micro nutrients.
  - Feeding Initiation.
  - Catch-up growth.
  - Sensory stimulation.
  - Prepare for follow up.

4. Abnormality in Renal Tubular Acidosis (RTA) with rickets is- *(PGMEE 2012-13)*

a. Loss of K+   b. Loss of Ca+

c. Loss of HCO₃–   d. All of the above

[Ref: Ghai 8th/e/p 499, Nelson 21st/e/pg. 2766]

Explanation

Vitamin D Resistant Rickets(X Linked Hypophosphatemia)-

- Usual mode of inheritance is X-linked Dominant.
- Clinical Manifestations-

- These patients have rickets, but abnormalities of the lower extremities and poor growth are the dominant features. Delayed dentition and tooth abscesses are also common. Some patients have hypophosphatemia and short stature without clinically evident bone disease.
- Laboratory Findings-
- Patients have high renal excretion of phosphate, hypophosphatemia, and increased alkaline phosphatase; PTH and serum calcium levels are normal. Hypophosphatemia normally upregulates renal 1α-hydroxylase and should lead to an increase in 1,25-D, but these patients have low or inappropriately normal levels of 1,25-D. Urinary Phosphate excretion is large, despite hypophosphatemia, indicating a defect in renal tubular Reabsorption.

Type of rickets/ Biochem parameter	Ser. Ca	Ser. Phosph.	Ser. Alk Phospha-tase	Ser. PTH	Ser. HCo3
Normal	9-10.5 mg/dl	3-4.5 mg/dl	30-120 IU	10-55 IU	21-30 meq/l
Hypophos-phatemic Rickets	N	↓	↑	N	N ↓ ↑
Vit D dependent Rickets	N/ ↓ (7.5-8)	N/ ↓ (7.5-8)	↑	↑	↑
Hyper-Parathyroid-ism	↑	↓	↑	↑	N
Nutritional rickets	↓	↓	↑	↑	N
Renal Tubular Acidosis -Distal	↓	N	↑	↑	N/↓
Renal Tubular Acidosis -Proximal	N	↓	↑	N	↓ ↓

5. How to assess Vit.D therapy in Rickets is- *(PGMEE 2012-13)*

a. Sr. Phosphatase

b. Sr. alkaline phosphatse

c. X-ray wrist

d. Sr. calcium

[Ref: Ghai 8th/e pg. 114, Nelson 21st/e/pg. 381]

6. Radiological features in rickets? *(PGMEE 2012-13)*
a. Cupping of distal end of radius
b. Fraying of the edge of metaphysis
c. Thickening of growth plate
d. All of the above

[Ref: Nelson 21st/e/pg. 377, Ghai 8th/e/p 113]

7. Flag sign is seen in- *(PGMEE 2013-14)*
a. Marasmus
b. Rickets
c. Kwashiorkor
d. Vitamin A deficiency

[Ref: O.P. Ghai 8th/e pg. 100, Nelson 21st/e/pg. 3589]

8. Niacin deficiency causes all except- *(PGMEE 2013-14)*
a. Diarrhoea
b. Dementia
c. Dactylitis
d. Dermatitis

[Ref: Ghai 8th/e pg. 118, Nelson 21st/e/pg. 367 table 62.1]

9. Exclusive breast feeding is advised till what age- *(PGMEE 2013-14)*
a. 3 months
b. 6 months
c. 9 months
d. 12 months

[Ref: Nelson 21st/e/pg. 1242 table 176.8, Ghai 8th/e/p 90]

10. The best parameter for assessment of chronic malnutrition is- *(PGMEE 2013-14, DNB pattern 2007)*
a. Weight for age
b. Weight for height
c. Height for age
d. Head circumference

[Ref: Nelson 21st/e/pg. 334; Park's PSM 22nd/e p. 60]

Explanation

- Waterlow's classification defines two groups of 'protein energy malnutrition';
  o Malnutrition with retarded growth, in which a drop in the **height/age ratio** points to a chronic condition-shortness, or stunting.
  o Malnutrition with a low weight for a normal height, in which the weight for height ratio is indicative of an acute condition of rapid weight loss, or wasting.
- Stunting (deficit in height for age) generally points towards a chronic course of malnutrition. – O.P.Ghai
- "Height is a stable measurement of growth as opposed to b ody weight. Whereas weight reflects only the present health status of the child, height indicates the event in the past also.

11. Hypervitaminosis A causes *(PGMEE 2013-14)*
a. Alopecia
b. Benign cranial hypertension (Pseudotumour cerebri)
c. Liver damage
d. All

[Ref: Nelson 21st/e/pg. 364]

12. Vitamin B$_6$ is used in treatment of- *(PGMEE 2013-14)*
a. Homocystinuria
b. Cystathionuria
c. Xanthourenic aciduria
d. All

[Ref: Nelson 21st/e/pg. 370]

13. Diagnosis of a child having diarrhea with perianal moist crust is- *(PGMEE 2013-14)*
a. Riboflavin deficiency
b. Acrodermatitis enteropathica
c. Pellagra
d. Menkes disease

[Ref: Nelson 21st/e/pg. 3587, Ghai 8th/e/p 121, 122]

Explanation

Acrodermatitis enteropathica

- Genetic AR disorder caused by mutation in the gene that encodes for a membrane protein that binds zinc.
- Characterized by periorificial dermatitis, alopecia, diarrhea.

14. Most potent form of vitamin D is- *(PGMEE 2013-14)*
a. 1, 25- dihydroxy cholecalciferol
b. 7-dehydro cholecalciferol
c. 25-hydroxy cholecalciferol
d. Ergocalciferol (Vit. D2)

[Ref: Harper 28th/e pg. 470]

15. Not seen in Kwashiorkor- *(PGMEE 2013-14)*
a. Increased transaminase
b. Apathy
c. Flaky paint dermatosis
d. Baggy pant appearance

[Ref: O.P. Ghai 8th/e/p 99, 100]

16. All are true about Wilson disease EXCEPT-
a. Raised copper level *(PGMEE 2013-14)*
b. Raised ceruloplasmin level
c. Kayser-Fleischer rings in the cornea
d. Autosomal Recessive

[Ref: Nelson 21st/e/pg. 2103, Ghai 8th/e/p 320]

17. All are seen in protein deficiency EXCEPT *(PGMEE 2013-14)*
a. Nail change
b. Cherry like skin
c. Stomatitis
d. Flaky paint like skin

[Ref: O.P. Ghai 8th/e pg 99, 100]

18. Breast milk at room temperature stored for- *(PGMEE 2012-13)*
a. 4 - 6 hrs
b. 8 - 12 hrs
c. 12 - 16 hrs
d. 24 - 48 hrs

[Ref: O.P. Ghai 7th/e pg. 127]

19. Exclusive breast feeding is at least till- *(PGMEE 2012-13)*
a. 4 month
b. 6 month
c. 8 month
d. 10 month

[Ref: Ghai 8th/e/p 150]

20. All are seen in Marasmus EXCEPT- *(PGMEE 2012-13)*
a. Hepatomegaly
b. Weight loss
c. Muscle wasting
d. Voracious appetite

[Ref: O.P. Ghai 8th/e pg. 99 table 6.10]

21. Kwashiorkor is diagnosed in a growth retarded children along with- *(PGMEE 2012-13)*
a. Edema and mental changes
b. Edema and hypopigmentation
c. Hypopigmentation and anemia
d. Hepatomegaly and good appetite

[Ref: O.P. Ghai 8th/e/p 99, 100]

22. Severe acute malnutrition as per who criteria- *(PGMEE 2019)*
a. Weight for age less than median plus – 2 SD
b. Weight for height less than median plus 2 SD
c. Weight for age less than median plus 3 SD
d. Weight for height less than median minus -3SD

[Ref: WHO SAM Guidelines; Nelson 20th/e pg. 301, 302]

6.	d
7.	c
8.	c
9.	b
10.	c
11.	d
12.	d
13.	b
14.	a
15.	d
16.	b
17.	b
18.	a
19.	b
20.	a
21.	a
22.	d

23. **Waterlow classification of malnutrition in children takes into account?** *(PGMEE 2013)*
    a. Percent of reference weight for age
    b. Weight for height (wasting) and height for age (stunting)
    c. Weight for height (wasting)
    d. Height for age (Stunting)

    [Ref: Nelson 21st/e/pg. 334 table 57.2]

24. **During treatment of malnutrition in child:** *(Recent Pattern June 2018)*
    a. Refeeding syndrome
    b. Thiamine is given at the end of feeding
    c. We have to look for electrolyte imbalance
    d. None of the above

    [Ref: O.P. Ghai 8th/e pg. 103,106]

25. **True about Gomez classification of malnutrition of children is?**
    a. Weight is compared with height
    b. Height is the only parameter
    c. Weight is the only parameter
    d. It doesn't take account of height and weight

    [Ref: Park PSM,Suraj Gupte (Recent Advances in Pediatrics-Child Nutrition]

Explanation

- Gomez Classification is based on weight retardation. The child is compared to normal child of same age with weight as parameter.The "Normal" reference child is teh 50th centile of the Boston Standards.The Advantages are since its a weight based classification which is widely used parameter.

Weight For Age (%)	Wt. of Childx 100/Wt. of child of same Age
90-110%	Normal.
75-89%	Mild Malnutrition(Ist Degree)
60-74%	Moderate MN(2nd Degree)
<60%	Severe MN(3rd Degree).

26. **In rickets all are EXCEPT:**
    a. Craniotabes
    b. Increased acid phosphatase
    c. Bow legs
    d. Increase alkaline phosphatase

    [Ref: Nelson 19th ,Ghai 7th]

Explanation

I. Skeletal Manifestations-

- Skull-
  - Craniotabes (pressure over Parietal/Occipetal bones give ping-pong ball like feeling)-Earliest Sign of Rickets.
  - Frontal/Parietal bossing;widened sutures,Delayed Closure of Ant. fontanel;Caput Quadratum(Hot Cross Bun skull-Widened sutures & thickening of bone edges around suture create a cruciate Pattern.
- Chest-
  - Rachitic Rosary,Pectus Carinatum(pigeon Breast), Harrisons Groove (Horizontal depression along lower border of chest Corresponding insertion of Diaphragm).
- Teeth-
  - Delayed eruptions, enamel Hypoplasia and dental Caries.
- Spine-
  - Thoracic Kyphosis(Rachitic Cat back),Increased Lumbar Lordosis,Scoliosis
- Limbs and Joints-
  - Bone pains and tenderness-MC manifestation;Coxa Vara,Genu Valgum/Varus;Bowing of tibia, Femur, Radius, Ulna;Widening of wrists,elbow, knee,ankle;
  - rachitic saber shins, Sausage like enlargement of ends of phalanges and metacarpals-String of Pearls deformity; Windswept deformity; Double Malleoli sign.
- Abdomen-
  - Rachitic Pot Belly-Marked hypotonia of abdominal wall muscles.

II.Systemic Manifestations-

- Growth retardation,Increased Sweating Over Fore-Head (Earliest symptom); Apathy,Listlessness, irritability, Ligament laxity, Hypotonia and Muscle Weakness; Tetany, laryngeal stridor, convulsions. Deficiency Of Vit D in early infancy may result in B/L Lamellar Cataracts.
- Biochemical Features-
- Vit D defi./Calcium Defi. rickets-
  - N/Decreased Calcium; Decreased Phosphate (except in Renal Osteodystrophy, where phosphate level is incresed because kidney is not able to excrete Calcium); Increased Parathormone; Increased Alk. Phosphatase.
- Phosphaturic/Hypophosphatemic Rickets-
  - Decreased Phosphate, Calcium Level is normal; Normal PTH; Increased Osteoblastic Acivity leads to Increased Alk. Phosphatase.

VITAMINS AND MINERALS

Described under Chapter "Vitamins and Minerals" Biochemistry.

23.	b
24.	c
25.	c
26.	b

PGMEE BASED ON THIS CHAPTER

Most of the questions from Organ Systems are given in their specific sections. Below given are only additional questions of systemic Pediatrics.

NERVOUS SYSTEM

1. True about childhood/infant neurological examination all EXCEPT *(PGMEE 2016-17)*

a. Papilledema is rare.

b. Frog like posture in hypotonic infant

c. Stroking patellar tendon of one side leads to extension of knee

d. Elbow cross midline during examination if passively done by examiner

[Ref: Nelson 21st/e/ch 608]

Explanation

Lets evaluate every option one by one:

- Papilloema is rare – true statement – Nelson 20th edition page 2793 states that Disc edema refers to swelling of the optic disc, and papilledema specifically refers to swelling that is secondary to increased ICP. Papilledema rarely occurs in infancy because the skull sutures can separate to accommodate the expanding brain

- Frog like posture in hypotonic infant – nelson page 2797, Hypotonic infants are floppy and typically presents in frog like posture.

- Stroking patellar tendon causes knee extension – classical knee reflex

- *Elbow crosses midline when done by examiner - When the upper extremity of a normal-term infant is pulled gently across the chest, the elbow does not quite reach the mid-sternum (scarf sign), whereas the elbow of a hypotonic infant extends beyond the midline with ease.*

2. Which of the following is MCC of syncope in children: *(Recent Pattern June 2018)*

a. Breath holding spell   b. Hypoglycemia

c. Hypocalcemia   d. Neurocardiogenic

[Ref: Nelson's 20th/e pg.515-516]

Explanation

- The vast majority of episodes are benign, and are due to neurocardiogenic syncope. Imp causes are:-
  - Vasovagal or neurocardiogenic syncope. A sudden drop in BP with or without a decrease in heart rate.
  - Arrhythmia
  - Structural heart disease (muscle or valve defects)
  - Orthostatic hypotension

NTDS

3. What is the best preventive measure for neural tube defects? *(PGMEE 2015)*

a. USG in 2nd trimester

b. Vitamin B12 supplementation to mother

c. BCG vaccination at birth

d. Folate supplementation to mother

[Ref: Ghai 8th/e/p 575, Nelson 21st/e/pg. 3066]

4. Neural tube defect present in all except *(PGMEE 2016-17)*

a. Mother diabetic

b. Maternal THFR deficiency

c. Antiepileptic drug intake

d. Maternal warfarin intake

[Ref: Ghai 8th/e/p 575, Nelson 21st/e/pg. 3066]

Explanation

Causes of NTD

- Maternal hyperthermia, drugs (valproic acid), malnutrition low RBC folate levels, chemical, maternal obesity, diabetes genetic factors (mutation in folate responses or folate - dependent enzyme pathways).

5. Most common birth defect in north India is?

a. Down's syndrome   *(PGMEE 2013)*

b. CTEV

c. Neural tube defects (Spina bifida)

d. Hemoglobinophathies

[Ref: Ghai 8th/e/p 575]

6. Which of the following is NOT true about encephalocoele? *(PGMEE 2015)*

a. It is protrusion of neural tissue through a defect

b. It is neural tube defect

c. Can be associated with hydrocephalus

d. Common in the frontal region

[Ref: Nelson's 21st/e/pg. 3068]

Explanation

- Two major forms of dysraphism affect the skull, resulting in protrusion of tissue through a bony midline defect, called cranium bifidum.
  - *A cranial meningocele* consists of a CSF-filled meningeal sac only, and
  - a *cranial encephalocele* contains the sac plus cerebral cortex, cerebellum, or portions of the brainstem.
- *The cranial defect occurs most commonly in the occipital region at or below the inion.*
- Some frontal lesions are associated with a cleft lip and palate.
- The etiology is presumed to be similar to that for anencephaly and myelomeningocele

1.	d
2.	d
3.	d
4.	d
5.	c
6.	d

- Infants with *a cranial encephalocele are at increased risk for developing hydrocephalus because of aqueductal stenosis, Chiari malformation, or the Dandy-Walker syndrome*
- Ultrasonography is most helpful in determining the contents of the sac. MRI or CT further helps define the spectrum of the lesion.
- Cranial encephalocele is often part of a syndrome. **Meckel-Gruber syndrome** is a rare AR condition that is characterized by an occipital encephalocele, cleft lip or palate, microcephaly, microphthalmia, abnormal genitalia, polycystic kidneys, and polydactyly.
- Determination of MSAFP levels and ultrasound measurement of the biparietal diameter, as well as identification of the encephalocele itself, can diagnose encephaloceles in utero.
- Fetal MRI can help define the extent of associated CNS anomalies and the degree of brain herniated into the encephalocele.

7. Medulloblastoma arises exclusively from the cells of-
a. Immature embryonal cells **(PGMEE 2015)**
b. Neurons
c. Ependymal cells
d. Spindle shaped cells

[Ref: Nelson's 21st/e/pg. 2674]

HYDROCEPHALUS

8. Triad of normal pressure hydrocephalus includes all except- **(PGMEE 2015)**
a. Headache   b. Gait disturbance
c. Urinary incontinence   d. Dementia

[Ref: Harrison's 19th/e/p 974]

9. Investigation of choice for hydrocephalus in neonates is- **(PGMEE 2015)**
a. CT Scan   b. Technitium-99 Scan
c. Skull Xray   d. MRI

[Ref: Nelson's 21st/e/pg. 3079, Ghai 8th//e/p 575]

10. True about Dandy walker syndrome is-
a. Cystic expansion of 4th ventricle **(PGMEE 2013-14)**
b. Cerebellar hypoplasia
c. Most have hydrocephalus
d. All

[Ref: Nelson's 21st/e/pg. 3072]

11. True regarding Dandy walker malformation
(PGMEE 2016)
a. Transillumination through skull is negative
b. Hydrocephalus is seen in <50% individuals
c. Cerebral hypoplasia
d. Enlargement posterior fossa

[Ref: Nelson's 21st/e/pg. 3077]

12. Common deformity in chiari II malformation is-
a. Meningomyelocele   (PGMEE 2013-14)
b. Hydrocephalus
c. Syringomyelia
d. All of above

[Ref: Nelson's 21st/e/ch. 609 pg. 3076, 77]

7.	a
8.	a
9.	d
10.	d
11.	d
12.	d
13.	d
14.	a
15.	d
16.	b
17.	b
18.	d

13. Most common cause of fetal ventriculomegaly is?
(PGMEE 2013)
a. Arnold Chiari malformation – I
b. Arnold Chiari malformation – II
c. Dandy Walker malformation
d. Aqueductal stenosis

[Ref: Nelson 21st/e/ch 609]

EPILEPSY/SEIZURES

14. Most common cause of convulsion on the First day of life in a newborn is- **(PGMEE 2012-13)**
a. Anoxia   b. Head Injury
c. Hypocalcemia   d. Hypoglycemia

[Ref: O.P. Ghai8th/e/p 168]

15. Initial drug of choice in a child with status epilepticus-
(PGMEE 2012-13)
a. Phenytoin   b. Phenobarbitone
c. Valproate   d. Lorazepam

[Ref: O.P. Ghai 8th/e/ pg. 555, Nelson's 21st/e/pg. 3117; AIIMS mole of p 86]

16. Drug of choice for juvenile myoclonic epilepsy is?
(PGMEE 2013)
a. Zonisamide   b. Valproate
c. Lamotrigine   d. Phenytoin

[Ref: Nelson's 21st/e/ch. 611.6 pg. 3104]

17. Best prognosis of neonatal seizures is in?
(PGMEE 2013)
a. Focal   b. Opsoclonus
c. Myoclonic   d. Tonic clonic

[Ref: Nelson's 21st/e/ch. 611]

18. A 6 year old child with acute onset of 104^0 fever. He was treated for febrile seizure in the past. To avoid recurrence of seizure attack what should be given?
(PGMEE 2013)
a. IV Diazepam infusion over 12 hourly
b. Paracetamol 400 mg and phenobarbitone
c. Paracetamol 400 mg 6 hourly
d. Oral diazepam 8 hourly

[Ref: Nelson's 21st/e/pg. 3094]

Explanation

Risk Factors For Recurrence of Febrile Seizures
MAJOR
Age <1yr
Duration of fever <24 hr
Fever 38-39^{0}C (100.4-102.2%)
MINOR
Family history of febrile seizures
Family history of epilepsy
Complex febrile seizure
Day-care
Mole gender
Lower serum sodium at time of presentation

Risk Factors For Occurrence of Subsequent Epilepsy After a Febrile Seizure	
Simple febrile seizure	1%
Recurrent febrile seizure	4%
Complex febrile seizures (more than 15 min duration recurrent within 24 hr)	6%
Fever <1hr before febrile seizure	11%
Family history of epilepsy	18%
Complex febrile seizure (focal)	29%
Neurodevelopmental abnormalities	33%

Treatment

- In general, antiepileptic therapy, continuous or intermittent, is not recommended for children with 1 or more simple febrile seizures
- If the seizure lasts for >5 min, acute treatment with diazepam, lorazepam, or midazolam is needed
- Rectal diazepam is often prescribed to be given at the time of reoccurrence of a febrile seizure lasting longer than 5 min. Alternatively, buccal or intranasal midazolam may be used and is often preferred by parents.
- Intravenous benzodiazepines, phenobarbital, phenytoin, or valproate may be needed in the case of febrile status epilepticus.
- *If the parents are very anxious concerning their child's seizures, intermittent oral diazepam (0.33 mg/kg every 8 hr during fever) or intermittent rectal diazepam (0.5 mg/kg administered as a rectal suppository every 8 hr), can be given during febrile illnesses.*
- In the vast majority of cases, it is not justified to use continuous therapy owing to the risk of side effects and lack of demonstrated long-term benefits, even if the recurrence rate of febrile seizures is expected to be decreased by these drugs.
- Chronic antiepileptic therapy may be considered for children with a high risk for later epilepsy.
- *Iron deficiency is associated with an increased risk of febrile seizures, and thus screening for that problem and treating it appears appropriate.*
- *Antipyretics can decrease the discomfort of the child but do not reduce the risk* of having a recurrent febrile seizure, probably because the seizure often occurs as the temperature is rising or falling.
- Meningitis should be considered in the differential diagnosis, and *lumbar puncture* should be performed for all infants younger than 6 mo of age who present with fever and seizure, or if the child is illappearing or at any age if there are clinical signs or symptoms of concern.
- Lumbar puncture is an option in a child 6-12 mo of age who is deficient in Haemophilus influenzae type b and Streptococcus pneumoniae immunizations or for whom immunization status is unknown
- An *EEG* should generally be restricted to suspected epilepsy cases and are used to delineate type of epilepsy rather than to predict its occurrence. EEG can also be helpful in patients who present with febrile status epilepticus because the presence of focal slowing present on the EEG obtained within 72 hr of the status has been shown to be highly associated with MRI evidence of acute hippocampal injury. EEG can help distinguish between ongoing seizure activity and a prolonged postictal period, sometimes termed a *nonepileptic twilight state.*

- *Neuroimaging* – only in neurologically abnormal children. Approximately 11% of children with febrile status epilepticus are reported to have (usually) *unilateral swelling of their hippocampus acutely*, which is followed by subsequent long-term hippocampal atrophy.

19. **Percent of children with simple febrile seizure developing epilepsy is-** *(PGMEE 2013-14)*
    a. 1-2%
    b. 2-5%
    c. 5-7%
    d. 7-10%

    [Ref: O.P. Ghai 8th/e/p 557]

20. **Generalised 3-4 spike and slow wave complex is seen in-**
    a. GTCS   *(PGMEE 2013-14)*
    b. Simple partial seizure
    c. Absence seizures
    d. Myoclonic epilepsy

    [Ref: O.P. Ghai 8th/e pg 550]

21. **Drug of choice for infantile Spasm-** *(PGMEE 2013-14)*
    a. ACTH   b. Vigabatrin
    c. Ethosuximide   d. Valproate

    [Ref: Nelson's 21st/e/pg. 3102]

22. **Rolando syndrome is best described by-**
    (PGMEE 2016-17)
    a. Type of epilepsy syndrome in children which begins near the central sulcus
    b. Type of Neural tube defect
    c. Type of Glycogen storage disease
    d. Defect in lipid metabolism

    [Ref: Nelson's 21st/e/ch. 611]

19.	a
20.	c
21.	a
22.	a
23.	b

Explanation

Rolando syndrome

- Is benign Rolandic epilepsy of childhood with centrotemporal spikes (BCECTS).
- It is the most common epilepsy syndrome in childhood.
- It starts around the age of 3-13 with a peak around 8-9 years and stops around age 14-18, hence the label benign.
- The seizures, sometimes referred to as **sylvian seizures**, start around the central sulcus of the brain (also called the centrotemporal area, located around the Rolandic fissure.

23. **Generalized 3-4 Hz spike and slow wave complexes on EEG are seen in?**
    a. Generalized tonic clonic seizure
    b. Absent seizure
    c. Temporal lobe epilepsy simple partial seizure
    d. Juvenile myoclonic epilepsy

    [Ref: Ghai 9th/e pg. 530]

Explanation

Absent seizures-EEG

- **Absent seizures-EEG** shows characteristic 3 per second spike and slow wave ("spike and Dome") pattern.
- Post-Ictal confusion and drowsiness do not occur and the pt can resume normal work soon after the seizures. Hyperventilation for 3 minutes can often precipitate the attack.Absence seizures may occur in multiples,every day. Attacks occuring in close succession indicate petit mal status or pyknolepsy.
- Other characteristic EEG findings are-

Type of Epilepsy	EEG findings
West Syndrome/Infantile Spasm	Diffuse high Voltage Spike, slow waves and Chaotic Activity "Hypsarrhythmia"
Lennaux Gestaut Syndrome	Very slow Background and slow generalised spike wave discharges(2 per second).
Juvenile Myoclonic Epilepsy	The EEG usually shows generalized 4-6 Hz polyspike–and–slow wave discharges
Absent seizures/Petit Mal	Generalized 3 Hz spike–and–slow wave discharges.

Drugs of choice-

Type of Epilepsy	DOC
G TCS (Grand Mal), Absence seizures (Petit Mal), Atonic Seizures, Myoclonic Epilepsy	Valproate
Partial Seizures	Carbamazepine/Ox-Carbazepine.
Status Eplilepticus	IV Lorazepam.
Febrile Seizures	Rectal Diazepam.
Seizures in Eclampsia	Magnesium sulfate.
Infantile Spasm	Vigabatrim.
Myoclonic Epilepsy	Valproic Acid.

MENINGITIS

24. **The most common causative agent of meningitis in the age group of 6 months-3 year amongst the following is-** *(PGMEE 2012-13)*
   a. N. gonorrhoeae   b. H. influenzae
   c. Streptococcus   d. Staphylococcus

   [Ref: Nelson's 21st/e/pg. 1390]

25. **In a small child diagnosed with H. influenza meningitis, what investigation must be done before discharging him from the hospital?** *(PGMEE 2013)*
   a. BERA   b. X-ray skull
   c. CT scan   d. MRI

   [Ref: Oski's pediatrics: Principles and practice by Julia A. Mc Millan]

24.	b
25.	a
26.	d
27.	a
28.	c
29.	a
30.	d
31.	d
32.	c

26. **The most common cause of meningitis in children aged 5 years is-** *(PGMEE 2013-14)*
   a. Staph. Meningitides   b. Strep. Pneumonia
   c. H-influenzae   d. N-meningitides

   [Ref: Nelson's 21st/e/pg. 3223]

27. **Most common cause of neonatal meningitis is-** *(PGMEE 2013-14)*
   a. E. coli   b. Pseudomonas
   c. Staph aureus   d. Pseudomonas

   [Ref: Nelson's 21st/e/ch. 621]

28. **In neonate with meningitis, test shows gram positive cocci having CAMP test positive. Most common source of infection is-** *(PGMEE 2013-14)*
   a. Respiratory tract   b. Hematogenous
   c. Genital tract   d. May be any

   [Ref: Nelson's 21st/e/pg. 998]

Explanation

- CAMP test positive for Group B streptococcus
- Negative CAMP test – Streptococcus Pyogenes
- Reverse CAMP test – to differentiate Clostridium perferingens from other clostridia

- Nelson writes that most common route of infection in case of GBS is ascending infection from genital tract of mother – leading to chorioamniotis. Most common source of infection is from maternal genital tract. Cut off of duration of membrane rupture has been taken as 18 hrs.

29. **Meningismus is:-** *(PGMEE 2016-17)*
   a. Meningeal irritation sign without meningitis
   b. Meningitis without meningeal irritation sign
   c. Headache leads to meningitis
   d. It occurs commonly in adults.

   [Ref: Nelson's 21st/e/ch. 621]

MISCELLANEOUS IN CNS

30. **Treatment of GBS in a child-** *(PGMEE 2012-13)*
   a. IV Ig   b. Plasmapharesis
   c. Ventilation   d. All of above

   [Ref: Nelson's 21st/e/ch. 634]

31. **Which is MC genetic cause of mental retardation-** *(PGMEE 2012-13)*
   a. Angel's syndrome   b. Cri-du-chat syndrome
   c. Tuberous sclerosis   d. Fragile-x-syndrome

   [Ref: Nelson 21st/e ch. 53]

32. **Aspirin is associated with-** *(PGMEE 2012-13)*
   a. Reiter Syndrome   b. Sjogren Syndrome
   c. Reye's Syndrome   d. William syndrome

   [Ref: Nelson's 21st/e/pg. 2126]

Explanation

Reye's Syndrome

- **Reye's Syndrome** → rapidly progressive encephalopathy
- Symptoms

○ Vomiting, personality changes, confusion, seizures, loss of consciousness, liver toxicity.
○ 5 stages
■ Cause
○ Unknown
○ In children 90% → Aspirin
○ Other → Shortly after recovery from viral infection (e.g. influenza, chickenpox), IEM etc.
■ T/t supportive. Mannitol can be used for cerebral edema

33. True about status marmoratus is all except-
(PGMEE 2013)
a. Have a marbled appearance
b. Associated with asphyxia
c. Unilateral
d. Present in basal ganglia

[Ref: Nelson's 21st/e/pg. 3170]

Explanation

Status marmoratus

■ It is a congenital condition due to maldevelopment of corpus stratum.
■ A/w choreoathetosis in which striate nuclei have marble like appearance caused by altered myelination in putamen, caudate & thalamus, which is as a result of acute total asphyxia in the basal nuclei in full term infants.

RESPIRATORY SYSTEM

34. Infant glottis is differentiated from adult glottis by:
(PGMEE 2016-17)
a. Larynx high up and narrowest area is glottis
b. Low larynx and narrowest area is glottis
c. Larynx high up and narrowest area is subglottis
d. Round epiglottis

[Ref: Dhingra 5th/e/p 303]

35. Chronic lung disease of infancy (Bronchopulmonary Dysplasia) is defined as-
(PGMEE 2015)
a. Tachypnoea > 50 breaths/min within 1 week of birth
b. Need for supplemental oxygen at 28 days postnatally
c. Presence of bilateral infiltrates on chest X-Ray for 2 weeks
d. Reticulogranular pattern on chest X-ray for 6 weeks

[Ref: Nelson's 21st/e/ch. 444 pg. 2324]

36. Most common cause of pneumonia in early onset sepsis in a neonate is-
(PGMEE 2015)
a. Pnemococcus
b. S. Pyogens
c. E Coli
d. S. Aureus

[Ref: O.P. Ghai 8th/e pg. 163, Care of the new born 6th/e Meharban Singh]

37. Fast breathing in a 3 year old child is?
(DNB December 2011)
a. > 30
b. > 50
c. > 40
d. > 60

[Ref: O.P. Ghai 8th/e pg. 759]

Explanation

Fast breathing in children:

Age group	Rate of breathing > than
< 2 months	60
2 -12 months	50
12- 60 months	40

38. Most common pulmonary tumor in children is-
(PGMEE 2012-13)
a. Small cell carcinoma
b. Carcinoid
c. Adeno carcinoma
d. Squamous cell carcinoma

[Ref: Nelson's 21st/e/ch. 438 pg. 2316]

39. Which of the following does NOT indicate respiratory distress in neonate?
(PGMEE 2012)
a. Grunt
b. Retraction
c. Tachypnea
d. Wheeze

[Ref: Nelson's 21st/e/pg. 870, Ghai 8th/e/p 138]

40. Most common cause of pneumonia in children is?
(PGMEE 2012)
a. RSV
b. Klebsiella
c. Staphylococcus aureus
d. Streptococcus pneumonae

[Ref: Nelson's 21st/e/pg. 2267]

41. Which of the following does not cause pneumonia:-
(PGMEE 2012)
a. Measles
b. Mumps
c. RSV
d. Influenza

[Ref: Nelson's 21st/e/pg. 2267; 19th/e chap 240]

Explanation

■ Viruses which commonly cause pneumonia in children are: - RSV,Influenza, adenovirus, rhinovirus and parainfluenza.
■ Bronchopneumonia is a common complication of Measles infection.

42. Which of the following vaccine does not prevent pneumonia in children:
(Recent Pattern June 2018)
a. Measles
b. Pneumococcal
c. Hib
d. Rubella

[Ref: Nelson's 20th/e pg. 1254]

Explanation

Vaccines which are known to prevent pneumonia include

■ PCV 13 (Pneumococcal)
■ H.influenzae type b (Hib)
■ Measles

43. In which disease, symptoms improve with crying-
(PGMEE 2013, 2012)
a. Bronchial asthma
b. Choanal atresia
c. Tetralogy of fallot
d. All of the above

[Ref: Nelson's 21st/e/pg. 2181, Ghai 8th/e/p 366]

33.	c
34.	c
35.	b
36.	c
37.	c
38.	b
39.	d
40.	d
41.	b
42.	d
43.	b

BRONCHIOLITIS

44. Most common cause of Bronchiolitis is?
(PGMEE 2013)

a. RSV
b. Mycoplasma
c. Parainfluenza
d. Adenovirus

[Ref: Nelson's 21st/e/pg. 2217]

45. Treatment of bronchiolitis includes all except-
(PGMEE 2012-13)

a. Bronchodilator
b. Humidified oxygen
c. Macrolides
d. None

[Ref: Ghai 8th/e pg. 382, Nelson's 21st/e/pg. 2219]

46. Which of the following is used for treatment of bronchiolitis? *(PGMEE 2012, PGMEE 2012-13)*

a. IVIG
b. Antibiotics
c. Ribavarin
d. Acyclovir

[Ref: Ghai 8th/e pg. 382, Nelson's 21st/e/pg. 22197]

GASTROINTESTINAL

47. Most common cause for acute infantile gastroenteritis is? *(DNB December 2011, PGMEE 2016-17)*

a. Adenovirus
b. Norwalk virus
c. E coli
d. Rota virus

[Ref: Nelson's 21st/e/pg. 1371; Ghai 8th/e/p 291; Microbiology by Ananthanarayan 6th/e pg. 529]

Explanation

Gastroenteritis in infants

- Viruses are the most common cause of Acute Infantile GE (Just like Acute Respiratory infections in children).
- "**Rotavirus** is recognized as the most common cause of diarrheal disease in infants and Children" (Ananthnarayan)
- Etiological agents for AGE in children are given below

Category	Agents
Viruses	Rota Virus, Adeno Virus, Calci Virus, Norwalk Virus, Astro Virus
Bacteria	EnteroToxic E.Coli(ETEC), Entero Invasive E. coli(EIEC), Shigella, Salmonella, Campylobacter, Aeromonas
Parasites	E.histolytica, Giardia, Cryptosporidium

48. Toddler diarrhea refers to- *(PGMEE 2016-17)*

a. Intermittent loose stools occurring in 1-3 years old
b. Loose stools during the night
c. Loose Stools after feeding
d. Loose stools after in neonates

[Ref: Nelson's 21st/e/pg. 1901]

49. Shape of cecum in newborn is- *(PGMEE 2015)*

a. Conical
b. Trapezoid
c. Ovoid
d. Globular

[Ref: Textbook of Human Anatomy By William James Hamilton p723]

Explanation

- Caecum is conical in shape in fetal life & saccular in adult life due to unequal development of its wall during postnatal life

50. A newborn fails to pass stools for the first 12 to 24 hours after birth presents with bilious vomiting and abdominal distension. Family history reveals presence of cystic fibrosis in sibling. What is the probable diagnosis? *(PGMEE 2016)*

a. Meconium Ileus
b. Meconium aspiration syndrome
c. Viral hepatitis
d. Regurgitation after feeding

[Ref: Nelson 20th/e/p 868]

Explanation

- Impaction of meconium causes intestinal obstructions and may be associated with CF.
- The absence of fetal pancreatic enzymes in CF limits normal digestive activities in the intestine, and meconium becomes viscid and mucilaginous. It clings to the intestinal wall and moves with difficulty.
- The inspissated and impacted meconium fills the intestinal canal but is most concentrated in the lower part of the ileum.
- Clinically, the pattern is that of congenital intestinal obstruction with or without intestinal perforation. Abdominal distention is prominent, and vomiting becomes persistent. Infrequently, 1 or more inspissated meconium stools may be passed shortly after birth.
- Patients with 2 copies of the F508del mutation have a 25% chance of presenting with meconium ileus.
- In families that already have at least 1 child with CF complicated by meconium ileus, there is a 39% recurrence rate for meconium ileus in subsequent children, which is more than the rates expected with autosomal recessive inheritance.
- In a twin study, 82% of monozygotic twins showed concordance for meconium ileus, whereas only 22% of dizygotic and 24% of 2 affected siblings showed concordance.

51. Treatment of choice in umbilical adenoma in a newborn is- *(PGMEE 2013-14)*

a. Surgery
b. Cauterisation
c. Strapping
d. Occlusion with coin

[Ref: SRB's Manual Of Surgery 4th/e/p 787]

52. Disease marker for early diagnosis of Hirschsprung disease is- *(PGMEE 2012-13)*

a. VIP
b. Adrenaline
c. Acetyl cholinesterase
d. None

[Ref: Nelson's 21st/e/pg. 1961]

44.	a
45.	c
46.	c
47.	d
48.	a
49.	a
50.	a
51.	b
52.	c

53. Gas under diaphragm on CXR in a 5 year old child is seen in- *(PGMEE 2012-13)*
a. Iatrogenic pneumoperitoneum
b. Chilaiditi's syndrome
c. Enteric fever with intestinal perforation
d. All

[Ref: Ghai 8th/e/ch 11]

54. Sandifer syndrome due to GERD in infants is confused with- *(PGMEE 2013)*
a. Acute otitis media   b. Sinusitis
c. Seizures   d. Recurrent vomiting

[Ref: Nelson's 21st/e/pg. 3125]

Explanation

- Gastroesophageal reflux in infants may cause paroxysmal episodes of generalized stiffening and opisthotonic posturing that may be accompanied by apnea, staring, and minimal jerking of the extremities which are often confused with seizures. Episodes often occur 30 min after a feed. In older children, this syndrome manifests with episodic dystonic or dyskinetic movements consisting of latero-, retro-, or torticollis, the exact pathophysiology of which remains elusive.

55. Common site of regional enteritis is- *(PGMEE 2012-13)*
a. Colon   b. Caecum
c. Distal ileum and colon d. Rectum

[Ref: Nelson's 21st/e/pg. 1981]

56. Most common cause of Acute Intestinal Obstruction in neonates is- *(PGMEE 2012-13)*
a. Acute Intussusception b. Malrotation
c. Jejunal atresia   d. Duodenal atresia

[Ref: Nelson's 21st/e/pg. 1950]

57. 6 year old boy presents with non-bilious vomiting. On examination he has palpable abdominal mass in the epigastrium. The clinical diagnosis is- *(PGMEE 2012-13)*
a. Pyloric stenosis
b. Oesophageal Atresia
c. Duodenal Atresia
d. Choledochal cyst

[Ref: Nelson's 21st/e/ch. 355.1 pg. 1946]

Explanation

- "Nonbilious vomiting" is the initial symptom of pyloric stenosis. The vomiting may or may not be projectile initially but is usually progressive, occurring immediately after a feeding. Emesis might follow each feeding, or it may be intermittent. The vomiting usually starts after 3 wk of age, but symptoms can develop as early as the 1st wk of life and as late as the 5th mo."
- Rest of the causes given as choices are well known for vomiting in a neonate soon after birth. Amniotic fluid gastritis is MC cause for vomiting in a neonate on day 1 of life.
- Ultrasound examination confirms the diagnosis in the majority of cases. Criteria for diagnosis include:-
  ○ pyloric thickness 3-4 mm,
  ○ an overall pyloric length 15-19 mm, and
  ○ pyloric diameter of 10-14 mm .

- Ultrasonography has a sensitivity of about 95%. When contrast studies are performed, they demonstrate an elongated pyloric channel (string sign), a bulge of the pyloric muscle into the antrum (shoulder sign), and parallel streaks of barium seen in the narrowed channel, producing a "double tract sign".
- Most Common volvulous in children is mid gut volvulous associated with Malrotation and small bowel is the MC part of GIT involved.Large Bowel and Colon volvulous are rare.

58. Chronic constipation in children is not seen in- *(PGMEE 2012-13)*
a. Stricture   b. Jejunal polyp
c. Hirschspring disease   d. Hypothyroidism

[Ref: Ghai 8th/e/p 284]

HEPATOBILIARY SYSTEM

59. Portal venous pressure in a child is- *(PGMEE 2012-13)*
a. 3-5 mm Hg   b. 4-6 mm Hg
c. 7-10 mm Hg   d. 10-15 mm Hg

[Ref: Nelson's 21st/e/pg. 2141]

60. False about neonatal hepatitis is - *(PGMEE 2012-13)*
a. May get positive family history
b. More common in preterm or IUGR baby
c. Caused by virus
d. Always conjugated hyperbilirubinemia

[Ref: Nelson's 21st/e/pg. 2093]

Explanation

- The term neonatal hepatitis implies intrahepatic cholestasis, which has various forms.
- Idiopathic neonatal hepatitis, which can occur in either a sporadic or a familial form, is a disease of unknown cause.
- Patients with the sporadic form presumably have a specific yet undefined metabolic or viral disease.
- Familial forms, on the other hand, presumably reflect a genetic or metabolic aberration; in the past, patients with α1-antitrypsin deficiency were included in this category.
- AAGENAES SYNDROME is a form of idiopathic familial intrahepatic cholestasis associated with lymphedema of the lower extremities. The relationship between liver disease and lymphedema is not understood and may be attributable to decreased hepatic lymph flow or hepatic lymphatic hypoplasia. Affected patients usually present with episodic cholestasis with elevation of serum aminotransferases, alkaline phosphatase, and bile acids. Between episodes, the patients are usually asymptomatic and biochemical indices improve. Compared to other types of hereditary neonatal cholestasis, patients with Aagenaes syndrome have a relatively good prognosis because more than 50% can expect a normal life span. The locus for Aagenaes syndrome is mapped to a 6.6 cM interval on chromosome 15q. JSJJVS
- OTHER causes include Zellweger syndrome, Neonatal Iron storage disorder – Alloimmune disorder with poor prognosis.

53.	d
54.	c
55.	c
56.	d
57.	a
58.	b
59.	c
60.	d

■ Can present initially with indirect hyperbilirubinemia which gradually progresses to conjugated hyperbilirubinemia.

61. All are true about kernicteres EXCEPT-
a. Opisthotonus   *(PGMEE 2012-13)*
b. Occurs with bilirubin more than 25 mg%
c. No long term effect
d. Deposition in basal ganglion

[Ref: Nelson's 21st/e/pg. 957]

62. Most common cause of portal hypertension in children is-   *(PGMEE 2012-13)*
a. Veno-occlusive disease
b. Post necrotic
c. Extrahepatic compression
d. Budd chiari syndrome

[Ref: Ghai 8th/e/p 319 ; GHAI pg 319 EPPVO MC in Indu Cirrho MC in WES]

63. Commonest cause of cholestatic jaundice in new born is-   *(PGMEE 2012-13)*
a. Physiological
b. Choledochal cyst
c. Hypoplasia of biliary tract
d. Neonatal hepatitis

[Ref: Nelson's 21st/e/pg. 2090-2092]

64. Congenital TB has primary focus most commonly in:
a. Lung   b. Liver   *(PGMEE 2016-17)*
c. Spleen   d. Kidney

[Ref: Nelson's 21st/e/pg. 1575]

65. In case of an infant having congenital tuberculosis, the most common site for the primary focus is:
a. Liver
b. Lung   *(PGMEE 2016-17)*
c. Umbilical artery
d. Umbilical vein

[Ref: Nelson's 21st/e/pg. 1575]

URINARY SYSTEM

CONGENITAL MALFORMATIONS OF URINARY TRACT

66. Unilateral renal agenesis is associated with-
a. Hypogonadism   *(PGMEE 2012-13)*
b. Single cyst and fibrosis
c. Imperforate anus
d. Tracheoesophageal fistula

[Ref: Nelson's 21st/e/pg. 2787]

67. Autosomal recessive Polycystic kidneys – all are true except-   *(PGMEE 2015)*
a. Defective gene is PKHD1
b. Seen in adults
c. Both kidneys show innumerable cysts
d. USG shows salt and pepper appearance

[Ref: Nelson's 21st/e/pg. 2744]

68. Potter's Facies is seen with-   *(PGMEE 2015)*
a. Kasbach Merritt Syndrome
b. Xanthogranulomatous pyelonephritis
c. Hepatic fibrosis
d. Bilateral renal agenesis

[Ref: Nelson's 21st/e/pg. 2787]

69. WAGR syndrome – which of the following is not a component -   *(PGMEE 2015)*
a. Aniridia
b. Renal agenesis
c. Mental Retardtion
d. Anomalies of the genitourinary tract

[Ref: Nelson's 21st/e/pg. 2989 table 600.1]

POSTERIOR URETHRAL VALVES AND PUJO

70. Which is not a feature of posterior urethral valve-
a. Hydronephrosis   *(PGMEE 2012-13)*
b. Recurrent UTI
c. Palpable bladder
d. Painful stress incontinence

[Ref: Nelson's 21st/e/pg. 2808; O.P. Ghai 8h/e pg. 506]

71. A male child presents with repeated urinary infections and failure to gain weight. A MCU was carried out as shown in image, most probable diagnosis is?
     (PGMEE 2013)

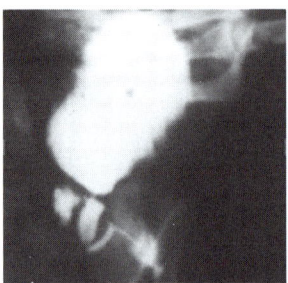

a. Post urethral valve   b. Meatal stenosis
c. Bladder polyp   d. Bladder diverticula

[Ref: Nelson's 21st/e/pg. 2808, Ghai 8th/e/ p506]

72. Most common anomaly of upper urogenital tract is-
a. Ureterocele   *(PGMEE 2012-13)*
b. Ectopic uretheral opening
c. Uretero pelvic junction stenosis
d. Ectopic ureter

[Ref: Nelson's 21st/e/pg. 2801]

URINARY TRACT INFECTION (UTI)

73. Most common cause of urinary tract infection in children is-   *(PGMEE 2015; 2012)*
a. Candida
b. Klebsiella sp.
c. E Coli
d. Psedomonas Aerognosa

[Ref: Nelson's 21st/e/pg. 2789, Ghai 8th/e/p 483]

61.	c
62.	c
63.	d
64.	b
65.	a
66.	d
67.	b
68.	d
69.	b
70.	d
71.	a
72.	c
73.	c

74. In children renal failure in terms of urine output is defined as? *(PGMEE 2013)*
   a. Less than 0.3 ml/kg/hr
   b. Less than 0.5 ml/kg/hr
   c. Less than 0.8 ml/kg/hr
   d. Less than 1 ml/kg/hr

   [Ref: Nelson's 21st/e/pg. 2770 table 550.1]

MISCELLANEOUS

75. Treatment of nocturnal enuresis in a 14 year old child is
   a. Desmopressin *(PGMEE 2013-14)*
   b. Punishment
   c. Bed alarm
   d. Positive reinforcement

   [Ref: Nelson's 21st/e/pg. 2821, Ghai 8th/e pg. 505]

76. All of the following are true about xanthogranulomatous pyelonephritis except- *(PGMEE 2015)*
   a. Proteus is most common organism
   b. It is form of chronic pyelonephritis
   c. Seen only in infancy
   d. Focal form is common in children

   [Ref: Internet (Medscape)]

MUSCULAR DYSTROPHIES: DMD, BMD

Described in Medicine Chap " Musculoskeletal Disorders & Myopathies" in Neurology

74.	b
75.	d
76.	c

1. Breast feeding is contraindicated in- *(PGMEE 2015)*
a. LBW infant
b. HIV positive mother
c. Hepatitis B positive mother
d. Tuberculosis history 2 years back

[Ref: Nelson 21st/e/pg. 322 table 56.2]

2. Which of the following is true about Kangaroo Mother Care? *(PGMEE 2015)*
a. Can be done by father also
b. Effective thermal control
c. Indicated for LBW babies
d. All of the above

[Ref: Ghai 8th/e/p. 148]

3. Which of the following is not a component of Kangaroo mother care (KMC): *(Recent Pattern June 2018)*
a. Skin to skin contact
b. Supplementary nutrition
c. Exclusive breast feeding
d. Early discharge and follow-up

[Ref: O.P. Ghai 8th/e pg. 148]

Explanation

Kangaroo mother care:

- KMC is care of preterm or LBW infants by placing skin-to-skin contact with the mother. The baby is placed in vertical position between the mother's breasts and under her clothes.
- Kangaroo nutrition: exclusive breast feeding
- KMC can be continuous or intermittent (at least 1-2 hour) when continuous KMC is not possible
- All mothers can provide KMC irrespective of age, parity, education, culture or religion
- Initiated in a facility and continued at home.
- Clinical benefits
  o Significantly increases milk production in mothers
  o Increases exclusive breast feeding rates
  o Reduces incidence of respiratory tract and nosocomial infection
  o Better cardiorespiratory stability
  o Fewer apneic episodes
  o Improved weight gain
  o Improves thermal protection in infants and there is a reduced chance of hypothermia
  o Improves emotional bonding between the infant and mothers
  o Reduces the duration of hospital stay
  o Improved survival in low resource setting
- KMC is indicated in all stable LBW babies, sick but hemodynamically stable babies

- When to stop KMC
  o >2500 g weight and a gestation of 37 weeks
  o A baby who upon being put in kangaroo position, tends to wriggle out, pull limbs out or cries, is not in need of KMC any more

4. All of the following are causes of neonatal bradycardia except- *(PGMEE 2015)*
a. BCG Vaccine   b. Head injury
c. Hypoxia   d. Hypothermia

[Ref: Nelson 21st/e/pg. 538]

5. 45 day old infant presents with seizures. Examination reveals he is icteric, having bulging fontanelles and opisthotonic posture. Treatment is all except- *(PGMEE 2015)*
a. Chlorpromazine   b. Exchange Transfusion
c. Intensive Phototherapy d. Phenobarbitone

[Ref: O.P. Ghai 8th/e p 175, Nelson 21st/e/pg. 123.3; Cloherty 8th edition, page 350]

Explanation

Bilirubin Toxicity & available treatments

- Unconjugated bilirubin that is not bound to albumin is a potential toxin that can enter the brain and cause apoptosis and/or necrosis. If the blood-brain barrier is disrupted by factors including hyperosmolarity, asphyxia, and hypercarbia, bilirubin can also enter the brain bound to albumin in preterm.
- Bilirubin-induced neurologic dysfunction (BIND). The brain regions typically affected by bilirubin toxicity include the basal ganglia, cerebellum, white matter, and the brainstem nuclei.
- Kernicterus refers to the chronic and permanent sequelae of bilirubin toxicity that develop during the first year of age.

6. Erythematous blotchy rash is seen on the abdomen, trunk and face of a 3 day old child along with yellowish papules. However the child feels well. What is the management? *(PGMEE 2015)*
a. Urgent intravenous antibiotics
b. No treatment
c. Steroids and antibiotic lotion
d. Steroids cream

[Ref: Nelson 21st/e/pg. 3454; Cloherty 8th/e/p 973]

Explanation

- Erythematous blotchy rashes over trunk indicates erythema toxicum.

Erythema Toxicum

- Scattering of macules, papules, and even some vesicles or small white or yellow pustules on erythematous base,

Answers

1. b
2. d
3. b
4. a
5. a
6. b

which usually occur on the trunk but also frequently appear on the extremities and face. It occurs in up to 70% of term newborns; occurs rarely in premature infants.

- Unknown etiology
- Vesicle contents when smeared and stained with Wright stain will show a predominance of eosinophils.
- **No treatment necessary**

7. Further investigation is essential in a newborn with which condition? *(PGMEE 2015)*

a. Lens opacity   b. Erythema toxicum
c. Mongolian spots   d. Vaginal bleeding

[Ref: Nelson 2th/e/ch 647]

Explanation

- Lens opacity in a new born may be because of congenital cataract which requires further investigations for various disorders like IEM, herediatry syndromes etc.
- Rest all option can be found in a normal newborn.

8. Female newborn presents with vaginal bleeding, 4 days after birth, what is to be done? *(PGMEE 2012)*

a. Blood transfusion
b. Surgery
c. Wait and watch
d. Clotting Factor deficiency to be ruled out

[Ref: Nelson 21st/e/pg. 704]

9. All of the following are features of Hypoxic Ischaemic encephalopathy except- *(PGMEE 2015)*

a. Increased tone
b. Decreased level of consciousness
c. Seizure
d. Apneic spells

[Ref: Ghai 8th/e/p 166-167]

Explanation

Sarnat & Sarnat staging of HIE

Stage	Tone
Stage 1	Normal
Stage 2	Hypo
Stage 3	Flaccid

10. Which of the drugs must be available in labor room while mother being given narcotics for pain: *(NEET Pattern 2017)*

a. Fentanyl   b. Naloxone
c. Pheneramine   d. Morphine

[Ref: Dutta's Obs. 8th / e, pg. 592; Holland Brew's Obs.4th / e, pg. 429; Williams Obs. 24th / e, pg. 507, 626]

Explanation

- Naloxone is narcotic antagonist - which reverses
- Reverses respiratory depression in fetus induced by opioid narcotics given to mother during labour
- Mechanism of action – displacement of narcotic from specific receptors in CNS
- Dose –
  - Mother – 0.4 mg IV in labour, may be repeated
  - Newborn – 10 µg/kg IM or IV, may be repeated when

neonate born with narcotic depression, given after adequate ventilation

- Indication – narcotic/opioid analgesics given to mother during labour
- Contraindication – newborn of a narcotic-addicted mother, may precipitate withdrawal symptoms

11. All of the following drugs can be used, in neonatal resuscitation except? *(PGMEE 2015)*

a. Adrenaline   b. Sodium Bicarbonate
c. Dopamine   d. Milrinone

[Ref: Nelson 21st/e/pg. 927]

12. A newborn presents with subconjunctival hemorrhage. The treatment is- *(PGMEE 2015)*

a. Vitamin C syrup
b. Antibiotic eye drops
c. No treatment
d. Antibiotic and steroid drops

[Ref: Nelson 21st/e/pg. 3364]

13. True about cephalohematoma is- *(PGMEE 2015)*

a. It is hemorrhage between the skull and periosteum
b. It is hemorrhage within the subcutaneous tissue around the skull
c. It is extraperiosteal bleeding in the skull
d. Crosses suture line.

[Ref: Ghai 8th/e/p 141, Nelson 21st/e/pg. 913]

14. False about cephalohematoma is *(PGMEE 2016-17)*

a. Maximum at birth then regresses
b. Cause is injury to periosteum
c. Exudative fluid present
d. Localized collection beneath periosteum

[Ref: Ghai 8th/e/p 141, Nelson 21st/e/pg. 913]

15. Apnea in a neonate is defined as- *(PGMEE 2015)*

a. Cessation of respiration for 15 seconds irrespective of bradycardia
b. Cessation of respiration for 20 seconds or more with bradycardia and cyanosis
c. Cessation of respiration for less than 20 seconds with bradycardia or cyanosis
d. Cessation of respiration for 30 seconds without bradycardia of cyanosis

[Ref: O.P. Ghai 8th/e/p 171]

16. Apnea of prematurity lasts for? *(PGMEE 2012)*

a. 10 seconds   b. 15 seconds
c. 20 seconds   d. 25 seconds

17. A baby born with thick meconium aspiration management *(PGMEE Nov. 2016)*

a. Suctioning   b. Intubation + suctioning
c. Intubation   d. ECMO

[Ref: Nelson 21st/e/pg. 941]

18. Gas reaches colonic end in a newborn by? *(DNB June 2011)*

a. 2-3 hours   b. 4-5 hours
c. 6-7 hours   d. 8-10 hours

[Ref: http://radiographics.rsna.org/content/19/5/1219.full by T.Berrocal et al]

7.	a
8.	c
9.	a
10.	b
11.	d
12.	c
13.	a
14.	a
15.	b
16.	c
17.	c
18.	d

Explanation

- "In a healthy neonate, air can usually be identified in the stomach within minutes of birth, and within 3 hours the entire small bowel usually contains gas. After 8–9 hours, healthy neonates demonstrate sigmoid gas"

Age Group	Colonic Transit Time
Newborn	8-10 hrs
1 year	10 hrs.
5-15 years	11 hrs.
Adult Male	12 hrs.
Adult Female	16 hrs

19. Which response is not seen in newborns as a measure of thermogenesis? *(DNB June 2011; PGMEE 2015)*
a. Shivering
b. Breakdown of brown fat
c. Increased physical activity/Universal flexion attitude
d. Cutaneous vasoconstrictions

[Ref: Ghai 8th/e/p 143]

Explanation

Non shivering thermogenesis in newborn

- Alawys remember that newborn cannot produce heat by shivering.A newborn is more prone for hypothermia because of large surface area per unit of body weight.
- Thermogenesis in Newborn-
- Cold stress leads to rapid increase in level of circulating Catecholamines,which in turn lead to
  1. Lipolysis and reesterification of brown fat leading to release of heat.
  2. Incresed Heart rate so as to increase more Oxygen to tissues.
  3. Peripheral vasoconstriction.
- *Role of Brown fat in Thermogenesis-*
  - In infants brown fat is an important site of thermogenesis.
  - It is located around adrenal gland,kidneys,nape of neck,interscapular and axillary regions.
  - Metabolism of brown fat produces heat. Blood flowing thru brown fat becomes warm and through circulation transfers heat to other parts of body, this is known as non-shivering thermogensis.

20. Large dose of vitamin-K in a newborn cause?
a. Hyperprothombinemia *(DNB June 2011)*
b. Hemolytic anemia
c. Convulsions
d. Bulging of posterior fontanel

[Ref: Nelson 21st/e/pg. 375; Ghai 7th/e pg 86]

Explanation

- Menadione/Kenadione are used in a dose of 1 mg i/m injections in anterolateral thigh in newborns as a routine at the time of birth.
- Menadione unsubstituted in the 3rd position causes toxicity in children expressed as **jaundice,hemolysis and kernicterus.**
- Phylloquinone is essentially non-toxic.

19. a
20. b
21. c

21. Management of 1 week old baby with imperforate anus and meconuria is? *(PGMEE 2012, 2011)*
a. Side window colostomy
b. Excision of pouch and permanent ileostomy
c. Diversion colostomy with sleeve resection followed by pull through
d. Dividing the fistula and end colostomy

[Ref: Nelson 21st/e/pg. 2057; Congenital Pouch colon ,then and Now;DK Gupta,shilpa Sharma, JIAPS,Jan-March-2007,Vol. 12,Issue 1,pp 5-12] Cloherty 8th edition, page 955, Nelson 20th edition – page 1896-97

Explanation

Congenital Pouch colon or Congenital short colon

- This is a specific type of Anorectal Malformation;seen mainly in Indian subcontinent. It is Known as Congenital Pouch colon or Congenital short colon. Here, a varying length of large colon is replaced by a large pouch which often opens into genito-Urinary tract by a fistulous communication associated with anorectal agenesis. The Diagnostic criteria are-
  1. There is anorectal agenesis.
  2. Total length of the colon is short.
  3. Colon has a pouch formation for a varying length-saccular or diverticular with collection of meconium and fecal matter.
  4. The blood supply to the pouch is abnormal.
  5. The colon wall is thick and muscular with hypertrophied mucosa.
  6. The fistula with genitourinary tract is large, muscular and long.It is closely adherent with the bladder wall.
  7. There is no transitional zone between the pouch coln and the normal bowel.The pattern changes suddenly and sharply.
- Clinical Features-
  - Most cases present in early neonatal period with an absent anal opening and distension of abdomen with or without meconuria.
  - The association of bilious vomitings with early gross distension of abdomen in a case of ARM is strongly suggestive.
- Management- Two stage procedure-
  1. A diversion colostomy at birth with sleeve resection of colonic pouch.
  2. Followed by pull through.
- Imperforate anus - Fifty percent have anomalies including those in the VACTERL association. Infants with imperforate anus may pass meconium if a rectovaginal or rectourinary fistula exists. A fistula is present in 80% to 90% of affected males and 95% of females. It may take 24 hours for the fistula to become evident. The presence or absence of a visible fistula at the perineum is the critical distinction in the diagnosis and management of imperforate anus. Of note, in order to prevent urinary tract infections, prophylactic antibiotics should be considered until the fistula can be definitively repaired.
  - **Perineal fistula.** Meconium may be visualized on the perineum. It may be found in the rugal folds or scrotum in boys and in the vagina in girls. This fistula may be dilated to allow passage of meconium to

temporarily relieve intestinal obstruction. When the infant is beyond the newborn period, the imperforate anus can generally be primarily repaired.

○ **No perineal fistula present**. There may be a fistula that enters the urinary tract or, for girls, the vagina. **The presence of meconium particles in the urine is diagnostic of a rectovesicular fistula.** Vaginal examination with a nasal speculum or cystoscope may reveal a fistula. A cystogram may show a fistula and document the level of the distal rectum, which can also be defined by ultrasonography. **A temporary colostomy may be necessary in neonates with an imperforate anus without a perineal fistula.** Primary repair of these infants without a colostomy is now being performed at some institutions.

Nelson writes:

- In children with a high lesion, a double-barrel colostomy is per formed.
- This effectively separates the fecal stream from the urinary tract. It also allows the performance of an augmented pressure colostogram before repair to identify the exact position of the distal rectum and the fistula.
- **The definitive repair or posterior sagittal anorecto plasty (PSARP) is performed at about 1 yr of age.**
- A midline incision is made, often splitting the coccyx and even the sacrum. Using a muscle stimulator, the surgeon stays strictly in the midline and divides the sphincter complex and identifies the rectum. The rectum is then opened in the midline and the fistula is identified from within the rectum. This allows a division of the fistula without injury to the urinary tract. The rectum is then dissected proximally until enough length is gained to suture it to an appropriate perineal position. The muscles of the sphincter complex are then sutured around (and especially behind) the rectum.
- Other operative approaches (such as an anterior approach) are used, but the most popular procedure is by laparoscopy. This operation allows division of the fistula under direct visualization and identification of the sphincter complex by transillumination of perineum.
- Usually, the colostomy can be closed 6 wks or more after the PSARP. Two weeks after any anal procedure, twice-daily dilatations are performed by the family. By doing frequent dilatations, each one is not so painful and there is less tissue trauma, inflammation, and scarring.
- Perineal fistula can be treated with simple progressive dilatations – dilated till dilator number 14 can be inserted.

22. APGAR stands for (*NEET Pattern 2017*)

a. Appearance, Pressure, Grimace, Activity respiration
b. Appearance, Pulse, Grimace, Activity, Respiration
c. Appearance, Pressure, Grimace, Activity Respiration
d. Awareness, Pulse, Grimace, Activity, Respiration

[Ref: Nelson 21st/e/ chl. 113.3pg. 872]

Explanation

APGAR Evaluation of Newborn Infants*

- Modified from Apgar V:A proposal for a new method of evaluation of the newborn infant, Res Anesth Analg 32:260-267, 1953.

Sign	0	1	2
Heart rate	Absent	Below 100	Over 100
Respiratory effort	Absent	Slow, irregular	Good, crying
Muscle tone	Limp	Some flexion of extremities	Active motion
Response to catheter in nostril (tested after oropharynx is clear)	No response	Grimace	Cough or sneeze
Color	Blue, pale	Body pink, extremities blue	Completely pink

Factors Affecting the Apgar Score

False-Positive (No Fetal Acidosis or Hypoxia; Low Apgar Score
Prematurity
Analgesics, narcotics, sedatives
Magnesium sulfate
Acute cerebral trauma
Precipitous delivery
Congenital myopathy
Congenital neuropathy
Spinal cord trauma
Central nervous system anomaly
Lung anomaly (diaphragmatic hernia)
Airway obstruction (choanal atresia)
Congenital pneumonia and sepsis
Previous episodes of fetal asphyxia (recovered)
Hemorrhage hypovolemia

False-Negative (Acidosis; Normal Apgar Score)
Maternal acidosis
High fetal catecholamine levels
Some full term infants

23. A neonate born with APGAR 6 at 1 min indicates: (*Recent Pattern June 2018*)

a. Newborn requiring routine post-delivery care
b. Newborn is mildly depressed and require some resuscitative measures
c. Newborn is severely depressed and need prompt action
d. Newborn is not depressed and require only ongoing care

[Ref: O.P. Ghai 8th/e pg. 126; Nelson's 20th/e pg. 798]

Explanation

Apgar Score

- APGAR score is quantitative method for assessing the infant's respiratory, circulatory and neurological status.
- APGAR is a acronym which includes 5 criteria:-
  ○ A - Appearance (colour)
  ○ P - Pulse rate (HR)
  ○ G - Grimace (reflex response to catheter in the nose)
  ○ A - Activity (muscle tone)
  ○ R - Respiratory efforts (Cry or breathing effort)

22.	b
23.	b

Score	0	1	2
1. Respiration (Breathing Efforts)	none	slow, irregular	good, crying
2. Heart rate (bpm)	Absent	< 100	> 100
3. Colour of the body	Blue or pale	Body pink extremities blue	pink
4. Muscle tone	flaccid	Some flexion of extremities	Actively moving
5. Reflex stimulation	No response	Grimace or sneeze	cries, coughs

[Remember that respiratory rate is **not** included in APGAR score]
- In delivery room APGAR is taken at 1, 5 and 10 minutes.
- At 1 minute:-
  ○ Normal baby will get a score of 7-10
  ○ In asphyxia score is 4-6 mild depression, 1-3 severe depression.
- *Action plan*
  ○ A normal Apgar score is 7 to 10 and means a newborn is in good to excellent condition, usually only requiring routine post-delivery care.
  ○ Babies scoring between 4 and 6 are in fair condition and **may require some resuscitative** measures. Depressed neonate (Apgar score < 7) usually improves in response to O$_2$ by hood/ facemask, with or without PPV of lungs.
  ○ Neonate with an Apgar score < 4 are in poor condition and need immediate medical attention.

24. Presence of grimace gets APGAR score of
a. 0   b. 1   *(PGMEE 2013-14)*
c. 2   d. 3

[Ref: Nelson 21st/e/pg. 872, Ghai 8th/e/p 126 table 8.2]

25. Apgar score at 1 minute is 3. This indicates that
a. Child is severely depressed   *(PGMEE 2019)*
b. Child is mildly depressed
c. Nothing to be done
d. Further resuscitation not needed

[Ref: NRP]

26. APGAR score is – include all except- *(PGMEE 2013-14)*
a. Color   b. Respiratory rate
c. Muscle tone   d. Heat rate

[Ref: Nelson 21st/e/pg. 872, Ghai 8th/e/p 126 table 8.2]

27. Most common cause of per rectal bleeding in infant is- *(PGMEE 2013-14)*
a. Anal fissure   b. Rectal polyp
c. Intussusception   d. Hypertension

[Ref: Nelson 21st/e/pg. 1910]

Explanation
- Anal fissure is m/c/ cause of GI bleeding in infants. (Ref. Medscape)

24.	b
25.	a
26.	b
27.	a
28.	d
29.	b
30.	a
31.	a
32.	b

28. Macrosomia is   *(PGMEE 2013-14)*
a. Big mouth   b. Large tongue
c. Large head   d. Large size baby

[Ref: Ghai 8th/e/p 778]

29. Very low birth weight is less than: *(Recent Pattern June 2018)*
a. 1000 gm   b. 1500 gm
c. 2000 gm   d. 2500 gm

[Ref: O.P. Ghai 8th/e pg. 125; Nelson's 20th/e pg. 789]

Explanation
- Low birth weight (LBW) is defined as a fetus that weighs < 2500 g (5 lb 8 oz) irrespective of gestational age.
- Very Low Birth Weight (VLBW) is <1500 g
- Extremely Low Birth Weight (ELBW) is <1000 g.
- Normal weight at term delivery is 2500 g - 4200 g.
- SGA is not a synonym of LBW, VLBW or ELBW. Small for gestational age (SGA) babies are those whose birth weight, length, or head circumference lies below the 10th percentile for that gestational age

30. Principle mode of heat exchange is an infant incubator is- *(PGMEE 2013-14)*
a. Convection   b. Conduction
c. Evaporation   d. Radiation

[Ref: Nelson 21st/e/ch. 114]

Explanation

Major mechanism of heat loss	
At birth	Evaporation
After birth in incubator	Radiation
Under radiation vomer	Conversion

- Most imp mechanism of heat gain/heat exchange in neonates
  ○ In incubator → convection
  ○ Under radiant wormer → Radiation

31. All are feature of prematurity in neonate except- *(PGMEE 2013-14)*
a. Thick ear cartilage   b. Abundant lanugo
c. Empty Scrotum   d. No crease on sole

[Ref: Nelson 21st/e/ch. 113.2 pg. 868]

32. In a delivery room a neonate delivered found to have HR <60 even after effective Positive Pressure Ventilation and no respiratory efforts. What is the line of action:- *(PGMEE 2018)*
a. Oxygen by mask
b. Start chest compression
c. Chest compression + adrenaline
d. Adrenaline

[Ref: Textbook of neonatal resuscitation – 7th edition]

Explanation

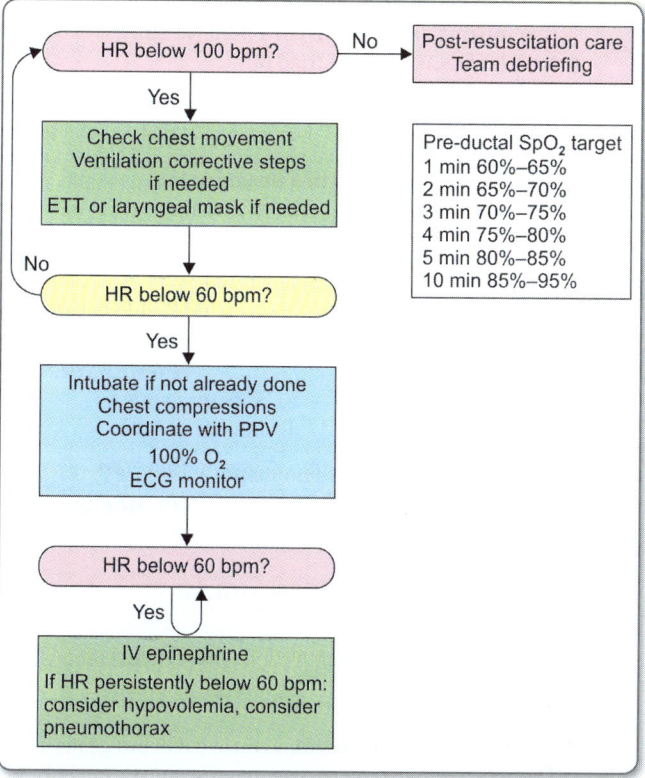

33. What is the initial stimulus for closure of PDA
a. Arterial oxygen tension **(PGMEE 2019)**
b. Prostaglandins
c. Both
d. None

34. Where is the probe placed to detect pre-ductal SpO2 at 3 minutes in a case of PDA **(PGMEE 2019)**
a. Right upper limb b. Left upper limb
c. Right lower limb d. Left lower limb

[Ref. Nelson 21st ed. Pg 2382]

35. Target Oxygen saturation in a preterm neonate is after initial stabilization? **(PGMEE 2013)**
a. 85-95% b. > 95%
c. 70-95% d. < 80%

[Ref: Ghai 8th/e/p 169]

36. How much pressure does a neonate require for first inflation? **(PGMEE 2012)**
a. 25 cm of Hg b. 25 mm of Hg
c. 25 mm of H2O d. 25cm of H2O

[Ref: Nelson 21st/e/pg. 925, Ghai 8th/e/p 130]

37. Normal value of fetal scalp blood pH is?
a. 7 b. 7.1 **(PGMEE 2012)**
c. 7.3 d. 7.25

[Ref: Nelson 21st/e/pg. 885]

38. In neonatal hyperglycemia the blood sugar is above? **(PGMEE 2012-13)**
a. 100 mg/dl b. 125 mg/dl
c. 150 mg/dl d. 175 mg/dl

[Ref: Indian Pediatrics 208; 45:29-38;CCOUER T_4 pg. 293]

39. Causes of conjugated hyperbilirubinemia is- **(PGMEE 2012-13)**
a. Breast milk jaundice b. Gilbert syndrome
c. Rotor syndrome d. Criglar Najjar

[Ref: Nelson 21st/e/pg. 2086, Ghai 8th/e/p 312]

40. MRP – 2 protein defect is seen in: **(PGMEE 2019)**
a. Criggler Nagger syndrome I
b. Criggler Nagger syndrome II
c. Dubin Johnson syndrome
d. Rotor's syndrome

Explanation

- The Dubin Johnson's Syndrome (DJS) is a rare, congenital, benign disorder characterized by mild conjugated hyperbilirubinemia and deposition of a dark pigment in the liver; it is now recognized as due to mutations in MRP2 leading to the loss of expression or function of MRP2 protein (Kartenbeck et al. 1996).

41. Which condition is fatal in infancy **(PGMEE 2019)**
a. Criggler Nagger syndrome I
b. Criggler Nagger syndrome II
c. Dubin Johnson syndrome
d. Gilbert syndrome

[Ref: Nelson 21st/e/pg. 2086, Ghai 8th/e/p 312]

42. Neonatal Jaundice first tissue appears in the 2nd week. Which of the following is NOT a cause? **(PGMEE 2012-13)**
a. Galactosemia b. Rh Incompatibility
c. Hypothyroidism d. Breast milk Jaundice

[Ref: Nelson 21st/e/pg. 967]

43. A 4-days-old neonate is brought by the mother to the pediatrician and is found to have a bilirubin of 18 mg%. What is the next step? **(NEET Pattern 2017)**
a. Stop breastfeeding
b. Start phototherapy and continue breastfeeding
c. Start phototherapy and stop breastfeeding
d. Exchange transfusion

[Ref: Nelson 21st/e/ch. 123.3]

Explanation

Breast milk jaundice (BMJ)

- Significant unconjugated hyperbilirubinemia (breast milk jaundice) develops in an ~ 2% of breast-fed term infants after the 7th day of life, with maximal bilirubin levels reached 10-30 mg/dL during the 2nd-3rd week.
- Continuation of breast-feeding decreases the bilirubin level gradually but hyperbilirubinemia may persist for 3-10 wk at lower levels.
- If nursing/breast feeding is discontinued, the bilirubin level falls rapidly, reaching normal range within a few days. **Phototherapy may be useful.** Kernicterus is uncommon with BMJ. **The etiology of BMJ is not very clear but may be attributed to the +nce of glucuronidase in some breast milk.**

Breast feeding jaundice (BFJ)

- BMJ syndrome should be distinguished from an early-onset, accentuated unconjugated hyperbilirubinemia known as *breast-feeding jaundice (BFJ)*, which usually

33.	a
34.	a
35.	a
36.	d
37.	d
38.	c
39.	c
40.	c
41.	a
42.	b
43.	b

occurs in the 1st week of life in breast-fed newborns, who normally have higher serum bilirubin levels than formula-fed newborns. Hyperbilirubinemia (>12 mg%) develops in 13% of breast-fed infants in the 1st wk of life and may be due to decreased milk intake with dehydration and/or reduced caloric intake.

- Prophylactic supplements of glucose water to breast-fed infants are a/w higher bilirubin levels, in part because of reduced intake of the higher–caloric density breast milk.
- **Frequent breast-feeding (>10/24 hr), rooming-in with night feeding, and lactation support decreases the incidence of early BFJ.** *Even when BFJ develops, breast-feeding should be continued if possible.* It is an option to temporarily interrupt breast-feedings and substitute with infant milk formula for 1-2 days.
- In addition, frequent feeding and supplementation with formula or expressed breast milk is appropriate if the intake seems inadequate, weight loss is excessive, or the infant appears dehydrated.

44. The dose of betamethasone in prenatal period to prevent respiratory distress syndrome is- *(PGMEE 2012-13)*
- a. 6 mg
- b. 4 mg stat
- c. 6 mg 12 hours
- d. 12 mg 24 hours apart

[Ref: Nelson 21st/e/ch. 115]

45. Meconium passage in utero leads to which of the following- *(PGMEE 2012-13)*
- a. Meconium ileus
- b. Obstructive emphysema
- c. Listeriosis
- d. Pathological jaundice

[Ref: Ghai 8th/e/p 170]

Explanation

Meconium passage in utero

Listerosis

→ MAS

→ Meconium particles in bronchi → Obstus Erpts

→ Obstructive emphysema

46. Premature baby presents with pain abdomen and blood in stool. X ray shown. Investigations are likely to show *(PGMEE 2019)*

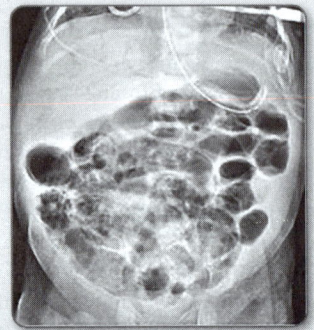

- a. Hyponatremia, Metabolic acidosis, Thrombocytopenia
- b. Hypernatremia, Metabolic alkalosis, Thrombocytosis
- c. Hypokalemia, Metabolic, alkalosis, Thrombocytopenia
- d. Hyperkalemia, metabolic acidosis, Thrombocytosis

[Ref: Nelson 20th/e pg. 870, 871]

Explanation

- The clinical picture and radiograph is typical of NEC (necrotizing enterocolitis) in a preterm baby.
- NEC is catarasized by a triad of:-
  ○ Hyponatremia
  ○ Metabolic acidosis
  ○ Thrombocytopenia

47. Gas reaches colonic end in a newborn by?
- a. 2-3 hours
- b. 4-5 hours
- c. 6-7 hours
- d. 8-10 hours

Ref: http://radiographics.rsna.org/content/19/5/1219. full by T.Berrocal et al

48. In asymmetrical IUGR which organ is not affected- *(PGMEE 2012-13)*
- a. Brain
- b. Subcutaneous fat
- c. Liver
- d. Muscle

[Ref: Nelson 20th/e/ p 823]

49. IUGR is caused by all except- *(PGMEE 2012-13)*
- a. Smoking
- b. Chronic renal failure
- c. Gestational Diabetes Mellitus (GDM)
- d. Alcohol

[Ref: Nelson 20th/e/p 823 table 87-4]

Explanation

- Pre gestational diabetes may cause IUGR but gestational Diabetes Mellitus may cause macrosomia (large baby).

50. A hymenal tag in a newborn is best treated by- *(PGMEE 2012-13)*
- a. Leaving it as such
- b. Surgery
- c. Steroids
- d. Cautery

[Ref: Internet]

51. Neonatal period extends upto- *(PGMEE 2012-13)*
- a. 21 days of life
- b. 24 days of life
- c. 28 days of life
- d. 30 days of life

[Ref: O.P. Ghai 8th/e/p 124]

52. In baby, stool followed by breastfeeding is attributed to? *(PGMEE 2014)*
- a. Rooting reflex
- b. Moro reflex
- c. Swallowing reflex
- d. Gastrocolic reflex

[Ref: Ghai 8th/e/p 135]

53. A 3 hour old preterm baby develops respiratory grunt and X-ray shows reticulonodular pattern. Diagnosis is- *(PGMEE 2012-13)*
- a. Meconium aspiration syndrome
- b. Transient tachypnea of newborn
- c. Hyaline membrane disease
- d. All

[Ref: Ghai 8th/e pg. 169, Nelson 21st/e/pg. 932; Cloherty 8th, page 438, chapter 33]

Explanation

Classic signs of RDS

- Low volume lungs
- Ground glass appearance of lung fields or Reticulogranular pattern in B/L lung fields

44.	d
45.	b
46.	a
47.	d
48.	a
49.	c
50.	a
51.	c
52.	d
53.	c

- Symmetric findings
- Air bronchograms

54. A neonate delivered at 32 weeks, is put on a ventilator, X-ray shows 'white out lung' and ABG reveals PO2 of 75. Ventilator settings are an, FiO2 of 70, and rate of 50/minute. Next step to be taken should be:
(Recent Pattern June 2018)
a. Increase rate to 60 per minute
b. Increase FiO2 to 80
c. Continue ventilation with the same settings
d. Weaning ventilator

[Ref: O.P. Ghai 8th/e pg. 169; Nelson's 20th/e pg. 858]

Explanation

- 'White - Out' CXR in a preterm neonate is a sign of Hyaline Membrane disease i.e. RDS.
  - ABG reveals pO2, of 75 : which is acceptable.
  - FiO2 (Fractional Inspiratory O2), here in the ventilator settings, is 75% well above the normal.
  - Respiratory Rate settings in the ventilator is 50/min : Normal for that age.
- The FiO2 being given is in the higher normal range, and increasing FiO2 as this carries a risk of ROP (Retinopathy of Prematurity).
- Rate of 50/min is OK in this neonate.
- Weaning from ventilator will start once the baby shows signs of overventilation or hyperoxygenation with the current settings, i.e. If pO2 in ABG goes up in the range of 120 .
- The answer here would be to continue the current settings till such time when the baby shows hyperoxygenation, and then slowly wean him off the ventilator

55. At risk infant are all except:
a. Birth order > 3
b. Twin
c. Birth weight < 2.5 kg weight
d. Artificial feeding

[Ref: Park 25th/e]

56. Which of the following is not a high risk infant:
a. Twins   *(Recent Pattern June 2018)*
b. With PEM
c. Working mother
d. With congenital malformation

[Ref: Park's 24th/e pg. 570]

Explanation

High Risk Infant

- "At risk" babies are major contributor of perinatal, neonatal & infant mortality. So it is very important identifying these babies.
- The basic criteria for identifying these babies include:-
  - Birth weight <2500 gm (LBW babies)
  - Twins
  - Birth order ≥ 5
  - Babies on artificial feeding
  - Weight < 70% of expected (malnutrion level II & III)
  - Children with PEM , diarrhoea
  - Failure to gain weight for 3 consecutive months (FTT)
  - Working mother/ single parent

57. Stools in breast feeding infants are: *(PGMEE 2016-17)*
a. Meconium colored
b. Greenish stools
c. Yellow stool
d. Colorless stools

[Ref: Ghai 8th/e/ch 8]

58. Lecithin-Sphingomyelin ratio (L:S ratio) is used for-
(PGMEE 2013-14)
a. Kidney maturity
b. Brain maturity
c. Age of infant
d. Lung maturity

[Ref: Nelson 21st/e/pg. 890]

59. Hypoglycemia in infants more than 24 hours of age is defined as blood glucose levels less than
a. 50mg/dl
b. 45ml/dl
c. 40mg/dl
d. 55mg/dl

Explanation

Age	Ser glucose Level
1-3 Hours	35 mg/dL
3-24 Hours	40 mg/dL
after 24 Hours	45 mg/dL

60. Severe hypothermia in a neonate is temperature?
a. < 35 C
b. < 34 C
c. < 33 C
d. < 32 C

Ref: Ghai pg 116

Explanation

- Hypothermia In Neonates-
- Nonshivering Thermogenesis
- Normal Axillary Temperature: 36.5 – 37.5°C
- Cold stress: 36.5 – 36.0°C
- Moderate hypothermia: 36 – 32°C
- Severe hypothermia < 32°C.

Neonate are more prone for hypothermia because of

- Large surface area/body weight ratio
- Decreased subcutaneous and brown fat/baby weight
- Immature/thin skin.

EXTRA EDGE

Definitions-

- **Appropriate for date/AGA-**Babies with birth wt. ranging between 10th-90th percentile of appropriate chart.
- **SGA/Small for dates-Babies** with birth wt less than 10th percentile.
- **LGA/Large for Dates-**Babies with Birth wt. more than 90th percentile.
- **Low Birth Wt-**Any neonate with Bwt. less than 2500gm irrespective of gestational age.
- **Very Low Birth** Wt-Any neonate with Bwt. less than 1500 gm irrespective of gestational age.
- **Extremly Low Birth Wt-**Any neonate with Bwt. less than 1000gm irrespective of gestational age.

54.	c
55.	a
56.	d
57.	c
58.	d
59.	b
60.	d

1. **Which of the following vaccine should not be given in patient with Egg allergy:** *(PGMEE 2015)*
   a. Varicella
   b. Measles
   c. MMR
   d. Influenza

   [Ref: Vaccine Safety, Canadian Immunization Guide.http://www.phac-aspc.gc.ca/publicat]

2. **Which of the following is the most common cause of Vaccine failure** *(PGMEE 2015)*
   a. Inappropriate manufacturing
   b. Improper storage
   c. Maternal antibodies
   d. Improper administration

   [Ref: Measles and Poliomyelitis: Vaccines, Immunization, and Control, Edouard Kurstak, p-80]

3. **Killed vaccine is** *(PGMEE 2013)*
   a. Measles
   b. BCG
   c. OPV
   d. Hepatitis A

   [Ref: K. Park, 23rd ed. p-103]

4. **Additional component of UIP PLUS does not include**
   a. Hepatitis B vaccine *(PGMEE 2013)*
   b. Diarrhea management
   c. Safe motherhood
   d. Acute repiratory infections

   [Ref: Textbook of Paediatric Nursing, Assuma Beevi.T.M, 1st ed. p-41, Unicef. Org/ immunization/ index_immunization plus.html]

5. **Strain used in Mumps vaccine is:** *(PGMEE 2012, 2013)*
   a. Jeryll lynn
   b. OKA
   c. DANISH 1331
   d. Edmonston

   [Ref: K. Park, 25th/e pg. 165]

6. **Hepatitis B vaccine, dose schedule in adult (in months)** *(PGMEE 2012)*
   a. 0,1,2 months
   b. 0,6,12 months
   c. 0,1,6 months
   d. 2,4,6 months

   [Ref: K. Park, 25th/e pg. 235, CDC website]

7. **Protection level of tetanus anti-toxin is:** *(PGMEE 2012)*
   a. >0.01 IU/ml
   b. >0.5 IU/ml
   c. >1.0 IU/ml
   d. >5 IU/ml

   [Ref: K. Park, 25th/e pg. 340]

8. **Which of the following is NOT a type of cholera vaccine?** *(PGMEE 2013)*
   a. CVD-103-Hgr
   b. mORC-Vax
   c. WC-rBS
   d. Ty21 A

   [Ref: K. Park, 25th/e pg. 256]

9. **Mass vaccination is ineffective in** *(PGMEE 2012)*
   a. Tetanus
   b. Measles
   c. Poliomyelitis
   d. None of the above

   [Ref: K. Park, 23rd ed. p-312. Mass vaccination: Global aspects- progress and obstacles. Stanley A Plotkins, P-3]

10. **A full course of immunization against Tetanus with 3 doses of Tetanus toxoid, confers immunity for how many years-** *(PGMEE 2008)*
    a. 5
    b. 10
    c. 15
    d. 20

    Explanation

    - A minimum of two doses of tetanus toxoid administered at least 1 month apart, with the last dose given at least 2 weeks before the estimated date of delivery, appears to provide protective levels of antibody for well above 80% of newborns. The second dose is preferably given 4 or more weeks before delivery to ensure high maternal antibody levels and maximal transplacental antibody transfer. The estimated duration of protection against NT from two TT doses is up to 3 years; after a third dose, protection lasts for up to 10 years. Efficacy above 80% and long-term protection are desired, so the WHO recommends a schedule of five properly spaced TT doses (administered over a minimum period of years, and preferably over 10 years) to protect the newborns of vaccinated women for the duration of their reproductive years. [Vaccines, 6th Edition By Stanley A. Plotkin, MD, Walter Orenstein, MD and Paul A. Offit, MD].

11. **Trivalent oral polio vaccine contains, type 3 virus** *(PGMEE 2012)*
    a. 100,000 TCID 50
    b. 200,000 TCID 50
    c. 300,000 TCID 50
    d. 400,000 TCID 50

    [Ref: K. Park, 23rd ed. p-206]

12. **Newborn child with HIV + and symptomatic, which vaccine will be given** *(PGMEE 2014)*
    a. Measles
    b. Live J.E
    c. BCG
    d. OPV vaccine

    [Ref:Infectious Disease in Children and Newer Vaccines, TK Ghosh, 1st ed., p-142, Nancy R. Immunization for children with HIV /AIDS, BIPAI]

13. **A child presented at 18 months of age who has never been vaccinated before. Which vaccines will you administer?** *(NEET Pattern 2017)*
    a. DPT Booster and OPV
    b. Pentavalent vaccine
    c. BCG and OPV
    d. Pentavalent, BCG, MMR, OPV

    Ref: Indian Academy of Pediatrics (IAP) Recommended Immunization Schedule for Children Aged 0 through 18 years — India, 2016 and Updates on Immunization.

1.	None
2.	c
3.	d
4.	a
5.	a
6.	c
7.	a
8.	d
9.	a
10.	b
11.	c
12.	a
13.	d

Explanation

BCG Vaccine

Routine vaccination:
- Should be given at birth or at first contact
- **Catch up vaccination**: may be given up to 5 years.

DPT/DPaT

- **Catch-up vaccination:**
- Catch-up schedule: The 2nd childhood booster is not required if the last dose has been given beyond the age of 4 years
- Catch up below 7 years: DTwP/DTaP at 0, 1 and 6 months;
- Catch up above 7 years: Tdap, Td, and Td at 0, 1 and 6 months.

HEP B Vaccine

- Catch-up vaccination:
- Administer the 3-dose series to those not previously vaccinated.
- In catch up vaccination use 0, 1, and 6 months schedule.

MMR Vaccine

- **Catch-up vaccination:**
- Ensure that all school-aged children and adolescents have had at least 2 doses of MMR vaccine (3 doses if the 1st dose is received before 12 months) ;
- The minimum interval between the 2 doses is 4 weeks.
- One dose if previously vaccinated with one dose (2 doses if the 1st dose is received before 12 months) ;
- 'Stand alone' measles/any measles-containing vaccine or MMR can be administered to infants aged 6 through 8 months during outbreaks. However, this dose should not be counted.

14. Live attenuated vaccine can be given to *(PGMEE 2014)*
a. Children under 8 years
b. Patients on radiation
c. Patients on steroids
d. HIV patients

15. Which type of vaccine is MMR? *(PGMEE 2010)*
a. Live attenuated   b. Killed
c. Toxoid   d. Subunit

[Ref: K. Park, 25th/e pg. 111 & 162]

16. Immunity starts after how many days of yellow fever vaccination- *(PGMEE 2015)*
a. 7-10 days   b. 2-3 months
c. 2-3 weeks   d. 4-5 weeks

[Ref: K. Park, 25th/e pg. 309]

17. Which of the following is not a killed vaccine?
a. IPV   *(PGMEE 2015)*
b. Cholera vaccine
c. Hepatitis A vaccine
d. Hepatitis B vaccine

[Ref: Park, 25th/e pg. 111; Ghai pg 169]

18. Not a freeze dried vaccine- *(PGMEE 2015)*
a. Rubella   b. JE
c. Yellow fever   d. DPT and OPV both

[Ref: Park, 25th/e pg. 117]

19. Most widely used vaccine, beside OPV- *(PGMEE 2015)*
a. TT   b. Pneumococcal
c. BCG   d. Influenza

[Ref: www.ncbi.nlm.mih.]

20. MMR is a type of:- *(PGMEE 2016-17)*
a. Live vaccine   b. Killed vaccine
c. Subunit vaccine   d. Immunoglobulin

[Ref: K. Park, 25th/e pg. 111]

21. Chicken pox is: *(PGMEE 2016-17)*
a. Live vaccine   b. Killed vaccine
c. Subunit vaccine   d. Immunoglobulin

[Ref: K. Park, 25th/e pg. 111]

22. Vaccine which is not given at Birth: *(PGMEE 2016-17)*
a. BCG   b. OPV
c. Hepatitis B   d. DPT

[Ref: K. Park, 25th/e pg. 935]

23. Recombinant vaccine is: *(PGMEE 2016-17)*
a. Rotavirus   b. Step B
c. Typhoid vaccine   d. Hep B

[Ref: K. Park, 25th/e pg. 111]

BCG

24. BCG is given over *(PGMEE 2015)*
a. Volar aspect of left forearm
b. Left deltoid
c. Dorsal aspect of left forearm
d. Right deltoid

[Ref: Park, 25th/e pg. 135 & 213]

25. Which of the following vaccine is given to newborn? *(PGMEE 2015)*
a. Hib   b. MMR
c. DPT   d. BCG

[Ref: Ghai 8th/e/ch 9; Park, 25th/e pg. 213]

DPT/ TT

26. A man falls from bike and sustains an injury to his foot. TT was last taken 12 years ago & his primary immunization status is unknown. What would you recommend? *(PGMEE 2015)*
a. TT complete course + Human Tetanus Immunoglobulin
b. Nothing required
c. TT 1 dose + Human Tetanus Immunoglobulin
d. TT 1 dose

[Ref: Park, 25th/e pg. 341]

27. Which Diptheria vaccine is recommended in a 14 years old girl? *(PGMEE 2015)*
a. DT   b. Tdap
c. DPT   d. dT

[Ref: www.tapcoi.com; Park, 25th/e pg. 175]

28. DPT vaccine is given- *(PGMEE 2015)*
a. Subcutaneous   b. Intradermal
c. Intramuscular   d. Intravenous

[Ref: Park 23rd/e p. 162; O.P Ghai 8th/e/p/193]

14.	a
15.	a
16.	a
17.	b
18.	d
19.	c
20.	a
21.	a
22.	d
23.	d
24.	b
25.	d
26.	a
27.	d
28.	c

29. Herd immunity threshold for diphtheria- *(PGMEE 2015)*

    a. 50%   b. 60%
    c. 85%   d. 95%

        [Ref: Park 23rd/e p. 161]

30. In DPT vaccine, rare adverse effect of pertussis is:- *(PGMEE 2016-17)*

    a. Cough   b. Fever
    c. Encephalopathy   d. Pain

        [Ref: Park, 25th/e pg. 175]

OPV AND IPV

31. VAPP develops how many days following OPV administration *(PGMEE 2015)*
    a. 7-14
    b. 20-70
    c. 60-90
    d. Immediately

[Ref: WHO Information sheet observed rate of vaccine reactions for polio vaccines; Park, 25th/e pg. 227]

32. OPV bivalent vaccine contains *(PGMEE 2012)*
    a. P1 and P2
    b. P2 and P3
    c. P1 and P3
    d. P1, P2 and P3

    [Ref: Global Polio Eradication Initiative www.polioeradication.org; Park, 25th/e pg. 226]

33. False regarding polio vaccination- *(PGMEE 2015)*
    a. First OPV is given at 4 weeks
    b. Both killed and live vaccines are available
    c. OPV induces both humoral and intestinal immunity
    d. IPV is given intramuscularly

    [Ref: Park, 25th/e pg. 226]

Explanation

Polio Vaccine schedule (Ref AIP Immunization update 2014)

Schedule	Schedule	Comment
Birth - OPV-0	6 mth - OPV-1	All doses of IPV may be replaced with OPV if administration of IPV is not feasible
6 week - IPV-1	9 mth - OPV-2	Additional doses of OPV on all SIA & 2 doses of IPV instead of 3 primary series if started at 8 week & 3 weeks internal h/n doses
10 w- IPV-2	16-18 mth IPV - B-1	
14 w - IPV-3	4=6 yr OPV-3	No clue should leave the fertility without potent vaccine (IPV/OPV) if indicated by school

34. Image of polio vaccine is given below. VVM indicates:- *(PGMEE 2016-17)*

    a. Vaccine can be used
    b. Vaccine is not safe to use
    c. Vaccine must be discarded
    d. Inconclusive

    [Ref: Immunization for medical officers. Ministry of health and family welfare. p 42; Park, 25th/e pg. 121]

35. Zero dose of Polio vaccine is given- *(DNB pattern 2007)*
    a. Before giving DPT
    b. At birth
    c. When child is having diarrhoea
    d. When child is having Polio

    [Park, 25th/e pg. 134]

Explanation

- The WHO EPI Global Advisory Committee has strongly recommended BCG and Polio vaccine to be given at birth or at first contact, in countries where tuberculosis and polio have not been controlled.

MEASLES

36. Strain of virus not used in measles vaccine is:
    a. Moraten strain   *(PGMEE 2015)*
    b. Edmondson Zagreb strain
    c. Schwartz strain
    d. Jeryll Lynn strain

[Ref: Park, 25th/e pg. 165; Community Medicine Recent Advances –Suryakanta, 3rd ed., p-319]

37. In measles outbreak, measles vaccine can be given within *(PGMEE 2013)*
    a. 2-3 months   b. 2 days
    c. 3-5 months   d. 6-9 months

    [Ref: K. Park, 25th/e pg. 162]

38. After taking MMR live vaccine, conception should not occur within- *(PGMEE 2015)*
    a. 2 weeks   b. 4 weeks
    c. 8 weeks   d. 10 weeks

    [Ref: CDC guidelines of vaccination in pregnancy]

39. Which of the following vaccine is given subcutaneously- *(PGMEE 2015)*
    a. BCG   b. Typhoid
    c. Measles   d. Live influenza

    [Ref: Park, 25th/e pg. 135]

MMR VACCINE

40. RA 27/3 vaccine is for- *(PGMEE 2016-17)*
    a. Measles   b. Mumps
    c. Rubella   d. Cholera

    [Ref: Park, 25th/e pg. 164]

29. c
30. c
31. a
32. c
33. a
34. a
35. b
36. d
37. d
38. b
39. c
40. c

OTHER VACCINES

41. The trivalent Influenza vaccine contains all strains of influenza virus except: *(PGMEE 2015)*
- a. H1N1
- b. H3N2
- c. H2N1
- d. Influenza B

[Ref:-Key Facts About Seasonal Flu Vaccine, CDC http://www.cdc.gov/flu/protect/keyfacts.htm]

42. Which vaccine to be given every year ? *(PGMEE 2019)*
- a. Hepatitis A
- b. Pneumococcal
- c. Influenza
- d. Chicken pox

[Ref. IAP Immunisation guidelines 2014]

43. What is the route of administration of live attenuated influenza vaccine? *(PGMEE 2015)*
- a. Subcutaneous
- b. Nasal
- c. Oral
- d. Intramuscular

[Ref: Nelson 21st/e/ch. 197 pg. 1347; Park, 25th/e pg. 171]

44. Regarding PPSV vaccine following is true- *(PGMEE 2015)*
- a. Commonly used
- b. Given at birth
- c. Obtained from cell wall polysaccharide
- d. Indicated in sickle cell disease

[Ref: Essentials of microbiology 3rd/e p. 391]

Explanation

PPSV (IAP Immunization update 2014)
- Minimum age 2 yr.
- Not recommended for routine use in healthy individuals.
- Recommended only for the vaccination of person with certain high risk condition.
- Administer PPSV at least 8 weeks after the last dose of PCV to children aged 2 yrs or older with certain underlying medical condition like anatomic or functional asplenia (including sickle cell disease) HIV infection, clcochlear implant or CSF leak.
- An additional dose of PPSV should be administered after 5 yrs to children with anatomic/functional asplenia or an immunocompromising candidate.
- PPSV should be never be used alone for prevention of pneumococcal disease among high risk individuals.

45. Following is true about Hib conjugate vaccine-
- a. Capsular polysaccharide *(PGMEE 2015)*
- b. PRP (polyribosylribitol phosphate) with carrier
- c. Capsular polysaccharide with carrier
- d. Cell wall polysaccharide

[Ref: Park, 25th/e pg. 173 & 185]

Explanation

Hib conjugate vaccine (Ref CDC gov)
- Polyribosylribitol phosphate (PRP) capsule of Hib is a major virulence factor for the organism. Antibody to PRP is the primary contributor to serum bacterial activity.

46. Japanese encephalitis vaccine in routine schedule is given in how many doses- *(PGMEE 2015)*
- a. Three doses with second dose 1 month and 3rd dose 6 months after the first dose
- b. Two doses 1 month apart with a booster after 1-2 years if needed
- c. Three doses 1 month apart followed by a booster if needed
- d. Single dose vaccine

[Ref: Park, 25th/e pg. 313]

47. Not true about Vi polysaccharide vaccine of typhoid:
- a. Single dose is given *(PGMEE 2015)*
- b. Given at birth
- c. Revaccination at 3 years
- d. Given subcutaneously

[Ref: Park, 25th/e pg. 260]

Explanation
- Vi Polysaccharide vaccine - given >2 yrs of age.
- Single dose at 2 year & revaccination of every 3 year.

41. c
42. c
43. b
44. d
45. b
46. b
47. b

1. **Dried blood spot test in neonates is used for:**
   (NEET Pattern 2017)
   a. Inborn error of metabolism
   b. Blood group
   c. Total cell count
   d. Creatinine and bilirubin

   [Ref: Avery diseases of newborn, 9th edition, chapter 27, page 316]

Explanation

Guthrie test

- Introduced by **Guthrie and Susi** (1963).
- The blood sample is obtained from lateral or the medial side of heel of the infant.
- Blood should be applied to only one side of the filter paper card, but it should saturate each circle on the card.
- **After obtaining blood, specimen should be dried in air at room temperature for at least 3 hours before being placed in an envelope.**
- *Timing of collection:* The optimal time for collection of the specimen is within 24 to 48 hours after birth.

Method – Tandem Mass Spectrometry

Disorders Screened

- Cystic fibrosis
- Galactosemia
- Aminoacid and fatty acid disorders
- Organic acidemias
- Congenital hypothyroidism
- Congenital adrenal hyperplasia
- Biotinidase deficiency
- G-6-PD and sickle cell disease

1.	**a**
2.	**c**
3.	**b**
4.	**d**
5.	**c**

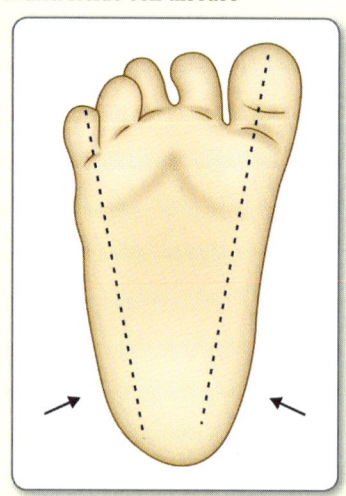

GALACTOSEMIA

2. **8 days old male child presents with pale stools, turmeric colored urine, yellow discolouration of sclera, H/O consanguineous marriage. On 3rd day after birth developed fever and sepsis which was treated with chloramphenicol broad spectrum antibiotic. Investigation of choice to be done is assays of:**
   (PGMEE 2014-15)
   a. β–glucosidase   b. β-galactosidase
   c. GALT   d. Alpha –glucosidase

   [Ref: Nelson 20th/e pg. 727]

3. **In children with classical galactosemia all are true EXCEPT:** *(PGMEE 2018)*
   a. E. coli sepsis is common
   b. Elimination of galactose in diet will NOT reverse cataract
   c. Patients with partial deficiency of transferase are generally asymptomatic
   d. Galactose is converted to galactitol which is toxic to brain & liver

   [Ref: Ref: Nelson 20th/e pg. 727]

DISORDERS OF AMINO ACID METABOLISM

4. **One year old male child with sparse blond hair, developmental delay and tremors, diagnosis-**
   (PGMEE 2013-14)
   a. Cerebral palsy   b. Infantile tremor syndrome
   c. Albinism   d. Phenylketonuria

   [Ref: Ghai 8th/e/ch 23]

5. **What is diet plan in phenylketonuria?** *(PGMEE 2015)*
   a. Complete restriction of phenylalanine
   b. Low tyrosine diet
   c. Low phenylalanine diet
   d. Complete restriction of tyrosine

   [Ref: Nelson 21st/e/pg. 697]

Explanation

- Start low phenylalanine diet if blood phenylalanine level is >10 mg/dL.
- Most Physicians advise phenylalanine restricted diet in patient with mild phenylalaninemia i.e. >6 mg/dL blood levels.
- Because phenylalanine is not synthesized endogenously, small amount of phenylalanine should be added to diet to prevent phenylalanine deficiency.

6. **Urine smells like 'sweaty feet' in?** *(PGMEE 2013-14)*
   a. Gaucher's Disease   b. Phenylketonuria
   c. Maple Syrup disease   d. Isovaleric acidemia

   [Ref: Nelson 21st/e/pg. 688]

7. **Enzyme deficient in phenylketonuria-**
   a. Tyrosine transaminase   *(PGMEE 2012-13)*
   b. Phenylalanine hydroxylase
   c. Homogentisic oxidase
   d. Tyrosinase

   [Ref: Nelson 21st/e/pg. 689]

8. **FeCl3 test in phenylketonuria will give which color?**
   (PGMEE 2012-13)
   a. Red   b. Purple
   c. Blue   d. Green

   [Ref: Nelson 21st/e/pg. 689]

9. **Mousy odour urine is seen in-**
   (PGMEE 2013-14, 2012-13)
   a. Alkaptonuria   b. Phenylketonuria
   c. Fabry's disease   d. Cystinuria

   [Ref: Nelson 21st/e/pg. 688 table]

10. **A baby, normal at birth, develops poor feeding and vomiting in the 1st week of life, and later becomes lethargic and comatose. Laboratory finding shows deficiency in branched chain α- ketoglutarate dehydrogenase. The disease is** *(PGMEE 2016)*
    a. Phenylketonuria
    b. Maple syprup urine disease
    c. Multiple carboxylase deficiency
    d. Tyrosinemia

    [Ref: Nelson 21st/e/pg. 708]

11. **Feature of cystinuria -** *(PGMEE 2013-14)*
    a. Autosomal recessive
    b. Impaired proximal tubular reabsorption of cystin
    c. Recurrent renal stone
    d. All of the above

    [Ref: Ghai 8th/e/p 503]

DISORDERS OF GLYCOGEN METABOLISM

12. **Which is NOT a Liver glycogenoses-** *(PGMEE 2012-13)*
    a. Von Gierke disease   b. Pompes disease
    c. Hers disease   d. Type III glycogenosis

    [Ref: Nelson 21st/e/pg. 777]

13. **Infant presents with hepatomegaly, hypoglycemia, hyperlipidemia and acidosis. Diagnosis is-**
    (PGMEE 2012-13)
    a. Tarui's disease   b. Pompe's disease
    c. Von Gierke's   d. All

    [Ref: Nelson 21st/e/pg. 777; 20th/e/pg. 717 table]

Explanation

- Ven Gierke disease is due to *Glucose 6 Phosphatase* enzyme deficiency.
- C/F- Growth retardation, hepatomegaly, hypoglycemia.
- Labs: elevated blood lactate, cholesterol, triglycerides & uric acid levels

14. **A 5 years old child presents with enlarged liver, uncontrolled hypoglycemia and ketosis. Most probable diagnosis is?** *(PGMEE 2012-13; 2011)*
    a. Diabetes mellitus
    b. Glycogen storage disease
    c. Lipid storage disorders
    d. Mucopolysacharidosis

    [Ref: Nelson 21st/e/pg. 777]

Explanation

- Recurrent hypoglycemic attacks with hepatomegaly are seen in Type I GSD (Von Gierke s disease)
- Glycogen Storage Diseases result from a hereditary deficiency of one of the enzyme involved in the synthesis or sequential degardation of Glycogen.
- Clinical features depend on type of enz involved and organ involvement.
- GSD can be divided into :-

Hepatic form of GSD (Liver Glycogenoses)

- Liver is the main organ in Glycogen metabolism.
- Inherited deficiency of hepatic enzymes leads to:-
  ○ Storage of Glycogen in Liver → Hepatomegaly.
  ○ Reduced blood sugar → Hypoglycemia.
- Examples are:-
  ○ Type I Glycogenosis→ Hypoglycemia is characteristic Glucose-6-Phosphatase deficiency.
  ○ Type III Glycogenosis → Debranching Enz deficiency.
  ○ Type IV Glycogenosis → Branching enzyme deficiency.
  ○ Type VI Glycogenosis → Liver Phosphorylase deficiency.
  ○ Type VII Tauri → Pompe

Myopathic form of GSD (Muscle Glycogenoses)

- In skeletal Muscles, glycogen is used primarily as energy source.This energy is derived by glycolysis, leading to formation of Lactate. Therfore enzyme deficiency leads to:-
  ○ Glycogen deposition in muscles.
  ○ Muscle cramps after exercise.
  ○ Exercise induced rise in blood lactate levels owing to block in glycolysis.
  ○ Myogobinemia may be associated.
- Examples include
  ○ Type II Glycogenosis → Phosphofructokinase deficiency (Pompe's disease)
  ○ Type V Glycogenosis → Phosphorylase defi(Mcardle's disease)
  ○ Type VII Glycogenosis → Tauri disease

  [Mnemonic for muscle GSD: PMT/ 2,5,7]

Miscellaneous types of GSDs

- Associted with Glycogen storage in many organs and death in early life.
- Examples include:-
  ○ Type II Glycogenosis → Acid Maltase deficiency (Pompe› s disease).

6.	d
7.	b
8.	d
9.	b
10.	b
11.	d
12.	b
13.	c
14.	b

1. **Highest cure rate is of-**   *(PGMEE 2012-13)*
   a. Wilm's Tumor   b. Rhabdomyosarcoma
   c. Retinoblastoma   d. All

   [Ref: Nelson 21st/e/pg. 2697]

Explanation

- Approximately 95% of children in US with retinoblastoma are cured, but if it progress to metastatic disease, mortality is over 50% cases.

2. **Diagnosis in a 2 year old boy having testicular lump with increased Alpha fetoprotein is-**   *(PGMEE 2013-14)*
   a. Teratoma   b. Choriocarcinoma
   c. Seminoma   d. Yolk sac tumor

   [Ref: Love and Bailey 26th/e/p 1385]

Explanation

- Yolk sac tumor is a rare malignant tumor of cells that line the yolk sac of embryo. These cells normally become ovaries or testes. These cells secrete α Fetoprotein (AFP) & HCG

3. **Not common in chidren-**   *(PGMEE 2013-14)*
   a. Osteosarcoma   b. Neuro blastoma
   c. Ewing's sarcoma   d. None of the above

   [Ref: Ghai 8th/e/ ch 20]

4. **A mass in the posterior cranial fossa of a child shows contrast medium– enhancing nodule within the wall of a cystic mass. Diagnosis is-**   *(PGMEE 2013-14)*
   a. Meningioma
   b. Hemangiocytic pericytoma
   c. Astrocytoma (polycystic)
   d. Ependymoma

   [Ref: Nelson 21st/e/pg. 2669]

Explanation

Polycystic astrocytoma

- Classic neuroradiological feature in PA is the presence of contrast enhancing nodule within the wall of a cystic mass.
- Presence of *Rosenthal fibres* (condensed masses of glial filaments occurring in compact areas) help in establishing the diagnosis.

5. **All are seen in first decade except-**   *(PGMEE 2012-13)*
   a. Ameloblastoma
   b. Retinoblastoma
   c. Neurobastoma
   d. Rhabdomyosarcoma

   [Ref: Ghai 8th/e ch 20]

6. **Most common tumor of newborn:**   *(PGMEE 2016-17)*
   a. Sacrococcygeal tumour
   b. Retinoblastoma
   c. Wilm's tumour
   d. Neuroblastoma

   [Ref: Nelson 21st/e/pg. 2698]

Explanation

Wilm's tumour

7. **All are true about Wilm's tumor EXCEPT:**
   a. Presents below 5 years of age
   b. Can be bilateral
   c. Presents as abdominal mass
   d. Spreads mainly through lymphatics

   [Ref: Ghai 7th pp592; Nelson 21st/e/pg. 2681]

Explanation

Wilm's tumour (WT)

- Aka nephroblastoma.
- M/c renal neoplasm in childhood.
- Peak incidence is between 2 and 5 yr of age. 80% of WT present under 5 yrs of age. The peak age diagnosis is 2-3 years.
- WT has also been encountered in neonates, adolescents, and adults. It can arise in one or both kidneys. The incidence of bilateral WT is 7%, and individuals with horseshoe kidney are at twice the risk for development of WT as the general population.
- Mostly sporadic;1-2% may have familial predisposition (inherited as Autosomal Dominant).
- Following Mutations are seen in Wilms-
  o Wilms Tumor Gene(WT1) on chromosome 11
  o CTNNB1 gene encoding the proto-oncogene beta carotene.
  o p53.
- *WT is associated with:-*

Syndrome	Association
WAGR syndrome	- Wilms tumor - Aniridia - Genital abnormalities (Male Pseudo-hermaphroditism) - Mental Retardation

Syndrome	Association
Beckwith wiedmann syndrome	■ Hemihypertrophy ■ BWS has high incidence of nephro and hepatoblastoma ■ Macrosomia and Macroglossia. ■ Midline abdominal wall defects (Omphalocele, Umbilical Hernia) ■ Ear creases/Pits. ■ Renal Medullary Cysts and adrenal cytomegaly. ■ Neonatal Hypoglycemia.
Denys-Drash Syndrome	■ Gonadal Dysgenesis (Male Pseudo-hermaphrodite) ■ Nephropathy (Mesangial Sclerosis) ■ Wilms Tumor

- Histologically mixed tumour
- M/c presentation is an *abdominal flank mass*, which is often asymptomatic.
- Other Features at presentation include
- Abdominal Pain (30%); Hypertension (25%); Hematuria (10- 25%); Fever (20%), Anorexia and vomiting.
- Spread :- M/c site lung and then liver.Brain is rare while Lymphatic spread is uncommon.
- Polycythemia may occur d/ to erythropoietin
- production. Poor Prognostic Factors-
- Unfavorable Histology, Hyperploidy, Large Tumor, Advanced Stage T/t - Nephrectomy, RT useful.

8. All are true about wilm's except:
   a. Present at 5 years of age
   b. Hematuria is the presenting symptom
   c. Presents as abdominal mass
   d. Most commonly metastasize to lung

   [Ref :Ghai 7th pp 591]

9. Most common thyroid tumor in children is?
   (PGMEE 2011)
   a. Papillary carcinoma
   b. Follicular carcinoma
   c. Medullary carcinoma
   d. Thyroid lymphoma

   [Ref: Nelson 21st/e/pg. 2934]

Explanation

- Histologically, the carcinomas are papillary or follicular variant of papillary carcinoma (88%), follicular (10%), medullary (2%), or mixed differentiated tumors.
- All of the thyroid cancers in a retrospective study of children with autoimmune thyroiditis were papillary carcinomas. Thyroid cancer in children is more likely to be multifocal, with spread to regional lymph nodes at presentation.
- The type of tumor and the natural course of disease in irradiated and nonirradiated patients are the same except that multicentricity is more common in irradiation-induced cancer.
- Undifferentiated (anaplastic) thyroid neoplasms are rare in children and usually have a rapidly fatal course. Lymphomas and teratomas of the thyroid are also reported in children.

8.   a
9.   a

1. Phocomelia is: *(PGMEE 2013-14)*
   a. Absence of long bones
   b. Reduplication of bones
   c. Absence of heart
   d. Absence of brain

[Ref: Nelson 21st/e/ch. 115.4, pg. 886]

2. True about Fragile X syndrome is- *(PGMEE 2019)*
   a. Triple nucleotide CAG Sequence mutation
   b. 10% Female carriers mentally retarded
   c. Males have iq 20-40
   d. Gain of function mutation

[Ref: Nelson 20th/e pg. 622, 623]

3. Fetal alcohol syndrome is characterized by all except: *(Recent Pattern June 2018)*
   a. Wide palpebral fissure
   b. Low intelligence
   c. Large proportionate body
   d. Septal defects of heart

[Ref: Nelson 20th/e pg. 894]

Explanation

Fetal alcohol syndrome

- Excess alcohol in pregnancy can be teratogenic to fetus, The condition is known as fetal alcohol syndrome.
- Some evidence suggests that alcohol may impair placental transfer of essential amino acids and zinc, both necessary for protein synthesis, which may account for IUGR
- Characteristics of fetal alcohol syndrome include : -
   ○ IUGR (not large proportionate body)
   ○ Microcephaly
   ○ Congenital heart defects (ASD, VSD)
   ○ Mental retardation
   ○ Facial dysmorphism → Short palpebral fissures, epicanthal folds, maxillary hypoplasia, micrognathia, low set ears, smooth philtrum, thin smooth upper lip
   ○ Minor joint anomalies
   ○ Hyperkinetic movements

4. Feature of Pierre Robin syndrome: *(PGMEE 2016-17)*
   a. Cleft lip, Retrognathia
   b. Cleft lip, glossoptosis
   c. Cleft palate, Retrognathia
   d. Cleft lip, cleft palate

[Ref: Nelson 21st/e/ch. 119, pg. 911 table 119.1]

5. Ponds fracture is most common in- *(PGMEE 2013-14)*
   a. Old age   b. Children
   c. Adult   d. No relation with age

[Ref: Maheshwari]

6. Satellite sequences during G$_0$ phase are seen in? *(PGMEE 2012)*
   a. Terminal centrioles   b. Nucleolus
   c. Kinetochore   d. Chromosome

[Ref: Lewin's essential genes by Jaceyn E. Krebs, Eliott S. Goldstein, Stephen T. Kilpatrick pg. 229]

7. Hypoglycemia in infants more than 24 hours of age is defined as blood glucose levels less than *(DNB June 2011)*
   a. 40mg/dl   b. 45ml/dl
   c. 50mg/dl   d. 55mg/dl

[Ref: Nelson 21st/e/ch. 111, pg. 848; 222X 245-50 mg/dlclouer t4 aiims protocx bgl gohgid nelson?]

8. Not seen in Refsum disease is- *(PGMEE 2013-14)*
   a. CCF   b. Retinitis pigmentosa
   c. Ataxia   d. Ichthyosis

[Ref: Nelson 21st/e/ch. 104.2, pg. 748]

9. Which of the following is correct about shock in child? *(PGMEE 2015)*
   a. Respiratory rate is more sensitive than heart rate as an indicator of early shock
   b. Tachycardia is a very sensitive indicator of depletion of intravascular volume
   c. Mottling of extremities is seen in early shock
   d. Confusion, stupor and coma are early signs

[Ref: Ghai 8th/e/p 716]

Explanation

Features of shock in child

- Heart rate is more sensitive indicator of shock than respiratory rate.
- Mottling of extremities, confusion, stupor, coma are late signs of shock.

10. Inotropic support for severely dehydrated child with dopamine is done at what rate- *(PGMEE 2015)*
   a. 0.1-0.5 microgram/kg/min
   b. 1-5 microgram/kg/min
   c. 1-5 mg/kg/min
   d. 10-15 mg/kg/min

[Ref: Ghai 8th/e/p 717]

11. Swiping of oral cavity not to done in foreign body ingestion in children as - *(PGMEE 2013-14)*
   a. Children do not allow swiping
   b. Oral cavity small, inability to clear
   c. Leads to in advertently pushing of foreign body
   d. Should be done forcibly

[Ref: Nelson 21st/e/pg. 1942]

1.	a
2.	c
3.	c
4.	c
5.	b
6.	c
7.	b
8.	a
9.	b
10.	b
11.	c

Explanation

- Swiping of oral cavity not to be done in foreign body ingestion in children as it leads to inadvertently pushing of foreign body & lodgment in inner airways
- Back thrust should be given instead.

12. Congenital rubella causes all except:
a. Deafness
b. Cataract
c. Cardiac defects
d. Hydrocephalus

[Ref: Nelson 21st/e/ch. 274, pg. 1676]

Explanation

Nerve deafness

- "Nerve deafness is the single most common finding among infants with CRS. Most infants have some degree of intrauterine growth restriction. Retinal findings described as salt-and-pepper retinopathy are the most common ocular abnormality but have little early effect on vision. Unilateral or bilateral cataracts are the most serious eye finding, occurring in about a third of infants. Cardiac abnormalities occur in half of the children infected during the 1st 8 wk of gestation. Patent ductus arteriosus is the most frequently reported cardiac defect, followed by lesions of the pulmonary arteries and valvular disease. Interstitial pneumonitis leading to death in some cases has been reported. Neurologic abnormalities are common and may progress following birth. Meningoencephalitis is present in 10-20% of infants with CRS and may persist for up to 12 mo. Longitudinal follow-up through 9-12 yr of infants without initial retardation revealed progressive development of additional sensory, motor, and behavioral abnormalities, including hearing loss and autism. PRP has also been recognized rarely after CRS. Subsequent postnatal growth retardation and ultimate short stature have been reported in a minority of cases. Rare reports of immunologic deficiency syndromes have also been described."
- Triad of CRS is
  1. Sensorineural Deafness
  2. Eye anomalies (Salt and pepper Retinopathy, Cataract,microphthalmia).
  3. Congenital Heart Dis. (specially PDA; others include VSD, PS-Peripheral, ASD-rarely). Microcephaly and Mental retardation is another imp association in CRS.

13. What is true of Vitamin D resistant rickets?
a. X linked recessive
b. No End organ resistance to 1, 25 (OH)2 D2
c. Defect in proximal tabular reabsorption
d. Hyperphosphatemia and high 1, 25 (OH)2 D3

Ref: Ghai 7th,pp 82-84;Nelsons 19th

IMNCI

14. Pink colour in IMNCI refers to *(PGMEE 2016)*
a. Home management
b. Reassurance
c. Urgent referral
d. OPD base Treatment

[Ref: Ghai 8th/e/p 752]

15. Which color is not used for categorizing an ill child in IMNCI? *(PGMEE 2016-17)*
a. Green
b. Red
c. Yellow
d. Pink

[Ref: Ghai 8th/e/p 752]

16. According to IMNCI 'Pneumonia' is: *(PGMEE 2016-17)*
a. Respiratory rate in 6 month old child 56 per minutes
b. Stridor in 9 month old child
c. Respiratory rate in 12 month old child 35 per minutes
d. Chest indrawing in 3 year old child

[Ref: Ghai 20th/e/ p 759]

17. Iron and folic acid requirement of 6 months to 10 years old children is?
a. 20 mg elemental iron and 100 microgram folic acid
b. 100 mg elemental iron and 500 microgram folic acid
c. 60 mg elemental iron and 500 microgram folic acid
d. 100 mg elemental iron and 1000 microgram folic acid

Ref: Park PSM 18th,pp 686

Explanation

- National Nutrition Anemia Control Programme is based on daily administration of iron and Folic acid to children.
- Adult/For mothers tab consists of 60mg elemental Iron and 500 microgram of Folic acid while for children it contains 20 mg iron and 100 microgram of Folic acid.

18. As per RCH II vitamin-A dosage at 9th month of age is?
a. 50,000 units
b. 1 lakh units
c. 1.5 lakh units
d. 2 lakh units

Ref: Ghai 7th pp 80.

Explanation

- Currently Vitamin A is given only to children less than 3 years old who are at greatest risk, and the administration of first two doses islinked with routine immunization to improve the coverage. A dose of 100,000 IU kis given along with measles vaccine at 9 months of age and 2,00,000 IU with DPT booster at fifteen months. subsequently 3 more doses are given (of 200,000 IU) at 24, 30 and 36 months of age.

MISCELLANEOUS

19. Not a common cause of meningitis in a child of age 8 years is:
a. S. pneumococci
b. H. influenza
c. S. aureus
d. Meningococci

[Ref: Nelson 21st/e/ch. 621.1, pg. 3223]

Explanation

- Meningitis due to Staph. aureus is associated with Cranial trauma and neurosurgical procedures and less frequently with endocarditis, parameningeal foci,diabetes mellitus or malignancy.
- H. influenzae type b causes meningitis between 2 months 3 years age group.

Meningitis in Children (Etiological agents)

- **Newborn:** GBS are the m/c cause f/b gram negative bacilli.

12.	d
13.	c
14.	c
15.	b
16.	a
17.	a
18.	b
19.	b,c

- Infancy: H. influenzae type B is the m/c cause in India. Meningococcal in developed countries.
- Child with complement deficiency (C5-C8): Recurrent meningococcal meningitis.
- CSF leak, cochlear implants predispose the child for: Pneumococcal meningitis.
- CSF shunt infection predispose the child for : Coagulase negative staphylococci
- A child with Lumbosacral dermal sinus and meningomyelocele: Staphylococci, Gram -ve enteric bacilli.
- A child with T-lymphocyte defect: Listeria monocytogenes.
- A child splenic dysfunction, SCD, asplenia is at risk of: Sepsis and meningitis with capsular organism (pneumococcal, Hib, meningococci)

20. Non immune hydrops is seen in?
   a. Alpha thalassemia major
   b. Rh incompatibility
   c. Bilateral renal agenesis
   d. Maternal rubella

Ref: Nelson 17th pg 616

Explanation

Hydrops Fetalis

- Hydrops Fetalis is defined as the accumulation of extracellular fluid in fetal body cavities like pleural. pericardial, scalp and body wall edema and ascitis

Imp causes of Non-Immune Hydrops fetalis

Maternal	Placental	Fetal
Anemia	Chorio-angioma	Hematological-Twin to twin TF; Ch. fetomaternal TF, Homozygous alpha Thalassemia.
Pre-eclampsia	Compression torsion of Umbilical cord	Cardiovascular- CHD-TOF, ASD,VSD, Hypoplasia cordis, Dysrhythmias, AV mf,
Hypo-albuninemia Infections-		TORCH, Parvovirus B 19, CMV, Coxsackie, syphilis, HSV, Leptospirosis
Diabetes mellitus		Renal-cong Neph. syndr, Obstructive uropathy, PCKD, Hypoplastic kidney, Prune Belly syndr

Maternal	Placental	Fetal
		GI Dis-Diaphragmatic hernia,mid gut volvulous,GI obstr,Meconium peritonitis,Hepatic disorders-Cirrhosis, necrosis.
		Pulmonary-Cong. cystadenomatoid mf, pulm lymphangiectasia, Pulm Leiomyosarcoma, Diaphragmat-ic hernia, Alveolar cell adenoma
		Chromosomal dis-Trisomies 21,18,13; Mosaicism, Turner syndr, unbalanced Translocations and triploidy. Metabolic Dis-Gauchers,Gangliosi dosis,MPS,Mucolipidosis.

21. All of the following cause proximal muscle weakness EXCEPT:
   a. Polymyositis
   b. Duchene muscular dystrophy
   c. Myotonic dystrophy
   d. Becker's muscular dystrophy

[Ref: Nelson 19th]

Explanation

- Myopathies in general have proximal muscle weakness, whereas neuropathies have Distal Muscle weakness; but Myotoni Dystrophy is an exception to this rule as it involves distal muscles mainly.
- Myopathy Vs Muscular Dystrophy-
  o Myopathy is a disease pathology which causes structural changes/functional impairment of muscle; whereas muscular dystrophy means abnormal growth of muscle. In fact, muscular dystrophy is a type of Myopathy and is characterised by-a. It is a primary myopathy. b. Its course is progressive. c. It has got genetic basis. d. Degeneration and Death of muscle fibres is associated with it.

20. a,d
21. c

CHAPTER 22

Psychiatry

APPROACH TO PSYCHIATRIC DISORDERS

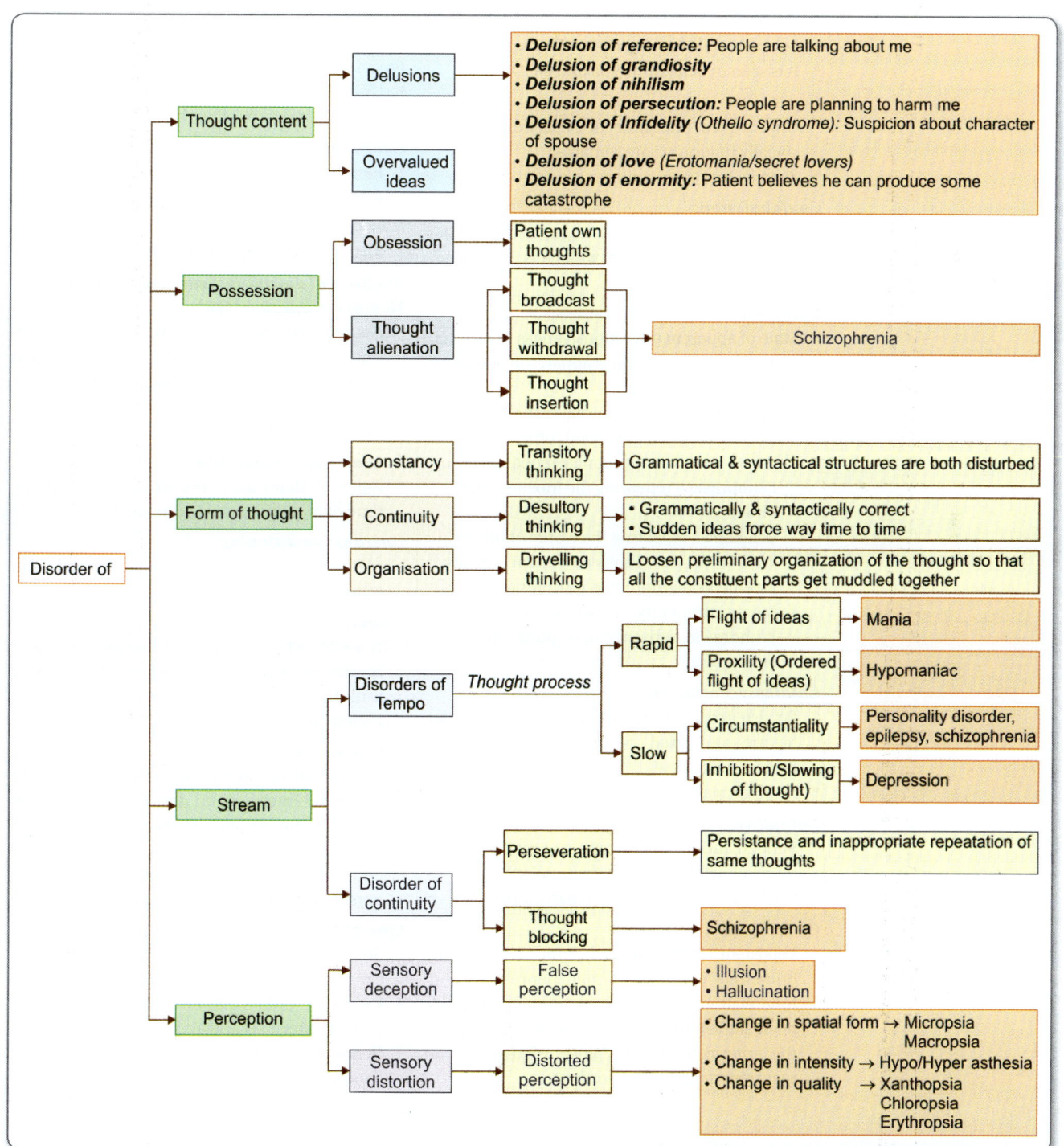

Abreaction:
- Expression and emotional discharge of unconscious material (such as a repressed idea or emotion) by verbalization.

Abulia:
- Inability to make decision.

Allodynia:
- Feeling pain to a normal non painful stimulus

Alexithymia:
- Inability to recognize and describe feelings.

Anhedonia:
- Loss of pleasure in previously pleasurable activities.

Ambivalence:
- Severe inability to decide for or against a point.
- It is seen in Schizophrenia and OCD.

Coprolalia:
- Unprovoked utterance of obscene words or socially inappropriate remarks.
- Seen in Tourette's syndrome

Confabulation:
- Defect in memory manifesting as unintentional filling of gaps of memory with facts that are not true.

Catatonia:
- State of apparent unresponsiveness to external stimuli in a person who is apparently awake.
- **Classical features:**
  - Mutism – absence of verbal response
  - Negativism such as Gegenhalten
  - Perseveration–inappropriate repetition of acts
  - Echopraxia – repeating the movement of others
  - Echolalia – repeating the words of others
  - Waxy flexibility – limbs are retained in any posture as manipulated by other person
  - Motor immobility – catalepsy, stupor
  - Withdrawal – absence of response to environment

Catalepsy/Posturing:
- Persistence maintenance of an uncomfortable, bizarre and fixed posture despite external resistance.
- Seen in catatonia.

Cataplexy:
- Sudden and transient loss of voluntary muscle tone following a strong emotional stimulus.
- Commonly associated with narcolepsy.

Cyclothymia:
- Persistent instability of mood, involving numerous episodes of mild depression and mild elation (hypomania), none of which has been sufficiently severe or prolonged to fulfill the criteria for bipolar affective disorder or recurrent depressive disorder.

Dysthymia:
- Mild depression with chronic course (≥2 years).

Delusion:
- False and firm belief based on misinterpretation of external reality that persists despite the evidence to the contrary.

Depersonalization:
- A change in the awareness of self in which the individual feels as if he is unreal.

Derealization:
- A change in the perception of the external world where the individual feels as if the surrounding is unreal.

Frigidity:
- Hypoactive sexual desire

Free Association:
- Uncensored expression of the ideas, impression, etc passing through the mind.

Hoarding:
- Persistent difficulty in discarding or parting with one's possession regardless of their worth.

Illusion:
- Misinterpretation of a sensory stimulus.

Intellectual disability/Learning disability/Mental retardation (MR):
- Neurodevelopmental disorder characterized by significantly impaired intellectual activity (such as learning, problem solving, judgment) and adaptive functioning (activities of daily life such as communication and independent living).

Involutional Melancholia:
- Agitated depression occurring at about the time of menopause or andropause

Operant Conditioning:
- Method of learning through reward and punishment

Stupor:
- Is a state where the patient though conscious, is unresponsive to his environment i.e. patient is mute and immobile (akinetic mutism).
- Patient appears awake.

Submissiveness:
- Adaptation of one's behavior to the actual or perceived interests and desires of others even when doing so anthithetical to one's own interests, needs, or desires.
- Submissiveness is a facet of the broad personality trait domain Negative Affectivity.

Synesthesia:
- Stimulus in one sensory modality produces sensation in other sensory modality.
- Example – Colors may be heard or sounds may be seen after LSD abuse.
- Reflex hallucination is a morbid form of Synesthesia.

Schizoaffective Disorders:
- Patient has features of both mood disorder (depression or mania) and schizophrenia (hallucination, delusion and distorted thinking).

Functional hallucination:
- Hallucinations are triggered by a stimulus in the same modality.
- E.g. auditory hallucination only on hearing sound of a rotating fan.

Hallucination:
- False perception without external stimulation.
- Arises from external objective space.
- Cannot be recognized as unreal by subject.

Pseudohallucination:
- Involuntary and false sensory perception.
- Arising from inner subjective space.
- It is recognized as unreal by subject.

Pseudocyesis:
- False belief of being pregnant

SCIENTISTS AND THEIR CONTRIBUTION

1 **Aaron Beck:** **C**ognitive theory/Cognitive model of depression
- Cognitive/negative triad:
  - Negative views about self
  - Negative views about world/experience
  - Negative views about future

2 **Abraham Maslow:** Theory of hierarchy of needs

3 **B.F. Skinner:** Theory of operant conditioning

4 **Emil Kraepelin:** Coined the term Dementia Praecox.

5 **Eugene Bleuler:**
- Coined the term Schizophrenia
- Proposed primary symptoms of schizophrenia known as 4 'A' of Schizophrenia
  - **A**utism → Withdrawal into self
  - **A**mbivalence → inability to decide
  - Loosening of **A**ssociation
  - **A**ffect disturbance

6 **Erik Erikson:** Theory of psychosocial personality development

7 **Hecker:** Coined the term Hebephrenia

8 **Ivan Pavlov:** Theory of classical conditioning (learning by association)

9 **Jean Piaget:** Theory of cognitive development

10 **Kahlbaum:** Catatonia

11 **Kubler Ross:** Described the 5 stages of death
- **D**enial, **A**nger, **B**argaining, **D**epression, **A**cceptance

12 **Kurt Schneider:** First rank symptoms of Schizophrenia
- Auditory hallucination
- Thought alienation phenomenon (insertion, withdrawal, broadcasting)
- Delusional perception
- Passivity phenomenon
  - Made act
  - Made impulse
  - Made affect
  - Somatic passivity

13 **Morel:** Coined the term 'Demence Precoce'

14 **Nancy Anderson:** **N**egative Schizophrenia

15 **Sigmund Freud:**
- Father of psychoanalysis
- Theory of Psychodynamics
- Theory of psychosexual development
- Structural theory of mind
- Free association
- Interpretation of dreams

16 **T.J. Crow:** **T**ype I and II of Schizophrenia

FACTS

- National Mental Health Program was launched in 1982
- World mental health day: 10th oct.
- Adding emotional weight to memories and sensory experience is a function of → Limbic system especially Amygdala
- PTSD is associated with overactivity of Amygdala
- Regulation of emotional drives → Frontal Lobe
- Formed visual Hallucination is seen in lesion of → Temporal lobe
- Pseudo community formation is seen in → Delusional disorders
- ↑ in suicidal behavior is due to → ↓ in serotonin.

- Psychodynamic theory of mental illness is based on → Unconscious internal conflict.
- Beck's cognitive triad of depression:
  - Helplessness
  - Worthlessness
  - Hopelessness
- Pseudo dementia and Nihilistic delusions seen in: depression
- Anniversary reaction is a type of: Grief reaction
- **Labella indifference** is seen in: Conversion disorder.
- Astasia – abasia pattern of gait is seen in: Conversion disorder.
- Type **D** personality has recently found to be a risk factor for → CA**D**

- Narcolepsy → Excessive daytime sleepiness
- Premature ejaculation is a sexual disorder of orgasm phase
- Hypersexuality in females → Nymphomania
- Hypersexuality in males → Satyriasis / Don Juanism
- IPC 377 is in reference of → Homosexuality
- Bruxism (tooth grinding) is commonly seen in Stage-II of NREM sleep.
- Maximum duration of time spent is in → NREM stage II
- *Physical dependence:*
  - ○ Least – Cannabis
  - ○ Max – Opioid
  - ○ None – LSD
- Acute Paranoid schizophrenia like symptoms are seen in intoxication of → Amphetamine > LSD.
- **Mc Evan's sign** (Pinching skin of face or neck would cause transient dilatation of pupil).
- Jellineck classification → for Alcohol use disorder
- Alcoholic seizures are usually **GTCS type** seen within 12-24 hrs of stopping alcohol.

- Confabulation is typically seen in → alcoholism
- Disulfiram inhibits enzyme → Aldehyde dehydrogenase
- **Ecstasy**: MDMA (3, 4 methylene dioxy-amphetamine)
- Acute intoxication with which drug can cause acute paranoid schizophrenia like syndrome → Amphetamine
- Typical anti-psychotics acts by → D_2 receptor antagonism
- Atypical antipsychotics act on 5 HT_2 and D_2 receptor blockade.
- Maximum risk of Metabolic syndrome → Olanzapine > Clozapine
- Minimal risk of Tardive dyskinesia (among Antipsychotics) → Clozapine
- Normal therapeutic level of lithium is → 0.7 - 1.1 mEq/L
- Best therapy suited to teach daily life skills to a mentally challenged child → Contingency
- Phototherapy is mode of treatment in seasonal affective disorder

Disorder of Sexual Development

Phases of Sexual Development		Disorders Resulting from Fixation
Oral phase	Birth – 1.5 years	▪ Alcohol and drug dependence ▪ Schizophrenia
Anal phase	1.5–3 years	▪ OCD
Phallic phase	3–5 years	▪ Oedipus/Electra complex ▪ Hysteria ▪ Castration anxiety in boys ▪ Penis envy in girls

Timeline

	Duration	Diagnosis
Psychotic symptoms	<1 month	Brief psychosis
	1-6 months	Schizophreniform disorder
	≥6 months	Schizophrenia
Depressive symptoms	>2 weeks	Depression
	>2 years	Dysthymia
Hyperarousal/ Flashback	<1 month	Acute stress disorder
	>1 month	Post Traumatic Stress Disorder

Withdrawal Features

Substance	Withdrawal Features
Alcohol	Hangover > Tremulousness > Insomnia, seizure
Cocaine	Hypersomnia, Vivid unpleasant dreams
Opioid	Insomnia with Yawning, ↑bodily secretion, body ache, pupillary dilatation

REMEMBER

Obsessive Compulsive and related disorders:
- OCD
- Body dysmorphic disorder
- Hoarding disorder
- Trichotillomania → repeated pulling of one's own hair
- Excoriation disorder

Body Dysmorphic Disorder:
- Preoccupation with an imagined defect in the physical appearance of oneself which causes marked anxiety and distress.

Impulse control disorders
- Pyromania
- Kleptomania → irresistible impulse to steal without regard of need or monetary profit.
- Intermittent explosive disorder
- **Oniomania**: Compulsive buying

Autism spectrum disorders:
- Autism
- Asperger syndrome
- Rett syndrome
- Childhood disintegration disorder

IQ Range and Degree of Intellectual Disability:
- 90-109 → Normal IQ
- 80-89 → Low normal IQ
- 70-79 → Borderline IQ
- 50-69 → Mild Intellectual disability (moron)
- 35-49 → Moderate Intellectual disability
- 20-34 → Severe Intellectual disability

Disability certificate are issued for:
- Schizophrenia
- Bipolar affective disorder
- OCD
- Dementia

Indications of ECT:
- Resistant depression
- Severe depression with suicidal risk
- Depression with psychotic features

MOST COMMON

- MC psychiatric disorder in the world → Depression.
- MC mental disorder leading to suicide → Depression.
- MC cause of premature death in schizophrenia → Suicide
- MC comorbidity associated with OCD → Anxiety disorder
- MC obsession in adults → Contamination.
- MC compulsions → Checking > Washing.
- MC type of schizophrenia → Paranoid
- MC hallucination in non-organic psychiatric disorder → Auditory Hallucination.

- MC perceptual disorder in schizophrenia → Auditory Hallucination.
- MC delusion in schizophrenia → Delusion of persecution
- MC dissociative disorder → Dissociative Amnesia
- MC eating disorder → Binge eating disorder
- MC cause of erectile dysfunction in middle aged men → Psychogenic
- MC drug of abuse in India → Tobacco.
- MC employed screening test for alcohol misuse → CAGE Questionnaire.

SYNDROMES

❶ Othello's syndrome:
- Aka Delusion of infidelity/Morbid jealousy
- Suspicion about the character of spouse

❷ Ganser syndrome
- Approximate answers or vorbeireden
- Clouding of Consciousness and disorientation
- Hallucination
- Episodic amnesia
- Seen in:
  - Prisoners (awaiting trial)
  - Army personnel going to war
  - Recent Head injury

❸ De Clérambault syndrome
- Aka Erotomanic delusion/Delusion of love
- Patient believes that a person of higher status or fame has fallen in love with him.

❹ Van Gogh syndrome
- Schizophrenia with self-mutilating behavior

❺ Pfropf schizophrenia
- Schizophrenia with mental retardation

❻ Ekbom's syndrome
- Delusion of parasite infestation

❼ Magnus syndrome
- Aka Cocaine bugs
- Tactile hallucination similar to worm crawling sensation in cocaine abusers

❽ Cotard syndrome
- Aka Delusion of Nihilism
- Patient holds a belief that he is already dead, has lost internal organs or they are putrefying.

Delusional Misidentification Syndromes

❶ Capgras syndrome (Delusion of double)
- Patient believes that a close relative or spouse has been replaced by an identical looking impostor i.e. a person has been replaced by an exact double

❷ Fregoli's syndrome
- Patient beliefs that various people he meets are actually the same person in disguise. i.e. single person has come disguised as different person.

❸ Intermetamorphosis
- A belief that people in the surrounding swap identities with each other while maintaining the same appearance.

❹ Syndrome of subjective doubles
- A belief that there is a double of him or herself carrying out independent actions.

❺ Mirrored self-misidentification
- A delusional belief that self-reflection in the mirror is that of another person.

PSYCHOSIS VS NEUROSIS

	Psychosis	Neurosis
Definition	▪ Major personality disorder which disturbs the emotional and mental aspect of life	▪ Mild mental disorder due to excessive anxiety or irrational behavior without underlying organic disease
Features	▪ Loss of insight ▪ Lack of subjective distress due to illness ▪ Complete alteration of personality ▪ Loss of contact with external reality ▪ Impaired judgement ▪ Hallucination and Delusion ++	▪ Insight present ▪ Subjective distress present due to symptoms ▪ Partial change in personality ▪ Contact with reality is preserved ▪ Normal judgement ▪ Hallucination and Delusion –
Treatment	▪ Antipsychotics, ECT	▪ Counselling, Behavior therapy, etc
Prognosis	▪ Bad	▪ Good

Examples	▪ Acute Psychotic disorders
	▪ Schizophrenia
	▪ Delusional disorder
	▪ Mood disorders:
	  ○ Mania
	  ○ Depression
	  ○ Bipolar disorders
		▪ Phobia
		▪ Conversion/Somatoform disorder
		▪ Dissociative disorders
		▪ Obsessive Compulsive Disorder
		▪ Anxiety
		  ○ Generalized Anxiety Disorder
		  ○ Panic disorders

SCHIZOPHRENIA

- Is a psychiatric illness that affects how people think, feel, and perceive
- Estimated lifetime prevalence is 1% worldwide.
- Psychiatric condition with maximum heritability
- Concordance rate for Monozygotic twins in schizophrenia → 47%
- If both parents have schizophrenia, chances in their child → 40%
- Schizophrenia is associated with chromosomal deletion → 22q11
- Peak age of onset – 2nd decade
- 1st symptom relieved with drugs → Auditory hallucinations.
- 1st symptom to reappear in treatment resistant schizophrenia: Auditory hallucinations.
- Defect of **C**onation is typically seen in → **C**atatonic schizophrenia.
- Maximum psychomotor features – Catatonic Schizophrenia

- *Risk factors:*
  - Genetics and family history
  - Low socioeconomic status
  - Industrialization
  - Drugs – amphetamine, cocaine, cannabis
- *Positive symptoms:*
  - Hallucinations – usually auditory
  - Delusions
  - Formal thought disorder
  - Disorganized speech and behavior
- *Negative symptoms:*
  - Affective flattening – decrease in emotional range
  - Alogia – poverty of speech
  - Anhedonia – loss of interests and drive
  - Avolition – inertia
- *Cognitive symptoms:*
  - Deficits in working memory and attention
- *Mood symptoms*:
  - Inappropriately cheerful or depressed

- *Diagnostic criteria* – at least 2 of the following symptoms must be present for ≥ 6 months:
  - Delusions
  - Hallucinations
  - Disorganized speech
  - Disorganized or catatonic behavior
  - Negative symptoms
- *MRI* – Enlarged ventricles, decrease volume in medial temporal lobe and hippocampus
- *Management*:
  - Antipsychotics for positive symptoms and to prevent relapses.
  - Most effective antipsychotics – Clozapine (but not first line)

- DOC for refractory schizophrenia – Clozapine
- *Poor Prognostic factors:*
  - Early onset of illness
  - Insidious onset
  - Family history
  - Male sex
  - Negative symptoms
  - Prominent cognitive symptoms
  - Absence of depression
  - Absence of stressor event
  - Structural brain disease
  - Hebephrenic type

Types

	Type 1	Type 2
Symptoms	▪ Positive symptoms	▪ Negative symptoms
Personality disorder	▪ Egosyntonic	▪ Egodystonic
CT scan	▪ Normal	▪ Structural brain abnormalities
Response to Rx and Prognosis	▪ Good	▪ Poor

Paranoid	Hebephrenic	Catatonic	Simple
▪ MC form ▪ Develops later in life ▪ Hallucination + ▪ Delusion +	▪ Early onset ▪ Disorganized behavior ▪ Disorganized speech ▪ Poor prognosis	▪ Rarest type ▪ Unusual motor movements ▪ Best prognosis	▪ Negative symptoms are most prominent ▪ Hallucination and delusion rare

DEPRESSION

- *Clinical signs:*
  - Veraguth sign – triangular folds of eyelids
  - Omega sign
  - Pseudo dementia
  - Paradox Suicide
- *Diagnostic criteria:* ≥5 of the following symptoms have been present during the same 2 week period
  - **S**leep disturbance – insomnia or hypersomnia
  - **W**eight change or appetite disturbance
  - **A**nhedonia

- Depressed or irritable **M**ood
- **I**ndecisiveness
- Feelings of worthlessness
- Lack of energy
- Recurrent suicidal ideation or **suicide** attempt

Mn: Depressed - SWAMI - feels worthless - but no energy - to commit suicide
- Best therapy – combination of medication and psychotherapy
- Transcranial magnetic stimulation and Vagus nerve stimulation - for treatment resistant major depression.

Depression with Melancholic Features

- Loss of pleasure in almost all activities
- Depression that is worse in the morning
- Waking up 2 hours earlier than usual

- Psychomotor retardation or agitation
- Significant weight loss or anorexia
- Excessive or inappropriate guilt

Atypical Depression

- Increased appetite or significant weight gain
- Mood reactivity
- Increased sleep

- Leaden paralysis – Feelings of heaviness in limbs
- Interpersonal rejection sensitivity

BIPOLAR DISORDER

- Bipolar disorder, or manic-depressive illness (MDI), is characterized by periods of prolonged depression that alternate with periods of mania (excessively elevated or irritable mood).
- Chromosome associated with bipolar disorders: 18, 22
- Manic episodes are characterized by mood disturbances (elation, irritability, or expansiveness) that last for at least 1 week.
- It must be associated with ≥3 of the following symptoms:
  - Grandiosity
  - Diminished need for sleep
  - Excessive talkativeness
  - Flight of ideas or racing thoughts
  - Easy distractibility
  - Increased level of goal focused activity
  - Excessive pleasurable activities
- Hypomanic episodes are characterized by an elevated, expansive, or irritable mood that last for ≥ 4 consecutive days
- Lithium is considered a first-line agent for long-term prophylaxis and maintenance in bipolar illness

Types

- Type I Bipolar disorders: Manic episodes alternating with depression.
- Type II Bipolar disorders: Hypomanic episode alternating with depression.

OBSESSIVE COMPULSIVE DISORDER

- An Obsession is defined as persistent and inappropriate thoughts, urges, or images which cause marked anxiety or distress. These thoughts are intrusive and subject attempts to suppress or ignore them.
- Compulsions are defined as repetitive behavior or mental acts performed in response to an obsession (e.g. hand washing, ordering, checking, counting, repeating words etc.)
- *Defense mechanism in OCD:*
  - Primary → Undoing, Reaction formation, Isolation
  - Secondary → Repression, Displacement
- OCD is associated with → Secondary Depression
- DOC for OCD – SSRI
- Refractory cases – Neurosurgery (anterior capsulotomy or deep brain stimulation)

NEUROTRANS MITTERS

Hormone	Schizophrenia	Depression	OCD	Mania	Delirium	Parkinsonism	Alzheimer
Dopamine	↑	↓	↑	↑	↑	↓	
Serotonin	↑	↓	↓				
Norepineph-rine	↓	↓		↑			↓
GABA	↓				↑		
Glutamate	↓				↑		
Acetylcholine	↓			↓	↓	↑	↓
Cortisol		↑					
Thyroid		↓					

ADJUSTMENT REACTION, GRIEF AND PTSD

	Adjustment Disorder	Grief/Bereavement	PTSD
Stressor	▪ Failure, losses ▪ Relationship issues	▪ Death	▪ Severe traumatic events ▪ Sexual assault like rape
Onset after the incident	▪ Within 3 months	▪ Usually immediately	▪ Within 6 months but may be delayed
Symptoms	▪ Symptoms of Depression like low mood, sadness, anxiety, anger, sleep disturbances	▪ Depressive – sadness, tearfulness, lack of sleep	▪ Emotional numbness ▪ Hyperarousal – impaired sleep ▪ Re-experience of trauma – Flashbacks and nightmares ▪ Avoidance
Duration	▪ ≤ 6 months after termination of stressor	▪ Usually resolve within 2 months	▪ Persist for ≥1 month ▪ If ≤1 month → Acute stress reaction

PERSONALITY DISORDERS

- PD is an permanent pattern of inner experience and behavior
- It is pervasive and inflexible
- It is Egosyntonic – acceptable and compatible with one's value/self-image

- Onset – adolescent or early adulthood
- Remains stable over time
- Borderline PD is aka Ambulatory Schizophrenia

Cluster	PD	Major Traits
A (Odd, Eccentric)	Paranoid PD	▪ Pervasive distrust and suspiciousness ▪ Preoccupied with unjustified doubts
	Schizoid PD	▪ Detachment from social relationship (E.g. *Sanyasi*) ▪ Restricted range of expression of emotions ▪ **Emotional coldness,** ▪ Preoccupation with fantasy and introspection ▪ Prefer solitary activities
	Schizotypal PD	▪ Odd thinking and perception, Vague stereotyped speech ▪ Odd belief and magical thinking, Superstitious ▪ May progress to schizophrenia, delusional disorder etc.
B (Dramatic, Emotional)	Antisocial PD *Diagnosed in individual ≥18 years	▪ Disregard and violation of the law ▪ Involvement in illegal activities ▪ Repeated lying and deception ▪ Lack of remorse
	Borderline PD (Emotionally unstable PD)	▪ Instability of interpersonal relationship ▪ Marked impulsivity ▪ Suicidal/Self-mutilating behavior ▪ Labile mood ▪ Unstable self-image ▪ Feeling of emptiness ▪ Micropsychotic episodes
	Narcissistic PD	▪ Grandiose, Exaggeration of self-achievements ▪ Lack of empathy, Envy of others
	Histrionic PD	▪ Needs to be center of attraction ▪ Inappropriate sexual behavior
C (Anxious, Fearful)	Avoidant PD	▪ Hypersensitive to criticism and rejection ▪ Anxiety, Avoidance of social activities
	Dependent PD	▪ Submissive and clinging behavior ▪ Difficulty in making independent decisions
	Obsessive Compulsive PD	▪ Perfectionism, Orderliness and controlling others ▪ Excessive devotion to work ▪ Inflexible, Stubbornness

SOMATIC SYMPTOMS

Diagnosis		Description
Somatic symptom disorder		▪ Significant anxiety, thoughts or feelings about ≥1 somatic symptoms which interrupt day to day activity
Illness anxiety disorder/ Hypochondriasis		▪ Preoccupation with fear of having a serious illness despite none or mild symptoms and consistently negative evaluations
Conversion disorders/ Functional neurological symptom disorder		▪ Alteration in ≥1 motor or sensory symptoms incompatible with recognized neurological conditions ▪ Acute in onset and often associated with stressor or precipitating conflict ▪ Patient derive both primary and secondary gain
Factitious disorder	Imposed on self (Munchausen's syndrome)	▪ Intentional falsification or deliberate induction of signs or symptoms on **self** with a primary goal of assuming a sick role
	Imposed on another (Munchausen by proxy)	▪ Intentional falsification or deliberate induction of signs or symptoms in **another** individual, usually a child
Malingering		▪ Intentional Falsification or gross exaggeration of symptoms done deliberately for a known external purpose ▪ Motive is to obtain secondary gain like leave, financial benefit etc.

DISSOCIATIVE DISORDERS

Disorders	Description
Dissociative amnesia	▪ Inability to recall important personal information
Dissociative fugue	▪ Unexpected travel + inability to recall past ± new identity
Dissociative identity disorder	▪ Existence of ≥2 personality traits or identities within a single individual
Depersonalization/Derealization disorder	▪ Depersonalization – feeling of detachment from one's self ▪ Derealization – feeling of detachment from the external world

EATING DISORDERS

	Anorexia Nervosa	Bulimia Nervosa
Prevalence in women	▪ 0.5-1%	▪ 1-3%
Onset	▪ Mid adolescence (13-18 years)	▪ Late adolescence
Body image	▪ May be distorted	▪ May be distorted
Weight	▪ Severe weight loss	▪ Usually normal
BMI	▪ Low	▪ Normal
Clinical features	▪ Dry skin, Lanugo body hair ▪ Hypothermia, Hypotension	▪ Dry skin, dehydration ▪ Bilateral parotid enlargement
Association	▪ Depression, phobia	▪ Depression
Appetite	▪ Normal	▪ Increased
Diet	▪ Very less / avoiding food	▪ Recurrent episode of binge eating
Compensation act	▪ In binge eating / purging type	▪ Self induced vomiting ▪ Use of purgatives or appetite suppressants
Blood glucose	▪ Low	▪ Normal
Lab	▪ Hypokalemia and alkalosis in purging type	▪ Electrolyte imbalance – hypokalemia
T3 and T4 levels	▪ Low normal	▪ Normal
LH and FSH levels	▪ Low	▪ Normal
Sex hormones level	▪ Low	▪ Normal
Cortisol	▪ Increased	▪ Normal
Menstruation	▪ Amenorrhoea	▪ Normal or oligomenorrhea
Screening tool	▪ SCOFF questionnaire	▪ SCOFF questionnaire
Treatment	▪ Behavior therapy	▪ SSRI

ANXIETY DISORDERS

	Panic Disorders	Social Anxiety Disorder	Generalized Anxiety Disorder

Features	▪ Recurrent Panic attack (abrupt onset of intense fear) associated with:
	  ○ Chest pain, Dyspnea, Palpitation
	  ○ Sweating, Trembling, fainting
	  ○ Fear of dying,
		▪ Fear of social situations or performances where an individual is likely to be judged by others
		▪ Avoidance of social or performance activities like speaking in public
			▪ Excessive anxiety and difficult to control worry about a number of events
			▪ Present for at least 6 months and are associated with restlessness, easy fatigability, irritability, sleep disturbances etc.

Treatment	▪ Panic attack – Benzodiazepines (DOC) ▪ Panic disorder – SSRI (DOC)	▪ DOC – SSRI ▪ Cognitive behavior therapy	▪ DOC – SSRI ▪ Cognitive behavior therapy

Specific Phobias

- Agoraphobia – fear of places from where escape is difficult
- Aerophobia – fear of flying
- Claustrophobia – fear of closed spaces
- Sitophobia – fear of eating

POSTPARTUM MOOD DISORDERS

	Postpartum Blues	Postpartum Depression	Postpartum Psychosis
Onset	▪ 2-3 days after delivery	▪ Within 12 weeks after delivery	▪ Within 2 weeks of delivery
Resolve	▪ Within 10 days	▪ Persist for >2 weeks	▪ After inpatient treatment
Symptoms	▪ Tearfulness, irritability, anxiety ▪ No thoughts of harming the baby	▪ Anhedonia, insomnia, decreased appetite ▪ Thoughts of harming the baby present	▪ Mania, delusion, hallucination ▪ Thoughts of harming the baby or self
Treatment	▪ Supportive care	▪ Non pharmacological and pharmacological	▪ Mood stabilizer and Antipsychotics

AUTISM SPECTRUM DISORDER

	Autism	Asperger Syndrome	Rett Syndrome
Age of diagnosis	▪ <3 years	▪ 7-8 years	▪ 2-4 years
Gender	▪ Boys > Girls	▪ Boys > Girls	▪ Girls > Boys
IQ	▪ Can have intellectual impairment	▪ Normal or high	▪ Can have intellectual impairment
Language	▪ Delay	▪ Normal	▪ Delay
Communication skill	▪ Impaired	▪ Normal	▪ Impaired
Social interaction	▪ Impaired	▪ Impaired	▪ Impaired
Stereotyped behavior	▪ +	▪ +	▪ +
Extra edge			▪ Associated with mutation in **MECP2** gene on X chromosome ▪ Deceleration in head growth ▪ Motor development delay

DELIRIUM VS DEMENTIA

	Delirium	Dementia
Hallmark	▪ Impaired consciousness	▪ Loss of memory
Onset	▪ Acute	▪ Insidious
Duration	▪ Days – weeks	▪ Months – years
Course	▪ Transient and fluctuating with lucid interval (Waxing and waning) ▪ Reversible	▪ Stable and progress gradually (downhill) ▪ Irreversible
Consciousness	▪ Altered	▪ Alert
Orientation	▪ Impaired	▪ Intact
Attention	▪ Impaired	▪ Normal; impaired in advanced stage
Perception	▪ Illusion +, Hallucination +	▪ Normal initially
Screening	▪ Confusion assessment method	
EEG	▪ Diffuse slow wave or low voltage activity	▪ Normal
Treatment	▪ Haloperidol – MC used drug	▪ Anticholinergics

TREATMENT MODALITIES

Disease	Non Pharmacological Therapy	Pharmacotherapy
Premature ejaculation	▪ Master's and Johnson's Squeeze technique	▪ SSRI (Dapoxetine)
Erectile dysfunction		▪ Sildenafil/Tadalafil ▪ Alprostadil (PGE$_1$ analogue) ▪ Phentolamine
Anorexia Nervosa	▪ Cognitive Behavior Therapy – **TOC** ▪ Dynamic psychotherapy	▪ Cyproheptadine (H$_1$ and 5HT$_2$ antagonist) ▪ Antidepressants
Bulimia Nervosa	▪ Cognitive Behavior Therapy ▪ Dynamic psychotherapy	▪ SSRI ▪ Imipramine
Generalised Anxiety Disorders (GAD)	▪ Cognitive Behavior Therapy ▪ Relaxation technique	▪ SSRI → **DOC** ▪ β-blockers ▪ Benzodiazepine ▪ Buspirone - 5HT$_{1A}$ partial agonist
Panic attack		▪ Low dose Benzodiazepine
Panic disorder	▪ Cognitive Behavior Therapy	▪ SSRI (**P**aroxetine → **DOC**)
Phobia	▪ Behavior Therapy – **TOC** ▪ Systemic desensitization ▪ Exposure and response prevention ▪ Relaxation technique	▪ SSRI: **DOC** ▪ BZD
OCD	▪ Cognitive Behavior therapy – **TOC** ▪ Exposure and response prevention ▪ Systemic desensitization ▪ Flooding	▪ SSRI: **DOC** ▪ ECT in resistant cases ▪ Deep brain stimulation ▪ Neurosurgery – Angulotomy, Capsulotomy
Post-traumatic stress disorder (PTSD)	▪ Cognitive Behavior therapy – **TOC** ▪ Eye movement desensitization and reprocessing (EMDR)	▪ SSRI
Narcolepsy		▪ Armodafinil, Modafinil
Nocturnal enuresis	▪ Behavior therapy: **TOC**	▪ Imipramine: **DOC** ▪ Desmopressin (Intranasal)
Nightmares	▪ Sleep hygiene ▪ Stimulus control therapy	▪ TCA, BZD, Sleep hygiene
Night terror		▪ Low dose BZD
Alcohol withdrawal seizures		▪ BZD (Long term anti-epileptic drugs are not indicated)
Delirium tremens		▪ BZD (Chlordiazepoxide is **DOC**, Lorazepam and Oxazepam in case of liver function derangement)
Alcohol Detoxification		▪ BZD (Chlordiazepoxide is **DOC**)
Acute opioid intoxication		▪ Naloxone
Prevention of opioid dependence		▪ Anticraving drug : Naltrexone
Prevention of alcohol dependence		▪ Naltrexone ▪ Baclofen ▪ Acamprosate
Borderline personality disorder	▪ Dialectical behavior therapy	
Schizophrenia		▪ Atypical antipsychotics (**DOC**)
Treatment resistant schizophrenia	▪ Family therapy to ↓ negative expressed emotions	▪ Clozapine: **DOC**

Contd...

Disease	Non Pharmacological Therapy	Pharmacotherapy

Depression	▪ **Physical therapy:**
	  ○ 10th and 5th CN stimulation
	  ○ Phototherapy
	  ○ ECT
	  ○ rTMS
		▪ **SSRI - DOC**
		▪ SNRI
		▪ TCA
		▪ Psychosurgery

Atypical depression		▪ MAOI (Moclobemide)

Hypomania/Mania		▪ Mood stabilizer
		  ○ Sodium valproate: **DOC**
		  ○ Lithium carbonate
		  ○ Carbamazepine

Bipolar affective disorder		▪ Prophylaxis with Li
Rapid Cyclers		▪ Na-Valproate: **DOC**
Neuroleptic induced acute akathisia		▪ β-blocker, BZD ▪ Lowering dose of anti-psychotic drugs
Opioid withdrawal symptoms		▪ Methadone: **DOC** ▪ Substitution therapy—buprenorphine + naloxone
Suicidal thoughts		▪ ECT
ADHD		▪ Dextroamphetamine ▪ Methylphenidate (**DOC**: age >6 years) ▪ Atomoxetine HCl, clonidine
Tic Disorder	▪ Habit reversal therapy	▪ Antipsychotics

MULTIPLE CHOICE QUESTIONS

CHAPTER 1: BASICS IN PSYCHIATRY

DISORDERS OF PERCEPTION

1. Hallucination is disorder of: (PGMEE 2012)
- a. Memory
- b. Perception
- c. Intelligence
- d. Thought

[Ref: Niraj Ahuja 7th/e/p 13]

Explanation
- ■ Hallucination: perception without an existing external stimulus.

2. All of the following are disorders of Perception, except: (PGMEE 2015-16)
- a. Delusion
- b. Hallucination
- c. Depersonalisation
- d. Illusion

[Ref: Psychiatry By Neel Burton (John Wiley and Sons) 2nd/e pg. 24, 25]

3. All are perceptional disorder EXCEPT? (PGMEE 2014)
- a. Illusion
- b. Hallucinations
- c. Delusion
- d. None

[Ref: Niraj Ahuja 7th/e/p 13]

4. Hallucinations are describes as: (PGMEE 2014)
- a. Alteration of perception of one's reality
- b. Misinterpretation of stimuli
- c. Feeling of familiarity with unfamiliar thing
- d. Perception without an existing external stimulus

[Ref: Niraj Ahuja 7th/e/p 13]

5. Visual hallucinations are seen in all except: (PGMEE 2013)
- a. Delirium
- b. Alcohol withdrawal
- c. Schizophrenia
- d. Depression

[Ref: Niraj Ahuja 7th/e/ch 6]

6. Hallucinations are not seen in: (PGMEE 2014)
- a. LSD
- b. Schizophrenia
- c. Seizure due to intracerebral space occupying lesions
- d. Anxiety

[Ref: Niraj Ahuja 7th/e/p 28 & 56]

7. Phantom limb is an example of disorder of: (PGMEE 2015)
- a. Cognition
- b. Perception
- c. Thought
- d. None of the above

[Ref: Niraj Ahuja 7th/e/p 13]

COGNITION & THOUGHT

8. Loosening of association is an example of: (PGMEE 2013)
- a. Concrete thinking
- b. Schneider's first symptoms
- c. Formal thought disorder
- d. Perseveration

[Ref: Niraj Ahuja 7th/e/p 12]

9. Expression of affect in a suppressed is called:- (PGMEE 2018)
- a. Free association
- b. Abreaction
- c. Hypnosis
- d. Avolition

Ref: (CTP, 10th ed)

Explanation
- ■ *Abreaction* (German: Abreagieren) is a psychoanalytical term for reliving an experience to purge it of its emotional excesses—a type of catharsis.
- ■ *Free association* is a practice in psychoanalytic therapy in which a client is asked to freely share thoughts, random words, and anything else that comes to mind, regardless of how coherent or appropriate the thoughts are i.
- ■ *Avolition* is the decrease in the motivation to initiate and perform self-directed purposeful activities. It is a symptom of various forms of psychopathology.
- ■ *Hypnosis* is the state of human consciousness involving focused attention and decreased peripheral awareness and an enhanced capacity to respond to suggestion.

10. Persistent belief in something which is not a fact is: (PGMEE 2014)
- a. Delirium
- b. Illusion
- c. Delusion
- d. Hallucination

[Ref: Niraj Ahuja 7th/e p. 83]

11. Cotard's syndrome has: (PGMEE 2013)
- a. Nihilistic delusions
- b. Religious delusions
- c. Persecutory delusions
- d. Hypochondrical delusion

[Ref: Niraj Ahuja 7th/e/ch 7]

12. Delusion is not seen in: (PGMEE 2014)
- a. Depression
- b. Mania
- c. Schizophrenia
- d. Anxiety

[Ref: Niraj Ahuja 7th/e/ch 8]

13. Which of the following is a Delusional misidentification syndrome: (PGMEE 2015-16)
- a. Othello Syndrome
- b. Ekbom's Syndrome
- c. Cotard's Syndrome
- d. Capgras Syndrome

[Ref: Kaplan's 11th/e pg. 336]

1.	b
2.	a
3.	c
4.	d
5.	d
6.	d
7.	b
8.	c
9.	b
10.	c
11.	a
12.	d
13.	d

14. **Patient with schizophrenia is admitted in psychiatry ward. On the appearance of nurse, the patient starts beating his wife on seeing the nurse and says that the wife is not his real wife but actually the nurse is, and accuses her of giving him wrong medication. What is the diagnosis?** *(NEET Pattern 2017)*
    a. Syndrome of subjection double
    b. Othello syndrome
    c. Capgras syndrome
    d. Fregoli syndrome

Explanation

- The delusional misidentification syndromes (DMS) are characterized by paranoia and hostility towards misidentified objects .
- Important DMS include:-
  - The Capgras delusion,
  - Fregoli syndrome,
  - The syndrome of Intermetamorphosis, and
  - The syndrome of Subjective Doubles.
- *Capgras syndrome or Imposter syndrome* → Irrational belief that a familial person /someone they know or recognize has been replaced by an imposter (exact double). Seen in **paranoid schizophrenia (m/c)**, delusional disorders, Lewy body dementia.

About Other Options

- *Othello syndrome* → Infidelity involving spouse.
- *Fregoli syndrome* → Person holds a delusional belief that different people are in fact a single person who changes his or her appearance or is in disguise.

15. **A man came to psychiatry OPD. He believed that he was the richest person in the world and that his family member and neighbor were plotting against his and planning to harm him but family members disagree with him. Which problem of content of thought is the patient is suffering from.** *(NEET Pattern 2017)*
    a. Delusion of grandeur
    b. Delusion of grandeur and persecution
    c. Delusion of grandeur, persecution and reference
    d. Delusion of persecution

Explanation

- Delusion of grandeur and persecution) **no clearcut description of delusion of reference (like; people talking about him, patient feel that they talk about him or make fun of him)**

16. **Erotomania is seen in:** *(PGMEE 2012)*
    a. Neurosis
    b. Unipolar mania
    c. Recurrent mania
    d. Bipolar depression

[Ref: Niraj Ahuja 7th/e/ch 6]

17. **A 80 year male gives same answers to all questions. Most likely diagnosis is:** *(PGMEE 2014)*
    a. Mania
    b. Organic Brain Disease
    c. Depression
    d. Convulsions

[Ref: Niraj Ahuja 7th/e/ch 3]

DELUSIONAL DISODERS

18. **Time interval between acute and persistent psychotic disease is:** *(PGMEE 2013)*
    a. 1 week
    b. 2 week
    c. 3 week
    d. 1 months

[Ref: Niraj Ahuja 7th/e/ch 7]

19. **Which is the most common type of persistent delusional disorder?** *(PGMEE 2015)*
    a. Delusion of jealousy
    b. Somatic delusion
    c. Delusion of persecution
    d. Delusion of grandeur

[Ref: Niraj Ahuja7th/e/ch 7]

20. **Which of the following is not true regarding delusional disorder?** *(PGMEE Jan 2019)*
    a. Early immigration
    b. Social isolation
    c. Sensory impairment
    d. Occurs at early age

21. **One female thinks that her boyfriend/lover do not love her:** *(PGMEE 2016-17)*
    a. Delusion of jealousy
    b. Delusion of love
    c. Delusion of persecution
    d. Delusion of reference

[Ref: Niraj Ahuja 7th/e/p 83]

Explanation

- Delusion of jealousy or Delusion of infidelity is a false belief that one's romantic partner, no more loves him/her, and is in romantic relationship with other/s.
- Delusion of love is a false belief that a specific person (classically a person higher in status) is in love with him/her.
- Delusion of persecution is a false belief that a person or a set of people are conspiring against him/her.
- Delusion of reference is a false belief that others are referring to him/her in their conversations or actions.

22. **Infidelity & jealousy involving spouse is called–**
    a. Declerambault's syndrome *(PGMEE 2014)*
    b. Capgras syndrome
    c. Hypochondrial paranomia
    d. Othello syndrome

[Ref: Niraj Ahuja 7th/e/ch7/ p. 84]

23. **Which of the following is a type of delusion:** *(PGMEE 2013)*
    a. Othello syndrome
    b. Clerambault's syndrome
    c. Both
    d. None

[Ref: Niraj Ahuja 7th/e p 84]

24. **Delusion of doubles is found in:** *(PGMEE 2013)*
    a. Reactive psychosis
    b. Capgras syndrome
    c. Paranoid schizophrenia
    d. Schizoaffective disorder

[Ref: Niraj Ahuja 7th/e p. 87]

14.	c
15.	c
16.	c
17.	b
18.	d
19.	c
20.	d
21.	a
22.	d
23.	c
24.	b

25. Acute and transient psychotic disorder, onset of symptoms: *(PGMEE 2013)*
   a. < 1 weeks
   b. < 2 weeks
   c. < 3 weeks
   d. < 4 weeks

[Ref: Niraj Ahuja 7th/e/p 85]

26. Folie-a-deux means: *(PGMEE 2013)*
   a. Sharing of delusion
   b. Delusion of persecution
   c. Delusion of double
   d. None

[Ref: Niraj Ahuja 7th/e/p 247]

Explanation
- Folie a-deux is a shared delusion (commonly between parent and children).

27. Doppel ganger is characterized by *(PGMEE 2013)*
   a. Indentification of stranger as familiar
   b. Feeling of double of oneself
   c. Shadow following person
   d. None of the above

[Ref: Neel Burton p22]

MEMORY

28. Confabulation is problem with: *(PGMEE 2014)*
   a. Concentration
   b. Intelligence
   c. Attention
   d. Memory

[Ref: Niraj Ahuja 7th/e/p 27]

29. Immediate memory is tested by: *(NEET Pattern 2017)*
   a. Digit span forward
   b. Digit span backward
   c. Subtraction test 20-1
   d. Subtraction test 100-7

Explanation
- Digit forward- test of attention.
- Digit backward- test of concentration.
- Serial subtraction (100-7/40-3/ 20-1)-test of concentration/working memory.

CLASSIFICATION

30. Which category of ICD is associated with schizophrenia? *(PGMEE 2015)*

   a. F0
   b. F10
   c. F20
   d. F21

[Ref: Niraj Ahuja 7th/e/p 3]

31. Which category of ICD is associated with mood disorders? *(PGMEE 2015)*
   a. F00
   b. F11
   c. F21
   d. F31

[Ref: Niraj Ahuja 7th/e/p 3]

32. Number of axes in DSM 4 are: *(PGMEE 2015)*
   a. 2
   b. 3
   c. 4
   d. 5

[Ref: Niraj Ahuja 7th/e p. 4]

PSYCHOSIS VS NEUROSIS

33. NOT seen in 'psychosis': *(PGMEE 2013)*
   a. Personality disturbances
   b. Loss of insight

   c. Preserved contact with reality
   d. Presence of delusions

[Ref: Niraj Ahuja 7th/e/ch 7/p 83]

34. All are features of neurosis except: *(PGMEE 2013)*
   a. Personality disturbance
   b. Contact with reality preserved
   c. Symptoms cause subjective distress
   d. Insight is maintained

[Ref: Niraj Ahuja 7th/e/ch 8/p 89]

35. What is a feature of Psychosis and not neurosis: *(PGMEE 2014)*

   a. Personality and behavior preserved
   b. Lack of insight
   c. Insight is preserved
   d. Contact with reality is preserved

[Ref: Niraj Ahuja 7th/e/ p 83 & 89]

PSYCHIATRIC TESTS

36. Rorschach test measures: *(PGMEE 2014)*
   a. Intelligence
   b. Neuroticism
   c. Personality
   d. Creativity

[Ref: Niraj Ahuja 7th/e/p 17]

37. Patient is asked to perform Serial subtraction. What is he getting tested for? *(PGMEE 2015)*
   a. Mathematical ability
   b. Long term memory
   c. Working memory
   d. Recall power

[Ref: Oxford Hankey's clinical neurology 2nd/e p. 23]

38. For what is the person tested if asked, 'what will he do if he sees his house on fire'? *(PGMEE 2015)*
   a. Personal judgement
   b. Social judgement
   c. Test judgement
   d. None of the above

[Ref: Niraj Ahuja, 7th/e/ch 2]

Explanation
- **Test Judgment:** Is assessed by response to patient's predicted behavior in certain virtual situations, like house set on fire, open envelop found on street, etc.
- **Social Judgment:** Is assessed by observing subtle manifestations in behavior that are contrary to acceptable social norms, pertinent to various situations
- **Personal Judgment:** Is assessed by response to questions regarding ability to sufficiently make realistic future plans, w.r.t. education, job, etc.

MISCELLANEOUS

39. Patient wants to scratch for itching in his amputated limb is an example of: *(PGMEE 2015)*
   a. Phantom limb hallucination
   b. Pseudohallucination
   c. Illusion
   d. Autoscopy hallucination

[Ref: Love & Bailey 26th/e/p 893]

40. Which is the highest rated insight? *(PGMEE 2015)*
   a. Intellectual
   b. Psychological
   c. Emotional
   d. Affective

[Ref: Niraj Ahuja 7th/e/ ch 2 pg 15]

25.	b
26.	a
27.	b
28.	d
29.	a
30.	c
31.	d
32.	d
33.	c
34.	a
35.	b
36.	c
37.	c
38.	c
39.	a
40.	c

1. **Organic brain lesion is suggested by which of the following–** *(PGMEE 2014)*
   a. Visual hallucinations
   b. Depression
   c. Formal thought disorder
   d. Auditory hallucinations

   [Ref: Niraj Ahuja 7th/e p. 28]

2. **Perseveration is described as:** *(DNB 2007)*
   a. Persistent repetition of the same words beyond their relevance
   b. When a patient feels very distressed about it
   c. Characteristic of schizophrenia
   d. Characteristic of obsessive compulsive disorder (OSD)

   [Ref: Niraj Ahuja 7th/e/p 56]

Explanation

- Perseveration is either a speech-language or a motor pathology where there is repetition of a particular response (such as a word, phrase, or gesture) either in the absence or cessation of a stimulus, after it has served its purpose.
- This term is used irrespective of whether the person feels distressed about it or not.
- Although may be present in schizophrenia and obsessive compulsive disorder, they are not characteristic of these disorders. They are characteristically indicate frontal lobe damage.

3. **Loss of Orientation occurs in which sequence:** *(PGMEE 2016-17)*
   a. Time-> place ->person
   b. Place->time->person
   c. Time->person->place
   d. Person->Time->Place

   [Ref: Niraj Ahuja 7th/e/p 14]

DELIRIUM

4. **Not a clinical feature of delirium–** *(PGMEE 2012)*
   a. Preserved attention
   b. Disturbed sleep
   c. Disorientation
   d. Hallucination

   [Ref: Niraj Ahuja 7th/e p. 20]

5. **All are features of delirium except:** *(PGMEE 2014)*
   a. Disorientation
   b. Loss of memory
   c. Confusion
   d. Hyperactivity

   [Ref: Niraj Ahuja 7th/e p. 20]

Explanation

- In Delirium, patients have ↓ attention span and short-term memory

6. **False regarding delirium tremens:** *(PGMEE 2013)*
   a. Tremors
   b. Clouding of consciousness
   c. Visual hallucination
   d. Opthalmoplegia

   [Ref: Niraj Ahuja 7th/e/p 38]

7. **Difference between delirium and dementia:** *(PGMEE 2018)*
   a. Clouding of consciousness
   b. Loss of orientation to time, place and person
   c. Loss of memory
   d. Fluctuating course

   [Ref: (DSM-5; P-596)]

Explanation

- Dementia and delirium can coexist in clinical setting. When they present independently in a patients the sole feature of clouding of consciousness differentiate the two condition. Clouding of consciousness remain the hallmark feature of delirious state due to any cause.

Characteristic	Delirium	Dementia
Cause	Fluctuating from hour to hours, "sundowning"	Progressive deterioration
Consciousness	Clouded	Intact

8. **Post cardiac surgery delirium is aggravated maximally by:** *(Recent Pattern June 2018)*
   a. Anti psychotic
   b. Anti depressants
   c. Benzodizipines
   d. Anticholinergics

   [Ref: Synopsis of Psychiatry by Kaplan & Sadock's 11th/e pg. 668]

Explanation

- Benzodizipines are the drugs commonly used during cardiac surgery for anxiolytic and sedative effect.
- Delirium associated with intoxication is seen more commonly with **benzodiazepines** or **barbiturates** if the dosage are sufficiently high.
- Delirium that is indistinguishable from delirium tremens associated with alcohol withdrawal is seen more commonly with barbiturate withdrawal.

9. **Confusion assessment scale used for which of the following?** *(PGMEE Jan 2019)*
   a. Schizophrenia
   b. Delirium
   c. Dementia
   d. Depression

DEMENTIA

10. **Catastrophic reaction is seen in:** *(PGMEE 2014)*
    a. Schizophrenia
    b. Delirium
    c. Dementia
    d. Anxiety

    [Ref: Niraj Ahuja 7th/e/p 22]

11. **Subcortical dementia is seen in all except:** *(PGMEE 2012)*
    a. Wilson's disease
    b. Parkinsonism
    c. Huntington's chorea
    d. Alzheimer's disease

    [Ref: Niraj Ahuja 7th/e p. 24]

1.	a
2.	a
3.	a
4.	a
5.	None
6.	d
7.	a
8.	c
9.	b
10.	c
11.	d

12. True about Alzeimer　　　　　*(PGMEE 2016-17)*
a. Most common cause of dementia
b. More common in Men
c. Increase in brain Acetyl Cholinesterase activity
d. Treatable cause of dementia

[Ref: Niraj Ahuja 7th/e/ch 3]

13. Symptoms of vascular dementia:　　*(PGMEE 2016-17)*
a. Disorientation
b. Visual Hallucination
c. Memory Deficit
d. All of the above

[Ref: Niraj Ahuja 7th/e/ch 3]

14. All are reversible causes of dementia except:
a. Meningoencephalitis　　　*(PGMEE 2013)*
b. Alzheimer's disease
c. Hypothyroidism
d. Hydrocephalus

[Ref: Niraj Ahuja 7th/e/p 23]

15. Dementia is seen in all except:　　*(PGMEE 2014)*
a. Huntington's chorea
b. Alzheimer's disease
c. Pick's ds.
d. Schizophrenia

[Ref: Niraj Ahuja 7th/e/p. 24]

16. Commonest cause of dementia in adult is:
　　　　　　　　　　　　　　(PGMEE 2015)
a. Alzheimer's　　　　b. Multiinfarct
c. Pick disease　　　　d. Metabolic cause

[Ref: Niraj Ahuja 7th/e/p. 23]

17. Pseudodementia is seen in:　　　*(PGMEE 2014)*
a. Schizophrenia　　　b. Depression
c. Alcoholism　　　　d. Mania

[Ref: Niraj Ahuja 7th/e/p. 23]

18. Which of the following is explicit memory:
　　　　　　　　　　　　　　(PGMEE 2013)
a. Sementic　　　　　b. Non-declarative
c. Procedural　　　　d. Working

19. Biochemical etiology in Alzheimer's disease is related to:　　　　　　　　*(PGMEE 2014)*
a. Acetyl choline　　　b. Dopamine
c. Serotonin　　　　d. GABA

[Ref: Niraj Ahuja 7th/e p 25]

Explanation

- The Central cholinergic deficit hypothesis suggests that a dysfunction of acetylcholine containing neurons in the brain contributes substantially to the cognitive decline observed in those with advanced age and Alzheimer's disease (AD).
- Classically, Dopamine, Serotonin and GABA are associated with psychotic, mood and anxiety disorders, respectively.

20. Rivastigmine and Donepezil are drugs used predominantly in the management of:　　*(PGMEE 2013)*
a. Delusion　　　　b. Dissociation
c. Depression　　　d. Dementia

[Ref: Niraj Ahuja 7th/e/25]

Explanation

- Best initial treatment: cholinesterase inhibitor (Donepezil, Rivastigmine and galantamine)

WERNICKE'S – KORSAKOFF'S PSYCHOSIS

21. A chronic alcoholic 36 hours after stopping alcohol presents with tremors, confusion and difficulty in vision. Most like diagnosis is:-　　*(PGMEE 2018)*
a. Wernickes Koroskoff's syndrome
b. Delirium tremens
c. Alcoholic hallucinosis
d. Obsessive compulsive disorder

[Ref: (CTP, 10 th ed)]

Explanation

- *Delirium tremens* – if in place of difficulty in vision there would be seizure, auditory/ visual hallucination (Lilliputian halluciantion).
- *Alcoholic hallucinosis*- pt with alcoholism with auditory hallucination in clear consciousness, there can be history of fearfulness because of those threating content of hallucination

22. Wernicke-encephalopathy is due to deficiency of:
a. Pyridoxine　　　　*(PGMEE 2013)*
b. Niacin
c. Thiamine
d. Folic acid

[Ref: Niraj Ahuja 7th/e p.27]

23. All are affected in Wernicke's disease except–
a. Thalamus　　　　*(PGMEE 2015)*
b. Hypothalamus
c. Hippocampus
d. Mammillary bodies

[Ref: Niraj Ahuja 7th/e/p 38]

24. All are associated with Wernicke's encephalopathy except:
a. Cog wheel rigidity　　　*(PGMEE 2012)*
b. Alteration in mental function
c. VIth nerve palsy
d. Ataxia

[Ref: Niraj Ahuja 7th/e p. 38]

25. Classical triad of global confusion, ataxia and ophthalmoplegia is seen in:　　*(PGMEE 2013)*
a. Wernicke's encephalopathy
b. Delirium tremors
c. Alzheimer's disease
d. Korsakoff psychosis

[Ref: Niraj Ahuja 7th/e p. 38]

26. Not present in Wernicke's encephalopathy:
　　　　　　　　　　　　　(PGMEE 2012)
a. Confusion　　　　b. Ataxia
c. Aphasia　　　　d. Nystagmus

[Ref: Niraj Ahuja 7th/e p. 38]

12.	a
13.	d
14.	b
15.	d
16.	a
17.	b
18.	a
19.	a
20.	d
21.	a
22.	c
23.	c
24.	a
25.	a
26.	c

27. **Not seen in Korsakoff's syndrome:** *(PGMEE 2014)*
    a. Confusion
    b. Confabulation
    c. Hallucinations
    d. Inability to learn new things

    [Ref: Niraj Ahuja 7th/e p.38]

28. **Earliest symptom amongst classical triad of Wernicke's encephalopathy showing improvement to thiamine therapy:** *(PGMEE 2013)*
    a. Ataxia
    b. Confusion
    c. Ophthalmoplegia
    d. All are equally responsive

    [Ref: Essential of clinical psychiatry 4th/e p. 340]

AMNESIA

29. **Total score in Mini Mental Status Examination [MMSE] is:** *(PGMEE 2012, MAH 10)*
    a. 25   b. 30
    c. 35   d. 40

    [Ref: Harrison Manual Of Medicine 19th/e p 947]

30. **Which of the following are sections of mental state examination?** *(PGMEE 2015)*
    a. Speech and language
    b. Mood and affects
    c. Cognition
    d. All the above

    [Ref: Niraj Ahuja 7th/e/p 11]

31. **Benzodiazepine causes which type of amnesia:** *(Recent Pattern June 2018)*
    a. Anterograde
    b. Psychogenic
    c. Biological
    d. None

    [Ref: Synopsis of Psychiatry by Kaplan & Sadock's 11th/ e. pg. 719]

Explanation

- Benzodiazepines can produce anterograde amnesia (i.e., a loss of memory for events occurring forward in time).
- Short-term memory is remains unaffected, but long-term memory is impaired.
- The memory loss may occur as the events are not transferred from short-term memory to long-term memory and thus not consolidated into memory storage.
- Information stored prior to the ingestion of a benzodiazepine is not affected.
- Memory impairment is more with BZDs with-
  ○ High receptor affinity,
  ○ BZDs that accumulate in the body,
  ○ BZDs that are given in high doses or intravenously, or that are eliminated slowly.

27.	c
28.	c
29.	b
30.	d
31.	a

CANNABIS

1. The withdrawal from all of the following may produce suicidal tendencies except: *(PGMEE 2014)*
a. Amphetamine   b. Alcohol
c. Cocaine   d. Cannabis

[Ref: Niraj Ahuja 7th/e p. 45]

Explanation
- Cannabis does not produce withdrawal symptoms.

2. Amotivational syndrome is seen in *(PGMEE 2014, PGMEE 2016-17)*
a. Amphetamine   b. Cocaine
c. Cannabis   d. LSD

[Ref: Niraj Ahuja 7th/e/p 46]

OPIOID

3. Most commonly abused opioid: *(PGMEE 2012)*
a. Bupremorphine   b. Oxycodone
c. Morphine   d. Diacetylmorphine

[Ref: Niraj Ahuja 7th/e/ch 4]

4. Piloerection is caused by withdrawal of which drug? *(PGMEE 2015)*
a. Smoking   b. Alcohol
c. Cannabis   d. Morphine

[Ref: Niraj Ahuja 7th/e/p 43]

5. Not a feature of heroin [smack] withdrawal: *(PGMEE 2014)*
a. Hypertension   b. Yawning
c. Hypersomnia   d. Muscle cramps

[Ref: Niraj Ahuja 6th/e/ ch 4]

6. Opiate withdrawal is treated with: *(PGMEE 2014)*
a. Pethidine   b. Nalorphine
c. CPZ   d. Methadone

[Ref: Niraj Ahuja 7th/e p. 44]

7. "Smack" is the "common" name for: *(PGMEE 2014)*
a. Opium   b. Cacaine
c. Heroin   d. None

[Ref: Niraj Ahuja 7th/e/ch 4]

ALCOHOL

8. Delirium tremens is seen in which condition: *(PGMEE 2012)*
a. Morphine poisoning   b. Alcohol overdoses
c. Alcohol withdrawal   d. Atropine poisoning

[Ref: Niraj Ahuja 7th/e/p 37]

Explanation
- Alcohol withdrawal symptoms
  ○ Tremors
  ○ Tachycardia
  ○ Hypertension

○ Delirium tremens (DTs)
○ Agitation
○ Malaise, Nausea
○ Seizure

9. Morbid jealousy is most often seen in patients taking: *(PGMEE 2014)*
a. LSD   b. Amphetamine
c. Alcohol   d. Cannabis

[Ref: Namboordiri 3rd/e p. 325]

10. Pupils in Alcohol intoxication are *(PGMEE 2016-17)*
a. Dilated pupils
b. Constricted pupil
c. Hippus reaction
d. No change in pupils

[Ref: Niraj Ahuja 7th/e/ch 4]

11. Alcoholic Paranoia is associated with: *(PGMEE 2013, 10)*
a. Hallucinations   b. Impulse agitation
c. Drowsiness   d. Fixed delusions

[Ref: Niaj Ahuja 7th/e/ch 4]

12. CAGE questionnaire is used for– *(PGMEE 2015)*
a. Alcoholism   b. Schizophrenia
c. Opioid abuse   d. Paranoid Psychosis

[Ref: Niraj Ahuja 7th/e/p 37]

13. A 55 year old male with history of regular alcohol intake for the last 15 years presents with seeing snakes all around the room, irrelevant talks, violent behavior, not recognizing of family members. He has not had alcohol for the past 3 days. What is this condition? *(PGMEE 2016-17)*
a. Delirium tremens
b. Korsakoff's psychosis
c. Wernicke's encephalopathy
d. Schizzophrenia

[Ref: Niraj Ahuja 7th/e/ch 4/ p 38]

Explanation
- Delirium tremens (DTs) is a rapid onset of confusion usually caused by withdrawal from alcohol, typically 2-4 days into the withdrawal. Characteristic symptoms are acute confusion, lack of orientation, tremors, insomnia, illusions and hallucinations, and autonomic instability.
- Wernicke encephalopathy is an acute neuropsychiatric sequala of chronic alcohol use disorder characterized by the triad – ophthalmoplegia, ataxia, and confusion.
- Korsakoff's syndrome, again a neuropsychiatric sequala of chronic alcohol use disorder characterized by memory impairments (with or without confabulation), confusion and personality changes. Together Wernicke encephalopathy and Korsakoff's syndrome is called Wernicke-Korsakoff syndrome.
- Hallucinations of schizophrenia occur in clear consciousness and full orientation.

1.	d
2.	c
3.	d
4.	d
5.	c
6.	d
7.	c
8.	c
9.	c
10.	a
11.	d
12.	a
13.	a

14. A 45 yr chronic alcoholic who has abstained from alcohol for last 10 yrs now present with 2 days loss of memory, confusion and ataxia. Likely diagnosis is:
(Recent Pattern June 2018)
a. Wernicke's syndrome
b. Delirium tremens
c. Korsakoff psychosis
d. Acquired hepato neuro degenerative disorder

[Ref: Synopsis of Psychiatry by Kaplan & Sadock's 11th/e. pg. 628]

Explanation

Alcohol withdrawal

- Classic signs of alcohol withdrawal is tremulousness. Spectrum of symptoms include psychotic and perceptual symptoms like delusions & hallucinations, seizures, and the symptoms of delirium tremens (DT) or alcoholic delirium.
  - Tremulousness (alcoholic shakes/jitters) develops 6-8 hours after the cessation of drinking
  - The psychotic & perceptual symptoms develop in 8-12 hours
  - Seizures in 12-24 hours

15. True about delirium tremens all EXCEPT
a. Quite a common complication in alcohol withdrawal
b. Auditory hallucination
c. Visual hallucination
d. ECG changes are seen

[Ref: Niraj Ahuja 7th/e/p 38]

16. All are seen in alcohol withdrawal syndrome EXCEPT–
(DNB Dec' 2009)
a. Hallucination   b. Tremors
c. Hypersomnolence   d. Autonomic hyperactivity

[Ref:Kaplan & Sadock's Synopsis of Psychiatry, 10th edn, pg-398]

Explanation

Diagnostic Criteria for Alcohol Withdrawal

- Cessation of (or reduction in) alcohol use that has been heavy and prolonged.
- 2 or more of the following, developing within several hours to a few days after Criterion A:
  - Autonomic hyperactivity (e.g., sweating or pulse rate greater than 100)
  - Increased hand tremor
  - Insomnia
  - Nausea or vomiting
  - Transient visual, tactile, or auditory hallucinations or illusions
  - Psychomotor agitation
  - Anxiety
  - Grand mal seizures
- The symptoms in Criterion B cause clinically significant distress or impairment in social, occupational, or other important areas of functioning.
- The symptoms are not due to a general medical condition and are not better accounted for by another mental disorder.

TREATMENT OF ALCOHOL DEPENDENCE

17. Drug of choice in delirium tremens is: *(PGMEE 2014)*
a. Chlordiazepoxide   b. Phenytoin
c. Morphine   d. Diazepalm

[Ref: Essential of clinical psychiatry 4th/e p. 421]

18. Deterrent agent used in alcohol dependence is–
(PGMEE 2013)
a. Naloxone   b. Nalterxone
c. Disulfiram   d. Acamprosate

[Ref: Niraj Ahuja 7th/e/p 41]

19. Hangover following alcohol consumption is treated by:
(PGMEE 2012)
a. NSAIDs and Hydration   b. Niacin
c. Riboflavin   d. Pyridoxine

[Ref: Niraj Ahuja 7th/e/p 40]

MISCELLANEOUS

20. Formication is seen with: *(PGMEE 2013)*
a. Cannabis poisoning
b. Chronic use of amphetamine
c. Alcohol withdrawal
d. Acute amphetamine intoxication

[Ref: Niraj Ahuja 7th/e/ch 4]

21. Magnan syndrome is:
a. Tactile hallucinations   b. Auditory hallucinations
c. Visual hallucinations   d. Gustatory hallucinations

[Ref: Niraj Ahuja 7th/e/ch 4]

22. Drug used for cocaine withdrawal symptoms is:
(PGMEE 2013)
a. Floxetine   b. No drug
c. Phenobarbital   d. Lorazepam

[Ref: Kaplan & Sadock 10th/e p. 427]

23. Schizophrenia like symptom & Paranoid psychosis can be seen with chronic use of: *(Recent Pattern June 2018)*
a. Cannabis Indica   b. Amphetamine
c. Chlorpromazine   d. Morphine

[Ref: Synopsis of Psychiatry by Kaplan & Sadock's 11th/e pg. 668,677]

Explanation

- Amphetamine is the most common cause of drug induced schizophrenia & paranoid delusions & hallucinations. Amphetamine use can also induce symptoms of anxiety disorders, such as GAD (Generalised anxiety disorder), panic disorder by increasing dopaminergic activity in CNS.
- Other drugs which can produce schizophrenia like state:-
  - LSD (5HT2 receptor agonist)
  - NMDA receptor antagonist & channel blockers. Phencyclidine and Ketamine Mescaline
  - Cocaine (release dopamine) * NMDA receptor agonist cycloserine reduce negative symptoms.
  - Alcohol
  - Barbiturate withdrawal
  - Belladonna

14.	b
15.	a
16.	c
17.	a
18.	c
19.	a
20.	b
21.	a
22.	b
23.	b

24. Paranoid hallucinations are produced by:

(PGMEE 2012)

- a. Chlorpromazine
- b. Parazetine
- c. Amphetamine
- d. Morphine

[Ref: Niraj Ahuja 7th/e/p 49]

25. All are seen in nicotine withdrawal except:

(PGMEE 2013, DNB pattern Dec'2011)

- a. Bradycardia
- b. Anxiety
- c. Hyperhydrosis
- d. Insomnia

[Ref: Kaplan & Sadock 10th/e p. 440]

Explanation

Criteria for Nicotine Withdrawal

- Daily use of nicotine for at least several weeks.
- Abrupt cessation of nicotine use, or reduction in the amount of nicotine used, followed within 24 hours by four (or more) of the following symptoms:
  - Marked dysphoric or depressed mood
  - Insomnia
  - Irritability, frustration, or anger
  - Anxiety
  - Difficulty in concentrating
  - Restlessness
  - Decreased heart rate
  - Increased appetite or weight gain

26. Which is not a feature of caffeine withdrawal?

(DNB pattern Dec'2011)

- a. Headache
- b. Weight gain
- c. Drowsiness
- d. Depression

[Ref: Kaplan & Sadock's Synopsis of Psychiatry, 10th edn, pg-415]

Explanation

Criteria for Caffeine Withdrawal

- Prolonged daily use of caffeine.
- Abrupt cessation of caffeine use, or reduction in the amount of caffeine used, closely followed by headache and one (or more) of the following symptoms:
  - Marked fatigue or drowsiness
  - Marked anxiety or depression
  - Nausea or vomiting

27. Etheroman refer to: *(PGMEE 2012)*

- a. Ether addiction
- b. Excessive ether use drug anaesthesia
- c. Acute psychosis post ether anaesthesia
- d. None

24.	c
25.	c
26.	b
27.	c

1. Incidence of Schizophrenia in US is:

(DNB pattern Dec'2011)

a. 0.5%
b. 1%
c. 1.5%
d. 2%

[Ref: Niraj Ahuja 7th/e/ch 5/ p 54]

Explanation

- In the United States, the lifetime prevalence of schizophrenia is about 1 percent, which means that about 1 person in 100 will develop schizophrenia during their lifetime.
- The Epidemiologic Catchment Area study sponsored by the National Institute of Mental Health reported a lifetime prevalence of 0.6 to 1.9 percent. According to DSM-IV-TR, the annual incidence of schizophrenia ranges from 0.5 to 5.0 per 10,000, with some geographic variation (e.g., the incidence is higher for persons born in urban areas of industrialized nations). Schizophrenia is found in all societies and geographical areas, and incidence and prevalence rates are roughly equal worldwide.

2. Schizophrenia word means: *(PGMEE 2015)*

a. Split thoughts
b. Split mood
c. Split mind
d. Split associations

[Ref: Niraj Ahuja 7th/e/ch 5/ p 54]

3. The term "Dementia precox" was coined by:

(PGMEE 2012, 08)

a. Kraepelin
b. Bleuler
c. Schneider
d. Freud

[Ref: Niraj Ahuja 7th/e/ch 5/ p 54]

4. Term schizophrenia was coined by: *(PGMEE 2014)*

a. Bleuler
b. Sigmund Freud
c. Erich muir
d. None

[Ref: Niraj Ahuja 7th/e/ch 5/ p. 54]

5. Most common neurotransmitter implicated in the etiology of schizophrenia is: *(PGMEE 2013)*

a. GABA
b. Norepinephrine
c. Dopamine
d. Serotonin

[Ref: Niraj Ahuja 7th/e/ch 5/ p 63]

6. Schizophrenia commonly seen in which socioeconomic strata: *(PGMEE 2013)*

a. Low
b. Middle
c. Upper middle
d. Upper

[Ref: Niraj Ahuja 7th/e/ch 5/ p 65]

7. Eugen Bleuler's criteria for schizophrenia includes all the following except: *(PGMEE 2015-16)*

a. Automatism
b. Ambivalence
c. Loosening of association
d. Inappropriate affect

[Ref: Kaplan & Sadock's 11th/e pg. 467; Niraj Ahuja 7th/e pg. 54, 55]

8. Most common hallucination in schizophrenia:

a. Auditory hallucination
(PGMEE 2016-17)
b. Visual hallucination
c. Tactile hallucination
d. Tactie hallucination

[Ref: Niraj Ahuja 7th/e/p 56]

9. All are true in schizophrenia EXCEPT:

(PGMEE 2016-17)

a. Term given by Eugen Bleuler,
b. It a type of psychosis
c. First rank symptoms are given by Kurt Schneider
d. It is a type of neurosis

[Ref: Niraj Ahuja 7th/e/ch 5]

10. All are false about schizophrenia EXCEPT:

(DNB Dec'2009)

a. It is the disorder of thought
b. It is an example of split personality
c. It is due to emotional turmoil
d. It is due to childhood trauma

[Ref: Kaplan & Sadock's Synopsis of Psychiatry, 10th edn, pg-234,277]

Explanation

- Thought can be divided into process (or form) and content. Process refers to the way in which a person puts together ideas and associations, the form in which a person thinks. Process or form of thought can be logical and coherent or completely illogical and even incomprehensible. Content refers to what a person is actually thinking about: ideas, beliefs, preoccupations, obsessions.

- *The list of formal thought disorder is as follows:*
  ○ **Circumstantiality**. Overinclusion of trivial or irrelevant details that impede the sense of getting to the point.
  ○ **Clang associations**. Thoughts are associated by the sound of words rather than by their meaning (e.g., through rhyming or assonance).
  ○ **Derailment**. (Synonymous with loose associations.) A breakdown in both the logical connection between ideas and the overall sense of goal-directedness. The words make sentences, but the sentences do not make sense.
  ○ **Flight of ideas**. A succession of multiple associations so that thoughts seem to move abruptly from idea to idea; often (but not invariably) expressed through rapid, pressured speech.
  ○ **Neologism**. The invention of new words or phrases or the use of conventional words in idiosyncratic ways.
  ○ **Perseveration**. Repetition of out of context of words, phrases, or ideas.

1.	b
2.	c
3.	a
4.	a
5.	c
6.	a
7.	a
8.	a
9.	d
10.	a

- ○ **Tangentiality.** In response to a question, the patient gives a reply that is appropriate to the general topic without actually answering the question. Example:
  - Doctor: Have you had any trouble sleeping lately?
  - Patient: usually sleep in my bed, but now I'm sleeping on the sofa
- ▪ **Thought blocking.** A sudden disruption of thought or a break in the flow of ideas.

SCHNEIDER'S FIRST RANK SYMPTOMS

11. First rank symptoms of schizophrenia are all except:
(PGMEE 2012)
- a. Somatic passivity
- b. Ambivalence
- c. Delusional perception
- d. Running commentary

[Ref: Niraj Ahuja 7th/e p. 55]

12. Ambivalence is most commonly associated with:
- a. Schizophrenia *(PGMEE 2014)*
- b. Generalized anxiety disorder
- c. Depression
- d. OCD

[Ref: Niraj Ahuja 7th/e/ch 5]

13. Which one of the following is not considered as first rank symptoms of schizophrenia? *(PGMEE 2014)*
- a. Delusional perceptions
- b. Insertion of thoughts
- c. Compulsive acts that relieve the tension
- d. Auditory hallucinations

[Ref: Niraj Ahuja 7th/e/ch 5/p. 55]

14. Schneider's First rank symptoms seen in:
(PGMEE 2014)
- a. Schizophrenia
- b. Delusion
- c. Schizoid personality
- d. Hallucination

[Ref: Niraj Ahuja 7th/e/ch 5/ p 55]

CLINICAL FEATURES OF SCHIZOPHRENIA

15. Catatonia is most commonly seen with:
- a. Schizophrenia *(PGMEE 2015)*
- b. Depression
- c. Anxiety disorder
- d. Obsessive compulsive disorder

[Ref: Niraj Ahuja 7th/e/ch 5]

16. Diagnostic symptoms of schizophrenic patient are all except: *(PGMEE 2013)*
- a. Disorganized speech
- b. Hallucinations
- c. Social withdrawal
- d. Catatonia

[Ref: Neeraj Ahuja 7th/e/ch 5]

17. Which of the following hallucinations is characteristic of schizophrenia: *(PGMEE 2014)*
- a. Auditory hallucinations commanding the patient
- b. Auditory hallucinations giving running commentary
- c. Auditory hallucinations criticizing the patient
- d. Auditory hallucinations talking to patient

[Ref: Niraj Ahuja 7th/e/ch 5/ p56]

18. Anhedonia is seen in which psychiatric condition?
(PGMEE 2016-17)
- a. Obsessive Compulsive Disorder
- b. Schizophrenia
- c. Panic Disorder
- d. Hypochondriasis

[Ref: Niraj Ahuja 7th/e/p 55-56]

19. Negative symptom of schizophrenia: *(PGMEE 2013)*
- a. Motor hyperactivity
- b. Delusion
- c. Hallucination
- d. Anhedonia

[Ref: Niraj Ahuja 7th/e/ch 5]

TYPES OF SCHIZOPHRENIA

20. In schizophrenia early onset with poor prognosis is seen in *(PGMEE 2014, PGMEE 2016-17)*
- a. Simple
- b. Paranoid
- c. Catatonic
- d. Hebephrenic

[Ref: Niraj Ahuja 7th/e p. 58]

21. Best prognosis is seen in: *(PGMEE 2014)*
- a. Paranoid schizophrenia
- b. Catatonic schizophrenia
- c. Hebephrenic schizophrenia
- d. Undifferentiated schizophrenia

[Ref: Niraj Ahuja 7th/e/ch 5/p 59]

22. In stuporous catatonia, all are seen except:
(PGMEE 2013)
- a. Mutism
- b. Ambitendency
- c. Akinesia
- d. Agitation

[Ref: Niraj Ahuja 7th/e/ch 5/p. 59]

23. All are features of catatonia except: *(PGMEE 2014)*
- a. Automatic obedience
- b. Cataplexy
- c. Mutism
- d. Negativism

[Ref: Niraj Ahuja 7th/e/ch 5 p. 59]

24. Waxy flexibility is characteristic of: *(PGMEE 2013)*
- a. OCD
- b. Stuporous cataonia
- c. Excitatory catatonia
- d. All

[Ref: Niraj Ahuja 7th/e p. 59]

25. Type of schizophrenia with mental retardation:
- a. Pfropf schizophrenia *(PGMEE 2012)*
- b. Von-Gogh syndrome
- c. Catatonic schizophrenia
- d. Paranoid schizophrenia

[Ref: Niraj Ahuja 7th/e/ch 5/p.61]

26. All are true about type I schizophrenia except:
(PGMEE 2013)
- a. Intellect maintained
- b. Acute illness
- c. Negative symptoms
- d. Good prognosis

[Ref: Niraj Ahuja 7th/e/ch 5/p 62]

27. All of the following are associated with good prognosis in schizophrenia except: *(PGMEE 2013)*
- a. Negative symptoms
- b. Married
- c. Late onset
- d. Acute onset

[Ref: Niraj Ahuja 7th/e/ch 5/ p 62]

11.	b
12.	a
13.	c
14.	a
15.	a
16.	c
17.	b
18.	b
19.	d
20.	d
21.	b
22.	d
23.	b
24.	b
25.	a
26.	c
27.	a

28. **Schizophrenia is associated with........ Personalities:**
    (PGMEE 2014)
    a. Pyknic
    b. Asthenic
    c. Atheletic
    d. All

29. **A patient who was taking Haloperidol for schizophernia for 10 years, now developed Parkinsonism like symptom which of the following drug will you give:**
    (Recent Pattern June 2018)
    a. Anti-muscarinic
    b. Anti-depressant
    c. Anti-cholinergic
    d. Anti-dopaminergic

    [Ref: Synopsis of Psychiatry by Kaplan & Sadock's 11th/e/pg. 924-925]

Explanation

Neurolept induced movement disorders

- As haloperidol is a high-potency neuroleptic . It tends to produce significant extrapyramidal side effects like:-
  ○ Acute akathisia (motor restlessness)
  ○ Acute dystonia (continuous spasms and muscle contractions)
  ○ Muscle rigidity
  ○ Parkinsonism (characteristic symptoms such as rigidity)
  ○ Neuroleptic malignant syndrome is a life threatening & often misdiagnosed condition.
  ○ Neurolept induced tardive dyskinesia is a late appearing adverse effect of neuroleptics

Treatment of Neurolept induced movement disorders

Drugs	Indication
Anticholinergics (Benztropine)	Acute dystonia, **parkinsonism**, akinesia, akathasia
Antihistamine	Acute dystonia, **parkinsonism**, akinesia, Rabbit syndrome
Beta antiadrenergics	Akathisia.
BZDs	Akathisia, Tardive dyskinesia.

- The Anticholinergics work by decreasing the activity of acetylcholine. The activity of acetylcholine and dopamine are linked, so if the activity of acetylcholine goes down, the activity of dopamine goes up. **Benztropine** and **trihexyphenidyl** are best anticholinergic options for drug-induced parkinsonism.
- The mainstay of treatment of Parkinson's disease is replacement of dopamine. It is not possible to administer dopamine directly because it does not cross the BBB Therefore, today most patients are given a combination of levodopa + carbidopa.
- Antidotes such as bromocriptine or ropinirole may be used to treat the extrapyramidal effects caused by haloperidol, acting as dopamine receptor agonists.
- Anticholinergics are most effective in Stage I and II patients suffering from tremor and sialorrhea.

28. b
29. c

DEPRESSION

1. Most common psychiatric illness: *(PGMEE 2015)*
   a. Mania
   b. Bipolar
   c. Depression
   d. Cyclothymia
   [Ref: Niraj Ahuja 7th/e/ ch 6]

2. Nihilistic delusions are seen in: *(PGMEE 2014)*
   a. Depression
   b. Schizophrenia
   c. Mania
   d. OCN
   [Ref: Niraj Ahuja 7th/e p. 71]

3. Classical triad symptoms of depression does not include– *(PGMEE 2013)*
   a. Distractibility
   b. Slowed thinking
   c. Depressed mood
   d. Psychomotor retardation
   [Ref: Niraj Ahuja 7th/e/p 71]

4. All are required to diagnose major depression except: *(PGMEE 2013)*
   a. Depressed mood
   b. Decreased concentration
   c. Nihlistic ideas
   d. Insomnia
   [Ref: Niraj Ahuja 7th/e/p 105]

5. Depression patients most prominently show which of the following feature: *(Recent Pattern June 2018)*
   a. Low mood
   b. Sleep disturbances
   c. Vague body aches
   d. Suicidal tendencies
   [Ref: Synopsis of Psychiatry by Kaplan & Sadock's 11th/e pg. 293]

Explanation

- Multiple physical symptoms (such as heaviness of head, vague body aches) are common in depression in elderly in developing countries (such as India)
  - MC psychiatric disorder in India: Depression
  - Neurotransmitter involved: Serotonin and NE
  - MC cause of suicide: Depression

Risk features of suicide in depression:

- Endogenous type of depression
- Psychotic depression
- MC type of post-puerperal psychosis: Depression
- Nihilistic ideas: Seen in depression

6. According to DSM – IV criteria for depression presence of symptoms should be for how many weeks:
   a. 1 week
   b. 2 weeks *(PGMEE 2012)*
   c. 3 weeks
   d. 4 weeks
   [Ref: Niraj Ahuja 7th/e/ch 6]

7. Young lady lost her job, loss of appetite, wakes up at 3 am What's diagnosis ? *(PGMEE 2014)*
   a. Schizophrenia
   b. Mania
   c. OCD
   d. Depression
   [Ref: Niraj Ahuja 7th/e/ch 6]

8. Defense mechanism used in depression: *(Recent Pattern June 2018)*
   a. Introjection
   b. Projection
   c. Altrusion
   d. All are correct
   [Ref: Synopsis of Psychiatry by Kaplan & Sadock's 11th/e pg. 162]

Explanation

- Defense mechanisms employed by depressed patients typically include denial, projection, idealization and devaluation, passive aggression, identification with the aggressor, and reaction formation

George Valliant's classification of Defense mechanism

- *Narcissistic defenses* are most primitive and appear in children & persons who are psychotically disturbed. Examples are:-
  - Projection
  - Denial
  - Distortion
- *Immature defenses* are seen in adolescents & some non-psychotic patients. Examples are:-
  - Acting out
  - Blocking
  - Hypochondriasis
  - Introjection
  - Passive aggressive behavior
  - Projection, regression
  - Schizoid fantasy, somatization
- *Neurotic defenses* are encountered in obsessive compulsive and hysterical patients. Examples are:- Controlling, displacement, dissociation, externalization, inhibition.
- *Mature defenses* are healthy and adaptive throughout the life cycle. Examples are:-
  - Altruism
  - Anticipation
  - Asceticism
  - Humour
  - Sublimation
  - Suppression

Mechanism	Features
Altrusion	The vicarious but constructive & instinctfully gratifying service to others, even to the detriment of the self.
Introjection	internalization of characteristic of the objects with the goal of ensuring closeness to object
Projection	Perceiving and reacting to unacceptable inner impulses and their derivatives as they were outside the self.

1. c
2. a
3. a
4. c
5. c
6. b
7. d
8. b

9. **Mr. A, comes to the psychiatry OPD with complaints of irritability, guilt of not being able to perform well in office and decreased interest in recreational activity since he left college 3 years back.** *(NEET Pattern 2017)*
   a. Adjustment disorder
   b. Dysthymia
   c. Cyclothymia
   d. Major depressive episode

Explanation

- Very long standing depression of mood which is never, or only very rarely, severe enough to fulfill the criteria for recurrent depressive disorder. The catch here is the affected person socio-occupational functioning was not impaired and is long standing in nature. Minimum duration criteria to diagnose dysthymia is 2 years.
- **Cyclothymia** is persistent instability of mood, involving numerous periods of mild depression & mild elation, none of which has been sufficiently severe or prolonged to fulfill the criteria for bipolar affective disorder or recurrent depressive disorder.

10. **A patient is depressed for past 3 years, do not go out of his house much and is cut off from society. But with normal sleep and normal weight. Most probable diagnosis is?**
    (DNB pattern Dec' 2011)
    a. Adjustment disorder   b. Dysthymia
    c. Cyclothymia   d. Major depressive episode

    [Ref: Kaplan & Sadock's Synopsis of Psychiatry, 10th edn, pg-563]

Explanation

- The DSM-IV-TR diagnosis criteria for dysthymic disorder stipulate the presence of a depressed mood most of the time for at least 2 years (or 1 year for children and adolescents).
- The essential features of primary dysthymic disorder include habitual gloom, brooding, lack of joy in life, and preoccupation with inadequacy. Dysthymic disorder then is best characterized as long-standing, fluctuating, low-grade depression, experienced as part of the habitual self and representing an accentuation of traits observed in the depressive temperament.

11. **Dysthymia is described as–** *(PGMEE 2015)*
    a. Chronic severe depression
    b. Personality disorder
    c. Bipolar disorder
    d. Chronic mild depression

    [Ref: Niraj Ahuja 7th/e/p 73]

12. **Cyclothymia is a type of:** *(PGMEE 2013)*
    a. Major depression
    b. Persistant mood disorder
    c. Dysthymia
    d. Bipolar mood disorder

    [Ref: Niraj Ahuja 7th/e/p 73]

13. **Diagnostic cut off for Dysthymia is** *(PGMEE 2016-17)*
    a. 3 year   b. 6 month
    c. 2 year   d. 1 year

    [Ref: Niraj Ahuja 7th/e/p 82]

14. **Alexithymia is:** *(PGMEE 2014)*
    a. Pathological sadness
    b. Affective flattening
    c. A feeling of intense rapture
    d. Inability to recognize and describe feelings

    [Ref: Niraj Ahuja 7th/e/p 246]

15. **For diagnosis of major depressive disorder which of the following must be present:** *(PGMEE 2014)*
    a. Loss of interest of pleasure
    b. Recurrent suicidal tendency
    c. Insomnia
    d. Indecisiveness

    [Ref: Niraj Ahuja 7th/e/p 105]

16. **Early morning awakening and reduced latency of REM sleep is suggestive of:** *(PGMEE 2014)*
    a. Schizophrenia   b. Depression
    c. Anxiety   d. Delirium

    [Ref: Niraj Ahuja 7th/e/p 72]

17. **Type of behavior therapy used in depression:**
    (Recent Pattern June 2018)
    a. Token economy procedure
    b. Aversion therapy
    c. Congnitive therapy
    d. Social skill training

    [Ref: Synopsis of Psychiatry by Kaplan & Sadock's 11th/e pg. 877, 1230]

Explanation

Behaviour therapy

Types	Uses
Systemic desensitization	Identifiable anxiety provoking stimulus e.g. phobia, obsession, compulsion
Interpersonal therapy, Cognitive behavior therapy	Modertae depression in children
Therapeutic graded exposure	Phobia
The token economy procedure	Schizophrenia
Participant modelling	Agoraphobia
Flooding (Implosion)	Phobias
Aversion therapy	Alcohol abuse, paraphilias, Impulse disorders

NEUROTRANSMITTERS IN DEPRESSION

18. **In depression, there is deficiency of which neurotransmitter:** *(PGMEE 2012)*
    a. 5-HT   b. Acetylcholine
    c. Dopamine   d. GABA

    [Ref: Niraj Ahuja 7th/e p.75]

19. **True about neurotransmitters in mania is–**
    a. Increased dopamine *(PGMEE 2013)*
    b. Increased norepinephrine
    c. Both "a" and "b"
    d. Decreased norepinephrine

    [Ref: Niraj Ahuja 7th/e p 75]

9.	b
10.	b
11.	d
12.	b
13.	c
14.	d
15.	a
16.	b
17.	c
18.	a
19.	c

CAUSES OF DEPRESSION

20. Endocrine disorders associated with depression are all except: *(PGMEE 2014)*
a. Hypothyroidism
b. Acromegaly
c. Pheochromocytona
d. Hyperthyroidism

[Ref: Niraj Ahuja 7th/e/p 75]

21. Depression is caused by all except: *(PGMEE 2014)*
a. Metronidazole
b. Levodopa
c. Clonazepam
d. Corticosteroid

[Ref: Niraj Ahuja 7th/e/ch 15]

TREATMENT OF DEPRESSION

22. What is the treatment of choice for endogenous depression with suicidal tendency: *(PGMEE 2014)*
a. Lithium
b. Psychoanalysis
c. ECT
d. Chlorpromazine

[Ref: Niraj Ahuja 7th/e p.77]

23. Treatment of choice in severe depression is: *(PGMEE 2014)*
a. Alprazolam
b. Fluoxetine
c. ECT
d. None

[Ref: Niraj Ahuja 7th/e p. 76]

24. Following are the somatic therapies used in depression except: *(PGMEE 2015)*
a. Transcranial magnetic stimulation
b. Deep brainstimulation
c. Electroconvulsive therapy
d. Ultrasound brain stem stimulation

25. Deep brain stimulation used in treatment of: *(PGMEE 2013)*
a. Dementia
b. Parkinsonism
c. Delirium
d. Resistant Depression & Parkinsonism both

[Ref: Niraj Ahuja 7th/e/ch 16]

Explanation

- Deep brain stimulation (DBS) is a surgical procedure used to treat several disabling neurological symptoms
  ○ Most commonly the debilitating motor symptoms of Parkinson's disease (PD), such as essential tremor, rigidity, stiffness, slowed movement, and walking problems.
  ○ Resistant Depression
  ○ OCD

26. SSRIs should be carefully used in the young for the management of depression due to increase in: *(PGMEE 2015)*
a. Suicidal ideation
b. Guilt ideation
c. Nihilism ideation
d. Envious ideation

[Ref: Managing depression in clinical practice by Edward S. Freidman p. 11]

20.	c
21.	a
22.	c
23.	b
24.	d
25.	d
26.	a
27.	b
28.	d
29.	a
30.	c
31.	d
32.	c
33.	d

MANIA AND BIPOLAR DISORDERS

MANIA

27. Characteristic of maniac episode is: *(PGMEE 2013)*
a. Increased sleep
b. Elevated mood
c. Grandiosity
d. Decreased appetite

[Ref: Niraj Ahuja 7th/e/p 70]

28. In mania, type of sleep disturbance: *(PGMEE 2016-17)*
a. In initiation
b. Early awakening
c. In maintenance
d. Decrease need for sleep

[Ref: Niraj Ahuja 7th/e/p 71]

29. All are features of mania except: *(PGMEE 2015)*
a. Disorientation
b. Pressure of speech
c. Granduer delusion
d. Insomnia

[Ref: Niraj Ahuja 7th/e p. 70, 71]

30. What type of disorder is mania?– *(PGMEE 2014)*
a. Neurotic disorder
b. Psychological disorders
c. Mood disorder
d. Obsessive disorder

[Ref: Niraj Ahuja 6th/e/ ch 6]

BIPOLAR DISORDERS

31. Bipolar disorder II is characterized by?: *(DNB Dec' 2009)*
a. Hypomania plus mania
b. Depression alone
c. Mania and depression
d. Hypomania and depression

[Ref: Kaplan & Sadock's Synopsis of Psychiatry, 10th edn, pg-544]

Explanation

- Bipolar I- mania & depression
- Bipolar II- hypomania & depression
- Dysthymia- at least 2 years of depressed mood that is not sufficiently severe to fit the diagnosis of major depressive episode.
- Cyclothymia- at least 2 years of frequently occurring hypomanic symptoms that cannot fit the diagnosis of manic episode and of depressive symptoms that cannot fit the diagnosis of major depressive episode.
- Cyclothymia and dysthymia are defined by DSM-IV-TR as disorders that represent less severe forms of bipolar disorder and major depression, respectively.

32. What is affected in bipolar disorders: *(PGMEE 2015)*
a. Personality
b. Perception
c. Emotions
d. Thought

[Ref: Niraj Ahuja 7th/e p 73]

33. The period of being normal between two episodes of psychosis is seen in– *(PGMEE 2014)*
a. Schizophrenia
b. Depression
c. Alcoholism
d. Manic depressive psyhosis (MDP)

[Ref: Niraj Ahuja 7th/e/p 73]

34. **Intense depression & misery without any cause is?**
    a. Melancholia   *(PGMEE Jan 2019)*
    b. Major depressive disorder
    c. Mania
    d. Schizophrenia

TREATMENT OF MANIA & BPD

35. **Drug of choice for prevention of episodes of bipolar mood disorder is–**   *(PGMEE 2012)*
    a. Buspirone
    b. Carbamazepine
    c. Imipramine
    d. Lithium carbonate

    [Ref: Niraj Ahuja 7th/e/p 78]

36. **DOC for rapid cycling Manic Depressive Psychosis:**
    a. Calcium channel blocker   *(PGMEE 2013)*
    b. Valproate
    c. Carbamazepine
    d. Li

    [Ref: Niraj Ahuja 7th/e/p 191-192]

37. **Not a predisposing factor for suicide:**   *(PGMEE 2014)*
    a. Depression   b. Living single person
    c. Female sex   d. Drug abuse

    [Ref: Niraj Ahuja 7th/e/p 223]

38. **Most common mental disorder as a cause of suicide:**
                                                     (PGMEE 2013)
    a. Alcohol dependence   b. Depression
    c. Mania   d. Schizophrenia

    [Ref: Niraj Ahuja 7th/e/p 222-224]

39. **All of the following factors increase the risk of suicide EXCEPT–**   *(PGMEE 2012)*
    a. Male   b. Depression
    c. Alone   d. Married person

    [Ref: Niraj Ahuja 7th/e p. 223]

MISCELLANEOUS

40. **The maximum DALY loss is for the following disease:**
    a. Bipolar depression   *(PGMEE 2012)*
    b. Schizophrenia
    c. Mania
    d. Unipolar depression

34.	a
35.	d
36.	b
37.	c
38.	b
39.	d
40.	d

ANXIETY DISORDERS

1. Most common of all psychiatric disorders are: *(PGMEE 2015)*
   a. Depression
   b. Schizophrenia
   c. Anxiety disorders
   d. Mania

   [Ref: Niraj Ahuja 7th/e/p 89]

2. Not an anxiety disorder– *(PGMEE 2013)*
   a. Phobia
   b. PTSD
   c. Conversion reaction
   d. OCD

   [Ref: Niraj Ahuja 7th/e/p 89]

3. Phobia is a type of: *(PGMEE 2014)*
   a. Mania   b. Depression
   c. Neurosis   d. Psychosis

   [Ref: Niraj Ahuja 7th/e/p 89]

4. Anxiety is a type of: *(PGMEE 2012)*
   a. Neurosis   b. Psychosis
   c. Personality   d. None

   [Ref: Niraj Ahuja 7th/e/p 89]

PANIC DISORDERS

5. Sudden onset pain in the chest, perspiration and feeling of impending doom can be seen with *(PGMEE 2016-17)*
   a. Asthenia
   b. Acute dystonia
   c. Panic attack
   d. Migraine

   [Ref: Niraj Ahuja 7th/e/p 90]

6. All of the following can be considered as treatment for anxiety except: *(PGMEE 2014)*
   a. Serotonin reuptake inhibitors
   b. Benzodiazepines
   c. Dopaminergic blockers
   d. Buspirone

   [Ref: Niraj Ahuja 7th/e/p 92]

7. A 25-year-old female presented with chest pain, palpitations perspiration when the deadline to submit the presentation was close. When investigated she was medically normal. The condition in: *(PGMEE 2016-17)*
   a. Anxiety
   b. Panic Attack
   c. Avoidant Personality
   d. Malingering

   [Ref. Niraj Ahuja 7th/e/ch 8]

PHOBIA

8. Phobia is defined as: *(PGMEE 2012)*
   a. Excessive unreasonable fear about a specific situation
   b. Palpitation on thinking about a definite entity
   c. Altered perception
   d. Perception without stimulation

   [Ref: Niraj Ahuja 7th/e/p 92]

9. Commonest phobia is: *(PGMEE 2014)*
   a. Photophobia
   b. Agoraphobia
   c. Thantophobia
   d. Acrophobia

   [Ref: Niraj Ahuja 7th/e/p 92]

10. Agoraphobia is described as: *(PGMEE 2014)*
   a. Fear of being in unfamiliar places
   b. Fear of closed spaces
   c. Fear of heights
   d. Fear of dogs

   [Ref: Niraj Ahuja 7th/e/p 89]

11. Agoraphobia is best described by: *(PGMEE 2016-17)*
   a. Fear of crowded places
   b. Fear of closed spaces
   c. Fear of open spaces
   d. Fear of both crowded and open spaces

   [Ref: Niraj Ahuja 7th/e/p 92]

12. Thanatophobia is defined as fear of: *(PGMEE 2013)*
   a. Closed spaces
   b. High places
   c. Flights
   d. Death

   [Ref: Internet]

13. A student unable to deliver speech before audience is suffering from: *(PGMEE 2013)*
   a. Agoraphobia   b. OCD
   c. Social phobia   d. Claustrophobia

   [Ref: Niraj Ahuja 7th/e/p 93]

14. Morbid fear of darkness *(PGMEE 2019)*
   a. Claustrophobia   b. Xenophobia
   c. Mysophobia   d. Nyctophobia

   [Ref: Kaplan & Sadock's 11th/e/p 403]

Explanation

- Nyctophobia is an extreme fear of night or darkness that can cause intense symptoms of anxiety and depression.
- A list of other important phobias is given below:-

1.	c
2.	c
3.	c
4.	a
5.	c
6.	c
7.	b
8.	a
9.	b
10.	a
11.	d
12.	d
13.	c
14.	d

Specific Phobias

Acrophobia	Fear of heights
Agoraphobia	Fear of open places
Ailurophobia	Fear of cats
Hydrophobia	Fear of water
Claustrophobia	Fear of closed spaces
Cynophobia	Fear of dogs
Mysophobia	Fear of dirt and germs
Pyrophobia	Fear of fire
Xenophobia	Fear of strangers
Zoophobia	Fear of animals
Amaxophobia	Fear of electromagnetic fields, of microwaves, and of society as a whole

15. **Flooding is a type of behavior therapy used in:**
    (PGMEE 2013)
    a. Mania
    b. Depression
    c. Phobia
    d. Schizophrenia

    [Ref: Niraj Ahuja 7th/e/p 94]

OBSESSIVE - COMPULSIVE DISORDERS (OCD)

16. **Irresistible urge to do a thing repeatedly is seen in:**
    a. Schizophrenia disorder   *(PGMEE 2014)*
    b. Schizophrenia
    c. Obsessive – compulsive disorder
    d. Depression

    [Ref: Niraj Ahuja 7th/e/p 95]

17. **OCD is associated with:**   *(PGMEE 2016-17)*
    a. Depression
    b. Ecstasy
    c. Mania
    d. Insomnia

    [Ref: Niraj Ahuja 7th/e/p 95]

18. **Repeated action done after an irrational impulse is called:**   *(PGMEE 2012)*
    a. Obsession
    b. Anxiety
    c. Compulsion
    d. None

    [Ref: Niraj Ahuja 7th/e/p 95]

19. **Which of the following statements differentiates the obsessional idea from delusions:**   *(PGMEE 2015)*
    a. The idea is not a conventional belief
    b. The idea is held on inadequate ground
    c. The idea is regarded as ego-alien by patient
    d. The idea is held inspite of contrary evidence

    [Ref: Niraj Ahuja 7th/e/p 95]

20. **Commonest symptom in obsessive compulsive disorder is:**   *(PGMEE 2015)*
    a. Compulsive checking
    b. Compulsive thinking about same
    c. Obsessive precision
    d. Compulsive washing of hand

    [Ref: Niraj Ahuja 7th/e/p 95]

21. **Fear of contamination and having to check and recheck are features characteristics of:**   *(PGMEE 2014)*
    a. Obsessive – compulsive disorder
    b. Agoraphobia
    c. Panic attacks
    d. Generalized anxiety disorder

    [Ref: Niraj Ahuja 7th/e/p 95]

22. **Which of the following type of OCD has the poor response Exposure and Response prevention?**
    (PGMEE Jan 2019)
    a. Magical thinking
    b. Dirt contamination
    c. Pathological doubt
    d. Hoarding

23. **Genetic link of development of anxiety is characteristically seen in which other psychiatric illness?**
    (PGMEE 2016-17)
    a. Obsessive compulsive disorders
    b. Depressive disorders
    c. Personality disorder
    d. Manic disorders

    [Ref: Niraj Ahuja 7th/e/p 96]

24. **Which transmitter is mainly involved in Obsessive Compulsive Disorder is:**   *(PGMEE 2014)*
    a. Dopamine
    b. NE
    c. Serotonin
    d. GABA

    [Ref: Niraj Ahuja 7th/e/ch 8]

25. **Characteristic of obsession are all EXCEPT:**
    (DNB Dec'2009)
    a. Compulsion
    b. Repetitive behavior
    c. Abstract thinking
    d. Ego dystonic

    [Ref: Kaplan & Sadock's Synopsis of Psychiatry, 10th edn, pg-604]

Explanation

- An obsession is a recurrent and intrusive thought, feeling, idea, or sensation. In contrast to an obsession, which is a mental event, a compulsion is a behavior. Specifically, a compulsion is a conscious, standardized, recurrent behavior, such as counting, checking, or avoiding. A patient with OCD realizes the irrationality of the obsession and experiences both the obsession and the compulsion as ego-dystonic (i.e., unwanted behavior).
- These recurrent obsessions or compulsions cause severe distress to the person. The obsessions or compulsions are time-consuming and interfere significantly with the person's normal routine, occupational functioning, usual social activities, or relationships. A patient with OCD may have an obsession, a compulsion, or both.
- Abstract thinking is the ability to deal with concepts. Patients can have disturbances in the manner in which they conceptualize or handle ideas. It is impaired in cases of Schizophrenia, mental retardation, post head injury personality change etc.

26. **The drug of choice for obsessive compulsive disorder:**
    (PGMEE 2014)
    a. Chlorpromazine
    b. Fluoxetine
    c. Benzodiazepine
    d. Imipramine

    [Ref: Niraj Ahuja 7th/e/p 98 and ch 15]

15.	c
16.	c
17.	a
18.	c
19.	c
20.	d
21.	a
22.	d
23.	a
24.	c
25.	c
26.	b

27. Psychosurgery is used in which of the following disease–
                                                    (PGMEE 2013)
  a. Phobia
  b. Depression
  c. OCD
  d. Generalized anxiety

[Ref: Niraj Ahuja 7th/e/p 98]

POST – TRAUMATIC STRESS DISODER

28. Post-traumatic stress syndrome is due to:
    (PGMEE 2014)
  a. Major life threatening events
  b. CVD
  c. Minor stress
  d. Head injury

[Ref: Niraj Ahuja 7th/e/p 112]

Explanation

Post traumatic stress disorder

- Diagnostic criteria for PTSD include: a history of exposure to a traumatic event that meets specific stipulations and symptoms from each of four symptom clusters:
  - Intrusion (Recurrent, involuntary, and intrusive memories, nightmares, flashbacks).
  - Avoidance (Trauma-related thoughts or feelings or external reminders (e.g., people, places, conversations, activities, objects, or situations),
  - Negative alterations in cognitions and mood (Inability to recall key features of the trauma, Overly negative thoughts, Exaggerated blame of self), and
  - Alterations in arousal and reactivity (Irritability or aggression, Risky or destructive behavior, Hypervigilance, Heightened startle reaction, Difficulty concentrating, Difficulty sleeping).
- Minimum duration: Symptoms last for more than 1 month.
- *Generalized anxiety disorder*: Presence of excessive anxiety and worry about a variety of topics, events, or activities. Worry occurs more often than not for at least 6 months and is clearly excessive. Excessive worry means worrying even when there is nothing wrong or in a manner that is disproportionate to the actual risk.

29. A 22 year old male who had suffered a road traffic accident 2 months back awakes in the night with fear. He is now having nightmares, afraid to drive and startles. Most likely cause of these symptoms is *(PGMEE 2018)*
  a. Generalized anxiety disorder
  b. Post traumatic stress disorder
  c. Panic attacks
  d. Psychosis

[Ref: (DSM-5, P 271)]

27. c
28. a
29. b

1. **All are true regarding somatization disorder except:** *(PGMEE 2014)*
   a. 1-Sexual symptoms
   b. 1-Pseudo neurological symptoms
   c. 4-Pain symptoms
   d. Maintain sick role

   [Ref: Niraj Ahuja 7th/e/p]

2. **Which of the following is FALSE about SOMATIZATION Syndrome:** *(PGMEE 2012)*
   a. Involves 2 sexual disturbance Symptoms
   b. Two GI symptoms
   c. Four pain symptoms
   d. Multiple recurrent symptoms

   [Ref: Internet]

3. **All are included in diagnosis criteria of somatization disorder except:** *(PGMEE 2013)*
   a. Visual Symptoms   b. Pain symptom
   c. GI symptom   d. Sexual symptom

   [Ref: Kaplan & Saddock's 10th/e p. 636]

DIFFERENTIAL DIAGNOSIS

4. **A patient has been seeking repeated admissions in various hospitals with a variety of symptoms. He had undergone appendicectomy, cholecystectomy, and other exploratory laparotomies on previous admission. The most likely diagnosis is:** *(PGMEE 2014)*
   a. Ganser's syndrome
   b. Conversion reaction
   c. Munchausen syndrome
   d. Hypochondriasis

   [Ref: Essential of clinical psychiatry 4th/e p. 897]

Explanation

- Ganser syndrome is a form of dissociative disorder where the person gives nonsensical or wrong answers to questions; other dissociative symptoms such as fugue, amnesia or conversion episodes, often with visual pseudohallucinations and a decreased state of consciousness are seen.
- Munchausen syndrome is a condition in which a person intentionally fakes, simulates, worsens, or self-induces an injury or illness for the main purpose of being treated like a medical patient.
- Conversion disorder is a mental condition in which a person has blindness, paralysis, or other nervous system (neurologic) symptoms that cannot be explained by medical evaluation.
- Hypochondriasis is a mental disorder characterized by excessive fear of or preoccupation with a serious illness, despite medical testing and reassurance to the contrary.

5. **All is true about Pseudocyesis except:** *(PGMEE 2015)*
   a. Labour pains at EDD
   b. Patient is pregnant
   c. Abdominal enlargement
   d. Amenorrhea

   [Ref: Kaplan & Saddock's Psychiatry p. 1801]

HYPOCHONDRIASIS

6. **Persistent preoccupation with serious illness and normal body function is called:** *(PGMEE 2013)*
   a. Obsession
   b. Conversion disorder
   c. Hypochondriasis
   d. Somatization

   [Ref: Kaplan & Saddock's 10th/e p. 642, 643]

7. **A 45-year-old man complains of gradual decrease in the size of his penis. He is afraid that it may disappear completely. The psychiatric disorder which presents with this phenomenon is:** *(PGMEE 2016-17)*
   a. Koro syndrome
   b. Dhat syndrome
   c. Malingering
   d. Hypochondriasis

   [Ref: Niraj Ahuja 7th/e/p 105]

Explanation

- Koro is a culture-bound syndrome in which an individual has an overvalued idea that one's genitalia are retracting and will disappear, despite evidence on the contrary.
- Dhat syndrome is another culture-bound syndrome, specifically found in the Indian subcontinent. Here male patients believe that they are passing semen in their urine and they suffer from premature ejaculation or impotence.
- Hypochondriasis is a mental disorder characterized by excessive fear of or preoccupation with a serious illness, despite medical testing and reassurance to the contrary.
- Malingering is the purposeful production of falsely or grossly exaggerated physical or psychological complaints with the goal of receiving a reward (such as- fraud financial compensation, avoiding school, work or military service, obtaining drugs, or as a mitigating factor for sentencing in criminal cases.

DISSOCIATIVE – CONVERSION DISORDER

8. **In conversion disorder all are found except:** *(PGMEE 2014)*
   a. Anaesthesia   b. Paralysis
   c. Abnormal gait   d. Jealousy

   [Ref: Niraj Ahuja 6th/e p. 106, 107]

1.	d
2.	a
3.	a
4.	c
5.	b
6.	c
7.	a,d
8.	d

9. La Belle Indifference is seen in: *(PGMEE 2015-16)*
   a. Mania
   b. Schizophrenia
   c. Depression
   d. Conversion disorder

   [Ref: Kaplan & Sadock's Synopsis of Psychiatry 11th/e pg. 475]

10. La bella indifference seen in: *(PGMEE 2015)*
   a. Multiple sclerosis
   b. Parietal lobe lesion
   c. Conversion disorder
   d. All of the above

   [Ref: Niraj Ahuja 6th/e p. 111]

11. Conversion disorder true statements are all except: *(PGMEE 2015)*

   a. La bella indifference is a feature
   b. There is primary and secondary gain
   c. Patient does not intentionally produce symptoms
   d. Autonomic nervous system involved

   [Ref: Niraj Ahuja 6th/e p. 106]

12. A 25 Year old woman suddenly collapsed on hearing a bad news. This phenomenon is known as: *(PGMEE 2015-16)*

   a. Catathrenia
   b. Catatonia
   c. Catalepsy
   d. Cataplexy

   [Ref: A Dictionary of Neurological Signs (Springer) 3rd/e pg. 74, 75]

13. A person laughs to a joke, and then suddenly loses tone of all his muscles. Most probable diagnosis of this condition is?: *(DNB Dec' 2009)*
   a. Cathrexix
   b. Catatonia
   c. Catalepsy
   d. Cataplexy

   [Ref: Kaplan & Sadock's Synopsis of Psychiatry, 10th edn, pg-274]

Explanation

- **Catalepsy:** Condition in which persons maintain the body position into which they are placed; observed in severe cases of catatonic schizophrenia.

- **Cataplexy:** Temporary sudden loss of muscle tone, causing weakness and immobilization; can be precipitated by a variety of emotional states and is often followed by sleep. Commonly seen in narcolepsy.
- **Cathexis**: In psychoanalysis, a conscious or unconscious investment of psychic energy in an idea, concept, object, or person.

14. Ataxia abasia is seen in: *(PGMEE 2013)*
   a. Conversion disorder
   b. Manic
   c. Depression
   d. PTSD

15. Differentiation of hysterical fits from epileptic fit:
   a. Incontinence *(PGMEE 2014)*
   b. Injuries to person
   c. Occurs in sleep
   d. Occurs when people are watching

   [Ref: Niraj Ahuja 6th/e p. 108; Kaplan & Saddock's 10th/e p. 640]

16. The most common form of dissociation hysteria is: *(PGMEE 2014)*

   a. Multiple personality
   b. Amnesia
   c. Somnambulism
   d. Fugue

   [Ref: Niraj Ahuja 6th/e p. 108]

17. Derealization & depersonalisation seen in which type of disorder: *(PGMEE 2012)*
   a. Mania
   b. Dissociative disorder
   c. Personality disorder
   d. None

   [Ref: Niraj Ahuja 6th/e p. 108, Namboodiri 3rd/e p. 221]

9.	d
10.	d
11.	d
12.	d
13.	d
14.	a
15.	d
16.	b
17.	b

1. **Schizoid Personality is classified in which of the following Clusters:** *(PGMEE 2015-16 & 2016-17)*
   a. Cluster A
   b. Cluster B
   c. Cluster C
   d. Cluster D

   [Ref: Niraj Ahuja 7th/e/p 113; Kaplan and Sadock's Synopsis of Psychiatry 11th/e pg. 742]

2. **Not a cluster B type of personality** *(PGMEE 2014)*
   a. Avoidant
   b. Narcissistic
   c. Antisocial
   d. Borderline

   [Ref: Niraj Ahuja 7th/e p. 113]

3. **Type C personality disorder consists of:** *(PGMEE 2012)*
   a. Narcissistic personality disorder
   b. Histrionic personality disorder
   c. Avoidant personality disorder
   d. Paranoid personality disorder

   [Ref: Niraj Ahuja 7th/e p. 113]

4. **Which of the following disorder appears in early childhood and continues in the adulthood?**
   a. Anxiety disorder *(PGMEE 2015)*
   b. Personality disorder
   c. Somatoform
   d. Mood disorder

   [Ref: Niraj Ahuja 7th/e/ch 9/ p 113]

5. **In personality disorder, features are all except:**
   a. Starts in childhood *(PGMEE 2013)*
   b. Disorder results in personal distress
   c. Behavior is maladaptive
   d. Ego dystonia

   [Ref: Niraj Ahuja 7th/e/ch 9/ p 113]

TYPES OF PERSONALITY DISORDERS

6. **Dramatic, emotional, well dressed person who has continuous longing for appreciation has which type of personality disorder?** *(PGMEE 2016-17)*
   a. Histrionic
   b. Schizoid
   c. Schizotypal
   d. Narcissistic

   [Ref: Niraj Ahuja 7th/e/p 116]

7. **What is the personality disorder with odd beliefs, unusual speech and perceptions:** *(PGMEE 2016-17)*
   a. Narcissistic
   b. Schizoid
   c. Schizotypal
   d. Histrionic

   [Ref: Niraj Ahuja 7th/e/p 115]

8. **Personality disorder having excessive sensitivity, self-importance and self- suspiciousness is:** *(PGMEE 2013)*
   a. Antisocial
   b. Histrionic
   c. Schizoid
   d. Paranoid

   [Ref: Niraj Ahuja 7th/e/p 114]

9. **Schizoid personality disorder all are seen except:** *(PGMEE 2012)*
   a. "Odd & detached"
   b. Prone to fantasy
   c. Suspicious
   d. Introspective

   [Ref: Niraj Ahuja 7th/e p. 114]

10. **An 18-year-old male having flat affect, excessive preoccupation with fantasy and introspection. Diagnosis:**
    a. Depression *(PGMEE 2014)*
    b. Schizophrenia
    c. Hysteria
    d. Schizoid personality disorder

    [Ref: Niraj Ahuja 7th/e/p 114]

Explanation

- These features are characteristic of schizoid personality disorder. Patients with depression have sad/depressed Affect with other symptoms such as fatigue, lack of concentration, inability to experience pleasure, decreased psychomotor activity, etc.
- Although schizophrenia patients my present with flat affect, they usually have other psychotic symptoms like delusions, hallucinations, disorganization, thought alienation, catatonia, etc.
- Hysteria is an older term for conversion disorder.

11. **What is the feature of antisocial personality:** *(PGMEE 2015)*
    a. Unstable interpersonal relationship
    b. Attention – seeking behavior
    c. Violation of rules of society
    d. Grandiose behavior

    [Ref: Niraj Ahuja 7th/e p. 115]

12. **Antisocial personality is associated with which of the following–** *(PGMEE 2014)*
    a. OCN
    b. Drug abuse
    c. Paranoid schizophrenia
    d. None

    [Ref: Niraj Ahuja 7th/e/p 115]

1.	a
2.	a
3.	c
4.	b
5.	d
6.	a
7.	c
8.	d
9.	c
10.	d
11.	c
12.	b

13. A lady is having unstable relationship with her husband. She always threatens him about committing suicide and has once consumed several sleeping pills. What type of personality is this? *(PGMEE 2013)*
a. Avoidant personality disorder
b. Depression
c. Borderline personality disorder
d. None

[Ref: Niraj Ahuja 7th/e/p 117]

Explanation

- Borderline personality disorder is characterized by an enduring pattern of unstable self-image and mood together with volatile interpersonal relationships, self-damaging impulsivity, recurrent suicidal threats or gestures and/or self-mutilating behavior.
- Avoidant personality disorder is characterized by excessive social discomfort, extreme sensitivity to negative perceptions of oneself, pervasive preoccupation with being criticized or rejected in social situations, and low self-esteem.
- Depression is not a personality disorder.

14. In which type of personality disorder, there are ideas of grandiosity and a need of constant praise from others?
a. Antisocial *(PGMEE 2015)*
b. Histrionic
c. Borderline
d. Narcissistic

[Ref: Niraj Ahuja 7th/e p. 116]

15. Bipolar disorder is associated with which other personality disorder? *(PGMEE 2013)*
a. Borderline   b. Anankastic
c. Antisocial   d. Narcissistic

[Ref: Niraj Ahuja 7th/e/p 117]

16. Borderline personality disorder is most effectively treated with which of the following? *(PGMEE 2012)*
a. Behavior therapy
b. Combination of both pharmacotherapy and behavioral therapy
c. Pharmacotherapy
d. None

[Ref: Niraj Ahuja 7th/e/p 117]

17. Obsessive Compulsive Disorder is associated with which personality: *(PGMEE 2013)*
a. Borderline
b. Histrionic
c. Narcissistic
d. Anankastic

[Ref: Niraj Ahuja 7th/e/p 118]

18. Which personality disorder/s can be a part of autistic spectrum of disorders? *(PGMEE 2015)*
a. Borderline
b. Schizotypical
c. Schizoid
d. Anti-social

19. What is the appropriate line of management for Borderline Personality Disorder: *(PGMEE 2016-17)*
a. Psychotherapy
b. Interpersonal therapy
c. Drug Therapy
d. Dialectical Behavior Therapy and Psychotherapy

[Ref: Niraj Ahuja 7th/e/p 117]

HABIT AND IMPULSE DOSORDERS

20. All are compulsive and habit forming disorder EXCEPT: *(PGMEE 2014)*
a. Nymphomania
b. Pyromania
c. Pathological gambling
d. Kleptomania

[Ref: Niraj Ahuja 7th/e/p 119]

21. Kleptomania means: *(PGMEE 2015)*
a. Compulsive hair pulling
b. Irresistible desire to steal things
c. Irresistible desire to set things on fire
d. Pathological gambling

[Ref: Niraj Ahuja 7th/e p. 119]

22. An-18-year old girl having noticeable hair loss due to persistent and recurrent failure to resist impulses to pullout hair is suffering from– *(PGMEE 2013)*
a. Depression
b. Phobia
c. OCD
d. Trichotillomania

[Ref: Niraj Ahuja 7th/e p. 119]

23. Trichotillomania refers to: *(PGMEE 2013)*
a. Compulsive hair pulling
b. Irresistible desire to steal things
c. Irresistible desire to set fire
d. Pathological gambling

[Ref: Niraj Ahuja 7th/e p. 119]

13.	c
14.	d
15.	d
16.	b
17.	d
18.	d
19.	d
20.	a
21.	b
22.	d
23.	a

SLEEP CYCLE & EEG

1. **Maximum duration of time is spent in which stage of NREM–** *(PGMEE 2012)*
   a. I
   b. II
   c. III
   d. IV

   [Ref: Niraj Ahuja 7th/e/p 133]

2. **EEG waves are also called:** *(PGMEE 2013)*
   a. Delta waves
   b. NERM rhythm
   c. REM rhythm
   d. Berger's waves

   [Ref: Internet]

3. **Pontogenitooccipital spike is characteristic of sleep stage:** *(PGMEE 2015)*
   a. Stage 1 NREM
   b. Stage 2 NREM
   c. Stage 4 NREM
   d. REM

   [Ref: Niraj Ahuja 7th/e/ch 11]

4. **A patient unable to sleep, undergoes a sleep study. The following EEG is obtained. What is stage of sleep?** *(NEET Pattern 2017)*

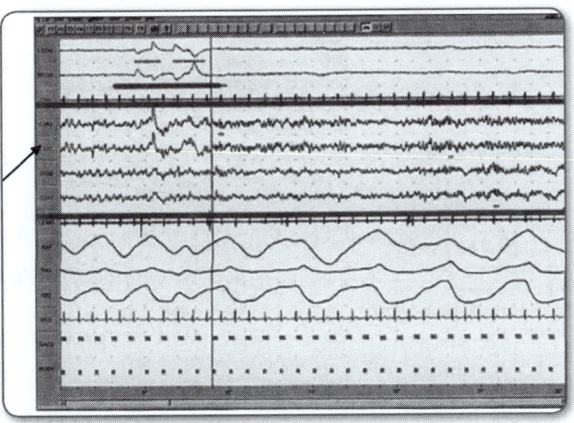

   a. NREM stage 4
   b. REM sleep
   c. NREM stage 2
   d. NREM stage 3

Explanation

- REM Sleep stage- Breathing becomes more rapid, irregular and shallow, eyes jerk rapidly and limb muscles are temporarily paralyzed. Brain waves during this stage increase to levels experienced when a person is awake. Also, heart rate increases, blood pressure rises, males develop erections and the body loses some of the ability to regulate its temperature.

SLEEP DISORDERS

5. **Bruxism is seen in:** *(PGMEE 2013)*
   a. NREM stage 1, 2
   b. NREM stage 3,4
   c. REM
   d. Any of the above

   [Ref: Niraj Ahuja 7th/e p. 140]

6. **What is bruxism?** *(PGMEE 2012)*
   a. Grinding of teeth during sleep
   b. Walking during sleep
   c. Sleep apnoea
   d. Nocturnal enuresis

   [Ref: Niraj Ahuja 7th/e p. 140]

7. **Parasomnia occurring in REM stage is–** *(PGMEE 2012)*
   a. Somniloquy
   b. Bruxism
   c. Night mares
   d. Night terror

   [Ref: Niraj Ahuja 7th/e p.140]

8. **Somnambulism is a term:** *(Recent Pattern June 2018)*
   a. Parasomnia of NREM Sleep
   b. Psychopathic disorder
   c. Some what between sleep and walking
   d. Used foe excessive daytime sleepiness

   [Ref: Synopsis of Psychiatry by Kaplan & Sadock's 11th/e pg. 539]

Explanation

Somnabulism

- Somnambulism or sleep walking is REM stage 4 parasomnia.
- It occurs during deepest type of non- REM sleep, stage 4 when delta waves (low-frequency, high-amplitude waveforms) appears in EEG.

REMEMBER

- Alpha waves are characteristic of relaxed wakefulness.
- Beta-like activity is characteristic of either alert wakefulness or REM sleep.
- Sleep spindles and K-complexes are characteristic of stage 2 sleep, which is a deeper sleep that occupies roughly 45% of the sleep cycle.

9. **Not true about somnambulism among the following is?** *(PGMEE Jan 2019)*
   a. Sleep walking.
   b. Patient consciousness is preserved
   c. Disorder of sleep arousal
   d. Low level motor skill/function is present.

1.	b
2.	d
3.	d
4.	b
5.	b
6.	a
7.	c
8.	a
9.	b

10. **Which of the following occurs in NREM Stage?**
    a. Night mares~ **(PGMEE 2014)**
    b. Narcolepsy
    c. Sleep paralysis
    d. Teeth grinding

    [Ref: Niraj Ahuja 7th/e/p 140]

NARCOLEPSY

11. **What is a feature of narcolepsy:** **(PGMEE 2015)**
    a. Bruxism
    b. Insomnia
    c. Somnambulism
    d. Hypersomnia at day time

    [Ref: Niraj Ahuja 7th/e p. 138]

12. **Narcolepsy all are true EXCEPT:**
    (Recent Pattern June 2018)
    a. Sudden loss of voluntary muscle control
    b. Excessive daytime sleepiness is the first symptom in most cases
    c. Familial, associated strongly with HLA DQ B1
    d. NREM sleep associated parasomnia

    [Ref: Synopsis of Psychiatry by Kaplan & Sadock's 11th/e pg. 548]

Explanation

Narcolepsy

- It is a sleep wake disorder most commonly present with irresistible sleep attacks of refreshing sleeps (REM type) in which patient abruptly falls asleep in inappropriate and even dangerous (eg while driving) situations.
- Age of onset **10-20 yr.**
- Each attack lasts **10-20 min.**
- There is onset of REM sleep within 15 minutes (average of **10-20**) of sleep onset.
- In up to **10%** of cases, there is a family history of the disorder.
- The classic symptoms are described as "*tetrad of narcolepsy*" which are:-
  ○ Cataplexy,
  ○ Sleep paralysis
  ○ Hypnagogic hallucinations, and
  ○ Excessive daytime sleepiness
- Treatment: Armodafinil is exclusively used

10.	d
11.	d
12.	d
13.	a
14.	d
15.	b
16.	c
17.	b
18.	b
19.	c

13. **What is the feature of narcolepsy:** **(PGMEE 2014)**
    a. Decreased REM sleep latency
    b. Increased sleep time
    c. Increase in muscle tone
    d. None of the above

    [Ref: Niraj Ahuja 7th/e/p 138]

14. **Narcolepsy is due to abnormality in:** **(PGMEE 2012)**
    a. Medulla oblongata
    b. Neocortex
    c. Cerebellum
    d. Hypothalamus

    [Ref: Niraj Ahuja 7th/e/ch 11]

15. **Night terror at start of sleep and no memory in morning occurs in which phase of sleep cycle? (PGMEE 2016-17)**
    a. REM   b. NREM
    c. Both   d. None

    [Ref: Niraj Ahuja 7th/e/p 140]

16. **Hypnogogic hallucinations are seen in which condition?**
    a. Schizophrenia **(PGMEE 2013)**
    b. Mania
    c. Narcolepsy
    d. Depression

    [Ref: Niraj Ahuja 7th/e/p 138]

17. **All are features of Narcolepsy EXCEPT–** **(PGMEE 2012)**
    a. Loss of muscle tone
    b. Sleep architecture normal
    c. Cataplexy
    d. Hallucination

    [Ref: Niraj Ahuja 7th/e/p 138]

18. **Not a feature of Narcolepsy–** **(PGMEE 2014)**
    a. Daytime sleepiness
    b. Catalepsy
    c. Cataplexy
    d. Hypnagogic hallucination

    [Ref: Niraj Ahuja 7th/e/p 138]

19. **Klein-Levin syndrome is characterised by–**
    a. Depression **(PGMEE 2012)**
    b. Insomnia
    c. Hypersomnia
    d. Anxiety

    [Ref: Niraj Ahuja 7th/e/p 139]

PREMATURE EJACULATION & ERECTILE DYSFUNCTION

1. Premature ejaculation is treated by: *(PGMEE 2013)*
a. Citalopram
b. Chlorpromazine
c. Dapoxetine
d. Escitalopram

[Ref: Niraj Ahuja 7th/e/p 130-131]

2. Men who have significant problems with premature ejaculation have difficulty in the phase of the sexual response cycle: *(Recent Pattern June 2018)*
a. Plateau phase
b. Orgasmic phase
c. Excitement phase
d. Resolution phase

[Ref: Synopsis of Psychiatry by Kaplan & Sadock's 11th/e pg. 568]

Explanation

Male sexual response cycle

Phase	Features	Dysfunction
1st (Excitement phase)	Lasts several minutes to hours CF: **Erection** due to congestion in corpora cavernosa	**Erectile dysfunction**, Female sexual arousal disorders & dyspareunia
2nd (Orgasmic phase)	3-15 seconds CF: Ejaculation	Premature ejaculation, Orgasmic disorder
3rd (Resolution phase)	Lasts 10-15 min, A sense of generalised relaxation	Post coital dysphoria & hedache

3. Psychological and organic erectile dysfunction are differentiated by presence of which of the following in psychological type? *(PGMEE 2012)*
a. PIPE therapy
b. Nocturnal penile tumescence
c. Slidenafil induced erection
d. Squeeze technique

[Ref: Niraj Ahuja 7th/e p. 128]

Explanation

- Pharmacologically induced penile erection (PIPE) therapy that includes use of drugs like oral sildenafil (sildenafil induced erection), intracavernosal papaverine, etc. is used for the treatment of Erectile dysfunction. Sildenafil induced erection test is used for assessment of the cavernous arteries' flow and to predict treatment response.
- Squeeze technique is a behavioral technique used in the treatment of Premature Ejaculation.
- Nocturnal penile tumescence (NPT) is the clinical name for several spontaneous physiological erections that men have while they sleep at night. An erection self-test is a procedure to determine if the cause of his erectile dysfunction is physical or psychological; presence of it clinical helps in excluding physiological/organic dysfunction.

4. Most accurate treatment of erectile dysfunction:
a. Master and Johnson technique *(PGMEE 2014)*
b. Sildenafil
c. Beta blockers
d. Papaverine

[Ref: Niraj Ahuja 7th/e/p 132]

5. What is Quod Hanc? *(PGMEE 2013)*
a. Male impotent to a particular woman
b. Women having high sexual desire
c. Passive partner in sexual intercourse
d. Men having high sexual desire

[Ref: K.S.N Reddy (synopsis of F.M.T) 25th/e/p 173]

Explanation

- Quod Hanc is a person who is impotent to one woman particularly but can perform sexual act successfully with another women.

MISCELLANEOUS

6. Well dressed man came for feeling of women trapped in man body is suffering from: *(PGMEE 2013)*
a. Frotteurism
b. Paraphilia
c. Gender identity disorder
d. Transverium

[Ref: Niraj Ahuja 6th/e p. 132-134]

1.	c
2.	c
3.	b
4.	b
5.	a
6.	C

1. **Pagophagia is compulsive eating of**   **(PGMEE 2013)**
   a. Salt
   b. Sand
   c. Ice
   d. Clay

2. **True about anorexia nervosa is all except:**
   a. Self-induced vomiting   **(PGMEE 2013)**
   b. Unknown in male
   c. Binge eating is common
   d. Amenorrhoea starts before severe loss of weight

   [Ref: Niraj Ahuja 7th/e/p 142]

3. **All are true about bulimia nervosa, except:**
   a. Bing eating   **(PGMEE 2013)**
   b. Purgative abuse
   c. Weight loss
   d. Self-induced vomiting

   [Ref: Niraj Ahuja 7th/e/p 144]

4. **More common in binge eating compared to bulimia nervosa is:**   **(PGMEE 2014)**
   a. Menstrual disorders
   b. Self induced vomiting
   c. Obesity
   d. Short duration

   [Ref: Niraj Ahuja 7th/e/p 144]

5. **A medical student comes with normal weight, parotid abscess and dental caries. She gets irritated by inquiry of her eating habit. Most probable diagnosis is?**
   (DNB pattern Dec' 2011)
   a. Adjustment disorder
   b. Bulimia
   c. Anorexia nervosa
   d. Conversion reaction

   [Ref: Kaplan & Sadock's Synopsis of Psychiatry, 10th edn, pg-736]

1. c
2. b
3. c
4. c
5. b

Explanation

Features	Anorexia Nervosa	Bulimia Nervosa
▪ Prevalence in women	0.5%	1-3%
▪ Age group/ Onset	Adolescent females	Early teens
▪ Onset	Mid adolescence	Late adolescence

Features	Anorexia Nervosa	Bulimia Nervosa
▪ Body image	Disturbed	Disturbed
▪ Cl/f	▪ Refusal to maintain body weight above normal, ▪ dry skin, lanugo hair	▪ Irresistible craving for food with episodes of over eating. Overperception of weight but weight is normal. ▪ Dry skin, hair loss, brittle nails
▪ Diet	Very less eating	**Binge eating (25-50%)** is f/b ▪ Self-induced vomiting ▪ Periods of starvation ▪ Use of purgatives and appetite suppressants
▪ Lab	–	Imbalanced electrolytes Hypokalemic hypochloremic alkalosis
▪ Weight	Markedly reduced, **Underweight** (85%)	usually normal
▪ LH & FSH levels ▪ Glucose levels	Low Low	usually normal usually normal
▪ Sex hormone levels	Low estrogen or testosterone	usually normal
▪ Thyroxine levels	Low normal	usually normal
▪ Cortisol levels	Increased	usually normal
▪ Menstruation	Absent (Amenorrhea in 100% cases)	usually normal or oligomenorrhea
▪ T/t	Behaviour therapy	Fluoxetine

- Patients of anorexia nervosa are vulnerable to sudden death from ventricular tachyarrhythmias.
- Diagnosis of Anorexia nervosa is made by all/e → Decreased appetite.

ADHD

1. **The treatment of choice in Attention deficit hyperactivity disorder is:** *(PGMEE 2012, 2016-17, 03)*
   a. Haloperidol
   b. Imipramine
   c. Methylphenidate
   d. Alprazolam

   [Ref: Niraj Ahuja 7th/e/p 167]

2. **Stimulant medication commonly is given to child for:**
   a. Speech development disorder *(PGMEE 2012)*
   b. ADHD
   c. Pervasive disorder
   d. Conduct disorder

   [Ref: Niraj Ahuja 7th/e/p 167]

3. **Tourette disorder is most commonly associated with:**
   a. ADHD *(PGMEE 2016-17)*
   b. Conduct disorder
   c. Antisocial personality disorder
   d. Autism spectrum disorders

   [Ref: Internet]

4. **Not an associated co-morbid condition in children with hyperkinetic attention deficit disorder (ADHD) is:** *(DNB pattern Dec'2010)*
   a. Elimination disorder
   b. Language disorder
   c. Anxiety disorder
   d. Sleep disorder

   [Ref: Kaplan & Sadock's Synopsis of Psychiatry, 10th edn, pg- 1206]

Explanation

- ADHD was associated with a substantially elevated prevalence of the following (all P<0.05):
  - Learning disabilities (46% versus 5% in other children, adjusted relative risk 7.79)
  - Conduct disorder (27% versus 2%, adjusted RR 12.58)
  - Anxiety (18% versus 2%, adjusted RR 7.45)
  - Depression (14% versus 1%, adjusted RR 8.04)
  - Speech problems (12% versus 3%, adjusted RR 4.42)

5. **Which of the following is not used for Attention Deficit Disorder:** *(PGMEE 2013)*
   a. Cognitive remediation therapy
   b. Cognitive behavioral therapy
   c. Flooding
   d. Cognitive enhancement therapy

   [Ref: Niraj Ahuja 7th/e/p 167]

Explanation

- Children with Attention deficit hyperactivity disorder (ADHD) find it hard to pay close attention like having trouble listening to what is being said in class. They appear easily distracted and have difficulty doing tasks from the beginning to end and are criticized for making careless mistakes. They often lose items, regardless of how expensive or important they are. They are always moving and "on the go", find it almost impossible to sit in a chair. When seated they tap feet or fidget or squirm. They run around and climb in order to burn energy.
- Although such symptoms may be fund in Mania, they are associated with acute presentation, elevated mood and related symptoms.
- In delirium, patients present with acute confusion and lack of orientation.
- Cerebral palsy has motor manifestations.

6. **Mother brings her 8 year old child to the OPD and complains that the child does not sit in class, keeps shifting from one task to other without finishing any, disturbs other students and does not listen to teachers. What is your diagnosis?** *(PGMEE 2016-17)*
   a. Attention deficit hyperactive disorder
   b. Cerebral Palsy
   c. Delirium
   d. Mania

   [Ref: Niraj Ahuja 7ᵗʰ/e/ch 14]

PERVASIVE DEVELOPMENT DISORDERS

7. **All are true about autism EXCEPT:-** *(DNB Dec' 2009)*
   a. Age between 18-24 months
   b. Child is able to interact
   c. Repetitive behaviour is seen
   d. Language is not well developed

   [Ref: Kaplan & Sadock's Synopsis of Psychiatry, 10th edn, pg-1191]

Explanation

- Autism is characterized by sustained impairment in comprehending and responding to social cues, aberrant language development and usage, and restricted, stereotypical behavioral patterns.
- Pervasive developmental disorders typically emerge in young children before the age of 3 years, and parents often become concerned about a child by 18 months as language development does not occur as expected. In about 25 percent of cases, some language develops and is subsequently lost. Children with pervasive developmental disorders often exhibit idiosyncratic intense interest in a narrow range of activities, resist change, and are not appropriately responsive to the social environment.

8. **Which of the following is not included in autism spectrum disorders:** *(Recent Pattern June 2018)*
   a. Asperger syndrome
   b. Autistic disorder
   c. Pragmatic communication disorder
   d. Pervasive developmental disorder

   [Ref: Synopsis of Psychiatry by Kaplan & Sadock's 11th/e pg. 1152]

1.	c
2.	b
3.	a
4.	a
5.	c
6.	a
7.	b
8.	c

Explanation

Autism spectrum disorders include

- Autism
- Asperger's syndrome
- Childhood disintegrative disorder
- Rett syndrome
- Pervasive developmental disorder

9. **Rett syndrome is characterized by all except:**
   a. Regression of acquired skills   *(PGMEE 2015)*
   b. Macrocephaly
   c. Autistic behavior
   d. Breath holding spells

   [Ref: Niraj Ahuja 7th/e/p 165]

10. **Asperger syndrome is:**   *(PGMEE 2016-17)*
    a. Pervasive Developmental disorder
    b. Hyperkinetic Disorder
    c. Speech Disorder
    d. Conduct Disorder

    [Ref: Niraj Ahuja 7th/e/p 165]

DYSLEXIA & CONDUCT DISORDERS

11. **Aggressive behavior and violation of social laws the condition is:**   *(PGMEE 2016-17)*
    a. Conduct disorder
    b. Pervasive Developmental Disorder
    c. Anxiety
    d. Psychosis

    [Ref: Niraj Ahuja 7th/e/p 167]

12. **A child has problems with reading and writing but has normal intelligence. The most likely diagnosis is:**
    a. Dyslexia   *(PGMEE 2016-17)*
    b. Rett's Disease
    c. Asperger's
    d. Mental Retardation

    [Ref: Niraj Ahuja 7th/e/ch 13 and 14]

MENTAL RETARDATION

13. **Normal IQ is:**   *(PGMEE 2014)*
    a. 45   b. 85
    c. 65   d. 100

    [Ref: Niraj Ahuja 7th/e/ch 13]

14. **IQ in severe mental retardation is:**   *(PGMEE 2012)*
    a. < 20   b. 20-35
    c. 35-50   d. 50-70

    [Ref: Niraj Ahuja 7th/e/p 156]

Explanation

- *Five major diagnostic axes for mental retardation:-*

Level	IQ
Mild	50-70
Moderate	49-35
Severe	34-20
Profound	Below 20

15. **I.Q. of 50 to 70 is:**   *(PGMEE 2016-17)*
    a. Mild mental retardation
    b. Moderate mental retardation
    c. Severe mental retardation
    d. Profound mental retardation

    [Ref: Niraj Ahuja 7th/e/p 156]

16. **Boy of 20 year old has mental age 9 year. His grade of mental retardation is:**   *(PGMEE 2016-17)*
    a. Mild   b. Moderate
    c. Severe   d. Profound

    [Ref: Niraj Ahuja 7th/e/p 156]

Explanation

- Mental retardation is now a days known as "intellectual disability or intellectual developmental disorder".
- Oligophrenia is an old word for mental retardation.

17. **Boy is not capable of learning math, drawing and also has cognitive disturbance. Diagnosis in this case is:**
    a. Learning disorder   *(PGMEE 2016-17)*
    b. Intellectual disorder
    c. ADHD
    d. Dyslexia

    [Ref: Niraj Ahuja 7th/e/ch 14]

Explanation

- Down syndrome is typically associated with delay in physical growth, characteristic facies and mild to moderate intellectual disability (Mental retardation)
- Oligophrenia is an old word for mental retardation.

18. **New term for mental retardation according to American psychiatric association :-**   *(PGMEE 2018)*
    a. Oligophrenia
    b. Mental subnormality
    c. Mild retardation
    d. Intellectual disability

    [Ref: (DSM-5, P 33)]

19. **Now a days Down's syndrome is referred to as:-**
    a. Oligophrenia   *(PGMEE 2018)*
    b. Submental disorder
    c. Mental madness
    d. Intellectual disability   *[Ref: (DSM-5, P 33)]*

Explanation

- *Tics* are sudden, rapid, recurrent, nonrhythmic motor movement or vocalization.
- *A stereotypy* is a repetitive or ritualistic movement, posture, or utterance.
  - Stereotypies may be either simple movements such as body rocking, or complex movements, such as self-caressing, crossing and uncrossing of legs, and marching in place.
  - They are found in people with intellectual disabilities, autism spectrum disorders, tardive dyskinesia.

9.	b
10.	a
11.	a
12.	a
13.	d
14.	b
15.	a
16.	b
17.	a
18.	d
19.	b

MISCELLANEOUS

20. Habit forming disorder among following are all EXCEPT:- *(PGMEE 2018)*
   a. Tics
   b. Thumb sucking
   c. Nail biting
   d. Tamper tantrum/Bruxism

Ref: (DSM-5; P-81)

Explanation

- *Tic-* is a sudden, rapid, recurrent, nonrhythmic motor movement or vocalization
- ***Childhood Habit Behaviors and Stereotypic Movement Disorder-*** These rarely require medical attention. In some children, a natural progression is seen, beginning with thumb or hand sucking and then progressing to body rocking and head banging and, later still, to nail biting and foot or finger tapping.
- E.g.- Thumb or hand sucking, Body rocking, Nail biting, Bruxism

21. Tics, hair pulling, nail biting can be treated by:- *(DNB Dec' 2011)*
   a. Mind fullness
   b. Social habit training
   c. Habit and response prevention
   d. No intervention required

[Ref: Kaplan & Sadock's Synopsis of Psychiatry, 10th edn, pg-783]

Explanation

- Successful behavioral treatments, such as biofeedback, self-monitoring, covert desensitization, and habit reversal, have been reported.

22. "Sterotypes" are: *(PGMEE 2018)*
   a. Mimicry
   b. Repetitive non-purposeful movements
   c. Tics
   d. Repetitive purposeful movements

Ref: DSM-5; P-829

20.	**a**
21.	**c**
22.	**b**

ECT

1. ECT is indicated in all EXCEPT– *(PGMEE 2013)*
a. Severe depression with suicidal risk
b. Sever manic attack
c. Severe psychosis
d. Catatonia schizophrenia

[Ref: Niraj Ahuja 7th/e/ch 16 page 199-200]

2. Electro convulsive therapy is most beneficial in:
a. Chronic schizophrenia *(PGMEE 2012, 2014)*
b. Mania
c. Hysteria
d. Depression with suicidal tendency

[Ref: Niraj Ahuja 7th/e/ch 16 page 199-203]

3. Absolute contraindication for Electro-Convulsive Therapy [ECT] is: *(PGMEE 2014)*
a. Vascular Dementia   b. Peripheral Neuropathy
c. Diabetic Retinopathy   d. Raised ICT

[Ref: Niraj Ahuja 7th/e p. 201]

4. Seizure lasting for __ minutes after ECT are called prolonged seizures according to American psychiatric association: *(Recent Pattern June 2018)*
a. > 90 sec.   b. > 3 min
c. > 1 min   d. > 30 min

[Ref: Kaplan & Sadock's 11th/e pg. 1071]

Explanation

Adverse effect of ECT:

■ An induced seizure lasting > 2 or 3 minutes is considered prolonged and can result in increased cognitive deficits.

PSYCHOLOGICAL TREATMENTS

5. Desensitization is a type of: *(PGMEE 2012)*
a. Behavior therapy   b. Psychotherapy
c. Psychoanalysis   d. None

[Ref: Niraj Ahuja 7th/e/p 214]

6. Pavlov's experiment is an example of: *(PGMEE 2013)*
a. Learned helplessness   b. Classical conditioning
c. Modeling   d. Operant conditioning

[Ref: Niraj Ahuja 7th/e/p 214]

PSYCHOANALYSIS

7. In which condition therapist is passive: *(PGMEE 2012)*
a. Psychoanalytic psycoanalysis
b. Classical psychoanalysis
c. Behavioral group therapy
d. Supportive group therapy

[Ref: Niraj Ahuja 7th/e/p 214]

8. Which of the following best represents the Stages of Change in Transtheoretical Model: *(PGMEE 2015-16)*
a. Contemplation - Preparation - Action - Maintenance
b. Preparation - Contemplation - Determination - Maintenance
c. Contemplation - Action - Determination - Maintenance
d. Preparation - Contemplation - Action - Maintenance

[Ref: Psychology By Passer pg. 516]

9. Patient & Psychotherapists, both participate actively in:
a. Psychoanalysis *(PGMEE 2013)*
b. Psychoanalytic psychotherapy
c. Psycodynamic psychotherapy
d. All of the above

[Ref: Niraj Ahuja 7th/e/p 214]

PHARMACOTHERAPY

10. A young schizophrenic who was recently started on a high potency antipsychotic, Haloperidol has developed neck rigidity. What is the diagnosis? *(PGMEE 2014)*
a. Tardive dyskinesia   b. Catatonia
c. Dystonia   d. Neuroleptic malignant synd

[Ref: KDT]

11. Drug used as antidepressant is: *(PGMEE 2016-17)*
a. Thioridazine   b. Thiothixine
c. Tianeptine   d. Trifluperidol

[Ref: Niraj Ahuja 7th/e/p 183]

MISCELLANEOUS

12. Drug used for narcoanalysis: *(PGMEE 2014)*
a. Propranolol   b. Scopolamine
c. Atropine   d. Naltrexone

[Ref: K.S.N Reddy (Synopsis of F.M.T) 25th/e/p.237]

13. Test based on the principle of suspect's reaction, if he witnesses an event then he behaves in a certain way is: *(PGMEE Jan 2019)*
a. Narcoanalysis   b. Brain mapping
c. Truth serum testing   d. Polygraph

14. Use of phototherapy in psychiatry is for: *(PGMEE 2015)*
a. Schizophrenia   b. Obsessive compulsive disorder
c. MR   d. Depression

[Ref: Niraj Ahuja 7th/e/p 82]

15. The most important Bright light treatment is:
a. Anorexia Nervosa *(PGMEE 2015-16)*
b. Schizophrenia
c. Obsessive Compulsive Disorder
d. Seasonal Affective Disorder

[Ref: Shorter Oxford Textbook of Psychiatry 6th/e pg. 565; Kaplan & Sadock's Concise Textbook of Clinical Psychiatry 3rd/e pg. 222; Oxford Handbook of Psychiatry 3rd/e pg. 298]

16. Psychosurgery is used in which condition? *(PGMEE 2013)*
a. Generalized anxiety   b. Depression
c. OCD   d. All

[Ref: Niraj Ahuja 7th/e/p 203-204]

17. Phototherapy is used for: *(PGMEE 2015)*
a. Mania   b. Schizophrenia
c. Sleep disorder   d. Sensory deprivation synd

1.	b
2.	d
3.	d
4.	b
5.	a
6.	b
7.	b
8.	a
9.	c
10.	c
11.	c
12.	b
13.	d
14.	d
15.	d
16.	c
17.	c

COGNITIVE DEVELOPMENT & THEORY OF MIND

1. Concrete thinking stage of cognitive development according to Jean Piaget occurs at– (PGMEE 2013)
a. 0-2 years
b. 2-5 years
c. 5-10 years
d. 10-15 years

[Ref: Niraj Ahuja 7th/e/p 153]

2. Ability to form a concept & generalize it, is known as: (PGMEE 2014)
a. Delusional thinking
b. Abstract thinking
c. Intellectual thinking
d. Concrete thinking

[Ref: Niraj Ahuja 7th/e/p 153]

3. Psychodynamic Theory of mental illness deals with–
a. Maladjusted reinforcement (PGMEE 2015)
b. Unconscious internal conflict
c. Organic neurological problem
d. Focus on teaching patient to restrain absurd thoughts

[Ref: Niraj Ahuja 7th/e/p90 & 93]

Explanation

- Maladgusted reinforcement is dealt under 'behavioral theory';
- Organic neurological problem is covered under 'biological theory' (i.e. organic neuropsychiatry);
- 'Cognitive theory' focuses on teaching patient to restrain absurd thoughts.
- Psychodynamic theory proposes internal/inner conflicts, where repressed behaviors and emotions surface into the patient's consciousness and present as mental illness.

4. Interpretation of dreams by Freud include all EXCEPT:-
(PGMEE 2018)
a. Condensation
b. Displacement
c. Sublimation
d. Consolidation

Ref: Kaplan and Sadock synopsis of Psychiatry, 11 th/ed pg. 154

Explanation

- Dream work involves the process of condensation, displacement, and secondary elaboration.
  - **Condensation:** Means unconscious impulses or wishes are converted into a single image.
  - **Symbolism:** Means an abstract concept can be represented by an image that symbolize it
  - **Displacement:** Transfer of energy from an original object to a neutral object.

- Topographical theory of mind was also given by Freud. In this he defined conscious, unconscious and subconscious thought process. **Unsoundness of mind** can be defined as a disease of the mind or the personality, in which there is derangement of the mental or emotional processes and impairment of behaviour control.

5. Information of repressed traumatic events can be brought into conscious mind by all except:
(PGMEE 2013)
a. Hypnosis
b. Focused attention
c. Dream and Abreaction
d. Somatic stimulation

[Ref: Niraj Ahuja 7th/e/ch 17]

6. The term 'id' was given by: (PGMEE 2012)
a. Wayker
b. Skinner
c. Freud
d. Blueler

[Ref: Niraj Ahuja 7th/e p. 206]

7. All of the following about "Aaron Becks cognitive theory of depression" is true, except:- (DNB pattern Dec'2010)
a. Negative thought of past
b. Negative thought of environment
c. Negative thought of future
d. Negative thought of self

[Ref: Kaplan & Sadock's Synopsis of Psychiatry, 10th edn, pg- 195]

Explanation

- From a cognitive perspective, depression can be explained by the cognitive triad, which explains that negative thoughts are about the self, the world, and the future.

DEFENSE MECHANISMS

8. Mature defense mechanism is: (PGMEE 2013)
a. Anticipation
b. Reaction formation
c. Projection
d. Denial

[Ref: Niraj Ahuja 7th/e/p 210]

Explanation

- George Vaillant introduced a four-level classification of defense mechanisms:
  - Level I – pathological defenses (e.g. psychotic denial, delusional projection)
  - Level II – immature defenses (e.g. fantasy, projection, passive aggression, acting out)
  - Level III – neurotic defenses (eg. intellectualization, reaction formation, dissociation, displacement, repression)
  - Level IV – mature defenses (e.g. humor, sublimation, suppression, altruism, anticipation)

1.	c
2.	b
3.	b
4.	d
5.	b
6.	c
7.	a
8.	a

9. **One of the important defense mechanism is:**

(PGMEE 2014)

a. Alienation
b. Suppression
c. Repression
d. Confabulation

[Ref: Niraj Ahuja 7th/e/ch 17]

PSYCHOSEXUAL DEVELOPMENT

10. **Oedipus complex is related to which phase of psycho-sexual development:** *(PGMEE 2013)*

a. Genital
b. Anal
c. Phallic
d. Oral

[Ref: Niraj Ahuja 7th/e p. 211]

11. **Theory of "Psychosexual development" was given by:**

(DNB pattern Dec'2010)

a. Anna Freud
b. Sigmond Freud
c. Jean Paiget
d. Skinner

[Ref: Kaplan & Sadock's Synopsis of Psychiatry, 10th edn, pg- 195]

Explanation

- Psychosexual development—first in the oral stage (exemplified by an infant's pleasure in nursing), then in the anal stage (exemplified by a toddler's pleasure in evacuating his or her bowels), then in the phallic stage. In the latter stage, Freud contended, male infants become fixated on the mother as a sexual object (known as the Oedipus Complex), a phase brought to an end by threats of castration, resulting in the Castration anxiety, the severest trauma in his young life.
- In his later writings Freud postulated an equivalent Oedipus situation for infant girls, the sexual fixation being on the father. Though not advocated by Freud himself, the term 'Electra complex' is sometimes used in this context. The repressive or dormant latency stage of psychosexual development preceded the sexually mature genital stage of psychosexual development. The child needs to receive the proper amount of satisfaction at any given stage in order to move on easily to the next stage of development; under or over gratification can lead to a fixation at that stage, which could cause a regression back to that stage later in life

9.	c
10.	c
11.	b
12.	b
13.	a
14.	d
15.	c
16.	d
17.	d
18.	d
19.	c

SCIENTISTS

12. **Psychoanalysis was founded by which of the following scientist:** *(PGMEE 2013)*

a. Jung
b. Freud
c. Adler
d. Eysenck

[Ref: Niraj Ahuja 7th/e p. 219]

13. **Topographic theory of mind was given by:**

a. Sigmond Freud *(PGMEE 2016-17)*
b. Kublor Ross
c. Beck
d. Kaplan

[Ref: Niraj Ahuja 7th/e/p 243]

14. **'Free association' is a term coined by:** *(PGMEE 2014)*

a. Juna
b. Adler
c. Erikson
d. Freud

[Ref: Niraj Ahuja 7th/e/p 243]

15. **Who is the 'Father of modern psychiatry'?**

(PGMEE 2013)

a. Bleuler
b. Kraepelin
c. Pinel
d. Freud

[Ref: Niraj Ahuja 7th/e/p 244]

16. **Term 'catatonia' was used by:** *(PGMEE 2014)*

a. Adolf meyer
b. Karen horney
c. Leo kanner
d. Karl Kahlbaum

[Ref: Niraj Ahuja 7th/e p. 244]

17. **Who coined the term 'psychiatry'?** *(PGMEE 2013)*

a. Moral
b. Pinel
c. Bleuler
d. Johann Reil

[Ref: Niraj Ahuja 7th/e/p 244]

18. **Extracampine hallucinations term was given by:**

a. William Harvey *(PGMEE 2015)*
b. Eden Speroff
c. Robert Macinoff
d. Eugene Bleuler

[Ref: Internet]

19. **Emile Durkheim's book is regarding which condition in psychiatry?** *(PGMEE 2015)*

a. Anxiety disorder
b. Obsessive compulsive disorder
c. Suicide
d. Schizophrenia